SEVENTH EDITION

Fields VIROLOGY:

DNA Viruses

SEVENTH EDITION

Fields VIROLOGY: DNA Viruses

EDITORS

Peter M. Howley, MD
Shattuck Professor of Pathological Anatomy
Departments of Immunology and Pathology
Harvard Medical School
Boston, Massachusetts

David M. Knipe, PhD
Higgins Professor of Microbiology and Molecular Genetics
Head, Harvard Program in Virology
Department of Microbiology
Blavatnik Institute
Harvard Medical School
Boston, Massachusetts

ASSOCIATE VOLUME EDITORS

Blossom Damania, PhD
Boshamer Distinguished Professor
Vice Dean for Research, School of Medicine
Department of Microbiology and Immunology
University of North Carolina at Chapel Hill
Chapel Hill, North Carolina

Jeffrey I. Cohen, MD
Chief, Laboratory of Infectious Diseases
National Institute of Allergy and Infectious Diseases
National Institutes of Health
Bethesda, Maryland

ASSOCIATE EDITORS

Sean P. J. Whelan, PhD
Marvin A. Brennecke Distinguished Professor
Chair, Molecular Microbiology
Washington University in Saint Louis, School of Medicine
Saint Louis, Missouri

Lynn Enquist, PhD
Henry L. Hillman Professor of Molecular Biology
Department of Molecular Biology
Princeton University
Princeton, New Jersey

Eric O. Freed, PhD
Director
HIV Dynamics and Replication Program Center for Cancer Research
National Cancer Institute
Frederick, Maryland

Wolters Kluwer

Philadelphia • Baltimore • New York • London
Buenos Aires • Hong Kong • Sydney • Tokyo

Acquisitions Editor: Sharon Zinner
Product Development Editor: Ariel S. Winter
Marketing Manager: Kirsten Watrud
Production Project Manager: Kirstin Johnson
Design Coordinator: Stephen Druding
Manufacturing Coordinator: Beth Welsh
Prepress Vendor: SPi Global

9 8 7 6 5 4 3 2

Printed in the United States of America

Cataloging in Publication data available on request from publisher

ISBN: 978-1-9751-1257-8

shop.lww.com

MPP0722

Contributors

Allison Abendroth, BSc (Hons I) PhD
Professor
Infection, Immunity and Inflammation
School of Medical Sciences
Faculty of Medicine and Health
The University of Sydney
New South Wales, Australia

Ann M. Arvin, MD
Lucile Salter Packard Professor of Pediatrics and Professor of Microbiology & Immunology
Stanford University
Stanford, California

William Britt, MD
Charles A. Alford Professor of Infectious Diseases
Departments of Pediatrics, Microbiology, and Neurobiology
University of Alabama School of Medicine
Birmingham, Alabama

Ethel Cesarman, MD, PhD
Professor and Vice-Chair for Education
Department of Pathology and Laboratory Medicine
Weill Cornell Medicine
New York, New York

Jeffrey I. Cohen, MD
Chief, Laboratory of Infectious Diseases
National Institute of Allergy and Infectious Diseases
National Institutes of Health
Bethesda, Maryland

Blossom Damania, PhD
Boshamer Distinguished Professor
Vice Dean for Research School of Medicine
Department of Microbiology and Immunology
University of North Carolina at Chapel Hill
Chapel Hill, North Carolina

Inger K. Damon, MD, PhD
Director, Division of High Consequence Pathogens and Pathology
National Center for Emerging and Zoonotic Infectious Diseases
Centers for Disease Control and Prevention
Atlanta, Georgia

James A. DeCaprio, MD
Professor of Medicine, Harvard Medical School
Chief, Division of Molecular and Cellular Oncology
Dana-Farber Cancer Institute
Boston, Massachusetts

Paul Dény, MD, PhD, HDR
Professor of Bacteriology-Virology
Service de Microbiologie Clinique, Groupe Hospitalier Universitaire Paris Seine Saint-Denis
Unité de Formation et Recherches Santé, Médecine, Biologie Humaine, Université Sorbonne Paris Nord, Bobigny, France
Cancer Research Center of Lyon
Lyon, France

Matthias G. Fischer, PhD
Research Group Leader
Department of Biomolecular Mechanisms
Max Planck Institute for Medical Research
Heidelberg, Germany

Louis Flamand, PhD, MBA
Professor and Chair
Department of Microbiology, Infectious Disease and Immunology
Faculty of Medicine, Université Laval
Québec City, Québec, Canada

Benjamin E. Gewurz, MD, PhD
Assistant Professor of Medicine
Division of Infectious Diseases
Department of Medicine
Brigham & Women's Hospital
Associate Chair
Harvard Graduate Program in Virology
Harvard Medical School
Boston, Massachusetts

Felicia Goodrum, PhD
Professor of Immunobiology
Department of Immunobiology
University of Arizona
Tucson, Arizona

Patrick Hearing, PhD
Professor
Department of Microbiology and Immunology
Renaissance School of Medicine
Stony Brook University
Stony Brook, New York

Ekaterina E. Heldwein, PhD
American Cancer Society (MA Division) Professor of Molecular Biology
Department of Molecular Biology and Microbiology
Tufts University School of Medicine
Boston, Massachusetts

Hans H. Hirsch, MD, MSc
FMH Infectious Diseases, FMH Internal Medicine, FAMH Med Microbiology
Professor, Medical Faculty
University of Basel
Department of Biomedicine
Transplantation & Clinical Virology Research
Director, Clinical Virology Diagnostics
Laboratory Medicine
University Hospital Basel
Senior Consultant
Infectious Diseases & Hospital Epidemiology Clinics
University Hospital Basel
Basel, Switzerland

Peter M. Howley, MD
Shattuck Professor of Pathological Anatomy
Departments of Immunology and Pathology
Harvard Medical School
Boston, Massachusetts

Yao-Wei Huang, PhD
Professor of Virology
Director, Department of Veterinary Medicine
Center for Veterinary Sciences
Zhejiang University
Hangzhou, Zhejiang Province, China

Michael J. Imperiale, PhD
Arthur F. Thurnau Professor
Department of Microbiology and Immunology
University of Michigan
Ann Arbor, Michigan

Christine Johnston, MD, MPH, FIDSA
Associate Professor
Department of Medicine
University of Washington
Seattle, Washington

David M. Knipe, PhD
Higgins Professor of Microbiology and Molecular Genetics
Head, Harvard Program in Virology
Department of Microbiology
Blavatnik Institute
Harvard Medical School
Boston, Massachusetts

Laurie T. Krug, PhD
Stadtman Investigator
HIV and AIDS Malignancy Branch
National Cancer Institute
Bethesda, Maryland

Thomas Lion, MD, PhD, MSc
Professor
Medical University of Vienna
Medical Director and CEO
Labdia Labordiagnostik
Head, Division of Molecular Microbiology
St. Anna Children's Cancer Research Institute
Vienna, Austria

Richard M. Longnecker, PhD
Dan and Bertha Research Professor
Department of Microbiology–Immunology
Lurie Comprehensive Cancer Center
Feinberg School of Medicine
Northwestern University
Chicago, Illinois

Douglas R. Lowy, MD
Chief, Laboratory of Cellular Oncology
Deputy Director, National Cancer Institute
National Institutes of Health
Bethesda, Maryland

William S. Mason, PhD
Professor
Fox Chase Cancer Center
Philadelphia, Pennsylvania

Alison A. McBride, PhD
Chief, DNA Tumor Virus Section
Laboratory of Viral Diseases
National Institute of Allergy and Infectious Diseases
National Institutes of Health
Bethesda, Maryland

Xiang-Jin Meng, MD, PhD
University Distinguished Professor and Director
Center for Emerging, Zoonotic and Arthropod-borne Pathogens
Department of Biomedical Sciences and Pathobiology
Virginia Polytechnic Institute and State University
Blacksburg, Virginia

Edward S. Mocarski, PhD
Robert W. Woodruff Professor of Microbiology and Immunology
Emory Vaccine Center
Department of Microbiology and Immunology
Emory University School of Medicine
Atlanta, Georgia
Professor Emeritus
Department of Microbiology and Immunology
Stanford University School of Medicine
Stanford, California

Ian J. Mohr, PhD
Professor
Department of Microbiology
New York University School of Medicine
New York, New York

Yasuko Mori, MD, PhD
Professor, Division of Clinical Virology
Centre for Infectious Diseases
Kobe University Graduate School of Medicine
Kobe, Japan

Bernard Moss, MD, PhD
NIH Distinguished Investigator
Chief, Genetic Engineering Section
Laboratory of Viral Diseases
National Institute of Allergy and Infectious Diseases
National Institutes of Health
Bethesda, Maryland

Colin R. Parrish, PhD
Professor of Virology
Baker Institute for Animal Health
Department of Microbiology and Immunology
College of Veterinary Medicine
Cornell University
Ithaca, New York

Philip E. Pellett, PhD
Professor and Chair
Department of Biochemistry, Microbiology and Immunology
Wayne State University School of Medicine
Detroit, Michigan

Panayampalli S. Satheshkumar, PhD
Lead, Immunodiagnostics and Proteomics Team
Poxvirus and Rabies Branch
Division of High Consequence Pathogens and Pathology
Centers for Disease Control and Prevention
Atlanta, Georgia

John T. Schiller, PhD
NIH Distinguished Investigator
Laboratory of Cellular Oncology
Center for Cancer Research
National Cancer Institute
National Institutes of Health
Bethesda, Maryland

Christoph Seeger, PhD
Professor
Fox Chase Cancer Center
Philadelphia, Pennsylvania

Geoffrey L. Smith, PhD
Head, Department of Pathology
University of Cambridge
Cambridge, United Kingdom

Catherine N. Sodroski
Harvard Program in Virology
Department of Microbiology
Harvard Medical School
Boston, Massachusetts

Camille Sureau, PhD
Senior Investigator
Molecular Virology Laboratory
Institut National de la Transfusion Sanguine
Paris, France

Richard J. Whitley, MD
Distinguished Professor
Loeb Eminent Scholar Chair in Pediatrics
Professor of Pediatrics, Microbiology, Medicine and Neurosurgery
University of Alabama at Birmingham
Birmingham, Alabama

William S. M. Wold, PhD
Professor and Chairman
Department of Molecular Microbiology and Immunology
Saint Louis University School of Medicine
St. Louis, Missouri

Danielle M. Zerr, MD, MPH
Professor
Pediatrics/Division of Infectious Diseases
University of Washington
Seattle, Washington

Fabien Zoulim, MD
Professor and Head of Laboratory
Viral Hepatitis Laboratory
INSERM U1052
Cancer Research Center of Lyon
Professor and Head of Department
Department of Hepatology
Hospices Civils de Lyon
Lyon, France

Preface

In the early 1980s, Bernie Fields originated the idea of a virology reference textbook that combined the molecular aspects of viral replication with the medical features of viral infections. This broad view of virology reflected Bernie's own research, which applied molecular and genetic analyses to the study of viral pathogenesis, providing an important part of the foundation for the field of molecular pathogenesis. Bernie led the publication of the first three editions of Virology, but he unfortunately died soon after the third edition went into production. The third edition became *Fields Virology* in his memory, and it is fitting that the book continues to carry his name. A number of changes and enhancements have now been introduced with the seventh edition of *Fields Virology*. The publication format of *Fields Virology* has been changed from a once every 5 to 6 years, two-volume book to an annual publication that comprises approximately one-fourth of the chapters organized by category. The annual publication provides both a physical book volume and importantly an e-book with an improved platform. Using an e-book format, our expectation is that individual chapters can be easily updated when major advances, outbreaks, etc., occur. The editorial board organized the four-volume series for the seventh edition to consist of volumes on Emerging Viruses, DNA Viruses, RNA Viruses, and Fundamental Virology, to be published on an annual basis, with the expectation that the topics will cycle approximately every 4 years creating an annualized, up-to-date publication. Each volume will contain approximately 20 chapters. The first volume of this seventh edition of *Fields Virology*, entitled Emerging Viruses and edited principally by Sean P. J. Whelan, was published in 2020. The second volume, DNA Viruses, has been principally edited by Jeffrey I. Cohen, Blossom Damania, Peter M. Howley, and David M. Knipe. There have been continued rapid advances in virology since the previous edition, and all of the chapters in the DNA Viruses volume are either completely new or have been significantly updated to reflect these advances. In this seventh edition, we have chosen to highlight important references published since the last edition while maintaining older classics. The main emphasis continues to be on viruses of medical importance and interest, but other viruses are described in specific cases where more is known about their mechanisms of replication or pathogenesis.

We wish to thank Patrick Waters of Harvard Medical School and all of the editorial staff members of Wolters Kluwer for their important contributions to the preparation of this book.

David M. Knipe, PhD
Peter M. Howley, MD
Jeffrey I. Cohen, MD
Blossom Damania, PhD
Lynn Enquist, PhD
Eric O. Freed, PhD
Sean P. J. Whelan, PhD

Introduction

DNA Viruses is the second volume of the seventh edition of *Fields Virology*. The first volume, Emerging Viruses, was published last year. The next two volumes, RNA Viruses and Fundamental Virology, will be published annually in subsequent years. There have been continued rapid advances in virology since the sixth edition that was published in 2013, and all of the chapters in the DNA Viruses volume are either completely new or have been significantly updated to reflect these advances. In this seventh edition, we have chosen to highlight important references published since the last edition while maintaining older classics.

This volume covers all of the DNA viruses of medical importance, including viruses that infect humans and animals. DNA viruses of plants, insects, and bacteria will be included in the fourth volume of the seventh edition, Fundamental Virology. In addition to DNA virus families, several thematic issues arise in the consideration of the DNA viruses in this volume. First, the smaller DNA viruses induce cell cycle progression because their genome replication is dependent on host cell DNA replication factors. When dysregulated, the viral activation of host cell DNA replication can lead to cellular proliferation and initiate oncogenic transformation pathways. In addition, some DNA viruses induce proliferation of the host cells and inhibit cellular differentiation in which they are persisting, thus expanding the number of persistently infected cells. Induction of cellular DNA replication factors and inhibition of cellular differentiation is often affected by the inhibition of tumor suppressor genes and pathways by specific DNA viral proteins encoded by these DNA tumor viruses. Indeed, just as oncogenic retroviruses led to the identification of cellular oncogenes, the DNA tumor viruses led to the identification of specific tumor suppressor genes, perhaps the best example being TP53. Second, DNA viruses manipulate the host transcriptional apparatus to allow efficient expression of their genes, and these regulatory systems have elucidated important mechanisms of eukaryotic gene expression. DNA viruses also encounter the host cell epigenetic silencing mechanisms and have evolved mechanisms to allow efficient gene expression for productive infection or silenced gene expression for latent infection, providing important model systems for the study of epigenetic regulation. Third, DNA viruses can often persist in the host cells by the establishment of persistent and sometimes latent infections. The mechanisms by which they do so vary somewhat among the different DNA viruses. The DNA genomes that persist in replicating cells are maintained in cells by the tethering of the viral genomes to cellular chromosomes by viral proteins that bind the viral genomes during mitosis. These systems have informed us about the mechanisms by which viruses can persist in the host organism. Fourth, many of the DNA viruses, including the parvoviruses, the adenoviruses, and some of the herpesviruses, have proven to be effective tools as vaccine platforms and as vectors in gene therapy and oncotherapy.

The organization of the chapters in this edition is similar to that of the previous editions. For most of the viruses, there is a single chapter that combines both the basic and clinical aspects of the virus. For several of the viruses, the basic virology related to viral replication and the viral pathogenesis are split between two chapters. In the DNA volume, this includes the papillomaviruses, the adenoviruses, the human herpesviruses, and the poxviruses. We are grateful to Jeff Cohen and Blossom Damania who joined us as the senior editors who participated in putting this volume together. We also are thankful to the chapter authors who have updated their chapters for this volume and to the new authors who have joined us in this continued endeavor to provide a comprehensive resource in virology.

Peter M. Howley
David M. Knipe

Contents

CHAPTER

1 Polyomaviridae

James A. DeCaprio • Michael J. Imperiale • Hans H. Hirsch

HISTORY

Polyomaviruses are found ubiquitously in a broad range of mammalian, avian, fish, and other species. These viruses can cause severe illness and death on an epidemic scale in birds and raccoons. By contrast, human polyomaviruses typically cause lifelong and asymptomatic infections but can lead to severe illness in immunocompromised patients. Recognition of the ubiquitous presence of polyomaviruses in their natural hosts as well as their disease-causing ability has prompted intensive research efforts.

Polyomaviruses are composed of nonenveloped capsids with a circular double-stranded DNA (dsDNA) genome of approximately 5,000 base pairs containing a single origin of replication and a bidirectional promoter that drives expression of messenger RNA (mRNA) transcripts encoding five to nine proteins. The small size of the polyomavirus (PyV) genome, comparable to a simple plasmid, and its limited number of genetic elements with potent biological activities have fostered research that continues to be at the forefront of biology in the fields of DNA replication, gene expression, signal transduction, and oncogenesis.

The history of PyV research began in the 1950s when Ludwig Gross noted that serial passage of mouse leukemia virus in mice occasionally led to the development of parotid gland tumors instead of leukemia.[112] He isolated this specific activity and demonstrated that the parotid agent differed from murine leukemia virus in its sedimentation, filtration, and heat stability properties. Stewart and colleagues observed the formation of more than 20 different tumor types in newborn mice inoculated with this agent and coined the name *polyomavirus*, derived from the Greek word *poly*, meaning many and *oma*, denoting tumor.[317] The mouse polyomavirus is often called simply "polyomavirus" but will be referred to as MPyV in this chapter, consistent with the most recent taxonomic classification (Table 1.1; Fig. 1.1).[230] Discovered at the same time as MPyV, murine pneumotropic virus (MPtV), also known as Kilham virus or K virus, can cause severe interstitial pneumonia in newborn mice.[110,167]

The next member of the PyV family to be isolated was simian virus 40 (SV40) by Sweet and Hilleman in 1960.[326] Poliovirus vaccine lots produced in rhesus monkey kidney cells were screened for the presence of contaminating viruses. SV40 was the 40th virus isolated from this screen and was notable for causing cytopathic or vacuolating effects in African green monkey kidney cells. It soon became evident that the early production batches of poliovirus vaccine were broadly contaminated with SV40. Although the Salk poliovirus vaccine was inactivated by formalin treatment, SV40 was relatively resistant to this treatment. The presence of potentially viable SV40 in the polio vaccine quickly became a public health concern when the ability of purified virus to cause tumors in newborn hamsters was reported.[104]

Since that time, many polyomaviruses have been isolated from a variety of mammalian, bird, and fish species. The first two human polyomaviruses, JC (JCPyV) and BK (BKPyV), were isolated in 1971 from immunocompromised patients.

TABLE 1.1 Polyomaviruses highlighted in this chapter are listed by genera. Informal and species names, abbreviation, and GenBank identification are provided

	Name	Species	Abbreviation	GenBank	Reference
Alpha					
	Merkel cell	HPyV5	MCPyV, MCV	HM011556.1	84
	Trichodysplasia spinulosa	HPyV8	TSPyV	GU989205.1	342
	HPyV9	HPyV9	HPyV9	HQ696595.1	294
	HPyV12 SaraPyV1	HPyV12 Sorex araneus	HPyV12 SaraPyV1	JX308829.1 MF374998	173 98
	New Jersey	HPyV13	NJPyV	KF954417.1	228
	Hamster	Mesocricetus auratus PyV1	HaPyV	JX036360.1	67
	Mouse	Mus musculus PyV1	MPyV, SE	AF442959.1	112
	Sumatran orangutan	Pongo abelii PyV1	OraPyV2, OraPyV-Sum	FN356901.1	111
	Bornean orangutan	Pongo pygmaeus PyV1	OraPyV1, OraPyV-Bor	FN356900.1	111
	Gorilla gorilla	Gorilla gorilla PyV1	GggPyV1, GgorgPyV1	HQ385752.1	185
	Chimpanzee	Pan troglodytes PyV1	ChPyV1	FR692334.1	68
	Raccoon	Procyon lotor PyV1	RacPyV	JQ178241.1	66
Beta					
	BK	HPyV1	BKPyV, BKV, BK	V01108.1	96
	JC	HPyV2	JCPyV, JCV, JC	J02226.1	252
	KI	HPyV3	KIPyV	EF127906.1	3
	WU	HPyV4	WUPyV	EF444549.1	97
	Simian virus 40	Macaca mulatta PyV1	SV40	J02400.1	326
	Mouse pneumotropic, Kilham, K	Mus musculus PyV2	MPtV	KT987216.1	167
	California sea lion	Zalophus californianus PyV1	SLPyV	GQ331138.1	55
	Squirrel monkey	Saimiri boliviensis PyV	SquiPyV	AM748741.2	347
Delta					
	HPyV6	HpyV6	HPyV6	HM011560.1	288
	HPyV7	HPyV7	HPyV7	HM011566.1	288
	Malawi	HPyV10	MWPyV	JQ898291.1	308
	St. Louis	HPyV11	STLPyV	JX463183.1	193
Gamma					
	Budgerigar fledgling disease virus	Aves PyV1	BFDV	AF241168.1	238
	Goose hemorrhagic	Anser anser PyV1	GHPV	AY140894.1	114
	Crow	Corvus monedula PyV1	CPyV	DQ192570.1	153
	Finch	Pyrrhula pyrrhula PyV1	FPyV	DQ192571.1	153
	Canary	Serinus canaria PyV1	CaPyV	GU345044.1	119
Unassigned					
	Bovine	Bos taurus PyV1	BPyV	NC_001442.1	291
	African green monkey, B-lymphotropic		LPyV AGMPyV	K02562.2	263
	Simian virus 12	Papio ursinus PyV	SA12	AY614708.1	338
	Lyon IARC Cat-associated Lyon-IARC polyomavirus		LIPyV	KY404016.1 MK898813.1	80,100

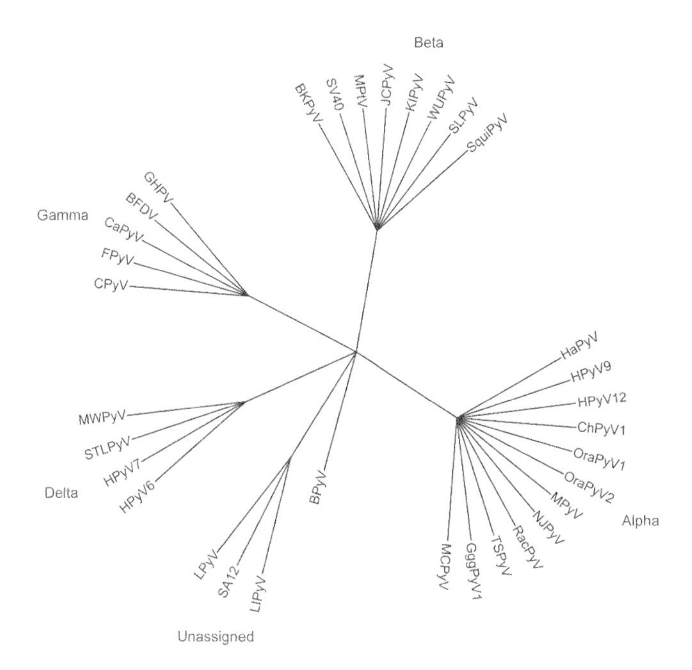

FIGURE 1.1 Taxonomy of polyomaviruses. Taxonomic tree of the family *Polyomaviridae* large T antigen proteins. Branch lengths do not correspond to phylogenetic distance. The genera Alphapolyomavirus, Betapolyomavirus, Deltapolyomavirus, Gammapolyomavirus, and unclassified polyomaviruses are labeled. See Table 1.1 for full names and GenBank Accession numbers. Figure courtesy of Jason Nomburg.

JCPyV was isolated by the transfer of brain tissue from a patient with progressive multifocal leukoencephalopathy (PML) into cultures of human fetal brain tissue.[252] BKPyV was isolated from the urine of a renal transplant patient after inoculating African green monkey kidney cells.[96]

The advent of advanced molecular biology techniques including polymerase chain reaction (PCR), rolling circle amplification, and next generation sequencing has led to the identification of at least 10 additional human polyomaviruses. WUPyV and KIPyV were isolated from respiratory secretions of young children by investigators at Washington University and the Karolinska Institute, respectively. The discovery of Merkel cell polyomavirus (MCPyV) reflected recognition that the incidence of Merkel cell carcinoma (MCC), a rare form of skin cancer, was more frequent in severely immunocompromised patients and suggestive of an infectious cause. MCPyV was initially detected in MCC specimens by digital transcriptome subtraction, a method that used high-throughput sequencing of cellular transcripts to identify sequences that did not match the human genome but were distantly related to BKPyV.[84]

Two additional human polyomaviruses, HPyV6 and HPyV7, were cloned from the skin or hair follicles of healthy adults using a technique called rolling circle amplification that takes advantage of the small circular nature of the polyomavirus dsDNA genome.[288] Using the same technique, trichodysplasia spinulosa–associated polyomavirus (TSPyV) was found in a patient with a rare skin disease named trichodysplasia spinulosa.[342] Although identification of novel polyomaviruses by DNA sequencing has become easier, isolation of infectious viruses or even virion particles remains a technical challenge.

Primate polyomaviruses from Old World monkeys include the simian agent 12 (SA12), isolated from a South African vervet monkey kidney culture, and B-lymphotropic polyomavirus (LPyV), isolated from an African green monkey lymphoblast cell line. Additional primate polyomaviruses directly isolated from animals include Bornean (OraPyV1) and Sumatran orangutan polyomavirus (OraPyV2), gorilla polyomavirus (GggPyV), and chimpanzee polyomavirus (CHPyV).[185] The first New World monkey polyomavirus (SquiPyV) isolated was from squirrel monkey.[347]

In addition to MPyV and MPtV, a number of nonprimate mammalian polyomaviruses have been identified. Hamster polyomavirus (HaPyV) was discovered in a spontaneously occurring hair follicle epithelioma from a Syrian hamster. This is an interesting member of the polyomavirus family because the behavior of the virus in the tumors most closely resembles that of the papillomaviruses in that viral particles can be found in the highly differentiated layers of the tissue. However, analysis of the HaPyV DNA sequence and its genome organization revealed that it is indeed a polyomavirus and most closely related to MPyV.[67] Bovine polyomavirus (BPyV) is among the smallest of the polyomavirus genomes with fewer than 4,700 base pairs. Sea lion polyomavirus (SLPyV) was isolated from a sick animal with kidney swelling, interstitial nephritis, and an intestinal lymphoma.[55] Raccoon polyomavirus (RacPyV) is associated with neuroglial brain tumors in the wild, with the seroprevalence of this virus in raccoons over 50% in some regions of the United States.[52,66]

Polyomaviruses have been isolated from several bird species. The first of these, budgerigar fledgling disease virus (BFDV), was isolated from a parakeet in 1986.[238] Unlike the narrow host range restriction of mammalian polyomaviruses, BFDV can infect and cause disease in a wide variety of bird species and is now referred to as *Aves polyomavirus 1*. Recently identified bird polyomaviruses include canary (CPyV), crow, finch (FPyV), and goose hemorrhagic polyomavirus (GHPV).[153] In general, the avian polyomaviruses cause a severe inflammatory illness that often results in death. Infection with GHPV causes hemorrhagic nephritis and enteritis.[152]

For many years, the polyomaviruses were studied principally as model systems for understanding basic eukaryotic cell processes including DNA replication, RNA transcription, splicing, and oncogenic transformation. The cloning and sequencing of the SV40 genome ushered in the era of recombinant DNA research. Several genetic elements from the SV40 genome, such as the origin of replication, the early promoter, the *STAG* (small t antigen) splice donor and acceptor, and the polyadenylation signal, are widely used in molecular biology laboratories throughout the world.[240,269,274]

Interest in the polyomaviruses as human pathogens lagged behind these more basic biological studies because for many years the incidence of polyomavirus-associated diseases was rare and not well recognized. The onset of the human immunodeficiency virus type 1 (HIV-1)/acquired immunodeficiency syndrome (AIDS) epidemic led to a dramatic rise in the incidence of PML, a JCPyV-induced disease. More recently, biological therapies for multiple sclerosis have also led to a significantly increased risk for developing JCPyV-associated PML. Advances in immunosuppressive regimens for hematopoietic stem cell and solid organ transplantation recipients and biological therapies for autoimmune diseases have led to increases in JCPyV, BKPyV, MCPyV, HPyV6, HPyV7, and potentially TSPyV-associated diseases. Furthermore, the transforming activity of MCPyV and its contribution to MCC and BKPyV association with urothelial carcinoma has generated further interest in the oncogenic activity of human polyomaviruses. However, while polyomaviruses share many features, there are many fundamental differences that can distinguish each member of this family.

CLASSIFICATION

Polyomaviruses were originally classified within the *Papovaviridae* family that included papillomavirus, polyomavirus, and vacuolating virus.[223] The vacuolating or cytopathic effect of SV40 virus on host cells during lytic infection led to this distinction (Fig. 1.2). Polyomaviruses and papillomaviruses are divided into separate families since 2000, after sequencing studies revealed that despite their similar physical appearance, the two groups of viruses have different genome organization. Several classifications have been proposed with the most recent report from the International Committee on Taxonomy of Viruses (ICTV) that includes four major categories (Alpha, Beta, Gamma, and Delta) plus an unclassified group containing several polyomaviruses isolated from fish (Table 1.1) (Fig. 1.1).[230] The human Alpha polyomaviruses comprise MCPyV, as well as TSPyV, HPyV9, and New Jersey (NJPyV). The Beta polyomaviruses include SV40 and the human JCPyV, BKPyV, KIPyV, and WUPyV polyomaviruses. The Gamma polyomaviruses contain species isolated from birds. Several polyomaviruses have not been officially classified within the family either because the complete viral genomic sequence is not available or they have significant differences in genome organization.

VIRION STRUCTURE

Polyomavirus virions are nonenveloped, 45- to 50-nm particles consisting of two or three virally encoded capsid proteins. All viruses have the major capsid protein Vp1 and the minor protein Vp2, and some also have Vp3 derived from an internal start site within the *VP2* gene.[286] The virions encapsidate a circular dsDNA genome wrapped with cellular histones H2A, H2B, H3, and H4.[331] The virion minichromosome exhibits the same nucleosome structure as cellular chromatin except for the absence of histone H1 that becomes associated with the viral genome in the infected cell. The particles have a T = 7 icosahedral symmetry and sediment at 240S in sucrose density gradients. The density of mature virions is 1.34 g/mL and of empty capsids is 1.29 g/mL, as determined by cesium chloride equilibrium gradient centrifugation (Fig. 1.3).[27] The polyomaviruses are relatively resistant to heat and formalin inactivation, as demonstrated by the isolation of viable SV40 from the Salk poliovirus vaccine.[319] Because polyomaviruses are nonenveloped, they are also resistant to lipid solvents. Similar to most viruses, preparations of polyomavirus virions often contain many different types of particles. For example, in addition to mature virions, one can find empty capsids or capsids that contain cellular DNA instead of viral DNA (Fig. 1.3). The ability of Vp1 and Vp2 to form pseudovirions has been exploited to generate not only infectious polyomavirus but also a variety of reporters.

The polyomavirus capsid contains 360 molecules of Vp1 arranged as 72 pentamers, each containing five molecules of Vp1 and one molecule of Vp2 or Vp3. Only the Vp1 molecule is exposed on the surface of the capsid. The icosahedral capsid has both five- and sixfold axes of symmetry, with 12 pentamers surrounded by 5 other pentamers and 60 pentamers surrounded by 6 pentamers (Fig. 1.4).[144,145,191,316] The recent cryo-EM analysis of BKPyV revealed the position of Vp2 and Vp3 under the Vp1 shell and contacts between the viral genome and the three capsid proteins (Fig. 1.5).[145] The C-terminus of each Vp1 molecule extends out of the pentamer and contacts the neighboring capsomere. This structure is flexible and thereby provides the means to form an icosahedron. Capsomere contacts are stabilized by the presence of calcium ions and mutations in residues that bind calcium result in unstable virions. Treatment of virus with EGTA under reducing conditions results in the dissociation of the capsid into Vp1 pentamers. In addition to Vp1, Vp2, and Vp3, APyV expresses Vp4 (agnoprotein 1a) that interacts with the C-terminus of Vp1 and may be incorporated into viral capsids.[302] The capsid also contains posttranslational modifications including disulfide bonds that form between the pentameric capsomeres. In addition, Vp2 undergoes myristoylation at its N-terminus. One

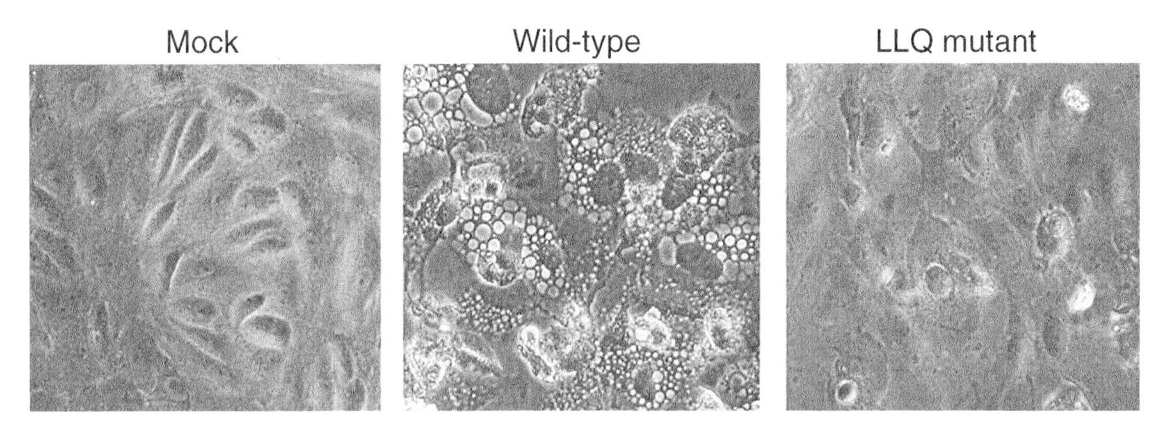

FIGURE 1.2 Interaction between simian virus 40 major capsid protein Vp1 and cell surface ganglioside GM1 triggers vacuole formation. CV-1 monkey cells were infected with wild-type SV40 or a GM1-binding defective (LLQ) Vp1 mutant. Phase-contrast images taken 72 hours postinfection.[204] (Adapted from Magaldi TG, Buch MH, Murata H, et al. Mutations in the GM1 binding site of simian virus 40 VP1 alter receptor usage and cell tropism. *J Virol* 2012;86(13): 7028–7042. Copyright © 2012 American Society for Microbiology. Amended with permission from American Society for Microbiology.)

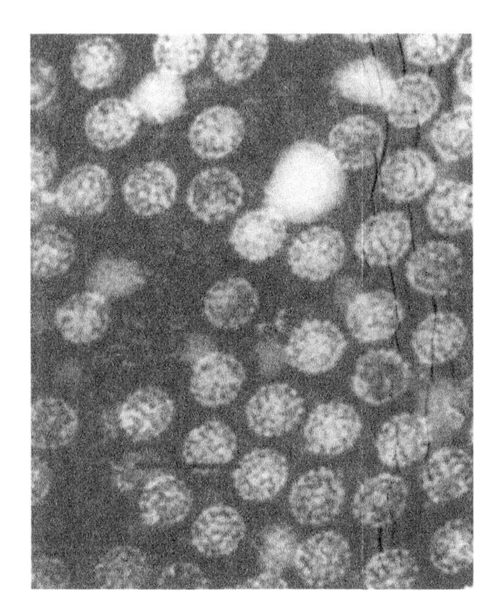
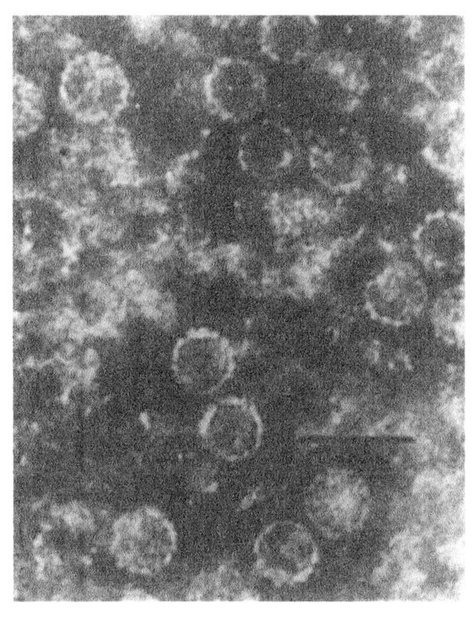

FIGURE 1.3 SV40 particles from full band density (left) and empty band density (right) isolated by density gradient centrifugation.[27] (Reprinted from Black PH, Crawford EM, Crawford LV. The purification of simian virus 40. *Virology* 1964;24(3):381–387. Copyright © 1964 Elsevier. With permission.)

report found a large number of posttranslational modifications on the BKPyV Vp1 protein, although the role of these modifications during infection is not known.[81]

GENOME STRUCTURE AND ORGANIZATION

The polyomavirus dsDNA circular genome contains approximately 5,000 base pairs and can be divided into three parts: the early viral gene region (EVGR) encoding genes that are expressed prior to the onset of DNA replication; the late viral gene region (LVGR) encoding genes expressed after viral DNA replication begins; and the regulatory region, also called noncoding control region (NCCR), containing the origin of viral DNA replication and the promoters and enhancers for early and late viral genes (Fig. 1.6). The early and late promoters give rise to primary transcripts from opposite strands of the DNA. The numbering system for the polyomavirus genome differs from virus to virus with nucleotide position 1 defined in different ways.[331] There has been precedent in recent years, however, to call the nucleotide preceding the A in the *LTAG* ATG nucleotide 1, with numbering proceeding in the late direction, that is, away from the *LTAG* open reading frame.

The small size of the polyomavirus genome made it amenable to classical genetic approaches.[331] Infection with temperature-sensitive mutants of SV40 led to the identification of five complementation groups, A, B, BC, C, and D. Mutations in group A mapped to the large T antigen (LTag) gene (*LTAG*); groups B, BC, and C to the *VP1* gene; and

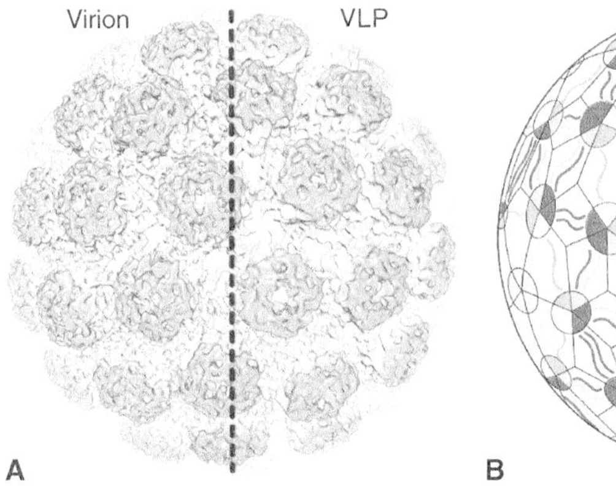

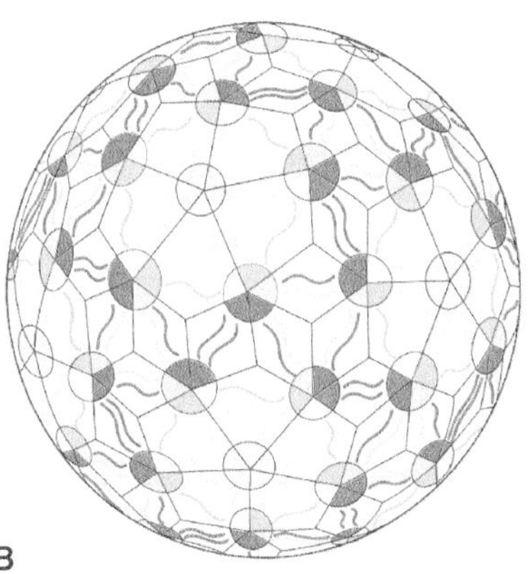

FIGURE 1.4 Cryo-EM structures of the BKPyV Virion and VLP. A: An external view of the virion (*left*) and VLP (*right*). **B:** The polyomavirus capsid built with 72 pentamers of Vp1. (Reprinted from Hurdiss DL, Morgan EL, Thompson RF, et al. New Structural Insights into the Genome and Minor Capsid Proteins of BK Polyomavirus using Cryo-Electron Microscopy. *Structure* 2016;24(4):528–536. https://creativecommons.org/licenses/by/4.0/.)

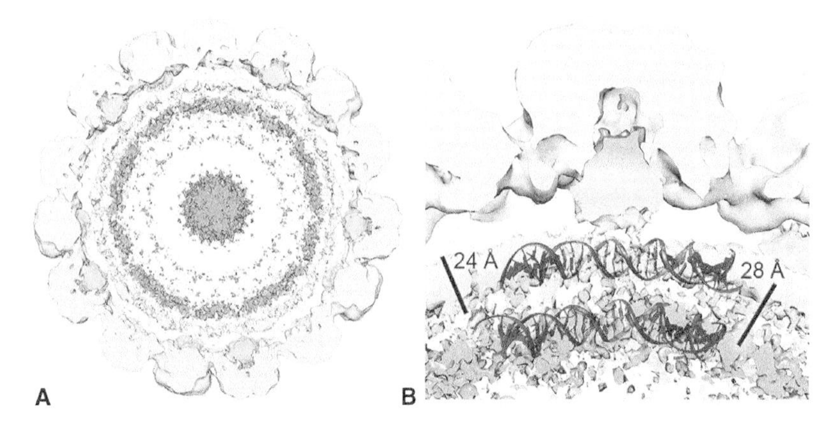

FIGURE 1.5 Minor capsid proteins and genome organization. A: A 40-Å thick slab through the unsharpened/unmasked virion map. Pyramidal density below each VP1 penton and two shells of electron density adjacent to the inner capsid layer can be seen. The density for SV40 Vp1 is colored *gray*. Density for Vp2 and Vp3 is colored *blue/green* and for packaged dsDNA *yellow/pink*. **B:** Enlarged view of the pyramidal density beneath a single VP1 penton of the virion.[145] Strands of dsDNA wrapped around a human histone octamer are shown. (Reprinted from Hurdiss DL, Morgan EL, Thompson RF, et al. New Structural Insights into the Genome and Minor Capsid Proteins of BK Polyomavirus using Cryo-Electron Microscopy. *Structure* 2016;24(4):528–536. https://creativecommons.org/licenses/by/4.0/.)

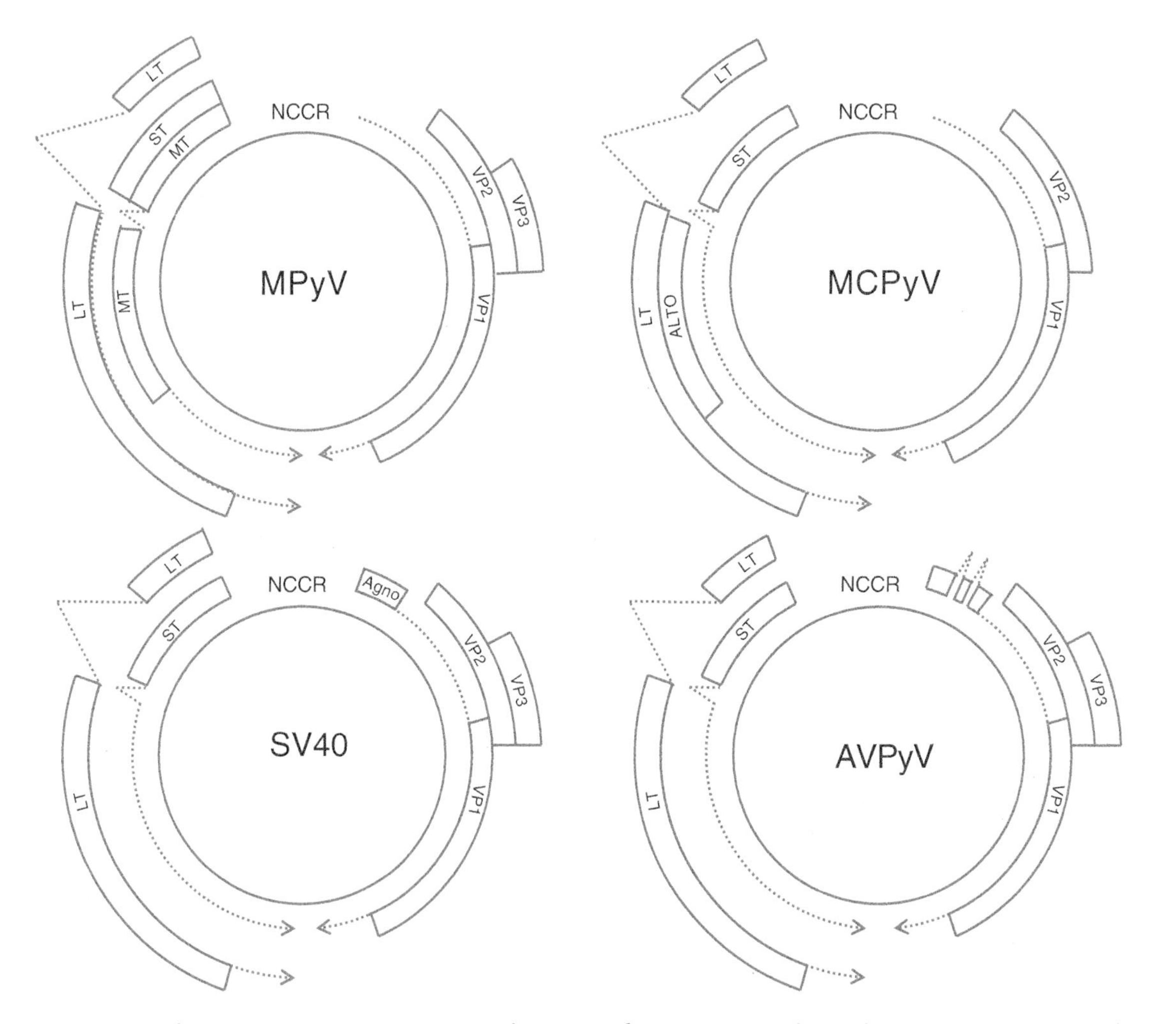

FIGURE 1.6 Polyomavirus Genome Organization depictions of major gene products of MPyV, MCPyV, SV40, and AVPyV. Noncoding control region (NCCR) controls bidirectional gene expression with early viral gene region (EVGR) shown in counterclockwise orientation and late viral gene region (LVGR) shown in clockwise orientation.

group D to the *VP2/3* gene. MPyV mutants were classified into similar complementation groups, although no standard nomenclature was developed for this virus. Other mutants of MPyV known as host range nontransforming (hr-t) mutants were selected for their ability to replicate but inability to transform cells. The hr-t mutations were later mapped to the middle T antigen (MTag) and small T antigen (STag) genes (*MTAG, STAG*) leaving an intact LTag.[309] The analysis of these early mutants set the stage for detailed and directed mutational studies enabled by recombinant DNA technology.

Another early genetic approach to the study of polyomaviruses was the selection for so-called evolutionary variants. In these experiments, viruses were passaged at high multiplicities of infection and variants were isolated. Many of these variants in SV40 and BKPyV had alterations in the NCCR involving partial sequence duplications, deletions, or combinations thereof.[184,229] The emergence of BKPyV NCCR rearrangements was partly dependent on the viral replication capacity in a given host cell. Of note, the NCCRs of BKPyV and JCPyV are frequently found to be rearranged when isolated from diseased tissues or patients' blood. These patient-derived rearranged NCCR variants also tend to replicate well in cell culture when compared to viruses containing the wild-type NCCR.[108,109]

The polyomavirus early and late promoters are contained within the NCCR and often overlap with each other as well as with the origin of replication. Transcription of the EVGR progresses from the early promoter around the genome in one direction. Transcription of the LVGR proceeds from the late promoter around the genome in the opposite direction. The EVGR mRNAs are produced by posttranscriptional processing at a polyadenylic acid or poly(A) site that is located about halfway around the circular genome from the start site and by removal of introns by the cellular splicing machinery. SV40 was one of the first experimental systems where it was demonstrated that RNA polymerase II transcribes past the 3′ end of the mature mRNA molecule, implying that the 3′ end, including the poly(A) tail, was generated posttranscriptionally.[88]

Each of the polyomaviruses encodes at least two early mRNAs by alternative splicing that are translated into the LTag and STag (Fig. 1.7). In addition, MPyV, HaPyV, and TSPyV produce a third alternatively spliced mRNA that codes for MTag.[340] The "T" in T antigen derives from the initial identification of these proteins as tumor antigens that were recognized by antisera from tumor-bearing animals inoculated with SV40. For many years, it was believed that the mRNAs encoding LTag, STag, and MTag were the only early transcripts,

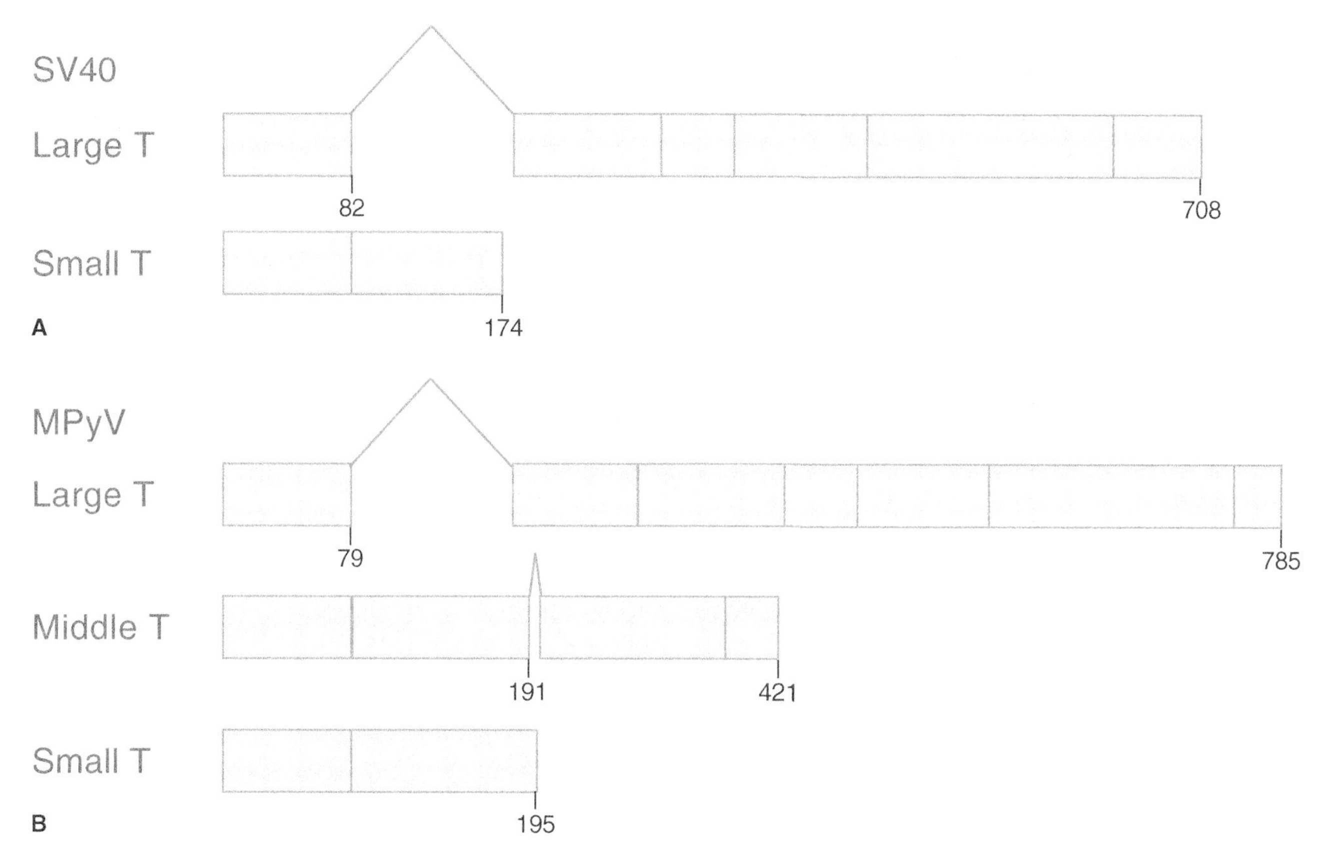

FIGURE 1.7 Simian virus 40 (SV40) (A) and mouse polyomavirus (MPyV) (B) T antigens. The N-terminal J domain is shared with all T antigens. SV40 expresses large and small T antigens, and MPyV expresses large, middle, and small T antigens. The large T antigens contain the LXCXE motif that binds directly to RB, a nuclear localization signal (NLS), a DNA-binding domain (DBD) that binds to the origin of replication, and a helicase domain. SV40 Large antigen contains a C-terminal host range (HR) domain. The small T antigens contain a unique domain not shared with large T antigen that binds to two Zn molecules. The MPyV middle T antigen shares the J domain and Zn-binding domain with small T antigen and also contains tyrosine and serine residues (YSY) that become phosphorylated, a proline-rich region, and a C-terminal hydrophobic domain. Figure courtesy of Camille Cushman.

but it has since been demonstrated that these viruses encode additional early mRNAs that differ in their splicing patterns. In SV40 and MPyV, an additional mRNA encodes a protein called 17KT and tiny T, respectively. Similarly, JCPyV produces a series of alternatively spliced mRNAs that encode proteins referred to as T′135, T′136, and T′165, while BKPyV encodes a molecule called truncated Tag, implicated in the induction of APOBEC3 activity in infected cells. MCPyV encodes a full-length, 816-residue LTag as well as an alternatively spliced T antigen called 57kT that corresponds to the first 440 and last 100 residues of the full-length LTag.[303] MCPyV and several other polyomaviruses encode an early protein called ALTO that is produced by overprinting of the second exon of the *LTAG* mRNA (Fig. 1.6).[43] TSPyV encodes ALTO as well as MTag in addition to LTag and STag.[344] The function of ALTO has not yet been elucidated. Of note, the Alpha polyomaviruses were previously grouped as Almi (ALTO or middle T) polyomaviruses.[43] The principle distinction in the LTag between the Alpha/Almi polyomaviruses with the Beta polyomaviruses is the number of residues between the end of the N-terminal J domain and the start of the origin binding domain. ALTO and MTag are encoded in the +1 reading frame of LTag exon 2.

The late mRNA is transcribed in the opposite direction from the early mRNAs. As with the early transcripts, the late transcript has a single poly(A) site approximately halfway around the genome and is alternatively spliced (Fig. 1.6). The LVGR of most polyomaviruses encodes three capsid proteins, Vp1, Vp2, and Vp3, although some, such as MCPyV, only encode Vp1 and Vp2.[286] Notably, Vp3 is translated in the same open reading frame as Vp2 but uses an alternate *AUG* start codon downstream of the *VP2* start codon and thereby shares all residues with Vp2. While it had been reported that SV40 encodes a Vp4 protein that uses an internal *AUG* start codon even further downstream from *VP3* and functions as a viroporin that promotes virus release from the infected cell, more recent studies found no effect of the start codon mutations on SV40 or BKPyV release, and failed to detect this protein.[125] The LVGR transcript from SV40, JCPyV, and BKPyV as well as SA12, BatPyV, BPyV, SLPyV, and SqPyV encode an additional protein called agnoprotein.

Avian polyomaviruses express early transcripts encoding LTag and STag, but the late transcripts have several distinct features (Fig. 1.6). There are two late transcription start sites, PL1 and PL2, that give rise to at least eight different transcripts by alternative splicing.[189] PL1 encodes two forms of Vp4 (agnoprotein 1a) and Vp4d (*VPD4*, agnoprotein 1b), while PL2 gives rise to two forms of agnoprotein 2a and 2b that use the same splice sites as *VP4* and *VP4d* but are translated in a different reading frame. Avian agnoprotein 2a and 2b bears some similarity to the SV40 agnoprotein. All of the late avian transcripts also encode for Vp1 or Vp2 and Vp3.

The LVGR transcript can also extend past the polyadenylation signal and give rise to a microRNA (miRNA) in several polyomaviruses.[46,323] The SV40 miRNA maps just 3′ of the late poly(A) site and appears to correspond to SAS (SV40-associated small RNA), a small RNA molecule identified 25 years earlier, albeit of then-unknown function.[4] These miRNAs are complementary to the early mRNAs, target the early mRNAs for degradation, and may serve to limit the expression levels of the T antigens. MiRNAs have been identified in SV40, BKPyV, JCPyV, MCPyV, SA12, and MPyV.[46] Based on both *in vivo* and *in vitro* data, the miRNAs of SV40, BKPyV, and MCPyV have been proposed to play an important role in persistent infection. How expression of the miRNA is controlled is poorly understood; in BKPyV, it has been suggested to be driven from the NCCR, while RNA-seq data from MCPyV suggests the possibility of an independent promoter.

Structure of T Antigens

Much of what is known about the protein structure of the polyomavirus T antigens comes from studies of SV40. All polyomavirus T antigens share an N-terminal region of approximately 80 residues that shows structural and sequence homology to the DnaJ or J domain found in host cell heat shock 40 (HSP40) homologs (Fig. 1.7). The J domain corresponds approximately to the first exon of *LTAG* and is also represented in the N-termini of all PyV STag and MTag. Full-length LTag is a nuclear phosphoprotein of approximately 700 residues. The molecule's atomic coordinates have been assembled from crystallography of isolated domains, including the J domain, the retinoblastoma protein (RB)-binding or LXCXE motif, the DNA-binding or origin-binding domain (DBD or OBD), and a central domain that contains the adenosine triphosphatase (ATPase) and helicase activities required for viral replication.[168,190] The C-terminus of SV40, BKPyV, and JCPyV LTag also contain a host range domain.[87] Studies using scanning transmission electron microscopy, negative staining with atomic force microscopy, and single-particle reconstruction of cryoelectron microscopy (cryo-EM) images revealed that LTag forms a double hexamer in a head-to-head arrangement when bound to the origin of DNA replication.[60]

A number of functional domains contained within LTag are required for viral replication. Functions intrinsic to SV40 LTag include the ATPase/helicase domain and the DBD that mediates direct interactions with specific DNA sequences at the origin of replication. In addition to these intrinsic functions, the SV40 LTag domains serve to recruit host factors important for viral replication (Fig. 1.8). For example, the N-terminal J domain, containing the canonical residues HPDK, binds and activates the ATPase activity of host cell HSC70.[40] The DBD binds to replication protein A (RPA), while the helicase domain binds to the DNA polymerase α/primase complex.[142] In addition, the helicase domains of many but not all polyomavirus LTags bind to p53. The outer surface of each SV40 LTag hexamer subunit can bind directly to the DBD of p53 (Fig. 1.9).[192] Similarly, the JCPyV, BKPyV, and MWPyV LTags can also bind to p53. However, MPyV and MCPyV LTag are notable exceptions among polyomaviruses because they do not bind to p53.[257]

Smaller functional motifs within LTags include the nuclear localization signal (NLS).[155,181] Mutations that disrupt the NLS result in the cytoplasmic localization of SV40 LTag and reduced ability to support the viral lytic life cycle. All mammalian polyomavirus LTag contain the conserved residues LXCXE (leucine-X-cysteine-X-glutamate, where X is any residue) that bind directly to the retinoblastoma family of tumor suppressor proteins including RB (RB1), p107 (RBL1), and p130 (RBL2).[65] The LTag and STag from GHPyV, CPyV, and

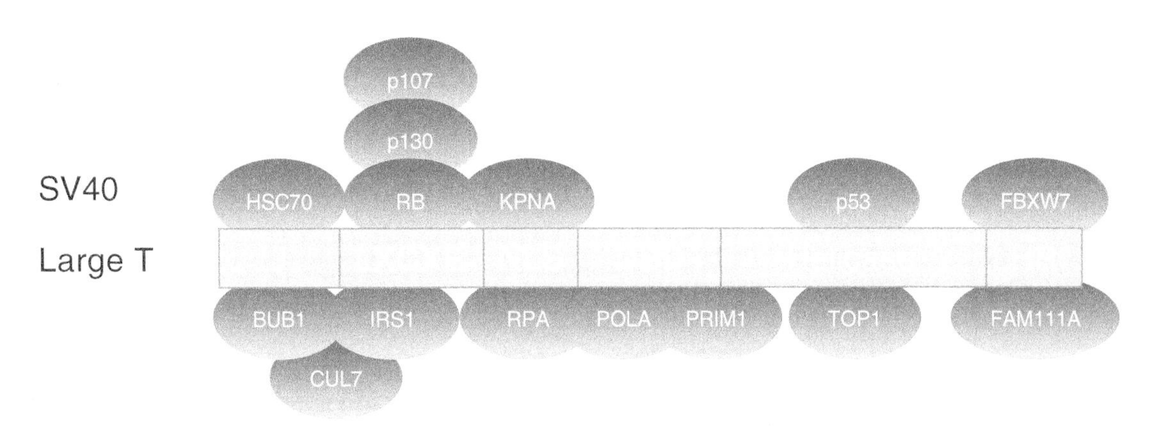

FIGURE 1.8 SV40 large T antigen interaction with host cell proteins. The J domain binds to HSC70, the LXCXE motif binds to RB and the RB-like p107 and p130, the helicase domain binds to TP53, the phosphorylated threonine residue 701 binds to FBXW7, and FAM111A binds to the host range (HR) domain. The cellular proteins BUB1, CUL7, and IRS1 bind to a region between the J domain and the LXCXE motif. Karyopherin (KPNA) binds to the nuclear localization sequence (NLS). Large T antigen recruits replication protein A (RPA), topoisomerase 1 (TOP1), DNA polymerase a (POLA), and primase (PRIM) to promote viral DNA replication. Figure courtesy of Camille Cushman.

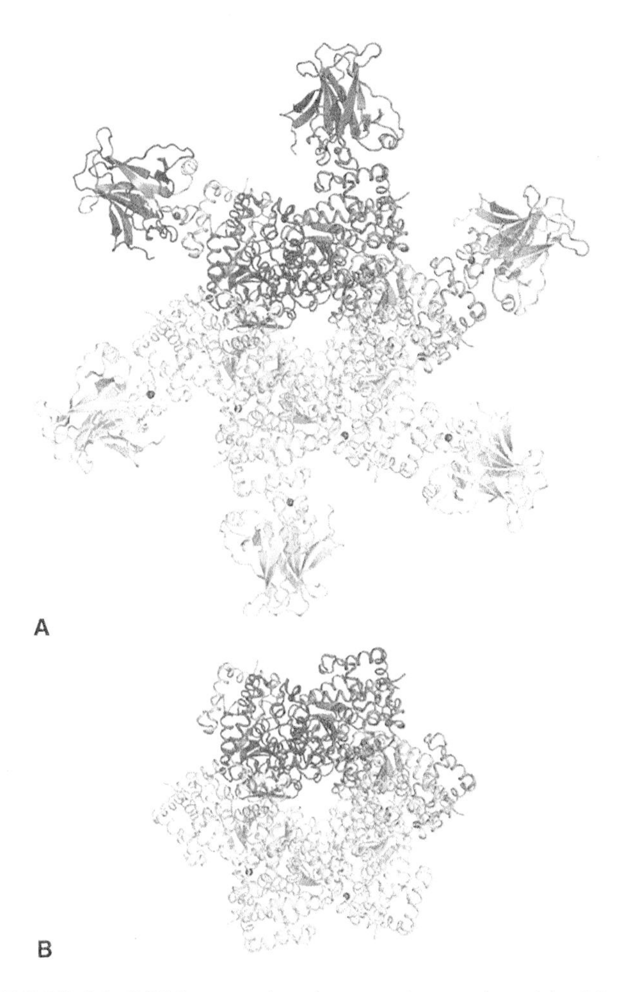

FIGURE 1.9 SV40 large antigen hexamer in complex with p53. The large T antigen hexamer in complex with p53 **(A)** and without p53 **(B).**[192] (Reprinted with permission from Lilyestrom W, Klein MG, Zhang R, et al. Crystal structure of SV40 large T-antigen bound to p53: interplay between a viral oncoprotein and a cellular tumor suppressor. *Genes Dev* 2006;20(17):2373–2382. Copyright © 2006 Cold Spring Harbor Laboratory Press.)

FPyV each contain the LXCXE motif, while those from APyV contain a related sequence, LXAXE. It is not known if any of the bird polyomavirus T antigens can bind to RB or p53.

SV40 LTag contains a series of posttranslational modifications, including phosphorylation, O-glycosylation, acylation, poly(ADP)-ribosylation, and acetylation. Phosphorylation regulates some of the functions of the molecule, including its subcellular localization and its ability to participate in the initiation of viral DNA synthesis. In addition, phosphorylation of C-terminally located threonine residues in SV40, BKPyV, and JCPyV LTag creates a phosphodegron motif (phospho-T-P-P-P) that binds directly to FBXW7, an F-box substrate adapter. LTag binding to FBXW7 interferes with FBXW7 binding to Cyclin E and thereby stabilizes it by reducing degradation by the SKP1–CUL1–FBXW7 ubiquitin ligase (Fig. 1.8).[355]

Polyomavirus STag is found in both the nucleus and cytoplasm. STag is a cysteine-rich protein ranging in size from 124 to 198 residues and shares its N-terminus with LTag (i.e., those residues encoded up to the 5′ LTag splice site) but contains a unique C-terminal region. STag contains the same N-terminal J domain as LTag and a unique C-terminal domain (Fig. 1.7). The unique domain of the mammalian polyomavirus STags contains a highly conserved set of cysteine and histidine residues that bind to two zinc molecules or iron–sulfur clusters.[335] These zinc-binding domains serve an important role in binding to the cellular protein phosphatase 2A (PP2A).[253] PP2A is a trimeric complex consisting of the scaffold A subunit and regulatory B subunit that bind to the catalytic C subunit. STag binds directly to the PP2A A subunit and thereby displaces or replaces the B subunit. SV40 STag binds specifically to the Aα (PPP2R1A) subunit, while MPyV and MCPyV STag binds to both the Aα and Aβ (PPP2R1B) subunits. The STag–PP2A complex contains also the Cα (PPP2CA) or Cβ (PPP2CB) catalytic subunit. There are at least 18 different B PP2A subunits identified in mammalian cells. At the very least, SV40 STag can displace the B56α (PPP2R5A), B56γ (PPP2R5C), and PR72/PR130 (PPP2R3A).[280] It is likely that the polyomavirus STag–PP2A complex not only serves to disrupt the cellular PP2A complexes but is also likely to retain specific phosphatase activity directed toward substrates. Notably, the bird polyomavirus STags do not contain the conserved cysteine/histidine residues, and it is not known if they are capable of PP2A binding.

The STags from several polyomaviruses can bind to cellular proteins in addition to PP2A. MCPyV STag can bind specifically to the MYC paralog MYCL (L-MYC) and the EP400 chromatin remodeling complex.[51] The MCPyV ST–MYCL–EP400 complex functions to transactivate a large number of genes that contribute to the oncogenic activity in MCC (Fig. 1.10). SV40 STag displaces common PP2A B subunits but also promotes A–C subunit interactions with alternative B subunits (B′, striatins) that are components of the striatin-interacting phosphatase and kinase (STRIPAK) complex. STag binding to STRN4, a component of the STRIPAK complex, facilitates PP2A-mediated dephosphorylation of MAP4K4 and induces cell transformation through the activation of the Hippo pathway effector YAP1 (Fig. 1.10).[169]

The MTag of MPyV shares its N-terminal J domain and PP2A-binding domain with STag (Fig. 1.7). The MPyV MTag and STag are identical for the N-terminal 191 residues until a splice junction that removes four nucleotides resulting in an additional 230 residues at the C-terminus of MTag. By contrast, STag contains only four unique amino acids after this intron. The unique MTag C-terminus is encoded by an alternate reading frame to that used for coding the second exon of LTag. Notably, MTag contains an N-terminal J domain in common with both LTag and STag, and like STag, binds to the A and C subunits of PP2A. The additional MPyV MTag residues mediate binding to several proteins involved in signal transduction, including the SRC tyrosine kinase, the SHC1 phosphotyrosine docking protein, 14-3-3, phospholipase C (PLCG1), and phosphatidylinositol 3-kinase (PIK3CA and PIK3R1) (Fig. 1.11).[284] MPyV MTag can also bind to the SRC-related tyrosine kinases YES1 and FYN. The C-terminus of MTag contains a 22-residue hydrophobic domain that moves the newly translated MTag from the cytoplasm through the endoplasmic reticulum (ER) to the inner plasma membrane. The combination of membrane localization with recruitment and activation of several enzymes enables MTag, which itself has no intrinsic enzymatic activity, to essentially function as a constitutively activated receptor tyrosine kinase that activates the RAS, MAPK, and AKT downstream signaling pathways.

STAGES OF REPLICATION

Mechanism of Attachment

Prior to the 21st century, the nature of the cell surface receptors for polyomaviruses was poorly understood. Early studies on SV40 indicated that it used the major histocompatibility complex (MHC) class I antigens to bind to cells. Supporting evidence for this model included observations that antibodies against MHC class I blocked virus binding to rhesus monkey kidney cells and the inability of virus to bind to human cells that do not express MHC class I, while experimentally induced expression of MHC class I in nonexpressing cells restored binding. Although the MHC class I antigens were implicated as the SV40 receptor, they were not sufficient to account for all binding. For example, virus binding occurred only on the apical surface of polarized monkey epithelial cells, while MHC class I antigens were expressed on both the apical and basolateral surfaces. In addition, expression of MHC class I on human kidney epithelial cells was not sufficient for SV40 infection.[203]

Subsequent results challenged the notion that SV40 uses a protein molecule as its receptor and demonstrated instead that it uses the branched ganglioside GM1 (Fig. 1.12).[334] This finding is more consistent with the route of entry of the virus through endosomes. In these studies, a cell line that did not express gangliosides and was unable to be infected by SV40 was rendered susceptible by preincubation with GM1. Gangliosides are glycosphingolipids that combine a sialylated oligosaccharide

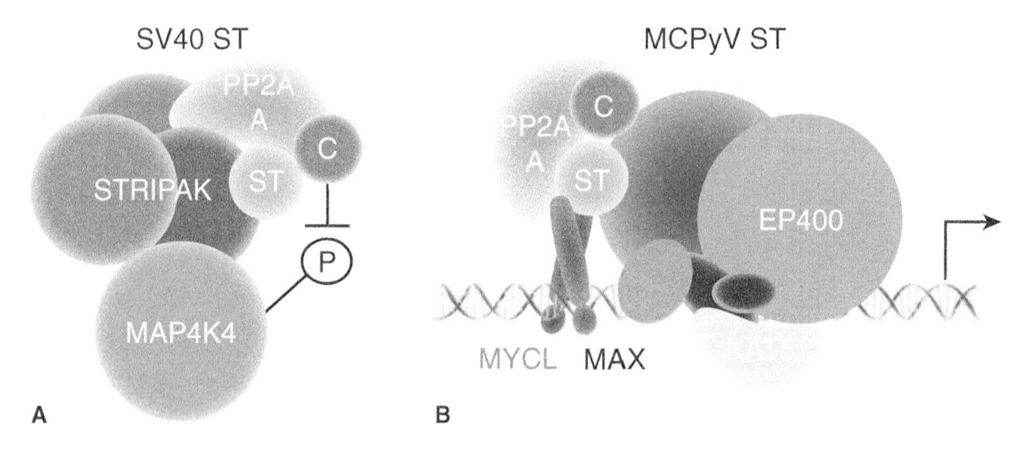

FIGURE 1.10 SV40 and MCPyV small T antigens form unique multiprotein complexes. A: SV40 small T antigen recruits the PP2A A and C subunits to the multiprotein STRIPAK complex and directs the dephosphorylation of MAP4K4 that leads to inhibition of the Hippo pathway and activation of YAP. (From Kim JW, Berrios C, Kim M, et al. STRIPAK directs PP2A activity toward MAP4K4 to promote oncogenic transformation of human cells. *Elife* 2020;9:e53003.) Ref.[169] **B:** The MCPyV small T antigen recruits the MYC paralog LMYC (MYCL) to the 15-component p400 complex containing EP400 and KAT5 to activate transcription. (From Cheng J, Park DE, Berrios C, et al. Merkel cell polyomavirus recruits MYCL to the EP400 complex to promote oncogenesis. *PLoS Pathog* 2017;13(10):e1006668. Ref.[51] Figure courtesy of Camille Cushman.)

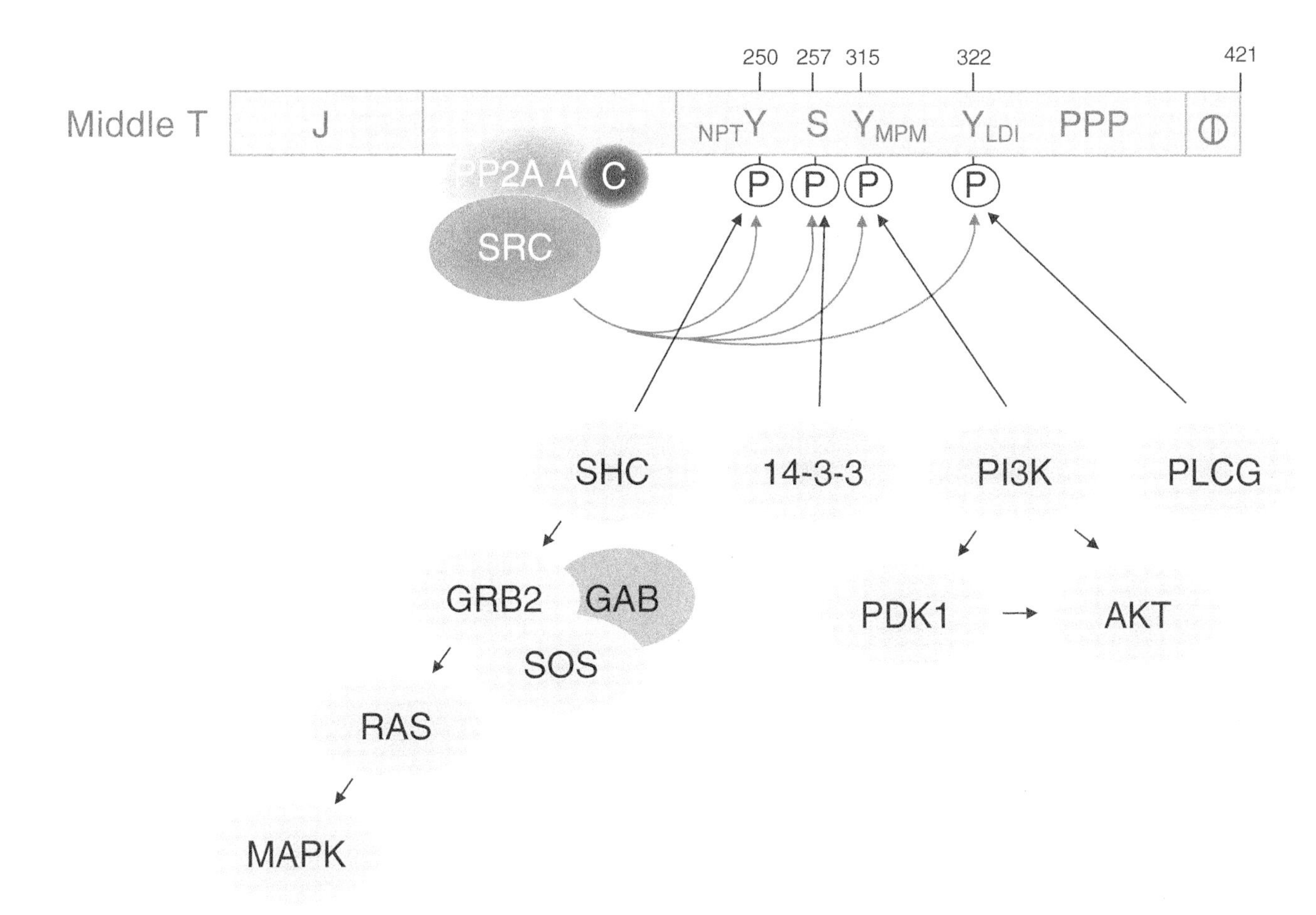

FIGURE 1.11 Mouse polyomavirus (MPyV) middle T antigen assembles an activated signaling complex. Tyrosine residues 250, 315, and 322 are phosphorylated by associated SRC kinase. Residues surrounding the phosphorylated tyrosine residues are required for specific association with SHC, 14-3-3, phosphoinositide 3-kinase (PI3K), and phospholipase C. PPP represents the proline-rich sequence. The C-terminus contains the hydrophobic membrane attachment site.[284] (Adapted from Schaffhausen BS, Roberts TM. Lessons from polyoma middle T antigen on signaling and transformation: a DNA tumor virus contribution to the war on cancer. *Virology* 2009;384(2):304–316. Copyright © 2008 Elsevier. With permission.)

with ceramide consisting of sphingosine and a fatty acid. The sialic acid is critical for virion binding to the cell. In addition to providing a binding site for the virus, the gangliosides direct the virus to the correct endocytic pathway. The efficiency of SV40 infection is dependent on the relative concentration of GM1 on the cell surface as well as its ability to activate focal adhesion kinase (PTK2).[311] Interaction of the SV40 Vp1 with GM1 contributes to the vacuolization phenotype observed with SV40 infection in cell culture (Fig. 1.2).[206] The crystal structures of various PyV Vp1 molecules with gangliosides have been solved (Fig. 1.13).[37,144,242]

Other polyomaviruses use distinct gangliosides as receptors (Fig. 1.12). For example, MPyV uses GT1b or GD1b.[334] After initial binding to the ganglioside, MPyV interacts with $\alpha4\beta1$ integrin that may serve as a secondary or cell type–specific receptor for viral entry.[249] BKPyV also uses gangliosides to enter the cell, as judged by restoration of infectivity to otherwise resistant cells upon preincubation with GT1a and GD1a. These branched gangliosides are found on the renal tubular epithelial cells that BKPyV normally infects. Another report indicated that an N-linked glycoprotein containing sialylated oligosaccharides can also mediate BKPyV binding. Both the glycolipid and glycoprotein contain sialic acid, consistent with early reports that BKPyV can hemagglutinate human red blood cells and that this activity was neuraminidase sensitive. There are various reports regarding the receptor for MCPyV, with some data indicating that MCPyV Vp1 capsomeres can bind the ganglioside GT1b, while pseudovirions can bind sulfated polysaccharides, such as heparan sulfates or chondroitin sulfates, to enter cells.[287] It has also been reported that BKPyV, SV40, and JCPyV can enter cells using nonsialylated glycosaminoglycans for infectious entry.[99]

JCPyV binds to lactoseries tetrasaccharide c (LTSc), a linear sialylated oligosaccharide that differs from the branched forms reported for other polyomaviruses (Fig. 1.12). LTSc is a pentasaccharide with the terminal sialic acid linked by an $\alpha2,6$ bond to the penultimate galactose. In addition, JCPyV uses the 5-hydroxytryptamine (serotonin) receptor 2A (HTR2A), perhaps as a cell type–specific receptor, for viral entry.[78] This receptor is expressed on glial cells, the major target cell for JCPyV. Antibodies to the HTR2A receptor as well as serotonin receptor antagonists such as mirtazapine block JCPyV infection, while expressing the receptor in otherwise noninfectible cells renders them susceptible to infection.

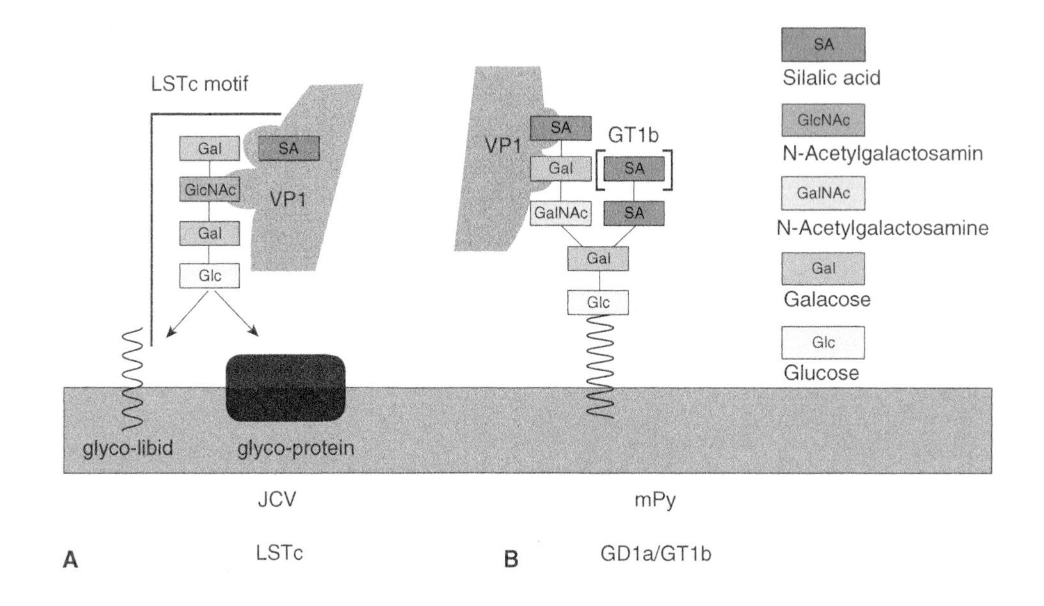

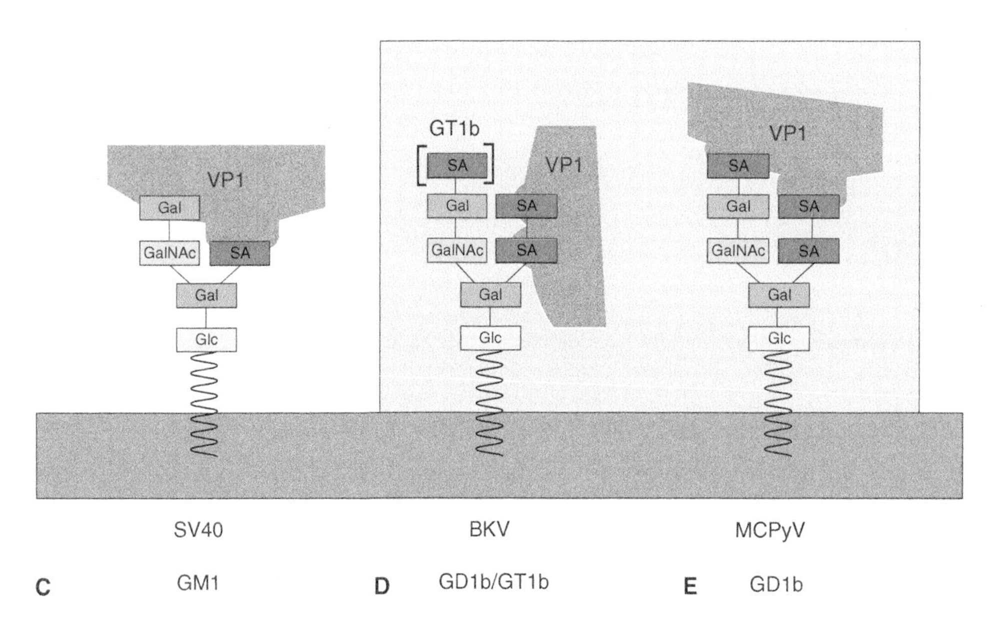

FIGURE 1.12 **Polyomavirus VP1–carbohydrate interaction. A:** JCV Vp1 binds to the LSTc pentasaccharide motif attached to either a protein or a lipid. **B:** MPyV Vp1 interacts with the SA-Gal motif attached to one branch of gangliosides GD1a or GT1b. **C:** SV40 VP1 engages the Gal and SA residues on both branches of ganglioside GM1. **D:** BKV Vp1 is predicted to bind to the di-SA motif of ganglioside GD1b or GT1b. **E:** MCPyV is postulated to interact with the SA on both branches of ganglioside GT1b. The shaded *light blue* area represents Vp1–sugar interactions for which there are only biochemical, but no crystal structure, data.[333] (Reprinted from Tsai B, Inoue T. A virus takes an "L" turn to find its receptor. *Cell Host Microbe* 2010;8(4):301–302. Copyright © 2010 Elsevier. With permission.)

Entry, Intracellular Trafficking, and Uncoating

The polyomaviruses use several pathways to enter into the cell and pass through the endosomes to the ER (Fig. 1.14). Although early studies indicated that SV40 and BKPyV enter the cell using a pathway involving caveolin, later studies indicated that caveolin was not essential.[374] Evidence also indicates that entry of SV40 and MPyV into the cell requires engagement of a signal transduction cascade through interactions at the cell surface.[137] Studies with various inhibitors of intracellular structures and processes have shed some light on how the virions travel within the cytosol after endocytosis. Molecules that interfere with microtubules and prevent movement of vesicles from the endosome to the ER interfere with SV40 infection. Infection can be blocked by the drug brefeldin A, which inhibits trafficking between the ER and the Golgi apparatus, and a number of other drugs that interfere with endosome maturation and trafficking to the ER.[248] A genome-wide siRNA screen revealed that BKPyV trafficking requires the Ras-related RAB18 protein and its associated factors syntaxin 18 and the NRZ complex to make its way to the ER.[372]

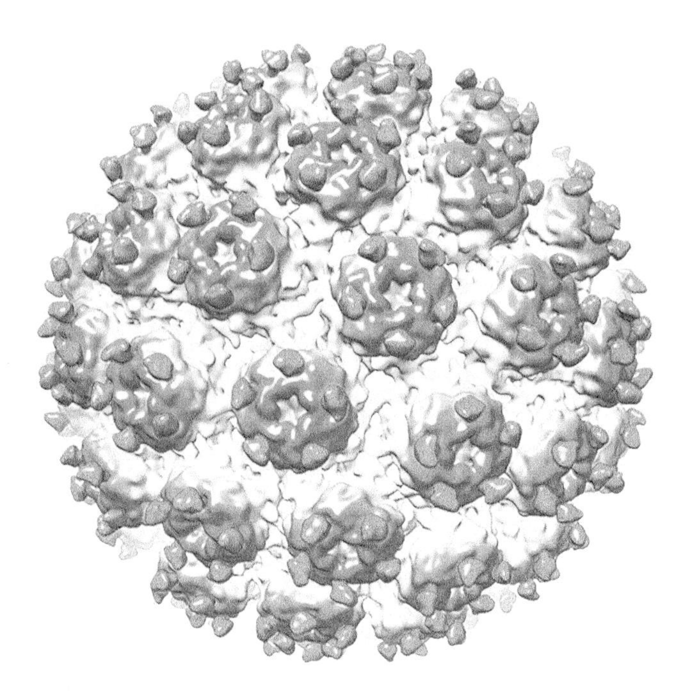

FIGURE 1.13 The structure of BKPyV and GT1b. Isosurface representation of the 3.4 Å structure of BKV, in complex with GT1b (*magenta*). (Reprinted from Hurdiss DL, Frank M, Snowden JS, et al. The Structure of an Infectious Human Polyomavirus and Its Interactions with Cellular Receptors. *Structure* 2018;26(6): 839–847.e3.https://creativecommons.org/licenses/by/4.0/.)

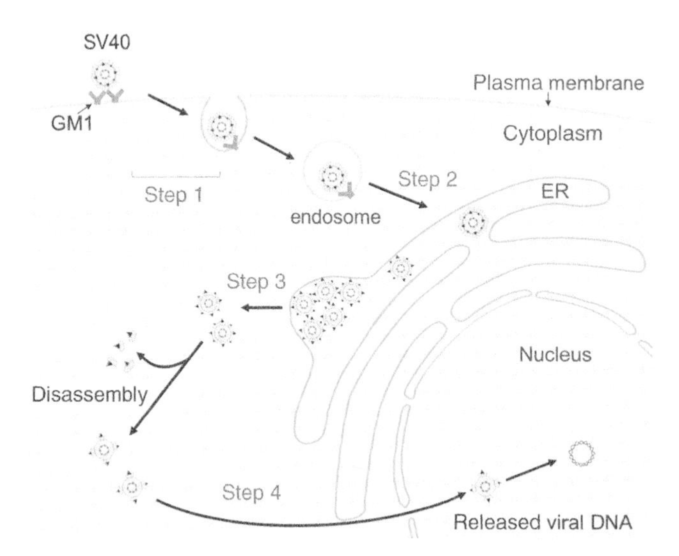

FIGURE 1.14 SV40 entry. *Step 1*: SV40 binds to the ganglioside GM1 host cell receptor at the plasma membrane. This event initiates receptor-mediated endocytosis that targets the virus to the endosomes. *Step 2*: SV40 is targeted to the ER from where it breaches the ER membrane to escape into the cytosol. *Step 3*: In the cytosol, the virus is mobilized into the nucleus. *Step 4*: The genome is released.[50] (Reprinted from Chen YJ, Liu X, Tsai B. SV40 Hijacks Cellular Transport, Membrane Penetration, and Disassembly Machineries to Promote Infection. *Viruses* 2019;11(10):917. https://creativecommons.org/licenses/by/4.0/.)

The polyomavirus capsid begins to disassemble in the ER. Evidence for this includes the appearance of epitopes on Vp2 and Vp3 that become accessible for immunostaining within the ER.[248] In addition, structural changes to the capsid, including disulfide bond reduction and isomerization mediated by ER-resident protein disulfide isomerases, can be detected biochemically at the point when the virus enters the ER. Furthermore, transmission EM experiments have detected changes in the morphology of virions that were isolated from the ER.[146] Evidence for a multistep disassembly process for SV40 includes the exposure of certain hydrophobic Vp2 and Vp3 epitopes in the ER, while further disassembly occurs later in the cytosol as evidenced by immunoassay detection of the viral genome. Similar to SV40, it has been shown that the conformation of the MPyV capsid begins to change in the ER due to the action of the endoplasmic reticulum protein 29 (ERP29) that plays a role in the processing of secretory proteins.[285,334] Capsid disassembly in the ER or the cytosol may be required because the viral particle is bigger than the functional capacity of the nuclear pore. The ER-associated degradation pathway, which functions to target misfolded cellular ER proteins for proteasome-mediated degradation, has also been implicated in polyomavirus disassembly and involves ER chaperone proteins.

The question of how the PyV genome gets transported to the nucleus remains to be answered. For SV40, it has been speculated that release from the vesicular compartment might involve Vp1, as noted earlier, or Vp2, by virtue of its myristoylated N-terminus inserting into the lipid bilayer.[248] Recent data have shown that a series of cellular factors, including BAG2, Erlin, dynein, kinesin, and SGTA can extract the particle from the ER and further facilitate disassembly.[50] An NLS in Vp2/Vp3 may mediate entry through the nuclear pore complex, since mutations in the NLS inhibit entry of the virion into the nucleus but do not affect capsid assembly or the production of new virions.

JCPyV enters the cell through clathrin-coated pits, as indicated by use of inhibitors of this pathway as well as the demonstration that JCPyV colocalizes with transferrin, known to use clathrin-mediated entry into the cell. Both microtubules and microfilaments play a role in trafficking of JCPyV to the nucleus. As with SV40, binding of JCPyV to its receptor induces a signal transduction cascade required for efficient entry that can be inhibited by genistein, a tyrosine kinase inhibitor. In addition, JCPyV appears to signal through the extracellular signal-regulated kinase (ERK) or mitogen-activated protein kinase (MAPK) pathway. Using fluorescently labeled virus-like particles (VLPs), it has been shown that JCPyV particles do not disassemble before they reach the nuclear pore and that the NLS of Vp1 is required for entry into the nucleus.

Transcription

After the polyomavirus genome enters the nucleus, it serves as a template for transcription by the cellular RNA polymerase II. Once inside the nucleus, the viral genome becomes wrapped in nucleosomes containing histone H1 in addition to the four core histones that are present in the virus particle.[345] Within the cell, the SV40 viral genome contains 24 nucleosomes with a nucleosome-free region of 400 base pairs encompassing the NCCR of early and late promoters and origin of replication. This is in contrast to the virion, where all regions of the SV40 genome are covered with nucleosomes devoid of H1. Chromatin immunoprecipitation can detect transcriptionally active chromatin, defined by the presence of RNA polymerase II, as early as 30 minutes postinfection with SV40.[10] The chromatin at this time also contains hyperacetylated histone H3 and H4, which have been associated with chromatin undergoing transcription initiation and elongation.[10]

Transcription of polyomavirus genes is governed by *cis*-acting sequences in the NCCR. The SV40 NCCR has been the most intensively studied and serves as a paradigm for the other polyomaviruses. Seminal studies involving SV40 include the demonstration that AT-rich sequences designated TATA boxes act to direct RNA polymerase II to the proper initiation site for transcription. The SV40 early promoter also contains a series of GC-rich sequences within the 21–base-pair repeat region. The host cell protein SP1, one of the first eukaryotic transcription factors to be cloned, binds to these sequences. The SV40 early promoter also contains a duplicated element called the 72–base-pair repeat, which was the first *cis*-acting DNA sequence to be deemed a transcriptional enhancer because it could activate transcription when placed several thousand base pairs distant from the transcription start site.[113,233] Interestingly, most clinical isolates of SV40 carry only a single copy of the 72–base-pair repeat, and it appears that duplication can be selected during passage in culture.[184]

In MPyV, the enhancer element consists of two neighboring enhancers called A and B, alternatively α and β, that can act independently. The activity of the MPyV enhancers is dependent on the cell environment, as viral variants that are selected for growth on differentiated or undifferentiated embryonal carcinoma cells have mutations that map to the enhancers. The MPyV early promoter is regulated by the cellular factors characterized as polyomavirus enhancer A–binding proteins (PEA) or RUNX1, CBFB, and ETV4 that are expressed when cells are growth stimulated with serum.

The JCPyV promoter shows a distinct tissue-specific activity that correlates with the sites of acute infection. While normal JCPyV virions can attach and enter many types of cells, its host range is restricted to those cells that express transcription factors that can bind to specific sequences in the JCPyV early promoter. These sequences include the TATA box as well as binding sites for the transcription factors SP1, YB1 (YBX1), Pur-alpha (PURA), AP-1, a heterodimer of JUN and FOS, nuclear factor 1 (NF1), NFAT, and NF-1 class X (NFIX). A nuclear factor-κB (NF-κB)-binding site that includes the NFAT site has been shown to be active for late transcription and contribute to positioning of other DNA-binding proteins to initiate efficient transcription.[94] NFAT consists of a family of proteins that are expressed in many cells but have multiple classes with tissue-specific expression. NFIX is highly expressed in human glial cells, stromal cells, B lymphocytes, and CD34+ stem cells that have all been reported to support JCPyV transcription and replication. Interactions between YB1 and PURA may also provide cell-specific regulation.

The BKPyV NCCR-mediated control of bidirectional EVGR and LVGR expression has been dissected in some detail by introducing discrete point mutations predicted to inactivate binding sites for a number of transcription factors and DNA-binding proteins including SP1, ETS1, NF1, YY1, and p53 (Fig. 1.15).[23] Assessing the bidirectional dual NCCR-reporter gene expression in human embryonic kidney HEK293 cells and replication activity of the corresponding BKPyV variants in primary human renal tubular epithelial cells led to identification of three phenotypic groups. Group-1 and group-2 mutations caused a strong and an intermediate level of activation of EVGR expression and viral replication, respectively, similar to NCCR rearrangements of clinical variants found in patients with BKPyV diseases,[109] whereas group-3 mutations reduced or failed reporter gene expression and viral replication.[23]

SP1 emerged as a key regulatory factor conferring either a group-1 or a group-3 phenotype, if mutating the binding site *SP1-2* close to the LVGR or *SP1-4* to the EVGR promoter, respectively.[22] Further mutational and sequence analysis indicated that the EVGR and the LVGR promoter partially overlapped in opposite outward directions in an imperfect rotational symmetry.[22] Thus, the EVGR bears the low-affinity *SP1-2* site proximal to a consensus promoter element consisting of a perfect *TATA*-box and one major initiator (Inr)/transcription start site (TSS) in a canonical distance of 31 bp, followed by a consensus downstream promoter element (DPE) at a distance of 28 bp. Thereby, the EVGR promoter of the BKPyV archetype NCCR fulfils the criteria of a developmental or regulated promoter with perfect *TATA*-box, focused TSS, and a low basal activity. By contrast, the LVGR promoter bears the high-affinity *SP1-4* partially overlapping with a potential transcription factor IIB (TFIIB) recognition element upstream (BREu), followed by two *TATA*-like elements, besides some dispersed TSSs, and potential DPEs. Thus, the archetype BKPyV LVGR promoter shows features of constitutive housekeeping or tissue-restricted genes, which changes from a focused transcription start to a dispersed type in the BKPyV Dunlop NCCR due to the deletions of the late promoter sequences.[22] Accordingly, the intertwined and imperfect symmetry of SP1 sites, *TATA*-box and -like elements, initiator, and DPEs in the BKPyV NCCR may contribute to maintenance of the archetypal focus on the LVGR side while repressing EVGR expression. At the same time, this organization permits an effective bidirectional system that is highly poised to shift the transcriptional balance to EVGR expression upon differential stimulation or group-1 type mutations.[22] Developing drugs preventing group-1 type activation or conferring group-3 type inactivation would be of interest for prevention and treatment of BKPyV replication.

The interaction of the human PyV NCCR with corresponding host cell makeup of transcription factors and DNA-binding proteins is predicted to play an important role for host cell permissiveness and likely depends on cellular differentiation and activation signals.[2] Two exploratory studies transfecting 13 HPyV NCCR reporter constructs into different cell lines derived from kidney, skin, lung, cervix, brain, and colon revealed host- and NCCR-attributable differences in EVGR and LVGR expression levels, reflecting a role for secondary host cell specificity with respect to viral gene expression and persistence.[2,231]

The MCPyV NCCR region is poorly characterized but represents an important opportunity to understand how this virus replicates normally and how it sustains LTag and STag expression in MCC. Of note, the entire NCCR region along with STag and the N-terminal region of LTag to the LXCXE, RB-binding, motif is conserved in MCC tumors containing integrated MCPyV viral DNA.[315] An early report indicated that the MCPyV early promoter could be activated by UV radiation, but no further studies have been reported.[232]

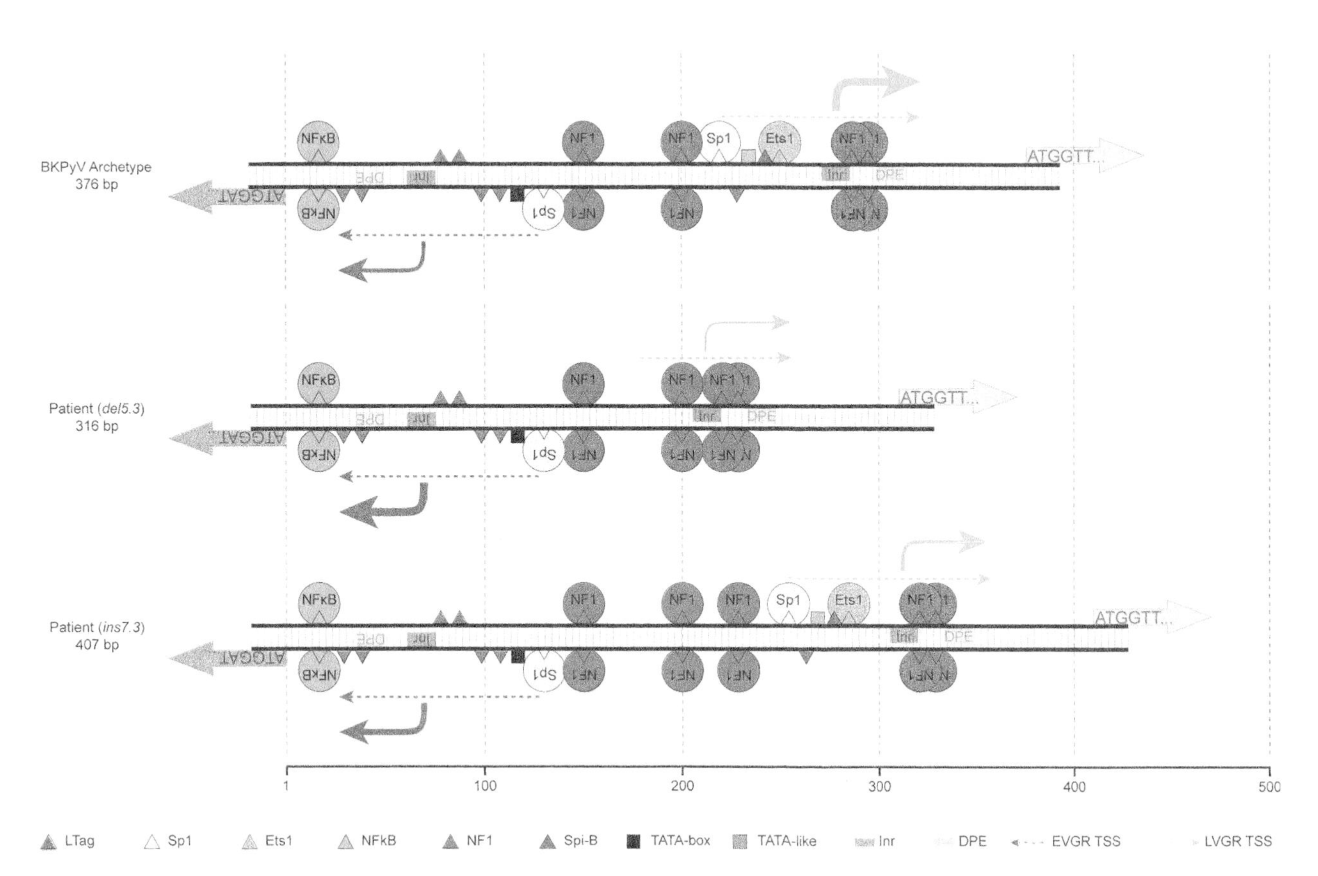

FIGURE 1.15 Bidirectional regulation from the BK polyomavirus NCCR. The transcription factors SP1, ETS1, and NF-1 determine the strength and direction of gene expression toward EVGR (early; *red arrow*) and LVGR (late; *green arrow*). **TOP:** The BKPyV archetype NCCR mediates basal activity with low EVGR expression (*dashed arrow*) and high LVGR expression (*green arrow*). SP1 and ETS1 contribute a directional effect on neighboring SP1 and ETS1, whereas NF1 has a stabilizing effect. **Middle:** Patient isolate del5.3 NCCR carries a deletion of SP1 and ETS1 transcription factor binding sites resulting in significantly increased EVGR expression and viral replication. **Bottom:** Patient isolate ins7.3 NCCR carries a partial duplication introducing additional NF1 binding sites in the center, which in an insulator-like fashion lower LVGR expression and confer significantly increased EVGR expression and viral replication.[23] (Modified after Bethge T, Hachemi HA, Manzetti J, et al. Sp1 sites in the noncoding control region of BK polyomavirus are key regulators of bidirectional viral early and late gene expression. *J Virol* 2015;89(6):3396–3411.)

Rearrangements in the NCCR have been found in BKPyV, JCPyV, and HPyV7-associated diseases.[35] The viral NCCRs referred to as archetype are thought to be associated with naturally circulating polyomaviruses, while rearranged NCCRs arise when high levels of viral replication emerge when cultured in the lab or during disease in patients with immunodeficiency. For example, direct cloning of the JCPyV NCCR from the CSF of HIV/AIDS patients with PML identified partial duplications, deletions, and other combinations that lead to increased EVGR expression and accelerated JCPyV replication in tissue culture.[108] BKPyV NCCR rearrangements have been shown to replace archetype virus in kidney transplant patients with high levels and prolonged duration of plasma BKPyV-DNAemia and histologically proven BKPyV-associated nephropathy.[109] These rearrangements may enable higher levels of LTag and viral replication that are tolerated by the patient's immunocompromised state.[108,109] Notably, an SV40/JCV hybrid virus containing JCPyV T antigen and Vp1, Vp2, and Vp3 coding sequences but a hybrid NCCR with elements of the SV40 enhancer grows with faster kinetics and to higher titers than wild-type JCPyV and has an expanded host range to human and monkey kidney cells as well as monkey glial cells.[337]

The SV40 early promoter undergoes negative feedback regulation by LTag.[328] When cells are infected with SV40 containing a temperature-sensitive LTag mutant at the nonpermissive or restrictive (elevated) temperature, early mRNAs are overproduced. The ability to repress early transcription is dependent on the binding of LTag to the promoter. Mutations that disrupt the DBD of LTag also typically lead to higher levels of LTag.[154] The SV40 NCCR contains three binding LTag-binding sites, referred to as sites I, II, and III, that are all involved in repression by LTag. Because site III overlaps the early promoter elements, it is possible that LTag-binding acts to prevent binding or displace other transcription factors to that region that may contribute to the ability of LTag to repress its own transcription. Furthermore, there is evidence for changes in repressive histone epigenetic marks as well as histone repositioning in SV40 chromosomes during the switch from early to late transcription.

Early gene expression in SV40 can also be down-regulated by miRNAs encoded by the LVGR.[323] Several other primate polyomaviruses have similar sequences that are predicted to form the characteristic hairpin structure of miRNA and have been detected during BKPyV and JCPyV infection in culture and patients. Somewhat surprisingly, an SV40 mutant virus lacking the miRNA does not produce more virus than wild type in cultured monkey kidney cells. However, cells infected with the miRNA-defective virus are more sensitive to killing by cytotoxic T lymphocytes *in vitro*. This observation led to the proposal that the miRNA serves to limit production of antigens recognized by the immune system and thereby protecting the infected cell.[323] Somewhat surprisingly, a mutant MPyV that cannot express its miRNA showed no difference in pathogenesis in animals.[324] More recently, it has been shown that the miRNA controls replication of BKPyV containing an archetype, but not rearranged, NCCR.[34] Moreover, the aforementioned SV40 miRNA mutant is less efficient than wild type in establishing a persistent infection in the Syrian hamster animal model, and the MCPyV miRNA also appears to control persistence.[329] Together, these findings support a model in which the relative amounts of expression of the early mRNAs and miRNAs, as governed by the structure of the NCCR, determine the outcome of infection.[34] Nonetheless, the role of the PyV miRNAs during infection remains to be fully elucidated.

Similar to the early promoter, the late promoter elements have been defined in a variety of *in vivo* and *in vitro* systems. In SV40, maximal late transcription requires sequences in the 21–base-pair GC repeats and the 72–base-pair enhancers. Late gene transcription occurs concomitantly with the onset of DNA replication, although replication is not required for activation of late transcription. LTag can promote viral replication as well as late gene expression. LTag can stimulate late transcription, although LTag binding the origin of replication is not required for this activity. Rather, transcription activation is accomplished through LTag interactions with components of the basal transcription machinery such as *TATA*-binding protein, a component of TFIID and TBP-associated factor 1 (TAF1), as well as transcription factors late SV40 factor (LSF, TFCP2), TEF-1 (TEAD1), and SP1. These interactions increase the binding of TBP and another basal transcription factor, TFIIA, to the *TATA* element.

The control of late gene expression in MPyV is more complicated. Host range or hr-t mutants that do not express functional STag or MTag produce equivalent amounts of late proteins, as does wild-type virus.[95] However, infection with a virus containing similar mutations in cells with a different genetic background demonstrated a stimulatory role of the two T antigens during the late phase. This does not appear to be solely due to amplification of the genome but may also involve direct activation of transcription. These same studies also indicated a role for MTag and STag in the induction of early gene expression. Notably, the MPyV differs from its primate counterparts in how its late primary RNA transcript is processed. The MPyV late poly(A) site is a relatively weak site, resulting in the RNA polymerase circling the viral genome multiple times. The first exon of the late transcript can therefore be spliced to itself multiple times, although the protein-coding sequence is only present once on each mature mRNA.

Translation

Limited studies have been performed to address perturbations in translation by the polyomaviruses. An important question in the polyomavirus life cycle is how and when does translation of Vp3 occur when the same reading frame on the late transcript encodes both Vp2 and Vp3. Vp3 uses an AUG sequence downstream of the Vp2 start codon. Mutagenesis of the SV40 LVGR between the Vp2 and Vp3 start codons revealed evidence for two internal ribosome entry sites (IRESs) that could potentially promote cap-independent translation of Vp3. This observation may be particularly important because SV40 infection leads to a decrease in cap-dependent translation.[369,370] SV40 STag leads to decreased phosphorylation of 4E-BP1 that in turn binds to and represses eIF4E, reducing cap-dependent translation. This inhibitory effect on phosphorylation 4E-BP1 required the SV40 STag PP2A-binding domain and was most evident at late times after infection.[370]

The ability of SV40 STag to reduce levels of 4E-BP1 phosphorylation during infection contrasts with the effects of MCPyV STag. As described later, part of the MCPyV genome is randomly integrated into the host cell chromosomes in a manner that includes the NCCR and permits expression of an intact STag and an N-terminal fragment of LTag.[84,315] In cell lines derived from MCC that express MCPyV STag, downstream targets of AKT and mTOR including 4E-BP1 were hyperphosphorylated, leading to increased cap-dependent translation.[304] This activity appeared to contribute to the transforming activity of MCPyV STag because a phosphorylation-resistant form of 4E-BP1 reduced cell growth in the MCC cell lines. Notably, this activity was independent of the MCPyV STag PP2A-binding domain, suggesting the possibility that this represents a unique function of MCPyV STag.

Replication of Viral Genomic DNA

To a great extent, PyV LTag orchestrates the viral life cycle. Studies of SV40 LTag led to groundbreaking insights into eukaryotic DNA replication including the role of its DNA-binding and helicase activities, culminating in the establishment of the first *in vitro* system for eukaryotic DNA replication. The history of these seminal discoveries and the scientists who made them is well described in a review.[82] While many of the insights into the molecular functions of polyomavirus LTag have come from studies on SV40, investigations into other polyomaviruses have also made substantial contributions to our understanding of viral replication.

The LTag binds directly to the viral origin of replication and functions as a helicase to unwind the viral dsDNA to enable replication. LTag also serves to recruit cellular proteins including RPA, DNA polymerase α/primase, and topoisomerases I and II to facilitate viral genome replication (Fig. 1.8). In addition, LTag induces changes in the cell to facilitate viral replication including the formation of viral replication centers within the nucleus (Fig. 1.16).

Polyomaviruses normally infect quiescent or growth-arrested cells that are not actively proliferating, yet they require the host cell's DNA synthetic machinery that is fully active during the S phase of the cell cycle. LTag plays a role in inducing exit from the quiescent state and entry into S phase by binding and inactivating the retinoblastoma tumor suppressor protein. LTag also functions to counter the cell's apoptotic responses induced by viral DNA replication by binding and inactivating the p53 tumor suppressor protein. The cellular DNA damage response to replicating viral genomes is triggered in part by LTag and appears to be required for efficient viral replication.

The SV40 origin of replication contains three regions, a core origin of 64 base pairs with four pentanucleotide (GAGGC) sequences organized as a pair of inverted repeats flanked by an early palindrome (EP) on the early side and an A/T-rich region on the late side.[310] The LTag DBD binds directly to the pentanucleotide sequence.[221] After two molecules of LTag bind to opposing inverted pentanucleotide sequences, they each recruit five additional molecules of LTag to form a hexamer. The two

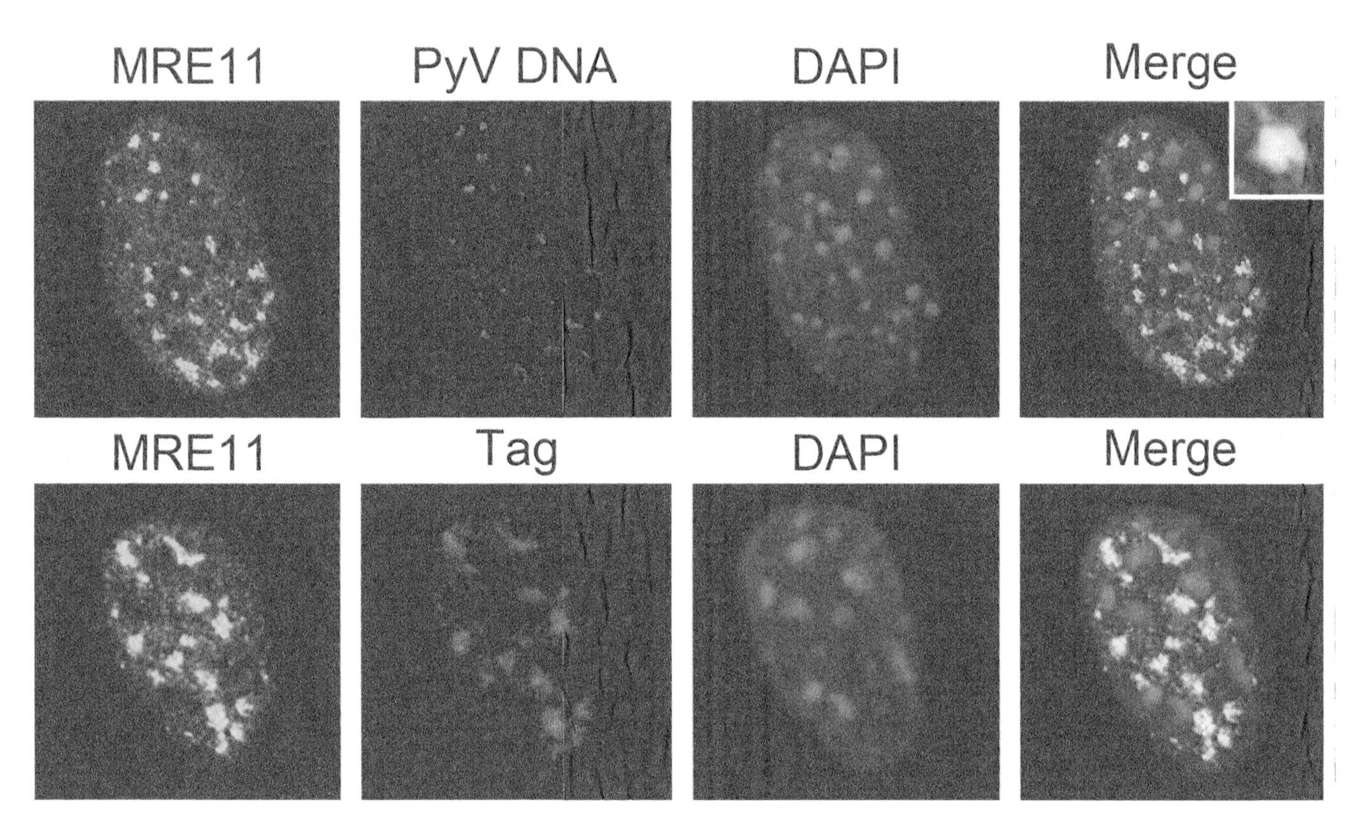

FIGURE 1.16 MPyV DNA and large T antigen form viral replication centers. C57 MEFs infected with MPyV were stained for MRE11 and PyV DNA (by FISH) or MRE11 and large T antigen.[79] (Reprinted from Erickson KD, Bouchet-Marquis C, Heiser K, et al. Virion assembly factories in the nucleus of polyomavirus-infected cells. *PLoS Pathog* 2012;8(4):e1002630. https://creativecommons.org/licenses/by/3.0/.)

hexamers face each other in a head-to-head orientation that surrounds the origin. After double-hexamer formation, LTag initiates melting of the DNA in the EP region and twisting of the A/T region. Viral DNA is opened to form single-stranded DNA (ssDNA) followed by LTag-recruiting RPA and topoisomerase I. The helicase domain of LTag recruits the DNA polymerase α/primase complex (POLA1, POLA2, PRIM1, PRIM2) that contributes to RNA Okazaki primer formation on the lagging strand.

Besides its role in initiation of DNA synthesis, LTag is also required for elongation of the growing chains. Elongation is carried out by DNA polymerase δ (POLD1, POLD2, POLD3, POLD4) in conjunction with its accessory factors, proliferating cell nuclear antigen (PCNA), and replication factor C (RF-C). The LTag translocates on ssDNA on the leading strand template in the 3′ to 5′ direction. LTag has an ATPase-dependent 3′ to 5′ helicase that advances each hexamer in opposite orientations along the viral DNA.[364] Replication occurs in a bidirectional manner and ends with the decatenation of the two linked circular molecules by topoisomerase II.

The bidirectional nature of SV40 DNA synthesis was demonstrated in two ways. First, Danna and Nathans performed an elegant experiment in which they pulse-labeled infected cells with^3 H-thymidine for 5 to 15 minutes, isolated fully replicated DNA molecules, and determined what parts of the genome were labeled.[62] The theory behind this approach is that the labeled thymidine would appear farthest from the origin of replication in cells that were labeled for the shortest time periods, because those were the closest to completion, and extend back toward the origin as the labeling time was extended. This allowed the mapping of the origin as well as the determination that replication was bidirectional. The second approach used shadowing of DNA with electron microscopy imaging of replicating SV40 and MPyV.[346] Here, replication forks were visualized and mapped in relation to the ends of the DNA molecules, which had been digested with a restriction endonuclease at a unique site on the chromosome.

Examination of the crystal structure of the LTag helicase domain when bound to adenosine triphosphate (ATP) or adenosine diphosphate (ADP) led to the proposal that ATP hydrolysis induces conformational changes that cause twisting of the hexamers resulting in expansion and constriction of the central channel that resembles the movement of an iris within an eye.[190] Using a variety of single-molecule assays, it was shown that after assembly of the SV40 LTag double hexamer on the origin, the hexamers separate to unwind DNA as a single hexamers that translocate in opposite directions on DNA in the 3′-to-5′ direction.[364]

Phosphorylation of LTag regulates its ability to drive DNA synthesis.[310] In SV40, phosphorylation of LTag threonine residue 124 by cyclin-dependent kinases enhances binding of the protein to the origin of replication, assembly of the double hexamers, and subsequent unwinding.[220] In MPyV, the corresponding LTag threonine residue 278 is also phosphorylated and mutation of this residue abolishes replication function. Conversely, phosphorylation of SV40 LTag serine residues 120 and 123 inhibits replication. These serine residues can be phosphorylated by casein kinase I and dephosphorylated by PP2A.

The N-terminal J domain of LTag contributes to viral DNA replication, functioning through binding to HSC70. While the J domain is not required for viral DNA replication *in vitro*, it plays a significant role *in vivo*.40 Notably, the J domain from the human HSP40 homolog HSJ-1 protein can support SV40 DNA replication when it was substituted for the homologous domain of LTag, suggesting that interaction of LTag with HSC70 and the host cell heat shock system facilitates viral replication. The mechanism by which the LTag J domain stimulates DNA replication is not known but may involve chaperone-mediated rearrangements of the initiation complex on the DNA.

An essential contribution of LTag to viral replication is to induce the cell to enter the cell cycle. Although polyomaviruses normally infect cells that are not actively dividing, they require the host cell's DNA synthetic machinery, produced and activated during S phase, for replication of the viral genome. LTag drives the resting cell into S phase by binding to RB and the RB-related proteins p107 (RBL1) and p130 (RBL2) (Fig. 1.8).[64] The RB tumor suppressor proteins, sometimes referred to as pocket proteins, inhibit entry into S phase through binding and repression of the E2F family of transcription factors.[71] During the quiescent (G0) and G1 phase of the cell cycle, RB and p130 form complexes with E2F on the promoters of genes required for DNA synthesis. Notably, p130 binds to the repressor E2F4/DP1 heterodimer and recruits the five-protein MuvB complex to the promoters of several hundred E2F-dependent, cell cycle–regulated genes.[196,281] The DREAM (DP1, RBL2, E2F4, and MuvB) complex is disrupted when LTag binds to p130, thereby releasing the MuvB core complex and enabling activation of E2F-dependent genes. When a cell is induced to divide physiologically, cyclin-dependent kinases serve to phosphorylate the RB family proteins, enabling their release from E2F and thereby permitting gene expression. LTag subverts this pathway by binding to RB family proteins and disrupting their binding to E2F. The LXCXE motif in LTag binds directly to the RB family proteins.[168] In addition, the LTag N-terminal J domain cooperates with the LXCXE motif binding of RB family proteins to facilitate their release from E2F. The SV40 LTag J domain also perturbs the phosphorylation status and stability of RB-related proteins, thereby contributing to loss of their E2F repression functions.[321,322]

In addition to causing the cell to enter S phase, SV40 LTag carries out another important role in establishing the proper cellular environment for replication. The inappropriate entry into S phase induced by LTag causes the cell to activate a p53-dependent growth arrest and proapoptotic response. The p53 tumor suppressor protein was first discovered by virtue of its being co-immunoprecipitated with SV40 LTag from cellular protein extracts.[180,195] SV40 LTag binds directly to the DBD of p53, thereby disrupting p53's ability to transactivate its target genes such as *p21* (*CDKN1A*), *PUMA*, and *MDM2* involved in cell cycle arrest, apoptosis, and autoregulation, respectively.

The ability of LTag to activate p53 is due, at least in part, to increased levels of ARF (alternate reading frame), a product of the *CDKN2A* gene that also expresses the CDK4 inhibitor p16 (*INK4A*). ARF functions to stabilize p53 by binding to and inhibiting the E3 ubiquitin ligase activity of MDM2 directed toward p53. Although normal cell cycle entry does not induce ARF expression, SV40 and MCPyV LTag and MPyV MTag induce expression of ARF.[236,257] Although LTag from many polyomaviruses can bind to p53 and thereby inactivate its growth inhibitory and apoptotic response, MPyV and MCPyV LTag are notable for their inability to bind directly to p53. Nonetheless, MPyV is able to counter the p53-mediated growth arrest by STag inhibition of ARF.[236] By contrast, MCPyV STag indirectly inhibits p53 function by contributing to increased levels of MDM2 and MDM4 that cooperatively function to degrade p53.[257]

Recent evidence indicates that the cellular DNA damage response (DDR) is required for SV40 MCPyV, MPyV, and BKPyV replication.[124,150,373] PyV infection induces a cellular DDR response that includes activation of the ATM and ATR kinases, resulting in phosphorylation of the specialized histone γ-H2AX and the checkpoint kinases CHK1 and CHK2. LTag colocalizes with phosphorylated ATM and γ-H2AX on DNA to form nuclear foci that include the MRN complex (Mre11, Rad50, and Nbs1) and 53BP1 (Fig. 1.16).[313] LTag alone without viral DNA can also induce the DDR, and this may be dependent on LTag interaction with BUB1. In addition to the replicative polymerases noted above, it is clear that DNA repair polymerases must also play an important role in polyomavirus genome replication, since inhibiting the cellular DDR, which is also induced by breaks on the viral genome resulting from replication fork stalling,[313] decreases the production of infectious viral genomes.[124,150] In addition, the DDR arrests cells to provide an environment that maximizes viral genome replication.

In addition to the DDR, much attention has focused on the role of nuclear structures called promyelocytic leukemia nuclear bodies (PML-NB) during replication and infection. In BKPyV infection, LTag colocalizes with PML-NB at very early times and, concomitant with the onset of viral DNA replication, induces a dramatic reorganization of PML-NB. It remains unclear if the changes in the PML-NB are a consequence or a requirement of viral replication. In MPyV-infected cells, PML-NB colocalize with structures that appear to be viral assembly factories.[79]

Assembly

Assembly of polyomaviruses begins with the translocation of Vp1, Vp2, and Vp3 into the nucleus and the formation of capsomeres. The Vp1, Vp2, and Vp3 from SV40 and MPyV each contain nuclear localization sequences. Vp2 and Vp3, in the absence of Vp1, do not accumulate in the nucleus but rather require Vp1 for nuclear transport, indicating that these proteins may be imported as a complex. The Vp2 or Vp3 NLS may be more important for trafficking of incoming virus from the ER to the nucleus than for import of the newly synthesized proteins during the late phase of the infection. This model fits with the data indicating that Vp2 and Vp3 become exposed as the virus transits through the ER.

It is unclear whether empty capsids are precursors to mature, DNA-containing virions or dead-end products, or whether the capsid assembles around the viral chromosome. While it has been reported that a *cis*-acting sequence in the origin region of SV40, *ses*, enhances DNA packaging, DNA molecules that lack this sequence element can still be encapsidated. The crystalline-like arrays of PyV virions present in nuclei may reflect the presence of viral factories. In this model, tubes comprised of Vp1, and possibly Vp2 and Vp3, can facilitate budding of virions containing viral DNA.[79] Examples of

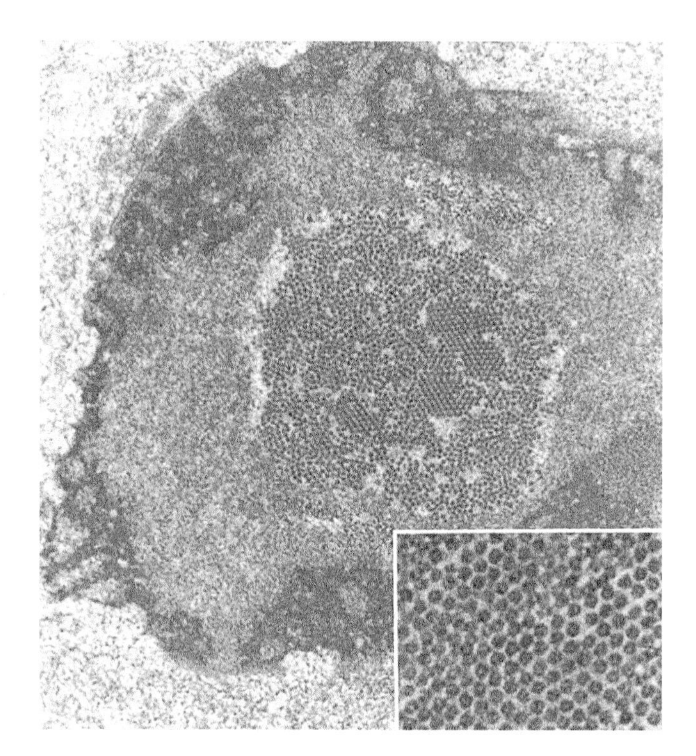

FIGURE 1.17 Crystalline-like arrays of virions in virus-associated trichodysplasia spinulosa. "Transmission electron micrograph showing clusters of intranuclear viral particles within the inner root sheath type cells (original magnification 320,000, **inset** 350,000)". (From Osswald SS, Kulick KB, Tomaszewski MM, et al. Viral-associated trichodysplasia in a patient with lymphoma: a case report and review. *J Cutan Pathol* 2007;34(9):721–725. Reprinted by permission of John Wiley & Sons, Inc.)

crystalline-like arrays of PyV virions have been observed in several diseases characterized by severe infection including PML, PyVAN, and trichodysplasia spinulosa (Fig. 1.17).

Purified recombinant Vp1, expressed in bacteria, yeast, or baculovirus-infected insect cells, can self-assemble into capsomeres. Under appropriate conditions, these capsomeres form capsid structures referred to as VLPs (Fig. 1.4). Therefore, viral DNA, Vp2, and Vp3 are not required for capsid formation. Changes in ionic strength and pH of the buffer can lead to formation of other structures including tubular moieties and T = 1 icosahedrons. It has been shown that chaperones such as HSP70 are required for efficient capsid assembly. VLPs are very similar to authentic virions and have been used for basic studies on receptor binding, virus entry, intracellular trafficking, and the immune response. VLPs have also been studied as vehicles for delivery of genes (i.e., as so-called pseudoviruses) and small molecules, and have been extensively used for serologic assessment of polyomavirus infection.

Release

The manner by which polyomaviruses leave the cell is poorly understood. While some studies indicate that the virus causes lysis of the cell, others indicate that virus can be shed from intact cells. For example, SV40 infection can cause a cytopathic effect (CPE) or vacuolating effect with destruction of the cell. The vacuolization effect requires interaction between SV40 Vp1 and binding to GM1 and is caused by the binding of released progeny viruses to GM1 (Fig. 1.2).[204] Alternatively, SV40 can leave polarized epithelial cells from the apical surface and can exit nonpolarized epithelial cells without killing them. A regulated virus exit process is suggested by the observation that SV40 can be detected in cytoplasmic membrane vesicles using electron microscopy, and release of virions is inhibited by monensin, which blocks vesicular transport.

JCPyV causes cell death through lytic infection of glial cells. Infection of astrocytes cultured *in vitro* supports a progressive JCPyV infection that leads to necrotic cell death and virion release. Notably, this model system did not yield any evidence for apoptosis by JCPyV infection.

The agnoprotein may also contribute to assembly and egress. SV40 isolates containing mutations in agnoprotein replicate with wild-type kinetics but produce plaques that are smaller than wild type due to inefficient release of mature virions from the cell. Other phenotypes of agnoprotein mutants that could account for inefficient viral replication include improper localization of Vp1. At the nuclear envelope, agnoprotein has been shown to dissociate heterochromatin protein 1 (HP1) from the lamin B receptor, resulting in destabilization of the envelope, perhaps explaining how agnoprotein could facilitate egress.[250] While some of the LTag host range mutations affect agnoprotein expression, the assembly defect in these mutants cannot be complemented by expression of agnoprotein *in trans*. Additional functions have been proposed for the JCPyV and BKPyV agnoprotein, including as a viroporin.[255] Recent studies demonstrate that the BKPyV agnoprotein allows the virus to evade innate immune sensing in the late viral replication phase by disrupting the mitochondrial network and membrane potential, and promoting p62/SQSTM1 mitophagy in renal tubular epithelial cells in vitro and in vivo.[214] JCPyV and SV40 infection similarly disrupt mitochondrial networks and aid in innate immune evasion by disrupting the mitochondrial network and by promoting mitophagy.

Most recently, it has been reported that, like a growing number other nonenveloped viruses, both BKPyV and JCPyV can be transmitted from cell to cell within extracellular vesicles.[234] Interestingly, JCPyV transmitted in vesicles is resistant to neutralizing antibodies, while BKPyV remains sensitive.[121,234]

PATHOGENESIS AND PATHOLOGY

Entry Into Host

The principal target cell for initial entry of polyomaviruses has been difficult to identify. However, it appears that, once exposed to a polyomavirus, an individual maintains a lifelong persistent infection as determined by specific serology to Vp1 or detection of the viral DNA on skin or in urine. For example, many polyomaviruses including SV40, BKPyV, and JCPyV are present in the urinary tract and excreted in the urine. Exposure to infected urine could be a source of infection for these polyomaviruses, although BKPyV rapidly loses its infectivity in urine.[107] There have been reports of JCPyV infection in human colonic epithelial cells and isolation of BKPyV and JCPyV from stool specimens.[30] Notably, BKPyV, JCPyV, MCPyV, KIPyV, and WUPyV have been frequently detected in sewage samples, while BPyV has been detected in farm wastewater samples.

JCPyV is able to productively infect tonsillar stromal cells in culture with efficiency nearly comparable to human glial cells. JCPyV DNA has also been found in lymphoid tissues including bone marrow and spleen. JCPyV DNA has been identified in tonsil stromal cells and in B cells isolated from tonsils. The ability of JCPyV to infect tonsillar stromal cells in culture and the presence of JCPyV DNA in tonsil tissue suggest the possibility that the initial infection could occur in these tissues as well.

BKPyV has been detected in lung tissue from one case of interstitial pneumonia in a hematopoietic stem cell transplant (HSCT) patient and in the respiratory tract and tonsil tissue in another, as well as in salivary glands, and can replicate in salivary cells in culture. This, together with the observation that the majority of the population in both developed and developing regions of the world seroconverts in early to mid-childhood, would support a respiratory or oropharyngeal–gastrointestinal route of transmission.[127] By the same token, it is surprising that other viruses were not reported, some of which had been proposed to be associated with respiratory symptoms or febrile tonsillitis such as BK virus and other polyomaviruses.

WUPyV and KIPyV can be detected in respiratory secretions that represent either the site of acute infection or persistence. For example, WUPyV is frequently detected in tonsils and nasopharyngeal lymphoid tissue from immunocompetent children. WUPyV and KIPyV were also found in plasma, urine, and respiratory samples of renal transplant patients.

For some polyomaviruses, there is evidence for maternal–fetal transmission. MPyV can be acquired vertically through transplacental transmission or direct contact as neonates.[371] By contrast, a recent study determined that the human polyomaviruses WUPyV, KIPyV, and MCPyV were not present in more than 500 fetal tissues, although serologic assessment indicated that nearly half of the mothers had been infected with MCPyV.[282]

Polyomavirus infection in birds spreads quickly in susceptible flocks. Avian polyomaviruses can be found in the urine and fecal matter in flocks, suggesting an oral route of transmission. Bird fledglings become viremic after being bitten by blowfly larvae and shed virus from their cloaca, thereby infecting the breeding adults.[268] In parrots, viremia was followed by cloacal shedding within 1 week of experimental infection.[266] Infected birds may harbor virus persistently throughout life, but acute infection can cause neurologic damage and death in younger birds.

Immune Response

Humoral immune responses occur in all animal species infected with polyomaviruses and show some cross-reactivity within rodent, primate, or avian families but not across those barriers unless immunized with laboratory-made virions or proteins. Antibody against polyomavirus is IgG, although a number of reports identified IgM and IgA responses with viral replication.[132,159] The Multicenter AIDS Cohort Study found that approximately 80% of all participants had immunoglobulin titers specific for MCPyV Vp1. Within the remaining group of seronegative participants, approximately 26% seroconverted in the following 4 years. Notably, no clinical signs or symptoms associated with acute MCPyV infection and subsequent seroconversion were appreciated.[330]

Measurements of cellular immune responses to JCPyV and BKPyV in infected individuals have identified CD8+ cytotoxic T lymphocytes (CTLs) that recognize epitopes on Vp1 and LTag. The epitope on BKPyV Vp1 amino acid residues 108 to 116 elicits a T-lymphocyte response that also recognizes JCPyV epitope Vp1 p100.[176] Using tetramer assays or CTL cell lysing assays, CD8+ T cells can be found in the peripheral circulation that are human leukocyte antigen (HLA) restricted to genotype A*02, B*07, and B*08, present in healthy blood donors and transplant patients.[76] Using overlapping 15mer peptide pools or immunodominant 9mers, JCPyV and BKPyV-specific CD4 and CD8 T cell responses have been detected in an HLA-independent manner in HIV, multiple sclerosis, or kidney transplant patients.[159] Viral-specific CD8+ T lymphocytes show a good correlation with time of survival in PML patients or with clearance of BKPyV in kidney transplant patients.

A CD8+ cytotoxic T-cell response was noted in an analysis of mRNA expression profiling of MCC.[261] Notably, patients with a better prognosis had a statistically significant increase in genes related to the CD8+ response. The response was most likely due to infiltrating CD8+ cells that were captured when the mRNA was prepared from the tumor.

There is also a T-cell–mediated immune response in SV40-infected monkeys and MPyV-infected mice that confers protection from infection and is thought to play a role in establishing viral persistence in SV40- and MPyV-infected animals. Stimulation of CD8+ CTLs in mice, however, affects different pathways involving CD28 and CD40 ligands during the course of either acute or persistent infection.[164]

The past few years have seen a growing interest in the innate immune response to polyomavirus infection. It was first shown that expression of LTags from SV40, JCPyV, and BKPyV induces the expression of interferon-stimulated genes (ISGs) in mouse embryonic fibroblasts.[102] Subsequently, experiments comparing BKPyV and JCPyV infection of primary human renal epithelial cells, a cell culture model first described in 2004 that has become the preferred model for these two human viruses, demonstrated that the ability of the two viruses to replicate was inversely correlated with induction of ISGs.[8] While both viruses induced interferon β, JCPyV-infected cells induced ISGs, correlating with poor replication, whereas BKPyV-infected cells had no ISG production, with robust levels of replication. On the other hand, BKPyV cannot replicate efficiently when exposed to type-1 interferons induced when infecting endothelial cells or when lacking wildtype agnoprotein.[5,214] The nature of the different responses in different cells, or even within the same cells in the presence of the two viruses, remains to be determined.

Persistence

One of the interesting biological characteristics of all the polyomaviruses is the maintenance of a chronic and lifelong infection in their hosts. Evidence for persistence of PyV infection in the urinary tract is supported by viral excretion in the urine of healthy individuals with remarkably high levels of virus, ranging from 10^3 to 10^8 copies per milliliter (c/mL). Virus can be detected in uroepithelial cells and in ductal pathways. However, there is no apparent pathology associated with such high levels of urinary excretion unless there is an underlying immune-compromised condition. There is no information, however, on the mechanisms of viral persistence other than the possible role of the PyV miRNA or innate immune response, as described above, or what triggers viral synthesis and multiplication and the consequences of lifelong virus shedding in the urine. There is no evidence that polyomaviruses enter a true latent state in which there is little or no viral gene expression or genome replication as with the herpesviruses.

For the human polyomaviruses, the kidney or urothelium is the primary location for BKPyV, whereas the kidney and lymphoid organs are locations for JCPyV with differing consequences of infection. The sites of persistence for WUPyV and KIPyV have not been determined, although viral DNA has been recovered from respiratory secretions. MCPyV, HPyV6, and HPyV7 DNA can be readily isolated from normal skin and MCPyV virions are shed from the skin.[288] Given the rarity of normal Merkel cells in skin, this raises the possibility that MCPyV is produced by the stratified epidermal keratinocytes rather than less abundant Merkel cells. Alternatively, dermal fibroblasts, capable of supporting MCPyV replication *in vitro*, could be a source for MCPyV isolated from the skin.[198,199]

Transformation

Since their initial discovery, polyomaviruses have been used to study the transformation of normal cells. The initial observations of the tumor-causing ability by MPyV followed by the observation that injection of SV40 into newborn hamsters led to tumor development heralded the potent transforming activities of polyomaviruses.[317] Since then, many more polyomaviruses have been identified and their transforming activity has been compared to MPyV and SV40.

The transforming activity of the polyomaviruses is limited to their T antigens. The Vp capsid proteins and agnoprotein do not have transforming activity. The LTag and STag of most mammalian polyomaviruses as well as MTag of MPyV, Rat, and HaPyV have transforming activities. The LTags of the different primate viruses have been shown to have different transformation efficiencies in cells in culture.[32,122] LTag transforms cells in part by binding to and inactivating the RB and p53 tumor suppressor proteins. The contribution of STag to transformation is dependent in part on binding to the protein phosphatase PP2A.[47] As noted above, SV40 STag recruitment of the STRIPAK complex and MCPyV STag recruitment of MYCL and the EP400 complex also contribute to their transforming potential.[51,169] MTag has unique transforming activities related to its ability to assemble and activate a tyrosine kinase signaling complex.[284]

The study of cellular transformation and its relationship to tumorigenesis was led by seminal studies of the polyomaviruses. Early studies on transformation included colony or focus formation studies of primary mouse embryo fibroblasts or established 3T3 cells. Using SV40, Risser and Pollack described a hierarchy of the transformed phenotype that began with immortalization of primary cells, followed by their growth in reduced serum conditions, anchorage-independent growth, and ultimately formation of xenograft tumors in mice.[276] The degree of transformation was dependent in part on the level of LTag expression; the higher level of LTag expressed enabled the more complete transformed phenotype.

The polyomaviruses have been used to study transformation and oncogenesis in a variety of ways. In addition to using the whole viral genome, expression vectors for the T antigens have been used to study transformation. Mammalian expression vectors that drive the expression of the EVGR containing *LTAG* and *STAG* or complementary DNAs (cDNAs) specific for *LTAG* or *STAG* have been used in cells as well as in transgenic mice.[117,118] The tsA58 temperature-sensitive allele of SV40 EVGR encoding an LTag mutant A438V has been used to study transformation and establish cell lines in vitro and from transgenic mice.[148,275]

A seminal breakthrough in the study of human carcinogenesis was made when it was demonstrated that the combination of just four genetic elements could fully transform normal human cells. Expression of the SV40 EVGR or separate cDNAs encoding for LTag and STag, an activated form of HRAS, plus the catalytic subunit of human telomerase reverse transcriptase (hTERT) could completely transform normal human cells, including the ability to form tumors as a xenograft in an animal.[117,118] This strategy was applied to transform a wide variety of human cell types including astrocytes, myoblasts, and epithelial cells derived from lung, breast, and prostate tissues. This approach was expanded by substitution of SV40 LTag and STag with human oncogenes and tumor suppressor genes that led to the establishment of a model system of human oncogenesis composed of completely human genetic elements.[47] This approach has been expanded to high-throughput screens of cDNAs for gain-of-function and short hairpin RNA interference (shRNAi) knockdown or CRISPR-Cas9 knockout for loss of function to identify cellular oncogenes and tumor suppressor genes.

The transforming activity of polyomaviruses is balanced by its capacity to lyse cells during infection. Polyomaviruses can transform cells and form tumors under circumstances when the T antigens are expressed but the virus does not undergo replication at sufficiently high levels to kill the cell. If the infected cell is permissive for virus replication, then it will be killed and not undergo transformation. Conversely, if a cell is restrictive for replication but enables T antigen expression, then it may undergo transformation. Typically, a restrictive cell undergoes transformation when the polyomavirus DNA becomes integrated into the host chromosomal DNA in a way that sustains expression of the T antigens. This situation occurs when MCPyV DNA becomes integrated into the host genome and contributes to the development of MCC. Integration of MCPyV DNA is typically accompanied by mutations in the EVGR that truncate LTag, eliminating the DNA binding and helicase domains, and rendering it incapable of supporting viral replication (Fig. 1.18). Alternatively, a cell can be semipermissive and sustain low levels of viral replication while expressing sufficient levels of T antigens to change the cellular growth characteristics.

The nonpermissive or restrictive environment is generally caused by species-specific differences in DNA replication factors. The best understood of these is the interaction of LTag with the DNA replication machinery including the DNA polymerase α/primase complex and recruitment to the viral origin of replication. SV40 cannot replicate its DNA in rodent cells, at least in part due to its inability to bind the DNA polymerase α/primase in these cells. BKPyV also cannot replicate in murine cells, although the cause of the restriction is multifactorial.

Another level of permissiveness involves the interaction between LTag and p53. Just as the LTag can affect p53 function, p53 has reciprocal effects on the ability of LTag to function as a replication factor.[90] A tissue-specific example of this restriction is found in the differential ability of SV40 to replicate in human fibroblasts and mesothelial cells.[29] SV40 replicates quite efficiently in fibroblasts, whereas replication is severely limited in mesothelial cells. The latter cells have higher steady-state levels of p53 than the former and decreasing p53 expression in mesothelial cells with antisense strategies increases viral replication. Changes in the viral NCCR can also change the outcome of the infection from lytic to nonlytic. Monkey kidney cells, permissive for SV40 replication, transduced with a viral

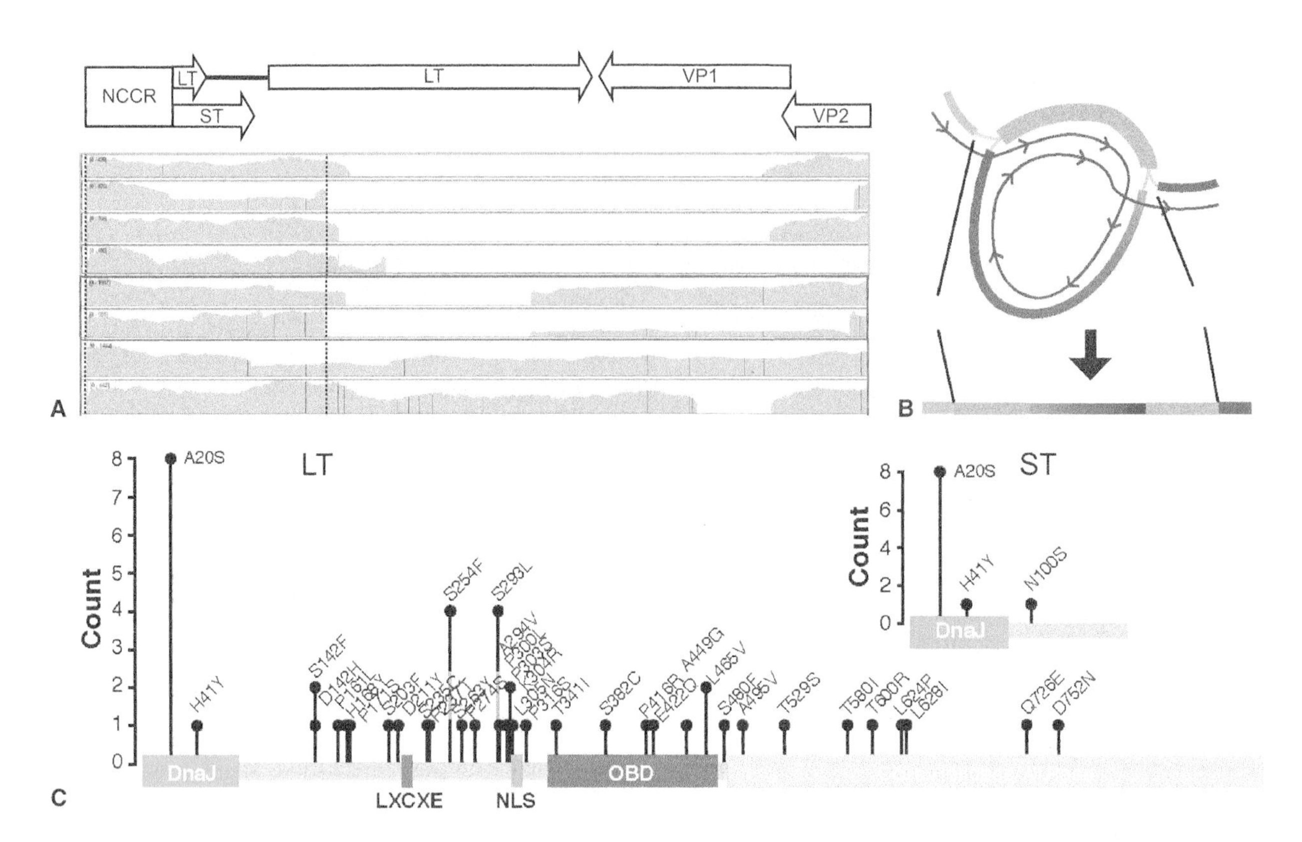

FIGURE 1.18 MCPyV Integration. A: MCPyV coverage and mutations from virus-positive cases. Read coverage for MCPyV in *gray*, and each plot represents a single patient. Scales for the coverage plots are set from 0 to the maximum read coverage per patient. The illustration above indicates relative position with MCPyV genome. Limits of minimal conserved region in MCCP tumors are indicated by dotted vertical lines. **B:** Representative assembly graph of partially duplicated MCPyV genome integrated into the tumor genome. Path for linearization of assembly graph shown by the *dark gray line*. **C:** Residue changes in MCPyV LT and ST (**inset**). Lollipop plot of LT missense mutations relative to the MCPyV reference with height reflecting the number of observations in cohort and residue change labeled above the position. LT and ST domains are highlighted by colored boxes. (Reprinted from Starrett GJ, Thakuria M, Chen T, et al. Clinical and molecular characterization of virus-positive and virus-negative Merkel cell carcinoma. *Genome Med* 2020;12(1):30. https://creativecommons.org/licenses/by/4.0/.)

genome containing a deletion of the SV40 origin of replication that disables replication are readily transformed while the wild-type virus causes lytic infection.[106] Some rearrangements in the BKPyV NCCR that cause a decrease in DNA replication efficiency can enhance the transforming ability of the virus.

A wide variety of transgenic mice lines have been generated that express polyomavirus EVGR or individual T antigens. Many of these animals develop tumors dependent on the specific promoter used. For example, the transgenic adenocarcinoma of the mouse prostate (TRAMP) model of prostate cancer uses the rat probasin promoter and pancreatic neuroendocrine tumors uses the rat insulin promoter (RIP) to drive expression of SV40 T antigens. MPyV MTag transgenic mice have been developed using a variety of promoters. Mice with MTag expression driven by the mouse mammary tumor virus long terminal repeat (MMTV-LTR) develop multifocal mammary adenocarcinomas that can become metastatic to the lung in 3 months. Several different strains of mice expressing MPyV MTag in the prostate tissues have been developed. Mice with MTag driven by the C3 promoter develop mouse prostatic intraepithelial neoplasia (mPIN). Another strain using the (ARR)2-Probasin promoter develop mPIN as early as 8 weeks of age that develops over time to become invasive cancer.

BKPyV induces different types of tumors dependent upon the rodent species and route of inoculation. Intracerebral inoculation of BKPyV in hamsters results in ependymomas, neuroblastomas, and pineal gland tumors. Intravenous inoculation causes pancreatic islet cell tumors, fibrosarcomas, and osteosarcomas. Mouse inoculations frequently result in fibrosarcomas, liposarcomas, nephroblastomas, gliomas, and choroid plexus tumors that are also common in SV40 LTag–expressing transgenic mice. BKPyV tumor induction shows some viral strain variation, with the prototype isolate, BKPyV Gardner, possessing the greatest oncogenic potential: this is probably related to the differences in transforming potential noted earlier between viruses carrying archetype and rearranged NCCRs. It is unclear whether *trans-* or *cis*-acting factors influence tumor formation frequency, but it is assumed that NCCR variations have a dominant role.

JCPyV inoculation into hamsters also results in multiple tumor types including medulloblastomas, glioblastomas, and pineocytomas. However, unlike BKPyV or SV40, JCPyV induces a grade 4 glioblastoma multiforme or malignant astrocytoma upon intracranial inoculation into owl and squirrel New World monkeys. By contrast, JCPyV does not induce tumors when inoculated into Old World macaques or rhesus or African green monkeys. Malignant brain tumors induced by JCPyV inoculation revealed that the viral genome was integrated into the cellular DNA.[226] The astrocytoma cells can be explanted and grown in culture. In some tumor cell explants, JCPyV LTag expression gradually diminishes upon continuous culture, and it enters into senescence. One owl monkey tumor, however, demonstrated unique properties, not only surviving in culture but also becoming transplantable back into other owl monkeys. JCPyV DNA in these tumor cells, termed 586, was both integrated in the cell chromosome and episomal in high copy number. JCPyV infectious virus was produced continually in culture, resulting in a persistent viral or carrier culture.[209]

EPIDEMIOLOGY

Members of the *Polyomaviridae* family are found throughout the world in bird, rodent, nonhuman primate, and human populations. The presence of polyomaviruses in the human population has been extensively studied. In one approach, evidence for prior infection by individual polyomaviruses has been performed with serum collected from individuals. For the most part, sera testing with viral particles or more recently using VLPs prepared from recombinant Vp1 corresponding to the different polyomaviruses enables determination of prior exposure. These serologic studies have revealed that infection with polyomavirus occurs as early as several months of age and increases in frequency until, by adulthood, several species of polyomaviruses have infected nearly all individuals (Fig. 1.19). In the second approach, sequencing of polyomavirus DNA collected from the urine or the skin enabled determination of the presence of various species of polyomaviruses. This approach has revealed that for the most part, an individual maintains a lifelong infection with polyomavirus. Although protective immunity against individual polyomaviruses may prevent reinfection, it may not be sufficient to prevent infection with a different strain of the same polyomavirus. In addition, these studies have revealed that polyomaviruses have coevolved along with the human population.

Evidence for prior infection with specific polyomaviruses can be determined in a sensitive enzyme-linked immunosorbent assay (ELISA). Recombinant forms of Vp1 from the corresponding polyomavirus are produced in bacteria or insect cells and spontaneously form VLPs. The purified VLPs are adhered to a plate and used to capture specific immunoglobulin molecules from sera. The relative amount of antibody captured is detected using anti-IgG– or anti-IgM–labeled secondary antibodies. In a useful variation of this assay, the recombinant VLP from a polyomavirus can be used to deplete the sera of antibodies specific for a given polyomavirus prior to exposure to the VLP attached to the plate. Depletion of immune sera with a polyomavirus-specific VLP permits determination of cross-reactivity of antibodies to different polyomaviruses. Using the VLP capture ELISA together with prior immunodepletion, evidence for infection with specific polyomaviruses can be obtained in a large collection of sera samples.

The VLP assay was initially used to detect evidence for prior infection with BKPyV and JCPyV in human sera and then expanded to search for evidence of prior infection with SV40. Some cross-reactivity in human sera has been observed between VLPs from BKPyV and SV40 and to a smaller degree between JCPyV and SV40.[163] Immune depletion of sera with BKPyV VLPs significantly reduces the titer of IgG-recognizing SV40 VLPs. Notably, reactivity of human sera against the African green monkey–derived lymphotropic polyomavirus (LPV) has been recognized for many years that was not appreciably depleted by preincubation with the VLP corresponding to SV40 or other known polyomaviruses. The discovery of human HPyV9, highly homologous to LPV, led to a direct comparison of sera reactivity for the two corresponding Vp1 proteins. Depletion with HPyV9 VLP removes most of the reactivity against monkey LPV.[332]

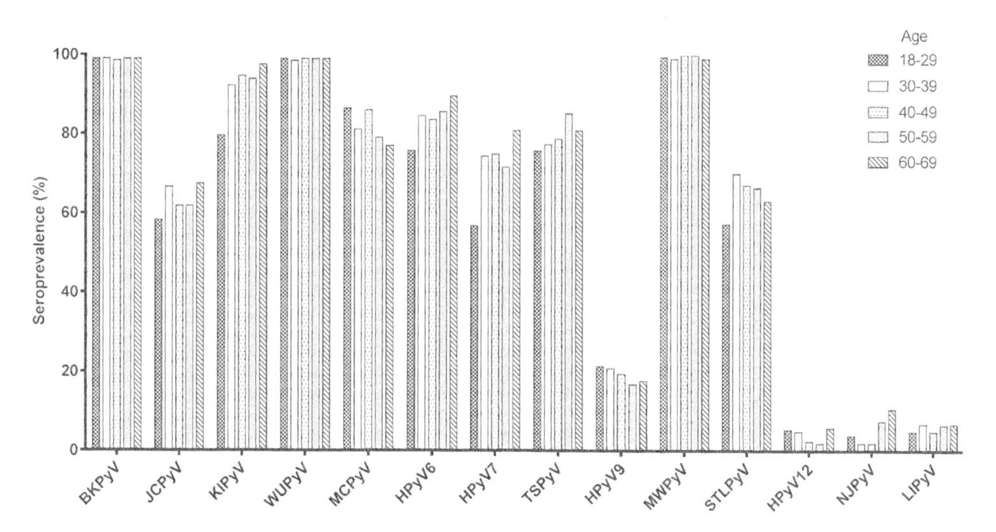

FIGURE 1.19 Seroprevalence of human polyomaviruses. "The percentage seropositivity of each polyomavirus is shown for the donor age categories 18–29".[156] (Reprinted from Kamminga S, van der Meijden E, Feltkamp MCW,et al. Seroprevalence of fourteen human polyomaviruses determined in blood donors. *PLoS One* 2018;13(10):e0206273. https://creativecommons.org/licenses/by/4.0/.)

VLP-based assays indicate that infection with human polyomaviruses can occur in the first few years of life. Serologic surveys of populations for the detection of antibodies specific for MCPyV and BKPyV indicate that seroconversion takes place early in life. Detection of maternal antibody in newborns begins to diminish within the first 3 months and is followed by evidence for newly acquired infection soon afterward and often within the first 2 years of life. Evidence for exposure continues to increase into adulthood, with titers corresponding to prior infection observed in approximately 50% to 80% of the sera tested (Fig. 1.19).[163,332] As evidenced by antibody titers, WUPyV and KIPyV infections can occur very early in life and then progressively become more common with age, with one report indicating 100% for KIPyV in healthy blood donors older than 50 years of age.[241]

Antibodies to both BKPyV and JCPyV are quite prevalent in populated countries but less prevalent in remote populations. In a study analyzing sera from Amerindian tribes from remote regions of South America, a low percentage of samples were positive, demonstrating low titers compared to a collection of Japanese samples with the majority positive with high antibody titers, particularly to JCPyV.[208] It also seemed that introduction of the human polyomaviruses into the Amerindian population occurred at the time of human contact from other countries.

In general, detection of viral DNA by PCR or direct sequencing is less sensitive than evidence for infection by serology-based testing. A comparison of evidence for infection using VLP assays, neutralization assays, and PCR-based detection of viral DNA isolated from the skin of more than 400 patients was performed. In this study, 65% had evidence for prior infection with MCPyV based on serology, but only 18% were positive by PCR amplification of DNA isolated from skin. This may be due to the inability of certain PCR primers to amplify all possible genomes of a given virus. Notably, nearly all patients with detectable amounts of MCPyV DNA on the skin had evidence for infection by serology against the virus.[83]

Because excretion of some human polyomaviruses in the urine is relatively common, a number of studies have tested urine for the prevalence of BKPyV and JCPyV. Sequencing of the polyomaviruses has revealed variation in all regions of the viral genome, especially the NCCR and the sequences encoding the C-termini of LTag and Vp1. Sequencing of BKPyV has identified four major subgroups with evidence for coevolution with known migration patterns of human hosts.[366] This approach demonstrated that excretion of the identical JCPyV virus occurred over 5 to 7 years in 19 different individuals and indicated persistent shedding rather than reinfection by different strains of JCPyV.[158] In addition, sequencing of JCPyV genomes revealed that the identical sequence was present in four of five families including parents and children, indicating that the virus spread horizontally within close quarters.[375]

Given that infection with JCPyV and BKPyV frequently occurs early in childhood among individuals living together, studies have been performed that reveal that polyomaviruses have coevolved with humans.[175,376] For example, a study collected urine samples from young and older individuals in Okinawa who had contact with American military and their families. The samples were analyzed using PCR to identify JCPyV DNA and nucleotide sequencing that could "type" variants of the DNA. One type was specific to Japan, while others were prominent in the United States. The results showed that none of the JCPyV DNA types found commonly in the American population were present in any age group in Japan, suggesting that virus is not easily transmitted between populations.[158] Additionally, urine samples collected from second- and third-generation Japanese Americans living in Los Angeles revealed that strains of JCPyV more commonly detected in Japan were present in the second- and third-generation Japanese American families.[325] A similar study of BKPyV found children to be infected with the local circulating strain, however, indicating transmission outside the family.[367]

Infection with MCPyV can also be traced back to childhood location by geographic areas based on sequences unique to specific polyomaviruses. Comparing the NCCR regions from different isolates revealed substitutions, small deletions, insertions, and duplications. Notably, strains detected in individuals from North America or Europe could be distinguished from those from Asia, supporting coevolution of viruses along with the host.[288]

CLINICAL FEATURES

Primary HPyV infections are assumed to occur without specific illness in the general population, either because of the subclinical course or because symptoms and signs are not specific and or usually self-limited. The natural route of transmission has not been defined for any HPyV. Person-to-person contact as well as environmental transmission of the nonenveloped virions are likely scenarios, via mucosal entry sites in the oropharyngeal, gastrointestinal, or respiratory tract.[215] Seroprevalence studies indicate that HPyV infections occur independently from one another, often during childhood and range from less than 30% to more than 90% in the general adult population, with an average of 6 to 8 different HPyV coinfections per person.[163] Detecting HPyV genomes by nucleic acid amplification testing (NAT) has been explored for identifying associations with clinical syndromes, such as KIPyV and WUPyV with respiratory tract disease. However, unequivocal evidence of proven disease by tissue pathology is currently only available for five HPyVs, plus one severe case of systemic vasculopathy associated with NJPyV (Table 1.2). In many cases, the affected patients were found to have inherited, acquired, or iatrogenic states of immunodeficiency. Thus, significant HPyV diseases must be considered opportunistic complications resulting from primary infection, secondary infection, or reactivation in immunocompromised hosts. However, inadequate HPyV-specific immune control does not appear to be sufficient for HPyV diseases but requires additional little understood local and systemic factors to account for their predilection to specific organs such as kidney, brain, or skin; clinical settings such as transplantation, HIV infection, or old age; and co-factors such as medication or UV light exposure.

Although initial infection of a host cell and placement of the viral genome into the host cell nucleus with subsequent viral gene expression underly any proven HPyV pathology, differences exist with respect to the leading contribution of virus replication–induced host cell loss, elicited inflammatory infiltrates, or host cell proliferative responses.[126] Prototypic examples for each of the three are PML in HIV/AIDS patients, PyV-associated nephropathy (PyVAN) in kidney transplant patients, and MCC in elderly immunocompromized persons, respectively. For PML in HIV/AIDS, the clinical and

TABLE 1.2 Polyomavirus associated diseases in humans. Site of infection, disease, risk factors for advanced illness, viral state, and pathologic features are provided

PyV	Infection	Disease, At-risk Population	Viral State	Pathologic Features
BKPyV	Kidney, urinary tract	PyV-associated nephropathy (PyVAN), kidney transplantation	Replicative	Lytic denudation, inflammation
		Hemorrhagic cystitis, hematopoietic stem cell transplantation (HSCT)	Replicative	Toxic damage, lytic denudation, inflammation
		Urothelial carcinoma, kidney transplantation with PyVAN	Nonreplicative, integrated	Oncogenic transformation
JCPyV	Brain, kidney, urinary tract	Progressive multifocal encephalopathy (PML), HIV/AIDS, multiple sclerosis	Replicative	Cytopathic
		PyVAN, kidney transplantation	Replicative	Lytic denudation, inflammation
MCPyV	Skin	Merkel cell carcinoma Elderly, sun exposure, immunocompromised	Nonreplicative, integrated, transformed	Neuroendocrine carcinoma
HPyV7	Skin	Pruritic hyperproliferative keratinopathy Solid organ transplantation recipient	Replicative, transforming	Proliferative, cytopathic
TSPyV	Skin	Trichodysplasia spinulosa Solid organ transplantation, CLL	Replicative, transforming	Proliferative, cytopathic
NJPyV	unknown	Systemic vasculopathy, pancreas transplantation	Replicative	Cytopathic

radiological presentation can be explained by oligodendrocyte loss from lytic JCPyV replication, causing progressive demyelination and neurological deficits in the absence of significant inflammatory infiltrates.[132,207] Conversely, significant BKPyV-induced renal tubular cell damage is nearly always marked by inflammatory infiltrates in the renal allograft, both of which contribute to declining renal function. MCC is characterized by host cell proliferation and metastasis resulting from chromosomally integrated viral genomes containing the NCCR persistently expressing MCPyV EVGR. However, the skin pathologies of *Trichodysplasia spinulosa* from TSPyV and pruritic hyperproliferative keratinopathy from HPyV7[41,138,219,342] can be placed between the extremes of replicative host cell lysis in JCPyV-PML and oncogenic transformation of MCPyV-carcinoma. In these syndromes, a prominent proliferative host cell pathology attributable to the HPyV early gene expression is followed by genome replication, Vp1 capsid protein expression, and lytic progeny release of TSPyV and HPyV7, respectively (Table 1.2).

Inflammatory responses play a mixed, often dynamic role of differing short- and long-term consequences. Following suppression of HIV replication in PML-AIDS by antiretroviral therapy (ART) effectively interrupting CD4 T cell loss, inflammatory responses become prominent as part of the immune reconstitution inflammatory syndrome (IRIS) leading to clinical and radiological aggravation, including unmasking of PML-IRIS.[132,210] Similarly, reducing immunosuppression for PyVAN in kidney transplantation can lead to functional worsening of renal function in an IRIS-like fashion, which is difficult to distinguish from acute cellular rejection.[73,225] In MCC, tumor-infiltrating lymphocytes have been associated with improved clinical outcomes, and their exhausted Tim-3 and PD-1 phenotype can be reinvigorated by immune checkpoint inhibitors PD-1 and PD-L1 to target the viral early antigens.[243] Appreciating details of the PyV pathology features is likely to be important for developing clinically successful antiviral and immunological prevention and treatment strategies.

BKPyV-Associated Diseases

BKPyV is recognized as the main etiological agent of polyomavirus-associated nephropathy (PyVAN), polyomavirus-associated hemorrhagic cystitis (PyVHC), and the increasingly recognized polyomavirus-associated urothelial cancer (PyVUC). BKPyV has also been implicated in rare cases of ureteric stenosis, pneumonitis, encephalitis, retinitis, vasculitis, and multiorgan involvement,[130] but little is known about their prevalence, risk factors, and pathogenesis.

Polyomavirus-Associated Nephropathy

Biopsy-proven PyVAN is encountered in 1% to 15% of kidney transplantations in the current era of immunosuppression across different programs and countries (Fig. 1.20).[129,134] While most cases of PyVAN are caused by BKPyV, fewer than 5% are caused by JCPyV.[140] Rarely, PyVAN has been diagnosed in the native kidneys of recipients after nonkidney solid organ transplantation (SOT) or allogeneic HSCT, or in patients with other forms of immune dysfunction including hyper-IgM syndrome, acute lymphocytic leukemia, or HIV/AIDS.[299] The common hallmark of PyVAN in these different clinical settings is uncontrolled lytic replication of BKPyV in renal tubular epithelial cells with associated inflammatory infiltrates that together compromise organ function.

The histopathology of PyVAN shows tubular epithelial cells with enlarged nuclei carrying ground-glass inclusions, resulting from numerous, often crystal-like, arrays of PyV virions of 40 to 45 nm diameter detectable by electron microscopy. The viral cytopathic effect causes cells to round up, slough off the tubular basement membrane, and undergo lysis thereby releasing free virions and virion aggregates. Early and late stages of the BKPyV replication cycle can be identified by immunohistochemistry showing LTag early gene expression alone or together with the late gene expression of Vp1 in the nucleus and agnoprotein in the cytoplasm, respectively.[187,296] BKPyV replication can be detected in the urothelial lining of the

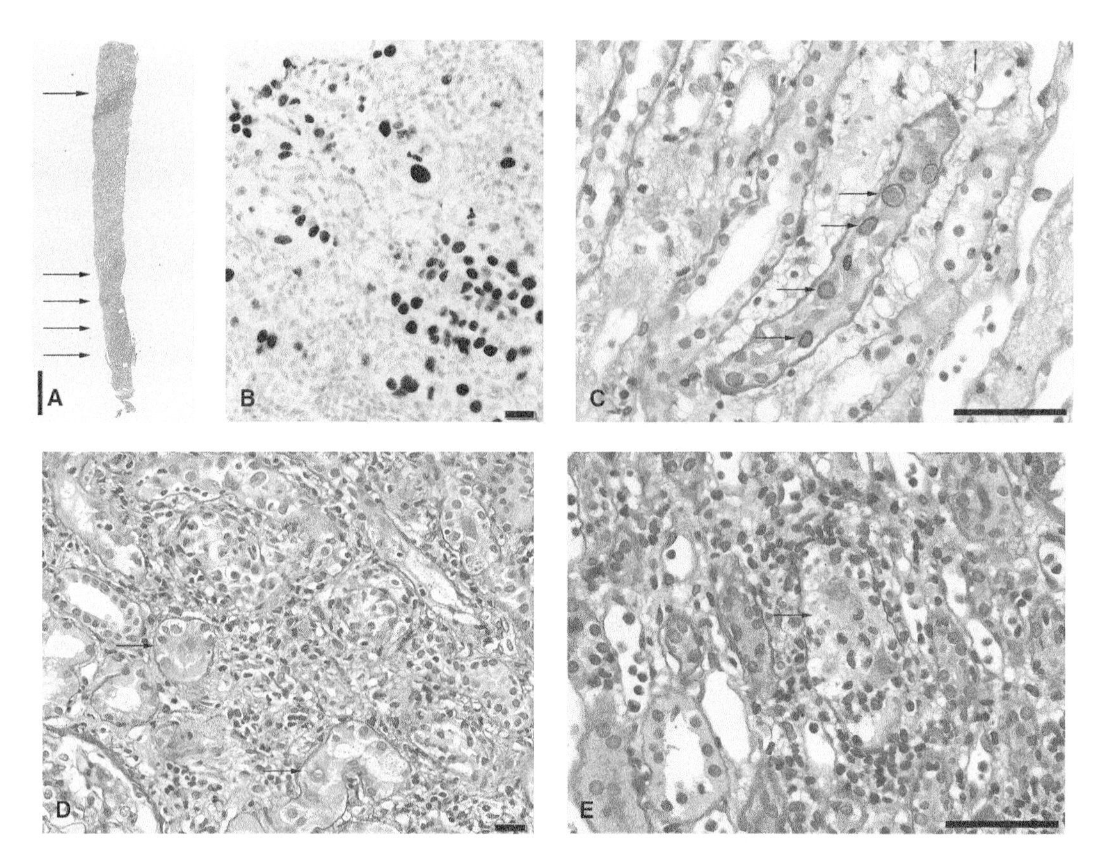

FIGURE 1.20 Histology of polyomavirus nephropathy. A: Kidney allograft biopsy showing focal involvement of cortex (*arrows*) at low magnification with striped interstitial inflammation (bar = 1 mm). **B:** PyV LTag-positive nuclei are detectable in the marked areas (bar = 20 μm). **C:** Early changes show some tubules containing virus-replicating cells (*arrows*) with little or no tubular damage or interstitial inflammation (bar = 50 μm). **D:** Florid PyVAN disease with tubular damage (*arrows*) and interstitial inflammation as prominent features, while virally infected cells are frequently more difficult to detect on routine stains (bar = 20 μm). **E:** After reducing immunosuppression, viral replication foci are cleared ("resolving PyVAN") that may be associated with dense inflammatory infiltrates and prominent intraepithelial lymphocytes in affected tubules (*arrow*, **E**, bar = 20 μm). **A, C-E:** PAS stain. **B:** PyV LTag immunohistochemistry with PAb416. Original magnifications: **A** 2.5×, **B** 20×, **C** 60×, **D** 40×, **E** 60×.

transitional cell layer in the renal pelvis, which contribute to the shedding of so-called decoy cells into the urine, and very high urine BKPyV loads of greater than 10^7 c/mL.[91,246] In early stages of PyVAN, isolated nephrons are affected, often located in the renal medulla and without prominent inflammatory infiltrates (denoted PyVAN-A), with little impact on renal function.[74] As BKPyV replication expands to multiple nephrons throughout the kidney, interstitial and tubular inflammatory infiltrates in response to cell lysis and tubular basement membrane denudation become dominant features (PyVAN-B). At this stage, declining renal function is progressively seen, which triggers renal biopsies for a histopathology diagnosis. This presentation is difficult to distinguish from acute cellular rejection, which requires increased, rather than lowered immunosuppression.

The interstitial infiltrates in PyVAN include mononuclear cells, granulocytes, and lymphocytes, specifically T cells and predominantly IgM-type plasma cells, which positively correlate with plasma IgM levels. Cellular regeneration failure characterized by tubular atrophy with only few BKPyV-replicating cells and extensive interstitial fibrosis are the hallmarks of end-stage disease (PyVAN-C). Thus, progressive viral tissue involvement, inflammation, tubular atrophy, and fibrosis have been associated with declining function and return to renal replacement therapy in 10% of patients with PyVAN-A, in 50% with PyVAN-B, and more than 80% with PyVAN-C.[74,135] Although most data have been obtained from kidney transplantation, histological changes similar to PyVAN-B and -C have been described in the failing native kidneys of patients suffering from other forms of immunodeficiency.[299]

Plasma DNA loads of BKPyV are a direct marker of renal involvement reflecting onset and clearance of PyVAN and have become the key diagnostic tool for screening and management of BKPyV in kidney transplant patients.[129,134] Plasma BKPyV loads are almost exclusively derived from nonencapsidated BKPyV DNA susceptible to DNase-I digestion rather than from circulating virions.[188] BKPyV-DNAemia is rarely found in nonkidney solid organ transplant (SOT) recipients except in case of proven PyVAN.

The diagnosis of proven PyVAN requires confirmation of tissue involvement. However, in kidney transplant patients with new onset of BKPyV-DNAemia and baseline renal allograft function, needle biopsies have a limited sensitivity, with false negative rates of 10% to 50%. However, in kidney transplant patients with new onset of BKPyV-DNAemia and baseline renal allograft function, needle biopsies have limited sensitivity, with false negative rates of 10% to 50%.[74] BKPyV-DNAemia serves an indicator of risk for developing biopsy-proven PyVAN, which is diagnosed in a subset of kidney transplant patients within another 2 to 6 weeks.[134] The detection rate of proven PyVAN in needle biopsies increases as plasma BKPyV loads rise above 10^4 to 10^6 c/mL, viral variants with rearranged NCCR emerge, or renal allograft function declines.[109] Conversely, in patients clearing proven PyVAN after reducing immunosuppression, the plasma BKPyV loads decline but clearance of BKPyV-DNAemia may lag several months behind the disappearance of LTag-positive cells in biopsies.[73] Upon surgical removal of the failing renal allograft with ongoing PyVAN, however, plasma BKPyV loads rapidly drop with a half-life of 1 to 2 hours to undetectable levels in less than 24 hours, even in patients on continued immunosuppression.[92] Thus, plasma BKPyV loads reflect the natural course of BKPyV complications involvement in the renal allograft and inform screening and management recommendations in renal transplant recipients.[129,134]

Importantly, BKPyV-IgG–seropositive immunocompetent healthy blood donors usually do not have detectable levels of BKPyV DNA in blood but can excrete viral DNA in urine. A small study of 20 healthy, nonpregnant, women over a 2-month period found episodic excretion of BKPyV in approximately 10% of samples tested.[77] Similar rates and levels of urinary shedding have been observed in donors and in recipients with residual urine production prior to kidney transplantation. Following intravenous induction and oral maintenance immunosuppression therapy, urinary BKPyV shedding in kidney transplant recipients increases to a cumulative incidence of 40% to 80% by 2 years posttransplant.[134,140] In approximately half of the cases, urine BKPyV loads increase to greater than 10^7 c/mL with "decoy cells" appearing in the urine.[74,134,136] Similar to high-level viruria and urinary decoy cell shedding, the detection of three-dimensional PyV virion aggregates in urine ("haufen") may appear, which have been reported to better correlate with advanced PyVAN and tissue injury. *Vp1* mRNA transcript levels of greater than 6.5×10^5 copies/ng total RNA in urinary sediments have been explored to identify and predict outcome of kidney transplant recipients with PyVAN.[61]

Risk factors for plasma BKPyV-DNAemia and proven PyVAN include characteristics of the donor such as BKPyV viruria, high BKPyV-IgG antibodies, higher number of HLA mismatches, and blood group incompatibilities; of the recipient including older age greater than 50 years among adults, younger age among children, male gender, low or absent BKPyV-IgG and neutralizing antibody titers, and low or absent BKPyV-specific T cells; and the type and intensity of immunosuppression such as high-dose corticosteroids for acute rejection, use of tacrolimus rather than cyclosporine, or mTOR inhibitors such as sirolimus or everolimus.[134,361]

In most, but not all cases, donor-type BKPyV is detected in the urine and blood of kidney transplant recipients.[293] Recipient low-level viruria before transplantation is not associated with an increased risk of developing high-level viruria or BKPyV-DNAemia after kidney transplantation, in line with the key role of BKPyV transmitted with the donor graft, but in some cases, recipient-type or non–donor-type BKPyV has been identified. Distinct genotypes of BKPyV have been reported to induce specific neutralizing antibodies in kidney transplant recipients immunity. Low-neutralizing antibodies have been associated with an increased risk of BKPyV-DNAemia and nephropathy posttransplant.[259,312] However, the immune effector mechanism may not be restricted neutralization, since induction of high titers is not sufficient for clearance.[159,201]

Antivirals for prophylaxis or treatment of BKPyV replication have not been successful in kidney transplant recipients or in other patients suffering from PyVAN. Compounds inhibiting BKPyV replication in cell culture such as cidofovir, brincidofovir (CMX001), leflunomide, fluoroquinolones, cyclosporine A, or mTOR inhibitors have been used in uncontrolled case series as adjuncts to reducing immunosuppression, hence obscuring their actual contribution to the often slow decline in BKPyV replication. This includes the use of intravenous immunoglobulin preparations, which may contain BKPyV-neutralizing antibody activities.[159,272] A recent meta-analysis was unable to identify a significant benefit of mTOR inhibitors in reducing BKPyV events in kidney transplant recipient.[212] A recent trial demonstrating the immunologic equivalence of the mTOR inhibitor everolimus together with a low-dosed calcineurin inhibitor regarding the transplant and reported less BKPyV events compared to the standard tacrolimus mycophenolate control arm but was limited by an overall underreporting of BKPyV events.[258] Dedicated randomized clinical trials are needed to evaluate the role of intravenous immunoglobulins, neutralizing monoclonal antibody preparations for prophylaxis or treatment of BKPyV replication in kidney transplantation. One properly conducted prospective randomized clinical trial concluded that levofloxacin use during the first 3 months had no impact on levels of BKPyV viruria or DNAemia.[171]

Current guidelines recommend monthly screening of all kidney transplant recipients for plasma BKPyV-DNAemia and reducing immunosuppression in case of BKPyV loads persisting greater than 10^3 c/mL for 3 weeks (probable PyVAN) or rising above 10^4 c/mL (presumptive PyVAN).[131,135] Since proven PyVAN is also treated by reducing immunosuppression, needle biopsy is not considered necessary unless there is a high suspicion of allograft rejection or another diagnosis. According to several larger prospective single-center cohorts, reducing immunosuppression alone has been associated with clearance rates of 50% to 100%, showing higher success rates when initiated promptly according to predefined indications. Different protocols have been applied consisting of first reducing the calcineurin inhibitor (tacrolimus, cyclosporine A) followed by the antimetabolite (mycophenolate, azathioprine), or alternatively by first reducing the antimetabolite followed by the calcineurin inhibitor. Subsequent acute rejection episodes have been observed in approximately 10% to 15% of cases, which mostly responded to antirejection treatment.[26] Based on in vitro studies and clinical observations, switching from tacrolimus/mycophenolate combinations to low-dose cyclosporine and mTOR inhibitors have been proposed.[159] However, direct comparisons of efficacy and tolerability are not available for any of the currently used approaches. Although most patients respond to reducing immunosuppression with clearance of BKPyV-DNAemia, patients with proven PyVAN appear to require more time and interventions.[26] The diagnosis of concurrent acute rejection is difficult and relies on detecting signs of endarteritis, fibrinoid vascular necrosis, glomerulitis, and C4d deposits along peritubular capillaries.[135] Molecular studies using comparative transcriptomics or proteomics failed to reveal significant differences between acute rejection and PyVAN other than the presence of BKPyV. In patients with sustained BKPyV-DNAemia and biopsy-proven acute rejection, a two-step approach of first treating acute rejection followed by reducing immunosuppression, for example, at 2 to 4 weeks after response is recommended.[135]

The outcome of BKPyV-DNAemia and PyVAN has significantly improved compared to historic reports.[271] Graft loss with ongoing BKPyV-DNAemia is seen in approximately 10% to 30% of cases.[73] However, even in patients with immunologically cleared BKPyV replication and disease, the renal graft survival is reduced due to the scarred nephrons lost shortening the time to renal replacement therapy. Further data are needed to identify the risk factors associated with an increased rate of antibody-mediated rejection after treatment.

Retransplantation after renal allograft loss secondary to BKPyV has been successfully performed with 3-year graft survival rates of 93.6%.[69,128] In most cases, immunosuppression was discontinued until retransplantation, which permitted BKPyV-specific immune recovery and clearing of BKPyV-DNAemia for at least 3 months. Surgical removal of the failing transplant or the native kidneys was not required for successful outcomes. However, in patients considered for preemptive retransplantation, a significant decline in plasma BKPyV loads of greater than 100-fold (2 log10) is recommended as indicator of emerging BKPyV-specific T cell control and preferentially combined with allograft nephrectomy.[25,128,183] Recurrence of plasma BKPyV DNAemia and PyVAN was observed after retransplantation, which responded to reducing immunosuppression in most cases.[69,128] Retransplantation has been successful in patients with other functioning allografts such as pancreas, although an increased risk of PyVAN recurrence and allograft loss has been reported.[227]

Polyomavirus-Associated Hemorrhagic Cystitis

BKPyV is the main etiological agent of PyVHC, which complicates 5% to 50% of allogeneic HSCT, but is rarely found in other types of transplantations or immunodeficiency conditions.[44] Because of the extensive urothelial damage and associated hemorrhagic bleeding, histology studies are rarely performed except in severe cases requiring therapeutic cystectomy. The diagnosis of PyVHC is based on the triad of symptoms of cystitis (dysuria, urge, lower abdominal discomfort), signs of macrohematuria (grade 2 or higher), and high urine BKPyV loads greater than 10^7 c/mL. Each component can occur alone and is not sufficient for the diagnosis of PyVHC. Other etiologies should be ruled out such as infections from other viruses including human adenovirus, cytomegalovirus, or herpes simplex. Hematuria can be due to urotoxic conditioning alone, coagulation disorders, malignancies, or mechanical factors such as catheters, and should be graded as microhematuria (grade 1) or macrohematuria (grade 2), with clots (grade 3), or renal failure (grade 4). Imaging studies of PyVHC using sonography or MRI may show thickened bladder walls and help to identify clots and postrenal obstruction or ureteric involvement.[247]

PyVHC is typically of late onset, occurring 2 to 12 weeks after engraftment and lasting for 3 to 5 weeks.[7,17] By contrast, hemorrhagic cystitis solely attributed to urotoxic conditioning is of early onset, mostly within 1 week after HSCT and lasting for just a few days.[7,17,295] In approximately half of the patients diagnosed with PyVHC, BKPyV DNA can be detected in serum or plasma with viral loads of greater than 10,000 c/mL. Following the widespread use of the chemoprotective agent mesna, hyperhydration, and forced diuresis during myeloablative conditioning to reduce bladder exposure to urotoxic metabolites such as acrolein, the rate and duration of early-onset hemorrhagic cystitis has declined, whereas late-onset PyVHC has remained as a significant complication.[17] Although milder forms exist, PyVHC after allogeneic HSCT frequently presents with immobilizing pain requiring generous analgesic treatment, hospital admission, and intensive nursing care.

PyVHC is rarely seen after kidney transplantation despite similarly high peak urine BKPyV loads in the order 10^8 to 10^{10} c/mL. This observation suggests that immune failure to control high-level BKPyV replication in the urothelial compartment is not sufficient to explain the prominent clinical features of massive inflammation and bleeding after HSCT. Instead, it is likely that urotoxic chemotherapy conditioning causes subclinical damage to the bladder epithelium.[24] High-level BKPyV replication during the fading immune control leads to extensive denudation of the urothelial lining and urine leakage into the hyperemic submucosa. Painful hemorrhagic exacerbation ensues with abundant inflammatory infiltrates coinciding with allogeneic stem cell engraftment, hence reminiscent of IRIS.[24] A role of *bona fide* IRIS in PyVHC pathogenesis is strongly suggested by two HIV/AIDS cases, not undergoing HSCT, following a rise in CD4 T cell count upon ART. One of these cases had cyclophosphamide exposure for treatment of non-Hodgkin lymphoma.[13,105]

The risk factors of PyVHC after HSCT are multiple and include myeloablative conditioning with cyclophosphamide, high-dose busulfan, and total body irradiation; T-cell depletion with antithymocyte globulin or alemtuzumab; male gender; unrelated, mismatched, and haplo-identical donors; umbilical cord grafts; as well as graft versus host disease. Higher BKPyV-specific antibodies pretransplant were correlated with the peak urine BKPyV loads and increased risk of PyVHC, supporting the view that PyVHC is primarily caused by BKPyV reactivation in the recipient.[7,360] However, many recipient populations with low or undetectable antibodies that develop high-level viruria have been reported as well as other factors including reinfection and nosocomial transmission. None of the risk factors have entered clinical routine protocols modifying the choice of donors or conditioning procedures. Routine screening for BKPyV replication has no impact on patient management since effective drugs for prophylaxis or treatment are not available.[44]

The treatment of PyVHC is based on unstinting pain relief and bladder irrigation combined with local urologic interventions as needed for anemic bleeding, clot removal, and renal failure. Platelet transfusion and local coagulation with fibrin glues are used as clinically indicated. Regaining BKPyV-specific immune control is thought to underly the spontaneous clearance but reducing or discontinuing immunosuppression is problematic due to the risk of precipitating or exacerbating graft versus host disease after allogeneic HSCT. Conversely, steroid treatment reducing the inflammatory component may cause transient relief but prolong the virus replicative denudation and bleeding.

A recent review of the available antiviral treatments concluded that off-label use of intravenous cidofovir is controversial due to limited efficacy and unclear benefits in the absence of randomized controlled trials.[44] This included administration of high doses of cidofovir as approved for the treatment of ganciclovir-resistant CMV retinitis. Uncontrolled case reports of successful responses following intravesical application of cidofovir, intravesical hyaluronate, intravenous immunoglobulins, leflunomide, levofloxacin, oxygen, or mesenchymal stem cells have been reported.[44] However, systemic and intravesical cidofovir were not effective in a pediatric study.[174] In the absence of randomized trials, a natural course with spontaneous resolution of PyVHC cannot be ruled out, coinciding with BKPyV-antibody increases has been reported in children.[174] This caveat also applies also to brincidofovir/CMX001, a lipid conjugate of cidofovir, which is approximately 400-fold more effective in inhibiting BKPyV replication in cell culture, but also showed cytostatic effects on the host cells. Recently, a randomized phase III trial investigating the role of oral brincidofovir for CMV prophylaxis in allogeneic HSCT but found no reduction in BKPyV events predefined as secondary end points.[217] In line with the role of virus-specific T cells in controlling BKPyV replication, adoptive transfer of BKPyV-specific T cells from stem donors or third-party donors may have promise as potential prophylactic or therapeutic modality for PyVHC.[336] Thus, significant efforts are needed to better understand the pathogenesis of PyVHC in order to develop effective prevention or therapies by targeting one or several components of the PyVHC triad.

BKPyV-associated cystitis with or without macrohematuria has been occasionally encountered in other immunocompromised hosts including in HIV/AIDS patients or in SOT recipients including kidney transplantation. In case of declining renal function in the absence of macrohematuria, ureteric stenosis or PyVAN should be considered in the differential diagnosis, in which case imaging studies and biopsies should be sought. Indeed, in some cases, BKPyV cystitis occurred together with proven PyVAN including patients after allogeneic HSCT.

Polyomavirus-Associated Urothelial Carcinoma

The host cell–transforming properties of the polyomavirus EVGR may contribute to the onset of PyVUC.[256] Morphological variations of PyVUC include transitional cell carcinoma, Bellini collecting duct carcinoma, and other intrarenal manifestations. PyVUC has been primarily encountered in patients with a history of prolonged BKPyV replication and PyVAN, most commonly after kidney transplantation or rarely in nonkidney SOT recipients. In a recent retrospective multicenter survey from the United States, approximately eight-fold more cases of urothelial carcinoma were reported among patients with prior PyVAN, although this association did not reach statistical significance.[277] Linking 55,697 kidney transplant recipients in the scientific registry of transplant recipients (SRTR) to 17 U.S. cancer registries, 584 incident renourinary malignancies were identified including 80 bladder cancers, a three-fold higher incidence for invasive bladder carcinoma among recipients previously treated for presumed or proven PyVAN compared to the control patients.[115] In a large single-center study, prolonged BKPyV replication and smoking were identified as independent risk factors for urothelial carcinoma.[197] Moreover, the donor origin of PyVUC pointed to a role of HLA mismatching in addition to immunosuppression, T cell depletion, and nonuse of mTOR inhibitors.[115]

The pathogenesis of PyVUC has been attributed to the immunologically uncensored high level of BKPyV replication leading to the occurrence of genetic accidents such as chromosomal genome integration of the BKPyV DNA, which disrupt or interfere with host cell–(onco-)lytic viral replication. NCCR rearrangements without genome integration might also play a role by favoring BKPyV EVGR expression without matching LVGR expression.[239] The role of BKPyV EVGR–encoded tumor antigen expression is supported by the absence of driver mutations in the top 50 genes found in non-BKPyV–associated cancers.[239] Replication of BKPyV is associated with induction of APOBEC3B, a single-stranded DNA cytosine deaminase that can induce C-to-T and C-to-G mutations in the viral and host genome. Prolonged high levels of BKPyV viruria can lead to significant changes in the host genome with a characteristic APOBEC mutational signature.[314] In some cases, chromosomal integration of BKPyV genomic sequences with rearranged NCCRs as single copies or concatemers or as nonintegrated viral episomes has been detected.[314]

PyVUC diagnosis relies on the surgical removal and histological analysis of the tumor, which is also considered therapeutic for in situ bladder cancers. Recurrence in immunocompromised patients and progression with metastatic lymph nodes or invasive disease are associated with a poor prognosis. Lasting remission of otherwise metastatic PyVUC has been observed after discontinuation of immunosuppression,[239] a maneuver not similarly feasible in nonkidney SOT patients.

Other BKPyV-Associated Diseases

Ureteric stenosis has been linked to BKPyV replication in kidney transplantation before the widespread emergence of PyVAN[56] but is rarely diagnosed in the current era despite the overall increased incidence of high-level BKPyV viruria. Less traumatic anastomosis surgery and routine ureteric stenting may account for this decline in events. Conversely, ureteric stents have been associated with an increased risk of BKPyV-DNAemia and PyVAN in some studies.[211] Local injury upon stent placement or removal has been suggested to cause local BKPyV reactivation, but ureteric stents clearly facilitate vesicoureteric reflux during bladder contraction and may cause accelerated retrograde spread to the renal allograft.[91,160] Stenosis resulting from inflamed ureters (ureteritis) after allogeneic HSCT has been described in the context of PyVHC. The clinical diagnosis is based on altered flux through the ureteric ostium or outright hydronephrosis in sonography or MRI studies together with high-level BKPyV viruria. Treatment involves urologic interventions including ureteric stenting, nephrostomas, and surgical reanastomosis to assure urinary drainage.

BKPyV encephalopathy is a rare, but well-documented entity in severely immunocompromised patients with disseminated replicative disease in the context of HIV/AIDS[33,339] or inherited immunodeficiency syndromes,[63] or hematopoietic disorders including chronic lymphatic leukemia, Hodgkin lymphoma, or allogeneic HSCT. Though not specifically documented, these conditions appear to combine T cell defects, absent or deficient antibody responses with chemotherapy and CD20 lymphocyte depletion using rituximab.[86,186] Focal neurological symptoms and signs reflect the areas of involvement and include visual disturbance, palsy, seizures, headache, nausea, ataxia, or cognitive deficits. Imaging studies using MRI may show edema with or without contrast-enhancing areas in the affected locations of the cortex, subcortical white matter, cerebellum, or brain stem. Thus, BKPyV encephalopathy is reminiscent of the more frequently encountered PML caused by JCPyV. Laboratory-confirmed cases of BKPyV encephalopathy combine clinical and imaging abnormalities with detectable BKPyV DNA in the cerebrospinal fluid (CSF), while JCPyV or other viral genomes by NAT are absent. CSF pleocytosis is rare and low, protein levels are normal or elevated, and glucose and lactate levels inconspicuous. In proven cases, stereotactic brain biopsy or autopsy tissue reveals very high tissue BKPV-DNA loads by NAT, LTag expression, and Vp1 capsid expression in the enlarged nuclei of infected cells by immunohistochemistry and intranuclear PyV virions of 40 nm diameter by electron microscopy.[63,339] Nonspecific monocytic and lymphocytic infiltrations have been described in the perivascular space, leptomeninges, cortex, and white matter, in addition to astrogliosis, reactive astrocytes with nuclear hyperchromatic changes, and oligodendroglia-like cells and occasional neurons with enlarged nuclei.[63] Where analyzed, the BKPyV NCCR was rearranged with deletions and duplications, which have been proposed to increase BKPyV replication in the CNS compartment.[63,318] In approximately half of the case reports of BKPyV encephalopathy, there was a significant preceding or coexisting pathology such as PyVAN[33,318,339] or PyVHC grade 4 suggesting dissemination of BKPyV from the renourinary tract with encephalopathy, meningoencephalitis, and retinitis.[33] However, BKPyV encephalopathy without involvement of another organ has been described in one apparently immunocompetent patient with serologically primary BKPyV replication who eventually recovered.[349]

The role of BKPyV in the CNS manifestations has been explored in a study of 124 children without known underlying disease presenting with suspected viral encephalitis. BKPyV, but not JCPyV DNA was been detected in the CSF of 3 (2.4%), all of whom were BKPyV seropositive, but JCPyV seronegative.[18] Among 42 immunocompetent adults presenting with meningoencephalitis, BKPyV DNA was found in the CSF of two (4.7%).[18] Thus, BKPyV should be considered in patients presenting with symptoms and signs of CNS involvement having undetectable JCPyV or other neurotropic viruses. Treatment of CNS disease caused by BKPyV has not been established. Given the dire prognosis of BKPyV encephalopathy in immunocompromised patients, some experts have administered intravenous cidofovir or high-dose intravenous immunoglobulins without changing outcome. Moreover, BKPyV CNS manifestations have been reported in patients receiving intravenous immunoglobulin prophylaxis, which raise questions about the efficacy and dosing.[63] Removing the underlying cause of immunodeficiency would be key and hence to consider adoptive T cell transfer alone or together with high-dose neutralizing antibodies.[336] Immune recovery in HIV/AIDS patients may be associated with paradoxical worsening of BKPyV CNS diseases, marked inflammation reminiscent of IRIS as well described for JCPyV-PML.

BKPyV pneumonia has been identified in a limited number but well-documented cases with mostly disseminated replication, all of which were fatal due to rapidly progressive respiratory failure. Postmortem studies showed diffuse alveolar damage, interstitial inflammatory infiltrates, cytopathically altered pneumocytes with enlarged nuclei, intranuclear inclusions staining positive for LTag, and PyV virions by electron microscopy.[93,339] The patients suffered from severe immunocompromising conditions such as HIV/AIDS,[339] allogeneic HSCT, or chronic lymphatic leukemia undergoing chemotherapy.[93,318] Steroids were used for treating graft versus host disease or for the complicating interstitial lung disease. In two-thirds of the cases, significant replicative BKPyV manifestations such as PyVAN or PyVHC preceded the pulmonary complications suggesting hematogenous viral spread and secondary multiorgan involvement including the CNS. In only one case of PyVHC grade 4, the diagnosis of BKPyV pneumonia was made antemortem, whereby the CT scan of the lungs showed diffuse ground glass infiltrates and typical cytopathic cells with enlarged nuclei harboring ground-glass inclusions in bronchoalveolar lavage samples.[363] Treatment attempts using cidofovir, vidarabine, or intravenous immunoglobulin were unsuccessful in all of these cases.

Other clinical entities with histologically proven involvement of BKPyV are rare and linked to exceptional presentations. This includes a profoundly immunosuppressed kidney transplant patient seropositive for BKPyV, who developed muscle weakness and a severe capillary leak syndrome with anasarca and died from myocardial infarction and circulatory arrest.[265] Postmortem, BKPyV replication was demonstrated in endothelial cells of the skeletal and heart muscle, but sparing the vasculature of the liver, lungs, and kidney.[265] The NCCR of the BKPyV was of archetype architecture but contained nucleotide substitutions[49] inactivating a conserved ETS1 transcription factor binding, which increased BKPyV EVGR expression and replication in cell culture similar to NCCR rearrangements.[23] Finally, BKPyV has been implicated in other clinical conditions including autoimmune disorders including systemic Lupus erythematosus[235] and sclerosing lymphocytic inflammatory salivary gland disease found in a subgroup of HIV-infected individuals. However, a role for BKPyV as a driver or bystander in these diseases and the role of immune dysfunction from immunogenetics, HIV coinfection, or immunosuppressive treatment have not been resolved.[245]

JCPyV-Associated Diseases

JCPyV is the main etiological agent of PML.[85,132,210,252,377] Other neurological manifestations are granule cell neuronopathy in the cerebellum, encephalopathy targeting cortical pyramidal neurons, as well as meningitis and encephalitis.[85,120,132] Despite its major tropism for the renourinary tract and persistent shedding in immunocompetent persons,[77] JCPyV is a rare cause of PyVAN in kidney transplant patients.[132] In addition, an association of JCPyV infection with malignancies in the brain, in lymph nodes, and in gastrointestinal tract has been reported.

JCPyV—Progressive Multifocal Leukoencephalopathy

The clinical entity of PML was first described in 1958 as a rare fatal demyelinating complication in immunocompromised patients exposed to chemotherapy and corticosteroids for treating hematological malignancies such as chronic lymphatic leukemia and Hodgkin lymphoma.[9] The histopathology is characterized by the loss of myelin-producing oligodendrocytes through lytic JCPyV replication, localizing predominantly to the subcortical white matter, but can extend into neurons in the cortical gray matter.[20,101] The expanding demyelinated areas show increased gliosis, surrounded by JCPyV-replicating oligodendrocytes with characteristic enlarged inclusion-bearing nuclei, reactive, partly multinucleated "bizarre" astrocytes, fat-loaded "foamy" macrophages, and variable numbers of infiltrating lymphocytes preferentially cuffing the perivascular space (Fig. 1.21).[350,353] JCPyV particles can be detected in the intranuclear inclusions of the oligodendrocytes by electron microscopy, but the specific diagnosis is commonly based on detecting intranuclear JCPyV genome by in situ hybridization or Vp1 capsid protein by immunohistochemistry.[151] NAT for JCPyV DNA is very sensitive and typically shows very high tissue viral loads with rearranged NCCRs that can be distinguished from latently persisting JCPyV in brain tissue.[132,210]

The incidence of PML in the general population is low and has been estimated to be less than 0.1 per 100,000 person years in North America and Europe, but at least 10- to 1,000-fold higher in patients with immunodeficiency states such as HIV/AIDS, allogeneic HSCT, SOT, or autoimmune diseases under therapy.[6] In addition, PML has been described in case reports of patients with less well-defined immunodeficiency including CD4 lymphocytopenia.[116] During the HIV/AIDS epidemic in the 1980s, a more than 10-fold overall increase in PML diagnoses was observed affecting 1% to 5% of HIV patients in the era before effective ART. Thereby, PML in HIV/AIDS patients became the classic reference with respect to risk, clinical presentation, imaging, pathology, and outcome.[132,210] HIV/AIDS patients with PML were JCPyV seropositive and had CD4 T cell counts falling below 100/μL blood,[165,222] implicating failing immune control and JCPyV reactivation in the CNS. Moreover, paradoxical clinical worsening as well as unmasking of PML by IRIS emerged as a novel manifestation of the disease following effective ART suppressing HIV-1 replication and reconstituting CD4 T-cell counts.[133,283] In the current era of early ART intervention, PML has practically disappeared among HIV-1–infected patients except for those presenting late but then still remains associated with significant morbidity and mortality.[6,165]

During the past decade, the decline of cases in HIV/AIDS has been replaced by a resurgence of PML among patients treated with novel drugs and antibody therapies targeting specific cells and pathways of the immune system for various underlying conditions.[42,103] The emerging therapeutics have been tentatively classified into four risk groups according to whether the underlying condition predisposes for PML in the absence of drug, the time from initiation of the drug to PML, and the frequency of PML.[19] Natalizumab represents the only class I agent conferring a high risk. Dimethyl fumarate and fingolimod are associated with low risk (class II). Class III agents confer very low or no risk and include alemtuzumab, mitoxantrone, rituximab, and teriflunomide and depend on the clinical context of previous or concurrent exposure to other drugs. Class IV drugs such as type-1 interferons have no risk.[19] Thus, PML in patients with refractory-remittent multiple sclerosis treated with natalizumab has provided novel insights with respect to the pathogenesis, risk assessment, presentation, and clinical management.[28,170]

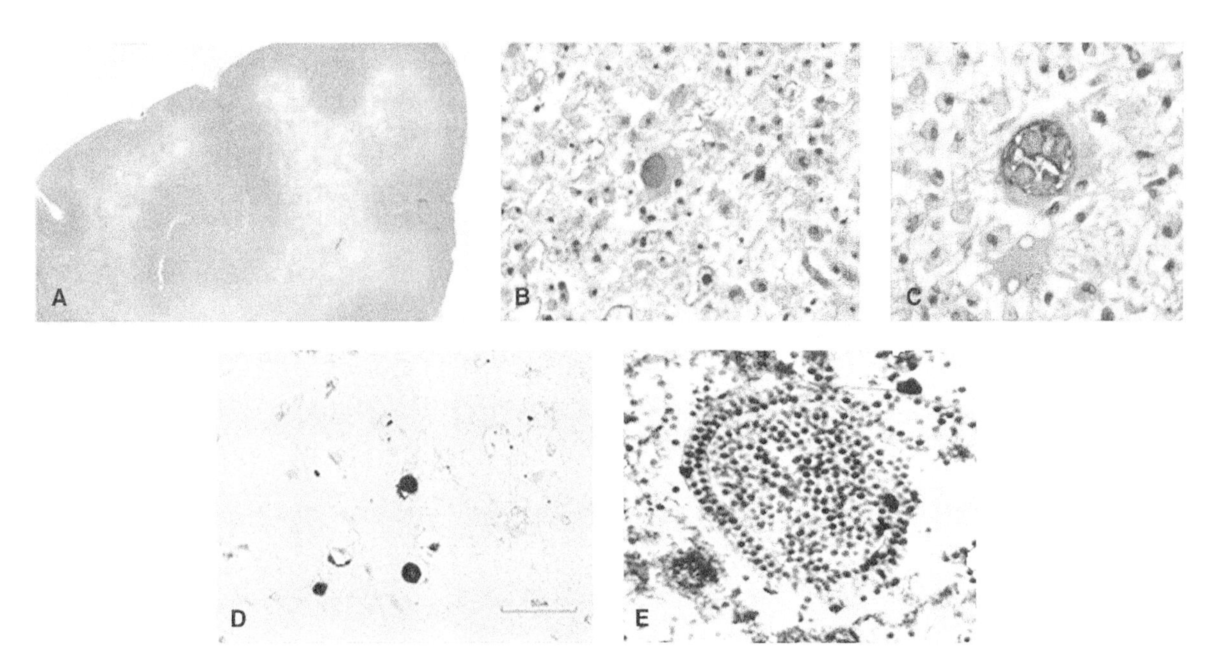

FIGURE 1.21 Histology of progressive multifocal leukoencephalopathy. A: Luxol fast blue staining with hematoxylin counterstain of the frontal lobe in a patient with progressive multifocal leukoencephalopathy (PML) shows extensive multifocal and confluent areas of demyelination. Small islands of demyelination coalesce to produce large confluent areas resulting in a "ground glass" bright appearance on T2-weighted MRI scan. **B:** Enlarged oligodendrocyte with a large inclusion-bearing nucleus is characteristic of PML. No discrete intranuclear inclusion is seen. **C:** A large bizarre astrocyte is depicted. **D:** Immunostaining with polyclonal antibody to JC virus from Abcam Inc. shows dark brown staining of nuclei of several oligodendrocytes. **E:** Electron micrograph of crystalline array of assembled JC virions in nuclei of infected oligodendrocyte in PML brain lesion. Virions measure 40 nm in diameter.[20] (Reprinted with permission from Berger JR, Aksamit AJ, Clifford DB, et al. PML diagnostic criteria: consensus statement from the AAN Neuroinfectious Disease Section. *Neurology* 2013;80(15):1430–1438. Copyright © 2013 American Academy of Neurology.)

The pathogenesis of PML appears to involve several steps associated with end-organ pathology caused by insufficient immune control over JCPyV replication in the CNS.[132,210] Since virtually all patients with PML are seropositive for JCPyV including those with HIV/AIDS or with multiple sclerosis treated with natalizumab, JCPyV replication in the CNS is viewed as the result of JCPyV reactivation. To reach the brain, JCPyV is delivered either by infected blood precursor cells from the bone marrow, by hematogenous spread during secondary viremia, or primary infection associated with viremia.[45,48,132,210] CD4 T cells appear to have a central role in JCPyV control, which involves the loss of helper functions needed for cytotoxic CD8 T cells to kill JCPyV-replicating cells, and for B cells to mount sufficient levels of neutralizing antibodies. Although the relative contributions are likely to differ depending on the underlying conditions, this notion is also consistent with PML cases associated with idiopathic CD4 T-cell lymphopenia and with lymphocyte depletion using antibody therapies such as OKT3, antithymocyte globulins, and rituximab, with therapies interfering with lymphocyte proliferation and function including homing to the sites of JCPyV replication in the CNS, and with high-dosed or prolonged corticosteroids exposure.[19,21,103] PML may arise following cancer immunotherapies by checkpoint inhibitor blockade targeting lymphocyte PD-1 exhaustion markers.[59,216] In HIV/AIDS, the systemic CD4 cell recovery after antiretroviral suppression of HIV replication has been associated with JCPyV-specific T-cell responses and PML survival.[75,165,194] Tissue studies reveal increasing inflammatory infiltrates including CD4 and CD8 T cells around active lesions suggesting that HLA class I and class II presentation via oligodendrocytes, astrocytes, and monocyte/macrophages is also locally operative.[149] Natalizumab treatment blocks $\alpha4\beta7$-integrin–dependent lymphocyte homing to active multiple sclerosis lesions in the CNS, without notably increasing the overall risk of opportunistic diseases. Hence, local failure of CNS immune surveillance must be viewed as a pivotal factor in PML pathogenesis.

The clinical presentation of PML depends on the location and the spread of the initially focal replication sites. Progressive neurological deficits in motor, visual, cognitive, and behavioral functions are noted as well as ataxia affecting everyday life activities including posture, movement, and speech. Epileptic episodes are rare in HIV/AIDS but have been more frequently noted in patients with leukocortical inflammation, particularly with PML-IRIS.[132,166]

Magnetic resonance imaging (MRI) of the CNS has become the key diagnostic procedure, while computed tomography of the CNS is neither sensitive nor specific to rule in or rule out PML. The most characteristic MRI pattern shows subcortical PML lesions of T2-hyperintense or fluid-attenuated inversion recovery (FLAIR) sequences, T1-hypointense, or demyelinated areas as hyperintense lesions in diffusion-weighted imaging (Fig. 1.22).[368] Gadolinium enhancement in T1-weighted imaging is seen in approximately half of the cases indicating inflammation and blood–brain barrier disruption and is less frequent in HIV/AIDS than in natalizumab-treated patients, but characteristic of IRIS-PML.[368] Although unilateral or bilateral involvement of the subcortical areas is frequent, infratentorial lesions can occur in the cerebellum or the brain stem with corresponding clinical deficits. A mass effect is usually not seen but may arise suddenly upon significant inflammation associated with PML-IRIS. Conversely, burned-out lesions can regress to atrophic areas, which correlate with persisting functional deficits. The differential diagnosis includes varicella zoster encephalopathy, CNS vasculitis, and various malignancies, which may sometimes coexist.[20] A challenging issue is distinguishing active multiple sclerosis and early PML, which may arise during the close MRI follow-up recommended in JCPyV-seropositive patients started on natalizumab.[354]

The clinical diagnosis of PML is graded according to the strength of criteria, whereby possible PML defines a case with typical clinical presentation and corresponding MRI results, but without the risk factor of known immunodeficiency. Probable PML is diagnosed in a typical case with the known risk of underlying immunodeficiency and corresponding MRI results. In such patients, detecting JCPyV-DNA in the CSF by highly sensitive NAT is recommended for a laboratory-confirmed (presumptive) diagnosis of PML.[20] However, even highly sensitive JCPyV-DNA assays detecting DNA as low as

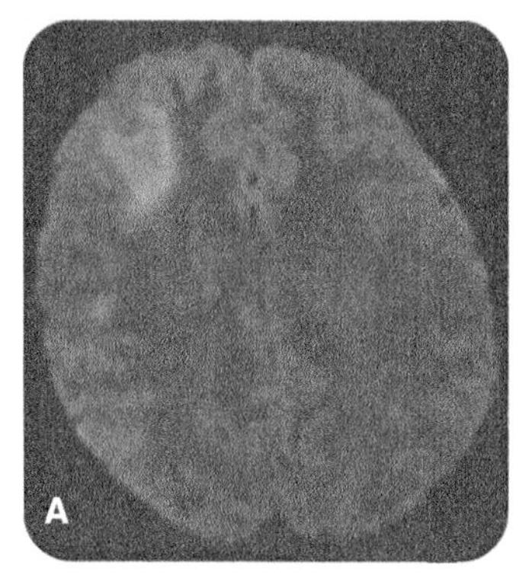

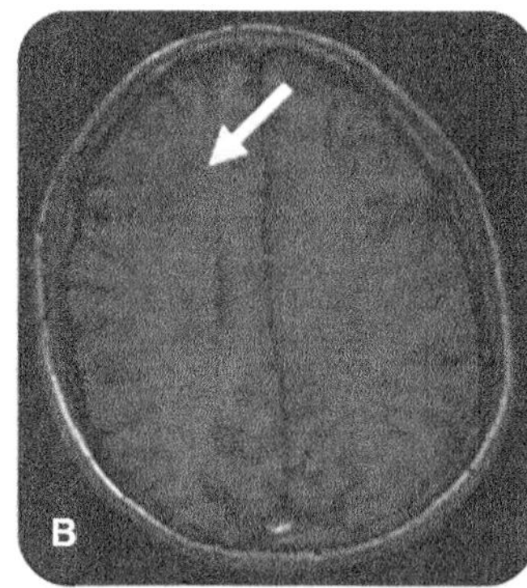

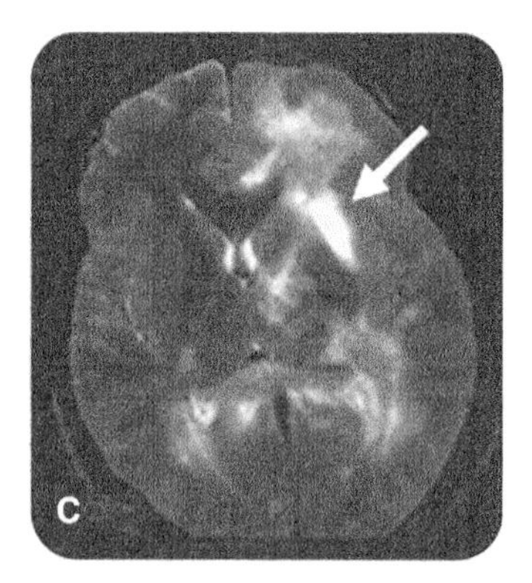

FIGURE 1.22 MRI in progressive multifocal leukoencephalopathy. A: Fluid-attenuated inversion recovery image with large subcortical lesion of right frontal lobe. A smaller lesion is observed posterior to this lesion. **B:** T1-weighted image shows hypointense lesion (*arrow*) in the right frontal lobe. **C:** T2-weighted image from another patient with extensive high signal intensity lesions in the white matter sparing the cortex. An area of hyperintensity similar to that of CSF suggests an area of cavitation. (Reprinted with permission from Berger JR, Aksamit AJ, Clifford DB, et al. PML diagnostic criteria: consensus statement from the AAN Neuroinfectious Disease Section. *Neurology* 2013;80(15):1430–1438. Copyright © 2013 American Academy of Neurology.[20])

10 to 50 c/mL CSF have been negative in approximately 25% of patients with histologically proven PML.[53] Thus, undetectable JCPyV-DNA in CSF does not exclude PML. A recent study suggested that the probability of detecting JCPyV-DNA in CSF increases with the volume of the PML lesions.[210,358] Thus, laboratory confirmation could be sought by repeating CSF testing for JCPyV-DNA[20,205] or by demonstrating intrathecal JCPyV-specific antibody titers.[20,352] In case of probable PML that cannot be resolved because of noninformative CSF results or because of suspicions of another etiology, the diagnosis should be sought by stereotactic brain tissue demonstrating the histopathologic triad of demyelination, oligodendrocytes with enlarged nuclei, reactive multinucleated astrocytes, and detection of JCPyV antigens or genome.[20]

Prevention of PML is difficult to achieve other than by avoiding the loss of functional virus-specific immune effectors in JCPyV-infected patients. For HIV-1 infected patients, this is achieved by the current strategy of early ART to prevent opportunistic infections that occur at lower CD4 cell counts.[279] Attempts to establish JCPyV-DNA detection in blood samples of HIV/AIDS patients taken 2 years to 6 months before PML diagnosis have been unsuccessful.[348] However, significant increases in JCPyV-specific antibody levels have been observed in HIV/AIDS patients at 6 months before the PML diagnosis.[165,348] For transplant patients, no specific predictors have been identified that could translate into prevention measures despite overall PML rates of 1.24 per 1,000 patient years among heart and lung transplant recipient and case fatality rates of more than 80%.[218] For multiple sclerosis patients, however, prolonged duration of natalizumab therapy of more than 18 months, prior exposure of immunosuppressive drugs, and a positive JCPyV serology status have led to risk stratification, monitoring, and counseling of the patients as the risk of PML increases more than 100-fold from 0.1 to 10–30 per 1,000 patient years.[28,210,267,292] As reported for HIV/AIDS patients,[132,165,348] the higher antibody levels are interpreted as an early marker of recent systemic exposure to JCPyV Vp1 capsid proteins, which are not consistently captured by viral DNA detection in blood. Notably, the level of JCPyV antibodies has been associated with a 10-fold higher risk when increased to high titers defined by a normalization index greater than 1.5 times higher than a reference serum as compared to low antibody levels with a normalization index less than 0.9.[210,267,292] To mitigate the devastating consequences of PML in the current absence of specific antiviral prophylaxis, the otherwise annual MRI of the CNS used to follow the multiple sclerosis lesions is recommended to be performed every 4 to 6 months to search for early radiological signs of presymptomatic PML in patients having or developing JCPyV antibody indices greater than 1.5, prior immunosuppression, and receiving natalizumab therapy for more than 18 months.[210,292,352] Small PML foci are often presymptomatic and have previously been overlooked unless becoming very large or impairing well-defined functions, for example, of the motor or visual cortex, cranial nerves or the cerebellum. Early diagnosis of presymptomatic or limited PML has been associated with better outcomes following discontinuation of natalizumab. The radiological diagnosis of probable PML in an asymptomatic multiple sclerosis patient at increased risk should be laboratory confirmed by testing for JCPyV DNA or intrathecal antibody in CSF. Thus, the risk stratification of multiple sclerosis patients has enabled the previously unknown diagnosis of asymptomatic or presymptomatic PML.

Treatment of PML is based on regaining specific immune control over JCPyV replication in the brain. In HIV/AIDS, this is achieved by rapidly suppressing HIV replication with potent ART typically including integrase inhibitors and nucleoside/nucleotide reverse transcriptase inhibitors. In patients on immunosuppressive therapies, the discontinuation of the respective drugs is attempted but is not always possible because of the underlying condition such as transplantation, acute rejection, graft versus host, or exacerbation of the autoimmune disorder. Similarly, adjuvant treatments with compounds improving immune recovery may have a role in patients with idiopathic CD4 lymphocytopenia and possibly HIV/AIDS including interleukin-7 and toll-like receptor-7 agonists. Given the potential role of PD-1 lymphocyte exhaustion, monoclonal blocking antibody therapy with the checkpoint inhibitor pembrolizumab has been reported to result in improvement or stabilization of at least two-thirds of PML patients.[59,139] As a more direct approach, adoptive cell therapy using JCPyV-specific or cross-reactive BKPyV-specific T cells has been explored for treatment of PML.[11,237] However, efficacy data from controlled clinical trials are lacking for any of these immunostimulatory therapies, and safety may be a limiting concern in transplant recipients and patients with autoimmune disorders. Finally, the emergence of PML in patients treated concomitantly with checkpoint inhibitors and corticosteroids suggests that immunosuppressive ablation of immune effectors overrides potential functional reconstitution. Conversely, corticosteroids may be lifesaving in severe cases of IRIS with increasing intracranial pressure,[327] but prolonged high-dose application should be avoided.[283]

Antivirals with documented or presumed inhibitory activity on JCPyV replication in cell culture have been used alone or in combinations with the hope to modify or ameliorate PML outcomes, but there is little evidence of clinical benefit. The list includes cytosine arabinoside, cidofovir, brincidofovir (CMX001), artesunate, and more recently mefloquine and mirtazapine. Intravenous immunoglobulins may deliver neutralizing activity and have been explored as an alternative to steroid treatment of PML-IRIS.[143,177,224] However, immunoglobulins penetrate poorly across the blood–brain barrier except in areas of inflammation.[39,54,177] The emergence of viral capsid escape mutants in PML necessitate dedicated clinical protocols and may include novel strategies for passive and active vaccination. Thus, either alone or together with immunological interventions, effective antivirals suppressing intracerebral JCPyV replication remain an unmet clinical need in prevention and treatment of PML.

Other JCPyV-Associated Diseases

JCPyV-associated granule cell neuronopathy has been proposed as a separate clinical entity from PML and is caused by lytic JCPyV replication in granule cell neurons of the cerebellum.[172,362] Clinically, the patients present with cerebellar ataxia as the leading sign, with corresponding active lesions in the gray matter without affecting the white matter identified by MRI. Accordingly, treatment faces the same challenges of regaining immune control, IRIS, and persisting atrophy. JCPyV replication of neuron in cortical and hippocampal areas has been described.[101,362]

JCPyV meningitis is a rare diagnosis presenting with the clinical signs of meningeal inflammation of neck stiffness, headache, and fever, with detectable JCPyV DNA in CSF in the absence of other pathogens. Pathology correlates are usually lacking,[132] though JCPyV replication with inflammation in the leptomeninges and the choroid plexus but sparing the brain parenchyma has been demonstrated in a fatal case of hydrocephalus.[1] A postmortem study identified leptomeningeal involvement in approximately 15% of fatal PML cases.[58]

JCPyV-associated nephropathy has been identified as a rare cause of renal allograft failure and graft loss affecting less than 1% of kidney transplant patients.[72,141] The patients have high urine JCPyV loads of more than 10^7 c/mL and decoy cell shedding, but unlike BKPyV DNAemia, JCPyV DNA is usually low or undetectable.[72] The clinical and histopathology features are indistinguishable from the more frequent BKPyVAN showing declining renal function and LTag staining in the enlarged nuclei of tubular epithelial cells. Since JCPyV may be detectable in native kidneys, specific diagnosis requires abundant detection of the JCPyV Vp1 capsid antigen or high genome tissue viral loads by in situ hybridization or NAT, while BKPyV genomes are typically absent or low.[72,182] Posttransplant screening is currently not recommended, but a high index of suspicion is warranted in patients with LTag-positive biopsy and undetectable BKPyV DNAemia or unexplained decline in renal function.[129,131] Successful treatment by reduced immunosuppression has been reported in cases of limited renal involvement, whereas direct or indirect graft failure was reported in other cases.[72,182] Serological studies in pediatric recipients indicate significant primary or secondary JCPyV exposure after kidney transplantation in 25% and 12.5%, respectively,[365] which result from reactivation or exogenous sources including the donor graft.[290] In a postmortem study of 111 HIV/AIDS patients, JCPyV has been identified in the native kidneys 7 (6.3%) cases, with limited tubuloepithelial signs of replication and damage in 4 (3.6%), but mostly little or no inflammation.

JCPyV-associated malignancies have been searched for ever since the initial demonstration of the transforming properties of JCPyV following nonlytic infection of nonpermissive cells and hosts.[132,359] In humans, malignancies with detectable JCPyV genomes, some with documented early viral gene expression have been described in the CNS such as oligodendroglioma, astrocytoma, medulloblastoma, ependymoma, and glioblastoma, primary CNS lymphoma as well as gastrointestinal carcinoma. However, other epidemiologic data are scarce. A recent study associated JCPyV with hematological malignancies and better survival,[202] while a meta-analysis covering 24 studies reported a four-fold increased risk of JCPyV detection in colorectal cancers but requires validation.[301] Mechanistically, JCPyV as driver or passenger needs to be addressed as well as a role of immunologically less surveyed anatomic locations, uncoupling of early versus late gene expression, and failure to immunologically clear EVGR-expressing tumor cells, as discussed.[132] Similar to PyVUC by BKPyV, a case of JCPyV-associated urothelial cancer has been reported occurring in a kidney transplant patient 5 years after JCPyV-associated nephropathy.[270]

Merkel Cell Polyomavirus and Merkel Cell Carcinoma

MCC is a highly aggressive, rapidly growing, neuroendocrine carcinoma of the skin that can quickly spread to lymph nodes and many other organs. The neuroendocrine features include a high nuclear–cytoplasmic ratio, giving it the appearance of a small blue cell tumor (Fig. 1.23). The chromatin pattern is typically open with few nucleoli, yielding a salt-and-pepper appearance. MCC typically presents on sun-exposed areas of elderly patients. Intense and lifelong UV exposure from the sun seems to be a particular risk for Caucasian patients, although MCC can occur in non–sun-exposed areas in young adults and children as well. Risk for developing MCC is increased in patients with severe immunocompromised conditions including HIV/AIDS, SOT, other cancers, and chemotherapy.[15]

Recognition of the increased risk for MCC in immunocompromised patients led to a focused search in the transcriptome of primary MCC tumors. The original report of the discovery MCPyV in MCC revealed many important insights reflective of polyomavirus biology.[84] In particular, the MCPyV viral DNA was found to be clonally integrated into the tumor genome. In one informative case, the integration pattern was identical in the primary tumor and a metastatic lymph node from the same patient. This indicates that the viral integration was an early event in the tumor formation. In addition, it has been repeatedly demonstrated that while the MCPyV is clonally integrated, the viral genome is highly mutated with preservation of the MCPyV NCCR and part of the EVGR leaving STag intact but deleting the C-terminal half of LTag (Fig. 1.18). Typically, the MCC-associated LTag contains the shared N-terminal J domain with STag and the LXCXE, RB-binding, motif. However, the LTag DBD and helicase domain are lost in most MCC tumors leaving it incapable of binding to the integrated origin of replication in the NCCR. The LVGR is often not present in the integrated viral genome and, if present, the *VP1* and *VP2* genes are not expressed. Notably, not all MCC tumors contain integrated copies of MCPyV. Some MCC tumors instead contain a high number of mutations with a characteristic UV mutational pattern reflective of chronic sun exposure. These UV-associated MCC tumors are histologically indistinguishable from virus-positive MCC tumors. By contrast, the MCPyV-positive tumors have a very low number of host genome mutations. The virus-positive MCC tumors show expression of MCPyV T antigens in every tumor cell (Fig. 1.23).

While antibodies to MCPyV Vp1 are widespread in the general population and may be significantly higher in MCC patients,[260] antibodies to LTag and STag are usually only detected in patients with MCPyV-positive MCC and can be used as a biomarker to follow the disease course.[262] Antibodies to STag are present initially in approximately 50% of all patients with MCC. Titers to STag drop within several months after the tumor has been successfully treated but can rise again if the tumor returns.

Other HPyV-Associated Diseases

Trichodysplasia Spinulosa

The clinical entity of *trichodysplasia spinulosa* has been described in 1995 in an adult kidney transplant recipient who developed widespread hair-like follicular spiny hyperkeratosis together with sebaceous gland hyperplasia.[147] Inner root sheath keratinocytes in the proliferative lesions were found to contain intranuclear arrays of polyomavirus-like particles, which sequencing revealed to be the eighth human polyomavirus.[123,251,342] Clinically, *trichodysplasia spinulosa* often affects the face with hair-like spiculae most visible around the nose, together with alopecia of the eyebrows and eyelashes, and thickening skin with increasing duration of disease (Fig. 1.24).

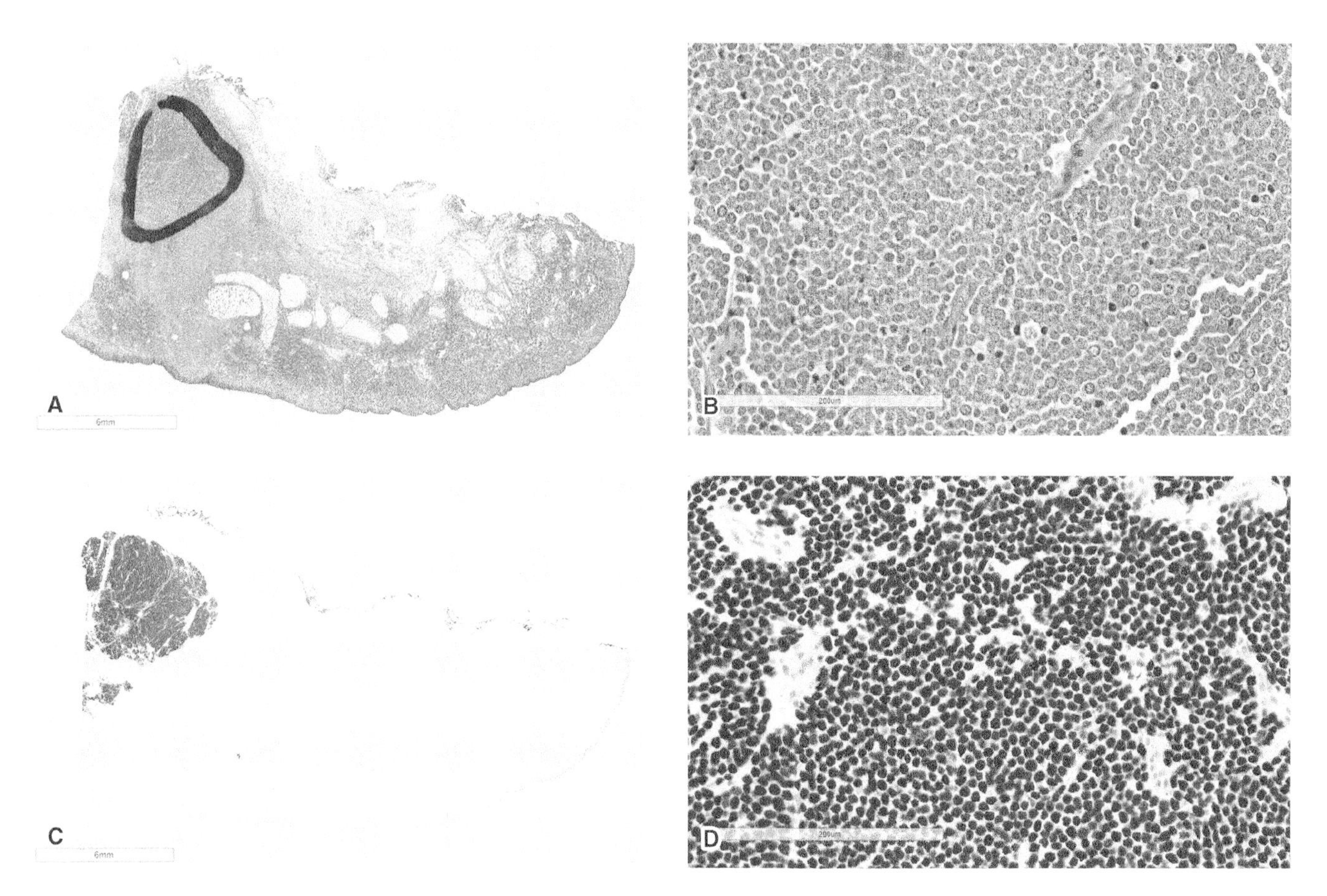

FIGURE 1.23 Merkel cell carcinoma. Hematoxylin and eosin **(A, B)** and immunohistochemistry with antibody specific for MCPyV LTag **(C, D)**. The low power H&E image **(A)** with pathologist's mark highlights the tumor in the dermal layer of the skin. The tumor appears *blue* due to the cellular high nuclear to cytoplasmic ratio. The high powered image shows the salt-and-pepper appearing chromatin pattern and high mitotic index. **C:** The low power IHC shows LTag-positive cells corresponding to the tumor only. **D:** The high power image highlights the appearance of LTag in the nuclei of each tumor cell with blood vessels unstained.

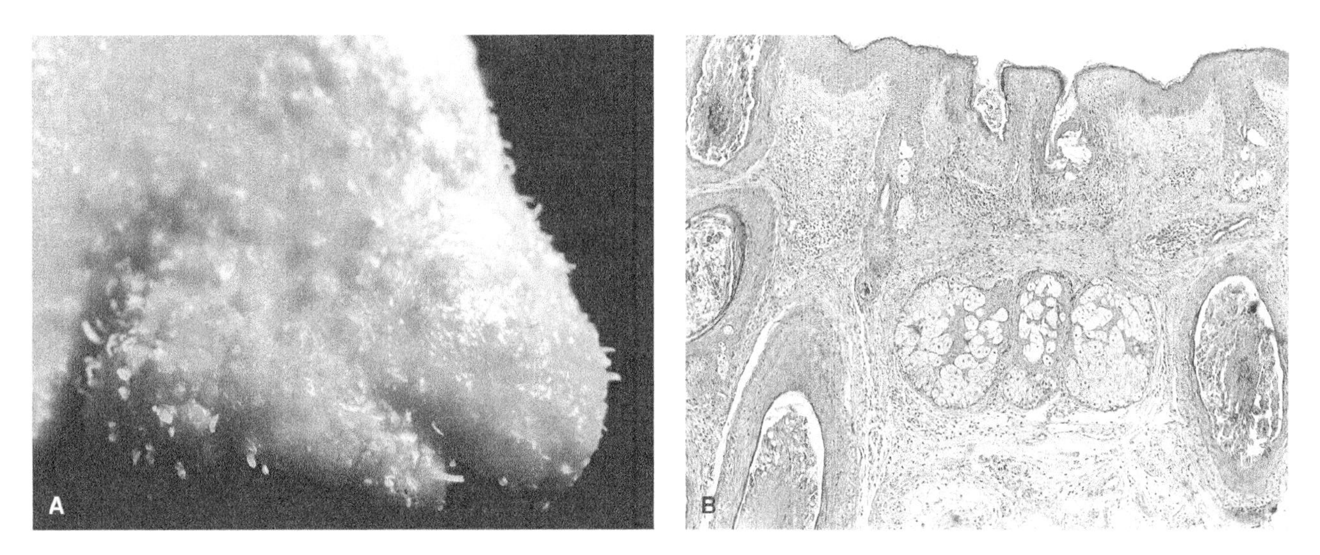

FIGURE 1.24 Trichodysplasia spinulosa. Affected nose with papules and spicules **(A)**. Biopsy of a hyperkeratotic follicular papule from the forehead. The epidermis reveals enlarged, hyperplastic hair bulbs and hypercornification within a distended follicular infundibulum (hematoxylin and eosin [H&E] stain, 10×) **(B)**.[342] (Reprinted from van der Meijden E, Janssens RW, Lauber C, et al. Discovery of a new human polyomavirus associated with trichodysplasia spinulosa in an immunocompromized patient. *PLoS Pathog* 2010;6(7):e1001024. https://creativecommons.org/licenses/by/3.0/.)

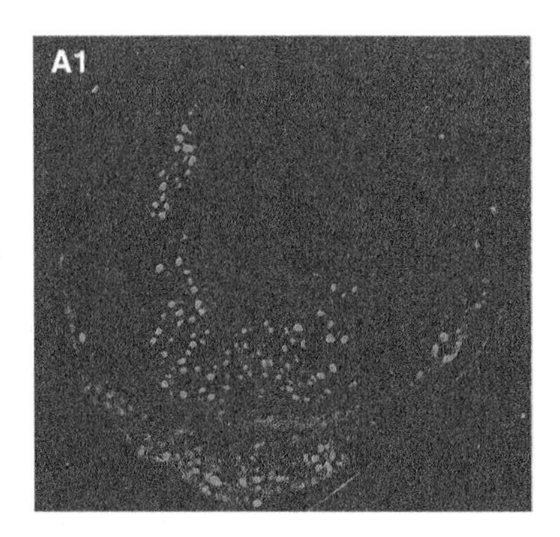

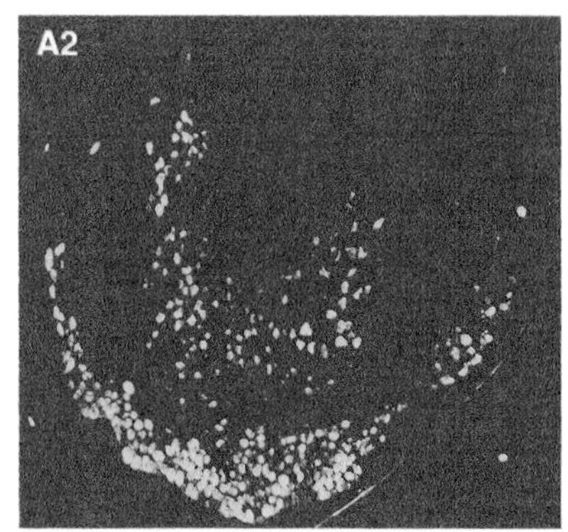

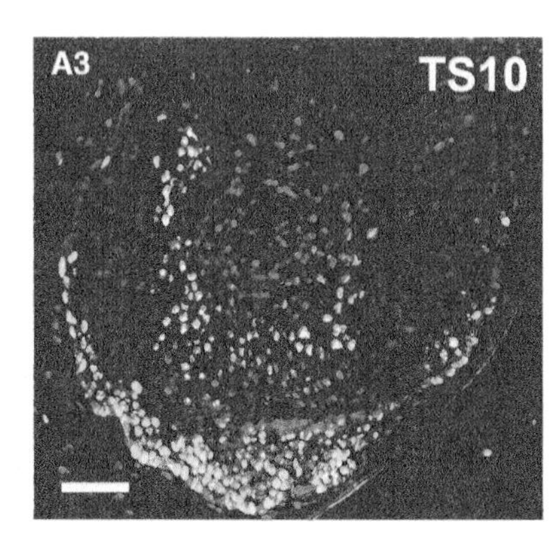

FIGURE 1.25 Immunohistopathology of TSPyV-associated trichodysplasia spinulosa. Colocalization of TSPyV large T antigen, Ki-67, and phosphorylated pRB. TSPyV LT-antigen (*red*) (A1) with Ki-67 (*green*) (A2) and merge (*yellow*) (A3) in a vertical section of hair follicle of TS10 is shown in the upper row.[162] (Reprinted from Kazem S, van der Meijden E, Wang RC, et al. Polyomavirus-associated Trichodysplasia spinulosa involves hyperproliferation, pRB phosphorylation and upregulation of p16 and p21. *PLoS One* 2014;9(10):e108947. https://creativecommons.org/licenses/by/4.0/.)

Extensive involvement of the skin of trunk and extremities has also been described with hypopigmented folliculocentric papules of 1-to 2 mm in diameter.[12,251] Histopathology studies reveal signs of activated inner root sheath cell proliferation and expression of the viral LTag, MTag, and capsid proteins, with enlarged trichohyalin cytoplasmic granules and minimal inflammation (Fig. 1.25).[351] Hair-shaft formation is missing or rudimentary with parakeratotic debris extending outward forming the hair-like spiculae. Although probably underreported, fewer than 50 cases have been described to date, all of which occurred in immunocompromised patients due to transplantation, hematological malignancy, or cancer chemotherapy.[161]

The pathogenesis of *trichodysplasia spinulosa* is not well understood. Person-to-person transmission of TSPyV mostly within families has been linked to the early rise in seroprevalence from 10% among children to more than 80% among adults, making TSPyV part of the normal adult skin microbiome.[89,343,357] Uncontrolled TSPyV reactivation has been proposed to occur in severely immunocompromised patients.[356] Alternatively, primary TSPyV infection in immunocompromised individuals has been proposed to explain the low rate of this complication despite the increasing number of profoundly immunocompromised people.[341] Detection of TSPyV DNA in noncutaneous specimens including blood and urine has been interpreted as marker of systemic dissemination.

The diagnosis of *trichodysplasia spinulosa* is based on the typical clinical presentation in an immunocompromised patient, which is supported by histopathology, and a high tissue TSPyV load of more than 10^6 c/μg DNA not found in other hyperkeratoses.[12,38] There is currently no specific prevention, screening, or prophylaxis for patients at risk. The treatment of *trichodysplasia spinulosa* is based on attempting to restore TSPyV-specific immunity, for example, by reducing immunosuppression, which is often limited or unsuccessful due to the underlying condition such as transplantation or hematological disorders. Cidofovir gel has been applied topically to target the TSPyV-replicating hyperproliferative cells, and responses to leflunomide, topical or systemic retinoic acid derivatives, and the physical removal of spiculae have been reported, likely by stimulating local inflammation and immune responses.[14,57,157,342]

HPyV7-Associated Pruritic Hyperproliferative Keratinopathy

New-onset, pruritic, brown hyperproliferative skin changes have been linked to HPyV7 replication in immunocompromised patients.[41,138] In the initial report, two lung transplant recipients developed highly pruritic velvety hyperproliferative plaques on the trunk, buttocks, and extremities several years after transplantation (Fig. 1.26).[138] On skin biopsy, the epidermal stratum corneum was thickened with cytopathic keratinocytes forming a peacock plumage pattern, with very little perivascular lymphocytic infiltrates in the dermis. By electron microscopy, intranuclear PyV inclusions were identified together with a high HPyV7 DNA load averaging 10^3 c/cell. Immunohistochemistry demonstrated early and late viral gene expression (Fig. 1.26). In both patients, HPyV7 DNA was detected in peripheral blood mononuclear cells. In one patient, pseudomembrane-like changes and glandular epithelium with viral inclusions of the gastric antrum mucosa was detected together with encapsidated DNase-resistant HPyV7 genomes in plasma suggesting hematogenous HPyV7 dissemination.[138] In both cases, the HPyV7 NCCRs were rearranged carrying a 16 bp-insertion and 12 bp-deletion, respectively, which conferred increased EVGR expression compared to the archetype NCCR.[2,138] Given the widespread exposure among adults[89] and the limited number of cases, risk factors and pathogenesis of HPyV7 skin disease are undefined other than profound immunodeficiency. Notably, mTOR inhibitors provided no protection while worsening following steroid exposure has been reported.

The clinical diagnosis is suggested by the expanding highly pruritic plaques in an immunocompromised patient and confirmed by histopathology on skin biopsy and high HPyV7 DNA loads by NAT. A similar clinical picture has been ascribed to HPyV6,[244] which should be tested in parallel. The differential diagnosis includes other infectious and noninfectious causes of pruritic hyperkeratoses, and specifically mTOR inhibitor toxicity.[264] Treatment attempts of HPyV7-associated pruritic hyperproliferative keratinopathy has been targeting the pruritus with little success using antihistamines, while limited improvement of the skin changes have been reported using topical or systemic cidofovir, except for one case of complete resolution following oral aciretin.[41]

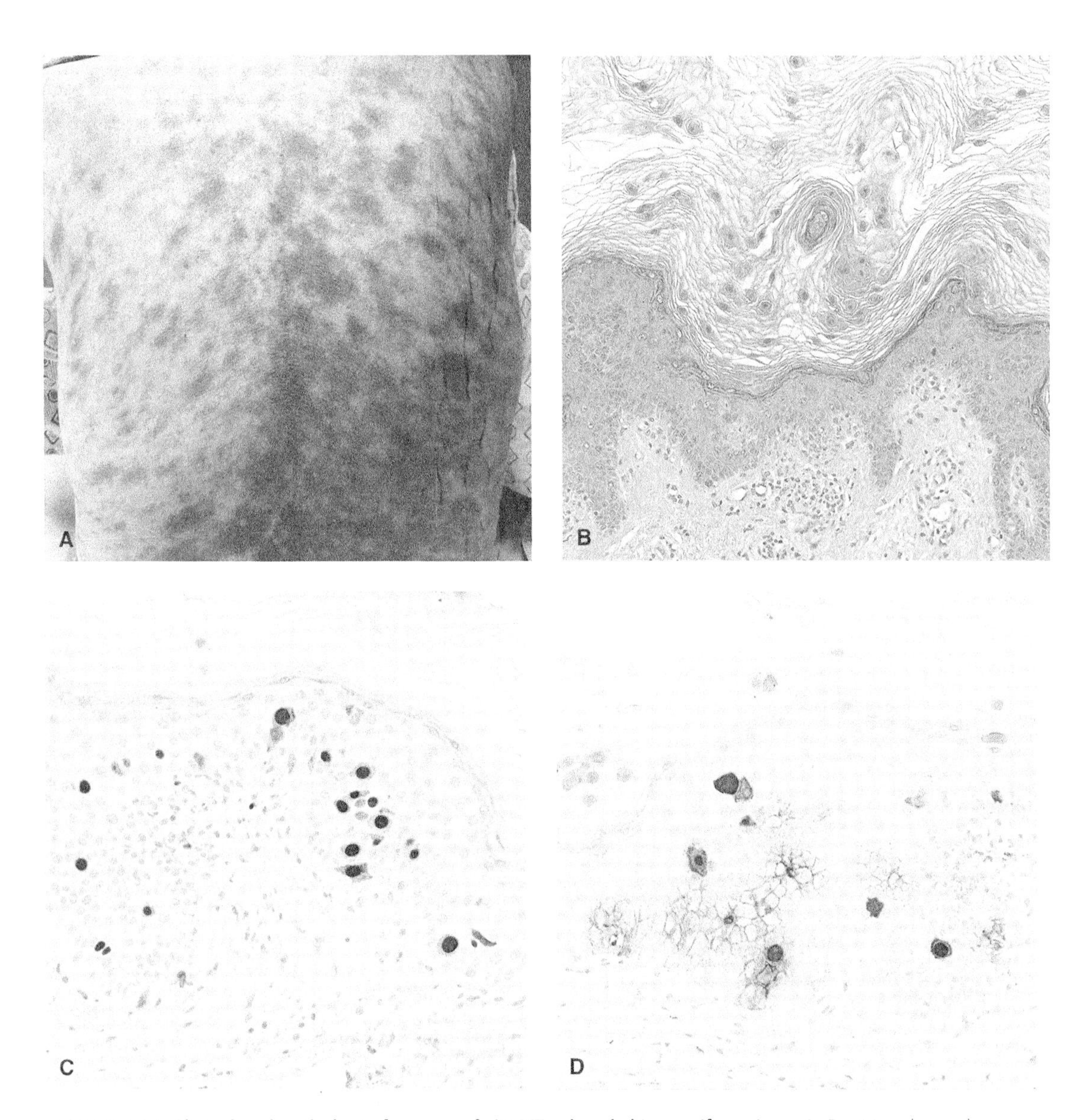

FIGURE 1.26 Clinical and pathologic features of HPyV7-related skin manifestations. A: Pruritic velvety plaques on the trunk. **B:** Viropathic keratinocytes in a peacock plumage pattern (original magnification, 20×; hematoxylin–eosin staining). **C:** Strong HPyV7 T antigen nuclear and cytoplasmic immunostaining in the keratinocytes (original magnification, 40×) **D:** HPyV7 viral capsid staining in the skin shows nuclear and cytoplasmic staining in keratinocytes, as well as a lacy pattern representing lysed virions in the intercellular space (original magnification, 40×).[138] (From Ho J, Jedrych JJ, Feng H, et al. Human polyomavirus 7-associated pruritic rash and viremia in transplant recipients. *J Infect Dis* 2015;211(10):1560–1565. Reproduced by permission of Oxford University Press.)

Other HPyV-Associated Manifestations

Explorative studies associating HPyVs with other clinical manifestations have largely been inconclusive with the possible exception of HPyV6 detection in approximately 50% of keratoacanthomas.[16] However, in a few cases, comprehensive histopathology and molecular studies supported an etiological or contributory role of HPyVs, which await independent confirmations. Thus, HPyV6 was detected in one case of BRAF inhibitor-induced epithelial proliferation, whereas no association with other dermatotropic HPyVs was detected.[289] HPyV6 has been described in a patient with angiolymphoid hyperplasia and eosinophilia (Kimura Disease).[273] HPyV13, also called NJPyV, was discovered in a kidney pancreas transplant patient presenting with localized necrotic skin and muscle disease due to viral replication in endothelial cells causing microthrombosis.[228] Cases of respiratory WUPyV replication[307] including subsequent disseminated multiorgan involvement were reported in allogeneic HSCT recipients.[306] KIPyV replication has also been documented in cases of pneumonia.[305] Both reports are consistent with the initial identification of KIPyV and WUPyV in respiratory fluids of patients with otherwise unidentified causes of pneumonia.[3,97] However, larger epidemiologic studies have not supported a consistent role for KIPyV and WUPyV in respiratory tract infectious diseases. KIPyV and WUPyV have been detected in fewer than 5% of patients with acute respiratory infectious disease including those requiring hospital admission, but frequently coexist with other respiratory pathogens. In a comprehensive study of 222 allogeneic HSCT recipients, the cumulative incidence of KIPyV and WUPyV detection during the first year posttransplant was 26% and 8%, respectively, and mostly involved co-detection of another respiratory virus.[178] The clinical presentations were mostly mild wheezing and sputum production. No association of either virus was found with acute graft versus host disease, lymphopenia, or death.[178] Thus, despite serological and molecular evidence of frequent exposure among immunocompetent and immunocompromised individuals, the contribution of KIPyV and WUPyV to human disease requires further study.

A recent report of a new human polyomavirus, Lyon IARC PyV (LIPyV), may have been isolated due to environmental exposure to domestic cats.[80,100] Similarly, HPyV12 may represent exposure to shrews.[98,173]

SV40 and Humans

From the mid-1950s to 1963, the simian polyomavirus SV40 was unknowingly introduced into more than 100 million people who had received contaminated poliovirus vaccines.[297] Because SV40 is tumorigenic in rodents and can transform human cells in culture, there has been concern about whether SV40 can contribute to cancer development in humans vaccinated with the contaminated polio vaccine or from other sources. There has also been controversy regarding whether SV40 can replicate and establish a productive infection in humans.

Follow-up studies from the initial polio vaccination efforts have concluded that there was not an increase in neoplasia over three decades in the population that was directly exposed to SV40 when compared with matched control populations not exposed to SV40.[298] A retrospective cohort study of data collected by programs designed to track tumor incidence in specific populations also did not find any association between SV40 exposure and increased risk.[320]

The FDA Office of Vaccine Research and Review convened a meeting of international authorities to discuss the topic of SV40 in the human population and the technical approaches needed to evaluate its presence as an infectious agent and role, if any, in human tumors.[36] The Institute of Medicine published a study concluding that the epidemiologic evidence regarding SV40 infections in humans was insufficient and recommended additional research.[319] There have been sporadic reports that SV40 DNA and LTag could be detected in human tumors such as ependymomas, osteosarcomas, mesotheliomas, and choroid plexus papillomas. However, unlike the presence of integrated MCPyV viral genome in MCC, there have been no reports of integrated SV40 viral genomes or expression of transcripts in human tumors. Instead, the frequent detection of SV40 viral DNA in human tumors may represent contamination in the laboratory with plasmids containing SV40 NCCR, splicing, polyadenylation, and other elements present in molecular biologic reagents.[200,213,269]

It is not certain if SV40 can establish a persistent infection in humans. While SV40 can replicate at very low levels in human fibroblasts and mesothelial cells in culture, it does not appear to be capable of replicating in lymphocytes.[29,300] Notably, while BKPyV and JCPyV are frequently detected in human sewage, the presence of SV40 has not been reported.[31] In addition, while some human sera are reactive against SV40 Vp1, suggesting a past infection, most of this activity can be depleted by preincubation with BKPyV or JCPyV Vp1.[163,278]

Avian Polyomavirus and Disease

Hemorrhagic nephritis and enteritis of geese develop rapidly after infection with GHPyV. Typical symptoms of infected birds include generalized edema, gout, hemorrhagic enteritis, interstitial nephritis following infection of the kidney tubular epithelium, and disruption of lung, feather follicle, and endothelial cells. Lymphoid tissues can become depleted of most lymphocytes. These features have been observed in naturally and experimentally infected birds.[179,254] In addition to GHPyV, infection with APyV, FPyV, and CPyV are associated with fatal disease often including hepatitis, ascites, enteritis, and nephritis.[153]

PERSPECTIVE

Since Ludwig Gross first described MPyV in 1953, polyomaviruses have proven to be relevant model systems for understanding fundamental biological processes in eukaryotic cells. In addition to the insights that have contributed to our understanding of transcription factors and enhancers, RNA splicing and polyadenylation, and DNA replication, the study of polyomaviruses has enriched our understanding of tumor suppressors, oncogenes, tyrosine kinase signaling, immunity, and tumorigenesis. The study of polyomavirus cell receptors, entry, and trafficking through the cell has brought remarkable insights that have challenged previously held models. Importantly, the information gained by study of polyomaviruses has enabled critical insights of human disease. As the population of immunosuppressed individuals increased due to HIV/AIDS and developments in transplantation medicine and the therapy of autoimmune diseases, the incidence of polyomavirus diseases continues to rise. A dramatic example of this has been the occurrence of JCPyV-induced PML in patients with multiple sclerosis or Crohn disease who were treated with an antibody that blocked lymphocytes from binding the VLA4 receptor through the α4 integrin molecule.

Continued investigation into the interaction between polyomaviruses and their hosts will be crucial for improving our ability to prevent and treat polyomavirus diseases in the future. Given new technology and model systems, it should be possible to develop high-throughput screens to identify more effective compounds that inhibit the viral life cycle. It is imperative that evidence-based clinical studies, guided by impeccable cellular and molecular studies, are implemented to benefit immunocompromised patients at risk for and suffering with polyomavirus diseases.

The contribution of MCPyV to MCC deserves special mention. To date, all studies indicate that expression of the MCPyV STag and a truncated form of LTag is present in approximately 80% of all MCCs. Consistent with the large body of literature on polyomavirus-mediated transformation, MCPyV is clonally integrated into the MCC cells in a manner that enables persistent expression of the T antigens. There are many questions that remain unanswered regarding the role of MCPyV T antigens in MCC. In addition, it is not understood what the contributions of age, UV exposure, and immunosuppression are to the risk for developing this cancer. Furthermore, it is not known what the normal host cell or tissue type for MCPyV is and what is the special relationship with Merkel cells. Also, the factors in the host and virus that sustain lifelong infection but permit reactivation of polyomavirus infection remain to be defined not only for MCPyV but also for all polyomaviruses.

The recent discoveries of new polyomaviruses in humans, primates, marsupials, and birds have brought renewed vigor to the field. It is likely that more polyomaviruses and related viral families will be discovered.[70] More importantly, it can be expected that further investigation of the new and previously studied polyomaviruses will continue to bring important new and fundamental insights into biology and disease. It can certainly be concluded that the polyomaviruses have paid huge dividends in the amount of knowledge they have yielded. Consequently, the future seems to hold great promise that study of polyomaviruses will continue to help us demystify fundamental cellular processes and give direct benefits to patients whose polyomavirus infection becomes organ and life threatening.

REFERENCES

1. Agnihotri SP, Wuthrich C, Dang X, et al. A fatal case of JC virus meningitis presenting with hydrocephalus in a human immunodeficiency virus-seronegative patient. *Ann Neurol* 2014;76(1):140–147.
2. Ajuh E, Wu Z, Kraus E, et al. Novel human polyomavirus non-coding control regions differ in bi-directional gene expression according to host cell, large T-antigen expression, and clinically occurring rearrangements. *J Virol* 2018;92:e02231-17.
3. Allander T, Andreasson K, Gupta S, et al. Identification of a third human polyomavirus. *J Virol* 2007;81(8):4130–4136.
4. Alwine JC, Dhar R, Khoury G. A small RNA induced late in simian virus 40 infection can associate with early viral mRNAs. *Proc Natl Acad Sci U S A* 1980;77(3):1379–1383.
5. An P, Saenz Robles MT, Duray AM, et al. Human polyomavirus BKV infection of endothelial cells results in interferon pathway induction and persistence. *PLoS Pathog* 2019;15(1):e1007505.
6. Anand P, Hotan GC, Vogel A, et al. Progressive multifocal leukoencephalopathy: a 25-year retrospective cohort study. *Neurol Neuroimmunol Neuroinflamm* 2019;6(6):e618.
7. Arthur RR, Shah KV, Baust SJ, et al. Association of BK viruria with hemorrhagic cystitis in recipients of bone marrow transplants. *N Engl J Med* 1986;315(4):230–234.
8. Assetta B, De Cecco M, O'Hara B, et al. JC polyomavirus infection of primary human renal epithelial cells is controlled by a type I IFN-induced response. *MBio* 2016;7(4):e00903-16.
9. Astrom KE, Mancall EL, Richardson EP Jr. Progressive multifocal leuko-encephalopathy; a hitherto unrecognized complication of chronic lymphatic leukaemia and Hodgkin's disease. *Brain* 1958;81(1):93–111.
10. Balakrishnan L, Milavetz B. Reorganization of RNA polymerase II on the SV40 genome occurs coordinately with the early to late transcriptional switch. *Virology* 2006;345(1):31–43.
11. Balduzzi A, Lucchini G, Hirsch HH, et al. Polyomavirus JC-targeted T-cell therapy for progressive multiple leukoencephalopathy in a hematopoietic cell transplantation recipient. *Bone Marrow Transplant* 2011;46(7):987–992.
12. Barone H, Brockman R, Johnson L, et al. Trichodysplasia spinulosa mimicking lichen nitidus in a renal transplant patient. *Pediatr Transplant* 2019;23(4):e13394.
13. Barouch DH, Faquin WC, Chen Y, et al. BK virus-associated hemorrhagic cystitis in a Human Immunodeficiency Virus-infected patient. *Clin Infect Dis* 2002;35(3):326–329.
14. Barton M, Lockhart S, Sidbury R, et al. Trichodysplasia spinulosa in a 7-year-old boy managed using physical extraction of keratin spicules. *Pediatr Dermatol* 2017;34(2):e74–e76.
15. Becker JC, Stang A, DeCaprio JA, et al. Merkel cell carcinoma. *Nat Rev Dis Primers* 2017;3:17077.
16. Beckervordersandforth J, Pujari S, Rennspiess D, et al. Frequent detection of human polyomavirus 6 in keratoacanthomas. *Diagn Pathol* 2016;11(1):58.
17. Bedi A, Miller CB, Hanson JL, et al. Association of BK virus with failure of prophylaxis against hemorrhagic cystitis following bone marrow transplantation. *J Clin Oncol* 1995;13(5):1103–1109.
18. Behzad-Behbahani A, Klapper PE, Vallely PJ, et al. BK virus DNA in CSF of immunocompetent and immunocompromised patients. *Arch Dis Child* 2003;88(2):174–175.
19. Berger JR. Classifying PML risk with disease modifying therapies. *Mult Scler Relat Disord* 2017;12:59–63.
20. Berger JR, Aksamit AJ, Clifford DB, et al. PML diagnostic criteria: consensus statement from the AAN neuroinfectious disease section. *Neurology* 2013;80(15):1430–1438.
21. Berger JR, Cree BA, Greenberg B, et al. Progressive multifocal leukoencephalopathy after fingolimod treatment. *Neurology* 2018;90(20):e1815–e1821.
22. Bethge T, Ajuh E, Hirsch HH. Imperfect symmetry of Sp1 and core promoter sequences regulates early and late virus gene expression of the bidirectional BK polyomavirus noncoding control region. *J Virol* 2016;90(22):10083–10101.
23. Bethge T, Hachemi HA, Manzetti J, et al. Sp1 sites in the noncoding control region of BK polyomavirus are key regulators of bidirectional viral early and late gene expression. *J Virol* 2015;89(6):3396–3411.
24. Binet I, Nickeleit, V, Hirsch HH. Polyomavirus infections in transplant recipients. *Curr Opin Organ Transplant* 2000;5:210–216.
25. Binggeli S, Egli A, Schaub S, et al. Polyomavirus BK-specific cellular immune response to VP1 and large T-antigen in kidney transplant recipients. *Am J Transplant* 2007;7(5):1131–1139.
26. Bischof N, Hirsch HH, Wehmeier C, et al. Reducing calcineurin inhibitor first for treating BK polyomavirus replication after kidney transplantation: long-term outcomes. *Nephrol Dial Transplant* 2019;34(7):1240–1250.
27. Black PH, Crawford EM, Crawford LV. The purification of simian virus 40. *Virology* 1964;24:381–387.
28. Bloomgren G, Richman S, Hotermans C, et al. Risk of natalizumab-associated progressive multifocal leukoencephalopathy. *N Engl J Med* 2012;366(20):1870–1880.
29. Bocchetta M, Di Resta I, Powers A, et al. Human mesothelial cells are unusually susceptible to simian virus 40-mediated transformation and asbestos cocarcinogenicity. *Proc Natl Acad Sci U S A* 2000;97(18):10214–10219.
30. Bofill-Mas S, Formiga-Cruz M, Clemente-Casares P, et al. Potential transmission of human polyomaviruses through the gastrointestinal tract after exposure to virions or viral DNA. *J Virol* 2001;75(21):10290–10299.
31. Bofill-Mas S, Pina S, Girones R. Documenting the epidemiologic patterns of polyomaviruses in human populations by studying their presence in urban sewage. *Appl Environ Microbiol* 2000;66(1):238–245.
32. Bollag B, Chuke WF, Frisque RJ. Hybrid genomes of the polyomaviruses JC virus, BK virus, and simian virus 40: identification of sequences important for efficient transformation. *J Virol* 1989;63(2):863–872.
33. Bratt G, Hammarin AL, Grandien M, et al. BK virus as the cause of meningoencephalitis, retinitis and nephritis in a patient with AIDS. *AIDS* 1999;13(9):1071–1075.
34. Broekema NM, Imperiale MJ. miRNA regulation of BK polyomavirus replication during early infection. *Proc Natl Acad Sci U S A* 2013;110(20):8200–8205.
35. Broekema NM, Abend JR, Bennett SM, et al. A system for the analysis of BKV noncoding control regions: application to clinical isolates from an HIV/AIDS patient. *Virology* 2010;407(2):368–373.
36. Brown F, Lewis AM. Simian virus 40 (SV40): a possible human polyomavirus. Symposium proceedings. Bethesda, Maryland, USA. January 27-28, 1997. *Dev Biol Stand* 1998;94:1–406.
37. Buch MH, Liaci AM, O'Hara SD, et al. Structural and functional analysis of murine polyomavirus capsid proteins establish the determinants of ligand recognition and pathogenicity. *PLoS Pathog* 2015;11(10):e1005104.
38. Caccetta TP, Dessauvagie B, McCallum D, et al. Multiple minute digitate hyperkeratosis: a proposed algorithm for the digitate keratoses. *J Am Acad Dermatol* 2012;67(1):e49–e55.
39. Calic Z, Cappelen-Smith C, Hodgkinson SJ, et al. Treatment of progressive multifocal leukoencephalopathy-immune reconstitution inflammatory syndrome with intravenous immunoglobulin in a patient with multiple sclerosis treated with fingolimod after discontinuation of natalizumab. *J Clin Neurosci* 2015;22(3):598–600.
40. Campbell KS, Mullane KP, Aksoy IA, et al. DnaJ/hsp40 chaperone domain of SV40 large T antigen promotes efficient viral DNA replication. *Genes Dev* 1997;11(9):1098–1110.
41. Canavan TN, Baddley JW, Pavlidakey P, et al. Human polyomavirus-7-associated eruption successfully treated with acitretin. *Am J Transplant* 2018;18(5):1278–1284.
42. Carson KR, Evens AM, Richey EA, et al. Progressive multifocal leukoencephalopathy after rituximab therapy in HIV-negative patients: a report of 57 cases from the Research on Adverse Drug Events and Reports project. *Blood* 2009;113(20):4834–4840.
43. Carter JJ, Daugherty MD, Qi X, et al. Identification of an overprinting gene in Merkel cell polyomavirus provides evolutionary insight into the birth of viral genes. *Proc Natl Acad Sci U S A* 2013;110(31):12744–12749.
44. Cesaro S, Dalianis T, Hanssen Rinaldo C, et al. ECIL guidelines for the prevention, diagnosis and treatment of BK polyomavirus-associated haemorrhagic cystitis in haematopoietic stem cell transplant recipients. *J Antimicrob Chemother* 2018;73(1):12–21.
45. Chapagain ML, Nerurkar VR. Human polyomavirus JC (JCV) infection of human B lymphocytes: a possible mechanism for JCV transmigration across the blood-brain barrier. *J Infect Dis* 2010;202(2):184–191.
46. Chen CJ, Kincaid RP, Seo GJ, et al. Insights into Polyomaviridae microRNA function derived from study of the bandicoot papillomatosis carcinomatosis viruses. *J Virol* 2011;85(9):4487–4500.
47. Chen W, Possemato R, Campbell KT, et al. Identification of specific PP2A complexes involved in human cell transformation. *Cancer Cell* 2004;5(2):127–136.
48. Chen Y, Bord E, Tompkins T, et al. Asymptomatic reactivation of JC virus in patients treated with natalizumab. *N Engl J Med* 2009;361(11):1067–1074.
49. Chen Y, Sharp PM, Fowkes M, et al. Analysis of 15 novel full-length BK virus sequences from three individuals: evidence of a high intra-strain genetic diversity. *J Gen Virol* 2004;85(Pt 9):2651–2663.
50. Chen YJ, Liu X, Tsai B. SV40 Hijacks cellular transport, membrane penetration, and disassembly machineries to promote infection. *Viruses* 2019;11(10):917.
51. Cheng J, Park DE, Berrios C, et al. Merkel cell polyomavirus recruits MYCL to the EP400 complex to promote oncogenesis. *PLoS Pathog* 2017;13(10):e1006668.
52. Church ME, Dela Cruz FN Jr, Estrada M, et al. Exposure to raccoon polyomavirus (RacPyV) in free-ranging North American raccoons (Procyon lotor). *Virology* 2016;489:292–299.
53. Cinque P, Dumoulin, A, Hirsch HH. Diagnosis of polyomavirus infection, replication and disease. In: Jerome K, ed. *Laboratory Diagnosis of Viral Infections* Vol 50 (Chapter 24). New York, NY: Informa Healthcare USA; 2009:401–424.
54. Clifford DB, De Luca A, Simpson DM, et al. Natalizumab-associated progressive multifocal leukoencephalopathy in patients with multiple sclerosis: lessons from 28 cases. *Lancet Neurol* 2010;9(4):438–446.
55. Colegrove KM, Wellehan JF Jr, Rivera R, et al. Polyomavirus infection in a free-ranging California sea lion (Zalophus californianus) with intestinal T-cell lymphoma. *J Vet Diagn Invest* 2010;22(4):628–632.
56. Coleman DV, Mackenzie EF, Gardner SD, et al. Human polyomavirus (BK) infection and ureteric stenosis in renal allograft recipients. *J Clin Pathol* 1978;31(4):338–347.
57. Coogle LP, Holland KE, Pan C, et al. Complete resolution of trichodysplasia spinulosa in a pediatric renal transplant patient: case report and literature review. *Pediatr Transplant* 2017;21(2):e12849.
58. Corbridge SM, Rice RC, Bean LA, et al. JC virus infection of meningeal and choroid plexus cells in patients with progressive multifocal leukoencephalopathy. *J Neurovirol* 2019;25(4):520–524.
59. Cortese I, Muranski P, Enose-Akahata Y, et al. Pembrolizumab treatment for progressive multifocal leukoencephalopathy. *N Engl J Med* 2019;380(17):1597–1605.

60. Cuesta I, Nunez-Ramirez R, Scheres SH, et al. Conformational rearrangements of SV40 large T antigen during early replication events. *J Mol Biol* 2010;397(5):1276–1286.
61. Dadhania D, Snopkowski C, Muthukumar T, et al. Noninvasive prognostication of polyomavirus BK virus-associated nephropathy. *Transplantation* 2013;96(2):131–138.
62. Danna KJ, Nathans D. Bidirectional replication of simian virus 40 DNA. *Proc Natl Acad Sci U S A* 1972;69(11):3097–3100.
63. Darbinyan A, Major EO, Morgello S, et al. BK virus encephalopathy and sclerosing vasculopathy in a patient with hypohidrotic ectodermal dysplasia and immunodeficiency. *Acta Neuropathol Commun* 2016;4(1):73.
64. DeCaprio JA. How the Rb tumor suppressor structure and function was revealed by the study of Adenovirus and SV40. *Virology* 2009;384(2):274–284.
65. DeCaprio JA, Ludlow JW, Figge J, et al. SV40 large tumor antigen forms a specific complex with the product of the retinoblastoma susceptibility gene. *Cell* 1988;54(2): 275–283.
66. Dela Cruz FN Jr, Giannitti F, Li L, et al. Novel polyomavirus associated with brain tumors in free-ranging raccoons, western United States. *Emerg Infect Dis* 2013;19(1):77–84.
67. Delmas V, Bastien C, Scherneck S, et al. A new member of the polyomavirus family: the hamster papovavirus. Complete nucleotide sequence and transformation properties. *EMBO J* 1985;4(5):1279–1286.
68. Deuzing I, Fagrouch Z, Groenewoud MJ, et al. Detection and characterization of two chimpanzee polyomavirus genotypes from different subspecies. *Virol J* 2010;7:347.
69. Dharnidharka VR, Cherikh WS, Neff R, et al. Retransplantation after BK virus nephropathy in prior kidney transplant: an OPTN database analysis. *Am J Transplant* 2010;10(5):1312–1315.
70. Dill JA, Camus AC, Leary JH, et al. Microscopic and molecular evidence of the first elasmobranch adomavirus, the cause of skin disease in a Giant Guitarfish, Rhynchobatus djiddensis. *MBio* 2018;9(3):e00185-18.
71. Dimova DK, Dyson NJ. The E2F transcriptional network: old acquaintances with new faces. *Oncogene* 2005;24(17):2810–2826.
72. Drachenberg CB, Hirsch HH, Papadimitriou JC, et al. Polyomavirus BK versus JC replication and nephropathy in renal transplant recipients: a prospective evaluation. *Transplantation* 2007;84(3):323–330.
73. Drachenberg CB, Papadimitriou JC, Chaudhry MR, et al. Histological evolution of BK virus-associated nephropathy: importance of integrating clinical and pathological findings. *Am J Transplant* 2017;17(8):2078–2091.
74. Drachenberg CB, Papadimitriou JC, Hirsch HH, et al. Histological patterns of polyomavirus nephropathy: correlation with graft outcome and viral load. *Am J Transplant* 2004;4(12):2082–2092.
75. Du Pasquier RA, Kuroda MJ, Zheng Y, et al. A prospective study demonstrates an association between JC virus-specific cytotoxic T lymphocytes and the early control of progressive multifocal leukoencephalopathy. *Brain* 2004;127(Pt 9):1970–1978.
76. Du Pasquier RA, Schmitz JE, Jean-Jacques J, et al. Detection of JC virus-specific cytotoxic T lymphocytes in healthy individuals. *J Virol* 2004;78(18):10206–10210.
77. Egli A, Infanti L, Dumoulin A, et al. Prevalence of polyomavirus BK and JC infection and replication in 400 healthy blood donors. *J Infect Dis* 2009;199:837–846.
78. Elphick GF, Querbes W, Jordan JA, et al. The human polyomavirus, JCV, uses serotonin receptors to infect cells. *Science* 2004;306(5700):1380–1383.
79. Erickson KD, Bouchet-Marquis C, Heiser K, et al. Virion assembly factories in the nucleus of polyomavirus-infected cells. *PLoS Pathog* 2012;8(4):e1002630.
80. Fahsbender E, Altan E, Estrada M, et al. Lyon-IARC polyomavirus DNA in feces of diarrheic cats. *Microbiol Resour Announc* 2019;8(29):e00550-19.
81. Fang CY, Chen HY, Wang M, et al. Global analysis of modifications of the human BK virus structural proteins by LC-MS/MS. *Virology* 2010;402(1):164–176.
82. Fanning E, Zhao K. SV40 DNA replication: from the A gene to a nanomachine. *Virology* 2009;384(2):352–359.
83. Faust H, Pastrana DV, Buck CB, et al. Antibodies to Merkel cell polyomavirus correlate to presence of viral DNA in the skin. *J Infect Dis* 2011;203(8):1096–1100.
84. Feng H, Shuda M, Chang Y, et al. Clonal integration of a polyomavirus in human Merkel cell carcinoma. *Science* 2008;319(5866):1096–1100.
85. Ferenczy MW, Marshall LJ, Nelson CD, et al. Molecular biology, epidemiology, and pathogenesis of progressive multifocal leukoencephalopathy, the JC virus-induced demyelinating disease of the human brain. *Clin Microbiol Rev* 2012;25(3):471–506.
86. Ferrari A, Luppi M, Marasca R, et al. BK virus infection and neurologic dysfunctions in a patient with lymphoma treated with chemotherapy and rituximab. *Eur J Haematol* 2008;81(3):244–245.
87. Fine DA, Rozenblatt-Rosen O, Padi M, et al. Identification of FAM111A as an SV40 host range restriction and adenovirus helper factor. *PLoS Pathog* 2012;8(10):e1002949.
88. Ford JP, Hsu MT. Transcription pattern of in vivo-labeled late simian virus 40 RNA: equimolar transcription beyond the mRNA 3' terminus. *J Virol* 1978;28(3):795–801.
89. Foulongne V, Sauvage V, Hebert C, et al. Human skin microbiota: high diversity of DNA viruses identified on the human skin by high throughput sequencing. *PLoS One* 2012;7(6):e38499.
90. Friedman PN, Kern SE, Vogelstein B, et al. Wild-type, but not mutant, human p53 proteins inhibit the replication activities of simian virus 40 large tumor antigen. *Proc Natl Acad Sci U S A* 1990;87(23):9275–9279.
91. Funk GA, Gosert, R., Comoli, P, et al. Polyomavirus BK replication dynamics in vivo and in silico to predict cytopathology and viral clearance in kidney transplants. *Am J Transplant* 2008;8:2368–2377.
92. Funk GA, Steiger J, Hirsch HH. Rapid dynamics of polyomavirus type BK in renal transplant recipients. *J Infect Dis* 2006;193(1):80–87.
93. Galan A, Rauch CA, Otis CN. Fatal BK polyoma viral pneumonia associated with immunosuppression. *Hum Pathol* 2005;36(9):1031–1034.
94. Gallia GL, Safak M, Khalili K. Interaction of the single-stranded DNA-binding protein Puralpha with the human polyomavirus JC virus early protein T-antigen. *J Biol Chem* 1998;273(49):32662–32669.
95. Garcea RL, Benjamin TL. Host range transforming gene of polyoma virus plays a role in virus assembly. *Proc Natl Acad Sci U S A* 1983;80(12):3613–3617.
96. Gardner SD, Field AM, Coleman DV, et al. New human papovavirus (B.K.) isolated from urine after renal transplantation. *Lancet* 1971;1(7712):1253–1257.
97. Gaynor AM, Nissen MD, Whiley DM, et al. Identification of a novel polyomavirus from patients with acute respiratory tract infections. *PLoS Pathog* 2007;3(5):e64.
98. Gedvilaite A, Tryland M, Ulrich RG, et al. Novel polyomaviruses in shrews (Soricidae) with close similarity to human polyomavirus 12. *J Gen Virol* 2017;98(12):3060–3067.
99. Geoghegan EM, Pastrana DV, Schowalter RM, et al. Infectious entry and neutralization of pathogenic JC polyomaviruses. *Cell Rep* 2017;21(5):1169–1179.
100. Gheit T, Dutta S, Oliver J, et al. Isolation and characterization of a novel putative human polyomavirus. *Virology* 2017;506:45–54.
101. Gheuens S, Wuthrich C, Koralnik IJ. Progressive multifocal leukoencephalopathy: why gray and white matter. *Annu Rev Pathol* 2013;8:189–215.
102. Giacobbi NS, Gupta T, Coxon AT, et al. Polyomavirus T antigens activate an antiviral state. *Virology* 2015;476:377–385.
103. Gieselbach RJ, Muller-Hansma AH, Wijburg MT, et al. Progressive multifocal leukoencephalopathy in patients treated with fumaric acid esters: a review of 19 cases. *J Neurol* 2017;264(6):1155–1164.
104. Girardi AJ, Sweet BH, Slotnick VB, et al. Development of tumors in hamsters inoculated in the neonatal period with vacuolating virus, SV-40. *Proc Soc Exp Biol Med* 1962;109:649–660.
105. Gluck TA, Knowles WA, Johnson MA, et al. BK virus-associated haemorrhagic cystitis in an HIV-infected man. *AIDS* 1994;8(3):391–392.
106. Gluzman Y, Ahrens B. SV40 early mutants that are defective for viral DNA synthesis but competent for transformation of cultured rat and simian cells. *Virology* 1982;123(1):78–92.
107. Goetsch HE, Zhao L, Gnegy M, et al. Fate of the urinary tract virus BK human polyomavirus in source-separated urine. *Appl Environ Microbiol* 2018;84(7).
108. Gosert R, Kardas P, Major EO, et al. Rearranged JC virus noncoding control regions found in progressive multifocal leukoencephalopathy patient samples increase virus early gene expression and replication rate. *J Virol* 2010;84(20):10448–10456.
109. Gosert R, Rinaldo CH, Funk GA, et al. Polyomavirus BK with rearranged noncoding control region emerge in vivo in renal transplant patients and increase viral replication and cytopathology. *J Exp Med* 2008;205(4):841–852.
110. Greenlee JE. Effect of host age on experimental K virus infection in mice. *Infect Immun* 1981;33(1):297–303.
111. Groenewoud MJ, Fagrouch Z, van Gessel S, et al. Characterization of novel polyomaviruses from Bornean and Sumatran orang-utans. *J Gen Virol* 2010;91(Pt 3):653–658.
112. Gross L. A filterable agent, recovered from Ak leukemic extracts, causing salivary gland carcinomas in C3H mice. *Proc Soc Exp Biol Med* 1953;83(2):414–421.
113. Gruss P, Dhar R, Khoury G. Simian virus 40 tandem repeated sequences as an element of the early promoter. *Proc Natl Acad Sci U S A* 1981;78(2):943–947.
114. Guerin JL, Gelfi J, Dubois L, et al. A novel polyomavirus (goose hemorrhagic polyomavirus) is the agent of hemorrhagic nephritis enteritis of geese. *J Virol* 2000;74(10):4523–4529.
115. Gupta G, Kuppachi S, Kalil RS, et al. Treatment for presumed BK polyomavirus nephropathy and risk of urinary tract cancers among kidney transplant recipients in the United States. *Am J Transplant* 2018;18(1):245–252.
116. Hadjadj J, Guffroy A, Delavaud C, et al. Progressive Multifocal Leukoencephalopathy in Primary Immunodeficiencies. *J Clin Immunol* 2019;39(1):55–64.
117. Hahn WC, Counter CM, Lundberg AS, et al. Creation of human tumour cells with defined genetic elements. *Nature* 1999;400(6743):464–468.
118. Hahn WC, Dessain SK, Brooks MW, et al. Enumeration of the simian virus 40 early region elements necessary for human cell transformation. *Mol Cell Biol* 2002;22(7):2111–2123.
119. Halami MY, Dorrestein GM, Couteel P, et al. Whole-genome characterization of a novel polyomavirus detected in fatally diseased canary birds. *J Gen Virol* 2010;91(Pt 12):3016–3022.
120. Haley SA, Atwood WJ. Progressive multifocal leukoencephalopathy: endemic viruses and lethal brain disease. *Annu Rev Virol* 2017;4(1):349–367.
121. Handala L, Blanchard E, Raynal PI, et al. BK polyomavirus hijacks extracellular vesicles for en bloc transmission. *J Virol* 2020;94(6):e01834-19.
122. Harris KF, Christensen JB, Imperiale MJ. BK virus large T antigen: interactions with the retinoblastoma family of tumor suppressor proteins and effects on cellular growth control. *J Virol* 1996;70(4):2378–2386.
123. Haycox CL, Kim S, Fleckman P, et al. Trichodysplasia spinulosa—a newly described folliculocentric viral infection in an immunocompromised host. *J Investig Dermatol Symp Proc* 1999;4(3):268–271.
124. Heiser K, Nicholas C, Garcea RL. Activation of DNA damage repair pathways by murine polyomavirus. *Virology* 2016;497:346–356.
125. Henriksen S, Hansen T, Bruun JA, et al. The presumed polyomavirus viroporin VP4 of simian virus 40 or human BK polyomavirus is not required for viral progeny release. *J Virol* 2016;90(22):10398–10413.
126. Hirsch HH. BK virus: opportunity makes a pathogen. *Clin Infect Dis* 2005;41(3):354–360.
127. Hirsch HH. Spatiotemporal virus surveillance for severe acute respiratory infections in resource-limited settings: how deep need we go? *Clin Infect Dis* 2019;68(7):1126–1128. https://doi.org/10.1093/cid/ciy663
128. Hirsch HH, Ramos E. Retransplantation after polyomavirus-associated nephropathy: just do it? *Am J Transplant* 2006;6(1):7–9.
129. Hirsch HH, Randhawa PS. Screening for BK polyomavirus DNAemia: what should be done? *Clin Transplant* 2019;33(10):e13672.
130. Hirsch HH, Steiger J. Polyomavirus BK. *Lancet Infect Dis* 2003;3(10):611–623.
131. Hirsch HH, Babel N, Comoli P, et al. European perspective on human polyomavirus infection, replication and disease in solid organ transplantation. *Clin Microbiol Infect* 2014;20 Suppl 7:74–88.
132. Hirsch HH, Kardas P, Kranz D, et al. The human JC polyomavirus (JCPyV): virological background and clinical implications. *APMIS* 2013;121:685–727.
133. Hirsch HH, Kaufmann G, Sendi P, et al. Immune reconstitution in HIV-infected patients. *Clin Infect Dis* 2004;38(8):1159–1166.
134. Hirsch HH, Knowles W, Dickenmann M, et al. Prospective study of polyomavirus type BK replication and nephropathy in renal-transplant recipients. *N Engl J Med* 2002;347(7):488–496.

135. Hirsch HH, Randhawa PS, AST Infectious Diseases Community of Practice. BK polyomavirus in solid organ transplantation—guidelines from the American Society of Transplantation Infectious Diseases Community of Practice. *Clin Transplant* 2019;33(9):e13528.
136. Hirsch HH, Vincenti F, Friman S, et al. Polyomavirus BK replication in de novo kidney transplant patients receiving tacrolimus or cyclosporine: a prospective, randomized, multicenter study. *Am J Transplant* 2013;13(1):136–145.
137. Hirsch HH, Yakhontova K, Lu M, et al. BK polyomavirus replication in renal tubular epithelial cells is inhibited by sirolimus, but activated by tacrolimus through a pathway involving FKBP-12. *Am J Transplant* 2016;16(3):821–832.
138. Ho J, Jedrych JJ, Feng H, et al. Human polyomavirus 7-associated pruritic rash and viremia in transplant recipients. *J Infect Dis* 2015;211(10):1560–1565.
139. Hoang E, Bartlett NL, Goyal MS, et al. Progressive multifocal leukoencephalopathy treated with nivolumab. *J Neurovirol* 2019;25(2):284–287.
140. Hocker B, Schneble L, Murer L, et al. Epidemiology of and risk factors for BK polyomavirus replication and nephropathy in pediatric renal transplant recipients: an International CERTAIN Registry Study. *Transplantation* 2019;103(6):1224–1233.
141. Hocker B, Tabatabai J, Schneble L, et al. JC polyomavirus replication and associated disease in pediatric renal transplantation: an international CERTAIN Registry study. *Pediatr Nephrol* 2018;33(12):2343–2352.
142. Huang H, Weiner BE, Zhang H, et al. Structure of a DNA polymerase alpha-primase domain that docks on the SV40 helicase and activates the viral primosome. *J Biol Chem* 2010;285(22):17112–17122.
143. Hughes R, Bensa S, Willison H, et al. Randomized controlled trial of intravenous immunoglobulin versus oral prednisolone in chronic inflammatory demyelinating polyradiculoneuropathy. *Ann Neurol* 2001;50(2):195–201.
144. Hurdiss DL, Frank M, Snowden JS, et al. The structure of an infectious human polyomavirus and its interactions with cellular receptors. *Structure* 2018;26(6):839–847 e833.
145. Hurdiss DL, Morgan EL, Thompson RF, et al. New structural insights into the genome and minor capsid proteins of BK polyomavirus using cryo-electron microscopy. *Structure* 2016;24(4):528–536.
146. Inoue T, Tsai B. A large and intact viral particle penetrates the endoplasmic reticulum membrane to reach the cytosol. *PLoS Pathog* 2011;7(5):e1002037.
147. Izakovic J, Buchner SA, Duggelin M, et al. [Hair-like hyperkeratoses in patients with kidney transplants. A new cyclosporin side-effect]. *Hautarzt* 1995;46(12):841–846.
148. Jat PS, Noble MD, Ataliotis P, et al. Direct derivation of conditionally immortal cell lines from an H-2Kb-tsA58 transgenic mouse. *Proc Natl Acad Sci U S A* 1991;88(12):5096–5100.
149. Jelcic I, Jelcic I, Kempf C, et al. Mechanisms of immune escape in central nervous system infection with neurotropic JC virus variant. *Ann Neurol* 2016;79(3):404–418.
150. Jiang M, Zhao L, Gamez M, et al. Roles of ATM and ATR-mediated DNA damage responses during lytic BK polyomavirus infection. *PLoS Pathog* 2012;8(8):e1002898.
151. Jochum W, Weber T, Frye S, et al. Detection of JC virus by anti-VP1 immunohistochemistry in brains with progressive multifocal leukoencephalopathy. *Acta Neuropathol* 1997;94(3):226–231.
152. Johne R, Muller H. The genome of goose hemorrhagic polyomavirus, a new member of the proposed subgenus Avipolyomavirus. *Virology* 2003;308(2):291–302.
153. Johne R, Wittig W, Fernandez-de-Luco D, et al. Characterization of two novel polyomaviruses of birds by using multiply primed rolling-circle amplification of their genomes. *J Virol* 2006;80(7):3523–3531.
154. Kalderon D, Smith AE. In vitro mutagenesis of a putative DNA binding domain of SV40 large-T. *Virology* 1984;139(1):109–137.
155. Kalderon D, Roberts BL, Richardson WD, et al. A short amino acid sequence able to specify nuclear location. *Cell* 1984;39(3 Pt 2):499–509.
156. Kamminga S, van der Meijden E, Feltkamp MCW, et al. Seroprevalence of fourteen human polyomaviruses determined in blood donors. *PLoS One* 2018;13(10):e0206273.
157. Kassar R, Chang J, Chan AW, et al. Leflunomide for the treatment of trichodysplasia spinulosa in a liver transplant recipient. *Transpl Infect Dis* 2017;19(4).
158. Kato A, Kitamura T, Sugimoto C, et al. Lack of evidence for the transmission of JC polyomavirus between human populations. *Arch Virol* 1997;142(5):875–882.
159. Kaur A, Wilhelm M, Wilk S, et al. BK polyomavirus-specific antibody and T-cell responses in kidney transplantation: update. *Curr Opin Infect Dis* 2019;32(6):575–583.
160. Kawanishi K, Honda K, Koike J, et al. A preliminary study into the significance of intrarenal reflux in BK virus nephropathy after kidney transplantation. *Transplant Direct* 2016;2(2):e64.
161. Kazem S, van der Meijden E, Feltkamp MC. The trichodysplasia spinulosa-associated polyomavirus: virological background and clinical implications. *APMIS* 2013;121:770–782.
162. Kazem S, van der Meijden E, Wang RC, et al. Polyomavirus-associated Trichodysplasia spinulosa involves hyperproliferation, pRB phosphorylation and upregulation of p16 and p21. *PLoS One* 2014;9(10):e108947.
163. Kean JM, Rao S, Wang M, et al. Seroepidemiology of human polyomaviruses. *PLoS Pathog* 2009;5(3):e1000363.
164. Kemball CC, Lee ED, Szomolanyi-Tsuda E, et al. Costimulation requirements for antiviral CD8+ T cells differ for acute and persistent phases of polyoma virus infection. *J Immunol* 2006;176(3):1814–1824.
165. Khanna N, Elzi L, Mueller NJ, et al., for the Swiss HIV Cohort Study. Incidence and outcome of progressive multifocal leukoencephalopathy in 20 years of the Swiss HIV Cohort Study. *Clin Infect Dis* 2009;48:1459–1466.
166. Khoury MN, Alsop DC, Agnihotri SP, et al. Hyperintense cortical signal on magnetic resonance imaging reflects focal leukocortical encephalitis and seizure risk in progressive multifocal leukoencephalopathy. *Ann Neurol* 2014;75(5):659–669.
167. Kilham L, Murphy HW. A pneumotropic virus isolated from C3H mice carrying the Bittner Milk Agent. *Proc Soc Exp Biol Med* 1953;82(1):133–137.
168. Kim HY, Ahn BY, Cho Y. Structural basis for the inactivation of retinoblastoma tumor suppressor by SV40 large T antigen. *EMBO J* 2001;20(1–2):295–304.
169. Kim JW, Berrios C, Kim M, et al. STRIPAK directs PP2A activity toward MAP4K4 to promote oncogenic transformation of human cells. *Elife* 2020;9:e53003.
170. Kleinschmidt-DeMasters BK, Tyler KL. Progressive multifocal leukoencephalopathy complicating treatment with natalizumab and interferon beta-1a for multiple sclerosis. *N Engl J Med* 2005;353(4):369–374.
171. Knoll GA, Humar A, Fergusson D, et al. Levofloxacin for BK virus prophylaxis following kidney transplantation: a randomized clinical trial. *JAMA* 2014;312(20):2106–2114.
172. Koralnik IJ, Wuthrich C, Dang X, et al. JC virus granule cell neuronopathy: a novel clinical syndrome distinct from progressive multifocal leukoencephalopathy. *Ann Neurol* 2005;57(4):576–580.
173. Korup S, Rietscher J, Calvignac-Spencer S, et al. Identification of a novel human polyomavirus in organs of the gastrointestinal tract. *PLoS One* 2013;8(3):e58021.
174. Koskenvuo M, Dumoulin A, Lautenschlager I, et al. BK polyomavirus-associated hemorrhagic cystitis among pediatric allogeneic bone marrow transplant recipients: treatment response and evidence for nosocomial transmission. *J Clin Virol* 2013;56(1):77–81.
175. Krumbholz A, Bininda-Emonds OR, Wutzler P, et al. Phylogenetics, evolution, and medical importance of polyomaviruses. *Infect Genet Evol* 2009;9(5):784–799.
176. Krymskaya L, Sharma MC, Martinez J, et al. Cross-reactivity of T lymphocytes recognizing a human cytotoxic T-lymphocyte epitope within BK and JC virus VP1 polypeptides. *J Virol* 2005;79(17):11170–11178.
177. Kuhle J, Gosert R, Buhler R, et al. Management and outcome of CSF-JC virus PCR-negative PML in a natalizumab-treated patient with MS. *Neurology* 2011;77(23):2010–2016.
178. Kuypers J, Campbell AP, Guthrie KA, et al. WU and KI polyomaviruses in respiratory samples from allogeneic hematopoietic cell transplant recipients. *Emerg Infect Dis* 2012;18(10):1580–1588.
179. Lacroux C, Andreoletti O, Payre B, et al. Pathology of spontaneous and experimental infections by Goose haemorrhagic polyomavirus. *Avian Pathol* 2004;33(3):351–358.
180. Lane DP, Crawford LV. T antigen is bound to a host protein in SV40-transformed cells. *Nature* 1979;278(5701):261–263.
181. Lanford RE, Butel JS. Construction and characterization of an SV40 mutant defective in nuclear transport of T antigen. *Cell* 1984;37(3):801–813.
182. Lautenschlager I, Jahnukainen T, Kardas P, et al. A case of primary JC polyomavirus infection-associated nephropathy. *Am J Transplant* 2014;14(12):2887–2892.
183. Leboeuf C, Wilk S, Achermann R, et al. BK polyomavirus-specific 9mer CD8 T cell responses correlate with clearance of BK viremia in kidney transplant recipients: first report from the Swiss Transplant Cohort Study. *Am J Transplant* 2017;17(10):2591–2600.
184. Lednicky JA, Butel JS. Simian virus 40 regulatory region structural diversity and the association of viral archetypal regulatory regions with human brain tumors. *Semin Cancer Biol* 2001;11(1):39–47.
185. Leendertz FH, Scuda N, Cameron KN, et al. African great apes are naturally infected with polyomaviruses closely related to Merkel cell polyomavirus. *J Virol* 2011;85(2):916–924.
186. Lesprit P, Chaline-Lehmann D, Authier FJ, et al. BK virus encephalitis in a patient with AIDS and lymphoma. *AIDS* 2001;15(9):1196–1199.
187. Leuenberger D, Andresen PA, Gosert R, et al. Human polyomavirus type 1 (BK virus) agnoprotein is abundantly expressed but immunologically ignored. *Clin Vaccine Immunol* 2007;14(8):959–968.
188. Leuzinger K, Naegele K, Schaub S, et al. Quantification of plasma BK polyomavirus loads is affected by sequence variability, amplicon length, and non-encapsidated viral DNA genome fragments. *J Clin Virol* 2019;121:104210.
189. Li J, Liu Q, Muller H, et al. Avian polyomavirus expression patterns of bicistronic late mRNAs. *Virology* 2009;388(1):42–48.
190. Li D, Zhao R, Lilyestrom W, et al. Structure of the replicative helicase of the oncoprotein SV40 large tumour antigen. *Nature* 2003;423(6939):512–518.
191. Liddington RC, Yan Y, Moulai J, et al. Structure of simian virus 40 at 3.8-A resolution. *Nature* 1991;354(6351):278–284.
192. Lilyestrom W, Klein MG, Zhang R, et al. Crystal structure of SV40 large T-antigen bound to p53: interplay between a viral oncoprotein and a cellular tumor suppressor. *Genes Dev* 2006;20(17):2373–2382.
193. Lim ES, Reyes A, Antonio M, et al. Discovery of STL polyomavirus, a polyomavirus of ancestral recombinant origin that encodes a unique T antigen by alternative splicing. *Virology* 2013;436(2):295–303.
194. Lima MA, Marzocchetti A, Autissier P, et al. Frequency and phenotype of JC virus-specific CD8+ T lymphocytes in the peripheral blood of patients with progressive multifocal leukoencephalopathy. *J Virol* 2007;81(7):3361–3368.
195. Linzer DI, Levine AJ. Characterization of a 54K dalton cellular SV40 tumor antigen present in SV40-transformed cells and uninfected embryonal carcinoma cells. *Cell* 1979;17(1):43–52.
196. Litovchick L, Sadasivam S, Florens L, et al. Evolutionarily conserved multisubunit RBL2/p130 and E2F4 protein complex represses human cell cycle-dependent genes in quiescence. *Mol Cell* 2007;26(4):539–551.
197. Liu S, Chaudhry MR, Berrebi AA, et al. Polyomavirus replication and smoking are independent risk factors for bladder cancer after renal transplantation. *Transplantation* 2017;101(6):1488–1494.
198. Liu P, Qiu Y, Xing C, et al. Detection and genome characterization of two novel papillomaviruses and a novel polyomavirus in tree shrew (Tupaia belangeri chinensis) in China. *Virol J* 2019;16(1):35.
199. Liu W, Yang R, Payne AS, et al. Identifying the target cells and mechanisms of Merkel cell polyomavirus infection. *Cell Host Microbe* 2016;19(6):775–787.
200. Lopez-Rios F, Illei PB, Rusch V, et al. Evidence against a role for SV40 infection in human mesotheliomas and high risk of false-positive PCR results owing to presence of SV40 sequences in common laboratory plasmids. *Lancet* 2004;364(9440):1157–1166.
201. Lorentzen EM, Henriksen S, Kaur A, et al. Early fulminant BK polyomavirus-associated nephropathy in two kidney transplant patients with low neutralizing antibody titers receiving allografts from the same donor. *Virol J* 2020;17(1):5.
202. Loutfy SA, Moneer MM, Salem SE, et al. Polyomavirus infections and its clinical relevance in cancer patients: a prospective study. *J Infect Public Health* 2017;10(1):22–30.
203. Low J, Humes HD, Szczypka M, et al. BKV and SV40 infection of human kidney tubular epithelial cells in vitro. *Virology* 2004;323(2):182–188.
204. Luo Y, Motamedi N, Magaldi TG, et al. Interaction between simian virus 40 major capsid protein VP1 and cell surface ganglioside GM1 triggers vacuole formation. *MBio* 2016;7(2):e00297.
205. Maas RP, Muller-Hansma AH, Esselink RA, et al. Drug-associated progressive multifocal leukoencephalopathy: a clinical, radiological, and cerebrospinal fluid analysis of 326 cases. *J Neurol* 2016;263(10):2004–2021.

206. Magaldi TG, Buch MH, Murata H, et al. Mutations in the GM1 binding site of simian virus 40 VP1 alter receptor usage and cell tropism. *J Virol* 2012;86(13):7028–7042.
207. Major EO. Progressive multifocal leukoencephalopathy lesions and JC virus: the limits and value of imaging. *JAMA Neurol* 2018;75(7):789–790.
208. Major EO, Neel JV. The JC and BK human polyoma viruses appear to be recent introductions to some South American Indian tribes: there is no serological evidence of cross-reactivity with the simian polyoma virus SV40. *Proc Natl Acad Sci U S A* 1998;95(26):15525–15530.
209. Major EO, Vacante DA, Traub RG, et al. Owl monkey astrocytoma cells in culture spontaneously produce infectious JC virus which demonstrates altered biological properties. *J Virol* 1987;61(5):1435–1441.
210. Major EO, Yousry TA, Clifford DB. Pathogenesis of progressive multifocal leukoencephalopathy and risks associated with treatments for multiple sclerosis: a decade of lessons learned. *Lancet Neurol* 2018;17(5):467–480.
211. Maliakkal JG, Brennan DC, Goss C, et al. Ureteral stent placement and immediate graft function are associated with increased risk of BK viremia in the first year after kidney transplantation. *Transpl Int* 2017;30(2):153–161.
212. Mallat SG, Tanios BY, Itani HS, et al. CMV and BKPyV infections in renal transplant recipients receiving an mTOR inhibitor-based regimen versus a CNI-based regimen: a systematic review and meta-analysis of randomized, controlled trials. *Clin J Am Soc Nephrol* 2017;12(8):1321–1336.
213. Manfredi JJ, Dong J, Liu WJ, et al. Evidence against a role for SV40 in human mesothelioma. *Cancer Res* 2005;65(7):2602–2609.
214. Manzetti J, Weissbach FH, Graf FE, et al. BK Polyomavirus evades innate immune sensing by disrupting the mitochondrial network and promotes mitophagy. *iScience* 2020;23:101257.
215. Martel-Jantin C, Pedergnana V, Nicol JT, et al. Merkel cell polyomavirus infection occurs during early childhood and is transmitted between siblings. *J Clin Virol* 2013;58(1):288–291.
216. Martinot M, Ahle G, Petrosyan I, et al. Progressive multifocal leukoencephalopathy after treatment with nivolumab. *Emerg Infect Dis* 2018;24(8):1594–1596.
217. Marty FM, Winston DJ, Chemaly RF, et al. A randomized, double-blind, placebo-controlled phase 3 trial of oral brincidofovir for cytomegalovirus prophylaxis in allogeneic hematopoietic cell transplantation. *Biol Blood Marrow Transplant* 2019;25(2):369–381.
218. Mateen FJ, Muralidharan R, Carone M, et al. Progressive multifocal leukoencephalopathy in transplant recipients. *Ann Neurol* 2011;70(2):305–322.
219. Matthews MR, Wang RC, Reddick RL, et al. Viral-associated trichodysplasia spinulosa: a case with electron microscopic and molecular detection of the trichodysplasia spinulosa-associated human polyomavirus. *J Cutan Pathol* 2011;38(5):420–431.
220. McVey D, Brizuela L, Mohr I, et al. Phosphorylation of large tumour antigen by cdc2 stimulates SV40 DNA replication. *Nature* 1989;341(6242):503–507.
221. Meinke G, Phelan P, Moine S, et al. The crystal structure of the SV40 T-antigen origin binding domain in complex with DNA. *PLoS Biol* 2007;5(2):e23.
222. Melliez H, Mary-Krause M, Bocket L, et al. Risk of progressive multifocal leukoencephalopathy in the combination antiretroviral therapy era in the French hospital database on human immunodeficiency virus (ANRS-C4). *Clin Infect Dis* 2018;67(2):275–282.
223. Melnick JL. Papova virus group. *Science* 1962;135(3509):1128–1130.
224. Mendell JR, Barohn RJ, Freimer ML, et al. Randomized controlled trial of IVIg in untreated chronic inflammatory demyelinating polyradiculoneuropathy. *Neurology* 2001;56(4):445–449.
225. Menter T, Mayr M, Schaub S, et al. Pathology of resolving polyomavirus-associated nephropathy. *Am J Transplant* 2013;13:1474–1483.
226. Miller NR, McKeever PE, London W, et al. Brain tumors of owl monkeys inoculated with JC virus contain the JC virus genome. *J Virol* 1984;49(3):848–856.
227. Mindlova M, Boucek P, Saudek F, et al. Kidney retransplantation following graft loss to polyoma virus-associated nephropathy: an effective treatment option in simultaneous pancreas and kidney transplant recipients. *Transpl Int* 2007;21:353–356.
228. Mishra N, Pereira M, Rhodes RH, et al. Identification of a novel polyomavirus in a pancreatic transplant recipient with retinal blindness and vasculitic myopathy. *J Infect Dis* 2014;210(10):1595–1599.
229. Moens U, Van Ghelue M. Polymorphism in the genome of non-passaged human polyomavirus BK: implications for cell tropism and the pathological role of the virus. *Virology* 2005;331(2):209–231.
230. Moens U, Calvignac-Spencer S, Lauber C, et al. ICTV virus taxonomy profile: polyomaviridae. *J Gen Virol* 2017;98(6):1159–1160.
231. Moens U, Van Ghelue M, Ludvigsen M, et al. Early and late promoters of BK polyomavirus, Merkel cell polyomavirus, Trichodysplasia spinulosa-associated polyomavirus and human polyomavirus 12 are among the strongest of all known human polyomaviruses in 10 different cell lines. *J Gen Virol* 2015;96(8):2293–2303.
232. Mogha A, Fautrel A, Mouchet N, et al. Merkel cell polyomavirus small T antigen mRNA level is increased following in vivo UV-radiation. *PLoS One* 2010;5(7):e11423.
233. Moreau P, Hen R, Wasylyk B, et al. The SV40 72 base repair repeat has a striking effect on gene expression both in SV40 and other chimeric recombinants. *Nucleic Acids Res* 1981;9(22):6047–6068.
234. Morris-Love J, Gee GV, O'Hara BA, et al. JC polyomavirus uses extracellular vesicles to infect target cells. *MBio* 2019;10(2).
235. Mortensen ES, Rekvig OP. Nephritogenic potential of anti-DNA antibodies against necrotic nucleosomes. *J Am Soc Nephrol* 2009;20(4):696–704.
236. Moule MG, Collins CH, McCormick F, et al. Role for PP2A in ARF signaling to p53. *Proc Natl Acad Sci U S A* 2004;101(39):14063–14066.
237. Muftuoglu M, Olson A, Marin D, et al. Allogeneic BK virus-specific T cells for progressive multifocal leukoencephalopathy. *N Engl J Med* 2018;379(15):1443–1451.
238. Muller H, Nitschke R. A polyoma-like virus associated with an acute disease of fledgling budgerigars (Melopsittacus undulatus). *Med Microbiol Immunol* 1986;175(1):1–13.
239. Muller DC, Ramo M, Naegele K, et al. Donor-derived, metastatic urothelial cancer after kidney transplantation associated with a potentially oncogenic BK polyomavirus. *J Pathol* 2018;244(3):265–270.
240. Mulligan RC, Berg P. Expression of a bacterial gene in mammalian cells. *Science* 1980;209(4463):1422–1427.
241. Neske F, Prifert C, Scheiner B, et al. High prevalence of antibodies against polyomavirus WU, polyomavirus KI, and human bocavirus in German blood donors. *BMC Infect Dis* 2010;10:215.
242. Neu U, Woellner K, Gauglitz G, et al. Structural basis of GM1 ganglioside recognition by simian virus 40. *Proc Natl Acad Sci U S A* 2008;105(13):5219–5224.
243. Nghiem PT, Bhatia S, Lipson EJ, et al. PD-1 blockade with pembrolizumab in advanced Merkel-cell carcinoma. *N Engl J Med* 2016;374(26):2542–2552.
244. Nguyen KD, Lee EE, Yue Y, et al. Human polyomavirus 6 and 7 are associated with pruritic and dyskeratotic dermatoses. *J Am Acad Dermatol* 2017;76(5):932–940 e933.
245. Nickeleit V, Singh HK. Polyomaviruses and disease: is there more to know than viremia and viruria? *Curr Opin Organ Transplant* 2015;20(3):348–358.
246. Nickeleit V, Hirsch HH, Binet IF, et al. Polyomavirus infection of renal allograft recipients: from latent infection to manifest disease. *J Am Soc Nephrol* 1999;10(5):1080–1089.
247. Nigo M, Marin D, Mulanovich VE. The first case of acute unilateral pan-ureteritis caused by BK polyomavirus in an allogeneic stem cell transplant patient. *Transpl Infect Dis* 2016;18(2):257–260.
248. Norkin LC, Anderson HA, Wolfrom SA, et al. Caveolar endocytosis of simian virus 40 is followed by brefeldin A-sensitive transport to the endoplasmic reticulum, where the virus disassembles. *J Virol* 2002;76(10):5156–5166.
249. O'Hara SD, Garcea RL. Murine polyomavirus cell surface receptors activate distinct signaling pathways required for infection. *MBio* 2016;7(6):e01836-16.
250. Okada Y, Suzuki T, Sunden Y, et al. Dissociation of heterochromatin protein 1 from lamin B receptor induced by human polyomavirus agnoprotein: role in nuclear egress of viral particles. *EMBO Rep* 2005;6(5):452–457.
251. Osswald SS, Kulick KB, Tomaszewski MM, et al. Viral-associated trichodysplasia in a patient with lymphoma: a case report and review. *J Cutan Pathol* 2007;34(9):721–725.
252. Padgett BL, Walker DL, ZuRhein GM, et al. Cultivation of papova-like virus from human brain with progressive multifocal leucoencephalopathy. *Lancet* 1971;1(7712):1257–1260.
253. Pallas DC, Shahrik LK, Martin BL, et al. Polyoma small and middle T antigens and SV40 small t antigen form stable complexes with protein phosphatase 2A. *Cell* 1990;60(1):167–176.
254. Palya V, Ivanics E, Glavits R, et al. Epizootic occurrence of haemorrhagic nephritis enteritis virus infection of geese. *Avian Pathol* 2004;33(2):244–250.
255. Panou MM, Prescott EL, Hurdiss DL, et al. Agnoprotein is an essential egress factor during BK polyomavirus infection. *Int J Mol Sci* 2018;19(3):902.
256. Papadimitriou JC, Randhawa P, Rinaldo CH, et al. BK polyomavirus infection and renourinary tumorigenesis. *Am J Transplant* 2016;16(2):398–406.
257. Park DE, Cheng J, Berrios C, et al. Dual inhibition of MDM2 and MDM4 in virus-positive Merkel cell carcinoma enhances the p53 response. *Proc Natl Acad Sci U S A* 2019;116(3):1027–1032.
258. Pascual J, Berger SP, Witzke O, et al. Everolimus with reduced calcineurin inhibitor exposure in renal transplantation. *J Am Soc Nephrol* 2018;29(7):1979–1991.
259. Pastrana DV, Brennan DC, Cuburu N, et al. Neutralization serotyping of BK polyomavirus infection in kidney transplant recipients. *PLoS Pathog* 2012;8(4):e1002650.
260. Pastrana DV, Wieland U, Silling S, et al. Positive correlation between Merkel cell polyomavirus viral load and capsid-specific antibody titer. *Med Microbiol Immunol* 2012;201:17–23.
261. Paulson KG, Iyer JG, Tegeder AR, et al. Transcriptome-wide studies of merkel cell carcinoma and validation of intratumoral CD8+ lymphocyte invasion as an independent predictor of survival. *J Clin Oncol* 2011;29(12):1539–1546.
262. Paulson KG, Lewis CW, Redman MW, et al. Viral oncoprotein antibodies as a marker for recurrence of Merkel cell carcinoma: a prospective validation study. *Cancer* 2017;123(8):1464–1474.
263. Pawlita M, Clad A, zur Hausen H. Complete DNA sequence of lymphotropic papovavirus: prototype of a new species of the polyomavirus genus. *Virology* 1985;143(1):196–211.
264. Peter Rout D, Nair A, Gupta A, et al. Epidermolytic hyperkeratosis: clinical update. *Clin Cosmet Investig Dermatol* 2019;12:333–344.
265. Petrogiannis-Haliotis T, Sakoulas G, Kirby J, et al. BK-related polyomavirus vasculopathy in a renal-transplant recipient. *N Engl J Med* 2001;345(17):1250–1255.
266. Phalen DN, Radabaugh CS, Dahlhausen RD, et al. Viremia, virus shedding, and antibody response during natural avian polyomavirus infection in parrots. *J Am Vet Med Assoc* 2000;217(1):32–36.
267. Plavina T, Subramanyam M, Bloomgren G, et al. Anti-JC virus antibody levels in serum or plasma further define risk of natalizumab-associated progressive multifocal leukoencephalopathy. *Ann Neurol* 2014;76(6):802–812.
268. Potti J, Blanco G, Lemus JA, et al. Infectious offspring: how birds acquire and transmit an avian polyomavirus in the wild. *PLoS One* 2007;2(12):e1276.
269. Poulin DL, DeCaprio JA. Is there a role for SV40 in human cancer? *J Clin Oncol* 2006;24(26):4356–4365.
270. Querido S, Fernandes I, Weigert A, et al. High-grade urothelial carcinoma in a kidney transplant recipient after JC virus nephropathy: the first evidence of JC virus as a potential oncovirus in bladder cancer. *Am J Transplant* 2020:20(4):1188–1191.
271. Randhawa PS, Finkelstein S, Scantlebury V, et al. Human polyoma virus-associated interstitial nephritis in the allograft kidney. *Transplantation* 1999;67(1):103–109.
272. Randhawa PS, Schonder K, Shapiro R, et al. Polyomavirus BK neutralizing activity in human immunoglobulin preparations. *Transplantation* 2010;89(12):1462–1465.
273. Rascovan N, Monteil Bouchard S, Grob JJ, et al. Human polyomavirus-6 infecting lymph nodes of a patient with an angiolymphoid hyperplasia with eosinophilia or Kimura disease. *Clin Infect Dis* 2016;62(11):1419–1421.
274. Reddy VB, Ghosh PK, Lebowitz P, et al. Simian virus 40 early mRNA's. I. Genomic localization of 3′ and 5′ termini and two major splices in mRNA from transformed and lytically infected cells. *J Virol* 1979;30(1):279–296.
275. Reynisdottir I, O'Reilly DR, Miller LK, et al. Thermally inactivated simian virus 40 tsA58 mutant T antigen cannot initiate viral DNA replication in vitro. *J Virol* 1990;64(12):6234–6245.

276. Risser R, Pollack R. A nonselective analysis of SV40 transformation of mouse 3T3 cells. *Virology* 1974;59(2):477–489.
277. Rogers R, Gohh R, Noska A. Urothelial cell carcinoma after BK polyomavirus infection in kidney transplant recipients: a cohort study of veterans. *Transpl Infect Dis* 2017;19(5).
278. Rollison DE, Helzlsouer KJ, Halsey NA, et al. Markers of past infection with simian virus 40 (SV40) and risk of incident non-Hodgkin lymphoma in a Maryland cohort. *Cancer Epidemiol Biomarkers Prev* 2005;14(6):1448–1452.
279. Saag MS, Benson CA, Gandhi RT, et al. Antiretroviral drugs for treatment and prevention of HIV infection in adults: 2018 recommendations of the International Antiviral Society-USA Panel. *JAMA* 2018;320(4):379–396.
280. Sablina AA, Hector M, Colpaert N, et al. Identification of PP2A complexes and pathways involved in cell transformation. *Cancer Res* 2010;70(24):10474–10484.
281. Sadasivam S, DeCaprio JA. The DREAM complex: master coordinator of cell cycle-dependent gene expression. *Nat Rev Cancer* 2013;13(8):585–595.
282. Sadeghi M, Riipinen A, Vaisanen E, et al. Newly discovered KI, WU, and Merkel cell polyomaviruses: no evidence of mother-to-fetus transmission. *Virol J* 2010;7:251.
283. Safdar A, Rubocki RJ, Horvath JA, et al. Fatal immune restoration disease in human immunodeficiency virus type 1-infected patients with progressive multifocal leukoencephalopathy: impact of antiretroviral therapy-associated immune reconstitution. *Clin Infect Dis* 2002;35(10):1250–1257.
284. Schaffhausen BS, Roberts TM. Lessons from polyoma middle T antigen on signaling and transformation: a DNA tumor virus contribution to the war on cancer. *Virology* 2009;384(2):304–316.
285. Schelhaas M, Malmstrom J, Pelkmans L, et al. Simian Virus 40 depends on ER protein folding and quality control factors for entry into host cells. *Cell* 2007;131(3):516–529.
286. Schowalter RM, Buck CB. The Merkel cell polyomavirus minor capsid protein. *PLoS Pathog* 2013;9(8):e1003558.
287. Schowalter RM, Pastrana DV, Buck CB. Glycosaminoglycans and sialylated glycans sequentially facilitate Merkel cell polyomavirus infectious entry. *PLoS Pathog* 2011;7(7):e1002161.
288. Schowalter RM, Pastrana DV, Pumphrey KA, et al. Merkel cell polyomavirus and two previously unknown polyomaviruses are chronically shed from human skin. *Cell Host Microbe* 2010;7(6):509–515.
289. Schrama D, Groesser L, Ugurel S, et al. Presence of human polyomavirus 6 in mutation-specific BRAF inhibitor-induced epithelial proliferations. *JAMA Dermatol* 2014;150(11):1180–1186.
290. Schreiber PW, Kufner V, Hubel K, et al. Metagenomic virome sequencing in living donor and recipient kidney transplant pairs revealed JC polyomavirus transmission. *Clin Infect Dis* 2019;69(6):987–994.
291. Schuurman R, Jacobs M, van Strien A, et al. Analysis of splice sites in the early region of bovine polyomavirus: evidence for a unique pattern of large T mRNA splicing. *J Gen Virol* 1992;73 (Pt 11):2879–2886.
292. Schwab N, Schneider-Hohendorf T, Melzer N, et al. Natalizumab-associated PML: challenges with incidence, resulting risk, and risk stratification. *Neurology* 2017;88(12):1197–1205.
293. Schwarz A, Linnenweber-Held S, Heim A, et al. Viral origin, clinical course, and renal outcomes in patients with BK virus infection after living-donor renal transplantation. *Transplantation* 2016;100(4):844–853.
294. Scuda N, Hofmann J, Calvignac-Spencer S, et al. A novel human polyomavirus closely related to the African green monkey-derived lymphotropic polyomavirus. *J Virol* 2011;85(9):4586–4590.
295. Seber A, Shu XO, Defor T, et al. Risk factors for severe hemorrhagic cystitis following BMT. *Bone Marrow Transplant* 1999;23(1):35–40.
296. Seemayer CA, Seemayer NH, Durmuller U, et al. BK virus large T and VP-1 expression in infected human renal allografts. *Nephrol Dial Transplant* 2008;23(12):3752–3761.
297. Shah K, Nathanson N. Human exposure to SV40: review and comment. *Am J Epidemiol* 1976;103(1):1–12.
298. Shah KV, Daniel RW, Kelly TJ Jr. Immunological relatedness of papovaviruses of the simian virus 40-polyoma subgroup. *Infect Immun* 1977;18(2):558–560.
299. Shah A, Kumar V, Palmer MB, et al. Native kidney BK virus nephropathy, a systematic review. *Transpl Infect Dis* 2019;21(4):e13083.
300. Shaikh S, Skoczylas C, Longnecker R, et al. Inability of simian virus 40 to establish productive infection of lymphoblastic cell lines. *J Virol* 2004;78(9):4917–4920.
301. Shavaleh R, Kamandi M, Feiz Disfani H, et al. Association between JC virus and colorectal cancer: systematic review and meta-analysis. *Infect Dis (Lond)* 2020;52(3): 152–160.
302. Shen PS, Enderlein D, Nelson CD, et al. The structure of avian polyomavirus reveals variably sized capsids, non-conserved inter-capsomere interactions, and a possible location of the minor capsid protein VP4. *Virology* 2011;411(1):142–152.
303. Shuda M, Feng H, Kwun HJ, et al. T antigen mutations are a human tumor-specific signature for Merkel cell polyomavirus. *Proc Natl Acad Sci U S A* 2008;105(42):16272–16277.
304. Shuda M, Kwun HJ, Feng H, et al. Human Merkel cell polyomavirus small T antigen is an oncoprotein targeting the 4E-BP1 translation regulator. *J Clin Invest* 2011;121(9):3623–3634.
305. Siebrasse EA, Nguyen NL, Smith C, et al. Immunohistochemical detection of KI polyomavirus in lung and spleen. *Virology* 2014;468–470C:178–184.
306. Siebrasse EA, Nguyen NL, Willby MJ, et al. Multiorgan WU polyomavirus infection in bone marrow transplant recipient. *Emerg Infect Dis* 2016;22(1):24–31.
307. Siebrasse EA, Pastrana DV, Nguyen NL, et al. WU polyomavirus in respiratory epithelial cells from lung transplant patient with Job syndrome. *Emerg Infect Dis* 2015;21(1):103–106.
308. Siebrasse EA, Reyes A, Lim ES, et al. Identification of MW polyomavirus, a novel polyomavirus in human stool. *J Virol* 2012;86(19):10321–10326.
309. Silver J, Schaffhausen B, Benjamin T. Tumor antigens induced by nontransforming mutants of polyoma virus. *Cell* 1978;15(2):485–496.
310. Simmons DT. SV40 large T antigen functions in DNA replication and transformation. *Adv Virus Res* 2000;55:75–134.
311. Snijder B, Sacher R, Ramo P, et al. Population context determines cell-to-cell variability in endocytosis and virus infection. *Nature* 2009;461(7263):520–523.
312. Solis M, Velay A, Porcher R, et al. Neutralizing antibody-mediated response and risk of BK virus-associated nephropathy. *J Am Soc Nephrol* 2018;29(1):326–334.
313. Sowd GA, Mody D, Eggold J, et al. SV40 utilizes ATM kinase activity to prevent non-homologous end joining of broken viral DNA replication products. *PLoS Pathog* 2014;10(12):e1004536.
314. Starrett GJ, Buck CB. The case for BK polyomavirus as a cause of bladder cancer. *Curr Opin Virol* 2019;39:8–15.
315. Starrett GJ, Thakuria M, Chen T, et al. Clinical and molecular characterization of virus-positive and virus-negative Merkel cell carcinoma. *Genome Med* 2020;12(1):30.
316. Stehle T, Gamblin SJ, Yan Y, et al. The structure of simian virus 40 refined at 3.1 A resolution. *Structure* 1996;4(2):165–182.
317. Stewart SE, Eddy BE, Borgese N. Neoplasms in mice inoculated with a tumor agent carried in tissue culture. *J Natl Cancer Inst* 1958;20(6):1223–1243.
318. Stoner GL, Alappan R, Jobes DV, et al. BK virus regulatory region rearrangements in brain and cerebrospinal fluid from a leukemia patient with tubulointerstitial nephritis and meningoencephalitis. *Am J Kidney Dis* 2002;39(5):1102–1112.
319. Stratton KR, Alamario DA, McCormick MC, Institute of Medicine (U.S.). Immunization Safety Review Committee. *Immunization safety review: SV40 contamination of polio vaccine and cancer*. Washington, DC: National Academies Press; 2003.
320. Strickler HD, Goedert JJ, Fleming M, et al. Simian virus 40 and pleural mesothelioma in humans. *Cancer Epidemiol Biomarkers Prev* 1996;5(6):473–475.
321. Stubdal H, Zalvide J, Campbell KS, et al. Inactivation of pRB-related proteins p130 and p107 mediated by the J domain of simian virus 40 large T antigen. *Mol Cell Biol* 1997;17(9):4979–4990.
322. Sullivan CS, Cantalupo P, Pipas JM. The molecular chaperone activity of simian virus 40 large T antigen is required to disrupt Rb-E2F family complexes by an ATP-dependent mechanism. *Mol Cell Biol* 2000;20(17):6233–6243.
323. Sullivan CS, Grundhoff AT, Tevethia S, et al. SV40-encoded microRNAs regulate viral gene expression and reduce susceptibility to cytotoxic T cells. *Nature* 2005;435(7042):682–686.
324. Sullivan CS, Sung CK, Pack CD, et al. Murine Polyomavirus encodes a microRNA that cleaves early RNA transcripts but is not essential for experimental infection. *Virology* 2009;387(1):157–167.
325. Suzuki M, Zheng HY, Takasaka T, et al. Asian genotypes of JC virus in Japanese-Americans suggest familial transmission. *J Virol* 2002;76(19):10074–10078.
326. Sweet BH, Hilleman MR. The vacuolating virus, S.V. 40. *Proc Soc Exp Biol Med* 1960;105:420–427.
327. Tan IL, McArthur JC, Clifford DB, et al. Immune reconstitution inflammatory syndrome in natalizumab-associated PML. *Neurology* 2011;77(11):1061–1067.
328. Tegtmeyer P, Schwartz M, Collins JK, et al. Regulation of tumor antigen synthesis by simian virus 40 gene A. *J Virol* 1975;16(1):168–178.
329. Theiss JM, Günther T, Alawi M, et al. A comprehensive analysis of replicating merkel cell polyomavirus genomes delineates the viral transcription program and suggests a role for mcv-miR-M1 in episomal persistence. *PLoS Pathog* 2015;11(7):e1004974.
330. Tolstov YL, Knauer A, Chen JG, et al. Asymptomatic primary Merkel cell polyomavirus infection among adults. *Emerg Infect Dis* 2011;17(8):1371–1380.
331. Tooze J, Acheson NH. *DNA Tumor Viruses* 2nd ed. Cold Spring Harbor, NY: Cold Spring Harbor Laboratory; 1981.
332. Trusch F, Klein M, Finsterbusch T, et al. Seroprevalence of human polyomavirus 9 and cross-reactivity to African green monkey-derived lymphotropic polyomavirus. *J Gen Virol* 2012;93(Pt 4):698–705.
333. Tsai B, Inoue T. A virus takes an "L" turn to find its receptor. *Cell Host Microbe* 2010;8(4):301–302.
334. Tsai B, Gilbert JM, Stehle T, et al. Gangliosides are receptors for murine polyoma virus and SV40. *EMBO J* 2003;22(17):4346–4355.
335. Tsang SH, Wang R, Nakamaru-Ogiso E, et al. The oncogenic small tumor antigen of Merkel cell polyomavirus is an iron-sulfur cluster protein that enhances viral DNA replication. *J Virol* 2016;90(3):1544–1556.
336. Tzannou I, Papadopoulou A, Naik S, et al. Off-the-shelf virus-specific T cells to treat BK virus, human herpesvirus 6, cytomegalovirus, Epstein-Barr virus, and adenovirus infections after allogeneic hematopoietic stem-cell transplantation. *J Clin Oncol* 2017;35(31):3547–3557.
337. Vacante DA, Traub R, Major EO. Extension of JC virus host range to monkey cells by insertion of a simian virus 40 enhancer into the JC virus regulatory region. *Virology* 1989;170(2):353–361.
338. Valis JD, Newell N, Reissig M, et al. Characterization of SA12 as a simian virus 40-related papovavirus of chacma baboons. *Infect Immun* 1977;18(1):247–252.
339. Vallbracht A, Lohler J, Gossmann J, et al. Disseminated BK type polyomavirus infection in an AIDS patient associated with central nervous system disease. *Am J Pathol* 1993;143(1):29–39.
340. van der Meijden E, Feltkamp M. The human polyomavirus middle and alternative T-antigens; thoughts on roles and relevance to cancer. Front Microbiol 2018;9:398.
341. van der Meijden E, Horvath B, Nijland M, et al. Primary polyomavirus infection, not reactivation, as the cause of trichodysplasia spinulosa in immunocompromised patients. *J Infect Dis* 2017;215(7):1080–1084.
342. van der Meijden E, Janssens RW, Lauber C, et al. Discovery of a new human polyomavirus associated with trichodysplasia spinulosa in an immunocompromized patient. *PLoS Pathog* 2010;6(7):e1001024.
343. van der Meijden E, Kazem S, Burgers MM, et al. Seroprevalence of trichodysplasia spinulosa-associated polyomavirus. *Emerg Infect Dis* 2011;17(8):1355–1363.
344. van der Meijden E, Kazem S, Dargel CA, et al. Characterization of T antigens, including middle T and alternative T, expressed by the human polyomavirus associated with trichodysplasia spinulosa. *J Virol* 2015;89(18):9427–9439.
345. Varshavsky AJ, Bakayev VV, Chumackov PM, et al. Minichromosome of simian virus 40: presence of histone HI. *Nucleic Acids Res* 1976;3(8):2101–2113.
346. Vasquez C, Kleinschmidt AK, Basilico C. Electron microscopic studies of polyoma DNA released in protein monolayers. *J Mol Biol* 1969;43(2):317–325.

347. Verschoor EJ, Groenewoud MJ, Fagrouch Z, et al. Molecular characterization of the first polyomavirus from a New World primate: squirrel monkey polyomavirus. *J Gen Virol* 2008;89(Pt 1):130–137.
348. Viscidi RP, Khanna N, Tan CS, et al. JC virus antibody and viremia as predictors of progressive multifocal leukoencephalopathy in human immunodeficiency virus-1-infected individuals. *Clin Infect Dis* 2011;53(7):711–715.
349. Voltz R, Jager G, Seelos K, et al. BK virus encephalitis in an immunocompetent patient. *Arch Neurol* 1996;53(1):101–103.
350. von Einsiedel RW, Fife TD, Aksamit AJ, et al. Progressive multifocal leukoencephalopathy in AIDS: a clinicopathologic study and review of the literature. *J Neurol* 1993;240(7):391–406.
351. Wanat KA, Holler PD, Dentchev T, et al. Viral-associated trichodysplasia: characterization of a novel polyomavirus infection with therapeutic insights. *Arch Dermatol* 2012;148(2):219–223.
352. Warnke C, von Geldern G, Markwerth P, et al. Cerebrospinal fluid JC virus antibody index for diagnosis of natalizumab-associated progressive multifocal leukoencephalopathy. *Ann Neurol* 2014;76(6):792–801.
353. Watanabe I, Preskorn SH. Virus-cell interaction in oligodendroglia, astroglia and phagocyte in progressive multifocal leukoencephalopathy. An electron microscopic study. *Acta Neuropathol* 1976;36(2):101–115.
354. Wattjes MP, Rovira A, Miller D, et al. Evidence-based guidelines: MAGNIMS consensus guidelines on the use of MRI in multiple sclerosis—establishing disease prognosis and monitoring patients. *Nat Rev Neurol* 2015;11(10):597–606.
355. Welcker M, Clurman BE. The SV40 large T antigen contains a decoy phosphodegron that mediates its interactions with Fbw7/hCdc4. *J Biol Chem* 2005;280(9):7654–7658.
356. Wiedinger K, Bitsaktsis C, Chang S. Reactivation of human polyomaviruses in immunocompromised states. *J Neurovirol* 2014;20(1):1–8.
357. Wieland U, Silling S, Hellmich M, et al. Human polyomaviruses 6, 7, 9, 10 and trichodysplasia spinulosa-associated polyomavirus in HIV-infected men. *J Gen Virol* 2014;95(Pt 4):928–932.
358. Wijburg MT, Kleerekooper I, Lissenberg-Witte BI, et al. Association of progressive multifocal leukoencephalopathy lesion volume with JC virus polymerase chain reaction results in cerebrospinal fluid of natalizumab-treated patients with multiple sclerosis. *JAMA Neurol* 2018;75(7):827–833.
359. Wollebo HS, White MK, Gordon J, et al. Persistence and pathogenesis of the neurotropic polyomavirus JC. *Ann Neurol* 2015;77(4):560–570.
360. Wong AS, Chan KH, Cheng VC, et al. Relationship of pretransplantation polyoma BK virus serologic findings and BK viral reactivation after hematopoietic stem cell transplantation. *Clin Infect Dis* 2007;44(6):830–837.
361. Wunderink HF, Haasnoot GW, de Brouwer CS, et al. Reduced risk of BK polyomavirus infection in HLA-B51-positive kidney transplant recipients. *Transplantation* 2019;103(3):604–612.
362. Wuthrich C, Batson S, Anderson MP, et al. JC virus infects neurons and glial cells in the hippocampus. *J Neuropathol Exp Neurol* 2016;75(8):712–717.
363. Yapa HM, McLornan DP, Raj K, et al. Pneumonitis post-haematopoietic stem cell transplant—cytopathology clinches diagnosis. *J Clin Virol* 2012;55(3):278–281.
364. Yardimci H, Wang X, Loveland AB, et al. Bypass of a protein barrier by a replicative DNA helicase. *Nature* 2012;492(7428):205–209.
365. Ylinen E, Miettinen J, Jalanko H, et al. JC polyomavirus-specific antibody responses in pediatric kidney transplant recipients. *Pediatr Transplant* 2019;23(8):e13586.
366. Yogo Y, Sugimoto C, Zhong S, et al. Evolution of the BK polyomavirus: epidemiological, anthropological and clinical implications. *Rev Med Virol* 2009;19(4):185–199.
367. Yogo Y, Zhong S, Suzuki M, et al. Occurrence of the European subgroup of subtype I BK polyomavirus in Japanese-Americans suggests transmission outside the family. *J Virol* 2007;81(23):13254–13258.
368. Yousry TA, Pelletier D, Cadavid D, et al. Magnetic resonance imaging pattern in natalizumab-associated progressive multifocal leukoencephalopathy. *Ann Neurol* 2012;72(5):779–787.
369. Yu Y, Alwine JC. 19S late mRNAs of simian virus 40 have an internal ribosome entry site upstream of the virion structural protein 3 coding sequence. *J Virol* 2006;80(13):6553–6558.
370. Yu Y, Kudchodkar SB, Alwine JC. Effects of simian virus 40 large and small tumor antigens on mammalian target of rapamycin signaling: small tumor antigen mediates hypophosphorylation of eIF4E-binding protein 1 late in infection. *J Virol* 2005;79(11):6882–6889.
371. Zhang S, McNees AL, Butel JS. Quantification of vertical transmission of Murine polyoma virus by real-time quantitative PCR. *J Gen Virol* 2005;86(Pt 10):2721–2729.
372. Zhao L, Imperiale MJ. Identification of Rab18 as an essential host factor for BK polyomavirus infection using a whole-genome RNA interference screen. *mSphere* 2017;2(4):e00291-17.
373. Zhao X, Madden-Fuentes RJ, Lou BX, et al. Ataxia telangiectasia-mutated damage-signaling kinase- and proteasome-dependent destruction of Mre11-Rad50-Nbs1 subunits in Simian virus 40-infected primate cells. *J Virol* 2008;82(11):5316–5328.
374. Zhao L, Marciano AT, Rivet CR, et al. Caveolin- and clathrin-independent entry of BKPyV into primary human proximal tubule epithelial cells. *Virology* 2016;492:66–72.
375. Zheng HY, Kitamura T, Takasaka T, et al. Unambiguous identification of JC polyomavirus strains transmitted from parents to children. *Arch Virol* 2004;149(2):261–273.
376. Zhong S, Randhawa PS, Ikegaya H, et al. Distribution patterns of BK polyomavirus (BKV) subtypes and subgroups in American, European and Asian populations suggest co-migration of BKV and the human race. *J Gen Virol* 2009;90(Pt 1):144–152.
377. Zurhein G, Chou SM. Particles resembling papova viruses in human cerebral demyelinating disease. *Science* 1965;148:1477–1479.

CHAPTER 2

Papillomaviridae: The Viruses and Their Replication

Alison A. McBride • Peter M. Howley

INTRODUCTION

The Papillomaviruses (PVs) comprise a group of nonenveloped epitheliotropic DNA viruses that induce benign squamous epithelial lesions in a variety of higher vertebrates. Some PVs are associated with cancers in their natural hosts including some of the human papillomaviruses (HPVs) that are the cause of human cervical cancer, other tumors of the urogenital tract, and head and neck oropharyngeal cancers. Indeed, 5% of human cancers are caused by oncogenic HPVs. In previous recent editions, the PVs were presented in a single chapter. Because of major advances in understanding the fundamental biology of the papillomaviruses, as well as advances due to the success of the preventive VLP-based vaccines, the PVs are covered by two separate chapters in this 7th Edition. This chapter will focus on fundamental aspects of the molecular biology and replication of the PVs and Chapter 3 by Schiller and Lowy will deal with more clinical aspects of the HPVs.

HISTORY

Warts were known to the ancient Greeks and Romans. Their infectious nature was recognized, but until the nineteenth century, genital warts were usually considered to be a form of syphilis or gonorrhea. The viral nature of human warts was demonstrated in the early 1900s when cell-free filtrates from lesions were shown to transmit the disease.[48] PVs were subsequently identified in a variety of vertebrate species in addition to humans.

The first animal PV was identified in the 1930s by Richard Shope, who characterized the transmissible nature of cutaneous papillomas arising in wild cottontail rabbits.[235] The Shope papillomavirus, now officially designated as *Sylvilagus floridanus* Papillomavirus 1 (SfPV1) but commonly called cottontail rabbit papillomavirus (CRPV), was the first DNA tumor virus identified. Shope's research also showed that although systemic injection with papilloma suspensions did not produce detectable infection, it could induce serum-neutralizing antibodies and protect rabbits against high-dose cutaneous viral challenge.[234] These findings laid the groundwork for believing that a preventive vaccine against a PV could be based on the induction of humoral immunity. In addition to causing benign papillomas, some warts induced by SfPV1/CRPV were observed to undergo malignant progression,[215,254] and for the next two decades, SfPV1/CRPV was an important model for the fundamental study of viral tumorigenesis.[143,253] However, its use as a model tumor virus was largely supplanted by the discovery in the late 1950s of the polyomaviruses, which could replicate in cultured cells and induce morphologic transformation *in vitro*, in contrast to SfPV1/CRPV, and were tumorigenic in experimental animals.

Although the PVs were studied less intensively in the 1950s and 1960s, that period was associated with some important advances, including the physicochemical analysis of PV virions, and the demonstration that PV replication was associated with the differentiation process of the infected epithelium.[216] However, it was the advent of molecular cloning in the 1970s that initiated more extensive studies of PVs. The cloning and sequencing of PV genomes led to the identification of open reading frames (ORFs) as putative viral genes and permitted investigators to determine the function of viral genes by reverse genetics, resulting in a much wider interest in PV research.[42,53,54] The bovine papillomavirus type 1 (BPV1) was the standard PV used for these studies because the virus induced focal transformation of established rodent cell lines.[21,74] The molecular cloning of the HPV genomes also led to the recognition that there were multiple HPV genotypes, and that a subset of these types was closely associated with human cancers. These included cervical cancer[25,73,190] and skin cancers in individuals with the primary immunodeficiency, epidermodysplasia verruciformis (EV).[190, p.461] The appreciation of their medical importance, combined with improved tools for analyzing PVs, further enhanced the utility of PVs as a model of viral tumorigenesis. Although the study of animal PVs continues to bring new information to the field, the medical importance of HPVs has shifted emphasis toward the analysis of HPV, especially when it was established that the biochemical properties of some nonstructural viral proteins differed from those of their BPV1 counterparts.

CLASSIFICATION

Initially, the PVs were classified together with the polyomaviruses as a single family, the *Papovaviridae*. Although the viruses share many similarities, including a double-stranded circular DNA genome, an icosahedral capsid composed of 72 pentamers, a nonenveloped virion, and the nucleus as the site of viral replication and virion assembly, they are genetically distinct virus families.

Hundreds of PVs (655 to date) have been isolated from diverse mammalian host species, birds, reptiles and fish, but thus far they have not been identified in nonvertebrates. PVs are species specific, and many different PV types can infect a given host species. HPVs have been analyzed most intensively; currently 440 different HPV types have been identified and classified, and there are likely more to be discovered (https://pave.niaid.nih.gov/).

PVs are named according to the host species they infect and are classified as individual types based on the DNA sequence of the L1 gene. The current International Committee on Taxonomy of Viruses (ICTV) classifies the *Papillomaviridae* family into two subfamilies, the *Firstpapillomavirinae* with more than 50 genera and 130 species, and the *Secondpapillomavirinae*, with a single genus containing fish papillomaviruses.[271, p.462] Within the PV community, the viruses are divided into the categories: subfamily, genus, species, type, and variant. The broadest category is a *genus*. PVs are divided into greater than 50 genera, each of which is designated by a letter of the Greek alphabet. Within a given *genus*, the L1 genes of all members share more than 60% identity. A *species* is designated for those PVs that share 60% to 70% identity within a given genus. A viral *type* has 71% to 89% identity with other types within the species, or conversely has an L1 DNA sequence that is at least 10% different from that of all other PV types. Within a type, there can be *variants*, which share more than 98% identity.[35] These variants have been studied intensively for viruses such as HPV16 because of its medical importance.[45,176]

The PV types can be organized into a phylogenetic tree based on the comparative homology of the L1 DNA sequence (Fig. 2.1). Similar (though not identical) phylogenetic relationships are also seen when homologies among other regions of the genome are compared. This is because different PV types appear to have arisen primarily from point mutations scattered throughout the genome, rather than from recombination between PVs.[41] These similarities are consistent with the conclusion that PVs have accompanied their host species during evolution and have evolved with them.[19,270]

Using this classification, HPVs are clustered among five of the greater than 50 genera: *Alpha-*, *Beta-*, *Gamma-*, *Mu-*, and *Nupapillomavirus*, while the other genera are occupied exclusively by animal PVs. The host species associated with each PV genus tend to be closely related evolutionarily. Thus, PVs that infect nonhuman primates are found within the genera that include HPVs, and some HPVs are more closely related to nonhuman primate viruses than to some of the other HPVs in the genus. The HPVs of greatest medical importance, that is, those that are associated with genital and mucosal cancers, are members of the *Alphapapillomavirus* genus. Most *Alphapapillomavirus* types primarily infect genital and nongenital mucosal surfaces and the external genitalia. This group of PVs is often referred to collectively as the "mucosal" types. The types that are associated with cervical cancer, often designated as high-risk types, are found in species 5, 6, 7, 9, and 11. HPV16, the type found most frequently in cervical cancer, is a member of species 9, while the next most common cancer-associated type, HPV18, is a member of species 7. HPV6, which causes most cutaneous genital warts, is a species 10 member.

In contrast to most species of the *Alphapapillomavirus* genus, members of *Alphapapillomavirus* species 4 (HPV2, 27, and 57) are primarily infectious for nongenital skin. The *Beta-*, *Gamma-*, *Mu*, and *Nupapillomavirus* viruses also infect nongenital skin. The *Betapapillomavirus* HPVs include those that are often designated EV specific, because they cause lesions, and cutaneous squamous cell carcinomas, mainly in patients with EV, a genetic susceptibility to widespread nongenital HPV lesions. Some PVs, including many members of the beta and gamma species, may behave as commensal agents, as they are frequently isolated from normal skin or plucked hair from humans and animals.[8,26]

The PVs in the *Deltapapillomavirus* genus, which includes BPV1 and other PVs of ungulates, cause fibropapillomas, rather than papillomas. This distinct pathology results from a proliferative dermal fibroblastic component under the epithelial portion of the lesion, because members of this genus induce nonproductive transformation of the fibroblasts, in addition to the productive infection of the overlying epithelium. The ability to transform nonepithelial cells is not species specific. This property can lead to the induction of nonproductive fibroblastic tumors in heterologous hosts under natural conditions, as in equine sarcoid of horses (from BPV1 or BPV2), or experimental hosts, such as hamsters. It also endows viruses such as BPV1 and BPV2 with the ability to induce focal transformation of cultured rodent cells.

VIRION STRUCTURE

PVs are small, nonenveloped, icosahedral DNA viruses that replicate in the nucleus of squamous epithelial cells. The PV particles are approximately 60 nanometers in diameter (Fig. 2.2). The virion particles consist of a single molecule of double-stranded circular DNA of about 8,000 base pairs (bp) in size, contained within a spherical protein coat, or capsid, composed of two viral proteins, L1, the major capsid protein, and L2, the minor capsid protein. The DNA constitutes approximately 12% of the virion by weight, accounting for their density in cesium chloride of 1.34 g/mL.[52]

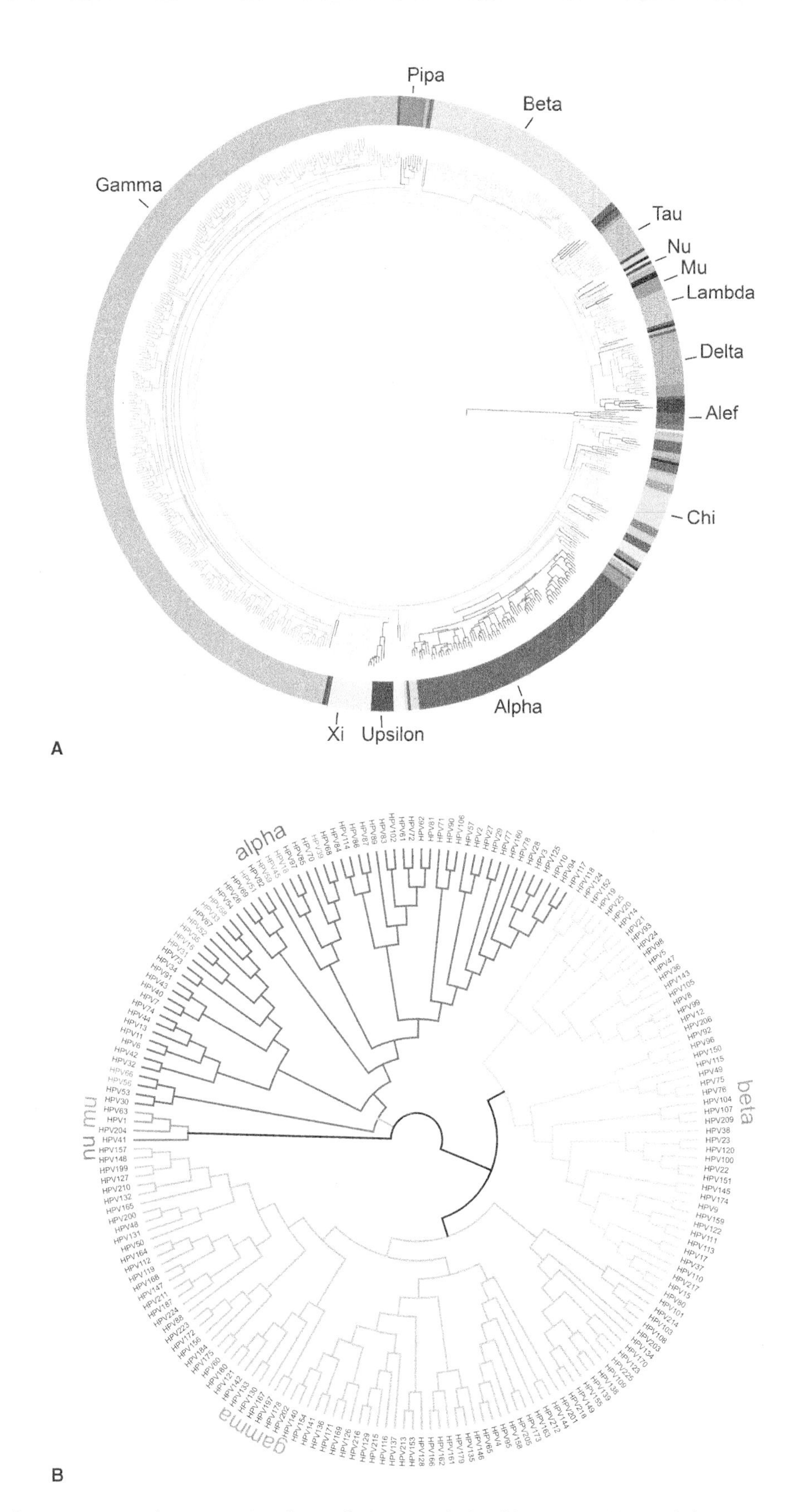

FIGURE 2.1 Phylogenetic trees demonstrating the evolutionary relationship among PVs. A: Phylogenetic tree based on the L1 sequence of 655 PVs characterized to date. This contains animal PVs, Reference HPVs (officially named by the HPV Reference center https://ki.se/en/labmed/international-hpv-reference-center) and Non-reference HPVs. The more common genera are indicated. **B:** Phylogenetic tree based on the L1 sequence of the Reference HPVs. HPVs are contained in five genera and each of them has different epithelial tropisms and disease associations. The *Alphapapillomavirus* HPVs include the low-risk mucosal types that cause genital warts, and the high-risk mucosal types associated with anogenital cancers (indicated in red text). Some *Betapapillomavirus* HPV types have been associated with nonmelanoma skin cancers (NMSC) in immunosuppressed individuals, and in individuals with epidermodysplasia verruciformis (EV).

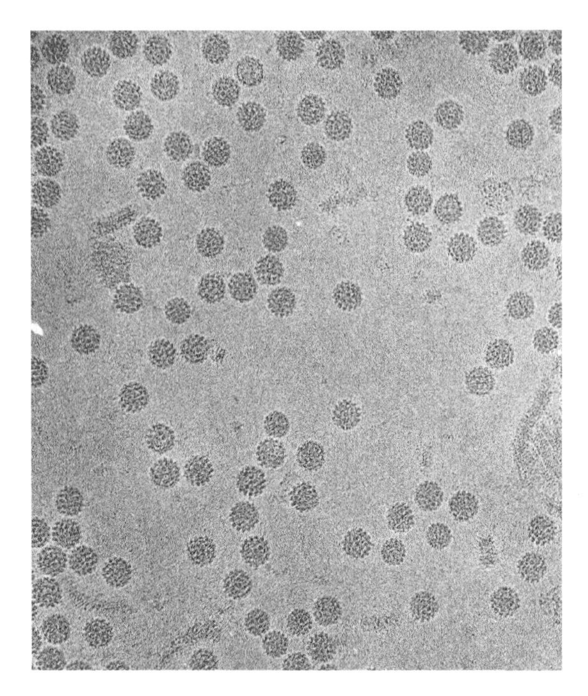

FIGURE 2.2 **Electron micrograph of BPV1 virion particles (55 nm in diameter).** (Reprinted from Baker TS, Newcomb WW, Olson NH, et al. Structures of bovine and human papillomaviruses—analysis by cryoelectron microscopy and three-dimensional image reconstruction. *Biophys J* 1991;60:1445–1456. Copyright © 1991 The Biophysical Society. With permission.)

Structural analysis by cryo-electron microscopy (cryo-EM) and three-dimensional image reconstruction techniques revealed that the viruses consist of 72 pentameric capsomers arranged on a $T = 7$ surface lattice.[10,267] The capsomers are composed of five L1 molecules with one L2 molecule occupying the axial lumen.[33] As with the polyomavirus capsids, the capsomers exist in two environments, one capable of making contact with six neighbors as observed in the 60 hexavalent capsomers and the other with 5 neighbors in the 12 pentavalent vertex capsomers (Fig. 2.3). Analysis of proteins in the virus particle showed that the viral DNA is associated with cellular histones to form a chromatin-like complex.[81,200]

Virus-like particles (VLPs) can be produced from different PVs by expressing L1 alone using mammalian or nonmammalian expression systems,[103,136,214] and these are the basis for the highly successful HPV vaccine (Chapter 3). The morphology of VLPs containing only L1 appears identical to intact virus particles in low resolution cryo-EM reconstructions,[102] but near atomic reconstructions reveal the putative location of the L2 protein.[100] The structure of a truncated $T = 1$ HPV16 L1 VLP containing 12 pentamers has been solved by x-ray crystallography to 3.5 Å resolution.[44] The structure of full-size BPV1 virions has been solved to 3.6 Å resolution using cryo-EM.[289]

GENOME STRUCTURE AND ORGANIZATION

To date, over 650 human and animal papillomavirus genomes have been sequenced in their entirety, and the overall genomic organization of each is very similar (https://pave.niaid.nih.gov/).[272] Each virus contains a regulatory region, approximately one kilobase in size, which contains the replication origin, transcriptional enhancers and repressor elements, and promoters. This region has been alternatively named the upstream regulatory region (URR), the long control region (LCR), or the noncoding region (NCR). The remainder of the genome is divided into the early and late coding regions. All viral ORFs are located on one strand, which serves as a template for transcription. The organization of an *Alphapapillomavirus* HPV genome is shown in Figure 2.4.

All PV genomes encode four core proteins; these are the replication proteins E1 and E2 (encoded in the early region), and the L1 and L2 capsid proteins (encoded by the late region, and expressed only in productively infected cells). Also encoded by almost all PVs are two fusion proteins expressed from spliced early mRNAs. E8^E2 contains a few amino acids encoded by the E8 ORF (overlaps E1) fused to the C-terminal half of the E2 protein. E1^E4 contains a few amino acids encoded by the

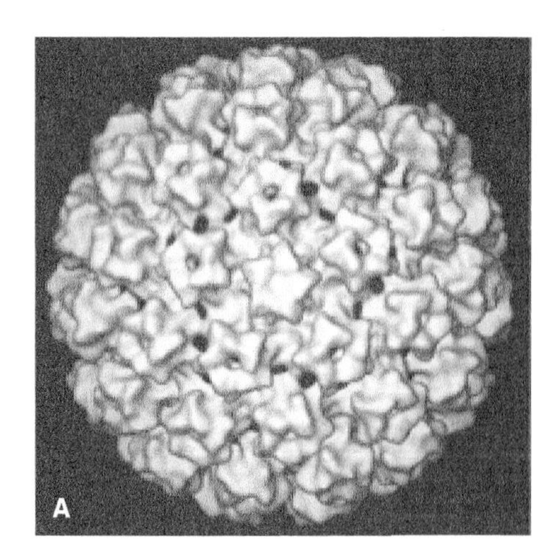

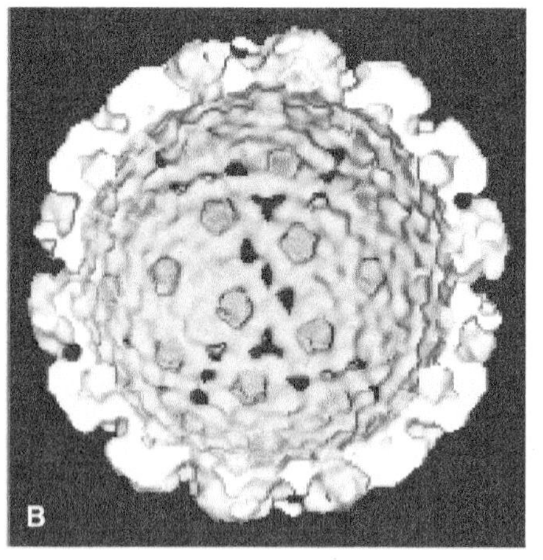

FIGURE 2.3 **A:** 3-D reconstruction of a BPV virion viewed down a 5-fold axis.[267] **B:** 3-D reconstruction of an interior/cutaway view of an HPV L1/L2 VLP with the L2 specific density shown in red. (Adapted from Buck CB, Cheng N, Thompson CD, et al. Arrangement of L2 within the papillomavirus capsid. *J Virol* 2008;82(11):5190–5197. Copyright © 2008 American Society for Microbiology. Amended with permission from American Society for Microbiology.)

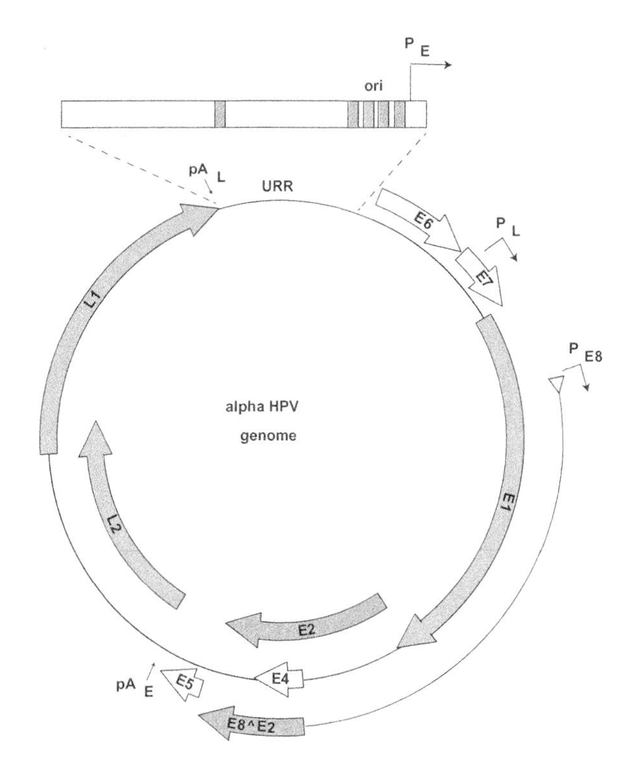

FIGURE 2.4 Oncogenic *Alphapapillomavirus* HPV genomic map. All HPVs have a circular dsDNA genome of approximately 7,000 to 8,000 bp. The location of early (E) and late (L) ORFs are shown. Only one strand is transcribed, and transcription initiates in the clockwise direction from three viral promoters P_E (early), P_{E8} (E8), and P_L (late) and terminates at one of two polyadenylation sites pA_E and pA_L. The URR is the Upstream Regulatory Region and contains the origin of DNA replication (ori). The orange boxes in the URR represent the four E2 binding sites and the blue box is the E1 binding site.

E1 ORF fused to E4, an ORF that overlaps the central portion of the E2 ORF.

Other PV genes (E5, E6, E7) are not encoded by all PVs and are likely evolutionary embellishments; these proteins help condition the cellular environment for optimal viral persistence and production. The functions of the individual ORFs are described in more detail in the relevant sections of this chapter. The E5 proteins are short hydrophobic polypeptides expressed from the ELR (early to late region) between the E2 and L2 ORFs. Notably, among the five genera of HPVs, only the *Alphapapillomavirus* HPVs encode E5 proteins. The E5 proteins encoded by different PVs can be evolutionarily unrelated, and occasionally more than one E5 is encoded by this region.[28] However, a few diverse PVs encode a hydrophobic E5-like protein that either replaces or overprints the E6 protein.[273] To avoid confusion with other ORFS, these have been designated E10 in the Papillomavirus Episteme.[272]

VIRUS REPLICATION

Papillomaviruses are highly species specific and have a specific tropism for squamous epithelial cells (reviewed in Ref.[66]). Productive infection of cells by the PVs can be divided into early, intermediate, and late stages, which are linked to the differentiation state of the epithelial cell. The tropism of the papillomaviruses for squamous epithelial cells is evidenced by the restriction of the late viral replication functions, such as vegetative viral DNA synthesis, the production of viral capsid proteins, and the assembly of virions, to differentiated epithelial cells. The close link of the papillomavirus life cycle with the differentiation program of the squamous epithelium is depicted in Figure 2.5.

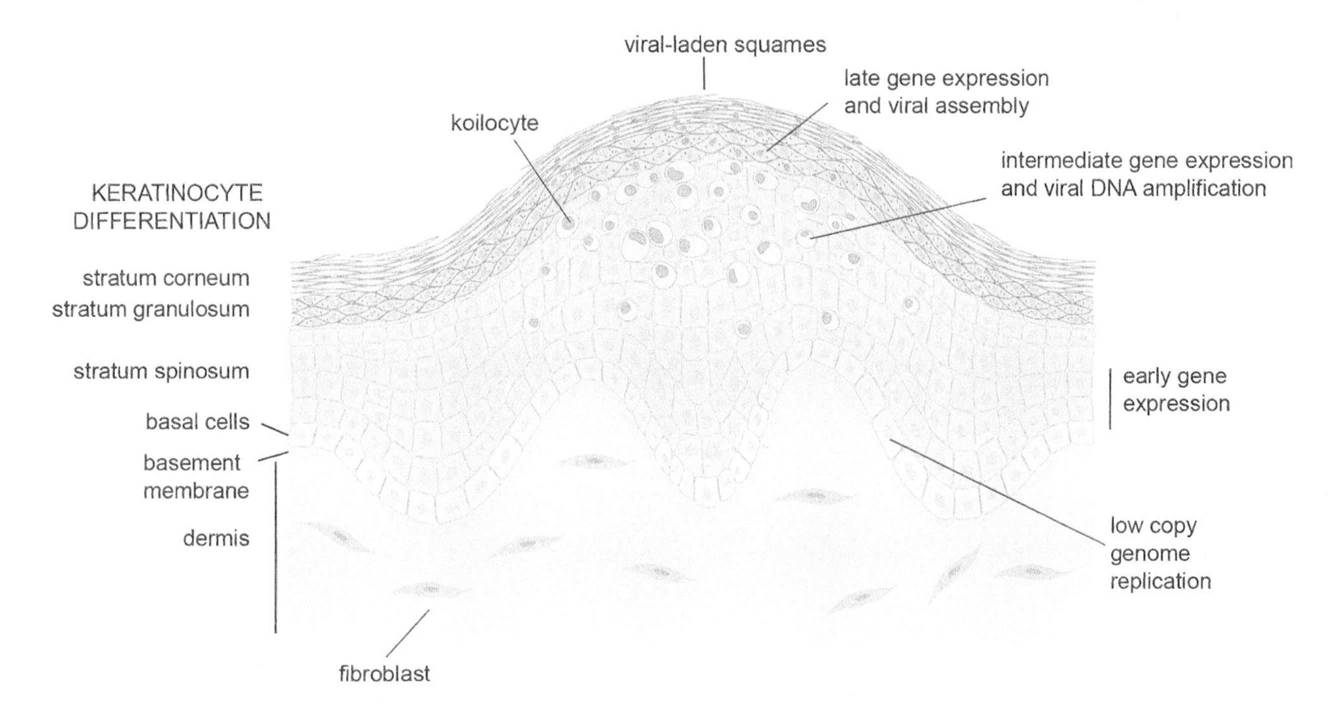

FIGURE 2.5 PV infection of cutaneous epithelia. Differentiation of normal and infected cutaneous squamous epithelium. The various epithelial strata are indicated on the left and the viral activities in the corresponding strata during productive infection are indicated. Koilocytes are atypical cells that are indicative of PV infection. Figure created with BioRender.com.

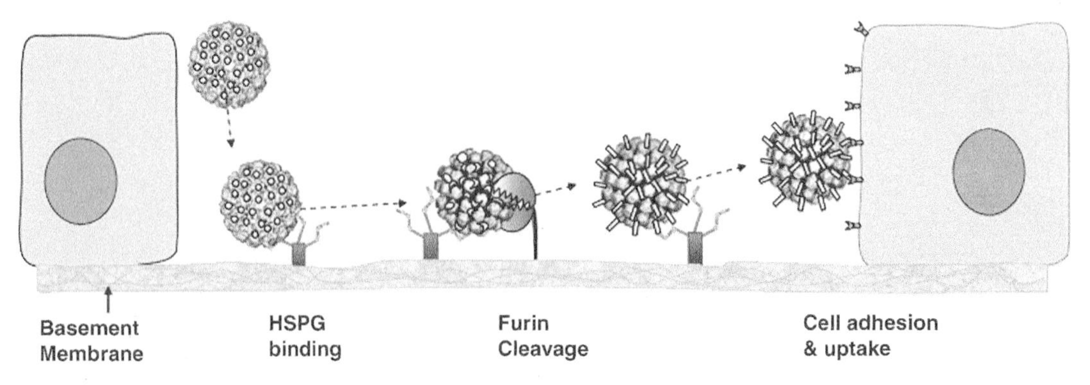

FIGURE 2.6 **Model of *in vivo* papillomavirus infection.** The virion first binds to HSPGs on the basement membrane exposed after disruption. This induces a conformational change exposing a site on L2 (depicted in *yellow*) susceptible to proprotein convertase (furin or PC5/6) cleavage. After L2 cleavage, an L2 neutralizing epitope is exposed and a previously unexposed region of L1 binds to an unidentified secondary receptor on the invading edge of the epithelial cells.

The basal cell is the only cell in the squamous epithelium capable of undergoing sustained cell division. Thus, the virus must infect the basal cell to establish a long-term, persistent infection. Only very low levels of viral DNA are found in the basal cells, but viral transcripts have been detected,[248] and at least some early viral proteins are found in basal cells.[4] Late gene expression, synthesis of capsid proteins, vegetative viral DNA synthesis, and assembly of virions occur only in terminally differentiating squamous epithelial cells.

Virion Attachment, Entry, and Trafficking

As noted above, persistent papillomavirus infection requires infection of the basal layer cells of the epithelium (reviewed in Ref.[66]). Because of the complex nature of the PV life cycle, most studies on viral entry have used *in vitro* generated virus and the following is a summary of those studies. To achieve selective infection of basal keratinocytes, the virions preferentially bind initially to heparan sulfate proteoglycans (HSPGs) on the basement membrane exposed at sites of epithelial trauma (Fig. 2.6).[127,212] This binding induces a conformational change in the capsid that exposes an N-terminal L2 peptide to cleavage by furin.[211] In one model, cleavage induces a conformational change that exposes a capsid-binding site (probably on an L1 surface) for a secondary, presently unknown, cell surface entry receptor on keratinocytes.[134] Alternatively, virions coated with HSPGs and growth factors interact with growth factor receptors, and this is essential for both cell entry and signaling of keratinocytes.[252]

Virions are internalized by endocytosis, and it was originally thought that low pH in the endosomal pathway caused disassembly of the capsid (Fig. 2.7). Recent findings, however,

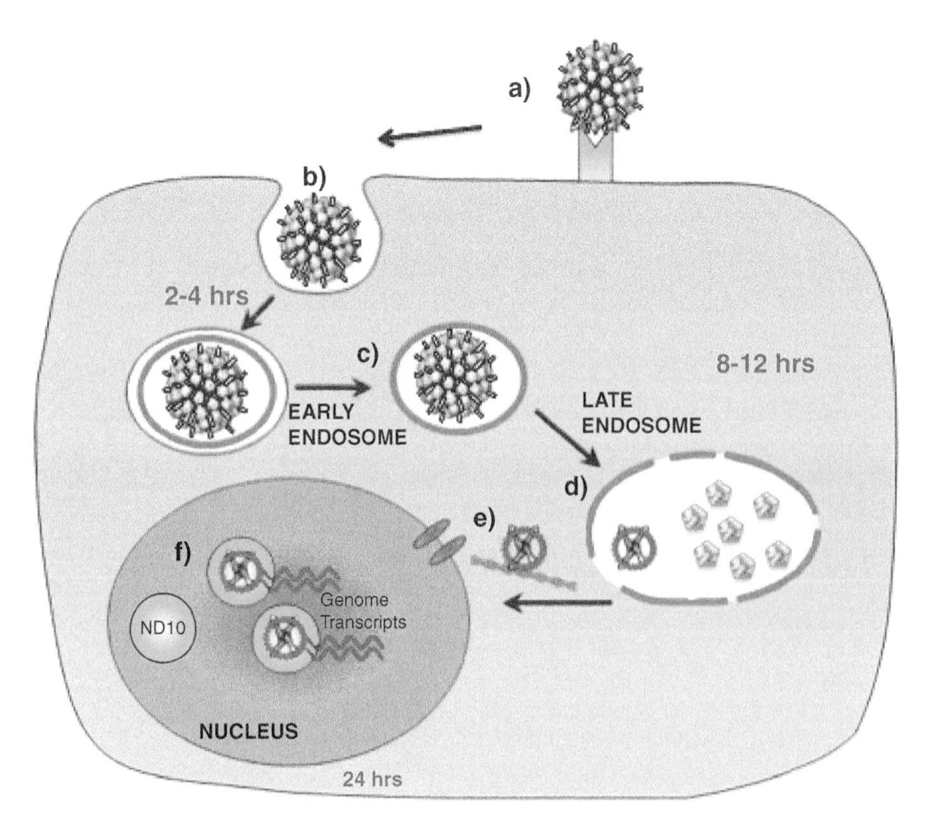

FIGURE 2.7 **Infectious process after cell binding.** After binding to a cell surface receptor (*a*), the virus enters the cell via an endocytic pathway (*b*) and within 4 hours localizes in the early endosome (*c*). By 12 hours, the virus uncoats within the late endosome and the viral genome complexed with L2 is released (*d*). The L2–genome complex traffics through the cytoplasm, perhaps via microtubules, and enters the nucleus by 24 hours (*e*). After nuclear entry, the complex colocalizes with ND10 and viral genome transcription begins (*f*).

show that the capsid-bound L2 protein undergoes further conformational changes and translocates across the endosomal membrane, resulting in intact virions enclosed in membrane vesicles.[130] The cytoplasmically exposed portion of L2 interacts with the retromer complex to traffic the viral containing vesicles to the trans-Golgi network (TGN).[61,205]

Entry of the HPV-containing vesicles into the nucleus requires nuclear envelope breakdown during mitosis, rather than active transport through nuclear pores.[208] During mitosis, the virion-containing membrane vesicles bind to condensed host mitotic chromosomes,[61] presumably to retain them in the nucleus until after the nuclear membrane reforms and prevent detection of cytoplasmic viral DNA by innate immune sensors. After cell division, specific nuclear condensates called PML nuclear bodies (PML-NBs) reform in association with the HPV containing vesicles.[101] PML-NBs are commonly hijacked by DNA viruses, and this localization promotes transcription of the HPV genome,[55] even though these structures contain antiviral factors that repress replication and transcription of incoming DNA viruses.[228] Not surprisingly, viruses counteract these repressive factors, and correspondingly HPV L2 displaces Sp100 repressors from the PML-NBs.[87]

Viral Transcription

Animal PV transcription has been studied extensively in a variety of different systems such as BPV1-infected bovine wart tissue, BPV1-infected rodent cells, MmuPV1-infected wart tissue, and SfPV1-induced lesions in cottontail rabbits. Viral transcripts have also been mapped in *Mupapillomavirus* HPVs (HPV1) and *Betapapillomavirus* HPVs (HPV5 and 8). However, best studied are those of the *Alphapapillomavirus* HPVs associated with genital tract lesions such as HPV11, HPV16, HPV18, and HPV31. Transcripts representing all stages of the infectious cycle have been identified in cervical carcinoma cell lines, differentiated organotypic culture systems, infected xenograft tissue in nude mice, and HPV-positive clinical lesions. Transcript maps for all papillomaviruses can be found at (https://pave.niaid.nih.gov/#explore/transcript_maps) (Fig. 2.8).

Viral RNAs and Promoters

Papillomavirus transcription is complex due to the presence of multiple promoters, alternate and multiple splice patterns, and the temporal synthesis of different mRNA species in differentiated cells (reviewed in Ref.[99]). In the oncogenic *Alphapapillomavirus* HPVs, transcription occurs in early, intermediate, and late phases, each dependent on the differentiation stage of the host keratinocyte. Early transcription occurs in the lower layers of a papilloma, intermediate transcription coincides with productive DNA replication, and late transcription generates the capsid proteins. A transcription map of an HPV is shown in Figure 2.8 and additional transcript maps for

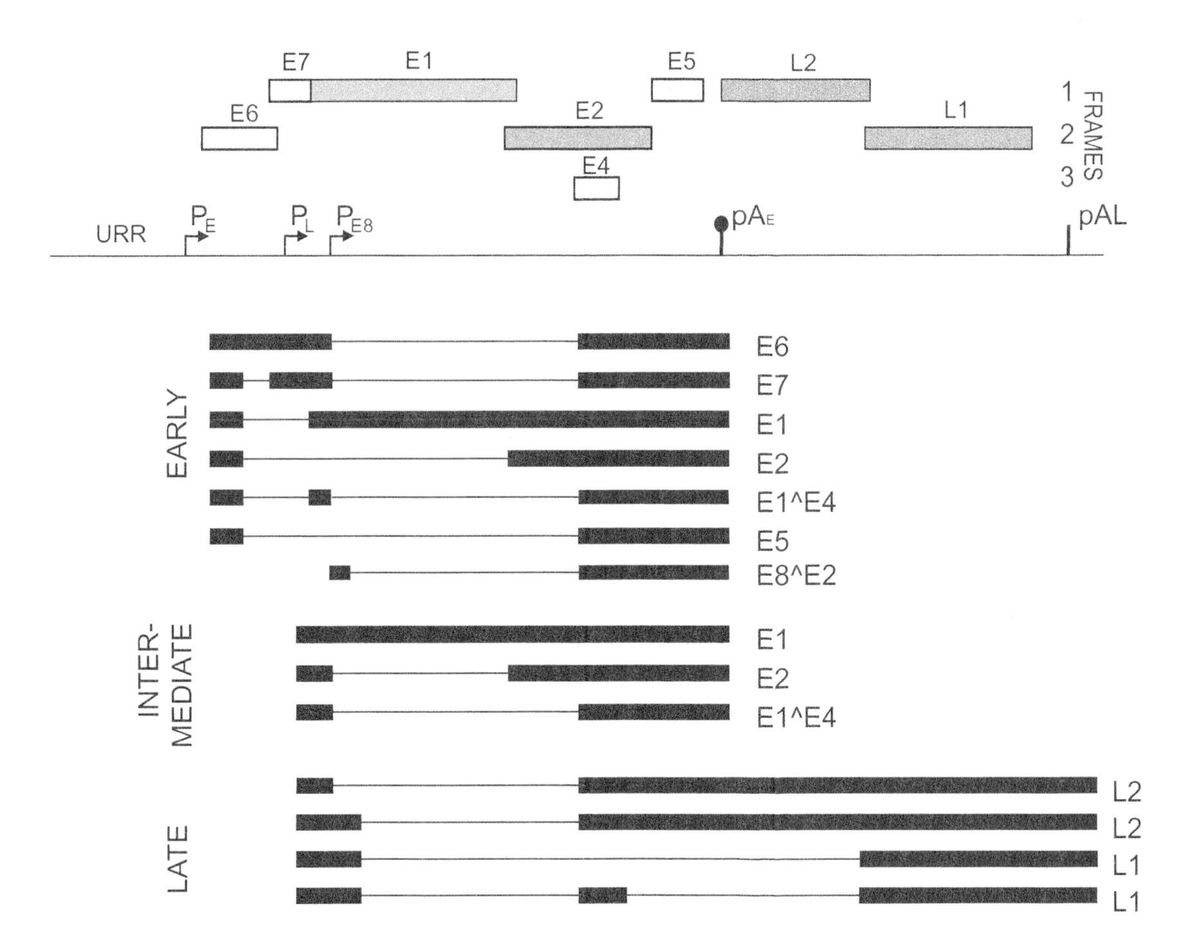

FIGURE 2.8 **Transcription map of an oncogenic *Alphapapillomavirus* HPV.** A linearized version of the viral genome is shown at the top. There are three phases of transcription depending on the differentiation status of the infected cells: Early transcripts use the early promoter (P_E) and polyadenylation site (pA_E); Intermediate transcripts use the late promoter (P_L) and early polyadenylation site (pA_E); and late transcripts use the late promoter and polyadenylation sites (P_L and pA_L).

other PVs can be found at http://pave.niaid.nih.gov/#explore/transcript_maps.

The oncogenic *Alphapapillomavirus* HPV genomes contain three promoters, P_E (early), P_{E8} (expresses the E8^E2 repressor), and P_L (late) as well as two polyadenylation sites, A_E (early) and A_L (late).[126] Multiple alternatively spliced early transcripts initiate from P_E and terminate at A_E; these express E6 and E7 as well as other early gene products. P_E is active immediately after infection whereas P_{E8} activity is delayed for several days, suggesting that E8^E2 expression might be important for maintaining low-level early transcription.[20] In the mid-layers of a papilloma, the late promoter, P_L, is activated but still uses the early polyadenylation site. This generates a series of intermediate transcripts that express high levels of E1, E2, and E4 to promote viral genome amplification.[126] At later stages of differentiation, the late promoter transcribes mRNAs that use the late polyadenylation site and encode the L1 and L2 capsid proteins.[126] Figure 2.5 shows these stages in a cutaneous papilloma.

There is an important difference in the structure and expression of the E6 and E7 mRNAs encoded by the "high-risk" and "low-risk" *Alphapapillomavirus* HPV types. The high-risk HPVs, such as HPV16 and HPV18, use a single promoter to synthesize alternatively spliced mRNAs that express E6, or E6*, and E7 proteins (Figs. 2.4 and 2.8). The E6-encoding mRNA is not able to synthesize E7 since there is insufficient spacing for translation reinitiation. The spliced E6* mRNA introduces a stop codon that allows reinitiation and translation of the E7 ORF. In contrast, the E6 and E7 genes of the low-risk HPVs such as HPV6 and HPV11 are expressed from two independent promoters.[241]

Regulation of Transcription (Cis Elements)

The URR (also known as LCR or NCR) of PVs contains enhancer elements that are responsive to cellular factors as well as to virally encoded transcriptional regulators. Each viral URR contains constitutive enhancer elements that determine tissue or cell type specificity. These constitutive enhancer elements play an important role in the initial expression of the viral genes after viral infection and may also be important for tissue tropism and maintenance of viral latency. A number of transcription factor binding sites have been identified in the URRs of multiple PVs, such as AP1, SP1, Oct-1, and YY1 (reviewed in Ref.[18]). In addition to the binding sites for cellular transcription factors, the URR contains binding sites for the virally encoded E2 proteins as well as the origin of DNA replication that contains binding sites for the E1 and E2 proteins.

E2 Regulatory Proteins

The papillomavirus E2 proteins regulate viral transcription and DNA replication and support long-term plasmid maintenance. E2 was first described as a transcriptional activator[244] capable of activating viral transcription through E2 responsive elements located within the viral genome. All E2 proteins contain two conserved domains: an N-terminal transactivation domain and a C-terminal sequence-specific DNA-binding and dimerization domain (reviewed in Ref.[168]). These domains are linked by a hinge region that is not well conserved in length or amino acid composition among different papillomaviruses. The dimeric E2 proteins bind the consensus sequence, $ACCN_6GGT$,[6,153] and regulate transcription from promoters containing E2 binding sites (reviewed in Ref.[168]).

The structure of the dimeric DNA-binding domain of E2 has been solved for many papillomaviruses and forms a previously unobserved DNA-binding fold of a dimeric antiparallel β barrel.[110] The structure of the N-terminal transactivation domain has also been solved for several PVs (https://pave.niaid.nih.gov/#explore/proteins/protein_structure_viewer/table_of_available_protein_structures/). It forms a cashew-shaped structure; the N-terminal portion consists of three antiparallel alpha-helices and is joined to a C-terminal antiparallel β-sheet structure by a region called the fulcrum[9] as shown in Figure 2.9.

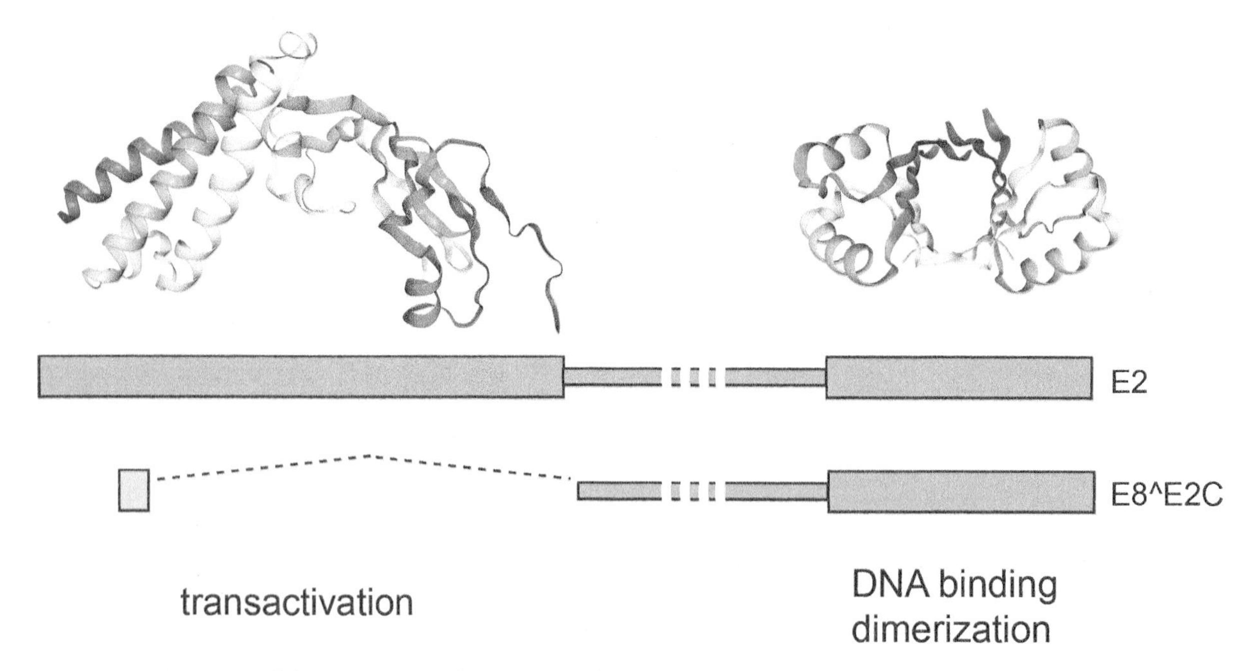

FIGURE 2.9 Structure of the E2 proteins. The structures of the HPV E2 and E8^E2 proteins are shown. The N-terminal transactivation domain is approximately 200 amino acids and is only present in the full-length form of E2 (HPV16 structure shown from 1DTO[9]).The C-terminal DNA-binding and dimerization domain is approximately 100 amino acids (HPV16 structure is shown Ref.[110]). These conserved domains are linked by a less well-conserved hinge of variable length and sequence.

In addition to the full-length E2 protein, all PVs encode a shorter repressor E2 protein named E8^E2 (reviewed in Refs.[69,168]). E8^E2 consists of a few amino acids encoded by the E8 ORF (overlaps E1) fused to the hinge and C-terminal domain of E2 (Fig. 2.9). These proteins antagonize both the replication and transcriptional regulatory functions by competing for DNA-binding sites and by forming inactive heterodimers with the full-length transactivator protein. E8^E2 proteins also recruit cellular corepressor complexes such as NCoR and SMRT.[68,207] The repressor functions of E8^E2 are important for maintaining low-level DNA replication and transcription as viruses that are mutated to eliminate E8^E2 expression spontaneously replicate to high copy number and synthesize high levels of viral DNA.[69] Some PVs, such as BPV1, encode two E2 repressor proteins, E2-TR and E8^E2.[69]

Full-length E2 proteins both activate and repress viral transcription, and this depends on the position of the cognate DNA-binding sites with respect to other promoter and enhancer elements. In the high-risk *Alphapapillomavirus* HPVs, there are four E2-binding sites in the URR that mediate this regulation (Fig. 2.4). The binding of *Alphapapillomavirus* HPV E2 to binding sites adjacent to the major early promoter results in its down-regulation.[259] Notably, this repression requires factors that interact with the transactivation domain of the full-length E2 protein, such as the Brd4 protein,[240,293] as well as the histone demethylase SMCX and components of the TIP60 complex including EP400.[240]

The interaction of E2 with Brd4 is also required for the transcriptional activation function of all PV E2 proteins.[120] Brd4 is a member of the BET family, proteins containing two bromodomains and one extra-terminal (ET) domain; the bromodomains bind acetylated lysines in histones and regulate transcriptional initiation and elongation.[63] Two highly conserved amino acid residues in the E2 transactivation domain interact with Brd4 and are required for E2 transactivation.

In addition to its role as a transcriptional regulator, E2 has critical roles in the initiation of viral DNA replication and long-term extrachromosomal maintenance of viral genomes within replicating cells, and this is described in detail below. The multiple functions of E2 are mediated by interactions with specific cellular factors, the best studied of which are listed in Table 2.1.

The late promoter (located in the E7 ORF in high-risk *Alphapapillomavirus* HPVs) is activated in early differentiating cells to generate transcripts that express high levels of E1^E4 and the E1 and E2 replication proteins. The late promoter is regulated by cellular activators and repressors that are modulated during keratinocyte differentiation.[39,291] Transcriptional elongation factors such as Brd4 provide further regulation of the late promoter.[243] The viral minichromosome contains a chromatin loop, mediated by CTCF and YY1, that suppresses viral enhancer activity.[197] Differentiation-dependent down-regulation of YY1 disrupts this loop and relieves suppression of the enhancer.[197]

Activation of late viral transcription occurs in terminally differentiated keratinocytes to express mRNA encoding the capsid proteins.[126] In fact, regulation of read-through of the early polyadenylation site constitutes the major switch from early to late gene expression.[126] True late mRNAs initiate at P_L and terminate at the late polyadenylation site, A_L. Late HPV mRNAs contain negative regulatory elements that reduce mRNA stability and inhibit RNA processing in undifferentiated cells (reviewed in Ref.[99]), and keratinocyte differentiation reduces levels of repressor proteins that bind these elements.

Virion Assembly and Release

Virion assembly takes place in the nuclei of terminally differentiated keratinocytes after vegetative viral genome amplification and expression of the capsid proteins.[64] *In vitro*, the L1 protein can self-assemble into VLPs, but L2 enhances packaging of viral DNA.[136,300] The viral genome does not require a sequence-specific packaging signal[34] and is assembled with host histones into a chromatinized minichromosome.[81] The capsids are further stabilized by the formation of disulfide bonds between conserved cysteines on adjacent L1 monomers induced by the oxidizing environment in the upper layers of a terminally differentiated squamous epithelium.[50] PVs are not cytolytic, and virions are released in squames that slough off the surface of the epithelium. E4-mediated collapse of cytokeratin filaments in these terminally differentiated cells might assist in virion release.[65]

Viral DNA Replication

The differentiation-dependent PV life cycle requires different modes of viral DNA replication at different stages (reviewed in Ref.[169]). Following infection of a basal keratinocyte, there is a limited amplification of the viral genome, which then becomes established as a stable, low copy plasmid. The viral genomes are maintained at a constant copy number in dividing cells and replicate on average once per cell cycle during S phase, in synchrony with host DNA replication.[96] This ensures persistent infection in the basal cells of the epidermis. Vegetative DNA replication occurs in the more differentiated cells of the infected epithelium. Such differentiated cells have exited the cell cycle and are no longer capable of supporting cellular DNA synthesis. Therefore, the virus activates the DNA damage response and uses DNA repair machinery to support vegetative viral DNA synthesis producing the genomes to be packaged into progeny virions.[179]

Origin of DNA Replication

Papillomavirus DNA replication requires the origin of DNA replication in cis and the viral E1 and E2 proteins in trans. The minimal origin of DNA replication contains an A/T rich region, an E1 binding site, and an E2 binding site.[269] E1 is an ATP-dependent helicase that binds and unwinds DNA at the replication origin.[80] E2 is a helicase loader that binds to E1 and facilitates binding of an E1–E2 complex to the replication origin.[247]

The E1 Protein

The E1 protein is well conserved among the PVs and is an origin-binding, ATP-dependent helicase. E1 contains four domains: an N-terminal regulatory domain, an origin DNA-binding domain, an oligomerization domain, and a helicase/ATPase domain and a C-terminal tail.[17,80] E1 binds to its cognate site in the origin with weak affinity; however, this binding is enhanced through its interaction with E2, which binds to adjacent DNA-binding motifs.[178,269] In addition to its interaction with E2, E1 has been shown to bind a number of cellular proteins such as Replication Protein A (RPA), DNA polymerase α-primase and DNA topoisomerase I (topo I) and thereby recruits the cellular

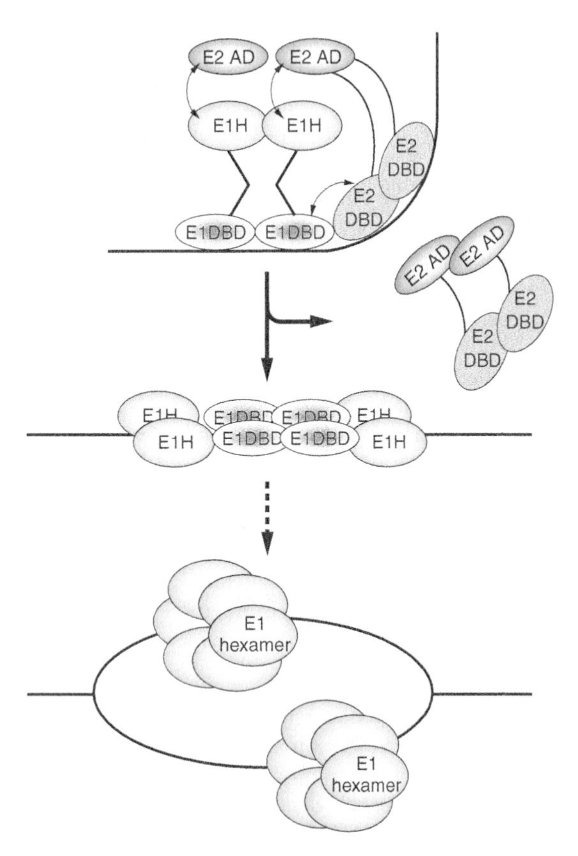

FIGURE 2.10 Proposed pathway for the assembly of an initiation-competent complex at the BPV origin of DNA replication. The E1 initiator binds cooperatively with E2 to the ori forming a specific E1$_2$E2$_2$–DNA complex. As a consequence of the interaction between the E1 and E2 DNA binding domains (DBDs), a sharp bend is induced in the ori DNA. The bend promotes the interaction between the E1 helicase domain (E1H) and the E2 transactivation domain (E2AD). The resulting highly sequence-specific complex serves to recognize the ori. In a reaction requiring ATP hydrolysis, E2 is displaced and additional E1 molecules are added to the complex, resulting in the formation of a complex where four molecules of E1 are bound to the ori. This complex can distort the DNA duplex and give rise to partially single stranded regions. Subsequently, additional E1 molecules are added. In a final step, E1 is assembled onto the exposed single strands forming a hexameric ring-like structure that constitutes the replicative helicase. This figure was graciously provided by Arne Stenlund and represents a modified version of a published figure.[79]

DNA replication initiation machinery to the viral replication origin (reviewed in Ref.[17]). After the E1/E2 complex binds the origin, E2 is displaced, and E1 ultimately forms a double hexameric structure that bidirectionally unwinds DNA (Fig. 2-10). The expression and intracellular localization of E1 is tightly regulated in dividing cells. The N-terminal domain contains nucleo–cytoplasmic shuttling elements that are regulated by phosphorylation to ensure that E1 localizes to the nucleus in a cell cycle–dependent manner (reviewed in Ref.[17]).

E2 Protein Replication Functions

E2 serves as an auxiliary factor that fosters the assembly of the preinitiation complex at the origin, but E2 itself plays no intrinsic role in viral DNA replication. E2 cooperatively binds with E1 to the replication origin (reviewed in Ref.[168]) and interacts with many cellular factors that can support and promote viral DNA replication (see Table 2.1).

Plasmid Maintenance Replication

E2 plays a critical role in viral DNA replication by supporting long-term maintenance of extrachromosomal viral genomes. This was first defined for BPV1, where it was shown that genome maintenance requires, in addition to the replication origin, a minichromosome maintenance element from the

TABLE 2.1 Cellular proteins interacting with papillomavirus E2 and E8^E2 proteins

Category	Examples of E2 Interacting Proteins	References
Nuclear matrix	MATR3; HNRNPU; HNRNPA1	(123)
Posttranslational modification	CSNK2A1, CSNK2A2, CSNK2B; SRPK1/2; PRMT5; PPP2CA/CB/R1A, BAZ1B	(123)
DNA replication/repair	RFC 2-5; ATAD5; WICH (BAZ1B, SMARCA5); TOPBP1; RINT1; CHLR1; ORC2	(24,38,60,123,191,222)
Transcription factor, chromatin binding, modifying, and remodeling	BRD4; Polycomb (E2F6, PCGF6, RNF2), NAP1, KDM1B; WDR5; WHSC (WHSC1/WHSCL1, SALL4); PRMT5; EHMT1; TTRAP/TIP60 (INO80, p400, TRRAP; NCOR1, HDAC, SAP18, KDM5C, GPS2 SWI/SNF (SMARCA4 and SMARCA2), NuRD (CHD4, SMARCA5, HDAC1/2, MTA1/2); WICH (BAZ1B, SMARCA5); TRRAP/TIP60 (INO80, EP400, TRRAP); NM1;	(13,123,147,180,222,239,240,293,295)
RNA processing	SRFS1, 2, 7, 10; C1QBP, CTCF	(123,180)
Chromosome structure	SMC5/6	(16,123,293)
Intracellular trafficking	VPS52, clathrin, RAB3IP, CDC20	(180)
Apoptosis	P53	(180,192)
E2 ubiquitylation	CUL3, SKP2	(15,180,299)
Papillomavirus E1 protein	Viral DNA replication	(178)
Papillomavirus L1 protein	Viral DNA replication, assembly	(236)

URR containing multiple E2-binding sites.[203] Both the E2 protein and viral genomes are observed in association with host mitotic chromosomes, leading to the model that E2 facilitates viral genome partitioning by interacting simultaneously with condensed mitotic chromatin and the viral genomes, thereby ensuring that viral genomes are contained within the nuclear envelope when it reforms during telophase.[121,238] The cellular protein Brd4 mediates the association of BPV1 E2 with mitotic chromosomes. The TA domain of BPV1 E2 associates with mitotic chromosomes and mutations that abrogate Brd4 binding also disrupt the tethering of E2 and viral genomes.[2,13,295] Brd4 may also be the tethering factor for some other PVs. Binding of E2 to Brd4 is conserved among all the papillomaviruses and plays an important role in the transcriptional activity of E2.[123,230,295]

Additional cellular factors are likely to be involved in E2-mediated tethering to mitotic chromosomes and PV genome maintenance. For instance, ChlR1 has been shown to be important for loading E2 onto mitotic chromosomes.[191] Also, the E2 proteins of some *Alphapapillomavirus* HPV types have been observed in association with the mitotic spindle rather than the chromosomes.[275] Finally, some E2 proteins bind at the ribosomal DNA loci on the short arm of acrocentric chromosomes.[189,204] Thus, the precise mechanism that ensure the stable maintenance of HPV genomes in host cells is still unresolved and will be a fruitful area for additional studies (reviewed in Ref.[51]).

Vegetative Viral DNA Replication

Vegetative replication of papillomavirus occurs only in the infected terminally differentiated keratinocytes and generates progeny genomes destined to be packaged in virions. These differentiated cells are no longer in S phase and need an alternative mode to synthesize DNA. Therefore, the virus expresses high levels of E1 and E2 and induces a DNA damage response that recruits numerous replication and repair factors to viral replication foci in the nucleus of infected cells.[88,179,221] There is evidence that replication switches from a bidirectional theta mode to a rolling circle, or recombination-directed replication mode late in infection.[86,220]

VIRAL TRANSFORMATION

BPV1 Transformation

Certain papillomaviruses are capable of inducing cellular transformation in tissue culture. The best studied of the transforming papillomaviruses is BPV1. Morphologic transformation in tissue culture was first described for BPV in the early 1960's.[21,23,262] In the late 1970's, a focus assay was developed using established cell lines to study BPV1 transformation.[74] In general, investigators have relied upon mouse C127 cells and NIH 3T3 cells for these transformation studies, although a variety of other rodent cells, including hamster and rat cells, are susceptible to BPV1-mediated transformation. Transformation of mouse C127 cells by BPV1 causes alterations in morphology, loss of contact inhibition, anchorage independence, and tumorigenicity in nude mice.[74]

One notable characteristic of BPV1-transformed rodent cells is that the viral DNA is maintained as a stable multicopy plasmid.[150] Integration of the viral genome is not required for either the initiation or maintenance of the transformed state. However, transformation is dependent upon the continued expression of viral genes as evidenced by the loss of the transformed phenotype in mouse cells that have been "cured" of the viral DNA by treatment with interferon.[268] Genetic studies mapped the BPV1 transforming genes to E5, E6, and E7.

BPV1 E5

The E5 gene is the major transforming gene of BPV1 in transformed cells. E5 encodes a small (44 amino acid) integral membrane protein that is sufficient for the transformation of certain established rodent cells in culture. E5 is highly conserved among the group of papillomaviruses that induce fibropapillomas in their natural host and have the capacity to induce fibroblastic tumors in hamsters. The E5 gene is believed to be responsible for the proliferation of dermal fibroblasts in fibropapillomas.

The E5 protein does not possess intrinsic enzymatic activity, and functions by altering the activity of cellular membrane proteins involved in proliferation. The first evidence that BPV1 E5 could activate growth factor receptors came from experiments that showed that E5 could cooperate with exogenously introduced EGF receptor or CSF1 receptor in the transformation of NIH3T3 cells.[163] Subsequent studies established the β-receptor for the platelet derived growth factor (PDGF) as the endogenous target for the BPV1 E5 protein in fibroblasts.[62,198] E5 activates the PDGF β receptor and transforms cells in a ligand-independent manner.[198,199] The mechanism of E5 activation of the PDGF β receptor involves complex formation with the receptor, thereby inducing receptor dimerization, trans-phosphorylation of tyrosine residues in the cytoplasmic domain of the receptor, and recruitment of cellular SH2 domain–containing proteins into a signal transduction complex.[62] Two transmembrane dimers of E5 clamp the PDGF β receptor in an active dimeric conformation.[132]

BPV1 E5 has also been shown to form a complex with the 16 kDa transmembrane channel-forming subunit of the vacuolar H^+-ATPase,[98] an abundant cellular protein located in the membranes of intracytoplasmic membranes and plasma membranes. Golgi acidification has been found to be impaired in cells transformed by the BPV1 E5 protein, due to the inhibition of the vacuolar H^+-ATPase.[223] It has not yet been shown directly that Golgi alkalinization plays a role in cellular transformation, but there is a good genetic correlation between the ability of specific E5 mutants to transform cells and Golgi alkalization.[223] Since many important growth regulatory proteins, including the PDGF β-receptor, transit through the Golgi apparatus, it is possible that the ability of E5 to perturb the pH of intracellular organelles might affect the activity of some of these proteins and in so doing, contribute to the transformed phenotype. It is additionally possible that the BPV1-mediated Golgi alkalinization may affect cellular functions unrelated to transformation that are important in the life cycle of the virus.

BPV1 E6

The BPV1 E6 and E7 genes also encode proteins with transforming activities. In mouse cells, the full transformed phenotype requires the expression of the E6 and E7 genes as well as E5.[184] The E6 and E7 genes of all the papillomaviruses encode proteins with conserved structural motifs. They contain domains of almost identically spaced CYS-X-X-CYS motifs (four in E6 and two in the carboxy-terminal portion of E7), that are involved in binding zinc.

No intrinsic enzymatic activities have been identified for BPV1 E6, and, like the oncogenic HPV E6 proteins, it likely functions through binding cellular targets. Several different cellular proteins have been found to interact with BPV1 E6 but the physiologic significance of a number of these putative cellular interacting proteins has not been established and may represent artifacts due to overexpression. There is, however, a good correlation between the transforming activities of BPV1 E6 and the binding to the focal adhesion protein paxillin.[265,276] This binding has also been shown to correlate with the disruption of the cellular actin cytoskeleton, a characteristic of transformed cells.[266] E6 binds to charged leucine motifs in paxillin known as LD motifs and in doing so competes with the ability of paxillin to bind to vinculin and the focal adhesion kinase.[266,276] Another cellular target of BPV1 E6 revealed by systematic proteomic studies is Mastermind-like 1 (MAML1).[32,217,256] MAML1 is a core component of the transcriptional activation complex that mediates the effects of the canonical Notch signaling pathway.[292] BPV1 as well as the *Betapapillomavirus* HPV E6 proteins repress Notch transcriptional activation, and this repression is dependent on an interaction with MAML1. Furthermore, the expression levels of endogenous Notch target genes are repressed by E6 proteins[256] interfering with keratinocyte differentiation.[175]

BPV1 E7

The E7 gene encodes a 127 amino acid zinc-binding protein that potentates the transforming activities of other BPV1 oncogenes. By itself, BPV1 E7 does not induce focus formation or anchorage independence, but enhances the transformation activity of BPV1 E5 and BPV1 E6.[22] When BPV1 E7 is coexpressed with either E5 or E6, it synergizes with these oncogenes to boost transformation efficiency four- to tenfold. Unlike the HPV E7 proteins, BPV1 E7 does not contain an LxCxE motif for binding the retinoblastoma tumor suppressor gene product (pRB), and it does not share the property of pRB binding and inactivation with the HPV E7 proteins.

BPV1 E7 binds the N-end rule E3 ligase UBR4 (initially referred to as p600),[59] and subsequently E7 binding to UBR4 was shown to be a characteristic of all the human HPVs.[286] For BPV1, the interaction between UBR4 and E7 correlates with the ability of E7 to enhance E6-mediated transformation.[58] BPV1 E7, similar to the HPV E7 proteins, also binds the nonreceptor protein tyrosine phosphatase PTPN14.[285] Similar to the HPV E7 proteins, BPV1 E7 causes the degradation of PTPN14, a process that is mediated by UBR-4.[285] This process and the cellular consequences are discussed below under the HPV E7 proteins.

HPV Immortalization and Transformation

The HPV16 and HPV18 genomes are not efficient at inducing transformation of established rodent cells; however, immortalization assays employing primary rodent cells, primary human fibroblast, and/or primary human keratinocytes have provided assays for studying their immortalization/transformation functions. In such assays, the high-risk HPVs, such as HPV16 and HPV18, are positive for immortalization or transformation, whereas the low-risk viruses, such as HPV6 and HPV11, are not.[229,249] These assays permitted the mapping of the E6 and E7 as viral oncogenes for the high-risk HPV types.

HPV E6

The HPV E6 proteins are approximately 150 amino acids in size and contain four Cys-X-X-Cys motifs that are involved in binding zinc. The first transforming activity identified for the high-risk alpha genus HPV E6 proteins (such as HPVs 16 and 18) was the ability to complement E7 in the immortalization of human keratinocytes.[109,182] This activity is explained at least in part by its ability to complex p53,[283] a property not possessed by the low-risk alpha genus HPV E6 proteins. The protein levels of p53 are generally quite low in HPV positive carcinoma cell lines and in cells immortalized by the HPV oncoproteins,[225] since high-risk HPV E6 proteins promote the ubiquitin-dependent degradation of p53.[227] Indeed the half-life of p53 is dramatically decreased in E6-expressing cells, and E6 dampens the p53 response when cells are challenged with genotoxic agents.[114,225] In targeting p53, the high-risk HPV E6 proteins inhibit DNA damage and oncogene-mediated cell death signals.[78,129,133]

HPV16 E6 induces p53 degradation by forming a complex with the cellular ubiquitin–protein ligase E6AP,[117,118] which is then able to bind and ubiquitylate p53 (Fig. 2.11).[224] E6AP is the founding member of a class of ubiquitin–protein ligases called HECT E3 proteins, which directly transfer ubiquitin to their substrates.[226] The catalytic domain of HECT proteins is a conserved 350 amino acid region defined by its *h*omology to the *E*6AP *c*arboxy *t*erminus (HECT).[116] The HECT domain binds to specific E2 enzymes and contains an active site cysteine residue that forms a thiolester bond with ubiquitin.[116,226] Structure studies have determined that the HECT domain is a bilobed structure, with a larger N-terminal lobe that interacts with the ubiquitin-conjugating enzyme, and a smaller C-terminal lobe containing the catalytic cysteine residue.[113]

Levels of p53 in E6 immortalized cells or in HPV-positive cervical carcinoma cells are, on average, two to three fold lower compared to primary cells.[225] In normal, non–HPV expressing cells, intracellular p53 levels increase significantly in response to DNA damage or genotoxic stress. Expression of the high-risk E7 proteins and their engagement of the pRB family of proteins causes a replication stress resulting in an increase in p53 protein levels within cells, which in turn transcriptionally activates the expression of cell cycle arrest genes and proapoptotic genes.[1,129] E7 also creates a signal that increases p53 levels by up-regulating expression of the long noncoding RNA DINO.[233] Higher levels of p53 can result in a G_1 growth arrest or apoptosis, as part of a cell defense mechanism that allows for either the repair of the DNA damage prior to the initiation of a new round of DNA replication or cell death. E6-expressing cells however do not manifest a p53-mediated cellular response to DNA damage,[133] indicating the ability of E6 to promote the degradation of p53 and prevent the p53 level to rise above a certain threshold level (Fig. 2.12). Under DNA-damaging conditions, the E6-stimulated degradation of p53 abrogates the negative growth regulatory effects of p53 and as such contributes to genomic instability. E6 hijacks E6AP to form a ternary complex with p53. E6AP does not normally regulate p53 protein stability in non–E6 expressing cells. Mdm2 is the major E3 ubiquitin ligase responsible for p53 degradation in the absence of E6.[108,145]

The E6AP protein is encoded by the UBE3A gene that is located in an imprinted region on chromosome 15q11-q13, and it has been linked to Angelman syndrome, a neurogenetic disorder characterized by severe mental retardation, ataxia, loss of speech, seizures, and other abnormalities.[137,167] An increase in UBE3A gene dosage has also been linked to autism spectrum disorders.[187] Although a number of E6AP interacting proteins and potential substrates, including RAD23A, UBQLN1/2, and the estrogen receptor have been described, the physiological

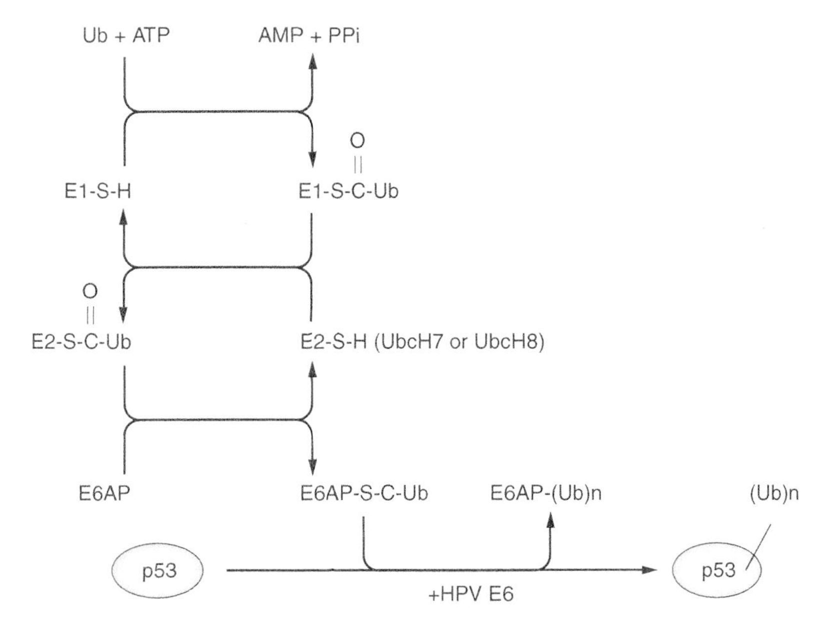

FIGURE 2.11 A ubiquitin thiolester cascade model for the HPV E6-dependent ubiquitination of p53. The E6 protein binds to the cellular protein E6-AP, and the complex together functions as an E3 (ubiquitin protein ligase) in facilitating the ubiquitination of p53.[224] The ubiquitination of a protein involves three cellular activities: E1 (ubiquitin activating enzyme), E2 (ubiquitin conjugating enzyme), and E3 (ubiquitin protein ligase). Ubiquitin is activated in an ATP-dependent manner and forms a high-energy thiolester with E1, which can then be transferred to the E2 through a thiolester linkage. Ubiquitin can then be transferred to a cysteine within the Hect domain of E6AP, again as a thiolester linkage,[226] through the direct binding of E6AP with UbcH7 or UbcH8.[148] In conjunction with HPV16 E6, E6AP then recognizes p53 and catalyses the formation of an isopeptide bond between the carboxy-terminal glycine of ubiquitin and a lysine side chain of p53.

relevance of some of these E6AP interactions is often uncertain.[140,149,152] E6AP is a component of a number of cellular complexes, including the proteasome and a 2MDa HUN complex that contains Herc2 and Neurl4.[164] E6 is recruited to each of these complexes by E6AP.

The crystal structure of the E6 protein bound to the 12-amino acid alpha helical LxxLL containing peptide of E6AP and the DNA binding domain of p53 was solved.[165] The binding of E6 to E6AP activates its E3 ligase activity and induces E6AP self-ubiquitylation.[131,257] The binding of E6 to E6AP

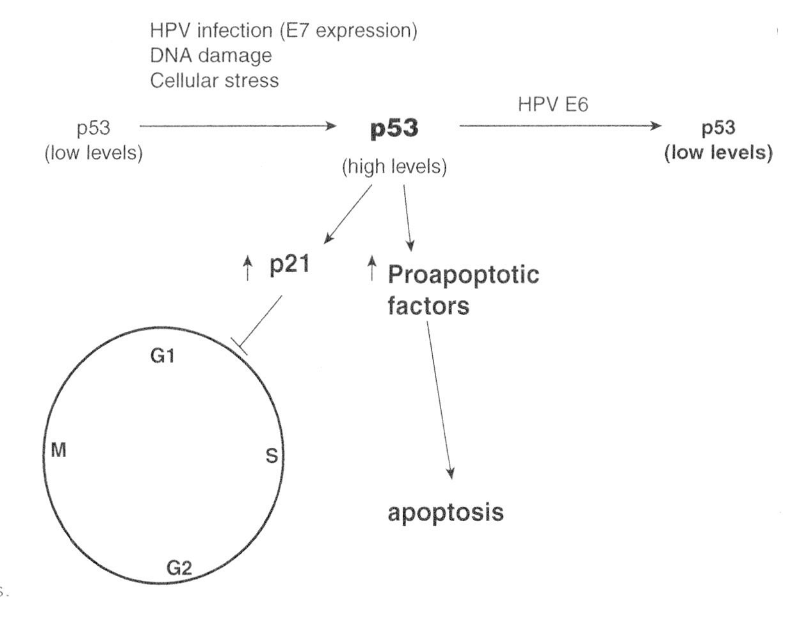

FIGURE 2.12 The level of p53 in primary cells is generally low. DNA damaging agents, viral infection, and expression of E7 increase the level of p53. Elevated levels of p53 can lead to either apoptosis or a cell cycle checkpoint arrest in G1 through the transcriptional activation of proapoptotic genes or p21^{cip1}. Viral oncoproteins may interfere with this negative growth regulatory function of p53, either by sequestering p53 into a stable, but nonfunctional complex (such as with SV40 TAg or the Ad5 55 kDa E1B protein) or by ubiquitylation and enhanced proteolysis as observed with the high-risk HPV E6 proteins.

causes a conformational change positioning E6 and p53 in the immediate vicinity of the catalytic center of E6AP.[219]

E6 encodes a number of p53-independent functions that are relevant to cellular transformation and immortalization. There are HPV16 E6 mutations that separate p53 degradation from cellular immortalization,[138,156] and it is possible that some of these p53-independent activities are still mediated by E6AP. One such function is its ability to activate telomerase in keratinocytes[141] through the transcriptional up-regulation of the rate-limiting catalytic subunit of human telomerase (hTERT).[138,188,277] Maintenance of telomere length is an important step in cellular immortalization and transformation, which occurs either through the transcriptional activation of hTERT expression or through the activation of the ALT recombination pathway. The mechanism of hTERT promoter activation by E6 is complex and controversial. Some studies have implicated c-Myc binding and activating the hTert promoter, and others show the E6AP-dependent degradation of the NFX1-91 transcriptional repressor of the hTERT promoter.[94,95] Interactions of E6 with E6AP as well as c-Myc have been shown to be important in the transcriptional activation of the hTERT promoter.[154,155,278,294]

Of note, the high-risk E6 oncoproteins contain a X-(S/T)-X-(V/I/L)-COOH motif at the extreme C-terminus that mediates binding with cellular PDZ domain–containing proteins. This PDZ binding motif (PBM) is unique in the high-risk HPV E6 proteins and is not present in the E6 proteins of the low-risk alpha genus HPV types. Although E6 could serve as a molecular bridge between these PDZ domain proteins and E6AP, facilitating their ubiquitylation and mediating their proteolysis, there is some evidence that the degradation of the PDZ domain–containing proteins may be E6AP independent.[166] Among the PDZ domain proteins implicated as E6 targets are hDlg, the human homologue of the Drosophila melanogaster Discs large tumor suppressor, and hScrib, the human homologue of the Drosophila Scribble tumor suppressor.[90,183] Additional PDZ domain proteins shown to be capable of binding to E6 are MAGI-1, MAGI-2, MAGI-3, MUPP1, and TIP-2/GIPC.[82,97,151,263] Several of the PDZ-containing proteins have been shown to be involved in negatively regulating cellular proliferation. Therefore, some of the p53-independent transforming activities of the high-risk E6 oncoproteins may be linked to their ability to bind and degrade some of these PDZ motif–containing proteins.[139,185]

Other activities of the hrHPV E6 proteins include the induction of genomic instability,[210,284] the maintenance of stable episomal replication during the viral life cycle,[194] and the immortalization of human mammary epithelial cells.[11,232] E6 has also been shown to up-regulate the expression of the innate immune DNA cytosine deaminase APOBEC3B.[279] The up-regulation of APOBEC3B is likely a significant source of genomic mutagenesis observed in multiple human cancers, including HPV-associated cancers. Recently, DNA damage response pathways have been shown to directly signal to the E6 PBM, resulting in Chk1- and Chk2-driven phosphorylation that can result in the enhanced ability of E6 to inhibit p53 transcriptional activity,[258] thus providing a link between the PBM and E6 regulation of p53 functions.

HPV16 E6 has also been reported to bind the transcriptional coactivator p300/CBP, a target also of Ad E1A and SV40 large T-antigen.[196,301] This interaction is limited to E6 proteins of high-risk HPVs associated with cervical cancer that have the capacity to repress p53-dependent transcription. The repression of p53 transcriptional activity by targeting the p53 coactivator CBP/p300 provides a second mechanism by which p53 can be inhibited. A subsequent study has shown that *in vitro*, E6 can inhibit p300-mediated acetylation on p53 and nucleosomal core histones.[264] A variety of other E6 cellular targets have been identified (Table 2.2); however, the physiologic

TABLE 2.2 Cellular targets of the papillomavirus E6 oncoproteins

Target	Function	Reference
E6-associated protein (E6AP) (alpha genus HPVs)	Ubiquitylation of associated proteins Ubiquitylation of E6	(224) (131)
MAML1 (beta genus HPVs)	Repress Notch transcription and signaling	(32,217,256)
p53	E6AP-dependent ubiquitylation and proteolysis	(227,283)
E6BP (Erc55)	Unknown	(43)
Paxillin	Disruption of the actin cytoskeleton	(266,276)
PDZ domain–containing proteins: HDlg, MUPP1, and hScrib (HR HPVs only)	E6AP-dependent ubiquitination and proteolysis	(90,151,183)
NHERF1	Degradation with activation of Wnt/β-catenin signaling	(70)
IRF-3	Inhibition of β-interferon induction	(213)
Clathrin adaptor complex AP-1	Unknown	(265)
Bak	Inhibition of Bak-induced apoptosis	(261)
CBP/p300	Inhibition of p53 transcriptional activity	(196,301)
Myc	Activation of cellular telomerase	(155)
NFX1-91	Activation of cellular telomerase	(94,95)
USP15	Stabilization of E6 Innate immune signaling	(280) (47)
USP46	Stabilization of Cdt2	(135)
ADA3	Transcriptional regulation	(146)
FADD/Caspase 8	Block apoptosis	(84,91)

relevance to the life cycle of the virus or to transformation or immortalization functions has not yet been elucidated for some of these interactions. Other p53-independent activities for the alpha genus HPV E6 proteins have been described in the literature, including the activation of cap-dependent translation.[245] Some recent reviews of HPV E6 will provide further details of these interactions.[104,111,281]

Most studies thus far on the molecular biology of the HPV E6 proteins have been on the alpha genus high-risk HPV types. Studies of the cutaneous HPVs are more limited, and less is known about the cellular activities of the cutaneous HPVs of the beta genus. Recently, the beta HPV E6 types as well as BPV1 E6 have been shown to bind Mastermind-like 1 (MAML1) and other members of the Notch transcription complex.[32,217,256] MAML1 and E6AP each complex E6 through LXXLL motifs, and the binding of MAML1 and E6AP to the various PV E6 proteins is mutually exclusive.[31,256] MAML1 is a core component of the transcriptional activation complex that mediates the effects of the canonical Notch signaling pathway. BPV1 and *Betapapillomavirus* HPV E6 repress Notch transcriptional activation, and this repression is dependent on an interaction with MAML1. Furthermore, the expression levels of endogenous Notch target genes are repressed by *Betapapillomavirus* HPV E6 proteins.[175,256]

Notch-dependent transcriptional programs are critical in the differentiation and cell cycle arrest of keratinocytes.[160,209] In addition, inactivating Notch pathway mutations have been recently reported in squamous cell carcinomas of the head and neck,[3,251] and the skin,[282] consistent with the notion that Notch signaling is a tumor suppressor pathway in squamous epithelial cells.[67] E6 binding to MAML1 provides novel mechanism of viral antagonism of the Notch signaling, and suggests that Notch signaling is an important epithelial cell pathway target for the *Betapapillomavirus* HPVs.

Interestingly, although most studies have focused on the high-risk alpha genus HPV, the cellular Na+/H+ Exchanger Regulatory Factor 1 (NHERF1) protein was found to bind E6 proteins of both high and low-risk E6 proteins as well as from diverse nonprimate mammalian species. The binding results in the degradation of NHERF1 resulting in the activation of canonical Wnt/β-catenin signaling, a key pathway that regulates cell growth and proliferation.[70]

HPV E7

The E7 protein encoded by the "high-risk" HPVs is a small nuclear protein of about 100 amino acids, has been shown to bind zinc, and is phosphorylated by casein kinase II (CK II). E7 is a multifunctional protein that shares some functional similarities with adenovirus (Ad) 12S E1A.[202] The HPV proteins also share important amino acid sequence similarity with portions of the AdE1A proteins and the SV40 large tumor antigen (TAg) (Fig. 2.13). These conserved regions are critical for some of the transforming activities in all three viral oncoproteins, and participate in the binding to the product of the retinoblastoma tumor suppressor gene pRB, and the related pocket proteins, p107 and p130.[56,76,287]

The retinoblastoma protein is a member of a family of cellular proteins that also includes p107 and p130, which are homologous in their binding "pockets" for E7, AdE1A, and SV40 TAg. The phosphorylation state of pRB is regulated through the cell cycle, being hypophosphorylated in G_0 and G_1 and phosphorylated during S, G_2, and M. pRB becomes phosphorylated at multiple serine residues by cyclin-dependent kinases at the G1/S boundary and remains phosphorylated until late M, when it becomes hypophosphorylated again through the action of a specific phosphatase (Fig. 2.14). The hypophosphorylated form represents the active form with respect to its ability to inhibit cell cycle progression. HPV16 E7, like SV40 TAg, binds preferentially to the hypophosphorylated form of pRB, resulting in the functional inactivation of pRB through the release of E2F transcription factors thus permitting progression S phase cell cycle progression. This property of the viral oncoproteins to complex pRB accounts, at least in part, for their ability to induce DNA synthesis and cellular proliferation.

The high-risk HPV E7 proteins associate with the pocket proteins and induce their proteasomal degradation.[27,129] The

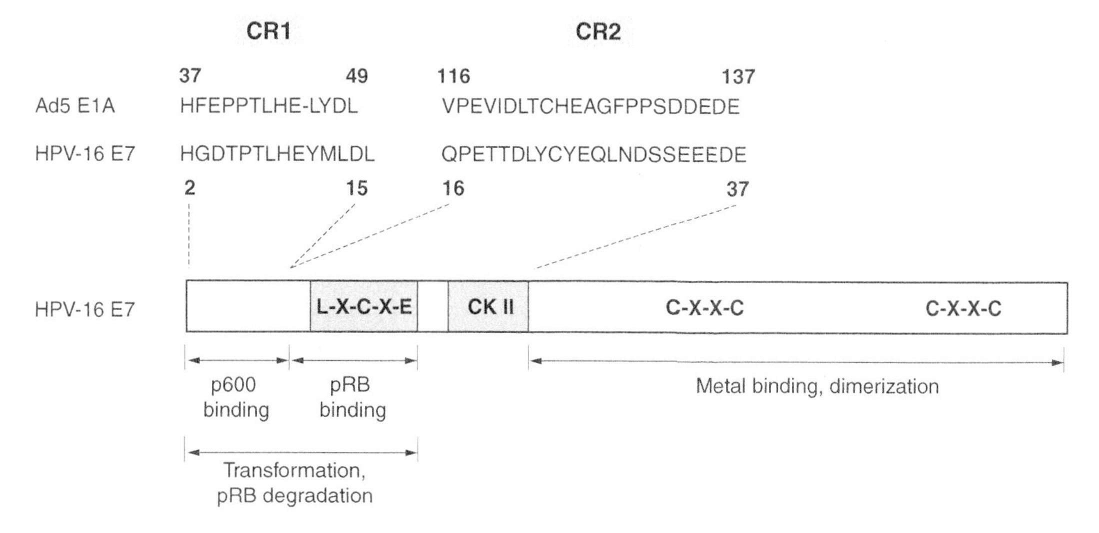

FIGURE 2.13 Amino acid sequence similarity between portions of conserved regions 1 and 2 (CR1, CR2) of the Ad5 E1A proteins and the amino terminal 38 amino acids of HPV16 E7. CR2 contains the pRB binding site and the casein kinase II (CKII) phosphorylation site of HPV16 E7.

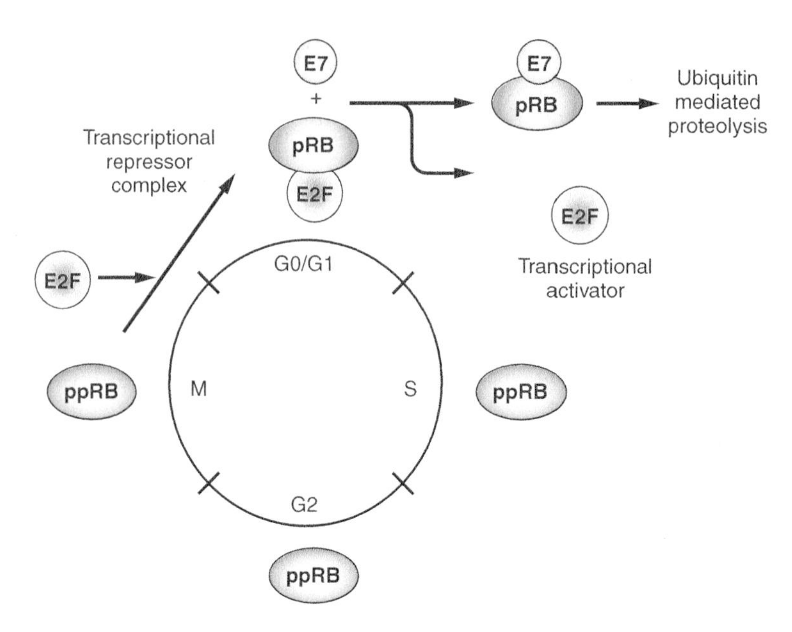

FIGURE 2.14 **E7 abrogates the cell cycle regulation mediated by pRB (as well as the related proteins p107 and p130) by complex formation.** During the cell cycle, pRB is differentially phosphorylated, and the underphosphorylated form is detected only in the G0/G1 phase. This underphosphorylated form is the active form of pRB, acting as a negative regulator of the cell cycle. During the transition to the S-phase, pRB is phosphorylated by cyclin-dependent kinases (cdk), resulting in the inactivation of its cell cycle regulatory functions. Members of the E2F family of cellular transcription factors are preferentially bound to the underphosphorylated form of pRB, and in complex with pRB cannot activate transcription. Phosphorylation of pRB or complex formation with E7 results in the release of the E2F factors allowing them to function as a transcriptional activators of cellular genes involved in cellular DNA synthesis and progression into the S phase of the cell cycle.

LXCXE motif within the CR2 homology domain of E7 is sufficient for pocket protein binding,[77,182] but additional sequences located in the immediate amino terminal CR1 homology domain of E7 are required for pocket protein degradation[129] and these sequences are also necessary for the transforming activities of E7.[201]

E7 targeting the pocket proteins, including pRB, is not sufficient to account for its immortalization and transforming functions, indicating that there are additional cellular targets of E7 that are relevant to cellular transformation.[124] Other E7 binding proteins that are important to its transformation activities are the E3 ligase UBR4 and protein tyrosine phosphatase PTPN14. Although all E7 proteins bind both these cellular proteins,[286] the high-risk HPV E7 proteins target the ubiquitin-dependent degradation of PTPN14 through its interaction with UBR4.[255,285] The degradation of PTPN14 by E7 impairs keratinocyte differentiation thus contributing to its oncogenic activity independent of its ability to target pRB.[106,107] The binding to UBR4 is also important in mediating some of the pRB independent functions of E7 such as modulating anoikis.[58] E7 can interact with cyclin-dependent kinase inhibitors. HPV16 E7 interacts with and abrogates the inhibitory activity of $p27^{kip1}$[295] and associates with $p21^{cip1}$ and abrogates its inhibition of cdks as well as its inhibition of PCNA-dependent DNA replication.[89,128] $p21^{cip1}$ is normally induced during keratinocyte differentiation,[177] and its inhibition by E7 may be critical in allowing papillomavirus viral DNA replication in differentiated squamous epithelial cells.[46]

Table 2.3 provides a list of various cellular targets with which HPV E7 has been shown to bind, although the physiologic relevance of some of these interactions remains unclear. Some recent reviews on E7 provide additional details of some of these interactions.[104,111,242]

E7 is necessary for the stable maintenance of HPV episomes in epithelial cells,[85,260] and sequences in E7 that contribute to cellular transformation are also important for the functions in the viral life cycle.[158,260] Hence, the ability of E7 proteins to induce DNA replication through the release of E2F transcription factor complexes and the inactivation of $p21^{CIP1}$[89,128] and $p27^{KIP1}$[296] is an essential component of the HPV replication strategy.

The high-risk HPV E7 proteins causes genomic instability in normal human cells.[284] HPV16 E7 induces G1/S and mitotic cell cycle checkpoint defects and uncouples synthesis of centrosomes from the cell division cycle.[181] This causes formation of abnormal multipolar mitoses, leading to chromosome missegregation and aneuploidy.[71] Moreover, there is an increased incidence of double-strand DNA breaks and anaphase bridges, suggesting that in addition to numerical abnormalities, high-risk E7 proteins also induce structural chromosome aberrations.[72] Abnormal centrosome duplication rapidly results in genomic instability and aneuploidy, one of the hallmarks of a cancer cell. This activity is therefore likely to be functionally relevant to the contribution of high-risk HPV to malignant progression.

The high-risk HPV E7 proteins have also been shown to reprogram cellular transcriptional programs.[172] The repressive H3K27 marks, which are necessary for binding of polycomb repressive complexes, are decreased in HPV16 E7-expressing cells due to the transcriptional induction of the KDM6A and KDM6B H3K27-specific demethylases.[170] The HPV16 E7-induction of p16(INK4A) is mediated by KDM6B.[170] Moreover, KDM6A- and KDM6B-responsive Homeobox genes are expressed at significantly higher levels, indicating that HPV16 E7 results in reprogramming of host epithelial cells. These effects are independent of the ability of E7 to inhibit the retinoblastoma tumor suppressor protein.

What are the roles of the E6 and E7 oncoproteins in the normal life cycle of an HPV infection? It is likely that they function to allow the replication of the viral DNA. The viral E1 and E2 proteins are necessary for the initiation of viral DNA replication, but the virus is otherwise totally dependent on host cell factors, including DNA polymerase α, thymidine kinase, PCNA, etc. for the replication of its DNA. These are proteins that are normally only expressed in S phase during cellular DNA replication in cycling cells. Vegetative DNA replication for the papillomaviruses, however, occurs only in the more differentiated cells of the epithelium that are no longer cycling

TABLE 2.3 Cellular targets of the human papillomavirus E7 oncoproteins

Associated Cellular Proteins	Functional Consequences	References
pRB, p107, p130	Disruption of E2F transcription factor complexes Degradation	(75,76) (27,129)
UBR4 and KCMF1	Inhibit anoikis	(59,115,286)
Cyclin-dependent kinase inhibitors (p21 and p27)	Inactivation of cdk inhibitory activity	(89,128,296)
Zer1 (HPV16 specific)	pRB ubiquitylation	(286)
PTPN14	Inhibition of keratinocyte differentiation	(255,285)
AP-1	Activation of c-jun transcriptional activation function	(7)
Centrosome components (gamma tubulin)	Aneuploidy	(185)
IGFBP-3	Inhibition of IGFBP-3 mediated apoptosis	(162)
E2F6	Prevent repression by E2F6 polycomb group complexes	(170,171)
HDAC	Activate transcription	(29,157,159)
IRF1 and p48	Block IFN response	(12,193)
Forkhead transcription factor MPP2	Activation of MPP2 transcriptional activity	(161)
RNF168	Affect host DNA damage response	(237)
Cullen 3	Not yet known	(286)

(see Fig. 2.5). Thus, the papillomaviruses have evolved a mechanism similar to that of the polyomaviruses and the adenoviruses, to activate the cellular genes necessary for the replication of their own DNA in otherwise quiescent cells. These viruses may do so through the E7 proteins and their ability to release the E2F transcription factors by binding the pocket proteins including pRB (Fig. 2.13). In addition, E7 binds and inhibits the cdk inhibitor $p21^{cip1}$ that is normally induced during keratinocyte differentiation, again presumably for the purpose of permitting viral DNA replication in a differentiated cell. The high-risk HPV E7 proteins, when expressed in the absence of E6, result in increased levels of p53 resulting in either a G1-mediated cell cycle arrest or apoptosis, depending upon the cell type. E7 creates a signal that increases p53 levels. E6, by promoting the degradation of p53, counters this activity of E7 and permits the E7-dependent activation of the cellular DNA replication genes required for viral DNA replication.

HPV E5

Many of the papillomaviruses that induce purely epithelial papillomas (such as CRPV and the HPVs) contain E5 genes with the potential to encode short hydrophobic peptides. The similarity of these peptides to the BPV1 E5 protein has prompted studies of the potential transforming activities of the HPV E5 genes. The E5 proteins of the HPVs are required for optimal growth.[83,92] In tissue culture, various HPV E5 genes have been shown to have some modest transforming activities and in transgenic mice HPV16 E5 expressed in basal keratinocytes can alter the growth and differentiation of stratified epithelia and induce epithelial tumors at a high frequency.[93] Furthermore, E5 has recently been implicated in the up-regulation of Met in human keratinocytes.[231]

Although the biochemical mechanisms by which the E5 genes of the epitheliotropic papillomaviruses exert their growth stimulatory effects have not yet been fully elaborated, they may involve interactions with the EGF receptor or the 16kD subunit of the vacuolar ATPase, each of which has been shown to bind HPV E5 proteins.[49,93,119,250,298] HPV E5 has also been shown to bind the A4 endoplasmic reticulum protein to regulate cellular proliferative activity.[142]

It should be noted, however, that the E5 gene is not expressed in most HPV-positive cancers, suggesting that if the E5 protein does stimulate cell proliferation *in vivo*, it presumably functions in benign papillomas and not in the cancers. It might also participate in the initiation of the carcinogenic process or in some other aspects of the viral/host cell interaction relevant to the pathogenesis of the HPV infection. Indeed there is also a report that would implicate E5 in the down-regulation of MHC class II antigen expression.[297]

Propagation and Assay in Cell Culture

PVs have proved difficult to propagate *in vitro* because the complete life cycle requires a stratified squamous epithelium, which is not mimicked in monolayer cultures. Most clinical identifications of PV infection, therefore, rely on techniques that identify the viral DNA, such as the polymerase chain reaction (PCR) or molecular hybridization, rather than isolation and assay of viral particles in cell culture.

Early to intermediate stages of the life cycle of many PVs can be studied in cells transfected with viral genomes derived from recombinant DNA. BPV1 can replicate in and transform mouse fibroblasts, though this species promiscuity is very unusual and because BPV1 is a fibropapillomavirus (a virus that replicates nonproductively in dermal fibroblasts as well as productively in the overlying keratinocytes). Human keratinocytes will support replication of transfected *Alphapapillomavirus* HPV genomes; HPVs from the Beta and Mu genera are more refractory to replication because of the strong repressive function of their viral E8^E2 protein.[69] HPV genome-containing keratinocytes can be induced to differentiate by treatment with high levels of calcium,[14] or by suspension in semisolid medium.[218] These treatments stimulate intermediate gene expression, viral

DNA amplification, and some late gene expression but not the production of viral particles

The complete virus life cycle can be recapitulated in cultured keratinocytes using an organotypic "raft" culture system. In this system, keratinocytes containing an HPV genome are cultured at the air–liquid interface on the surface of a dermal equivalent (e.g., a collagen gel containing fibroblasts).[174] This induces the formation of a completely stratified squamous epithelium that can be used to analyze various aspects of PV biology, genetics, and biochemistry, and to produce HPV virions (Fig. 2.15).

The species specificity of PVs has limited the study of HPV in animal models, but an early approach for HPV propagation was to expose primary cultured epithelial cells to virus and place them under the renal capsule of nude mice.[112] This immunologically protected site can support the growth of heterologous cells and foster formation of a multilayer epithelium that resembles a stratified squamous epithelium. The xenograft approach led to the successful propagation of several HPV types, although it is too cumbersome for routine virus isolation or for the molecular or biochemical analysis of virus replication.

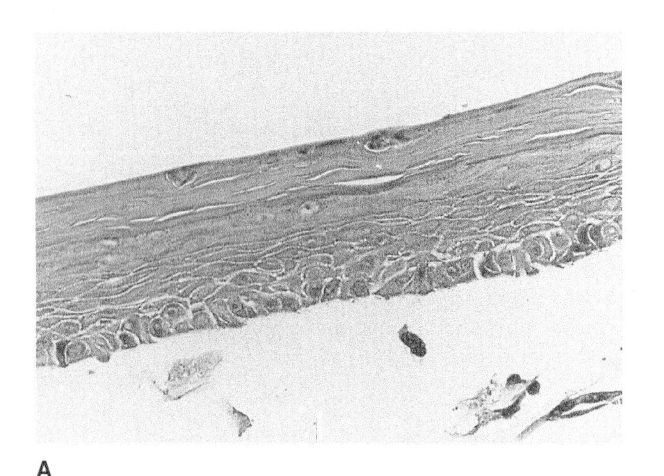

A

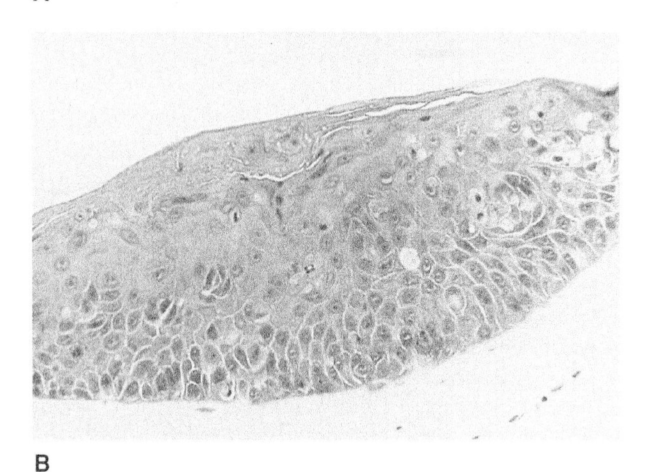

B

FIGURE 2.15 Raft cultures showing normal keratinocytes **(A)** and keratinocytes transfected with the full-length HPV16 genome **(B)**. The normal keratinocytes stratify and differentiate with an increase in the cytoplasmic–nuclear ratio in cells of the upper half of the epithelium and a prominent granular layer. In keratinocytes transfected with HPV16, while stratification takes place, differentiation is abnormal. There is hyperplasia of cells in the parabasal layer, and mitotic figures are observed in the upper half of the epithelium. No granular layer is seen, and the cytoplasmic–nuclear ratio does not change throughout the stratified epithelium. This morphology is similar to cervical intraepithelial neoplasia (CIN). Courtesy of D. McCance.

Papillomavirus gene transfer vectors, also known as pseudovirions, have been developed and are widely used for studies of viral entry and *in vitro* neutralization assays.[34] The most widely employed procedure involves cotransfection of plasmids expressing codon-modified L1 and L2 genes along with a reporter plasmid containing the SV40 origin of replication into SV40 T antigen expressing cells (usually 293TT). The L1 and L2 proteins efficiently package the amplified reporter plasmids, and the purified pseudoviruses (expressing marker genes such as GFP or secreted alkaline phosphatase) are widely used for studying the infectious process.

An extension of this technique is to transfect 293TT cells with recombinant papillomavirus genomes in addition to the L1 and L2 expression vector. The resulting viral particles contain HPV genomes and are called "quasivirus".[206] Quasiviruses can be used as a substitute for lesion-derived virions in basic virologic studies; they have the added advantage that they can contain mutated genomes and could not otherwise be produced.

Marker-PV genomes are related to both pseudoviruses and quasiviruses. These are recombinant PV genomes in which the late region has been replaced by genes encoding GFP, drug selectable markers, or shRNA.[57,274] Early and persistent stages of infection can be studied in cells infected or transfected with these genomes, but they are unable to complete the viral life cycle in the absence of the late genes.

PAPILLOMAVIRUS INFECTION OF EXPERIMENTAL ANIMALS

The species-specific nature of PV has thus far prevented adaptation of authentic HPV infection to experimental animals. However animal PV models have been played important roles in understanding PV pathogenesis.

Wild cottontail rabbits (*Sylvilagus floridanus*) represent the natural host for the CRPV.[235] Experimental studies of SfPV1/CRPV can be carried out in the natural host, but difficulties in maintaining cottontail rabbits under typical cage conditions have led to most SfPV1/CRPV studies being carried out in closely related domestic rabbits (*Oryctolagus cuniculus*).[30] SfPV1/CRPV can readily induce papillomas in domestic rabbits, where their persistence and progression to cutaneous cancer occurs more frequently than in cottontails. Although papillomas in cottontails usually contain large amounts of infectious SfPV1/CRPV, the lesions in domestic rabbits contain little or no infectious virus. Papillomas can also be induced by application of naked SfPV1/CRPV genomic DNA, permitting mutational analyses of the viral life cycle in this model.[144] SfPV1/CRPV genomes have also been incorporated into the L1/L2 capsids of other papillomavirus types and the resulting pseudovirions used to assess the protective capacity of HPV prophylactic vaccines.[173]

Rabbit oral papillomavirus (OcPV1) is a mucosotropic PV that was isolated from domestic rabbits.[195,288] Although SfPV1/CRPV and OcPV1/ROPV are closely related phylogenetically, they are sufficiently distinct antigenically that resistance to one virus does not confer resistance to the other. The canine oral papillomavirus (CPV1 or COPV) is another mucosotropic PV that has been studied.[186] CPV1 papillomas usually regress one to two months after infection, which makes this model well suited to studying aspects of host defense mechanisms against PV infection.[122]

Bovine PV1 (BPV1) is the prototype of a group of animal PVs, found in ungulates, that cause fibropapillomas.[36] The ability of these PVs to induce nonproductive transformation of dermal fibroblasts leads to their having a wider host range than other PVs, although the increased host range may be limited to fibroblasts. Benign dermal tumors known as equine sarcoid appear to arise following accidental dermal infection of horses with BPV1 or BPV2.[40] An experimental counterpart is the ability to induce nonneuronal tumors in hamsters inoculated intracerebrally with BPV1.

Bovine PV4 can induce oral mucosal lesions in cattle, as well as esophageal papillomas.[36] When cattle are fed bracken fern that contains chemical carcinogens, it can lead to esophageal cancers. One interesting feature of these cancers is that, although the BPV4 infection plays a role in their induction, the tumors themselves do not contain detectable BPV4 DNA.[37] This represents a rare instance of virally induced tumors that arise via a "hit-and-run" mechanism.

A rhesus papillomavirus (MmPV1/RhPV1) has been described that appears to be sexually transmitted between monkeys and to be associated with the development of cervical cancer.[290] MmPV1 and HPV16 are highly homologous, which suggests this animal model might have many similarities with human cervical infection with HPV. Infectious RhPV has not yet been isolated or propagated, however, severely limiting experimental analysis of this potentially useful model. The ability to generate RhPV quasivirions in cultured cells might increase the utility of this model.

Cervicovaginal infection by mucosatropic HPVs can be assessed using a pseudovirus-based mouse intravaginal challenge model.[212] Infection is generally monitored by whole animal luminescence imaging after inoculation with luciferase-expressing pseudovirions. Similar models have been developed to examine cutaneous infection.[5]

The first and only laboratory mouse PV, designated MmuPV1, was identified in a colony of immunodeficient inbred mice that spontaneously developed papillomas at cutaneous surfaces near the mucocutaneous junctions of the nose and mouth.[125] This has been an important advance in the field as it provides an infection-based model to study papillomavirus disease pathogenesis. Although phylogenetically distinct from the HPVs as a member of the *Pipapillomavirus* genus, MmuPV1 affords opportunities to study malignant progression following infection and the immunologic responses to infections in the mouse.[246] Another animal model that has received some attention is the African rodent *Mastomys coucha* that offers a model for skin-related cancers.[105]

ACKNOWLEDGMENTS

We are grateful to Karl Münger for providing a thoughtful and critical review of this chapter. AM is funded by the Intramural Research Program of the National Institute of Allergy and Infectious Diseases, National Institutes of Health.

REFERENCES

1. Abban CY, Meneses PI. Usage of heparan sulfate, integrins, and FAK in HPV16 infection. *Virology* 2010;403(1):1–16.
2. Abroi A, Ilves I, Kivi S, et al. Analysis of chromatin attachment and partitioning functions of bovine papillomavirus type 1 E2 protein. *J Virol* 2004;78:2100–2113.
3. Agrawal N, Frederick MJ, Pickering CR, et al. Exome sequencing of head and neck squamous cell carcinoma reveals inactivating mutations in NOTCH1. *Science* 2011;333(6046):1154–1157.
4. Alderborn A, Jareborg N, Burnett S. Evidence that the transcriptional trans-activating function of the bovine papillomavirus type 1 E2 gene is not required for viral DNA amplification in division-arrested cells. *J Gen Virol* 1992;73 (Pt 10):2639–2651.
5. Alphs HH, Gambhira R, Karanam B, et al. Protection against heterologous human papillomavirus challenge by a synthetic lipopeptide vaccine containing a broadly cross-neutralizing epitope of L2. *Proc Natl Acad Sci U S A* 2008;105(15):5850–5855.
6. Androphy EJ, Lowy DR, Schiller JT. Bovine papillomavirus E2 trans-activating gene product binds to specific sites in papillomavirus DNA. *Nature* 1987;325:70–73.
7. Antinore MJ, Birrer MJ, Patel D, et al. The human papillomavirus type 16 E7 gene product interacts with and trans-activates the AP1 family of transcription factors. *EMBO J* 1996;15:1950–1960.
8. Antonsson A, Erfurt C, Hazard K, et al. Prevalence and type spectrum of human papillomaviruses in healthy skin samples collected in three continents. *J Gen Virol* 2003;84(Pt 7):1881–1886.
9. Antson AA, Burns JE, Moroz OV, et al. Structure of the intact transactivation domain of the human papillomavirus E2 protein. *Nature* 2000;403:805–809.
10. Baker TS, Newcomb WW, Olson NH, et al. Structures of bovine and human papillomaviruses—analysis by cryoelectron microscopy and three-dimensional image reconstruction. *Biophys J* 1991;60:1445–1456.
11. Band V, DeCaprio JA, Delmolino L, et al. Loss of p53 protein in human papillomavirus type 16 E6-immortalized human mammary epithelial cells. *J Virol* 1991;65:6671–6676.
12. Barnard P, McMillan NA. The human papillomavirus E7 oncoprotein abrogates signaling mediated by interferon-alpha. *Virology* 1999;259:305–313.
13. Baxter MK, McPhillips MG, Ozato K, et al. The mitotic chromosome binding activity of the papillomavirus E2 protein correlates with interaction with the cellular chromosomal protein, Brd4. *J Virol* 2005;79:4806–4818.
14. Bedell MA, Hudson JB, Golub TR, et al. Amplification of human papillomavirus genomes in vitro is dependent on epithelial differentiation. *J Virol* 1991;65(5):2254–2260.
15. Bellanger S, Tan CL, Nei W, et al. The human papillomavirus type 18 E2 protein is a cell cycle-dependent target of the SCFSkp2 ubiquitin ligase. *J Virol* 2010;84:437–444.
16. Bentley P, Tan MJA, McBride AA, et al. The SMC5/6 complex interacts with the papillomavirus E2 protein and influences maintenance of viral episomal DNA. *J Virol* 2018;92(15):e00356-18.
17. Bergvall M, Melendy T, Archambault J. The E1 proteins. *Virology* 2013;445(1–2):35–56.
18. Bernard HU. Regulatory elements in the viral genome. *Virology* 2013;445(1–2):197–204.
19. Bernard HU, Calleja-Macias IE, Dunn ST. Genome variation of human papillomavirus types: phylogenetic and medical implications. *Int J Cancer* 2006;118(5):1071–1076.
20. Bienkowska-Haba M, Luszczek W, Myers JE, et al. A new cell culture model to genetically dissect the complete human papillomavirus life cycle. *PLoS Pathog* 2018;14(3):e1006846.
21. Black PH, Hartley JW, Rowe WP. Transformation of bovine tissue culture cells by bovine papillomavirus. *Nature* 1963;199:1016–1018.
22. Bohl J, Hull B, Vande Pol SB. Cooperative transformation and coexpression of bovine papillomavirus type 1 E5 and E7 proteins. *J Virol* 2001;75(1):513–521.
23. Boiron M, Levy JP, Thomas M, et al. Some properties of bovine papilloma virus. *Nature* 1964;201:423–424.
24. Boner W, Taylor ER, Tsirimonaki E, et al. A Functional interaction between the human papillomavirus 16 transcription/replication factor E2 and the DNA damage response protein TopBP1. *J Biol Chem* 2002;277(25):22297–22303.
25. Boshart M, Gissman L, Ikenberg H, et al. A new type of papillomavirus DNA, its presence in genital cancer biopsies and in cell lines derived from cervical cancer. *EMBO J* 1984;3:1151–1157.
26. Boxman IL, Berkhout RJ, Mulder LH, et al. Detection of human papillomavirus DNA in plucked hairs from renal transplant recipients and healthy volunteers. *J Invest Dermatol* 1997;108(5):712–715.
27. Boyer SN, Wazer DE, Band V. E7 protein of human papilloma virus-16 induces degradation of retinoblastoma protein through the ubiquitin-proteasome pathway. *Cancer Res* 1996;56:4620–4624.
28. Bravo IG, Alonso A. Mucosal human papillomaviruses encode four different E5 proteins whose chemistry and phylogeny correlate with malignant or benign growth. *J Virol* 2004;78(24):13613–13626.
29. Brehm A, Nielsen SJ, Miska EA, et al. The E7 oncoprotein associates with Mi2 and histone deacetylase activity to promote cell growth. *EMBO J* 1999;18:2449–2458.
30. Breitburd F, Salmon J, Orth G. The rabbit viral skin papillomas and carcinomas: a model for the immunogenetics of HPV-associated carcinogenesis. *Clin Dermatol* 1997;15(2):237–247.
31. Brimer N, Drews CM, Vande Pol SB. Association of papillomavirus E6 proteins with either MAML1 or E6AP clusters E6 proteins by structure, function, and evolutionary relatedness. *PLoS Pathog* 2017;13(12):e1006781.
32. Brimer N, Lyons C, Wallberg AE, et al. Cutaneous papillomavirus E6 oncoproteins associate with MAML1 to repress transactivation and NOTCH signaling. *Oncogene* 2012;31:4639–4646.
33. Buck CB, Cheng N, Thompson CD, et al. Arrangement of L2 within the papillomavirus capsid. *J Virol* 2008;82(11):5190–5197.
34. Buck CB, Pastrana DV, Lowy DR, et al. Efficient intracellular assembly of papillomaviral vectors. *J Virol* 2004;78(2):751–757.
35. Burk RD, Harari A, Chen Z. Human papillomavirus genome variants. *Virology* 2013;445(1–2):232–243.

36. Campo MS. Animal models of papillomavirus pathogenesis. *Virus Res* 2002;89:249–261.
37. Campo MS, Moar MH, Sartirana ML, et al. The presence of bovine papillomavirus type 4 DNA is not required for the progression to, or maintenance of, the malignant state in cancers of the alimentary tract in cattle. *EMBO J* 1985;4:1819–1825.
38. Campos-Leon K, Wijendra K, Siddiqa A, et al. Association of human papillomavirus 16 E2 with Rad50-interacting protein 1 enhances viral DNA replication. *J Virol* 2017;91(5).
39. Carson A, Khan SA. Characterization of transcription factor binding to human papillomavirus type 16 DNA during cellular differentiation. *J Virol* 2006;80(9):4356–4362.
40. Chambers G, Ellsmore VA, O'Brien PM, et al. Association of bovine papillomavirus with the equine sarcoid. *J Gen Virol* 2003;84(Pt 5):1055–1062.
41. Chan SY, Delius H, Halpern AL, et al. Analysis of genomic sequences of 95 papillomavirus types: uniting typing, phylogeny, and taxonomy. *J Virol* 1995;69:3074–3083.
42. Chen EY, Howley PM, Levinson AD, et al. The primary structure and genetic organization of the bovine papillomavirus type 1 genome. *Nature* 1982;299:529–534.
43. Chen JJ, Reid CE, Band V, et al. Interaction of papillomavirus E6 oncoproteins with a putative calcium-binding protein. *Science* 1995;269:529–531.
44. Chen XS, Garcea RL, Goldberg I, et al. Structure of small virus-like particles assembled from the L1 protein of human papillomavirus 16. *Mol Cell* 2000;5:557–567.
45. Chen Z, Terai M, Fu L, et al. Diversifying selection in human papillomavirus type 16 lineages based on complete genome analyses. *J Virol* 2005;79(11):7014–7023.
46. Cheng S, Schmidt-Grimminger DC, Murant T, et al. Differentiation-dependent upregulation of the human papillomavirus E7 gene reactivates cellular DNA replication in suprabasal differentiated keratinocytes. *Genes Dev* 1995;9:2335–2349.
47. Chiang C, Pauli EK, Biryukov J, et al. The human papillomavirus E6 oncoprotein targets USP15 and TRIM25 to suppress RIG-I-mediated innate immune signaling. *J Virol* 2018;92(6): e01737-17.
48. Ciuffo G. Innesto positivo con filtrato di verruca volgare. *Gior Ital Mal Venereol* 1907;48:12–17.
49. Conrad M, Bubb VJ, Schlegel R. The human papillomavirus type 6 and 16 E5 proteins are membrane-associated proteins which associate with the 16-kilodalton pore-forming protein. *J Virol* 1993;67:6170–6178.
50. Conway MJ, Alam S, Ryndock EJ, et al. Tissue-spanning redox gradient-dependent assembly of native human papillomavirus type 16 virions. *J Virol* 2009;83(20):10515–10526.
51. Coursey TL, McBride AA. Hitchhiking of viral genomes on cellular chromosomes. *Annu Rev Virol* 2019;6(1):275–296.
52. Crawford LV, Crawford EM. A comparative study of polyoma and papilloma viruses. *Virology* 1963;21:258–263.
53. Danos O, Engel LW, Chen EY, et al. Comparative analysis of the human type 1a and bovine type 1 papillomavirus genomes. *J Virol* 1983;46:557–566.
54. Danos O, Katinka M, Yaniv M. Human papillomavirus la complete DNA sequence: a novel type of genome organization among Papovaviridae. *EMBO J* 1982;1:231–236.
55. Day PM, Baker CC, Lowy DR, et al. Establishment of papillomavirus infection is enhanced by promyelocytic leukemia protein (PML) expression. *Proc Natl Acad Sci U S A* 2004;101(39):14252–14257.
56. DeCaprio JA, Ludlow JW, Figge J, et al. SV40 large tumor antigen forms a specific complex with the product of the retinoblastoma susceptibility gene. *Cell* 1988;54:275–283.
57. Delcuratolo M, Fertey J, Schneider M, et al. Papillomavirus-associated tumor formation critically depends on c-Fos expression induced by viral protein E2 and bromodomain protein Brd4. *PLoS Pathog* 2016;12(1):e1005366.
58. DeMasi J, Chao MC, Kumar AS, et al. Bovine papillomavirus E7 oncoprotein inhibits anoikis. *J Virol* 2007;81(17):9419–9425.
59. DeMasi J, Huh KW, Nakatani Y, et al. Bovine papillomavirus E7 transformation function correlates with cellular p600 protein binding. *Proc Natl Acad Sci U S A* 2005;102(32):11486–11491.
60. DeSmet M, Kanginakudru S, Rietz A, et al. The replicative consequences of papillomavirus E2 protein binding to the origin replication factor ORC2. *PLoS Pathog* 2016;12(10):e1005934.
61. DiGiuseppe S, Luszczek W, Keiffer TR, et al. Incoming human papillomavirus type 16 genome resides in a vesicular compartment throughout mitosis. *Proc Natl Acad Sci U S A* 2016;113(22):6289–6294.
62. DiMaio D, Lai CC, Mattoon D. The platelet-derived growth factor beta receptor as a target of the bovine papillomavirus E5 protein. *Cytokine Growth Factor Rev* 2000;11(4):283–293.
63. Donati B, Lorenzini E, Ciarrocchi A. BRD4 and cancer: going beyond transcriptional regulation. *Mol Cancer* 2018;17(1):164.
64. Doorbar J. The papillomavirus life cycle. *J Clin Virol* 2005;32(Suppl 1):S7–S15.
65. Doorbar J, Ely S, Sterling J, et al. Specific interaction between HPV-16 E1-E4 and cytokeratins results in collapse of the epithelial cell intermediate filament network. *Nature* 1991;352:824–827.
66. Doorbar J, Quint W, Banks L, et al. The biology and life-cycle of human papillomaviruses. *Vaccine* 2012;30(Suppl 5):F55–F70.
67. Dotto GP. Notch tumor suppressor function. *Oncogene* 2008;27(38):5115–5123.
68. Dreer M, Fertey J, van de Poel S, et al. Interaction of NCOR/SMRT repressor complexes with papillomavirus E8^E2C proteins inhibits viral replication. *PLoS Pathog* 2016;12(4):e1005556.
69. Dreer M, van de Poel S, Stubenrauch F. Control of viral replication and transcription by the papillomavirus E8^E2 protein. *Virus Res* 2017;231:96–102.
70. Drews CM, Case S, Vande Pol SB. E6 proteins from high-risk HPV, low-risk HPV, and animal papillomaviruses activate the Wnt/beta-catenin pathway through E6AP-dependent degradation of NHERF1. *PLoS Pathog* 2019;15(4):e1007575.
71. Duensing S, Lee LY, Duensing A, et al. The human papillomavirus type 16 E6 and E7 oncoproteins cooperate to induce mitotic defects and genomic instability by uncoupling centrosome duplication from the cell division cycle. *Proc Natl Acad Sci U S A* 2000;97:10002–10007.
72. Duensing S, Munger K. The human papillomavirus type 16 E6 and E7 oncoproteins independently induce numerical and structural chromosome instability. *Cancer Res* 2002;62(23):7075–7082.
73. Durst M, Gissmann L, Idenburg H, et al. A papillomavirus DNA from a cervical carcinoma and its prevalence in cancer biopsy samples from different geographic regions. *Proc Natl Acad Sci U S A* 1983;80:3812–3815.
74. Dvoretzky I, Shober R, Chattopadhyay SK, et al. A quantitative in vitro focus assay for bovine papilloma virus. *Virology* 1980;103:369–375.
75. Dyson N, Guida P, Munger K, et al. Homologous sequences in adenovirus E1A and human papillomavirus E7 proteins mediate interaction with the same set of cellular proteins. *J Virol* 1992;66:6893–6902.
76. Dyson N, Howley PM, Munger K, et al. The human papillomavirus-16 E7 oncoprotein is able to bind the retinoblastoma gene product. *Science* 1989;243:934–937.
77. Edmonds C, Vousden KH. A point mutational analysis of human papillomavirus type 16 E7 protein. *J Virol* 1989;63:2650–2656.
78. Eichten A, Rud DS, Grace M, et al. Molecular pathways executing the "trophic sentinel" response in HPV-16 E7-expressing normal human diploid fibroblasts upon growth factor deprivation. *Virology* 2004;319:81–93.
79. Enemark EJ, Chen G, Vaughn DE, et al. Crystal structure of the DNA binding domain of the replication initiation protein E1 from papillomavirus. *Mol Cell* 2000;6:149–158.
80. Enemark EJ, Joshua-Tor L. Mechanism of DNA translocation in a replicative hexameric helicase. *Nature* 2006;442(7100):270–275.
81. Favre M, Breitburd F, Croissant O, et al. Chromatin-like structures obtained after alkaline disruption of bovine and human papillomaviruses. *J Virol* 1977;21(3):1205–1209.
82. Favre-Bonvin A, Reynaud C, Kretz-Remy C, et al. Human papillomavirus type 18 E6 protein binds the cellular PDZ protein TIP-2/GIPC, which is involved in transforming growth factor beta signaling and triggers its degradation by the proteasome. *J Virol* 2005;79:4229–4237.
83. Fehrmann F, Klumpp DJ, Laimins LA. Human papillomavirus type 31 E5 protein supports cell cycle progression and activates late viral functions upon epithelial differentiation. *J Virol* 2003;77(5):2819–2831.
84. Filippova M, Parkhurst L, Duerksen-Hughes PJ. The human papillomavirus 16 E6 protein binds to Fas-associated death domain and protects cells from Fas-triggered apoptosis. *J Biol Chem* 2004;279(24):25729–25744.
85. Flores ER, Allen-Hoffmann BL, Lee D, et al. The human papillomavirus type 16 E7 oncogene is required for the productive stage of the viral life cycle. *J Virol* 2000;74(14):6622–6631.
86. Flores ER, Lambert PF. Evidence for a switch in the mode of human papillomavirus DNA replication during the viral life cycle. *J Virol* 1997;71:7167–7179.
87. Florin L, Schafer F, Sotlar K, et al. Reorganization of nuclear domain 10 induced by papillomavirus capsid protein l2. *Virology* 2002;295(1):97–107.
88. Fradet-Turcotte A, Bergeron-Labrecque F, Moody CA, et al. Nuclear accumulation of the papillomavirus E1 helicase blocks S-phase progression and triggers an ATM-dependent DNA damage response. *J Virol* 2011;85(17):8996–9012.
89. Funk JO, Waga S, Harry JB, et al. Inhibition of CDK activity and PCNA-dependent DNA replication by p21 is blocked interaction with the HPV-16 E7 oncoprotein. *Genes Dev* 1997;11:2090–2100.
90. Gardiol D, Kuhne C, Glaunsinger B, et al. Oncogenic human papillomavirus E6 proteins target the discs large tumour suppressor for proteasome-mediated degradation. *Oncogene* 1999;18:5487–5496.
91. Garnett TO, Filippova M, Duerksen-Hughes PJ. Accelerated degradation of FADD and procaspase 8 in cells expressing human papilloma virus 16 E6 impairs TRAIL-mediated apoptosis. *Cell Death Differ* 2006;13(11):1915–1926.
92. Genther SM, Sterling S, Duensing S, et al. Quantitative role of the human papillomavirus type 16 E5 gene during the productive stage of the viral life cycle. *J Virol* 2003;77(5):2832–2842.
93. Genther Williams SM, Disbrow GL, Schlegel R, et al. Requirement of epidermal growth factor receptor for hyperplasia induced by E5, a high-risk human papillomavirus oncogene. *Cancer Res* 2005;65:6534–6542.
94. Gewin L, Galloway DA. E box-dependent activation of telomerase by human papillomavirus type 16 E6 does not require induction of c-myc. *J Virol* 2001;75(15):7198–7201.
95. Gewin L, Myers H, Kiyono T, et al. Identification of a novel telomerase repressor that interacts with the human papillomavirus type-16 E6/E6-AP complex. *Genes Dev* 2004;18(18):2269–2282.
96. Gilbert DM, Cohen SN. Bovine papilloma virus plasmids replicate randomly in mouse fibroblasts throughout S phase of the cell cycle. *Cell* 1987;50:59–68.
97. Glaunsinger BA, Lee SS, Thomas M, et al. Interactions of the PDZ-protein MAGI-1 with adenovirus E4-ORF1 and high-risk papillomavirus E6 oncoproteins. *Oncogene* 2000;19:5270–5280.
98. Goldstein DJ, Schlegel R. The E5 oncoprotein of bovine papillomavirus binds to a 16 kd cellular protein. *EMBO J* 1990;9(1):137–145.
99. Graham SV. Keratinocyte differentiation-dependent human papillomavirus gene regulation. *Viruses* 2017;9(9):245.
100. Guan J, Bywaters SM, Brendle SA, et al. Cryoelectron microscopy maps of human papillomavirus 16 reveal L2 densities and heparin binding site. *Structure* 2017;25(2): 253–263.
101. Guion L, Bienkowska-Haba M, DiGiuseppe S, et al. PML nuclear body-residing proteins sequentially associate with HPV genome after infectious nuclear delivery. *PLoS Pathog* 2019;15(2):e1007590.
102. Hagensee ME, Olson NH, Baker TS, et al. Three-dimensional structure of vaccinia virus-produced human papillomavirus type 1 capsids. *J Virol* 1994;68:4503–4505.
103. Hagensee ME, Yaegashi N, Galloway DA. Self-assembly of human papillomavirus type 1 capsids by expression of the L1 protein alone or by coexpression of the L1 and L2 capsid proteins. *J Virol* 1993;67:315–322.
104. Harden ME, Munger K. Human papillomavirus molecular biology. *Mutat Res Rev Mutat Res* 2017;772:3–12.
105. Hasche D, Rosl F. Mastomys species as model systems for infectious diseases. *Viruses* 2019;11(2):182.

106. Hatterschide J, Bohidar AE, Grace M, et al. PTPN14 degradation by high-risk human papillomavirus E7 limits keratinocyte differentiation and contributes to HPV-mediated oncogenesis. *Proc Natl Acad Sci U S A* 2019;116(14):7033–7042.
107. Hatterschide J, Brantly AC, Grace M, et al. A conserved amino acid in the C terminus of human papillomavirus E7 mediates binding to PTPN14 and repression of epithelial differentiation. *J Virol* 2020;94(17).
108. Haupt Y, Maya R, Kazaz A, et al. Mdm2 promotes the rapid degradation of p53. *Nature* 1997;387:296–299.
109. Hawley-Nelson P, Vousden KH, Hubbert NL, et al. HPV16 E6 and E7 proteins cooperate to immortalize human foreskin keratinocytes. *EMBO J* 1989;8:3905–3910.
110. Hedge RS, Rossman SR, Laimins LA, et al. Crystal structure at 1.7A of the bovine papillomavirus-1 E2 DNA-binding domain bound to its DNA target. *Nature* 1992;359: 505–512.
111. Hoppe-Seyler K, Bossler F, Braun JA, et al. The HPV E6/E7 oncogenes: key factors for viral carcinogenesis and therapeutic targets. *Trends Microbiol* 2018;26(2): 158–168.
112. Howett MK, Christensen ND, Kreider JW. Tissue xenografts as a model system for study of the pathogenesis of papillomaviruses. *Clin Dermatol* 1997;15(2):229–236.
113. Huang L, Kinnucan E, Wang G, et al. Structure of an E6AP-UbcH7 complex: insights into ubiquitination by the E2-E3 enzyme cascade. *Science* 1999;286:1321–1326.
114. Hubbert NL, Sedman SA, Schiller JT. Human papillomavirus type 16 E6 increases the degradation rate of p53 in human keratinocytes. *J Virol* 1992;66:6237–6241.
115. Huh KW, DeMasi J, Ogawa H, et al. Association of the human papillomavirus type 16 E7 oncoprotein with the 600-kDa retinoblastoma protein-associated factor, p600. *Proc Natl Acad Sci U S A* 2005;102(32):11492–11497.
116. Huibregtse JM, Scheffner M, Beaudenon S, et al. A family of proteins structurally and functionally related to the E6-AP ubiquitin-protein ligase. *Proc Natl Acad Sci U S A* 1995;92:2563–2567.
117. Huibregtse JM, Scheffner M, Howley PM. A cellular protein mediates association of p53 with the E6 oncoprotein of human papillomavirus types 16 or 18. *EMBO J* 1991;10:4129–4135.
118. Huibregtse JM, Scheffner M, Howley PM. Cloning and expression of the cDNA for E6-AP: a protein that mediates the interaction of the human papillomavirus E6 oncoprotein with p53. *Mol Cell Biol* 1993;13:775–784.
119. Hwang ES, Nottoli T, DiMaio D. The HPV 16 E5 protein: expression, detection, and stable complex formation with transmembrane proteins in COS cells. *Virology* 1995;211:227–233.
120. Iftner T, Haedicke-Jarboui J, Wu SY, et al. Involvement of Brd4 in different steps of the papillomavirus life cycle. *Virus Res* 2017;231:76–82.
121. Ilves I, Kivi S, Ustav M. Long-term episomal maintenance of bovine papillomavirus type 1 plasmids is determined by attachment to host chromosomes, which is mediated by the viral E2 protein and its binding sites. *J Virol* 1999;73:4404–4412.
122. Jain S, Moore RA, Anderson DM, et al. Cell-mediated immune responses to COPV early proteins. *Virology* 2006;356(1–2):23–34.
123. Jang MK, Anderson DE, van Doorslaer K, et al. A proteomic approach to discover and compare interacting partners of papillomavirus E2 proteins from diverse phylogenetic groups. *Proteomics* 2015;15(12):2038–2050.
124. Jewers RJ, Hildebrandt P, Ludlow JW, et al. Regions of human papillomavirus type 16 E7 oncoprotein required for immortalization of human keratinocytes. *J Virol* 1992;66:1329–1335.
125. Joh J, Jenson AB, King W, et al. Genomic analysis of the first laboratory-mouse papillomavirus. *J Gen Virol* 2011;92(Pt 3):692–698.
126. Johansson C, Schwartz S. Regulation of human papillomavirus gene expression by splicing and polyadenylation. *Nat Rev Microbiol* 2013;11(4):239–251.
127. Johnson KM, Kines RC, Roberts JN, et al. Role of heparan sulfate in attachment to and infection of the murine female genital tract by human papillomavirus. *J Virol* 2009;83(5):2067–2074.
128. Jones DL, Alani RM, Münger K. The human papillomavirus E7 oncoprotein can uncouple cellular differentiation and proliferation in human keratinocytes by abrogating p21cip1-mediated inhibition of cdk2. *Genes Dev* 1997;11:2101–2111.
129. Jones DL, Thompson DA, Munger K. Destabilization of the RB tumor suppressor protein and stabilization of p53 contribute to HPV type 16 E7-induced apoptosis. *Virology* 1997;239:97–107.
130. Kamper N, Day PM, Nowak T, et al. A membrane-destabilizing peptide in capsid protein L2 is required for egress of papillomavirus genomes from endosomes. *J Virol* 2006;80(2):759–768.
131. Kao WH, Beaudenon SL, Talis AL, et al. Human papillomavirus type 16 E6 induces self-ubiquitination of the E6AP ubiquitin-protein ligase. *J Virol* 2000;74:6408–6417.
132. Karabadzhak AG, Petti LM, Barrera FN, et al. Two transmembrane dimers of the bovine papillomavirus E5 oncoprotein clamp the PDGF beta receptor in an active dimeric conformation. *Proc Natl Acad Sci U S A* 2017;114(35):E7262–E7271.
133. Kessis TD, Slebos RJ, Nelson WG, et al. Human papillomavirus 16 E6 expression disrupts the p53-mediated cellular response to DNA damage. *Proc Natl Acad Sci U S A* 1993;90:3988–3992.
134. Kines RC, Thompson CD, Lowy DR, et al. The initial steps leading to papillomavirus infection occur on the basement membrane prior to cell surface binding. *Proc Natl Acad Sci U S A* 2009;106(48):20458–20463.
135. Kiran S, Dar A, Singh SK, et al. The deubiquitinase USP46 is essential for proliferation and tumor growth of HPV-transformed cancers. *Mol Cell* 2018;72(5):823–835 e5.
136. Kirnbauer R, Booy F, Cheng N, et al. Papillomavirus L1 major capsid protein self-assembles into virus-like particles that are highly immunogenic. *Proc Natl Acad Sci U S A* 1992;89:12180–12184.
137. Kishino T, Lalande M, Wagstaff J. UBE3A/E6-AP mutations cause Angelman syndrome. *Nat Genet* 1997;15:70–73.
138. Kiyono T, Foster SA, Koop JI, et al. Both Rb/p16INK4a inactivation and telomerase activity are required to immortalize human epithelial cells. *Nature* 1998;396:84–88.
139. Kiyono T, Hiraiwa A, Fujita M, et al. Binding of high-risk human papillomavirus E6 oncoproteins to the human homologue of the Drosophila discs large tumor suppressor protein. *Proc Natl Acad Sci U S A* 1997;94(21):11612–11616.
140. Kleijnen MF, Shih AH, Zhou P, et al. The hPLIC proteins may provide a link between the ubiquitination machinery and the proteasome. *Mol Cell* 2000;6(2):409–419.
141. Klingelhutz AJ, Foster SA, McDougall JK. Telomerase activation by the E6 gene product of human papillomavirus type 16. *Nature* 1996;380:79–81.
142. Kotnik Halavaty K, Regan J, Mehta K, et al. Human papillomavirus E5 oncoproteins bind the A4 endoplasmic reticulum protein to regulate proliferative ability upon differentiation. *Virology* 2014;452–453:223–230.
143. Kreider JW. The Shope papilloma to carcinoma complex of rabbits: a model system of neoplastic progression and spontaneous regression. *Adv Cancer Res* 1981;35:81–110.
144. Kreider JW, Cladel NM, Patrick SD, et al. High efficiency induction of papillomas in vivo using recombinant cottontail rabbit papillomavirus DNA. *J Virol Methods* 1995;55(2):233–244.
145. Kubbutat MHG, Jones SN, Vousden KH. Regulation of p53 stability by Mdm2. *Nature* 1997;387:299–303.
146. Kumar A, Zhao Y, Meng G, et al. Human papillomavirus oncoprotein E6 inactivates the transcriptional coactivator human ADA3. *Mol Cell Biol* 2002;22:5801–5812.
147. Kumar RA, Naidu SR, Wang X, et al. Interaction of papillomavirus E2 protein with the Brm chromatin remodeling complex leads to enhanced transcriptional activation. *J Virol* 2007;81(5):2213–2220.
148. Kumar S, Kao WH, Howley PM. Physical interaction between specific E2 and Hect E3 enzymes determines functional cooperativity. *J Biol Chem* 1997;272:13548–13554.
149. Kumar S, Talis AL, Howley PM. Identification of HHR23A as a substrate for E6-associated protein-mediated ubiquitination. *J Biol Chem* 1999;274:18785–18792.
150. Law M-F, Lowy DR, Dvoretzky I, et al. Mouse cells transformed by bovine papillomavirus contain only extrachromosomal viral DNA sequences. *Proc Natl Acad Sci U S A* 1981;78:2727–2731.
151. Lee SS, Glaunsinger B, Mantovani F, et al. Multi-PDZ domain protein MUPP1 is a cellular target for both adenovirus E4-ORF1 and high-risk papillomavirus type 18 E6 oncoproteins. *J Virol* 2000;74:9680–9693.
152. Li L, Li Z, Howley PM, et al. E6AP and calmodulin reciprocally regulate estrogen receptor stability. *J Biol Chem* 2006;281(4):1978–1985.
153. Li R, Knight J, Bream G, et al. Specific recognition nucleotides and their context determine the affinity of E2 protein for 17 binding sites in the BPV-1 genome. *Genes Dev* 1989;3:510–526.
154. Liu X, Dakic A, Zhang Y, et al. HPV E6 protein interacts physically and functionally with the cellular telomerase complex. *Proc Natl Acad Sci U S A* 2009;106(44): 18780–18785.
155. Liu X, Yuan H, Fu B, et al. The E6AP ubiquitin ligase is required for transactivation of the hTERT promoter by the human papillomavirus E6 oncoprotein. *J Biol Chem* 2005;280:10807–10816.
156. Liu Y, Chen JJ, Gao Q, et al. Multiple functions of human papillomavirus type 16 E6 contribute to the immortalization of mammary epithelial cells. *J Virol* 1999;73:7297–7307.
157. Longworth MS, Laimins LA. The binding of histone deacetylases and the integrity of zinc finger-like motifs of the E7 protein are essential for the life cycle of human papillomavirus type 31. *J Virol* 2004;78:3533–3541.
158. Longworth MS, Laimins LA. Pathogenesis of human papillomaviruses in differentiating epithelia. *Microbiol Mol Biol Rev* 2004;68(2):362–372.
159. Longworth MS, Wilson R, Laimins LA. HPV31 E7 facilitates replication by activating E2F2 transcription through its interaction with HDACs. *EMBO J* 2005;24(10):1821–1830.
160. Lowell S, Jones P, Le Roux I, et al. Stimulation of human epidermal differentiation by delta-notch signalling at the boundaries of stem-cell clusters. *Curr Biol* 2000;10(9):491–500.
161. Luscher-Firzlaff JM, Westendorf JM, Zwicker J, et al. Interaction of the fork head domain transcription factor MPP2 with the human papilloma virus 16 E7 protein: enhancement of transformation and transactivation. *Oncogene* 1999;18(41):5620–5630.
162. Mannhardt B, Weinzimer SA, Wagner M, et al. Human papillomavirus type 16 E7 oncoprotein binds and inactivates growth-inhibitory insulin-like growth factor binding protein 3. *Mol Cell Biol* 2000;20:6483–6495.
163. Martin P, Vass WC, Schiller JT, et al. The bovine papillomavirus E5 transforming protein can stimulate the transforming activity of EGF and CSF-1 receptors. *Cell* 1989;59(1):21–32.
164. Martinez-Noel G, Galligan JT, Sowa ME, et al. Identification and proteomic analysis of distinct UBE3A/E6AP protein complexes. *Mol Cell Biol* 2012;32(15):3095–3106.
165. Martinez-Zapien D, Ruiz FX, Poirson J, et al. Structure of the E6/E6AP/p53 complex required for HPV-mediated degradation of p53. *Nature* 2016;529(7587):541–545.
166. Massimi P, Shai A, Lambert P, et al. HPV E6 degradation of p53 and PDZ containing substrates in an E6AP null background. *Oncogene* 2008;27(12):1800–1804.
167. Matsuura T, Sutcliffe JS, Fang P, et al. *De novo* truncating mutations in E6AP ubiquitin-protein ligase gene (UBE3A) in Angelman syndrome. *Nat Genet* 1997;15:74–77.
168. McBride AA. The papillomavirus E2 proteins. *Virology* 2013;445(1–2):57–79.
169. McBride AA. Mechanisms and strategies of papillomavirus replication. *Biol Chem* 2017;398(8):919–927.
170. McLaughlin-Drubin ME, Crum CP, Munger K. Human papillomavirus E7 oncoprotein induces KDM6A and KDM6B histone demethylase expression and causes epigenetic reprogramming. *Proc Natl Acad Sci U S A* 2011;108(5):2130–2135.
171. McLaughlin-Drubin ME, Huh KW, Munger K. Human papillomavirus type 16 E7 oncoprotein associates with E2F6. *J Virol* 2008;82(17):8695–8705.
172. McLaughlin-Drubin ME, Meyers J, Munger K. Cancer associated human papillomaviruses. *Curr Opin Virol* 2012;2(4):459–466.
173. Mejia AF, Culp TD, Cladel NM, et al. Preclinical model to test human papillomavirus virus (HPV) capsid vaccines in vivo using infectious HPV/cottontail rabbit papillomavirus chimeric papillomavirus particles. *J Virol* 2006;80(24):12393–12397.
174. Meyers C, Frattini MG, Hudson JB, et al. Biosynthesis of human papillomavirus from a continuous cell line upon epithelial differentiation. *Science* 1992;257:971–973.

175. Meyers JM, Spangle JM, Munger K. The human papillomavirus type 8 E6 protein interferes with NOTCH activation during keratinocyte differentiation. *J Virol* 2013;87(8):4762–4767.
176. Mirabello L, Yeager M, Yu K, et al. HPV16 E7 genetic conservation is critical to carcinogenesis. *Cell* 2017;170(6):1164–1174 e6.
177. Missero C, Calautti E, Eckner R, et al. Involvement of the cell-cycle inhibitor Cip1/WAF1 and the E1A-associated p300 protein in terminal differentiation. *Proc Natl Acad Sci U S A* 1995;92:5451–5455.
178. Mohr IJ, Clark R, Sun S, et al. Targeting the E1 replication protein to the papillomavirus origin of replication by complex formation with the E2 transactivator. *Science* 1990;250:1694–1699.
179. Moody CA, Laimins LA. Human papillomaviruses activate the ATM DNA damage pathway for viral genome amplification upon differentiation. *PLoS Pathog* 2009;5(10):e1000605.
180. Muller M, Jacob Y, Jones L, et al. Large scale genotype comparison of human papillomavirus E2-host interaction networks provides new insights for e2 molecular functions. *PLoS Pathog* 2012;8(6):e1002761.
181. Münger K, Baldwin A, Edwards KM, et al. Mechanisms of human papillomavirus-induced oncogenesis. *J Virol* 2004;78(21):11451–11460.
182. Münger K, Phelps WC, Bubb V, et al. The E6 and E7 genes of the human papillomavirus type 16 together are necessary and sufficient for transformation of primary human keratinocytes. *J Virol* 1989;63:4417–4421.
183. Nakagawa S, Huibregtse JM. Human scribble (vartul) is targeted for ubiquitin-mediated degradation by the high-risk papillomavirus E6 proteins and the E6AP ubiquitin-protein ligase. *Mol Cell Biol* 2000;20:8244–8253.
184. Neary K, DiMaio D. Open reading frames E6 and E7 of bovine papillomavirus type 1 are both required for full transformation of mouse C127 cells. *J Virol* 1989;63(1):259–266.
185. Nguyen CL, Eichwald C, Nibert ML, et al. Human papillomavirus type 16 E7 oncoprotein associates with the centrosomal component gamma-tubulin. *J Virol* 2007;81(24):13533–13543.
186. Nicholls PK, Stanley MA. The immunology of animal papillomaviruses. *Vet Immunol Immunopathol* 2000;73(2):101–127.
187. Noor A, Dupuis L, Mittal K, et al. 15q11.2 duplication encompassing only the UBE3A gene is associated with developmental delay and neuropsychiatric phenotypes. *Hum Mutat* 2015;36(7):689–693.
188. Oh ST, Kyo S, Laimins LA. Telomerase activation by human papillomavirus type 16 E6 protein: induction of human telomerase reverse transcriptase expression through Myc and GC-rich Sp1 binding sites. *J Virol* 2001;75:5559–5566.
189. Oliveira JG, Colf LA, McBride AA. Variations in the association of papillomavirus E2 proteins with mitotic chromosomes. *Proc Natl Acad Sci U S A* 2006;103(4):1047–1052.
190. Orth G, Favre M, Jablonska S, et al. Viral sequences related to a human skin papillomavirus in genital warts. *Nature* 1978;275:334–336.
191. Parish JL, Bean AM, Park RB, et al. ChlR1 is required for loading papillomavirus E2 onto mitotic chromosomes and viral genome maintenance. *Mol Cell* 2006;24:867–876.
192. Parish JL, Kowalczyk A, Chen HT, et al. E2 proteins from high- and low-risk human papillomavirus types differ in their ability to bind p53 and induce apoptotic cell death. *J Virol* 2006;80(9):4580–4590.
193. Park JS, Kim EJ, Kwon HJ, et al. Inactivation of interferon regulatory factor-1 tumor suppressor protein by HPV E7 oncoprotein. Implication for the E7-mediated immune evasion mechanism in cervical carcinogenesis. *J Biol Chem* 2000;275:6764–6769.
194. Park RB, Androphy EJ. Genetic analysis of high-risk e6 in episomal maintenance of human papillomavirus genomes in primary human keratinocytes. *J Virol* 2002;76(22):11359–11364.
195. Parsons RJ, Kidd JG. Oral papillomatosis of rabbits: a virus disease. *J Exp Med* 1943;77:233–250.
196. Patel D, Huang SM, Baglia LA, et al. The E6 protein of human papillomavirus type 16 binds to and inhibits co-activation by CBP and p300. *EMBO J* 1999;18:5061–5072.
197. Pentland I, Campos-Leon K, Cotic M, et al. Disruption of CTCF-YY1-dependent looping of the human papillomavirus genome activates differentiation-induced viral oncogene transcription. *PLoS Biol* 2018;16(10):e2005752.
198. Petti L, DiMaio D. Stable association between the bovine papillomavirus E5 transforming protein and activated platelet-derived growth factor receptor in transformed mouse cells. *Proc Natl Acad Sci U S A* 1992;89:6736–6740.
199. Petti L, DiMaio D. Specific interaction between the bovine papillomavirus E5 transforming protein and the b receptor for platelet-derived growth factor in stably transformed and acutely transfected cells. *J Virol* 1994;68:3582–3592.
200. Pfister H, Gissman L, zur Hausen H. Partial characterization of proteins of human papilloma viruses (HPV) 1-3. *Virology* 1977;83:131–137.
201. Phelps WC, Münger K, Yee CL, et al. Structure-function analysis of the human papillomavirus type 16 E7 oncoprotein. *J Virol* 1992;66:2418–2427.
202. Phelps WC, Yee CL, Münger K, et al. The human papillomavirus type 16 E7 gene encodes transactivation and transformation functions similar to those of adenovirus E1A. *Cell* 1988;53:539–547.
203. Piirsoo M, Ustav E, Mandel T, et al. Cis and trans requirements for stable episomal maintenance of the BPV-1 replicator. *EMBO J* 1996;15:1–11.
204. Poddar A, Reed SC, McPhillips MG, et al. The human papillomavirus type 8 E2 tethering protein targets the ribosomal DNA loci of host mitotic chromosomes. *J Virol* 2009;83:640–650.
205. Popa A, Zhang W, Harrison MS, et al. Direct binding of retromer to human papillomavirus type 16 minor capsid protein L2 mediates endosome exit during viral infection. *PLoS Pathog* 2015;11(2):e1004699.
206. Porter SS, McBride AA. Human papillomavirus quasivirus production and infection of primary human keratinocytes. *Curr Protoc Microbiol* 2020;57(1):e101.
207. Powell ML, Smith JA, Sowa ME, et al. NCoR1 mediates papillomavirus E8;E2C transcriptional repression. *J Virol* 2010;84(9):4451–4460.
208. Pyeon D, Pearce SM, Lank SM, et al. Establishment of human papillomavirus infection requires cell cycle progression. *PLoS Pathog* 2009;5(2):e1000318.
209. Rangarajan A, Talora C, Okuyama R, et al. Notch signaling is a direct determinant of keratinocyte growth arrest and entry into differentiation. *EMBO J* 2001;20(13):3427–3436.
210. Reznikoff CA, Belair C, Savelieva E, et al. Long-term genome stability and minimal genotypic and phenotypic alterations in HPV-16 E7-, but not E6-immortalized human uroepithelial cells. *Genes Dev* 1994;8:2227–2240.
211. Richards RM, Lowy DR, Schiller JT, et al. Cleavage of the papillomavirus minor capsid protein, L2, at a furin consensus site is necessary for infection. *Proc Natl Acad Sci U S A* 2006;103(5):1522–1527.
212. Roberts JN, Buck CB, Thompson CD, et al. Genital transmission of HPV in a mouse model is potentiated by nonoxynol-9 and inhibited by carrageenan. *Nat Med* 2007;13(7):857–861.
213. Ronco LV, Karpova AY, Vidal M, et al. The human papillomavirus 16 E6 oncoprotein binds to interferon regulatory factor-3 and inhibits its transcriptional activity. *Genes Dev* 1998;12:2061–2072.
214. Rose RC, Bonnez W, Reichman RC, et al. Expression of human papillomavirus type 11 L1 protein in insect cells: in vivo and in vitro assembly of virus like particles. *J Virol* 1993;67:1936–1944.
215. Rous P, Beard JW. The progression to carcinoma of virus-induced rabbit papillomas (Shope). *J Exp Med* 1935;62:523–548.
216. Rowson KEK, Mahy BWJ. Human papova (wart) virus. *Bacteriol Rev* 1967;31:110–131.
217. Rozenblatt-Rosen O, Deo RC, Padi M, et al. Interpreting cancer genomes using systematic host network perturbations by tumour virus proteins. *Nature* 2012;487(7408):491–495.
218. Ruesch MN, Laimins LA. Human papillomavirus oncoproteins alter differentiation-dependent cell cycle exit on suspension in semisolid medium. *Virology* 1998;250:19–29.
219. Sailer C, Offensperger F, Julier A, et al. Structural dynamics of the E6AP/UBE3A-E6-p53 enzyme-substrate complex. *Nat Commun* 2018;9(1):4441.
220. Sakakibara N, Chen D, McBride AA. Papillomaviruses use recombination-dependent replication to vegetatively amplify their genomes in differentiated cells. *PLoS Pathog* 2013;9(7):e1003321.
221. Sakakibara N, Mitra R, McBride AA. The papillomavirus E1 helicase activates a cellular DNA damage response in viral replication foci. *J Virol* 2011;85(17):8981–8995.
222. Sankovski E, Abroi A, Ustav M Jr, et al. Nuclear myosin 1 associates with papillomavirus E2 regulatory protein and influences viral replication. *Virology* 2018;514:142–155.
223. Schapiro F, Sparkowski J, Adduci A, et al. Golgi alkalinization by the papillomavirus E5 oncoprotein. *J Cell Biol* 2000;148(2):305–315.
224. Scheffner M, Huibregtse JM, Vierstra RD, et al. The HPV-16 E6 and E6-AP complex functions as a ubiquitin-protein ligase in the ubiquitination of p53. *Cell* 1993;75:495–505.
225. Scheffner M, Munger K, Byrne JC, et al. The state of the p53 and retinoblastoma genes in human cervical carcinoma cell lines. *Proc Natl Acad Sci U S A* 1991;88:5523–5527.
226. Scheffner M, Nuber U, Huibregtse J. Protein ubiquitination involving an E1-E2-E3 enzyme ubiquitin thioester cascade. *Nature* 1995;373(6509):81–83.
227. Scheffner M, Werness BA, Huibregtse JM, et al. The E6 oncoprotein encoded by human papillomavirus types 16 and 18 promotes the degradation of p53. *Cell* 1990;63:1129–1136.
228. Scherer M, Stamminger T. Emerging Role of PML Nuclear Bodies in Innate Immune Signaling. *J Virol* 2016;90(13):5850–5854.
229. Schlegel R, Phelps WC, Zhang YL, et al. Quantitative keratinocyte assay detects two biological activities of human papillomavirus DNA and identifies viral types associated with cervical carcinoma. *EMBO J* 1988;7:3181–3187.
230. Schweiger MR, You J, Howley PM. Bromodomain protein 4 mediates the papillomavirus E2 transcriptional activation function. *J Virol* 2006;80:4276–4285.
231. Scott ML, Coleman DT, Kelly KC, et al. Human papillomavirus type 16 E5-mediated upregulation of Met in human keratinocytes. *Virology* 2018;519:1–11.
232. Shamanin VA, Androphy EJ. Immortalization of human mammary epithelial cells is associated with inactivation of the p14ARF-p53 pathway. *Mol Cell Biol* 2004;24(5):2144–2152.
233. Sharma S, Munger K. KDM6A-Mediated Expression of the Long Noncoding RNA DINO Causes TP53 Tumor Suppressor Stabilization in Human Papillomavirus 16 E7-Expressing Cells. *J Virol* 2020;94(12):e02178-02119.
234. Shope RE. Immunization of rabbits to infectious papillomatosis. *J Exp Med* 1937;65:219–231.
235. Shope RE, Hurst EW. Infectious papillomatosis of rabbits; with a note on the histopathology. *J Exp Med* 1933;58:607–624.
236. Siddiqa A, Leon KC, James CD, et al. The human papillomavirus type 16 L1 protein directly interacts with E2 and enhances E2-dependent replication and transcription activation. *J Gen Virol* 2015;96(8):2274–2285.
237. Sitz J, Blanchet SA, Gameiro SF, et al. Human papillomavirus E7 oncoprotein targets RNF168 to hijack the host DNA damage response. *Proc Natl Acad Sci U S A* 2019;116(39):19552–19562.
238. Skiadopoulos MH, McBride AA. Bovine papillomavirus type 1 genomes and the E2 transactivator protein are closely associated with mitotic chromatin. *J Virol* 1998;72:2079–2088.
239. Smith JA, Haberstroh FS, White EA, et al. SMCX and components of the TIP60 complex contribute to E2 regulation of the HPV E6/E7 promoter. *Virology* 2014;468–470:311–321.
240. Smith JA, White EA, Sowa ME, et al. Genome-wide siRNA screen identifies SMCX, EP400, and Brd4 as E2-dependent regulators of human papillomavirus oncogene expression. *Proc Natl Acad Sci U S A* 2010;107:3752–3757.
241. Smotkin D, Prokoph H, Wettstein FO. Oncogenic and nononcogenic human genital papillomaviruses generate the E7 mRNA by different mechanisms. *J Virol* 1989;63(3):1441–1447.
242. Songock WK, Kim SM, Bodily JM. The human papillomavirus E7 oncoprotein as a regulator of transcription. *Virus Res* 2017;231:56–75.
243. Songock WK, Scott ML, Bodily JM. Regulation of the human papillomavirus type 16 late promoter by transcriptional elongation. *Virology* 2017;507:179–191.
244. Spalholz BA, Yang Y-C, Howley PM. Transactivation of a bovine papillomavirus transcriptional regulatory element by the E2 gene product. *Cell* 1985;42:183–191.
245. Spangle JM, Ghosh-Choudhury N, Munger K. Activation of cap-dependent translation by mucosal human papillomavirus E6 proteins is dependent on the integrity of the LXXLL binding motif. *J Virol* 2012;86(14):7466–7472.
246. Spurgeon ME, Lambert PF. Mus musculus Papillomavirus 1: a new frontier in animal models of papillomavirus pathogenesis. *J Virol* 2020;94(9).

247. Stenlund A. E1 initiator DNA binding specificity is unmasked by selective inhibition of non-specific DNA binding. *EMBO J* 2003;22(4):954–963.
248. Stoler MH, Broker TR. In situ hybridization detection of human papilloma virus DNA and messenger RNA in genital condylomas and a cervical carcinoma. *Hum Pathol* 1986;17:1250–1258.
249. Storey A, Pim D, Murray A, et al. Comparison of the in vitro transforming activities of human papillomavirus types. *EMBO J* 1988;6:1815–1820.
250. Straight SW, Hinkle PM, Jewers RJ, et al. The E5 oncoprotein of human papillomavirus type 16 transforms fibroblasts and effects downregulation of the epidermal growth factor receptor in keratinocytes. *J Virol* 1993;67:4521–4532.
251. Stransky N, Egloff AM, Tward AD, et al. The mutational landscape of head and neck squamous cell carcinoma. *Science* 2011;333(6046):1157–1160.
252. Surviladze Z, Dziduszko A, Ozbun MA. Essential roles for soluble virion-associated heparan sulfonated proteoglycans and growth factors in human papillomavirus infections. *PLoS Pathog* 2012;8(2):e1002519.
253. Syverton JT. The pathogenesis of the rabbit papilloma-to-carcinoma sequence. *Ann N Y Acad Sci* 1952;54:1126–1140.
254. Syverton JT, Berry GP. Carcinoma in the cottontail rabbit following spontaneous virus papilloma (Shope). *Proc Soc Exp Biol Med* 1935;33:399–400.
255. Szalmas A, Tomaic V, Basukala O, et al. The PTPN14 tumor suppressor is a degradation target of human papillomavirus E7. *J Virol* 2017;91(7):e00057-17.
256. Tan MJ, White EA, Sowa ME, et al. Cutaneous beta-human papillomavirus E6 proteins bind Mastermind-like coactivators and repress Notch signaling. *Proc Natl Acad Sci U S A* 2012;109(23):E1473–E1480.
257. Thatte J, Banks L. Human papillomavirus 16 (HPV-16), HPV-18, and HPV-31 E6 override the normal phosphoregulation of E6AP enzymatic activity. *J Virol* 2017;91(22):e01390-17.
258. Thatte J, Massimi P, Thomas M, et al. The human papillomavirus E6 PDZ binding motif links DNA damage response signaling to E6 inhibition of p53 transcriptional activity. *J Virol* 2018;92(16):e00465-18.
259. Thierry F, Yaniv M. The BPV1 E2 trans-acting protein can be either an activator or a repressor of the HPV18 regulatory region. *EMBO J* 1987;6:3391–3397.
260. Thomas JT, Hubert WG, Ruesch MN, et al. Human papillomavirus type 31 oncoproteins E6 and E7 are required for the maintenance of episomes during the viral life cycle in normal human keratinocytes. *Proc Natl Acad Sci U S A* 1999;96:8449–8454.
261. Thomas M, Banks L. Inhibition of Bak-induced apoptosis by HPV-18 E6. *Oncogene* 1998;17(23):2943–2954.
262. Thomas M, Boiron M, Tanzer J, et al. In vitro transformation of mice by bovine papillomavirus. *Nature* 1964;202:709–710.
263. Thomas M, Laura R, Hepner K, et al. Oncogenic human papillomavirus E6 proteins target the MAGI-2 and MAGI-3 proteins for degradation. *Oncogene* 2002;21(33):5088–5096.
264. Thomas MC, Chiang CM. E6 oncoprotein represses p53-dependent gene activation via inhibition of protein acetylation independently of inducing p53 degradation. *Mol Cell* 2005;17(2):251–264.
265. Tong X, Boll W, Kirschhausen T, et al. Interaction of the bovine papillomavirus E6 protein with the clathrin adaptor complex AP-1. *J Virol* 1998;72:476–482.
266. Tong X, Howley PM. The bovine papillomavirus E6 oncoprotein interacts with paxillin and disrupts the actin cytoskeleton. *Proc Natl Acad Sci U S A* 1997;94:4412–4417.
267. Trus BL, Roden RB, Greenstone HL, et al. Novel structural features of bovine papillomavirus capsid revealed by a three-dimensional reconstruction to 9 A resolution. *Nat Struct Biol* 1997;4(5):413–420.
268. Turek LP, Byrne JC, Lowy DR, et al. Interferon induces morphologic reversion with elimination of extrachromosomal viral genomes in bovine papillomavirus-transformed mouse cells. *Proc Natl Acad Sci U S A* 1982;79:7914–7918.
269. Ustav M, Ustav E, Szymanski P, et al. Identification of the origin of replication of bovine papillomavirus and characterization of the viral origin recognition factor E1. *EMBO J* 1991;10:4321–4329.
270. Van Doorslaer K. Evolution of the papillomaviridae. *Virology* 2013;445(1–2):11–20.
271. Van Doorslaer K, Chen Z, Bernard H, et al. ICTV virus taxonomy profile: Papillomaviridae. *J Gen Virol* 2018;99:989–990.
272. Van Doorslaer K, Li Z, Xirasagar S, et al. The Papillomavirus Episteme: a major update to the papillomavirus sequence database. *Nucleic Acids Res* 2017;45(D1):D499–D506.
273. Van Doorslaer K, McBride AA. Molecular archeological evidence in support of the repeated loss of a papillomavirus gene. *Sci Rep* 2016;6:33028.
274. Van Doorslaer K, Porter S, McKinney C, et al. Novel recombinant papillomavirus genomes expressing selectable genes. *Sci Rep* 2016;6:37782.
275. Van Tine BA, Dao LD, Wu SY, et al. Human papillomavirus (HPV) origin-binding protein associates with mitotic spindles to enable viral DNA partitioning. *Proc Natl Acad Sci U S A* 2004;101:4030–4035.
276. Vande Pol SB, Brown MC, Turner CE. Association of bovine papillomavirus type 1 E6 oncoprotein with the focal adhesion protein paxillin through a conserved protein interaction motif. *Oncogene* 1998;16:43–52.
277. Veldman T, Horikawa I, Barrett JC, et al. Transcriptional activation of the telomerase hTERT gene by human papillomavirus type 16 E6 oncoprotein. *J Virol* 2001;75(9): 4467–4472.
278. Veldman T, Liu X, Yuan H, et al. Human papillomavirus E6 and Myc proteins associate in vivo and bind to and cooperatively activate the telomerase reverse transcriptase promoter. *Proc Natl Acad Sci U S A* 2003;100:8211–8216.
279. Vieira VC, Leonard B, White EA, et al. Human papillomavirus E6 triggers upregulation of the antiviral and cancer genomic DNA deaminase APOBEC3B. *MBio* 2014;5(6).
280. Vos RM, Altreuter J, White EA, et al. The ubiquitin-specific peptidase USP15 regulates human papillomavirus type 16 E6 protein stability. *J Virol* 2009;83(17):8885–8892.
281. Wallace NA, Galloway DA. Novel functions of the human papillomavirus E6 oncoproteins. *Annu Rev Virol* 2015;2(1):403–423.
282. Wang NJ, Sanborn Z, Arnett KL, et al. Loss-of-function mutations in Notch receptors in cutaneous and lung squamous cell carcinoma. *Proc Natl Acad Sci U S A* 2011;108(43):17761–17766.
283. Werness BA, Levine AJ, Howley PM. Association of human papillomavirus types 16 and 18 E6 proteins with p53. *Science* 1990;248:76–79.
284. White A, Livanos EM, Tlsty TD. Differential disruption of genomic integrity and cell cycle regulation in normal human fibroblasts by the HPV oncoproteins. *Genes Dev* 1994;8: 666–677.
285. White EA, Munger K, Howley PM. High-risk human papillomavirus E7 proteins target PTPN14 for degradation. *MBio* 2016;7(5).
286. White EA, Sowa ME, Tan MJ, et al. Systematic identification of interactions between host cell proteins and E7 oncoproteins from diverse human papillomaviruses. *Proc Natl Acad Sci U S A* 2012;109(5):E260–E267.
287. Whyte P, Buchkovich KJ, Horowitz JM, et al. Association between an oncogene and an anti-oncogene: the adenovirus E1A proteins bind to the retinoblastoma gene product. *Nature* 1988;334(124):124–129.
288. Wilgenburg BJ, Budgeon LR, Lang CM, et al. Characterization of immune responses during regression of rabbit oral papillomavirus infections. *Comp Med* 2005;55(5): 431–439.
289. Wolf M, Garcea RL, Grigorieff N, et al. Subunit interactions in bovine papillomavirus. *Proc Natl Acad Sci U S A* 2010;107(14):6298–6303.
290. Wood CE, Chen Z, Cline JM, et al. Characterization and experimental transmission of an oncogenic papillomavirus in female macaques. *J Virol* 2007;81(12):6339–6345.
291. Wooldridge TR, Laimins LA. Regulation of human papillomavirus type 31 gene expression during the differentiation-dependent life cycle through histone modifications and transcription factor binding. *Virology* 2008;374(2):371–380.
292. Wu L, Aster JC, Blacklow SC, et al. MAML1, a human homologue of Drosophila mastermind, is a transcriptional co-activator for NOTCH receptors. *Nat Genet* 2000;26(4): 484–489.
293. Wu SY, Lee AY, Hou SY, et al. Brd4 links chromatin targeting to HPV transcriptional silencing. *Genes Dev* 2006;20:2383–2396.
294. Xu M, Luo W, Elzi DJ, et al. NFX1 interacts with mSin3A/histone deacetylase to repress hTERT transcription in keratinocytes. *Mol Cell Biol* 2008;28(15):4819–4828.
295. You J, Croyle JL, Nishimura A, et al. Interaction of the bovine papillomavirus E2 protein with Brd4 tethers the viral DNA to host mitotic chromosomes. *Cell* 2004;117: 349–360.
296. Zerfass-Thome K, Zwerschke W, Mannhardt B, et al. Inactivation of the cdk inhibitor p27KIP1 by the human papillomavirus type 16 E7 oncoprotein. *Oncogene* 1996;13:2323–2330.
297. Zhang B, Li P, Wang E, et al. The E5 protein of human papillomavirus type 16 perturbs MHC class II antigen maturation in human foreskin keratinocytes treated with interferon-gamma. *Virology* 2003;310(1):100–108.
298. Zhang B, Srirangam A, Potter DA, et al. HPV16 E5 protein disrupts the c-Cbl-EGFR interaction and EGFR ubiquitination in human foreskin keratinocytes. *Oncogene* 2005;24(15):2585–2588.
299. Zheng G, Schweiger M-R, Martinez-Noel G, et al. Brd4 regulation of papillomavirus E2 protein stability. *J Virol* 2009;83:8683–8692.
300. Zhou J, Sun XY, Stenzel DJ, et al. Expression of vaccinia recombinant HPV 16 L1 and L2 ORF proteins in epithelial cells is sufficient for assembly of HPV virion-like particles. *Virology* 1991;185:251–257.
301. Zimmermann H, Degenkolbe R, Bernard HU, et al. The human papillomavirus type 16 E6 oncoprotein can down-regulate p53 activity by targeting the transcriptional coactivator CBP/p300. *J Virol* 1999;73:6209–6219.

CHAPTER 3 Papillomaviruses

John T. Schiller • Douglas R. Lowy

The Papillomaviruses (PVs) comprise a widely dispersed group of nonenveloped epitheliotropic viruses of vertebrates that characteristically induce benign hyperproliferative lesions of the skin (warts) and mucous membranes (condylomata).[100] More than 200 genotypes (types) have been identified in humans.[43] All PVs have small double-stranded circular DNA genomes of approximately 8 kilobases, and all transcripts are derived from the same DNA strand (Fig. 3.1). They generally contain about eight distinct protein coding regions, which through alternatively spliced mRNAs can generate multiple protein species. The proteins function as virion structural proteins (L1 and L2), as regulators of viral genome transcription and replication (E1 and E2), and as determinants that perturb the normal physiology of host cell in ways that promote the virus productive life cycle (E4, E5, E6, E7, and E8). Productive infection occurs only in a stratified squamous epithelium, with the highly regulated expression of the viral genes being closely tied to the differentiation state of the keratinocytes (Fig. 3.2). In rare cases, the normal viral life cycle of a small subset of PV types goes awry, leading to the development of various epithelial malignancies, which are manifested in humans as cancer of the uterine cervix, as well as other cancers in the anogenital tract and the upper airway. An accompanying chapter details the basic molecular biology of PVs. This chapter will focus primarily on the epidemiology of human papillomaviruses (HPVs), the neoplastic diseases that they cause, and interventions to prevent or treat these diseases.

PAPILLOMAVIRUSES AND CANCER

Whereas most PVs do not appear to have oncogenic potential, a subset of PV is clearly implicated in the development of malignancy in humans and animals[403] (Table 3.1). In humans, approximately 5% of all cancers are attributable to HPV infection, with cervical cancer being the most important from a global public health perspective (Fig. 3.3).[81] HPVs are also implicated in other anogenital cancers, including anal cancer, vulvar cancer, and penile cancer, as well as in oropharyngeal and laryngeal cancers (Fig. 3.3). HPV infection is associated with virtually all cases of cervical cancer, the vast majority of cases of anal cancer, and many of the other forms of cancer (Fig. 3.3).[81,82] There may be concordant HPV infection at multiple mucosal sites,[58] and patients who have had one HPV-associated cancer may have an increased risk of a second HPV-associated cancer.[59]

In the developing world, cervical cancer accounts for more than 90% of the HPV-associated cancers,[81,82] while the noncervical cancers constitute at least one-half of the HPV-associated cancers in the United States and some other industrialized countries (Fig. 3.4).[320] This difference is attributable to substantial reductions in the incidence of cervical cancer brought about by Pap smear screening, as well as an increasing incidence of HPV-positive anal cancer and, especially, HPV-positive oropharyngeal cancer (OPC).[361] In the developing world, fewer than 10% of HPV-associated cancers occur in males,[81] while in the United States, more than 40% of them arise in males.[320]

A subset of skin-tropic HPV, especially HPV-5 and 8, is involved in the cutaneous squamous cell cancers that develop in association with epidermodysplasia verruciformis (EV), a rare inherited genodermatosis characterized by excessive flat

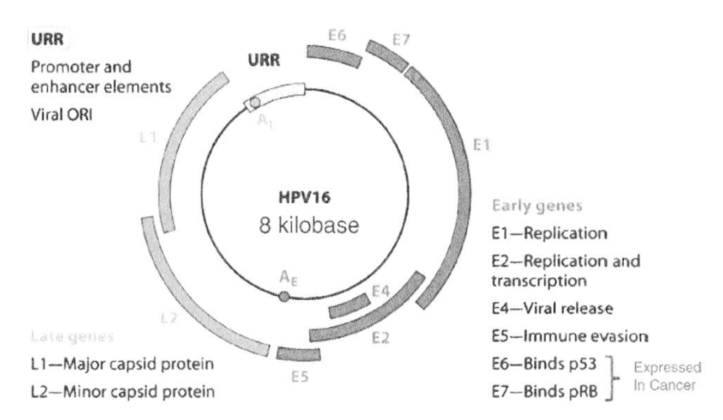

FIGURE 3.1 Schematic of the 8 kilobase double-stranded DNA genome of HPV-16. The open reading frames encoding viral polypeptides are shown in blue and green. The upstream regulatory region (URR) is depicted in yellow. A_E and A_L are the polyadenylation sites for the early and late transcripts, respectively. E6 and E7 bind multiple cellular proteins, in addition to p53 and pRB. (Figure from Stanley MA. Epithelial cell responses to infection with human papillomavirus. *Clin Microbiol Rev* 2012;25:215–222. Copyright © 2012 American Society for Microbiology. Reproduced with permission from American Society for Microbiology.)

wart-like papules.[243] These same types have been implicated in cutaneous squamous cell cancers in the general population or in immunosuppressed individuals, but their contribution to skin cancers in these populations remains unclear.[328] Some claims have been made of an association of HPV with several other common cancers, including those of the lung, breast, esophagus, colon, rectum, and prostate, but a consistent causal relationship has not been demonstrated.[68] Where detected, the HPV genome copy number has generally been found to be much lower than one per cancer cell in these cancers. As HPVs have an exceptional tropism for infecting cancer cells compared to intact normal tissues,[179] the possibility of reverse causality, that is, that infection is the result rather than the cause of the cancer, should be considered in these cases.

In the most well-studied examples of human cancers attributable to HPV, the tumors develop in a stratified squamous epithelium, they do not occur until many years after the

TABLE 3.1 Major clinical associations of HPVs by type

Clinical Association	Viral Type(s)
Skin	
Common warts	HPV-2, 27, 57
Plantar and palmar warts	HPV-1a**, 2, 27, 57
Flat warts	HPV-3, 10
Squamous cell cancer	HPV-5*, 8*
Genital tract	
Exophytic condyloma (any site)	HPV-6, 11
Flat condyloma (especially cervix)	HPV-6, 11, 16, 18, 31
Bowenoid papulosis	HPV-16, 18
Giant condyloma	HPV-6, 11
Cervical cancer	
Strong association	HPV-16, 18, 31, 45
Moderate association	HPV-33, 35, 39, 51, 52, 56, 58, 59, 68
Weak or no association	HPV-6, 11, 26, 42, 43, 44, 53, 54, 55, 62, 66
Vulvar and vaginal cancer	HPV-16
Penile cancer	HPV-16
Anal cancer	HPV-16
Recurrent respiratory papillomas	HPV-6, 11
Conjunctival papillomas	HPV-6, 11
Oral cavity	
Focal epithelial hyperplasia	HPV-13, 32
Infection with genital HPV	HPV-6, 11, 16
Lesions on lip	HPV-2
Oropharyngeal cancer	HPV-16

All list types belong to the Alpha genus unless otherwise designated.
* = Beta.
** = Mu.

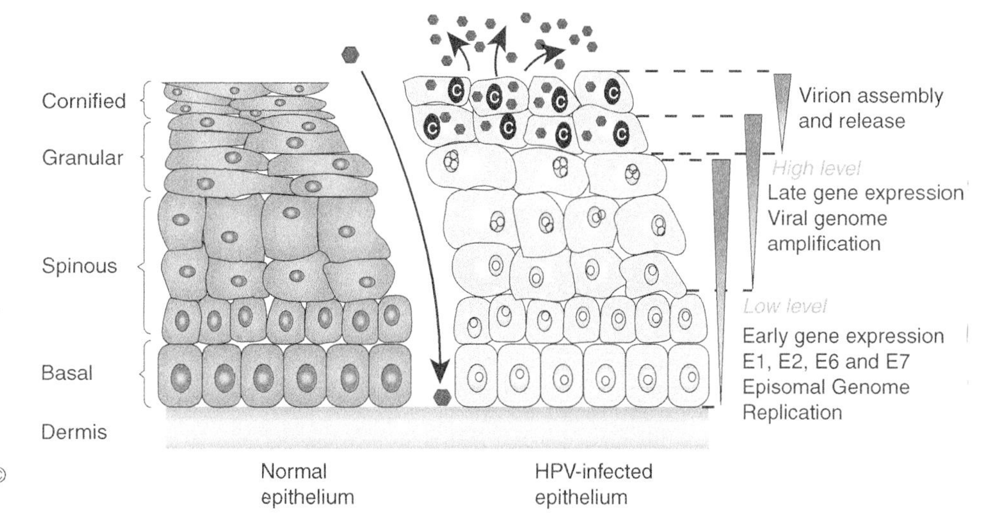

FIGURE 3.2 The HPV life cycle in a stratified squamous epithelium. Normal and infected epithelium are shown on the *left* and *right*, respectively. *Small circles* depict the viral genome in the nucleus and "C" indicates production of the virion capsid proteins. (Reprinted by permission from Nature: Moody CA, Laimins LA. Human papillomavirus oncoproteins: pathways to transformation. *Nat Rev Cancer* 2010;10:550–560. Copyright © 2010 Springer Nature.)

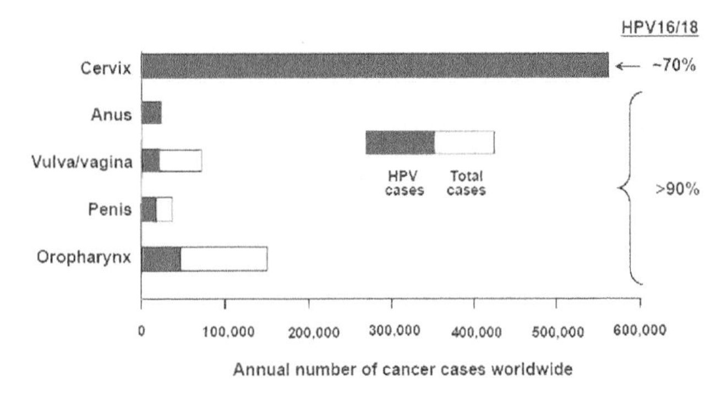

FIGURE 3.3 Worldwide annual incidence of HPV-associated cancers and attributable fraction of total cancers in 2018. The number of HPV-attributable cases is indicated in *blue* and HPV-independent cases in *white*. The approximate percent of attributable cases caused by HPV-16 or HPV-18 is indicated at the *right*. (Data derived from de Martel C, Georges D, Bray F, et al. Global burden of cancer attributable to infections in 2018: a worldwide incidence analysis. *Lancet Glob Health* 2020;8(2):e180–e190.)

initial infection, persistent infection is required for progression to invasive cancer, and maintenance of the transformed phenotype depends on the continued expression of at least some viral genes, especially E6 and E7.[125] On the other hand, most infections, even those caused by the HPV types implicated in cancer, have a benign outcome, because they either are self-limited or do not progress to cancer even when they are persistent.

The long interval between the initial infection and the development of cancer implies that, in addition to persistent infection by an appropriate HPV type, additional environmental and/or host factors contribute to malignant progression. Immune status is one important host parameter, with impaired cellular immune function being associated with a greater risk of persistent infection and cancer.[340] Adult patients with Fanconi anemia, an inherited disease with defective DNA repair, have been reported to have a greater than 100-fold increased risk of developing HPV-associated tumors.[177] Exogenous exposure of PV-induced lesions to cocarcinogens may represent an environmental mechanism. For example, most cutaneous cancers in EV occur on sun-exposed skin, which implies that UV light is serving as a cocarcinogen.[352]

Most HPV-associated cancers appear to depend on the continuous expression of viral genes (e.g., E6 and E7). However, it remains possible that viral gene expression may not be obligatory at all stages for some HPV-induced cancers.[315] In a small minority of cervical cancers that contain HPV DNA, the viral oncogenes are not expressed. Development of esophageal cancer in cattle by BPV-4 and the carcinogen in bracken fern is associated with complete loss of the viral genome in the malignant tumors.[44] A hit-and-run mechanism has been postulated to explain the generally low viral copy number in skin carcinomas.[315] A hit-and-run phenomenon suggests that, in these instances, the virus is required for tumor induction, but that its continued presence is consistently selected against, either biologically or immunologically, in progressed lesions. One plausible scenario is that antiapoptotic viral activities allow genetically damaged cells to survive and proliferate, permitting further genetic and/or epigenetic changes to accumulate that overcome the need for continued viral gene expression.

HUMAN PAPILLOMAVIRUS INFECTIONS OF THE GENITAL TRACT

HPV infection of the anogenital tract represents the most important medical burden from infection with this group of agents. In women, infection affects the genital skin and mucosa, including the vulva, vaginal tract, cervix, and anal canal. Most of these infections are sexually transmitted, which means that their prevalence is usually correlated with measures of sexual activity, such as the number of lifetime sexual partners, a recent change in sexual partner(s), and a history of other sexually transmitted infections.[40,327]

HPV infection of the anogenital tract is extremely common, with a wide range of clinical manifestations and outcomes, varying from asymptomatic and self-limited to persistent and associated with malignant progression. Viral factors and host factors each contribute to determining the outcome. The alpha-HPVs cause most anogenital infections, and the majority of oncogenic HPV types are from the alpha-7 and alpha-9 species, which together are often considered "high-risk" HPV types (Table 3.1).[310]

Cervical Cancer

Cervical cancer is the fourth most common malignancy among women worldwide, with an estimated 570,000 cases and 311,000 deaths in 2018.[9] Despite its worldwide distribution, the frequency of cervical cancer varies considerably, being about 10 times more common in some developing countries than in most industrialized ones.[82] More than 85% of cervical cancer occurs in developing countries, where it is frequently the most common cancer of women, accounting for as many as one-quarter of female cancers. Pap smear screening, which identifies cytologic abnormalities induced by persistent HPV infection,

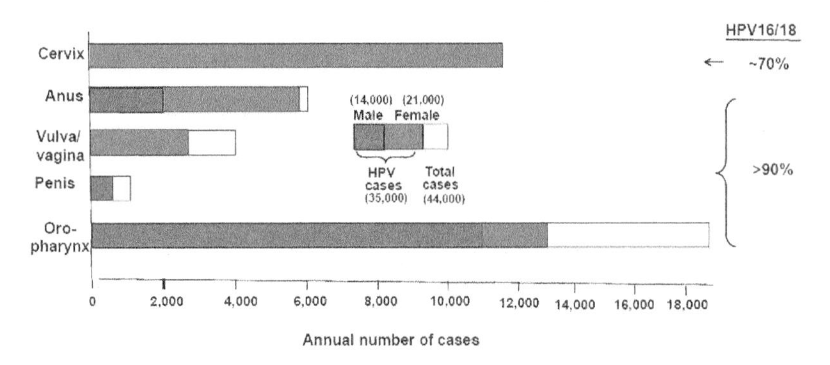

FIGURE 3.4 United States annual incidence of HPV-associated cancer in 2012–2016 and attributable fraction by gender. HPV-attributed cases in females are shown in *red*, HPV-attributable cases in males in *gray* and HPV-independent cases in *white*. The approximate percent of attributable cases caused by HPV-16 or HPV-18 is indicated at the *right*. (Data derived from Senkomago V, Henley SJ, Thomas CC, et al. Human papillomavirus-attributable cancers—United States, 2012–2016. *MMWR Morb Mortal Wkly Rep* 2019;68:724–728.)

has dramatically decreased the frequency of cervical cancer in many industrialized countries. In the United States, approximately 10,000 new cases are diagnosed annually, and about one-third of these women will die of their malignant disease.[320] The incidence of cervical cancer in the United States varies considerably among ethnic and, especially, socioeconomic groups.[22]

More than 90% of these cancers occur in the transformation zone of the cervix, where the columnar cells of the endocervix form a junction with the stratified squamous epithelium of the exocervix[42] (Fig. 3.5). About 85% of cervical cancers are squamous cell cancers. Most of the other cases are adenocarcinomas, with a small number being small cell neuroendocrine tumors.

Lesions that become malignant squamous cell carcinomas typically undergo a series of dysplastic changes over many years.[307] The severity of the lesion is determined by the degree to which the squamous epithelium is replaced by basaloid cells, with the entire thickness being replaced in the most severe dysplasias (Fig. 3.6). In the histologic classification of cervical intraepithelial dysplasia (CIN), grades 1, 2, and 3 correspond, respectively, to mild dysplasia, moderate dysplasia, and severe dysplasia or carcinoma *in situ*. The cervical dysplasias have their counterpart in the exfoliated cells present in the Papanicolaou (Pap) smear, as evidenced by the presence of koilocytes (evidence of virion production) and basaloid cells (evidence of dysplasia). In the binary cytologic Bethesda system,[196] abnormalities are classified as low-grade and high-grade squamous intraepithelial lesions (SIL), with low grade corresponding to mild cytologic abnormalities and high grade encompassing the more severe abnormalities (Fig. 3.6). CIN1 and LSIL are now

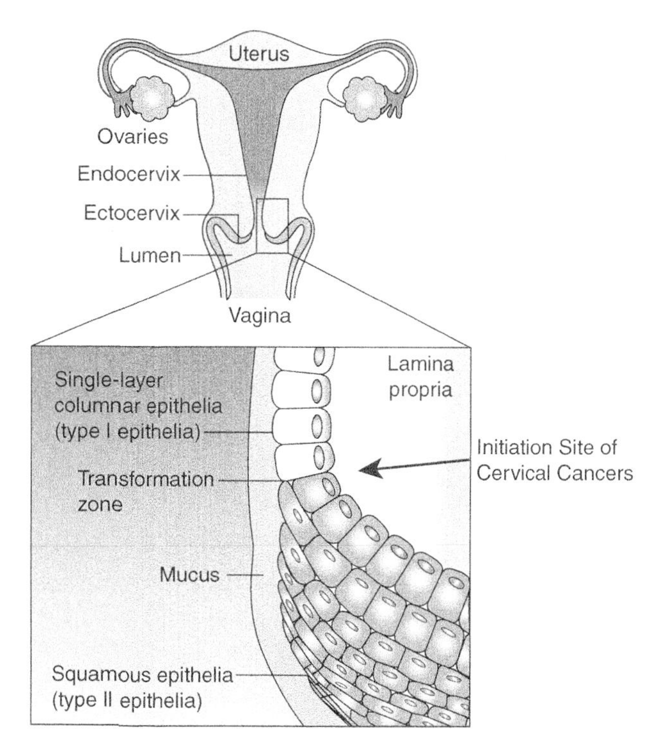

FIGURE 3.5 Female reproductive tract anatomy and histology. (Reprinted by permission from Nature: Iwasaki A. Antiviral immune responses in the genital tract: clues for vaccines. *Nat Rev Immunol* 2010;10:699–711. Copyright © 2010 Springer Nature. Ref.[164].)

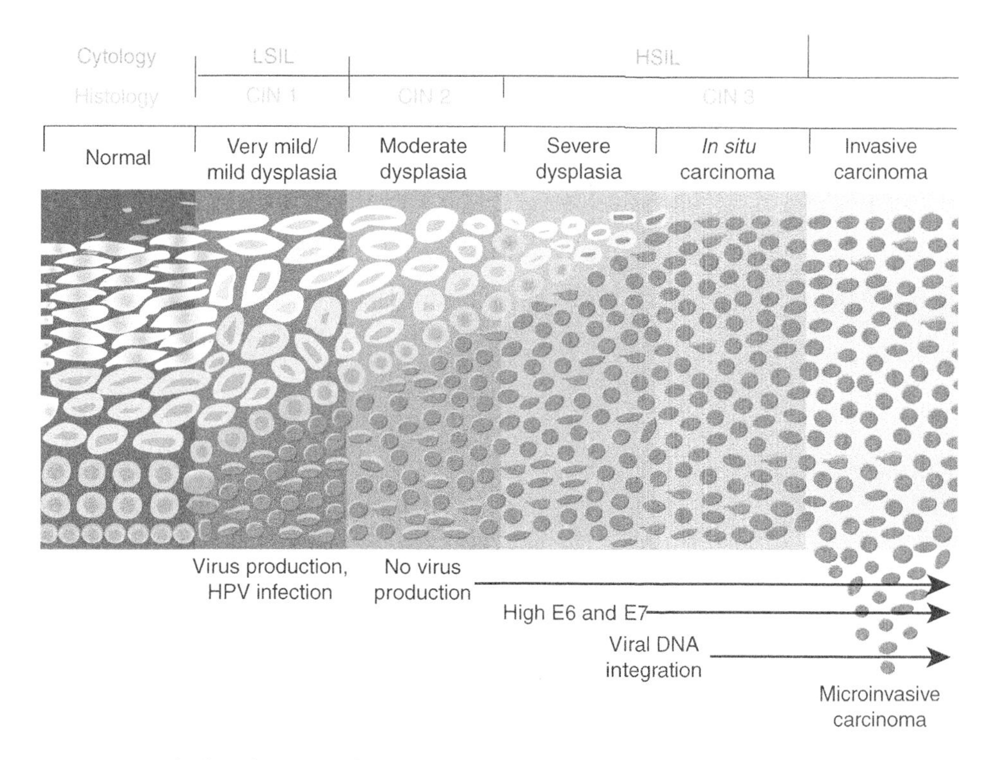

FIGURE 3.6 The histologic, cytologic, and virologic changes during progression from initial infection to cervical cancer. CIN, cervical intraepithelial neoplasia; LSIL, low-grade squamous intraepithelial neoplasia; HSIL, high-grade cervical intraepithelial neoplasia. (Modified with permission of American Society for Clinical Investigation from Lowy DR, Schiller JT. Prophylactic human papillomavirus vaccines. *J Clin Invest* 2006;116:1167–1173. Permission conveyed through Copyright Clearance Center, Inc. Ref.[214]).

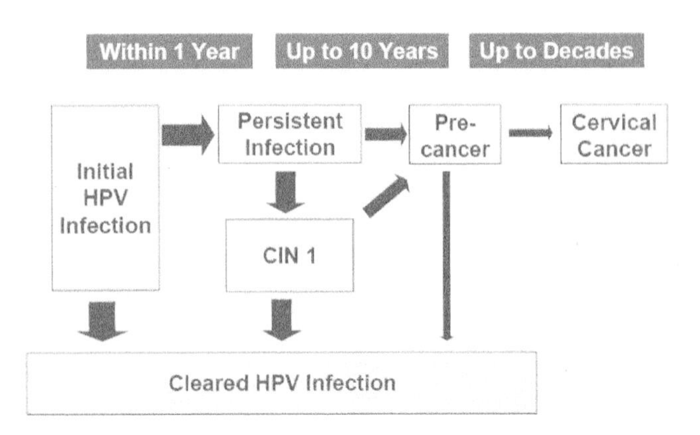

FIGURE 3.7 Natural history of oncogenic HPV infection and progression to cervical cancer. The bolder the *arrow*, the more frequent the transition between states. CIN 1, cervical intraepithelial neoplasia grade 1.

considered normal manifestations of productive HPV infection. Atypical squamous cytology of undetermined significance (ASCUS) is the cytologic designation for equivocal lesions; the risk of HPV-positive ASCUS lesions progressing to HSIL is similar to that of LSIL, while the risk of HPV-negative ASCUS lesions is about fourfold lower.[90]

Most dysplasias do not progress and, in fact, resolve spontaneously, but the likelihood of their resolution decreases with the severity of the dysplasia (Fig. 3.7). Severe dysplasias (also designated "precancers"), however, generally arise from less dysplastic lesions after several years,[210] although some precancers can develop rapidly, apparently without passing through a low-grade stage,[186] perhaps due to high-risk HPV infection of a uniquely susceptible subset of morphologically distinct cells residing in the squamocolumnar junction.[149] Because of the long interval between the development of cervical dysplasia and invasive cancer, follow-up of Pap smear abnormalities or positive results in newer virologic-based screens (discussed below) can identify most premalignant lesions. Appropriate follow-up of women with these abnormalities, together with appropriate treatment, can thereby prevent the development of most cases of cervical cancer.[89,276] In some countries with screening programs, however, the incidence of adenocarcinoma and adenosquamous cell carcinoma has been increasing, suggesting that Pap smear screening has been less effective in identifying the precursors to these tumor types.[359]

Role of HPV in Cervical Cancer

Cervical cancer was recognized for decades to behave as a sexually transmitted disease, long before sexually transmitted HPV infection was implicated in its pathogenesis. In the mid-1970s, Meisels and Fortin[231] recognized, on morphologic grounds, that HPV infection of the cervix occurred frequently, often with the histologic characteristics of mild CIN. These observations coincided with the proposal by zur Hausen[402] that HPV infection might be the putative sexually transmitted agent responsible for cervical cancer. During this period, the detection of HPV-5 or HPV-8 in skin cancer in patients with EV strongly suggested that some HPVs might have malignant potential.[257] Only a subset of the HPV types isolated from patients with EV was found in the skin cancers, implying that HPV types might vary in their oncogenicity. The molecular cloning of HPV-16 and HPV-18 from cervical cancer biopsies by zur Hausen and colleagues in the early 1980s[31,105] provided the field with the HPV types that were subsequently shown to be present in approximately two-thirds of cervical cancers worldwide. Using lower stringency hybridization techniques, other HPV types were later identified in cervical tumors.[403] Subsequent studies, carried out by many investigators, have sought to understand the natural history of HPV infection of the genital tract, determine the biological properties of different HPV types, elucidate the role of the virus in the pathogenesis of cervical disease, and identify nonviral factors that may influence the outcome of HPV infection.

More than 50 HPV types, mostly from the alpha genus, infect the genital tract.[317] Only a dozen of these types, however, are found regularly in cervical cancers, and in a higher proportion than in controls, leading these types to be designated as "high risk" (Table 3.1). On the other hand, HPV types that are detected relatively frequently in controls, but rarely in cancers, are designated "low risk." A worldwide study of almost 1,000 cervical cancers, from paraffin-embedded sections, indicated that more than 90% contain HPV DNA.[30] Although more than 20 HPV types were found in the tumors, two types from the alpha-7 (types 18 and 45) and two types from alpha-9 (types 16 and 31) species accounted for close to 80% of the HPV-positive cancers. Conversely, low-risk HPV (e.g., HPV-6 and HPV-11) was found in only two of these cancers. In all areas of the world, HPV-16 is the most common type found in the cancers. A follow-up evaluation of the cancers in this study that were initially believed to be HPV negative indicated either that they were false-negative results or that the DNA in the specimens was too degraded for the negative results to be deemed reliable.[372] The conclusion from this study was that at least 99.9% of cervical cancers contain HPV DNA and, therefore, that HPV infection is a necessary cause of cervical cancer, the first etiologic agent for a cancer to be so designated.

In a worldwide meta-analysis of 14,595 cervical cancers, of which 89.7% were HPV positive, HPV-16 and HPV-18 were detected in 70%, while no other type was found in no more than 4.4% (Fig. 3.8).[333] It seems likely that most cases reported as being HPV DNA negative represent false-negative findings. Some regional variation exists in the specific proportion of HPV types in cervical cancer, and also in CIN3, but this variation is relatively minor and is less than the wider variation that exists among asymptomatic infections or low-grade dysplasias.[49] In one recently identified racially associated susceptibility, HPV-35 appears to be more carcinogenic in women with African ancestry.[279]

Prospective population-based studies that evaluated progression from asymptomatic infection to CIN3 or worse (CIN3+) confirmed that HPV-16 is the most oncogenic type. In a recent Danish study, the 8-year absolute risk of progression of a single persistent HPV-16 infection to CIN3 was 55%.[304] The next most virulent types appear to be HPV-33, -18, and -31 with absolute risks of 33%, 32%, and 31%, respectively (Fig. 3.9). By contrast, HPV-56, considered a high-risk type, had an absolute risk of progression to CIN3 of only 3%.

Whereas most studies have focused on the more common squamous cell cancers, most cervical adenocarcinomas, adenosquamous carcinomas, and those carcinomas with neuroendocrine differentiation also contain HPV DNA. In an international analysis that pooled eight case–control studies,

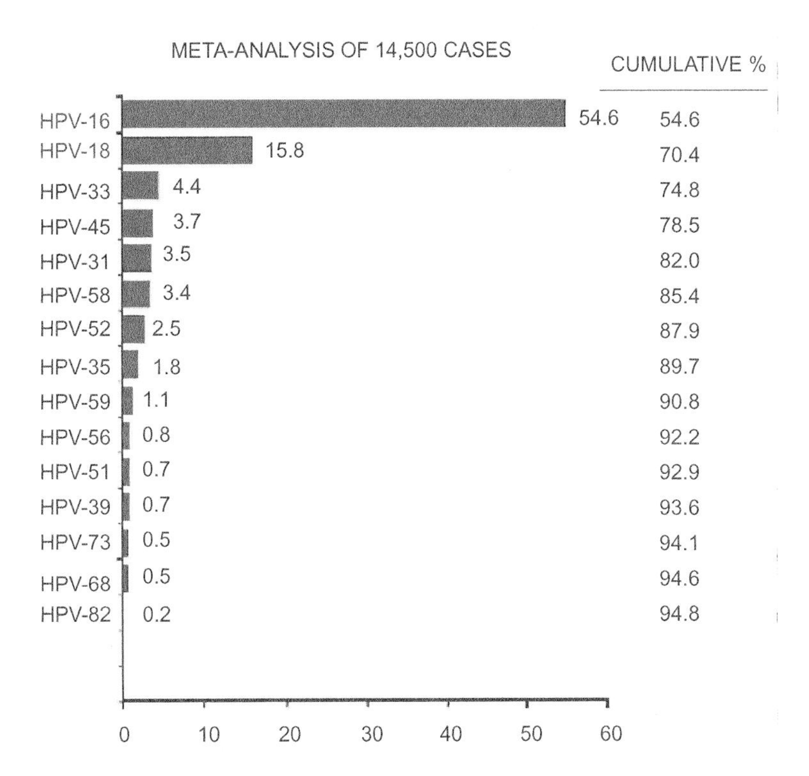

FIGURE 3.8 Worldwide percentages of cervical cancer attributed to the most frequent HPV types. (Data from Smith JS, Lindsay L, Hoots B, et al. Human papillomavirus type distribution in invasive cervical cancer and high-grade cervical lesions: a meta-analysis update. *Int J Cancer* 2007;121:621–632.)

the adjusted odds ratio of adenocarcinoma for HPV-positive women was 81.3 (95% CI 42.0 to 157.1), and HPV-16 and HPV-18 accounted for 82% of these tumors.[50] A larger proportion of these tumors are associated with HPV-18, compared with squamous cell carcinomas, and in some studies, the number of HPV-18–associated tumors was greater than that associated with HPV-16. Low-risk HPV types may rarely be associated with cervical cancer and other cancers.[86] In addition, some HPV types, such as HPV-26, might be more oncogenic in an immunocompromised host.[141] It should also be recognized that this classification may not apply to HPV infections in all sites. For example, the Buschke-Löwenstein tumor, which is a low-grade squamous cell carcinoma of the external genitalia, is usually associated with the low-risk HPV-6 or HPV-11.[137]

Natural History of Genital Human Papillomavirus Infection

Genital HPV infection is considered the most common sexually transmitted viral infection, with an estimated lifetime risk in U.S. women and men with at least one opposite sex partner of 85% and 91%, respectively.[61] The estimated prevalence of infection varies with the age of the population and depends on the sensitivity of the HPV assay employed. A population-based study of cervical infection in the United States, which used a very sensitive DNA-based test, found 42.5% of women 14 to 59 were HPV positive, with those 20 to 24 having the highest prevalence, 53.8%, decreasing to 38.8% in women 50 to 59.[142] The infections were divided approximately equally between high-risk and low-risk types. Since sexually active women 19 or younger

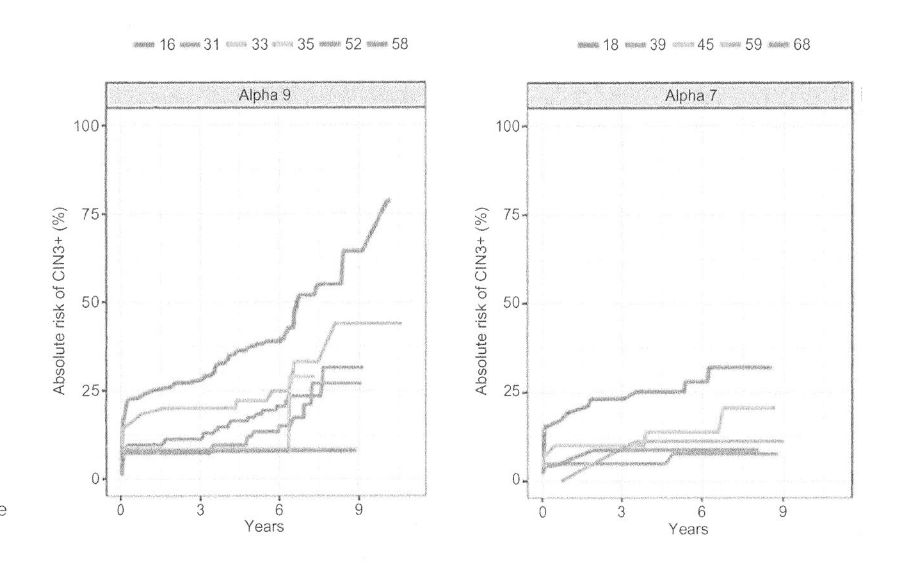

FIGURE 3.9 Absolute risk of a single persistent HPV infection progressing to CIN3 over time according to type. Alpha 9 and Alpha 7 refer to the two species of the genus that include the major oncogenic types.

acquire genital HPV infection at a high rate,[389] the comparatively low prevalence of 32.9% among those 14 to 19 probably arises because many in this age group are not yet sexually active. The decreasing prevalence of HPV infection beyond age 24 results from a combination of the self-limited nature of most infections, decreasing HPV exposure with age, and resistance to reinfection. It has been estimated that approximately 75% of the high-risk HPV infections leading to cervical cancer are acquired by age 30.[41] Genital HPVs can establish latency, but it is not clear whether reactivation from latency is a substantial risk factor for progression to cervical or other anogenital cancers.[131]

The natural history of genital HPV infection in men has been studied less systematically than that in women, with only one large prospective multicentric study.[327] As with women, infections in men are very common, and most are self-limited. In males, however, prevalence does not tend to decrease with age.[126] Penile infection is detected in 16% to 69% of healthy men depending on the population, sampling method, and HPV detection method.[95] When controlled for lifetime number of sexual partners, male circumcision has been identified as an important negative risk factor for prevalent penile infection in the men and for cervical cancer in their current sexual partners, although this association may be attenuated when multiple sites on the male genitalia are sampled.[5,6] Circumcision also reduced high-risk HPV acquisition and prevalence by approximately one-third in two randomized control trials in adult males.[132,351]

Although most women with HPV infection of the genital tract do not have detectable cytologic abnormalities, the epidemiology of genital HPV infection appears to account for the epidemiology of cervical neoplasia, including the dysplasias that precede cervical carcinoma (Fig. 3.6).[29] Following the development of validated HPV DNA assays in the early 1990s,[337] many studies have consistently shown that infection with high-risk HPV represents the major risk factor for high-grade cervical dysplasias and invasive cancer.[312] In cytologically normal women, being positive for a high-risk HPV places them at much higher risk for developing cytologic abnormalities compared with women who are HPV negative.[182,308] In addition, results of a serologic assay based on antibodies to HPV-16 L1 virus-like particles (VLPs) that can identify currently and previously infected individuals implicated HPV-16–related viruses prospectively in the development of cervical cancer.[138,204]

As noted above, most genital infections are self-limited, with the majority of incident infections clearing within 12 months and approximately 90% within 2 years, as operationally defined as the inability to detect HPV DNA in a sensitive assay.[240,386] Clearance of HPV infection appears to return an individual to the same low risk of CIN3 or invasive cancer as an individual in whom HPV has not been detected previously. Low-grade dysplasia may be caused by infection with either low-risk or high-risk HPV. Persistent (i.e., long-term) infection with a high-risk HPV type, which occurs in a minority of infected women, is by far the single most important risk factor for developing CIN3 or invasive cancer (CIN3+). However, the magnitude of the risk depends on the HPV type (Fig. 3.9), and even on the variant within a given type.[235,311] In practical terms, persistence is usually defined as meaning that the same HPV type has been identified in two or more genital samples taken over a certain period, with the interval usually being at least 4 to 12 months. Persistent infections may clear spontaneously but are less likely to do so the longer they persist. Conversely, only some persistent infections progress to CIN3, and only some CIN3 progress to invasive cancer (Fig. 3.7). HPV-16 infections are more likely to persist than infection by other HPV types.[211] However, persistence *per se* is not sufficient for progression to high-grade dysplasia, because low-risk HPV types that persist are much less likely to progress than high-risk types.[309] The distinct biological activities of high-risk E6 and E7 (discussed in Chapter 2) are likely to represent at least partial explanations of the differences in the likelihood of progression.

Molecular Pathogenesis of Cervical Cancer

High-risk HPV types can infect the genital skin, the vaginal tract, or the cervix. If the cervix is not infected initially, the virus can spread locally, presumably by autoinoculation, to the cervix.[386] Cervical neoplastic lesions can be single or multiple. The production of progeny virions is usually limited to asymptomatic or low-grade lesions, as the full viral replication cycle is tied to the differentiation process (Fig. 3.2).[98,238] A subset of cuboidal cervical cells in the transformation zone that expresses specific embryologic markers may be particularly susceptible to malignant progression when they become infected (Fig. 3.5).[148,149]

In high-grade dysplasias and cancers, a restricted number of the viral genes are expressed, primarily E6 and E7, and their expression is now detected throughout the lesion, in contrast to most of their expression being in suprabasal cells during productive infection (Fig. 3.6).[98] Both genes are expressed from a single promoter, with alternate splicing determining their relative level of expression,[349] and progression to high-grade disease may be associated with a splicing pattern that favors E7 production. As discussed in detail in the accompanying chapter by McBride and Howley, E6 and E7 each interacts with multiple cellular factors, most notably p53 and pRb, respectively, to drive progression to high-grade dysplasia and cancer. Methylation of the HPV-16 viral genome appears to influence progression to moderate- and high-grade neoplasia, with methylation of CpG sites in L1, L2, and E2/E4 being associated with an increased risk of precancer, while methylation of upstream regulatory region (URR) sites is associated with a decreased risk.[33]

Integration of HPV DNA is strongly associated with malignant progression. In one study of 155 samples, integration was not detected in any asymptomatic infections or CIN1 lesions but was present in 5% of CIN2 lesions, in 16% of CIN3 lesions, and in 87% of invasive cancer.[184] The frequency of viral DNA integration may vary with the HPV type. In an analysis of The Cancer Genome Atlas (TCGA) data set, 76% of HPV-16–positive samples had integrated copies, whereas all HPV-18–positive cases had integrated viral genomes.[45] Viral DNA integration can occur at many sites throughout the genome, but it is clonal for a given lesion and is found preferentially at transcriptionally active and genomically fragile sites. In a given lesion, it usually involves only one locus or a few loci, and the viral genome can be integrated as a single copy or as tandem repeats.[229] The conclusion that a proportion of cancers contains both extrachromosomal and integrated viral genomes has recently been challenged.[239] These cancers may instead harbor circular replicons containing both viral and host DNA segments.

Viral genome integration drives malignant progression primarily because it can increase the expression of the E6 and E7 oncogenes, which can occur via several mechanisms. Integration can disrupt the expression of E2, which is a negative regulator of E6/E7 transcription in undifferentiated cells. Alternatively, integration can generate E6/E7 transcripts with 3′ cellular sequences that stabilize the mRNAs,[107] or it can increase transcription by occurring in the vicinity of cellular enhancer elements.[229] Clonal outgrowth of cells with integrated viral genomes exemplifies the selective advantage conferred by E6/E7 overexpression in neoplastic progression, and studies in cervical cancer–derived cell lines indicate that continued expression of E6 and E7 is necessary for their continued viability and proliferative ability.[88] However, integration offers no selective vantage for the virus *per se,* since integrated genomes are unable to produce progeny virions. In cancers where only episomal copies are detected, E2 is often inactivated, frequently by mutation or epigenetic silencing, resulting in dysregulation of E6/E7 expression.[52]

It has been postulated that the viral genome can also contribute to carcinogenesis by insertional mutagenesis via integration in the vicinity of cellular protooncogenes or tumor suppressor genes, activating and repressing their expression, respectively. Viral DNA integration near the c-Myc protooncogene has been observed in up to 10% of cervical cancer in some case series and was associated with its increased expression.[104,376] However, current evidence suggests that insertional mutagenesis is not obligatory for malignant progression and functions in only a minority of cervical cancers.

It is noteworthy that HPV-16– and HPV-18–positive cell lines derived from cervical and anal cancers harbor wild-type versions of p53 and pRb, in contrast to HPV-negative tumor-derived cell lines, many of which have mutations in p53- and pRb-related pathways.[242] This observation implies that there is sufficient functional inactivation of p53 and pRb by HPV E6 and E7, respectively, and that there is virtually no selective pressure for the genetic inactivation of the *p53* and *pRb* genes. Another consistent feature of dysplasias and cancer is that most cells express the p16 tumor suppressor, as a cellular response to the E7-dependent inactivation of pRb,[25] again in contrast to many tumors not associated with HPV, in which p16 tends to be silenced. Immunostaining for p16 has frequently been used as a surrogate marker for elevated HPV E7 expression.

The E7s of high-risk HPVs stimulate DNA replication stress that leads to DNA breakage and chromosomal instability.[185] In addition, high-risk HPVs induce abnormal centrosome duplication, which can result in genomic instability and aneuploidy.[102] The deregulation of this mitotic event appears to depend on both E6 and E7, with the latter protein being more responsible for the effect.[185] In a study that compared the incidence of aneuploidy and viral DNA integration, both were associated with increasing dysplasia.[232] Although 95% (19/20) of lesions with integrated viral DNA were aneuploid, only 59% (19/32) of aneuploid lesions had integrated viral genomes. As aneuploidy was found significantly more frequently than integration, it was concluded that deregulated viral oncogene expression results first in chromosomal instability and aneuploidization, which are subsequently followed by viral DNA integration.

Although the E5 gene, which can potentiate signaling through growth factor receptors and promote immune evasion (discussed below), is considered an oncogene, the studies mentioned above imply a central role for high-risk E6 and E7 in cervical cancer pathogenesis, and tumors that contain only integrated HPV DNA have usually lost expression of E5. However, some evidence suggests that, in HPV-16–associated tumors that retain extrachromosomal copies of the viral genome, E5 may also contribute to their pathogenesis. In one study, HPV-16 E5 protein was detected in 12/20 (60%) of invasive cancers.[53] A more recent study confirmed the loss of E5 transcription with integration of HPV-16 or HPV-18 genomes in cervical cancers and further found no association between E5 expression and overall survival of the patients.[19]

Cellular Events in Cervical Cancer

Although infection with high-risk HPV may be necessary for the development of cervical cancer, or other cancers attributable to HPV infection, it is clearly not sufficient. Cancers arise long after initial infection and only after other factors have collaborated with the infection. As discussed above, some changes (e.g., integration) may be virus specific. Other changes associated with progression include genetic and epigenetic alteration of cellular genes that complement the activities of high-risk HPV E6 and E7. A genomic characterization of 228 primary cervical cancers with whole genome sequencing and RNAseq analyses by The Cancer Genome Atlas (TCGA) Research Network found that mutations characteristic of ABOBEC3 cytidine deaminase activity predominated.[45] This finding is consistent with the observation that ABOBEC3, a mutagenic cellular antiviral protein, is activated in response to many viral infections, including HPV.[335] ABOBEC3B is consistently elevated in HPV-associated cancers. The mechanism of its activation by high-risk HPV infection is uncertain. It may involve the interactions of E6 with p53 and E7 with pRB, but infection by HPV pseudovirions, which do not encode the viral oncogenes or other viral genes, also induces ABOBEC3 expression.[275] It is also uncertain whether this induction has evolved primarily as a host strategy to limit HPV replication, a viral strategy to promote adaptation and immune escape by increasing sequence diversity in the viral genomes, a viral strategy to suppress virus induction of host LINE element transposition, or some combination thereof.[373] Regardless, it is clear that a cellular mechanism that has evolved to restrict replication of a broad range of viruses plays a key role in the progression of HPV-associated cancers.

The mutations, amplifications, and deletions observed in the TCGA analyses result in a spectrum of down-regulation of tumor suppressor and proapoptotic genes and up-regulation of proto-oncogenes and antiapoptotic genes. For example, potentially drug targetable activation in receptor tyrosine kinases, PI3 kinase, and MAP kinase pathways were frequently detected.[45] In addition, gene inactivation in pathways downstream of TGF beta, a growth-suppressive and proapoptotic factor in normal cells, was notably common, including inactivation of the TGF-beta receptor, CREB-binding protein, and the SMAD4 transcription factor. Epigenetic silencing, including DNA methylation and histone acetylation, of numerous genes is also seen in cervical cancers and has been reported to precede cancer development. For example, in one recent study, a cancer-like cellular DNA methylation pattern was detected in 72% of CIN3 and 55% of CIN2 but was virtually absent in high-risk HPV-positive asymptomatic infections.[363]

Other Cofactors in Cervical Cancer

Because only a small percentage of women infected with high-risk HPV have a malignant outcome, host and environmental factors have been examined for their possible influence on the incidence of cervical cancer and its precursor lesions.[55] When controlled for the presence of HPV infection, consistent association of increased risk has been found for smoking, oral contraceptives, early age of pregnancy, and multiparity.[51,162,163] Nutrition, micronutrients, and sexually transmitted diseases other than HPV were also associated with increased risk in some studies.[332,334] In addition, studies using next-generation sequencing of bacterial 16S rRNA have linked elements of the vaginal microbiome with persistence of HPV infection and progression to precancer or cancer.[198,358] In particular, increased disease severity was linked to increased bacterial diversity and low levels of *Lactobacillus* species.[236] In most instances, it is not clear how these cofactors contribute to dysplasia and carcinogenesis, or even if they are causally related. Possibilities include increasing the risk of establishing infection, decreasing local or systemic immunity, stimulating the growth of HPV-infected tissue, and inducing mutations in infected tissue. Furthermore, it is important to note that, where associations between these factors and cervical cancer were observed, the odds ratios were relatively low, generally in the range of 1.5 to 4.0. In comparison, the odds ratios associated with high-risk HPV infection were often over 100.[29]

Human Papillomavirus in Other Genital Sites

Anogenital Warts (Condylomas)

As with cervical HPV infection, condylomas, that is, anogenital warts (GW), are most prevalent among young, sexually active adults, and their frequency usually parallels that of other sexually transmitted conditions.[17,267] The estimated prevalence in the United States is 1% of the sexually active population aged 15 to 49, with about 7% of women and 4% of men giving history of at least one episode.[93] A survey conducted in the United Kingdom in 2010–2012 found that 3.8% and 4.6% of 16- to 44-year-old sexually experienced men and women, respectively, self-reported a GW diagnosis.[338] A similar proportion of reported GWs was found in a parallel survey in 1999–2001. In a worldwide survey, the median annual incidence of GW was 137 and 126 per 100,000 in men and women, respectively.[270] About 90% of genital warts are caused by HPV-6 or HPV-11, which are closely related to each other, with HPV-6 predominating.[106,133] Other HPV types, including HPV-16, may also be found in these lesions.

Condylomas are usually exophytic lesions that are frequently multiple. They can arise anywhere on the external genitalia and can be found simultaneously in multiple sites. In men, they occur most commonly on the penis and anus, and in women on the perineum and anus. The anus can develop multiple lesions that coalesce to surround the anal canal. Condylomas are usually self-limited, regressing spontaneously or after local treatment, but some lesions can persist for years.[272] As with other HPV infections, GWs, when they arise in patients with impaired cellular immunity, can be highly refractory to treatment. They can also increase in size and number during pregnancy and regress following delivery.[241] This sequence of events may be a reflection of the immune suppression associated with pregnancy.

GWs in children commonly result from virus inoculation at birth or from incidental spread from cutaneous warts,[233,345] although some GWs in children may be sexually transmitted, secondary to sexual abuse.[292] In contrast to anogenital lesions in adults, a significant proportion of GWs in children contain HPV types that are usually isolated from nongenital warts, perhaps because, compared with adults, the genital skin in children is more susceptible to infection with these nongenital HPV types.[167]

Bowenoid papulosis is a related entity.[134] The lesions usually consist of multiple small papules that histologically resemble Bowen disease or squamous cell carcinoma *in situ*. Most of these lesions contain HPV-16, but the rate of transition to frank malignancy appears to be much lower for the external genitalia than for the cervix.

Vulvar, Vaginal, and Penile Malignancy

Genital HPV can routinely infect other genital areas that contain stratified squamous epithelium. The risk of malignant progression associated with HPV infection at non-cervical sites is less than that of cervical infection, perhaps because these tissues lack a defined transformation zone from simple columnar to stratified squamous epithelium. High-risk HPVs, most often HPV-16, are associated with a subset of cancers of the vulva, vagina, and penis. Worldwide HPV attributable fractions for 2018 were estimated to be 25%, 78% and 53%, respectively (Fig. 3.3).[81] Giant condyloma acuminatum, also called the *Buschke-Löwenstein tumor*, is a low-grade, locally invasive squamous cell carcinoma that involves the external genitalia, most frequently the penis. It is associated with low-risk HPV types, such as 6 and 11.[137]

In squamous cell carcinoma of the vulva, most HPV-positive invasive tumors are designated morphologically as being warty or basaloid, tend to arise in younger women, and have a better prognosis than HPV-negative cancers, which tend to have a keratinizing morphology.[252,384] HPV-16 predominates in vulvar and vaginal cancers (>75%) and high-grade dysplasias (VIN2/3 and VAIN2/3), but a broader range of low-risk and high-risk types is detected in low-grade lesions (VIN1 and VAIN1).[87] Risk factors for vulvar and vaginal cancers are similar to those for cervical cancer and include immunosuppression, irradiation, smoking, and infection with herpes simplex virus type 2.[161] Vulvar and vaginal (and also anal) high-grade dysplasia and cancers occur more frequently in women with a previous history of cervical HPV infection or dysplasia.[27] Some evidence, based on virus–host DNA junction analysis, suggests that, in some instances, dysplastic cells may actually have been self-transplanted from the cervix to these sites.[368] Family history is also a risk factor for vulvar, vaginal, and penile cancer.[397]

The incidence of penile cancer, almost all of which are squamous cell carcinomas, is low in most highly developed countries, generally less than 1/100,000 but may be four times higher is some developing countries. In a systematic review in which 48% of penile cancer was HPV positive, the most frequently detected types were HPV-16 (30.8%), HPV-6 (6.7%), and HPV-18 (6.6%).[15] In addition to sexual activity, risk factors include smoking, phimosis, and lack of circumcision.[234]

Anal Cancer

Anal cancer shares important similarities with cervical cancer, as well as some differences. The disease is more frequent in women than in men, with about 19,000 HPV-attributable annual cases in women and 9,000 annual cases in men worldwide.[81] Its incidence has been gradually increasing in the United States since the mid-1980s, with a similar rate of increase in men and women between 1992 and 2004.[169] Anal HPV infection appears to be sexually transmitted in most instances, and a history of receptive anal intercourse in women and of homosexual activity in men is associated with an increased risk for this cancer.[114] Such a history is often lacking, however, which makes it likely that many anal infections have spread from other genital areas. Consistent with this interpretation, simultaneous cervical and anal infection, often with the same HPV type, is common, and the prevalence and type distribution of anal infection by high-risk HPVs in women appears to be similar to that of cervical infection.[258] However, in spite of the fact that cervical cancer incidences have decreased dramatically in countries with comprehensive screening programs, the worldwide incidence of cervical cancer remains 30-fold higher than that of anal cancer.[81] As with cervical cancer, high-risk HPV has been found in almost all anal cancers, with an even greater preponderance of HPV-16 than in cervical cancer, and most anal cancers arise in the transition zone between columnar and squamous epithelium. However, the anal transformation zone does not harbor the distinctive monolayer of undifferentiated embryonic cells seen in the cervical transformation zone, which might make it less susceptible to malignant progression after high-risk HPV infection.[392]

The risk of anal cancer among individuals who are human immunodeficiency virus (HIV) positive is much greater than that in the general population, with especially high rates for HIV-positive men who have sex with men (MSMs).[69] In a U.S. study from 1996 to 2012, the standardized incidence ratio in HIV-positive individuals overall was 19.1, but was 38.7 for HIV-positive MSMs, which translates to an incidence rate of 89.0 per 100,000 person-years. This rate is approximately twice the rate of cervical cancer in women in high-incidence low-income countries that lack organized screening programs.[9] HIV-positive heterosexual males and females had incidence rates of 11.4 and 7.9, respectively. These differences largely reflect differences in the prevalence of high-risk HPV infection and associated dysplasia.[85]

HPV INFECTIONS OF THE AERODIGESTIVE TRACT

Infections of the Oral Cavity

Benign HPV infections of the oral cavity occur commonly.[123,346] They may be asymptomatic or associated with single or multiple lesions in any part of the oral cavity. Genital–mucosal HPV types, especially HPV-6, HPV-11, and HPV-16, have frequently been recovered from oral tissue. HPV is usually identified in at least one-half of papillomatous lesions in the oral cavity lesions. HPV-6 and HPV-11 seem to be responsible for most benign HPV oral lesions, although HPV-16 may also be found. In a systematic review, 4.5% of healthy subjects were positive for any HPV, 3.5% had high-risk HPV, and 1.3 % had HPV-16.[188] The overall detection rates were similar in men and women. Infections can be transmitted by multiple routes, including perinatal, saliva, and oral sex. The fraction of oral infections by genital mucosal high-risk types due to sexual versus nonsexual transmission is debatable and likely to vary across cohorts.[76,288]

Focal epithelial hyperplasia (FEH) is a familial disorder with autosomal-recessive inheritance that occurs only in the oral mucosa, most often in childhood and adolescence.[282] It is characterized by multiple benign papules, plaques, or nodules. Most cases of FEH are attributed to HPV-13 or HPV-32, two types that appear predominantly to infect the oral cavity.[302] FEH has a worldwide distribution, but it is most prevalent in the indigenous populations of Central and South America and of Alaska and Greenland. In Greenlandic Eskimos, the prevalence in different localities varied between 7% and 36%. By contrast, the prevalence among Caucasian residents in the same localities was less than 1 in 300.

Head and Neck Cancers

Cigarette smoking and alcohol consumption are two well-known risk factors for head and neck cancers. Although HPV does not appear to be involved in most cancers in the oral cavity, consistent data indicate that a subset of head and neck cancers are attributable to HPV infection, with HPV-16 accounting for about 90% of them.[48,189] The attributable fraction varies widely depending on the proportion of cancer from specific anatomical sites in the case series, country of origin, and the relative importance of other risk factors. Most of these HPV-associated cancers are located in the oropharynx, which includes the tonsils, tonsillar fossa, base of the tongue, and soft palette. It is not understood why the HPV-positive tumors preferentially develop in the oropharynx. The worldwide yearly cases attributed to HPV infection are 42,000, 5,900, and 4,100 for OPCs, other oral cancers, and laryngeal cancers, respectively.[81] In comparison to HPV-negative OPCs, HPV-positive cases tend to develop at an early age and respond better to treatment, although the prognostic advantage associated with HPV positivity attenuates with age.

There is accumulating evidence for a global time trend of increased OPC incidence, most notably in North America and northern Europe.[124] In the United Sates, the incidence of OPCs increased more than threefold between 1988 and 2004,[57] and these trends are expected to continue through the current decade.[353] Most of the increase has been in white men, who account for about three-quarters of OPC cases[124] (Fig. 3.10). Coupled with a decreasing incidence in cervical cancer (due to screening programs), there are now more OPCs than cervical cancer in the U.S. (18,900 vs. 11,800) and two-thirds of the OPCs are HPV positive,[361] although the incidence of oral high-risk HPV infection is an order of magnitude lower than that of anogenital infection.[123,142,278] The higher OPC rates in U.S. men than in women are correlated with the three- to fivefold higher prevalence of HPV-16 and other high-risk types in the oral cavity of men.[123] This difference in oral prevalence may be due to lower rates of seroconversion after genital infection in men than in women and therefore less protection against subsequent oral infections.[215]

Many behavioral risk factors for developing HPV-positive OPC are similar to those for anogenital HPV-positive cancers.[75] In addition, the risk of oral HPV positivity appears to be greatly influenced by the lifetime number of oral sex partners.[124,147] However, the alternative hypothesis that mother-to-child transmission *in utero* or early in life, leading to dysregulation of virus-specific T-cell immunity, is the primary risk factor was recently proposed.[347]

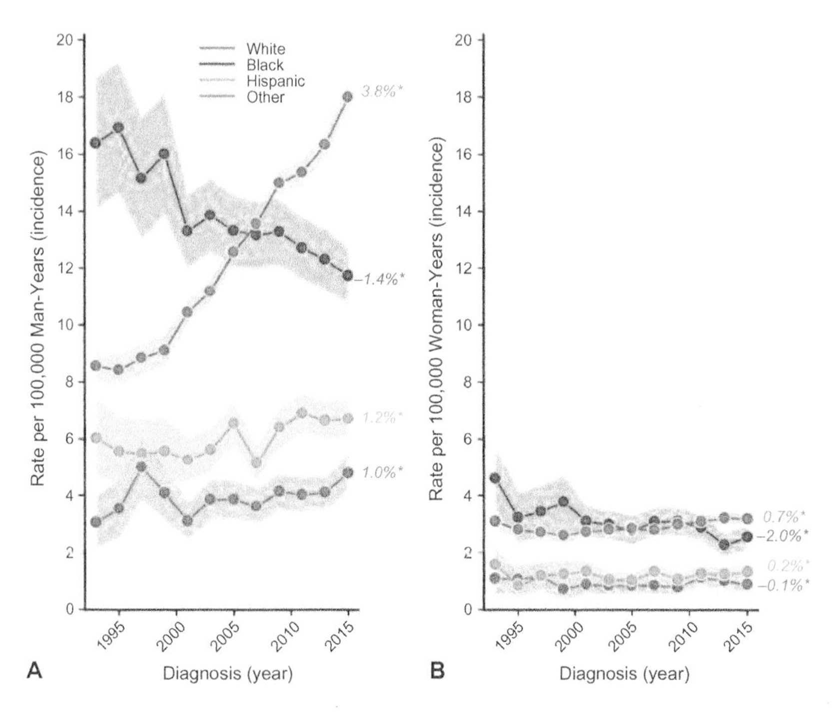

FIGURE 3.10 Incidence trends in oropharynx cancers in the United States stratified by race and sex. Panel A depicts incidence trends in men and **Panel B** the trends in women. (*) indicates statistically significant trend ($p < 0.05$). (Reprinted with permission from Tota JE, Best AF, Zumsteg ZS, et al. Evolution of the oropharynx cancer epidemic in the United States: moderation of increasing incidence in younger individuals and shift in the burden to older individuals. *J Clin Oncol* 2019;37:1538–1546. Copyright © 2019 by American Society of Clinical Oncology.)

HPV-positive OPC tumors share many molecular features with those of HPV-positive anogenital tumors.[26] Specifically, they preferentially express E6 and E7, their p53 and pRb genes are usually wild type, and the vast majority of them express p16.[168] By contrast, the HPV-negative tumors tend to have mutant p53 and to be p16 negative. Most studies suggest that tobacco and alcohol increase the risk of both HPV-negative and HPV-positive tumors.[56] Despite the similarities with HPV-positive anogenital cancers, there is thus far no clearly identifiable premalignant oropharyngeal lesion for HPV-positive tumors, many of which may form deep in the tonsillar crypts. Interestingly, viral genome integration has been detected in only a minority of HPV-associated oropharyngeal cancers,[117,255] and some of the circular replicons consist of virus and human DNA hybrids.[239]

Recurrent Respiratory Papillomatosis (Laryngeal Papillomatosis)

Laryngeal papillomatosis, which is also called recurrent respiratory papillomatosis (RRP), is a rare condition whose papillomas can severely compromise the airway, particularly in young children.[110] Most lesions are caused by genital HPV types that are also associated with external genital warts, with HPV types 6 and 11 being responsible for more than 90%. High-risk HPV types, including 16, 18, 31, and 33, are infrequently detected in RRP. The vocal cords of the larynx are the site most commonly affected, but the papillomas can arise at other sites, including the trachea, lungs, nose, and oral cavity, even without laryngeal involvement.[348] Lesions can be single or multiple. Symptomatic papillomas are generally treated surgically, with the goal of debulking the lesion without damaging the normal tissue.[382] However, the recurrent nature of the disease means that periodic surgical treatment may be required. It is important to avoid the necessity of performing a tracheostomy in patients with RRP, because papillomas often grow along the tissues involved in the tracheostomy, resulting in severe morbidity. A number of case series have suggested that vaccination with the prophylactic HPV vaccines after surgery can decrease disease recurrence, decrease disease burden, and/or increase intersurgical intervals,[94] although these findings have not been verified in a randomized controlled trial.

Epidemiologic studies suggest that RRP can develop by at least two mechanisms.[200] One primarily affects young children and the other when RRP is first diagnosed in older individuals. The incidence of RRP is approximately 4 per 100,000 in children and 2 per 100,000 in adults.[110] RRP may occur at any age, but the risk of developing it decreases after 5 years of age. In children below this age, a maternal history of genital warts is a risk factor for RRP, and infection is thought to usually occur at birth during passage through an infected genital tract. In a population-based study in Denmark, close to 1% of children whose mothers had a history of genital warts developed RRP, which represented a 231 times higher risk of RRP relative to women without a history of genital warts.[330] *In utero* transmission also occurs but is uncommon, so RRP is extremely rare in children delivered by cesarean delivery.[321] First pregnancy and young age of the mother are associated with an increased risk, whereas cesarean section carries a lower risk.[322] HLA antigen class II polymorphism may also be a contributing factor.[118] A history of oral sex may be a risk factor in adult RRP.[200]

Although HPV-6 causes genital warts more frequently than HPV-11, the reverse is true of RRP, and HPV-11 infections tend to be more aggressive than RRP associated with HPV-6.[96,381] Patients less than 3 years of age also tend to have more extensive and aggressive disease. Given the presumed single exposure to HPV during vaginal delivery, the long and variable latent period of up to 5 years for childhood RRP remains to be explained. Latency has been shown in the larynx of patients with RRP who are in remission.[223]

RRP is associated with a low risk of spread to the bronchi and lungs, progression to severe dysplasia, and even to cancer.[121] The rates of malignant progression are estimated to be lower than 1% in children and 5% in adults. The risk of such progression is increased if the papillomas have been subjected to smoking, cytotoxic drugs, or X-irradiation, which was a common treatment of RRP in the 1940s.[110] In contrast to cervical cancer, HPV-6 and HPV-11 in RRP are clearly associated with severe dysplasia and cancer, with HPV-11 predominating, although most HPV-positive laryngeal cancers arise in patients without RRP and contain a high-risk HPV, especially HPV-16.[103]

HUMAN PAPILLOMAVIRUS AND THE NONGENITAL SKIN

Nongenital Skin Warts

Three classes of nongenital skin papillomas are generally distinguished based on morphological criteria. Common warts (verruca vulgaris) are exophytic papules that are found on many skin surfaces, most often the dorsal hands and fingers.[115] Although many HPV types are detected in common warts, often more than one within a single lesion, a recent causal estimation based on viral loads has implicated types 2, 27, and 57 in about three-quarters of cases.[35] Plantar and palmar warts are generally endophytic papules, and, in recent studies, more than 90% of cases appear to be caused by HPV-1a, 2, 27, or 57[83] (Table 3.1). Both classes of papillomas occur frequently in older children and young adults, with a peak prevalence at 9 to 10 years and point prevalence estimates of 3% to 30%.[80,329] The third morphologic class consists of flat warts (verruca plana), which are slightly elevated smooth papules, most often on the upper extremities and the face, and are most often caused by HPV-3 or HPV-10.[393]

HPV can remain infectious in the environment for extended periods,[298] and transmission via fomites is thought to commonly occur.[119] Because of the apparent need for HPV to reach the basement membrane underlying the epithelium and subsequently infect basal cells at the time of inoculation,[290] maceration of the skin predisposes to cutaneous infection. Multiple lesions are most common, and they can be distributed symmetrically or be unilateral. Lesions involving apposing areas of skin or mucous membrane, as occurs frequently, probably develop by autoinoculation.

Most skin warts persist for several months and regress in the absence of treatment. A recent retrospective study in children found that 65% of common skin warts spontaneously regressed within 2 years and 80% within 4 years.[197] Regression of lesions is thought to be mediated immunologically. When most lesions regress spontaneously, there may be a mild mononuclear cell infiltrate, although regression of flat warts can be associated with an erythematous reaction around the lesions in association with an intense inflammatory infiltrate. The lower incidence of warts in older individuals[281] likely implies that immune mechanisms have rendered them relatively resistant to reinfection.

Epidermodysplasia Verruciformis

EV is a rare genodermatosis in which affected individuals have a unique susceptibility to cutaneous HPV infections.[219,256] More recently, an "acquired" form of EV has been reported in some immunocompromised patients. The warts in "genetic" EV usually develop in childhood, become widespread, do not tend to regress, and, in some instances, may progress to squamous cell cancers. Two predominant types of lesions are seen, which can occur in the same patient. Some lesions have the appearance of flat warts, whereas others are flat, scaly, red-brown macules. The flat warts are caused by the same HPV types that induce flat warts in the general population, usually HPV-3 or HPV-10. The scaly lesions are associated with a range of beta-HPV types, especially HPV-5 and HPV-8. Patients with EV are frequently infected with several HPV types. The lesions in patients with EV are resistant to usual treatment modalities.

Genetic EV has been divided into "classical" and "nonclassical" categories.[157] Both classes display autosomal recessive inheritance and many families with EV have a history of parental consanguinity. Classical EV is associated with mutations in the EVER1/TMC6 or EVER2/TMC8 genes and accounts for three-quarters of genetic EV cases.[171] These genes are expressed in T cells and other leukocytes, and EV patients exhibit minor impairment in some cell-mediated immune functions such as cutaneous anergy to common skin test antigens.[273] The genes are also expressed in keratinocytes, where they control zinc efflux. The characteristic feature of classical EV is that patient pathologies are limited to increased susceptibility to clinical manifestations of skin infections by EV-associated HPV types but, surprisingly, they do not have increases in lesions caused by mucosatropic or common wart HPV types.

Nonclassical EV has been linked to mutations in a number of genes that have the common feature of impairing cell-mediated immunity, and patients often present with a variety of other infections and diseases.[157] Genes linked to nonclassical EV include RHOH, an atypical Rho GTPase specific for hematopoietic cells, MST1, a hepatocyte growth factor-like protein implicated in T-cell survival and migration, and CORO1A, an actin-binding protein involved in phagocytosis and a cause of severe combined immunodeficiency.[283] In addition, the genetic defect for a subset of EV patients remains to be determined.

Acquired EV is not associated with a family history of the disease or early onset but rather with immunosuppression, regardless of age, yet clinically, it closely resembles genetic EV. It was first described in organ transplant recipients on immunosuppressive drugs. It is also a rare manifestation of HIV infection, although, surprisingly, lesion development is not correlated with viral load or $CD4^+$ T-cell count.[166]

About one-third of EV patients develop skin cancers in association with their lesions. Most of the malignant tumors remain local, but regional and distant metastases may occur. The risk of malignant progression is limited to the pityriasis-like lesions, which are the lesions that contain the EV-associated types. HPV-5 and HPV-8 are considered the most oncogenic, because most of the skin cancers contain one of these two types.[256] The skin cancers usually develop on sun-exposed areas, implying that carcinoma develops in EV by a combination of infection by an oncogenic EV HPV type plus the cocarcinogenic effects of UV light. p53 mutations are common in EV-associated cancers,[261] in contrast to the mucosal cancers associated with alpha HPV types.

Nonmelanoma Skin Cancer

Nonmelanoma skin cancers (NMSC), which are extremely common, are generally subdivided into basal cell carcinomas (BCC) and squamous cell carcinomas (SCC). They generally arise on exposed areas of skin, most commonly in light-skinned individuals. Sunlight exposure is a predominant risk factor, and tumors associated with sun exposure are usually locally invasive, but only rarely metastasize. The skin of immunosuppressed individuals is at high risk of developing warts as well as premalignant lesions and NMSC, especially SCC, in sun-exposed areas.[136,155]

The known oncogenic potential of at least some HPV types and the consistent finding of certain beta genus HPV types in SCC associated with EV make HPV infection an attractive etiologic agent for at least some NMSC in individuals who do not have EV.[293] Beta HPVs are known to encode E6 and E7 oncoproteins that can interfere with UV-induced apoptosis in cultured cells, which might allow keratinocytes with UV-induced mutations to survive and progress to carcinomas.[352] They also promote skin carcinogenesis in transgenic mouse models.[144,224,365]

Beta HPV DNA is frequently detected in SCC using sensitive PCR-based detection methods, but it is also frequently detected in normal skin.[32,374] Furthermore, the genome copy number is usually much lower than one copy per tumor cell, in contrast to HPV-associated anogenital and oral cancers. A study employing an unbiased analysis involving high-throughput sequencing of randomly primed mRNAs detected virtually no HPV transcripts in SCC specimens.[12] A recent prospective study evaluating the association between beta HPVs and SCC in over 500 organ transplant recipients for more than a decade found significant associations for detecting five or more beta types in plucked eyebrow hairs and for high beta HPV viral loads. However, the hazard ratios were rather weak, 1.7 and 1.8, respectively. In addition, there was no association between SCC and serum antibodies to beta HPV antigens.[32]

Overall, the association between HPV infection and NMSC in the absence of EV must be considered tentative at present, since continuous expression of predominant HPV types has not been as clearly identified in NMSC in the general population, as it is in EV-associated cancers or mucosal cancers associated with HPV. In addition, the HPV-positive tumors are not clinicopathologically distinct from the HPV-negative ones, in contrast to vulvar or oral cancer. Therefore, it remains possible that the detection of HPV DNA may be an epiphenomenon. This latter possibility needs to be seriously considered, because healthy skin often contains HPV DNA, especially beta types, and removal of the superficial layers of NMSC lesions has been reported to result in a drastic reduction in the proportion of HPV-positive tumors.[109]

However, it remains formally possible that cutaneous HPVs may induce SCC but are not required for their maintenance, secondary to a putative strong biological or immunological selection for their loss during progression.[122] This scenario is referred to as "hit-and-run" carcinogenesis. Interestingly, such a hit-and-run mechanism has been documented in the induction of alimentary carcinomas in cattle infected with bovine papillomavirus type 4 and in an HPV-38 E6/E7 transgenic mouse model, where skin expression of the oncoproteins (and long-term UV exposure) was required for SCC initiation but not for maintenance.[365] Based primarily on observations of reduced UV or chemical-induced skin carcinogenesis in mice colonized with MmuPV1, an alternative hypothesis that cell-mediated immunity to HPV infections of the skin might actually protect against skin cancers has been proposed.[341]

HUMAN IMMUNODEFICIENCY VIRUS AND HUMAN PAPILLOMAVIRUS INFECTIONS

The interaction between HIV and genital HPV infections centers on two interrelated questions. First, does HPV infection potentiate acquisition of HIV? Second, does HIV infection increase risk of HPV-induced cancers? The effect of HPV infection on risk of HIV acquisition remains uncertain. An increased risk of HIV seroconversion with existing or incident HPV infection was reported in two meta-analyses, but the association was not strong, as the odds ratio was 1.9, and it is difficult to exclude residual confounding biases, especially since the infections share the same primary risk factor, sexual transmission.[154,212] Two mechanisms have been proposed of how HPV infection would increase HIV acquisition. First, HPV infections can increase the local tissue concentration of T cells, including T helper cells, a primary target for HIV.[355] Second, *in vitro* studies have reported that HPV-16 E7 down-regulates E-cadherin, an epithelial adhesion molecule and might thereby increase HIV virion access to underlying dermal T cells that are thought to play a role in initiating infection in the anogenital tract.[203]

By contrast, there is considerable evidence that HIV infection potentiates HPV carcinogenesis. However, the magnitude of the increased risk is difficult to generalize, because CD4 T-cell counts inversely correlate with the magnitude of risk, and they vary considerably in study populations, primarily based on access to active retroviral therapy (ART).[174] In addition, more intense screening in HIV positives in some setting can increase the detection of premalignant lesions and subsequent treatment can decrease cancer incidences. Finally, the aforementioned common risk factors for acquisition of the two viruses can bias toward stronger associations. A large retrospective study of a U.S. cohort over the period from 1980 to 2004 (spanning the institution of ART) observed an increase in all major HPV-associated cancer in person diagnosed with HIV/AIDS. The standardized incident ratios (SIRs) and 95% CIs were 5.6 (4.8 to 6.5) for cervical cancer, 34.6 (20.8 to 38.8) for anal cancer, 8.4 (3.8 to 16.0) for vaginal or vulvar cancer, 4.4 (1.9 to 8.7) for penile cancer, and 1.6 (1.2 to 2.1) for OPC.[60]

There is biological plausibility, and mounting evidence, that HIV infection potentiates several steps in the process of HPV carcinogenesis, most notably persistence of infection and progression to cancer.[244] A higher prevalence of genital high-risk HPV infection, and particularly multiple infections, is generally observed in HIV positives versus negatives in a given population. For example, in a cohort of HIV-infected and uninfected Ghanaian women, the prevalence of genital HPV infection was 75.0% versus 42.6%, respectively.[254] Prevalence is a function of both acquisition rate and persistence of the HPV infections, and both parameters are higher in HIV-infected women. For example, in a U.S.-based cohort, the 8-year cumulative detection of cervical high-risk HPV DNA was 67% in HIV-seropositive women versus 36% for HIV-seronegative women ($p = 0.001$).[228] In a similar cohort, 24.1% of the HPV infections in HIV-positive women persisted, as defined by HPV DNA positivity in cervical samples taken 3 to 12 months apart, versus 3.9% in HIV-negative women.[343] Many subsequent studies have documented that cervical infections tend to persist longer in HIV-positive women.

HIV-positive women also progress from normal cytology or LSIL to HSIL more rapidly than do their HIV-negative counterparts. For example, in a 10-year U.S. study, the rate of progression to HSIL was 5.3 versus 1.3 per 1,000 person-years, respectively.[227] HIV status can also influence HPV type distribution in HSIL/CIN3, with HPV-16 infections less dominant in HIV-positive women (OR 0.6, 95% CI 0.4 to 0.7).[67]

As discussed below, it is likely that T cells play a critical role in clearing HPV infection, so the increased persistence and progression of HPV infection are likely attributable to the well-documented T-cell dysfunction induced by HIV infection. Consistent with this conjecture, risk of cervical cancer tends to increase with decreases in CD4 counts. In a large North American study of HIV-infected women, the rate of invasive cervical cancer was 7.7, 3.0, and 2.3 times greater in women with CD4 counts of less than 200, 200 to 349, greater than 350 cell per mL, respectively, compared to HIV-uninfected women (p(trend) = 0.001).[1] There is evidence that initiation of antiretroviral therapies that improve CD4 counts modestly increases the rate of cervical lesion regression and decreases the rates of progression approximately twofold.[2]

Immunity

A defining feature of HPV infections is their persistence, implying that they successfully evade elimination by host immunity. Although some infections, particularly with some species of the HPV beta genus, may persist lifelong in an occult fashion, most HPV infections are nevertheless cleared, or controlled to undetectable levels, within months or years. For example, up to 90% of anogenital HPV infections clear within 2 years.[152] In addition, incident infection rates tend to decline with age after they peak, consistent with the acquisition of effective immunity, and adaptive T-cell immunity is implicated in clearance/control. Individuals with conditions that affect T-cell immunity, such as pregnancy, immunosuppressive chemotherapy, or HIV infection, are at increased risk of HPV infection that persists, as well as an increased risk of HPV-associated cancers.[11,113] At least some of these infections likely represent reactivation of latent infection, rather than being secondary to new exogenous exposure. Even benign HPV infections in immunosuppressed patients are notoriously difficult to treat, and reduction of the immune suppression may be associated with the spontaneous improvement of the HPV-induced lesions.[286] Consistent with the critical role of adaptive T-cell responses in control of HPV infections, specific class I and class II human leukocyte antigen (HLA) alleles have been associated with increased or decreased risk of persistent genital HPV infection, or progression to precancer and cancer.[260] By contrast, defects in B-cell immunity do not appear to greatly influence the course of HPV infections once established.

HPVs evade effective immune responses by three broad mechanisms: maintenance of immune ignorance, suppression of innate immune responses, and inhibition of effective adaptive immune responses.[217,379,399] As detailed in the accompanying chapter on basic PV biology, the PV life cycle appears to have evolved specifically to promote immune ignorance. It takes place entirely within a stratified epithelium, with no significant viremia to expose the viral antigens to the systemic immune system.[97] Furthermore, viral gene expression in the epithelium is regulated in a way that limits exposure to local intraepithelial immunity. Only low levels of the nonstructural proteins are expressed in the lower levels of epithelium where the infection is maintained and where immune surveillance is active. High-level expression of viral genes and production of virions occur only in the terminally differentiating keratinocytes of the upper layers of the epithelium, which are under limited immune monitoring (Fig. 3.2). Cell lysis is not induced during productive infection, so there is no release of cellular danger signals to alert the immune system of its presence. Rather the virions are released from or in the desquamating cells in the upper most layers of the epithelium. Low intrinsic immunogenicity of the viral proteins does not seem to play a role. For instance, the capsids can be highly immunogenic when exposed to the systemic immune system, as exemplified by the VLP vaccine studies discussed below.

In part because of this effective maintenance of ignorance, the immune responses to infections are typically delayed and muted. Virion antibody responses have been best characterized for genital infections in women. Systemic antibodies are generally not detected until months after initial infection, and the titers induced are modest.[91] Responses may be somewhat more robust for genital wart types than high-risk types.[47] Many infections clear without the induction of a measurable systemic antibody response. The fact that PVs have evolved into hundreds of genotypes that are essentially distinct serotypes that cannot be effectively cross-neutralized by antibodies induced by natural infection or VLP vaccination strongly implies that such antibodies play an important role in virus/host interactions.[360] It is unlikely that virion antibodies play a role in clearing infections because the virion proteins are not expressed on the surface of living cells, so they are not susceptible to known antibody-mediated mechanism of immune regression, and virion antibodies at the time of detection of prevalent infection are not associated with persistent/clearance of genital HPV-16 infection.[354] However, neutralizing antibodies induced by infection likely play a role in preventing successive rounds of autoinoculation, reinfection from an external source, and perhaps spread to another host. The latter can be readily envisioned for female genital mucosal infections where the virions are shed into mucus that can also contain virion-neutralizing antibodies.[247]

There is some disagreement in the literature over whether virion antibodies measured after natural infection can protect from reinfection.[299,354,369] It seems quite likely that women with higher-than-average virion antibody titers to mucosal types in their serum are afforded at least partial protection from type-specific reinfection.[300] A meta-analysis of studies up to 2016 reported that antibodies to HPV-16 capsids were associated with protection in women (pooled RR, 0.65; 95% CI 0.50 to 0.80) but not in men (pooled RR, 1.22; 95% CI 0.67 to 1.77).[20] However, the interpretation of these studies is confounded by difficulties in distinguishing reinfection from reactivation of latent infection, in distinguishing low level of virion-specific from nonspecific antibodies, and by the possibility that antibody responses might often be a surrogate marker for protective cell-mediated immune responses.

Most adults are seropositive for L1 antibodies to one or more cutaneous HPVs, and the antibody responses tend to persist.[8] The role of these antibodies in the natural history of cutaneous HPV infection is not well understood.

Specific antibody responses to the early (nonstructural) viral proteins are seldom detected, except in the case of invasive cancers.[21] In cervical cancers, responses to E6 and/or E7 are detected in approximately half of the patients.[370] An exception appears to be HPV-16–associated OPCs, where approximately one-third of patients have detectable HPV-16 E6 antibodies up to 10 years prior to cancer diagnosis.[192] The preferential development of these cancers in tonsillar crypts juxtaposed to lymphoid tissues might explain the more frequent antibody response in subjects who subsequently develop OPC.

The cell-mediated immune effector mechanisms and viral antigens involved in lesion regression and prevention of reactivation are not well defined. Descriptive studies of cell-mediated immune responses have mostly focused on genital infections in women. Until recently, most studies have evaluated systemic responses, whereas local mucosal responses are likely to be the critical determinants. Many healthy individuals develop relatively strong systemic type 1 (IFNγ, TNFα, IL2 producing) T-cell responses to L1, but they are unlikely to be protective, since L1 is not detectably expressed in the basal layers of the epithelium, where the infection is maintained. More modest systemic CD4+ and CD8+ cytotoxic T-cell (CTL) responses to E6 and E7 are often also detected in women with previous or current cervical genital HPV infections.[245] Interestingly, failure to clear HPV-16 infection was associated with lack of induction of CTL to E6, but not to E7.[246] In women with HPV-16–associated CIN1, CD4 T-cell responses to E2 and E6 were most frequently detected, and Th1-type CD4 responses to these viral proteins are also most frequently detected in women without infection.[79,375] In a prospective study, the presence of HPV-16 E2-specific responses in an IFNγ ELISPOT assay correlated with lack of progression of HPV-16–associated lesions.[388]

In some studies, the local tissue responses in regressing cervical lesions have also been characterized. Granzyme B–expressing CD8 T cells predominated, and a higher ratio of CD8 and Foxp3-negative CD4 cells over CD4 Foxp3-positive (regulatory) CD4 T cells was detected.[259,387] By contrast, the infiltrates in persistent and progressing lesions were associated with a suppressive environment, including granzyme B–negative and PD-1–expressing T cells (a sign of immune exhaustion) and high numbers of Foxp3+ Tregs, and macrophages.[140,165] There is a shift from a Th1 to a Th2 response in persistent infections, and a greater number of Th17 cells are seen in higher grade lesions. In a prospective study of high-grade HPV-16–associated CIN lesions, infiltration of CD8+ T cells into the epithelium was observed in lesions destined to regress.[355] They were excluded from the epithelium in lesions that persisted, although infiltrates in the submucosa adjacent to the lesions were frequently observed. The results suggest that dysregulation of T-cell trafficking and/or adhesion plays a role in viral immune evasion.

HPVs actively inhibit innate immune recognition of infected keratinocytes by multiple mechanisms. Suppression of innate immune responses to its double-stranded DNA genome occurs by at least three mechanisms. First, the viral genome appears to be shielded from host foreign DNA sensors by remaining enclosed in the virion coat proteins within a membrane-bound vesicle during infectious entry until it is delivered to the nucleus.[78] Second, viral proteins interfere with the activity of the DNA pattern recognition receptor (PRR) TLR9, which can trigger downstream inflammatory cascades. For example, HPV-16 E7 down-regulates TLR9 expression by recruiting histone demethylase JARID1B and histone deacetylase HDAC1 to the TLR9 promoter.[143] Third, the E7 proteins of both HPV-16 and HPV-18 have been shown to block the activity of STING, a cytosolic protein that induces inflammatory responses after recognition of cytosolic DNA that has been converted into cyclic diGMP/AMP by cyclic GMP/AMP synthase (cGAS).[201,216] Yet to be explained is why the latter mechanism has evolved if the viral genome replicates in the nucleus and seems to avoid cytoplasmic exposure during infectious entry. One possibility is that, during cell division, segregation of the multicopy viral genome to daughter nuclei is not always complete, leaving some copies in the cytoplasm where they would otherwise be recognized by the cGAS/STING sensing mechanism. In addition, the HPV E6 proteins of a number of high-risk and low-risk alpha HPVs, and also beta HPVs, inhibit activation of retinoic acid–inducible gene-1 (RIG-1), a cytoplasmic sensor of viral RNA that can activate the production of antiviral interferons.[62]

Viral proteins also more directly evade the innate immune activities of type 1 IFNs, mainly IFNα and IFNβ, by inhibiting their production and their activities. HPV-16 E6 binds to interferon regulatory factor (IRF)-3 and thereby prevents its ability to activate the IFN promoters,[296] while HPV-16 E7 inactivates IRF-1, also leading to inhibition of IFN gene transcription.[266] In addition, HPV infection induces up-regulation of the deubiquitinating enzyme ubiquitin C-terminal hydrolase L1 (UCHL1), which results in the inhibition of TRAF3, a protein that transmits the signals from activated TLRs to the IRFs involved in type 1 IFN production. HPV E6 and E7 also inhibit the activities of the IFNs that are produced in response to infection by interfering with signaling through the IFNα/β receptor (IFNAR). They do this via multiple mechanisms focused on inhibiting the transcriptional activation of the IFN genes by STAT1 and/or STAT2 (Fig. 3.11) by decreasing their expression, phosphorylation, and nuclear translocation.[16,54,209,248]

High-risk HPV infections also down-regulate the NF-κB pathway, a signaling pathway involved in activating the expression of multiple genes of innate immunity, such as IFNs, cytokines, and defensins, as well as genes involved in antigen presentation in adaptive immunity. As with the STATs, they do so by multiple mechanisms. Both E6 and E7 bind nuclear cofactors, for example p300 and CBP, that activate NF-κB.[158,269,401] In addition, up-regulation of UCHL1 leads to increased degradation of an essential modulator of NF-κB, which decreases NF-κB phosphorylation and its downstream signaling.[172]

Lastly, it was shown that HPV-16 E6 directly down-regulates protein levels of IL-1β, a key proinflammatory cytokine of innate immunity.[249] It does so by inducing the ubiquitin-dependent degradation of pro-IL-1β upon formation of a complex with it, p53, and E6-AP, the ubiquitin ligase involved in E6-mediated p53 degradation (Fig. 3.11).

HPVs have also evolved multiple mechanisms to evade recognition by the adaptive immune systems (Fig. 3.11).[18] E5 of multiple high-risk and low-risk types reduces cell surface expression of MHC I molecules on keratinocytes by interacting with their cellular transport proteins and thereby sequestering the MHC I molecules in the Golgi and ER, leading to reduced recognition by CD8 T cells.[14,135] HPV-16 and HPV-6 E5 also sequester CD1d in the ER, which inhibits its cell surface expression. CD1d is the invariant MHC-like molecule that

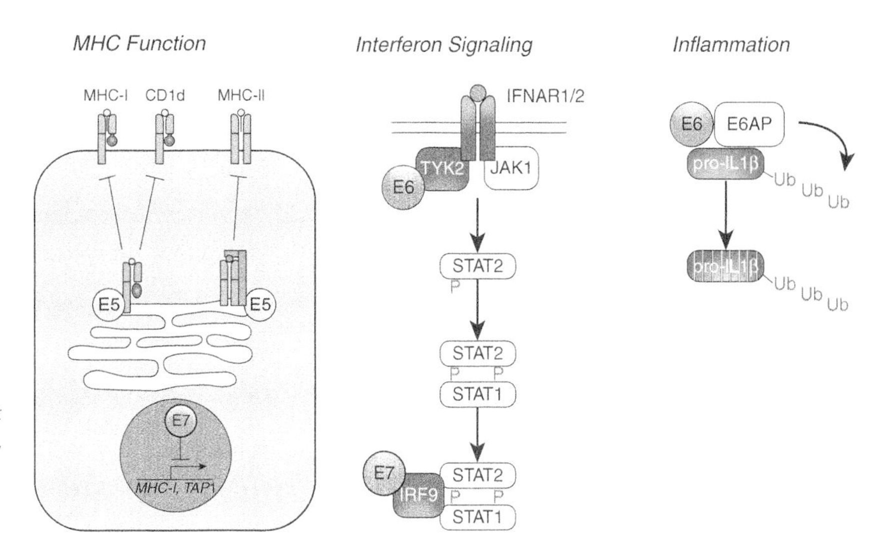

FIGURE 3.11 HPV oncoproteins inhibit immune responses by multiple mechanisms. Mechanisms that inhibit antigen presentation, type 1 interferon signaling, and degradation of proinflammatory cytokines are depicted from *left* to *right*. (Reprinted from Westrich JA, Warren CJ, Pyeon D. Evasion of host immune defenses by human papillomavirus. *Virus Res* 2017;231:21–33. Copyright © 2016 Elsevier. With permission.)

presents lipid antigens to natural killer cells (NKTs), suggesting that NKTs may function in controlling HPV infection.[237] High-risk E7s repress MHC expression by recruiting histone deacetylases to their promoter (Fig. 3.11).[120,208] By a similar mechanism, E7 also inhibits transcription of TAP1 and LMP2, which are critical components in loading peptides on MHC I molecules.[120]

HPVs of the alpha and several other genera decrease the local concentration of tissue Langerhans cells (LCs), a primary antigen-presenting cell type in the epithelium, which may create an environment permissive for viral persistence by helping to prevent the priming of an adaptive immune response to the virus.[207] Two explanations for the lower LC density in infected tissues have been proposed. First, E-cadherin is involved in retention of LC in the epithelium, and its expression is reduced in infected lesions.[159] Second, CCL20 is a chemokine that recruits LC to sites of inflammation, and E6 and E7 downregulate its expression by the previously described inhibition of the NF-κB signaling pathways.

The above discussion on immune evasion was focused on immune deviation in normal keratinocytes during productive infections within an epithelium. However, the normal tissue architecture is disrupted in invasive HPV-induced cancers, and they are therefore subject to same selective pressures of systemic immunity as other carcinomas. Nevertheless, many of the mechanisms described above that reduce innate immunity and inhibit induction of adaptive immunity, especially those that are E6/E7 mediated, which have evolved to promote viral persistence during their normal life cycle, are also likely to function in inhibiting effective immune responses after progression to cancer. A presentation of the complexities of the immune responses observed in HPV-associated cancers is beyond the scope of this chapter, but they are critically discussed in several recent reviews.[336,357,399]

DIAGNOSIS AND TREATMENT

Human Papillomavirus Diagnosis

The approach used for the diagnosis of HPV infection may depend to a considerable degree on the underlying goal for making the diagnosis. These goals can include a determination of whether HPV is present, whether an active infection is present, which HPV type is associated with the infection, and the degree of cellular atypia associated with the infection. If routine *in vitro* propagation of HPV from clinical samples was available, its isolation from productive infections, theoretically, would be possible. No such assays exist, however, and their utility would be limited by the fact that high-grade dysplasias and cancers do not produce infectious virus. The potential use of virus-specific antibodies to detect infected cells in tissue sections or extracts is limited by analogous considerations. L1 and E4 proteins can be expressed at high levels in productive lesions, but not in high-grade dysplasias and cancers.[99] The expression of E6 or E7 proteins is higher in advanced lesions, and the clinical utility of detecting the E6 proteins of high-risk types remains an area of active investigation.[284]

Serologic assays in an ELISA format that monitor the antibody response to L1 in VLPs have utility for population-based research studies to measure relative lifetime infection by specific types, although not all infected individuals seroconvert.[47,91,251] More recently, multiplex assays that permit simultaneous detection of antibodies to multiple HPV VLP types have been developed and employed in natural history studies and vaccine trials.[289] Various *in vitro* neutralization assays, based on L1/L2 pseudovirion transducing marker gene plasmids, have also been developed and exhibit sensitivities similar to ELISAs.[268,319] However, these assays, which measure both current and past infection, are not sufficiently sensitive to be used for routine clinical diagnosis. Invasive cervical cancers, but not the premalignant lesions, are associated with serum antibodies against E6 and/or E7; however, approximately one-third of patients were negative for antibodies to the type corresponding to the HPV DNA type in their cancer.[70] Unlike cervical cancer, virtually all patients with HPV-16–positive OPC have detectable anti-E6 serum antibodies.[153,199]

In contrast to serology, sensitive, reproducible, and robust molecular assays have been developed to detect HPV DNA and RNA in cervical swabs and biopsy samples, several of which have been approved by the FDA.[74,313,398] Approaches for such assays include PCR consensus primers (or alternative amplification systems) that can be used in conjunction with a reverse line blot for specific hybridization, synthetic RNA probes that capture viral DNA, real-time PCR, and microarrays. Some assays detect L1 DNA sequences, whereas others detect E6 or E7 DNA or RNA. More recently, assays based on high-throughput next-generation DNA sequencing have been developed and validated. Because they can determine the entire viral genome sequence, they provide variant, as well as type-specific, information.[371] The highest analytical sensitivity may be preferred if the goal is to detect as many infections as possible. However, as discussed below, a lower sensitivity threshold may be more useful clinically, as it can increase the specificity for identifying high-risk lesions.

CANCER SCREENING

For cervical cancer screening, the goal is to maximize identification of those infections associated with high-grade abnormalities (true positives), which usually should be treated, while excluding as many infections with no or only low-grade abnormalities (false positives) as possible, which should not be treated because most are destined to clear spontaneously (Fig. 3.7). Achieving this balance means that the signal used for screening must exceed a certain threshold, in order to reduce the number of false positives, while still identifying the vast majority of true positives.

Since its introduction in the 1950s, cytologic screening with Pap smears, whose goal is to prevent cancer by identifying premalignant lesions that can then be treated, has been the principal test for assessing cervical cancer risk.[23] Coupled with colposcopic follow-up of high-grade findings and ablation of histologically confirmed CIN2/3, its use has led to a greater than 70% reduction in cervical cancer mortality in developed countries with high-quality testing at regular intervals.[301] However, Pap-based screening has proven difficult to implement in most low-resource settings, because it is difficult to initially establish a program requiring well-trained cytologists, quality control can be challenging, and a single Pap test has relatively low sensitivity in identifying premalignant lesions, which means the test must be repeated on a regular basis.

HPV-based assays have greater sensitivity than cytology, which gives them several advantages, including greater negative predictive value, which can permit longer intervals between screens, and a greater sensitivity in detecting cervical adenocarcinoma precursors, which cytologic screening tends to miss.[23,173,287,295] However, the specificity of HPV DNA for cervical precancer can be relatively low, particularly in younger women, because they generally have relatively high rates of infection and high rates of subsequent clearance. To avoid excessive follow-up and overtreatment of infections destined to regress, HPV-based testing is generally not recommended for younger women, under 30 in the United States. However, co-testing with cytology and HPV has been adopted for women over 25 to 30 in some countries. The U.S. Preventative Services Task Force cervical cancer screening guidelines now recommend cytology-based screening every 3 years for women 21 to 65 years of age or co-testing with cytology and an FDA-approved HPV test every 5 years for women 30 to 65.[318] HPV testing is also recommended for women with equivocal (ASCUS) Pap smears.

Hybrid Capture II (Digene), a signal amplification test, was the first HPV test approved by the FDA, in 2003. Since then, four additional signal and nucleic acid amplification–based tests have been approved: Cervista HPV HR (Hologic), Cervista HPV 16/18 (Hologic), Cobas HPV test (Roche Molecular Systems), and APTIMA HPV, which detects HPV E6/E7 mRNA (Gen-Probe). Some assays use a cocktail that can detect more than 10 high-risk HPV types in aggregate, while other assays report type-specific results. The greater oncogenicity of HPV-16, and HPV-18 and 45 to a lesser extent, argues for the importance of knowing whether a patient is infected with these HPV types. In 2014, the FDA approved the Roche Cobas test for primary screening in women starting at age 24. It is likely that primary HPV screening will become the standard of care in many countries in the coming decade.

Recent guidelines for follow-up of positive HPV tests, or co-tests with cytology, are based on estimates of the absolute risk that the result predicts a precancer (Fig. 3.12).[89,276] Therefore, follow-up varies by HPV type identified, based on the relative risk of the infection reflecting the presence of a precancer (Table 3.2). For example, the U.S. guidelines recommend immediate referral to colposcopy of HPV-16 or 18 DNA–positive results, while referral to cytology is recommended for positive results for other high-risk HPV types.[160]

A challenge for the future will be to adjust screening recommendation in populations with high vaccine coverage.[178] The positive predictive value of programs will decrease as the number of true positives (CIN2+ detections) will decrease because of a large reduction in infection by the major high-risk HPV types, while the number of false positives will likely remain constant, particularly in the case of cytology-based screening.[342]

HPV-based assays have great potential for translation to low-resource settings, because they would require only one or two lifetime tests to substantially reduce cervical cancer death rates[305] and because self-sampling could be employed. Multiple studies have shown that patient and health care worker–collected samples generate comparable sensitivities and specificities.[145] Based on these considerations, the WHO currently recommends HPV testing, if feasible, over cytology as the primary screening method. The main impediments to implementation of HPV screening in low-resource settings are the cost of the tests and, because of its relative insensitivity for CIN2+, the need to follow up relatively large numbers of positive women. However, lower cost and rapid point of care tests have been and are being developed, including careHPV (QIAGEN) and Ampfire (Atila Bio Systems).[350]

A number of biomarkers, in addition to cytology, are being evaluated as triage tests, to distinguish between those HPV infections associated with precancer and those that are not. The most advanced test, which has been FDA approved, uses immunostaining for p16INK4a, which is elevated in response to the inactivation of pRb by E7 of high-risk viruses, plus costaining for the Ki67 cell cycle entry marker (CINtech Plus Cytology, Roche). Methylated viral DNA or methylation of specific cellular genes, as well as other markers, such as microRNA profiling, is also being evaluated.[73,213,325]

Visual inspection of the cervix after staining with acetic acid (VIA) or Lugol iodine (VILI) followed by ablation of suspicious lesions has been investigated in trials in multiple settings as a simple low-cost point of care "see-and-treat" approach.[306] VIA has now been implemented in national or regional cervical cancer prevention programs in several South Asian and

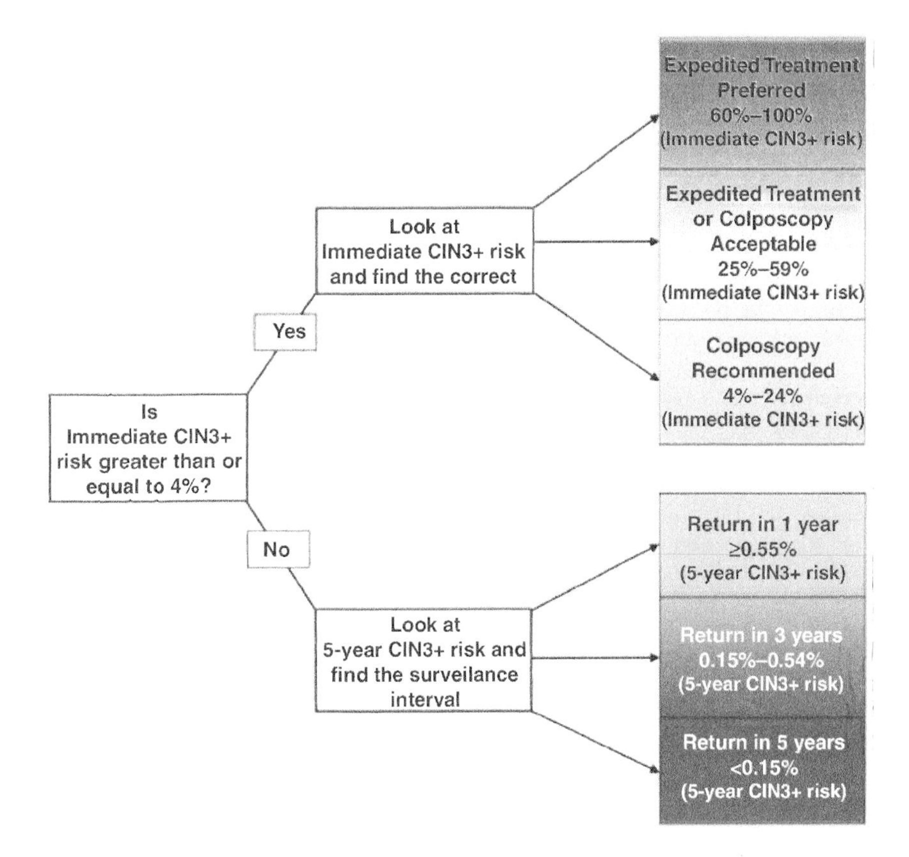

FIGURE 3.12 **Decision tree from the American Society of Colposcopy and Cervical Pathology for management of women with a positive cervical cancer screening test.** (Reprinted with permission from Perkins RB, Guido RS, Castle PE, et al. 2019 ASCCP risk-based management consensus guidelines for abnormal cervical cancer screening tests and cancer precursors. *J Low Genit Tract Dis* 2020;24:102–131.)

sub-Saharan Africa countries.[3] However, the positive predictive value of VIA for CIN2+ is approximately 10%, which, in the absence of a triage test, results in considerable overtreatment. To address this issue, artificial intelligence–generated software has been developed based on a training set of photographs of histologically confirmed cervical lesions and was shown to markedly increase the positive predictive value of visual inspection.[156] The use of cell phones for digital imaging and data transmission to a central computer could make this approach amenable to many low-resource settings.

While population-wide screening efforts are directed toward cervical cancer, the more limited anal cancer screening activities have been focused on high-risk groups, including men who have sex with men, HIV-positive men and women, and patients with other forms of immunosuppression.[7] The high risk of anal cancer among HIV positives, especially MSMs, has led the CDC to recommend annual digital rectal exams in HIV positives, especially those with a history of receptive anal intercourse.[390] Visual inspection by anoscopy after application of acetic acid is currently considered the most sensitive and specific test for high-grade anal dysplasia but, as with cervical colposcopy, it is too expense to use as a primary screening tool. Therefore, anal cytology, similar to the cervical Pap smear test and available for high-risk populations at some clinical centers, is generally used as the initial test.[263] Recommendations for screening high-risk groups do not normally include HPV testing, because of the high prevalence of anal HPV infections in cytologically normal individuals in these populations and hence the relatively low predictive value for high-grade anal dysplasias.[367] At this time, treatment of anal HSIL has not been formally proven to reduce the incidence of anal cancer, although it seems likely based on the analogy to cervical disease, and a clinical trial to examine this question is well under way, with an estimated completion date of 2026 (ClinicalTrials.gov Indentifier: NCT02135419).

TABLE 3.2 Risk of CIN3+ by HPV genotyping and cytology with no prior HPV testing history

Current HPV	Current Cytology	CIN3+ Immediate Risk, %	CIN3+ 5 Year Risk, %
HPV-16	NILM	5.3	8.8
HPV-18	NILM	3.0	4.5
HR12	NILM	1.3	2.2
HPV-16	LSIL	11	15
HPV-18	LSIL	3.1	3.9
HR12	LSIL	3.7	4.7
HPV-16	HSIL	60	64
HPV-18	HSIL	30	30
HR12	HSIL	35	37

NILM, negative for intraepithelial lesions or malignancy; LSIL, low-grade squamous intraepithelial neoplasia; HSIL, high-grade squamous intraepithelial neoplasia; HR12, 12 high-risk HPV types excluding HPV-16 and HPV-18. Data extracted from Demarco M, Egemen D, Raine-Bennett TR, et al. A study of partial human papillomavirus genotyping in support of the 2019 ASCCP risk-based management consensus guidelines. *J Low Genit Tract Dis* 2020;24:144–147.

Screening for HPV-associated OPC risk is not recommended, even though the cancers typically present at a late stage with lymph node involvement, and the rate of HPV-associated OPC is starting to exceed the rate of cervical cancer in the U.S. and some Western European countries.[194] There are multiple reasons for this situation. First, long-term survival of HPV-associated OPCs remains high, so the measurable outcome of early detection would more likely be a reduction in morbidity associated with treatment rather than reduced mortality. In addition, the precursor lesions of OPC have not been identified, although oral HPV DNA is more frequently detected in OPC patients than in controls. In one study, oral HPV-16 prevalence was detected in approximately 20% of OPC cases an average of 6 years prior to diagnosis versus 1% in controls.[4] However, the relative low rate of OPC in the general population would mean that most positive results would be false positive for OPC. In addition, there are few prospective studies that relate detection of oral HPV and subsequent risk of OPC, that is, establish the positive predictive value. Surprisingly, antibody responses to HPV-16 E6 appear to be a sensitive and specific marker for HPV-16–associated OPC. In several studies, 25% to 50% of OPC patients were seropositive HPV-16 E6 (vs. 0.4%-0.7% in controls), which is similar to the fraction of cases attributable to HPV-16 in these study cohorts. There was 100% concordance between positivity for HPV-16 antibodies and oral HPV-16 DNA in the limited number of cases that could be evaluated, and the antibodies were detected in sera many years prior to cancer diagnosis.[190,194] However, as with HPV DNA testing, this level of specificity would result in many more false positive than true positive tests. More acceptable false positive rates might be obtained if testing were limited to higher risk individuals, for example males, populations with a high HPV-16–attributable fraction, smokers, or those with high-risk sexual behavior profiles. In addition, an effective triage test to further risk stratify HPV-16 antibody or DNA-positive individuals might need to be developed and validated before general screening for HPV-associated OPCC would be practical.

Treatment

In cervical HPV infection, treatment of low-grade dysplasia is not usually warranted, given that most of these lesions will clear spontaneously. High-grade dysplasias represent precancerous lesions that are unlikely to resolve spontaneously, and their treatment is recommended to prevent cervical cancer. Depending on the setting, treatment of cervical dysplasia can be surgical, with cryotherapy, via loop electrosurgical excision, or by laser. More recently, thermocoagulation has generated promising results in comparison to cryotherapy for treatment in see-and-treat trials in low-resource settings.[63] In most instances, these approaches prevent cervical cancer. HPV testing can be used to evaluate treatment effectiveness, because most successfully treated cases become negative for HPV DNA, whereas incompletely treated cases may remain positive,[400] although this follow-up testing is not routinely done. Cervical cancer is treated by surgery, radiotherapy, and chemotherapy, with early-stage tumors having a better prognosis than more advanced tumors.[226]

Treatments of anal HSIL include imiquimod, fluorouracil, infrared photocoagulation, thermal ablation, and laser therapy. None are considered optimal, and they are associated with a high recurrence rate and with more morbidity than treatment of cervical HSIL.[129]

Therapeutic vaccines have been under active development for decades, yet none have proven effective enough to warrant commercialization.[66,112] Most have targeted HPV-16 and HPV-18 E6 and/or E7 with the aim of generating cell-mediated immune responses that would induce regression of CIN2+ lesions, or in some cases high-grade vulvar lesions. Various vaccine strategies have been tested, including those based on peptides, whole proteins, naked DNA, and viral or bacterial vectors.[391] While many have induced detectable T-cell responses, they have mostly been directed at generation of systemic T cells, although the targeted lesions are intraepithelial, raising the question of whether the circulating T cells efficiently traffic across the basement membrane into the tissue where the lesion resides.[71]

CIN2+ may represent a relatively high bar for a therapeutic vaccine, both commercially and immunologically. Current ablative therapies for it are generally well tolerated and effective, making it difficult to improve on standard of care. In addition, CIN2+ are persistent lesions that have likely already undergone considerable immune selection, so they might be resistant to vaccine-induced cell-mediated immune responses. By contrast, persistent high-risk HPV infection/CIN1 may prove to be a more attractive target. With the transition to HPV-based screening, increasing large numbers of women are being informed that that they have a sexually transmitted infection by an oncovirus, but there is no treatment available. These infections are also less likely to have undergone immune selection and might therefore be more likely to respond to the vaccine. However, the vaccine would have to be very well tolerated and effective, since 90% of low-grade infections will spontaneously resolve, and so trials would have to be large and the primary end points probably based on time to clearance rather than ultimate rate of clearance.[72]

Given what is now known about key molecular events in HPV infection, considerable potential exists for developing antiviral therapies against HPV in addition to immunotherapy.[111,262] An antiviral that targeted a molecular activity common to all HPV types, or at least to a large number of them, such as the interaction between high-risk E6 and E6AP, might have the theoretical advantage of being active against multiple types, in contrast to the predominantly type-specificity of most viral antigens. However, development of antivirals targeting the viral oncoproteins has proven difficult, in part because they lack, with the exception of E1, enzymatic activities.

Antisense and ribozyme approaches may also have some potential, but their activity is likely to be type specific. Alternatively, the use of genome-editing technologies to inactivate E6/E7 genes can be envisioned. Both transcription activator-like effector nuclease (TALEN) and clustered regulatory interspaced short palindromic repeats (CRISPR)–Cas9 based systems were shown to induce cell death *in vitro* and reduce tumor growth *in vivo* of HPV-16– and HPV-18–derived cervical cancer cell lines.[176,323,394] However, efficient delivery to infected cells within the lesions remains a substantial hurdle to clinical application.

Two immunomodulatory agents, interferon and imiquimod, are approved for use against genital warts, although destructive therapy is often used to treat these lesions.[395] In placebo-controlled trials, intralesional and parenteral interferon therapy was active against refractory genital warts,[378] and topical imiquimod, which activates TLR7 and induces interferons and other cytokines, was also effective.[377] Neither agent, however, cures more than two-thirds of treated patients.

Surgery remains the principal therapeutic modality for RRP, although it is seldom curative.[195] Intralesional cidofovir, an antiviral that inhibits DNA polymerases, has been used as an adjuvant therapy to surgery, but it showed no significant efficacy in a randomized control trial.[230] Interferon therapy of RRP has been less successful than that of genital warts, and treatment is associated with serious side effects, including leukopenia and thrombocytopenia.[146] More recently, intralesional or systemic Bevacizumab, an anti-VEGF monoclonal antibody, and intramuscular injection of Gardasil, the prophylactic HPV vaccine, have been evaluated as RRP treatments.[195] While both have yielded some promising results, the findings are derived from individual cases or small case series. Larger randomized control studies will be needed to critically evaluate their effectiveness.

As with other HPV infections, no specific antiviral therapy is available for nongenital warts. Most treatments are aimed at destroying the lesional tissue while causing as little long-term damage to the surrounding normal tissue. No single therapeutic modality will cure all warts, which has led to the wide range of therapies. At least partial regression can be obtained with many therapies, but even complete clearance that is then followed by recurrence is usually of limited clinical value. Treatment of cutaneous warts is based on destruction and/or immunostimulation. The most common destructive treatments are cryotherapy, laser therapy, and salicylic acid. Cryotherapy and salicylic acids have similar cure rates, about 50% compared to 25% for placebo control.[38,298] Immunostimulatory treatments include imiquimod (a TLR 7 agonist), 5-fluorouracil, and intralesional injection of tuberculin protein, Candida antigen or the measles/mumps/rubella vaccine. They generate clearance rates of 25% to 95%.[108] However, it is likely that destructive treatments also function, at least in part, by immunostimulatory mechanisms, via induction of local inflammation and promoting exposure of viral antigens to the immune system.

PREVENTION

Interruption of Transmission

As noted above, the epidemiology of various forms of HPV infection can differ drastically. Therefore, approaches to control genital HPV infection would be distinct from those to control nongenital infections. Optimal Pap smear and/or HPV-based screening programs can prevent most cervical cancers, which represent the most serious public health consequence of HPV infection, but screening is complex and expensive and presumably does not have appreciable impact on transmission.

Public health efforts that can prevent other sexually transmitted infections should, in principle, also be effective in preventing genital HPV infection. Indeed, decreased sexual promiscuity on the part of both sexual partners should reduce the likelihood of exposure to genital HPV.[362] In the absence of specific treatment that would eradicate genital infections, investigation of sexual partners of infected individuals would not be expected to have much impact on HPV transmission, although it may help identify infected individuals who otherwise might not realize that they are infected.

Although HPV can infect genital areas that are not covered by condoms, condom use may reduce the incidence of genital HPV infection. Consistent with this possibility, several studies in men have reported that condom use is associated with fewer genital HPV infections and a shorter duration of infection in those men who were infected.[250] For women, a meta-analysis found no consistent evidence that condom use in their sexual partners reduced the risk of acquisition of cervical HPV infection, but it was associated with some protection against genital warts, CIN2, CIN3, and cervical cancer.[221] However, in a well-conducted prospective study, consistent condom use by their partners reduced cervicovaginal HPV infection in young women by two-thirds.[385]

As another possible intervention measure, circumcision of adult men was shown to reduce their acquisition of high-risk HPV infection by almost one-half after 2 years.[130,351] A recent meta-analysis reported that male circumcision reduces the odds of penile HPV infection in HIV-positive MSMs (OR 0.71, 95% CI 0.51 to 0.99) but was not significantly protective in HIV-negative MSMs (OR 0.86, 95%CI 0.53 to 1.41). Circumcision was not found to protect against anal infection in MSMs, regardless of HIV status.[396]

HPV topical microbicides are under active evaluation. Carrageenan, a complex polysaccharide derived from red algae, is a potent and broadly active inhibitor of cultured cell infection by alpha HPV types.[39] *In vivo*, it mitigates the potentiating effects on cervicovaginal HPV pseudovirus infection induced by nonoxonol 9 containing over-the-counter spermicides in mouse and macaque models.[290,291] Carrageenans are widely used in food and cosmetic products and are the main gelling agent in some over-the-counter sexual lubricants. In a trial designed to test the efficacy of a carrageenan gel in the prevention of HIV infection, some protection against HPV infection at the exit visit was observed, but only in the subgroup that was most compliant with use instructions.[222] Clinical trials designed to formally evaluate carrageenan gels as HPV microbicides in women and MSMs are under way.[202,274]

Epidemiologic findings, discussed earlier, suggest that most cases of juvenile-onset RRP that arise in infants and young children have been transmitted from exposure to the mother's HPV during vaginal delivery. This hypothesis raises the possibility that the use of cesarean section for the delivery of infants of mothers with known genital HPV infection would reduce the risk of HPV exposure. The incidence of genital HPV infection is high, however, whereas that of RRP is low, which means that many cesarean sections would be needed to prevent each case of RRP. These considerations suggest that the morbidity and mortality risk to the mother associated with cesarean section may, in most situations, be greater than the risk of RRP to the baby, which has led some investigators to argue against the widespread use of this procedure to prevent RRP. However, because the risk of RRP is greater for younger women and for first pregnancies, a subset of HPV-positive women may exist for whom the cost-to-benefit analysis might favor cesarean section.[321] HPV vaccination in Australia with Gardasil (or Gardasil 9), which prevents genital HPV-6 and HPV-11 infections (discussed below), has been reported to result in a more than fivefold reduction in RRP compared with historic controls.[253]

Prophylactic Vaccination

The important public health consequences of genital HPV infection made it highly desirable to develop effective vaccines against those HPV infections associated with cancer, especially cervical cancer. Vaccines to prevent oncogenic HPV infections could potentially prevent the full spectrum of HPV-associated cancers, in contrast to current screening programs, which are mainly effective in preventing squamous carcinoma of the cervix. Although it would be ideal if a vaccine could both treat established infection and induce long-term protection against incident infection, therapeutic and prophylactic vaccines generally have distinct effector mechanisms, cell-mediated immunity and antibodies, respectively, so they have largely been pursued separately. As noted above, efforts to develop therapeutic vaccines have thus far had limited success in human clinical trials, and there are no commercial therapeutic HPV vaccines. By contrast, initiatives to develop HPV prophylactic vaccines have followed the success of preventive vaccines against other viral diseases[280] and have led to the commercial licensing of four distinct vaccines.

Early studies with CRPV indicated that systemic injection with papilloma suspensions that did not produce detectable infection could induce serum-neutralizing antibodies and protect rabbits against high-dose cutaneous viral challenge.[326] Intradermal injection of a vaccine composed of formalin-inactivated COPV virions was shown to protect against COPV-induced oral lesions under field conditions.[24] This result demonstrated that systemic immunization can induce protective immunity against natural transmission of a mucosal PV infection. However, the viral determinants that conferred protection were not definitively identified in these studies.

The inability to produce preparative amounts of HPV virions, together with the presence of oncogenes in the viral genomes, suggested that a subunit vaccine would be a preferred approach. A key observation in the development of a prophylactic vaccine was finding that L1 can self-assemble into VLPs, which are empty capsids that closely resemble those of authentic virions morphologically and immunologically.[139,181,297] As with authentic virions, L1 VLPs were highly immunogenic, inducing high titers of neutralizing antibodies that recognize conformation-dependent virion epitopes.[181] In several animal PV models, systemic immunization with L1 VLPs induced strong protection against high-dose experimental challenge by the homologous virus.[34,65,180,344] Protection was type specific, was of long duration, and could be passively transferred with immune IgG, implying that neutralizing antibodies were sufficient for protection. L2 also contains neutralization epitopes, but they are not exposed in the context of the mature virion.[316] Therefore, while co-expression of L1 and L2 in cells results in L1/L2 VLPs, these VLPs were neither more immunogenic nor more protective than L1 VLPs.[34] Human trials, therefore, went forward with L1 VLPs, with the main focus on HPV-16 and HPV-18, the two most oncogenic HPV types. Despite the excellent results with the preclinical models, none represented a genital infection, and it was unclear how relevant these models would be to genital infection under natural conditions. In addition, most vaccines protect against systemic infection that has a viremic phase, which exposes the virus in contact with antibodies in the blood, whereas HPV induces an infection that is confined to the epithelium.

Four commercial prophylactic HPV vaccines have been developed (Table 3.3). GlaxoSmithKline's Cervarix is a bivalent vaccine composed of L1 VLPs of HPV-16 and HPV-18; Merck's Gardasil is a quadrivalent vaccine composed of L1 VLPs of HPV-6, 11, 16, and 18; Merck's Gardasil 9 contains the four types in Gardasil plus VLPs of five additional high-risk types; and Cecolin is a bivalent vaccine composed of HPV-16 and HPV-18 VLPs. In addition to their valency, the vaccines differ in production system, adjuvant, and recommended injection

TABLE 3.3 Characteristics of HPV VLP prophylactic vaccines

	Cervarix	Gardasil	Gardasil-9	Cecolin
Manufacturer	GlaxoSmithKline	Merck		
VLP types	HPV-16/18	HPV-6/11/16/18	HPV-6/11/16/18/ 31/33/45/52/58	HPV-16/18
Dose of L1 protein	20/20 μg	20/40/40/20 μg	30/40/60/40/ 20/20/20/20/20 μg	40/20 μg
Producer cells	*Trichoplusia ni* (Hi 5) insect cell line infected with L1 recombinant baculovirus	*Saccharomyces cerevisiae* (baker's yeast) expressing L1	*Saccharomyces cerevisiae* (baker's yeast) expressing L1	*E. coli*
Adjuvant	500 μg aluminum hydroxide, 50 μg 3-*O*-deacylated-4′-monophosphoryl lipid A	225 μg aluminum hydroxyphosphate sulfate	500 μg aluminum hydroxyphosphate sulfate	208 μg aluminum hydroxide
Injection schedule	0, 1, 6 months	0, 2, 6 months	0, 2, 6 months	0, 1, 6 months
Licensure	Many countries	Many countries	Many countries	China

Gardasil® and Gardasil-9® (Merck & Co., Whitehouse Station, NJ, USA).
Cervarix® (GlaxoSmithKline Biologicals, Rixensart, Belgium).
Cecolin® (Xiamen Innovax Biotech Co., Xiamen, China).
HPV, human papillomavirus; VLP, virus-like particle.

TABLE 3.4 Four-year efficacy of HPV VLP vaccines against vaccine-targeted types according to protocol analyses of phase III clinical trials

Study	Vaccine	Sex/Age	End Point	Efficacy[a]	95% CI	Reference
PATRICA	Cervarix	Females 15–25	CIN2+	94.9%	87.7–98.4	205
FUTURE I/II	Gardasil	Females 15–26	CIN2+	100%	94.7–100	183
FUTURE I/II	Gardasil	Females 15–26	VIN2+/VaIN2+	100%	82.6–100	183
FUTURE I/II	Gardasil	Females 15–26	Genital warts	99.0%	96.2–99.9	92
CVT	Cervarix	Female 18–25	6 month persist. infect.	90.9%	82.0–95.9	150
CVT	Cervarix	Females 18–25	Anal infection at exit	83.6%[b]	66.7–92.8	191
Merck 020	Gardasil	Males 16–26	Genital warts	89.4%	65.5–97.9	127
Merck 020	Gardasil	Males 16-26	6 month persist. infect.	85.6%	73.4–92.9	127
Merck 020	Gardasil	Males 16–26	AIN2+	74.9%	8.8–95.4	264
V503-001	Gardasil-9	Females 16–26	CIN/VIN/VaIN2+ HPV-31/33/45/52/58	96.7%	80.9–99.8	170
HPV-PRO-003	Cecolin	Females 18–45	CIN2+/persistent infection	100%/97.8%	55.6–100/87.1–99.9	285

[a]Efficacy against vaccine-targeted types per protocol cohorts.
[b]Subjects were cervical HPV-16/18 DNA negative at entry but anal HPV not evaluated at entry.
95% CI, ninety-five percent confidence interval; PATRICIA, Papilloma TRial against Cancer In young Adults; FUTURE, Females United To Unilaterally Reduce Endo/Ecocervical Disease; CVT, Costa Rica Vaccine Trial; CIN2+, cervical intraepithelial neoplasia grade two or worse; VIN2+, vulvar intraepithelial neoplasia grade two or worse; VaIN2+, vaginal intraepithelial neoplasia grade two or worse.

schedule (Table 3.3). The vaccines were generally safe and able to consistently induce high titers of capsid-reactive antibodies in early-phase trials. In phase III clinical trials of young women in which three dose of the vaccine were administered by intramuscular injection over 6 months, all four vaccines were also highly effective at preventing acquisition of persistent cervical infection and high-grade CIN caused by the types targeted by the vaccine (Table 3.4).[10,285] These results have led to worldwide licensure of Cervarix, Gardasil, and Gardasil 9, while Cecolin is licensed exclusively in China. The vaccines have been licensed for prevention of CIN and cervical cancer caused by the vaccine-targeted types.

Unexpectedly, both Cervarix and Gardasil appear to induce a high level of protection against persistent cervical infection up to a decade postvaccination even after administration of only one dose of the vaccine.[380] However, these findings are based on post hoc analyses that were not designed to evaluate one dose efficacy. Formal randomized trials comparing one versus two doses of Cervarix and Gardasil 9 are now underway.[303]

The vaccines also induced modest but durable protection against cervical infection caused by specific nonvaccine types closely related to HPV-16 or HPV-18.[220] For instance, both Cervarix and Gardasil induced partial protection against persistent infection by HPV-31. Cervarix, but not Gardasil, also induced substantial protection against HPV-45, and borderline protection against HPV-35 and HPV-58.[356]

Gardasil was also highly effective at preventing genital warts, and vulvar and vaginal intraepithelial neoplasia, and it has been licensed for these indications[92,183] (Table 3.4). Cervarix was not evaluated for these end points, apparently because it does not target HPV-6 and HPV-11, the types that cause most genital warts. Neither vaccine induced significant clearance of established infections or regression of established lesions, so they are not licensed for treatment of HPV infection or disease.[116,151]

Consistent with the observation of ongoing protection for more than a decade, neutralizing antibody titers induced by the vaccines have remained essentially stable, even after a single dose, and above the levels induced by natural infection, supporting optimistic projections for long-term, perhaps lifelong, protection without the need for booster immunizations (Fig. 3.13).[13,193] Cross-neutralizing antibodies against related types, when they are detected, appear to recognize subdominant epitopes, as their titers are much lower than the titers against the vaccine-targeted types,[175] but they appear to be as durable as type-specific antibody responses.[128] The remarkably high, consistent, and durable antibody response to the vaccines may in large part be attributed to the strong signaling through the B-cell receptors after their engagement of the dense repetitive array of epitopes on the VLP surface. In addition, their repetitive and particular nature promotes their phagocytosis by antigen-presenting cells for generation of strong T helper responses and the binding of natural IgM and complement that promotes their acquisition by follicular dendritic cells for presentation to B cells in lymph nodes.[314]

Gardasil was also tested for efficacy in men. Strong protection from genital warts was documented[127] (Table 3.4). Relatively few penile intraepithelial lesions were detected in the trials, so the trial was unable to critically evaluate this end point. The subset of the men who had sex with men was concurrently enrolled in a study of anal infection and anal intraepithelial neoplasia (AIN).[264] Excellent protection against vaccine type–related anal infection and AIN was observed (Table 3.4). The findings led to licensure for these indications and for preven-

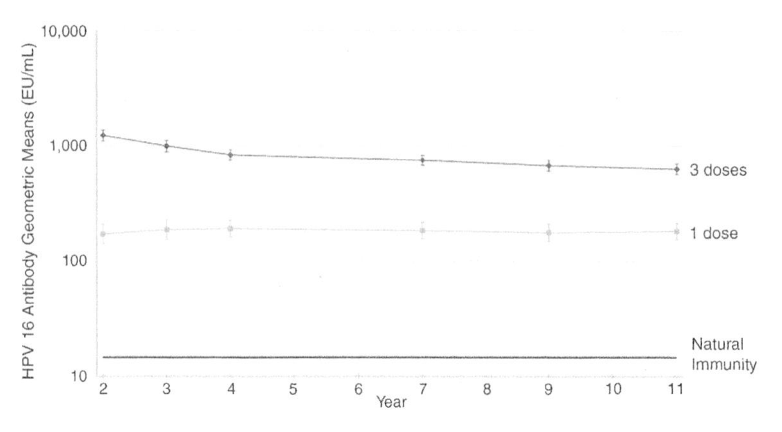

FIGURE 3.13 Durability of the serum antibody responses by doses of Cervarix received, as measured in an HPV-16 VLP ELISA. (Data derived from the long term follow up of the Costa Rican Vaccine Trial (CVT) Kreimer AR, Sampson JN, Porras C, et al. Evaluation of durability of a single-dose of the bivalent HPV vaccine: the CVT Trial. *J Natl Cancer Inst* 2020;112:1038–1046. The results were similar for HPV18.)

tion of AIN and anal cancer in the United States and elsewhere. Licensure was extended to anal neoplasia and anal cancer in women based on the argument that AIN and anal cancer are indistinguishable in the two sexes. Licensure of Gardasil 9 was based on immunological noninferiority for the four VLP types it shares with Gardasil, together with strong protection against CIN2+ caused by the five additional high-risk types in Gardasil 9. Although Cervarix has not been evaluated for prevention of AIN in either sex, it was shown to significantly reduce the prevalence of anal HPV infection at the end of a 4-year trial in young women.[191]

The above trials were conducted in young women and men ages 15 to 26 years, with the exception of Cecolin, where the women were 18 to 45. Immunobridging studies were used to extend licensure to 9- to 14-year-olds. Antibody responses to both Cervarix and Gardasil were significantly higher (two- to threefold) in the younger vaccinees compared with the older age groups.[28,271] The higher responses in children led to a comparison of two- and three-dose vaccination protocols. For both vaccines, the antibody responses of children after two doses given 6 months apart were not inferior to the responses of young adults to three doses given according to the recommended schedules.[187,294] These findings have led most national programs to adopt a two-dose schedule for adolescents younger than 15 years of age.

Although highly immunogenic, both vaccines were well tolerated in both sexes. The primary side effects attributable to the vaccines were short-term pain, swelling, and erythema at injection site and low-grade fever and/or headache.[364,366] No pattern of serious adverse events was associated with vaccination in either the clinical trials or subsequently in immunization programs.[277,324,383]

Neutralizing antibodies are believed to be the primary, if not exclusive, immune effectors for the VLP vaccines, although a formal immune correlate of protection has not been determined.[314] In part, this shortcoming is due to the remarkably small number of vaccine failures to date and the inability to definitively distinguish incident infection from emergence or reactivation of infections present at the time of vaccination. Antibodies induced by systemic VLP vaccination could reach the anogenital sites of infection by two mechanisms. One mechanism is transudation of serum IgG, which is especially pronounced at the cervix.[247] Alternatively, systemic antibodies could be directly exudated at the site of trauma required for initiating infection.[290] The second mechanism appears to be fully able to prevent infection, since strong protection was observed against genital warts on external genitalia, sites not normally exposed to transudated antibodies in mucus. In a mouse cervicovaginal challenge model, VLP-induced antibodies were shown to protect from keratinocyte infection by two distinct mechanisms.[77] At high concentrations, the antibodies prevented binding of the capsids to the basement membrane of the cervicovaginal epithelium. At lower concentrations that were nonetheless effective at preventing infection, the capsids were able to bind the basement membrane and undergo the conformational change that exposes L2 N-terminal epitopes. However, they were subsequently unable to stably associate with the cervicovaginal keratinocytes. Two possible explanations for these observations are that lower antibody occupancy is needed to prevent capsid binding to the keratinocyte surface receptor than binding to the heparan sulfate proteoglycans of the basement membrane or that the capsids are efficiently phagocytosed by neutrophils and other phagocytic cells via interaction between their Fc receptors and the capsid/antibody complexes.

Since their initial approval in 2006, HPV vaccines have been introduced into the national programs of approximately 120 countries.[84] However, few countries have approached the WHO goal of 90% coverage rates, as stated in the WHO's call for cervical cancer elimination.[46] National programs are mostly centered on vaccination of preadolescent or adolescent girls, ages 9 to 15 years, since worldwide more than 90% of HPV-associated cancers occur in women,[81] genital HPV infections are often acquired soon after initiating sexual activity, and children responded better than adults to the vaccines. However, the evidence that Gardasil protects young men from genital warts and anal cancer precursors has provided additional support for considering male vaccination programs, and about 20 countries have adopted gender-neutral vaccination programs.

The HPV vaccines have now also shown impressive effectiveness in national immunization programs,[37,101] and this effectiveness is particularly evident in analysis of women from cohorts vaccinated prior to sexual debut and in countries with high coverage rates, such as Scotland and Australia (Fig. 3.14).[101] In the Scottish program, which until recently employed Cervarix, an 89% (95% CI 81% to 94%) reduction in CIN3 diagnoses, independent of causal HPV type, was observed in young women vaccinated at age 12 to 13.[265] In 18- to 24-year-old Australian women, the prevalence of vaccine-targeted type infections

FIGURE 3.14 Changes in CIN2+ in screened females after vaccine introduction in countries with at least 50% coverage according to the age at screening. (Reprinted from Drolet M, Benard E, Perez N, et al.; HPV Vaccination Impact Study Group. Population-level impact and herd effects following the introduction of human papillomavirus vaccination programmes: updated systematic review and meta-analysis. *Lancet* 2019;394:497–509. Copyright © 2019 Elsevier. With permission.)

before initiation of their Gardasil vaccination program in 2007 was 22.5% in contrast to 1.5% 9 years after its initiation.[218] Interestingly, the reduction in CIN2+ detection in Australia was comparable in women who received one, two, or three doses of vaccine at age 15 or younger.[36] Clear evidence of herd immunity has emerged in female vaccination programs, even in countries with modest coverage rates. For example, in the decade since the introduction of the vaccines in the U.S. in 2007, the prevalence of vaccine-targeted types in women age 20 to 24 at the time of screening decreased from 13.1% in 2007 to 1.3% in 2015–2016 in vaccinated women, but also decreased to 5.8% in unvaccinated women (Fig. 3.15).[225] The decrease in HPV prevalence was less dramatic in 25- to 29-year-olds, presumably because more of them were infected prior to vaccination. There is also clear evidence that the vaccines induce herd immunity in men. For example, there was a reduction of penile infections by the vaccine-targeted types in young men from 2004 to 2015 (prior to the initiation of a male vaccination program in Australia) from 22% (95% CI 14% to 33%) to 6% (3% to 10%).[64]

Because progression from incident infection to cancer generally takes at least a decade, there is limited evidence that the HPV vaccines prevent cervical or other HPV-induced cancers. However, a recent study based on the Swedish health registry reported that there has been a significant reduction in cervical cancer in women under 31 years[206] since the initiation of the Swedish vaccination program in 2006. The incident ratio was 0.47 (95% CI 0.27 to 0.75) in women vaccinated at age 17 to 30 and 0.12 (95% CI 0.00 to 0.34) for women vaccinated before the age of 17. In addition, modeling exercises indicate that there is great potential for cancer prevention worldwide if coverage rates could be improved.[331] There is an urgent need to expand vaccine coverages of girls, especially in low- and middle-income countries, because few will likely have the opportunity to participate in cervical cancer screening programs as adults. As an illustration of the unmet potential of the vaccines, it has been estimated that, in the absence of vaccination, there would be 19 million cases and 10 million deaths from cervical cancer worldwide in females who were age 14 to 29 in 2014. To date, only 365,000 cases and 150,000 deaths have been averted by vaccination, and almost all of these are in higher income countries (Fig. 3.16) with well-established vaccination programs.

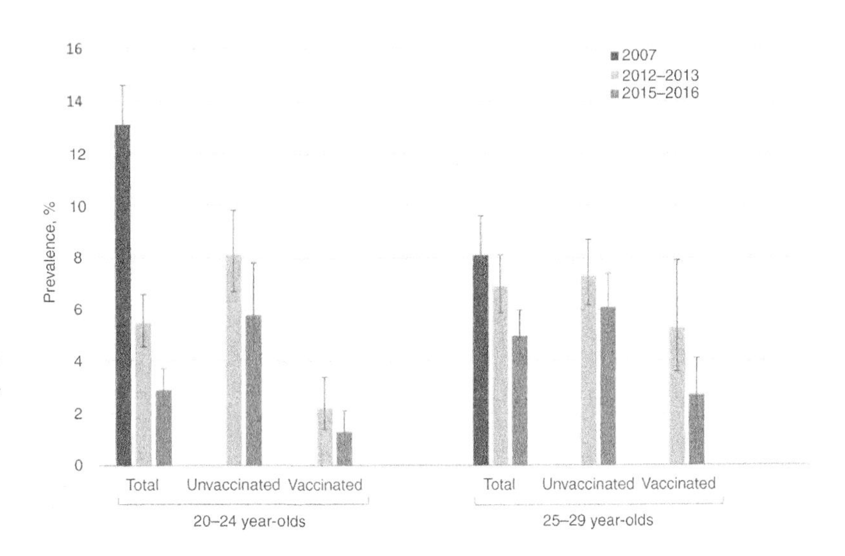

FIGURE 3.15 Decline in vaccine-type HPV prevalence in U.S. women receiving at least one vaccine dose and screened for cervical cancer since vaccine licensure in 2007: evidence of direct and herd effects of vaccination. (Reprinted from Markowitz LE, Naleway AL, Lewis RM, et al. Declines in HPV vaccine type prevalence in women screened for cervical cancer in the United States: evidence of direct and herd effects of vaccination. *Vaccine* 2019;37:3918–3924. Copyright © 2019 Elsevier. With permission.)

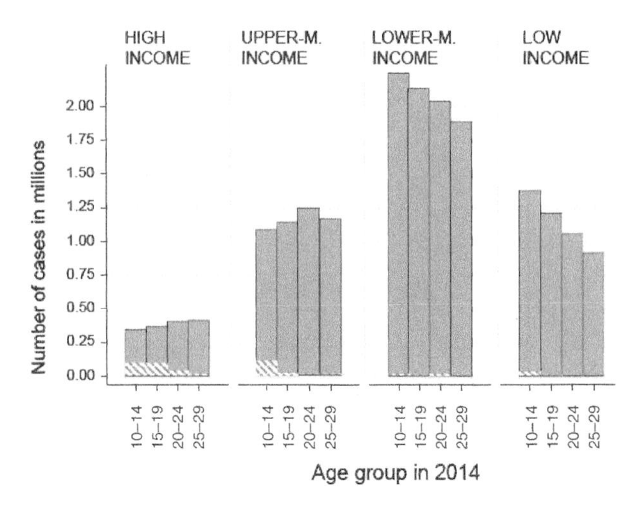

FIGURE 3.16 **Estimated number of cumulative cases of cervical cancer over the next 65 years by age in 2014 and country income level in the absence of HPV vaccines (*blue bars*) and the number of cancers that have been averted by vaccination (*red stripe bars*).** (Reprinted with permission from Bruni L . Global vaccine uptake and projected cervical cancer disease reductions. 2017. www.HPVWorld.com. Data from Bruni L, Diaz M, Barrionuevo-Rosas L, et al. Global estimates of human papillomavirus vaccination coverage by region and income level: a pooled analysis. *Lancet Glob Health* 2016;4(7):e453–e463. doi: 10.1016/S2214-109X(16)30099-7.)

REFERENCES

1. Abraham, AG, D'Souza G, Jing Y, et al. Invasive cervical cancer risk among HIV-infected women: a North American multicohort collaboration prospective study. *J Acquir Immune Defic Syndr* 2013;62:405–413.
2. Adler DH, Kakinami L, Modisenyane T, et al. Increased regression and decreased incidence of human papillomavirus-related cervical lesions among HIV-infected women on HAART. *AIDS* 2012;26:1645–1652.
3. Adsul P, Manjunath N, Srinivas V, et al. Implementing community-based cervical cancer screening programs using visual inspection with acetic acid in India: a systematic review. *Cancer Epidemiol* 2017;49:161–174.
4. Agalliu I, Gapstur S, Chen Z, et al. Associations of oral alpha-, beta-, and gamma-human papillomavirus types with risk of incident head and neck cancer. *JAMA Oncol* 2016;2:599–606.
5. Albero G, Castellsague X, Giuliano AR, et al. Male circumcision and genital human papillomavirus: a systematic review and meta-analysis. *Sex Transm Dis* 2012;39:104–113.
6. Albero G, Castellsague X, Lin HY, et al. Male circumcision and the incidence and clearance of genital human papillomavirus (HPV) infection in men: the HPV Infection in men (HIM) cohort study. *BMC Infect Dis* 2014;14:75.
7. Albuquerque A, Rios E, Schmitt F. Recommendations favoring anal cytology as a method for anal cancer screening: a systematic review. *Cancers (Basel)* 2019;11:1942.
8. Antonsson A, Green AC, Mallitt KA, et al. Prevalence and stability of antibodies to 37 human papillomavirus types—a population-based longitudinal study. *Virology* 2010;407:26–32.
9. Arbyn M, Weiderpass E, Bruni L, et al. Estimates of incidence and mortality of cervical cancer in 2018: a worldwide analysis. *Lancet Glob Health* 2020;8(2):e191–e203.
10. Arbyn M, Xu L. Efficacy and safety of prophylactic HPV vaccines. A Cochrane review of randomized trials. *Expert Rev Vaccines* 2018;17:1085–1091.
11. Arends MJ, Benton EC, McLaren KM, et al. Renal allograft recipients with high susceptibility to cutaneous malignancy have an increased prevalence of human papillomavirus DNA in skin tumours and a greater risk of anogenital malignancy. *Br J Cancer* 1997;75:722–728.
12. Arron ST, Ruby JG, Dybbro E, et al. Transcriptome sequencing demonstrates that human papillomavirus is not active in cutaneous squamous cell carcinoma. *J Invest Dermatol* 2011;131:1745–1753.
13. Artemchuk H, Eriksson T, Poljak M, et al. Long-term antibody response to human papillomavirus vaccines: up to 12 years of follow-up in the Finnish maternity cohort. *J Infect Dis* 2019;219:582–589.
14. Ashrafi GH, Haghshenas MR, Marchetti B, et al. E5 protein of human papillomavirus type 16 selectively downregulates surface HLA class I. *Int J Cancer* 2005;113:276–283.
15. Backes DM, Kurman RJ, Pimenta JM, et al. Systematic review of human papillomavirus prevalence in invasive penile cancer. *Cancer Causes Control* 2009;20:449–457.
16. Barnard P, McMillan NA. The human papillomavirus E7 oncoprotein abrogates signaling mediated by interferon-alpha. *Virology* 1999;259:305–313.
17. Baseman JG, Koutsky LA. The epidemiology of human papillomavirus infections. *J Clin Virol* 2005;32(Suppl 1):S16–S24.
18. Bashaw AA, Leggatt GR, Chandra J, et al. Modulation of antigen presenting cell functions during chronic HPV infection. *Papillomavirus Res* 2017;4:58–65.
19. Basto DL, Chaves CBP, Felix SP, et al. The papillomavirus E5 gene does not affect EGFR transcription and overall survival in cervical cancer. *J Med Virol* 2020;92(8):1283–1289.
20. Beachler DC, Jenkins G, Safaeian M, et al. Natural acquired immunity against subsequent genital human papillomavirus infection: a systematic review and meta-analysis. *J Infect Dis* 2016;213:1444–1454.
21. Beachler DC, Waterboer T, Pierce Campbell Ch M, et al. HPV16 E6 seropositivity among cancer-free men with oral, anal or genital HPV16 infection. *Papillomavirus Res* 2016;2:141–144.
22. Beavis AL, Gravitt PE, Rositch AF. Hysterectomy-corrected cervical cancer mortality rates reveal a larger racial disparity in the United States. *Cancer* 2017;123:1044–1050.
23. Bedell SL, Goldstein LS, Goldstein AR, et al. Cervical cancer screening: past, present, and future. *Sex Med Rev* 2020;8:28–37.
24. Bell JA, Sundberg JP, Ghim SJ, et al. A formalin-inactivated vaccine protects against mucosal papillomavirus infection: a canine model. *Pathobiology* 1994;62:194–198.
25. Bergeron C, Ronco G, Reuschenbach M, et al. The clinical impact of using p16(INK4a) immunochemistry in cervical histopathology and cytology: an update of recent developments. *Int J Cancer* 2015;136:2741–2751.
26. Berman TA, Schiller JT. Human papillomavirus in cervical cancer and oropharyngeal cancer: one cause, two diseases. *Cancer* 2017;123:2219–2229.
27. Bertoli HK, Thomsen LT, Iftner T, et al. Risk of vulvar, vaginal and anal high-grade intraepithelial neoplasia and cancer according to cervical human papillomavirus (HPV) status: a population-based prospective cohort study. *Gynecol Oncol* 2020;157(2):456–462.
28. Block SL, Nolan T, Sattler C, et al. Comparison of the immunogenicity and reactogenicity of a prophylactic quadrivalent human papillomavirus (types 6, 11, 16, and 18) L1 virus-like particle vaccine in male and female adolescents and young adult women. *Pediatrics* 2006;118:2135–2145.
29. Bosch FX, Lorincz A, Munoz N, et al. The causal relation between human papillomavirus and cervical cancer. *J Clin Pathol* 2002;55:244–265.
30. Bosch FX, Manos MM, Munoz N, et al. Prevalence of human papillomavirus in cervical cancer: a worldwide prospective. *J Nat Cancer Inst* 1995;87:796–802.
31. Boshart M, Gissmann L, Ikenberg H, et al. A new type of papillomavirus DNA, its presence in genital cancer biopsies and in cell lines derived from cervical cancer. *EMBO J* 1984;3:1153–1157.
32. Bouwes Bavinck JN, Feltkamp MCW, Green AC, et al. Human papillomavirus and post-transplantation cutaneous squamous cell carcinoma: a multicenter, prospective cohort study. *Am J Transplant* 2018;18:1220–1230.
33. Bowden SJ, Kalliala I, Veroniki AA, et al. The use of human papillomavirus DNA methylation in cervical intraepithelial neoplasia: a systematic review and meta-analysis. *EBioMedicine* 2019;50:246–259.
34. Breitburd F, Kirnbauer R, Hubbert NL, et al. Immunization with virus-like particles from cottontail rabbit papillomavirus (CRPV) can protect against experimental CRPV infection. *J Virol* 1995;69:3959–3963.
35. Breznik V, Fujs Komlos K, Hosnjak L, et al. Determination of causative human papillomavirus type in tissue specimens of common warts based on estimated viral loads. *Front Cell Infect Microbiol* 2020;10:4.
36. Brotherton JM, Budd A, Rompotis C, et al. Is one dose of human papillomavirus vaccine as effective as three?: A national cohort analysis. *Papillomavirus Res* 2019;8:100177.
37. Brotherton JML, Bloem PN. Population-based HPV vaccination programmes are safe and effective: 2017 update and the impetus for achieving better global coverage. *Best Pract Res Clin Obstet Gynaecol* 2018;47:42–58.
38. Bruggink SC, Gussekloo J, Berger MY, et al. Cryotherapy with liquid nitrogen versus topical salicylic acid application for cutaneous warts in primary care: randomized controlled trial. *CMAJ* 2010;182:1624–1630.
39. Buck CB, Thompson CD, Roberts JN, et al. Carrageenan is a potent inhibitor of papillomavirus infection. *PLoS Pathog* 2006;2:e69.
40. Burchell AN, Winer RL, de Sanjose S, et al. Chapter 6: Epidemiology and transmission dynamics of genital HPV infection. *Vaccine* 2006;24(Suppl 3):S3/52–61.
41. Burger EA, Kim JJ, Sy S, et al. Age of acquiring causal human papillomavirus (HPV) infections: leveraging simulation models to explore the natural history of HPV-induced cervical cancer. *Clin Infect Dis* 2017;65:893–899.
42. Burghardt E, Ostor AG. Site and origin of squamous cervical cancer: a histomorphologic study. *Obstet Gynecol* 1983;62:117–127.
43. Bzhalava D, Eklund C, Dillner J. International standardization and classification of human papillomavirus types. *Virology* 2015;476:341–344.
44. Campo MS, O'Neil BW, Barron RJ, et al. Experimental reproduction of the papilloma-carcinoma complex of the alimentary canal in cattle. *Carcinogenesis* 1994;15:1597–1601.
45. Cancer Genome Atlas Research Network, Albert Einstein College of Medicine, Analytical Biological Services, et al. Integrated genomic and molecular characterization of cervical cancer. *Nature* 2017;543:378–384.
46. Canfell K, Kim JJ, Brisson M, et al. Mortality impact of achieving WHO cervical cancer elimination targets: a comparative modelling analysis in 78 low-income and lower-middle-income countries. *Lancet* 2020;395:591–603.
47. Carter JJ, Koutsky LA, Hughes JP, et al. Comparison of human papillomavirus types 16, 18, and 6 capsid antibody responses following incident infection. *J Infect Dis* 2000;181:1911–1919.
48. Castellsague X, Alemany L, Quer M, et al. HPV involvement in head and neck cancers: comprehensive assessment of biomarkers in 3680 patients. *J Natl Cancer Inst* 2016;108:djv403.
49. Castellsague X, Ault KA, Bosch FX, et al. Human papillomavirus detection in cervical neoplasia attributed to 12 high-risk human papillomavirus genotypes by region. *Papillomavirus Res* 2016;2:61–69.
50. Castellsague X, Diaz M, de Sanjose S, et al. Worldwide human papillomavirus etiology of cervical adenocarcinoma and its cofactors: implications for screening and prevention. *J Natl Cancer Inst* 2006;98:303–315.
51. Castellsague X, Munoz N. Chapter 3: Cofactors in human papillomavirus carcinogenesis—role of parity, oral contraceptives, and tobacco smoking. *J Natl Cancer Inst Monogr* 2003;20–28.

52. Chaiwongkot A, Vinokurova S, Pientong C, et al. Differential methylation of E2 binding sites in episomal and integrated HPV 16 genomes in preinvasive and invasive cervical lesions. *Int J Cancer* 2013;132:2087–2094.
53. Chang JL, Tsao YP, Liu DW, et al. The expression of HPV-16 E5 protein in squamous neoplastic changes in the uterine cervix. *J Biomed Sci* 2001;8:206–213.
54. Chang YE, Laimins LA. Microarray analysis identifies interferon-inducible genes and Stat-1 as major transcriptional targets of human papillomavirus type 31. *J Virol* 2000;74:4174–4182.
55. Chattopadhyay K. A comprehensive review on host genetic susceptibility to human papillomavirus infection and progression to cervical cancer. *Indian J Hum Genet* 2011;17:132–144.
56. Chaturvedi AK, D'Souza G, Gillison ML, et al. Burden of HPV-positive oropharynx cancers among ever and never smokers in the US population. *Oral Oncol* 2016;60:61–67.
57. Chaturvedi AK, Engels EA, Pfeiffer RM, et al. Human papillomavirus and rising oropharyngeal cancer incidence in the United States. *J Clin Oncol* 2011;29:4294–4301.
58. Chaturvedi AK, Katki HA, Hildesheim A, et al. Human papillomavirus infection with multiple types: pattern of coinfection and risk of cervical disease. *J Infect Dis* 2011;203:910–920.
59. Chaturvedi AK, Kleinerman RA, Hildesheim A, et al. Second cancers after squamous cell carcinoma and adenocarcinoma of the cervix. *J Clin Oncol* 2009;27:967–973.
60. Chaturvedi AK, Madeleine MM, Biggar RJ, et al. Risk of human papillomavirus-associated cancers among persons with AIDS. *J Natl Cancer Inst* 2009;101:1120–1130.
61. Chesson HW, Dunne EF, Hariri S, et al. The estimated lifetime probability of acquiring human papillomavirus in the United States. *Sex Transm Dis* 2014;41:660–664.
62. Chiang C, Pauli EK, Biryukov J, et al. The human papillomavirus E6 oncoprotein targets USP15 and TRIM25 to suppress RIG-I-mediated innate immune signaling. *J Virol* 2018;92:e01737-17.
63. Chigbu CO, Onwudiwe EN, Onyebuchi AK. Thermo-coagulation versus cryotherapy for treatment of cervical precancers: A prospective analytical study in a low-resource African setting. *J Obstet Gynaecol Res* 2020;46:147–152.
64. Chow EPF, Machalek DA, Tabrizi SN, et al. Quadrivalent vaccine-targeted human papillomavirus genotypes in heterosexual men after the Australian female human papillomavirus vaccination programme: a retrospective observational study. *Lancet Infect Dis* 2017;17:68–77.
65. Christensen ND, Reed CA, Cladel NM, et al. Immunization with virus-like particles induces long-term protection of rabbits against challenge with cottontail rabbit papillomaviruses. *J Virol* 1996;70:960–965.
66. Clark KT, Trimble CL. Current status of therapeutic HPV vaccines. *Gynecol Oncol* 2020;156:503–510.
67. Clifford GM, Goncalves MA Franceschi S; HPV and HIV Study Group. Human papillomavirus types among women infected with HIV: a meta-analysis. *AIDS* 2006;20:2337–2344.
68. Cobos C, Figueroa JA, Mirandola L, et al. The role of human papilloma virus (HPV) infection in non-anogenital cancer and the promise of immunotherapy: a review. *Int Rev Immunol* 2014;33:383–401.
69. Colon-Lopez V, Shiels MS, Machin M, et al. Anal cancer risk among people with HIV infection in the United States. *J Clin Oncol* 2018;36:68–75.
70. Combes JD, Pawlita M, Waterboer T, et al. Antibodies against high-risk human papillomavirus proteins as markers for invasive cervical cancer. *Int J Cancer* 2014;135:2453–2461.
71. Cuburu N, Graham BS, Buck CB, et al. Intravaginal immunization with HPV vectors induces tissue-resident CD8+ T cell responses. *J Clin Invest* 2012;122:4606–4620.
72. Cuburu N, Schiller JT. Moving forward with human papillomavirus immunotherapies. *Hum Vaccin Immunother* 2016;12:2875–2880.
73. Cuschieri K, Ronco G, Lorincz A, et al. Eurogin roadmap 2017: triage strategies for the management of HPV-positive women in cervical screening programs. *Int J Cancer* 2018;143:735–745.
74. Cuzick J, Cadman L, Mesher D, et al. Comparing the performance of six human papillomavirus tests in a screening population. *Br J Cancer* 2013;108:908–913.
75. D'Souza G, Kreimer AR, Viscidi R, et al. Case–control study of human papillomavirus and oropharyngeal cancer. *N Engl J Med* 2007;356:1944–1956.
76. D'Souza G, Wentz A, Kluz N, et al. Sex differences in risk factors and natural history of oral human papillomavirus infection. *J Infect Dis* 2016;213:1893–1896.
77. Day PM, Kines RC, Thompson CD, et al. In vivo mechanisms of vaccine-induced protection against HPV infection. *Cell Host Microbe* 2010;8:260–270.
78. Day PM, Weisberg AS, Thompson CD, et al. Human papillomavirus 16 capsids mediate nuclear entry during infection. *J Virol* 2019;93.
79. de Jong A, van der Burg SH, Kwappenberg KM, et al. Frequent detection of human papillomavirus 16 E2-specific T-helper immunity in healthy subjects. *Cancer Res* 2002;62:472–479.
80. de Koning MN, Quint KD, Bruggink SC, et al. High prevalence of cutaneous warts in elementary school children and the ubiquitous presence of wart-associated human papillomavirus on clinically normal skin. *Br J Dermatol* 2015;172:196–201.
81. de Martel C, Georges D, Bray F, et al. Global burden of cancer attributable to infections in 2018: a worldwide incidence analysis. *Lancet Glob Health* 2020;8(2):e180–e190.
82. de Martel C, Plummer M, Vignat J, et al. Worldwide burden of cancer attributable to HPV by site, country and HPV type. *Int J Cancer* 2017;141:664–670.
83. de Planell-Mas E, Martinez-Garriga B, Zalacain AJ, et al. Human papillomaviruses genotyping in plantar warts. *J Med Virol* 2017;89:902–907.
84. de Sanjose S, Brotons M, LaMontagne DS, et al. Human papillomavirus vaccine disease impact beyond expectations. *Curr Opin Virol* 2019;39:16–22.
85. de Sanjose S, Palefsky J. Cervical and anal HPV infections in HIV positive women and men. *Virus Res* 2002;89:201–211.
86. de Sanjose S, Serrano B, Tous S, et al. Burden of human papillomavirus (HPV)-related cancers attributable to HPVs 6/11/16/18/31/33/45/52 and 58. *JNCI Cancer Spectr* 2018;2:pky045.
87. De Vuyst H, Clifford GM, Nascimento MC, et al. Prevalence and type distribution of human papillomavirus in carcinoma and intraepithelial neoplasia of the vulva, vagina and anus: a meta-analysis. *Int J Cancer* 2009;124:1626–1636.
88. DeFilippis RA, Goodwin EC, Wu L, et al. Endogenous human papillomavirus E6 and E7 proteins differentially regulate proliferation, senescence, and apoptosis in HeLa cervical carcinoma cells. *J Virol* 2003;77:1551–1563.
89. Demarco M, Egemen D, Raine-Bennett TR, et al. A study of partial human papillomavirus genotyping in support of the 2019 ASCCP risk-based management consensus guidelines. *J Low Genit Tract Dis* 2020;24:144–147.
90. Demarco M, Lorey TS, Fetterman B, et al. Risks of CIN 2+, CIN 3+, and cancer by cytology and human papillomavirus status: the Foundation of Risk-Based Cervical Screening Guidelines. *J Low Genit Tract Dis* 2017;21:261–267.
91. Dillner J. The serological response to papillomaviruses. *Semin Cancer Biol* 1999;9:423–430.
92. Dillner J, Kjaer SK, Wheeler CM, et al. Four year efficacy of prophylactic human papillomavirus quadrivalent vaccine against low grade cervical, vulvar, and vaginal intraepithelial neoplasia and anogenital warts: randomised controlled trial. *BMJ* 2010;341:c3493.
93. Dinh, TH, Sternberg M, Dunne EF, et al. Genital warts among 18- to 59-year-olds in the United States, national health and nutrition examination survey, 1999–2004. *Sex Transm Dis* 2008;35:357–360.
94. Dion GR, Teng S, Boyd LR, et al. Adjuvant human papillomavirus vaccination for secondary prevention: a systematic review. *JAMA Otolaryngol Head Neck Surg* 2017;143:614–622.
95. Diorio GJ, Giuliano AR. The role of human papilloma virus in penile carcinogenesis and preneoplastic lesions: a potential target for vaccination and treatment strategies. *Urol Clin North Am* 2016;43:419–425.
96. Donne AJ, Hampson L, Homer JJ, et al. The role of HPV type in recurrent respiratory papillomatosis. *Int J Pediatr Otorhinolaryngol* 2010;74:7–14.
97. Doorbar J. The papillomavirus life cycle. *J Clin Virol* 2005;32(Suppl 1):S7–S15.
98. Doorbar J, Egawa N, Griffin H, et al. Human papillomavirus molecular biology and disease association. *Rev Med Virol* 2015;25(Suppl 1):2–23.
99. Doorbar J, Elston RC, Napthine S, et al. The E1E4 protein of human papillomavirus type 16 associates with a putative RNA helicase through sequences in its C terminus. *J Virol* 2000;74:10081–10095.
100. Doorbar J, Quint W, Banks L, et al. The biology and life-cycle of human papillomaviruses. *Vaccine* 2012;30(Suppl 5):F55–F70.
101. Drolet M, Benard E, Perez N, et al.; HPV Vaccination Impact Study Group. Population-level impact and herd effects following the introduction of human papillomavirus vaccination programmes: updated systematic review and meta-analysis. *Lancet*. 2019;394:497–509.
102. Duensing S, Munger K. Centrosome abnormalities, genomic instability and carcinogenic progression. *Biochim Biophys Acta* 2001;2:M81–M88.
103. Duray A, Descamps G, Arafa M, et al. High incidence of high-risk HPV in benign and malignant lesions of the larynx. *Int J Oncol* 2011;39:51–59.
104. Dürst M, Croce CM, Gissmann L, et al. Papillomavirus sequences integrate near cellular oncogenes in some cervical carcinomas. *Proc Natl Acad Sci USA* 1987;84:1070–1074.
105. Dürst M, Gissmann L, Ikenberg H, et al. A papillomavirus DNA from a cervical carcinoma and its prevalence in cancer biopsy samples from different geographic regions. *Proc Natl Acad Sci USA* 1983;80:3812–3815.
106. Egawa N, Doorbar J. The low-risk papillomaviruses. *Virus Res* 2017;231:119–127.
107. Ehrig F, Hafner N, Driesch C, et al. Differences in stability of viral and viral-cellular fusion transcripts in HPV-induced cervical cancers. *Int J Mol Sci* 2019;21:112.
108. Fields JR, Saikaly SK, Schoch JJ. Intralesional immunotherapy for pediatric warts: a review. *Pediatr Dermatol* 2020;37:265–271.
109. Forslund O, Lindelof B, Hradil E, et al. High prevalence of cutaneous human papillomavirus DNA on the top of skin tumors but not in "Stripped" biopsies from the same tumors. *J Invest Dermatol* 2004;123:388–394.
110. Fortes HR, von Ranke FM, Escuissato DL, et al. Recurrent respiratory papillomatosis: a state-of-the-art review. *Respir Med* 2017;126:116–121.
111. Fradet-Turcotte A, Archambault J. Recent advances in the search for antiviral agents against human papillomaviruses. *Antivir Ther* 2007;12:431–451.
112. Frazer IH, Chandra J. Immunotherapy for HPV associated cancer. *Papillomavirus Res* 2019;8:100176.
113. Frisch M, Biggar RJ, Goedert JJ. Human papillomavirus-associated cancers in patients with human immunodeficiency virus infection and acquired immunodeficiency syndrome. *J Natl Cancer Inst* 2000;92:1500–1510.
114. Frisch M, Glimelius B, van den Brule AJ, et al. Sexually transmitted infection as a cause of anal cancer. *N Engl J Med* 1997;337:1350–1358.
115. Fuller C, Hudgins E, Finelt N. Human-papillomavirus-related disease in pediatrics. *Curr Opin Pediatr* 2018;30:169–174.
116. FUTURE II Study Group. Prophylactic efficacy of a quadrivalent human papillomavirus (HPV) vaccine in women with virological evidence of HPV infection. *J Infect Dis* 2007;196:1438–1446.
117. Gao G, Johnson SH, Kasperbauer JL, et al. Mate pair sequencing of oropharyngeal squamous cell carcinomas reveals that HPV integration occurs much less frequently than in cervical cancer. *J Clin Virol* 2014;59:195–200.
118. Gelder CM, Williams OM, Hart KW, et al. HLA class II polymorphisms and susceptibility to recurrent respiratory papillomatosis. *J Virol* 2003;77:1927–1939.
119. Gentles JC, Evans EG. Foot infections in swimming baths. *Br Med J* 1973;3:260–262.
120. Georgopoulos NT, Proffitt JL, Blair GE. Transcriptional regulation of the major histocompatibility complex (MHC) class I heavy chain, TAP1 and LMP2 genes by the human papillomavirus (HPV) type 6b, 16 and 18 E7 oncoproteins. *Oncogene* 2000;19:4930–4935.
121. Gerein V, Rastorguev E, Gerein J, et al. Incidence, age at onset, and potential reasons of malignant transformation in recurrent respiratory papillomatosis patients: 20 years experience. *Otolaryngol Head Neck Surg* 2005;132:392–394.
122. Gheit T. Mucosal and cutaneous human papillomavirus infections and cancer biology. *Front Oncol* 2019;9:355.
123. Gillison ML, Broutian T, Pickard RK, et al. Prevalence of oral HPV infection in the United States, 2009–2010. *JAMA* 2012;307:693–703.
124. Gillison ML, Chaturvedi AK, Anderson WF, et al. Epidemiology of human papillomavirus-positive head and neck squamous cell carcinoma. *J Clin Oncol* 2015;33:3235–3242.
125. Gillison ML, Shah KV. Chapter 9: Role of mucosal human papillomavirus in nongenital cancers. *J Natl Cancer Inst Monogr* 2003;57–65.
126. Giuliano AR, Lee JH, Fulp W, et al. Incidence and clearance of genital human papillomavirus infection in men (HIM): a cohort study. *Lancet* 2011;377:932–940.

127. Giuliano AR, Palefsky JM, Goldstone S, et al. Efficacy of quadrivalent HPV vaccine against HPV infection and disease in males. *N Engl J Med* 2011;364:401–411.
128. Godi A, Panwar K, Haque M, et al. Durability of the neutralizing antibody response to vaccine and non-vaccine HPV types 7 years following immunization with either Cervarix(R) or Gardasil(R) vaccine. *Vaccine* 2019;37:2455–2462.
129. Goldstone SE, Johnstone AA, Moshier EL. Long-term outcome of ablation of anal high-grade squamous intraepithelial lesions: recurrence and incidence of cancer. *Dis Colon Rectum* 2014;57:316–323.
130. Grabowski MK, Kong X, Gray RH, et al. Partner human papillomavirus viral load and incident human papillomavirus detection in heterosexual couples. *J Infect Dis* 2016;213:948–956.
131. Gravitt PE, Winer RL. Natural history of HPV infection across the lifespan: role of viral latency. *Viruses* 2017;9:267.
132. Gray RH, Serwadda D, Kong X, et al. Male circumcision decreases acquisition and increases clearance of high-risk human papillomavirus in HIV-negative men: a randomized trial in Rakai, Uganda. *J Infect Dis*. 2010;201:1455–1462.
133. Greer CE, Wheeeler CM, Lander MB, et al. Human papillomavirus (HPV) type distribution and serological response to HPV 6 virus-like particle in patients with genital warts. *J Clin Microb* 1995;33:2058–2063.
134. Gross G, Hagedorn M, Ikenberg H, et al. Bowenoid papulosis. Presence of human papillomavirus (HPV) structural antigens and of HPV 16-related DNA sequences. *Arch Dermatol* 1985;121:858–863.
135. Gruener M, Bravo IG, Momburg F, et al. The E5 protein of the human papillomavirus type 16 down-regulates HLA-I surface expression in calnexin-expressing but not in calnexin-deficient cells. *Virol J* 2007;4:116.
136. Grulich AE, Vajdic CM. The epidemiology of cancers in human immunodeficiency virus infection and after organ transplantation. *Semin Oncol* 2015;42:247–257.
137. Grussendorf-Conen EI. Anogenital premalignant and malignant tumors (including Buschke-Lowenstein tumors). *Clin Dermatol* 1997;15:377–388.
138. Gutierrez-Xicotencatl L, Salazar-Pina DA, Pedroza-Saavedra A, et al. Humoral immune response against human papillomavirus as source of biomarkers for the prediction and detection of cervical cancer. *Viral Immunol* 2016;29:83–94.
139. Hagensee ME, Yaegashi N, Galloway DA. Self-assembly of human papillomavirus type 1 capsids by expression of the L1 protein alone or by coexpression of the L1 and L2 capsid proteins. *J Virol* 1993;67:315–322.
140. Hammes LS, Tekmal RR, Naud P, et al. Macrophages, inflammation and risk of cervical intraepithelial neoplasia (CIN) progression—clinicopathological correlation. *Gynecol Oncol* 2007;105:157–165.
141. Handisurya A, Rieger A, Bankier A, et al. Human papillomavirus type 26 infection causing multiple invasive squamous cell carcinomas of the fingernails in an AIDS patient under highly active antiretroviral therapy. *Br J Dermatol* 2007;157:788–794.
142. Hariri S, Unger ER, Sternberg M, et al. Prevalence of genital human papillomavirus among females in the United States, the National Health and Nutrition Examination Survey, 2003–2006. *J Infect Dis* 2011;204:566–573.
143. Hasan UA, Zannetti C, Parroche P, et al. The human papillomavirus type 16 E7 oncoprotein induces a transcriptional repressor complex on the Toll-like receptor 9 promoter. *J Exp Med* 2013;210:1369–1387.
144. Hasche D, Stephan S, Braspenning-Wesch I, et al. The interplay of UV and cutaneous papillomavirus infection in skin cancer development. *PLoS Pathog* 2017;13:e1006723.
145. Hawkes D, Keung MHT, Huang Y, et al. Self-collection for cervical screening programs: from research to reality. *Cancers (Basel)* 2020;12:1053.
146. Healy GB, Gelber RD, Trowbridge AL, et al. Treatment of recurrent respiratory papillomatosis with human leukocyte interferon. Results of a multicenter randomized clinical trial. *N Engl J Med* 1988;319:401–407.
147. Heck JE, Berthiller J, Vaccarella S, et al. Sexual behaviours and the risk of head and neck cancers: a pooled analysis in the International Head and Neck Cancer Epidemiology (INHANCE) consortium. *Int J Epidemiol* 2010;39:166–181.
148. Herfs M, Soong TR, Delvenne P, et al. Deciphering the multifactorial susceptibility of mucosal junction cells to HPV infection and related carcinogenesis. *Viruses* 2017;9:85.
149. Herfs M, Yamamoto Y, Laury A, et al. A discrete population of squamocolumnar junction cells implicated in the pathogenesis of cervical cancer. *Proc Natl Acad Sci U S A* 2012;109:10516–10521.
150. Herrero R, Wacholder S, Rodriguez AC, et al. Prevention of persistent human papillomavirus infection by an HPV16/18 vaccine: a community-based randomized clinical trial in Guanacaste, Costa Rica. *Cancer Discov* 2011;1:408–419.
151. Hildesheim A, Herrero R, Wacholder S, et al. Effect of human papillomavirus 16/18 L1 viruslike particle vaccine among young women with preexisting infection: a randomized trial. *JAMA* 2007;298:743–753.
152. Ho GY, Bierman R, Beardsley L, et al. Natural history of cervicovaginal papillomavirus infection in young women. *N Engl J Med* 1998;338:423–428.
153. Holzinger D, Wichmann G, Baboci L, et al. Sensitivity and specificity of antibodies against HPV16 E6 and other early proteins for the detection of HPV16-driven oropharyngeal squamous cell carcinoma. *Int J Cancer* 2017;140:2748–2757.
154. Houlihan CF, Larke NL, Watson-Jones D, et al. Human papillomavirus infection and increased risk of HIV acquisition. A systematic review and meta-analysis. *AIDS* 2012;26:2211–2222.
155. Howley PM, Pfister HJ. Beta genus papillomaviruses and skin cancer. *Virology* 2015;479–480:290–296.
156. Hu L, Bell D, Antani S, et al. An observational study of deep learning and automated evaluation of cervical images for cancer screening. *J Natl Cancer Inst* 2019;111:923–932.
157. Huang S, Wu JH, Lewis DJ, et al. A novel approach to the classification of epidermodysplasia verruciformis. *Int J Dermatol* 2018;57:1344–1350.
158. Huang SM, McCance DJ. Down regulation of the interleukin-8 promoter by human papillomavirus type 16 E6 and E7 through effects on CREB binding protein/p300 and P/CAF. *J Virol* 2002;76:8710–8721.
159. Hubert P, Caberg JH, Gilles C, et al. E-cadherin-dependent adhesion of dendritic and Langerhans cells to keratinocytes is defective in cervical human papillomavirus-associated (pre)neoplastic lesions. *J Pathol* 2005;206:346–355.
160. Huh WK, Ault KA, Chelmow D, et al. Use of primary high-risk human papillomavirus testing for cervical cancer screening: interim clinical guidance. *Gynecol Oncol* 2015;136:178–182.
161. Hussain SK, Sundquist J, Hemminki K. Familial clustering of cancer at human papillomavirus-associated sites according to the Swedish Family-Cancer Database. *Int J Cancer* 2008;122:1873–1878.
162. International Collaboration of Epidemiological Studies of Cervical Cancer; Appleby P, Beral V, Berrington de Gonzalez A, et al. Carcinoma of the cervix and tobacco smoking: collaborative reanalysis of individual data on 13,541 women with carcinoma of the cervix and 23,017 women without carcinoma of the cervix from 23 epidemiological studies. *Int J Cancer* 2006;118:1481–1495.
163. International Collaboration of Epidemiological Studies of Cervical Cancer; Appleby P, Beral V, Berrington de Gonzalez A, et al. Cervical cancer and hormonal contraceptives: collaborative reanalysis of individual data for 16,573 women with cervical cancer and 35,509 women without cervical cancer from 24 epidemiological studies. *Lancet* 2007;370:1609–1621.
164. Iwasaki A. Antiviral immune responses in the genital tract: clues for vaccines. *Nat Rev Immunol* 2010;10:699–711.
165. Jaafar F, Righi E, Lindstrom V, et al. Correlation of CXCL12 expression and FoxP3+ cell infiltration with human papillomavirus infection and clinicopathological progression of cervical cancer. *Am J Pathol* 2009;175:1525–1535.
166. Jacobelli S, Laude H, Carlotti A, et al. Epidermodysplasia verruciformis in human immunodeficiency virus-infected patients: a marker of human papillomavirus-related disorders not affected by antiretroviral therapy. *Arch Dermatol* 2011;147:590–596.
167. Jayasinghe Y, Garland SM. Genital warts in children: what do they mean? *Arch Dis Child* 2006;91:696–700.
168. Jordan RC, Lingen MW, Perez-Ordonez B, et al. Validation of methods for oropharyngeal cancer HPV status determination in US cooperative group trials. *Am J Surg Pathol* 2012;36:945–954.
169. Joseph DA, Miller JW, Wu X, et al. Understanding the burden of human papillomavirus-associated anal cancers in the US. *Cancer* 2008;113:2892–2900.
170. Joura EA, Giuliano AR, Iversen OE, et al. A 9-valent HPV vaccine against infection and intraepithelial neoplasia in women. *N Engl J Med* 2015;372:711–723.
171. Kalinska-Bienias A, Kowalewski C, Majewski S. The EVER genes—the genetic etiology of carcinogenesis in epidermodysplasia verruciformis and a possible role in non-epidermodysplasia verruciformis patients. *Postepy Dermatol Alergol* 2016;33:75–80.
172. Karim R, Tummers B, Meyers C, et al. Human papillomavirus (HPV) upregulates the cellular deubiquitinase UCHL1 to suppress the keratinocyte's innate immune response. *PLoS Pathog* 2013;9:e1003384.
173. Katki HA, Wentzensen N. How might HPV testing be integrated into cervical screening? *Lancet Oncol* 2012;13:8–10.
174. Kelly H, Weiss HA, Benavente Y, et al.; ART and HPV Review Group. Association of antiretroviral therapy with high-risk human papillomavirus, cervical intraepithelial neoplasia, and invasive cervical cancer in women living with HIV: a systematic review and meta-analysis. *Lancet HIV* 2018;5:e45–e58.
175. Kemp TJ, Hildesheim A, Safaeian M, et al. HPV16/18 L1 VLP vaccine induces cross-neutralizing antibodies that may mediate cross-protection. *Vaccine* 2011;29:2011–2014.
176. Kennedy EM, Kornepati AV, Goldstein M, et al. Inactivation of the human papillomavirus E6 or E7 gene in cervical carcinoma cells by using a bacterial CRISPR/Cas RNA-guided endonuclease. *J Virol* 2014;88:11965–11972.
177. Khoury R, Sauter S, Butsch Kovacic M, et al. Risk of human papillomavirus infection in cancer-prone individuals: what we know. *Viruses* 2018;10:47.
178. Kim JJ, Burger EA, Sy S, et al. Optimal cervical cancer screening in women vaccinated against human papillomavirus. *J Natl Cancer Inst* 2017;109.
179. Kines RC, Cerio RJ, Roberts JN, et al. Human papillomavirus capsids preferentially bind and infect tumor cells. *Int J Cancer* 2016;138:901–911.
180. Kirnbauer R, Chandrachud L, O'Neil B, et al. Virus-like particles of bovine papillomavirus type 4 in prophylactic and therapeutic immunization. *Virology* 1996;219:37–44.
181. Kirnbauer R, Taub J, Greenstone H, et al. Efficient self-assembly of human papillomavirus type 16 L1 and L1-L2 into virus-like particles. *J Virol* 1993;67:6929–6936.
182. Kjaer SK, Frederiksen K, Munk C, et al. Long-term absolute risk of cervical intraepithelial neoplasia grade 3 or worse following human papillomavirus infection: role of persistence. *J Natl Cancer Inst* 2010;102:1478–1488.
183. Kjaer SK, Sigurdsson K, Iversen OE, et al. A pooled analysis of continued prophylactic efficacy of quadrivalent human papillomavirus (Types 6/11/16/18) vaccine against high-grade cervical and external genital lesions. *Cancer Prev Res (Phila)* 2009;2:868–878.
184. Klaes R, Woerner SM, Ridder R, et al. Detection of high-risk cervical intraepithelial neoplasia and cervical cancer by amplification of transcripts derived from integrated papillomavirus oncogenes. *Cancer Res* 1999;59:6132–6136.
185. Korzeniewski N, Spardy N, Duensing A, et al. Genomic instability and cancer: lessons learned from human papillomaviruses. *Cancer Lett* 2011;305:113–122.
186. Koutsky LA, Holmes KK, Critchlow CW, et al. A cohort study of the risk of cervical intraepithelial neoplasia grade 2 or 3 in relation to papillomavirus infection. *N Engl J Med* 1992;327:1272–1278.
187. Krajden M, Cook D, Yu A, et al. Human papillomavirus 16 (HPV 16) and HPV 18 antibody responses measured by pseudovirus neutralization and competitive Luminex assays in a two- versus three-dose HPV vaccine trial. *Clin Vaccine Immunol* 2011;18:418–423.
188. Kreimer AR, Bhatia RK, Messeguer AL, et al. Oral human papillomavirus in healthy individuals: a systematic review of the literature. *Sex Transm Dis* 2010;37:386–391.
189. Kreimer AR, Clifford GM, Boyle P, et al. Human papillomavirus types in head and neck squamous cell carcinomas worldwide: a systematic review. *Cancer Epidemiol Biomarkers Prev* 2005;14:467–475.
190. Kreimer AR, Ferreiro-Iglesias A, Nygard M, et al. Timing of HPV16-E6 antibody seroconversion before OPSCC: findings from the HPVC3 consortium. *Ann Oncol* 2019;30:1335–1343.
191. Kreimer AR, Gonzalez P, Katki HA, et al. Efficacy of a bivalent HPV 16/18 vaccine against anal HPV 16/18 infection among young women: a nested analysis within the Costa Rica Vaccine Trial. *Lancet Oncol* 2011;12:862–870.

192. Kreimer AR, Johansson M, Waterboer T, et al. Evaluation of human papillomavirus antibodies and risk of subsequent head and neck cancer. *J Clin Oncol* 2013;31:2708–2715.
193. Kreimer AR, Sampson JN, Porras C, et al. Evaluation of durability of a single-dose of the bivalent HPV vaccine: the CVT Trial. *J Natl Cancer Inst* 2020;112:1038–1046.
194. Kreimer AR, Shiels MS, Fakhry C, et al. Screening for human papillomavirus-driven oropharyngeal cancer: considerations for feasibility and strategies for research. *Cancer* 2018;124:1859–1866.
195. Kumar N, Preciado D. Airway papillomatosis: new treatments for an old challenge. *Front Pediatr* 2019;7:383.
196. Kurman RJ, Henson DE, Herbst AL, et al. Interim guidelines for management of abnormal cervical cytology. The 1992 National Cancer Institute Workshop. *JAMA* 1994;271:1866–1869.
197. Kuwabara AM, Rainer BM, Basdag H, et al. Children with warts: a retrospective study in an outpatient setting. *Pediatr Dermatol* 2015;32:679–683.
198. Kyrgiou M, Mitra A, Moscicki AB. Does the vaginal microbiota play a role in the development of cervical cancer? *Transl Res* 2017;179:168–182.
199. Lang Kuhs KA, Pawlita M, Gibson SP, et al. Characterization of human papillomavirus antibodies in individuals with head and neck cancer. *Cancer Epidemiol* 2016;42:46–52.
200. Larson DA, Derkay CS. Epidemiology of recurrent respiratory papillomatosis. *APMIS* 2010;118:450–454.
201. Lau L, Gray EE, Brunette RL, et al. DNA tumor virus oncogenes antagonize the cGAS-STING DNA-sensing pathway. *Science* 2015;350:568–571.
202. Laurie C, El-Zein M, Tota J, et al.; LIMIT-HPV Study Group. Lubricant Investigation in Men to Inhibit Transmission of HPV Infection (LIMIT-HPV): design and methods for a randomised controlled trial. *BMJ Open* 2020;10:e035113.
203. Laurson J, Khan S, Chung R, et al. Epigenetic repression of E-cadherin by human papillomavirus 16 E7 protein. *Carcinogenesis* 2010;31:918–926.
204. Lehtinen M, Dillner J, Knekt P, et al. Serologically diagnosed infection with human papillomavirus type 16 and risk for subsequent development of cervical carcinoma: nested case–control study. *BMJ* 1996;312:537–539.
205. Lehtinen M, Paavonen J, Wheeler CM, et al. Overall efficacy of HPV-16/18 AS04-adjuvanted vaccine against grade 3 or greater cervical intraepithelial neoplasia: 4-year end-of-study analysis of the randomised, double-blind PATRICIA trial. *Lancet Oncol* 2012;13:89–99.
206. Lei J, Ploner A, Elfstrom KM, et al. HPV vaccination and the risk of invasive cervical cancer. *N Engl J Med* 2020;383:1340–1348.
207. Leong CM, Doorbar J, Nindl I, et al. Loss of epidermal Langerhans cells occurs in human papillomavirus alpha, gamma, and mu but not beta genus infections. *J Invest Dermatol* 2010;130:472–480.
208. Li H, Ou X, Xiong J, et al. HPV16E7 mediates HADC chromatin repression and down-regulation of MHC class I genes in HPV16 tumorigenic cells through interaction with an MHC class I promoter. *Biochem Biophys Res Commun* 2006;349:1315–1321.
209. Li S, Labrecque S, Gauzzi MC, et al. The human papilloma virus (HPV)-18 E6 oncoprotein physically associates with Tyk2 and impairs Jak-STAT activation by interferon-alpha. *Oncogene* 1999;18:5727–5737.
210. Liaw KL, Glass AG, Manos MM, et al. Detection of human papillomavirus DNA in cytologically normal women and subsequent cervical squamous intraepithelial lesions. *J Natl Cancer Inst* 1999;91:954–960.
211. Liaw KL, Hildesheim A, Burk RD, et al. A prospective study of human papillomavirus (HPV) type 16 DNA detection by polymerase chain reaction and its association with acquisition and persistence of other HPV types. *J Infect Dis* 2001;183:8–15.
212. Lissouba P, Van de Perre P, Auvert B. Association of genital human papillomavirus infection with HIV acquisition: a systematic review and meta-analysis. *Sex Transm Infect* 2013;89:350–356.
213. Lorincz AT, Brentnall AR, Scibior-Bentkowska D, et al. Validation of a DNA methylation HPV triage classifier in a screening sample. *Int J Cancer* 2016;138:2745–2751.
214. Lowy DR, Schiller JT. Prophylactic human papillomavirus vaccines. *J Clin Invest* 2006;116:1167–1173.
215. Lu B, Viscidi RP, Wu Y, et al. Prevalent serum antibody is not a marker of immune protection against acquisition of oncogenic HPV16 in men. *Cancer Res* 2012;72:676–685.
216. Luo X, Donnelly CR, Gong W, et al. HPV16 drives cancer immune escape via NLRX1-mediated degradation of STING. *J Clin Invest* 2020;130:1635–1652.
217. Ma W, Melief CJ, van der Burg SH. Control of immune escaped human papilloma virus is regained after therapeutic vaccination. *Curr Opin Virol* 2017;23:16–22.
218. Machalek DA, Garland SM, Brotherton JML, et al. Very low prevalence of vaccine human papillomavirus types among 18- to 35-year old Australian women 9 years following implementation of vaccination. *J Infect Dis* 2018;217:1590–1600.
219. Majewski S, Jablonska S, Orth G. Epidermodysplasia verruciformis. Immunological and nonimmunological surveillance mechanisms: role in tumor progression. *Clin Dermatol* 1997;15:321–334.
220. Malagon T, Drolet M, Boily MC, et al. Cross-protective efficacy of two human papillomavirus vaccines: a systematic review and meta-analysis. *Lancet Infect Dis* 2012;12:781–789.
221. Manhart LE, Koutsky LA. Do condoms prevent genital HPV infection, external genital warts, or cervical neoplasia? A meta-analysis. *Sex Transm Dis* 2002;29:725–735.
222. Marais D, Gawarecki D, Allan B, et al. The effectiveness of Carraguard, a vaginal microbicide, in protecting women against high-risk human papillomavirus infection. *Antivir Ther* 2011;16:1219–1226.
223. Maran A, Amella CA, Di Lorenzo TP, et al. Human papillomavirus type 11 transcripts are present at low abundance in latently infected respiratory tissues. *Virology* 1995;212:285–294.
224. Marcuzzi GP, Hufbauer M, Kasper HU, et al. Spontaneous tumour development in human papillomavirus type 8 E6 transgenic mice and rapid induction by UV-light exposure and wounding. *J Gen Virol* 2009;90:2855–2864.
225. Markowitz LE, Naleway AL, Lewis RM, et al. Declines in HPV vaccine type prevalence in women screened for cervical cancer in the United States: evidence of direct and herd effects of vaccination. *Vaccine* 2019;37:3918–3924.
226. Martin-Hirsch PL, Wood NJ. Cervical cancer. *BMJ Clin Evid* 2011;2011:0818.
227. Massad LS, Seaberg EC, Wright RL, et al. Squamous cervical lesions in women with human immunodeficiency virus: long-term follow-up. *Obstet Gynecol* 2008;111:1388–1393.
228. Massad LS, Xie X, Burk R, et al. Long-term cumulative detection of human papillomavirus among HIV seropositive women. *AIDS* 2014;28:2601–2608.
229. McBride AA, Warburton A. The role of integration in oncogenic progression of HPV-associated cancers. *PLoS Pathog* 2017;13:e1006211.
230. McMurray JS, Connor N, Ford CN. Cidofovir efficacy in recurrent respiratory papillomatosis: a randomized, double-blind, placebo-controlled study. *Ann Otol Rhinol Laryngol* 2008;117:477–483.
231. Meisels A, Fortin R. Condylomatous lesions of the cervix and vagina. I. Cytologic patterns. *Acta Cytol* 1976;20:505–509.
232. Melsheimer P, Vinokurova S, Wentzensen N, et al. DNA aneuploidy and integration of human papillomavirus type 16 e6/e7 oncogenes in intraepithelial neoplasia and invasive squamous cell carcinoma of the cervix uteri. *Clin Cancer Res* 2004;10:3059–3063.
233. Merckx M, Liesbeth WV, Arbyn M, et al. Transmission of carcinogenic human papillomavirus types from mother to child: a meta-analysis of published studies. *Eur J Cancer Prev* 2013;22:277–285.
234. Minhas S, Manseck A, Watya S, et al. Penile cancer—prevention and premalignant conditions. *Urology* 2010;76:S24–S35.
235. Mirabello L, Yeager M, Cullen M, et al. HPV16 sublineage associations with histology-specific cancer risk using HPV whole-genome sequences in 3200 women. *J Natl Cancer Inst* 2016;108:djw100.
236. Mitra A, MacIntyre DA, Lee YS, et al. Cervical intraepithelial neoplasia disease progression is associated with increased vaginal microbiome diversity. *Sci Rep* 2015;5:16865.
237. Miura S, Kawana K, Schust DJ, et al. CD1d, a sentinel molecule bridging innate and adaptive immunity, is downregulated by the human papillomavirus (HPV) E5 protein: a possible mechanism for immune evasion by HPV. *J Virol* 2010;84:11614–11623.
238. Moody CA, Laimins LA. Human papillomavirus oncoproteins: pathways to transformation. *Nat Rev Cancer* 2010;10:550–560.
239. Morgan IM, DiNardo LJ, Windle B. Integration of human papillomavirus genomes in head and neck cancer: is it time to consider a paradigm shift? *Viruses* 2017;9:208.
240. Moscicki AB, Schiffman M, Burchell A, et al. Updating the natural history of human papillomavirus and anogenital cancers. *Vaccine* 2012;30(Suppl 5):F24–F33.
241. Mullegger RR, Haring NS, Glatz M. Skin infections in pregnancy. *Clin Dermatol* 2016;34:368–377.
242. Munger K. The role of human papillomaviruses in human cancers. *Front Biosci* 2002;7:d641–d649.
243. Myers DJ, Fillman EP. Epidermodysplasia verruciformis. In: *StatPearls*. Treasure Island, FL; 2019.
244. Myers KO, Ahmed NU. The role of HIV in the progression through the stages of the human papillomavirus to cervical cancer pathway. *AIDS Rev* 2018;20:94–1043.
245. Nakagawa M, Stites DP, Palefsky JM, et al. CD4-positive and CD8-positive cytotoxic T lymphocytes contribute to human papillomavirus type 16 E6 and E7 responses. *Clin Diagn Lab Immunol* 1999;6:494–498.
246. Nakagawa M, Stites DP, Patel S, et al. Persistence of human papillomavirus type 16 infection is associated with lack of cytotoxic T lymphocyte response to the E6 antigens. *J Infect Dis* 2000;182:595–598.
247. Nardelli-Haefliger D, Wirthner D, Schiller JT, et al. Specific antibody levels at the cervix during the menstrual cycle of women vaccinated with human papillomavirus 16 virus-like particles. *J Natl Cancer Inst* 2003;95:1128–1137.
248. Nees M, Geoghegan JM, Hyman T, et al. Papillomavirus type 16 oncogenes downregulate expression of interferon-responsive genes and upregulate proliferation-associated and NF-kappaB-responsive genes in cervical keratinocytes. *J Virol* 2001;75:4283–4296.
249. Niebler M, Qian X, Hofler D, et al. Post-translational control of IL-1beta via the human papillomavirus type 16 E6 oncoprotein: a novel mechanism of innate immune escape mediated by the E3-ubiquitin ligase E6-AP and p53. *PLoS Pathog* 2013;9:e1003536.
250. Nielson CM, Harris RB, Nyitray AG, et al. Consistent condom use is associated with lower prevalence of human papillomavirus infection in men. *J Infect Dis* 2010;202:445–451.
251. Nonnenmacher B, Kruger Kjaer S, Svare E, et al. Seroreactivity to HPV16 virus-like particles as a marker for cervical cancer risk in high risk populations. *Int J Cancer* 1996;68:704–709.
252. Nooij LS, Ter Haar NT, Ruano D, et al. Genomic characterization of vulvar (pre)cancers identifies distinct molecular subtypes with prognostic significance. *Clin Cancer Res* 2017;23:6781–6789.
253. Novakovic D, Cheng ATL, Zurynski Y, et al. A prospective study of the incidence of juvenile-onset recurrent respiratory papillomatosis after implementation of a National HPV Vaccination Program. *J Infect Dis* 2018;217:208–212.
254. Obiri-Yeboah D, Akakpo PK, Mutocheluh M, et al. Epidemiology of cervical human papillomavirus (HPV) infection and squamous intraepithelial lesions (SIL) among a cohort of HIV-infected and uninfected Ghanaian women. *BMC Cancer* 2017;17:688.
255. Olthof NC, Speel EJ, Kolligs J, et al. Comprehensive analysis of HPV16 integration in OSCC reveals no significant impact of physical status on viral oncogene and virally disrupted human gene expression. *PLoS One* 2014;9:e88718.
256. Orth G. Host defenses against human papillomaviruses: lessons from epidermodysplasia verruciformis. *Curr Top Microbiol Immunol* 2008;321:59–83.
257. Orth G, Jablonska S, Favre M, et al. Characterization of two types of human papillomaviruses in lesions of epidermodysplasia verruciformis. *Proc Natl Acad Sci USA* 1978;75:1537–1541.
258. Ortiz AP, Romaguera J, Perez CM, et al. Prevalence, genotyping, and correlates of anogenital HPV infection in a population-based sample of women in Puerto Rico. *Papillomavirus Res* 2016;2:89–96.
259. Ovestad IT, Gudlaugsson E, Skaland I, et al. Local immune response in the microenvironment of CIN2-3 with and without spontaneous regression. *Mod Pathol* 2010;23:1231–1240.
260. Paaso A, Jaakola A, Syrjanen S, et al. From HPV infection to lesion progression: the role of HLA alleles and host immunity. *Acta Cytol* 2019;63:148–158.
261. Padlewska K, Ramoz N, Cassonnet P, et al. Mutation and abnormal expression of the p53 gene in the viral skin carcinogenesis of epidermodysplasia verruciformis. *J Invest Dermatol* 2001;117:935–942.

262. Pal A, Kundu R. Human papillomavirus E6 and E7: the cervical cancer hallmarks and targets for therapy. *Front Microbiol* 2019;10:3116.
263. Palefsky JM. Screening to prevent anal cancer: current thinking and future directions. *Cancer Cytopathol* 2015;123:509–510.
264. Palefsky JM, Giuliano AR, Goldstone S, et al. HPV vaccine against anal HPV infection and anal intraepithelial neoplasia. *N Engl J Med* 2011;365:1576–1585.
265. Palmer T, Wallace L, Pollock KG, et al. Prevalence of cervical disease at age 20 after immunisation with bivalent HPV vaccine at age 12–13 in Scotland: retrospective population study. *BMJ* 2019;365:l1161.
266. Park JS, Kim EJ, Kwon HJ, et al. Inactivation of interferon regulatory factor-1 tumor suppressor protein by HPV E7 oncoprotein. Implication for the E7-mediated immune evasion mechanism in cervical carcinogenesis. *J Biol Chem* 2000;275:6764–6769.
267. Partridge JM, Koutsky LA. Genital human papillomavirus infection in men. *Lancet Infect Dis* 2006;6:21–31.
268. Pastrana DV, Buck CB, Pang YY, et al. Reactivity of human sera in a sensitive, high-throughput pseudovirus-based papillomavirus neutralization assay for HPV16 and HPV18. *Virology* 2004;321:205–216.
269. Patel D, Huang SM, Baglia LA, et al. The E6 protein of human papillomavirus type 16 binds to and inhibits co-activation by CBP and p300. *EMBO J* 1999;18:5061–5072.
270. Patel H, Wagner M, Singhal P, et al. Systematic review of the incidence and prevalence of genital warts. *BMC Infect Dis* 2013;13:39.
271. Pedersen C, Petaja T, Strauss G, et al. Immunization of early adolescent females with human papillomavirus type 16 and 18 L1 virus-like particle vaccine containing AS04 adjuvant. *J Adolesc Health* 2007;40:564–571.
272. Pennycook KB, McCready TA. Condyloma acuminata. In: *StatPearls*. Treasure Island, FL; 2020.
273. Pereira de Oliveira WR, Carrasco S, Neto CF, et al. Nonspecific cell-mediated immunity in patients with epidermodysplasia verruciformis. *J Dermatol* 2003;30:203–209.
274. Perino A, Consiglio P, Maranto M, et al. Impact of a new carrageenan-based vaginal microbicide in a female population with genital HPV-infection: first experimental results. *Eur Rev Med Pharmacol Sci* 2019;23:6744–6752.
275. Periyasamy M, Singh AK, Gemma C, et al. p53 controls expression of the DNA deaminase APOBEC3B to limit its potential mutagenic activity in cancer cells. *Nucleic Acids Res* 2017;45:11056–11069.
276. Perkins RB, Guido RS, Castle PE, et al. 2019 ASCCP risk-based management consensus guidelines for abnormal cervical cancer screening tests and cancer precursors. *J Low Genit Tract Dis* 2020;24:102–131.
277. Phillips A, Patel C, Pillsbury A, et al. Safety of human papillomavirus vaccines: an updated review. *Drug Saf* 2018;41:329–346.
278. Pickard RK, Xiao W, Broutian TR, et al. The prevalence and incidence of oral human papillomavirus infection among young men and women, aged 18–30 years. *Sex Transm Dis* 2012;39:559–566.
279. Pinheiro M, Gage JC, Clifford GM, et al. Association of HPV35 with cervical carcinogenesis among women of African ancestry: evidence of viral-host interaction with implications for disease intervention. *Int J Cancer* 2020;147:2677–2686.
280. Plotkin SA. Correlates of protection induced by vaccination. *Clin Vaccine Immunol* 2010;17:1055–1065.
281. Plunkett A, Merlin K, Gill D, et al. The frequency of common nonmalignant skin conditions in adults in central Victoria, Australia. *Int J Dermatol* 1999;38:901–908.
282. Premoli-De-Percoco G, Cisternas JP, Ramirez JL, et al. Focal epithelial hyperplasia: human-papillomavirus-induced disease with a genetic predisposition in a Venezuelan family. *Hum Genet* 1993;91:386–388.
283. Przybyszewska J, Zlotogorski A, Ramot, Y. Re-evaluation of epidermodysplasia verruciformis: reconciling more than 90 years of debate. *J Am Acad Dermatol* 2017;76:1161–1175.
284. Qiao YL, Jeronimo J, Zhao FH, et al. Lower cost strategies for triage of human papillomavirus DNA-positive women. *Int J Cancer* 2014;134:2891–2901.
285. Qiao YL, Wu T, Li RC, et al. Efficacy, safety, and immunogenicity of an *Escherichia coli*-produced bivalent human papillomavirus vaccine: an interim analysis of a randomized clinical trial. *J Natl Cancer Inst* 2020;112:145–153.
286. Reusser NM, Downing C, Guidry J, et al. HPV carcinomas in immunocompromised patients. *J Clin Med* 2015;4:260–281.
287. Rijkaart DC, Berkhof J, van Kemenade FJ, et al. HPV DNA testing in population-based cervical screening (VUSA-Screen study): results and implications. *Br J Cancer* 2012;106:975–981.
288. Rintala M, Grenman S, Puranen M, et al. Natural history of oral papillomavirus infections in spouses: a prospective Finnish HPV Family Study. *J Clin Virol* 2006;35:89–94.
289. Robbins HA, Li Y, Porras C, et al. Glutathione S-transferase L1 multiplex serology as a measure of cumulative infection with human papillomavirus. *BMC Infect Dis* 2014;14:120.
290. Roberts JN, Buck CB, Thompson CD, et al. Genital transmission of HPV in a mouse model is potentiated by nonoxynol-9 and inhibited by carrageenan. *Nat Med* 2007;13:857–861.
291. Roberts JN, Kines RC, Katki HA, et al. Effect of Pap smear collection and carrageenan on cervicovaginal human papillomavirus-16 infection in a rhesus macaque model. *J Natl Cancer Inst* 2011;103:737–743.
292. Rogstad KE, Wilkinson D, Robinson A. Sexually transmitted infections in children as a marker of child sexual abuse and direction of future research. *Curr Opin Infect Dis* 2016;29:41–44.
293. Rollison DE, Viarisio D, Amorrortu RP, et al. An emerging issue in oncogenic virology: the role of beta human papillomavirus types in the development of cutaneous squamous cell carcinoma. *J Virol* 2019;93:e01003-e01018.
294. Romanowski B, Schwarz TF, Ferguson LM, et al. Immunogenicity and safety of the HPV-16/18 AS04-adjuvanted vaccine administered as a 2-dose schedule compared to the licensed 3-dose schedule: results from a randomized study. *Hum Vaccin* 2011;7:1374–1386.
295. Ronco G, Giorgi-Rossi P, Carozzi F, et al. Efficacy of human papillomavirus testing for the detection of invasive cervical cancers and cervical intraepithelial neoplasia: a randomised controlled trial. *Lancet Oncol* 2010;11:249–257.
296. Ronco LV, Karpova AY, Vidal M, et al. Human papillomavirus 16 E6 oncoprotein binds to interferon regulatory factor-3 and inhibits its transcriptional activity. *Genes Dev* 1998;12:2061–2072.
297. Rose RC, Bonnez W, Reichman RC, et al. Expression of human papillomavirus type 11 L1 protein in insect cells: in vivo and in vitro assembly of viruslike particles. *J Virol* 1993;67:1936–1944.
298. Ryndock EJ, Meyers C. A risk for non-sexual transmission of human papillomavirus? *Expert Rev Anti Infect Ther* 2014;12:1165–1170.
299. Safaeian M, Castellsague X, Hildesheim A, et al.; Costa Rica HPV Vaccine Trial and the PATRICIA study groups. Risk of HPV-16/18 infections and associated cervical abnormalities in women seropositive for naturally acquired antibodies: pooled analysis based on control arms of two large clinical trials. *J Infect Dis* 2018;218:84–94.
300. Safaeian M, Porras C, Schiffman M, et al. Epidemiological study of anti-HPV16/18 seropositivity and subsequent risk of HPV16 and −18 infections. *J Natl Cancer Inst* 2010;102:1653–1662.
301. Safaeian M, Solomon D, Castle PE. Cervical cancer prevention–cervical screening: science in evolution. *Obstet Gynecol Clin North Am* 2007;34:739–760, ix.
302. Said AK, Leao JC, Fedele S, et al. Focal epithelial hyperplasia—an update. *J Oral Pathol Med* 2013;42:435–442.
303. Sampson JN, Hildesheim A, Herrero R, et al. Design and statistical considerations for studies evaluating the efficacy of a single dose of the human papillomavirus (HPV) vaccine. *Contemp Clin Trials* 2018;68:35–44.
304. Sand FL, Munk C, Frederiksen K, et al. Risk of CIN3 or worse with persistence of 13 individual oncogenic HPV types. *Int J Cancer* 2019;144:1975–1982.
305. Sankaranarayanan R, Nene BM, Shastri SS, et al. HPV screening for cervical cancer in rural India. *N Engl J Med* 2009;360:1385–1394.
306. Sauvaget C, Fayette JM, Muwonge R, et al. Accuracy of visual inspection with acetic acid for cervical cancer screening. *Int J Gynaecol Obstet* 2011;113:14–24.
307. Schiffman M, Castle PE, Jeronimo J, et al. Human papillomavirus and cervical cancer. *Lancet* 2007;370:890–907.
308. Schiffman M, Glass AG, Wentzensen N, et al. A long-term prospective study of type-specific human papillomavirus infection and risk of cervical neoplasia among 20,000 women in the Portland Kaiser Cohort Study. *Cancer Epidemiol Biomarkers Prev* 2011;20:1398–1409.
309. Schiffman M, Herrero R, Desalle R, et al. The carcinogenicity of human papillomavirus types reflects viral evolution. *Virology* 2005;337:76–84.
310. Schiffman M, Kjaer SK. Chapter 2: Natural history of anogenital human papillomavirus infection and neoplasia. *J Natl Cancer Inst Monogr* 2003;14–19.
311. Schiffman M, Rodriguez AC, Chen Z, et al. A population-based prospective study of carcinogenic human papillomavirus variant lineages, viral persistence, and cervical neoplasia. *Cancer Res* 2010;70:3159–3169.
312. Schiffman M, Wentzensen N. Human papillomavirus infection and the multistage carcinogenesis of cervical cancer. *Cancer Epidemiol Biomarkers Prev* 2013;22:553–560.
313. Schiffman M, Wentzensen N, Wacholder S, et al. Human papillomavirus testing in the prevention of cervical cancer. *J Natl Cancer Inst* 2011;103:368–383.
314. Schiller J, Lowy D. Explanations for the high potency of HPV prophylactic vaccines. *Vaccine* 2018;36:4768–4773.
315. Schiller JT, Buck CB. Cutaneous squamous cell carcinoma: a smoking gun but still no suspects. *J Invest Dermatol* 2011;131:1595–1596.
316. Schiller JT, Day PM, Kines RC. Current understanding of the mechanism of HPV infection. *Gynecol Oncol* 2010;118:S12–S17.
317. Schmitt M, Depuydt C, Benoy I, et al. Prevalence and viral load of 51 genital human papillomavirus types and three subtypes. *Int J Cancer* 2013;132:2395–2403.
318. Screening for Cervical Cancer: Recommendation Statement. *Am Fam Physician* 2019;99:Online.
319. Sehr P, Rubio I, Seitz H, et al. High-throughput pseudovirion-based neutralization assay for analysis of natural and vaccine-induced antibodies against human papillomaviruses. *PLoS One* 2013:8:e75677.
320. Senkomago V, Henley SJ, Thomas CC, et al. Human papillomavirus-attributable cancers—United States, 2012–2016. *MMWR Morb Mortal Wkly Rep* 2019;68:724–728.
321. Shah K, Kashima H, Polk BF, et al. Rarity of cesarean delivery in cases of juvenile-onset respiratory papillomatosis. *Obstet Gynecol* 1986;68:795–799.
322. Shah KV, Stern WF, Shah FK, et al. Risk factors for juvenile onset recurrent respiratory papillomatosis. *Pediatr Infect Dis J* 1998;17:372–376.
323. Shankar S, Prasad D, Sanawar R, et al. TALEN based HPV-E7 editing triggers necrotic cell death in cervical cancer cells. *Sci Rep* 2017;7:5500.
324. Shimabukuro TT, Su JR, Marquez PL, et al. Safety of the 9-valent human papillomavirus vaccine. *Pediatrics* 2019;144:e20191791.
325. Shiraz A, Crawford R, Egawa N, et al. The Early Detection of Cervical Cancer. The current and changing landscape of cervical disease detection. *Cytopathology* 2020;31:258–270.
326. Shope RE. Immunization of rabbits to infectious papillomatosis. *J Exp Med* 1937;65:219–231.
327. Sichero L, Giuliano AR, Villa LL. Human papillomavirus and genital disease in men: what we have learned from the HIM study. *Acta Cytol* 2019;63:109–117.
328. Sichero L, Rollison DE, Amorrortu RP, et al. Beta human papillomavirus and associated diseases. *Acta Cytol* 2019;63:100–108.
329. Silverberg JI, Silverberg NB. The U.S. prevalence of common warts in childhood: a population-based study. *J Invest Dermatol* 2013;133:2788–2790.
330. Silverberg MJ, Thorsen P, Lindeberg H, et al. Condyloma in pregnancy is strongly predictive of juvenile-onset recurrent respiratory papillomatosis. *Obstet Gynecol* 2003;101:645–652.
331. Simms KT, Steinberg J, Caruana M, et al. Impact of scaled up human papillomavirus vaccination and cervical screening and the potential for global elimination of cervical cancer in 181 countries, 2020–99: a modelling study. *Lancet Oncol* 2019;20:394–407.
332. Smith JS, Herrero R, Bosetti C, et al. Herpes simplex virus-2 as a human papillomavirus cofactor in the etiology of invasive cervical cancer. *J Natl Cancer Inst* 2002;94:1604–1613.
333. Smith JS, Lindsay L, Hoots B, et al. Human papillomavirus type distribution in invasive cervical cancer and high-grade cervical lesions: a meta-analysis update. *Int J Cancer* 2007;121:621–632.
334. Smith JS, Munoz N, Herrero R, et al. Evidence for Chlamydia trachomatis as a human papillomavirus cofactor in the etiology of invasive cervical cancer in Brazil and the Philippines. *J Infect Dis* 2002;185:324–331.

335. Smith NJ, Fenton TR. The APOBEC3 genes and their role in cancer: insights from human papillomavirus. *J Mol Endocrinol* 2019;62:R269–R287.
336. Smola S. Immune deviation and cervical carcinogenesis. *Papillomavirus Res* 2019;7:164–167.
337. Snijders PJ, Heideman DA, Meijer CJ. Methods for HPV detection in exfoliated cell and tissue specimens. *APMIS* 2010;118:520–528.
338. Sonnenberg P, Tanton C, Mesher D, et al. Epidemiology of genital warts in the British population: implications for HPV vaccination programmes. *Sex Transm Infect* 2019;95:386–390.
339. Stanley MA. Epithelial cell responses to infection with human papillomavirus. *Clin Microbiol Rev* 2012;25:215–222.
340. Stanley MA, Sterling JC. Host responses to infection with human papillomavirus. *Curr Probl Dermatol* 2014;45:58–74.
341. Strickley JD, Messerschmidt JL, Awad ME, et al. Immunity to commensal papillomaviruses protects against skin cancer. *Nature* 2019;575:519–522.
342. Sultana F, Winch K, Saville M, et al. Is the positive predictive value of high-grade cytology in predicting high-grade cervical disease falling due to HPV vaccination? *Int J Cancer* 2019;144:2964–2971.
343. Sun XW, Kuhn L, Ellerbrock TV, et al. Human papillomavirus infection in women infected with the human immunodeficiency virus. *N Engl J Med* 1997;337:1343–1349.
344. Suzich JA, Ghim S, Palmer-Hill FJ, et al. Systemic immunization with papillomavirus L1 protein completely prevents the development of viral mucosal papillomas. *Proc Natl Acad Sci USA* 1995;92:11553–11557.
345. Syrjanen S. Current concepts on human papillomavirus infections in children. *APMIS* 2010;118:494–509.
346. Syrjanen S. Oral manifestations of human papillomavirus infections. *Eur J Oral Sci* 2018;126(Suppl 1):49–66.
347. Syrjanen S, Syrjanen K. HPV in head and neck carcinomas: different HPV profiles in oropharyngeal carcinomas—why? *Acta Cytol* 2019;63:124–142.
348. Taliercio S, Cespedes M, Born H, et al. Adult-onset recurrent respiratory papillomatosis: a review of disease pathogenesis and implications for patient counseling. *JAMA Otolaryngol Head Neck Surg* 2015;141:78–83.
349. Tang S, Tao M, McCoy JP Jr, et al. The E7 oncoprotein is translated from spliced E6*I transcripts in high-risk human papillomavirus type 16- or type 18-positive cervical cancer cell lines via translation reinitiation. *J Virol* 2006;80:4249–4263.
350. Tang YW, Lozano L, Chen X, et al. An isothermal, multiplex amplification assay for detection and genotyping of human papillomaviruses in formalin-fixed, paraffin-embedded tissues. *J Mol Diagn* 2020;22:419–428.
351. Tobian AA, Serwadda D, Quinn TC, et al. Male circumcision for the prevention of HSV-2 and HPV infections and syphilis. *N Engl J Med* 2009;360:1298–1309.
352. Tommasino M. HPV and skin carcinogenesis. *Papillomavirus Res* 2019;7:129–131.
353. Tota JE, Best AF, Zumsteg ZS, et al. Evolution of the oropharynx cancer epidemic in the United States: moderation of increasing incidence in younger individuals and shift in the burden to older individuals. *J Clin Oncol* 2019;37:1538–1546.
354. Triglav T, Artemchuk H, Ostrbenk A, et al. Effect of naturally acquired type-specific serum antibodies against human papillomavirus type 16 infection. *J Clin Virol* 2017;90:64–69.
355. Trimble CL, Clark RA, Thoburn C, et al. Human papillomavirus 16-associated cervical intraepithelial neoplasia in humans excludes CD8 T cells from dysplastic epithelium. *J Immunol* 2010;185:7107–7114.
356. Tsang SH, Sampson JN, Schussler J, et al. Durability of cross-protection by different schedules of the bivalent HPV vaccine: the CVT trial. *J Natl Cancer Inst* 2020;112(10):1030–1037.
357. Tummers B, Burg SH. High-risk human papillomavirus targets crossroads in immune signaling. *Viruses* 2015;7:2485–2506.
358. Usyk M, Zolnik CP, Castle PE, et al. Cervicovaginal microbiome and natural history of HPV in a longitudinal study. *PLoS Pathog* 2020;16:e1008376.
359. van der Horst J, Siebers AG, Bulten J, et al. Increasing incidence of invasive and in situ cervical adenocarcinoma in the Netherlands during 2004–2013. *Cancer Med* 2017;6:416–423.
360. Van Doorslaer K, Bernard HU, Chen Z, et al. Papillomaviruses: evolution, Linnaean taxonomy and current nomenclature. *Trends Microbiol* 2011;19:49–50; author reply 50–51.
361. Van Dyne EA, Henley SJ, Saraiya M, et al. Trends in human papillomavirus-associated cancers—United States, 1999–2015. *MMWR Morb Mortal Wkly Rep* 2018;67:918–924.
362. Veldhuijzen NJ, Snijders PJ, Reiss P, et al. Factors affecting transmission of mucosal human papillomavirus. *Lancet Infect Dis* 2010;10:862–874.
363. Verlaat W, Van Leeuwen RW, Novianti PW, et al. Host-cell DNA methylation patterns during high-risk HPV-induced carcinogenesis reveal a heterogeneous nature of cervical pre-cancer. *Epigenetics* 2018;13:769–778.
364. Verstraeten T, Descamps D, David MP, et al. Analysis of adverse events of potential autoimmune aetiology in a large integrated safety database of AS04 adjuvanted vaccines. *Vaccine* 2008;26:6630–6638.
365. Viarisio D, Muller-Decker K, Accardi R, et al. Beta HPV38 oncoproteins act with a hit-and-run mechanism in ultraviolet radiation-induced skin carcinogenesis in mice. *PLoS Pathog* 2018;14:e1006783.
366. Vichnin M, Bonanni P, Klein NP, et al. An overview of quadrivalent human papillomavirus vaccine safety: 2006 to 2015. *Pediatr Infect Dis J* 2015;34:983–991.
367. Viciana P, Milanes-Guisado Y, Fontillon M, et al. High-risk human papilloma virus testing improves diagnostic performance to predict moderate- to high-grade anal intraepithelial neoplasia in human immunodeficiency virus-infected men who have sex with men in low-to-absent cytological abnormalities. *Clin Infect Dis* 2019;69:2185–2192.
368. Vinokurova S, Wentzensen N, Einenkel J, et al. Clonal history of papillomavirus-induced dysplasia in the female lower genital tract. *J Natl Cancer Inst* 2005;97:1816–1821.
369. Viscidi RP, Schiffman M, Hildesheim A, et al. Seroreactivity to human papillomavirus (HPV) types 16, 18, or 31 and risk of subsequent HPV infection: results from a population-based study in Costa Rica. *Cancer Epidemiol Biomarkers Prev* 2004;13:324–327.
370. Viscidi RP, Sun Y, Tsuzaki B, et al. Serological response in human papillomavirus-associated invasive cervical cancer. *Int J Cancer* 1993;55:780–784.
371. Wagner S, Roberson D, Boland J, et al. Development of the TypeSeq assay for detection of 51 human papillomavirus genotypes by next-generation sequencing. *J Clin Microbiol* 2019;57:e01794-18.
372. Walboomers JM, Jacobs MC, Manos MM, et al. Human papillomavirus is a necessary cause of invasive cervical cancer worldwide. *J Pathol* 1999;189:12–19.
373. Wallace NA, Munger K. The curious case of APOBEC3 activation by cancer-associated human papillomaviruses. *PLoS Pathog* 2018;14:e1006717.
374. Weissenborn S, Neale RE, Waterboer T, et al. Beta-papillomavirus DNA loads in hair follicles of immunocompetent people and organ transplant recipients. *Med Microbiol Immunol* 2012;201:117–125.
375. Welters MJ, de Jong A, van den Eeden SJ, et al. Frequent display of human papillomavirus type 16 E6-specific memory t-Helper cells in the healthy population as witness of previous viral encounter. *Cancer Res* 2003;63:636–641.
376. Wentzensen N, Vinokurova S, von Knebel Doeberitz M. Systematic review of genomic integration sites of human papillomavirus genomes in epithelial dysplasia and invasive cancer of the female lower genital tract. *Cancer Res* 2004;64:3878–3884.
377. Werner RN, Westfechtel L, Dressler C, et al. Self-administered interventions for anogenital warts in immunocompetent patients: a systematic review and meta-analysis. *Sex Transm Infect* 2017;93:155–161.
378. Westfechtel L, Werner RN, Dressler C, et al. Adjuvant treatment of anogenital warts with systemic interferon: a systematic review and meta-analysis. *Sex Transm Infect* 2018;94:21–29.
379. Westrich JA, Warren CJ, Pyeon D. Evasion of host immune defenses by human papillomavirus. *Virus Res* 2017;231:21–33.
380. Whitworth HS, Gallagher KE, Howard N, et al. Efficacy and immunogenicity of a single dose of human papillomavirus vaccine compared to no vaccination or standard three and two-dose vaccination regimens: a systematic review of evidence from clinical trials. *Vaccine* 2020;38:1302–1314.
381. Wiatrak BJ, Wiatrak DW, Broker TR, et al. Recurrent respiratory papillomatosis: a longitudinal study comparing severity associated with human papilloma viral types 6 and 11 and other risk factors in a large pediatric population. *Laryngoscope* 2004;114:1–23.
382. Wilcox LJ, Hull BP, Baldassari CM, et al. Diagnosis and management of recurrent respiratory papillomatosis. *Pediatr Infect Dis J* 2014;33:1283–1284.
383. Willame C, Gadroen K, Bramer W, et al. Systematic review and meta-analysis of postlicensure observational studies on human papillomavirus vaccination and autoimmune and other rare adverse events. *Pediatr Infect Dis J* 2020;39:287–293.
384. Williams A, Syed S, Velangi S, et al. New directions in vulvar cancer pathology. *Curr Oncol Rep* 2019;21:88.
385. Winer RL, Hughes JP, Feng Q, et al. Condom use and the risk of genital human papillomavirus infection in young women. *N Engl J Med* 2006;354:2645–2654.
386. Winer RL, Hughes JP, Feng Q, et al. Early natural history of incident, type-specific human papillomavirus infections in newly sexually active young women. *Cancer Epidemiol Biomarkers Prev* 2011;20:699–707.
387. Woo YL, Sterling J, Damay I, et al. Characterising the local immune responses in cervical intraepithelial neoplasia: a cross-sectional and longitudinal analysis. *BJOG* 2008;115:1616–1621; discussion 1621–1622.
388. Woo YL, van den Hende M, Sterling JC, et al. A prospective study on the natural course of low-grade squamous intraepithelial lesions and the presence of HPV16 E2-, E6- and E7-specific T-cell responses. *Int J Cancer* 2010;126:133–141.
389. Woodman CB, Collins S, Winter H, et al. Natural history of cervical human papillomavirus infection in young women: a longitudinal cohort study. *Lancet* 2001;357:1831–1836.
390. Workowski KA, Bolan GA; Centers for Disease Control and Prevention. Sexually transmitted diseases treatment guidelines, 2015. *MMWR Recomm Rep* 2015;64:1–137.
391. Yang A, Farmer E, Lin J, et al. The current state of therapeutic and T cell-based vaccines against human papillomaviruses. *Virus Res* 2017;231:148–165.
392. Yang EJ, Quick MC, Hanamornroongruang S, et al. Microanatomy of the cervical and anorectal squamocolumnar junctions: a proposed model for anatomical differences in HPV-related cancer risk. *Mod Pathol* 2015;28:994–1000.
393. Yoo H, Won SS, Choi HC, et al. Detection and identification of human papillomavirus types isolated from Korean patients with flat warts. *Microbiol Immunol* 2005;49:633–638.
394. Yoshiba T, Saga Y, Urabe M, et al. CRISPR/Cas9-mediated cervical cancer treatment targeting human papillomavirus E6. *Oncol Lett* 2019;17:2197–2206.
395. Yuan J, Ni G, Wang T, et al. Genital warts treatment: beyond imiquimod. *Hum Vaccin Immunother* 2018;14:1815–1819.
396. Yuan T, Fitzpatrick T, Ko NY, et al. Circumcision to prevent HIV and other sexually transmitted infections in men who have sex with men: a systematic review and meta-analysis of global data. *Lancet Glob Health* 2019;7:e436–e447.
397. Zhang L, Hemminki O, Chen T, et al. Familial clustering, second primary cancers and causes of death in penile, vulvar and vaginal cancers. *Sci Rep* 2019;9:11804.
398. Zheng R, Heller DS. High-risk human papillomavirus identification in precancerous cervical intraepithelial lesions. *J Low Genit Tract Dis* 2020;24:197–201.
399. Zhou C, Tuong ZK, Frazer IH. Papillomavirus immune evasion strategies target the infected cell and the local immune system. *Front Oncol* 2019;9:682.
400. Zielinski GD, Bais AG, Helmerhorst TJ, et al. HPV testing and monitoring of women after treatment of CIN 3: review of the literature and meta-analysis. *Obstet Gynecol Surv* 2004;59:543–553.
401. Zimmermann H, Degenkolbe R, Bernard HU, et al. The human papillomavirus type 16 E6 oncoprotein can down-regulate p53 activity by targeting the transcriptional coactivator CBP/p300. *J Virol* 1999;73:6209–6219.
402. zur Hausen H. Condylomata acuminata and human genital cancer. *Cancer Res* 1976;36:794.
403. zur Hausen H. Papillomaviruses in the causation of human cancers—a brief historical account. *Virology* 2009;384:260–265.

CHAPTER

4 *Adenoviridae*: The Viruses and Their Replication

Patrick Hearing

Adenoviruses were first isolated and characterized in the 1950s. In 1953, Rowe and colleagues observed spontaneous cytopathic effect in primary cultures of human adenoids.[254] In 1954, Hilleman and Werner isolated an agent from respiratory secretions of military recruits during an epidemic of respiratory disease.[120] The viruses discovered by the two groups were found to be related and named *adenoviruses*. Human adenoviruses cause acute respiratory disease among the military and in infants and the elderly, but they are responsible for a small portion of respiratory morbidity in the general population and for 5% to 10% of respiratory illnesses in children.[188] Due to significant morbidity caused by adenovirus infections among the military, a vaccine directed against Ad4 and Ad7 was redeveloped and currently is in use.[163]

Besides respiratory disease, adenoviruses cause epidemic conjunctivitis and infantile gastroenteritis, and less frequently pneumonia or myocarditis.[188] With immunocompetent individuals, adenovirus infection is clinically inapparent or generally associated with mild and self-limiting disease. With immunosuppressed patients, however, adenovirus infections can lead to severe, life-threatening disease including fulminant pneumonia, hepatitis, encephalitis, and/or systemic infection.[175] Patients undergoing immunosuppressive therapy, including organ transplant patients and hematopoietic stem cell transplant recipients, and AIDS patients are included in this category. Adenoviruses have been identified that infect all vertebrates. With humans, over 100 types (serotypes/genotypes) have been identified, with many recent isolates corresponding to intra- and intertypic recombinants.[175] Adenoviruses contain a linear, double-stranded DNA (dsDNA) genome packaged within an icosahedral capsid.

In 1962, Trentin and colleagues made the seminal discovery that human adenovirus type 12 induces malignant tumors after inoculation into newborn hamsters.[303] This was the first time that a human virus was discovered to be oncogenic. No compelling epidemiologic evidence was reported linking adenoviruses with cancers in humans despite extensive studies.[201] Nevertheless, the ability of adenovirus to induce tumors in animals and to transform primary cells in culture established an important model system for studying oncogenesis.

Adenoviruses provide a highly tractable model system for studying virus–host interactions. In general, human adenoviruses may be propagated to high titer and used to establish synchronous infections in cultured cells. With the advent of recombineering, the viral genome may be readily manipulated to generate highly specific viral mutants, facilitating the study of adenovirus gene functions.[283] Studies of adenovirus have provided fundamental insights into the identification and our understanding of numerous cellular processes including the regulation of viral and cellular gene expression and DNA replication, cell cycle control and oncogenic transformation, translational control, and the regulation of innate and adaptive immune responses to infection. Perhaps the most recognized contribution of the adenovirus system to modern biology was the discovery of messenger RNA (mRNA) splicing,[23] but seminal observations were made in many areas using adenovirus as a model system. Adenoviruses also are currently being utilized in a wide variety of gene therapy settings, including as oncolytic and vaccine vectors.[326] This chapter overviews the structure of the adenovirus particle, the adenovirus replication cycle in human cells, and adenovirus interactions with the host cell and organism.

CLASSIFICATION

Adenoviruses belong to the *Adenoviridae* family. *Adenoviridae* have been isolated from all vertebrates. Currently there are five genera: *Mastadenovirus* originate from mammals, including all human adenoviruses; *Aviadenovirus* originate from birds;

TABLE 4.1 Classification schemes for human adenoviruses (HAdVs, Genus *Mastadenovirus*)

		Oncogenic Potential			
Species	Representative Types	Tumors in Animals	Transformation In Culture	% GC	Hemagglutination Group
A	12	High	Positive	46–47	IV (little or none)
B	3, 7, 35	Moderate	Positive	49–51	I (complete for monkey erythrocytes)
C	2, 5	Low or none	Positive	55	II (partial for rat erythrocytes)
D	9, 17	Mammary tumors	Positive	55–57	III (complete for rat erythrocytes)
E	4	Low or none	Positive	58	III
F	40, 41	Unknown	Negative	51	III
G	52	Unknown	Unknown	55	Unknown

Atadenovirus have a broader range of hosts including reptiles, birds, a marsupial, and mammals; *Siadenovirus* originate from reptiles and birds; and *Ichtadenovirus* originate from fish.[64] Over 100 human adenovirus types have been isolated that fall into one of seven species (A–G) based on serology, hemagglutination, oncogenicity in rodents, transformation of cultured primary cells, and genome sequencing[70] (http://hadvwg.gmu.edu/) (Table 4.1). Over half of human adenoviruses are species D, followed by species B; one to only a few human adenoviruses are species E, F, or G. Human adenoviruses are identified based on their species and type designation; for example, HAdV-C5 is human adenovirus species C type 5. Adenoviruses were previously categorized by antigenic serotypes, but the current nomenclature also includes definition based on genotype.[7] Serotypes are defined based on the antigenicity of the major capsid protein hexon, which contains the prominent neutralizing epitopes. Novel human adenoviruses may arise by intra- and interspecies recombination, resulting in chimeric viral genomes; this occurs most frequently with adenovirus species D.[175] The tropism of human adenoviruses is diverse, with a variety of tissues and organs infected. Generally, adenoviruses within a species cause infections at particular sites in body, including ocular infections with species B and D; enteric infections with species A, F, and G; and respiratory infections with species B, C, and E.[175] Less common adenovirus infections include hemorrhagic cystitis and central nervous system infections with species B.

VIRION STRUCTURE

Adenoviruses are complex, nonenveloped, icosahedral particles approximately 95 nm in diameter, *pseudo* T = 25 triangulation number[258] (Fig. 4.1). The major capsid proteins include hexon (protein II) constituting the facets, penton base (protein III) constituting the vertices, and fiber (protein IV) projecting from each vertex (Fig. 4.2). Adenovirus particles have a mass of 150 MDa and contain DNA (13% of mass), protein (87% of mass), no membrane or lipid, and trace amounts of carbohydrate, because the virion fiber protein is modified by glucosamine.[132] Virions consist of a protein shell (capsid) surrounding a DNA-containing core. A single adenovirus particle contains 240 trimers of hexon, 12 pentamers of penton base, 12 trimers of fiber, and a number of other capsid proteins that serve to stabilize the virion and function as core proteins associated with the viral DNA[258] (Fig. 4.3, Table 4.2). The virion also contains a protease (AVP, adenovirus-associated protease), protein IVa2, and terminal protein covalently attached at each 5' end of the genome.

The first high-resolution structures of an intact HAdV-C5 virion were reported in 2010 and included a 3.6Å resolution cryoelectron microscopic (cryoEM) structure[178] (Fig. 4.1) and a 3.5Å resolution x-ray crystallographic structure.[244] The cryoEM structure was reinterpreted several years later to include the structures and locations of the virion cement proteins IIIa, VI, VIII, and IX.[245] Additionally, a segment of core protein V was visualized in association with protein VI. The revised crystal structure of a pseudo-typed HAdV-C5/D17 virion was recently reported that is consistent with the models of minor capsid proteins determined by cryoEM.[162] In addition to these structures of intact virus particles, a number of high-resolution crystal structures have been reported for capsid proteins, including a hexon trimer (2.5Å resolution)[256] (Fig. 4.4), penton base (3.3Å resolution)[350] (Fig. 4.5), fiber shaft (2.4Å resolution),[243] and fiber knob (1.5Å resolution)[242] (Fig. 4.5). The structures of minor capsid proteins VI and VII were determined by cryoEM[61] (Fig. 4.6).

Only the basal portions of the fibers were visualized in the cryoEM structure (Fig. 4.1).[178] However, full-length fiber proteins were evident in negatively stained transmission electron micrographs of single virions (Fig. 4.2) and in the x-ray crystal structure (Fig. 4.5). Most human adenoviruses encode a single fiber protein. However, HAdV-F40, HAdV-F41, and HAdV-G52 encode two fiber proteins, with one or the other bound to each penton base.[139,148] Because the fiber knob interacts with a cellular receptor, the incorporation of two different fiber proteins may extend the range of cell types to which these viruses bind. The fiber shaft of human adenoviruses is composed of repeats of an approximately 15-residue structural motif, and the length of the shaft varies among types from six repeating units in HAdV-B3 to 21 in HAdV-C2 and HAdV-C5.[243] A symmetry mismatch occurs in the interaction between the fivefold symmetric penton base and the threefold symmetric trimeric fiber. This interaction is mediated by a hydrophobic ring around a central pore on the top surface of the penton base, hydrophobic residues on the bottom of the

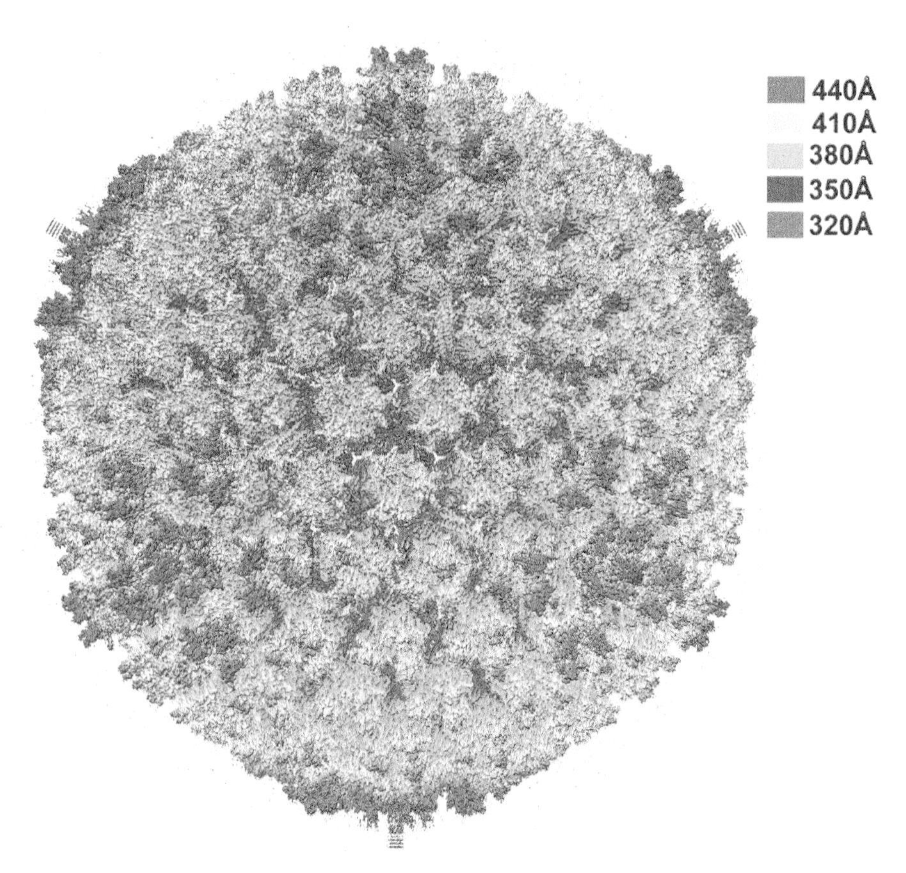

FIGURE 4.1 **The HAdV-C5 virion.** Color coding (*upper right*) represents distance from the center of the virion in angstroms. (Courtesy of Z. Hong Zhou; from Liu H, Jin L, Koh SB, et al. Atomic structure of human adenovirus by cryo-EM reveals interactions among protein networks. *Science* 2010;329:1038–1043.)

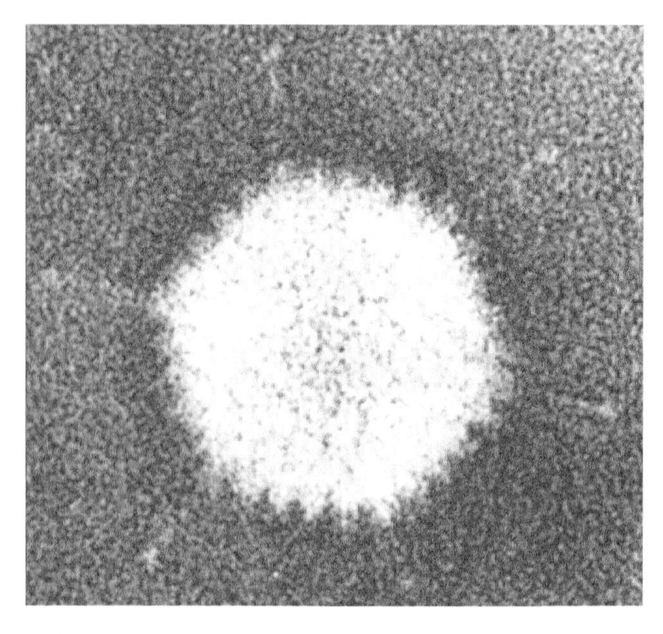

FIGURE 4.2 **Visualization of adenovirus fibers in a negatively stained transmission electron micrograph.** (Courtesy of Robley C. Williams).

fiber shaft, and flexible N-terminal tails of the fiber monomers (Fig. 4.5) that insert into three of five available grooves formed by neighboring subunits of the penton base.[182] The N-terminal residues of the fiber monomers extend to the bases of penton loops containing RGD sequences that bind to integrins on the target cell plasma membrane, triggering endocytosis of the virion (see Mechanisms of Entry, Uncoating, and Intracellular Trafficking).

Minor capsid proteins IIIa, VIII, and IX stabilize nonequivalent interactions between hexon trimers, allowing the same hexon trimer to be used in four different chemical environments on the surface of the capsid[178,244] (Figs. 4.6 and 4.7). Networks of interactions between the minor capsid proteins stabilize two groups of capsomeres and hold them together. On the outside surface of the virus particle, 240 copies of protein IX bind between adjacent hexons to stabilize the facets of the virion. On the inside surface of the virus particle at each of the vertices, five copies of protein IIIa bridge each penton base with adjacent hexons. Additionally, 120 copies of protein VIII per virion stabilize hexon–hexon interactions at the threefold and fivefold axes of symmetry[178,245] (Fig. 4.7).

The core of the virion contains seven known viral proteins and the viral genome. Polypeptide VII (174 amino acids), the major core protein with 500 to 800 copies per virion,

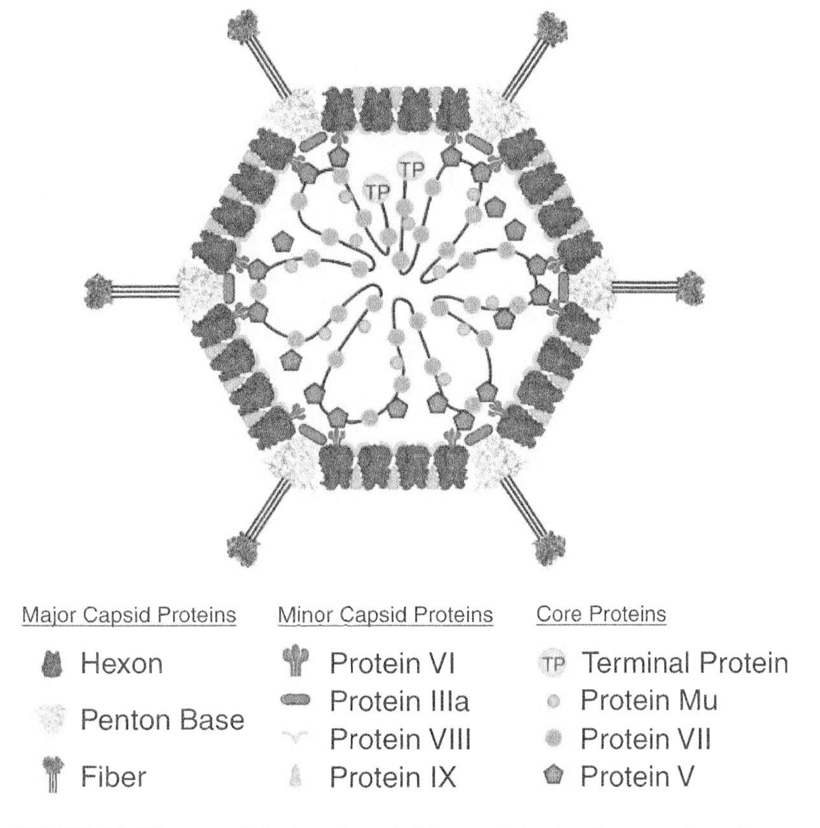

FIGURE 4.3 Diagram of the location of virion proteins in a human adenovirus particle. A schematic diagram of the adenovirus virion is shown with major and minor capsid proteins depicted and core proteins identified (Reprinted Nemerow GR, Pache L, Reddy V, et al. Insights into adenovirus host cell interactions from structural studies. *Virol* 2009;384:380–388. Copyright © 2008 Elsevier. With permission.)

TABLE 4.2 HAdV-C5 structural proteins

Polypeptide	Amino Acid Residues	Copies in Virion
II (Hexon)	952	240 trimers
III (Penton base)	571	12 pentamers
pIIIa	585	60 monomers
IV (Fiber)	581	12 trimers
IVa2	449	5
V	368	150–160
pVI	250	60 hexamers
pVII	174	500–800
pVIII	227	100–120
pIX	140	240
pμ (pX)	36	100–300

Adapted from Chen PH, Ornelles DA, Shenk T. The adenovirus L3 23-kilodalton proteinase cleaves the amino-terminal head domain from cytokeratin 18 and disrupts the cytokeratin network of HeLa cells. *J Virol* 1993;67:3507–3514.

polypeptide V (368 amino acids; 150 copies/virion), and μ (36 amino acids; 100 to 300 copies/virion)[17,218] are basic, arginine-rich proteins that contact the viral DNA.[4,44] Adenovirus core protein VII condenses DNA in clusters and bundles within the capsid.[199] The adenovirus DNA–protein core lacks symmetry and precise order but exists in numerous, defined spheres (adenosomes) that may be visualized by cryoelectron tomography[234] (Fig. 4.8). Remarkably, Ad5 particles are efficiently assembled and visually appear normal in the complete absence of core protein VII.[226] Adenovirus particles that lack core protein VII exhibit increased internal pressure, indicating that VII reduces repulsive DNA–DNA interactions.[199]

Protein VI associates with a cavity on the inner surface of hexon trimers[61,178,245] (Fig. 4.7) and with protein V,[200] tethering the highly ordered capsid to the less ordered DNA–protein core. A basic 115-residue disordered region in the middle of each polypeptide VI is proposed to contribute to an interaction with the core.[257] The N terminus of each penton base monomer also interacts with the core, and the C terminus of protein IIIa may as well,[178] consistent with reports that these proteins also interact with protein V[272] and that IIIa is responsible for type-specific packaging of viral DNA into virions.[190] Protein IVa2 is present in only a few copies at one

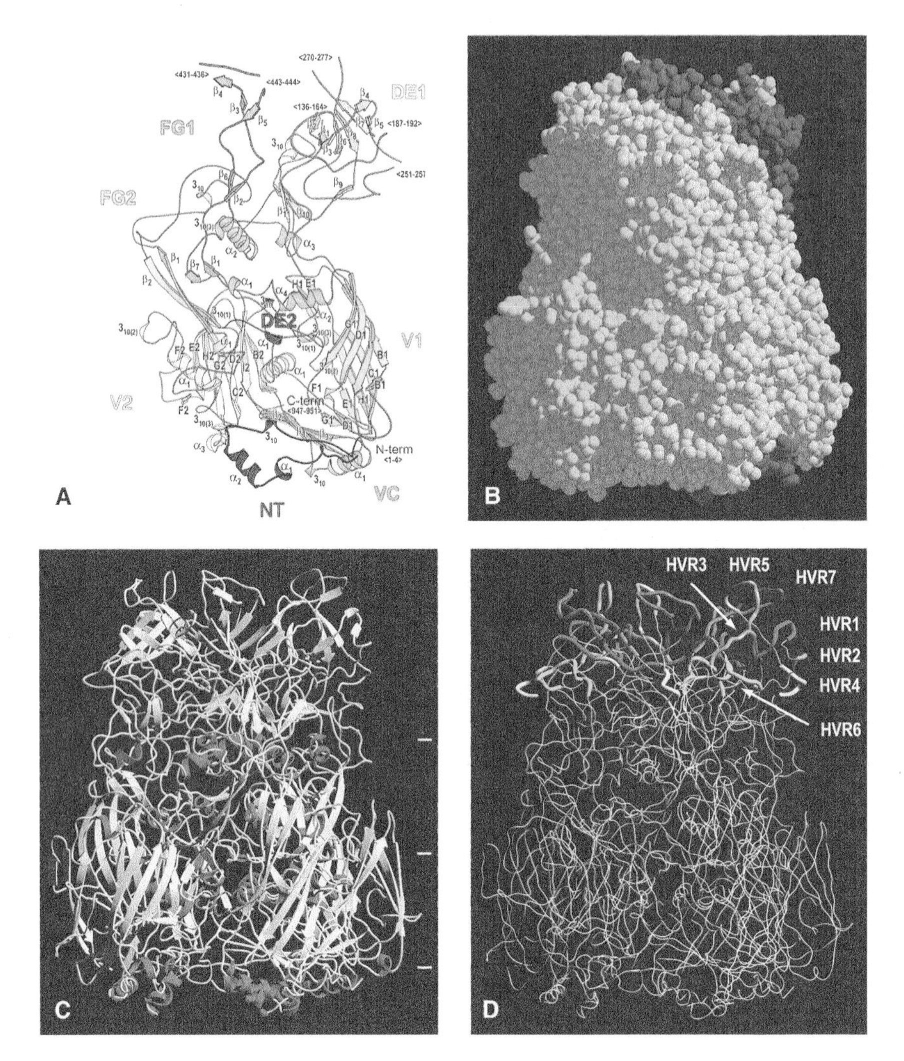

FIGURE 4.4 HAdV-C5 hexon structure. A: Ribbon diagram of a hexon monomer. View from the inside of the trimer. Loops DE1, FG1, and FG2 constitute the outer surface of hexon in the virion. DE2 is a small loop in the hexon monomer interface. **B:** Space-filling model of the hexon trimer. Subunits of the trimer are colored *red, green,* and *yellow.* **C:** Ribbon diagram of the hexon trimer. Structural elements are colored with β-strands in *yellow* and α-helices in *red.* **D:** The seven hypervariable regions (HVRs) that contain serotype-specific residues in HAdV-C5 hexon are shown on the trimeric hexon structure. The HVRs correspond to *red,* HVR1 (aa 137–181); *orange,* HVR2 (aa 187–193); *blue,* HVR3 (aa 211–218); *yellow,* HVR4 (aa 247–260); *tan,* HVR5 (aa 267–282); *green,* HVR6 (aa 304–315); and *magenta,* HVR7 (aa 421–449). (Reprinted with permission Rux JJ, Burnett RM. Type-specific epitope locations revealed by X-ray crystallographic study of adenovirus type 5 hexon. *Mol Ther* 2000;1(1):18–30. Copyright © 2000 American Society for Gene Therapy)

vertex of the icosahedron,[52] binds to the packaging domain at the left end of the viral genome, and is required for packaging viral DNA into the capsid (see Virion Assembly). The sixth protein in the core is terminal protein, which is covalently attached to the 5′ ends of the viral DNA and therefore present in only two copies per virion. The core also contains approximately 10 molecules of the viral cysteine protease AVP that functions to cleave precursors of a number of virion proteins during maturation of the virion and in virus escape from endosomes during the infection process[194] (see Virion Assembly and Mechanisms of Entry, Uncoating, and Intracellular Trafficking).

GENOME STRUCTURE AND ORGANIZATION

Adenovirus genomes are linear dsDNAs ranging in size from 26,000 to 45,000 base pairs (bp).[64] Adenovirus terminal protein is covalently attached to the 5′ end of each strand and serves as a protein primer of DNA replication (see Viral DNA Replication). Homologous genes shared by all adenoviruses encode the three viral proteins required for viral DNA replication, the preterminal protein (pTP), viral DNA polymerase (Ad-Pol), the viral single-stranded DNA-binding

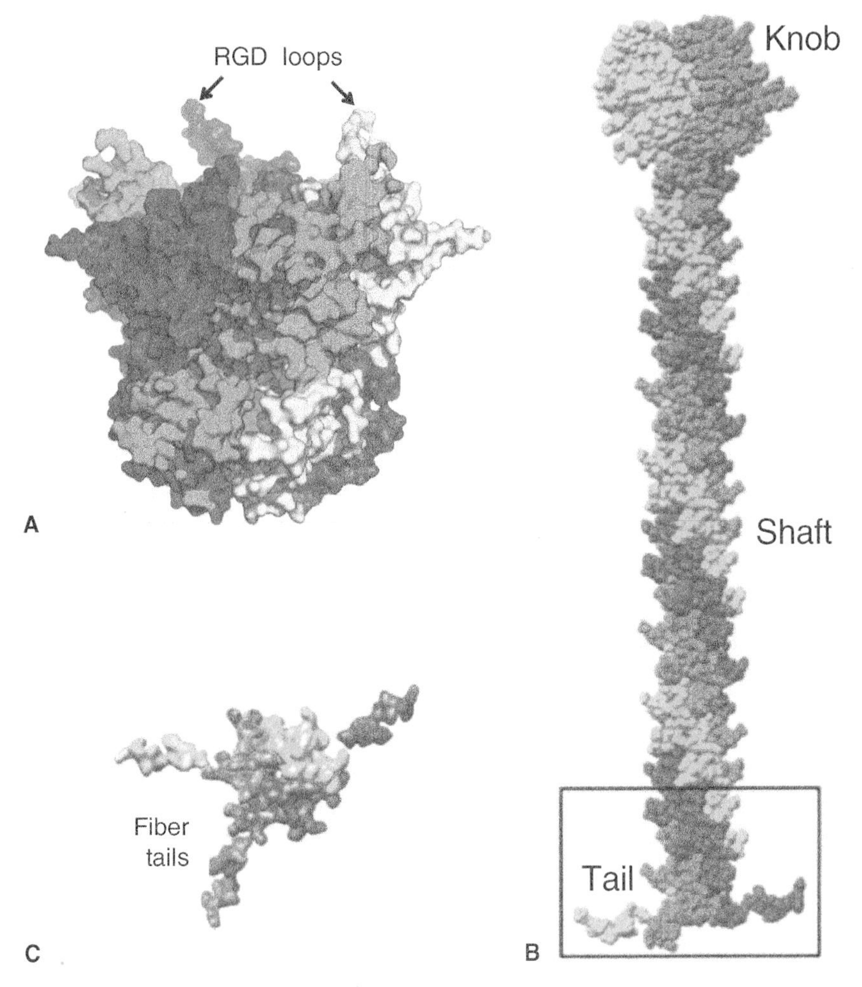

FIGURE 4.5 **Structures of HAdV-C2 penton base and fiber. A:** Space-filling model of a penton base. Each of the five penton base subunits is shown in a separate color. RGD loops are indicated. **B:** Model of fiber shaft and knob. Each of the three fiber subunits is shown in a separate color. **C:** View of the fiber shaft from the bottom with three fiber N-terminal tails that fit into three of five grooves between the subunits at the top of the penton base. (**A**: Reprinted from Zubieta C, Schoehn G, Chroboczek J, et al. The structure of the human adenovirus 2 penton. *Mol Cell* 2005;17:121–135. Copyright © 2005 Elsevier. With permission. **B, C** Reprinted from Liu HL, Wu L, Zhou ZH. Model of the trimeric fiber and its interactions with the pentameric penton base of human adenovirus by cryo-electron microscopy. *J Mol Biol* 2011;406:764–774. Copyright © 2010 Elsevier. With permission.)

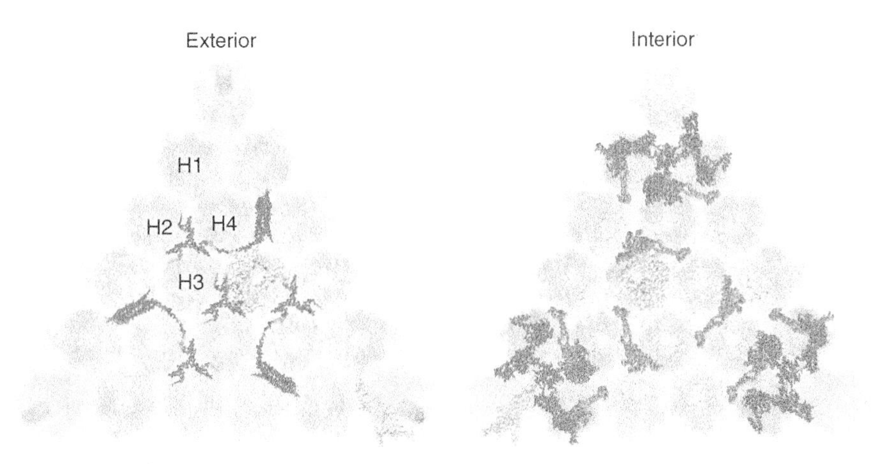

FIGURE 4.6 **Four different chemical environments of HAdV-C5 hexon trimers and locations of minor cement proteins.** Models of one of the twenty facets of an Ad5 icosahedron viewed from outside (*Exterior*) and inside (*Interior*) the virion. Penton bases with the base of a fiber trimer are at the three corners of the triangular facet. Hexon trimers are in four distinct chemical environments, each shown in a different color shade: (H1) two hexon trimers neighboring each penton base; (H2) two hexon trimers on the edges of each facet between the penton base–associated hexon trimmers; (H3) three hexon trimers at the center of each facet; and (H4) three hexon trimers between the central hexon trimers and the penton-associated hexon trimers. These nonequivalent interactions are stabilized by protein IX (*purple*) between hexon trimers, visible from the exterior surface, and proteins IIIa (*red*) and VIII (*blue*) on the inner surface. (Courtesy of Z. Hong Zhou; from Liu H, Jin L, Koh SB, et al. Atomic structure of human adenovirus by cryo-EM reveals interactions among protein networks. *Science* 2010;329:1038–1043.)

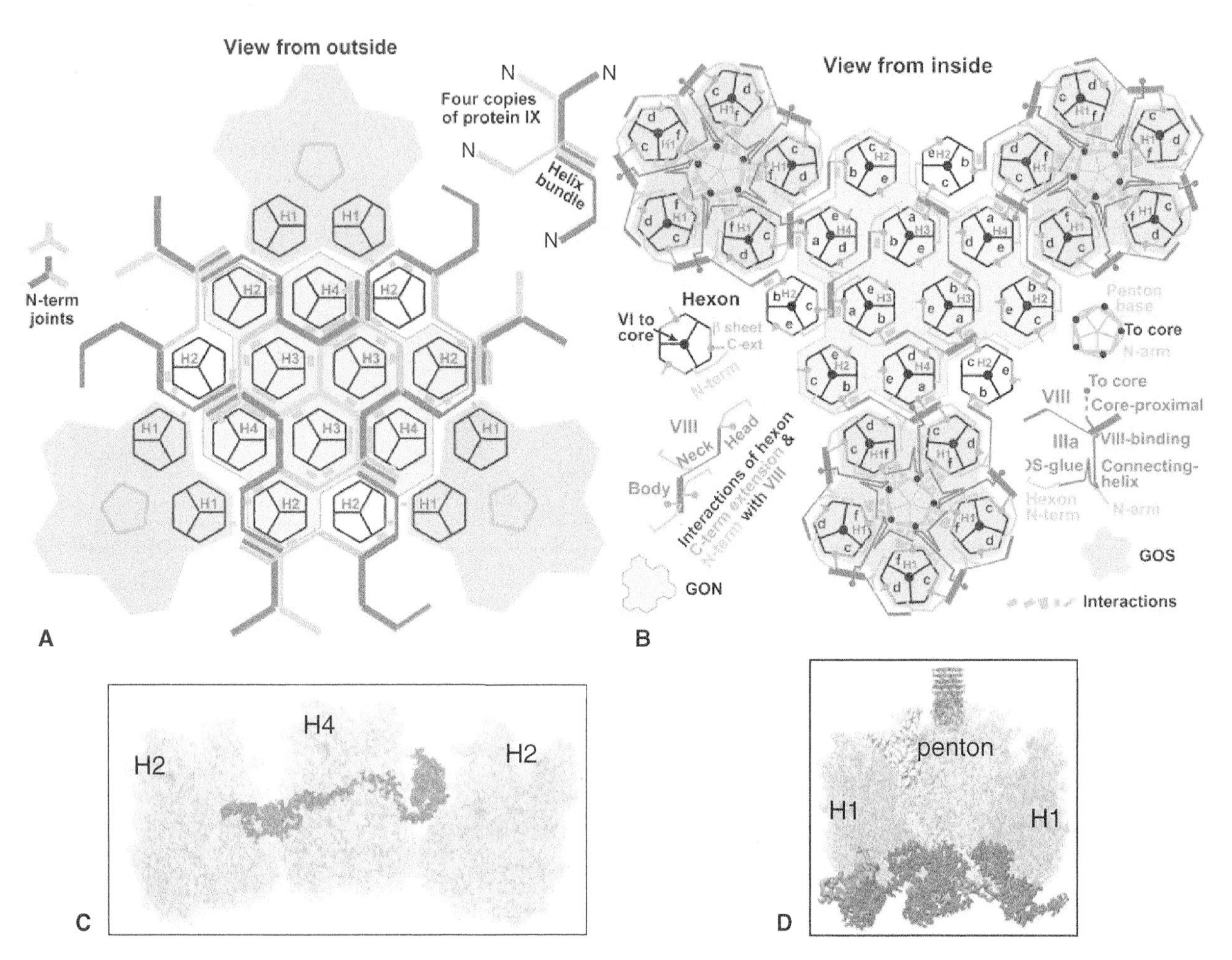

FIGURE 4.7 Diagram of the interactions of minor proteins IIIa, VIII, and IX that stabilize nonequivalent hexon trimer interactions. A: Hexon trimers are labeled H1 to H4 as described in Figure 4.6. The diagram at the upper right represents four different conformations of protein IX shown in different colors. N indicates their amino termini. These link hexon trimers in a group of nine (*gray*), and link groups of nine from neighboring facets. Groups-of-nine hexon trimers are released when virions are disrupted under mild conditions. **B:** Letters *a* through *f* indicate hexon monomers with distinct conformations of their extended N- and C-termini. As diagrammed at the lower left, three hexon C-termini and four hexon N-termini interact with one protein VIII. At each vertex of the icosahedron, five copies of protein IIIa link five hexon trimers to the central penton base, forming groups-of-six capsomeres (GOS, *shaded in blue*). Protein VIII links groups-of-nine hexon trimers (GON, *shaded in gray*) to groups-of-nine hexon trimers in neighboring facets and groups-of-nine hexon trimers to groups-of-six capsomeres at the vertices. Protein VI binds in a central cavity on the inner surface of hexon trimers, represented as a *black circle*. **C:** Side view of protein IX (*purple*) inlaid into the canyons between hexon trimers. **D:** Side view of proteins IIIa (*red*) interacting with penton base and H1 hexons and protein VIII (*blue*) interacting with H1 hexons on the inner surface of the capsid shell. (Courtesy of Z. Hong Zhou. Adapted from Liu H, Jin L, Koh SB, et al. Atomic structure of human adenovirus by cryo-EM reveals interactions among protein networks. *Science* 2010;329:1038–1043.)

protein (DBP), and the major structural components of the virion described above (see Virion Structure), except that core protein V is found only with *Mastadenoviruses* isolated from mammals.[64] These conserved genes are encoded in the central portion of the genome. Additional genes specific to adenoviruses from different vertebrates are encoded primarily near the ends of the genome. The genomes of all adenoviruses have inverted terminal repeat (ITR) sequences ranging in size from 36 to over 200 bp.[64] The ITRs function as DNA replication origins (see Viral DNA Replication). Most human adenovirus genomes encode homologous genes represented by the extensively studied and closely related HAdV-C2 and HAdV-C5. HAdV-C2 DNA was the first adenovirus genome to be completely sequenced[249] with a length of 35,937 base pairs bp. This chapter will concentrate on the human adenoviruses, all having the same general genome organization.

The human adenovirus genome contains a *cis*-acting packaging domain at the left end that is required for encapsidation of the viral genome into the virion at late times after infection.[224] The packaging domain is located just upstream of the E1A coding region and within the E1A transcriptional enhancer region. The human adenovirus genome contains five early transcription units (E1A, E1B, E2, E3, and E4), four intermediate transcription units transcribed around the time of onset of viral DNA replication (pIX, IVa2, L4 intermediate, and E2-late), and one major late transcription unit that is processed to generate five families of late mRNAs (L1–L5) (Fig. 4.9). These transcription units are all transcribed by

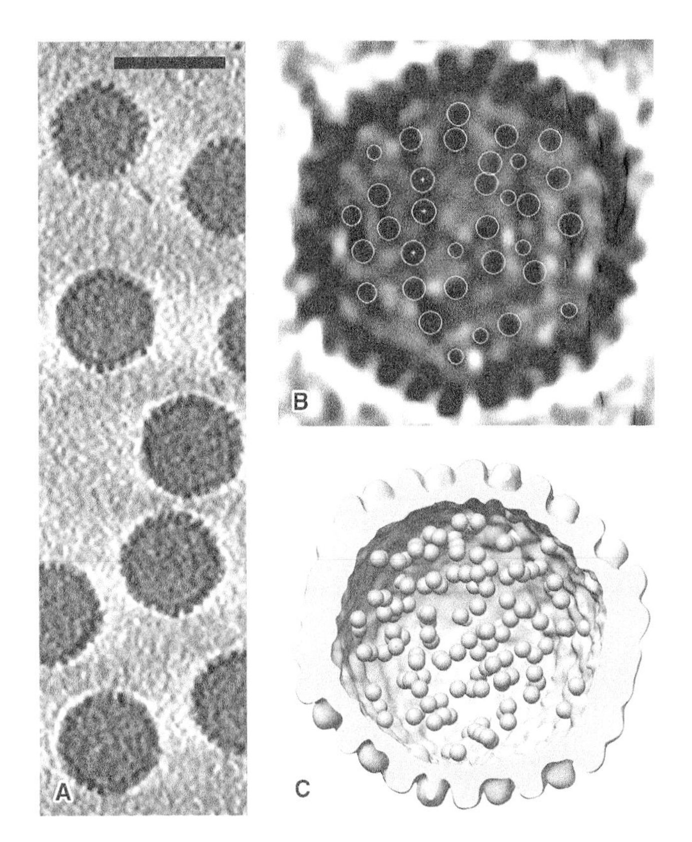

FIGURE 4.8 CryoEM modeling of HAdV-C5 adenosomes within a virion particle. A: CryoEM tomogram of adenovirus particles. The bar = 100 nm. **B:** A single virus particle is shown with the highest density regions in *black*. Adenosomes are circled in *white*. **C:** Surface rendering showing an HAdV-C5 capsid cross section; adenosomes are indicated in blue. (From Pérez-Berná AJ, Marion S, Chichón FJ, et al. Distribution of DNA-condensing protein complexes in the adenovirus core. *Nucl Acids Res* 2015;43:4274–4283. Reproduced by permission of Oxford University Press.)

host RNA polymerase II. The major late promoter (MLP) is transcribed at a low level during the early phase of infection, generating only the L1 family of mRNAs encoding the L1-52/55-kD protein. After the onset of viral DNA replication, transcripts are generated from all five late regions (L1–L5). In addition, the E2 transcription unit is transcribed from an alternative promoter, the E2-late promoter, as well as from the E2-early promoter. The adenovirus genome encodes one or two (depending on the type) virus-associated (VA) RNAs transcribed by host RNA polymerase III. By convention, the adenovirus genome map is drawn with the E1A gene at the left end (Fig. 4.9). Both strands of the viral DNA are transcribed, with the rightward reading strand as the template for the E1A, E1B, pIX, major late, VA RNA, and E3 transcription units, and the leftward reading strand as the template for the E4, E2, and IVa2 transcription units.

Except for the IVa2 and pIX transcription units, each of the adenovirus genes transcribed by RNA polymerase II gives rise to multiple mRNAs generated by alternative pre-mRNA splicing, and in the case of the major late, E2, and E3 transcription units, by the use of alternative polyadenylation sites as well. The L4 intermediate mRNAs shown in Figure 4.9 encode proteins L4-22K and L4-33K expressed from an intermediate phase promoter.[207]

Some of the proteins generated from the same transcription unit share amino acid sequences, such as the two major polypeptides encoded by the E1A region (Fig. 4.10) and the L4-22K and L4-33K proteins of the L4 region (Fig. 4.11). Other proteins encoded by a specific transcription unit have no sequences in common, such as the two major E1B-encoded proteins (Fig. 4.10) and the L4-100K, L4-22K, and L4-pVIII proteins (Fig. 4.11). Unfortunately, no consistent terminology has been adopted for naming adenovirus proteins: the E1A proteins are named large and small E1A and are often referred to by the sedimentation coefficient of the mRNAs that encode them (13S and 12S) or their amino acid composition (289aa and 243aa). The E1B and E3 proteins are designated by their apparent molecular mass estimated from SDS gel electrophoresis (although specific acronyms now have been assigned to certain E3 gene products). The E2 proteins are named for their functions, and the E4 proteins are named by their reading frames. Proteins encoded by the major late transcription unit are named for the virion proteins discussed above (see Virion Structure) and based on their relative mobilities by SDS-PAGE. Various historical names of viral polypeptides are used in this chapter, generally preceded by the name of the transcription unit or family of late mRNAs that encodes them (e.g., E4 ORF6, L4-100K).

Many of the individual adenovirus transcription units encode a series of polypeptides with related functions. As will be discussed, the E1A unit encodes two principal proteins that activate transcription and induce the host cell to enter S phase of the cell cycle. E1B encodes two proteins that block apoptosis. E2 encodes three proteins that function in viral DNA replication. E3 encodes products that modulate the innate and adaptive immune responses to infection. The late family of mRNAs encodes proteins primarily involved in the production and assembly of viral capsids. Only the E4 unit encodes proteins with a disparate set of functions. E4 products mediate transcriptional, RNA splicing, and translational regulation, mediate mRNA nuclear export, modulate DNA replication and apoptosis, and counteract innate responses to infection.

STAGES OF REPLICATION

The replication cycle is divided by convention into two phases, early and late, that are separated by the onset of viral DNA replication (Fig. 4.12). Early events commence as soon as the infecting virus interacts with the host cell. These include adsorption, penetration, movement of partially uncoated virus particles to a nuclear pore complex (NPC), transport of viral DNA through the NPC into the nucleus, and the expression of early genes. Early viral gene products promote further viral gene expression and viral DNA replication, induce cell cycle progression, block apoptosis, and antagonize a variety of host antiviral measures. The length of the early phase of infection varies depending on the cell type and multiplicity of infection but generally lasts 6 to 12 hours. Concomitant with the onset of viral DNA replication, the late phase begins with the expression of late viral genes and the assembly of progeny virions. The infectious cycle generally is completed 30 to 72 hours after infection, depending on parameters listed above. By the end of the lytic replication cycle, approximately 10^5 progeny

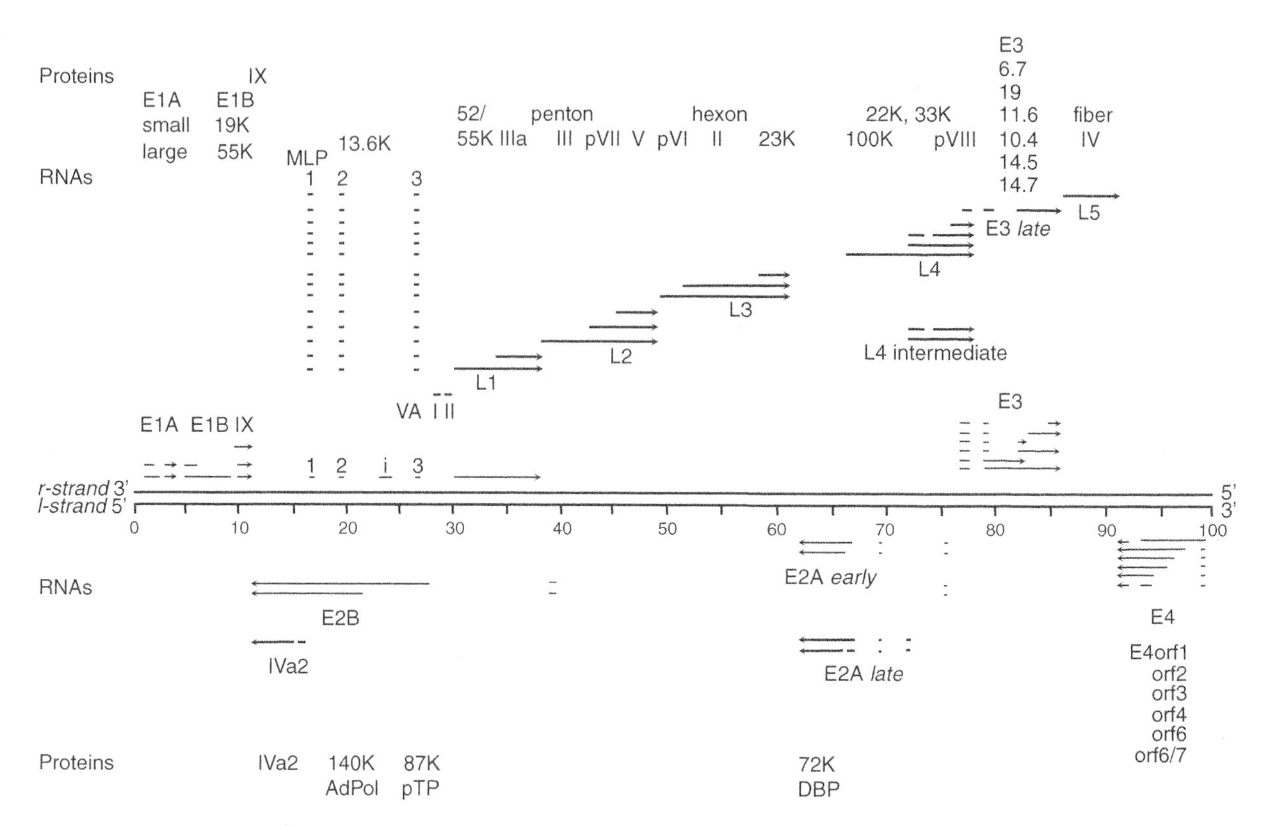

FIGURE 4.9 **HAdV-C2 and HAdV-C5 genomes.** The 35,937 bp genome of HAdV-C2 is divided into 100 map units. Early mRNAs are E1A, E1B, E2A-*early*, E2B, E3, and E4. Late mRNAs are L1, L2, L3, L4, and L5. Intermediate RNAs are IX, IVa2, L4 intermediate, and E2A-*late*. *Arrowheads* represent polyadenylated 3′ ends. Most late mRNAs originate at the major late promoter (MLP) at 16.8 map units and contain the tripartite leader (TPL) whose exons are labeled 1, 2, and 3. Proteins translated from the mRNAs transcribed to the right and left are named along the top and along the bottom of the diagram, respectively. Penton base is also designated virion protein III. Hexon is also designated virion protein II. Fiber is also designated virion protein IV. pVI, pVII, and pVIII refer to precursor polypeptides that are cleaved during virion maturation.

virus particles per cell are produced, along with the synthesis of a substantial excess of viral proteins and DNA that are not assembled into virions.

Studies of the human adenovirus replication cycle have focused primarily on the closely related HAdV-C2 and HAdV-C5 (Ad2, Ad5) viruses. These closely related types have been favored because they are easily grown in the laboratory and an extensive collection of mutant viruses have been developed. When other human adenovirus types have been studied, their growth strategies generally have proved similar to the paradigm established for these prototypes, although unique aspects are evident.

Mechanisms of Attachment

Adenoviruses use distinct cellular receptors for attachment and internalization. Initial attachment of HAdVs in species A and

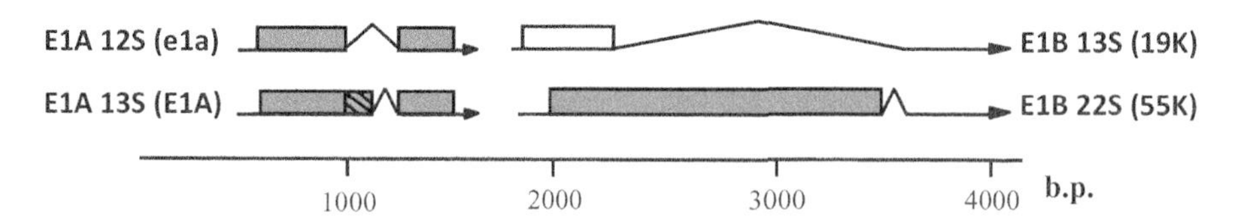

FIGURE 4.10 **HAdV-C2 and HAdV-C5 major E1A and E1B mRNAs and proteins expressed during the early phase of infection and in transformed cells.** The small e1a and large E1A proteins, 243R and 289R, respectively, are translated from spliced mRNAs with single introns having alternative 5′ donor splice sites and the same 3′ acceptor splice site (12S and 13S E1A mRNAs). Translation starts at the first AUG of both mRNAs, and the second exon of both mRNAs is translated in the same reading frame. Consequently, the E1A 243R and 289R proteins are identical with the exception of the unique 43 aa central region in 289R (hatched). E1B proteins of 19K and 55K proteins are translated from the first and second AUG in alternative reading frames of the 22S E1B mRNA. E1B 19K also is expressed from the first AUG of the smaller 13S E1B mRNA.

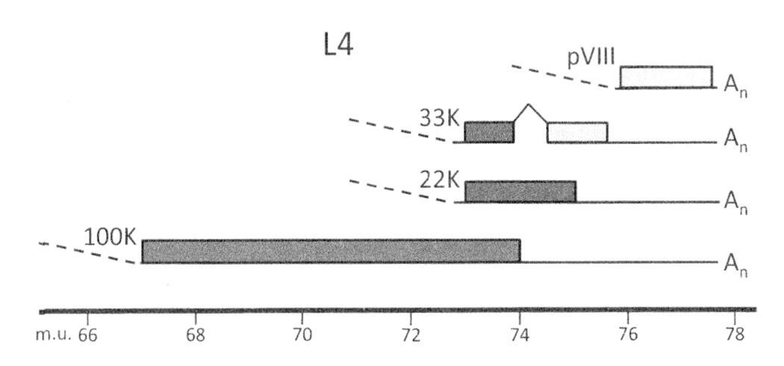

FIGURE 4.11 HAdV-C5 mRNAs and proteins from the L4 region. The coding sequences of the L4-100K, L4-22K, L4-33K, and L4-pVIII proteins shown. *Dashed lines* at the left represent splicing to the third exon of the tripartite leader.

C–F (but not species B) is mediated by high-affinity binding of the fiber knob domain to the host–cell transmembrane CAR protein (coxsackie B, adenovirus receptor)[20,250,300] (Fig. 4.13). Human CAR (345 amino acids) is a transmembrane protein of epithelial cell tight junctions with extracellular domains in the immunoglobulin (Ig) superfamily.[53] CAR is abundantly expressed in a number of tissues (brain, heart, lung, intestine, pancreas, liver, and kidney), but little or no CAR is expressed on hematopoietic cells or adult muscle.[165] Infection does not require the CAR cytoplasmic domain, implying that CAR function in infection is primarily as an anchor for high-affinity virus binding.[313] The finding that most CAR is localized below the apical surface of polarized epithelial cells, on the basolateral surface, raises the question of how adenoviruses that utilize CAR infect from the lumen of the airway since the apical and basolateral surfaces are excluded from each other by tight junctions. The resolution of this question lies in the expression of an alternatively spliced isoform of CAR, CAR(Ex8), that localizes to the apical membrane of epithelia.[78] Interestingly, CAR(Ex8) apical expression is stimulated by the host innate immune response to infection suggesting that adenoviruses may utilize innate signaling pathways to promote epithelial cell infection.[158]

The x-ray crystal structure of a complex between the HAdV-A12 fiber knob and the extracellular N-terminal Ig-like domain (D1) of CAR showed that three CAR molecules bind to the three interfaces between fiber knob monomers through the same surface used by CAR for homotypic interactions.[24] The avidity generated from the three independent interactions generates a high-affinity binding with a $K_D \approx 1$ nM.[185] Free fiber proteins produced during the late phase of infection in excess over fiber proteins incorporated into virions are released with progeny virions from the basolateral surfaces of infected airway epithelial cells and interfere with CAR oligomerization at tight junctions. This promotes release of progeny virions to the airway lumen.[311] In this way, the fiber protein serves two functions: initial attachment of virions to CAR on host cells during infection and disruption of CAR-mediated intercellular binding to promote virus escape.

Species B adenoviruses and species D HAdV-D37 bind CD46, a regulator of the complement cascade present on the plasma membrane of most cell types, including hematopoietic cells.[90,268] As with CAR binding, three extracellular domains of CD46 are bound by three fiber monomer interfaces in the fiber knob.[237] HAdV-F40 and HAdV-F41 incorporate one of two different fibers at each vertex of the virion. The longer of these binds to CAR. The receptor for the shorter fiber protein of HAdV-F40 and HAdV-F41 is not known, but it is postulated to contribute to the tropism of these viruses for intestinal epithelium.[56] In addition to CAR and CD46, a number of other cell surface molecules serve as receptors for different human adenoviruses, including desmoglein 2 (DSG2, species B), scavenger receptor A-II (species C), heparan sulfate proteoglycans (species A–D), and sialylated glycoproteins (species D).[165]

Infection by adenoviruses elicits a potent, long-term humoral immune response. While most neutralizing antibodies bind to the major virion protein hexon and are primarily responsible for the classification of HAdVs into serotypes,[92,301] neutralizing antibodies to fiber are also generated[79] and neutralize synergistically with antibodies to penton base,[91] which interacts with the secondary HAdV receptor.

Mechanisms of Entry, Uncoating, and Intracellular Trafficking

Following high-affinity binding of the HAdV-C5 fiber knob to CAR, the RGD loop domains of penton base subunits associate with αvβ3 and αvβ5 integrins on the host cell surface with 50-fold lower affinity than the interaction of fiber with CAR[319] (Fig. 4.13). Integrins are abundant heterodimeric transmembrane proteins involved in cell adhesion to the extracellular matrix and neighboring cells via RGD peptide motifs in the bound extracellular protein and are exploited by many viruses for cell entry.[287] At saturation, approximately 4 integrins are bound to the pentameric penton base.[50] Neutralizing antibodies that bind loops on the outer surface of penton block association with integrins.[122] Interaction of the penton base with integrins is presumably facilitated by their high local concentration resulting from high-affinity binding of the fiber knob to transmembrane CAR. Clustering of integrins through binding to the subunits of a pentameric penton base triggers integrin transmembrane signaling, leading to activation of phosphoinositide-3-OH kinase (PI3K), p130CAS, and Rho family GTPases.[172] This results in the localized actin polymerization required for endocytosis of the virion via clathrin-coated pits in classic receptor-mediated endocytosis that involves clathrin adapters and the large GTPase dynamin[101] (Fig. 4.13). Dynamin multimerizes into a spiral-shaped structure that promotes the membrane fusion required for separating an endosome from the plasma membrane.[93,314]

By contrast, species B adenoviruses, with CD46 as the primary receptor, enter cells through a penton base interaction with αv integrins that stimulates an alternative, clathrin-independent mechanism of endocytosis termed macropinocytosis.[3,141] Macropinocytosis requires integrins, F-actin, protein kinase C, and small G proteins of the Rho family, but not dynamin.[203] Species C HAdVs also stimulate macropinocytosis but do not use this process as a primary route of infection.[3]

Uncoating of the virion begins at the cell surface (Fig. 4.13). The interaction of penton base with integrins at the cell surface and during endocytosis leads to detachment of fibers, and fiberless virions are endocytosed.[212] Following endocytosis of clathrin-coated vesicles containing HAdV-C2, the vesicles

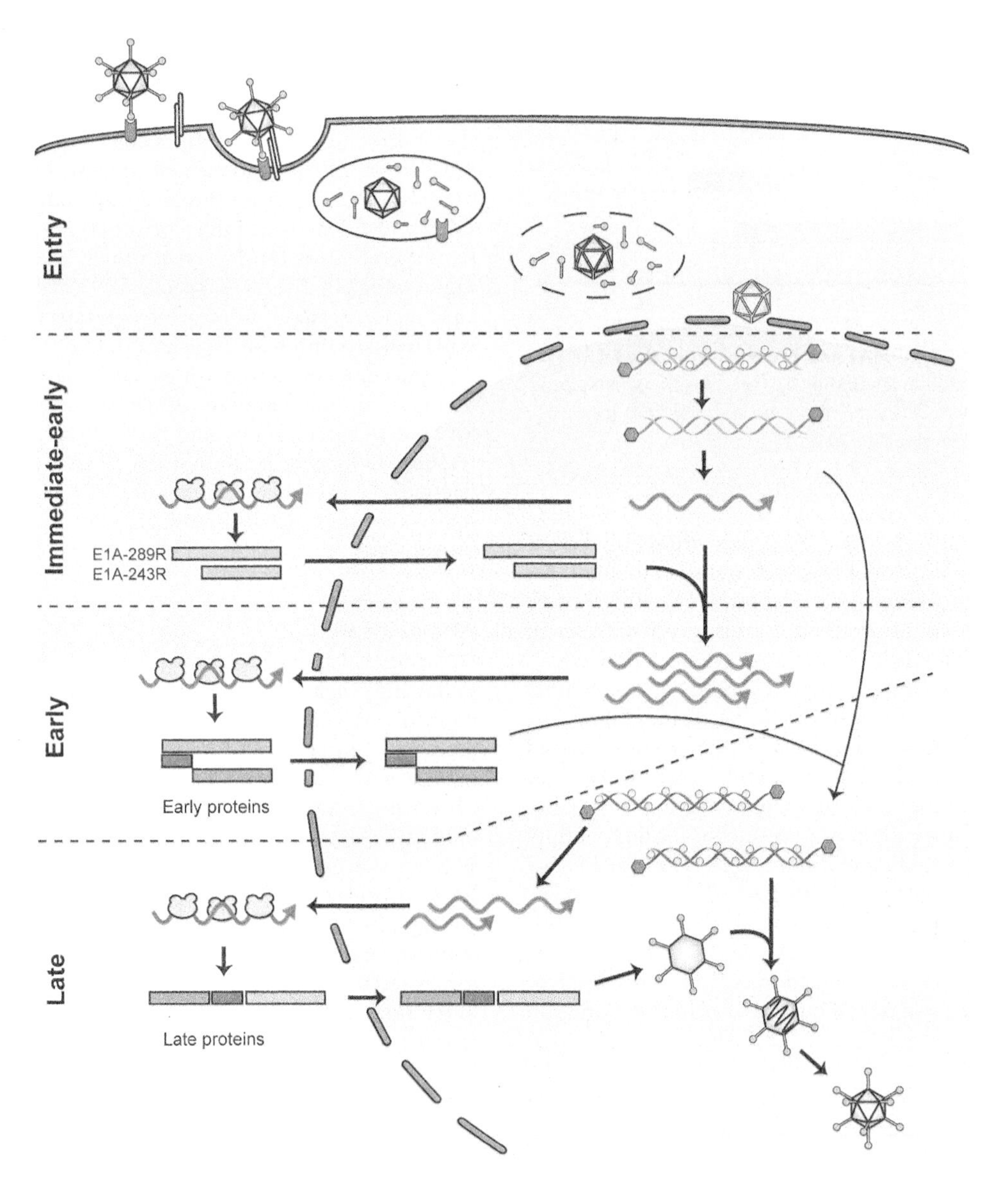

FIGURE 4.12 The HAdV-C5 life cycle. HAdV-C5 attachment to the cell is initiated by the fiber protein interacting with the cellular CAR receptor (*purple shape*), followed by interaction between the Ad penton base and cellular integrins (*yellow shapes*). Ad enters the cell through the endocytic pathway, where the viral particle is partially degraded inside the endosome, before being released into the cytosol. At the nuclear pore complex, the viral particle is disassembled. The Ad DNA–terminal protein (*orange hexagons*)–core protein VII (*yellow circles*) complex is transported through the nuclear pore; VII is released from viral genome during the early phase on infection. Immediate early E1A proteins are expressed first during infection and induce the expression of other early genes that facilitate viral replication and counteract cellular antiviral responses. Viral DNA replication proceeds, which triggers activation of the major late promoter and late gene expression. Progeny viruses are then assembled. Following encapsidation of the viral genome, the viral protease proteolyzes multiple viral proteins inside the virus particle to generate a mature virion that is released from the infected cell.

mature into early endosomes. Release of penton base, peripentoneal hexon trimers, and the internal capsid proteins IIIa, VI, and VIII occurs in the endosome.[104] Lysis of the endosome and release of partially uncoated virions into the cytosol is mediated by an N-terminal amphipathic helical, membrane lytic domain of protein VI.[321] Protein VI binds the internal side of the endosomal membrane and induces positive curvature strain that leads to membrane fragmentation.[192]

For adenovirus species A, B, C, and D, release of penton base and protein VI and lysis of endosomes are blocked by α-defensins, antimicrobial cysteine-rich peptides released from host neutrophils.[214,274] CryoEM and other studies indicate that thousands of defensin molecules bind to HAdV species A, B, C, and D (but not E or F) virions. Defensins bound at the interface between fiber and penton base are particularly important for inhibiting infection, by preventing the loss of the vertex

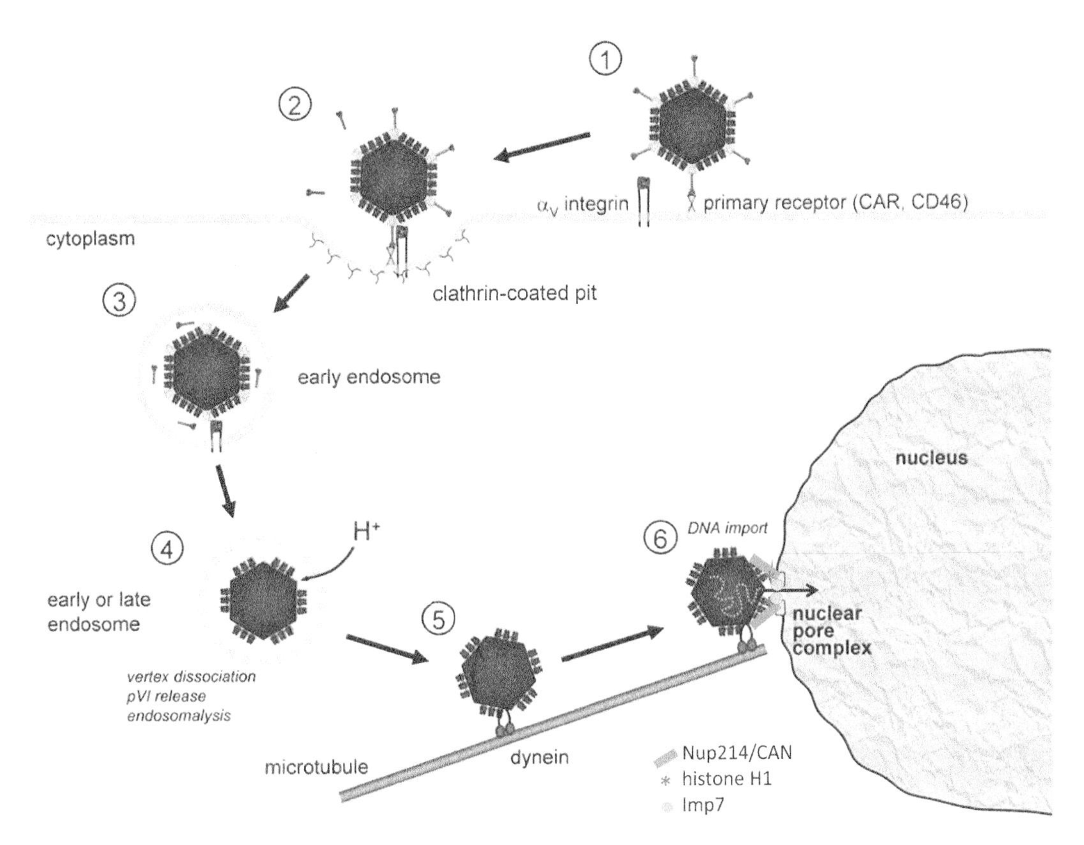

FIGURE 4.13 HAdV attachment, internalization, uncoating, intracellular transport. (1) The fiber knob binds to the primary cellular receptor, CAR (HAdV species A, C, D, E, F) or CD46 (HAdV species B); (2) The RGD loops of penton monomers (Fig. 4.5A) bind α_v integrins and stimulate endocytosis in clathrin-coated vesicles for species C; (3) Fibers begin to dissociate from pentons at the plasma membrane and completely dissociate in early endosomes; (4) The vertices of the particle composed of penton base and peripentoneal hexon trimers dissociate in endosomes, and the internal capsid proteins IIIa, VI, and VIII are released. Protein VI lyses the endosome, releasing the partially uncoated particle into the cytosol; (5) where it is transported on microtubules by dynein motor proteins to the microtubule organizing center and then associates with the cytoplasmic filament nucleoporin NUP214/CAN (6). The viral DNA bound by protein VII is then imported through the nuclear pore complex. (Reprinted from Nemerow GR, Pache L, Reddy V, et al. Insights into adenovirus host cell interactions from structural studies. *Virol* 2009;384:380–388. Copyright © 2008 Elsevier. With permission.)

region and therefore preventing escape of protein VI and endosome lysis.[274] As a consequence, virion-containing endosomes mature into late endosomes and fuse with lysosomes where virion proteins and DNA are degraded.[274]

In the absence of these host defenses, endosomal lysis occurs. The subvirion particles released into the cytosol are transported to the nucleus on microtubules[170,191] (Fig. 4.13). Fluorescently labeled virion particles were observed with live cell imaging to switch rapidly between minus-ended microtubule motility toward the juxtanuclear microtubule organizing center (MTOC) and plus-ended motility away from the nucleus. But transient activation of protein kinase A (PKA) by integrin signaling and activation of the p38 MAP kinase and its target MAPKAP kinase 2 (MK2) increased the frequency and velocity of minus-end directed movement of subviral particles by the dynein motor protein complex[293] until they reach the MTOC.[13] A neutralizing monoclonal antibody to hexon does not interfere with endosome lysis but rather blocks infection by inhibiting the association of virions with microtubules, suggesting that it is hexon that binds to microtubule motors.[273]

From the juxtanuclear MTOC, subvirion particles associate with NPCs[102] via an interaction between hexon trimers and the Phe-Gly repeat–containing domain of NPC cytoplasmic filament protein CAN/Nup214.[304] Surprisingly, the activity of exportin 1 (CRM1), a nuclear export factor, is required for this association with the cytoplasmic side of NPCs, since association of subvirion particles with NPCs is blocked by leptomycin B and ratjadone A, highly specific inhibitors of exportin 1, and by small interfering RNA (siRNA) to exportin 1.[291] How exportin 1 functions in this process is unclear.

The diameter of subviral particles bound to the NPC (~90 nm) is too large to pass through diffusional channels in the pore, approximately 5 to 9 nm.[2] Viral uncoating occurs at the nuclear pore as shown by exposure of core polypeptide VII and hexon epitopes that are hidden in intact virions.[102] FRET experiments with fluorescently labeled virions indicate that the half-time for disassembly of the icosahedral capsid, probably coincident with unpackaging at the NPC, is approximately 60 minutes.[198] Blocking NPC binding by microinjection of wheat germ agglutinin or specific antibodies that bind to central domains of the NPC blocks exposure of the VII and hexon epitopes, indicating that an interaction with the NPC is required to trigger final capsid disassembly.[102] This mechanism assures that viral DNA is released only at the NPC in preparation for transport into the nucleus. Nuclear import of the viral DNA core requires histone H1 and H1 import factors.[304]

Viral DNA bound by the major basic core protein VII enters the nucleus, while most hexon and protein IX remain associated with NPCs, indicating that the viral DNA–protein VII complex separates from the partially dissociated capsid during the nuclear import process.[43,102,281,333] The protein VII–viral DNA complex is imported into the nucleus in a Ran-dependent mechanism involving protein VII binding to the importin transportin.[121,324] Experiments with HAdV-C2 containing a green fluorescent protein V fusion protein indicate that core protein V remains on the cytoplasmic side of the NPC and does not enter the nucleus with the protein VII–viral DNA complex.[239] Protein VII remains associated with viral DNA during the early phase of infection and may be dissociated by transcription of the viral genome,[45] although this idea and how viral DNA is converted from a VII-bound state to a cellular histone–associated chromatin state are controversial.[97]

Adenovirus infection activates components of the innate immune response that recognize pathogen-associated molecular patterns (PAMPs), specifically endosomal and cytoplasmic viral DNA. Binding of purified recombinant HAdV-C5 fiber knob to the CAR receptor of human A549 lung carcinoma cells causes an increase in MAP kinases ERK1/2 and JNK activities minutes after addition to cells and NF-κB translocation to nuclei thereafter.[294] This is associated with the induction of proinflammatory chemokine gene expression. Toll-like receptor 9 (TLR9) is activated by viral DNA within endosomes in plasmacytoid dendritic cells (pDCs), resulting in the secretion of interferon alpha (IFNα).[15,39,130,348] Adenovirus DNA recognition in non-pDCs is TLR independent, via cytoplasmic sensing of viral DNA.[348] In some human cell lines, cytoplasmic viral DNA induces the activation of cGAS/STING, resulting in the phosphorylation and activation of TBK1 and IRF3 and the subsequent induction of IFNβ gene expression.[164] In human THP1 monocyte cells, infection with species B or C adenoviruses triggers the activation of the NLRP3 inflammasome to promote an innate response and IL-1β secretion.[210] Many studies have used murine models of human adenovirus infection. In mice, adenovirus infection induces the production of high levels of type I IFNs by pDCs, conventional DCs, and macrophages.[348] Additionally, adenovirus infection of murine antigen-presenting cells (APCs) and primary lung fibroblasts stimulates IRF3-mediated IFN and proinflammatory responses through a TLR-independent DNA-sensing mechanism[215] dependent on the cGAS-STING pathway.[164,348] These data demonstrate that in a cell type–specific manner, adenovirus uncoating stimulates innate antiviral cellular responses that induce IFN and inflammatory signaling pathways.

Early Gene Transcription

Core protein VII serves the crucial role of suppressing activation of the cellular DNA damage response (DDR) when the viral DNA first enters the nucleus.[146] In the absence of such protection, the cellular Mre11-Rad50-Nbs1 complex is activated by the termini of the viral DNA; if unabated, a DDR significantly inhibits viral DNA replication[317] (discussed below). Protein VII interacts with the cellular chromatin remodeling factor, template activating factor-I (TAF-I/SET), during the early phase of infection.[110,111,333] TAF-I/SET is a histone-binding chromatin remodeling factor. TAF-I/SET knockdown in adenovirus-infected cells results in a delay in transcription of early genes.[111] It is proposed that TAF-I/SET promotes the remodeling of the adenovirus protein VII–DNA complex into cellular histone–containing chromatin. Chromatin immunoprecipitation assays indicate that cellular histones replace much of protein VII early in infection, generating viral genomes bound by both VII and acetylated nucleosomes.[154] The DNA of an HAdV-C5 gene therapy vector is assembled into physiologically spaced nucleosomes containing histone H3.3, the isotype associated with transcribed cellular genes, dependent on the activity of the histone chaperone HIRA.[251] Protein VII-SET interaction also contributes to the ability of protein VII to inhibit DDR signaling pathways.[9] Protein VII interacts with cellular nucleosomes and alters chromatin composition and accessibility.[10] This includes proteins of the high-mobility group protein B (HMGB) family. HMGB1 is released in response to inflammatory stimuli and serves as a danger signal to trigger immune responses. Protein VII binds directly to HMGB1, sequesters HMGB1 in cellular chromatin, and inhibits its activity to block extracellular immune signaling.[10] Thus, core protein VII plays multiple important roles at early and late times after adenovirus infection.

The E1A region is the first region to be transcribed following infection[213] due to a constitutive transcriptional enhancer region located upstream of the E1A promoter.[117] The major cellular transcription factor that activates E1A expression via the enhancer is GABP, but a number of other transcription factors interact with this and flanking sequences including members of the ATF family, SP1, and E2F transcription factors to stimulate E1A expression.[35,114,176] Two major E1A mRNAs and encoded proteins are expressed early after infection by alternative splicing of a primary transcript, using either one of two 5′ donor splice sites and the same 3′ acceptor splice site[236] (Fig. 4.10, 13S and 12S E1A mRNAs). The protein encoded by the longer E1A mRNA has been termed large E1A, E1A 13S protein, and E1A 289R (289 amino acid residues). The protein encoded by the shorter E1A mRNA has been termed small e1a, E1A 12S protein, and E1A 243R. E1A 289R and E1A 243R will be used henceforth.

The E1A 289R protein transactivates the early region E1B, E2-early, E3, and E4 promoter regions (discussed below). The E1B transcription unit is located immediately to the right of the E1A region (Fig. 4.9). The E1B promoter is composed primarily of an SP1 transcription factor–binding site closely juxtaposed to a TATA box.[328] Additional transcription factor–binding sites in the 3′-end of the E1A transcription unit stimulate E1B transcription further.[230] Transcription of the E2 region peaks after the other early regions,[213] and while the other early regions continue to be transcribed throughout the late phase of infection, E2 transcription reaches much higher levels than the other early regions, in part because of the activation of a second E2 promoter, the E2-late promoter (Fig. 4.9). The E2-early promoter is composed of two binding sites for the E2F family of transcription factors in inverted orientation upstream of a TATA box and a binding site for the ATF family of transcription factors located upstream of the E2F sites.[159,169] The E2-late promoter extends upstream from the transcription start site and includes a TATA box, binding sites for two SP1 transcription factors, and two sites that bind CAAT box–binding factors.[25] The E3 promoter consists of a TATA box and upstream binding sites for transcription factors NF1, AP1, and ATFs.[129] In lymphoid cells, an upstream NF-κB site is critical for E3 expression.[322] The E3 region expresses a number of alternatively spliced mRNAs encoding proteins that inhibit innate and acquired immune responses to viral infection (discussed below). Consequently, activation of E3 by NF-κB, which activates multiple cellular genes involved in innate and acquired immune responses, likely functions in a regulatory feedback loop that protects virus-infected cells from host antiviral mechanisms. The E4 promoter region contains a TATA box and binding sites for multiple transcription factors including E4F, E4TF1, ATFs, and GABP.[35,169,315] The E1A enhancer region also activates all of the adenovirus early promoter regions *in cis*.[118]

Although early and late are conventional terms for events that occur during the replication cycle, the functional distinction between early and late genes is often blurred. Early genes continue to be expressed at late times after infection, and the promoter controlling expression of the major late transcription unit directs a low level of transcription early after infection. Also, the viral genes encoding proteins IVa2, pIX, L4-22K, and L4-33K are expressed at an intermediate time, thus forming a delayed-early or intermediate expression category.

Functions of Adenovirus Early Proteins

E1A

There are three main outcomes of adenovirus early gene expression. First, the host cell is induced to enter S phase of the cell cycle, providing an optimal environment for viral replication. E1A and E4 gene products play roles in this process. Second, various antiviral defenses of the host cell and organism are inhibited. The E1A, E1B, E3, and VA RNA genes contribute to these defenses. Third, viral gene products required for viral DNA replication are synthesized. E2 encodes the viral replication proteins.

Both E1A 289R and 243R proteins share regions that are conserved across adenovirus species and include conserved region 1 (CR1) and CR2 in the 5′ exon and CR4 in the 3′ exon (Fig. 4.14). In addition, E1A 289R contains CR3 corresponding to the unique sequences in this protein. Three additional, alternatively spliced E1A mRNA species designated 9S, 10S, and 11S accumulate at later times in the infectious cycle that contains the same 3′ exon but have additional sequences spliced out of the 5′ exons.[285] However, no functions have been described for products of these mRNAs.

The E1A 289R and E1A 243R proteins can each stimulate G_0- and G_1-arrested cells to enter S phase in the absence of other mitogenic signals via the conserved sequences that they share.[211,241,282] Presumably, this reflects the situation when HAdV-C2 and HAdV-C5 infect differentiated, G_0-arrested upper respiratory tract epithelial cells. Induction of cellular DNA synthesis requires E1A protein interactions with the abundant, closely related nuclear lysine acetyl transferases p300 and CBP (KAT3B, KAT3A) and the retinoblastoma family proteins pRb (RB1), p107 (RBL1), and p130 (RBL2).[151] E1A proteins interact with p300/CBP via sequences at the N terminus and CR1 and bind RB family proteins via CR1 and CR2 (Fig. 4.13). E1A binds to Rb family members using sequences in CR1 and a conserved LXCXE motif in CR2 that interacts

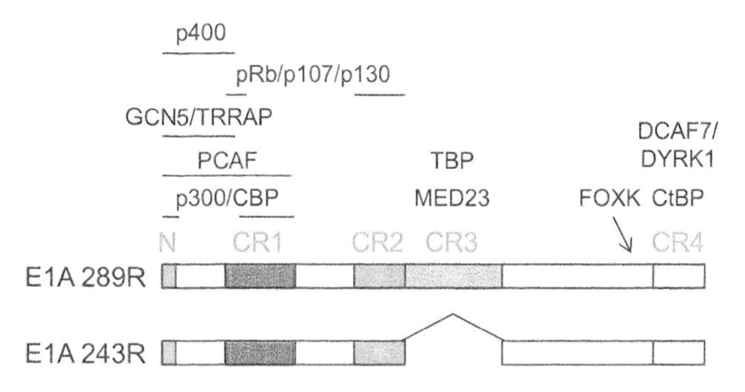

FIGURE 4.14 Protein–protein interaction domains of the E1A protein. Extensively conserved amino acid sequences in the primate adenoviruses are designated CR1 (*red*), CR2 (*blue*), CR3 (*orange*), and CR4 (*yellow*) and the conserved N-terminal region is indicated (*green*). N-terminal, CR1, and CR2 sequences that mediate interactions with cellular binding proteins are indicated by horizontal lines with the proteins listed above. MED23 and TBP bind to CR3. CtBP and DYRK1/DCAF7 bind to CR4 and FOXK protein interacts with sequences just N-terminal of CR4.

with the pocket domain of Rb family proteins (Fig. 4.15).[73] The transforming proteins of other DNA tumor viruses, polyomavirus large T antigen and papillomavirus E7 proteins, use the same conserved sequence for interactions with Rb family proteins.[151] The E2F family of transcription factors control genes required for entry into S phase.[147] Rb family proteins interact with E2F transactivators via the central Rb pocket domain and the C-terminal regions of E2Fs, which contain the transactivation domain. Rb proteins mask the E2F transactivation domain and recruit transcriptional repressors (e.g., HDACs) to promoter regions.[66] E1A binds to the Rb pocket region with high affinity and displaces Rb family proteins from E2Fs by competitive interaction with the same Rb pocket sequences that bind to the E2F transactivation domain[12] (Fig. 4.15). The interactions of E1A with p300/CBP and Rb family members induce cell proliferation and are required for transformation of primary cells,[74,124,318] and these E1A protein interactions induce global changes in the localization of these transcriptional regulators throughout the host cell genome to alter cellular gene expression patterns.[81]

A series of reports have defined how the adenovirus E1A proteins positively and negatively regulate cellular gene expression. In quiescent mouse cells, the promoter regions of the cell cycle–regulated genes Cdc6 and cyclin A are bound by E2F4 associated with p130 and the histone deacetylation complex HDAC1/2–mSin3B to repress gene expression.[96] These promoter regions also are associated with the Suv39H1 histone methylase transferase, which methylates histone H3 lysine 9 (H3K9), generating binding sites for the repressive heterochromatin protein 1 (HP1).[96,269] E1A expression leads to the loss of repressive E2F4–p130 complexes and replacement with activating E2Fs 1, 2, and 3 and the acetylation of H3K9.[96,269] This was not observed with an E1A CR2 mutant that does not bind Rb family proteins.[96] An N-terminal E1A mutant that does not bind the histone acetyl transferase/chromatin remodeling complex containing TRRAP–PCAF–p400[89] displaces the E2F4–p130 corepressor complex but does not induce acetylation of H3K9, transcription of the Cdc6 and cyclin A genes, and entry into S phase.[269] These results demonstrate that E1A induces cells to enter S phase by reconfiguring chromatin structure on

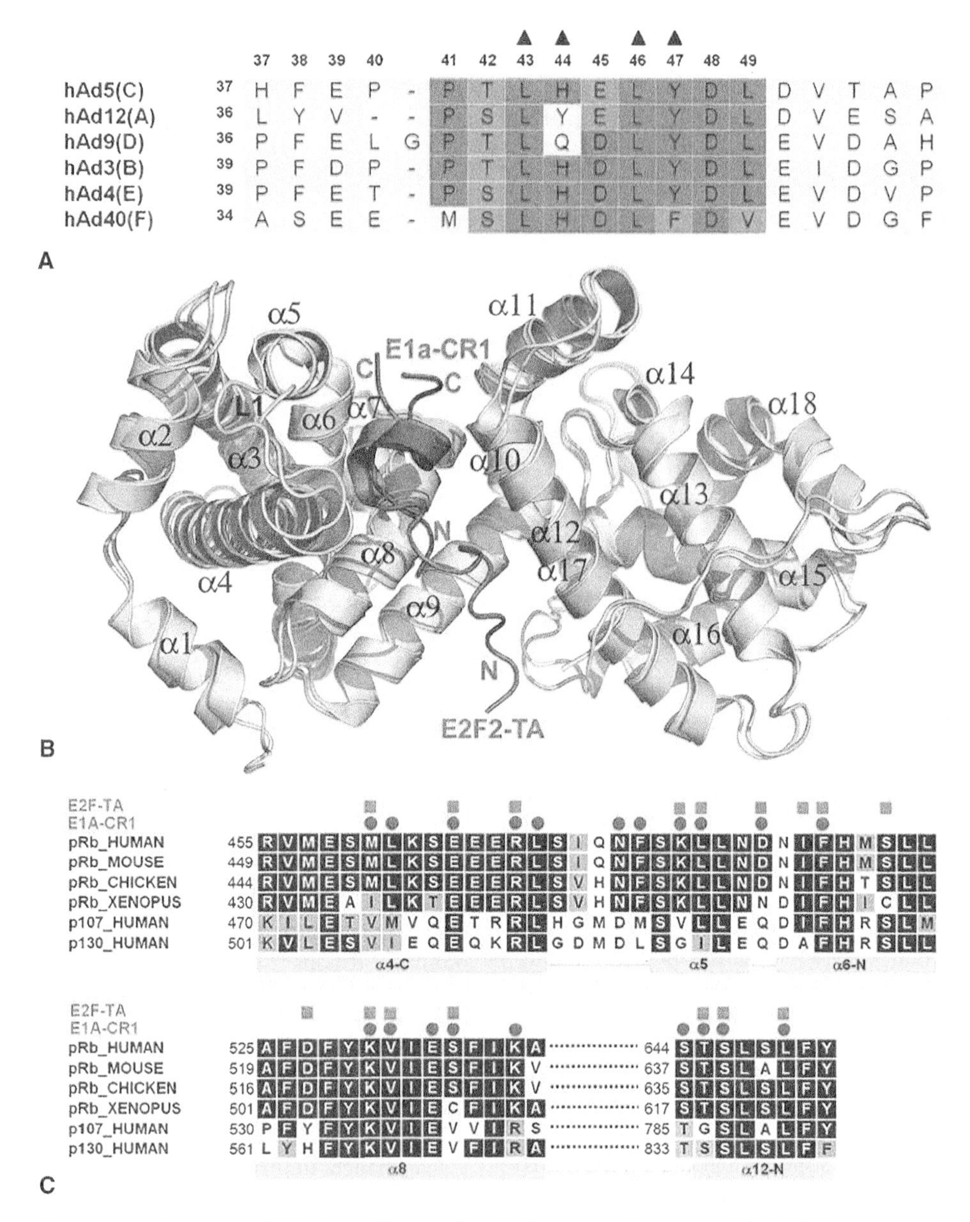

FIGURE 4.15 **Structure of the E1A–Rb complex. A:** Sequence alignment of E1A CR1 from different adenovirus types/species. Invariant and conserved CR1 residues are highlighted in *dark* and *light purple*, respectively. Residues indicated by *solid triangles* are involved in pRb interaction. **B:** Ribbon diagram of the E1A CR1–Rb and E2F2-TA–Rb structures with E1A CR1 and E2F2-TA are shown in *purple* and *red*, respectively. **C:** Sequence alignment of human pRb paralogs and pRb orthologs from selected species. Residues that mediate interaction with E1A CR1 and E2F2-TA are marked with *purple* circles and *red* squares, respectively. (Reprinted with permission from Liu X, Marmorstein R. Structure of the retinoblastoma protein bound to adenovirus E1A reveals the molecular basis for viral oncoprotein inactivation of a tumor suppressor. *Genes Devel* 2007:21:2711–2716, with permission. Copyright © 2007 Cold Spring Harbor Laboratory Press.)

specific cellular promoter regions both by displacing repressive E2F4 complexes via interaction with Rb family proteins and by inducing H3 acetylation using the TRRAP–PCAF–p400 complex.[96,269]

Genomic studies with an HAdV-C5 mutant virus that expresses the E1A 243R but not the E1A 289R protein revealed that, remarkably, E1A 243R associated with the promoters of most cellular genes in a specific temporal order, either activating or inhibiting their expression.[81] In quiescent primary human fibroblasts, the E1A 243R protein was associated with the promoter regions of genes involved in cell cycle, and DNA, RNA, and protein synthesis, amounting to approximately 30% of all cellular genes. The E1A 243R protein directed the enrichment of p300/CBP and PCAF, the depletion of Rb family proteins, and the acetylation of histone H3K18 at these genes, resulting in their transcriptional activation.[81] Induction of many of these genes also was observed in quiescent human fibroblasts infected with HAdV-C5.[204] The E1A 243R protein was also associated with the promoters of genes involved in inflammation and other defenses against pathogens (~20% of cellular genes) causing the enrichment for pRb, p130, the acetylation of histone H4K16, and transcriptional repression.[81] Repression of genes involved in innate immune responses, inhibition of cell cycle progression, and induction of genes involved in metabolic pathways contributing to cell growth also were observed after infection of HeLa cells with HAdV-C2.[99,345] At later times after infection of growth-arrested primary human fibroblasts, E1A 243R and p107 associated with the remaining approximately 50% of genes involved in differentiated cell functions and repressed their transcription.[81] The E1A 243R protein represses the expression of a specific set of cellular genes (e.g., cytokine signaling pathway genes such as TGFβ and TNF) via an E1A–p300–pRb complex that specifically interacts within the transcribed sequences of these genes.[80] The E1A–p300–pRb complex condenses cellular chromatin dependent on the lysine acetyl transferase activity of p300 associated with E1A and pRb acetylation.[80] These novel and important results revealed specific epigenetic reprogramming of cellular gene expression by the E1A 243R protein dependent on interactions with p300/CBP and Rb family proteins. Further, the results suggested that after E1A dissociates Rb family proteins from E2F4 and other transcription factors to induce cell proliferation, it also exploits the same Rb family proteins to repress antiviral response genes and differentiated cell functions that may otherwise inhibit virus replication.

The E1A 289R protein autoactivates transcription of the E1A region approximately fivefold and stimulates transcription from the E1B, E2 early, E3, and E4 regions from tenfold (E1B) to hundredfold (E2-early, E3, and E4).[206] Activation requires a stable, highly specific interaction of E1A CR3 with the MED23 subunit of the human mediator transcription complex.[31,286] E1A CR3 transcriptional activation domain interaction with MED23 both increases the assembly of preinitiation complexes on promoters and stimulates transcriptional elongation.[36,312] The zinc finger in E1A CR3 binds to the TATA-binding protein, TBP, and other components of the TFII-D general transcription factor complex, stimulating the formation of an RNA polymerase II preinitiation complex.[94,95] The E1A 289R protein does not bind to DNA directly but may be recruited to promoter regions via interaction with several cellular transcription factors, including members of the ATF family, AP1, USF, and SP1.[176,177,290] E1A may recruit positive (e.g., p300/CBP) or negative (e.g., Rb family members) regulators of transcription in conjunction with these cellular factors, activating or repressing gene expression, respectively. In addition, a glutamic acid–proline repeat, AR1, immediately C terminal to CR3 in HAdV-C2 and HAdV-C5 E1A, is essential for E1A 289R activation of the early adenovirus promoters.[290]

E1A CR4 (Fig. 4.14) contains a nuclear localization signal (NLS) at the very C terminus.[189] The E1A 243R protein is sufficient to immortalize primary rodent cells *in vitro* and promote oncogenic transformation in conjunction with another oncogene such as Ad E1B 55K or activated H-Ras.[255] Sequences in the C-terminal exon of the E1A 243R protein reduce transformation in these assays, since specific CR4 mutant proteins displayed augmented transformation properties.[49] The C-terminal region of the E1A proteins binds to a number of cellular proteins including forkhead transcription factors FOXK1/K2, protein kinase DYRK1A and cofactor DCAF7, and the transcriptional repressor C-terminal–binding protein (CtBP). DYRK1A/DCAF7 and CtBP bind to sequences within CR4, while FOXK1/K2 interacts with sequences just N terminal of CR4. The C-terminal transformation repression function was originally attributed to interaction with CtBP, which binds to the highly conserved sequence PXDLS present in all primate adenoviruses.[49] CtBP is a transcriptional corepressor. A complex picture has emerged concerning the regulation of E1A immortalization and transformation functions by these C-terminal–binding proteins. Initially, the interaction of E1A CR4 with CtBP was found to be important for transformation of primary rodent cells by HAdV-C2 E1A and E1B, whereas CtBP binding negatively regulated E1A-mediated tumorigenesis and metastasis in cooperation with oncogenic H-Ras.[49] More recent studies have presented somewhat divergent views of these processes, with one report suggesting that E1A–CtBP interaction suppresses both immortalization and oncogenic H-Ras transformation of primary rodent cells without significantly affecting tumorigenicity,[292] whereas another study concluded that the interaction of E1A with DYRK1A/DCAF7 plays an important role in E1A 243R suppression of transformation by activated H-Ras while CtBP was not involved.[54] A third study concluded that E1A interaction with either FOXK1/K2 or DYRK1A/DCAF7 decreases oncogenic transformation.[155] These discrepancies may reflect differences in the types of transformation and oncogenicity assays used as well as differences in specific E1A C-terminal mutants. The results may indicate functional redundancy in the interaction of E1A with the three different cellular protein complexes FOXK1/K2, DYRK1A/DCAD7, and CtBP. Finally, the interaction of E1A with CtBP was shown to enhance replication during HAdV-C5 infection of normal human bronchial epithelial cells, and consistent with this result, CtBP knockdown in human U2OS osteosarcoma cancer cells also augmented the virus replication cycle.[292]

In a separate study, the role of E1A CR4–binding partners in the regulation of cellular gene expression was examined.[339] Growth-arrested primary human epithelial cells were infected with HAdV-C5 E1A CR4 mutant viruses containing specific amino acid substitutions individually within the FOXK1/K2, DYRK1A/DCAF7, or CtBP-binding sites and RNA-seq was conducted to analyze changes in cellular gene expression compared to wild-type HAdV-C5. Comparing E1A CR4 mutant viruses to wild-type HAdV-C5, only a small number of genes showed altered expression, but of those genes, a large overlap was observed with genes that were overexpressed with all three individual CR4 mutants.[339] Some of these genes encode proteins that have antiviral functions, and their promoter regions are enriched for IFN-stimulated response elements. Further analyses showed that the E1A CR4 mutant viruses activate transcription of a subset of IFN-stimulated genes (ISGs). Expression of these ISGs was mediated by an increase in protein levels of the transcription factor IRF3 and IRF3 bound to the promoters of the activated ISGs.[339] CR4 mutant viruses with combinations of these mutations displayed the same phenotype as did the individual mutants, indicating that all three CR4 cellular proteins function as a complex. This idea was supported by protein biochemical experiments.[339] These results demonstrate that wild-type E1A suppresses the expression of ISGs and that the CR4 mutants are not able to do so. Further, the results suggest that FOXK1/K2, DYRK1A/DCAF7, and CtBP bind coordinately to the C-terminal region of E1A and that disruption of any one interaction relieves E1A repression of all three activities.

The adenovirus E1A proteins are well characterized for their ability to block IFN signaling pathways and the induction of ISG expression. Early studies in cancer cell lines demonstrated that HAdV-C5 infection, or HAdV-C5 E1A expression alone, blocked the induction of ISG expression by IFNα.[246] This was the result of reduced formation of the ISGF3 complex due to decreased levels of its constituent proteins.[108,142] Inhibition of ISG expression also correlated with E1A binding to p300/CBP.[252] Different results were found in primary human airway epithelial cells, in which E1A blocked IFN-induced ISG expression by direct interaction with STAT1 via E1A N-terminal sequences.[184] E1A expression also resulted in down-regulation of STAT1 phosphorylation.[184] Cancer cell lines have altered signal transduction pathways and likely respond to viral infection in different ways compared to primary cells. Recently, E1A was found to inhibit ISG expression via the cellular DNA-dependent ATPase RuvBL1.[217] The RVB complex is required for efficient activation of ISG expression during type I IFN signaling.[98] The C-terminal region of E1A binds RuvBL1, and E1A–RuvBL1 complexes bind to the promoter regions of ISGs to repress their activation.[217]

Modification of histones by ubiquitin marks transcriptionally active chromatin.[332] In a study to analyze if HAdV-C5 regulates histone modification, global ubiquitylated histone 2B levels were compared for wild-type HAdV-C5 and an E1A-null mutant virus.[84] The HAdV-C5 E1A mutant virus strongly induced H2B ubiquitylation at lysine 120 (H2B-K120) in primary and transformed human cells, but wild-type HAdV-C5 did not. A similar induction of H2B ubiquitin levels was observed following type I IFN treatment; E1A expression alone reversed this effect.[84] Human Bre1/RNF20 is an E3 ubiquitin ligase that monoubiquitylates H2B-K120. The N-terminal region of E1A binds to hBre1/RNF20 and blocks the interaction between hBre1 and the ubiquitin conjugase catalytic subunit Ube2b.[84] This results in the inhibition of histone 2B monoubiquitylation at ISG promoter regions and an inhibition of ISG induction following type I IFN treatment. Subsequent studies showed that E1A also utilizes hBre1 to recruit the RNA polymerase II transcription elongation factor hPaf1 to adenovirus early promoter regions, stimulating viral gene expression.[83] These studies demonstrated how the E1A proteins co-opt cellular transcriptional regulators to promote viral gene expression and inhibit the expression of cellular genes involved during innate responses to infection, in this case specifically during type I IFN signaling.

While the E1A proteins were originally described as activators of viral early gene expression, it is clear that an important effect of the E1A proteins is the down-regulation of innate cellular responses to infection, particularly with respect to different aspects of IFN signaling. E1A proteins block cytoplasmic IFN signaling pathways, inhibiting the cellular response to infection, and they down-regulate mechanisms that are used by the cell to promote ISG expression in the nucleus. In addition, a recent study suggests that IFN inhibition of viral gene expression may promote persistent adenoviral infection.[347]

E1B

The E1B region encodes two abundant spliced mRNAs (13S and 22S), encoding proteins commonly referred to as E1B 19K and E1B 55K (Fig. 4.10). The level and activity of the tumor suppressor p53 are induced by the abnormal stimulation of the cell cycle induced by the E1A proteins.[65,186] The E1B 19K and E1B 55K proteins inhibit p53-dependent induction of apoptosis by different mechanisms. E1B 19K is homologous to cellular BCL-2 family of proteins and functions as a viral mimic of MCL-1, an antiapoptotic member of the BCL-2 family.[58] MCL-1 binds to the proapoptotic BCL-2 family members BAK and BAX, preventing them from co-oligomerizing and forming pores in the outer mitochondrial membrane. Apoptosis is induced following infection with an E1B 19K mutant virus because the critical cellular antiapoptotic BCL-2 family member MCL-1 is degraded by the proteasome.[57] In the absence of E1B 19K, formation of such BAK–BAX pores in the outer mitochondrial membranes of infected cells releases apoptogenic proteins such as cytochrome c and Smac/DIABOLO, leading to the activation of caspase-9 and caspase-3 and the ensuing apoptotic program.[58] This pathway is blocked in wild-type virus-infected cells by the sequestration of activated BAK and BAX by E1B 19K.

p53 function is directly inhibited by the E1B 55K protein through multiple mechanisms. Like SV40 large T antigen, the E1B 55K protein binds the tumor suppressor p53.[22] E1B 55K binds to the amino terminus of p53, which also contains the p53 activation domain and the region bound by MDM2, the major ubiquitin ligase controlling p53 proteasomal degradation.[145,174] As a result, p53 is stabilized and transcriptional activation by p53 is inhibited.[334,335] The E1B 55K protein functions as an E3 SUMO1 (small ubiquitin-like modifier) ligase for p53,[232] resulting in the sumoylation of approximately 1% of p53 and association of the complex with promyelocytic leukemia protein (PML) nuclear bodies.[208,232] Sumoylation of a small fraction of a nuclear protein can result in the association of nearly all of the nuclear protein with PML nuclear bodies, based on higher-order protein–protein interactions.[115] In the case of the E1B 55K–p53 complex, this can be explained by the formation of a large network of p53 tetramers cross-linked by the binding of E1B 55K dimers[197] and the binding of sumoylated E1B 55K[75,323] to SUMO-interaction motifs in the PML protein within PML nuclear bodies. Association of E1B 55K–SUMO1 complexes with PML nuclear bodies promotes E1B 55K nuclear export by exportin 1 (CRM1).[149,160,232] In cells transformed by E1A and E1B, or when E1B 55K is expressed in the absence of other viral proteins, E1B 55K–p53 complexes exported to the cytoplasm are transported on microtubules by dynein motor proteins to the microtubule organizing center (MTOC) where they accumulate, forming large cytoplasmic inclusion bodies,[338] termed aggresomes, and are targeted for degradation.[180,232]

The HAdV-C5 E1B 55K protein also forms a complex with the E4 ORF6 protein. This complex associates with cellular proteins elongins B and C, cullin 5, and Rbx1 to form an E3 ubiquitin ligase that polyubiquitinates p53, leading to its proteasomal degradation[109,240] (Fig. 4.16). E1B 55K also binds the host cell Mre11-Rad50-Nbs1 (MRN) complex through a distinct region from the E1B 55K region that binds p53.[267] The MRN complex functions as a sensor of DNA damage, activating a DDR and cell cycle checkpoint signaling.[317] If activated, a cellular DDR significantly inhibits adenovirus DNA replication and results in an abortive viral infection. The E1B 55K–E4 ORF6 ubiquitin ligase complex plays a pivotal role among all species of adenoviruses to prevent a DDR from occurring.[317] E1B 55K–MRN complexes also associate with PML nuclear

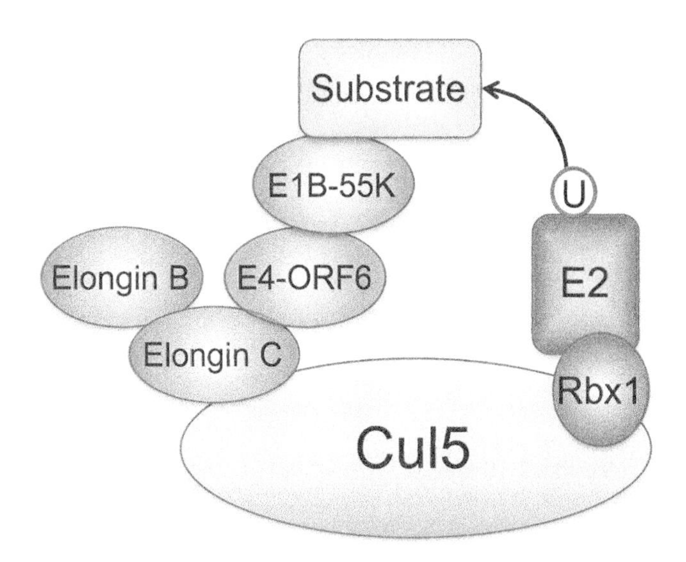

FIGURE 4.16 **The HAdV-C5 E1B 55K–E4 ORF6 ubiquitin ligase complex.** The E1B 55K–E4 ORF6 ubiquitin ligase complex is depicted with Cul5, elongins B and C, Rbx1, E4 ORF6, E1B 55K, ubiquitin (U), and substrate shown. The model of the E1B 55K–E4 ORF6 ubiquitin ligase complex is hypothetical and based on the crystal structure of the Cul1-Rbx1-Skp1-F boxSkp2 SCF[346] ubiquitin ligase complex.

bodies and subsequently are exported to aggresomes at the MTOC.[180] The HAdV-C5 E1B 55K–E4 ORF6–elongin B/C–cullin 5–Rbx1 ubiquitin ligase also polyubiquitinates subunits of the MRN complex, inducing their proteasomal degradation.[288] During infection, MRN complex components and p53 are first inhibited by being sequestered into PML nuclear bodies and then by their nuclear export and proteasomal degradation. This prevents them from interacting with nuclear substrates, and transport to the MTOC accelerates the rate of their degradation; proteasomes and components of the ubiquitination pathway are concentrated at the MTOC.[180] The E1B 55K–E4 ORF6 ubiquitin ligase complex also targets other proteins involved in the DNA damage response, including DNA ligase IV[14] and the Bloom helicase.[219] The interaction of these two proteins with the termini of adenovirus genomes would be expected to interfere with viral DNA replication. Integrin α3 was identified as another substrate of this viral ubiquitin ligase.[63] Additional substrates targeted for degradation by the E1B 55K–E4 ORF6 ubiquitin ligase complex include Tankyrase 1–binding protein 1, Tip60, SPOC1, ATRX, SMARCAL1, ALCAM, EPHA2, and PTPRF.[279] Interestingly, the E1B 55K–E4 ORF6 proteins of other Ad serotypes form ubiquitin ligase complexes with either Cul2 or Cul5, which directs their substrate specificity; all of the E1B 55K–E4 ORF6 complexes target components of the DNA damage response, ensuring efficient viral DNA replication.[47,48,86] In an E4 ORF6–independent manner, HAdV-C5 E1B 55K targets the chromatin remodeling factor Daxx for proteasomal degradation.[266] While it is not clear why all of these substrates are targeted for degradation, several of them (Tip60, SPOC1, and Daxx/ATRX) function as intrinsic cellular activities that limit viral early gene expression and virus replication.

The E1B 55K–E4 ORF6 ubiquitin ligase complex is required for the inhibition of host mRNA nuclear export and the nuclear export of viral late mRNAs during the late phase of infection,[29,327] but the relevant substrate involved in nuclear export of cellular and viral mRNAs remains to be identified. Finally, E1B 55K counteracts the inhibition of Ad replication by type I IFNs in normal human cells by inhibiting ISG induction.[41] This function requires the transcriptional repression domain of E1B 55K[40] but is independent of the formation of the E1B 55K–E4 ORF6 ubiquitin ligase complex.[41] In the absence of E1B 55K, type I IFNs inhibit viral DNA replication, although viral replication protein expression is similar compared to that of the wild-type virus.[41]

E2

E2 encodes the three viral proteins required for adenovirus DNA replication, pTP, Ad-Pol, and DBP. DBP, encoded in the E2A region, is required in much larger amounts than the Ad-Pol or the pTP encoded in the E2B region (Fig. 4.9). Greater levels of E2A mRNAs, which encode DBP, are expressed than the E2B mRNAs as the result of alternative polyadenylation of the E2 primary transcript, most frequently at the E2A polyadenylation site near 62 map units. Some E2 primary transcripts are spliced to exons at 39 and then 29 map units to generate pTP mRNAs or to exons at 39 and then 23 map units to generate Ad-Pol mRNAs (Fig. 4.9). The E2B mRNAs utilize the same polyadenylation site as the IVa2 mRNA expressed at intermediate times postinfection. The mechanism of Ad DNA replication is discussed below.

E3

The proteins encoded by the E3 region provide protection of infected cells from innate and adaptive host immune responses[173] (Fig. 4.17). The HAdV-C2 and HAdV-C5 E3-gp19K protein is a type I glycoprotein localized in the endoplasmic reticulum (ER). E3-gp19K binds to major histocompatibility complex class I (MHC-I) heavy chain in the ER, prevents transport of MHC-I to the cell surface by virtue of an ER-retrieval signal on E3-gp19K, and prevents killing of Ad-infected cells by cytotoxic T lymphocytes.[173] E3-gp19K and its function are conserved among all human adenovirus species, except species A,[88] in which the E1A proteins cause down-regulation of MHC-I expression.[138] E3-gp19K binds with higher affinity to HLA-A than it does to HLA-B, and it binds poorly if at all to HLA-C.[88] E3-gp19K binds via a domain conserved among adenovirus serotypes to the outer surface of the peptide-binding groove on MHC-I molecules.[181] E3-gp19K also binds to TAP (transporter associated with processing), prevents formation of the TAP–tapasin complex, and limits the inclusion of TAP into the peptide-loading complex of antigenic peptide, MHC-I, and chaperones.[19] This property of E3-gp19K could retard cell surface expression of MHC-I in individuals with HLA-B and HLA-C MHC-I molecules. Reduced expression of MHC-I could render infected cells susceptible to killing by natural killer (NK) cells. Further, the E1A proteins up-regulate ligands recognized by the NKG2D receptor on NK cells and sensitize the E1A-expressing cells to NK cell–mediated cell lysis.[202,253] Multiple ligands for NKG2D are known, including the MHC-I chain–related A (MICA) and B (MICB) proteins. As is the case with MHC-I, E3-gp19K causes retention of MICA and MICB in the ER, prevents their transport to the cell surface, and reduces killing of E3-gp19K–expressing cells by NK cells.[202]

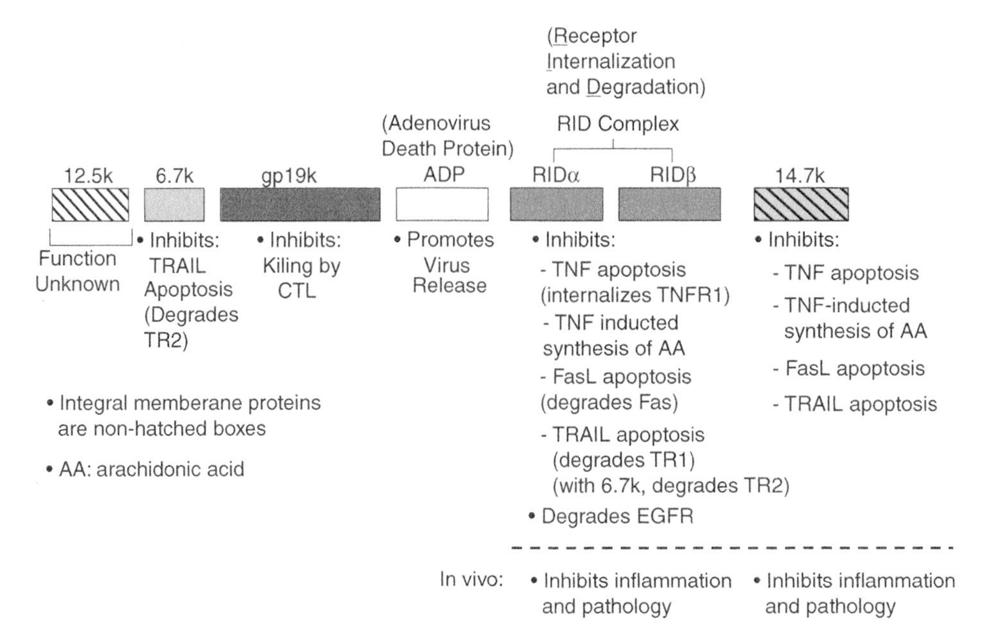

FIGURE 4.17 Schematic illustrating the E3 proteins and their functions. Each colored bar represents a protein with the name of the protein given above. Colored bars without hatches designate integral membrane proteins.

The E3-14.7K protein inhibits TNF-induced cytolysis of adenovirus-infected cells.[173] E3-14.7K binds to cellular IKKγ/NEMO, modulating NF-κB activity and inhibiting TNF-induced apoptosis, and it also binds to caspase 8 (FLICE) and inhibits Fas ligand–induced apoptosis.[173] In addition, E3-14.7K inhibits internalization of TNF receptor 1 and the formation of the death-signaling complex (DISC) that is required for TNF-induced apoptosis.[265] E3-14.7K also inhibits the activity of cytoplasmic phospholipase A2 blocking TNF-induced cell lysis and TNF-induced release of arachidonic acid,[173] a property that might be important in reducing inflammation.

The E3-10.4K protein and the E3-10.4K/E3-14.5K complex clear the epidermal growth factor receptor (EGFR) from the cell surface.[173] The E3-10.4K and E3-14.5K proteins were later renamed RIDα and RIDβ (receptor internalization and degradation), respectively, when it was shown that these proteins also cause the internalization and lysosomal degradation of not only EGFR but also cell surface Fas, TRAIL receptor 1, and TNF receptor 1.[173] RID inhibits cytolysis induced by Fas ligand and TNF. RID, functioning in concert with the E3-6.7K protein, also down-regulates TRAIL receptor 2 from the cell surface.[173] RID inhibits TNF-induced translocation of cytosolic phospholipase A_2 to membranes from where arachidonic acid is generated,[173] and it inhibits lipopolysaccharide- and interleukin-1β–mediated signaling responses.[68] Thus, both RID and E3-14.7K might function *in vivo* to inhibit inflammatory responses associated with infection. RIDα has been reported to function independently of RIDβ to down-regulate EGFR.[173]

The E3-6.7K protein alone inhibits apoptosis induced through Fas, TNF receptor, and TRAIL receptors and prevents TNF-induced release of arachidonic acid.[205] Further, E3-6.7K interacts with calcium modulator and cyclophilin ligand (CAML), a calcium-modulating protein, preventing calcium efflux from the ER, maintaining calcium homeostasis and inhibiting apoptosis induced by thapsigargin, which inhibits calcium uptake by the ER.[205]

The E3 adenovirus death protein (ADP) is an 11.6-kD integral membrane, palmitoylated glycoprotein that is expressed most abundantly at late times after infection from the major late promoter; ADP promotes the efficient lysis of cells late after infection, allowing virus release and dissemination.[173]

E4

The HAdV-5 E4 region encodes six identified proteins named based on their open reading frame numbers (E4 ORF1, E4 ORF2, E4 ORF3, E4 ORF4, E4 ORF6, and E4 ORF6/7) (Fig. 4.18). The E4 proteins have a variety of functions. HAdV-D9 induces mammary fibroadenoma tumors in female rats[135] and the E4 region is required.[136] The HAdV-D9 E4 ORF1 protein is an oncogene and transforms cells in culture and promotes mammary tumors in rats.[134] The oncogenic properties of E4 ORF1 map in part, to a C-terminal PDZ-binding domain that interacts with cellular PDZ-containing proteins such as DLG, MUPP1, MAGI1, and ZO2.[137] E4 ORF1 proteins from adenoviruses of species A–D were found to activate PI3K, but only HAdV-D9 E4 ORF1 both transforms cells in culture and promotes tumors in animals; E4 ORF1 proteins from species A–C have limited transformation potential.[87] The E4 ORF1 PDZ-binding domain is required for PI3K activation, which stimulates activation of downstream effector protein kinases PKB and S6K.[87] HAdV-D9 E4 ORF1, DLG1, and PI3K form a ternary protein complex that localizes to the plasma membrane to activate PI3K, and the ability of E4 ORF1 to transform human epithelial cells in culture is ablated by a PDZ-domain mutation that blocks DLG1 and PI3K binding and by inhibitors of PI3K activity.[156] Interestingly, the ability of E4 ORF1 to activate PI3K via DLG1 binding and membrane localization is a conserved function with adenoviruses of species A–D, although the oncogenic potential for mammary

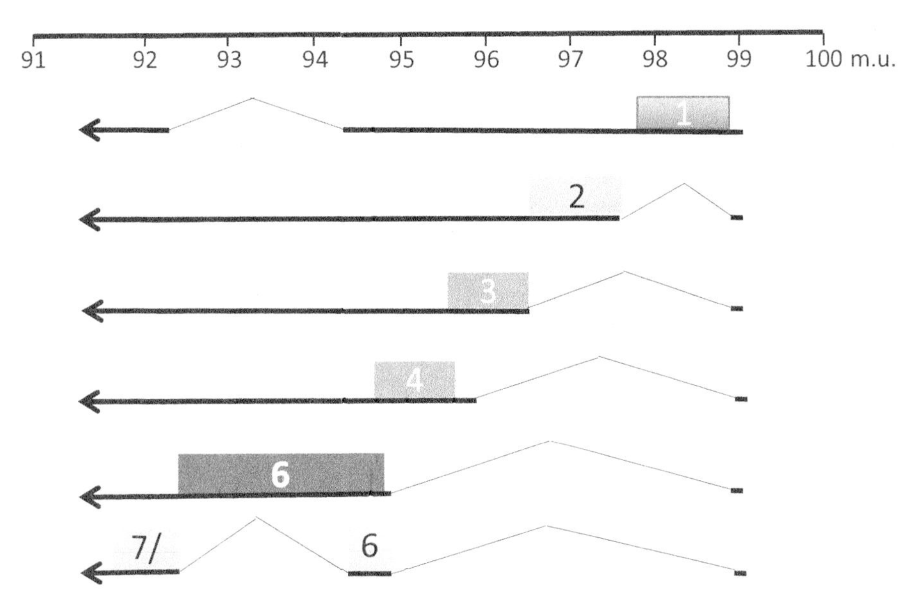

FIGURE 4.18 HAdV-C2 E4 mRNAs and proteins. The E4 open reading frames are designated above the ORFs. Alternative pre-mRNA splicing locates the first AUG of each E4 open reading frame near the 5′ end of the respective mRNA. E4 ORF7 is translated as a fusion with the N-terminal part of ORF6 fused in-frame with ORF7. Additional mRNAs not shown encoding E4 ORF1, –ORF3, and -ORF4 additionally are spliced to remove the intron that fuses ORFs 6 and 7.

tumor formation is unique to the HAdV-D9 E4 ORF1 protein.[161] The lack of oncogenic potential of the E4 ORF1 protein of nonspecies D adenoviruses may be due to poor protein expression in rat cells with species A–C E4 ORF1 proteins.[316]

The HAdV-C5 E4 ORF1 and E4 ORF4 proteins activate the protein kinase mTOR in the absence of nutrient and mitogenic signaling.[221] Activated mTOR stimulates protein synthesis by phosphorylating and inhibiting 4EBP1, an inhibitor of the eIF4E cap-binding translation initiation factor.[259] Activated mTOR also phosphorylates and activates S6K, which stimulates translation by phosphorylating ribosomal protein S6 and additional targets, leading to increased synthesis of ribosomes and translation factors.[259] Mitogens activate mTOR by activating PI3K through a pathway involving AKT and PKB, the tumor suppressor complex TSC1–TSC2, and the Ras-family GTPase Rheb that ultimately leads to mTOR activation.[259] E4 ORF1 stimulates PI3K, resulting in Rheb-GTP loading and mTOR activation.[221] Human epithelial cells infected with wild-type HAdV-C5, but not a complete E4-null virus, have increased glycolytic metabolism with elevated glucose consumption and lactate production, and decreased oxygen consumption.[296] The E4 ORF1 protein is sufficient to induce this glycolytic flux. Surprisingly, this effect does not require the PDZ-binding domain of E4 ORF1, indicating that this effect is independent of PI3K activation.[296] E4 ORF1 binds to the transcription factor MYC in the nucleus and augments MYC binding to promoters of glycolytic genes resulting in their elevated expression.[296] An HAdV-C5 E4 ORF1 mutant (D68A) was identified that did not enhance glycolytic metabolism. By comparing cells infected with the E4 ORF1 D68A mutant virus to wild-type HAdV-C5 infection, increased glycolytic metabolism was found to significantly enhance viral DNA replication, possibly due to increased nucleotide pools.[296] Subsequently, HAdV-C5 infection was found to alter host cell glutamine utilization and increase expression of glutamine transporters and glutamine catabolism enzymes.[297] Consequently, there were increased intracellular levels of both essential and nonessential amino acids in HAdV-C5–infected cells compared to those in uninfected cells or cells infected with the E4 ORF1 D68A mutant virus.[297] This effect required E4 ORF1, MYC activation, and it promoted optimal adenovirus replication.[297] The ability of E4 ORF1 to activate constitutive epidermal growth factor and insulin receptor signaling contributes to MYC activation, a function that is conserved among different adenovirus species.[157] Collectively, these results show how adenovirus infection subverts cellular metabolism, similar to that which occurs in cancer cells, to optimize conditions for viral replication.

There is no functional activity to date linked with E4 ORF2.

The E4 ORF3 protein is multifunctional. It functions by forming a multimeric protein scaffold in the nucleus of infected cells and sequestering cellular proteins into these structures to block their activities. These E4 ORF3 filamentous structures have often been referred to as nuclear tracks. This was first described with the reorganization of PML nuclear bodies (PML-NB), also known as PML oncogenic domains (PODs), or ND10,[37,72] where E4 ORF3 is both necessary and sufficient for this to occur (Fig. 4.19). The reorganization of PML-NB requires higher-order multimerization by E4 ORF3.[228,231] E4 ORF3 interacts with PML isoform II, mediating PML-NB disruption and inhibiting the activity of PML-II as part of an innate response to infection.[8,123] PML-NB have antiviral properties, particularly with DNA viruses, both intrinsically and following induction by IFNs.[262] E4 ORF3 inhibits PML-NB antiviral activity.[307,308]

The E4 ORF3 protein of species C adenoviruses inhibits a DDR. In this way, E4 ORF3 and E4 ORF6 display redundant activities, since inhibition of a DDR is the most critical aspect of E4 function *in vitro*.[33,126] E4 ORF3 directs the relocalization of MRN complex proteins into PML-containing nuclear tracks

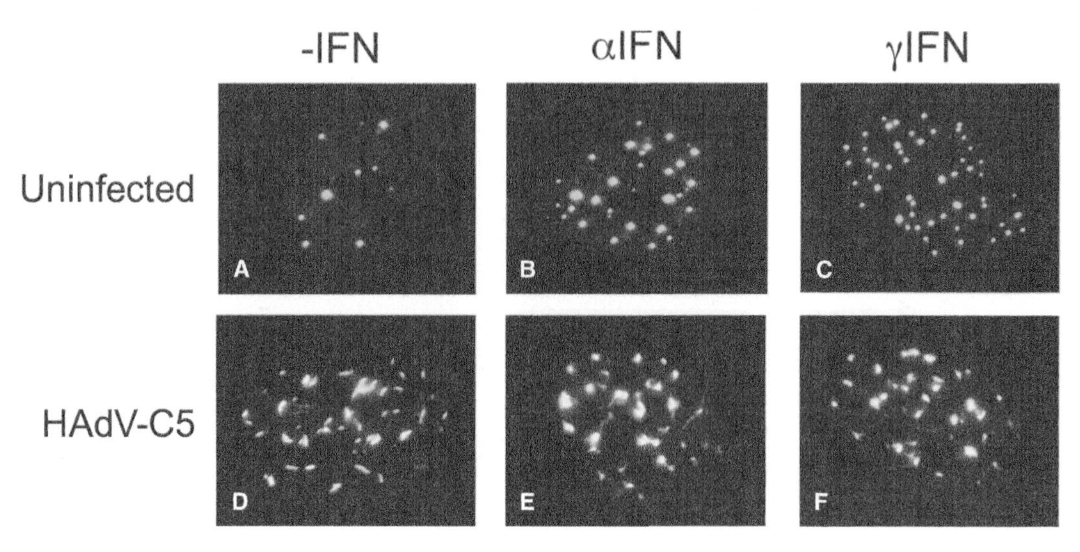

FIGURE 4.19 **HAdV-C5 E4 ORF3 rearranges PML-NB during an IFN response.** Vero cells seeded onto coverslips and were untreated **(A, D)**, or pretreated with IFNα **(B, E)** or IFNγ **(C, F)** for 24 h. Subsequently, the cells were left uninfected **(A–C)** or infected with HAdV-C5 **(D–F)**. At 18 h after infection, the cells were immunostained for PML (FITC, *green*) and E4 ORF3 (TRITC, *red*). The images represent a merge of compressed, deconvolved Z stacks. (Adapted from Ullman AJ, Reich NR, Hearing P. The adenovirus E4 ORF3 protein inhibits the interferon-mediated antiviral response. *J Virol* 2007;81:4744–4752.)

to sequester and block their activity.[77,288,289] It is curious that this function is only conserved among species C E4 ORF3 proteins, since inhibition of a DDR is so crucial for viral replication, although this activity is redundant with MRN degradation by the E1B 55K–E4 ORF6 ubiquitin ligase complex that is more widely conserved. The E4 ORF3 protein inhibits p53 signaling by inducing the formation of heterochromatin at p53-induced promoter regions, thereby blocking p53 DNA binding and transactivation.[280] Once again, this E4 ORF3 activity parallels, and perhaps complements, the inhibition of p53 by E1B 55K alone and the E1B 55K–E4 ORF6 complex.

E4 ORF3 induces SUMO modification of Mre11 and Nbs1 in virus-infected cells.[277] Protein sumoylation regulates diverse processes including protein–protein interaction, subcellular localization, protein stability, and enzymatic activity.[343] Ad infection, or E4 ORF3 expression alone, causes a dramatic reorganization of endogenous SUMO1 and SUMO2/SUMO3 into nuclear tracks.[277] A proteomic study identified multiple cellular proteins whose sumoylation is increased upon Ad5 E4 ORF3 expression.[276] Many of the E4 ORF3 SUMO substrates are involved in a DDR. Like ubiquitylation, sumoylation is carried out by a cascade of enzymatic steps.[343] Biochemical studies using an *in vitro* SUMO conjugation assay demonstrated that E4 ORF3 functions as a SUMO E3 ligase.[278] Several substrates whose sumoylation is increased by E4 ORF3 (e.g., TFII-I and TIF-1γ) are subsequently degraded by the ubiquitin–proteasome pathway in the absence of any other viral proteins.[34,85] E4 ORF3 SUMO ligase activity is conserved across the human adenovirus species.[275] The E4 ORF3 protein does not possess any of the typical domains of SUMO E3 ligases, but E4 ORF3 interacts with the SUMO E2 conjugation enzyme UBC9 along with noncovalently bound SUMO. E4 ORF3 oligomerization is critical for this ternary binding to occur, and this interaction correlates directly with E4 ORF3 E3 SUMO ligase activity.[275] These results are consistent with a model whereby E4 ORF3 serves as a platform for SUMO modification by mediating colocalization of components of the SUMO conjugation machinery with target substrate proteins.

The E4 ORF4 protein regulates multiple different aspects of the adenovirus replication cycle including viral and cellular gene expression,[18,30] alternative pre-mRNA splicing[76,144] (see Regulation of RNA Splicing During the Late Phase), protein translation,[209,221] and cell death.[171,271] The E4 ORF4 protein binds to the substrate-binding β subunits of the trimeric protein phosphatase PP2A family,[153] and all E4 ORF4 activities are attributed to this interaction. PP2A is a highly abundant serine/threonine protein phosphatase with broad-based activity affecting metabolism, RNA splicing, translation, development, and cell cycle progression. E4 ORF4 induces death in transformed cells that is independent of p53 and involves noncanonical programmed cell death.[167,195,270] E4 ORF4 is redundant with E4 ORF1 in stimulating mTOR activity, and this requires PP2A binding, although E4 ORF4 does not affect Rheb-GTP levels, and mTOR activation is independent of PI3K and AKT.[221] How this interaction leads to mTOR activation is not understood, but it seems likely that alterations in the substrate specificity or activity of PP2A are involved.[342] Finally, the E4 ORF4 reduces the phosphorylation of the DDR effector protein kinases ATM and ATR, inhibiting a DDR in adenovirus-infected cells, and consequently sensitizes cells to DNA-damaging agents.[32]

The E4 ORF6 protein was discussed earlier in the context of E1B 55K and the E1B 55K–E4 ORF6 ubiquitin ligase complex (Fig. 4.16). E4 ORF6 also has unique functions. E4 ORF6 interacts with and inhibits p53 independently of E1B 55K.[71] E4 ORF6, but not E1B 55K, also can bind to p73 and inhibit p73 function.[119,196,284,320] The p73 protein is a member of the p53 family that is able to activate transcription through p53 response elements. p73 is transcriptionally induced by the E1A 243R protein, probably through E2F-binding sites associated with one of its two alternative promoters.[82] Thus, E4 ORF6 antagonizes the function of both p53 and p73, blocking their potential inhibitory effects on viral replication. Finally, HAdV-A12 E4 ORF6 targets DNA topoisomerase II–binding protein 1 (TOPBP1), a DDR protein, for CUL2-based degradation independent of E1B 55K.[27]

E4 ORF7 is expressed as a fusion with the N-terminal region of E4 ORF6 by alternative pre-mRNA splicing and results in the translation of a protein called E4 ORF6/7 (Fig. 4.18). E4 ORF6/7 forms a dimer that binds to E2F transcription factors, greatly increasing their affinity for the E2-early promoter by cooperative binding to inverted E2F-binding sites.[127] This serves as an important transcriptional activator of the E2-early promoter.[131] E4 ORF6/7 also can displace Rb family proteins from E2Fs by competitive binding with the E2F–pRb interface and functionally substitute for this E1A activity, stimulating viral replication.[216] Finally, E4 ORF6/7 also can activate the cellular E2F-1 promoter by the same mechanism.[261]

Viral DNA Replication

Adenovirus DNA replication occurs by a mechanism requiring a minimal set of viral replication proteins: pTP, Ad-Pol, and DBP. The ITRs serve as the replication origins. Viral DNA replication takes place in two stages[168] (Fig. 4.20). First, synthesis is initiated at either terminus of the linear DNA and proceeds in a continuous fashion to the other end of the genome. The products of this stage of replication are a duplex consisting of a parental and daughter strand plus a displaced single strand of parental DNA. In the second stage, a complement to the displaced single strand is synthesized. The single-stranded template circularizes through annealing of its self-complementary ITRs. The resulting duplex "panhandle," in the otherwise single-stranded circle, has the same structure as the termini of the duplex viral genome. This structure is recognized by the same initiation machinery that operates in the first stage of replication, and complementary strand synthesis generates a second completed duplex consisting of one parental and one daughter strand.

Three functional domains have been defined within the terminal 51 bp of species C adenovirus ITRs.[42] Nucleotides 1 to 18 contain the minimal core sequences sufficient for origin function, although at low levels of activity. The sequence between base pairs 9 to 18 (5′-ATAATATACC-3′) is conserved among different human adenovirus species, and a complex of pTP and Ad-Pol binds to this region.[295] Nucleotides 19 to 40 and 41 to 51 contain binding sites for cellular proteins NFI (CTF, CCAAT box transcription factor) and NFIII (Oct-1, octamer-binding protein 1), respectively. These cellular transcription factors significantly stimulate core origin activity. The DNA-binding domain of NFI interacts with Ad-Pol, and the DNA-binding domain of Oct-1 binds to pTP.[140] The binding of NFI is stimulated by DBP.[140] The resulting protein–DNA and protein–protein interactions stabilize binding and properly position the pTP–Ad-Pol complex at the genome termini. pTP is synthesized as an 80-kD polypeptide that is active in the initiation of DNA replication. It is subsequently processed by AVP proteolysis at three sites during assembly of virions to generate a 55-kD fragment (TP) that is covalently attached to the genome within the viral capsid. Ad-Pol is a 140-kD protein in the eukaryotic Polα family.[179] Like other Polαs, Ad-Pol contains both 5′ to 3′ DNA polymerase activity and 3′ to 5′ exonuclease activity; the latter serves a proofreading function during DNA replication.[150] The error rate of Ad-Pol is estimated at 1.3×10^{-7} per bp per infection cycle.[248]

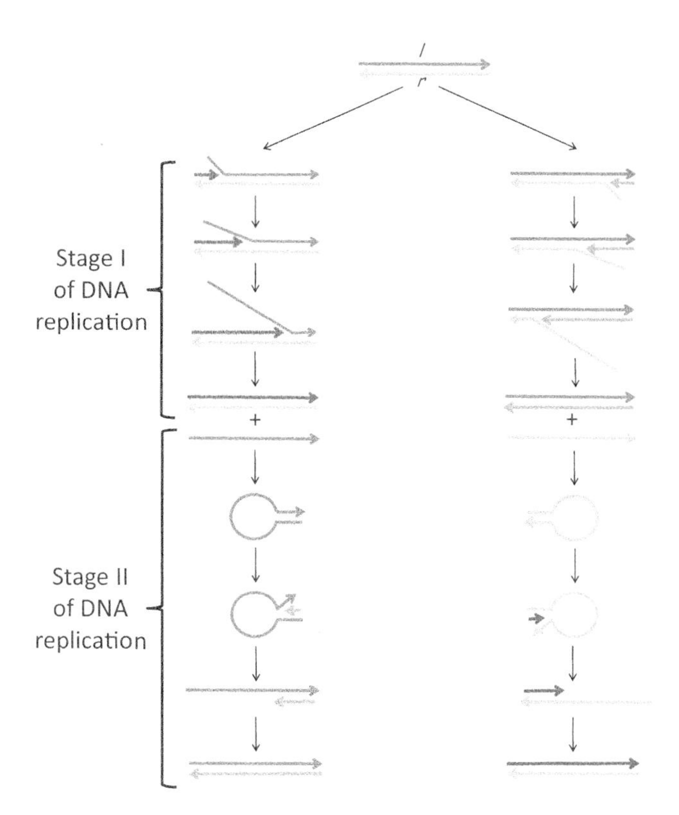

FIGURE 4.20 Mechanism of adenovirus DNA replication. With molecules where replication is initiated at the right end, the *l* parental strand is replicated displacing the *r* parental strand; with molecules where replication is initiated at the left end, the *r* parental strand is replicated displacing the *l* parental strand. Replication beginning at the left end is shown on the left column and beginning at the right end is shown on the right column. Replication occurs in two stages: synthesis of the entire length of one strand (Stage 1), followed by synthesis of the entire length of the complementary strand (Stage 2). Replication is primed by the pTP protein (not shown) covalently attached to dCMP whose 3′-OH group is extended by Ad-Pol. One entire strand is displaced as ssDNA. A "panhandle" structure is formed when the left end and right end ITRs of this molecule base pair generating a double-stranded ITR identical to that contained in the parental genome. Note that unlike the mechanism for replication of most other DNA molecules, lagging-strand synthesis does not occur as short Okazaki fragments that are ligated together. (Adapted from Lechner RL, Kelly TJ Jr. The structure of replicating adenovirus 2 DNA molecules. *Cell* 1977;12:1007–1020. Copyright © 1977 Elsevier. With permission.)

As a protein primer, pTP preserves the integrity of the viral genome termini during multiple rounds of DNA replication. The priming reaction begins with the formation of an ester bond catalyzed by the Ad-Pol between the β-OH of serine residue 580 in pTP and the α-phosphoryl group of deoxycytidine monophosphate (dCMP), the first residue at the 5′ end of the DNA chain.[42] pTP melts the end of the DNA duplex, allowing the template strand to enter the active site of the polymerase. The 3′-OH group of the pTP–dCMP complex then serves to prime synthesis of the nascent strand by Ad-Pol.[42] Replication and late transcription take place in large nuclear domains called replication compartments or replication centers.[238] pTP association with the insoluble nuclear matrix fraction[260] may help to localize the viral replication centers. In addition, pTP binds to the multiprotein pyrimidine biosynthesis enzyme CAD (carbamyl phosphate synthetase, aspartate transcarbamylase, and dihydroorotase).[6] CAD colocalizes with pTP and viral replication compartments on the nuclear matrix.[6] pTP–CAD interaction may anchor viral genomes at the nuclear matrix and in proximity to nucleotides and other factors required for replication.

Chain elongation requires viral Ad-Pol, DBP, and cellular topoisomerase I.[42] DBP binds tightly and cooperatively in a sequence-independent fashion to single-stranded DNA. The three-dimensional structure of the C-terminal DBP DNA-binding domain sufficient for *in vitro* replication was determined by x-ray crystallography.[305] The DBP C-terminal domain has a flexible hinge that hooks onto an adjacent DNA-binding protein monomer. This drives the formation of long, multimeric DBP chains bound to single-stranded DNA. Polymerization of the DNA-binding protein on single-stranded DNA drives strand separation, consistent with the lack of a requirement for a DNA helicase to unwind the double-stranded template at the growing fork in reconstituted DNA replication reactions.[67] In the presence of DBP, Ad-Pol is highly processive and can travel the entire length of the chromosome after it has separated from pTP.[42] Topoisomerase I enhances the synthesis of nascent chains greater than 9 kbp long; hence, it must be needed to overcome a DNA structural problem that arises only after extensive replication.

Late Gene Transcription

Adenovirus late genes begin to be actively expressed at the onset of viral DNA replication. The adenovirus late coding regions are organized into a single large transcription unit with the major late promoter (MLP) directing the initiation of an approximately 28 kb pre-mRNA.[349] The MLP exhibits low activity early after infection but becomes several hundred-fold more active on a per DNA molecule basis at late times. This primary transcript is processed by differential use of five polyadenylation sites to generate late mRNA families L1–L5 and extensive alternative splicing to generate multiple distinct mRNA sites[349] (Fig. 4.9). The mechanism that prevents RNA polymerase II elongation past the L1 region during the early phase is poorly understood, as is the mechanism that relieves this inhibition during the late phase. The processed L1–L5 mRNAs all contain a 201-nucleotide (nt) untranslated tripartite leader (TPL) sequence generated from the splicing of three short exons[21,51] (Fig. 4.9). Different open reading frames in each late mRNA family are accessed by alternative RNA splicing of donor splice sites at the 3′ end of the third tripartite leader exon to different splice acceptor sites within L1–L5 that define the 5′ end of the protein-coding exon(s) (Fig. 4.9). There appear to be at least two distinct components that contribute to the delayed activation of the major late promoter during infection: a *cis*-acting change in the viral chromosome dependent on viral DNA replication[299] and transactivation by two viral proteins, IVa2 and L4-22K, synthesized at intermediate times postinfection.[336] The IVa2 and L4-22K proteins stimulate transcription from the MLP by binding to sites in the first intron between TPL exons 1 and 2.[336] These two proteins also bind cooperatively to repeated sequences at the left end of the genome to promote packaging of viral DNA into capsids (see Virion Assembly).

Regulation of RNA Splicing During the Late Phase

Three viral proteins, E4 ORF4[76,144] and the L4-33K and L4-22K proteins,[26] remodel the host cell splicing machinery, regulating the splicing of viral pre-mRNAs, and likely cellular pre-mRNAs, during the late phase of infection. During the late phase, alternative splicing of the L1 pre-mRNA is regulated by L4-33K, shifting expression from the L1-52/55K protein to L1-IIIa.[302] The L4-33K protein regulates this splicing via the sequence immediately upstream of the L1-IIIa 3′ acceptor splice site, functioning as a splicing enhancer that induces splicing to this site.[302] Early during infection, host cell SR proteins bind to a sequence just upstream from the IIIa splicing branch point, blocking binding of the U2 snRNP to the L1-IIIa 3′ acceptor splice site.[143] Dephosphorylation of host SR proteins dependent on E4 ORF4 relieves this inhibition of L1-IIIa splicing.[144] Since the phosphorylation of serine–arginine–rich (SR) proteins is required for their association with consensus splicing signals, the dephosphorylation and inactivation of SR proteins may contribute to the inhibition of host cell gene expression during the late phase.[144] Several other 3′ acceptor splice sites in the MLP pre-mRNA with short polypyrimidine tracts also are activated during the late phase of infection, probably through similar mechanisms to the control of the L1-IIIa splice site.[1] Finally, during the intermediate stage of infection, the L4-22K protein (Fig. 4.11) is translated from an mRNA expressed from the L4P promoter, termed L4P, that is embedded in the upstream coding region of L4-100K[207] (Fig. 4.9). The L4-22K protein directs splicing of the L4-33K pre-mRNA.[105] As described above, the L4-33K protein in turn regulates splicing of other adenovirus late transcripts. Analysis of an HAdV-C5 L4-22K mutant virus demonstrated that only L4-33K transcripts, and transcripts for the adjacent L4-pVIII protein, are regulated by L4-22K.[105] Thus, while both L4 proteins are splicing regulators, they clearly have different targets. There is an exquisite level of regulation that takes place during the late phase of adenovirus infection that precisely coordinates the cascade of late viral gene expression. This represents an elegant feedback loop that finely tunes the temporal switch of gene expression patterns during the late phase of infection.

Regulation of Translation

During the early phase of infection, viral early mRNAs are translated along with the continued translation of host cell mRNAs. During the late phase of infection, however, translation of host cell mRNAs is significantly inhibited, and virtually all translation is dedicated to late viral mRNAs, especially mRNAs containing the TPL sequence.[60] In addition to their facilitated transport from the nucleus to the cytoplasm, viral late mRNAs are preferentially translated when they reach the cytoplasm.[16] During this period, when viral mRNAs constitute about 20% of the total cytoplasmic mRNA pool, they are translated to the exclusion of host mRNAs.[11] The inhibition of host mRNA translation results from the inhibition of cap-dependent translation. eIF4E, the translation initiation factor that binds the 5′-^{m7}GpppN cap structure on most cellular mRNAs, is dephosphorylated at late times after adenovirus infection.[128] eIF4E is a subunit of eIF4F multiprotein complex, which functions as a cap-dependent RNA helicase to unwind secondary structures at the 5′ ends of mRNAs and promote recruitment of the 40S ribosomal subunit and scanning to the translation initiation codon.[133] Dephosphorylation of eIF4E inhibits the interaction of the eIF4F complex with capped mRNAs, thus inhibiting all cap-dependent translation.[128]

In uninfected cells, eIF4E is phosphorylated by the protein kinase Mnk1, which is thought to allow tighter binding to cap structures.[133] During the late phase of adenovirus infection, the L4-100K protein binds to eIF4G, displacing Mnk1 kinase and resulting in reduced eIF4E phosphorylation.[59] Late viral mRNAs transcribed from the major late promoter continue to be translated because of the 5′ TPL.[183] The TPL promotes cap-independent translation by two mechanisms. First, the TPL promotes an alternative form of translation initiation referred to as ribosome shunting.[337] Rather than scanning from the 5′ cap to the initiation codon, the 40S ribosomal subunit binds the TPL and is translocated to the translation initiation codon without scanning the 5′ untranslated region. Ribosome shunting is largely dependent on three regions of the TPL that are complementary to the 3′ end of 18S rRNA, evoking a mechanism of translation initiation similar to that in bacteria.[337] Similar complementarity between the 5′ untranslated region of the IVa2 mRNA and 18S ribosomal RNA also promotes ribosome shunting and maintains IVa2 translation during the late phase.[337] In addition to the structure of the TPL, L4-100K is required for the stimulation of translation by the TPL during the late phase of infection.[116] L4-100K binds both the TPL and the eIF4G scaffolding subunit of eIF4F, thereby directly stimulating ribosome shunting.[331] The TPL also stimulates late mRNA export from the nucleus during the late phase, possibly through an interaction with L4-100K.[125]

VA RNAs

The small, abundant VA RNAs were named when their viral origin was still uncertain. Different adenovirus species encode one or two VA RNAs; HAdV-C2 and HAdV-C5 encode two VA RNAs termed VAI and VAII. The VA RNAs are each about 160 nt in length, are GC rich, adopt stable secondary structures that are important for their function, and are transcribed by host cell RNA polymerase III.[309] VA RNA synthesis begins during the early phase of infection and dramatically accelerates during the late phase as the viral DNA template is amplified. VAI accumulates to about 10^8 molecules per infected HeLa cell, roughly the abundance of ribosomes, and VAII reaches about 10^7 molecules per cell.[309]

The function of VA RNAs was first discovered by analysis of a mutant HAdV-C5 virus in which the VAI gene was deleted.[298] The VAI mutant virus grew poorly and displayed greatly reduced levels of viral late proteins. Further studies identified a defect in protein initiation[264] resulting from phosphorylation of the eukaryotic initiation factor-2 (eIF-2) α subunit.[247,263] eIF-2 binds to guanosine triphosphate (GTP) and the initiator tRNA to form a ternary complex, which then interacts with the 40S ribosomal subunit. When the 40S ribosomal subunit binds the initiation codon, eIF-2 hydrolyzes the GTP to GDP and leaves the 40S subunit with the initiator tRNA in the ribosomal P site. Subsequent steps in the initiation process involving additional factors result in the binding of the 60S ribosomal subunit and chain elongation.[133] For eIF-2 to participate in another round of translation initiation, GDP must be replaced with GTP in a reaction catalyzed by eIF-2B, a guanosine nucleotide exchange factor. This exchange reaction is inhibited by phosphorylation of the eIF-2 α subunit. Phosphorylated eIF-2-α forms a tight complex with eIF-2B, preventing it from cycling and catalyzing the exchange reaction.[133] As a result, global translation initiation is inhibited when about one-third to one-half of eIF-2 is phosphorylated, trapping all available eIF-2B.

Phosphorylation of eIF-2 is mediated by the cellular protein kinase PKR. Synthesis of an inactive form of PKR is induced by IFN and the latent PKR enzyme phosphorylates eIF-2α when activated by dsRNA.[309] It is presumed that the symmetrical transcription of the adenovirus genome gives rise to dsRNA. PKR is activated by transautophosphorylation when two molecules of PKR interact with one molecule of dsRNA.[309] The highly abundant VAI RNA adopts a tertiary structure with extensive base pairing (Fig. 4.21) that binds PKR in monomeric form and blocks PKR activation by preventing PKR dimerization.[152] VAI RNA thereby blocks the antiviral effect of dsRNA and the antiviral effect of IFN. In contrast to VAI, an HAdV-C5 VAII mutant virus grows normally.[298]

Both VAI and VAII RNAs inhibit the processing of cellular microRNAs (miRNAs).[5,187] miRNAs are approximately 22 nucleotide RNAs incorporated into RNA silencing complexes (RISC) that inhibit translation of mRNAs to which they base pair with a small number of base-pair mismatches.[310] They are transcribed as long precursors called pri-miRNAs and processed by the nuclear enzyme Drosha into approximately 65 nucleotide stem-loop RNAs called pre-miRNAs. pre-miRNAs are exported from the nucleus to the cytoplasm where they are further processed by the ribonuclease Dicer into the approximately 22 nucleotide miRNAs incorporated into RISC complexes.[310] RISC complexes can also be programmed by siRNAs that have the characteristics of products of Dicer digestion: approximately 22 bp dsRNAs with two base 3′ single-stranded regions. When the siRNA in an RISC complex hybridizes to perfectly complementary regions of an mRNA in vertebrate cells, the RISC complex cleaves the mRNA, initiating its rapid degradation by exonucleases.[310]

VA RNAs are synthesized in the nucleus and transported into the cytoplasm by the same exportin that transports pre-miRNAs. During the late phase of adenovirus infection, the abundantly expressed VA RNAs interfere with the nuclear export of pre-miRNAs by competing with them for binding to exportin-5.[187] VA RNAs in the cytoplasm also bind to Dicer and competitively inhibit pre-miRNA processing.[5,187] The competitive inhibition of pre-miRNA nuclear export and cytoplasmic processing by VA RNAs interferes with the expression of cellular miRNAs. Since Dicer is a critical enzyme in processing dsRNA into miRNAs and siRNAs, the VA RNAs are expected to interfere with endogenous miRNA activities and siRNA interference that might result from adenovirus-specific dsRNAs. Deep RNA sequencing during the course of HAdV-C2 infection of normal, quiescent human lung fibroblasts demonstrated the deregulation of cellular miRNA expression during different phases of infection with both up-regulation and down-regulation of specific cellular miRNAs.[344] A number of these miRNAs are associated with the control of cell growth, but the functional consequences of these changes remain to be determined.

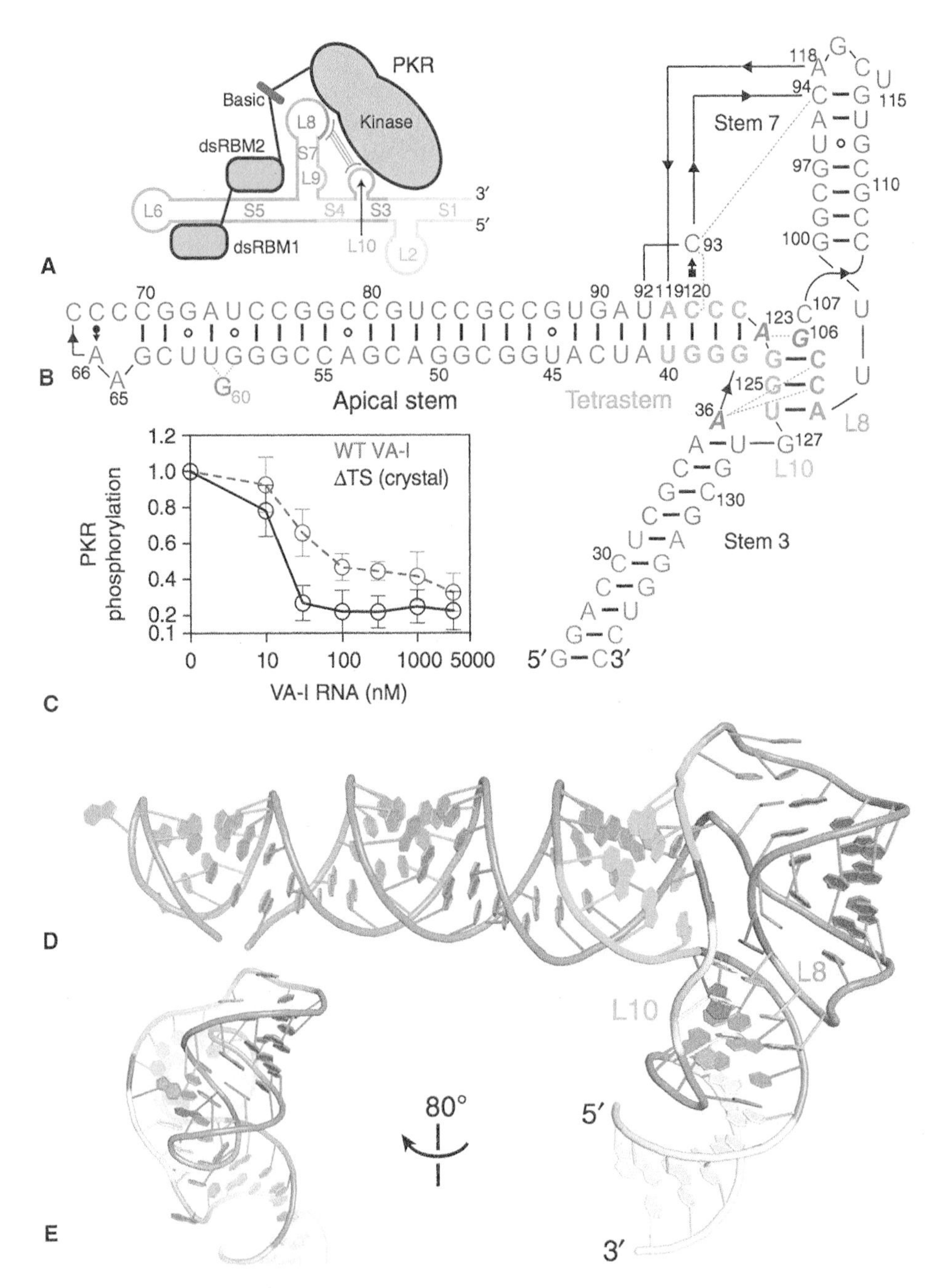

FIGURE 4.21 **HAdV-C2 VA RNA. A:** Schematic diagram of HAdV-C2 VA RNAI and binding to PKR. Stem structures are indicated by S designations and loops are indicated by L designations. S1 and L2 are absent from the VAI crystal structure. Double-stranded RNA-binding motifs are labeled dsRBM1 and dsRBM2. Base pairing between loops 8 and 10 is indicated by *triple red lines*. **B:** VAI RNA secondary structure derived from the crystal structure. Base pairing is indicated by lines and open circles between individual bases. Arrows designate adjacent residues. Base pairing between residues in loop 8 (*violet*) and loop 10 (*orange*) are shown with helix capping residues indicated in *red*. Wild type VAI residues are shown in blue; synthetic sequences used for the replacement of S1 and L2 are shown in *gray*. **C:** Inhibition of PKR phosphorylation by wild-type VAI and the truncated VAI used for crystallography. **D and E:** Ribbon diagram of the three-dimensional structure of HAdV-C2 VAI RNA. (Reprinted from Hood IV, Gordon JM, Bou-Nader C, et al. Crystal structure of an adenovirus virus-associated RNA. *Nature Commun* 2019:10:2871. https://creativecommons.org/licenses/by/4.0/.)

Virion Assembly

The replication of viral DNA, coupled with the production of large quantities of the adenovirus structural and assembly proteins, sets the stage for virion production. The multifunctional L4-100K protein functions as a chaperone in the folding of the trimeric hexon protein.[38] Penton capsomeres consisting of a pentameric penton base and trimeric fiber assemble in the cytoplasm, subsequently joining to form a complete penton capsomere. Hexon and penton capsomeres are imported into the nucleus, where assembly of the virion occurs.

The adenovirus genome is packaged into capsids in a polarized manner starting at the left end of the genome.[224] Extensive mutational analysis of the HAdV-C5 genome showed that seven AT-rich sequences, termed A repeats, with the consensus sequence 5′-TTTG-N_8-CG-3′ and located between nt 200 and 400 function as *cis*-acting packaging sequences.[224] This approximately 200 nt packaging domain functions in virion assembly when placed at the right end of the genome and in an inverted orientation at the left end but must be located within approximately 500 bp of an end.[224] Results from mutational studies of the packaging sequences, *in vitro* protein–DNA binding studies, and chromatin immunoprecipitation assays of infected cells demonstrate that the viral IVa2, L1-52/55K, and L4-22K proteins bind the packaging domain and promote viral DNA packaging into capsids.[223,227,235,306,330,340] Viral mutants in the IVa2, L1-52/55K, and L4-22K proteins are defective for genome packaging and produce empty virion particles.[106,113,222,330,341] Mutation of the L4-33K and L1-IIIa proteins also results in the formation of empty capsids,[69,329] but the L4-33K protein does not interact directly with the packaging sequences,[329] and L1-IIIa binds weakly to this region.[190] The L1-IIIa protein binds directly to the L1-52/55K and this interaction mediates, at least in part, serotype specificity that is observed with adenovirus packaging.[190,325] The IVa2 and L4-22K proteins mediate the sequence specificity by binding to the conserved packaging motifs, specifically the GC motif with IVa2 and the TTTG motif with L4-22K, and bind to these sites in a cooperative manner.[223,227,235,306,340] The L1-52/55K protein is brought into this complex by interaction with IVa2, and L1-IIIa is recruited by L1-52/55K binding.[107,190]

Analysis of the IVa2 sequence from human and nonhuman adenoviruses showed that they contain conserved Walker A box and B box consensus sequences found in ATPases. Consistent with this, HAdV-C5 IVa2 binds ATP,[225] and mutation of the conserved lysine in the Walker A box required for activity of ATPases resulted in loss of viability.[229] The IVa2 protein is associated with one vertex of the mature virion particle,[52] consistent with a potential role in a portal complex for viral DNA encapsidation. A long-standing model for adenovirus assembly hypothesizes that viral DNA is inserted into an empty capsid using a unique portal vertex and a packaging motor, as found with DNA-containing bacteriophages.[224] DNA-containing bacteriophages package naked DNA by the direct contact between the DNA phosphate backbone of the viral genome and the portal motor complex.[224] As described above, the Ad genome within the mature capsid is associated with viral core proteins raising the question if naked adenovirus DNA, or a preformed DNA–protein complex, is the packaging substrate. If an adenovirus DNA–core protein complex is encapsidated via a portal vertex, then a new type of packaging motor would have to be invoked compared to those used by bacteriophages. Recent results suggest that adenovirus assembly occurs by an alternative mechanism using a concerted process whereby virus particles assemble around the DNA in the nucleus at the periphery of replication compartments.[55] Such a model requires verification but more easily accommodates the assembly of virions containing a preformed DNA–core protein complex.

The final step in virion maturation involves numerous proteolytic cleavages of internal capsid proteins by the adenovirus protease, AVP. AVP is a cysteine protease that requires viral DNA and a C-terminal peptide of pVI (pVIc) as cofactors for cleavage of the precursor proteins.[193] pVIc forms a disulfide bond with AVP.[100] The AVP–pVIc complex binds to and slides along DNA, with pVIc serving as a molecular sled.[28] It is hypothesized that as AVP–pVIc complexes slide on DNA, they encounter and process the virion precursor proteins in proximity to the DNA.[28] AVP cleaves seven internal capsid proteins, including pIIIa, pVI, pVII, pVIII, pμ (pX), pTP, and L1-52/55K.[194] These cleavages are absolutely essential for the formation of fully infectious particles. AVP cleavage of internal capsid proteins increases the internal pressure within the virion, which has been proposed to promote virus disassembly following infection.[220] AVP cleavage of pVI also exposes the N-terminal amphipathic helix region that is required for virus escape from the endosome (see Mechanisms of Entry, Uncoating, and Intracellular Trafficking). Finally, AVP activity is required for the exit of the L1-52/55K protein from maturing capsids.[112,233] A mutant virus with a temperature-conditional AVP accumulates noninfectious virion particles that fail to escape the endosome because they contain unprocessed polypeptides.[103] The requirement of DNA and a pVI fragment for activation of AVP prevents AVP from processing precursors until the protease, DNA, and precursor proteins are incorporated into maturing virion particles.

Virus Release

There are several processes that facilitate the release of progeny virions from infected cells and the spread of progeny virus in infected tissues. Late in the infectious cycle, AVP cleaves the cellular cytokeratin K18.[46] This cleavage occurs at amino acid 74 of the cytokeratin, creating a "headless" protein that is not able to polymerize and form filaments; rather, it accumulates in cytoplasmic clumps. A normal intermediate filament system helps to maintain the mechanical integrity of cells, and perturbations to the network would be expected to make the infected cell more susceptible to lysis. The E3-ADP protein facilitates the release of progeny virions by the induction of cell death (see Functions of E3 Proteins). The E1B 55K–E4 ORF6 ubiquitin ligase complex induces the degradation of integrin α3, which appears to decrease attachment of infected cells to their substratum.[62] This likely increases virus spread in the respiratory tract. The interaction of E4 ORF1 protein with PDZ-domain–containing members of the membrane-associated guanylate kinase protein family disrupts tight junctions between epithelial cells and likely aids in progeny virus dissemination.[137,166] Finally, tight junctions are also disrupted by free fiber trimers released from infected cells that interfere with CAR oligomerization.[311] This likely promotes the release of progeny virions into the airway lumen in the respiratory tract.

PERSPECTIVES

Since their discovery nearly seven decades ago, adenoviruses have maintained their status as a fertile ground for revealing fundamental insights into multiple aspects of animal cell biology and human antiviral defenses. Successively deeper understanding of the structure and assembly of the virion provides exquisite examples of macromolecular interactions and assembly. It also allows the design of novel adenovirus gene therapy vectors with engineered receptor-binding domains to direct cell type–specific viral infection and with genetic alterations to promote replication in specific cell types such as cancer cells. Adenovirus evolution has led to the expression of multiple proteins that interact with a variety of cellular effectors, each of which has a profound effect on the biology of the cell. Through these interactions, adenoviruses help to identify cellular proteins and protein complexes that are nodes in the regulation of cellular processes. Adenoviral proteins provide us with molecular tools for exploring cell biology. The large number of recent references in this chapter demonstrates that research on adenoviruses continues to provide fundamental advances in all aspects of biology and that adenovirus research continues to be a productive and rewarding area of discovery.

ACKNOWLEDGMENTS

I am very grateful to Dr. Arnold J. Berk who provided the *Adenoviridae* chapter from the previous edition of this book as a reference for the current chapter and to Dr. William S.M. Wold who provided the section on E3 proteins from the previous edition of this book. I thank Dr. Yueting Zheng who created Figure 4.12.

REFERENCES

1. Akusjarvi G. Temporal regulation of adenovirus major late alternative RNA splicing. *Front Biosci* 2008;13:5006–5015.
2. Alber F, Dokudovskaya S, Veenhoff LM, et al. The molecular architecture of the nuclear pore complex. *Nature* 2007;450:695–701.
3. Amstutz B, Gastaldelli M, Kalin S, et al. Subversion of CtBP1-controlled macropinocytosis by human adenovirus serotype 3. *EMBO J* 2008;27:956–969.
4. Anderson CW, Young ME, Flint SJ. Characterization of the adenovirus 2 virion protein, mu. *Virology* 1989;172:506–512.
5. Andersson MG, Haasnoot PC, Xu N, et al. Suppression of RNA interference by adenovirus virus-associated RNA. *J Virol* 2005;79:9556–9565.
6. Angeletti PC, Engler JA. Adenovirus preterminal protein binds to the CAD enzyme at active sites of viral DNA replication on the nuclear matrix. *J Virol* 1998;72:2896–2904.
7. Aoki K, Benko M, Davison AJ, et al. Toward an integrated human adenovirus designation system that utilizes molecular and serological data and serves both clinical and fundamental virology. *J Virol* 2011;85:5703–5704.
8. Atwan Z, Wright J, Woodman A, et al. Promyelocytic leukemia protein isoform II inhibits infection by human adenovirus type 5 through effects on HSP70 and the interferon response. *J Gen Virol* 2016;97:1955–1967.
9. Avgousti DC, Della Fera AN, Otter CJ, et al. Adenovirus core protein VII downregulates the DNA damage response on the host genome. *J Virol* 2017;91. pii: e01089-17.
10. Avgousti DC, Herrmann C, Kulej K, et al. A core viral protein binds host nucleosomes to sequester immune danger signals. *Nature* 2016;535:173–177.
11. Babich A, Feldman LT, Nevins JR, et al. Effect of adenovirus on metabolism of specific host mRNAs: transport control and specific translational discrimination. *Mol Cell Biol* 1983;3:1212–1221.
12. Bagchi S, Raychaudhuri P, Nevins JR. Adenovirus E1A proteins can dissociate heteromeric complexes involving the E2F transcription factor: a novel mechanism for E1A trans-activation. *Cell* 1990;62:659–669.
13. Bailey CJ, Crystal RG, Leopold PL. Association of adenovirus with the microtubule organizing center. *J Virol* 2003;77:13275–13287.
14. Baker A, Rohleder KJ, Hanakahi LA, et al. Adenovirus E4 34k and E1b 55k oncoproteins target host DNA ligase IV for proteasomal degradation. *J Virol* 2007;81:7034–7040.
15. Basner-Tschakarjan E, Gaffal E, O'Keeffe M, et al. Adenovirus efficiently transduces plasmacytoid dendritic cells resulting in TLR9-dependent maturation and IFN-alpha production. *J Gene Med* 2006;8:1300–1306.
16. Beltz GA, Flint SJ. Inhibition of HeLa cell protein synthesis during adenovirus infection. Restriction of cellular messenger RNA sequences to the nucleus. *J Mol Biol* 1979;131:353–373.
17. Benevento M, Di Palma S, Snijder J, et al. Adenovirus composition, proteolysis, and disassembly studied by in-depth qualitative and quantitative proteomics. *J Biol Chem* 2014;289:11421–11430.
18. Ben-Israel H, Sharf R, Rechavi G, et al. Adenovirus E4orf4 protein downregulates MYC expression through interaction with the PP2A-B55 subunit. *J Virol* 2008;82:9381–9388.
19. Bennett EM, Bennink JR, Yewdell JW, et al. Cutting edge: adenovirus E19 has two mechanisms for affecting class I MHC expression. *J Immunol* 1999;162:5049–5052.
20. Bergelson JM, Cunningham JA, Droguett G, et al. Isolation of a common receptor for Coxsackie B viruses and adenoviruses 2 and 5. *Science* 1997;275:1320–1323.
21. Berget SM, Moore C, Sharp PA. Spliced segments at the 5' terminus of adenovirus 2 late mRNA. *Proc Natl Acad Sci U S A* 1977;74:3171–3175.
22. Berk AJ. Recent lessons in gene expression, cell cycle control, and cell biology from adenovirus. *Oncogene* 2005;24:7673–7685.
23. Berk AJ. Discovery of RNA splicing and genes in pieces. *Proc Natl Acad Sci U S A* 2016;113:801–805.
24. Bewley MC, Springer K, Zhang YB, et al. Structural analysis of the mechanism of adenovirus binding to its human cellular receptor, CAR. *Science* 1999;286:1579–1583.
25. Bhat G, SivaRaman L, Murthy S, et al. In vivo identification of multiple promoter domains of adenovirus EIIA-late promoter. *EMBO J* 1987;6:2045–2052.
26. Biasiotto R, Akusjarvi G. Regulation of human adenovirus alternative RNA splicing by the adenoviral L4-33K and L4-22K proteins. *Int J Mol Sci* 2015;16:2893–2912.
27. Blackford AN, Patel RN, Forrester NA, et al. Adenovirus 12 E4orf6 inhibits ATR activation by promoting TOPBP1 degradation. *Proc Natl Acad Sci U S A* 2010;107:12251–12256.
28. Blainey PC, Graziano V, Perez-Berna AJ, et al. Regulation of a viral proteinase by a peptide and DNA in one-dimensional space: IV. Viral proteinase slides along DNA to locate and process its substrates. *J Biol Chem* 2013;288:2092–2102.
29. Blanchette P, Kindsmuller K, Groitl P, et al. Control of mRNA export by adenovirus E4orf6 and E1B55K proteins during productive infection requires E4orf6 ubiquitin ligase activity. *J Virol* 2008;82:2642–2651.
30. Bondesson M, Ohman K, Manervik M, et al. Adenovirus E4 open reading frame 4 protein autoregulates E4 transcription by inhibiting E1A transactivation of the E4 promoter. *J Virol* 1996;70:3844–3851.
31. Boyer TG, Martin ME, Lees E, et al. Mammalian Srb/Mediator complex is targeted by adenovirus E1A protein. *Nature* 1999;399:276–279.
32. Brestovitsky A, Nebenzahl-Sharon K, Kechker P, et al. The adenovirus E4orf4 protein provides a novel mechanism for inhibition of the DNA damage response. *PLoS Pathog* 2016;12:e1005420.
33. Bridge E, Ketner G. Redundant control of adenovirus late gene expression by early region 4. *J Virol* 1989;63:631–638.
34. Bridges RG, Sohn SY, Wright J, et al. The adenovirus E4-ORF3 protein stimulates SUMOylation of general transcription factor TFII-I to direct proteasomal degradation. *MBio* 2016;7:e02184.
35. Bruder JT, Hearing P. Nuclear factor EF-1A binds to the adenovirus E1A core enhancer element and to other transcriptional control regions. *Mol Cell Biol* 1989;9:5143–5153.
36. Cantin GT, Stevens JL, Berk AJ. Activation domain-mediator interactions promote transcription preinitiation complex assembly on promoter DNA. *Proc Natl Acad Sci U S A* 2003;100:12003–12008.
37. Carvalho T, Seeler JS, Ohman K, et al. Targeting of adenovirus E1A and E4-ORF3 proteins to nuclear matrix-associated PML bodies. *J Cell Biol* 1995;131:45–56.
38. Cepko CL, Sharp PA. Assembly of adenovirus major capsid protein is mediated by a nonvirion protein. *Cell* 1982;31:407–415.
39. Cerullo V, Seiler MP, Mane V, et al. Toll-like receptor 9 triggers an innate immune response to helper-dependent adenoviral vectors. *Mol Ther* 2007;15:378–385.
40. Chahal JS, Gallagher C, DeHart CJ, et al. The repression domain of the E1B 55-kilodalton protein participates in countering interferon-induced inhibition of adenovirus replication. *J Virol* 2013;87:4432–4444.
41. Chahal JS, Qi J, Flint SJ. The human adenovirus type 5 E1B 55 kDa protein obstructs inhibition of viral replication by type I interferon in normal human cells. *PLoS Pathog* 2012;8:e1002853.
42. Challberg MD, Kelly TJ Jr. Adenovirus DNA replication in vitro. *Proc Natl Acad Sci U S A* 1979;76:655–659.
43. Chatterjee PK, Vayda ME, Flint SJ. Adenoviral protein VII packages intracellular viral DNA throughout the early phase of infection. *EMBO J* 1986;5:1633–1644.
44. Chatterjee PK, Vayda ME, Flint SJ. Identification of proteins and protein domains that contact DNA within adenovirus nucleoprotein cores by ultraviolet light cross-linking of oligonucleotides 32P-labelled in vivo. *J Mol Biol* 1986;188:23–37.
45. Chen J, Morral, N, Engel DA. Transcription releases protein VII from adenovirus chromatin. *Virology* 2007;369:411–422.
46. Chen PH, Ornelles DA, Shenk T. The adenovirus L3 23-kilodalton proteinase cleaves the amino-terminal head domain from cytokeratin 18 and disrupts the cytokeratin network of HeLa cells. *J Virol* 1993;67:3507–3514.
47. Cheng CY, Gilson T, Dallaire F, et al. The E4orf6/E1B55K E3 ubiquitin ligase complexes of human adenoviruses exhibit heterogeneity in composition and substrate specificity. *J Virol* 2011;85:765–775.
48. Cheng CY, Gilson T, Wimmer P, et al. Role of E1B55K in E4orf6/E1B55K E3 ligase complexes formed by different human adenovirus serotypes. *J Virol* 2013;87:6232–6245.
49. Chinnadurai, G. Modulation of oncogenic transformation by the human adenovirus E1A C-terminal region. *Curr Top Microbiol Immunol* 2004;273:139–161.
50. Chiu CY, Mathias, P Nemerow GR, et al. Structure of adenovirus complexed with its internalization receptor, alphavbeta5 integrin. *J Virol* 1999;73:6759–6768.
51. Chow, LT, Gelinas, RE, Broker, TR, et al. An amazing sequence arrangement at the 5' ends of adenovirus 2 messenger RNA. *Cell* 1977;12:1–8.
52. Christensen JB, Byrd SA, Walker AK, et al. Presence of the adenovirus IVa2 protein at a single vertex of the mature virion. *J Virol* 2008;82:9086–9093.

53. Cohen CJ, Shieh JT, Pickles RJ, et al. The coxsackievirus and adenovirus receptor is a transmembrane component of the tight junction. *Proc Natl Acad Sci U S A* 2001;98:15191–15196.
54. Cohen MJ, Yousef AF, Massimi P, et al. Dissection of the C-terminal region of E1A redefines the roles of CtBP and other cellular targets in oncogenic transformation. *J Virol* 2013;87:10348–10355.
55. Condezo GN, San Martin C. Localization of adenovirus morphogenesis players, together with visualization of assembly intermediates and failed products, favor a model where assembly and packaging occur concurrently at the periphery of the replication center. *PLoS Pathog* 2017;13:e1006320.
56. Croyle MA, Stone M, Amidon GL, et al. In vitro and in vivo assessment of adenovirus 41 as a vector for gene delivery to the intestine. *Gene Ther* 1998;5:645–654.
57. Cuconati A, Mukherjee C, Perez D, et al. DNA damage response and MCL-1 destruction initiate apoptosis in adenovirus-infected cells. *Genes Dev* 2003;17:2922–2932.
58. Cuconati A, White E. Viral homologs of BCL-2: role of apoptosis in the regulation of virus infection. *Genes Dev* 2002;16:2465–2478.
59. Cuesta R, Xi Q, Schneider RJ. Adenovirus-specific translation by displacement of kinase Mnk1 from cap-initiation complex eIF4F. *EMBO J* 2000;19:3465–3474.
60. Cuesta R, Xi Q, Schneider RJ. Preferential translation of adenovirus mRNAs in infected cells. *Cold Spring Harb Symp Quant Biol* 2001;66:259–267.
61. Dai X, Wu L, Sun R, et al. Atomic structures of minor proteins VI and VII in human adenovirus. *J Virol* 2017;91. pii: e00850-17.
62. Dallaire F, Blanchette P, Branton PE. A proteomic approach to identify candidate substrates of human adenovirus E4orf6-E1B55K and other viral cullin-based E3 ubiquitin ligases. *J Virol* 2009;83:12172–12184.
63. Dallaire F, Blanchette P, Groitl P, et al. Identification of integrin alpha3 as a new substrate of the adenovirus E4orf6/E1B 55-kilodalton E3 ubiquitin ligase complex. *J Virol* 2009;83:5329–5338.
64. Davison AJ, Benko M, Harrach B. Genetic content and evolution of adenoviruses. *J Gen Virol* 2003;84:2895–2908.
65. Debbas M, White E. Wild-type p53 mediates apoptosis by E1A, which is inhibited by E1B. *Genes Dev* 1993;7:546–554.
66. DeCaprio, JA. How the Rb tumor suppressor structure and function was revealed by the study of Adenovirus and SV40. *Virology* 2009;384:274–284.
67. Dekker J, Kanellopoulos PN, Loonstra AK, et al. Multimerization of the adenovirus DNA-binding protein is the driving force for ATP-independent DNA unwinding during strand displacement synthesis. *EMBO J* 1997;16:1455–1463.
68. Delgado-Lopez F, Horwitz MS. Adenovirus RIDalphabeta complex inhibits lipopolysaccharide signaling without altering TLR4 cell surface expression. *J Virol* 2006;80:6378–6386.
69. D'Halluin JC, Milleville M, Boulanger PA, et al. Temperature-sensitive mutant of adenovirus type 2 blocked in virion assembly: accumulation of light intermediate particles. *J Virol* 1978;26:344–356.
70. Dhingra A, Hage E, Ganzenmueller T, et al. Molecular evolution of human adenovirus (HAdV) species C. *Sci Rep* 2019;9:1039.
71. Dobner T, Horikoshi N, Rubenwolf S, et al. Blockage by adenovirus E4orf6 of transcriptional activation by the p53 tumor suppressor. *Science* 1996;272:1470–1473.
72. Doucas V, Ishov AM, Romo A, et al. Adenovirus replication is coupled with the dynamic properties of the PML nuclear structure. *Genes Dev* 1996;10:196–207.
73. Dyson N, Guida P, McCall C, et al. Adenovirus E1A makes two distinct contacts with the retinoblastoma protein. *J Virol* 1992;66:4606–4611.
74. Egan C, Bayley ST, Branton PE. Binding of the Rb1 protein to E1A products is required for adenovirus transformation. *Oncogene* 1989;4:383–388.
75. Endter C, Kzhyshkowska J, Stauber R, et al. SUMO-1 modification required for transformation by adenovirus type 5 early region 1B 55-kDa oncoprotein. *Proc Natl Acad Sci U S A* 2001;98:11312–11317.
76. Estmer Nilsson C, Petersen-Mahrt S, Durot C, et al. The adenovirus E4-ORF4 splicing enhancer protein interacts with a subset of phosphorylated SR proteins. *EMBO J* 2001;20:864–871.
77. Evans JD, Hearing P. Relocalization of the Mre11-Rad50-Nbs1 complex by the adenovirus E4 ORF3 protein is required for viral replication. *J Virol* 2005;79:6207–6215.
78. Excoffon KJ, Gansemer ND, Mobily ME, et al. Isoform-specific regulation and localization of the coxsackie and adenovirus receptor in human airway epithelia. *PLoS One* 2010;5:e9909.
79. Fender P, Kidd AH, Brebant R, et al. Antigenic sites on the receptor-binding domain of human adenovirus type 2 fiber. *Virology* 1995;214:110–117.
80. Ferrari R, Gou D, Jawdekar G, et al. Adenovirus small E1A employs the lysine acetylases p300/CBP and tumor suppressor Rb to repress select host genes and promote productive virus infection. *Cell Host Microbe* 2014;16:663–676.
81. Ferrari R, Pellegrini M, Horwitz GA, et al. Epigenetic reprogramming by adenovirus e1a. *Science* 2008;321:1086–1088.
82. Flinterman M, Guelen L, Ezzati-Nik S, et al. E1A activates transcription of p73 and Noxa to induce apoptosis. *J Biol Chem* 2005;280:5945–5959.
83. Fonseca GJ, Cohen MJ, Nichols AC, et al. Viral retasking of hBre1/RNF20 to recruit hPaf1 for transcriptional activation. *PLoS Pathog* 2013;9:e1003411.
84. Fonseca GJ, Thillainadesan G, Yousef AF, et al. Adenovirus evasion of interferon-mediated innate immunity by direct antagonism of a cellular histone posttranslational modification. *Cell Host Microbe* 2012;11:597–606.
85. Forrester NA, Patel RN, Speiseder T, et al. Adenovirus E4orf3 targets transcriptional intermediary factor 1gamma for proteasome-dependent degradation during infection. *J Virol* 2012;86:3167–3179.
86. Forrester NA, Sedgwick GG, Thomas A, et al. Serotype-specific inactivation of the cellular DNA damage response during adenovirus infection. *J Virol* 2011;85:2201–2211.
87. Frese KK, Lee SS, Thomas DL, et al. Selective PDZ protein-dependent stimulation of phosphatidylinositol 3-kinase by the adenovirus E4-ORF1 oncoprotein. *Oncogene* 2003;22:710–721.
88. Fu J, Li L, Bouvier M. Adenovirus E3-19K proteins of different serotypes and subgroups have similar, yet distinct, immunomodulatory functions toward major histocompatibility class I molecules. *J Biol Chem* 2011;286:17631–17639.
89. Fuchs M, Gerber J, Drapkin R, et al. The p400 complex is an essential E1A transformation target. *Cell* 2001;106:297–307.
90. Gaggar A, Shayakhmetov DM, Lieber A. CD46 is a cellular receptor for group B adenoviruses. *Nat Med* 2003;9:1408–1412.
91. Gahery-Segard H, Farace F, Godfrin D, et al. Immune response to recombinant capsid proteins of adenovirus in humans: antifiber and anti-penton base antibodies have a synergistic effect on neutralizing activity. *J Virol* 1998;72:2388–2397.
92. Gall JG, Crystal RG, Falck-Pedersen E. Construction and characterization of hexon-chimeric adenoviruses: specification of adenovirus serotype. *J Virol* 1998;72:10260–10264.
93. Gastaldelli M, Imelli N, Boucke K, et al. Infectious adenovirus type 2 transport through early but not late endosomes. *Traffic* 2008;9:2265–2278.
94. Geisberg JV, Chen JL, Ricciardi RP. Subregions of the adenovirus E1A transactivation domain target multiple components of the TFIID complex. *Mol Cell Biol* 1995;15:6283–6290.
95. Geisberg JV, Lee WS, Berk AJ, et al. The zinc finger region of the adenovirus E1A transactivating domain complexes with the TATA box binding protein. *Proc Natl Acad Sci U S A* 1994;91:2488–2492.
96. Ghosh MK, Harter ML. A viral mechanism for remodeling chromatin structure in G0 cells. *Mol Cell* 2003;12:255–260.
97. Giberson AN, Davidson AR, Parks RJ. Chromatin structure of adenovirus DNA throughout infection. *Nucleic Acids Res* 2012;40:2369–2376.
98. Gnatovskiy L, Mita P, Levy DE. The human RVB complex is required for efficient transcription of type I interferon-stimulated genes. *Mol Cell Biol* 2013;33:3817–3825.
99. Granberg F, Svensson C, Pettersson U, et al. Modulation of host cell gene expression during onset of the late phase of an adenovirus infection is focused on growth inhibition and cell architecture. *Virology* 2005;343:236–245.
100. Graziano V, Luo, G Blainey PC, et al. Regulation of a viral proteinase by a peptide and DNA in one-dimensional space: II. Adenovirus proteinase is activated in an unusual one-dimensional biochemical reaction. *J Biol Chem* 2013;288:2068–2080.
101. Greber UF, Flatt JW. Adenovirus entry: from infection to immunity. *Annu Rev Virol* 2019;6:177–197.
102. Greber, UF, Suomalainen, M, Stidwill, RP, et al. The role of the nuclear pore complex in adenovirus DNA entry. *EMBO J* 1997;16:5998–6007.
103. Greber UF, Webster P, Weber J, et al. The role of the adenovirus protease on virus entry into cells. *EMBO J* 1996;15:1766–1777.
104. Greber UF, Willetts M, Webster P, et al. Stepwise dismantling of adenovirus 2 during entry into cells. *Cell* 1993;75:477–486.
105. Guimet D, Hearing P. The adenovirus L4-22K protein has distinct functions in the posttranscriptional regulation of gene expression and encapsidation of the viral genome. *J Virol* 2013;87:7688–7699.
106. Gustin KE, Imperiale MJ. Encapsidation of viral DNA requires the adenovirus L1 52/55-kilodalton protein. *J Virol* 1998;72:7860–7870.
107. Gustin KE, Lutz P, Imperiale MJ. Interaction of the adenovirus L1 52/55-kilodalton protein with the IVa2 gene product during infection. *J Virol* 1996;70:6463–6467.
108. Gutch MJ, Reich NC. Repression of the interferon signal transduction pathway by the adenovirus E1A oncogene. *Proc Natl Acad Sci U S A* 1991;88:7913–7917.
109. Harada JN, Shevchenko A, Shevchenko A, et al. Analysis of the adenovirus E1B-55K-anchored proteome reveals its link to ubiquitination machinery. *J Virol* 2002;76:9194–9206.
110. Haruki H, Gyurcsik B, Okuwaki M, et al. Ternary complex formation between DNA-adenovirus core protein VII and TAF-Ibeta/SET, an acidic molecular chaperone. *FEBS Lett* 2003;555:521–527.
111. Haruki H, Okuwaki, M, Miyagishi M, et al. Involvement of template-activating factor I/SET in transcription of adenovirus early genes as a positive-acting factor. *J Virol* 2006;80:794–801.
112. Hasson TB, Ornelles DA, Shenk T. Adenovirus L1 52- and 55-kilodalton proteins are present within assembling virions and colocalize with nuclear structures distinct from replication centers. *J Virol* 1992;66:6133–6142.
113. Hasson TB, Soloway PD, Ornelles DA, et al. Adenovirus L1 52- and 55-kilodalton proteins are required for assembly of virions. *J Virol* 1989;63:3612–3621.
114. Hatfield L, Hearing P. Redundant elements in the adenovirus type 5 inverted terminal repeat promote bidirectional transcription in vitro and are important for virus growth in vivo. *Virology* 1991;184:265–276.
115. Hay RT. SUMO: a history of modification. *Mol Cell* 2005;18:1–12.
116. Hayes BW, Telling GC, Myat MM, et al. The adenovirus L4 100-kilodalton protein is necessary for efficient translation of viral late mRNA species. *J Virol* 1990;64:2732–2742.
117. Hearing P, Shenk T. The adenovirus type 5 E1A transcriptional control region contains a duplicated enhancer element. *Cell* 1983;33:695–703.
118. Hearing P, Shenk T. The adenovirus type 5 E1A enhancer contains two functionally distinct domains: one is specific for E1A and the other modulates all early units in cis. *Cell* 1986;45:229–236.
119. Higashino F, Pipas JM, Shenk T. Adenovirus E4orf6 oncoprotein modulates the function of the p53-related protein, p73. *Proc Natl Acad Sci U S A* 1998;95:15683–15687.
120. Hilleman MR, Werner JH. Recovery of new agent from patients with acute respiratory illness. *Proc Soc Exp Biol Med* 1954;85:183–188.
121. Hindley CE, Lawrence FJ, Matthews DA. A role for transportin in the nuclear import of adenovirus core proteins and DNA. *Traffic* 2007;8:1313–1322.
122. Hong SS, Bardy M, Monteil M, et al. Immunoreactive domains and integrin-binding motifs in adenovirus penton base capsomer. *Viral Immunol* 2000;13:353–371.
123. Hoppe A, Beech SJ, Dimmock J, et al. Interaction of the adenovirus type 5 E4 Orf3 protein with promyelocytic leukemia protein isoform II is required for ND10 disruption. *J Virol* 2006;80:3042–3049.

124. Howe JA, Mymryk JS, Egan C, et al. Retinoblastoma growth suppressor and a 300-kDa protein appear to regulate cellular DNA synthesis. *Proc Natl Acad Sci U S A* 1990;87:5883–5887.
125. Huang W, Flint SJ. The tripartite leader sequence of subgroup C adenovirus major late mRNAs can increase the efficiency of mRNA export. *J Virol* 1998;72:225–235.
126. Huang MM, Hearing P. Adenovirus early region 4 encodes two gene products with redundant effects in lytic infection. *J Virol* 1989;63:2605–2615.
127. Huang MM, Hearing P. The adenovirus early region 4 open reading frame 6/7 protein regulates the DNA binding activity of the cellular transcription factor, E2F, through a direct complex. *Genes Dev* 1989;3:1699–1710.
128. Huang JT, Schneider RJ. Adenovirus inhibition of cellular protein synthesis involves inactivation of cap-binding protein. *Cell* 1991;65:271–280.
129. Hurst HC, Jones NC. Identification of factors that interact with the E1A-inducible adenovirus E3 promoter. *Genes Dev* 1987;1:1132–1146.
130. Iacobelli-Martinez M, Nemerow GR. Preferential activation of Toll-like receptor nine by CD46-utilizing adenoviruses. *J Virol* 2007;81:1305–1312.
131. Imperiale MJ, Hart RP, Nevins JR. An enhancer-like element in the adenovirus E2 promoter contains sequences essential for uninduced and E1A-induced transcription. *Proc Natl Acad Sci U S A* 1985;82:381–385.
132. Ishibashi M, Maizel JV Jr. The polypeptides of adenovirus. VI. Early and late glycopolypeptides. *Virology* 1974;58:345–361.
133. Jackson RJ, Hellen CU, Pestova TV. The mechanism of eukaryotic translation initiation and principles of its regulation. *Nat Rev Mol Cell Biol* 2010;11:113–127.
134. Javier RT. Adenovirus type 9 E4 open reading frame 1 encodes a transforming protein required for the production of mammary tumors in rats. *J Virol* 1994;68:3917–3924.
135. Javier R, Raska K Jr, Macdonald GJ, et al. Human adenovirus type 9-induced rat mammary tumors. *J Virol* 1991;65:3192–3202.
136. Javier R, Raska K Jr, Shenk T. Requirement for the adenovirus type 9 E4 region in production of mammary tumors. *Science* 1992;257:1267–1271.
137. Javier RT, Rice AP. Emerging theme: cellular PDZ proteins as common targets of pathogenic viruses. *J Virol* 2011;85:11544–11556.
138. Jiao J, Guan H, Lippa AM, et al. The N terminus of adenovirus type 12 E1A inhibits major histocompatibility complex class I expression by preventing phosphorylation of NF-kappaB p65 Ser276 through direct binding. *J Virol* 2010;84:7668–7674.
139. Jones MS II, Harrach B, Ganac RD, et al. New adenovirus species found in a patient presenting with gastroenteritis. *J Virol* 2007;81:5978–5984.
140. de Jong RN, van der Vliet PC. Mechanism of DNA replication in eukaryotic cells: cellular host factors stimulating adenovirus DNA replication. *Gene* 1999;236:1–12.
141. Kalin S, Amstutz B, Gastaldelli M, et al. Macropinocytotic uptake and infection of human epithelial cells with species B2 adenovirus type 35. *J Virol* 2010;84:5336–5350.
142. Kalvakolanu DV, Bandyopadhyay SK, Harter ML, et al. Inhibition of interferon-inducible gene expression by adenovirus E1A proteins: block in transcriptional complex formation. *Proc Natl Acad Sci U S A* 1991;88:7459–7463.
143. Kanopka A, Muhlemann O, Akusjarvi G. Inhibition by SR proteins of splicing of a regulated adenovirus pre-mRNA. *Nature* 1996;381:535–538.
144. Kanopka A, Muhlemann O, Petersen-Mahrt S, et al. Regulation of adenovirus alternative RNA splicing by dephosphorylation of SR proteins. *Nature* 1998;393:185–187.
145. Kao CC, Yew PR, Berk AJ. Domains required for in vitro association between the cellular p53 and the adenovirus 2 E1B 55K proteins. *Virology* 1990;179:806–814.
146. Karen KA, Hearing P. Adenovirus core protein VII protects the viral genome from a DNA damage response at early times after infection. *J Virol* 2011;85:4135–4142.
147. Kent LN, Leone G. The broken cycle: E2F dysfunction in cancer. *Nat Rev Cancer* 2019;19:326–338.
148. Kidd AH, Chroboczek J, Cusack S, et al. Adenovirus type 40 virions contain two distinct fibers. *Virology* 1993;192:73–84.
149. Kindsmuller K, Groitl P, Hartl B, et al. Intranuclear targeting and nuclear export of the adenovirus E1B-55K protein are regulated by SUMO1 conjugation. *Proc Natl Acad Sci U S A* 2007;104:6684–6689.
150. King AJ, Teertstra WR, Blanco L, et al. Processive proofreading by the adenovirus DNA polymerase. Association with the priming protein reduces exonucleolytic degradation. *Nucleic Acids Res* 1997;25:1745–1752.
151. King CR, Zhang A, Tessier TM, et al. Hacking the cell: network intrusion and exploitation by adenovirus E1A. *MBio* 2018;9. pii: e00390-18.
152. Kitajewski J, Schneider RJ, Safer B, et al. Adenovirus VAI RNA antagonizes the antiviral action of interferon by preventing activation of the interferon-induced eIF-2 alpha kinase. *Cell* 1986;45:195–200.
153. Kleinberger T, Shenk T. Adenovirus E4orf4 protein binds to protein phosphatase 2A, and the complex down regulates E1A-enhanced junB transcription. *J Virol* 1993;67:7556–7560.
154. Komatsu T, Haruki H, Nagata K. Cellular and viral chromatin proteins are positive factors in the regulation of adenovirus gene expression. *Nucleic Acids Res* 2011;39:889–901.
155. Komorek J, Kuppuswamy M, Subramanian T, et al. Adenovirus type 5 E1A and E6 proteins of low-risk cutaneous beta-human papillomaviruses suppress cell transformation through interaction with FOXK1/K2 transcription factors. *J Virol* 2010;84:2719–2731.
156. Kong K, Kumar M, Taruishi M, et al. The human adenovirus E4-ORF1 protein subverts discs large 1 to mediate membrane recruitment and dysregulation of phosphatidylinositol 3-kinase. *PLoS Pathog* 2014;10:e1004102.
157. Kong K, Kumar M, Taruishi M, et al. Adenovirus E4-ORF1 dysregulates epidermal growth factor and insulin/insulin-like growth factor receptors to mediate constitutive Myc expression. *J Virol* 2015;89:10774–10785.
158. Kotha PL, Sharma P, Kolawole AO, et al. Adenovirus entry from the apical surface of polarized epithelia is facilitated by the host innate immune response. *PLoS Pathog* 2015;11:e1004696.
159. Kovesdi I, Reichel R, Nevins JR. Identification of a cellular transcription factor involved in E1A trans-activation. *Cell* 1986;45:219–228.
160. Kratzer F, Rosorius O, Heger P, et al. The adenovirus type 5 E1B-55K oncoprotein is a highly active shuttle protein and shuttling is independent of E4orf6, p53 and Mdm2. *Oncogene* 2000;19:850–857.
161. Kumar M, Kong K, Javier RT. Hijacking Dlg1 for oncogenic phosphatidylinositol 3-kinase activation in human epithelial cells is a conserved mechanism of human adenovirus E4-ORF1 proteins. *J Virol* 2014;88:14268–14277.
162. Kundhavai Natchiar S, Venkataraman S, Mullen TM, et al. Revised crystal structure of human adenovirus reveals the limits on protein IX quasi-equivalence and on analyzing large macromolecular complexes. *J Mol Biol* 2018;430:4132–4141.
163. Kuschner RA, Russell KL, Abuja M, et al. A phase 3, randomized, double-blind, placebo-controlled study of the safety and efficacy of the live, oral adenovirus type 4 and type 7 vaccine, in U.S. military recruits. *Vaccine* 2013;31:2963–2971.
164. Lam E, Stein S, Falck-Pedersen E. Adenovirus detection by the cGAS/STING/TBK1 DNA sensing cascade. *J Virol* 2014;88:974–981.
165. Lasswitz L, Chandra N, Arnberg N, et al. Glycomics and proteomics approaches to investigate early adenovirus-host cell interactions. *J Mol Biol* 2018;430:1863–1882.
166. Latorre IJ, Roh MH, Frese KK, et al. Viral oncoprotein-induced mislocalization of select PDZ proteins disrupts tight junctions and causes polarity defects in epithelial cells. *J Cell Sci* 2005;118:4283–4293.
167. Lavoie JN, Nguyen M, Marcellus RC, et al. E4orf4, a novel adenovirus death factor that induces p53-independent apoptosis by a pathway that is not inhibited by zVAD-fmk. *J Cell Biol* 1998;140:637–645.
168. Lechner RL, Kelly TJ Jr. The structure of replicating adenovirus 2 DNA molecules. *Cell* 1977;12:1007–1020.
169. Lee KA, Hai TY, SivaRaman L, et al. A cellular protein, activating transcription factor, activates transcription of multiple E1A-inducible adenovirus early promoters. *Proc Natl Acad Sci U S A* 1987;84:8355–8359.
170. Leopold PL, Kreitzer G, Miyazawa N, et al. Dynein- and microtubule-mediated translocation of adenovirus serotype 5 occurs after endosomal lysis. *Hum Gene Ther* 2000;11:151–165.
171. Li S, Brignole C, Marcellus R, et al. The adenovirus E4orf4 protein induces G2/M arrest and cell death by blocking protein phosphatase 2A activity regulated by the B55 subunit. *J Virol* 2009;83:8340–8352.
172. Li E, Stupack D, Klemke R, et al. Adenovirus endocytosis via alpha(v) integrins requires phosphoinositide-3-OH kinase. *J Virol* 1998;72:2055–2061.
173. Lichtenstein DL, Toth K, Doronin K, et al. Functions and mechanisms of action of the adenovirus E3 proteins. *Int Rev Immunol* 2004;23:75–111.
174. Lin J, Chen J, Elenbaas B, et al. Several hydrophobic amino acids in the p53 amino-terminal domain are required for transcriptional activation, binding to mdm-2 and the adenovirus 5 E1B 55-kD protein. *Genes Dev* 1994;8:1235–1246.
175. Lion T. Adenovirus infections in immunocompetent and immunocompromised patients. *Clin Microbiol Rev* 2014;27:441–462.
176. Liu F, Green MR. A specific member of the ATF transcription factor family can mediate transcription activation by the adenovirus E1a protein. *Cell* 1990;61:1217–1224.
177. Liu F, Green MR. Promoter targeting by adenovirus E1a through interaction with different cellular DNA-binding domains. *Nature* 1994;368:520–525.
178. Liu H, Jin L, Koh SB, et al. Atomic structure of human adenovirus by cryo-EM reveals interactions among protein networks. *Science* 2010;329:1038–1043.
179. Liu H, Naismith JH, Hay RT. Adenovirus DNA replication. *Curr Top Microbiol Immunol* 2003;272:131–164.logan
180. Liu Y, Shevchenko A, Shevchenko A, et al. Adenovirus exploits the cellular aggresome response to accelerate inactivation of the MRN complex. *J Virol* 2005;79:14004–14016.
181. Liu H, Stafford WF, Bouvier M. The endoplasmic reticulum lumenal domain of the adenovirus type 2 E3-19K protein binds to peptide-filled and peptide-deficient HLA-A*1101 molecules. *J Virol* 2005;79:13317–13325.
182. Liu H, Wu L, Zhou ZH. Model of the trimeric fiber and its interactions with the pentameric penton base of human adenovirus by cryo-electron microscopy. *J Mol Biol* 2011;406:764–774.
183. Logan J, Shenk T. Adenovirus tripartite leader sequence enhances translation of mRNAs late after infection. *Proc Natl Acad Sci U S A* 1984;81:3655–3659.
184. Look DC, Roswit WT, Frick AG, et al. Direct suppression of Stat1 function during adenoviral infection. *Immunity* 1998;9:871–880.
185. Lortat-Jacob H, Chouin E, Cusack S, et al. Kinetic analysis of adenovirus fiber binding to its receptor reveals an avidity mechanism for trimeric receptor-ligand interactions. *J Biol Chem* 2001;276:9009–9015.
186. Lowe SW, Ruley HE. Stabilization of the p53 tumor suppressor is induced by adenovirus 5 E1A and accompanies apoptosis. *Genes Dev* 1993;7:535–545.
187. Lu S, Cullen BR. Adenovirus VA1 noncoding RNA can inhibit small interfering RNA and MicroRNA biogenesis. *J Virol* 2004;78:12868–12876.
188. Lynch JP III, Kajon AE. Adenovirus: epidemiology, global spread of novel serotypes, and advances in treatment and prevention. *Semin Respir Crit Care Med* 2016;37:586–602.
189. Lyons RH, Ferguson BQ, Rosenberg M. Pentapeptide nuclear localization signal in adenovirus E1a. *Mol Cell Biol* 1987;7:2451–2456.
190. Ma HC, Hearing P. Adenovirus structural protein IIIa is involved in the serotype specificity of viral DNA packaging. *J Virol* 2011;85:7849–7855.
191. Mabit H, Nakano MY, Prank U, et al. Intact microtubules support adenovirus and herpes simplex virus infections. *J Virol* 2002;76:9962–9971.
192. Maier O, Galan DL, Wodrich H, et al. An N-terminal domain of adenovirus protein VI fragments membranes by inducing positive membrane curvature. *Virology* 2010;402:11–19.
193. Mangel WF, McGrath WJ, Toledo DL, et al. Viral DNA and a viral peptide can act as cofactors of adenovirus virion proteinase activity. *Nature* 1993;361:274–275.
194. Mangel WF, San Martin C. Structure, function and dynamics in adenovirus maturation. *Viruses* 2014;6:4536–4570.
195. Marcellus RC, Lavoie JN, Boivin D, et al. The early region 4 orf4 protein of human adenovirus type 5 induces p53-independent cell death by apoptosis. *J Virol* 1998;72:7144–7153.
196. Marin MC, Jost CA, Irwin MS, et al. Viral oncoproteins discriminate between p53 and the p53 homolog p73. *Mol Cell Biol* 1998;18:6316–6324.
197. Martin ME, Berk AJ. Adenovirus E1B 55K represses p53 activation in vitro. *J Virol* 1998;72:3146–3154.

198. Martin-Fernandez M, Longshaw SV, Kirby I, et al. Adenovirus type-5 entry and disassembly followed in living cells by FRET, fluorescence anisotropy, and FLIM. *Biophys J* 2004;87:1316–1327.
199. Martin-Gonzalez N, Hernando-Perez M, Condezo GN, et al. Adenovirus major core protein condenses DNA in clusters and bundles, modulating genome release and capsid internal pressure. *Nucleic Acids Res* 2019;47:9231–9242.
200. Matthews DA, Russell WC. Adenovirus core protein V is delivered by the invading virus to the nucleus of the infected cell and later in infection is associated with nucleoli. *J Gen Virol* 1998;79:1671–1675.
201. McLaughlin-Drubin ME, Munger K. Viruses associated with human cancer. *Biochim Biophys Acta* 2008;1782:127–150.
202. McSharry BP, Burgert HG, Owen DP, et al. Adenovirus E3/19K promotes evasion of NK cell recognition by intracellular sequestration of the NKG2D ligands major histocompatibility complex class I chain-related proteins A and B. *J Virol* 2008;82:4585–4594.
203. Meier O, Greber UF. Adenovirus endocytosis. *J Gene Med* 2004;6(Suppl 1):S152–S163.
204. Miller DL, Myers CL, Rickards B, et al. Adenovirus type 5 exerts genome-wide control over cellular programs governing proliferation, quiescence, and survival. *Genome Biol* 2007;8:R58.
205. Moise AR, Grant JR, Vitalis TZ, et al. Adenovirus E3-6.7K maintains calcium homeostasis and prevents apoptosis and arachidonic acid release. *J Virol* 2002;76:1578–1587.
206. Montell C, Fisher EF, Caruthers MH, et al. Resolving the functions of overlapping viral genes by site-specific mutagenesis at a mRNA splice site. *Nature* 1982;295:380–384.
207. Morris SJ, Scott GE, Leppard KN. Adenovirus late-phase infection is controlled by a novel L4 promoter. *J Virol* 2010;84:7096–7104.
208. Muller S, Dobner T. The adenovirus E1B-55K oncoprotein induces SUMO modification of p53. *Cell Cycle* 2008;7:754–758.
209. Muller U, Kleinberger T, Shenk T. Adenovirus E4orf4 protein reduces phosphorylation of c-Fos and E1A proteins while simultaneously reducing the level of AP-1. *J Virol* 1992;66:5867–5878.
210. Muruve DA, Petrilli V, Zaiss AK, et al. The inflammasome recognizes cytosolic microbial and host DNA and triggers an innate immune response. *Nature* 2008;452:103–107.
211. Nakajima T, Masuda-Murata M, Hara E, et al. Induction of cell cycle progression by adenovirus E1A gene 13S- and 12S-mRNA products in quiescent rat cells. *Mol Cell Biol* 1987;7:3846–3852.
212. Nakano MY, Boucke K, Suomalainen M, et al. The first step of adenovirus type 2 disassembly occurs at the cell surface, independently of endocytosis and escape to the cytosol. *J Virol* 2000;74:7085–7095.
213. Nevins JR, Ginsberg HS, Blanchard JM, et al. Regulation of the primary expression of the early adenovirus transcription units. *J Virol* 1979;32:727–733.
214. Nguyen EK, Nemerow GR, Smith JG. Direct evidence from single-cell analysis that human {alpha}-defensins block adenovirus uncoating to neutralize infection. *J Virol* 2010;84:4041–4049.
215. Nociari M, Ocheretina O, Murphy M, et al. Adenovirus induction of IRF3 occurs through a binary trigger targeting Jun N-terminal kinase and TBK1 kinase cascades and type I interferon autocrine signaling. *J Virol* 2009;83:4081–4091.
216. O'Connor RJ, Hearing P. The E4-6/7 protein functionally compensates for the loss of E1A expression in adenovirus infection. *J Virol* 2000;74:5819–5824.
217. Olanubi O, Frost JR, Radko S, et al. Suppression of type I interferon signaling by E1A via RuvBL1/Pontin. *J Virol* 2017;91. pii: e02484-16.
218. van Oostrum J, Burnett, RM. Molecular composition of the adenovirus type 2 virion. *J Virol* 1985;56:439–448.
219. Orazio NI, Naeger CM, Karlseder J, et al. The adenovirus E1b55K/E4orf6 complex induces degradation of the Bloom helicase during infection. *J Virol* 2011;85:1887–1892.
220. Ortega-Esteban A, Condezo GN, Perez-Berna AJ, et al. Mechanics of viral chromatin reveals the pressurization of human adenovirus. *ACS Nano* 2015;9:10826–10833.
221. O'Shea C, Klupsch K, Choi S, et al. Adenoviral proteins mimic nutrient/growth signals to activate the mTOR pathway for viral replication. *EMBO J* 2005;24:1211–1221.
222. Ostapchuk P, Almond M, Hearing P. Characterization of empty adenovirus particles assembled in the absence of a functional adenovirus IVa2 protein. *J Virol* 2011;85:5524–5531.
223. Ostapchuk P, Anderson ME, Chandrasekhar S, et al. The L4 22-kilodalton protein plays a role in packaging of the adenovirus genome. *J Virol* 2006;80:6973–6981.
224. Ostapchuk P, Hearing P. Control of adenovirus packaging. *J Cell Biochem* 2005;96:25–35.
225. Ostapchuk P, Hearing P. Adenovirus IVa2 protein binds ATP. *J Virol* 2008;82:10290–10294.
226. Ostapchuk P, Suomalainen M, Zheng Y, et al. The adenovirus major core protein VII is dispensable for virion assembly but is essential for lytic infection. *PLoS Pathog* 2017;13:e1006455.
227. Ostapchuk P, Yang J, Auffarth E, et al. Functional interaction of the adenovirus IVa2 protein with adenovirus type 5 packaging sequences. *J Virol* 2005;79:2831–2838.
228. Ou HD, Kwiatkowski W, Deerinck TJ, et al. A structural basis for the assembly and functions of a viral polymer that inactivates multiple tumor suppressors. *Cell* 2012;151:304–319.
229. Pardo-Mateos A, Young CS. A 40 kDa isoform of the type 5 adenovirus IVa2 protein is sufficient for virus viability. *Virology* 2004;324:151–164.
230. Parks CL, Banerjee S, Spector DJ. Organization of the transcriptional control region of the E1b gene of adenovirus type 5. *J Virol* 1988;62:54–67.
231. Patsalo V, Yondola MA, Luan B, et al. Biophysical and functional analyses suggest that adenovirus E4-ORF3 protein requires higher-order multimerization to function against promyelocytic leukemia protein nuclear bodies. *J Biol Chem* 2012;287:22573–22583.
232. Pennella MA, Liu Y, Woo JL, et al. Adenovirus E1B 55-kilodalton protein is a p53-SUMO1 E3 ligase that represses p53 and stimulates its nuclear export through interactions with promyelocytic leukemia nuclear bodies. *J Virol* 2010;84:12210–12225.
233. Perez-Berna AJ, Mangel WF, McGrath WJ, et al. Processing of the L1 52/55k protein by the adenovirus protease: a new substrate and new insights into virion maturation. *J Virol* 2014;88:1513–1524.
234. Perez-Berna AJ, Marion S, Chichon FJ, et al. Distribution of DNA-condensing protein complexes in the adenovirus core. *Nucleic Acids Res* 2015;43:4274–4283.
235. Perez-Romero P, Tyler RE, Abend JR, et al. Analysis of the interaction of the adenovirus L1 52/55-kilodalton and IVa2 proteins with the packaging sequence in vivo and in vitro. *J Virol* 2005;79:2366–2374.
236. Perricaudet M, Akusjarvi G, Virtanen A, et al. Structure of two spliced mRNAs from the transforming region of human subgroup C adenoviruses. *Nature* 1979;281:694–696.
237. Persson BD, Reiter DM, Marttila M, et al. Adenovirus type 11 binding alters the conformation of its receptor CD46. *Nat Struct Mol Biol* 2007;14:164–166.
238. Pombo A, Ferreira J, Bridge E, et al. Adenovirus replication and transcription sites are spatially separated in the nucleus of infected cells. *EMBO J* 1994;13:5075–5085.
239. Puntener D, Engelke MF, Ruzsics Z, et al. Stepwise loss of fluorescent core protein V from human adenovirus during entry into cells. *J Virol* 2011;85:481–496.
240. Querido E, Blanchette P, Yan Q, et al. Degradation of p53 by adenovirus E4orf6 and E1B55K proteins occurs via a novel mechanism involving a Cullin-containing complex. *Genes Dev* 2001;15:3104–3117.
241. Quinlan MP, Grodzicker T. Adenovirus E1A 12S protein induces DNA synthesis and proliferation in primary epithelial cells in both the presence and absence of serum. *J Virol* 1987;61:673–682.
242. van Raaij MJ, Louis N, Chroboczek J, et al. Structure of the human adenovirus serotype 2 fiber head domain at 1.5 A resolution. *Virology* 1999;262:333–343.
243. van Raaij MJ, Mitraki A, Lavigne G, et al. A triple beta-spiral in the adenovirus fibre shaft reveals a new structural motif for a fibrous protein. *Nature* 1999;401:935–938.
244. Reddy VS, Natchiar SK, Stewart PL, et al. Crystal structure of human adenovirus at 3.5 A resolution. *Science* 2010;329:1071–1075.
245. Reddy VS, Nemerow GR. Structures and organization of adenovirus cement proteins provide insights into the role of capsid maturation in virus entry and infection. *Proc Natl Acad Sci U S A* 2014;111:11715–11720.
246. Reich N, Pine R, Levy D, et al. Transcription of interferon-stimulated genes is induced by adenovirus particles but is suppressed by E1A gene products. *J Virol* 1988;62:114–119.
247. Reichel PA, Merrick WC, Siekierka J, et al. Regulation of a protein synthesis initiation factor by adenovirus virus-associated RNA. *Nature* 1985;313:196–200.
248. Risso-Ballester J, Cuevas JM, Sanjuan R. Genome-wide estimation of the spontaneous mutation rate of human adenovirus 5 by high-fidelity deep sequencing. *PLoS Pathog* 2016;12:e1006013.
249. Roberts RJ, O'Neill KE, Yen CT. DNA sequences from the adenovirus 2 genome. *J Biol Chem* 1984;259:13968–13975.
250. Roelvink PW, Lizonova A, Lee JG, et al. The coxsackievirus-adenovirus receptor protein can function as a cellular attachment protein for adenovirus serotypes from subgroups A, C, D, E, and F. *J Virol* 1998;72:7909–7915.
251. Ross PJ, Kennedy MA, Christou C, et al. Assembly of helper-dependent adenovirus DNA into chromatin promotes efficient gene expression. *J Virol* 2011;85:3950–3958.
252. Routes JM, Li H, Bayley ST, et al. Inhibition of IFN-stimulated gene expression and IFN induction of cytolytic resistance to natural killer cell lysis correlate with E1A-p300 binding. *J Immunol* 1996;156:1055–1061.
253. Routes JM, Ryan S, Morris K, et al. Adenovirus serotype 5 E1A sensitizes tumor cells to NKG2D-dependent NK cell lysis and tumor rejection. *J Exp Med* 2005;202:1477–1482.
254. Rowe WP, Huebner RJ, Gilmore LK, et al. Isolation of a cytopathogenic agent from human adenoids undergoing spontaneous degeneration in tissue culture. *Proc Soc Exp Biol Med* 1953;84:570–573.
255. Ruley HE. Adenovirus early region 1A enables viral and cellular transforming genes to transform primary cells in culture. *Nature* 1983;304:602–606.
256. Rux JJ, Burnett RM. Type-specific epitope locations revealed by X-ray crystallographic study of adenovirus type 5 hexon. *Mol Ther* 2000;1:18–30.
257. Saban SD, Silvestry M, Nemerow GR, et al. Visualization of alpha-helices in a 6-angstrom resolution cryoelectron microscopy structure of adenovirus allows refinement of capsid protein assignments. *J Virol* 2006;80:12049–12059.
258. San Martin C. Latest insights on adenovirus structure and assembly. *Viruses* 2012;4:847–877.
259. Saxton RA, Sabatini DM. mTOR signaling in growth, metabolism, and disease. *Cell* 2017;169:361–371.
260. Schaack J, Ho, WY Freimuth P, et al. Adenovirus terminal protein mediates both nuclear matrix association and efficient transcription of adenovirus DNA. *Genes Dev* 1990;4:1197–1208.
261. Schaley J, O'Connor RJ, Taylor LJ, et al. Induction of the cellular E2F-1 promoter by the adenovirus E4-6/7 protein. *J Virol* 2000;74:2084–2093.
262. Scherer M, Stamminger T. Emerging role of PML nuclear bodies in innate immune signaling. *J Virol* 2016;90:5850–5854.
263. Schneider RJ, Safer B, Munemitsu SM, et al. Adenovirus VAI RNA prevents phosphorylation of the eukaryotic initiation factor 2 alpha subunit subsequent to infection. *Proc Natl Acad Sci U S A* 1985;82:4321–4325.
264. Schneider RJ, Weinberger C, Shenk T. Adenovirus VAI RNA facilitates the initiation of translation in virus-infected cells. *Cell* 1984;37:291–298.
265. Schneider-Brachert W, Tchikov V, Merkel O, et al. Inhibition of TNF receptor 1 internalization by adenovirus 14.7K as a novel immune escape mechanism. *J Clin Invest* 2006;116:2901–2913.
266. Schreiner S, Wimmer P, Sirma H, et al. Proteasome-dependent degradation of Daxx by the viral E1B-55K protein in human adenovirus-infected cells. *J Virol* 2010;84:7029–7038.
267. Schwartz RA, Lakdawala SS, Eshleman HD, et al. Distinct requirements of adenovirus E1b55K protein for degradation of cellular substrates. *J Virol* 2008;82:9043–9055.
268. Segerman A, Atkinson JP, Marttila M, et al. Adenovirus type 11 uses CD46 as a cellular receptor. *J Virol* 2003;77:9183–9191.
269. Sha J, Ghosh MK, Zhang K, et al. E1A interacts with two opposing transcriptional pathways to induce quiescent cells into S phase. *J Virol* 2010;84:4050–4059.
270. Shtrichman R, Kleinberger T. Adenovirus type 5 E4 open reading frame 4 protein induces apoptosis in transformed cells. *J Virol* 1998;72:2975–2982.
271. Shtrichman R, Sharf R, Kleinberger T. Adenovirus E4orf4 protein interacts with both Balpha and B' subunits of protein phosphatase 2A, but E4orf4-induced apoptosis is mediated only by the interaction with Balpha. *Oncogene* 2000;19:3757–3765.
272. Silvestry M, Lindert S, Smith JG, et al. Cryo-electron microscopy structure of adenovirus type 2 temperature-sensitive mutant 1 reveals insight into the cell entry defect. *J Virol* 2009;83:7375–7383.

273. Smith JG, Cassany A, Gerace L, et al. Neutralizing antibody blocks adenovirus infection by arresting microtubule-dependent cytoplasmic transport. *J Virol* 2008;82:6492–6500.
274. Smith JG, Silvestry M, Lindert S, et al. Insight into the mechanisms of adenovirus capsid disassembly from studies of defensin neutralization. *PLoS Pathog* 2010;6:e1000959.
275. Sohn SY, Hearing P. Mechanism of adenovirus E4-ORF3-mediated SUMO modifications. *MBio* 2019;10. pii: e00022-19.
276. Sohn SY, Bridges RG, Hearing P. Proteomic analysis of ubiquitin-like posttranslational modifications induced by the adenovirus E4-ORF3 protein. *J Virol* 2015;89:1744–1755.
277. Sohn SY, Hearing P. Adenovirus regulates sumoylation of Mre11-Rad50-Nbs1 components through a paralog-specific mechanism. *J Virol* 2012;86:9656–9665.
278. Sohn SY, Hearing P. The adenovirus E4-ORF3 protein functions as a SUMO E3 ligase for TIF-1gamma sumoylation and poly-SUMO chain elongation. *Proc Natl Acad Sci U S A* 2016;113:6725–6730.
279. Sohn SY, Hearing P. Adenoviral strategies to overcome innate cellular responses to infection. *FEBS Lett* 2019;593:3484–3495. doi: 10.1002/1873-3468.13680.
280. Soria C, Estermann FE, Espantman KC, et al. Heterochromatin silencing of p53 target genes by a small viral protein. *Nature* 2010;466:1076–1081.
281. Spector DJ, Johnson JS, Baird NL, et al. Adenovirus type 5 DNA-protein complexes from formaldehyde cross-linked cells early after infection. *Virology* 2003;312:204–212.
282. Stabel S, Argos P, Philipson L. The release of growth arrest by microinjection of adenovirus E1A DNA. *EMBO J* 1985;4:2329–2336.
283. Stanton RJ, McSharry BP, Armstrong M, et al. Re-engineering adenovirus vector systems to enable high-throughput analyses of gene function. *Biotechniques* 2008;45:659–662, 664–668.
284. Steegenga WT, Shvarts A, Riteco N, et al. Distinct regulation of p53 and p73 activity by adenovirus E1A, E1B, and E4orf6 proteins. *Mol Cell Biol* 1999;19:3885–3894.
285. Stephens C, Harlow E. Differential splicing yields novel adenovirus 5 E1A mRNAs that encode 30 kd and 35 kd proteins. *EMBO J* 1987;6:2027–2035.
286. Stevens JL, Cantin GT, Wang G, et al. Transcription control by E1A and MAP kinase pathway via Sur2 mediator subunit. *Science* 2002;296:755–758.
287. Stewart PL, Nemerow GR. Cell integrins: commonly used receptors for diverse viral pathogens. *Trends Microbiol* 2007;15:500–507.
288. Stracker TH, Carson CT, Weitzman MD. Adenovirus oncoproteins inactivate the Mre11-Rad50-NBS1 DNA repair complex. *Nature* 2002;418:348–352.
289. Stracker TH, Lee DV, Carson CT, et al. Serotype-specific reorganization of the Mre11 complex by adenoviral E4orf3 proteins. *J Virol* 2005;79:6664–6673.
290. Strom AC, Ohlsson P, Akusjarvi G. AR1 is an integral part of the adenovirus type 2 E1A-CR3 transactivation domain. *J Virol* 1998;72:5978–5983.
291. Strunze S, Trotman LC, Boucke K, et al. Nuclear targeting of adenovirus type 2 requires CRM1-mediated nuclear export. *Mol Biol Cell* 2005;16:2999–3009.
292. Subramanian T, Zhao LJ, Chinnadurai G. Interaction of CtBP with adenovirus E1A suppresses immortalization of primary epithelial cells and enhances virus replication during productive infection. *Virology* 2013;443:313–320.
293. Suomalainen M, Nakano MY, Boucke K, et al. Adenovirus-activated PKA and p38/MAPK pathways boost microtubule-mediated nuclear targeting of virus. *EMBO J* 2001;20:1310–1319.
294. Tamanini A, Nicolis E, Bonizzato A, et al. Interaction of adenovirus type 5 fiber with the coxsackievirus and adenovirus receptor activates inflammatory response in human respiratory cells. *J Virol* 2006;80:11241–11254.
295. Temperley SM, Hay RT. Recognition of the adenovirus type 2 origin of DNA replication by the virally encoded DNA polymerase and preterminal proteins. *EMBO J* 1992;11:761–768.
296. Thai M, Graham NA, Braas D, et al. Adenovirus E4ORF1-induced MYC activation promotes host cell anabolic glucose metabolism and virus replication. *Cell Metab* 2014;19:694–701.
297. Thai M, Thaker SK, Feng J, et al. MYC-induced reprogramming of glutamine catabolism supports optimal virus replication. *Nat Commun* 2015;6:8873.
298. Thimmappaya B, Weinberger C, Schneider RJ, et al. Adenovirus VAI RNA is required for efficient translation of viral mRNAs at late times after infection. *Cell* 1982;31:543–551.
299. Thomas GP, Mathews MB. DNA replication and the early to late transition in adenovirus infection. *Cell* 1980;22:523–533.
300. Tomko RP, Xu R, Philipson L. HCAR and MCAR: the human and mouse cellular receptors for subgroup C adenoviruses and group B coxsackieviruses. *Proc Natl Acad Sci U S A* 1997;94:3352–3356.
301. Toogood CI, Crompton J, Hay RT. Antipeptide antisera define neutralizing epitopes on the adenovirus hexon. *J Gen Virol* 1992;73:1429–1435.
302. Tormanen H, Backstrom E, Carlsson A, et al. L4-33K, an adenovirus-encoded alternative RNA splicing factor. *J Biol Chem* 2006;281:36510–36517.
303. Trentin JJ, Yabe Y, Taylor G. The quest for human cancer viruses. *Science* 1962;137:835–841.
304. Trotman LC, Mosberger N, Fornerod M, et al. Import of adenovirus DNA involves the nuclear pore complex receptor CAN/Nup214 and histone H1. *Nat Cell Biol* 2001;3:1092–1100.
305. Tucker PA, Tsernoglou D, Tucker AD, et al. Crystal structure of the adenovirus DNA binding protein reveals a hook-on model for cooperative DNA binding. *EMBO J* 1994;13:2994–3002.
306. Tyler RE, Ewing SG, Imperiale MJ. Formation of a multiple protein complex on the adenovirus packaging sequence by the IVa2 protein. *J Virol* 2007;81:3447–3454.
307. Ullman AJ, Hearing P. Cellular proteins PML and Daxx mediate an innate antiviral defense antagonized by the adenovirus E4 ORF3 protein. *J Virol* 2008;82:7325–7335.
308. Ullman AJ, Reich NC, Hearing P. Adenovirus E4 ORF3 protein inhibits the interferon-mediated antiviral response. *J Virol* 2007;81:4744–4752.
309. Vachon VK, Conn GL. Adenovirus VA RNA: an essential pro-viral non-coding RNA. *Virus Res* 2016;212:39–52.
310. Valencia-Sanchez MA, Liu J, Hannon GJ, et al. Control of translation and mRNA degradation by miRNAs and siRNAs. *Genes Dev* 2006;20:515–524.
311. Walters RW, Freimuth P, Moninger TO, et al. Adenovirus fiber disrupts CAR-mediated intercellular adhesion allowing virus escape. *Cell* 2002;110:789–799.
312. Wang G, Balamotis MA, Stevens JL, et al. Mediator requirement for both recruitment and postrecruitment steps in transcription initiation. *Mol Cell* 2005;17:683–694.
313. Wang X, Bergelson JM. Coxsackievirus and adenovirus receptor cytoplasmic and transmembrane domains are not essential for coxsackievirus and adenovirus infection. *J Virol* 1999;73:2559–2562.
314. Wang K, Huang S, Kapoor-Munshi A, et al. Adenovirus internalization and infection require dynamin. *J Virol* 1998;72:3455–3458.
315. Watanabe H, Imai T, Sharp PA, et al. Identification of two transcription factors that bind to specific elements in the promoter of the adenovirus early-region 4. *Mol Cell Biol* 1988;8:1290–1300.
316. Weiss RS, Lee SS, Prasad BV, et al. Human adenovirus early region 4 open reading frame 1 genes encode growth-transforming proteins that may be distantly related to dUTP pyrophosphatase enzymes. *J Virol* 1997;71:1857–1870.
317. Weitzman MD, Ornelles DA. Inactivating intracellular antiviral responses during adenovirus infection. *Oncogene* 2005;24:7686–7696.
318. Whyte P, Williamson NM, Harlow E. Cellular targets for transformation by the adenovirus E1A proteins. *Cell* 1989;56:67–75.
319. Wickham TJ, Mathias P, Cheresh DA, et al. Integrins alpha v beta 3 and alpha v beta 5 promote adenovirus internalization but not virus attachment. *Cell* 1993;73:309–319.
320. Wienzek S, Roth J, Dobbelstein M. E1B 55-kilodalton oncoproteins of adenovirus types 5 and 12 inactivate and relocalize p53, but not p51 or p73, and cooperate with E4orf6 proteins to destabilize p53. *J Virol* 2000;74:193–202.
321. Wiethoff CM, Wodrich H, Gerace L, et al. Adenovirus protein VI mediates membrane disruption following capsid disassembly. *J Virol* 2005;79:1992–2000.
322. Williams JL, Garcia J, Harrich D, et al. Lymphoid specific gene expression of the adenovirus early region 3 promoter is mediated by NF-kappa B binding motifs. *EMBO J* 1990;9:4435–4442.
323. Wimmer P, Schreiner S, Everett RD, et al. SUMO modification of E1B-55K oncoprotein regulates isoform-specific binding to the tumour suppressor protein PML. *Oncogene* 2010;29:5511–5522.
324. Wodrich H, Cassany A, D'Angelo MA, et al. Adenovirus core protein pVII is translocated into the nucleus by multiple import receptor pathways. *J Virol* 2006;80:9608–9618.
325. Wohl BP, Hearing P. Role for the L1-52/55K protein in the serotype specificity of adenovirus DNA packaging. *J Virol* 2008;82:5089–5092.
326. Wold WS, Toth K. Adenovirus vectors for gene therapy, vaccination and cancer gene therapy. *Curr Gene Ther* 2013;13:421–433.
327. Woo JL, Berk AJ. Adenovirus ubiquitin-protein ligase stimulates viral late mRNA nuclear export. *J Virol* 2007;81:575–587.
328. Wu L, Berk A. Constraints on spacing between transcription factor binding sites in a simple adenovirus promoter. *Genes Dev* 1988;2:403–411.
329. Wu K, Guimet D, Hearing P. The adenovirus L4-33K protein regulates both late gene expression patterns and viral DNA packaging. *J Virol* 2013;87:6739–6747.
330. Wu K, Orozco D, Hearing P. The adenovirus L4-22K protein is multifunctional and is an integral component of crucial aspects of infection. *J Virol* 2012;86:10474–10483.
331. Xi Q, Cuesta R, Schneider RJ. Tethering of eIF4G to adenoviral mRNAs by viral 100k protein drives ribosome shunting. *Genes Dev* 2004;18:1997–2009.
332. Xiao T, Kao CF, Krogan NJ, et al. Histone H2B ubiquitylation is associated with elongating RNA polymerase II. *Mol Cell Biol* 2005;25:637–651.
333. Xue Y, Johnson JS, Ornelles DA, et al. Adenovirus protein VII functions throughout early phase and interacts with cellular proteins SET and pp32. *J Virol* 2005;79:2474–2483.
334. Yew PR, Berk AJ. Inhibition of p53 transactivation required for transformation by adenovirus early 1B protein. *Nature* 1992;357:82–85.
335. Yew PR, Liu X, Berk AJ. Adenovirus E1B oncoprotein tethers a transcriptional repression domain to p53. *Genes Dev* 1994;8:190–202.
336. Young CS. The structure and function of the adenovirus major late promoter. *Curr Top Microbiol Immunol* 2003;272:213–249.
337. Yueh A, Schneider RJ. Selective translation initiation by ribosome jumping in adenovirus-infected and heat-shocked cells. *Genes Dev* 1996;10:1557–1567.
338. Zantema A, Fransen JA, Davis-Olivier A, et al. Localization of the E1B proteins of adenovirus 5 in transformed cells, as revealed by interaction with monoclonal antibodies. *Virology* 1985;142:44–58.
339. Zemke NR, Berk AJ. The adenovirus E1A C terminus suppresses a delayed antiviral response and modulates RAS signaling. *Cell Host Microbe* 2017;22:789–800.e5.
340. Zhang W, Imperiale MJ. Interaction of the adenovirus IVa2 protein with viral packaging sequences. *J Virol* 2000;74:2687–2693.
341. Zhang W, Imperiale MJ. Requirement of the adenovirus IVa2 protein for virus assembly. *J Virol* 2003;77:3586–3594.
342. Zhang Z, Mui MZ, Chan F, et al. Genetic analysis of B55alpha/Cdc55 protein phosphatase 2A subunits: association with the adenovirus E4orf4 protein. *J Virol* 2011;85:286–295.
343. Zhao X. SUMO-mediated regulation of nuclear functions and signaling processes. *Mol Cell* 2018;71:409–418.
344. Zhao H, Chen M, Tellgren-Roth C, et al. Fluctuating expression of microRNAs in adenovirus infected cells. *Virology* 2015;478:99–111.
345. Zhao H, Granberg F, Elfineh L, et al. Strategic attack on host cell gene expression during adenovirus infection. *J Virol* 2003;77:11006–11015.
346. Zheng N, Schulman BA, Song L, et al. Structure of the Cul1-Rbx1-Skp1-F boxSkp2 SCF ubiquitin ligase complex. *Nature* 2002;416:703–709.
347. Zheng Y, Stamminger T, Hearing P. E2F/Rb family proteins mediate interferon induced repression of adenovirus immediate early transcription to promote persistent viral infection. *PLoS Pathog* 2016;12:e1005415.
348. Zhu J, Huang X, Yang Y. Innate immune response to adenoviral vectors is mediated by both Toll-like receptor-dependent and -independent pathways. *J Virol* 2007;81:3170–3180.
349. Ziff, EB. Transcription and RNA processing by the DNA tumour viruses. *Nature* 1980;287:491–499.
350. Zubieta C, Schoehn G, Chroboczek J, et al. The structure of the human adenovirus 2 penton. *Mol Cell* 2005;17:121–135.

CHAPTER

5 Adenoviruses

Thomas Lion • William S. M. Wold

INTRODUCTION

Since the first isolation from adenoidal tissue over 60 years ago,[571] human adenoviruses (HAdVs; *adén, gen.adénos = gland*) have provided continuous challenges in a variety of clinical settings. In addition to their well-established role as infectious agents, adenoviral genomes were also shown to contain potent oncogenes, and the ability of certain types of the virus to induce tumor growth has been demonstrated in different mammalian animal models in the early 1960s.[250,297,677] Despite a number of studies addressing the possible role of HAdVs in human malignant disease, their putative oncogenicity in man has remained enigmatic.[367,368,583] The investigation of adenovirus (AdV) biology has led to Nobel Prize–winning discoveries in mRNA splicing and to important progress in the understanding of antigen presentation to T cells.[208] Moreover, the ability of adenoviruses to infect many cell types facilitated their exploitation as vectors for gene delivery to generate new tools for innovative treatments of important diseases such as cancer and cardiovascular disorders.[136,137,473,610,738] Hence, adenoviruses are highly versatile organisms with a broad spectrum of clinical roles and applications. They are an important cause of infections in both immunocompetent and immunocompromised individuals, and continue to provide clinical challenges pertaining to diagnostics and treatment. The growing number of HAdV types identified by genomic analysis, as well as the improved understanding of the sites of viral persistence and reactivation, require continuous adaptations of diagnostic approaches to facilitate timely detection and monitoring of HAdV infections. In view of the clinical relevance of life-threatening HAdV diseases in the immunocompromised setting, there is an urgent need for highly effective treatment modalities lacking major side effects. A major focus of this chapter will therefore be the recent progress in the understanding and management of HAdV infections, including pertinent recent literature. Some of the earlier literature can be found in previous Editions of Fields Virology.[724,725]

HISTORY

During attempts to establish tissue culture lines from tonsils and adenoidal tissue surgically removed from children, Rowe and colleagues recognized that a transmissible agent was causing degeneration of the epithelial-like cells, and adenoviruses were first cultured and reported as distinct viral agents in 1953.[571] A nomenclature for HAdVs was adopted in 1956, and reclassification was performed in 1999.[686] The family of *Adenoviridae* included four genera, each corresponding to an independent evolutionary lineage that supposedly coevolved with the respective vertebrate hosts: *Mastadenovirus* (mastós = breast) from mammals, *Aviadenovirus* (avis = bird) from birds, *Atadenovirus* (the prefix stands for adenine and thymine, acknowledging the high AT content in the genomes of the first recognized members of this genus) and *Siadenovirus* (the prefix stands for sialidase, reflecting the presence of a putative sialidase homolog in members of this genus) from a broad range of hosts.[39,117,686] A fish adenovirus falls into a fifth clade, the more recently established genus *Ichtadenovirus* (ichthýs = fish).[226] In turtles, members of a sixth AdV lineage have been discovered, pending official recognition as an independent genus.[226] Human AdVs are divided into seven species termed A, B, C, D, E, F, and G, based on serum neutralizing and hemagglutination epitopes, genome sequence and function, oncogenic properties in newborn hamsters, and pathology in humans. These species were previously referred to as groups or subgroups.

Historically, human AdV isolates were designated as serotypes, based on neutralization of productive infection by homologous sera.[39] More recently, with the advent of high-throughput AdV genome sequencing and bioinformatic analysis, new insights into AdV genome structure and taxonomy have been obtained.[117,224] Evolution of AdVs seems to have been driven not only by sequence divergence but also by frequent recombination between different (sero)types.[436,441,557,559,560,607,707–709] Researchers have taken the view that AdV isolates should be designated as "types" rather than "serotypes," as per definitions of the International Committee on Taxonomy of Viruses. Two similar but not exact proposals have been advanced to characterize AdVs.[18,605] With one proposal, for example, human AdV serotype 1 will be designated "type HuAdV-1," with the "1" referring to hexon (the major capsid protein) identity. The rationale is that hexon should remain the major identifier "because it contains the major neutralizing epitope, which is targeted in molecular diagnosis".[18] With the other proposal, human AdV serotype 1 will become "type HAdV-C1," with the "C" referring to species C.[605] In the current article, "type" rather than "serotype" will be used to reflect the important impact of genomic analysis on the identification of novel variants during the last decade.[605] According to current standard nomenclature, "H" (for Human) should precede the species and type number, for example, HAdV-C5.

The first 51 HAdV types belonging to the species A-F were identified by serotyping, and were therefore originally referred to as serotypes (Table 5.1). Species B was further divided based on their genome similarities and restriction enzyme analysis into subspecies B1 (HAdV B3, B7, B16, B21, B50) and B2 (HAdV B11, B14, B34, B35, B55).[759] The first HAdV type identified by genomic analysis, which had been isolated from a patient with gastroenteritis, was assigned to the newly established species G in 2007, and was termed HAdV-G52.[307] All subsequent HAdV types, generally representing intraspecies recombinants, were identified by whole genome sequencing (WGS) and computational analysis[133,219,220,284,325,422,423] (Table 5.1). Furthermore, the genome sequence of the HAdV-C5 reference material (ARM) was published as a reference strain for vectors based on this HAdV type.[643] The genomes of different types within a species are usually highly related, but the divergence between different species can be considerable, and may therefore also affect the specificity of molecular detection.[422,423]

TABLE 5.1 Current spectrum of known human adenoviruses

Species	Types (Serotypes/Genotypes)
A	12, 18, 31, 61
B	3, 7, 11, 14, 16, 21, 34, 35, 50, 55, 66, 68, 76–79
C	1, 2, 5, 6, 57, 89, 104
D	8-10, 13, 15, 17, 19, 20, 22-30, 32, 33, 36–39, 42-49, 51, 53, 54, 56, 58, 59, 60, 63, 64, 65, 67, 69–75, 80–88, 90–103
E	4
F	40, 41
G	52

The HAdV species (A–G) and types (1–103) belonging to individual species are indicated. While the types 1–51 were identified by serotyping, all subsequently identified types (52–103) were identified by genomic sequencing and computational analysis.

From Lion T. Adenovirus persistence, reactivation, and clinical management. *FEBS Lett* 2019;593(24):3571–3582. Copyright © 2019 Federation of European Biochemical Societies. Reprinted by permission of John Wiley & Sons, Inc. Ref.[423]

INFECTIOUS AGENT

Propagation and Assay in Cell Culture

A number of cell lines including the primary human embryonic kidney (HEK) cells or continuous epithelial lines, such as HEp-2, HeLa, KB, HEK 293, and A549, have been used for propagation of HAdVs. The viruses in monolayer cell culture have a characteristic cytopathic effect (CPE). The cells round up, swell, and detach from the culture surface into grape-like clusters, and the nuclei become enlarged. Eventually the cells lyse, leaving cell debris. This CPE is the result of the infection passing into the "late" stage of infection, when adenoviral DNA, mRNA, and proteins are being made in large quantities, and virions are assembling in the cell nucleus. HAdVs increase glycolysis in continuous cell lines, thereby stimulating the cells to produce large quantities of acid. Rapid cytopathology can be induced within several hours of inoculating concentrated crude virus preparations, and the effect is not related to viral replication. Rather, it is caused by the penton base component of the free viral penton capsomere. Nuclear morphologic changes in infected cells have also been used for diagnostic purposes.[725]

Biological Characteristics

A general description of the biological characteristics including the structural proteins and the genomic structure is outlined in the preceding chapter.

Phylogeny and Human Adenoviral Species

The marked overall pattern of host specificity suggests that tight long-term association with their hominine hosts has governed HAdV evolution. However, there is evidence for natural host switches mediated by cross-species transmission, supporting the zoonotic origin of some HAdVs.[47,123,124] Studies in fecal samples from wild African great apes and humans, involving ancestral host reconstruction, support the notion that HAdV-B, in particular, originated in gorillas, and individual recombinants were transmitted to other apes and humans, presumably via the fecal–oral route, more than 100,000 years ago. However, while HAdV-B, -E, and -C have a high prevalence in gorilla and chimpanzee populations, HAdV-D has never been detected in great apes.[260,261] However, there is not only evidence for anthropozoonosis (transmission from animals to humans), but also for zooanthroponosis (transmission from humans to animals), indicating that adenoviruses are continuously crossing host/species barriers.[47]

Together with other mammalian adenoviruses, HAdVs are classified into the genus *Mastadenovirus*, and are further parsed into seven species termed A-G, with further subdivision of species B into subspecies B1 and B2, as briefly outlined above.[307,426,561,606,708,759] Species designation depends on several of the following characteristics: phylogenetic distance (>5% to 15%, based primarily on distance matrix analysis of the DNA polymerase amino acid sequence), genome organization (characteristically in the E3 region), nucleotide composition (G + C%), oncogenicity in rodents, host range, cross-neutralization, ability to recombine, number of VA RNA genes, and hemagglutination.[225] More than 30 simian (simia = monkey, ape) adenoviruses (SAdVs) display a sequence identity to their human counterparts to such an extent that they have also been included in the taxonomy of HAdVs within species B, C, E, and G.[225] Previously, HAdVs were identified, characterized, and classified by serum neutralization (SN) and hemagglutination inhibition (HI) assays, but more recently genomic and bioinformatic analysis of the entire viral genome has superseded serological methods for the typing of novel viruses.[18,225,307,426,561,606,708] The viruses belonging to individual HAdV species display high similarity to each other at the nucleotide level and do not commonly recombine with members of other species. The grouping into different species reflects, in part, the general cell tropism of the viruses and the resulting diseases and symptoms. Examples of common associations of individual HAdV species with infections at specific locations include gastroenteritis (HAdV-F and -G), pneumonia (HAdV-B, -C, -E), hepatitis (HAdV-C), meningoencephalitis (HAdV-A, -B, -D), cystitis (HAdV-B), and keratoconjunctivitis (HAdV-B, -D), but other HAdV species may also occur at the indicated sites of infection.[149,307,560]

(Sero)typing of Human Adenoviruses

HAdV subtyping below the level of species by SN and HI assays has led to the identification of 51 serotypes (Table 5.1). The hypervariable loops (L1 and L2) of the hexon protein form the SN epitope and are the main determinants of serologic reactivity, while the fiber protein is responsible for HI typing and is a major determinant of tropism. The combination of the SN and HI tests facilitates more complete virus identification than does either method alone. The first HAdV identified on the basis of genetic analysis was also classified as a novel species (HAdV-G), and received the chronological number 52.[307] Because all subsequently identified novel HAdVs were detected and characterized using computational analysis of genomic data (Table 5.1), it has been agreed to replace the term "serotype" by "type," and criteria for the assignment of new types have been established.[18,605]

Current Status of HAdV Types and Evolution of Human Adenoviruses

The number of HAdVs has been steadily expanding and currently includes more than 100 different types within the species A-G (Table 5.1) (http://hadvwg.gmu.edu/). Novel HAdV types reportedly arise from intra- or interspecies recombination events most frequently occurring within species D, the largest of all HAdV species, presently including over 70 different types. As outlined in Table 5.1, HAdV types 1 to 51 were characterized by serotyping, while the remaining types identified since 2007 were detected and described by genomic and bioinformatic analysis.[307,453,562]

Homologous recombination (HR) and mutation are important evolutionary processes driving genetic variation within HAdV genomes.[562] They are favored by the immune pressure of the host and environmental bottlenecks. In HAdV species B, mutations seem to play a more important role, whereas among the largest HAdV species D, HR between two or more virus types infecting the same cell(s) is the predominant mechanism contributing to genomic diversity.[287,475,562] While rapid selection of novel capsid gene sequences is apparently the main factor for the diversity in HAdV species B, recombinant types have also been described.[133,285,747]

HR of tumorigenic adenoviruses *in vitro* has been documented already in the 1970s,[655,719] and it was shown to occur predominantly between HAdV types belonging to the same species, within regions of high sequence homology.[560] The recent availability of WGS and bioinformatics has permitted the description of recombination events within genomes of HAdV species A, B, and D, particularly within the penton base, hexon, and fiber genes.[436,559,561,706] Recombination of capsid protein genes may diversify the tissue tropism of novel HAdV types, thereby potentially enhancing the pathogenicity and virulence of the new viruses.[133,229] In HAdV species C, recombination events between the genes encoding major capsid proteins are rare, and the recently identified recombinant type HAdV-C89, displaying a novel penton base sequence, has remained an exceptional observation.[133] The evolution of HAdV-C has mostly occurred at the subtype level, because the early gene regions E1 and E4 implicated in recombination events within this species are not considered in the type definition. Nevertheless, such recombinations at the subtype level may influence the virulence of HAdV-C strains.[133] The requirements for recombination events appear to include coinfection of individual cells with at least two different adenoviruses displaying very similar nucleotide sequences at the recombination hotspots in the genome, and long-term viral persistence in the host.[362,460,696] In bacteria, a signal for recombination between homologous DNA is the *c*rossover *h*otspot *i*nstigator (Chi) nucleotide sequence. This was first identified in bacteriophage lambda and then in bacterial DNA and later was shown to mediate recombination between them. The octanucleotide Chi sequence in *Escherichia coli* induces the conversion of the RecBCD enzyme from a helicase to an exonuclease, producing single-stranded (ss)DNA that can invade homologous double-stranded (ds)DNA during recombination. Chi-like nucleotide sequences adjacent to the junction of conserved and hypervariable gene segments in HAdV-D may therefore be an important signal for HR. This notion supports the concept that local bacterial flora might enhance natural recombination mediated by Chi-like nucleotide sequence motifs at HAdV-D recombination hotspots.[287] Indeed, recent experimental evidence indicated that coinfection with two different HAdV-D types in the presence of *E. coli* lysate increased the recombination. This effect was attributed to the bacterial RecA protein, which binds to the Chi-like adenoviral sequences located directly adjacent to the coding sequence for penton base hypervariable region 2.[393] The viruses may therefore repurpose the bacterial recombination machinery, and the authors proposed that free Rec proteins present in the gastrointestinal (GI) tract upon bacterial cell death could facilitate the evolution of HAdV species by HR. This concept supports the occurrence of transkingdom interactions between bacteria of the intestinal microbiome and enteric viruses.[393] The emergence of new HAdV-D types in patients with AIDS indicates a role of multiple persisting viruses under impaired immune surveillance.[113,562] HAdV-D genomes seem to recombine more frequently than do other human adenoviral species, and several of the currently more than 70 HAdV-D types have apparently emerged via recombination between hexon and fiber coding regions.[562] The majority of novel HAdV types identified by genomic analysis belong to species D, and they were shown to include sequences derived from multiple other types from the same species. For example, HAdV-D53 resulted from recombination in penton, hexon, and fiber regions of HAdV-D22, D37, and D8, respectively. Similarly, HAdV-D67 was identified as a recombinant between HAdV-D9, D25, D26, D33, and D46.[325,453] The latest additions to the rapidly evolving genus D include the types HAdV-D100 (a recombinant of hexon D17, fiber D30, and a novel penton base recombined from D38 [HVR1] and D48 [HVR2]), HAdV-D101 (a recombinant of hexon D37, fiber D45, and a novel penton base recombined from D59 [HVR1] and D67 [HRV2]), HAdV-D102 (a recombinant of hexon D38, fiber D30, and a novel penton base recombined from D62 [HVR1] and D54 [HRV2]), and HAdV-D103 (a recombinant of hexon D33, fiber D30, and a novel penton base recombined from D37 [HVR1] and D48 [HRV2]) (Table 5.1; http://hadvwg.gmu.edu).

Moreover, current data provide evidence for the occurrence of recombination between different HAdV species, and even between human and simian adenoviruses (SAdVs).[123,717] Computational analysis of HAdV-E4, the only representative of species E, indicated that this virus is of zoonotic origin and has evolved through two interspecies recombination events with lateral partial gene transfer. HAdVE-4 contains 97% SAdV-E26-like genome chassis with a hexon containing the L1 and L2 regions from a HAdV-B16-like virus, which may provide compatibility with the new host.[123,667] Adaptation of the virus to the new host could also be related to a further recombination event leading to the acquirement of a NF-1 binding site motif, which is required for efficient viral replication.

Molecular evolution of HAdVs by HR can result in new viruses displaying different tissue tropism and increased virulence. Improved knowledge of HR might therefore facilitate prediction of potential emerging HAdV types. In addition to their role in the evolution of novel HAdV types, it is important to understand the recombination mechanisms, if adenoviral vectors are to be used in human patients who might coincidentally be infected with a wild-type virus. Moreover, the occurrence of viral recombinants with lateral DNA and epitope transfers between HAdVs and SAdVs must be borne in mind when chimpanzee adenoviruses are considered as vectors for gene delivery in human patients to exploit the lack of immunoreactivity to these viruses (see below).

Key Antigens

The clinically important HAdV antigens include primarily the three capsid proteins: hexon, penton base, and fiber. Most early studies indicated that the hexon, and to a lesser extent the fiber proteins, contain most of the epitopes recognized by neutralizing antibodies, but the penton base displays neutralizing epitopes as well.[96,257,440] The neutralization properties of polyclonal antibodies are often concordant with the inhibition of HAdV-induced hemagglutination (HA) of red blood cells. However, the HA functions are a property of the fiber,[497] which apparently must be linked to the penton base for complete HA to occur. Because of recombination within species in clinical isolates, it is not uncommon to isolate a virus that demonstrates discordant reactions in the neutralization and HA inhibition reactions.

Studies in naturally infected humans found that the majority of neutralizing antibodies were directed against the hypervariable regions of hexon, but some were also directed against the fiber and possibly the penton base.[558,646] In contrast, other published data suggest that HAdV-C5 neutralizing antibodies to fiber are more common than those to hexon in the naturally infected population, but immunization with a replication-defective HAdV-C5-based vector raised more neutralizing antibodies to capsid proteins other than fiber.[96] Most studies in animal models investigating infections with HAdV-C5-based vectors found that the predominant neutralizing antibodies are directed at hypervariable hexon regions.[385,558,750] Mechanisms by which neutralizing antibodies function include virus aggregation, virus destabilization, blocking virus–receptor interactions, and integrin-mediated internalization.[626] One study provided evidence that the HAdV-C5 neutralizing antihexon monoclonal antibody 9C12 inhibits adenovirus infection by blocking microtubule-dependent translocation of the virus to the microtubule-organizing center following endosome penetration.[626] Another study based on using the same monoclonal antibody as well as polyclonal HAdV-C5 neutralizing antibodies concluded that the cellular cytosolic protein TRIM21 binds to the antibody in the internalized antibody–virus complex, and targets the virus to the proteasome for degradation.[446]

There are species- and type-specific epitopes on both hexon and fiber. Type-specific domains have been mapped to unique sequences in loop 1 (amino acids 281 to 292) and loop 2 (amino acids 441 to 455) of the hexon by generating neutralizing antibodies to peptides from each of these regions, and this epitope is referred to as the ε determinant.[440] Loops 1 and 2 had previously been shown by crystallography to be on the surface of the virion. Differences in the HA properties of rhesus and vervet monkey erythrocytes for two important subtypes of HAdV-B11 (HAdV-B11p and HAdV-B11a) have been related to nucleotide sequence differences in the shaft and knob region of fiber. The knob region of fiber, which has HA properties that are used for HI tests, includes the γ determinant. The subtypes HAdV-B11p and B11a display some differences in tissue tropism in that B11p can persist in the urinary tract and B11a causes acute respiratory tract infections. These properties may be related to the changes in fiber polypeptides, otherwise displaying identity for 92.3% of their amino acids.[440] There are antibodies apparently reacting with conserved hexon domains from all human types, as determined by the complement fixation (CF) test and serologic techniques, such as immunofluorescent (IF) antibody and enzyme-linked immunosorbent assays (ELISA).

HAdV-specific CD4+ T lymphocytes have been detected in peripheral blood in nearly all naturally infected humans of all ages.[61,84,274,397,500] When peripheral blood mononuclear cells (PBMCs) were stimulated in bulk culture (e.g., by incubation with intact HAdV particles, HAdV-infected cell extracts, purified HAdV proteins, or with pools of peptides that span various HAdV proteins), CD4+ T lymphocytes specific to hexon were identified in healthy donors.[174,600,752] Other studies using peptides corresponding to parts of several HAdV proteins identified a number of CD4+ T-cell epitopes, including the dominant HLA DP4-restricted H910-924 epitope, located in the base of the hexon protein, which is conserved among HAdV types and detectable in PBMCs from the majority of healthy adults analyzed.[601] Many other CD4+ T-cell epitopes located in the conserved regions of HAdV-C5 hexon that are conserved across HAdV types have been identified.[398,399,600,751] In a study that analyzed PBMCs from 44 healthy donors, 10 CD4+ T-cell immunodominant hexon epitopes were detected in more than 50% of subjects examined, and the HLA restriction element for some of these peptides is known.[600,751] In addition to the more frequently observed HAdV- and hexon-specific CD4+ T cells, hexon-specific CD8+ T cells have also been detected in PBMCs from healthy donors. These cells are cross-reactive with various HAdV types, secrete IFNγ (interferon gamma), and display cytolytic activity in culture.[274,308,398,751] CD4+ and CD8+ T cells specific for HAdV proteins other than hexon, including penton base and DNA polymerase, have also been identified.[174,308,399] There is increasing evidence that hexon-specific cytotoxic T lymphocytes (CTLs) are protective in humans.[398] Indeed, mixtures of CD4+ and CD8+ cells specific for hexon and other HAdV proteins were shown to be effective upon adoptive cell transfer for infections by various HAdV types in allogeneic hematopoietic stem cell transplant (SCT) recipients or in primary immunodeficiencies.[2,173,194,310,336,399,400,537,595,751] The therapeutic effect is believed to be mediated by the coordinated action of the adoptively transferred CD4+ and CD8+ T cells.[751]

Infection of Experimental Animals

Similar to other mammalian or avian AdV species, HAdVs are mostly host specific in their replication cycle, and even nonhuman primates are poor hosts for HAdVs. HAdV species C can replicate in the lung of cotton rats, permitting to study the pathogenesis of HAdV-mediated pneumonia in these animals.[531] An ocular model of infection with either HAdV-C5 or HAdV-D8 has been described in cotton rats, and the clinical manifestations, including subepithelial corneal opacities, were similar to epidemic keratoconjunctivitis (EKC).[327] The animals shed the virus, developed specific antibodies to the infecting virus, and were able to transmit the infection to control cotton rats. A similar ocular model was reported in New Zealand white rabbits after topical or intrastromal inoculations of HAdV-C5.[103,569] The virus appeared to replicate, and most of the animals developed a humoral immune response. There were findings of blepharitis, conjunctivitis, iritis, corneal edema, and subepithelial corneal infiltrates that were consistent with immune-mediated clinical disease. The HAdV-C5 New Zealand white rabbit model has been used to evaluate the antiviral activity of several compounds including cidofovir, 2′-3′ dideoxycytidine, *N*-chlorotaurine, and dexamethasone povidone–iodine, and the results provided a basis for ensuing clinical trials.[101,103,517,568,569]

A number of groups have explored mouse models for studying HAdV-mediated pathogenesis to evaluate oncolytic (replication-competent) HAdV vectors for cancer gene therapy. HAdVs can infect cells of virtually all mammalian species including murine cells, especially if high multiplicities of infection are used (~100 plaque forming units per cell). Early HAdV proteins are expressed at good levels, and HAdV-C5 DNA replication was documented in Syrian hamsters, indicating that these animals are a suitable permissive immunocompetent model for HAdV pathogenesis and testing of oncolytic HAdV vectors, in contrast to mice where no evidence of vector replication has been obtained.[662,727,745] HAdV-C5 replicates modestly in cotton rat cells,[638] canine cells,[661] and porcine cells.[304] In three Syrian hamster cancer cell lines, the burst size (virus yield per cell) was about 1,000, only 10-fold less than in A549 cells.[662] Moreover, Syrian hamsters displayed HAdV-C5 replication in the liver following intravenous administration, and efficient (~4-log) replication in the lungs following intranasal or intratracheal administration.[662,745] Due to the permissiveness of Syrian hamster tissues for HAdV-C5 and the availability of numerous Syrian hamster cancer cell lines, these animals have been used as a model to investigate the toxicology and antitumor efficacy of oncolytic HAdV-C5-based vectors.[59,131,672,674,675,744] Immunocompetent and immunosuppressed (by treatment with cyclophosphamide) hamsters bearing subcutaneous tumors formed by injection with various Syrian hamster cancer cell lines were treated by intratumoral injection with a variety of oncolytic HAdV vectors.[48,129,130,132,330,634,748] In general, these studies showed that oncolytic HAdV-C5-based vectors suppress the tumor growth, and that a rapid adaptive immune response to the vector appears to eliminate the vector from the tumor.[617] Syrian hamsters have also been used to study the biodistribution and toxicity of oncolytic HAdV-C5-based vectors in advance of clinical trials.[351,456,631,745] Immunocompetent, newborn, and immunosuppressed Syrian hamsters have been used to evaluate compounds inhibiting HAdV replication, and a mouse model was used to test the virostatic compound cidofovir against disseminated murine AdV type 1 infection.[135,673,726] HAdVs inoculated into a variety of rodent species cause a number of tumors. Pronounced oncogenicity in newborn Syrian hamsters has been demonstrated for HAdV types A12, A18, and A31, and much has been learned about the mechanism of action of the genes in the E1A and E1B regions from these viral models. The integrated HAdV-A12 sequences in these hamster tumors are a model for understanding epigenetic consequences of foreign DNA integration.[140,141] In addition to rodent animal models,[411,450,579] porcine cells were recently shown to provide a valuable model for preclinical testing of engineered oncolytic chimeric HAdV-C5/3 vectors[361] (see section on Adenoviruses as Vectors for further details).

PATHOGENESIS AND PATHOLOGY

Entry into the Host

Adenoviruses enter susceptible hosts by oral, nasopharyngeal, or ocular infection. Experimental data have identified several receptors, attachment factors, and facilitators as HAdV binding partners, which display steric features complementary to components of the viral capsid or to virions in complex with host proteins.[163,177,209,386,497,718,729] Currently known receptor molecules include the coxsackie and adenovirus receptor (CAR), CD46, desmoglein-2 (DSG2), integrins, sulfated glycosaminoglycans (GAG), and sialic acid–containing oligosaccharides, including the disialylated GD1 glycan as well as polysialylated glycoproteins[86–88,405,499,637,642,711] (Fig. 5.1). Additionally, two related proteins, CD80 and CD86, co-stimulatory molecules from the immunoglobulin superfamily that are present on mature dendritic cells and B lymphocytes, were shown to serve as attachment receptors for members of HAdV species B via the fiber knob domain, and can be utilized for infection of otherwise nonpermissive cells.[618] The diversity of HAdV receptors contributes to the broad tropism of these viruses, and structural studies are thus an important source of information on HAdV–host cell interactions. Moreover, studies in murine models identified the macrophage scavenger receptor SR-A6 (MARCO) as an adenovirus type–specific virus entry receptor involved in the sensing of infection with HAdV and recombinant adenoviral vectors. This receptor is important for production of IFN type I, and may therefore play a role in innate antiviral immunity.[445,641]

The CAR receptor is a 46-kDa transmembrane protein involved in the formation of tight junctions of polarized cells, where it mediates cell-to-cell adhesion. Moreover, it was recently shown to also regulate synaptic transmission in neuronal communication, and to play an important role both in controlling recruitment of immune cells and in tumorigenesis.[505,578,730] It mediates recognition of the fiber knobs protruding from the viral capsid, thereby anchoring the virus to the cell. This high-affinity receptor interaction, which operates in most HAdVs, with the exception of representatives of species B, is unable to promote virus entry into cells.[111] HAdVs of species B can be differentiated based on their receptor usage. Members of HAdV subspecies B1 predominantly utilize CD46 as a receptor. The binding is mediated by fiber knobs of the virus, which recognize the receptor with different affinities. The membrane protein CD46 is expressed on virtually all cells, where it acts as a cofactor for inactivation of different complement components. Members of HAdV subspecies B2 utilize DSG2 as their high-affinity receptor, a calcium-binding transmembrane glycoprotein from the cadherin protein family, but HAdV-B11 was shown to use either CD46 or DSG2.[711,712,714] When the HAdV fiber binds to DSG2, opening of intercellular junctions results in increased access to receptors trapped deep within the junction, but the dissociation of the intercellular junctions may also facilitate the lateral viral spread in epithelial cells and, potentially, the penetration into subepithelial cell layers and the bloodstream.[711] The fiber protein on HAdVs mediates viral entry via interaction of its most distal structure with host cell receptors, and phylogenetic analysis of HAdV-D types associated with EKC revealed that they form a unique clade characterized by a shared amino acid composition of the fiber knob.[286] Proteotyping analysis showed that it is possible to predict human corneal cell tropism by identifying specific amino acids at a critical position of the fiber knob, with evidence for positive selection.[287] Different representatives of HAdV species D associated with EKC appear to bind to α2,3-linked sialic acid present in the GD1a ganglioside on the corneal cell surface.[28,499]

Unlike the great majority of HAdVs, HAdV-G52 displays a long and a short fiber protein. While the long fiber binds to the CAR receptor, the short fiber knob forms transient electrostatic interactions with long chains of polysialic acid (polySia), rendering CAR and polySia the most efficient attachment factors for HAdV-G52.[404] The fiber knob can also interact with

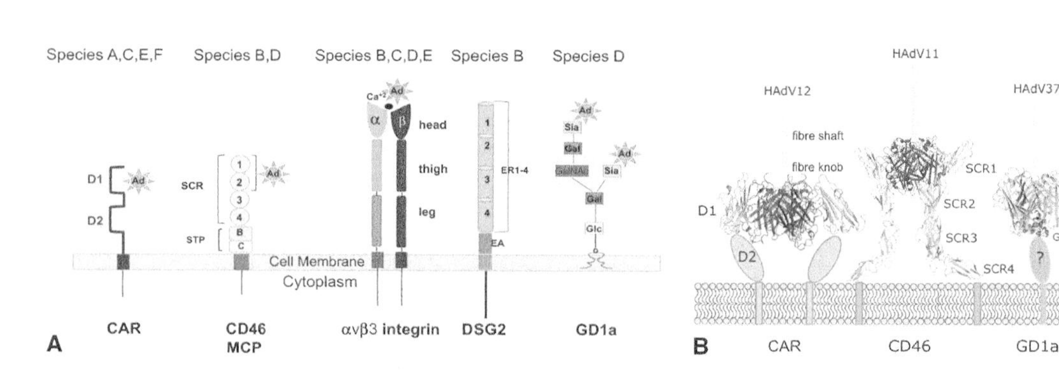

FIGURE 5.1 Cell receptors for adenovirus attachment and internalization. A: The diagram indicates the HAdV species using the CAR, complement receptor (CD46/MCP), vitronectin-binding integrin αvβ5, the glycolipid-anchored receptor GD1a, or desmoglein 2 (DSG2). Sialic acid residues on certain receptors have been shown to be the actual site of virus fiber interaction. **B:** Structural view of HAdV binding types to attachment receptors (examples of individual HAdV types). The trimeric knob is shown in shades of purple; the trimeric fiber shaft is represented by a yellow line (length not to scale). Domains not featured in structures are represented with cartoon shapes. ([Panel A] from Nemerow G, Flint J. Lessons learned from adenovirus (1970-2019). *FEBS Lett* 2019;593(24):3395–3418. Copyright © 2019 Federation of European Biochemical Societies. Reprinted by permission of John Wiley & Sons, Inc. [Panel B] from Stasiak AC, Stehle T. Human adenovirus binding to host cell receptors: a structural view. *Med Microbiol Immunol* 2020;209(3):325–333. https://creativecommons.org/licenses/by/4.0/.)

monosialylated and disialylated glycans, albeit with lower affinity. Only polySia-containing glycoproteins on target cells therefore appear to serve as efficient receptors for HAdV-G52.[405] Since polySia is highly expressed on various cancer cell types displaying very aggressive and invasive properties, exploitation of HAdV-G52 might provide the basis for developing oncolytic vectors (see below) targeting particularly tumors characterized by elevated polySia expression. The low seroprevalence and reduced liver tropism of this HAdV type further support this notion.[405]

A recently described additional receptor-independent mechanism of HAdV entry into cells is the use of exosomes.[110,111,621] Exosomes are nano-sized, membrane-bound vesicles with a diameter of 30 to 150 nm that are generated during endosome maturation,[81] and are secreted into the extracellular environment by many eukaryotic cell types.[110,306] They act as carriers of nucleic acids, lipids, and proteins, and their composition reflects the subcellular origin and the physiology of the parent cells.[110,306] Exosomes can carry viral genomes and act as vehicles for viruses facilitating entry into host cells, thereby providing a mechanism of evasion from the immune system.[111] It has been demonstrated that HAdV-C5 can exploit exosomes for cellular entry in CAR-deficient cells by binding to these particles and entering cells via phosphatidylserine or different binding proteins.[621] The exploitation of exosomes loaded with HAdVs would be advantageous for therapeutic applications in cancer treatment owing to the evasion from host immune response and broader tropism of virus delivery. However, prior to moving towards clinical application, several challenges need to be met, including the low production yield and short half-life of the vesicles as well as the lack of knowledge about their possible immunogenic properties or toxic effects.[111,281,347,768]

It is necessary to consider that the administration of HAdV-based vectors *in vivo* may display different modes of cell entry, as suggested by studies in murine models proposing a CAR-independent mechanism, but it is unclear whether this pathway also operates in humans. The coagulation factor X (FX) binds to the adenovirus capsid and protects the virion from natural antibody and classical complement-mediated neutralization in both mice and humans.[145] The findings in murine models indicated that infection of hepatic cells occurred through HAdV binding to FX, directing the complexes to hepatocellular receptors, including heparin sulfate proteoglycans[700,701] (Fig. 5.2). The high-affinity interaction of several HAdVs with FX may facilitate bridging of the hexon protein in the viral capsid to heparin sulfate proteoglycans expressed on the surface of hepatocytes. The virus complexed with FX binds to the cell surface through the serine protease domain of FX rather than through a direct interaction of the virus with the cell surface.[323,700] Once bound to the cell surface, efficient and rapid intracellular transport of the virus remains dependent upon engagement of α_v integrins via the penton base protein.[51] Virus internalization, facilitated by a secondary interaction with cellular integrins, is mediated by the loops of viral penton base proteins containing an Arg-Gly-Asp (RGD) motif.[493,756] If the CAR receptor is involved, the fiber shaft may need to undergo strong flexion to facilitate simultaneous engagement of the virus with CAR and integrin receptors to form the tethered ligand assembly.[175,177,434,731,756]

After the interaction with host cell receptors and integrin-mediated endocytosis, the virus particles undergo uncoating, with dissolution of the viral capsid in the endosome. The removal of various scaffolding proteins is important for virulence. Thereafter, the virus is transferred through the cytoplasm along microtubules into the nucleus by dynein (cytoskeletal motor protein)-dependent translocation.[340]

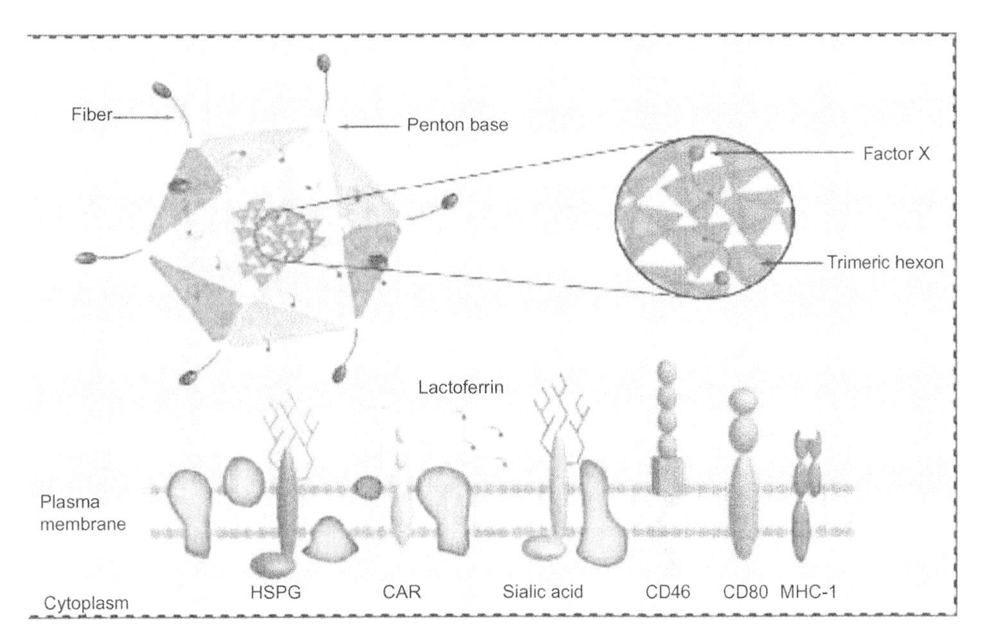

FIGURE 5.2 Coagulation factor X–mediated HAdV binding to liver cell receptors including heparin sulfate proteoglycans (HSPG). While the receptors are generally membrane proteins, other ligands are present in a soluble form, such as lactoferrin and coagulation factor X, which are used as a bridge between the virus and the cell, to target the liver. The receptor usage depends on the HAdV type and the targeted tissue.

Sites of Primary Replication and Spread of the Virus

The original observation of HAdVs in tonsils and adenoids indicate that these tissues of the oropharynx are an initial site of entry and replication. Initial replication of HAdV types causing respiratory disease most likely occurs in the nonciliated respiratory epithelium, although some limited replication and persistence can also occur within lymphocytes.[422] The apical surfaces of ciliated respiratory epithelium in the lower airways do not display the CAR receptor and are therefore difficult to infect by HAdV types requiring this molecule for cellular attachment. However, disruption of the integrity of cell-to-cell contact can facilitate basolateral infection of such polarized epithelial cells via this receptor.[712] Manifestations of HAdV infection are often topically restricted to the eyes or the pharynx, but contiguous extension into the lungs can occur. A possible molecular mechanism facilitating spread of the virus over respiratory epithelia can be mediated by the fiber protein, which is synthesized in great abundance in the infected cells and binds to CAR on the basolateral surface upon release from lysed cells. This binding disrupts the CAR homodimers in tight junctions, thus increasing paracellular permeability.[612] This, in turn, allows the virus to escape onto the apical surface of the respiratory epithelium, thereby making it possible to infect other areas of the respiratory tract. While various HAdV types (e.g., HAdV-C5) are mainly associated with upper respiratory tract infections, a few pneumotropic HAdV types (E4, B3, B7, B14p1) can cause severe lower respiratory tract infections like pneumonia and acute respiratory distress syndrome (ARDS), even in immunocompetent patients. The highly pathogenic HAdV-B14p1 virus was shown to infect differentiated human bronchial epithelial cells efficiently from the apical surface using the DSG2 receptor and to induce proinflammatory cytokines as potential virulence factors. Infectious virus progeny is also released via the apical surface, thereby promoting endobronchial dissemination of the infection from the upper to the lower respiratory tract.[383] Moreover, dissociation of the intercellular junctions by binding to DSG2 may facilitate spread of the virus locally and into deeper tissue layers, mediating access to the bloodstream.[711] The occurrence of systemic infection characterized by viremia, which is observed particularly in the immunocompromised patient setting, is discussed below. Since CAR is expressed on endothelial cells, viremia caused by HAdV types utilizing this receptor might be promoted by the fiber protein via the mechanism described above.[409,549] The successful use of oral, live, microencapsulated HAdV vaccines by the military to prevent ARDS suggests that, if the respiratory tract can be physically bypassed by the viruses, intestinal virus replication causes an immunizing rather than a virulent infection.[93,552] While some HAdV types including particularly F40 and F41 are a common cause of intestinal disease, various HAdV types can replicate in the intestine without causing gastroenteritis.

Tissue Tropism in the Host

The general affinity of HAdV species to individual tissues is outlined above, but members of the largest species D show particularly great variability in their tropism ranging from growth in ocular to GI and respiratory tissues.[288,362,561,706] Adenoviral keratoconjunctivitis, which is a major cause of ocular morbidity, is most commonly caused by representatives of species D, including types D8, D19, and D37, but can also be mediated by HAdV-E4, C5, B3, B7, B11, and B14.[437] GI manifestations are mainly associated with HAdV-F40 and F41, but G52 and different members of species D have also been observed.[307,422,437,452,453] Respiratory tract involvement has been associated mainly with HAdV-B3, B7, B16 and B21, E4, and various members of species C.[467] The knowledge about the basis of tissue tropism has been expanding,[386,565,623,637] and the indicated examples demonstrate that certain adenoviruses have a strong tropism to specific tissues. However, the same clinical manifestations can also be caused by other HAdV types and species, thus requiring diagnostic screening methods with broad specificity.

Chemical Defense and Immune Response

In the airways, the virus must penetrate the surface fluid, and sialic acid present in the mucus may bind and inhibit HAdV species D types that use sialic acid as a receptor.[499] The virus must also survive chemical defenses of the host. These include a large variety of antimicrobial peptides that are able to neutralize microbes directly. Among these peptides are the defensins, a family of small cationic amphipathic peptide molecules divided into two classes, α- and β-defensins.[234,252,720,721] The α-defensins HNP1 and HD5 were to shown to neutralize HAdV types of species A, B1, B2, C, and E but not species D and F.[627,628] The defensins bind HAdV particles outside the cell, block uncoating of the virion, and restrict the release of virions from endocytic vesicles.[627] Thousands of α-defensin molecules bind to sensitive virus types, and neutralization of the virus depends on binding to critical determinants in a region spanning the fiber and penton base proteins. Binding to these determinants is proposed to prevent the release of fiber from the virion, the first step in the uncoating process within the endosome.[628] HNP1 is expressed primarily in neutrophils, monocytes, lymphocytes, and natural killer (NK) cells, while HD5 is expressed mainly by Paneth cells in the intestine.[234,253] The role of defensins in HAdV infections has recently been demonstrated in human enteroids representing a primary intestinal cell culture system, which indicated potent HAdV-type restricted neutralization by the enteric human alpha-defensin HD5.[254]

Similar to other viral infections, HAdV is controlled by innate and adaptive immune responses.[23,24,106,240,516,617] The first steps of immune response include the activation of a systemic proinflammatory state by the release of various cytokines, and the attraction of immune cells to the sites of infection.[23] Innate effector cells, particularly NK cells, which can destroy virus-infected cells in a nonspecific fashion, are recruited and activated.[69,240] Moreover, rapid secretion of antiviral cytokines such as IFNγ, TNF (tumor necrosis factor), IL (interleukin)-1, IL-2, and macrophage inflammatory proteins (MIPs) is triggered by HAdV and targets different steps in the viral life cycle, thereby limiting the amplification and spread of the virus. The presence of specific cytokine signatures was reported in pediatric SCT recipients with localized and invasive HAdV infection. Patients with invasive infections had increased levels of the proinflammatory cytokines IL-1β, IL-6, IL-8, IL-12, IFNγ, and TNFα. Simultaneous release of other cytokines associated with invasive HAdV infection includes also IL-17, IL-18, OSM, MIP1α, and IP10.[233] Induction of IL-6 and IL-8 does not require HAdV gene expression and likely occurs via interaction of the virion with integrins on the cell surface. Early proteins of HAdV derived from E1A, E1B, E3, and E4 as well as the virus-associated (VA) noncoding RNAs are able to antagonize innate immune responses of the host.[240] The E1A proteins block the assembly of IFN-induced transcription factors, and VA-I, a 159 nucleotide noncoding RNA, binds to the double-stranded RNA-dependent protein kinase R (PKR). This kinase mediates antiviral activity by attenuation of viral protein translation, and inhibition of the kinase by VA-I RNA enables HAdVs to evade this defense mechanism.[146,682,702] Moreover, HAdVs display different mechanisms enabling them to counteract the induction of type I IFNs (IFNα and β), which are an important part of the innate response to viral infection. For example, the HAdV-encoded E1B 55 kDa protein mediates transcriptional repression of IFN-inducible genes, thereby facilitating viral replication.[80] Another example includes the E3-19K transmembrane glycoprotein encoded in the E3 region, which is localized in the endoplasmic reticulum and binds to newly synthesized MHC (major histocompatibility complex) class I molecules. This leads to inhibition of intracellular transport and cell surface expression of class I molecules, thereby impairing antigen presentation to CD8+ cytotoxic T cells. In this way, HAdV-infected cells can evade recognition and T-cell attack. Furthermore, the E3 14.7K protein is a potent inhibitor of TNF-mediated apoptosis.

In addition to providing the first line of defense, the innate immune system supports proliferation and differentiation of the adaptive immune response mediated by T and B lymphocytes. The generation of HAdV-specific T cells facilitates lysis of infected cells by a perforin-dependent mechanism.[235] Although the large number of existing HAdV types implies that the expression of antigens representing potential T-cell targets can be expected to be highly polymorphic, T cells raised against HAdV, including the CD4 and CD8 subsets, were shown to display cross-reactivity against different adenoviral species.[398] These observations indicate that such T cells recognize conserved sequences of amino acid residues from a structural protein of HAdV.[335] Although the HAdV-derived penton protein was identified as a relevant target of the anti-HAdV immune response, the hexon protein, which contains generic antigenic components common to all adenoviral species, has been regarded as one of the most important immunodominant T-cell targets.[600,669] Hence, HAdV exposure during the childhood and the ensuing generation of cross-reactive cytotoxic T cells is believed to lead to broad HAdV immunity in adults.[273] Neutralizing antibodies (see section on Key Antigens) are protective against disease manifestation in the previously infected host or against reinfection with the same HAdV type, but do not eliminate the carrier state.[170,664]

Healthy individuals usually carry HAdV-specific T cells, which can be identified by various methods, such as IFNγ secretion assays, cytokine flow cytometry, or MHC class I multimers.[195,600] The absence of HAdV-specific T cells has a negative impact on the course of HAdV infections, and conversely, reconstitution of HAdV-specific T-cell response correlates with viral clearance.[173,751] The findings that many CD4- or CD8-restricted hexon epitopes are shared among different species and types of the virus suggest that T cells with such specificities can be protective against most, if not all, HAdVs. This fact can be exploited for vaccine-based or adoptive T-cell transfer immunotherapy for treating HAdV infections, as outlined in the Therapy section below.[310]

Virulence

The emergence of novel HAdV types and strains can present with altered patterns of tropism and virulence. While the severity of HAdV-E4 infections in outbreaks appears to depend more on preexisting conditions in patients than on genetically determined viral virulence factors, the increased viral pathogenesis conveyed by HAdV-B7 has been attributed to a genetic change.[547] Studies performed in HAdV-B7 isolates from an outbreak among students in China revealed a mutation in the VA RNA gene associated with increased expression of the viral packaging protein L1 52/55K. This viral genetic change apparently mediated faster viral growth leading to increased clinical virulence.[740]

In addition to mutations, intraspecies and, less commonly, interspecies HAdV recombination increases the rate of molecular evolution, and results in novel HAdV types that could theoretically have increased viral fitness, altered cell tropism, and increased virulence. However, HAdV recombination often remains unnoticed because of the self-limited nature of the infections.[107] Mutations or recombinations resulting in a more pathogenic HAdV genotype causing outbreaks of more severe disease facilitate the identification of such genetic changes, as demonstrated for the emerging variant HAdV-B14p1.[15,548] It was shown that infection of primary human bronchial epithelial cells with HAdV-B14p1 resulted in increased expression of IP-10 and I-TAC, two proinflammatory chemokines implicated in ARDS, and the authors suggested that these molecules are potential virulence factors related to infection by this highly pneumotropic virus.[383]

In order to understand the reasons for increased transmission and the mechanisms of increased pathogenicity and virulence of outbreak strains, epidemiological and clinical studies must be coupled with appropriate research approaches. Sequencing and bioinformatics studies can assess viral genes and the encoded structural proteins that might result in altered sensitivity of the emerging virus to preexistent neutralizing antibodies in a given population and identify potential mechanisms of altered biological properties.[107] Differences in the knob domain of the fiber gene and the L1 loop domain of the hexon gene have been implicated as determinants of tissue tropism and virulence in HAdVs. The fiber protein is of great importance for virus–cell interactions, thus explaining its importance as a virulence factor. Recent studies in an emerging, highly pathogenic fowl adenovirus confirmed the important role of fiber and hexon genes as determinants of virulence.[761]

Persistence and Latency

HAdVs are capable of establishing persistent infections, similar to herpesviruses and other viral species.[193,367,422,521,547,572] Due to their ability to enter different cell types via a number of receptors discussed above, persistence of HAdV infections has been reported for a variety of sites such as tonsillar or adenoidal T lymphocytes, lung epithelial cells, brain tissue, and, very importantly, intestinal lymphocytes, as addressed in more detail below.[366,367,422] A recent study reported the presence of persistent nonproductive HAdV infection with representatives of species C, B, and E in the majority of children with hypertrophic adenoids and palatine tonsils, while epithelial and subepithelial tonsillar cells seem to be critical for virus production and shedding in nasopharyngeal secretions.[532] Studies in a humanized mouse model suggested the presence of persistent cellular reservoirs in the bone marrow,[564] but this observation has not been confirmed in the human clinical setting. Attempts to model HAdV latency in different human lymphocyte cell lines using representatives of species C indicated permissiveness for HAdV infection in both T- and B-cell lines, and showed the ability to maintain the infected cell lines for long periods, with production of small amounts of infectious virus in two of the cell lines tested (BJAB, Ramos). Based on their observations, the authors concluded that quiescent viral genome could persist in nondividing lymphocytes indefinitely and, in dividing lymphocytes, the viral genome could persist by replicating sufficiently to compensate for loss due to dilution.[758] A study using human tonsil and adenoid tissues indicated that the presence of viral DNA from different HAdV-C types peaks at 4 years of age and declines thereafter. Viral DNA replication occurred in most donor samples by lymphocyte stimulation in culture, suggesting that HAdV-C types can establish latent infections in mucosal lymphocytes, and that stimulation of these cells can cause viral reactivation resulting in infectious virus production.[193] This notion was supported by a study in pediatric allogeneic SCT recipients suggesting that the observed HAdV-associated complications were attributable to reactivation of persistent virus rather than to infection *de novo*.[690]

Owing to their genetic heterogeneity, HAdVs display broad tissue tropism and can infect several cell types. Not surprisingly, therefore, currently available evidence indicates that they can persist in a latent state in a variety of susceptible cells following primary infection. Latency is characterized by expression of viral proteins by the host cell without replication of a complete virus. In addition to the persistence in tonsillar lymphocytes,[193,572] latent HAdV infections were described to occur in intestinal T lymphocytes and in lung epithelial cells, where they seem to play a role in the pathogenesis of obstructive airway disease.[249] Evidence for long-term HAdV persistence in the ocular surface following conjunctivitis has been provided,[333] and the central nervous system (CNS) was identified as a sanctuary for adenoviral persistence.[367] Importantly, the entire GI tract is a common location of HAdV persistence in children.[366] Other sites of HAdV persistence have also been suggested, but the experimental evidence is limited.[212,407,766] Evasion from immune surveillance is a prerequisite for the establishment of persistent infections in permissive cells and tissues. Immune escape of adenoviruses can be mediated by different mechanisms. Specific viral proteins can block responses to anti-inflammatory and cytolytic cytokines, intrinsic cellular apoptosis, as well as innate and adaptive cellular immune responses.[590,723] Moreover, proteins encoded by the E3 region in the HAdV genome can protect infected cells from Fas ligand–induced apoptosis and from destruction by cytotoxic T cells. The T-cell attack is reduced or prevented by E3-mediated down-regulation of MHC class I molecules, thereby affecting antigen presentation.[222,415,462,503,533,603] Recent evidence indicates that the HAdV early genes required for viral replication can be repressed by IFN-mediated binding of E2F/Rb proteins to the E1A enhancer region, thus leading to inhibition of immediate early viral transcription. Both IFNα and IFNβ were demonstrated to suppress lytic viral replication and to promote persistent infection.[767] It is conceivable therefore that intrinsic IFN production provides the basis for the commonly observed establishment of HAdV persistence in lymphocytes.[192,193,362,366]

Persistence and Reactivation in the Gastrointestinal Tract

Rising Adenovirus Copy Numbers in Stool Precede Invasive Infection

Although different cells and tissues had been reported in the literature to carry persistent adenoviruses,[193,366,367,564,572] the notion that the GI tract is a very important site for persistence of these viruses has been considered common knowledge for many years, despite the fact that there was no direct evidence providing proof for this concept. More than a decade ago, screening data assessing the presence of HAdVs at different sites in pediatric transplant recipients revealed that patients who develop viremia test positive in stool samples before the virus becomes detectable in peripheral blood (PB).[424,425] This observation has stimulated a systematic study addressing the correlation of HAdV appearance and quantity in stool with the risk for invasive infection in children undergoing allogeneic SCT. The study included more than 130 pediatric transplant recipients and indicated that the observation of viremia is almost invariably preceded by HAdV positivity in serial stool specimens.[425] However, the proportion of patients with HAdV positivity in stool exceeded by far the percentage of patients who developed invasive infection (37% vs. 12% in the indicated study). Molecular analysis by a quantitative PCR-based approach covering the entire spectrum of HAdV types known at that time suggested that the kinetics, and ultimately the passing of a certain threshold of HAdV copy numbers in stool, permit the identification of patients at high risk for invasive infection. Rapidly increasing HAdV copy numbers exceeding the threshold of 10E6 copies/g of stool were shown to indicate a greater than 70% risk for viremia, while none of the patients displaying maximum HAdV copy numbers in stool below this threshold experienced viremia during the entire observation period.[425] The ability to differentially assess the risk for ensuing viremia by serial monitoring of stool samples, using the indicated threshold level of HAdV copy numbers, was statistically highly significant.[425] Very similar observations were subsequently made by several other investigators, thereby confirming the tight correlation between HAdV positivity in stool and subsequently in PB.[114,167,269,300,402,635] The virtually invariable presence of increasing virus levels in serial stool samples prior to invasive infection in the pediatric transplant setting indicated that the GI tract apparently serves as the most important compartment for HAdV expansion, and further supported the notion of the intestine being the central site of HAdV persistence and reactivation in children.[369]

Adenoviruses Persist in Mucosal Lymphocytes and Replicate Effectively in Epithelial Cells

To investigate whether and where HAdV persistence might occur in the intestine, biopsy material derived from more than 140 largely immunocompetent children, who had undergone elective diagnostic endoscopy of the upper and lower GI tract for a variety of clinical indications, was investigated. Analysis by a pan-HAdV PCR assay indicated presence of the virus along the entire GI tract, with the highest prevalence in the ileum, in approximately one-third of the individuals tested[366] (Fig. 5.3). Analysis of the biopsy specimens by *in situ* hybridization or immunohistochemistry revealed virus signals in mucosal lymphocytes, while the epithelial cells in

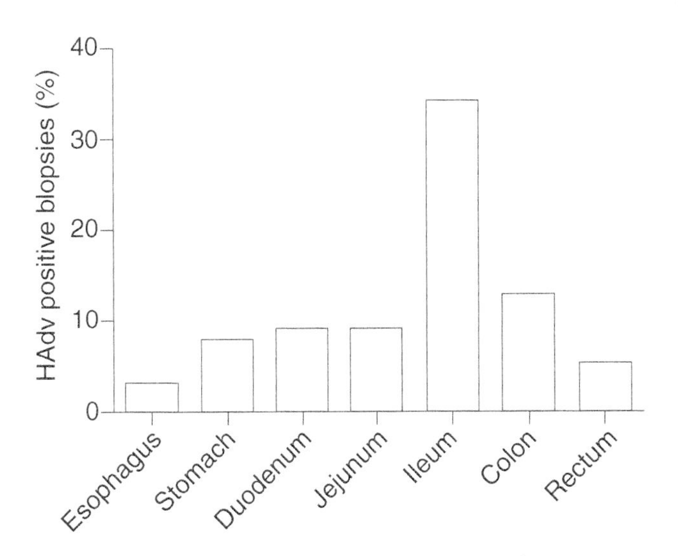

FIGURE 5.3 Distribution of HAdV persistence in the gastrointestinal tract of children. Distribution of HAdV persistence in the gastrointestinal tract of children.

this cohort were essentially free of virus signals (Fig. 5.4A and C). When the same analyses were performed in pediatric transplant recipients with documented HAdV reactivation, who underwent diagnostic endoscopy for suspected intestinal graft versus host disease, *in situ* hybridization and immunohistochemistry performed on biopsy sections showed massive signal accumulation in the epithelial cells (Fig. 5.4B and D).[366] These studies provided the basis for a conceptual model suggesting that intestinal lymphocytes facilitate long-term persistence of the virus but do not provide an environment conducive for efficient viral replication, possibly due to their IFN production.[767] Rather, viruses leaking from these cells could enter and replicate in intestinal epithelial cells, and subsequently become detectable in stool. If the immune surveillance is severely impaired, HAdVs can massively expand in the entire intestinal epithelium, leading to rapidly rising virus copy numbers in stool. This concept is in line with the clinical observation of extremely high virus levels in the stool of pediatric transplant recipients, which can exceed 10E11 copies/g.[422,425]

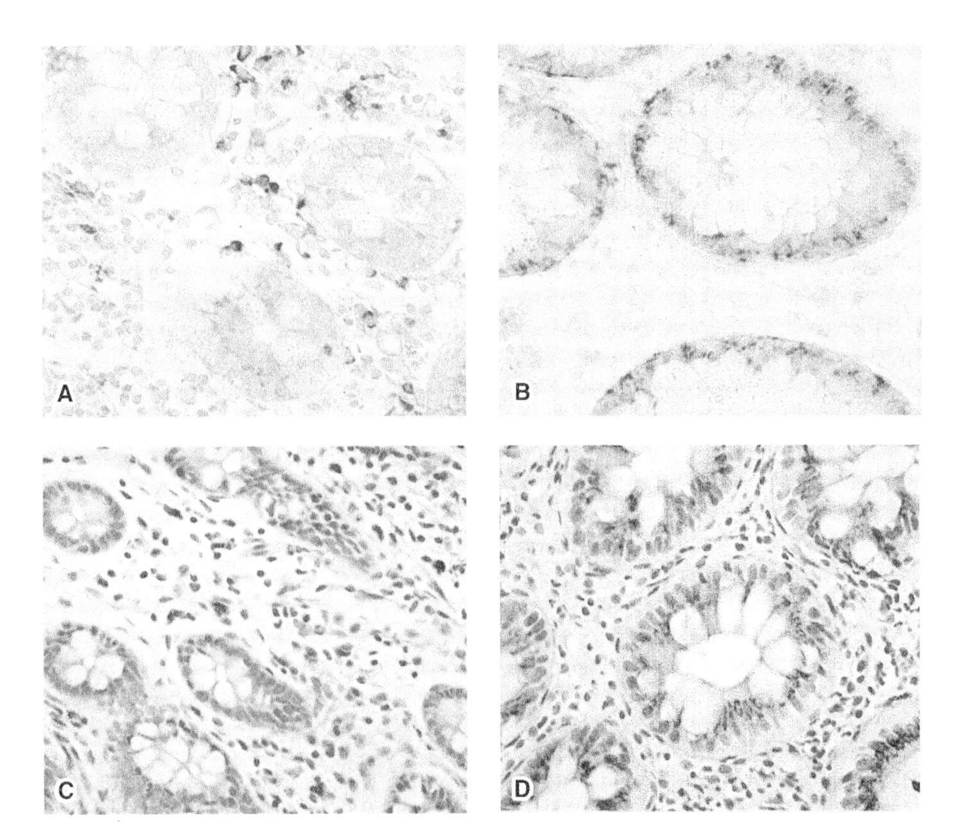

FIGURE 5.4 Detection of adenovirus persistence and reactivation in the gastrointestinal tract. Upper panels: *In situ* hybridization of GI tract biopsies for HAdV DNA performed by using biotinylated adenovirus probes and detection via alkaline phosphatase. **A:** Biopsies from immunocompetent children revealed scattered signals in individual lymphoid cells of the lamina propria (*dark blue signals*), while epithelial cells showed no signals. **B:** Biopsies from children with HAdV reactivation posttransplant show dense signals in the intestinal epithelium (*dark blue signals*). **Lower panels:** Immunohistochemistry on GI tract biopsies for detection of HAdV protein. **C:** Biopsies from immunocompetent children revealed scattered signals in individual lymphoid cells of the lamina propria (*brown signals*), while epithelial cells showed no signals. **D:** Biopsies from children with HAdV reactivation posttransplant show dense signals in the intestinal epithelium (*brown signals*). Hence, the distribution of signals reflecting HAdV DNA or protein in panels **A**, **C**, **B**, and **D**, respectively, was identical. (Magnification 400x). (Adapted from Kosulin K, Geiger E, Vécsei A, et al. Persistence and reactivation of human adenoviruses in the gastrointestinal tract. *Clin Microbiol Infect* 2016;22(4):381.e1–381.e8. Copyright © 2015 European Society of Clinical Microbiology and Infectious Diseases. With permission. Ref.[366])

Intestinal Adenovirus Persistence May Correlate With the Risk of Posttransplant Reactivation

The documented persistence of adenoviruses in lymphoid cells of the intestinal lamina propria in the pediatric setting may be related to the observation that primary exposure to these viruses generally occurs already at a very young age.[269,366] The proportion of children displaying HAdV persistence in intestinal biopsies and the percentage of pediatric allogeneic SCT recipients showing viral reactivation during the posttransplant period were quite similar in the studies performed.[366,425] This observation supported the notion that HAdV persistence in the GI tract may directly correlate with the occurrence of virus reactivation in the intestine upon the onset of severe immunosuppression. Further support for this concept is provided by the fact that the distribution of HAdV species found in children with intestinal persistence of the virus was virtually identical to that observed in patients displaying reactivation after allogeneic SCT.[366]

By contrast, there is no evidence for intestinal HAdV persistence in adult individuals at the present time, and it is conceivable that the GI tract might not play a central role as the main site of HAdV reactivation and expansion in the adult immunocompromised setting. Although life-threatening invasive HAdV infections occur in adult SCT recipients (Table 5.2), they appear to be less frequent than in pediatric patients, and the main source of virus reactivation remains enigmatic.[423,653]

Intestinal Shedding of Adenoviruses Before Stem Cell Transplantation Is Prognostically Relevant

The documentation of intestinal HAdV persistence in a considerable proportion of children raised the question whether shedding of the virus into the stool commonly occurs already prior to the onset of severe immunosuppression related to pretransplant conditioning and, if so, whether it might have an impact on the occurrence of invasive infections during the posttransplant period. These questions were addressed by analyzing a cohort of more than 300 pediatric patients who underwent allogeneic SCT at a single center.[364] Intestinal HAdV shedding prior to transplantation was documented in 14% of the individuals analyzed, and there was a highly significant correlation with ensuing HAdV-related complications in this subset of patients. Detection of HAdV positivity in stool before SCT correlated with a rapid rise of virus copy numbers very early posttransplant and a significantly more frequent occurrence of adenoviremia. The incidence of viremia within the first 100 days posttransplant in patients displaying HAdV positivity in stool prior to SCT, in comparison to individuals who tested negative for the virus before transplantation (33% vs. 7%), was statistically highly significant. Moreover, patients with pretransplant intestinal HAdV shedding developed adenoviremia already at early time points after allografting.[364] An early onset of invasive infection is clinically relevant, because it implies longer duration of systemic exposure to the virus, while the patients are still heavily immunosuppressed. From the therapeutic perspective,

TABLE 5.2 Incidence and lethal outcome of HAdV viremia after SCT

Year	Reference	Adults		Children	
		Viremia % of Patients	Lethal Cases	Viremia % of Patients	Lethal Cases
2019	Ali et al.[12]			10.5%	4/19
2018	Fisher et al.[176]			26.2%	13/50
2017	Ramsay et al.[550]	1.5%	3/10		
2015	Feghoul et al.[167]			25%	7/18
2013	Hiwarkar et al.[244]			15%	n.r.
2012	Sive et al.[625]	12%	1/14		
2012	Taniguchi et al.[659]	9%	4/10		
2012	Watson et al.[716]			16%	2/7
2011	Öhrmalm et al.[502]	3%	0/2	15%	0/3
2010	Lion et al.[425]			10%	8/16
2009	de Pagter et al.[122]			31%	3/19
2008	Gustafson et al.[216]	15%	2/4	15%	1/2
2007	Sivaprakasam et al.[624]			11%	3/8
2007	Kalpoe et al.[321]	5%	1/5	14%	3/8
2006	Yusuf et al.[749]			21%	1/37
2005	van Tol et al.[687]			6%	7/21
2005	Walls et al.[704]			42%	2/7
2004	Avivi et al.[27]	14%	3/3		

The actual number of lethal cases in relation to the total number of patients with viremia in the respective studies is indicated.

From Lion T. Adenovirus persistence, reactivation, and clinical management. *FEBS Lett* 2019;593(24):3571–3582. Ref.[423]

TABLE 5.3 Current recommendations for HAdV diagnostic screening and monitoring in the allogeneic SCT setting

STOOL		PERIPHERAL BLOOD	
Children	Adults	Children	Adults
Screening for intestinal shedding on ≥2 different days 1–2 weeks prior to conditioning (B II[a])	n.r.	**Screening ≥1×/week post SCT** (A II[a])	**Screening ≥1×/week post SCT** (B III[a])
Screening post SCT 1×/week (A II[a])	n.r.	**Monitoring of virus levels 1–2×/week** in patients testing positive for HAdV in peripheral blood (A II[a])	**Monitoring of virus levels 1–2×/week** in patients testing positive for HAdV in peripheral blood (A II[a])
Monitoring of virus levels 1–2×/week in the presence of virus levels in stool above the critical threshold, in the absence of viremia; in pediatric patients receiving preemptive anti-HAdV treatment (A III[a])	n.r.	**Monitoring of virus levels 1–2×/week** in patients with viremia undergoing antiviral treatment (A II[a])	**Monitoring of virus levels 1–2×/week** in patients with viremia undergoing antiviral treatment (A II[a])

[a]Strength of recommendation (Grades A–D, A being the strongest recommendation for use) and Quality of evidence (Levels I–III, I being the highest level) according to the ECIL-6 scoring system.[245]
n.r., no recommendation.
From Lion T. Adenovirus persistence, reactivation, and clinical management. *FEBS Lett* 2019;593(24):3571–3582. Copyright © 2019 Federation of European Biochemical Societies. Reprinted by permission of John Wiley & Sons, Inc. Ref.[423]

it implies the need to bridge a longer time period until immune reconstitution.[423] The apparent prognostic role of pretransplant intestinal HAdV shedding has led to pertinent recommendations for diagnostic monitoring (Table 5.3).

EPIDEMIOLOGY

Although adenoviruses in general are not mutually pathogenic across humans and animals, simian species were occasionally shown to display antibodies to human AdVs and antibodies to simian AdVs were detected in human sera, in line with the occurrence of anthropozoonosis and vice versa (see above).[158] Indeed, cross-species transmission of a novel simian AdV, causing a lethal outbreak in a closed monkey colony, to a researcher who was in close contact with the animals has been described,[95] and other similar cases of anthropozoonosis could be documented.[99,717] There is substantial evidence indicating that AdVs have previously crossed host/species barriers and will continue to do so.[47] The high degree of asymptomatic shedding of live AdV in nonhuman primates and the evidence for zoonotic transmissions require caution in close interaction with such animals.[573] Similarly, season-independent respiratory or intestinal HAdV shedding by asymptomatic persons has been documented, and represents a source of infections by different routes.[42,267,362,743]

Most HAdV epidemics in immunocompetent individuals are observed in winter and early spring, but infections in immunocompromised patients occur throughout the year.[289,471,615,741,764] Epidemiological data indicate that the majority of primary HAdV infections occur during the first 5 years of life due to the lack of humoral immunity. In children, HAdV infections account for up to 15% of upper respiratory tract and about 5% of lower respiratory tract inflammatory diseases.[258] In immunocompetent individuals, the infections are mostly mild and self-limiting, but severe and even fatal courses have been reported, as specified below.[70,585,620]

HAdV infections are readily spread within human populations, and outbreaks have been described in crowded settings including medical facilities, such as hospitals and nursing homes,[55,324,580,710] military bases,[320,510,566] and schools.[36] The HAdVs-associated outbreaks can cause GI disease,[506] pharyngoconjunctival fever,[410] febrile respiratory illness,[746] and/or keratoconjunctivitis.[166,201,414] Individuals infected with HAdV are extremely contagious during the incubation period, which typically ranges from 4 to 8 days but can last up to 24 days, depending on the HAdV type involved.[422] The HAdV types commonly linked to outbreaks include HAdV-B3, E4, B7, D8, B14, and B55, and these viruses are regarded as more virulent and likely to spread.[70,196,223,340,382,438,541,597,733] The predominant HAdV types detected in association with disease differ among different geographic regions and countries and change over time by spreading across continents and replacing hitherto dominant strains, as documented by the abundance of globally occurring outbreaks.[111,438,652,760]

Transmission

Transmission can occur from an infected person to other individuals via respiratory routes, fecal–oral contamination, and/or direct contact, such as shaking hands. Respiratory transmission via coughing or sneezing is a predominant mode of transmission, but fecal–oral transmission can occur through contaminated food or water, including for example, public swimming pools due to ineffective chlorine treatment[46] (see also section Stability and Inactivation). Hence, infections in the immunocompetent host are typically caused by exposure to infected individuals via inhalation of aerosolized droplets or direct conjunctival inoculation, but transmission may also occur by fecal–oral spread including recreational freshwater or tap water, contact with infected tissue, airflow filters, contaminated fomites, or environmental surfaces, due to the stability of HAdVs in the environment.[406,410,574,630,710,769]

Although exogenous infection by nosocomial or community acquisition in the inpatient setting is a rather rare cause of HAdV-related diseases, outbreaks of infections on hematology or transplant wards as well as in eye clinics resulting in closures have been documented.[77,377,384,457,482,507] Many reports described HAdV spread via local outbreaks in common areas, such as camps, playgrounds, dormitories, and schools.[89,238,280,414,763] Appropriate control measures, including frequent hand washing, sanitizing surfaces, staying at home when ill, avoiding close contact with people who are sick, and covering nose and mouth when sneezing or coughing, may therefore be pertinent to minimize the transmission of HAdV infections and prevent outbreaks.[111]

The transmission dynamics and the high levels of morbidity caused by HAdV infections in military camps have been documented by various investigators.[41,317] Interestingly, HAdV infections do not commonly spread to civilian personnel in contact with the military, and HAdV-related acute respiratory disease (ARD) was far less frequent in similarly congregated college students, suggesting that additional factors affecting young recruits, such as more crowded sleeping conditions or the fatigue associated with basic training, could be factors contributing to the pronounced morbidity in this setting. A study performed in military recruits after discontinuation of the vaccination program, which lasted more than a decade (1999–2011), revealed an increase in the percentage of soldiers seropositive for HAdV-E4 from 34% at enrollment to 97% by the end of the study. Potential sources of HAdV transmission included the presence of virus on surfaces in living quarters, including pillows, lockers, and rifles as well as extended pharyngeal viral shedding over the course of several days. The introduction of recruits, who were still shedding adenovirus, into new training groups was also documented.[574] Because of the crowded setting in military living quarters and easy transmission of infections, vaccination against the most prevalent HAdV types E4, B7, and B14 in military recruits has been highly recommended and reintroduced in 2011[54,318,320] (see section Vaccine).

Prevalence of HAdV Species and Types

Most HAdV species appear to circulate globally, but predominant types differ between countries or geographic regions and change over time.[14,219,318,337,343,417–419,496,615,739,757] Transmission of new strains across continents may occur and lead to replacement of hitherto dominant HAdV types.[319] The adenoviruses reported to be most commonly associated with human disease worldwide are HAdV-C1, C2, C5, B3, B7, B21, E4, and F41,[13,20,33,90,437,543,741,760,764] with great predominance of the HAdV types F41 and F40 in patients with gastroenteritis.[29,376,413,540]

Epidemic forms of HAdV-related disease involving primarily types E4 and B7 have been extensively described in military recruits, including also recent reports on outbreaks,[36,358] but the reintroduction of vaccination programs has greatly improved the situation (see section Vaccines).

In immunocompromised patients in the transplant setting, some of the most commonly reported adenovirus types include HAdV-C1, C2, C5, A12, A31, B3, B11, B16, B34, and B35, with strong predominance of species C in most but not all instances.[328,425,461,486,534] Transplant centers from different geographic regions reported a prevalence of HAdV species C in the range of 80% of all adenoviral infections observed.[150,372,422,424,425] Sequential or concomitant coinfections with different adenoviruses from the same or from different species are quite commonly observed both in the immunocompetent and immunocompromised patient settings[206,379,654] (Figs. 5.5 and 5.6), and may thus play a role in the generation of recombinant HAdV types.

Serological surveys have provided estimates for the prevalence of specific HAdV infections. Neutralizing antibodies against HAdV-C5 were found in the great majority (>70% to 100%) of the populations in Sub-Saharan Africa, Northern India, Thailand, China, and Brazil, while the indicated prevalence

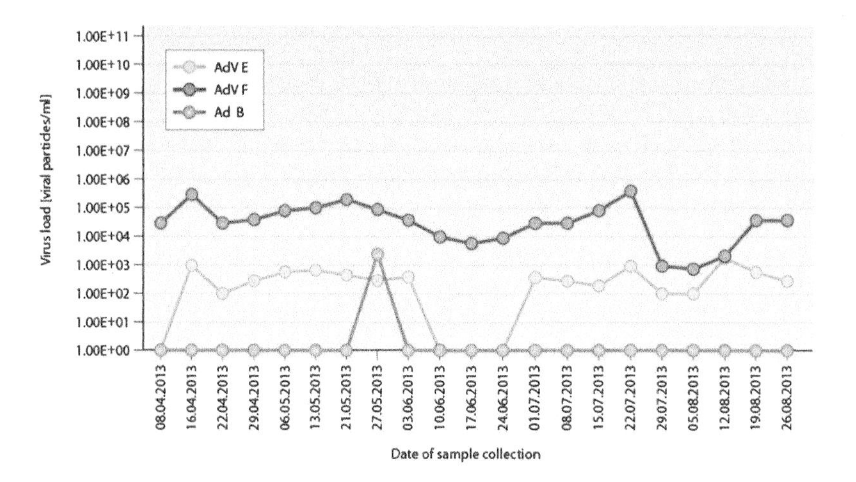

FIGURE 5.5 Adenoviremia with multiple HAdV species. Different HAdV types or species can be detected in peripheral blood and/or other sites, both concomitantly and sequentially. The example displayed shows a rare constellation with invasive infection associated with HAdV species E, F, and occasionally B, during the posttransplant course (x-axis) of a pediatric patient. This observation highlights the fact that very unusual findings are possible, which must be accounted for by the implementation of appropriate diagnostic techniques for HAdV detection and monitoring. The *y*-axis indicates the virus copy number per mL of blood determined by real-time PCR. (Reprinted from Lion T. Adenovirus infections in immunocompetent and immunocompromised patients. *Clin Microbiol Rev* 2014;27(3):441–462. Ref.[422])

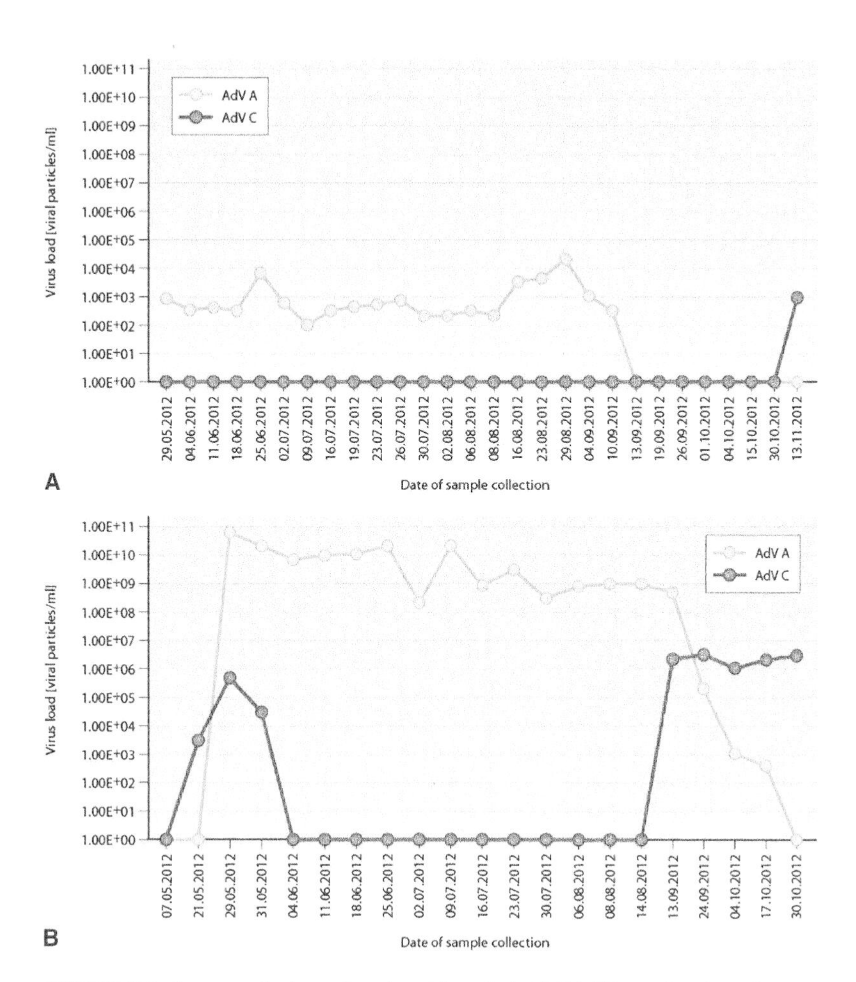

FIGURE 5.6 Course of adenoviremia with switch of HAdV species A to C. Kinetics of HAdV viremia during the posttransplant course in a pediatric patient revealing disappearance of DNAemia caused by HAdV species A below the detection level of real-time PCR, and recurrence of HAdV positivity in peripheral blood after about 6 weeks of negative PCR findings with HAdV species C **(A)**. The switch observed in peripheral blood was preceded by corresponding kinetics of HAdV viral loads in serial stool specimens **(B)**. (Reprinted from Lion T. Adenovirus infections in immunocompetent and immunocompromised patients. *Clin Microbiol Rev* 2014;27(3):441–462. Ref.[422])

in Japan, Europe and the United States was somewhat lower (40% to 70%).[32,94,144,158,296,451,522,648,663] Neutralizing antibodies against HAdV-C6, which has been evaluated as an alternative vaccine vector, have been identified in about half of subjects tested, but the titers were mostly low.[34,451] A study performed in the United States found a seroprevalence of HAdV-C2 of greater than 80%.[22] Seroprevalence studies have also been conducted for less common HAdV types, also to assess their potential exploitability as vectors, and provided variable results in different geographic regions. For example, antibodies against HAdV-B35 were found at low frequencies (0% to 10%) in Europe and the United States, a somewhat higher (<20%) prevalence was detected in Japan, Thailand, and Sub-Saharan Africa,[22,32] and the findings for HAdV-B11 revealed a seroprevalence of 10% to 30% in sub-Saharan Africa and Japan.[255,663] For HAdV-D26 and D28, the seroprevalence in the United States was determined to be ≤10% with low titers, but the percentage for D26 was considerably higher in countries such as Brazil or Thailand, and reached 60% to 80% in sub-Saharan Africa.[32,94,158,312,451] The indicated examples highlight the regional differences in the seroprevalence of specific HAdVs, possibly affecting the broad applicability of vectors based on individual HAdV types. It should be noted that the serological studies described above refer primarily to neutralizing antibodies, and the total prevalence of HAdV antibodies is higher. Further, a very high proportion of adult humans carry HAdV-specific T cells, including primarily $CD4^+$ but also $CD8^+$ subsets, which appear to display broad reactivity due to cross-reactive (often hexon-derived) epitopes.[61,94,274]

Stability and Inactivation of Adenovirus

As nonenveloped viruses with a well-organized capsid and a double-stranded DNA genome, HAdVs are expected to be stable. They can survive for long time periods in liquid and have been identified as the most prevalent enteric viruses in environmental waters worldwide.[523] They also remain stable on surfaces in a desiccated state and can retain their infectious properties even after several weeks in moisture-free environments. It was shown that HAdV titers are not lost after shipment of simulated conjunctival samples to a reference laboratory, even after several days at ambient temperatures.[567] The stability of the virus at low pH is a matter of debate, but HAdVs are resistant to gastric and biliary secretions and can therefore be detected at high loads in feces.[454]

The long-term stability of HAdVs in surface and ground water is well recognized,[556] and a study on the prevalence and quantity of HAdV in drinking water and river water in South Africa revealed presence of the virus in greater than 5% of drinking water samples, with predominance of HAdV species D, and in greater than 20% of river water samples, with predominance of enteric types of the virus.[684] Urban wastewaters in Italy were shown to commonly contain different HAdV types including mostly F41, and considerably less often the types B3, A12, and C5, with implications for waterborne HAdV–related health risks.[277] Adenoviruses were also identified in recreational waters in Brazil including freshwater and sea beaches, with common detection of viable HAdV species C and F.[197,199,215] Similar findings were also made in a number of other geographic areas.[5,263,309,359,439]

The risks of infection in swimming pool water were recently reviewed.[46] Based on the observation that HAdVs are the most UV-resistant viruses, their detection has become a key indicator of water quality, and environmental protection agencies and water-treatment companies are developing and employing protocols for adequate detection and elimination of adenoviral contamination in water sources and systems.[153,164,242,647]

As nonenveloped viruses, HAdVs are resistant to many disinfectants. Effective decontamination of surfaces and equipment is of paramount importance, particularly in transplant and intensive care units to prevent this mode of transmission in immunosuppressed patients.[62] A study addressing the efficacy of germicides examined 21 different products for their ability to inactivate HAdV-D8 and concluded that the disinfectants to be used for effective environmental surface disinfection may include products providing approximately 1,900 parts per million (ppm) available free chlorine, 65% ethanol with 0.63% quaternary ammonium compound (QAC), 79.6% ethanol with 0.1% QAC, or 70% ethanol. These disinfectants should be allowed to contact all environmental surfaces for at least 1 minute.[575] For disinfecting ophthalmological equipment, the authors recommend 70% ethanol or approximately 5,000 ppm chlorine. High-level disinfectants such as 0.55% *ortho*-phthaldehyde, ≥2.4% glutaraldehyde, or 0.2% peracetic acid (PAA) may also be used, but equipment must be compatible and rinsed thoroughly.[575] The virus-inactivating properties of different surface disinfectants including PAA-based, QAC-based, and 2-propanol-based products have recently been tested, and the virucidal efficacy of the PAA-based wipe was deemed most efficient.[37] Moreover, potassium peroxymonosulfate has been successfully evaluated as a disinfectant for prevention of EKC acquired by nosocomial infections in ophthalmological clinics.[230]

A number of studies have employed ultraviolet light to inactivate microbial pathogens including HAdV.[191,408,539] Photochemical treatment (PCT) has also been used to prevent transfusion-transmitted disease resulting from viral contamination. The photosensitizing compound 8-Methoxypsoralen (8-MOP) combined with long-wavelength ultraviolet irradiation (UVA) inactivates many viruses, but toxicity limits its use in animals and humans. The toxicological and photosensitizing properties of riboflavin (vitamin B2) make it suitable for virus inactivation in preparations for biological use.[63] The combination of amotosalen-HCl and UVA for cross-linking of pathogen-derived DNA has also been successfully used to inactivate a wide range of pathogens including viruses in platelet concentrates and other blood products.[416,484,584,622] A system based on using the frangible anchor linker effector (FRALE) compound amustaline (S-303) with labile alkylating activity revealed a robust pathogen reduction profile, permitting efficient elimination of HAdV titers (by 5-logs) in whole blood products.[53,67,481] Ultraviolet light–based inactivation of enteric adenoviruses was also shown to be feasible in water, although HAdV-F species are among the most UV-resistant water-borne viruses.[138,539]

Ozone is a powerful disinfectant against all types of waterborne pathogens, including viruses, and was shown to be also effective against HAdV when applied in water and wastewater.[728] Moreover, the virucidal potential of gamma radiation against HAdV may be exploited for disinfection treatment of sustainable water supplies or polluted waters.[523,524] Chlorine is, however, the most widely used disinfection product for water,[200,313,490] and the required chlorination doses for disinfection of water from enteric viruses, including HAdV, have been recently reviewed.[544] However, chlorine-based disinfection can produce toxic byproducts, rendering the search for alternative agents a relevant task. In this context, various natural and synthetic compounds including *N*-chlorotaurine (NCT), bromamine-T (BAT), and grape seed extract (GSE) were recently tested for inactivation of HAdV in water, and showed promising results.[190]

CLINICAL FEATURES

HAdVs were initially isolated mainly from military recruits with acute febrile respiratory disease, and were subsequently associated with a number of clinical manifestations including upper and lower respiratory tract infections, keratoconjunctivitis, gastroenteritis, cystitis, meningoencephalitis, myocarditis, and hepatitis but also with noninflammatory conditions such as obesity.[97,121,160,437,447] HAdV infections are readily transmittable and in some instances highly contagious. Although the clinical courses are usually mild and self-limiting, infections may cause local outbreaks with severe courses, occasionally leading to lethal outcomes even in immunocompetent individuals.[10,40,92,585] However, adenoviruses play a particularly important role in patients with strongly impaired immune response, where viral disease is associated with high morbidity and mortality, and infections in this setting are an important focus of the present chapter.

HAdVs can commonly infect and replicate at various sites of the respiratory tract as well as in the eye and the GI tract.

Less frequently, HAdVs can infect the urinary bladder, the liver, and occasionally the pancreas, the myocardium, or the CNS. Many HAdV infections are subclinical and result in antibody formation conveying protection against exogenous reintroduction of the same HAdV type. Common illnesses associated with various HAdVs are described in the following paragraphs. It is important to bear in mind, however, that detection of HAdV in clinical specimens does not necessarily imply a cause and effect relationship with the disease, particularly when highly sensitive molecular detection methods are used, and screening is restricted to a limited number of common viral pathogens.

Respiratory Diseases

Endemic Adenovirus Infections in Young Children

About 7% of upper respiratory tract infection cases in children below 5 years of age are attributable to HAdV.[292,515] The usual symptoms include nasal congestion, coryza, and cough. Other patients may have an exudative tonsillitis that may be clinically indistinguishable from disease caused by streptococcus A infection. The respiratory symptoms are often accompanied by systemic manifestations, such as generalized malaise, fever, chills, myalgia, and headache. Commonly observed types of the virus include HAdV-C1, C2, C5, and C6, and less frequently B3 and B7, which are endemic in most populations.[31,64,161,337,412,489,632,713,736,764] Sporadic cases may reveal symptoms indiscernible from other viral respiratory infections, such as influenza, parainfluenza, or respiratory syncytial virus.[515] If conjunctivitis accompanies the signs and symptoms already described, the disease is designated as *pharyngoconjunctival fever*, most commonly associated with HAdV types B3, B7, and B14. HAdVs also cause lower respiratory tract infections in children, and are probably responsible for about 10% of pneumonias in the pediatric setting.[516] Moreover, HAdVs were identified as the most common pathogens associated with a pertussis-like syndrome, and coinfections by *Bordetella pertussis* were identified in a proportion of patients.[442,576]

Acute Respiratory Disease in Adults

In adults, HAdV types from subspecies B1, including B3, B7, B16, B21, and B50, as well as HAdV-E4, are commonly associated with ARD, whereas representatives of subspecies B2, including B11, B14, B34, and B35, have been more frequently associated with urinary tract and opportunistic infections in immunocompromised patients.[611] Without significant circulation in North America, HAdV-B14 emerged as a significant cause of acute and sometimes severe ARD in 2006 and was subsequently characterized by genomic and bioinformatic analysis.[606] Initially, the infection was recognized in three military bases under continuous systematic surveillance,[468] but widespread outbreaks associated with several deaths were demonstrated thereafter in North America and several other geographic areas.[70,75,76,159,262,319,469] The only unique characteristic identified in the HAdV-B14p1 variant implicated in several documented outbreaks was a deletion of two amino acids in the knob region of the fiber protein.[319] Low antibody titers against HAdV-B14 in recruits sampled at admission to training camp and initial detection of HAdV-14p1 in cities on the US West Coast, which represent major ports of entry into the country from Asia, suggest that travel and commerce played a major role in the introduction of this HAdV variant into the United States.[319] Older age, chronic underlying condition, low absolute lymphocyte counts, and elevated creatinine levels were associated with severe illness. In most instances, no epidemiological link could be established between individual cases.[159] Adenoviral pneumonia can present with severe radiological findings,[79,511,657] and has been associated particularly with the HAdV-B types including B3, B7, B14, B21, B55, HAdV-C types C1, C2, C5, and HAdV-E4.[76,90,317,318,597,658,762] A number of reports on HAdV-associated respiratory disease with severe courses and sometimes fatal outcome have been recently published.[74,198,762]

Acute Respiratory Disease in Military Recruits

In many respects, ARD is similar to the description of respiratory infection in children. The syndrome was predominantly associated with HAdV-E4 (92.8% in a study conducted 2004–2006),[206] and less commonly with HAdV-B7. After 2005, coincidently with similar findings in civilian populations, simultaneous emergence of diverse infections attributable to HAdV-B3, B7, B14, and B21 was observed.[468] Some cases of ARD in young military recruits had a fatal outcome related to the pneumonitis that may accompany and complicate other, milder, respiratory symptoms. A significant increase in severe and fatal cases was observed upon emergence of HAdV-B14 infections in US military facilities,[468,495] but the prominent role of this HAdV type could not be confirmed by another study in US military recruits with HAdV-associated pneumonia.[691] Further aspects of this disease are discussed in the sections Epidemiology and Vaccines. In recent studies, HAdV was shown to be the most common viral pathogen identified in Korean military hospitals in soldiers displaying pneumonia, with the highest prevalence of HAdV-B55 and HAdV-E4.[241,358]

Ocular Infections

EKC is a major cause of ocular morbidity in developed and developing countries, and no efficacious therapeutic options are currently available. Epidemiologically, ocular infections can occur sporadically or affect large groups of contacts. When the source of infection is recreational water, the number of affected individuals may be high. The incubation period of EKC ranges from 2 days to 2 weeks. Patients are contagious after the onset of symptoms and for up to 2 weeks thereafter.[352] The infection presents as follicular conjunctivitis with edema of the eyelids, pain, lacrimation, and photophobia, often followed by corneal subepithelial infiltrates. The infection is often unilateral with hypertrophy of the draining preauricular lymph nodes, but may be associated with multiple lymph node involvement and symptoms of systemic infection, with flu-like symptoms such as myalgia and fever. It can lead to the development of corneal opacities, blurred vision, and other sequelae, which can persist for months or even years. The infection is highly contagious and responsible for outbreaks around the globe, highlighting the importance of accurate diagnosis and rapid containment. The infection has been associated with various HAdV-D types including particularly D8, D37, and D64 (previously designated as 19a), and the recombinant types D53, D54, and D56 were recently identified by molecular typing strategies as emerging etiologic agents of EKC infections worldwide. Recombination events among circulating HAdV-D types represent a source of new infectious disease threats, and the growing number of HAdV types permitted genomic and phenotypic analyses to determine EKC-related pathological properties.[202,287,305]

In a recent study on HAdV-positive EKC patients, species D was most common (63% of the cases), but as many as four species including also HAdV-B, E, and C, and a total of 21 different types were detected.[392] The findings are largely in line with an earlier study that revealed the presence of HAdV-B3 and B7, HAdV-E4, and HAdV-C2 in addition to a variety of HAdV-D types.[763] Differential diagnosis and discrimination from infections by other agents, such as *Chlamydia trachomatis*, HSV1 (herpes simplex virus), EV70 (Enterovirus 70), or CVA24v (Coxsackievirus group type A24) can be difficult.[326]

Recent observations suggest that distinct innate immune responses to HAdV infection of the conjunctiva and cornea involving, for example, NK cells and IFN type 1 may be mediated by stimulation of specific pattern recognition receptors dependent on the cell entry and trafficking. While it was generally believed that HAdVs enter host cells via dynamin-dependent, clathrin-mediated endocytosis before trafficking along microtubules to the nucleus for replication, recent data revealed that the viruses utilize a variety of entry mechanisms, including macropinocytosis and caveolin-mediated pathways. The specific mechanism of entry appears to depend largely on the specific pairing of cell and virus type, and multiple pathways can be exploited. Novel insights into ocular surface immunology may provide the basis for therapies manipulating immune responses to infection with the aim of improving clinical outcomes.[86–88,98,516]

Hemorrhagic Cystitis

Hemorrhagic cystitis (HC) is a significant cause of morbidity and occasionally even mortality in SCT or organ transplant recipients. The reported incidences range from 6% to 30% in patients undergoing SCT, and are related to the use of chemotherapeutic agents, such as cyclophosphamide or busulfan, or to viral infections involving the human polyomaviruses BKV and JCV, HAdVs, and rarely other viral pathogens. Clinical manifestations of HC include microscopic to gross hematuria with clot formation that can lead to urinary tract obstruction and sometimes renal failure.[477] Infections involving HAdVs were reported to account for 3.9% and 9.8% of HC cases among pediatric and adult HCT recipients, respectively,[204,477] involving particularly different HAdV-B types, such as B7, B11, B21, B34, B35, and less commonly other HAdV species and types.[182] Transplanting organs from HAdV-seropositive donors to seronegative recipients appears to be a potential risk factor for severe disease, and donor-transmitted infection in kidney transplant recipients has been associated with HC, allograft tubulointerstitial nephritis and graft loss. Moreover, disseminated HAdV infections with fatal outcome have been described in renal transplant recipients.[182,371,688] Rising HAdV levels detected by PCR screening in peripheral blood and urine correlate with HC, but no clear threshold for diagnosis could be established.[355] Standardized monitoring and treatment of HAdV infections in the organ transplant setting has not been established, and the treatment modalities employed include supportive care measures such as hyperhydration, forced diuresis, continuous bladder irrigation, and/or blood transfusions.[477] In patients not responding to reduction of immunosuppression, cidofovir is commonly used for treatment of HAdV-related disease, although evidence provided by randomized clinical trials is missing.[182]

Meningoencephalitis

Although HAdV has been recognized as a relevant viral pathogen implicated in neurological diseases, particularly in immunocompromised patients, it has been rarely observed in infectious syndromes of the CNS.[121,520,693] In immunocompetent individuals, including particularly children, HAdVs are a rare cause of CNS disease. The disease spectrum is variable, ranging from mild aseptic meningitis and fully reversible encephalopathy to severe, potentially fatal, acute necrotizing encephalopathy.[577,596] The HAdV species and types isolated from cerebrospinal fluid (CSF) in patients with CNS infections were quite diverse. Reported cases include HAdV-A31, B3, B7, C2, D26, and D49.[143,186] Moreover, HAdV-F41 was identified in a recently published case of neonatal meningoencephalitis.[656] Presentations of HAdV infections as isolated CNS disease involving species C and D, without detectable viremia, were documented in two children after SCT.[186] Cidofovir infusions (5 mg/kg weekly) were administered with concomitant reduction of the immunosuppressive treatment, and this regimen was successful in one of the patients. It is necessary to bear in mind, however, that intravenously administered cidofovir does not seem to cross the blood–brain barrier efficiently.[186] HAdV-related meningoencephalitis appears to be a rare event, which is not associated with typical clinical or radiological signs. Because of the severity of such infections, systematic PCR-based HAdV-screening in the CSF is required in cases of unexplained neurological symptoms in severely immunocompromised patients, even if PCR testing of blood samples remains negative.[186]

Gastrointestinal Diseases

Diarrhea is a major cause of death in the pediatric population worldwide, particularly among children below five, and even more so below 2 years of age, affecting mainly low- and middle-income countries.[43,428,540,703] Infections by viruses play a leading role, and a variety of viral pathogens have been implicated in gastroenteritis, including rotavirus, norovirus, adenovirus, sapovirus, astrovirus, parechovirus, and bocavirus, which occurred alone or in combination, involving both viral and bacterial pathogens.[4,82,108,268,301,339] In most studies, rotavirus and norovirus predominated, while HAdVs accounted for less than 1% to 30% of pediatric cases of acute diarrhea, often accompanied by vomiting and fever.[4,82,105,376,381,429,530] The adenoviruses most commonly observed in fecal specimens of patients with gastroenteritis across many studies were HAdV-F40 and F41, which are therefore referred to as enteric HAdVs,[29,105,376,381,479,530,636] but the variety of HAdV species and types reported in this clinical setting is very high, including HAdV-A types 12, 18, 31, and 61; HAdV-B types 3, 7, 11, 14, 16, and 21; HAdV-C types 1, 2, 5, and 6; HAdV-D types 8 to 10, 19, 26, 28, 29, 30, 32, 37, 43 to 46, 64, and 70; and HAdV-G52.[4,113,307,376,381,429,479,530,540] Some geographic regions such as Sub-Saharan Africa appear to have a very high prevalence and diversity of HAdV-D types associated with various infections including gastroenteritis, and subclinical infections with prolonged shedding have been documented, particularly in immunocompromised hosts.[514] Seasonal distribution of HAdV infections remains a controversial topic. The reported seasonal peaks of HAdV infections varied depending on the geographical region and weather patterns of the country. A number of studies, including some of those cited above, reported a seasonal occurrence of GI HAdV infections (e.g., during the rainy season), but others did not identify any seasonal distribution pattern,[127,128,376,636] and long-term intestinal HAdV shedding is known to occur also in asymptomatic children.[422,425,479] The clinical importance of HAdV shedding in the context of allogeneic SCT is discussed below. One of the complications occurring in patients with GI HAdV infections is intussusception, a condition caused by a segment of the intestine invaginating into an adjacent segment. The classical clinical symptoms include intermittent abdominal pain, currant jelly stool, palpable mass and vomiting. The resulting small bowel obstruction, which may ultimately lead to necrosis, perforation, and sepsis, is a life-threatening complication. There are several, also recent, reports on the association of HAdV-related gastroenteritis as a trigger of intussusception, but this condition is likely to be multifactorial.[60,295,348,394]

Celiac Disease

Infectious agents have been implicated in the pathogenesis of many autoimmune diseases. Celiac disease (CD) is an autoimmune disorder affecting patients with a specific genetic predisposition (HLA-DQ2, HLA-DQ8) who are exposed to gluten, the major storage protein of wheat and similar grains. An environmental factor, such as an infectious agent, is thought to precipitate the disease via various pathogenic mechanisms, such as molecular mimicry, resulting in modulation of the host's immune tolerance.[526] It has been shown that partial amino acid sequence homology between alpha-gliadin, a component of gluten, and an early region protein (E1B-58 kDa) of HAdV-A12 results in immunological cross-reaction. This led to the proposal that prior infection by HAdV-A12 could be associated with the development of CD, possibly by immunological cross-reactivity between antigenic determinants shared by the viral protein and alpha-gliadins.[311] However, the results of an ensuing study suggested that persistent HAdV-A12 infection is not a major component in the pathogenesis of CD.[443] By contrast, the only prospective study on CD and viral infection indicated that frequent rotavirus infections might increase the risk of development of CD antibodies in a cohort at high risk,[640] while other studies with retrospective designs have studied adenovirus, enterovirus, and orthoreovirus as potential triggers of CD with conflicting or inconclusive results.[49,311,443] A recent study revealed that frequent exposure to enterovirus during early childhood was associated with increased risk of CD, suggesting that the interaction between enteroviruses and higher gluten intake may lead to a cumulative effect of these factors in CD development.[421] These observations were confirmed in another recent longitudinal study, which indicated that a higher frequency of enterovirus, but not adenovirus, during early childhood was associated with later CD.[314]

Myocarditis

Myocarditis is an inflammatory disease of the cardiac muscle tissue caused by myocardial infiltration of immunocompetent cells following different kinds of cardiac injury. Infectious causes include a variety of microorganisms including many different viruses, bacteria, protozoa, or fungi, but most frequently the myocardial inflammatory process is directed against viral pathogens.[17,38,458,678,685] The viruses most commonly associated with myocarditis were enteroviruses (EV), such as coxsackieviruses A and B, echovirus, and poliovirus, but during the past decades, a shift was observed to parvovirus B19 (B19V) and human herpesvirus 6 (HHV6) as the most frequently detected cardiotropic viruses in endomyocardial biopsies (EMBs).[125,685,692] Nevertheless, other herpesviruses including CMV and EBV also play a role in this clinical context,[17,125] and prominent involvement of adenoviruses in myocarditis is well established, particularly in children.[585] Coinfections with different viruses have been reported to occur in 12% of acute myocarditis cases.[17] Various studies indicated a prevalence of HAdV in EMB analyzed by PCR in 0% to 23% of patients with acute viral myocarditis.[38,50,125,614] A study based on EMB in pediatric heart transplant patients revealed HAdV genome presence in 9.6% of patients, and viral sequences detectable by PCR were associated with decreased graft survival.[478]

The diagnosis can be challenging, because various clinical methods including imaging techniques can be misleading if infectious agents are involved. Accurate diagnosis requires simultaneous histological, immunohistochemical, and molecular biological workup of the tissue, with strong reliance on EMB-based tools as the gold standard.[17,38,374,554] However, a significant limitation of cardiac biopsy is the observation that the myocardium may be affected in a patchy fashion, thus hampering the exclusion of myocarditis by negative biopsy results.[228]

In addition to supportive care, patients with active myocarditis can receive immunosuppressive treatment upon exclusion of viral persistence in the myocardium, but immunosuppression is contraindicated in EV- or HAdV-positive patients.[66,685] Other treatment approaches include immunomodulation by IFNβ, immunoglobulins, and the anti-inflammatory compounds colchicine and canakinumab.[38,685] Moreover, inhibiting the pro-inflammatory cytokine IL-1 (interleukin-1) by blocking the IL-1 receptor with the naturally occurring compound anakinra was demonstrated to be effective against both myocardial inflammation and contractile dysfunction, and was shown to be suitable for treatment of critically ill myocarditis patients.[72,73] Another immunomodulatory approach relying on the use of adoptive regulatory T-cell transfer was shown to improve coxsackievirus B3–induced myocarditis, and mesenchymal stromal cells (MSCs) were demonstrated to be cardioprotective in myocarditis induced by this viral pathogen, by suppressing inflammasome activation in experimental models.[472,509]

Hepatitis

The liver is one of the organs that can be severely affected by HAdV infections in immunocompromised individuals, including particularly pediatric liver transplant or allogeneic SCT recipients, and patients with malignant disorders receiving chemotherapy. In patients with HAdV-associated hepatitis, histological sections of biopsies revealed localized or massive hepatocyte necrosis, often with absence of associated inflammation. The clinical courses can be fulminant, resulting in acute liver failure with high mortality.[512,570,587]

Adenovirus Infections During Pregnancy

A report on the occurrence of hydrops fetalis and fetal tachyarrhythmia associated with intrauterine HAdV infection documented by PCR in a preterm baby[551] sparked the question whether the virus needs to be regarded a fetal pathogen. This notion was assessed by a prospective observational study indicating that echogenic liver lesions with or without hydrops and neural tube defects were significantly more common in the presence of HAdV detectable by PCR in amniotic fluid. The prevalence and seasonal variation of HAdV detection was similar in sonographically normal and abnormal pregnancies, thus raising questions regarding the significance of these findings.[35] Another study addressing the prevalence of virus isolation in amniotic fluid samples revealed HAdV in 1.3% of fetuses with anomalies, while structurally normal fetuses did not show any evidence for this virus.[519] Asymptomatic fetal viral infection in amniotic fluid tested after the second trimester of pregnancy did not increase the risk for adverse perinatal outcome,[470] and recent studies addressing the risks associated with viral infections during pregnancy did not identify HAdV as an important pathogen in this clinical context.[518,545,619] Nevertheless, adeno-associated virus-2 (AAV-2) has been reported to cause trophoblast dysfunction, and placental AAV-2 infections were associated with preeclampsia.[21]

Obesity

Infection with HAdV-D36 has been associated with obesity in humans. This notion is supported by experimental infections in animals including mice, rats, chickens, and monkeys revealing increases in body fat in a large proportion of instances.[134,476] Moreover, studies on HAdV-D36 infections in humans indicated the presence of antibodies to this virus type in approximately 30% of pediatric and adult individuals around the globe, with a wide range of percentages, but the prevalence in nonobese persons was found to be lower.[8,25,629,735] Infection with HAdV-D36 apparently increases adipogenesis in animals and humans, and the E4orf1 protein derived from HAdV-D36 is responsible for increasing glucose upt ake.[7,134,168,613] Inflammation induced by the virus was shown to contribute to angiogenesis in adipose tissues, thereby maintaining proper glycemic control and metabolic robustness, and the virus was reported to regulate adipose stem cell differentiation and glucolipid metabolism.[302,349]

The prevention of obesity in mice by an anti-HAdV-D36 vaccine supported the notion of employing a vaccination strategy to prevent obesity in humans as well.[487] It is necessary to consider, however, that obesity is a multifactorial, complex phenomenon influenced by genetic, metabolic, cultural, environmental, and lifestyle-related factors, influencing the propensity for obesity apparently conveyed by HAdV-D36 infection.[30,341] A study performed in military staff failed to show any correlation of HAdV-D36 infection status with increase of the BMI (body mass index), and other variables such as high calorie intake and sedentary lifestyle are important components of the multifactorial basis for obesity.[480,697] Other risk factors for obesity include comorbidities such as diabetes mellitus, hypertension, dyslipidemia, endocrine disorders, genetic factors, or certain medications, for example, antihyperglycemics, antidepressants, antipsychotics, and hormones.[142,165,341,373,390] A possible explanation for the apparent association between HAdV-D36 infection and obesity could be an increased susceptibility of obese individuals to viral infections in general, as suggested by different studies.[139,276,332] Indeed, different viral pathogens including, for example, herpesviruses have also been associated with obesity.[665,698] These observations provide a basis for additional studies addressing the correlation between metabolic processes and immune response, including particularly the role of IFNs as key immune regulators against viral infections and in autoimmunity, which are emerging as pivotal players in the regulation of adipogenesis.[341,665]

DISEASES ASSOCIATED WITH IMMUNOCOMPROMISED PATIENTS

In contrast to many other community-acquired viruses, adenoviral infections can occur both by exogenous acquisition and by reactivation of persistent virus[513]; however, the latter appears to be far more prevalent in immunocompromised individuals.[422] Recipients of allogeneic SCT represent one of the most vulnerable patient groups due to the severely impaired function of their immune system.[266,395,422,423] This is mainly attributable to the lack of functional CD4 and CD8 T lymphocytes in the early posttransplant period, particularly during the first 100 days after allografting. In this setting, exogenous exposure or viral reactivation can result in invasive infections potentially conferring high morbidity and mortality rates, particularly in children.[424] The reported frequency of invasive HAdV infections in the allogeneic SCT setting is considerably higher in pediatric patients (6% to 42%) than in adults (1.5% to 15%) (Table 5.2), but the clinical manifestations can be equally severe.[12,45,338,389,423,598] Differences in the observed frequencies might be related to the permanent circulation of HAdV among children[705] but could also be attributable to the more prevalent persistence of the virus in the childhood, providing a constantly available source of reactivation. In immunocompromised patients, HAdV infection can cause a variety of clinical syndromes including asymptomatic viremia, localized acute respiratory illness, gastroenteritis, conjunctivitis, urinary tract infection, or disseminated disease. In this population of patients (and less commonly in immunocompetent individuals), HAdV infections can be very severe, and can cause respiratory failure, HC, neurologic disease, and disseminated infection with lethal failure of individual or multiple organs.[41,422,608]

Risk Factors

Major factors conferring a high risk of invasive HAdV infection and disseminated disease include allogeneic stem cell (or organ) transplantation and any severe immunosuppression with lack of cellular antiadenoviral activity. More specifically, the most prominent risk factors include allogeneic transplantations with *in vivo* and/or *ex vivo* T-cell depletion, grafts from unrelated donors or cord blood, treatment with the anti-CD52 antibody alemtuzumab (Campath™) or antithymocyte globulin (ATG), and presence of graft versus host disease (GvHD) grades III-IV associated with the use of immunosuppressive age nts.[78,114,244,388,420,457,659] Additionally, severe lymphopenia with CD3+ cell counts below 300/μL PB, and absence of HAdV-specific T cells play an important role in the development of viral disease.[172,213,485,751,752] In contrast to allogeneic SCT recipients, donor-positive/recipient-negative HAdV serostatus appears to be a risk factor for severe courses of infection in patients undergoing solid organ transplantation (SOT).[16,290,422,455]

Evidence from pediatric populations indicates that persistent HAdV infection is a risk factor for viral reactivation and ensuing disease with life-threatening clinical manifestations during phases of severe immunosuppression, including particularly allogeneic SCT and, to some extent, SOT recipients.[45,156,247,364,366,424,512] In individuals displaying invasive infection during the posttransplant course, the risk of multiple organ involvement leading to fatal outcome can be high, depending on a variety of parameters such as the level of immunosuppression, the time of onset, or the treatment options available.[422]

Incidence of HAdV Infections in Immunocompromised Adult and Pediatric Patients

In individuals with various congenital immunodeficiencies, particularly in association with severe combined immunodeficiency (SCID) syndrome, severe and recurrent pulmonary HAdV infections and even lethal disseminated disease are not uncommon,[11,437] with reported fatality rates reaching up to 55%.[149] By contrast, life-threatening disease currently appears to be relatively rare in acquired immunodeficiency associated with HIV, where HAdV infections are mostly associated with acute diarrhea only.[3,491] Other clinical manifestations in this setting have become rather exceptional, which is attributable to the availability of highly effective antiretroviral treatment strategies.[272,694] Before the era of effective antiretroviral therapy, a number of authors reported severe and fatal cases in patients with HIV/AIDS associated with pneumonia, hepatitis, nephritis, meningoencephalitis, and disseminated disease.[342,592]

In patients undergoing chemotherapy for malignant diseases, respiratory infections caused by HAdV have been documented during phases of neutropenia, and lethal HAdV disease has been reported in children receiving chemotherapy for acute lymphoblastic or myeloid leukemia and in adults treated with alemtuzumab or receiving chemotherapy.[303,555,563,639] In SOT recipients, HAdV infections can be asymptomatic, but prolonged and severe courses impacting morbidity, graft loss, and mortality may occur.[56,57,156,180,183,184,239,248,444,465,512,602,604,737] Infections can be acquired *de novo* or via reactivation of latent virus from the recipient or the transplanted organ.[271] The occurrence of adenoviremia has been reported in less than 10% of adult patients after kidney, heart, or liver transplantation. Although the symptoms of HAdV infection were usually mild, and invasive infection did not correlate with organ rejection, severe and even fatal courses have also been described.[182,231,271,587,715] Studies in patients undergoing lung transplantation showed that pulmonary infection with HAdV can correlate with significantly elevated rates of rejection, bronchiolitis obliterans, and mortality.[102,699] In line with the epidemiology of HAdV infections, detection of this virus appears to be more common in pediatric SOT,[248,478] with reported rates of HAdV infection ranging from 3.5% to 38% after liver transplantation,[120,155] 7% to 50% after lung and heart transplantation,[427,431,616] and 4% to 57% after intestinal or multivisceral transplantation.[181,465,525] In children after small bowel transplantation, biopsies often revealed the presence of HAdV, but the occurrence of virus-related disease seemed to correlate primarily with the intensity of immunosuppressive treatment.[181] Adenovirus was the most common infectious agent in this context, and enterocolitis, sometimes mimicking rejection, may occur.[360] In the autologous SCT setting, HAdV infections seem to be a rare event,[1,345,742] while allogeneic SCT represents a major risk factor. In allogeneic SCT recipients, young age was shown to confer an elevated risk of HAdV infection,[687] and life-threatening disease was invariably associated with adenoviremia, or more precisely HAdV-DNAemia, because the detection is generally based on PCR-based analysis.[157,424]

De novo Infection and Viral Reactivation in Transplant Recipients

In the allogeneic transplantation setting, adenoviral complications can arise from *de novo* infection or reactivation of persistent endogenous HAdV. Exogenous infection can occur by virus transmission from the donor via the graft or from the environment.[690] The occurrence of outbreaks on transplant wards documents the role of environmental sources for HAdV spread.[457,650] However, endogenous reactivation of persistent HAdV appears to be the predominant cause of HAdV-associated disease in severely immunocompromised patients. This notion is supported by the absence of a seasonal pattern of infections in this setting and the finding that the HAdV strain detected prior to allogeneic SCT is generally identical to the strain isolated during the posttransplant period.[687,690] The presence of high neutralizing antibody titers against specific HAdV types before allogeneic SCT permitted prediction of reactivation and viral disease caused by the same HAdV type.[690] Detection of HAdV DNA in feces or nasopharyngeal aspirates in the recipient prior to SCT has been reported as a risk factor for viral dissemination posttranplant.[122,425] Although HAdV reactivation in the immunocompromised setting could conceivably occur at different sites, observations in pediatric allogeneic SCT recipients made over a period of more than 15 years suggest that massive viral replication preceding invasive infection occurs almost invariably in the GI tract.[366,424,425] The monitoring of viral load in serial stool samples during the posttransplant period therefore permits timely assessment of impending disseminated disease,[422,423,425] as outlined below.

Definitions of Adenoviral Infection and Disease

In the past, different groups have proposed definitions of localized and disseminated adenovirus infection, probable and proven/definite adenovirus disease, which were based on various technical approaches to virus detection.[178,425,649] Owing to the fact that highly sensitive techniques based primarily on PCR have become the gold standard for the detection and monitoring of HAdV infections, the ECIL (European Conference on Infections in Leukemia) group has recommended the following definitions[455]:

- Local infection: positive HAdV PCR, virus isolation, or antigen detection in biopsy material or fluids other than peripheral blood
- Systemic (invasive) infection: positive HAdV PCR (viremia/DNAemia), virus isolation, or antigen detection in peripheral blood
- Probable disease: HAdV infection plus corresponding symptoms and signs without histological confirmation
- Proven disease: HAdV infection plus corresponding symptoms related to the infection and histological confirmation of HAdV in the appropriate location

In extension of the above criteria, prospective studies defined intestinal adenovirus disease as reproducible detection of HAdV in stool specimens at levels detectable and quantifiable by real-time PCR together with enteritis, in the absence of other infections or GvHD, while mere presence of HAdV in stool was regarded as virus shedding only. Disseminated HAdV disease was defined as multiple organ involvement (e.g., hepatitis, encephalitis, retinitis) in the presence of two or more HAdV-positive PCR assays in peripheral blood and other sites tested (e.g., CSF, bronchoalveolar lavage, respiratory secretions, urine), in absence of other identifiable causes. HAdV-associated death was defined as multiple organ failure in the presence of increasing or persisting adenoviral load in peripheral blood, in association with HAdV detection from multiple other sites.[422,425]

Clinical Presentation and Outcome of HAdV Infections in Solid Organ and Allogeneic Stem Cell Transplantation

The most common occurrence of HAdV disease is observed between 2 and 3 months posttransplant, and the first symptoms include fever, enteritis, elevated liver enzymes, and secondary pancytopenia.[454] In SOT recipients, the transplanted organ is often the primary site of HAdV-related disease. Clinical manifestations reported in patients receiving lung, liver, kidney, or small bowel transplantations include pneumonia, hepatitis, nephritis, HC, enteritis, and disseminated disease.[289] The manifestations tend to be more severe in pediatric transplant populations, with reported mortality rates occasionally exceeding 50%,[422] and surveillance of HAdV load in peripheral blood may be instrumental in identifying patients requiring antiviral treatment, in order to prevent fatal disease.[155,715] In adult patients undergoing SOT, the incidence of viremia is lower, often transient and self-limited, with asymptomatic clinical courses. Routine surveillance of HAdV by PCR therefore does not seem to be indicated in adult organ transplant recipients.[270,271]

Data on HAdV infections in the hematopoietic SCT setting are far more abundant. In allogeneic SCT recipients, the spectrum of HAdV-associated disease can range from mild gastroenteric or respiratory symptoms to severe manifestations including hemorrhagic enteritis or cystitis, pneumonia, hepatitis, nephritis, encephalitis, myocarditis, and occasionally, concomitant involvement of several organs, which may lead to lethal outcome with multi-organ failure, as outlined above.[321,422,423,504] Postmortem investigation of the affected organs, including particularly the liver, reveals massive replication of the virus with lysis of the infected cells and release of viral particles into peripheral blood,[185] underlining the diagnostic relevance of viremia. In a study performed in the pediatric allogeneic SCT setting, transplant-related mortality associated with HAdV reached 6% of the entire patient cohort investigated,[424,425] but fatal disease attributable to HAdV infection has been reported in up to 50% of patients with DNAemia.[425,659] The majority of transplant-related deaths attributable to HAdV infection occur within the first 100 days posttransplant.[422,423,425]

It is important to emphasize that the occurrence and overall mortality of HAdV infections is apparently lower in adult patients undergoing allogeneic SCT (<1%), but can also be very high in the presence of HAdV-DNAemia[27,216,659] (Table 5.2). Fatal outcome is particularly frequent in cases of DNAemia associated with disseminated disease, with reported lethality rates reaching up to 60% to 80% both in children and in adults.[188,380,422,423] Clinical observations indicate that the courses of invasive HAdV infection in children undergoing allogeneic SCT can be fulminant, with fatal outcome within a few days after onset of the first clinical symptoms of viral disease.[425] Timely onset of treatment is important for successful control of HAdV infections in immunocompomised patients, but immediate availability of effective therapeutic strategies is still limited. Rapid and reliable diagnosis of impending HAdV disease is therefore of paramount importance (see section Diagnosis).

EVIDENCE LINKING ADENOVIRUSES TO HUMAN CANCER

The WHO (World Health Organization) estimated that more than 15% of all cancers are attributable to infections, and nearly 10% are linked to viruses.[527] Viruses can contribute to the biology of multistep oncogenesis, and have been implicated in several hallmarks of cancer.[466] To identify viruses contributing to cancer via direct or indirect oncogenesis, the following characteristics were proposed: (a) presence and persistence of viral DNA in tumor biopsies; (b) growth-promoting activity of viral genes in model systems; (c) dependence of malignant phenotype on continuous viral oncogene expression or modification of host genes; and (d) epidemiological evidence that a virus represents a major risk for development of cancer.[770] In contrast to the concept that persistence of virus-specific oncogenes is required to maintain the transformed cellular phenotype, the "hit-and-run" hypothesis raises the notion that viruses can mediate cellular transformation through an initial hit attributable to their mutagenic potential, while maintenance of the transformed state may be compatible with the loss of viral molecules.[494]

Several decades ago, it was demonstrated that HAdV-A12 can induce various tumors in newborn Syrian hamsters, and similar observations were later made in different experimental rodent models with other HAdV types belonging particularly to the species A, B, and D.[205,250,298] The mechanism of malignant transformation has been attributed to the early adenoviral proteins E1A and E1B, which act as transcription factors interfering with important tumor suppressor proteins such as Rb (retinoblastoma) or p53, as well as proteins of the DNA repair machinery, chromatin remodeling, and ubiquitination.[44,354,483] The E1A, E1B, and other regions were found to be integrated into cellular DNA, and the viral genes were expressed as proteins mediating the transformed state. Moreover, the adenoviral E3 and E4 proteins were shown to block the host immune response and the onset of apoptosis.[153,593] The E4 region encodes the products of E4orf6 and E4orf3 acting as oncoproteins, which cooperate with E1A proteins to transform primary rodent cells.[494] These observations indicated a rather complex pattern of interactions between early adenoviral proteins and important cellular control mechanisms, which may contribute to malignant transformation. The well-established tumorigenic properties of different HAdVs in experimental mammalian animal models,[722] and their ability to persist in different cell types in the human host raised questions pertaining to HAdV oncogenicity in human cancer.[367] Nevertheless, the evidence for a possible association of HAdV with human malignancies has remained scarce over many years, although it has been demonstrated that multipotent human mesenchymal stem cells can be reproducibly transformed by the E1A/E1B oncogenes derived from HAdV-C5.[633]

High prevalence of HAdV sequences has been documented in a variety of malignant neoplasms including particularly brain tumors, such as oligodendroglioma, glioblastoma, or ependymoma.[367] Control samples of nonmalignant counterparts of HAdV-positive brain tumors, including specimens of ependymal cells, plexus choroideus, and periventricular white matter also revealed the presence of HAdV DNA in most specimens tested. The identification of HAdV types detected both in malignant and nonmalignant brain tissue specimens revealed predominantly representatives of species B and D and, less commonly, C. The presence of contamination as a possible cause of false-positive results was excluded by confirmatory results obtained by *in situ* hybridization. The CNS was shown to represent a common site of HAdV infection with virus persistence, thus providing evidence for the possible contribution of HAdVs to the multistep process of tumor pathogenesis in brain tissue.[367]

Epidemiological studies indicated a link between *in utero* infection with viruses and ALL (acute lymphoblastic leukemia),[207] and screening of amniotic fluid samples in the second trimester of pregnancy revealed DNA from different viruses detectable by PCR, suggesting that infections *in utero*, including HAdV, are fairly common.[470] Adenovirus DNA was detected at an elevated frequency in Guthrie cards from children who developed ALL,[217] but in subsequent studies the frequency was regarded as too low to permit an association between HAdV and the development of leukemia.[259,689] In a more recent study focusing on lymphoid malignancies including various types of lymphocytic leukemia, malignant lymphoma, and multiple myeloma, adenoviral DNA was only detected in a high proportion of mantle cell lymphoma specimens. The presence of adenoviral sequences identified by pan-adenovirus PCR screening was confirmed in individual cells by FISH (fluorescence in-situ hybridization), and the most prevalent HAdV species detected was C, and less commonly B.[370]

A recent study based on WGS and RNA-seq (RNA sequencing) in a large spectrum of tumor entities revealed adenoviral sequences in several tumor types including renal cell carcinoma, breast adenocarcinoma, prostate adenocarcinoma, head and neck carcinoma, and hepatocellular carcinoma.[753] Samples testing positive for HAdV were identified both in the tumor and in the adjacent nonmalignant tissue, possibly indicating viral persistence in the respective tissues. Virus positivity was observed in nearly half of the renal carcinoma cases investigated, and the virus was detectable by WGS, but escaped detection by RNA-seq, in line with absent or very low expression of viral genes during latent phases.[498] Interestingly, driver gene mutations commonly occurring in renal cancer did not co-occur with HAdV detection, raising the hypothesis that the virus might contribute to cancer development independently from the well-known driver genes. Of note, the outcome of patients with HAdV-positive renal tumors was significantly better than that of individuals displaying virus-negative tumors.[753] Rather surprisingly, these data were not included in a more recently published version of the study.[754]

Although the associations with various malignant tumors are intriguing, it was not possible thus far to provide clear indications for a causal relationship between HAdV infection and tumorigenicity in humans.[533] It is important to emphasize, however, that the studies discussed above addressing HAdV-induced cancer in humans do not rule out a "hit and run" mechanism in which the virus causes changes in cells eventually leading to cancer, but the viral genome is not retained by the cells.[282] This mechanism of transformation has been reported in primary rat cells,[494] raising the possibility that even tumors lacking any detectable virus-specific molecules can display viral pathogenesis. This notion may require consideration when using adenoviral vectors for gene therapy. At present, the putative implication of HAdVs in human cancer continues posing an intriguing enigma.

DIAGNOSIS

Infections of the upper and lower respiratory tract caused by HAdVs are clinically difficult to distinguish from other respiratory viruses and even some bacterial infections. The appearance of tonsils in small children can be similar to streptococcal or herpesvirus infections. Differential diagnostic considerations also apply to HAdV-mediated (kerato)conjunctivitis, which usually begins unilaterally, with moderate enlargement of the preauricular lymph node, and sometimes with subsequent involvement of the contralateral eye. The symptoms of hemorrhagic manifestations of the urinary tract caused by HAdV infections in immunosuppressed patients can be similar to bacterial infections or drug toxicity affecting the bladder. Due to the difficult clinical diagnosis, laboratory tests are required for reliable HAdV identification, and previously common approaches including viral isolation, cell culture, immunofluorescence-based detection of HAdV-specific antibodies, serological analysis by HI and SN tests, as well as examination by light or electron microscopy were addressed in some detail in the previous Editions of Fields Virology.[724,725] Due to the present dominance of molecular diagnostic approaches, the current chapter is focused on these techniques. The molecular methods employed for qualitative HAdV screening by broad-spectrum (pan-adenoviral) PCR assays, quantitative monitoring by real-time PCR tests, and typing at the levels of species, types and strains, based on specific PCR tests and sequencing techniques, are used in both the immunocompetent and immunocompromised patient settings. In this chapter, the emphasis is placed on HAdV diagnosis and monitoring in patients with severely impaired immune response displaying a high risk for invasive infections.

Diagnosis in the Immunocompromised Setting

Invasive infection defined by the presence of adenoviremia/DNaemia renders serial diagnostic monitoring of PB samples during the posttransplant course of paramount importance. It has been demonstrated that HAdV detection and documentation of rising virus levels in plasma by quantitative PCR (qPCR)-based monitoring precede the onset of clinical symptoms of organ involvement by several weeks,[424] thus offering the possibility for preemptive initiation of treatment. The observation that patients can succumb to disseminated HAdV disease within a few days after presenting with symptoms of systemic infection highlights the need for careful diagnostic monitoring and early implementation of therapeutic measures.[424] Although lethal HAdV infections have been described in both adult and pediatric allogeneic SCT recipients, the reported frequency of invasive infections with severe clinical courses is considerably higher in children, as indicated in Table 5.2.[12,27,122,167,176,216,244,321,425,502,550,624,625,659,687,704,755] Different groups have tried to define thresholds of HAdV levels in plasma as a trigger for the initiation of antiviral treatment,[388,420,660] but the assessment of absolute virus copy numbers greatly depends on the method used, and published data cannot be readily transferred to other centers without complete harmonization of the technical approaches used. In this regard, the documentation of rising virus copy numbers may be a more universal parameter, which is rather independent of the particular methodological approach used, as long as a quantitative (at present predominantly molecular) technique is employed. Nevertheless, clinical experience in the pediatric setting has indicated that the initiation of treatment at the stage of invasive HAdV infection, as documented by the presence of viremia, may not prevent disseminated disease with lethal outcome in a number of insta nces.[422–425,755] These observations have stimulated the search for diagnostic options facilitating early assessment of the risk for systemic infections, and the GI tract was demonstrated to represent the most important compartment for expansion of the virus prior to dissemination in pediatric SCT recipients.[366,425] Although the importance of serial monitoring of stool samples in children during the posttransplant period has not yet been fully recognized by the latest ECIL recommendations,[455] there is now ample evidence supporting the role of intestinal HAdV shedding for early detection of impending invasive infection,[167,269,300,364,425] and the recent recommendations published on behalf of the IDWP (Infectious Disease Working Party) of the EBMT (European Society of Blood and Marrow Transplantation) strongly suggest the inclusion of serial monitoring of stool specimens in the routine diagnostic program in pediatric allogeneic SCT[245] (Table 5.3). In the adult SCT setting, there is currently no indication supporting the role of the GI tract for HAdV expansion before the infection becomes invasive, and testing of PB specimens is therefore the preferred approach for patient surveillance.[245] Although the presence of adenoviremia is reportedly correlated with a high risk of lethal disseminated disease,[422] the appropriate timing for the initiation of treatment is still a matter of debate.

Predictive Value of Viremia and HAdV Replication in the Gastrointestinal Tract

Since spread of the virus into peripheral blood is a characteristic sign of disseminated HAdV disease, and viral load values correspond to the severity of organ pathology,[236] quantitative monitoring in plasma or serum has become an essential screening tool after allogeneic SCT, as specified in more detail below. Additionally, there is growing evidence that HAdV detection and surveillance of virus proliferation kinetics in stool provide early information on impending invasive infection and HAdV disease.[300,401,425] Viral persistence in the GI tract and shedding of HAdV into feces is a common finding, which reportedly occurs in more than one-third of pediatric patients after allogeneic SCT, and may not necessarily be associated with clinical symptoms of intestinal infection.[366,422,423] Detection and quantitative surveillance of HAdV in serial stool samples revealed two distinct patterns indicating the risk of invasive infection. Patients displaying very slow or absent proliferation kinetics in serial analyses, with maximum HAdV loads below 10E6 virus copies/g of stool, apparently have a very low risk of adenoviremia. By contrast, patients showing rapid proliferation exceeding the threshold of 10E6 virus copies/g, and sometimes revealing extremely high viral loads of more than 10E11 copies/g, have a very high risk of experiencing viremia and disseminated disease (see section Persistence and Reactivation in the GI Tract).[425] These observations were largely confirmed by other groups,[114,167,269,300,402,635] and will expectedly have important implications for future diagnostic and treatment strategies.

Diagnostic Screening

Conventional approaches to HAdV detection at affected sites such as peripheral blood, stool, urine, bronchoalveolar lavage, and nasopharyngeal aspirates or swabs formerly included primarily immunofluorescent staining for antigen detection and viral culture.[149,289,344,387] However, due to the limited sensitivity and, in case of viral culture, rather long time to readout, these methods have been largely supplanted in routine clinical diagnostics by molecular screening approaches generally relying on PCR-based techniques.[289,363,365,425] Owing to the superior sensitivity and specificity of molecular tests facilitating equally effective detection of all HAdV types in any diagnostic material, PCR assays have become a standard screening tool.[455] Despite the predominance of certain HAdV species in specific clinical settings including immunocompromised patients, employment of broad-spectrum HAdV screening assays is necessary in order to permit reliable detection even of rarely occurring HAdV species and types with adequate sensitivity (Fig. 5.5). Several groups have established such "pan-adenoviral" assays based on PCR, exploiting the sequence information available at the respective points in time.[148,150,237,265,363] The HAdV screening assays target conserved regions within the HAdV genome, most commonly within the hexon gene, but the inclusion of additional target regions, for example, within the fiber gene, may be required to ensure reliable detection of all known types with comparable sensitivity.[148,363,365] Due to the fact that the spectrum of newly identified HAdV types identified by the implementation of genomic analyses has been expanding, established assays need to be updated in order to facilitate reliable coverage of the entire range of HAdVs.[363] Since the newly identified HAdV types generally result from recombination events within the same or different human species of the virus,[562] the target regions of established PCR assays are preserved in most instances, thus permitting equally sensitive detection of the new recombinants. Nevertheless, this issue requires careful attention, as exemplified by one of the early HAdV screening assays based on the sequence information accessible at that time.[148] The test was originally demonstrated to cover all 51 known HAdV (sero)types with comparable detection limits. Alignment with genomic sequences of subsequently published HAdV types revealed that the primer/probe combinations of this real-time PCR assay can be expected to reliably cover nearly all hitherto identified HAdV types, with two exceptions. The sequence of HAdV-A61 revealed a few mismatches in the target region of the downstream primer, possibly affecting the sensitivity of detection. This finding required the addition of an appropriately modified primer to the reaction, and subsequent confirmation of this adaption *in vitro*. The second exception was HAdV-G52, which displays the greatest similarity to a simian adenovirus (SAdV-1), and would not be reliably covered by the assay. This example highlights the need to control and adequately adapt established diagnostic assays based on newly identified HAdV types, if the test is expected to serve for "pan-adenoviral" screening.[363] The availability of complete genomic sequences of all currently known HAdV types greatly facilitates appropriate modifications of established assays and the development of novel tests. The same requirements apply to commercial HAdV assays that are FDA approved in the United States and/or CE marked in Europe. A number of such kits have been introduced including the Adenovirus R-gene™ kit (BioMérieux, Lyon, France), ELITe MGB®Kit kit (ELITech Group Molecular Diagnostics, Puteaux, France), FilmArray® RP (BioFire Diagnostics, Inc, Salt Lake City, UT, United States), eSensor RVP (GenMark Diagnostics, Carlsbad, CA, United States), xTAG RVP *FAST* and xTAG RVPv1 (Luminex Molecular Diagnostics, Toronto, Canada), Prodesse ProAdeno™+ Assay (Hologic Gen-Probe, San Diego, CA, United States), and Anyplex II RV16 (Seegene, South Korea), and the list is probably not exhaustive. Most of the indicated kits cover multiple viruses and are only approved for qualitative analysis of respiratory specimens. Studies comparing the performance of such kits indicated a particularly high variability for HAdV detection, and inadequate identification of certain HAdV types by some of the tests.[109,350,528] The monitoring of patients in the immunocompromised setting requires tests permitting reliable detection of all potentially relevant HAdV types in different clinical specimens, and accurate quantitative assessment of viral loads. Among the currently available commercial kits, this requirement appears to be met by the Adenovirus R-gene kit,[299,365] and possibly by the ELITe MGB® kit, although the latter seems to be approved for whole blood analysis only.

It is important to emphasize that the lower detection limit for HAdV detection in clinical specimens, including particularly peripheral blood, should be in the range of 10E2 virus copies/mL in order to prevent false-negative test results, and to permit early initiation of treatment according to some of the published guidelines.[420]

Relevance of HAdV Detection and Quantification at Specific Sites

A prospective study in pediatric patients undergoing allogeneic SCT, which focused on screening of HAdV at different sites including throat, stool, urine, peripheral blood, and occasionally other sites, revealed that detection of adenovirus at multiple (i.e., more than 2) sites reflects the presence of invasive infection. However, at that time detection of HAdV in peripheral blood was the only site permitting risk assessment of disseminated disease.[424] A number of studies provided similar findings,[150,157,188,216,321] rendering peripheral blood the most important source for clinical surveillance of HAdV infections in the immunocompromised setting. The time point of HAdV DNAemia may be of prognostic relevance: some studies showed that patients showing DNAemia before day 100 after allogeneic SCT developed life-threatening disseminated disease in more than 60% of instances despite antiadenoviral treatment, whereas later onset of viremia did not seem to be associated with disseminated HAdV disease.[424,425] Interestingly, other reports suggested that HAdV detection in nasopharyngeal aspirates of children prior to allogeneic SCT is a strong predictor for ensuing adenoviremia and may therefore provide an indication for postponement of transplantation, if possible.[122,420] In fact, HAdV may be persistently detectable in nasopharyngeal secretions in some pediatric patients,[291,322] and these observations therefore require careful consideration.

Despite the clear diagnostic and prognostic relevance of HAdV DNAemia, only a proportion of high-risk patients with this finding develop overt disease. A number of groups have therefore attempted to identify virus load levels that could serve as a rational basis for the onset of preemptive antiviral treatment. However, the thresholds suggested by different authors were highly divergent, ranging from 10E2 (in individuals with high risk) to greater than 10E6 copies/mL,[157,188,216,388,420,660] thus rendering generally applicable conclusions difficult. Moreover, the measured absolute values are, at least to some extent, dependent on the individual technique used, and in absence of appropriate interlaboratory standardization, the values cannot be readily adopted by or exchanged between centers. Other authors have shown that rapidly rising viral loads are detectable in peripheral blood prior to onset of clinical symptoms of HAdV disease, suggesting that the monitoring of viral titer kinetics may be a more readily applicable parameter.[424,599] Moreover, in addition to facilitating prediction of HAdV-related disease, surveillance of HAdV copy number kinetics in peripheral blood is also instrumental for assessment of the response to therapy.[189,420,425] In some studies, a decrease in viral load by at least one log within 2 to 3 weeks of antiviral treatment was regarded as a minimum requirement for adequate response,[424,425] but there are no generally accepted guidelines for diagnostic definitions of response at the present time.

The relevance of HAdV replication kinetics and peak load levels in stool specimens of pediatric allogeneic SCT recipients for risk assessment of invasive infection has already been indicated above. Since timely onset of antiviral therapy appears to be critical in this setting, and starting treatment upon detection of HAdV viremia may be too late in a number of instances,[173,369,424,425] it is essential to identify the earliest possible time points for rational initiation of therapy. In view of the high risk of invasive infection and disseminated disease in children displaying rapid HAdV proliferation kinetics in serial stool specimens with peak levels exceeding 10E6 virus copies/g, systematic screening of intestinal excretions should be part of the diagnostic routine during the posttransplant period. The median time span between detection of HAdV loads in stool exceeding the indicated threshold and first appearance of the virus in peripheral blood was 11 days in one of the studies performed,[425] thus providing a rational window of opportunity for early onset of therapy, with the aim to prevent invasive infection (Fig. 5.7).

Adenovirus Typing

Identification of adenoviruses at the level of species, (sero) types, and even strains is of relevance for epidemiological studies and for precise documentation of nosocomial outbreaks. For the selection of optimal treatment, HAdV typing is currently of lesser importance because, with the exception of ribavirin (see below), available therapeutic strategies are independent from the HAdV species present. However, in view of the fact that different HAdV species and types may occur contemporaneously or sequentially in individual patients[151,372,460,696,766] (Figs. 5.5 and 5.6), typing may permit better understanding of the dynamics and evolution of HAdV infection.

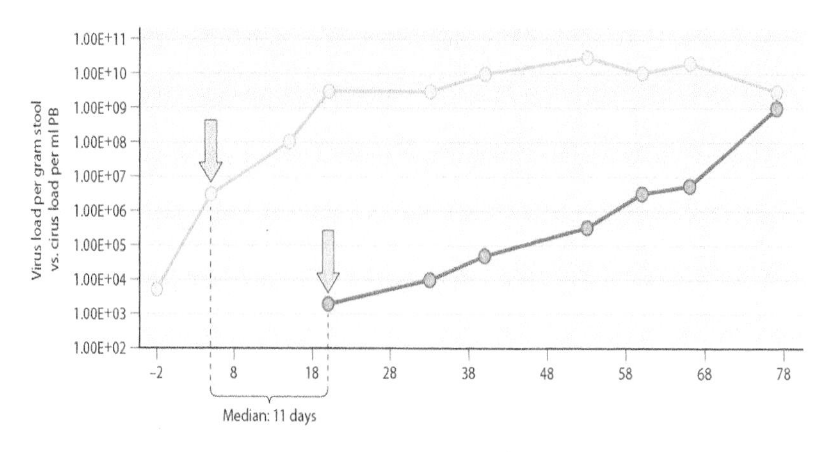

FIGURE 5.7 Temporal correlation between intestinal HAdV infection and viremia. The median time span between the observation of rapidly rising HAdV copy numbers in serial stool specimens (*blue line*) exceeding the threshold of 10E6 virus copies/g of stool (*left arrow*) and the first detection of viremia (*right arrow; red line*) was 11 days, providing a rational basis for early onset of treatment. (Reprinted from Lion T. Adenovirus infections in immunocompetent and immunocompromised patients. *Clin Microbiol Rev* 2014;27(3):441–462. Ref.[422])

Typing was traditionally performed by serological methods, but these approaches have mostly been replaced by molecular techniques based on PCR amplification of specific target regions coupled with different detection formats such as fragment length analysis, hybridization to species-specific probes, or sequencing.[147,315,553,764] Molecular typing methods are more rapid, are readily applicable, and can provide better discriminating capacity. Owing to the decreasing costs of next generation sequencing (NGS) approaches, whole genome analysis[307] may become the method of choice for detailed HAdV typing in the foreseeable future even in the routine diagnostic setting.

Molecular HAdV Detection and Monitoring of Viral Load

The importance of appropriate diagnostic HAdV monitoring is underlined by the fact that the morbidity and mortality in immunocompromised patients with invasive infection can be very high, in both the pediatric and adult settings (Table 5.2). In such patients, particularly in the pediatric allogeneic SCT setting, adenoviruses can be detected in a variety of clinical materials.[422–424] Although it has been reported that HAdV detection in respiratory specimens of pediatric transplant recipients is of prognostic relevance for invasive infection,[122] there is strong evidence supporting the essential role of serial stool monitoring for early prediction of impending adenoviremia.[114,167,269,288,300,402,425,635] Hence, monitoring of stool specimens has been widely adopted as a routine diagnostic tool in children undergoing allogeneic SCT.[203] Moreover, monitoring of PB specimens is generally employed in both the pediatric and adult allogeneic SCT settings to identify patients at high risk for HAdV-related systemic disease and to assess the response to antiviral treatment approaches[203] (Table 5.3).

Technical Considerations for Diagnostic Testing

From the diagnostic perspective, it is important to emphasize that the technical approach, which mostly relies on quantitative PCR testing, needs to cover the entire known spectrum of HAdV species and types, in order to prevent missing any potentially life-threatening infections by these viruses. Essentially, any HAdV species can occur in the severely immunocompromised setting, but geographic differences in the distribution of HAdV species exist, based on reports of invasive infections from different centers.[422] In many regions, representatives of HAdV species C predominate, followed by species A and B, while members of other HAdV species are rather rare in immunosuppressed patients, and often occur only in combination with one of the more common species.[422] However, different HAdV species or types can occur concomitantly or sequentially, underlining the need to employ diagnostic tests displaying very broad specificity for quantitative HAdV detection (Figs. 5.5 and 5.6). Due to the permanent expansion of the HAdV spectrum (Table 5.1), it is necessary to monitor and potentially adjust the assays used, as pointed out previously.[365,422]

Patient Surveillance Based on the Monitoring of Stool

Recent recommendations published on behalf of the European Bone Marrow Transplant Association (EBMT) have highlighted the importance of HAdV detection and monitoring in stool samples of pediatric SCT recipients[245] (Table 5.3). The relevance of pretransplant assessment of intestinal HAdV shedding has been recognized, and molecular screening at specific time points has been suggested by the expert panel (Table 5.3). Moreover, based on initial data highlighting the importance of HAdV monitoring in stool in the pediatric SCT setting,[425] which were corroborated by several other investigators,[114,167,269,300,635] pertinent recommendations for diagnostic surveillance have been provided (Table 5.3). It is necessary to bear in mind, however, that HAdV levels above 10E6 virus copies/g of stool, which were originally described as the critical threshold for the risk of impending invasive infection,[425] may need to be adjusted according to the quantitative readout of the specific method used. By contrast, the use of rapidly increasing HAdV copy numbers in serial stool specimens as a dynamic parameter may be applicable regardless of the particular quantitative technique employed. Data obtained from serial monitoring of stool specimens may provide a basis for early initiation of antiviral treatment, with the aim to reduce HAdV-related morbidity and prevent invasive infection. However, due to the current lack of data on systematic stool monitoring in the adult SCT setting, the recommendations for diagnostic exploitation of feces are presently restricted to pediatric transplant recipients only (Table 5.3).

Patient Surveillance Based on the Monitoring of Peripheral Blood

In adult organ transplant recipients, viremia is often asymptomatic, and the risk of progression to adenoviral disease in the presence of HAdV DNAemia with or without specific cutoff values for viral loads remains unknown.[180] Routine screening for HAdV is therefore not recommended at present, although adenovirus infections in this setting can be severe and affect morbidity, mortality, and graft survival, particularly in young children.[180]

In line with the latest ECIL recommendations for HAdV diagnostics in SCT recipients and patients with leukemia, monitoring of PB specimens by quantitative PCR, based on the presence of a defined risk profile, is regarded as the cornerstone of diagnostic surveillance.[12,455] Indeed, prior to the identification of the important role of stool monitoring in the pediatric SCT setting, a decade ago,[425] HAdV surveillance in transplant recipients was largely based on PB monitoring only, and different investigators tried to define thresholds of HAdV copy numbers requiring the initiation of treatment. The indicated thresholds varied, as outlined above, also depending on the individual risk profile.[210,388,420,660] However, as indicated, the virus quantity determined depends on the specific method employed, and the numbers therefore cannot be easily transferred between centers without aligning the methodological approaches. It has been shown that increasing HAdV copy numbers can be detected in PB prior to the onset of clinical symptoms indicative of organ involvement, and the average time span between the first log increase in viral load and the appearance of disseminated disease was several weeks.[424] These observations indicated that a dynamic parameter of documented viral expansion in PB might be a more universally applicable approach to identifying patients who require treatment, which would be independent of using completely harmonized molecular methods. However, the reported mortality in SCT recipients with adenoviremia is high (Table 5.2), and it is questionable therefore whether the initiation of antiviral treatment in this setting should be triggered by specific thresholds or dynamic parameters of viral expansion. In view of the limited efficacy of current treatment options, it might be reasonable to initiate treatment upon HAdV detection in PB at any level, upon consideration of the individual risk for disseminated disease.

The IDWP-EBMT recommendations for the employment of PB monitoring in the SCT setting are outlined in Table 5.3.[245] Recent studies have addressed the prognostic role of diagnostic parameters including HAdV peak levels (PL) and the time-averaged area under the curve (AAUC) of virus copy numbers in PB. The latter parameter reflects the overall exposure to the virus by assessing the viral burden over time, and was therefore presumed to provide potentially more reliable prognostic information. The predictive value for patient outcome reflected by all-cause, nonrelapse, or HAdV-related mortality was determined, and was significant for the parameters tested.[369,755] However, since nonrelapse mortality also encompasses death attributable to graft versus host disease, treatment-related toxicity, and other infections, and all-cause mortality also includes disease relapse, correlation with these criteria may overestimate the actual contribution of HAdV to lethal outcome. In one of the studies looking at HAdV-related mortality, peak virus levels in PB below 10E4 copies/mL and low AAUC levels correlated with a low probability of succumbing to the viral infection,[369] thereby providing diagnostic markers of potential prognostic relevance.

PREVENTION AND TREATMENT

Approaches to Antiadenoviral Treatment in Immunocompromised Patients

The optimal time point for initiation of antiadenoviral treatment in the immunocompromised setting has been a matter of discussion, and certainly depends on the individual risk situation and the treatment options available. Prophylactic therapy against HAdV infections is not performed due to the limited efficacy and toxicity of currently available antiviral agents,[455] but preemptive treatment is warranted due to the unfavorable outcome of symptomatic disease.[245] In pediatric SCT recipients, HAdV detection in stool prior to SCT has been associated with an elevated risk for early onset of invasive infection, and it was suggested that postponing elective transplantations and providing early preemptive treatment might be a sensible option in high-risk constellations.[364] Moreover, in the pediatric SCT setting, an algorithm has been proposed suggesting the onset of preemptive therapy based on the detection of expanding HAdV copy numbers in stool exceeding the threshold of 10E6 virus copies/g, which had been identified as critical for the risk of invasive infection.[422] The presence of low-level viremia can reportedly resolve spontaneously, particularly in the presence of established or incipient immune reconstitution (lymphocyte count >300/mL). However, treatment strategies aiming at the prevention of invasive infection appear to be reasonable, due to the considerable proportion of severe or even lethal courses of infection in patients displaying adenoviremia[245,388] (Table 5.2). Based on these considerations, the recent recommendations published on behalf of the Infectious Diseases Working Party of the EBMT suggest the initiation of antiadenoviral treatment in patients with rapidly rising HAdV levels in stool above the threshold defined as critical[245] (Table 5.3). This recommendation is applicable in pediatric SCT recipients, where intestinal HAdV reactivation and expansion is a virtually invariable finding prior to systemic infection.[422] Additionally, it is strongly recommended to start treatment in the presence of adenoviremia greater than 10E3/mL in lymphopenic patients with less than 25 CD3+ T cells/μL PB[245] (Table 5.3). Due to the important role of immunosuppression as a risk factor for potentially life-threatening HAdV infection, the first therapeutic measure should be tapering of any immunosuppressive treatment, whenever clinically possible.

Current Treatment Modalities

Present recommendations for treatment of HAdV infections focus on immunocompromised patients including particularly allogeneic transplant recipients who apparently carry the greatest risk of severe and life-threatening clinical courses. The approaches pursued may include prophylaxis, preemptive treatment based on virus detection prior to the onset of clinical symptoms, sometimes linked to specific thresholds of viral load, or therapeutic (symptomatic) treatment in the presence of virus-related disease. At present, there is little evidence for a beneficial effect of HAdV prophylaxis, and the ECIL does not recommend prophylactic antiviral therapy with currently available virostatic drugs.[455] In SOT recipients, the indication for therapy in mild or asymptomatic HAdV infection in not clear, since prospective studies have shown that adenoviremia may be present without any clinical symptoms, and may clear spontaneously.[271] Some authors therefore recommend antiviral treatment only in symptomatic patients.[437] By contrast, in patients undergoing allogeneic SCT, preemptive treatment is strongly advocated by all major guidelines in order to inhibit or slow down viral replication, with the aim to prevent overt disease until immune reconstitution from the allograft permits clearance of the infection.[245,420,455] The principal options for preemptive treatment include (a) the tapering of immunosuppressive therapy, which should be performed whenever possible, (b) antiviral drugs, and (c) immunotherapy in case of failure of the previous lines of treatment.

Antiviral Drugs

Most abundant evidence for the *in vivo* efficacy of antiviral therapy against HAdV in the preemptive or symptomatic settings is available for cidofovir,[16,71,179,187,214,357,420,433,435] but the clinical effect of the drug as treatment for overt viral disease is apparently limited.[346,391] The compound is a nucleotide analog of cytosine inhibiting preferentially viral DNA polymerase and viral replication by more efficient competitive incorporation into DNA.[85] Since cidofovir is already a monophosphate, it shows poor oral bioavailability but does not require a viral enzyme (e.g., thymidine kinase) for its phosphorylation, which is required to phosphorylate ganciclovir (see below), and cidofovir can be converted to the di- and triphosphate forms by cellular enzymes. These triphosphorylated acyclic nucleoside phosphonates have a generally higher affinity for viral DNA polymerases than for cellular DNA polymerases, thereby providing specificity for virus-infected cells. They act as inhibitors of the viral DNA polymerase, for which the triphosphate is a substrate, and they function as DNA synthesis chain terminators through a variety of mechanisms.[118] Although resistant mutants have been described *in vitro*, cidofovir apparently displays efficacy against all HAdV species,[85,168] and is currently the primary anti-HAdV agent for preemptive therapy, although it is not approved for this application.[119,420,422,423,425] Cidofovir is a substrate of OAT1 (organic anion transporter 1), which is prevalent in renal tubules, and prolonged exposure of the kidney to the compound leads to nephrotoxicity.[726] The drug is used as induction therapy at a dose of 5 mg/kg/wk for 2 weeks and at 2-week intervals thereafter.[455] Alternatively, a schedule of 1 mg/kg three times a week in combination with hyperhydration and probenecid has been suggested to reduce renal toxicity,[245,420] and the required duration of therapy is linked to the clinical and molecular response, determined by a rather individually defined reduction of viral load.[420,425] Clinical results of preemptive treatment with cidofovir in the context of allogenic SCT are controversial, with studies reporting success rates of approximately 70% or more, and others reporting rather poor responses.[420,425,651] The efficacy in transplant recipients has been shown to depend on at least partial immune recovery.[243,455,695,755] The limitations of treatment with cidofovir include its low bioavailability and poor correlation of pharmacologic effects with the prescribed dose.[112] Moreover, the nephrotoxicity mediated by cidofovir can be dose limiting and sometimes severe, and frequent monitoring of renal and tubular function as well as concomitant hydration and uroprotection with probenecid are recommended.[420,455] The use of intravesical cidofovir for HC in SCT recipients, applied at 1 to 5 mg/kg in 100 mL saline via an indwelling catheter for 1 hour, revealed good efficacy and low toxicity.[6,246,591]

Ribavirin is a nucleoside analog of guanosine displaying *in vitro* activity against DNA and RNA viruses, and the mechanisms of action may include inhibition of viral polymerases, viral RNA capping, and increased mutation rates in newly synthesized DNA.[403,488] Analysis of HAdV isolates revealed consistent sensitivity of all types belonging to species C only, and the evidence for therapeutic efficacy of the compound *in vivo* is controversial.[256,488,671] Ribavirin is therefore not generally recommended for treatment of HAdV infections.[353,455] However, despite the conflicting results on the activity against HAdV *in vivo*, the low nephrotoxicity of ribavirin and the documented *in vitro* efficacy against HAdV species C may justify its use in specific clinical situations.[52,423] Oral, intravenous, and aerosol therapy with ribavirin has been used,[115,609] and the compound has been applied in a clinical study at a dose of 20 mg/kg in combination with cidofovir as preemptive therapy in the presence of infections caused by representatives of HAdV species C in the pediatric allogeneic SCT setting.[425] However, the actual clinical benefit of this treatment remains unclear.

Ganciclovir is a synthetic analog of 2′-deoxy-guanosine, which requires phosphorylation to ganciclovir monophosphate by a viral kinase, and subsequently, formation of ganciclovir diphosphate and triphosphate catalyzed by cellular kinases. Ganciclovir triphosphate is a competitive inhibitor of deoxyguanosine triphosphate (dGTP) incorporation into DNA, and preferentially inhibits viral rather than cellular DNA polymerases. Moreover, it is a poor substrate for chain elongation, thereby disrupting viral DNA synthesis. A possible benefit of ganciclovir against HAdV infections in allogeneic SCT recipients has been suggested.[58] However, since adenoviruses (in contrast to members of the herpesvirus family) lack viral thymidine kinase, and cellular kinases are inefficient in phosphorylating the compound, the anti-HAdV efficacy of ganciclovir is predictably modest,[488] although some HAdV types reportedly displayed EC_{50} values less than 10 μM *in vitro*.[91] Based on current data, there appears to be no justification for recommending the use of this drug for systemic HAdV treatment,[420,425,455] but the compound used in an ophthalmic gel showed efficacy against HAdV types associated with EKC.[264]

Among other antiviral agents tested, the pyrophosphate analog foscarnet was demonstrated to display no activity against HAdV.[91,488]

A rather recently introduced compound termed brincidofovir (1-*O*-hexadecyloxypropyl-cidofovir, formerly CMX001) is an orally bioavailable lipid conjugate of cidofovir displaying substantially less nephrotoxicity than the parent drug, and considerably higher anti-HAdV efficacy, with EC_{50} values in the submicromolar range.[91] The largely absent nephrotoxicity is attributable to the fact that brincidofovir, in contrast to cidofovir, is not a substrate for OAT1 in the renal tubules.[668] The compound is effective against a variety of DNA viruses, and has been successfully employed for treatment of viral infections in allogeneic SCT recipients and other settings, although resistant mutations may arise.[294] Clinical observations on the efficacy against HAdV showed promising results, and several reports on severely affected immunocompromised patients highlighted the lifesaving potential of this agent.[26,65,114,464,550,645,683] Brincidofovir provided orally at a recommended dose of 2 mg/kg (and a maximum of 100 mg) twice weekly permitted clearance of the virus in a substantial proportion of patients, even in the absence of immune reconstitution, with GI symptoms as the main toxic side effect.[210,243,755] The clinical symptoms and the histological findings in colon biopsies, including edema of the lamina propria, epithelial apoptosis, and crypt injury, are similar to the damages caused by GvHD, infection, or toxicity of the immunosuppressive agent MMF (mycophenolate mofetil).[126] The differential diagnosis is clinically important, however, because of the different treatment modalities required in each setting. A possible solution could be the use of an intravenous formulation of the drug, which did not show any GI toxicity in early studies.[395] Brincidofovir is currently regarded as the most effective antiadenoviral agent, and a recent preclinical study indicated that its combination with valganciclovir (an orally bioavailable valyl ester prodrug of ganciclovir) was more efficacious than either drug alone, permitting substantial dose reduction of both compounds for better control of toxic side effects.[676]

Development of Novel Antiadenoviral Compounds

The lack of safe and efficacious drugs approved for treatment of HAdV infections has stimulated the search for new antiviral compounds including not only novel developments but also the testing of agents currently employed in other clinical contexts for their efficacy against HAdVs.[449] Repurposing of drugs already approved by the regulatory agencies for other indications is an attractive approach due to lower risks and costs in comparison to new developments.[726] In addition to the virostatic agents discussed above, other nucleoside analogs are currently in development. For example, USC-087, an *N*-alkyl tyrosinamide phosphonate ester prodrug of HPMPA (hydroxyphosphonylmethoxypropyl-adenine),[542] the adenine analog of cidofovir, was shown to be highly effective against multiple HAdV types in cell culture, and promising activity was also documented in a Syrian hamster model after oral administration. The compound was therefore deemed eligible as a candidate for further clinical development as an anti HAdV drug.[675] Furthermore, additional lipid ester derivatives were tested *in vitro* and showed anti-HAdV efficacy, particularly against the pneumotropic type B14.[375] Some other nucleoside analogs investigated *in vitro* include N4-derivatives of 6-azacytidine, which were shown to provide high anti-HAdV activity and low toxicity,[9] and filociclovir (cyclopropavir) displaying questionable activity against HAdVs.[91,227]

Besides different nucleoside analogs, a variety of unrelated compounds displaying anti-HAdV potential has been investigated. In a recent study, three salicylanilide-based anthelminthic drugs including niclosamide, rafoxanide, and oxyclozanide, were shown to display anti-HAdV activity at low concentrations and apparently low toxicity. The mechanism of action of the former two compounds is interference with the transport of HAdV particles from the endosome to the nuclear membrane, while the latter compound targets transcription of the E1A gene, and individual pairwise combinations of these agents displayed strong synergistic effects. Based on these observations, the compounds will be tested in Syrian hamster models of HAdV infection to further investigate their efficacy and safety.[448] Moreover, various salicylamide derivatives related to the lead compound niclosamide are potent inhibitors of HAdV infection, displaying differential activity at various stages of the infectious process, including virus entry, DNA replication, or postreplication steps.[734] The same group also showed that the synthetic steroid drug mifepristone (a progesterone and glucocorticoid receptor antagonist used for treatment of secondary hyperglycemia and for medical abortion during pregnancy) displays pronounced anti-HAdV activity *in vitro*, apparently by interfering with nuclear entry of the virus.[448] Piperazines are a broad class of chemical compounds containing a core piperazine functional group (a six-membered ring containing two nitrogen atoms at opposite positions), and different phenyl as well as urea/thiourea derivatives were shown to display anti-HAdV activity at low concentrations and with low cytotoxicity, thus displaying potential for further development as anti-HAdV drugs.[459,582]

The cardiotonic steroids, digoxin and digitoxin, which are used in clinical treatment of cardiac insufficiency, were demonstrated to display potent inhibitory effects against multiple HAdV species. The compounds alter the cascade of adenoviral gene expression, acting after initiation of early gene expression to block viral DNA replication and synthesis of viral structural proteins. Adenoviruses are dependent on the host RNA splicing machinery for alternative assembly of primary transcripts, and antiviral activity mediated by these steroids could be related to interference with this host cell function. However, the exact mechanism by which the compounds inhibit HAdV replication has yet to be fully characterized.[211]

Examples of other approaches to developing novel anti-HAdV treatment options include synthetic quinazoline–dione, pyrrole, and pyrrolopyrimidine compounds,[329,474] plant-derived compounds such as phenols from black tea or dioscin from air potato,[331,430] RNA interference-based methodologies,[278,279,356,529,586] or inhibition of protein kinases involved in the virus–host interaction, such as the cyclin-dependent protein kinase 7 (CDK7) inhibitor LDC4297 or the clinically approved CDK4/6 inhibitor palbociclib.[275,767] While the development of novel anti-HAdV compounds is a task of paramount importance, repurposing drugs that are well established in the clinical setting for other applications, such as nitazoxanide[162] and various agents indicated above, might represent an interesting alternative or complementary treatment modality for HAdV infections.

Immunotherapy

Measures supporting T-cell immunity play an important role in the armamentarium against invasive HAdV infections.[213,581,751] This is attributable to the current limitations of antiviral chemotherapy and the evidence that T-cell recovery, with reconstitution of HAdV-specific immune response, is essential for effective clearance of invasive infections in immunocompromised patients. The initial steps of antiviral treatment should therefore include tapering of immunosuppressive treatment, whenever possible.[245]

The proportion of HAdV-reactive T cells within the entire lymphocyte population of individuals who had been exposed to the virus is low. Administration of unselected donor lymphocyte infusion (DLI) can still provide antiviral immunity, but the potentially high frequency of alloreactive T cells and the ensuing side effects are a major impediment to this approach.[420,679] Alternative strategies might consider NK cell–based immunotherapy to abrogate T cell–mediated alloreactivity.[68,218,293,334,588,732] In order to greatly reduce or prevent alloreactivity, isolation of HAdV-specific T cells from peripheral blood of the original stem cell donor has been exploited for treatment of HAdV infections in allogeneic SCT recipients not responding to antiviral chemotherapy, and different approaches to the generation of such cells have been established. Regardless of the HAdV species the donor has been exposed to, the HAdV-reactive T cells are expected to be cross-reactive with all HAdV types because the hexon, the main constituent of the viral capsid, is the immunodominant T-cell target containing several epitopes conserved among adenoviruses.[398] One of the early successful attempts of adoptive T-cell transfer was based on the isolation of donor-derived mononuclear cells, their stimulation *ex vivo* with HAdV antigen, and magnetic separation of reactive T cells secreting IFNγ, which included both CD4+ and CD8+ T cells. The cells were infused without further *in vitro* expansion, and the results indicated that the efficacy of this treatment does not depend on the dose of infused cells, because even very low numbers of HAdV-specific donor-derived T cells expand easily *in vivo* in the presence of constant antigen challenge mediated by the viral infection.[173] The most critical parameter for the success of treatment was appropriate timing, that is, the early T-cell transfer upon detection of viremia.[173] These observations indicated that rapid availability of T cells for adoptive transfer by methods requiring only short or no *in vitro* expansion is important. Based on this notion, a number of different approaches to selection of HAdV-specific T cells have been introduced. The considerable variety of approaches includes, for example, different types of MHC multimers facilitating clinical-grade enrichment of HAdV-specific or multivirus-specific T cells displaying low or absent alloreactivity.[589,670] The MHC multimer technology requires knowledge of immunodominant HLA-restricted peptide epitopes and facilitates the isolation of antigen-specific CD8+ T cells (MHC class I multimers) or CD4+ T cells (MHC class II multimers) of high purity.[152] Short-term *in vitro* expansion under GMP (good manufacturing practice) conditions can render adoptive T-cell transfer available in less than 2 weeks.[83,195,681]

Adoptive transfer of HAdV-specific T cells has been used for more than a decade against invasive HAdV infections failing to respond to virostatic agents.[173,283,537,538,594,595] In view of the apparent importance of timely treatment onset for successful control of the infection,[173] different sources of access to appropriate immune cells have been investigated.

In addition to various approaches to isolating HAdV-specific T cells from the respective SCT donors,[171,173,194,195,508] other sources of virus-specific T cells including third party donors have emerged.[232,536,644,752] Allogeneic third party donors are a particularly important alternative option in cord blood recipients, in patients allografted from HAdV-seronegative donors, and in SOTs from cadaveric donors where donor blood is not available. Healthy seropositive individuals have been exploited to generate partially human leukocyte antigen (HLA)-matched virus-specific T cells for adoptive immunotherapy.[19,152] However, clinical implementation of this approach requires the availability of a large pool of HLA-typed healthy donors, and the use of incompletely HLA-matched T cells bears the risk of complications resulting from alloreactive side effects.[535] Despite the existing concerns, this approach appears to be feasible, and current clinical results are encouraging.[644] Another methodology pursued is the generation of virus-specific T-cell (VST) lines established from healthy donors with common HLA polymorphisms.[396,680] The employment of banked third-party-derived VSTs was demonstrated to represent an additional safe and readily applicable strategy for rapidly available treatment of severe viral infections in allogeneic SCT recipients,[396] thus further expanding the spectrum of clinical options for effective immunotherapy in immunocompromised patients. It is necessary to bear in mind, however, that the persistence of VSTs derived from peripheral blood is reportedly 14 to 90 days, thus potentially requiring multiple infusions.[501,680] By contrast, virus-specific T cells isolated from cord blood (CB) and expanded *ex vivo* showed long-term persistence after infusion and a decreased risk of GvHD owing to lower alloreactivity.[2,116] Moreover, CB-derived T cells have longer telomeres than do cells from adult donors, thus providing greater proliferative potential. This property coupled with extended *in vivo* persistence might obviate the need for multiple infusions.[116] Due to the large number of global inventories of frozen CB units, development of VST products derived from CB might be exploited as a novel platform for third-party antiviral T cells.[116] Owing to the fact that CB contains predominantly naïve T cells, the process of *ex vivo* VST generation currently takes approximately 1 month.[2] Since rapid availability of HAdV-specific T cells is apparently of great relevance, concepts providing off-the-shelf access to these cells certainly represent an attractive option.[116,221,310,680] However, in pediatric SCT recipients it was shown in a prospective study that the average time span between HAdV expansion in serial stool specimens above the critical threshold and the first appearance of adenoviremia was as long as 11 days[425] (Fig. 5.7). During this time span, it is also feasible to isolate and expand donor-derived HAdV-specific T cells to permit adoptive transfer before or upon the onset of viremia.[194] Alternatively, it may be conceivable, particularly in high-risk constellations, to generate virus-specific T cells already prior to allogeneic SCT, to ensure timely availability of targeted immune therapy. At the present time, due to the current limitations of treatment by virostatic agents, immune therapeutic approaches are an important asset in the armamentarium against HAdV infections in the immunocompromised setting. Adoptive transfer of HAdV-specific T cells is currently one of the most promising treatment approaches in high-risk patient populations,[455] which should ideally be performed in the context of clinical trials in specialized centers.

Vaccines

Outbreaks of HAdV infections, commonly caused by types E4 and B7 in closed or crowded environments such as military recruit camps, have led to fatal courses of pneumonia or myocarditis.[41,317,585] Such events have provided the basis for the establishment of vaccination programs for select HAdV types targeting specific high-risk cohorts of healthy individuals, with a focus on military personnel.[54] Vaccination programs in U.S. military trainees covering the most commonly occurring HAdV types E4 and B7 have been discontinued for more than a decade (see Clinical features-ARD in military recruits), and were resumed with a newly available FDA-approved live oral vaccine against these two HAdV types in 2011, to control the increased incidence of pulmonary infections during the cessation of vaccination. The vaccine comes as two tablets to be taken at the same time and is compatible with concomitant performance of other vaccinations. The viruses replicate once they reach the intestine, and the localized infection is usually asymptomatic, while mediating good systemic neutralizing antibody responses. Reintroduction of the vaccine resulted in a dramatic decline in HAdV disease burden within the first 2 to 3 years.[104,546] It is recommended by the Department of Defense in enlisted soldiers entering basic training but may also be encouraged in other military personnel at high risk for adenovirus infection.[463] The vaccine is reported to prevent illness caused by these two virus types with an efficacy of 99.3% (95% CI, 96.0 99.9; $p < 0.001$), and the virus isolation rates have fallen dramatically after reinitiation of the vaccination program.[100,251,378] Updates on the vaccine are available on the Web site of the Centers for Disease Control and Prevention (www.cdc.gov/vaccines). The vaccine has only been approved for use in military personnel. This restriction might be attributable to the fact that the vaccine contains live, apparently not attenuated, HAdV strains that can be excreted to the environment and lead to an increased risk of clinically symptomatic transmission, thereby limiting broad applicability in the general population.[93]

As outlined above in the sections Epidemiology and Clinical features, HAdV types other than E4 and B7 have also been associated with febrile ARD in the military, including the types B14 (B14p1), B21, and B55.[93,316] In fact, HAdV-B14 became more common in the US military after reintroduction of the vaccination program covering the types E4 and B7,[546] and the types B14 and B55 have reemerged as prevalent strains worldwide among both military recruits and civilians. There is thus considerable interest in developing innovative HAdV vaccines based, for example, on the use of inactived or replication-defective viruses applicable in the general population.[93] Recently, recombinant trivalent and tetravalent live vaccines directed against the HAdV types B3, B7, and B55 ± B14 were successfully tested in mouse models, where high titers of neutralizing antibodies and effective protection against these virus types could be documented.[432,666] Optimization of the candidate vaccines could, in future, help in preventing respiratory diseases caused by these HAdV types.

ADENOVIRUSES AS VECTORS FOR VACCINATION, GENE THERAPY, AND CANCER TREATMENT

Please see the ebook for this section.

PERSPECTIVES

The exploitation of AdV-based vectors for cancer therapy and vaccination will expectedly play an increasingly important role in the future, provided that ongoing studies reveal adequate efficacy and safety. With regard to the clinical management of HAdV infections, particularly in the immunocompromised setting, recent insights emanating from studies on intestinal HAdV persistence and the role of virus shedding into the stool can set the stage for improved diagnostic approaches. Consequently, optimized diagnostics will greatly affect the rational and timely onset of antiviral treatment, which was shown to be a prerequisite for successful therapy facilitating improved control of adenoviral infections. The encouraging data provided by studies testing brincidofovir in SCT recipients with adenoviremia are hampered by the fact that the producer has terminated clinical development of the drug, because the stringent requirements for clinical approval have not been met by the data available to date. Currently, the drug is still available on the basis of compassionate use, but the long-term supply is more than questionable. Due to the urgent need for effective treatment of HAdV infections in immunocompromised patients, loss of this therapeutic option in the future would have a negative impact on the ability to successfully control life-threatening infections by adenoviruses. This unexpected circumstance should stimulate experimental research directed towards the development of novel antiviral agents and/or towards repurposing compounds approved for other applications to expand the anti-HAdV treatment options. Combined and dose-adapted therapies will possibly improve the efficacy of treatment and reduce the toxicity of some commonly prescribed virostatic drugs. Detailed understanding of the mechanisms mediating HAdV reactivation and the transition from persistent to lytic infection during immunosuppression might provide the basis for rationally designed innovative therapeutic strategies.

If the safety, efficacy, and feasibility of HAdV-specific or multivirus-specific T-cell transfer can be firmly established, it is reasonable to envision that this treatment will be successfully employed not only in the settings of preemptive and symptomatic therapy but also as prophylaxis in high-risk patients to prevent severe viral diseases. The establishment of allogeneic T-cell donor registries of HLA-typed healthy donors tested for the presence of virus-specific T cells could serve as a rapidly available source for adoptive immunotherapy in immunocompromised patients lacking a suitable T-cell donor. Such T-cell donor registries might provide readily available off-the-shelf products facilitating rapid initiation of immunotherapy in patients carrying a high risk of life-threatening viral infections. Broad availability of banked third-party virus-specific T cells and/or virus-specific T-cell lines could mark the beginning of a new era in combating the threats of viral infections in immunocompromised patients in the foreseeable future. Finally, the omics revolution has advanced our knowledge about the

HAdV and host-cell interplay at the RNA and protein levels, and novel insights gained from this research will expectedly lay the grounds for additional innovative treatment options.[765]

REFERENCES

1. Abinun M, Flood TJ, Cant AJ, et al. Autologous T cell depleted haematopoietic stem cell transplantation in children with severe juvenile idiopathic arthritis in the UK (2000-2007). *Mol Immunol* 2009;47:46–51.
2. Abraham AA, John TD, Keller MD, et al. Safety and feasibility of virus-specific T cells derived from umbilical cord blood in cord blood transplant recipients. *Blood Adv* 2019;3:2057–2068.
3. Adeyemi OA, Yeldandi AV, Ison MG. Fatal adenovirus pneumonia in a person with AIDS and Burkitt lymphoma: a case report and review of the literature. *AIDS Read* 2008;18:196–198, 201–202, 206–207.
4. Afrad MH, Avzun T, Haque J, et al. Detection of enteric- and non-enteric adenoviruses in gastroenteritis patients, Bangladesh, 2012-2015. *J Med Virol* 2018;90:677–684.
5. Ahmed W, Hamilton KA, Lobos A, et al. Quantitative microbial risk assessment of microbial source tracking markers in recreational water contaminated with fresh untreated and secondary treated sewage. *Environ Int* 2018;117:243–249.
6. Aitken SL, Zhou J, Ghantoji SS, et al. Pharmacokinetics and safety of intravesicular cidofovir in allogeneic HSCT recipients. *J Antimicrob Chemother* 2016;71:727–730.
7. Akheruzzaman M, Hegde V, Dhurandhar NV. Twenty-five years of research about adipogenic adenoviruses: a systematic review. *Obes Rev* 2019;20:499–509.
8. Aldhoon-Hainerova I, Zamrazilova H, Atkinson RL, et al. Clinical and laboratory characteristics of 1179 Czech adolescents evaluated for antibodies to human adenovirus 36. *Int J Obes (Lond)* 2014;38:285–291.
9. Alexeeva I, Nosach L, Palchykovska L, et al. Synthesis and comparative study of anti-adenoviral activity of 6-azacytidine and its analogues. *Nucleosides Nucleotides Nucleic Acids* 2015;34:565–578.
10. Alharbi S, Van Caeseele P, Consunji-Araneta R, et al. Epidemiology of severe pediatric adenovirus lower respiratory tract infections in Manitoba, Canada, 1991-2005. *BMC Infect Dis* 2012;12:55.
11. Al-Herz W, Moussa MA. Survival and predictors of death among primary immunodeficient patients: a registry-based study. *J Clin Immunol* 2012;32:467–473.
12. Ali S, Krueger J, Richardson SE, et al. The yield of monitoring adenovirus in pediatric hematopoietic stem cell transplant patients. *Pediatr Hematol Oncol* 2019;36:161–172.
13. Alkhalaf MA, Guiver M, Cooper RJ. Genome stability of adenovirus types 3 and 7 during a simultaneous outbreak in Greater Manchester, UK. *J Med Virol* 2015;87:117–124.
14. Ampuero JS, Ocana V, Gomez J, et al. Adenovirus respiratory tract infections in Peru. *PLoS One* 2012;7:e46898.
15. Anderson BD, Barr KL, Heil GL, et al. A comparison of viral fitness and virulence between emergent adenovirus 14p1 and prototype adenovirus 14p strains. *J Clin Virol* 2012;54:265–268.
16. Anderson EJ, Guzman-Cottrill JA, Kletzel M, et al. High-risk adenovirus-infected pediatric allogeneic hematopoietic progenitor cell transplant recipients and preemptive cidofovir therapy. *Pediatr Transplant* 2008;12:219–227.
17. Andreoletti L, Leveque N, Boulagnon C, et al. Viral causes of human myocarditis. *Arch Cardiovasc Dis* 2009;102:559–568.
18. Aoki K, Benko M, Davison AJ, et al. Toward an integrated human adenovirus designation system that utilizes molecular and serological data and serves both clinical and fundamental virology. *J Virol* 2011;85:5703–5704.
19. Arasaratnam RJ, Leen AM. Adoptive T cell therapy for the treatment of viral infections. *Ann Transl Med* 2015;3:278.
20. Arashkia A, Bahrami F, Farsi M, et al. Molecular analysis of human adenoviruses in hospitalized children <5 years old with acute gastroenteritis in Tehran, Iran. *J Med Virol* 2019;91:1930–1936.
21. Arechavaleta-Velasco F, Ma Y, Zhang J, et al. Adeno-associated virus-2 (AAV-2) causes trophoblast dysfunction, and placental AAV-2 infection is associated with preeclampsia. *Am J Pathol* 2006;168:1951–1959.
22. Aste-Amezaga M, Bett AJ, Wang F, et al. Quantitative adenovirus neutralization assays based on the secreted alkaline phosphatase reporter gene: application in epidemiologic studies and in the design of adenovector vaccines. *Hum Gene Ther* 2004;15:293–304.
23. Atasheva S, Shayakhmetov DM. Adenovirus sensing by the immune system. *Curr Opin Virol* 2016;21:109–113.
24. Atasheva S, Yao J, Shayakhmetov DM. Innate immunity to adenovirus: lessons from mice. *FEBS Lett* 2019;593:3461–3483.
25. Atkinson RL. A personal look at the past and future of obesity science. *Eur J Clin Nutr* 2020;74(2):215–219.
26. Averbuch D, Safadi R, Dar D, et al. Successful brincidofovir treatment of metagenomics-detected adenovirus infection in a severely Ill signal transducer and activator of transcription-1-deficient patient. *Pediatr Infect Dis J* 2019;38:297–299.
27. Avivi I, Chakrabarti S, Milligan DW, et al. Incidence and outcome of adenovirus disease in transplant recipients after reduced-intensity conditioning with alemtuzumab. *Biol Blood Marrow Transplant* 2004;10:186–194.
28. Baker AT, Mundy RM, Davies JA, et al. Human adenovirus type 26 uses sialic acid-bearing glycans as a primary cell entry receptor. *Sci Adv* 2019;5:eaax3567.
29. Banerjee A, De P, Manna B, et al. Molecular characterization of enteric adenovirus genotypes 40 and 41 identified in children with acute gastroenteritis in Kolkata, India during 2013-2014. *J Med Virol* 2017;89:606–614.
30. Baranowski T, Motil KJ, Moreno JP. Multi-etiological perspective on child obesity prevention. *Curr Nutr Rep* 2019;8:1–10.
31. Barnadas C, Schmidt DJ, Fischer TK, et al. Molecular epidemiology of human adenovirus infections in Denmark, 2011-2016. *J Clin Virol* 2018;104:16–22.
32. Barouch DH, Kik SV, Weverling GJ, et al. International seroepidemiology of adenovirus serotypes 5, 26, 35, and 48 in pediatric and adult populations. *Vaccine* 2011;29:5203–5209.
33. Barrero PR, Valinotto LE, Tittarelli E, et al. Molecular typing of adenoviruses in pediatric respiratory infections in Buenos Aires, Argentina (1999-2010). *J Clin Virol* 2012;53:145–150.
34. Barry MA, Weaver EA, Chen CY. Mining the adenovirus "virome" for systemic oncolytics. *Curr Pharm Biotechnol* 2012;13:1804–1808.
35. Baschat AA, Towbin J, Bowles NE, et al. Is adenovirus a fetal pathogen? *Am J Obstet Gynecol* 2003;189:758–763.
36. Bautista-Gogel J, Madsen CM, Lu X, et al. Outbreak of respiratory illness associated with human adenovirus type 7 among persons attending Officer Candidates School, Quantico, Virginia, 2017. *J Infect Dis* 2020;221(5):697–700.
37. Becker B, Henningsen L, Paulmann D, et al. Evaluation of the virucidal efficacy of disinfectant wipes with a test method simulating practical conditions. *Antimicrob Resist Infect Control* 2019;8:121.
38. Bejiqi R, Retkoceri R, Maloku A, et al. The diagnostic and clinical approach to pediatric myocarditis: a review of the current literature. *Open Access Maced J Med Sci* 2019;7:162–173.
39. Benko M, Harrach B, Both GW, et al. Family adenoviridae. In: Fauquet CM, Mayo MA, Maniloff J, et al., eds. *Virus Taxonomy.* San Diego, CA: Elsevier Academic Press; 2005:213–228.
40. Berciaud S, Rayne F, Kassab S, et al. Adenovirus infections in Bordeaux University Hospital 2008-2010: clinical and virological features. *J Clin Virol* 2012;54:302–307.
41. Binder AM, Biggs HM, Haynes AK, et al. Human adenovirus surveillance—United States, 2003-2016. *MMWR Morb Mortal Wkly Rep* 2017;66:1039–1042.
42. Birger R, Morita H, Comito D, et al. Asymptomatic shedding of respiratory virus among an ambulatory population across seasons. *mSphere* 2018;33(6):e00667–18.
43. Black RE, Cousens S, Johnson HL, et al. Global, regional, and national causes of child mortality in 2008: a systematic analysis. *Lancet* 2010;375:1969–1987.
44. Blackford AN, Grand RJ. Adenovirus E1B 55-kilodalton protein: multiple roles in viral infection and cell transformation. *J Virol* 2009;83:4000–4012.
45. Boge CLK, Fisher BT, Petersen H, et al. Outcomes of human adenovirus infection and disease in a retrospective cohort of pediatric solid organ transplant recipients. *Pediatr Transplant* 2019;23(6):e13510.
46. Bonadonna L, La Rosa G. A review and update on waterborne viral diseases associated with swimming pools. *Int J Environ Res Public Health* 2019;16(2):166.
47. Borkenhagen LK, Fieldhouse JK, Seto D, et al. Are adenoviruses zoonotic? A systematic review of the evidence. *Emerg Microbes Infect* 2019;8:1679–1687.
48. Bortolanza S, Bunuales M, Otano I, et al. Treatment of pancreatic cancer with an oncolytic adenovirus expressing interleukin-12 in Syrian hamsters. *Mol Ther* 2009;17:614–622.
49. Bouziat R, Hinterleitner R, Brown JJ, et al. Reovirus infection triggers inflammatory responses to dietary antigens and development of celiac disease. *Science* 2017;356:44–50.
50. Bowles NE, Ni J, Kearney DL, et al. Detection of viruses in myocardial tissues by polymerase chain reaction. evidence of adenovirus as a common cause of myocarditis in children and adults. *J Am Coll Cardiol* 2003;42:466–472.
51. Bradshaw AC, Parker AL, Duffy MR, et al. Requirements for receptor engagement during infection by adenovirus complexed with blood coagulation factor X. *PLoS Pathog* 2010;6:e1001142.
52. Breuer S, Rauch M, Matthes-Martin S, et al. Molecular diagnosis and management of viral infections in hematopoietic stem cell transplant recipients. *Mol Diagn Ther* 2012;16:63–77.
53. Brixner V, Kiessling AH, Madlener K, et al. Red blood cells treated with the amustaline (S-303) pathogen reduction system: a transfusion study in cardiac surgery. *Transfusion* 2018;58:905–916.
54. Broderick M, Myers C, Balansay M, et al. Adenovirus 4/7 vaccine's effect on disease rates is associated with disappearance of adenovirus on building surfaces at a military recruit base. *Mil Med* 2017;182:e2069–e2072.
55. Brown JR, Shah D, Breuer J. Viral gastrointestinal infections and norovirus genotypes in a paediatric UK hospital, 2014-2015. *J Clin Virol* 2016;84:1–6.
56. Bruminhent J, Apiwattanakul N, Hongeng S, et al. Absolute lymphocyte count and human adenovirus-specific T-cell immune restoration of human adenovirus infection after kidney transplantation. *J Med Virol* 2019;91:1432–1439.
57. Bruminhent J, Athas DM, Hess BD, et al. Disseminated adenovirus disease in heart transplant recipient presenting with conjunctivitis. *Transpl Infect Dis* 2015;17:125–128.
58. Bruno B, Gooley T, Hackman RC, et al. Adenovirus infection in hematopoietic stem cell transplantation: effect of ganciclovir and impact on survival. *Biol Blood Marrow Transplant* 2003;9:341–352.
59. Bunuales M, Garcia-Aragoncillo E, Casado R, et al. Evaluation of monocytes as carriers for armed oncolytic adenoviruses in murine and Syrian hamster models of cancer. *Hum Gene Ther* 2012;23:1258–1268.
60. Burnett E, Kabir F, Van Trang N, et al. Infectious etiologies of intussusception among children <2 years old in 4 Asian countries. *J Infect Dis* 2020;221(9):1499–1505.
61. Calcedo R, Vandenberghe LH, Roy S, et al. Host immune responses to chronic adenovirus infections in human and nonhuman primates. *J Virol* 2009;83:2623–2631.
62. Calkavur S, Olukman O, Ozturk AT, et al. Epidemic adenoviral keratoconjunctivitis possibly related to ophthalmological procedures in a neonatal intensive care unit: lessons from an outbreak. *Ophthalmic Epidemiol* 2012;19:371–379.
63. Callahan SM, Wonganan P, Obenauer-Kutner LJ, et al. Controlled inactivation of recombinant viruses with vitamin B2. *J Virol Methods* 2008;148:132–145.
64. Calvo C, Garcia-Garcia ML, Sanchez-Dehesa R, et al. Eight year prospective study of adenoviruses infections in hospitalized children. Comparison with other respiratory viruses. *PLoS One* 2015;10:e0132162.
65. Camargo JF, Morris MI, Abbo LM, et al. The use of brincidofovir for the treatment of mixed dsDNA viral infection. *J Clin Virol* 2016;83:1–4.
66. Camargo PR, Okay TS, Yamamoto L, et al. Myocarditis in children and detection of viruses in myocardial tissue: implications for immunosuppressive therapy. *Int J Cardiol* 2011;148:204–208.

67. Cancelas JA, Gottschall JL, Rugg N, et al. Red blood cell concentrates treated with the amustaline (S-303) pathogen reduction system and stored for 35 days retain post-transfusion viability: results of a two-centre study. *Vox Sang* 2017;112:210–218.
68. Cardoso Alves L, Berger MD, Koutsandreas T, et al. Non-apoptotic TRAIL function modulates NK cell activity during viral infection. *EMBO Rep* 2020;21:e48789.
69. Carlin CR. New insights to adenovirus-directed innate immunity in respiratory epithelial cells. *Microorganisms* 2019;7(8):216.
70. Carr MJ, Kajon AE, Lu X, et al. Deaths associated with human adenovirus-14p1 infections, Europe, 2009-2010. *Emerg Infect Dis* 2011;17:1402–1408.
71. Caruso Brown AE, Cohen MN, Tong S, et al. Pharmacokinetics and safety of intravenous cidofovir for life-threatening viral infections in pediatric hematopoietic stem cell transplant recipients. *Antimicrob Agents Chemother* 2015;59:3718–3725.
72. Cavalli G, Foppoli M, Cabrini L, et al. Interleukin-1 receptor blockade rescues myocarditis-associated end-stage heart failure. *Front Immunol* 2017;8:131.
73. Cavalli G, Pappalardo F, Mangieri A, et al. Treating life-threatening myocarditis by blocking interleukin-1. *Crit Care Med* 2016;44:e751–e754.
74. Cederwall S, Pahlman LI. Respiratory adenovirus infections in immunocompetent and immunocompromised adult patients. *Epidemiol Infect* 2020;147:e328.
75. Centers for Disease Control and Prevention. Acute respiratory disease associated with adenovirus serotype 14—four states, 2006-2007. *MMWR Morb Mortal Wkly Rep* 2007;56: 1181–1184.
76. Centers for Disease Control and Prevention. Outbreak of adenovirus 14 respiratory illness—Prince of Wales Island, Alaska, 2008. *MMWR Morb Mortal Wkly Rep* 2010;59:6–10.
77. Centers for Disease Control and Prevention. Adenovirus-associated epidemic keratoconjunctivitis outbreaks—four states, 2008-2010. *MMWR Morb Mortal Wkly Rep* 2013;62: 637–641.
78. Cesar Pereira Santos H, Nunes Vieira Almeida T, Souza Fiaccadori F, et al. Adenovirus infection among allogeneic stem cell transplant recipients. *J Med Virol* 2017;89:298–303.
79. Cha MJ, Chung MJ, Lee KS, et al. Clinical features and radiological findings of adenovirus pneumonia associated with progression to acute respiratory distress syndrome: a Single Center Study in 19 adult patients. *Korean J Radiol* 2016;17:940–949.
80. Chahal JS, Gallagher C, DeHart CJ, et al. The repression domain of the E1B 55-kilodalton protein participates in countering interferon-induced inhibition of adenovirus replication. *J Virol* 2013;87:4432–4444.
81. Chahar HS, Bao X, Casola A. Exosomes and their role in the life cycle and pathogenesis of RNA viruses. *Viruses* 2015;7:3204–3225.
82. Chaimongkol N, Khamrin P, Suantai B, et al. A wide variety of diarrhea viruses circulating in pediatric patients in Thailand. *Clin Lab* 2012;58:117–123.
83. Chakupurakal G, Onion D, Bonney S, et al. HLA-peptide multimer selection of adenovirus-specific T cells for adoptive T-cell therapy. *J Immunother* 2013;36:423–431.
84. Chakupurakal G, Onion D, Cobbold M, et al. Adenovirus vector-specific T cells demonstrate a unique memory phenotype with high proliferative potential and coexpression of CCR5 and integrin alpha4beta7. *AIDS* 2010;24:205–210.
85. Chamberlain JM, Sortino K, Sethna P, et al. Cidofovir diphosphate inhibits adenovirus 5 DNA polymerase via both nonobligate chain termination and direct inhibition, and polymerase mutations confer cidofovir resistance on intact virus. *Antimicrob Agents Chemother* 2019;63(1):e01925-18.
86. Chandra N, Frangsmyr L, Arnberg N. Decoy receptor interactions as novel drug targets against EKC-causing human adenovirus. *Viruses* 2019;11(3):242.
87. Chandra N, Frangsmyr L, Imhof S, et al. Sialic acid-containing glycans as cellular receptors for ocular human adenoviruses: implications for tropism and treatment. *Viruses* 2019;11:(5):395.
88. Chandra N, Liu Y, Liu JX, et al. Sulfated glycosaminoglycans as viral decoy receptors for human adenovirus type 37. *Viruses* 2019;11(3):247.
89. Chang SY, Lee CN, Lin PH, et al. A community-derived outbreak of adenovirus type 3 in children in Taiwan between 2004 and 2005. *J Med Virol* 2008;80:102–112.
90. Chehadeh W, Al-Adwani A, John SE, et al. Adenovirus types associated with severe respiratory diseases: a retrospective 4-year study in Kuwait. *J Med Virol* 2018;90:1033–1039.
91. Chemaly RF, Hill JA, Voigt S, et al. In vitro comparison of currently available and investigational antiviral agents against pathogenic human double-stranded DNA viruses: a systematic literature review. *Antiviral Res* 2019;163:50–58.
92. Chen SP, Huang YC, Chiu CH, et al. Clinical features of radiologically confirmed pneumonia due to adenovirus in children. *J Clin Virol* 2013;56:7–12.
93. Chen S, Tian X. Vaccine development for human mastadenovirus. *J Thorac Dis* 2018;10:S2280–S2294.
94. Chen H, Xiang ZQ, Li Y, et al. Adenovirus-based vaccines: comparison of vectors from three species of adenoviridae. *J Virol* 2010;84:10522–10532.
95. Chen EC, Yagi S, Kelly KR, et al. Cross-species transmission of a novel adenovirus associated with a fulminant pneumonia outbreak in a new world monkey colony. *PLoS Pathog* 2011;7:e1002155.
96. Cheng C, Gall JG, Nason M, et al. Differential specificity and immunogenicity of adenovirus type 5 neutralizing antibodies elicited by natural infection or immunization. *J Virol* 2010;84:630–638.
97. Chhabra P, Payne DC, Szilagyi PG, et al. Etiology of viral gastroenteritis in children <5 years of age in the United States, 2008-2009. *J Infect Dis* 2013;208:790–800.
98. Chigbu DI, Labib BA. Pathogenesis and management of adenoviral keratoconjunctivitis. *Infect Drug Resist* 2018;11:981–993.
99. Chiu CY, Yagi S, Lu X, et al. A novel adenovirus species associated with an acute respiratory outbreak in a baboon colony and evidence of coincident human infection. *MBio* 2013;4:e00084.
100. Choudhry A, Mathena J, Albano JD, et al. Safety evaluation of adenovirus type 4 and type 7 vaccine live, oral in military recruits. *Vaccine* 2016;34:4558–4564.
101. Cinal A. Randomized, controlled, phase 2 trial of povidone-iodine/dexamethasone ophthalmic suspension for treatment of adenoviral conjunctivitis. *Am J Ophthalmol* 2019;197:184.
102. Clark NM, Lynch JP III, Sayah D, et al. DNA viral infections complicating lung transplantation. *Semin Respir Crit Care Med* 2013;34:380–404.
103. Clement C, Capriotti JA, Kumar M, et al. Clinical and antiviral efficacy of an ophthalmic formulation of dexamethasone povidone-iodine in a rabbit model of adenoviral keratoconjunctivitis. *Invest Ophthalmol Vis Sci* 2011;52:339–344.
104. Clemmons NS, McCormic ZD, Gaydos JC, et al. Acute respiratory disease in US army trainees 3 years after reintroduction of adenovirus vaccine (1). *Emerg Infect Dis* 2017;23:95–98.
105. Colak M, Bozdayi G, Altay A, et al. Detection and molecular characterisation of adenovirus in children under 5 years old with diarrhoea. *Turk J Med Sci* 2017;47:1463–1471.
106. Coll RC. Role reversal: adaptive immunity instructs inflammasome activation for anti-viral defence. *EMBO J* 2019;38:e103533.
107. Cook J, Radke J. Mechanisms of pathogenesis of emerging adenoviruses. *F1000Res* 2017;6:90.
108. Corcoran MS, van Well GT, van Loo IH. Diagnosis of viral gastroenteritis in children: interpretation of real-time PCR results and relation to clinical symptoms. *Eur J Clin Microbiol Infect Dis* 2014;33:1663–1673.
109. Couturier MR, Barney T, Alger G, et al. Evaluation of the FilmArray® Respiratory Panel for clinical use in a large children's hospital. *J Clin Lab Anal* 2013;27:148–154.
110. Crenshaw BJ, Gu L, Sims B, et al. Exosome biogenesis and biological function in response to viral infections. *Open Virol J* 2018;12:134–148.
111. Crenshaw BJ, Jones LB, Bell CR, et al. Perspective on adenoviruses: epidemiology, pathogenicity, and gene therapy. *Biomedicines* 2019;7(3):61.
112. Cundy KC. Clinical pharmacokinetics of the antiviral nucleotide analogues cidofovir and adefovir. *Clin Pharmacokinet* 1999;36:127–143.
113. Curlin ME, Huang ML, Lu X, et al. Frequent detection of human adenovirus from the lower gastrointestinal tract in men who have sex with men. *PLoS One* 2010;5:e11321.
114. Dailey Garnes NJM, Ragoonanan D, Aboulhosn A. Adenovirus infection and disease in recipients of hematopoietic cell transplantation. *Curr Opin Infect Dis* 2019;32:591–600.
115. Darr S, Madisch I, Heim A. Antiviral activity of cidofovir and ribavirin against the new human adenovirus subtype 14a that is associated with severe pneumonia. *Clin Infect Dis* 2008;47:731–732.
116. Dave H, Luo M, Blaney JW, et al. Toward a rapid production of multivirus-specific T cells targeting BKV, adenovirus, CMV, and EBV from umbilical cord blood. *Mol Ther Methods Clin Dev* 2017;5:13–21.
117. Davison AJ, Benko M, Harrach B. Genetic content and evolution of adenoviruses. *J Gen Virol* 2003;84:2895–2908.
118. De Clercq E. The clinical potential of the acyclic (and cyclic) nucleoside phosphonates: the magic of the phosphonate bond. *Biochem Pharmacol* 2011;82:99–109.
119. De Clercq E, Li G. Approved antiviral drugs over the past 50 years. *Clin Microbiol Rev* 2016;29:695–747.
120. De Mezerville MH, Tellier R, Richardson S, et al. Adenoviral infections in pediatric transplant recipients: a hospital-based study. *Pediatr Infect Dis J* 2006;25:815–818.
121. De Ory F, Avellon A, Echevarria JE, et al. Viral infections of the central nervous system in Spain: a prospective study. *J Med Virol* 2013;85:554–562.
122. De Pagter AP, Haveman LM, Schuurman R, et al. Adenovirus DNA positivity in nasopharyngeal aspirate preceding hematopoietic stem cell transplantation: a very strong risk factor for adenovirus DNAemia in pediatric patients. *Clin Infect Dis* 2009;49: 1536–1539.
123. Dehghan S, Seto J, Liu EB, et al. Computational analysis of four human adenovirus type 4 genomes reveals molecular evolution through two interspecies recombination events. *Virology* 2013;443:197–207.
124. Dehghan S, Seto J, Liu EB, et al. A zoonotic adenoviral human pathogen emerged through genomic recombination among human and nonhuman simian hosts. *J Virol* 2019;93(18):e00564-19.
125. Dennert R, Crijns HJ, Heymans S. Acute viral myocarditis. *Eur Heart J* 2008;29:2073–2082.
126. Detweiler CJ, Mueller SB, Sung AD, et al. Brincidofovir (CMX001) toxicity associated with epithelial apoptosis and crypt drop out in a hematopoietic cell transplant patient: challenges in distinguishing drug toxicity from GVHD. *J Pediatr Hematol Oncol* 2018;40:e364–e368.
127. Dey SK, Hoq I, Okitsu S, et al. Prevalence, seasonality, and peak age of infection of enteric adenoviruses in Japan, 1995-2009. *Epidemiol Infect* 2013;141:958–960.
128. Dey SK, Shimizu H, Phan TG, et al. Molecular epidemiology of adenovirus infection among infants and children with acute gastroenteritis in Dhaka City, Bangladesh. *Infect Genet Evol* 2009;9:518–522.
129. Dhar D, Spencer JF, Toth K, et al. Effect of preexisting immunity on oncolytic adenovirus vector INGN 007 antitumor efficacy in immunocompetent and immunosuppressed Syrian hamsters. *J Virol* 2009;83:2130–2139.
130. Dhar D, Spencer JF, Toth K, et al. Pre-existing immunity and passive immunity to adenovirus 5 prevents toxicity caused by an oncolytic adenovirus vector in the Syrian hamster model. *Mol Ther* 2009;17:1724–1732.
131. Dhar D, Toth K, Wold WS. Syrian hamster tumor model to study oncolytic Ad5-based vectors. *Methods Mol Biol* 2012;797:53–63.
132. Dhar D, Toth K, Wold WS. Cycles of transient high-dose cyclophosphamide administration and intratumoral oncolytic adenovirus vector injection for long-term tumor suppression in Syrian hamsters. *Cancer Gene Ther* 2014;21:171–178.
133. Dhingra A, Hage E, Ganzenmueller T, et al. Molecular evolution of human adenovirus (HAdV) species C. *Sci Rep* 2019;9:1039.
134. Dhurandhar NV. Infections and body weight: an emerging relationship? *Int J Obes Relat Metab Disord* 2002;26:745–746.
135. Diaconu I, Cerullo V, Escutenaire S, et al. Human adenovirus replication in immunocompetent Syrian hamsters can be attenuated with chlorpromazine or cidofovir. *J Gene Med* 2010;12:435–445.
136. Diaconu I, Cerullo V, Hirvinen ML, et al. Immune response is an important aspect of the antitumor effect produced by a CD40L-encoding oncolytic adenovirus. *Cancer Res* 2012;72:2327–2338.
137. Dicks MD, Spencer AJ, Edwards NJ, et al. A novel chimpanzee adenovirus vector with low human seroprevalence: improved systems for vector derivation and comparative immunogenicity. *PLoS One* 2012;7:e40385.

138. Ding N, Craik SA, Pang X, et al. Assessing UV inactivation of adenovirus 41 using integrated cell culture real-time qPCR/RT-qPCR. *Water Environ Res* 2017;89:323–329.
139. Dobner J, Kaser S. Body mass index and the risk of infection—from underweight to obesity. *Clin Microbiol Infect* 2018;24:24–28.
140. Doerfler W. Epigenetic consequences of genome manipulations: caveats for human germline therapy and genetically modified organisms. *Epigenomics* 2019;11:247–250.
141. Doerfler W, Weber S, Naumann A. Inheritable epigenetic response towards foreign DNA entry by mammalian host cells: a guardian of genomic stability. *Epigenetics* 2018;13:1141–1153.
142. Druce MR, Wren AM, Park AJ, et al. Ghrelin increases food intake in obese as well as lean subjects. *Int J Obes (Lond)* 2005;29:1130–1136.
143. Dubberke ER, Tu B, Rivet DJ, et al. Acute meningoencephalitis caused by adenovirus serotype 26. *J Neurovirol* 2006;12:235–240.
144. Dudareva M, Andrews L, Gilbert SC, et al. Prevalence of serum neutralizing antibodies against chimpanzee adenovirus 63 and human adenovirus 5 in Kenyan children, in the context of vaccine vector efficacy. *Vaccine* 2009;27:3501–3504.
145. Duffy MR, Doszpoly A, Turner G, et al. The relevance of coagulation factor X protection of adenoviruses in human sera. *Gene Ther* 2016;23:592–596.
146. Dzananovic E, Astha, Chojnowski G, et al. Impact of the structural integrity of the three-way junction of adenovirus VAI RNA on PKR inhibition. *PLoS One* 2017;12:e0186849.
147. Ebner K, Rauch M, Preuner S, et al. Typing of human adenoviruses in specimens from immunosuppressed patients by PCR-fragment length analysis and real-time quantitative PCR. *J Clin Microbiol* 2006;44:2808–2815.
148. Ebner K, Suda M, Watzinger F, et al. Molecular detection and quantitative analysis of the entire spectrum of human adenoviruses by a two-reaction real-time PCR assay. *J Clin Microbiol* 2005;43:3049–3053.
149. Echavarria M. Adenoviruses in immunocompromised hosts. *Clin Microbiol Rev* 2008;21: 704–715.
150. Echavarria M, Forman M, van Tol MJ, et al. Prediction of severe disseminated adenovirus infection by serum PCR. *Lancet* 2001;358:384–385.
151. Echavarria M, Maldonado D, Elbert G, et al. Use of PCR to demonstrate presence of adenovirus species B, C, or F as well as coinfection with two adenovirus species in children with flu-like symptoms. *J Clin Microbiol* 2006;44:625–627.
152. Eiz-Vesper B, Maecker-Kolhoff B, Blasczyk R. Adoptive T-cell immunotherapy from third-party donors: characterization of donors and set up of a T-cell donor registry. *Front Immunol* 2012;3:410.
153. Elmahdy MEI, Magri ME, Garcia LA, et al. Microcosm environment models for studying the stability of adenovirus and murine norovirus in water and sediment. *Int J Hyg Environ Health* 2018;221:734–741.
154. Endter C, Dobner T. Cell transformation by human adenoviruses. *Curr Top Microbiol Immunol* 2004;273:163–214.
155. Engelmann G, Heim A, Greil J, et al. Adenovirus infection and treatment with cidofovir in children after liver transplantation. *Pediatr Transplant* 2009;13:421–428.
156. Engen RM, Huang ML, Park GE, et al. Prospective assessment of adenovirus infection in pediatric kidney transplant recipients. *Transplantation* 2018;102:1165–1171.
157. Erard V, Huang ML, Ferrenberg J, et al. Quantitative real-time polymerase chain reaction for detection of adenovirus after T cell-replete hematopoietic cell transplantation: viral load as a marker for invasive disease. *Clin Infect Dis* 2007;45:958–965.
158. Ersching J, Hernandez MI, Cezarotto FS, et al. Neutralizing antibodies to human and simian adenoviruses in humans and New-World monkeys. *Virology* 2010;407:1–6.
159. Esposito DH, Gardner TJ, Schneider E, et al. Outbreak of pneumonia associated with emergent human adenovirus serotype 14—Southeast Alaska, 2008. *J Infect Dis* 2010;202: 214–222.
160. Esposito S, Preti V, Consolo S, et al. Adenovirus 36 infection and obesity. *J Clin Virol* 2012;55:95–100.
161. Esposito S, Zampiero A, Bianchini S, et al. Epidemiology and clinical characteristics of respiratory infections due to adenovirus in children living in Milan, Italy, during 2013 and 2014. *PLoS One* 2016;11:e0152375.
162. Esquer Garrigos Z, Barth D, Hamdi AM, et al. Nitazoxanide is a therapeutic option for adenovirus-related enteritis in immunocompromised adults. *Antimicrob Agents Chemother* 2018;62:e01937-18.
163. Excoffon KJ, Bowers JR, Sharma P. 1. Alternative splicing of viral receptors: a review of the diverse morphologies and physiologies of adenoviral receptors. *Recent Res Dev Virol* 2014;9:1–24.
164. Farkas K, Cooper DM, McDonald JE, et al. Seasonal and spatial dynamics of enteric viruses in wastewater and in riverine and estuarine receiving waters. *Sci Total Environ* 2018;634:1174–1183.
165. Farooqi IS, Wangensteen T, Collins S, et al. Clinical and molecular genetic spectrum of congenital deficiency of the leptin receptor. *N Engl J Med* 2007;356:237–247.
166. Fedaoui N, Ayed NB, Yahia AB, et al. Genetic variability of human adenovirus type 8 causing epidemic and sporadic cases of keratoconjunctivitis. *Arch Virol* 2016;161:1469–1476.
167. Feghoul L, Chevret S, Cuinet A, et al. Adenovirus infection and disease in paediatric haematopoietic stem cell transplant patients: clues for antiviral pre-emptive treatment. *Clin Microbiol Infect* 2015;21:701–709.
168. Feghoul L, Mercier-Delarue S, Salmona M, et al. Genetic diversity of the human adenovirus species C DNA polymerase. *Antiviral Res* 2018;156:1–9.
169. Feizy Z, Peddibhotla S, Khan S, et al. Nanoparticle-mediated in vitro delivery of E4orf1 to preadipocytes is a clinically relevant delivery system to improve glucose uptake. *Int J Obes (Lond)* 2020;44(7):1607–1616.
170. Feng Y, Sun X, Ye X, et al. Hexon and fiber of adenovirus type 14 and 55 are major targets of neutralizing antibody but only fiber-specific antibody contributes to cross-neutralizing activity. *Virology* 2018;518:272–283.
171. Feucht J, Opherk K, Lang P, et al. Adoptive T-cell therapy with hexon-specific Th1 cells as a treatment of refractory adenovirus infection after HSCT. *Blood* 2015;125:1986–1994.
172. Feuchtinger T, Lang P, Handgretinger R. Adenovirus infection after allogeneic stem cell transplantation. *Leuk Lymphoma* 2007;48:244–255.
173. Feuchtinger T, Matthes-Martin S, Richard C, et al. Safe adoptive transfer of virus-specific T-cell immunity for the treatment of systemic adenovirus infection after allogeneic stem cell transplantation. *Br J Haematol* 2006;134:64–76.
174. Feuchtinger T, Richard C, Joachim S, et al. Clinical grade generation of hexon-specific T cells for adoptive T-cell transfer as a treatment of adenovirus infection after allogeneic stem cell transplantation. *J Immunother* 2008;31:199–206.
175. Findlay JS, Cook GP, Blair GE. Blood coagulation factor X exerts differential effects on adenovirus entry into human lymphocytes. *Viruses* 2018;10(1):20.
176. Fisher BT, Boge CLK, Petersen H, et al. Outcomes of human adenovirus infection and disease in a retrospective cohort of pediatric hematopoietic cell transplant recipients. *J Pediatric Infect Dis Soc* 2019;8(4):317–324.
177. Flatt JW, Butcher SJ. Adenovirus flow in host cell networks. *Open Biol* 2019;9:190012.
178. Flomenberg P, Babbitt J, Drobyski WR, et al. Increasing incidence of adenovirus disease in bone marrow transplant recipients. *J Infect Dis* 1994;169:775–781.
179. Florescu DF, Chambers HE, Qiu F, et al. Cidofovir in pediatric solid organ transplant recipients: University of Nebraska experience. *Pediatr Infect Dis J* 2015;34:47–51.
180. Florescu DF, Hoffman JA; AST Infectious Diseases Community of Practice. Adenovirus in solid organ transplantation. *Am J Transplant* 2013;13(Suppl 4):206–211.
181. Florescu DF, Islam MK, Mercer DF, et al. Adenovirus infections in pediatric small bowel transplant recipients. *Transplantation* 2010;90:198–204.
182. Florescu MC, Miles CD, Florescu DF. What do we know about adenovirus in renal transplantation? *Nephrol Dial Transplant* 2013;28:2003–2010.
183. Florescu DF, Schaenman JM; AST Infectious Diseases Community of Practice. Adenovirus in solid organ transplant recipients: guidelines from the American Society of Transplantation Infectious Diseases Community of Practice. *Clin Transplant* 2019;33(9):e13527.
184. Florescu DF, Stohs EJ. Approach to infection and disease due to adenoviruses in solid organ transplantation. *Curr Opin Infect Dis* 2019;32:300–306.
185. Forstmeyer D, Henke-Gendo C, Brocker V, et al. Quantitative temporal and spatial distribution of adenovirus type 2 correlates with disease manifestations and organ failure during disseminated infection. *J Med Virol* 2008;80:294–297.
186. Frange P, Peffault de Latour R, Arnaud C, et al. Adenoviral infection presenting as an isolated central nervous system disease without detectable viremia in two children after stem cell transplantation. *J Clin Microbiol* 2011;49:2361–2364.
187. Ganapathi L, Arnold A, Jones S, et al. Use of cidofovir in pediatric patients with adenovirus infection. *F1000Res* 2016;5:758.
188. Ganzenmueller T, Buchholz S, Harste G, et al. High lethality of human adenovirus disease in adult allogeneic stem cell transplant recipients with high adenoviral blood load. *J Clin Virol* 2011;52:55–59.
189. Ganzenmueller T, Heim A. Adenoviral load diagnostics by quantitative polymerase chain reaction: techniques and application. *Rev Med Virol* 2012;22:194–208.
190. Garcia LAT, Boff L, Barardi CRM, et al. Inactivation of adenovirus in water by natural and synthetic compounds. *Food Environ Virol* 2019;11:157–166.
191. Garcia LA, Nascimento MA, Barardi CR. Effect of UV light on the inactivation of recombinant human adenovirus and murine norovirus seeded in seawater in shellfish depuration tanks. *Food Environ Virol* 2015;7:67–75.
192. Garnett CT, Erdman D, Xu W, et al. Prevalence and quantitation of species C adenovirus DNA in human mucosal lymphocytes. *J Virol* 2002;76:10608–10616.
193. Garnett CT, Talekar G, Mahr JA, et al. Latent species C adenoviruses in human tonsil tissues. *J Virol* 2009;83:2417–2428.
194. Geyeregger R, Freimuller C, Stemberger J, et al. First-in-man clinical results with good manufacturing practice (GMP)-compliant polypeptide-expanded adenovirus-specific T cells after haploidentical hematopoietic stem cell transplantation. *J Immunother* 2014;37:245–249.
195. Geyeregger R, Freimuller C, Stevanovic S, et al. Short-term in-vitro expansion improves monitoring and allows affordable generation of virus-specific T-cells against several viruses for a broad clinical application. *PLoS One* 2013;8:e59592.
196. Ghebremedhin B. Human adenovirus: viral pathogen with increasing importance. *Eur J Microbiol Immunol (Bp)* 2014;4:26–33.
197. Girardi V, Demoliner M, Gularte JS, et al. 'Don't put your head under water': enteric viruses in Brazilian recreational waters. *New Microbes New Infect* 2019;29:100519.
198. Girardi V, Gregianini TS, Gularte JS, et al. Temporal dynamics of Human mastadenovirus species in cases of respiratory illness in southern Brazil. *Braz J Microbiol* 2019;50: 677–684.
199. Girardi V, Mena KD, Albino SM, et al. Microbial risk assessment in recreational freshwaters from southern Brazil. *Sci Total Environ* 2019;651:298–308.
200. Girones R, Carratala A, Calgua B, et al. Chlorine inactivation of hepatitis E virus and human adenovirus 2 in water. *J Water Health* 2014;12:436–442.
201. Gong T, Wang HG, Shi Y, et al. The epidemic genotypes of human adenovirus in outpatient children with adenoviral conjunctivitis from 2011 to 2012 in Jiangxi, China. *Intervirology* 2019;62:30–36.
202. Gonzalez G, Yawata N, Aoki K, et al. Challenges in management of epidemic keratoconjunctivitis with emerging recombinant human adenoviruses. *J Clin Virol* 2019;112: 1–9.
203. Gonzalez-Vicent M, Verna M, Pochon C, et al. Current practices in the management of adenovirus infection in allogeneic hematopoietic stem cell transplant recipients in Europe: the AdVance study. *Eur J Haematol* 2019;102:210–217.
204. Gorczynska E, Turkiewicz D, Rybka K, et al. Incidence, clinical outcome, and management of virus-induced hemorrhagic cystitis in children and adolescents after allogeneic hematopoietic cell transplantation. *Biol Blood Marrow Transplant* 2005;11:797–804.
205. Graham FL, Rowe DT, McKinnon R, et al. Transformation by human adenoviruses. *J Cell Physiol Suppl* 1984;3:151–163.
206. Gray GC, McCarthy T, Lebeck MG, et al. Genotype prevalence and risk factors for severe clinical adenovirus infection, United States 2004-2006. *Clin Infect Dis* 2007;45:1120–1131.
207. Greaves M. Infection, immune responses and the aetiology of childhood leukaemia. *Nat Rev Cancer* 2006;6:193–203.

208. Greber UF, Arnberg N, Wadell G, et al. Adenoviruses—from pathogens to therapeutics: a report on the 10th International Adenovirus Meeting. *Cell Microbiol* 2013;15:16–23.
209. Greber UF, Flatt JW. Adenovirus entry: from infection to immunity. *Annu Rev Virol* 2019;6:177–197.
210. Grimley MS, Chemaly RF, Englund JA, et al. Brincidofovir for asymptomatic adenovirus viremia in pediatric and adult allogeneic hematopoietic cell transplant recipients: a randomized placebo-controlled phase II trial. *Biol Blood Marrow Transplant* 2017;23:512–521.
211. Grosso F, Stoilov P, Lingwood C, et al. Suppression of adenovirus replication by cardiotonic steroids. *J Virol* 2017;91(3):e01623-16.
212. Guarner J, de Leon-Bojorge B, Lopez-Corella E, et al. Intestinal intussusception associated with adenovirus infection in Mexican children. *Am J Clin Pathol* 2003;120:845–850.
213. Guerin-El Khourouj V, Dalle JH, Pedron B, et al. Quantitative and qualitative CD4 T cell immune responses related to adenovirus DNAemia in hematopoietic stem cell transplantation. *Biol Blood Marrow Transplant* 2011;17:476–485.
214. Guerra Sanchez CH, Lorica CD, Arheart KL, et al. Virologic response with 2 different cidofovir dosing regimens for preemptive treatment of adenovirus DNAemia in pediatric solid organ transplant recipients. *Pediatr Transplant* 2018:e13231.
215. Gularte JS, Girardi V, Demoliner M, et al. Human mastadenovirus in water, sediment, sea surface microlayer, and bivalve mollusk from southern Brazilian beaches. *Mar Pollut Bull* 2019;142:335–349.
216. Gustafson I, Lindblom A, Yun Z, et al. Quantification of adenovirus DNA in unrelated donor hematopoietic stem cell transplant recipients. *J Clin Virol* 2008;43:79–85.
217. Gustafsson B, Huang W, Bogdanovic G, et al. Adenovirus DNA is detected at increased frequency in Guthrie cards from children who develop acute lymphoblastic leukaemia. *Br J Cancer* 2007;97:992–994.
218. Gyurova IE, Ali A, Waggoner SN. Natural killer cell regulation of B cell responses in the context of viral infection. *Viral Immunol* 2019;33(4):334–341.
219. Hage E, Espelage W, Eckmanns T, et al. Molecular phylogeny of a novel human adenovirus type 8 strain causing a prolonged, multi-state keratoconjunctivitis epidemic in Germany. *Sci Rep* 2017;7:40680.
220. Hage E, Gerd Liebert U, Bergs S, et al. Human mastadenovirus type 70: a novel, multiple recombinant species D mastadenovirus isolated from diarrhoeal faeces of a haematopoietic stem cell transplantation recipient. *J Gen Virol* 2015;96:2734–2742.
221. Hanley PJ. Build a bank: off-the-shelf virus-specific T cells. *Biol Blood Marrow Transplant* 2018;24:e9–e10.
222. Hansen TH, Bouvier M. MHC class I antigen presentation: learning from viral evasion strategies. *Nat Rev Immunol* 2009;9:503–513.
223. Haque E, Banik U, Monowar T, et al. Worldwide increased prevalence of human adenovirus type 3 (HAdV-3) respiratory infections is well correlated with heterogeneous hypervariable regions (HVRs) of hexon. *PLoS One* 2018;13:e0194516.
224. Harrach B, Benko M. Phylogenetic analysis of adenovirus sequences. *Methods Mol Med* 2007;131:299–334.
225. Harrach B, Benkö M, Both GW, et al. Family—adenoviridae. In: King AMQ, Adams MJ, Carstens EB, et al., eds. *Virus Taxonomy—Ninth Report of the International Committee on Taxonomy of Viruses*. Oxford, UK: Elsevier; 2012:125–141.
226. Harrach B, Tarjan ZL, Benko M. Adenoviruses across the animal kingdom: a walk in the zoo. *FEBS Lett* 2019;593:3660–3673.
227. Hartline CB, Keith KA, Eagar J, et al. A standardized approach to the evaluation of antivirals against DNA viruses: orthopox-, adeno-, and herpesviruses. *Antiviral Res* 2018;159:104–112.
228. Hartyanszky I Jr, Tatrai E, Laszik A, et al. Patchy myocardial pattern of virus sequence persistence in heart transplant recipients—possible role of sampling error in the etiology. *Transplant Proc* 2011;43:1285–1289.
229. Hashimoto S, Gonzalez G, Harada S, et al. Recombinant type Human mastadenovirus D85 associated with epidemic keratoconjunctivitis since 2015 in Japan. *J Med Virol* 2018;90:881–889.
230. Hashizume M, Aoki K, Ohno S, et al. Disinfectant potential in inactivation of epidemic keratoconjunctivitis-related adenoviruses by potassium peroxymonosulfate. *Eur J Ophthalmol* 2019:1120672119891408.
231. Hatlen T, Mroch H, Tuttle K, et al. Disseminated adenovirus nephritis after kidney transplantation. *Kidney Int Rep* 2018;3:19–23.
232. Haveman LM, Bierings M, Klein MR, et al. Selection of perforin expressing CD4+ adenovirus-specific T-cells with artificial antigen presenting cells. *Clin Immunol* 2013;146:228–239.
233. Haveman LM, de Jager W, van Loon AM, et al. Different cytokine signatures in children with localized and invasive adenovirus infection after stem cell transplantation. *Pediatr Transplant* 2010;14:520–528.
234. Hazlett L, Wu M. Defensins in innate immunity. *Cell Tissue Res* 2011;343:175–188.
235. Heemskerk B, van Vreeswijk T, Veltrop-Duits LA, et al. Adenovirus-specific CD4+ T cell clones recognizing endogenous antigen inhibit viral replication in vitro through cognate interaction. *J Immunol* 2006;177:8851–8859.
236. Heim A. Advances in the management of disseminated adenovirus disease in stem cell transplant recipients: impact of adenovirus load (DNAemia) testing. *Expert Rev Anti Infect Ther* 2011;9:943–945.
237. Heim A, Ebnet C, Harste G, et al. Rapid and quantitative detection of human adenovirus DNA by real-time PCR. *J Med Virol* 2003;70:228–239.
238. Heindl LM, Augustin AJ, Messmer EM; ADVISE study group. ADenoVirus Initiative Study in Epidemiology (ADVISE)-results of a multicenter epidemiology study in Germany. *Graefes Arch Clin Exp Ophthalmol* 2019;257:249–251.
239. Hemmersbach-Miller M, Bailey ES, Kappus M, et al. Disseminated adenovirus infection after combined liver-kidney transplantation. *Front Cell Infect Microbiol* 2018;8:408.
240. Hendrickx R, Stichling N, Koelen J, et al. Innate immunity to adenovirus. *Hum Gene Ther* 2014;25:265–284.
241. Heo JY, Noh JY, Jeong HW, et al. Molecular epidemiology of human adenovirus-associated febrile respiratory illness in soldiers, South Korea(1). *Emerg Infect Dis* 2018;24:1221–1227.
242. Hijnen WA, Beerendonk EF, Medema GJ. Inactivation credit of UV radiation for viruses, bacteria and protozoan (oo)cysts in water: a review. *Water Res* 2006;40:3–22.
243. Hiwarkar P, Amrolia P, Sivaprakasam P, et al. Brincidofovir is highly efficacious in controlling adenoviremia in pediatric recipients of hematopoietic cell transplant. *Blood* 2017;129:2033–2037.
244. Hiwarkar P, Gaspar HB, Gilmour K, et al. Impact of viral reactivations in the era of pre-emptive antiviral drug therapy following allogeneic haematopoietic SCT in paediatric recipients. *Bone Marrow Transplant* 2013;48:803–808.
245. Hiwarkar P, Kosulin K, Cesaro S, et al. Management of adenovirus infection in patients after haematopoietic stem cell transplantation: state-of-the-art and real-life current approach: a position statement on behalf of the Infectious Diseases Working Party of the European Society of Blood and Marrow Transplantation. *Rev Med Virol* 2018;28:e1980.
246. Ho QY, Tan CS, Thien SY, et al. The use of intravesical cidofovir for the treatment of adenovirus-associated haemorrhagic cystitis in a kidney transplant recipient. *Clin Kidney J* 2019;12:745–747.
247. Hoffman JA. Adenoviral disease in pediatric solid organ transplant recipients. *Pediatr Transplant* 2006;10:17–25.
248. Hoffman JA. Adenovirus infections in solid organ transplant recipients. *Curr Opin Organ Transplant* 2009;14:625–633.
249. Hogg JC. Role of latent viral infections in chronic obstructive pulmonary disease and asthma. *Am J Respir Crit Care Med* 2001;164:S71–S75.
250. Hohlweg U, Dorn A, Hosel M, et al. Tumorigenesis by adenovirus type 12 in newborn Syrian hamsters. *Curr Top Microbiol Immunol* 2004;273:215–244.
251. Hoke CH Jr, Snyder CE Jr. History of the restoration of adenovirus type 4 and type 7 vaccine, live oral (Adenovirus Vaccine) in the context of the Department of Defense acquisition system. *Vaccine* 2013;31:1623–1632.
252. Holly MK, Diaz K, Smith JG. Defensins in viral infection and pathogenesis. *Annu Rev Virol* 2017;4:369–391.
253. Holly MK, Smith JG. Paneth cells during viral infection and pathogenesis. *Viruses* 2018;10(5):225.
254. Holly MK, Smith JG. Adenovirus infection of human enteroids reveals interferon sensitivity and preferential infection of goblet cells. *J Virol* 2018;92(9):e00250-18.
255. Holterman L, Vogels R, van der Vlugt R, et al. Novel replication-incompetent vector derived from adenovirus type 11 (Ad11) for vaccination and gene therapy: low seroprevalence and non-cross-reactivity with Ad5. *J Virol* 2004;78:13207–13215.
256. Homma M, Inoue Y, Hasegawa Y, et al. Blood ribavirin concentration in high-dose ribavirin for adenovirus-induced haemorrhagic cystitis—a case report. *J Clin Pharm Ther* 2008;33:75–78.
257. Hong SS, Habib NA, Franqueville L, et al. Identification of adenovirus (ad) penton base neutralizing epitopes by use of sera from patients who had received conditionally replicative ad (addl1520) for treatment of liver tumors. *J Virol* 2003;77:10366–10375.
258. Hong JY, Lee HJ, Piedra PA, et al. Lower respiratory tract infections due to adenovirus in hospitalized Korean children: epidemiology, clinical features, and prognosis. *Clin Infect Dis* 2001;32:1423–1429.
259. Honkaniemi E, Talekar G, Huang W, et al. Adenovirus DNA in Guthrie cards from children who develop acute lymphoblastic leukaemia (ALL). *Br J Cancer* 2010;102:796–798.
260. Hoppe E, Pauly M, Gillespie TR, et al. Multiple cross-species transmission events of human adenoviruses (HAdV) during hominine evolution. *Mol Biol Evol* 2015;32:2072–2084.
261. Hoppe E, Pauly M, Robbins M, et al. Phylogenomic evidence for recombination of adenoviruses in wild gorillas. *J Gen Virol* 2015;96:3090–3098.
262. Houng HS, Gong H, Kajon AE, et al. Genome sequences of human adenovirus 14 isolates from mild respiratory cases and a fatal pneumonia, isolated during 2006-2007 epidemics in North America. *Respir Res* 2010;11:116.
263. Huang WC, Chou YP, Kao PM, et al. Nested-PCR and TaqMan real-time quantitative PCR assays for human adenoviruses in environmental waters. *Water Sci Technol* 2016;73:1832–1841.
264. Huang J, Kadonosono K, Uchio E. Antiadenoviral effects of ganciclovir in types inducing keratoconjunctivitis by quantitative polymerase chain reaction methods. *Clin Ophthalmol* 2014;8:315–320.
265. Huang ML, Nguy L, Ferrenberg J, et al. Development of multiplexed real-time quantitative polymerase chain reaction assay for detecting human adenoviruses. *Diagn Microbiol Infect Dis* 2008;62:263–271.
266. Hubmann M, Fritsch S, Zoellner AK, et al. Occurrence, risk factors and outcome of adenovirus infection in adult recipients of allogeneic hematopoietic stem cell transplantation. *J Clin Virol* 2016;82:33–40.
267. Huh K, Kim I, Jung J, et al. Prolonged shedding of type 55 human adenovirus in immunocompetent adults with adenoviral respiratory infections. *Eur J Clin Microbiol Infect Dis* 2019;38:793–800.
268. Huh JW, Kim WH, Moon SG, et al. Viral etiology and incidence associated with acute gastroenteritis in a 5-year survey in Gyeonggi province, South Korea. *J Clin Virol* 2009;44:152–156.
269. Hum RM, Deambrosis D, Lum SH, et al. Molecular monitoring of adenovirus reactivation in faeces after haematopoietic stem-cell transplantation to predict systemic infection: a retrospective cohort study. *Lancet Haematol* 2018;5:e422–e429.
270. Humar A, Doucette K, Kumar D, et al. Assessment of adenovirus infection in adult lung transplant recipients using molecular surveillance. *J Heart Lung Transplant* 2006;25:1441–1446.
271. Humar A, Kumar D, Mazzulli T, et al. A surveillance study of adenovirus infection in adult solid organ transplant recipients. *Am J Transplant* 2005;5:2555–2559.
272. Huppmann AR, Orenstein JM. Opportunistic disorders of the gastrointestinal tract in the age of highly active antiretroviral therapy. *Hum Pathol* 2010;41:1777–1787.
273. Hutnick NA, Carnathan D, Demers K, et al. Adenovirus-specific human T cells are pervasive, polyfunctional, and cross-reactive. *Vaccine* 2010;28:1932–1941.
274. Hutnick NA, Carnathan DG, Dubey SA, et al. Vaccination with Ad5 vectors expands Ad5-specific CD8 T cells without altering memory phenotype or functionality. *PLoS One* 2010;5:e14385.

275. Hutterer C, Eickhoff J, Milbradt J, et al. A novel CDK7 inhibitor of the Pyrazolotriazine class exerts broad-spectrum antiviral activity at nanomolar concentrations. *Antimicrob Agents Chemother* 2015;59:2062–2071.
276. Huttunen R, Syrjanen J. Obesity and the risk and outcome of infection. *Int J Obes (Lond)* 2013;37:333–340.
277. Iaconelli M, Valdazo-Gonzalez B, Equestre M, et al. Molecular characterization of human adenoviruses in urban wastewaters using next generation and Sanger sequencing. *Water Res* 2017;121:240–247.
278. Ibrisimovic M, Kneidinger D, Lion T, et al. An adenoviral vector-based expression and delivery system for the inhibition of wild-type adenovirus replication by artificial microRNAs. *Antiviral Res* 2013;97:10–23.
279. Ibrisimovic M, Lion T, Klein R. Combinatorial targeting of 2 different steps in adenoviral DNA replication by herpes simplex virus thymidine kinase and artificial microRNA expression for the inhibition of virus multiplication in the presence of ganciclovir. *BMC Biotechnol* 2013;13:54.
280. Ikonen N, Savolainen-Kopra C, Enstone JE, et al. Deposition of respiratory virus pathogens on frequently touched surfaces at airports. *BMC Infect Dis* 2018;18:437.
281. Ingato D, Lee JU, Sim SJ, et al. Good things come in small packages: overcoming challenges to harness extracellular vesicles for therapeutic delivery. *J Control Release* 2016;241:174–185.
282. Ip WH, Dobner T. Cell transformation by the adenovirus oncogenes E1 and E4. *FEBS Lett* 2020;594(12):1848–1860.
283. Ip W, Silva JMF, Gaspar H, et al. Multicenter phase 1/2 application of adenovirus-specific T cells in high-risk pediatric patients after allogeneic stem cell transplantation. *Cytotherapy* 2018;20:830–838.
284. Ishiko H, Aoki K. Spread of epidemic keratoconjunctivitis due to a novel serotype of human adenovirus in Japan. *J Clin Microbiol* 2009;47:2678–2679.
285. Ismail AM, Cui T, Dommaraju K, et al. Genomic analysis of a large set of currently-and historically-important human adenovirus pathogens. *Emerg Microbes Infect* 2018;7:10.
286. Ismail AM, Lee JS, Dyer DW, et al. Selection pressure in the human adenovirus fiber knob drives cell specificity in epidemic keratoconjunctivitis. *J Virol* 2016;90:9598–9607.
287. Ismail AM, Lee JS, Lee JY, et al. Adenoviromics: mining the human adenovirus species D genome. *Front Microbiol* 2018;9:2178.
288. Ismail AM, Zhou X, Dyer DW, et al. Genomic foundations of evolution and ocular pathogenesis in human adenovirus species D. *FEBS Lett* 2019;593:3583–3608.
289. Ison MG. Adenovirus infections in transplant recipients. *Clin Infect Dis* 2006;43:331–339.
290. Ison MG, Green M; AST Infectious Diseases Community of Practice. Adenovirus in solid organ transplant recipients. *Am J Transplant* 2009;9(Suppl 4):S161–S165.
291. Jaggi P, Kajon AE, Mejias A, et al. Human adenovirus infection in Kawasaki disease: a confounding bystander? *Clin Infect Dis* 2013;56:58–64.
292. Jain S, Williams DJ, Arnold SR, et al. Community-acquired pneumonia requiring hospitalization among U.S. children. *N Engl J Med* 2015;372:835–845.
293. Jaiswal SR, Chakrabarti S. Natural killer cell-based immunotherapy with CTLA4Ig-primed donor lymphocytes following haploidentical transplantation. *Immunotherapy* 2019;11:1221–1230.
294. James SH, Price NB, Hartline CB, et al. Selection and recombinant phenotyping of a novel CMX001 and cidofovir resistance mutation in human cytomegalovirus. *Antimicrob Agents Chemother* 2013;57:3321–3325.
295. Jang J, Lee YJ, Kim JS, et al. Epidemiological correlation between fecal adenovirus subgroups and pediatric intussusception in Korea. *J Korean Med Sci* 2017;32:1647–1656.
296. Jaoko W, Karita E, Kayitenkore K, et al. Safety and immunogenicity study of Multiclade HIV-1 adenoviral vector vaccine alone or as boost following a multiclade HIV-1 DNA vaccine in Africa. *PLoS One* 2010;5:e12873.
297. Javier RT. Adenovirus type 9 E4 open reading frame 1 encodes a transforming protein required for the production of mammary tumors in rats. *J Virol* 1994;68:3917–3924.
298. Javier R, Raska K Jr, Macdonald GJ, et al. Human adenovirus type 9-induced rat mammary tumors. *J Virol* 1991;65:3192–3202.
299. Jeulin H, Salmon A, Bordigoni P, et al. Comparison of in-house real-time quantitative PCR to the Adenovirus R-Gene kit for determination of adenovirus load in clinical samples. *J Clin Microbiol* 2010;48:3132–3137.
300. Jeulin H, Salmon A, Bordigoni P, et al. Diagnostic value of quantitative PCR for adenovirus detection in stool samples as compared with antigen detection and cell culture in haematopoietic stem cell transplant recipients. *Clin Microbiol Infect* 2011;17:1674–1680.
301. Jiang Y, Fang L, Shi X, et al. Simultaneous detection of five enteric viruses associated with gastroenteritis by use of a PCR assay: a single real-time multiplex reaction and its clinical application. *J Clin Microbiol* 2014;52:1266–1268.
302. Jiao Y, Liang X, Hou J, et al. Adenovirus type 36 regulates adipose stem cell differentiation and glucolipid metabolism through the PI3K/Akt/FoxO1/PPARgamma signaling pathway. *Lipids Health Dis* 2019;18:70.
303. Joffe M, Wagner SD, Tang JW. Case report: a fatal case of disseminated adenovirus infection in a non-transplant adult haematology patient. *BMC Infect Dis* 2018;18:58.
304. Jogler C, Hoffmann D, Theegarten D, et al. Replication properties of human adenovirus in vivo and in cultures of primary cells from different animal species. *J Virol* 2006;80:3549–3558.
305. Jonas RA, Ung L, Rajaiya J, et al. Mystery eye: human adenovirus and the enigma of epidemic keratoconjunctivitis. *Prog Retin Eye Res* 2019;76:100826.
306. Jones LB, Bell CR, Bibb KE, et al. Pathogens and their effect on exosome biogenesis and composition. *Biomedicines* 2018;6(3):79.
307. Jones MS II, Harrach B, Ganac RD, et al. New adenovirus species found in a patient presenting with gastroenteritis. *J Virol* 2007;81:5978–5984.
308. Joshi A, Zhao B, Romanowski C, et al. Comparison of human memory CD8 T cell responses to adenoviral early and late proteins in peripheral blood and lymphoid tissue. *PLoS One* 2011;6:e20068.
309. Kaas L, Ogorzaly L, Lecellier G, et al. Detection of human enteric viruses in french polynesian wastewaters, environmental waters and giant clams. *Food Environ Virol* 2019;11:52–64.
310. Kaeuferle T, Krauss R, Blaeschke F, et al. Strategies of adoptive T-cell transfer to treat refractory viral infections post allogeneic stem cell transplantation. *J Hematol Oncol* 2019;12:13.
311. Kagnoff MF, Paterson YJ, Kumar PJ, et al. Evidence for the role of a human intestinal adenovirus in the pathogenesis of coeliac disease. *Gut* 1987;28:995–1001.
312. Kahl CA, Bonnell J, Hiriyanna S, et al. Potent immune responses and in vitro pro-inflammatory cytokine suppression by a novel adenovirus vaccine vector based on rare human serotype 28. *Vaccine* 2010;28:5691–5702.
313. Kahler AM, Cromeans TL, Metcalfe MG, et al. Aggregation of adenovirus 2 in source water and impacts on disinfection by chlorine. *Food Environ Virol* 2016;8:148–155.
314. Kahrs CR, Chuda K, Tapia G, et al. Enterovirus as trigger of coeliac disease: nested case-control study within prospective birth cohort. *BMJ* 2019;364:l231.
315. Kajan GL, Lipiec A, Bartha D, et al. A multigene typing system for human adenoviruses reveals a new genotype in a collection of Swedish clinical isolates. *PLoS One* 2018;13:e0209038.
316. Kajon AE, Hang J, Hawksworth A, et al. Molecular epidemiology of adenovirus type 21 respiratory strains isolated from US military trainees (1996-2014). *J Infect Dis* 2015;212:871–880.
317. Kajon AE, Lamson DM, Bair CR, et al. Adenovirus type 4 respiratory infections among civilian adults, Northeastern United States, 2011-2015(1). *Emerg Infect Dis* 2018;24:201–209.
318. Kajon AE, Lamson DM, St George K. Emergence and re-emergence of respiratory adenoviruses in the United States. *Curr Opin Virol* 2019;34:63–69.
319. Kajon AE, Lu X, Erdman DD, et al. Molecular epidemiology and brief history of emerging adenovirus 14-associated respiratory disease in the United States. *J Infect Dis* 2010;202:93–103.
320. Kajon AE, Moseley JM, Metzgar D, et al. Molecular epidemiology of adenovirus type 4 infections in US military recruits in the postvaccination era (1997-2003). *J Infect Dis* 2007;196:67–75.
321. Kalpoe JS, van der Heiden PL, Barge RM, et al. Assessment of disseminated adenovirus infections using quantitative plasma PCR in adult allogeneic stem cell transplant recipients receiving reduced intensity or myeloablative conditioning. *Eur J Haematol* 2007;78:314–321.
322. Kalu SU, Loeffelholz M, Beck E, et al. Persistence of adenovirus nucleic acids in nasopharyngeal secretions: a diagnostic conundrum. *Pediatr Infect Dis J* 2010;29:746–750.
323. Kalyuzhniy O, Di Paolo NC, Silvestry M, et al. Adenovirus serotype 5 hexon is critical for virus infection of hepatocytes in vivo. *Proc Natl Acad Sci U S A* 2008;105:5483–5488.
324. Kandel R, Srinivasan A, D'Agata EM, et al. Outbreak of adenovirus type 4 infection in a long-term care facility for the elderly. *Infect Control Hosp Epidemiol* 2010;31:755–757.
325. Kaneko H, Aoki K, Ishida S, et al. Recombination analysis of intermediate human adenovirus type 53 in Japan by complete genome sequence. *J Gen Virol* 2011;92:1251–1259.
326. Kaneko H, Maruko I, Iida T, et al. The possibility of human adenovirus detection from the conjunctiva in asymptomatic cases during nosocomial infection. *Cornea* 2008;27:527–530.
327. Kaneko H, Mori S, Suzuki O, et al. The cotton rat model for adenovirus ocular infection: antiviral activity of cidofovir. *Antiviral Res* 2004;61:63–66.
328. Kang JM, Park KS, Kim JM, et al. Prospective monitoring of adenovirus infection and type analysis after allogeneic hematopoietic cell transplantation: a single-center study in Korea. *Transpl Infect Dis* 2018;20:e12885.
329. Kang D, Zhang H, Zhou Z, et al. First discovery of novel 3-hydroxy-quinazoline-2,4(1H,3H)-diones as specific anti-vaccinia and adenovirus agents via 'privileged scaffold' refining approach. *Bioorg Med Chem Lett* 2016;26:5182–5186.
330. Kangasniemi L, Parviainen S, Pisto T, et al. Effects of capsid-modified oncolytic adenoviruses and their combinations with gemcitabine or silica gel on pancreatic cancer. *Int J Cancer* 2012;131:253–263.
331. Karimi A, Moradi MT, Alidadi S, et al. Anti-adenovirus activity, antioxidant potential, and phenolic content of black tea (Camellia sinensis Kuntze) extract. *J Complement Integr Med* 2016;13:357–363.
332. Kaspersen KA, Pedersen OB, Petersen MS, et al. Obesity and risk of infection: results from the Danish Blood Donor Study. *Epidemiology* 2015;26:580–589.
333. Kaye SB, Lloyd M, Williams H, et al. Evidence for persistence of adenovirus in the tear film a decade following conjunctivitis. *J Med Virol* 2005;77:227–231.
334. Keib A, Gunther PS, Faist B, et al. Presentation of a conserved adenoviral epitope on HLA-C*0702 allows evasion of natural killer but not T cell responses. *Viral Immunol* 2017;30:149–156.
335. Keib A, Mei YF, Cicin-Sain L, et al. Measuring antiviral capacity of T cell responses to adenovirus. *J Immunol* 2019;202:618–624.
336. Keller MD, Bollard CM. Virus specific T-cell therapies for patients with primary immune deficiency. *Blood* 2020;135(9):620–628.
337. Kenmoe S, Vernet MA, Le Goff J, et al. Molecular characterization of human adenovirus associated with acute respiratory infections in Cameroon from 2011 to 2014. *Virol J* 2018;15:153.
338. Keyes A, Mathias M, Boulad F, et al. Cutaneous involvement of disseminated adenovirus infection in an allogeneic stem cell transplant recipient. *Br J Dermatol* 2016;174:885–888.
339. Khamrin P, Malasao R, Chaimongkol N, et al. Circulating of human bocavirus 1, 2, 3, and 4 in pediatric patients with acute gastroenteritis in Thailand. *Infect Genet Evol* 2012;12:565–569.
340. Khanal S, Ghimire P, Dhamoon AS. The repertoire of adenovirus in human disease: the innocuous to the deadly. *Biomedicines* 2018;6(1):30.
341. Khanal S, Ghimire P, Dhamoon AS. Reply to the Comment on: Subrat Khanal et al. The repertoire of adenovirus in human disease: the innocuous to the deadly. Biomedicines 2018, 6, 30. *Biomedicines* 2019;7(1):10.
342. Khoo SH, Bailey AS, de Jong JC, et al. Adenovirus infections in human immunodeficiency virus-positive patients: clinical features and molecular epidemiology. *J Infect Dis* 1995;172:629–637.
343. Killerby ME, Rozwadowski F, Lu X, et al. Respiratory illness associated with emergent human adenovirus genome type 7d, New Jersey, 2016-2017. *Open Forum Infect Dis* 2019;6:ofz017.

344. Kim YJ, Boeckh M, Englund JA. Community respiratory virus infections in immunocompromised patients: hematopoietic stem cell and solid organ transplant recipients, and individuals with human immunodeficiency virus infection. *Semin Respir Crit Care Med* 2007;28:222–242.
345. Kim NJ, Hyun TS, Pergam SA, et al. Disseminated adenovirus infection after autologous stem cell transplant. *Transpl Infect Dis* 2020;22(1):e13238.
346. Kim SJ, Kim K, Park SB, et al. Outcomes of early administration of cidofovir in non-immunocompromised patients with severe adenovirus pneumonia. *PLoS One* 2015;10:e0122642.
347. Kim OY, Lee J, Gho YS. Extracellular vesicle mimetics: novel alternatives to extracellular vesicle-based theranostics, drug delivery, and vaccines. *Semin Cell Dev Biol* 2017;67:74–82.
348. Kim JS, Lee SK, Ko DH, et al. Associations of adenovirus genotypes in Korean acute gastroenteritis patients with respiratory symptoms and intussusception. *Biomed Res Int* 2017;2017:1602054.
349. Kim J, Na H, Kim JA, et al. What we know and what we need to know about adenovirus 36-induced obesity. *Int J Obes (Lond)* 2020;44(6):1197–1209.
350. Kim HK, Oh SH, Yun KA, et al. Comparison of Anyplex II RV16 with the xTAG respiratory viral panel and Seeplex RV15 for detection of respiratory viruses. *J Clin Microbiol* 2013;51:1137–1141.
351. Kim KH, Ryan MJ, Estep JE, et al. A new generation of serotype chimeric infectivity-enhanced conditionally replicative adenovirals: the safety profile of ad5/3-Delta24 in advance of a phase I clinical trial in ovarian cancer patients. *Hum Gene Ther* 2011;22:821–828.
352. Kimura R, Migita H, Kadonosono K, et al. Is it possible to detect the presence of adenovirus in conjunctiva before the onset of conjunctivitis? *Acta Ophthalmol* 2009;87:44–47.
353. Kinchington PR, Romanowski EG, Jerold Gordon Y. Prospects for adenovirus antivirals. *J Antimicrob Chemother* 2005;55:424–429.
354. King CR, Zhang A, Tessier TM, et al. Hacking the cell: network intrusion and exploitation by adenovirus E1A. *MBio* 2018;9(3):e00390-18.
355. Klein J, Kuperman M, Haley C, et al. Late presentation of adenovirus-induced hemorrhagic cystitis and ureteral obstruction in a kidney-pancreas transplant recipient. *Proc (Bayl Univ Med Cent)* 2015;28:488–491.
356. Kneidinger D, Ibrisimovic M, Lion T, et al. Inhibition of adenovirus multiplication by short interfering RNAs directly or indirectly targeting the viral DNA replication machinery. *Antiviral Res* 2012;94:195–207.
357. Ko JH, Lim JU, Choi JY, et al. Early cidofovir administration might be associated with a lower probability of respiratory failure in treating human adenovirus pneumonia: a retrospective cohort study. *Clin Microbiol Infect* 2020;26(5):646.e9–646.e14.
358. Ko JH, Woo HT, Oh HS, et al. Ongoing outbreak of human adenovirus-associated acute respiratory illness in the Republic of Korea military, 2013 to 2018. *Korean J Intern Med* 2021;36(1):205–213.
359. Kokkinos P, Karayanni H, Meziti A, et al. Assessment of the virological quality of marine and running surface waters in NW Greece: a case study. *Food Environ Virol* 2018;10:316–326.
360. Koo J, Dawson DW, Dry S, et al. Allograft biopsy findings in patients with small bowel transplantation. *Clin Transplant* 2016;30:1433–1439.
361. Koodie L, Robertson MG, Chandrashekar M, et al. Rodents versus pig model for assessing the performance of serotype chimeric Ad5/3 oncolytic adenoviruses. *Cancers (Basel)* 2019;11(2):198.
362. Kosulin K. Intestinal HAdV infection: tissue specificity, persistence, and implications for antiviral therapy. *Viruses* 2019;11(9):804.
363. Kosulin K, Berkowitsch B, Lion T. Modified pan-adenovirus real-time PCR assay based on genome analysis of seventy HAdV types. *J Clin Virol* 2016;80:60–61.
364. Kosulin K, Berkowitsch B, Matthes S, et al. Intestinal adenovirus shedding before allogeneic stem cell transplantation is a risk factor for invasive infection post-transplant. *EBioMedicine* 2018;28:114–119.
365. Kosulin K, Dworzak S, Lawitschka A, et al. Comparison of different approaches to quantitative adenovirus detection in stool specimens of hematopoietic stem cell transplant recipients. *J Clin Virol* 2016;85:31–36.
366. Kosulin K, Geiger E, Vecsei A, et al. Persistence and reactivation of human adenoviruses in the gastrointestinal tract. *Clin Microbiol Infect* 2016;22:381 e1–e8.
367. Kosulin K, Haberler C, Hainfellner JA, et al. Investigation of adenovirus occurrence in pediatric tumor entities. *J Virol* 2007;81:7629–7635.
368. Kosulin K, Hoffmann F, Clauditz TS, et al. Presence of adenovirus species C in infiltrating lymphocytes of human sarcoma. *PLoS One* 2013;8:e63646.
369. Kosulin K, Pichler H, Lawitschka A, et al. Diagnostic parameters of adenoviremia in pediatric stem cell transplant recipients. *Front Microbiol* 2019;10:414.
370. Kosulin K, Rauch M, Ambros PF, et al. Screening for adenoviruses in haematological neoplasia: high prevalence in mantle cell lymphoma. *Eur J Cancer* 2014;50:622–627.
371. Kozlowski T, Nickeleit V, Andreoni K. Donor-transmitted adenovirus infection causing kidney allograft nephritis and graft loss. *Transpl Infect Dis* 2011;13:168–173.
372. Kroes AC, de Klerk EP, Lankester AC, et al. Sequential emergence of multiple adenovirus serotypes after pediatric stem cell transplantation. *J Clin Virol* 2007;38:341–347.
373. Krude H, Biebermann H, Schnabel D, et al. Obesity due to proopiomelanocortin deficiency: three new cases and treatment trials with thyroid hormone and ACTH4-10. *J Clin Endocrinol Metab* 2003;88:4633–4640.
374. Kuhl U, Schultheiss HP. Viral myocarditis. *Swiss Med Wkly* 2014;144:w14010.
375. Kumaki Y, Woolcott JD, Roth JP, et al. Inhibition of adenovirus serotype 14 infection by octadecyloxyethyl esters of (S)-[(3-hydroxy-2-phosphonomethoxy)propyl]- nucleosides in vitro. *Antiviral Res* 2018;158:122–126.
376. Kumthip K, Khamrin P, Ushijima H, et al. Enteric and non-enteric adenoviruses associated with acute gastroenteritis in pediatric patients in Thailand, 2011 to 2017. *PLoS One* 2019;14:e0220263.
377. Kuo IC. More than meets the eye: adenoviral conjunctivitis in healthcare settings. *Infect Control Hosp Epidemiol* 2017;38:1358–1360.
378. Kuschner RA, Russell KL, Abuja M, et al. A phase 3, randomized, double-blind, placebo-controlled study of the safety and efficacy of the live, oral adenovirus type 4 and type 7 vaccine, in U.S. military recruits. *Vaccine* 2013;31:2963–2971.
379. Kwon HJ, Rhie YJ, Seo WH, et al. Clinical manifestations of respiratory adenoviral infection among hospitalized children in Korea. *Pediatr Int* 2013;55:450–454.
380. La Rosa AM, Champlin RE, Mirza N, et al. Adenovirus infections in adult recipients of blood and marrow transplants. *Clin Infect Dis* 2001;32:871–876.
381. La Rosa G, Della Libera S, Petricca S, et al. Genetic diversity of human adenovirus in children with acute gastroenteritis, Albania, 2013-2015. *Biomed Res Int* 2015;2015:142912.
382. Lafolie J, Mirand A, Salmona M, et al. Severe pneumonia associated with adenovirus type 55 infection, France, 2014. *Emerg Infect Dis* 2016;22:2012–2014.
383. Lam E, Ramke M, Warnecke G, et al. Effective apical infection of differentiated human bronchial epithelial cells and induction of proinflammatory chemokines by the highly pneumotropic human adenovirus type 14p1. *PLoS One* 2015;10:e0131201.
384. Lamson Bs DM, Kajon AE, Shudt M, et al. Molecular typing and whole genome next generation sequencing of human adenovirus 8 strains recovered from four 2012 outbreaks of keratoconjunctivitis in New York State. *J Med Virol* 2018;90:1471–1477.
385. Lasaro MO, Ertl HC. New insights on adenovirus as vaccine vectors. *Mol Ther* 2009;17:1333–1339.
386. Lasswitz L, Chandra N, Arnberg N, et al. Glycomics and proteomics approaches to investigate early adenovirus-host cell interactions. *J Mol Biol* 2018;430:1863–1882.
387. Lee J, Choi EH, Lee HJ. Comprehensive serotyping and epidemiology of human adenovirus isolated from the respiratory tract of Korean children over 17 consecutive years (1991-2007). *J Med Virol* 2010;82:624–631.
388. Lee YJ, Chung D, Xiao K, et al. Adenovirus viremia and disease: comparison of T cell-depleted and conventional hematopoietic stem cell transplantation recipients from a single institution. *Biol Blood Marrow Transplant* 2013;19:387–392.
389. Lee YJ, Huang YT, Kim SJ, et al. Adenovirus viremia in adult CD34(+) selected hematopoietic cell transplant recipients: low incidence and high clinical impact. *Biol Blood Marrow Transplant* 2016;22:174–178.
390. Lee YS, Jun HS. Anti-diabetic actions of glucagon-like peptide-1 on pancreatic beta-cells. *Metabolism* 2014;63:9–19.
391. Lee M, Kim S, Kwon OJ, et al. Treatment of adenoviral acute respiratory distress syndrome using cidofovir with extracorporeal membrane oxygenation. *J Intensive Care Med* 2017;32:231–238.
392. Lee CS, Lee AY, Akileswaran L, et al. Determinants of outcomes of adenoviral keratoconjunctivitis. *Ophthalmology* 2018;125:1344–1353.
393. Lee JY, Lee JS, Materne EC, et al. Bacterial RecA protein promotes adenoviral recombination during in vitro infection. *mSphere* 2018;3.
394. Lee YH, Lin LH, Hung SP. Simultaneous intussusception associated with adenovirus infection in monozygotic twins: a case report. *Medicine (Baltimore)* 2019;98:e18294.
395. Lee YJ, Prockop SE, Papanicolaou GA. Approach to adenovirus infections in the setting of hematopoietic cell transplantation. *Curr Opin Infect Dis* 2017;30:377–387.
396. Leen AM, Bollard CM, Mendizabal AM, et al. Multicenter study of banked third-party virus-specific T cells to treat severe viral infections after hematopoietic stem cell transplantation. *Blood* 2013;121:5113–5123.
397. Leen AM, Bollard CM, Myers GD, et al. Adenoviral infections in hematopoietic stem cell transplantation. *Biol Blood Marrow Transplant* 2006;12:243–251.
398. Leen AM, Christin A, Khalil M, et al. Identification of hexon-specific CD4 and CD8 T-cell epitopes for vaccine and immunotherapy. *J Virol* 2008;82:546–554.
399. Leen AM, Christin A, Myers GD, et al. Cytotoxic T lymphocyte therapy with donor T cells prevents and treats adenovirus and Epstein-Barr virus infections after haploidentical and matched unrelated stem cell transplantation. *Blood* 2009;114:4283–4292.
400. Leen AM, Myers GD, Sili U, et al. Monoculture-derived T lymphocytes specific for multiple viruses expand and produce clinically relevant effects in immunocompromised individuals. *Nat Med* 2006;12:1160–1166.
401. Legoff J, Feghoul L, Mercier-Delarue S, et al. Broad-range PCR-electrospray ionization mass spectrometry for detection and typing of adenovirus and other opportunistic viruses in stem cell transplant patients. *J Clin Microbiol* 2013;51:4186–4192.
402. Legoff J, Resche-Rigon M, Bouquet J, et al. The eukaryotic gut virome in hematopoietic stem cell transplantation: new clues in enteric graft-versus-host disease. *Nat Med* 2017;23:1080–1085.
403. Lenaerts L, De Clercq E, Naesens L. Clinical features and treatment of adenovirus infections. *Rev Med Virol* 2008;18:357–374.
404. Lenman A, Liaci AM, Liu Y, et al. Human adenovirus 52 uses sialic acid-containing glycoproteins and the coxsackie and adenovirus receptor for binding to target cells. *PLoS Pathog* 2015;11:e1004657.
405. Lenman A, Liaci AM, Liu Y, et al. Polysialic acid is a cellular receptor for human adenovirus 52. *Proc Natl Acad Sci U S A* 2018;115:E4264–E4273.
406. Lessa FC, Gould PL, Pascoe N, et al. Health care transmission of a newly emergent adenovirus serotype in health care personnel at a military hospital in Texas, 2007. *J Infect Dis* 2009;200:1759–1765.
407. Leung AY, Chan M, Cheng VC, et al. Quantification of adenovirus in the lower respiratory tract of patients without clinical adenovirus-related respiratory disease. *Clin Infect Dis* 2005;40:1541–1544.
408. Li X, Cai M, Wang L, et al. Evaluation survey of microbial disinfection methods in UV-LED water treatment systems. *Sci Total Environ* 2019;659:1415–1427.
409. Li P, Liu Y, Maynard J, et al. Use of adenoviral vectors to target chemotherapy to tumor vascular endothelial cells suppresses growth of breast cancer and melanoma. *Mol Ther* 2010;18:921–928.
410. Li J, Lu X, Sun Y, et al. A swimming pool-associated outbreak of pharyngoconjunctival fever caused by human adenovirus type 4 in Beijing, China. *Int J Infect Dis* 2018;75:89–91.
411. Li X, Wang P, Li H, et al. The efficacy of oncolytic adenovirus is mediated by T-cell responses against virus and tumor in syrian hamster model. *Clin Cancer Res* 2017;23:239–249.

412. Li L, Woo YY, de Bruyne JA, et al. Epidemiology, clinical presentation and respiratory sequelae of adenovirus pneumonia in children in Kuala Lumpur, Malaysia. *PLoS One* 2018;13:e0205795.
413. Li P, Yang L, Guo J, et al. Circulation of HAdV-41 with diverse genome types and recombination in acute gastroenteritis among children in Shanghai. *Sci Rep* 2017;7:3548.
414. Li D, Zhou JN, Li H, et al. An outbreak of epidemic keratoconjunctivitis caused by human adenovirus type 8 in primary school, southwest China. *BMC Infect Dis* 2019;19:624.
415. Lichtenstein DL, Toth K, Doronin K, et al. Functions and mechanisms of action of the adenovirus E3 proteins. *Int Rev Immunol* 2004;23:75–111.
416. Lin L, Hanson CV, Alter HJ, et al. Inactivation of viruses in platelet concentrates by photochemical treatment with amotosalen and long-wavelength ultraviolet light. *Transfusion* 2005;45:580–590.
417. Lin GL, Lu CY, Chen JM, et al. Molecular epidemiology and clinical features of adenovirus infection in Taiwanese children, 2014. *J Microbiol Immunol Infect* 2019;52:215–224.
418. Lin YC, Lu PL, Lin KH, et al. Molecular epidemiology and phylogenetic analysis of human adenovirus caused an outbreak in Taiwan during 2011. *PLoS One* 2015;10:e0127377.
419. Lin MR, Yang SL, Gong YN, et al. Clinical and molecular features of adenovirus type 2, 3, and 7 infections in children in an outbreak in Taiwan, 2011. *Clin Microbiol Infect* 2017;23:110–116.
420. Lindemans CA, Leen AM, Boelens JJ. How I treat adenovirus in hematopoietic stem cell transplant recipients. *Blood* 2010;116:5476–5485.
421. Lindfors K, Lin J, Lee HS, et al. Metagenomics of the faecal virome indicate a cumulative effect of enterovirus and gluten amount on the risk of coeliac disease autoimmunity in genetically at risk children: the TEDDY study. *Gut* 2020;69(8):1416–1422.
422. Lion T. Adenovirus infections in immunocompetent and immunocompromised patients. *Clin Microbiol Rev* 2014;27:441–462.
423. Lion T. Adenovirus persistence, reactivation and clinical management. *FEBS Lett* 2019;593(24):3571–3582.
424. Lion T, Baumgartinger R, Watzinger F, et al. Molecular monitoring of adenovirus in peripheral blood after allogeneic bone marrow transplantation permits early diagnosis of disseminated disease. *Blood* 2003;102:1114–1120.
425. Lion T, Kosulin K, Landlinger C, et al. Monitoring of adenovirus load in stool by real-time PCR permits early detection of impending invasive infection in patients after allogeneic stem cell transplantation. *Leukemia* 2010;24:706–714.
426. Liu EB, Ferreyra L, Fischer SL, et al. Genetic analysis of a novel human adenovirus with a serologically unique hexon and a recombinant fiber gene. *PLoS One* 2011;6:e24491.
427. Liu M, Mallory GB, Schecter MG, et al. Long-term impact of respiratory viral infection after pediatric lung transplantation. *Pediatr Transplant* 2010;14:431–436.
428. Liu L, Oza S, Hogan D, et al. Global, regional, and national causes of under-5 mortality in 2000-15: an updated systematic analysis with implications for the Sustainable Development Goals. *Lancet* 2016;388:3027–3035.
429. Liu L, Qian Y, Zhang Y, et al. Adenoviruses associated with acute diarrhea in children in Beijing, China. *PLoS One* 2014;9:e88791.
430. Liu C, Wang Y, Wu C, et al. Dioscin's antiviral effect in vitro. *Virus Res* 2013;172:9–14.
431. Liu M, Worley S, Arrigain S, et al. Respiratory viral infections within one year after pediatric lung transplant. *Transpl Infect Dis* 2009;11:304–312.
432. Liu T, Zhou Z, Tian X, et al. A recombinant trivalent vaccine candidate against human adenovirus types 3, 7, and 55. *Vaccine* 2018;36:2199–2206.
433. Lopez SMC, Michaels MG, Green M. Adenovirus infection in pediatric transplant recipients: are effective antiviral agents coming our way? *Curr Opin Organ Transplant* 2018;23:395–399.
434. Lopez-Gordo E, Doszpoly A, Duffy MR, et al. Defining a novel role for the coxsackievirus and adenovirus receptor in human adenovirus serotype 5 transduction in vitro in the presence of mouse serum. *J Virol* 2017;91.
435. Lugthart G, Oomen MA, Jol-van der Zijde CM, et al. The effect of cidofovir on adenovirus plasma DNA levels in stem cell transplantation recipients without T cell reconstitution. *Biol Blood Marrow Transplant* 2015;21:293–299.
436. Lukashev AN, Ivanova OE, Eremeeva TP, et al. Evidence of frequent recombination among human adenoviruses. *J Gen Virol* 2008;89:380–388.
437. Lynch JP III, Fishbein M, Echavarria M. Adenovirus. *Semin Respir Crit Care Med* 2011;32:494–511.
438. Lynch JP III, Kajon AE. Adenovirus: epidemiology, global spread of novel serotypes, and advances in treatment and prevention. *Semin Respir Crit Care Med* 2016;37:586–602.
439. Mackowiak M, Leifels M, Hamza IA, et al. Distribution of *Escherichia coli*, coliphages and enteric viruses in water, epilithic biofilms and sediments of an urban river in Germany. *Sci Total Environ* 2018;626:650–659.
440. Madisch I, Harste G, Pommer H, et al. Phylogenetic analysis of the main neutralization and hemagglutination determinants of all human adenovirus prototypes as a basis for molecular classification and taxonomy. *J Virol* 2005;79:15265–15276.
441. Mahadevan P, Seto J, Tibbetts C, et al. Natural variants of human adenovirus type 3 provide evidence for relative genome stability across time and geographic space. *Virology* 2010;397:113–118.
442. Mahmoudi S, Banar M, Pourakbari B, et al. Identification of etiologic agents of the pertussis-like syndrome in children by real-time PCR method. *Prague Med Rep* 2018;119:61–69.
443. Mahon J, Blair GE, Wood GM, et al. Is persistent adenovirus 12 infection involved in coeliac disease? A search for viral DNA using the polymerase chain reaction. *Gut* 1991;32:1114–1116.
444. Majorant D, Qiu F, Kalil AC, et al. Adenovirus—a deadly disease in the solid organ transplant population: risk factors and outcomes. *Transplant Proc* 2018;50:3769–3774.
445. Maler MD, Nielsen PJ, Stichling N, et al. Key role of the scavenger receptor MARCO in mediating adenovirus infection and subsequent innate responses of macrophages. *MBio* 2017;8(4):e00670-17.
446. Mallery DL, McEwan WA, Bidgood SR, et al. Antibodies mediate intracellular immunity through tripartite motif-containing 21 (TRIM21). *Proc Natl Acad Sci U S A* 2010;107:19985–19990.
447. Mameli C, Zuccotti GV. The impact of viral infections in children with community-acquired pneumonia. *Curr Infect Dis Rep* 2013;15:197–202.
448. Marrugal-Lorenzo JA, Serna-Gallego A, Berastegui-Cabrera J, et al. Repositioning salicylanilide anthelmintic drugs to treat adenovirus infections. *Sci Rep* 2019;9:17.
449. Martinez-Aguado P, Serna-Gallego A, Marrugal-Lorenzo JA, et al. Antiadenovirus drug discovery: potential targets and evaluation methodologies. *Drug Discov Today* 2015;20:1235–1242.
450. Martinez-Velez N, Xipell E, Vera B, et al. The oncolytic adenovirus VCN-01 as therapeutic approach against pediatric osteosarcoma. *Clin Cancer Res* 2016;22:2217–2225.
451. Mast TC, Kierstead L, Gupta SB, et al. International epidemiology of human pre-existing adenovirus (Ad) type-5, type-6, type-26 and type-36 neutralizing antibodies: correlates of high Ad5 titers and implications for potential HIV vaccine trials. *Vaccine* 2010;28:950–957.
452. Matsushima Y, Shimizu H, Kano A, et al. Novel human adenovirus strain, Bangladesh. *Emerg Infect Dis* 2012;18:846–848.
453. Matsushima Y, Shimizu H, Kano A, et al. Genome sequence of a novel virus of the species human adenovirus d associated with acute gastroenteritis. *Genome Announc* 2013;1:e00068-12.
454. Matthes-Martin S, Boztug H, Lion T. Diagnosis and treatment of adenovirus infection in immunocompromised patients. *Expert Rev Anti Infect Ther* 2013;11:1017–1028.
455. Matthes-Martin S, Feuchtinger T, Shaw PJ, et al. European guidelines for diagnosis and treatment of adenovirus infection in leukemia and stem cell transplantation: summary of ECIL-4 (2011). *Transpl Infect Dis* 2012;14:555–563.
456. Matthews K, Noker PE, Tian B, et al. Identifying the safety profile of Ad5.SSTR/TK.RGD, a novel infectivity-enhanced bicistronic adenovirus, in anticipation of a phase I clinical trial in patients with recurrent ovarian cancer. *Clin Cancer Res* 2009;15:4131–4137.
457. Mattner F, Sykora KW, Meissner B, et al. An adenovirus type F41 outbreak in a pediatric bone marrow transplant unit: analysis of clinical impact and preventive strategies. *Pediatr Infect Dis J* 2008;27:419–424.
458. May LJ, Patton DJ, Fruitman DS. The evolving approach to paediatric myocarditis: a review of the current literature. *Cardiol Young* 2011;21:241–251.
459. Mazzotta S, Marrugal-Lorenzo JA, Vega-Holm M, et al. Optimization of piperazine-derived ureas privileged structures for effective antiadenovirus agents. *Eur J Med Chem* 2020;185:111840.
460. McCarthy T, Lebeck MG, Capuano AW, et al. Molecular typing of clinical adenovirus specimens by an algorithm which permits detection of adenovirus coinfections and intermediate adenovirus strains. *J Clin Virol* 2009;46:80–84.
461. McMillen T, Lee YJ, Kamboj M, et al. Limited diagnostic value of a multiplexed gastrointestinal pathogen panel for the detection of adenovirus infection in an oncology patient population. *J Clin Virol* 2017;94:37–41.
462. McNees AL, Gooding LR. Adenoviral inhibitors of apoptotic cell death. *Virus Res* 2002;88:87–101.
463. McNeil MM, Paradowska-Stankiewicz I, Miller ER, et al. Adverse events following adenovirus type 4 and type 7 vaccine, live, oral in the Vaccine Adverse Event Reporting System (VAERS), United States, October 2011-July 2018. *Vaccine* 2019;37:6760–6767.
464. Meena JP, Phillips RS, Kinsey S. Brincidofovir as a salvage therapy in controlling adenoviremia in pediatric recipients of hematopoietic stem cell transplant. *J Pediatr Hematol Oncol* 2019;41:e467–e472.
465. Mehta V, Chou PC, Picken MM. Adenovirus disease in six small bowel, kidney and heart transplant recipients; pathology and clinical outcome. *Virchows Arch* 2015;467:603–608.
466. Mesri EA, Feitelson MA, Munger K. Human viral oncogenesis: a cancer hallmarks analysis. *Cell Host Microbe* 2014;15:266–282.
467. Metzgar D, Gibbins C, Hudson NR, et al. Evaluation of multiplex type-specific real-time PCR assays using the LightCycler and joint biological agent identification and diagnostic system platforms for detection and quantitation of adult human respiratory adenoviruses. *J Clin Microbiol* 2010;48:1397–1403.
468. Metzgar D, Osuna M, Kajon AE, et al. Abrupt emergence of diverse species B adenoviruses at US military recruit training centers. *J Infect Dis* 2007;196:1465–1473.
469. Mi Z, Butt AM, An X, et al. Genomic analysis of HAdV-B14 isolate from the outbreak of febrile respiratory infection in China. *Genomics* 2013;102:448–455.
470. Miller JL, Harman C, Weiner C, et al. Perinatal outcomes after second trimester detection of amniotic fluid viral genome in asymptomatic patients. *J Perinat Med* 2009;37:140–143.
471. Mitchell LS, Taylor B, Reimels W, et al. Adenovirus 7a: a community-acquired outbreak in a children's hospital. *Pediatr Infect Dis J* 2000;19:996–1000.
472. Miteva K, Pappritz K, Sosnowski M, et al. Mesenchymal stromal cells inhibit NLRP3 inflammasome activation in a model of Coxsackievirus B3-induced inflammatory cardiomyopathy. *Sci Rep* 2018;8:2820.
473. Miura Y, Yamasaki S, Davydova J, et al. Infectivity-selective oncolytic adenovirus developed by high-throughput screening of adenovirus-formatted library. *Mol Ther* 2013;21:139–148.
474. Mohamed MS, Abd El-Hameed RH, Sayed AI, et al. Novel antiviral compounds against gastroenteric viral infections. *Arch Pharm (Weinheim)* 2015;348:194–205.
475. Mohamed Ismail A, Zhou X, Dyer DW, et al. Genomic foundations of evolution and ocular pathogenesis in human adenovirus species D. *FEBS Lett* 2019;593:3583–3608.
476. Montes-Galindo DA, Espiritu-Mojarro AC, Melnikov V, et al. Adenovirus 5 produces obesity and adverse metabolic, morphological, and functional changes in the long term in animals fed a balanced diet or a high-fat diet: a study on hamsters. *Arch Virol* 2019;164:775–786.
477. Mori Y, Miyamoto T, Kato K, et al. Different risk factors related to adenovirus- or BK virus-associated hemorrhagic cystitis following allogeneic stem cell transplantation. *Biol Blood Marrow Transplant* 2012;18:458–465.
478. Moulik M, Breinholt JP, Dreyer WJ, et al. Viral endomyocardial infection is an independent predictor and potentially treatable risk factor for graft loss and coronary vasculopathy in pediatric cardiac transplant recipients. *J Am Coll Cardiol* 2010;56:582–592.

479. Moyo SJ, Hanevik K, Blomberg B, et al. Prevalence and molecular characterisation of human adenovirus in diarrhoeic children in Tanzania; a case control study. *BMC Infect Dis* 2014;14:666.
480. Mozaffarian D, Hao T, Rimm EB, et al. Changes in diet and lifestyle and long-term weight gain in women and men. *N Engl J Med* 2011;364:2392–2404.
481. Mufti NA, Erickson AC, North AK, et al. Treatment of whole blood (WB) and red blood cells (RBC) with S-303 inactivates pathogens and retains in vitro quality of stored RBC. *Biologicals* 2010;38:14–19.
482. Muller MP, Siddiqui N, Ivancic R, et al. Adenovirus-related epidemic keratoconjunctivitis outbreak at a hospital-affiliated ophthalmology clinic. *Am J Infect Control* 2018;46:581–583.
483. Muncheberg S, Hay RT, Ip WH, et al. E1B-55K-mediated regulation of RNF4 SUMO-targeted ubiquitin ligase promotes human adenovirus gene expression. *J Virol* 2018;92.
484. Musso D, Richard V, Broult J, et al. Inactivation of dengue virus in plasma with amotosalen and ultraviolet A illumination. *Transfusion* 2014;54:2924–2930.
485. Myers GD, Bollard CM, Wu MF, et al. Reconstitution of adenovirus-specific cell-mediated immunity in pediatric patients after hematopoietic stem cell transplantation. *Bone Marrow Transplant* 2007;39:677–686.
486. Mynarek M, Ganzenmueller T, Mueller-Heine A, et al. Patient, virus, and treatment-related risk factors in pediatric adenovirus infection after stem cell transplantation: results of a routine monitoring program. *Biol Blood Marrow Transplant* 2014;20:250–256.
487. Na HN, Nam JH. Proof-of-concept for a virus-induced obesity vaccine; vaccination against the obesity agent adenovirus 36. *Int J Obes (Lond)* 2014;38:1470–1474.
488. Naesens L, Lenaerts L, Andrei G, et al. Antiadenovirus activities of several classes of nucleoside and nucleotide analogues. *Antimicrob Agents Chemother* 2005;49:1010–1016.
489. Nakamura H, Fujisawa T, Suga S, et al. Species differences in circulation and inflammatory responses in children with common respiratory adenovirus infections. *J Med Virol* 2018;90:873–880.
490. Nascimento MA, Magri ME, Schissi CD, et al. Recombinant adenovirus as a model to evaluate the efficiency of free chlorine disinfection in filtered water samples. *Virol J* 2015;12:30.
491. Nebbia G, Chawla A, Schutten M, et al. Adenovirus viraemia and dissemination unresponsive to antiviral therapy in advanced HIV-1 infection. *AIDS* 2005;19:1339–1340.
492. Nemerow G, Flint J. Lessons learned from adenovirus (1970-2019). *FEBS Lett* 2019;593:3395–3418.
493. Nestic D, Uil TG, Ma J, et al. $\alpha_v\beta_5$ Integrin is required for efficient infection of epithelial cells with human adenovirus type 26. *J Virol* 2019;93(1):e01474-18.
494. Nevels M, Tauber B, Spruss T, et al. "Hit-and-run" transformation by adenovirus oncogenes. *J Virol* 2001;75:3089–3094.
495. Neville JS, Bunning M, Lyons A, et al. Challenges associated with the emergence of adenovirus type 14 at US military training centers. *Mil Med* 2008;173:iv–vii.
496. Niang MN, Diop NS, Fall A, et al. Respiratory viruses in patients with influenza-like illness in Senegal: focus on human respiratory adenoviruses. *PLoS One* 2017;12:e0174287.
497. Nicklin SA, Wu E, Nemerow GR, et al. The influence of adenovirus fiber structure and function on vector development for gene therapy. *Mol Ther* 2005;12:384–393.
498. Nicoll MP, Hann W, Shivkumar M, et al. The HSV-1 latency-associated transcript functions to repress latent phase lytic gene expression and suppress virus reactivation from latently infected neurons. *PLoS Pathog* 2016;12:e1005539.
499. Nilsson EC, Storm RJ, Bauer J, et al. The GD1a glycan is a cellular receptor for adenoviruses causing epidemic keratoconjunctivitis. *Nat Med* 2011;17:105–109.
500. O'Brien KL, Liu J, King SL, et al. Adenovirus-specific immunity after immunization with an Ad5 HIV-1 vaccine candidate in humans. *Nat Med* 2009;15:873–875.
501. O'Reilly RJ, Prockop S, Hasan AN, et al. Virus-specific T-cell banks for 'off the shelf' adoptive therapy of refractory infections. *Bone Marrow Transplant* 2016;51:1163–1172.
502. Ohrmalm L, Lindblom A, Omar H, et al. Evaluation of a surveillance strategy for early detection of adenovirus by PCR of peripheral blood in hematopoietic SCT recipients: incidence and outcome. *Bone Marrow Transplant* 2011;46:267–272.
503. Oliveira ERA, Bouvier M. Immune evasion by adenoviruses: a window into host-virus adaptation. *FEBS Lett* 2019;593:3496–3503.
504. Omar H, Yun Z, Lewensohn-Fuchs I, et al. Poor outcome of adenovirus infections in adult hematopoietic stem cell transplant patients with sustained adenovirus viremia. *Transpl Infect Dis* 2010;12:465–469.
505. Ortiz-Zapater E, Santis G, Parsons M. CAR: a key regulator of adhesion and inflammation. *Int J Biochem Cell Biol* 2017;89:1–5.
506. Osborne CM, Montano AC, Robinson CC, et al. Viral gastroenteritis in children in Colorado 2006-2009. *J Med Virol* 2015;87:931–939.
507. Oyong K, Killerby M, Pan CY, et al. Outbreak of epidemic keratoconjunctivitis caused by human adenovirus type D53 in an eye care clinic—Los Angeles County, 2017. *MMWR Morb Mortal Wkly Rep* 2018;67:1347–1349.
508. Papadopoulou A, Gerdemann U, Katari UL, et al. Activity of broad-spectrum T cells as treatment for AdV, EBV, CMV, BKV, and HHV6 infections after HSCT. *Sci Transl Med* 2014;6:242ra83.
509. Pappritz K, Savvatis K, Miteva K, et al. Immunomodulation by adoptive regulatory T-cell transfer improves Coxsackievirus B3-induced myocarditis. *FASEB J* 2018:fj201701408R.
510. Park JY, Kim BJ, Lee EJ, et al. Clinical features and courses of adenovirus pneumonia in healthy young adults during an outbreak among Korean military personnel. *PLoS One* 2017;12:e0170592.
511. Park CK, Kwon H, Park JY. Thin-section computed tomography findings in 104 immunocompetent patients with adenovirus pneumonia. *Acta Radiol* 2017;58:937–943.
512. Patel RR, Hodinka RL, Kajon AE, et al. A case of adenovirus viremia in a pediatric liver transplant recipient with neutropenia and lymphopenia: who and when should we treat? *J Pediatric Infect Dis Soc* 2015;4:e1–e5.
513. Paulsen GC, Danziger-Isakov L. Respiratory viral infections in solid organ and hematopoietic stem cell transplantation. *Clin Chest Med* 2017;38:707–726.
514. Pauly M, Hoppe E, Mugisha L, et al. High prevalence and diversity of species D adenoviruses (HAdV-D) in human populations of four Sub-Saharan countries. *Virol J* 2014;11:25.
515. Pavia AT. Viral infections of the lower respiratory tract: old viruses, new viruses, and the role of diagnosis. *Clin Infect Dis* 2011;52 Suppl 4:S284–S289.
516. Pennington MR, Saha A, Painter DF, et al. Disparate entry of adenoviruses dictates differential innate immune responses on the ocular surface. *Microorganisms* 2019;7(9):351.
517. Pepose JS, Ahuja A, Liu W, et al. Randomized, controlled, phase 2 trial of povidone-iodine/dexamethasone ophthalmic suspension for treatment of adenoviral conjunctivitis. *Am J Ophthalmol* 2018;194:7–15.
518. Pereira L. Congenital viral infection: traversing the uterine-placental interface. *Annu Rev Virol* 2018;5:273–299.
519. Petrikovsky BM, Lipson SM, Kaplan MH. Viral studies on amniotic fluid from fetuses with and without abnormalities detected by prenatal sonography. *J Reprod Med* 2003;48:230–232.
520. Pham NT, Ushijima H, Thongprachum A, et al. Multiplex PCR for the detection of 10 viruses causing encephalitis/encephalopathy and its application to clinical samples collected from Japanese children with suspected viral. *Clin Lab* 2017;63:91–100.
521. Piatti G. Pre-transplant screening for latent adenovirus in donors and recipients. *Open Microbiol J* 2016;10:4–11.
522. Pilankatta R, Chawla T, Khanna N, et al. The prevalence of antibodies to adenovirus serotype 5 in an adult Indian population and implications for adenovirus vector vaccines. *J Med Virol* 2010;82:407–414.
523. Pimenta AI, Guerreiro D, Madureira J, et al. Tracking human adenovirus inactivation by gamma radiation under different environmental conditions. *Appl Environ Microbiol* 2016;82:5166–5173.
524. Pimenta AI, Margaca FMA, Cabo Verde S. Virucidal activity of gamma radiation on strawberries and raspberries. *Int J Food Microbiol* 2019;304:89–96.
525. Pinchoff RJ, Kaufman SS, Magid MS, et al. Adenovirus infection in pediatric small bowel transplantation recipients. *Transplantation* 2003;76:183–189.
526. Plot L, Amital H. Infectious associations of Celiac disease. *Autoimmun Rev* 2009;8:316–319.
527. Plummer M, de Martel C, Vignat J, et al. Global burden of cancers attributable to infections in 2012: a synthetic analysis. *Lancet Glob Health* 2016;4:e609–e616.
528. Popowitch EB, O'Neill SS, Miller MB. Comparison of the Biofire FilmArray RP, Genmark eSensor RVP, Luminex xTAG RVPv1, and Luminex xTAG RVP fast multiplex assays for detection of respiratory viruses. *J Clin Microbiol* 2013;51:1528–1533.
529. Pozzuto T, Roger C, Kurreck J, et al. Enhanced suppression of adenovirus replication by triple combination of anti-adenoviral siRNAs, soluble adenovirus receptor trap sCAR-Fc and cidofovir. *Antiviral Res* 2015;120:72–78.
530. Primo D, Pacheco GT, Timenetsky M, et al. Surveillance and molecular characterization of human adenovirus in patients with acute gastroenteritis in the era of rotavirus vaccine, Brazil, 2012-2017. *J Clin Virol* 2018;109:35–40.
531. Prince GA, Porter DD, Jenson AB, et al. Pathogenesis of adenovirus type 5 pneumonia in cotton rats (Sigmodon hispidus). *J Virol* 1993;67:101–111.
532. Proenca-Modena JL, de Souza Cardoso R, Criado MF, et al. Human adenovirus replication and persistence in hypertrophic adenoids and palatine tonsils in children. *J Med Virol* 2019;91:1250–1262.
533. Prusinkiewicz MA, Mymryk JS. Metabolic reprogramming of the host cell by human adenovirus infection. *Viruses* 2019;11(2):141.
534. Przybylski M, Rynans S, Waszczuk-Gajda A, et al. Sequence typing of human adenoviruses isolated from Polish patients subjected to allogeneic hematopoietic stem cell transplantation—a single center experience. *Hematology* 2018;23:633–638.
535. Qasim W, Derniame S, Gilmour K, et al. Third-party virus-specific T cells eradicate adenoviraemia but trigger bystander graft-versus-host disease. *Br J Haematol* 2011;154:150–153.
536. Qasim W, Gilmour K, Zhan H, et al. Interferon-gamma capture T cell therapy for persistent adenoviraemia following allogeneic haematopoietic stem cell transplantation. *Br J Haematol* 2013;161:449–452.
537. Qian C, Campidelli A, Wang Y, et al. Curative or pre-emptive adenovirus-specific T cell transfer from matched unrelated or third party haploidentical donors after HSCT, including UCB transplantations: a successful phase I/II multicenter clinical trial. *J Hematol Oncol* 2017;10:102.
538. Qian C, Wang Y, Reppel L, et al. Viral-specific T-cell transfer from HSCT donor for the treatment of viral infections or diseases after HSCT. *Bone Marrow Transplant* 2018;53:114–122.
539. Qiu Y, Li Q, Lee BE, et al. UV inactivation of human infectious viruses at two full-scale wastewater treatment plants in Canada. *Water Res* 2018;147:73–81.
540. Qiu FZ, Shen XX, Li GX, et al. Adenovirus associated with acute diarrhea: a case-control study. *BMC Infect Dis* 2018;18:450.
541. Qiu FZ, Shen XX, Zhao MC, et al. A triplex quantitative real-time PCR assay for differential detection of human adenovirus serotypes 2, 3 and 7. *Virol J* 2018;15:81.
542. Quenelle DC, Collins DJ, Pettway LR, et al. Effect of oral treatment with (S)-HPMPA, HDP-(S)-HPMPA or ODE-(S)-HPMPA on replication of murine cytomegalovirus (MCMV) or human cytomegalovirus (HCMV) in animal models. *Antiviral Res* 2008;79:133–135.
543. Qurei L, Seto D, Salah Z, et al. A molecular epidemiology survey of respiratory adenoviruses circulating in children residing in Southern Palestine. *PLoS One* 2012;7:e42732.
544. Rachmadi AT, Kitajima M, Kato T, et al. Required chlorination doses to fulfill the credit value for disinfection of enteric viruses in water: a critical review. *Environ Sci Technol* 2020;54(4):2068–2077.
545. Racicot K, Mor G. Risks associated with viral infections during pregnancy. *J Clin Invest* 2017;127:1591–1599.
546. Radin JM, Hawksworth AW, Blair PJ, et al. Dramatic decline of respiratory illness among US military recruits after the renewed use of adenovirus vaccines. *Clin Infect Dis* 2014;59:962–968.
547. Radke JR, Cook JL. Human adenovirus infections: update and consideration of mechanisms of viral persistence. *Curr Opin Infect Dis* 2018;31:251–256.
548. Radke JR, Yong SL, Cook JL. Low-level expression of the E1B 20-kilodalton protein by adenovirus 14p1 enhances viral immunopathogenesis. *J Virol* 2016;90:497–505.

549. Rahimi N. Defenders and challengers of endothelial barrier function. *Front Immunol* 2017;8:1847.
550. Ramsay ID, Attwood C, Irish D, et al. Disseminated adenovirus infection after allogeneic stem cell transplant and the potential role of brincidofovir—case series and 10 year experience of management in an adult transplant cohort. *J Clin Virol* 2017;96:73–79.
551. Ranucci-Weiss D, Uerpairojkit B, Bowles N, et al. Intrauterine adenoviral infection associated with fetal non-immune hydrops. *Prenat Diagn* 1998;18:182–185.
552. Ratto-Kim S, Yoon IK, Paris RM, et al. The US military commitment to vaccine development: a century of successes and challenges. *Front Immunol* 2018;9:1397.
553. Rayne F, Wittkop L, Bader C, et al. Rapid Adenovirus typing method for species identification. *J Virol Methods* 2017;249:156–160.
554. Razzano D, Fallon JT. Myocarditis: somethings old and something new. *Cardiovasc Pathol* 2020;44:107155.
555. Renzi S, Ali S, Portwine C, et al. Adenovirus infection in children with acute myeloid leukemia: a report from the Canadian Infection in Acute Myeloid Leukemia Research Group. *Pediatr Infect Dis J* 2018;37:135–137.
556. Rigotto C, Hanley K, Rochelle PA, et al. Survival of adenovirus types 2 and 41 in surface and ground waters measured by a plaque assay. *Environ Sci Technol* 2011;45:4145–4150.
557. Rivailler P, Mao N, Zhu Z, et al. Recombination analysis of Human mastadenovirus C whole genomes. *Sci Rep* 2019;9:2182.
558. Roberts DM, Nanda A, Havenga MJ, et al. Hexon-chimaeric adenovirus serotype 5 vectors circumvent pre-existing anti-vector immunity. *Nature* 2006;441:239–243.
559. Robinson CM, Rajaiya J, Walsh MP, et al. Computational analysis of human adenovirus type 22 provides evidence for recombination among species D human adenoviruses in the penton base gene. *J Virol* 2009;83:8980–8985.
560. Robinson CM, Seto D, Jones MS, et al. Molecular evolution of human species D adenoviruses. *Infect Genet Evol* 2011;11:1208–1217.
561. Robinson CM, Singh G, Henquell C, et al. Computational analysis and identification of an emergent human adenovirus pathogen implicated in a respiratory fatality. *Virology* 2011;409:141–147.
562. Robinson CM, Singh G, Lee JY, et al. Molecular evolution of human adenoviruses. *Sci Rep* 2013;3:1812.
563. Roch N, Salameire D, Gressin R, et al. Fatal adenoviral and enteroviral infections and an Epstein-Barr virus positive large B-cell lymphoma after alemtuzumab treatment in a patient with refractory Sezary syndrome. *Scand J Infect Dis* 2008;40:343–346.
564. Rodriguez E, Ip WH, Kolbe V, et al. Humanized mice reproduce acute and persistent human adenovirus infection. *J Infect Dis* 2017;215:70–79.
565. Rodriguez E, Romero C, Rio A, et al. Short-fiber protein of ad40 confers enteric tropism and protection against acidic gastrointestinal conditions. *Hum Gene Ther Methods* 2013;24:195–204.
566. Rogers AE, Lu X, Killerby M, et al. Outbreak of acute respiratory illness associated with adenovirus type 4 at the U.S. Naval Academy, 2016. *MSMR* 2019;26:21–27.
567. Romanowski EG, Bartels SP, Vogel R, et al. Feasibility of an antiviral clinical trial requiring cross-country shipment of conjunctival adenovirus cultures and recovery of infectious virus. *Curr Eye Res* 2004;29:195–199.
568. Romanowski EG, Gordon YJ. Update on antiviral treatment of adenoviral ocular infections. *Am J Ophthalmol* 2008;146:635–637.
569. Romanowski EG, Yates KA, Gordon YJ. The in vitro and in vivo evaluation of ddC as a topical antiviral for ocular adenovirus infections. *Invest Ophthalmol Vis Sci* 2009;50:5295–5299.
570. Ronan BA, Agrwal N, Carey EJ, et al. Fulminant hepatitis due to human adenovirus. *Infection* 2014;42:105–111.
571. Rowe WP, Huebner RJ, Gilmore LK, et al. Isolation of a cytopathogenic agent from human adenoids undergoing spontaneous degeneration in tissue culture. *Proc Soc Exp Biol Med* 1953;84:570–573.
572. Roy S, Calcedo R, Medina-Jaszek A, et al. Adenoviruses in lymphocytes of the human gastro-intestinal tract. *PLoS One* 2011;6:e24859.
573. Roy S, Vandenberghe LH, Kryazhimskiy S, et al. Isolation and characterization of adenoviruses persistently shed from the gastrointestinal tract of non-human primates. *PLoS Pathog* 2009;5:e1000503.
574. Russell KL, Broderick MP, Franklin SE, et al. Transmission dynamics and prospective environmental sampling of adenovirus in a military recruit setting. *J Infect Dis* 2006;194:877–885.
575. Rutala WA, Peacock JE, Gergen MF, et al. Efficacy of hospital germicides against adenovirus 8, a common cause of epidemic keratoconjunctivitis in health care facilities. *Antimicrob Agents Chemother* 2006;50:1419–1424.
576. Saiki-Macedo S, Valverde-Ezeta J, Cornejo-Tapia A, et al. Identification of viral and bacterial etiologic agents of the pertussis-like syndrome in children under 5 years old hospitalized. *BMC Infect Dis* 2019;19:75.
577. Sakrani N, Almazrouei S, Mohan S, et al. Adenovirus as a rare cause of acute necrotising encephalitis. *BMJ Case Rep* 2019;12(12):e232338.
578. Salinas S, Junyent F, Core N, et al. What is CAR doing in the middle of the adult neurogenic road? *Neurogenesis (Austin)* 2017;4:e1304790.
579. Salzwedel AO, Han J, LaRocca CJ, et al. Combination of interferon-expressing oncolytic adenovirus with chemotherapy and radiation is highly synergistic in hamster model of pancreatic cancer. *Oncotarget* 2018;9:18041–18052.
580. Sammons JS, Graf EH, Townsend S, et al. Outbreak of adenovirus in a neonatal intensive care unit: critical importance of equipment cleaning during inpatient ophthalmologic examinations. *Ophthalmology* 2019;126:137–143.
581. Sanchez-Cespedes J, Marrugal-Lorenzo JA, Martin-Gandul C, et al. T-cells immune response controls the high incidence of adenovirus infection in adult allogenic hematopoietic transplantation recipients. *Haematologica* 2021;106(1):275–278.
582. Sanchez-Cespedes J, Martinez-Aguado P, Vega-Holm M, et al. New 4-acyl-1-phenylaminocarbonyl-2-phenylpiperazine derivatives as potential inhibitors of adenovirus infection. synthesis, biological evaluation, and structure-activity relationships. *J Med Chem* 2016;59:5432–5448.
583. Sanchez-Prieto R, de Alava E, Palomino T, et al. An association between viral genes and human oncogenic alterations: the adenovirus E1A induces the Ewing tumor fusion transcript EWS-FLI1. *Nat Med* 1999;5:1076–1079.
584. Santa Maria F, Laughhunn A, Lanteri MC, et al. Inactivation of Zika virus in platelet components using amotosalen and ultraviolet A illumination. *Transfusion* 2017;57:2016–2025.
585. Savon C, Acosta B, Valdes O, et al. A myocarditis outbreak with fatal cases associated with adenovirus subgenera C among children from Havana City in 2005. *J Clin Virol* 2008;43:152–157.
586. Schaar K, Roger C, Pozzuto T, et al. Biological antivirals for treatment of adenovirus infections. *Antivir Ther* 2016;21:559–566.
587. Schaberg KB, Kambham N, Sibley RK, et al. Adenovirus hepatitis: clinicopathologic analysis of 12 consecutive cases from a single institution. *Am J Surg Pathol* 2017;41:810–819.
588. Schmidt S, Tramsen L, Rais B, et al. Natural killer cells as a therapeutic tool for infectious diseases—current status and future perspectives. *Oncotarget* 2018;9:20891–20907.
589. Schmitt A, Tonn T, Busch DH, et al. Adoptive transfer and selective reconstitution of streptamer-selected cytomegalovirus-specific CD8+ T cells leads to virus clearance in patients after allogeneic peripheral blood stem cell transplantation. *Transfusion* 2011;51:591–599.
590. Schneider-Brachert W, Tchikov V, Merkel O, et al. Inhibition of TNF receptor 1 internalization by adenovirus 14.7K as a novel immune escape mechanism. *J Clin Invest* 2006;116:2901–2913.
591. Schneidewind L, Neumann T, Schmidt CA, et al. Comparison of intravenous or intravesical cidofovir in the treatment of BK polyomavirus-associated hemorrhagic cystitis following adult allogeneic stem cell transplantation—a systematic review. *Transpl Infect Dis* 2018;20:e12914.
592. Schnurr D, Bollen A, Crawford-Miksza L, et al. Adenovirus mixture isolated from the brain of an AIDS patient with encephalitis. *J Med Virol* 1995;47:168–171.
593. Schreiner S, Burck C, Glass M, et al. Control of human adenovirus type 5 gene expression by cellular Daxx/ATRX chromatin-associated complexes. *Nucleic Acids Res* 2013;41:3532–3550.
594. Schultze-Florey RE, Tischer S, Kuhnau W, et al. Persistent recipient-derived human adenovirus (HAdV)-specific T cells promote HAdV control after allogeneic hematopoietic stem cell transplantation. *Bone Marrow Transplant* 2017;52:609–611.
595. Schultze-Florey RE, Tischer-Zimmermann S, Heuft HG, et al. Transfer of Hexon and Penton selected adenovirus-specific T cells for refractory adenovirus infection after haploidentical stem cell transplantation. *Transpl Infect Dis* 2020;22(1):e13201.
596. Schwartz KL, Richardson SE, MacGregor D, et al. Adenovirus-associated central nervous system disease in children. *J Pediatr* 2019;205:130–137.
597. Scott MK, Chommanard C, Lu X, et al. Human adenovirus associated with severe respiratory infection, Oregon, USA, 2013-2014. *Emerg Infect Dis* 2016;22:1044–1051.
598. Sedlacek P, Petterson T, Robin M, et al. Incidence of adenovirus infection in hematopoietic stem cell transplantation recipients: findings from the AdVance Study. *Biol Blood Marrow Transplant* 2019;25:810–818.
599. Seidemann K, Heim A, Pfister ED, et al. Monitoring of adenovirus infection in pediatric transplant recipients by quantitative PCR: report of six cases and review of the literature. *Am J Transplant* 2004;4:2102–2108.
600. Serangeli C, Bicanic O, Scheible MH, et al. Ex vivo detection of adenovirus specific CD4+ T-cell responses to HLA-DR-epitopes of the Hexon protein show a contracted specificity of T(HELPER) cells following stem cell transplantation. *Virology* 2010;397:277–284.
601. Seregin SS, Aldhamen YA, Appledorn DM, et al. Use of DAF-displaying adenovirus vectors reduces induction of transgene- and vector-specific adaptive immune responses in mice. *Hum Gene Ther* 2011;22:1083–1094.
602. Serrano RM, Darragh RK, Parent JJ. Successful treatment of disseminated adenovirus infection with cidofovir and intravenous immunoglobulin in an infant following heart transplant. *Cardiol Young* 2018;28:888–889.
603. Sester M, Koebernick K, Owen D, et al. Conserved amino acids within the adenovirus 2 E3/19K protein differentially affect downregulation of MHC class I and MICA/B proteins. *J Immunol* 2010;184:255–267.
604. Sester M, Leboeuf C, Schmidt T, et al. The "ABC" of virus-specific T cell immunity in solid organ transplantation. *Am J Transplant* 2016;16:1697–1706.
605. Seto D, Chodosh J, Brister JR, et al.; Members of the Adenovirus Research Community. Using the whole-genome sequence to characterize and name human adenoviruses. *J Virol* 2011;85:5701–5702.
606. Seto J, Walsh MP, Mahadevan P, et al. Genomic and bioinformatics analyses of HAdV-14p, reference strain of a re-emerging respiratory pathogen and analysis of B1/B2. *Virus Res* 2009;143:94–105.
607. Seto J, Walsh MP, Metzgar D, et al. Computational analysis of adenovirus serotype 5 (HAdV-C5) from an HAdV coinfection shows genome stability after 45 years of circulation. *Virology* 2010;404:180–186.
608. Shachor-Meyouhas Y, Hadash A, Kra-Oz Z, et al. Adenovirus respiratory infection among immunocompetent patients in a pediatric intensive care unit during 10-year period: co-morbidity is common. *Isr Med Assoc J* 2019;21:595–598.
609. Shah DP, Ghantoji SS, Mulanovich VE, et al. Management of respiratory viral infections in hematopoietic cell transplant recipients. *Am J Blood Res* 2012;2:203–218.
610. Shang Q, Wang H, Song Y, et al. Serological data analyses show that adenovirus 36 infection is associated with obesity: a meta-analysis involving 5739 subjects. *Obesity (Silver Spring)* 2014;22:895–900.
611. Sharma A, Li X, Bangari DS, et al. Adenovirus receptors and their implications in gene delivery. *Virus Res* 2009;143:184–194.
612. Sharma P, Martis PC, Excoffon K. Adenovirus transduction: more complicated than receptor expression. *Virology* 2017;502:144–151.
613. Shastri AA, Hegde V, Peddibhotla S, et al. E4orf1: a protein for enhancing glucose uptake despite impaired proximal insulin signaling. *PLoS One* 2018;13:e0208427.
614. Shauer A, Gotsman I, Keren A, et al. Acute viral myocarditis: current concepts in diagnosis and treatment. *Isr Med Assoc J* 2013;15:180–185.
615. Shen CF, Wang SM, Wang JR, et al. Comparative study of clinical and epidemiological characteristics of major pediatric adenovirus epidemics in southern Taiwan. *BMC Infect Dis* 2019;19:681.

616. Shirali GS, Ni J, Chinnock RE, et al. Association of viral genome with graft loss in children after cardiac transplantation. *N Engl J Med* 2001;344:1498–1503.
617. Shirley JL, de Jong YP, Terhorst C, et al. Immune responses to viral gene therapy vectors. *Mol Ther* 2020;28:709–722.
618. Short JJ, Vasu C, Holterman MJ, et al. Members of adenovirus species B utilize CD80 and CD86 as cellular attachment receptors. *Virus Res* 2006;122:144–153.
619. Silasi M, Cardenas I, Kwon JY, et al. Viral infections during pregnancy. *Am J Reprod Immunol* 2015;73:199–213.
620. Siminovich M, Murtagh P. Acute lower respiratory tract infections by adenovirus in children: histopathologic findings in 18 fatal cases. *Pediatr Dev Pathol* 2011;14:214–217.
621. Sims B, Gu L, Krendelchtchikov A, et al. Neural stem cell-derived exosomes mediate viral entry. *Int J Nanomedicine* 2014;9:4893–4897.
622. Singh Y, Sawyer LS, Pinkoski LS, et al. Photochemical treatment of plasma with amotosalen and long-wavelength ultraviolet light inactivates pathogens while retaining coagulation function. *Transfusion* 2006;46:1168–1177.
623. Singh G, Zhou X, Lee JY, et al. Recombination of the epsilon determinant and corneal tropism: human adenovirus species D types 15, 29, 56, and 69. *Virology* 2015;485:452–459.
624. Sivaprakasam P, Carr TF, Coussons M, et al. Improved outcome from invasive adenovirus infection in pediatric patients after hemopoietic stem cell transplantation using intensive clinical surveillance and early intervention. *J Pediatr Hematol Oncol* 2007;29:81–85.
625. Sive JI, Thomson KJ, Morris EC, et al. Adenoviremia has limited clinical impact in the majority of patients following alemtuzumab-based allogeneic stem cell transplantation in adults. *Clin Infect Dis* 2012;55:1362–1370.
626. Smith JG, Cassany A, Gerace L, et al. Neutralizing antibody blocks adenovirus infection by arresting microtubule-dependent cytoplasmic transport. *J Virol* 2008;82:6492–6500.
627. Smith JG, Nemerow GR. Mechanism of adenovirus neutralization by human alpha-defensins. *Cell Host Microbe* 2008;3:11–19.
628. Smith JG, Silvestry M, Lindert S, et al. Insight into the mechanisms of adenovirus capsid disassembly from studies of defensin neutralization. *PLoS Pathog* 2010;6:e1000959.
629. Sohrab SS, Kamal MA, Atkinson RL, et al. Viral infection and obesity: current status and future prospective. *Curr Drug Metab* 2017;18:798–807.
630. Soller JA, Bartrand T, Ashbolt NJ, et al. Estimating the primary etiologic agents in recreational freshwaters impacted by human sources of faecal contamination. *Water Res* 2010;44:4736–4747.
631. Sonabend AM, Ulasov IV, Han Y, et al. Biodistribution of an oncolytic adenovirus after intracranial injection in permissive animals: a comparative study of Syrian hamsters and cotton rats. *Cancer Gene Ther* 2009;16:362–372.
632. Song E, Wang H, Kajon AE, et al. Diagnosis of pediatric acute adenovirus infections: is a positive PCR sufficient? *Pediatr Infect Dis J* 2016;35:827–834.
633. Speiseder T, Hofmann-Sieber H, Rodriguez E, et al. Efficient transformation of primary human mesenchymal stromal cells by adenovirus early region 1 oncogenes. *J Virol* 2017;91:e01782-16.
634. Spencer JF, Sagartz JE, Wold WS, et al. New pancreatic carcinoma model for studying oncolytic adenoviruses in the permissive Syrian hamster. *Cancer Gene Ther* 2009;16:912–922.
635. Srinivasan A, Klepper C, Sunkara A, et al. Impact of adenoviral stool load on adenoviremia in pediatric hematopoietic stem cell transplant recipients. *Pediatr Infect Dis J* 2015;34:562–565.
636. Sriwanna P, Chieochansin T, Vuthitanachot C, et al. Molecular characterization of human adenovirus infection in Thailand, 2009-2012. *Virol J* 2013;10:193.
637. Stasiak AC, Stehle T. Human adenovirus binding to host cell receptors: a structural view. *Med Microbiol Immunol* 2020;209(3):325–333.
638. Steel JC, Morrison BJ, Mannan P, et al. Immunocompetent syngeneic cotton rat tumor models for the assessment of replication-competent oncolytic adenovirus. *Virology* 2007;369:131–142.
639. Steiner I, Aebi C, Ridolfi Luthy A, et al. Fatal adenovirus hepatitis during maintenance therapy for childhood acute lymphoblastic leukemia. *Pediatr Blood Cancer* 2008;50:647–649.
640. Stene LC, Honeyman MC, Hoffenberg EJ, et al. Rotavirus infection frequency and risk of celiac disease autoimmunity in early childhood: a longitudinal study. *Am J Gastroenterol* 2006;101:2333–2340.
641. Stichling N, Suomalainen M, Flatt JW, et al. Lung macrophage scavenger receptor SR-A6 (MARCO) is an adenovirus type-specific virus entry receptor. *PLoS Pathog* 2018;14:e1006914.
642. Storm RJ, Persson BD, Skalman LN, et al. Human adenovirus type 37 uses $\alpha_V\beta_1$ and $\alpha_3\beta_1$ integrins for infection of human corneal cells. *J Virol* 2017;91(5):e02019-16.
643. Sugarman BJ, Hutchins BM, McAllister DL, et al. The complete nucleotide acid sequence of the adenovirus type 5 reference material (ARM) genome. *BioProcess J* 2003;2:27–33.
644. Sukdolak C, Tischer S, Dieks D, et al. CMV-, EBV- and ADV-specific T cell immunity: screening and monitoring of potential third-party donors to improve post-transplantation outcome. *Biol Blood Marrow Transplant* 2013;19:1480–1492.
645. Sulejmani N, Nagai S, Safwan M, et al. Brincidofovir as salvage therapy for adenovirus disease in intestinal transplant recipients. *Pharmacotherapy* 2018;38:470–475.
646. Sumida SM, Truitt DM, Lemckert AA, et al. Neutralizing antibodies to adenovirus serotype 5 vaccine vectors are directed primarily against the adenovirus hexon protein. *J Immunol* 2005;174:7179–7185.
647. Sun S, Shi Y, Tong HI, et al. Effective concentration, recovery, and detection of infectious adenoviruses from environmental waters. *J Virol Methods* 2016;229:78–85.
648. Sun C, Zhang Y, Feng L, et al. Epidemiology of adenovirus type 5 neutralizing antibodies in healthy people and AIDS patients in Guangzhou, southern China. *Vaccine* 2011;29:3837–3841.
649. Suparno C, Milligan DW, Moss PA, et al. Adenovirus infections in stem cell transplant recipients: recent developments in understanding of pathogenesis, diagnosis and management. *Leuk Lymphoma* 2004;45:873–885.
650. Swartling L, Allard A, Torlen J, et al. Prolonged outbreak of adenovirus A31 in allogeneic stem cell transplant recipients. *Transpl Infect Dis* 2015;17:785–794.
651. Symeonidis N, Jakubowski A, Pierre-Louis S, et al. Invasive adenoviral infections in T-cell-depleted allogeneic hematopoietic stem cell transplantation: high mortality in the era of cidofovir. *Transpl Infect Dis* 2007;9:108–113.
652. Takahashi K, Gonzalez G, Kobayashi M, et al. Pediatric infections by human mastadenovirus C Types 2, 89, and a recombinant type detected in Japan between 2011 and 2018. *Viruses* 2019;11(12):1131.
653. Takamatsu A, Tagashira Y, Hasegawa S, et al. Disseminated adenovirus infection in a patient with a hematologic malignancy: a case report and literature review. *Future Sci OA* 2019;5:FSO412.
654. Takayama R, Hatakeyama N, Suzuki N, et al. Quantification of adenovirus species B and C viremia by real-time PCR in adults and children undergoing stem cell transplantation. *J Med Virol* 2007;79:278–284.
655. Takemori N. Genetic studies with tumorigenic adenoviruses. 3. Recombination in adenovirus type 12. *Virology* 1972;47:157–167.
656. Tamiya M, Komatsu H, Hirabayashi M, et al. Neonatal meningoencephalitis caused by human adenovirus species F infection. *Pediatr Int* 2019;61:99–101.
657. Tan D, Fu Y, Xu J, et al. Severe adenovirus community-acquired pneumonia in immunocompetent adults: chest radiographic and CT findings. *J Thorac Dis* 2016;8:848–854.
658. Tan D, Zhu H, Fu Y, et al. Severe community-acquired pneumonia caused by human adenovirus in immunocompetent adults: a multicenter case series. *PLoS One* 2016;11:e0151199.
659. Taniguchi K, Yoshihara S, Tamaki H, et al. Incidence and treatment strategy for disseminated adenovirus disease after haploidentical stem cell transplantation. *Ann Hematol* 2012;91:1305–1312.
660. Teramura T, Naya M, Yoshihara T, et al. Adenoviral infection in hematopoietic stem cell transplantation: early diagnosis with quantitative detection of the viral genome in serum and urine. *Bone Marrow Transplant* 2004;33:87–92.
661. Ternovoi VV, Le LP, Belousova N, et al. Productive replication of human adenovirus type 5 in canine cells. *J Virol* 2005;79:1308–1311.
662. Thomas MA, Spencer JF, La Regina MC, et al. Syrian hamster as a permissive immunocompetent animal model for the study of oncolytic adenovirus vectors. *Cancer Res* 2006;66:1270–1276.
663. Thorner AR, Vogels R, Kaspers J, et al. Age dependence of adenovirus-specific neutralizing antibody titers in individuals from sub-Saharan Africa. *J Clin Microbiol* 2006;44:3781–3783.
664. Tian X, Fan Y, Liu Z, et al. Broadly neutralizing monoclonal antibodies against human adenovirus types 55, 14p, 7, and 11 generated with recombinant type 11 fiber knob. *Emerg Microbes Infect* 2018;7:206.
665. Tian Y, Jennings J, Gong Y, et al. Viral infections and interferons in the development of obesity. *Biomolecules* 2019;9(11):726.
666. Tian X, Jiang Z, Fan Y, et al. A tetravalent vaccine comprising hexon-chimeric adenoviruses elicits balanced protective immunity against human adenovirus types 3, 7, 14 and 55. *Antiviral Res* 2018;154:17–25.
667. Tian X, Wu H, Zhou R. Molecular evolution of human adenovirus type 16 through multiple recombination events. *Virus Genes* 2019;55:769–778.
668. Tippin TK, Morrison ME, Brundage TM, et al. Brincidofovir is not a substrate for the human organic anion transporter 1: a mechanistic explanation for the lack of nephrotoxicity observed in clinical studies. *Ther Drug Monit* 2016;38:777–786.
669. Tischer S, Geyeregger R, Kwoczek J, et al. Discovery of immunodominant T-cell epitopes reveals penton protein as a second immunodominant target in human adenovirus infection. *J Transl Med* 2016;14:286.
670. Tischer S, Kaireit T, Figueiredo C, et al. Establishment of the reversible peptide-major histocompatibility complex (pMHC) class I Histamer technology: tool for visualization and selection of functionally active antigen-specific CD8(+) T lymphocytes. *Int Immunol* 2012;24:561–572.
671. Tollefson AE, Spencer JF, Ying B, et al. Cidofovir and brincidofovir reduce the pathology caused by systemic infection with human type 5 adenovirus in immunosuppressed Syrian hamsters, while ribavirin is largely ineffective in this model. *Antiviral Res* 2014;112:38–46.
672. Tollefson AE, Ying B, Spencer JF, et al. Pathology in permissive syrian hamsters after infection with species C human adenovirus (HAdV-C) is the result of virus replication: HAdV-C6 replicates more and causes more pathology than HAdV-C5. *J Virol* 2017;91:e00284-17.
673. Toth K, Spencer JF, Dhar D, et al. Hexadecyloxypropyl-cidofovir, CMX001, prevents adenovirus-induced mortality in a permissive, immunosuppressed animal model. *Proc Natl Acad Sci U S A* 2008;105:7293–7297.
674. Toth K, Spencer JF, Ying B, et al. HAdV-C6 is a more relevant challenge virus than HAdV-C5 for testing antiviral drugs with the immunosuppressed Syrian Hamster model. *Viruses* 2017;9(6):147.
675. Toth K, Spencer JF, Ying B, et al. USC-087 protects Syrian hamsters against lethal challenge with human species C adenoviruses. *Antiviral Res* 2018;153:1–9.
676. Toth K, Tollefson AE, Spencer JF, et al. Combination therapy with brincidofovir and valganciclovir against species C adenovirus infection in the immunosuppressed Syrian hamster model allows for substantial reduction of dose for both compounds. *Antiviral Res* 2017;146:121–129.
677. Trentin JJ, Yabe Y, Taylor G. The quest for human cancer viruses. *Science* 1962;137:835–841.
678. Tschope C, Muller I, Xia Y, et al. NOD2 (Nucleotide-Binding Oligomerization Domain 2) is a major pathogenic mediator of Coxsackievirus B3-induced myocarditis. *Circ Heart Fail* 2017;10:e003870.
679. Tzannou I, Leen AM. Preventing stem cell transplantation-associated viral infections using T-cell therapy. *Immunotherapy* 2015;7:793–810.
680. Tzannou I, Papadopoulou A, Naik S, et al. Off-the-shelf virus-specific T cells to treat BK virus, human herpesvirus 6, cytomegalovirus, epstein-barr virus, and adenovirus infections after allogeneic hematopoietic stem-cell transplantation. *J Clin Oncol* 2017;35:3547–3557.
681. Uhlin M, Gertow J, Uzunel M, et al. Rapid salvage treatment with virus-specific T cells for therapy-resistant disease. *Clin Infect Dis* 2012;55:1064–1073.
682. Vachon VK, Conn GL. Adenovirus VA RNA: an essential pro-viral non-coding RNA. *Virus Res* 2016;212:39–52.
683. Van Genechten T, van Heerden J, Bauters T, et al. Successful treatment of adenovirus infection with brincidofovir in an immunocompromised patient after hematological stem cell transplantation. *Case Rep Infect Dis* 2020;2020:5981289.

684. Van Heerden J, Ehlers MM, Heim A, et al. Prevalence, quantification and typing of adenoviruses detected in river and treated drinking water in South Africa. *J Appl Microbiol* 2005;99:234–242.
685. Van Linthout S, Tschope C. Viral myocarditis: a prime example for endomyocardial biopsy-guided diagnosis and therapy. *Curr Opin Cardiol* 2018;33:325–333.
686. Van Regenmortel MHV, Fauquet CM, Bishop DHL, et al. *Virus Taxonomy: Classification and Nomenclature of Viruses. Seventh Report of the International Committee on Taxonomy of Viruses Family Adenoviridae*. San Diego, CA: Academic Press; 2000:227–237.
687. Van Tol MJ, Kroes AC, Schinkel J, et al. Adenovirus infection in paediatric stem cell transplant recipients: increased risk in young children with a delayed immune recovery. *Bone Marrow Transplant* 2005;36:39–50.
688. Varma MC, Kushner YB, Ko DS, et al. Early onset adenovirus infection after simultaneous kidney-pancreas transplant. *Am J Transplant* 2011;11:623–627.
689. Vasconcelos GM, Kang M, Pombo-de-Oliveira MS, et al. Adenovirus detection in Guthrie cards from paediatric leukaemia cases and controls. *Br J Cancer* 2008;99:1668–1672.
690. Veltrop-Duits LA, van Vreeswijk T, Heemskerk B, et al. High titers of pre-existing adenovirus serotype-specific neutralizing antibodies in the host predict viral reactivation after allogeneic stem cell transplantation in children. *Clin Infect Dis* 2011;52:1405–1413.
691. Vento TJ, Prakash V, Murray CK, et al. Pneumonia in military trainees: a comparison study based on adenovirus serotype 14 infection. *J Infect Dis* 2011;203:1388–1395.
692. Verdonschot J, Hazebroek M, Merken J, et al. Relevance of cardiac parvovirus B19 in myocarditis and dilated cardiomyopathy: review of the literature. *Eur J Heart Fail* 2016;18:1430–1441.
693. Vidal LR, de Almeida SM, Cavalli BM, et al. Human adenovirus meningoencephalitis: a 3-years' overview. *J Neurovirol* 2019;25:589–596.
694. Vincentelli C, Schniederjan MJ, Brat DJ. 35-year-old HIV-positive woman with Basal forebrain mass. *Brain Pathol* 2010;20:265–268.
695. Vora SB, Brothers AW, Englund JA. Renal toxicity in pediatric patients receiving cidofovir for the treatment of adenovirus infection. *J Pediatric Infect Dis Soc* 2017;6:399–402.
696. Vora GJ, Lin B, Gratwick K, et al. Co-infections of adenovirus species in previously vaccinated patients. *Emerg Infect Dis* 2006;12:921–930.
697. Voss JD, Burnett DG, Olsen CH, et al. Adenovirus 36 antibodies associated with clinical diagnosis of overweight/obesity but not BMI gain: a military cohort study. *J Clin Endocrinol Metab* 2014;99:E1708–E1712.
698. Voss JD, Dhurandhar NV. Viral infections and obesity. *Curr Obes Rep* 2017;6:28–37.
699. Vu DL, Bridevaux PO, Aubert JD, et al. Respiratory viruses in lung transplant recipients: a critical review and pooled analysis of clinical studies. *Am J Transplant* 2011;11:1071–1078.
700. Waddington SN, McVey JH, Bhella D, et al. Adenovirus serotype 5 hexon mediates liver gene transfer. *Cell* 2008;132:397–409.
701. Waddington SN, Parker AL, Havenga M, et al. Targeting of adenovirus serotype 5 (Ad5) and 5/47 pseudotyped vectors in vivo: fundamental involvement of coagulation factors and redundancy of CAR binding by Ad5. *J Virol* 2007;81:9568–9571.
702. Wakabayashi K, Machitani M, Tachibana M, et al. A MicroRNA derived from adenovirus virus-associated RNAII promotes virus infection via posttranscriptional gene silencing. *J Virol* 2019;93(2):e01265-18.
703. Walker CLF, Rudan I, Liu L, et al. Global burden of childhood pneumonia and diarrhoea. *Lancet* 2013;381:1405–1416.
704. Walls T, Hawrami K, Ushiro-Lumb I, et al. Adenovirus infection after pediatric bone marrow transplantation: is treatment always necessary? *Clin Infect Dis* 2005;40:1244–1249.
705. Walls T, Shankar AG, Shingadia D. Adenovirus: an increasingly important pathogen in paediatric bone marrow transplant patients. *Lancet Infect Dis* 2003;3:79–86.
706. Walsh MP, Chintakuntlawar A, Robinson CM, et al. Evidence of molecular evolution driven by recombination events influencing tropism in a novel human adenovirus that causes epidemic keratoconjunctivitis. *PLoS One* 2009;4:e5635.
707. Walsh MP, Seto J, Jones MS, et al. Computational analysis identifies human adenovirus type 55 as a re-emergent acute respiratory disease pathogen. *J Clin Microbiol* 2010;48:991–993.
708. Walsh MP, Seto J, Liu EB, et al. Computational analysis of two species C human adenoviruses provides evidence of a novel virus. *J Clin Microbiol* 2011;49:3482–3490.
709. Walsh MP, Seto J, Tirado D, et al. Computational analysis of human adenovirus serotype 18. *Virology* 2010;404:284–292.
710. Wan GH, Huang CG, Huang YC, et al. Surveillance of airborne adenovirus and *Mycoplasma pneumoniae* in a hospital pediatric department. *PLoS One* 2012;7:e33974.
711. Wang H, Li ZY, Liu Y, et al. Desmoglein 2 is a receptor for adenovirus serotypes 3, 7, 11 and 14. *Nat Med* 2011;17:96–104.
712. Wang H, Li Z, Yumul R, et al. Multimerization of adenovirus serotype 3 fiber knob domains is required for efficient binding of virus to desmoglein 2 and subsequent opening of epithelial junctions. *J Virol* 2011;85:6390–6402.
713. Wang YF, Shen FC, Wang SL, et al. Molecular epidemiology and clinical manifestations of adenovirus respiratory infections in taiwanese children. *Medicine (Baltimore)* 2016;95:e3577.
714. Wang H, Tuve S, Erdman DD, et al. Receptor usage of a newly emergent adenovirus type 14. *Virology* 2009;387:436–441.
715. Watcharananan SP, Avery R, Ingsathit A, et al. Adenovirus disease after kidney transplantation: course of infection and outcome in relation to blood viral load and immune recovery. *Am J Transplant* 2011;11:1308–1314.
716. Watson T, MacDonald D, Song X, et al. Risk factors for molecular detection of adenovirus in pediatric hematopoietic stem cell transplantation recipients. *Biol Blood Marrow Transplant* 2012;18:1227–1234.
717. Wevers D, Metzger S, Babweteera F, et al. Novel adenoviruses in wild primates: a high level of genetic diversity and evidence of zoonotic transmissions. *J Virol* 2011;85:10774–10784.
718. Wiethoff CM, Nemerow GR. Adenovirus membrane penetration: tickling the tail of a sleeping dragon. *Virology* 2015;479–480:591–599.
719. Williams J, Grodzicker T, Sharp P, et al. Adenovirus recombination: physical mapping of crossover events. *Cell* 1975;4:113–119.
720. Wilson SS, Wiens ME, Holly MK, et al. Defensins at the mucosal surface: latest insights into defensin-virus interactions. *J Virol* 2016;90:5216–5218.
721. Wilson SS, Wiens ME, Smith JG. Antiviral mechanisms of human defensins. *J Mol Biol* 2013;425:4965–4980.
722. Wimmer P, Tauber B, Spruss T, et al. Adenovirus type 5 early encoded proteins of the E1 and E4 regions induce oncogenic transformation of primary rabbit cells. *J Gen Virol* 2010;91:1828–1833.
723. Wold WS, Doronin K, Toth K, et al. Immune responses to adenoviruses: viral evasion mechanisms and their implications for the clinic. *Curr Opin Immunol* 1999;11:380–386.
724. Wold WSM, Horwitz MS. Adenoviruses. In: Fields BN, Knipe DM, Howley PM, eds. *Fields Virology*. 5th ed. Philadelphia, PA: Lippincott Williams & Wilkins; 2007:2395–2436.
725. Wold WSM, Ison MG. Adenovirus. In: Knipe DM, Howley PH, eds. *Fields Virology*. 6th ed. Philadelphia, PA: Lippincott Williams & Wilkins; 2013:1732–1767.
726. Wold WSM, Tollefson AE, Ying B, et al. Drug development against human adenoviruses and its advancement by Syrian hamster models. *FEMS Microbiol Rev* 2019;43:380–388.
727. Wold WS, Toth K. Chapter three—Syrian hamster as an animal model to study oncolytic adenoviruses and to evaluate the efficacy of antiviral compounds. *Adv Cancer Res* 2012;115:69–92.
728. Wolf C, von Gunten U, Kohn T. Kinetics of inactivation of waterborne enteric viruses by ozone. *Environ Sci Technol* 2018;52:2170–2177.
729. Wolfrum N, Greber UF. Adenovirus signalling in entry. *Cell Microbiol* 2013;15:53–62.
730. Wrackmeyer U, Kaldrack J, Juttner R, et al. The cell adhesion protein CAR is a negative regulator of synaptic transmission. *Sci Rep* 2019;9:6768.
731. Wu E, Nemerow GR. Virus yoga: the role of flexibility in virus host cell recognition. *Trends Microbiol* 2004;12:162–169.
732. Wu Z, Subramanian N, Jacobsen EM, et al. NK Cells from RAG- or DCLRE1C-deficient patients inhibit HCMV. *Microorganisms* 2019;7:546.
733. Xie L, Zhang B, Xiao N, et al. Epidemiology of human adenovirus infection in children hospitalized with lower respiratory tract infections in Hunan, China. *J Med Virol* 2019;91:392–400.
734. Xu J, Berastegui-Cabrera J, Chen H, et al. Structure-activity relationship studies on diversified salicylamide derivatives as potent inhibitors of human adenovirus infection. *J Med Chem* 2020;63(6):3142–3160.
735. Xu MY, Cao B, Wang DF, et al. Human adenovirus 36 infection increased the risk of obesity: a meta-analysis update. *Medicine (Baltimore)* 2015;94:e2357.
736. Xu L, Liu J, Liu C, et al. Case-control study of the epidemiological and clinical features of human adenovirus 55 and human adenovirus 7 infection in children with acute lower respiratory tract infections in Beijing, China, 2008-2013. *BMC Infect Dis* 2018;18:634.
737. Xu J, Patel KV, Dsouza M, et al. Disseminated adenovirus infection in heart and kidney transplant. *Turk Kardiyol Dern Ars* 2018;46:231–233.
738. Yamasaki S, Miura Y, Davydova J, et al. Intravenous genetic mesothelin vaccine based on human adenovirus 40 inhibits growth and metastasis of pancreatic cancer. *Int J Cancer* 2013;133:88–97.
739. Yang J, Mao N, Zhang C, et al. Human adenovirus species C recombinant virus continuously circulated in China. *Sci Rep* 2019;9:9781.
740. Yang X, Wang Q, Liang B, et al. An outbreak of acute respiratory disease caused by a virus associated RNA II gene mutation strain of human adenovirus 7 in China, 2015. *PLoS One* 2017;12:e0172519.
741. Yao LH, Wang C, Wei TL, et al. Human adenovirus among hospitalized children with respiratory tract infections in Beijing, China, 2017-2018. *Virol J* 2019;16:78.
742. Yasuda S, Najima Y, Konishi T, et al. Disseminated adenovirus infection in a patient with relapsed refractory multiple myeloma undergoing autologous stem cell transplantation and pomalidomide/dexamethasone as salvage regimens. *J Infect Chemother* 2019;25:371–375.
743. Ye S, Whiley DM, Ware RS, et al. Detection of viruses in weekly stool specimens collected during the first 2 years of life: a pilot study of five healthy Australian infants in the rotavirus vaccine era. *J Med Virol* 2017;89:917–921.
744. Ying B, Spencer JF, Tollefson AE, et al. Male Syrian hamsters are more susceptible to intravenous infection with species C human adenoviruses than are females. *Virology* 2018;514:66–78.
745. Ying B, Toth K, Spencer JF, et al. INGN 007, an oncolytic adenovirus vector, replicates in Syrian hamsters but not mice: comparison of biodistribution studies. *Cancer Gene Ther* 2009;16:625–637.
746. Yoo H, Gu SH, Jung J, et al. Febrile respiratory illness associated with human adenovirus type 55 in South Korea military, 2014-2016. *Emerg Infect Dis* 2017;23:1016–1020.
747. Yoshitomi H, Sera N, Gonzalez G, et al. First isolation of a new type of human adenovirus (genotype 79), species Human mastadenovirus B (B2) from sewage water in Japan. *J Med Virol* 2017;89:1192–1200.
748. Young BA, Spencer JF, Ying B, et al. The role of cyclophosphamide in enhancing antitumor efficacy of an adenovirus oncolytic vector in subcutaneous Syrian hamster tumors. *Cancer Gene Ther* 2013;20:521–530.
749. Yusuf U, Hale GA, Carr J, et al. Cidofovir for the treatment of adenoviral infection in pediatric hematopoietic stem cell transplant patients. *Transplantation* 2006;81:1398–1404.
750. Zaiss AK, Vilaysane A, Cotter MJ, et al. Antiviral antibodies target adenovirus to phagolysosomes and amplify the innate immune response. *J Immunol* 2009;182:7058–7068.
751. Zandvliet ML, Falkenburg JH, van Liempt E, et al. Combined CD8+ and CD4+ adenovirus hexon-specific T cells associated with viral clearance after stem cell transplantation as treatment for adenovirus infection. *Haematologica* 2010;95:1943–1951.
752. Zandvliet ML, van Liempt E, Jedema I, et al. Simultaneous isolation of CD8(+) and CD4(+) T cells specific for multiple viruses for broad antiviral immune reconstitution after allogeneic stem cell transplantation. *J Immunother* 2011;34:307–319.
753. Zapatka M, Borozan I, Brewer DS, et al., Lichter P on behalf of the PCAWG Pathogens Working Group, and the ICGC/TCGA PanCancer Analysis of Whole Genomes Network. The landscape of viral associations in human cancers. *bioRxiv* 2018. doi: https://doi.org/10.1101/465757.
754. Zapatka M, Borozan I, Brewer DS, et al. The landscape of viral associations in human cancers. *Nat Genet* 2020;52:320–330.

755. Zecca M, Wynn R, Dalle JH, et al. Association between adenovirus viral load and mortality in pediatric allo-HCT recipients: the multinational AdVance study. *Bone Marrow Transplant* 2019;54(10):1632–1642.
756. Zhang Y, Bergelson JM. Adenovirus receptors. *J Virol* 2005;79:12125–12131.
757. Zhang W, Huang L. Genome analysis of a novel recombinant human adenovirus type 1 in China. *Sci Rep* 2019;9:4298.
758. Zhang Y, Huang W, Ornelles DA, et al. Modeling adenovirus latency in human lymphocyte cell lines. *J Virol* 2010;84:8799–8810.
759. Zhang Q, Jing S, Cheng Z, et al. Comparative genomic analysis of two emergent human adenovirus type 14 respiratory pathogen isolates in China reveals similar yet divergent genomes. *Emerg Microbes Infect* 2017;6:e92.
760. Zhang J, Kang J, Dehghan S, et al. A survey of recent adenoviral respiratory pathogens in Hong Kong reveals emergent and recombinant human adenovirus type 4 (HAdV-E4) circulating in civilian populations. *Viruses* 2019;11(2):129.
761. Zhang Y, Liu R, Tian K, et al. Fiber2 and hexon genes are closely associated with the virulence of the emerging and highly pathogenic fowl adenovirus 4. *Emerg Microbes Infect* 2018;7:199.
762. Zhang SY, Luo YP, Huang DD, et al. Fatal pneumonia cases caused by human adenovirus 55 in immunocompetent adults. *Infect Dis (Lond)* 2016;48:40–47.
763. Zhang L, Zhao N, Sha J, et al. Virology and epidemiology analyses of global adenovirus-associated conjunctivitis outbreaks, 1953-2013. *Epidemiol Infect* 2016;144:1661–1672.
764. Zhao MC, Guo YH, Qiu FZ, et al. Molecular and clinical characterization of human adenovirus associated with acute respiratory tract infection in hospitalized children. *J Clin Virol* 2020;123:104254.
765. Zhao H, Punga T, Pettersson U. Adenovirus in the omics era—a multipronged strategy. *FEBS Lett* 2020;594(12):1879–1890.
766. Zheng X, Lu X, Erdman DD, et al. Identification of adenoviruses in specimens from high-risk pediatric stem cell transplant recipients and controls. *J Clin Microbiol* 2008;46:317–320.
767. Zheng Y, Stamminger T, Hearing P. E2F/Rb Family proteins mediate interferon induced repression of adenovirus immediate early transcription to promote persistent viral infection. *PLoS Pathog* 2016;12:e1005415.
768. Zhu X, Badawi M, Pomeroy S, et al. Comprehensive toxicity and immunogenicity studies reveal minimal effects in mice following sustained dosing of extracellular vesicles derived from HEK293T cells. *J Extracell Vesicles* 2017;6:1324730.
769. Zhu Z, Zhang Y, Xu S, et al. Outbreak of acute respiratory disease in China caused by B2 species of adenovirus type 11. *J Clin Microbiol* 2009;47:697–703.
770. zur Hausen H. Oncogenic DNA viruses. *Oncogene* 2001;20:7820–7823.

CHAPTER

6 Parvoviridae

Colin R. Parrish

INTRODUCTION AND HISTORY

Parvoviruses are small, nonenveloped viruses with a linear, single-strand DNA (ssDNA) genome of about 5,000 bases. The family *Parvoviridae* (Table 6.1) contains two subfamilies: *Parvovirinae* and *Densovirinae*.[91] The latter infect invertebrates and will not be described in detail in this chapter. The *Parvovirinae* are divided into eight genera: *Amdoparvovirus*, *Aveparvovirus*, *Bocaparvovirus*, *Copiparvovirus*, *Dependoparvovirus*, *Erythroparvovirus*, *Protoparvovirus*, and *Tetraparvovirus*. The adeno-associated viruses (AAVs) among the dependoparvoviruses require coinfection with a helper virus for productive infection. The others are autonomous, and although most require the host cell to go through S phase for viral DNA replication but do not induce cell division, some may be able to replicate in nonmitotic cells by other mechanisms related to the DNA damage response.[107] The AAV helper virus is most commonly an adenovirus, but herpesviruses have also been shown to help productive replication.

In the 1920s and 1930s, feline and raccoon diseases characterized by enteritis, panleukopenia, and cerebellar ataxia were recognized as being of viral origin. In the late 1940s, a similar disease was noted in mink; in 1952, it was determined that those diseases were caused by similar small, DNA-containing viruses.[363] Parvoviruses were isolated from rats (Kilham rat virus),[196] and the H-1 virus isolated from human tumor tissue–infected hamsters.[362] Between 1960 and 1962, small particles were observed within adenovirus preparations by electron microscopy, and AAV was identified that depended on coinfection of the cells with adenovirus for replication[21,163,277] or on herpesviruses.[54] The human parvovirus B19 was first identified in 1974 during screening of a diagnostic blood sample (with the code B19). The B19 virus is associated with transient aplastic crisis in patients with sickle cell disease, with the childhood "fifth" disease, and with postinfection arthralgia in older patients. In 1978, a new virus of dogs (canine parvovirus [CPV]) caused myocarditis and enteritis in dogs, and that was derived from a preexisting virus similar to feline panleukopenia virus (FPV).[378] Many additional parvoviruses have been isolated from animals and cell cultures, and by discovery of viral DNA using cloning or sequencing approaches.[186,187,332] Many of the viruses grow poorly or not at all in cultured cells, and many also have not been associated with overt disease in their natural hosts.

BIOLOGY OF THE PARVOVIRUSES

The parvoviruses have small (~26 nm diameter) and structurally stable capsids that bind host cell receptors and small ssDNA genomes with few genes that control their interactions with their hosts, and they replicate in dividing cells, in association with a DNA damage response, or in the presence of a helper virus. Parvoviruses are widespread, and sequencing of DNA shows that several parvoviruses are likely to be infecting most invertebrate and vertebrate animals. The presence of integrated viral DNA fragments in the genomes of many different vertebrate

TABLE 6.1 Classification of *Parvoviridae*

Subfamily: *Parvovirinae*
Genus: *Protoparvovirus*
Members:
Minute Virus of Mice
Chicken parvovirus
Feline panleukopenia virus
H-1 parvovirus
HB parvovirus
Kilham rat virus
Lapine parvovirus
Lulll virus
Mouse parvovirus 1
Porcine parvovirus
RT parvovirus
Tumor virus X

Genus: *Erythroparvovirus*
Members:
Human parvovirus B19
Pig-tailed macaque parvovirus
Rhesus macaque parvovirus
Simian parvovirus

Genus: *Dependoparvovirus*
Members:
Adeno-associated virus-2
Adeno-associated virus-1
Adeno-associated virus-3
Adeno-associated virus-4
Adeno-associated virus-5
Avian adeno-associated virus
Bovine adeno-associated virus
Canine adeno-associated virus
Duck parvovirus
Equine adeno-associated virus
Goose parvovirus
Ovine adeno-associated virus

Genus: *Bocaparvovirus*
Members:
Bovine parvovirus
Canine minute virus

Genus: *Amdoparvovirus*
Member:
Aleutian mink disease virus

Subfamily: *Densovirinae*
Genus: *Ambidensovirus*
Members:
Junonia coenia densovirus
Galleria mellonella densovirus

Genus: *Iteradensovirus*
Member:
Bombyx mori densovirus

Genus: *Brevidensovirus*
Members:
Aedes aegypti densovirus
Aedes albopictus densovirus

Genus: *Pefuambidensovirus*
Member:
Periplaneta fuliginosa densovirus

and invertebrate animals also indicates that related viruses have been infecting animals for millions of years.[34,57,186,189,221,281] The viruses transmit between hosts by routes that include fecal–oral, urine, and respiratory spread, and the capsids are stable in the environment and readily transmitted by contaminated fomites. Entry into the body likely involves infection of dividing epithelial or lymphoid cells of the upper respiratory tract, oropharynx, or intestine. The viruses are structurally and genetically simple, and do not induce the host cell to proliferate, and generally appear not to manipulate the host immune responses to high levels. Where the mechanisms have been defined, the host and tissue tropisms are determined by the requirement for dividing cells of the autonomous parvoviruses, by host receptor binding, or by the cell-specific controls of viral gene expression.

AAVs are cryptic viruses and are not clearly associated with any pathology. The AAVs are widespread, and natural hosts appear to include most vertebrates (see Table 6.1). Viral persistence is likely related to the ability of the entire viral genomic DNA to integrate into the host genome, and AAV DNA sequences may be found in many tissues.[134,304] If AAV infects a healthy cell in the absence of a helper virus, the viral genome does not replicate but may establish a persistent infection by chromosomal integration or by forming stable extrachromosomal concatemers of AAV genomes[119]. The integrated AAV genome may be rescued by superinfection of the cells with a helper virus.[76] Extrachromosomal or integrated latency is likely functionally equivalent if the infected cell does not divide; however, in dividing cells, the nonreplicating extrachromosomal AAV DNA would be diluted out. Stressing host cells may allow some limited AAV replication, and this can be achieved by exposure of the cell to genotoxic conditions that include ultraviolet irradiation, ionizing radiation, and cycloheximide.[323,393]

There are complex two-way relationships between AAVs and their helper viruses. AAVs can inhibit the replication of adenovirus in a process that depends on the relative amounts of the two viruses and on the temporal relationship of the coinfection.[68,69] Adenovirus inhibition likely results from AAV Rep protein inhibition of heterologous promoters, and that inhibition is also seen in coinfections of AAV and SV40, papillomavirus, and some herpesviruses.[159,198,209,396]

TAXONOMY AND CLASSIFICATION

The Family *Parvoviridae* has unenveloped capsids of about 25 nm diameter with icosahedral symmetry composed of 60 copies of the capsid proteins. The nucleic acid is single-stranded linear DNA between 4 and 6 kb in length. The classification is frequently updated with changes in the nomenclature.[91] The two subfamilies, *Parvovirinae* and *Densovirinae*, are distinguished mostly on their abilities to infect vertebrate versus invertebrate hosts, respectively. The *Parvovirinae* are subdivided into ten genera: *Amdoparvovirus*, *Artiparvovirus*, *Aveparvovirus*, *Bocaparvovirus*, *Copiparvovirus*, *Dependoparvovirus*, *Erythroparvovirus*, *Loriparvovirus*, *Protoparvovirus*, and *Tetraparovirus*. The *Densovirinae* are subdivided into eight genera (see examples in Table 6.1). Genera are defined by their genomic and biological properties and by their DNA sequence relatedness, biological host ranges, and/or capsid antigenicity.

There is significant variation in the details of the viral genomes and gene expression. Protoparvoviruses may package mostly one DNA strand, or package both DNA strands in variable proportions, and the ssDNA genome has different hairpin structures at each end. There are generally two messenger RNA (mRNA) promoters and a single polyadenylation site near the 3′ end of the -ve strand DNA. The Erythroparvoviruses are related to the B19 human parvovirus, and mature virions contain equivalent proportions of positive and negative sense ssDNA, the DNA molecules contain inverted terminal repeats (ITRs), and there is a single transcriptional promoter and two polyadenylation signals. Amdoparvoviruses are related to the Aleutian mink disease virus (AMDV), whereas the bocaparvoviruses are related to bovine parvovirus and the canine minute virus and include many viruses of humans and other hosts. Dependovirus virions package equivalent numbers of positive- or negative-strand ssDNA genomes, with ITRs of approximately 145 nucleotides—of which the first approximately 125 nucleotides form a palindromic sequence.

Structure of Capsid and General Properties

The particle has a molecular weight (MW) of 5.5 to 6.2 × 10^6 daltons. The buoyant density of the intact virion in cesium chloride (CsCl) is 1.39 to 1.42 g/cm^3,[359] and the sedimentation coefficient of the virion in neutral sucrose gradients is 110 to 122. The virions are resistant to inactivation, even for 60 minutes at pHs between 3 and 9, or at 56°C, but can be inactivated

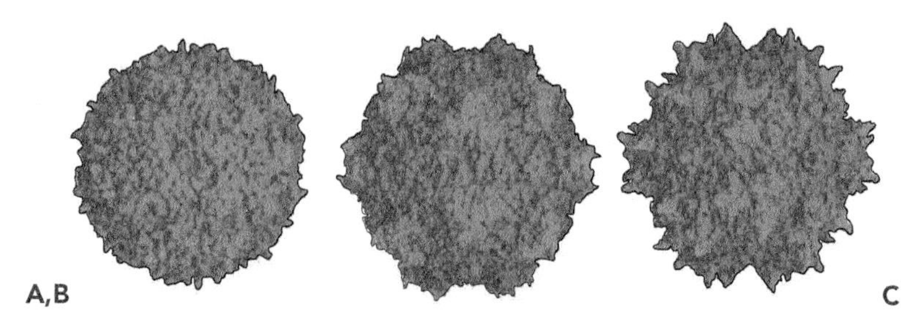

FIGURE 6.1 **Surface topologies of the capsids of various members of the *Parvoviridae*, calculated from the atomic structures of the viruses. A:** The insect-infecting densonucleosis virus Galleria mellonella densovirus (GmDNV). **B:** The autonomous parvovirus minute virus of mice. **C:** The dependovirus adeno-associated virus type 2. (Courtesy of Agbandje-McKenna, University of Florida.)

by formalin, β-propiolactone, hydroxylamine, and oxidizing agents. The capsids have T = 1 icosahedral structures and are assembled from 60 copies of between 2 and 4 forms of a single structural protein (with varying names, but generally virus protein [VP]: VP1, VP2, and VP3), which package the linear, ssDNA genome[365] (Fig. 6.1). The capsid structures of all of the parvoviruses share an overall similar structure[4,192,335,365,376,391] (see Fig. 6.1). An eight-stranded, antiparallel β-barrel constitutes around one-third of the sequence of the structural protein, and some of the large loops connecting the strands of the β-barrel make up the capsid surface. The capsid surface determines host and tissue interactions, forms receptor-binding sites, and makes up the epitopes recognized by antibodies. Antiparallel β-ribbons form a cylinder about the icosahedral fivefold axes, with a channel through the capsid in many viruses.[96,122,192] N-terminal sequences of some VP molecules (VP2 in the Protoparvoviruses) are externalized through that channel, and they may be cleaved by host or other proteases to a shorter form (VP3 in the Protoparvoviruses). DNA packaging also occurs through the channel at one fivefold axis, leaving a short sequence (~20 nucleotides) of the 5′ end of the genome outside the capsid after the genome is packaged, and that has the replication protein (NS1) attached.[95,96,291] The capsid surface structures vary, but they often include one large or three smaller spike-like protrusions surrounding the icosahedral threefold axes of symmetry, depressions about the fivefold axes, and dimple-like depressions at the icosahedral twofold axes[73,365,391] (Fig. 6.1).

Conformation-dependent epitopes are important targets of neutralizing antibodies on the exposed surface of the capsids of all of the viruses of vertebrates, and where it has been examined much of the capsid surface appears to bind antibodies, apart from the depressed regions.[151,319,349,366,384,400] Linear epitopes recognized by antibodies include the exposed N-terminus of VP2 of parvovirus full capsids and the N-terminus of VP1 for the B19 parvovirus.[113,213,257]

Functions of the Capsid Proteins

Most autonomous parvovirus and AAV capsids contain combinations of three overlapping proteins—MWs of 80,000 to 86,000 (VP1), 64,000 to 75,000 (VP2), and 60,000 to 62,000 (VP3)—although AMDV, B19, and simian parvovirus assemble from only VP1 and VP2. For the autonomous viruses, VP1 and VP2 are generally derived from alternatively spliced viral messages, and VP3 is generated in DNA-containing capsids by proteolytic cleavage of VP2.

The unique regions of VP1 of most or all parvoviruses contain a calcium-dependent phospholipase A_2 (PLA_2) enzymatic activity that is thought to be buried within the capsid after assembly, but which becomes exposed during cell entry.[123,354,403] The VP1 unique sequence is exposed on the surface of B19 capsids, which may reflect a difference in the structure of that virus.[113(p1),114] The PLA_2 activities of the different viruses differ significantly.[58] Peptides near the N-terminus of VP1 contain basic amino acid motifs that likely function as nuclear localization motifs during cell entry and capsid assembly.[165,224,371,383]

Genome Structures and Organizations

All parvoviruses of vertebrates have similar genome structures, with terminal repeats required for DNA replication, nonstructural protein genes on the left half of the genome (the 3′ end of the –ve strand DNA), and capsid protein genes on the right half of the genome (Fig. 6.2). Smaller proteins are produced by alternative splicing of some viruses and include the NS2 protein

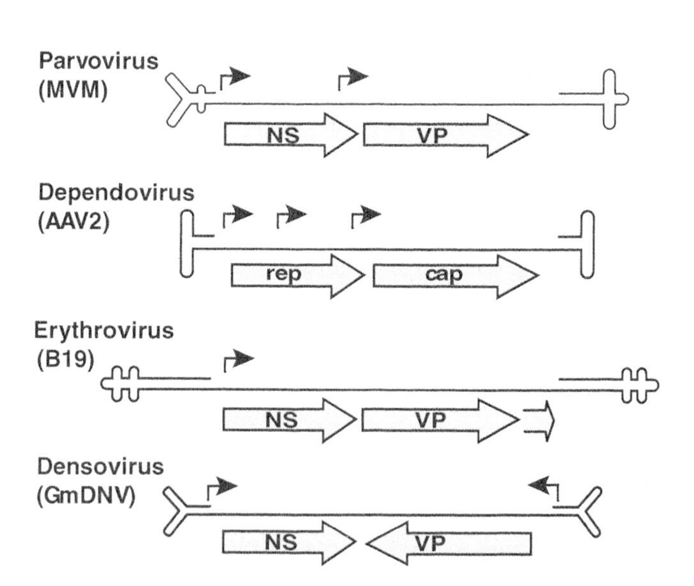

FIGURE 6.2 **The genome structures of different members of the *Parvoviridae*, showing genomes of three of the nine genera, the parvoviruses, the dependoviruses, and the erythroviruses, indicating the promoters and open reading frames of the major genes, nonstructural and viral protein.** The terminal hairpins are magnified approximately 20-fold relative to the intervening single-stranded sequences.

in the viruses similar to minute virus of mice (MVM) and the NP1 protein in the bocaviruses (see later discussion). The functions of the noncoding sequences between the capsid protein and the 5′ terminal hairpin of the autonomous parvoviruses are less well understood; however, in the B19 viruses, there is a short open reading frame (ORF) encoding a protein (p11), and that region may also be involved in regulating the packaging of the viral DNA.[96,97] The smaller ORFs include the NP1 protein in several viruses, the 11 kDa protein in the B19 human parvovirus, and small ORFs that overlaps the VP1 and VP2 N-terminal sequence in an alternative reading frame—the small alternatively translated (SAT) protein of many autonomous parvoviruses, and the assembly activating peptide of the AAV-like viruses.[145,261,345] Other alternatively spliced RNA products have been identified for many viruses, although the predicted proteins produced have generally not been characterized.

Epidemiology and Antiviral Immunity

Many autonomous parvoviruses, including CPV, FPV, porcine parvovirus (PPV), and B19 human parvovirus, cause acute infections of their hosts that last for fewer than 10 days. The virus is cleared by the host immunity, and infectious virus is not subsequently shed, although viral DNA may persist in many tissues,[13,164,342] and even in bones recovered from archeological sites.[255] Some parvoviruses show prolonged replication and persistence: Rodent parvoviruses may persist in the kidneys and be shed in the urine, although that is mostly seen in immune deficient mouse strains, while AMDV persists in mink when antibodies are present and may replicate for the life of the animal.[10,43,178,293] For B19 in humans, rare chronic persistent infections occur in individuals who are immunosuppressed, or who do not develop effective immunity.[128,206]

The mechanisms of transmission among the parvoviruses vary and in many cases are not well defined. Carnivore parvoviruses such as CPV and FPV are spread by fecal–oral transmission.[235,236,278] Some rodent parvoviruses also replicate in the intestine as well as systemically, and may also be transmitted through urine after replication in the kidney.[25(p),157,174,215] The human B19 virus replicates primarily in the bone marrow but develops a very high level viremia—and it is thought to be transmitted by respiratory routes after virus is shed into the lungs or other respiratory secretions.[50,51]

Cell-mediated immunity likely assists in recovery from infection; however, humoral immunity alone can protect animals against infection and is also important for recovery from infection, as immune immunoglobulin G (IgG) can arrest CPV replication in dogs and can terminate chronic human infections by the B19 parvovirus.[51] Antibodies produced in mink reduce titers of AMDV but do not eliminate the virus, thus allowing the persistent infection to occur.[8,10,43,178]

No clear role for antigenic variation in the epidemiology of the parvoviruses has been revealed. Viruses of different genera or species are distinguished by polyclonal sera, but little antigenic variation has been demonstrated within most virus species, and any epidemiologic significance is not known. Some changes altering the antigenic structure of a virus may also alter host range or other properties so that multiple selections may be occuring.[14,72,214,260,314] For MVM, antigenic variants were readily selected with neutralizing monoclonal antibodies in tissue culture or in persistent infections of SCID mice,[225] although it is not known whether similar variation occurs in nature.

Genetic Variation and Evolution

These DNA viruses are replicated by host cell DNA polymerases, but the error rates are likely much higher than seen for the host genomic DNA. The single-stranded DNA genome may make it susceptible to modification, and the mode of DNA replication may lead to significant sequence variation. The temporal rates of sequence variation may be high (>4 × 10^{-4} variations per site per year) when measured over defined periods.[22,229,330,331,375] MVM mutant strains grown persistently in immune deficient mice or under monoclonal antibody selection showed variation at several sites owing to host or immune selection.[314] Recombination is likely quite common among the parvoviruses.[232,329]

All parvoviruses are related through a distant common ancestor, and the sequences can be subdivided into several clades that show some correlations with the hosts of origin,[232] although there are many variants. Parvovirus-related sequences are integrated into the genomes of many vertebrate and invertebrate animals, mostly as partial or degenerate sequences, which would not generate infectious virus and are less likely to recombine productively with infectious viral sequences.[34,57,161,186,187,221] Despite the high rates of variation seen among contemporary viruses, the genomes of viruses that share significant homology may have diverged millions of years ago. This is seen in the finding of syntenic integrated parvoviral sequences in related mammals, showing that integration occurred prior to the host evolutionary divergence, often 10s of millions of years.

Several different parvoviruses likely infect most host species, and there are numerous examples of viral DNA of otherwise unknown parvoviruses in human or animal tissues and feces[44,126,341] —although fecal viruses may also derive from materials in the diet. For example, within cows, three parvovirus sequences were discovered by searching for nonhost DNAs[11], several erythroviruses have been identified in humans and other primates, and those are related to a chipmunk parvovirus.[75,164,179,332] Sequences of multiple viruses were identified in rodents, bats, opossums, birds, and cattle in Brazil[346], and similar numbers of variant viruses were found in different wild birds in Australia[370] The human B19-like parvoviruses include three distinct clades that differ by 5% to 20% in sequence; within each clade, the viruses differ by less than 1% to 4%[132,328], and viral sequences recovered from skeletal remains suggest a slower evolution over longer time periods.[255] Many parvovirus strains have worldwide distributions, although geographic clustering may occur.[55,253,375] Significant variation (of up to 16%) was seen in the genomes of AMDV isolates, perhaps owing to the cocirculation and coinfection of animals with variant virus strains.[318,373] Because that virus can form persistent infections with continuously circulating virus, and antibodies appear not to protect, mixed and super infections likely occur.[269]

Infection Pathways

Parvoviruses bind to one or more cell surface receptors, are endocytosed and then traffic within the endosomal system, and are released into the cytoplasm in the vicinity of the nucleus, and the DNA with or without the capsids enters the nucleus. There appear to be no substantial differences between the general features of the infection pathways used by the autonomous viruses and AAVs (Fig. 6.3).

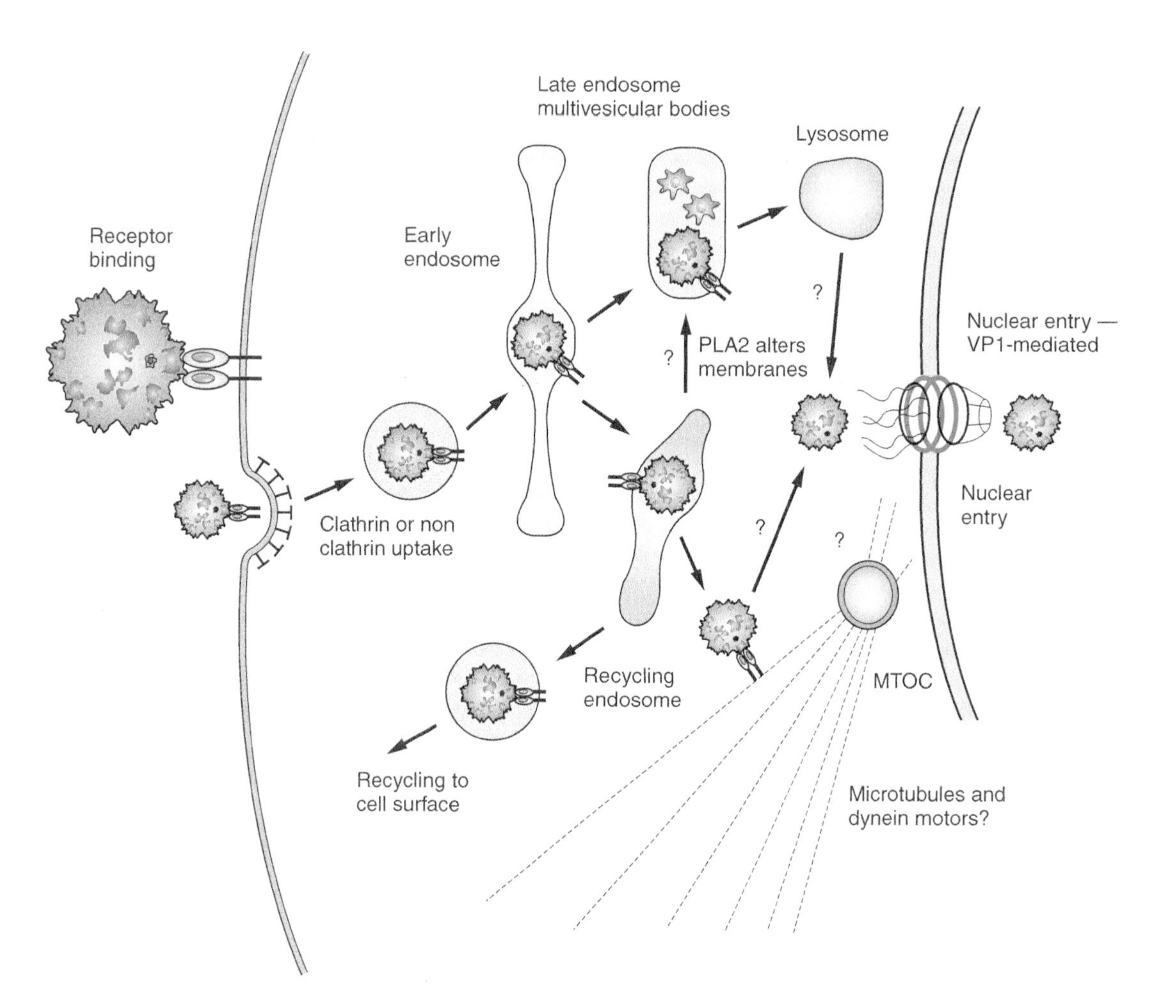

FIGURE 6.3 A general summary of the known or proposed infection pathways of viral capsids from the cell surface to the nucleus, as exemplified by the canine parvovirus binding to the transferrin receptor and being taken up by clathrin-mediated endocytosis. The later steps of the pathway, including sorting the endosomal system of the cell and trafficking within the cytoplasm and into the nucleus, may vary between viruses and are still not completely defined.

Capsid Structures and Cell Infection

The parvovirus capsid is a stable sphere of about 26 nm in diameter (see Fig. 6.1). Flexibility is required during infection to allow genome release and to expose protein structures from within the capsid. The VP1 unique region (between 40 and 230 residues long, depending on the virus) is not required for capsid formation or DNA packaging,[368,371] but that sequence includes a basic amino acid motif, which likely acts as a nuclear localization sequence (NLS), and a phospholipase A2 (PLA_2) enzyme structure, which is active when released from the capsid.[224,239,311,354,371,403] The PLA_2 activity varies widely, with that of PPV showing approximately 100-fold higher PLA_2 activity than the AAV2 or the human B19 parvovirus.[58] The PLA_2 modification of the lipid components of the endosome may allow more efficient viral release.[123] The VP1 unique region has also been reported to contain a proteinase activity.[204]

The capsids show various surface features, including raised regions around the threefold axis of symmetry, a depressed region spanning the twofold axis, and in many cases a pore at the fivefold axis of symmetry that runs through the capsid (e.g., Refs.[5,249,290,335,336,365]) (see Fig. 6.1). The parvoviruses infecting invertebrates show a relatively smooth surface.[191,282] The host ranges and tissue tropisms of CPV and FPV, and of MVM variants, are controlled by a small number of residues on the capsid surface.[3,5,26,185,214]

Variability and flexibility in the capsid structure are important for viral infectivity and capsid functions—in particular, the externalization of VP1 and VP2 N-terminal sequences. Flexibility of surface loops occurs in CPV, FPV, MVM, and AAV capsids at different pHs, and after removal of Ca^{++} or other ions from capsids.[94,321,334] For many parvoviruses and AAVs, the VP1 or VP2 N-terminal regions can be exposed to the exterior in DNA-containing capsids, or after certain mild treatments, and that exposure was increased by changes of residues surrounding the fivefold axis of icosahedral symmetry.[67,93,122,203,291,371]

Cell Receptor Binding

Various molecules mediate parvovirus cell binding and infection. One cellular receptor for parvovirus B19 is globoside or erythrocyte P antigen (glycosphingolipid tetrahexoseceramide), and people who genetically lack P antigen (p phenotype) appear to resist parvovirus B19 infection.[39,48,49,190] However, the role of globoside binding is not well understood, and in some studies capsids did not bind the globoside *in vitro*, and its role may occur after cellular uptake[39]. The α5β1 integrin has been reported as a receptor for infection of erythroid progenitor cells.[380]

Transferrin receptor type 1 (TfR) is used by CPV and FPV for cell infection, and receptor binding controls differences in the host ranges of those viruses.[167,275] Capsids bind through contacts between the TfR apical domain and the capsid threefold spike.[56,214,274] CPV and FPV also bind to some forms of sialic acid but that binding appears not to mediate infection.[223] MVM capsids bind sialic acids, primarily *N*-acetyl neuraminic acid, and hemagglutinate mouse erythrocytes, and cell infection can be blocked by neuraminidase treatment of the cells prior to virus binding.[95] Differences in affinity of binding result in different pathogenicity in mice.[5,152,226]

The AAVs have broad cellular tropisms and infect many hosts. Infection may require more than one cell surface molecule, and different viral strains use different receptors. Different AAVs have been reported to bind sialic acids, heparan sulfate proteoglycan,[194,357] growth factor receptors,[289,298,382] and integrins.[356] Tropisms of AAV serotypes are at least in part associated with receptors on target cells, and retargeting AAV capsids to alternative receptors may allow transduction of additional cell types.[156,222,258,283,390]

Endocytosis and Endosomal Release

Parvoviruses require receptor-mediated endocytosis for cell infection. Capsids of CPV, H1, and MVM are taken up rapidly into cells by clathrin-mediated endocytosis, and are associated with clathrin-coated pits and vesicles after uptake.[101,220,276] Infection is inhibited by treatment of cells with lysosomotropic agents ammonium chloride (NH_4Cl), chloroquine, or bafilomycin A1, indicating that low endosomal pH is required for infection.[30,276,311] After uptake, capsids may be detected in endosomes by antibody staining or *in situ* hybridization for a number of hours.[154,276,355] The infectious process may be slow, and CPV infection could be blocked by anticapsid antibodies injected into the cytoplasm of cells 4 or more hours after virus uptake.[371,372]

Uptake and endocytosis of the AAV capsids follow similar pathways, and infection may require signaling after receptor binding.[108,288,322,404] Many studies have been aimed at improving the uptake and transduction of cells by use of variant AAVs, or by various approaches to capsid engineering.[65,217,303] Infection is influenced by the activity of the proteasome system, as proteosomal inhibitors can enhance the infection of many AAV vectors.[240,395] The capsids may be retained for long periods in the endosomal system, with some models indicating transport to the trans-Golgi compartment, and there may be a delay before the capsids escape into the cytoplasm.[29,36,109,117,404]

The mechanisms of capsid escape from endocytic vesicles into the cytosol are not well understood, but those likely involve the PLA_2 activity of the VP1 unique region, which enhances the release of the capsids into the cytoplasm, perhaps by modifying the endosomal membrane.[58,113,141]

Transport Within the Cytoplasm

Capsids are released into the cytoplasm from vesicles in a perinuclear location, and further processing and trafficking events likely occur before transport to the nucleus. Cell infection by MVM is affected by the activity of the proteasome, because infection can be reduced by proteasome inhibitors of the chymotrypsin-like activity (*N*-tosyl-L-phenylalanine chloromethyl ketone and aclarubin) but not by inhibitors of the trypsin-like activity, but without clear evidence for ubiquitination or of direct proteolytic digestion of the capsids.[312] Active mechanisms may also transport capsids from other regions of the cytoplasm to the vicinity of the nucleus. Endosomal vesicles transport the incoming virions to the vicinity of the nucleus, and that process, or possible direct transport of capsids, may be blocked by treatment of cells with nocodazole to depolymerize microtubules or by injection of an antibody against the intermediate chain of dynein.[234,353,371,372] By electron microscopy, capsids have been seen to associate with tubulin and dynein structures *in vitro*, and viral capsids may be precipitated from infected cells along with intermediate chain of dynein.

Nuclear Transport

Nuclear transport is thought to involve the viral capsid or DNA passing through the nuclear pore complex, although injection of MVM capsids into the cytoplasm of *Xenopus* oocytes showed possible permeabilization of the nuclear envelope.[88] Other studies show varying results after injection of parvovirus capsids into the cytoplasm of cells—some show them remaining in the cytoplasm, while others suggest passage through the nuclear pore.[234,372] Nuclear entry may require modification of the capsid to expose NLSs in the VP1 unique region. A VP1-derived peptide mediates nuclear transport when conjugated to bovine serum albumin (BSA),[371] that peptide is exposed on virions entering the cells, and antibodies to the VP1 unique region blocked infection when injected into cells around the time of virus inoculation.[371] MVM capsids have NLS motifs in both VP1 and VP2 (Fig. 6.4). A VP1 unique region that could mediate nuclear transport is required for efficient cell infection by MVM capsids.[224,367]

Viral DNA Release From the Capsid and Initiation of Replication

The viral DNA genome is released from the capsid for replication, but the process is not fully understood. The DNA may be extracted from the capsid without particle disassembly. DNA-containing capsids have 20 to 30 nucleotides of the 5′ end of the viral genome exposed on the outside of the capsid, with NS1 or Rep protein covalently attached to the 5′ end of that DNA in newly produced capsids. The 3′ end of the viral DNA may also become exposed outside the capsid without capsid disintegration[93,94], and that may initiate DNA replication by the host cell DNA polymerase, which could remove the DNA without capsid disassembly.

Autonomous Virus DNA Replication

The autonomous parvovirus genome is a linear ssDNA with terminal palindromes (Fig. 6.5), and many viruses have different palindromes at each end[20,306] and many primarily package the minus DNA strand.[97] DNA replication has been most extensively studied for the rodent protoparvoviruses. Only two nonstructural (NS) proteins are encoded by most parvoviruses. Replication depends on the DNA replication machinery of the cell and various cellular proteins, and in most cases the cell must pass through S phase.[358,386]

NS1 is the major parvovirus regulatory protein involved in DNA replication and gene regulation. It is a helicase, adenosine triphosphatase (ATPase), and site-specific nickase, and it

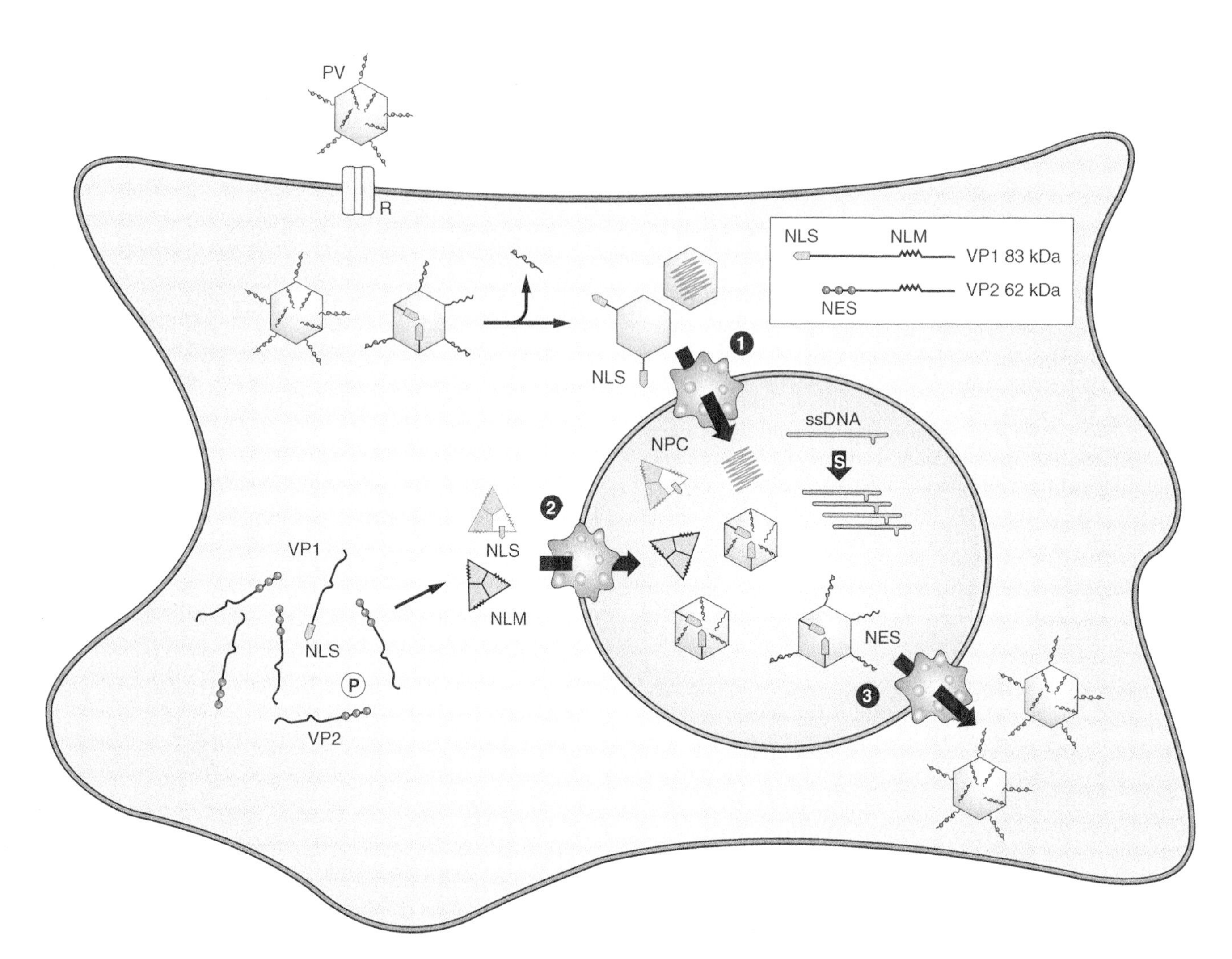

FIGURE 6.4 **The nuclear transport of the parvoviral capsid proteins and capsids in the life cycle.** Part *(1)* shows the processes include the cleavage of the VP2 N-terminal sequences containing a nuclear export sequence (NES) from the incoming particle and exposure of the N-terminal sequences of the VP1 protein containing a nuclear localization sequence (NLS). Part *(2)* shows association between the VP1 and phosphorylated VP2 results in translocation into the nucleus as timers, where the particles assemble. Part *(3)* shows how the newly assembled particles are transported out of the nucleus and into the cytoplasm using the phosphorylated N-terminus of the VP2 protein as an NES. (Adapted from Valle N, Riolobos L, Almendral JM. Synthesis, post-translational modification and trafficking of the parvovirus structural polypeptides. In: Kerr JR, Cotmore SF, Bloom ME, et al., eds. *Parvoviruses*. London: Hodder Arnold; 2006:291–304. Copyright © 2005 by Taylor & Francis Group, LLC. Reproduced by permission of Taylor and Francis Group, LLC, a division of Informa plc.)

becomes covalently attached to the 5′ side of the nick through residue Y210,[23,85,92,95,267] within a motif characteristic of proteins involved in rolling circle replication (RCR motif).[170] NS1 cleaves within the extended duplex form of oriL in the dimer bridge and within the hairpinned form of the right end palindrome, but not the hairpinned form of the left terminal palindrome (see Figs. 6.5–6.7). The left end palindrome contains a short sequence that is not complementary; when extended in the dimer bridge, there is a 5′GA/TC to the right of the axis of symmetry and a 5′GAA/CTT to the left, and cleavage occurs at the 5′GA/TC site and involves a cellular protein (parvovirus initiation factor [PIF]).[81,83] The interaction between NS1 and PIF allows ATP hydrolysis so that the DNA double helix can be unwound and NS1 cleavage of its single-stranded substrate (see Fig. 6.5). PIF is a cellular transcriptional factor of the KDWK motif family, which functions as a heterodimer with subunits of 96 and 79 kDa.[84]

Other cellular proteins are required or assist in MVM DNA replication, including phosphokinase C (PKC), PKC eta, which is required for NS1 to function in RCR, while PKC lambda phosphorylates NS1 at T435 and S473 so that NS1 can function as a helicase.[89,210,266] Cyclin A is required for DNA replication. MVM replication evokes a DNA damage response, and H2AX, Nbs1, RPA32, Chk2, and p53 are all phosphorylated and recruited to MVM replication centers.[2,316] Parvovirus DNA replication takes place in discrete subnuclear structures (called parvovirus-associated replication structures [PARs]), which contain DNA polymerases α and δ.[31,103,169]

Autonomous parvovirus DNA replication involves a complex series of specific single-stranded cleavages, extensions from base-paired 3′ ends, and the base pairing and resolution of terminal palindromic structures—as shown in Figures 6.6 and 6.7. The 3′ terminal hairpin of the viral genome serves as a primer for complementary strand synthesis (see step 1, Fig. 6.6).

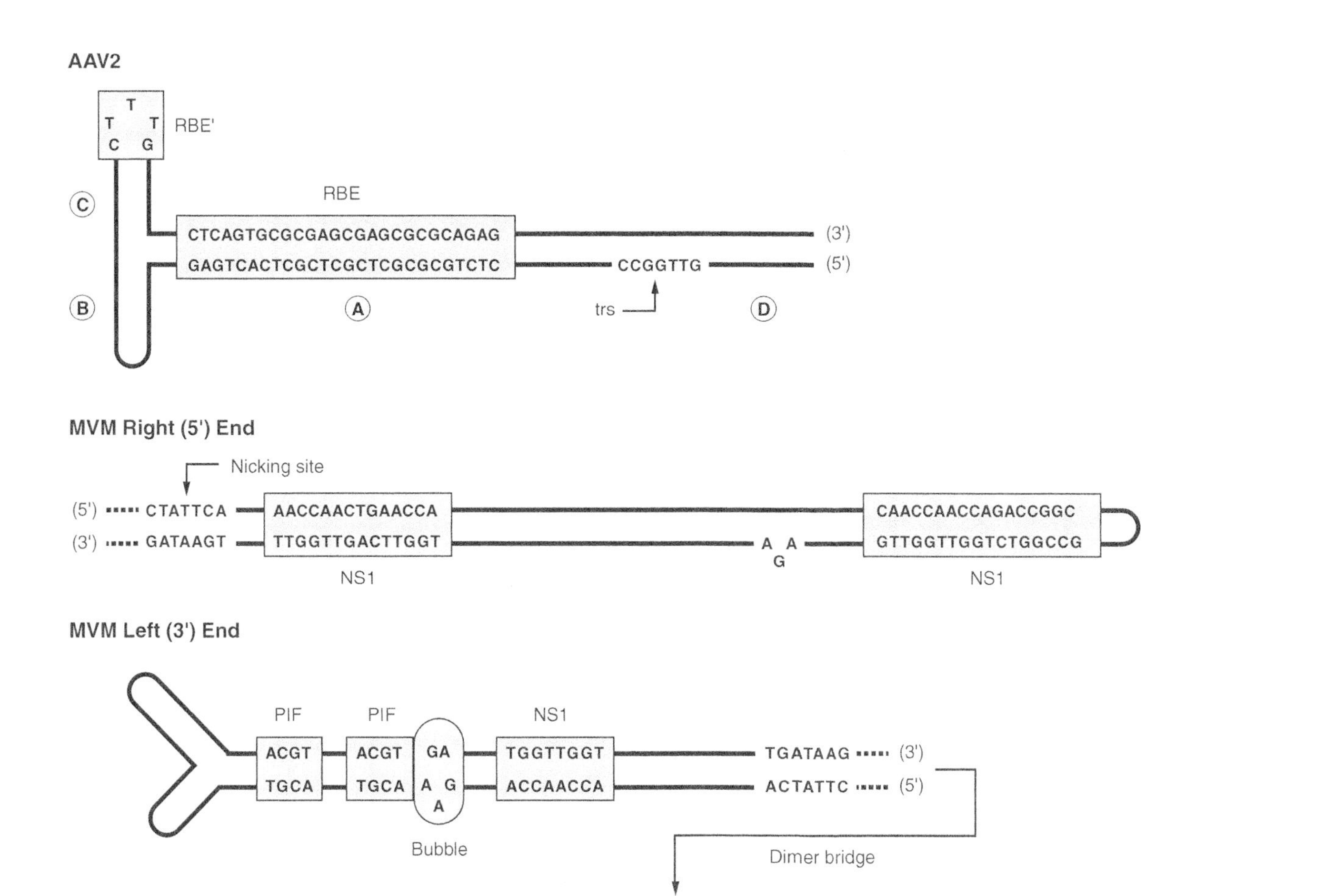

FIGURE 6.5 **Comparison of the 3′ and 5′ terminal palindromic sequences of minute virus of mice (MVM) DNA with the adeno-associated virus (AAV) terminal repeat, which is identical at both ends.** Also shown is the 3′ dimer bridge that is formed in a dimer replicative intermediate during MVM replication. In each case, the key sequence elements are indicated that area required for AAV Rep nicking at the terminal resolution site (TRS), of NS1 nicking at the 5′ (right end) hairpin, or in the 3′ (left end) dimer bridge. The hairpin sequences are shown in their most stable secondary structure. In the AAV hairpin, B and C by convention are the small internal palindromes flanked by the A palindrome that forms the stem of the first 125 bases. The D sequence comprises the remaining 20 bases of the terminal repeats that are inboard of the TRS.

The elongating strand is covalently linked to the hairpinned form of the 5′ end of the template to form a linear duplex molecule covalently cross-linked at both ends by DNA hairpins (see step 2, Fig. 6.6). The hairpin at the right end is nicked on the newly synthesized strand by NS1 at a site 18 nucleotides downstream from the original 5′ end, with the NS1 becoming covalently linked to the 5′ end released (see step 3, Fig. 6.6). The 3′ OH released by this cleavage is used as a primer for repair synthesis to fill the gap, so that the right end of the intermediate is now a double-stranded extended form of the original 5′ palindrome, with NS1 covalently linked to the 5′ end of the parental strand. The restored 5′ end is 18 nucleotides longer than the 5′ end of virion DNA (step 4, Fig. 6.6). The extended form of the right end palindromic sequence is denatured so that both strands can form hairpins (see step 5, Fig. 6.6), and the 3′ OH primes DNA synthesis through both strands of the linear duplex monomer, forming a linear duplex dimer (see step 7, Fig. 6.6). The palindromic sequence at the center of the dimer intermediate is termed the dimer bridge, and three sites in the dimeric intermediate are potentially susceptible to single-strand nicking by NS1: two in the covalently closed right end hairpins at each end of the intermediate and a third on the right side of the dimer bridge at GA/TC (nicked at TC; the GAA/TCC sequence on the left side of the dimer bridge is not cleaved)[98] (see Figs. 6.6 and 6.7). Nicking at TC leaves NS1 covalently linked to the 5′ side of the nick and a free 3′ OH, and the bound NS1 unwinds the helix in the 3′ to 5′ direction, allowing the palindromic sequence of the dimer bridge to form a cruciform structure that can function as a template for the synthesis. When the newly synthesized strand extends beyond the GA bubble sequence, there is a template strand switch where the newly synthesized strand is displaced from the template, forms

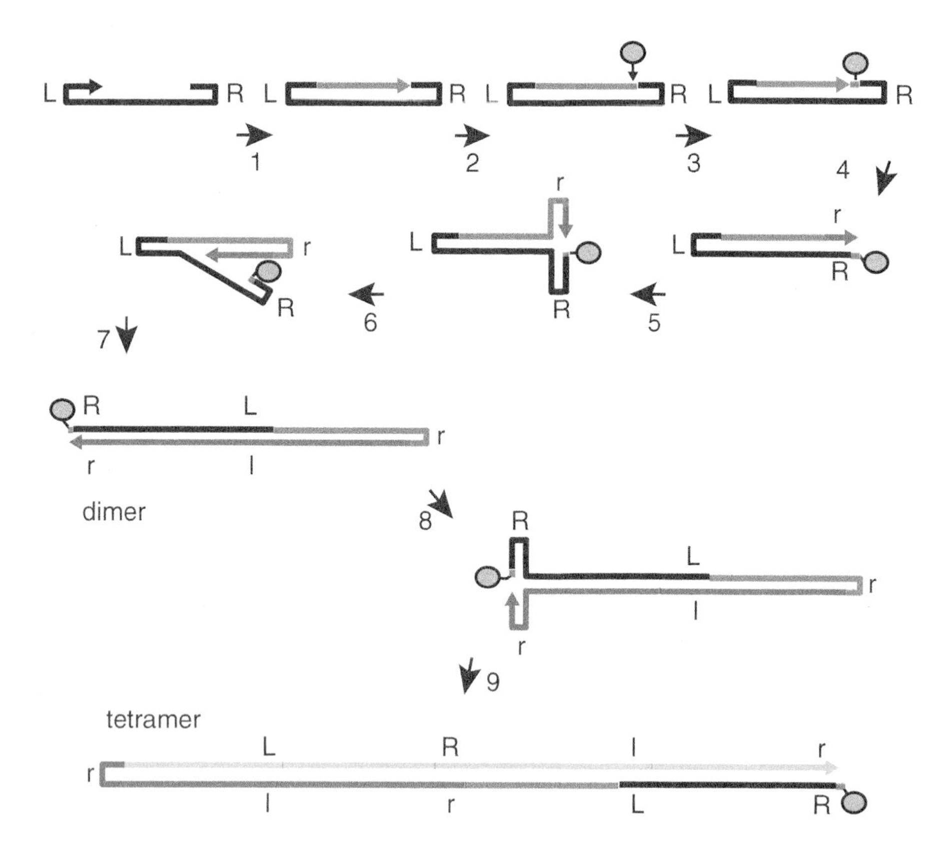

FIGURE 6.6 **The replication cycle of the autonomous parvovirus DNA, based on the rolling hairpin model for minute virus of mice (MVM).** The viral genome is represented by a continuous line (shaded *black* for the original genome and different colors for the newly synthesized DNAs); the 3′ end is indicated by an *arrowhead.* The letters L and R represent the left-end and right-end palindromic sequences, respectively. Upper and lower case represent the "flip" and "flop" versions of the sequences, which are inverted complements of each other. (Reprinted with permission from Cotmore SF, Tattersall P. Parvovirus DNA replication. In: DePamphilis ML, ed. *DNA Replication in Eukaryotic Cells.* Plainview, NY: Cold Spring Laboratory Press; 1996: 801. Copyright © 1996 Cold Spring Harbor Laboratory Press.)

a hairpin, and copies the strand to the right of the dimer bridge. This creates a new left terminal palindrome in the original flip orientation and displaces a single-stranded monomer equivalent, which is still linked to a duplex, unit length component. This proposed synthesis involves two template strand switches. The duplex molecule created is cross-linked at one end by the right palindrome and could go through multiple rounds of displacement synthesis to produce minus strands with the original flip orientation of the left palindrome for packaging into the virion, as seen for MVM.[97] In this model, NS1 cannot cleave oriL when the left end palindrome is in the hairpin conformation but can in the extended duplex form of the dimer bridge in the RF. However, NS1 can nick oriR when the right end palindrome is hairpinned. The genomic ssDNA is generated and packaged only when capsids are present.[96,97]

Adeno-Associated Virus DNA Replication

The AAV genomes vary in size (between 4,500 and 5,000 nucleotides long) and have palindromic terminal sequences that serve as the primers for DNA replication of AAV (see Fig. 6.5). AAVs have several forms of the NS1 equivalent protein (called Rep) with multiple functions in DNA replication, while DNA polymerase, ssDNA-binding protein, and additional factors are supplied by either the helper virus or the cell. Because of the AAV ITR and the evidence for inversion of the palindromic sequences at both termini, replication can occur by single-strand displacement (Fig. 6.8). The 3′ terminal repeats fold over to form hairpin structures[233] that serve as primers for DNA synthesis[350] (see Fig. 6.8). Complementary strand synthesis forms a linear duplex molecule cross-linked at one end by the terminal hairpin, or the growing end of the complementary strand may become covalently linked to the hairpinned form of the ITR at the 5′ end of the parental strand template to form a linear duplex cross-linked at both ends. Resolution is achieved by Rep 68 or 78 binding to the hairpin via a Rep binding sequence [RBS], as well as a secondary binding site on one of the cross-arms, (see Fig. 6.5) and nicking the original parental strand at the terminal resolution site (TRS), which is opposite the phosphodiester bond between the 3′OH of the primer and the 5′PO_4 of the first nucleotide inserted into the progeny strand.[45,77,241,317] Rep covalently binds to the 5′ end released by the nick, while the 3′ end serves as a primer for synthesis, filling in the resultant gap at the 5′ end of the parental strand using the displaced hairpin sequence as the template.[171,337] Thus, the original 3′ end of the parental strand is transferred to become the 5′ end of the new strand, and the terminal palindromic sequence is inverted. The 3′ end of the newly synthesized strand may now fold over to prime synthesis of another new strand to produce a linear, duplex dimer-length molecule.[262] The structure of the initial primer strand may be either a linear single strand with a hairpinned 3′ end or a single-stranded circle held together by H-bonding between the ITRs (see Fig. 6.8).

The functional complex of Rep is a pentamer.[160] The large Rep proteins introduce site-specific nicks at the TRS, and their helicases cause hairpin unwinding during resolution of the termini, while the two smaller Rep 52/40 proteins can bind ATP, have helicase activity, and may be involved in packaging of ssDNA strands into preformed capsids.[172,337,340] Rep 40 does not bind specifically to RBS but does bind ssDNA.[399] The site-specific DNA binding and endonuclease activities are functions of the N-terminal domain of the larger Rep 68/78 proteins.[338] The RBS is a tandem repeat of four copies of GAGC, but only two of the GAGC are required to bind Rep.[77,241,317]

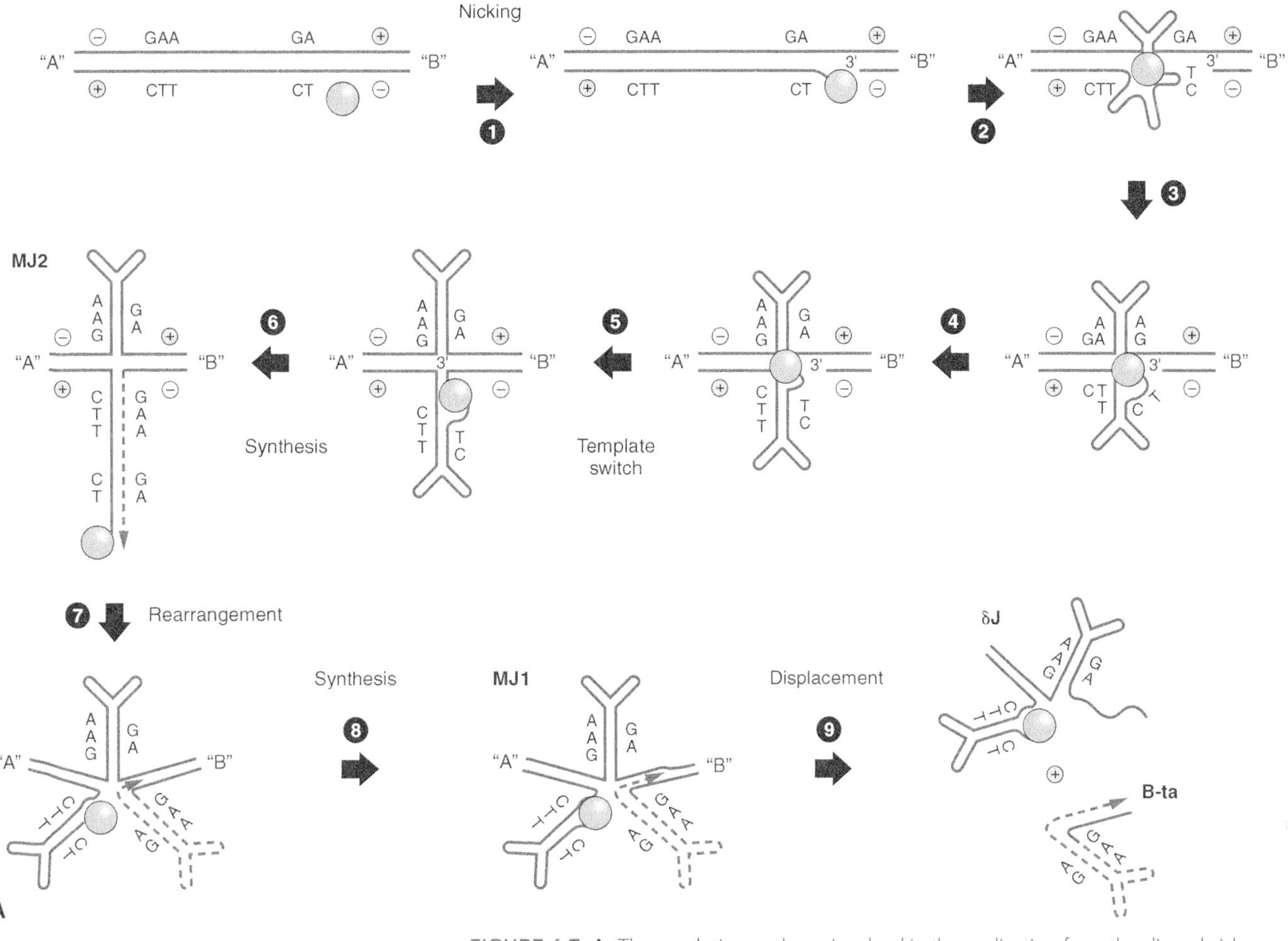

δJ "A" "B"

"A" "B"

"A" GAA GA

B CTT CT

FIGURE 6.7 A: The resolution pathway involved in the replication from the dimer bridge during the replication of minute virus of mice. After nicking the initiation site in the B arm of the dimer bridge (step i), NS1 associates with RPA to function as a 3′-to-5′ helicase (step ii), unwinding the lower strand of the palindrome and allowing the exposed single strands to fold back on themselves, creating a cruciform intermediate (step iii). Branch migration proceeds (step iv), eventually passing the inactive initiation site in the A arm. At this point, the exposed 3′ nucleotide can switch templates and anneal to its complement in the lower cruciform arm (step v). A replication fork assembling at this time will copy and unwind the cruciform arm, synthesizing a palindrome in the flip orientation on the end of the negative sense B strand (step vi). This heterocruciform structure corresponds to the MJ2 intermediate. In a second duplex-to-hairpin transition, the palindromic heterocruciform arm of MJ2 is then melted out and both strands fold back on themselves (step vii), allowing the exposed 3′ end to base pair with inboard sequences in the B arm. A replication fork established at this 3′ end would copy the lower strand of the B arm (step viii), creating the MJ1 intermediate and progressively displacing the upper strand, leading to the eventual release of a newly synthesized B turnaround form (step ix). The residual δJ intermediate is partially single stranded, having an intact upper strand paired to an NS1-associated lower strand from the A arm. Because this complex carries the active helicase, it is presumed to be a dynamic structure in which the bridge palindrome is periodically reconfigured into a cruciform structure, as shown. **B:** Introduction of a single-strand nick and resolution of the δJ intermediate. The initiation site in the A arm of the palindrome is periodically exposed as a single strand during duplex-to-hairpin rearrangements of δJ (step i). This allows NS1 to attack the initiation site in $OriL_{GAA}$ without the help of a cofactor (step ii). Nicking leads to the release of a positive sense B strand and leaves a base-paired 3′ nucleotide on the A arm (step iii) to prime assembly of a fork that will copy the hairpin, creating an extended form of the A arm (step iv). (Adapted from Cotmore SF, Tattersall P. Resolution of parvovirus dimer junctions proceeds through a novel heterocruciform intermediate. *J Virol* 2003;77(11):6245–6254. Copyright © 2003 American Society for Microbiology. Amended with permission from American Society for Microbiology.)

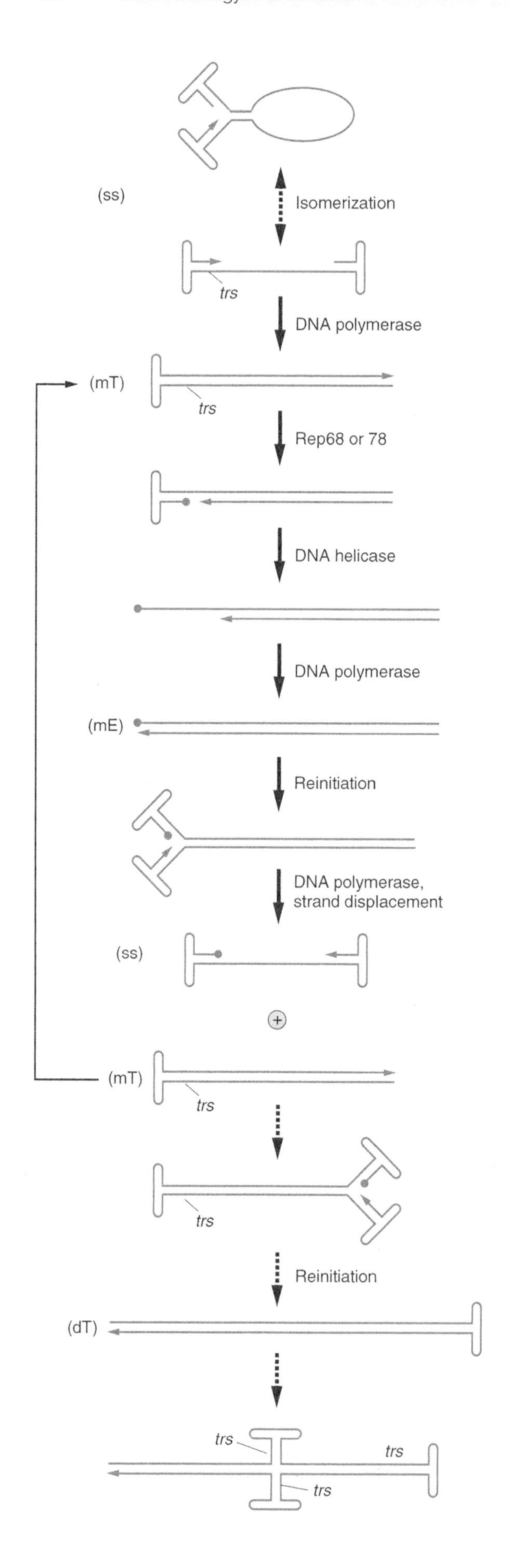

Rep 68/78 functions as a multimeric complex that binds to the RBS in the stem of the T-shaped structure of the folded ITR and also to a second site (RBS′, GTTTC) at the tip of the cross arm farthest removed from the TRS[46,317] (see Fig. 6.5). The TRS consists of a seven-base sequence (3′CCGGT/TG5′) recognized only on the correct strand.[46] Once bound to the hairpin, Rep unwinds the stem of the ITR in a reaction that requires ATP hydrolysis to generate a single-stranded TRS,[105,339] and then tyrosine 156 of Rep is linked to the 5′ phosphate end of the nick.[172,338] Rep remains covalently bound until after packaging occurs.[296]

AAV DNA replication requires both cellular and helper virus components. Although adenovirus encodes a DNA polymerase, AAV replication primarily uses cellular DNA polymerase δ. Other cellular factors required included replication factor 3, proliferating cell nuclear antigen (PCNA), and the so-called minichromosome maintenance complex. The herpes simplex virus (HSV) DNA polymerase may be used for AAV replication.[252,381] Several other helper virus gene products are required for AAV DNA replication. Adenovirus ssDNA-binding protein enhances AAV DNA replication.[66,177] HSV gene products include UL30/UL42 HSV DNA polymerase; the helicase–primase complex of UL5, UL8, and UL52; and the UL29 product ICP8, the HSV ssDNA-binding protein[252,381] AAV DNA replication colocalizes with helper viral ssDNA-binding proteins and with replication protein A (RPA), the cellular ssDNA-binding protein, and proteins associated with the DNA damage response.[327] In adenovirus coinfected cells, AAV replication can be associated with PML bodies, but those are not seen with the HSV helper.[125] Cellular proteins associated with AAV DNA replication include replication factor C (RFC), PCNA, RPA, Mre 11/rad50/Nbs1 complex, Ku70 and -86, and other mismatch repair proteins.[262,263] Nuclear high mobility group protein 1 (HMG1) binds to cruciform DNA[90] and binds to AAV hairpins and Rep to stimulate Rep nicking, ATPase activity, and repression of AAV gene expression from the P5 promoter. The 52 kDa FK 506 binding protein FKBP52 binds to the single-stranded form of the D region of the ITR, the 20 nucleotide of the ITR beyond the palindrome.[238,299] The phosphorylated form of the protein binds and inhibits DNA replication, whereas when the nonphosphorylated form binds, synthesis can occur. Phosphorylation is controlled by the epidermal growth factor receptor tyrosine kinase and correlates with the ability of AAV vectors to transduce cells in the absence of a helper virus.

FIGURE 6.8 The replication cycle of the adeno-associated viral DNA. The single-stranded DNA released from the virion after uncoating (top two possible forms) is extended from the 3′ end of the hairpin to form a full-length hairpin. The hairpin is nicked at the terminal recognition site by Rep68 or rep78, leaving the Rep protein attached to the end of the DNA. The hairpinned end is unwound, and the 3′ end formed by Rep cleavage is extended to the end of the template strand. The ends of each strand refold into their alternative self-base pairing hairpin structures, and full-length DNA synthesis from the 3′ primer on the left end of the genome produces one single-stranded genome and one duplex structure, which can each serve as a substrate for additional round of replication. mT, monomer turnaround; dT, dimer turnaround replicative form; ss, single-strand viral DNA; mE, monomer extended replicative form, TRS, terminal recognition site.

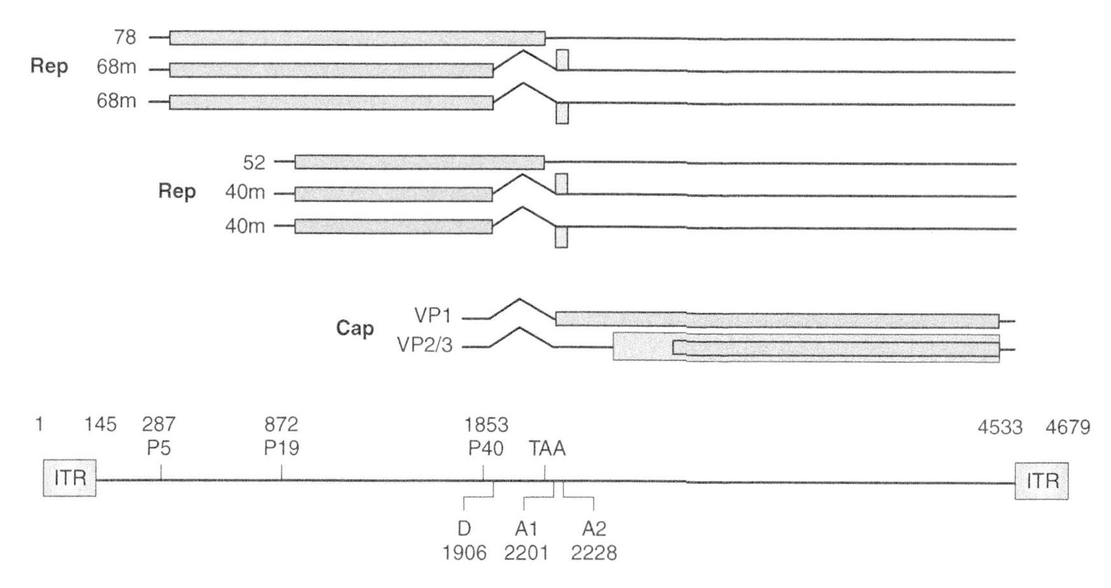

FIGURE 6.9 Transcriptional maps of the autonomous parvovirus minute virus of mice. The three major transcript classes (R1, R2, and R3) are shown relative to the viral genome, and the P4 and P38 promoters are indicated. The proteins encoded are shown as NS1, NS2, VP1/2, and the SAT proteins. The alternative open reading frames used are shown as different shading patterns. (Adapted from Pintel DJ, Gersappe A, Haut D, et al. Determinants that govern alternative splicing of parvovirus pre-mRNAs. *Semin Virol* 1995;6(5):283–290. Copyright © 1995 Elsevier. With permission.)

Transcription

Autonomous Parvovirus Transcription

The transcriptional schemes of the autonomous parvoviruses are both complex and variable (Figs. 6.9 and 6.10). Many use promoters around map positions 4 and 38 to generate two primary transcripts, along with one polyadenylation signal near the right end of the genome, and most have multiple additional messages generated primarily by alternative splicing.[181,254] A small intron is generally found between map positions 44 and 46, and a large intron between map positions 10 and 39. For MVM, all messengers have the small intron spliced, although alternative splice donor and acceptor sites are used. Half of the P4 transcripts also have the larger intron spliced at alternative splice donor and splice acceptor sites, producing at least nine mRNAs.[181,254] Where the P38 transcript uses the upstream splice donor site, the mRNA is translated to VP1, while the downstream donor site gives VP2. The erythroparvoviruses have one promoter at map position 6 but produce at least 12 different messages.[133] Those include two polyadenylation signals—near the middle of the genome and at the right end[147,272] (see Fig. 6.10). Read-through of the internal polyA site occurs only with genome replication, and the large transcript is translated into the capsid protein.[148] The Amdoparvoviruses have promoters at map positions 3 and 36, and the mRNAs have complex splicing patterns.[300,347] The Bocaparvoviruses have promoters at map positions 4.5, 13, and 39; NS proteins and VPs are encoded in large ORFs in the left and right sides of the genome, and a small ORF that overlaps the 3′ terminus of the NS ORF encodes NP1.[74,112(p1)]

Regulation of transcription and posttranscriptional modification is complex. For MVM, splicing of the large intron (map units 10 to 39) depends on splicing of the small intron

FIGURE 6.10 Transcription map of the B19 genome, showing the level of complexity of the RNAs produced by alternative splicing and polyadenylation. The main features shown include the viral promoter (P6), the various splice donors (D1 and D2) and acceptors (A1-1, A1-2, A2-1, A2-2), and the polyadenylation sites (pA). Other features shown are the open reading frames (*open* or *closed boxes*) and the products likely generated from each transcript. (Adapted from Guan W, Cheng F, Huang Q, et al. Inclusion of the central exon of parvovirus B19 precursor mRNA is determined by multiple splicing enhancers in both the exon and the downstream intron. *J Virol* 2011;85(5):2463–2468. Copyright © 2011 American Society for Microbiology. Amended with permission from American Society for Microbiology.)

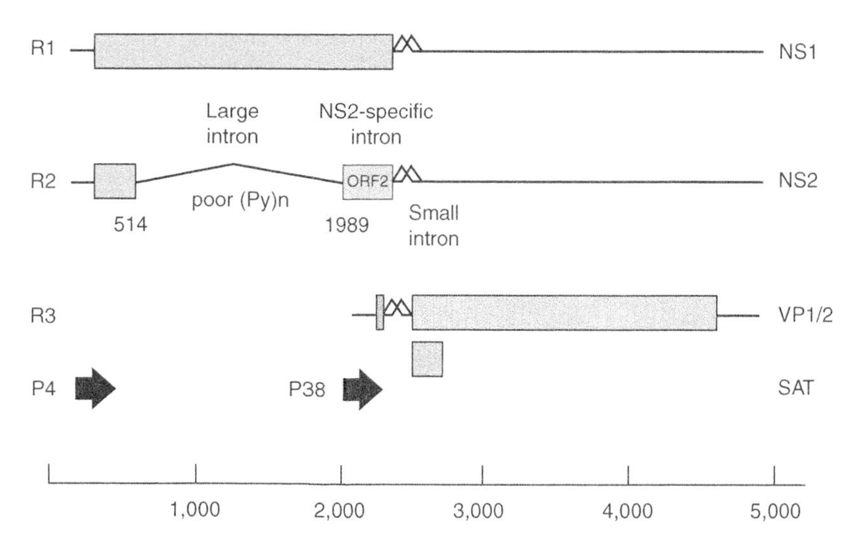

(44 to 46), and NS1 transactivates P39 transcription.[111,405] Three *cis*-active genomic sequences near P39 are required for transactivation—the tar (transactivation response element) to which NS1 binds in a reaction that is ATP dependent, an Sp1 site, and the TATA box.[6,82,230,231] NS1 can also interact with CBP, Sp1, TBP (TATA-binding protein), and TFIIA in the absence of DNA.[201,231] The promoter contains binding sites for Sp1, CREB/ATF, E2F, and NF-Y, and several regulatory mechanisms link MVM expression and replication to the cell cycle.[106,130,285] The viral NS2 interacts with the nuclear export protein Crm-1 and mutations altering MVMi NS2 binding to Crm-1 influence replication in different cells.[78,250]

AAV Transcription

The AAV genome contains three transcription units with promoters at map positions 5, 19, and 40 (Fig. 6.11), and one polyadenylation signal is at map position 96, so that all three transcripts cover the 3′ half of the plus strand.[301,352] A single intron lies just beyond mp 40, and the ratio of spliced to unspliced mRNA species depends on binding of Rep 78/68 to the transcription template.[301,302] Four mRNAs cover all or part of the ORF in the left half of the genome, two of which initiate at the P5 (mp5) promoter; one is spliced and produces Rep 68, and the other is not spliced and forms Rep 78. The P19 promoter also produces two mRNAs producing Rep 52 and

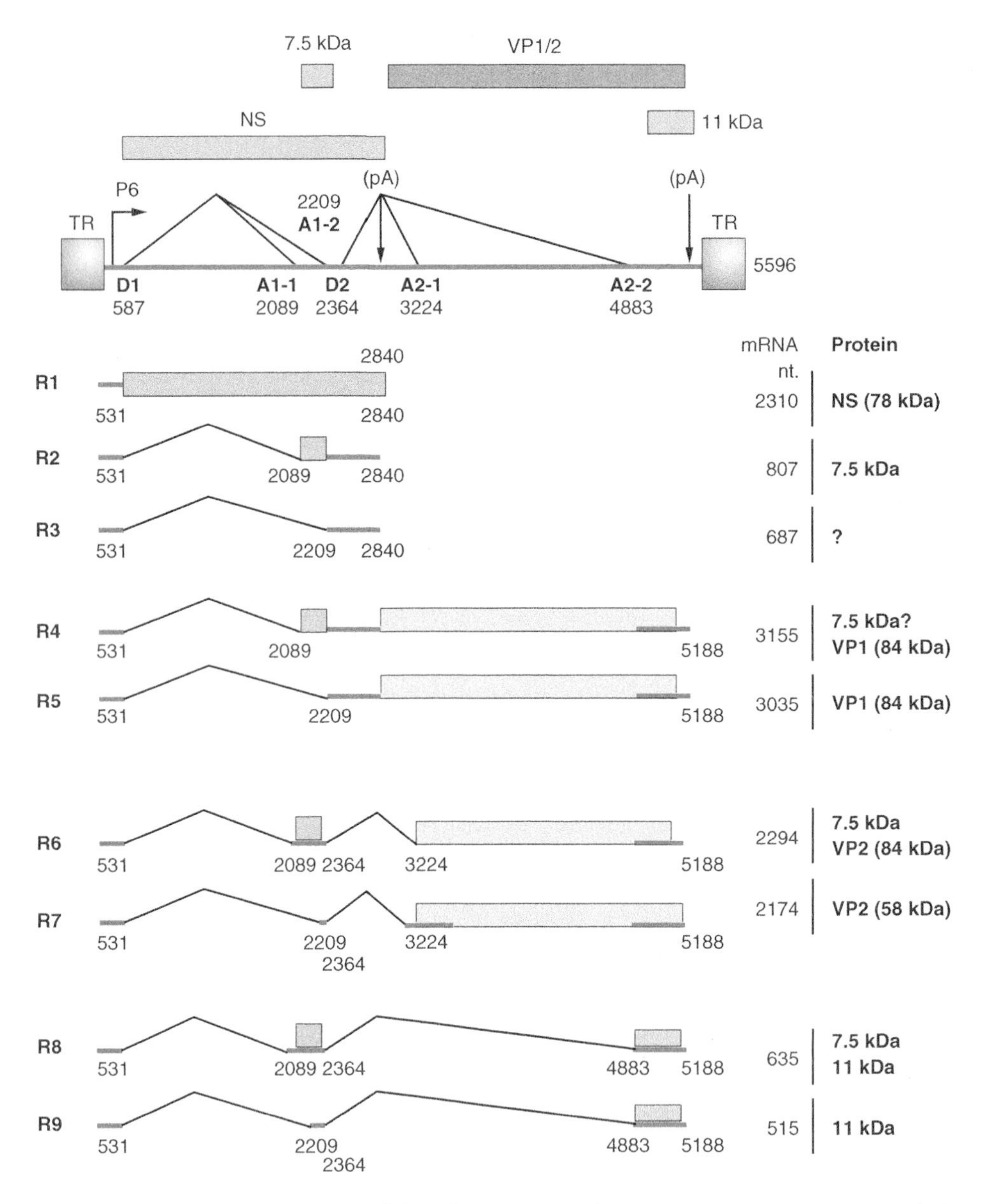

FIGURE 6.11 Transcriptional map of the adeno-associated virus type 2 (AAV2) genome, which includes three promoters (P5, P19, P40), the small intron donor (D), and acceptors (A1 and A2), the termination sites of the Rep and Cap messages. The major transcripts and the proteins they encode are shown, and the different open reading frames used are shown with different shading. (Adapted from Qiu J, Yoto Y, Tullis G, et al. Parvovirus RNA processing strategies. In: Kerr JR, Cotmore SF, Bloom ME, et al., eds. *Parvoviruses*. London: Hodder Arnold; 2006:253–274. Copyright © 2005 by Taylor & Francis Group, LLC. Reproduced by permission of Taylor and Francis Group, LLC, a division of Informa plc.)

Rep 40. The P40 produces two major mRNAs splice variants; one encodes VP1, and when the VP1 initiator codon is spliced out, an ACG initiator codon is used to translate VP2, and the first AUG in phase is used as the initiator codon for VP3.[256] An additional protein encoded by an alternative ORF within the *cap* gene has the initiator codon CTG, and the 23-kd protein promotes capsid formation.[261,345] In AAV5, most transcripts originating from P7 and P19 are polyadenylated at a site in the intron.[301,397]

AAV represses its own transcription and DNA replication in the absence of a helper virus, but limited Rep expression results in establishment of latent infection. Adenovirus helper factors include early regions (E) 1A, 1B, 2A, and 4 (ORF 6).[7,307] The ICP0 gene product of HSV-1 turns on AAV transcription and can activate transcription from an integrated latent viral genome.[137] Cellular transcriptional regulatory elements control AAV RNA synthesis, and the P5 promoter sequence contains binding sites for cellular, helper, and AAV transcriptional factors.[208,284]

Protein Synthesis

Autonomous Parvovirus Proteins

Protein synthesis depends on transcription, and NS protein transcripts appear earliest in the course of infection, and NS proteins regulate gene expression.[86,110,218] NS1 dimerizes prior to nuclear localization,[268,297] MVM NS2 is required for efficient virus growth in a host-dependent manner and is essential for growth in mouse cell lines and in animals.[104,228,259,316]

Adeno-Associated Virus Proteins

AAV protein amounts correspond to the levels of their transcripts. Rep78 and 68 are predominantly found in the nucleus, while Rep52 and 40 are also found in the cytoplasm.[244] Rep78 represses the p5 promoter, while Rep68 and Rep52 are less repressive, while either Rep78 or 68 may transactivate the p40 promoter.[166] VP1 to VP3 are translated from alternatively spliced p40 mRNAs, with VP2 starting from an ACG codon and VP3 from a downstream AUG, and VP1 is translated from the low-abundance spliced p40 message [256](see Fig. 6.11).

Virion Assembly

Capsid proteins translated in the cytoplasm are transported to the nucleus, where they assemble[309] (see Fig. 6.4). The major capsid proteins can assemble alone into capsids that are structurally similar to normal capsids, which can package DNA,[315,367,402] but the other capsid proteins (VP1 and VP3) are required for infectivity, likely due to the PLA_2 and nuclear localization functions of the VP1.[123,141,315,321,371] VP2 assembly requires nuclear transport, and multiple NLS appear to be present, and it is enhanced by the expression of an assembly activating protein.[165,261,390]

Viral ssDNA is inserted into the preassembled capsid and requires the helicase activity of the NS1 to translocate the ssDNA into the capsid[96,116,291,406] (Fig. 6.12). The polarity of DNA packaging of some viruses results from differences in the use of sequences at each end of the genome for initiating replication.[97] Capsids may be retained within the nucleus, translocated into the cytoplasm, or transported out of the cell in a process regulated at least in part by the phosphorylation state of the capsid proteins and the activity of gelsolin in the cytoplasm[28,120,224,385,402] (see Fig. 6.4).

Adeno-Associated Virus Latent Infection

AAV can establish a latent infection, apparently allowing the genome to persist until conditions allow replication. In cell culture AAV latent infection requires inoculation of a high multiplicity of infection in the absence of helper, but the genomes may persist for many cell passages.[286] The AAV genome can integrate into the cell genome: wild-type AAV2 integrated to a higher level at a specific site (AAVS1) on the q arm of human chromosome 19 (q13.4), which included a 33-nucleotide sequence containing the RBS and the TRS separated by an 11-nucleotide spacer.[168,219,245,320] (Fig. 6.13). Expression of Rep 78/68 was required in *trans*, and viral DNA was mostly integrated as a concatemer.[76,140,168,175,286] Integration occurs approximately randomly without Rep expression.[243] The AAV genome may also survive for prolonged periods as an extrachromosomal element and be expressed in the absence of a Rep gene. The unusual ends of the genome allow it to resist intracellular exonucleases and may prevent DNA modification, which would turn off expression. The extrachromosomal forms of AAV DNA are concatemers that are thought to be circular.[344] Many people likely harbor viral DNA sequences that can be reactivated.[129] No negative consequences of AAV DNA persistence have been demonstrated.

PATHOGENESIS AND CONTROL OF TISSUE TROPISM

Parvoviruses likely infect most vertebrates and invertebrates, and many appear not to be commonly associated with disease.[126,180,341] Some major vertebrate pathogens are listed in Table 6.2. Autonomous parvoviruses mostly require S phase of the cell cycle for their replication, so there is an age dependence to many diseases. However, only some tissues containing dividing cells are targeted for high levels of infection, and there are additional controls of tropism.[278] Viral genes, including the capsid and NS2 sequences, govern the host range or pathogenicity of parvoviruses.[26(p),42,56,104,227]

Fetal and Neonatal Infections

Fetal and newborn animals are highly susceptible to infection owing to the large number of dividing cells, and several parvoviruses cause fetal death or abortion. However, maternal immunity completely protects the fetus, and maternal antibodies generally also protect the newborn for some weeks after birth. Fetal or neonatal infections in animals lacking maternal immunity can be caused by PPV,[102,351] bovine parvovirus,[348] goose and duck parvovirus,[265] parvovirus B19,[70,270] and AMDV.[8] Some infections are fatal, or the surviving fetus may suffer severe sequelae, such as congenital cerebellar ataxia by infecting cells in the developing cerebellum.[195,305] Neonatal dogs infected with CPV may develop myocarditis.[216] MVM and other parvoviruses may infect renal vascular endothelial cells and lymphocytes in mice.[53,215] Newborn mink infected with AMDV develop severe respiratory distress due to infection of type 2 alveolar pneumocytes, which proliferate in the neonatal period.[10,374]

Older Animals

Parvoviral diseases in older animals result from the direct effects of virus infection on target tissues, and sometimes from the subsequent immune responses. Direct infections of the target

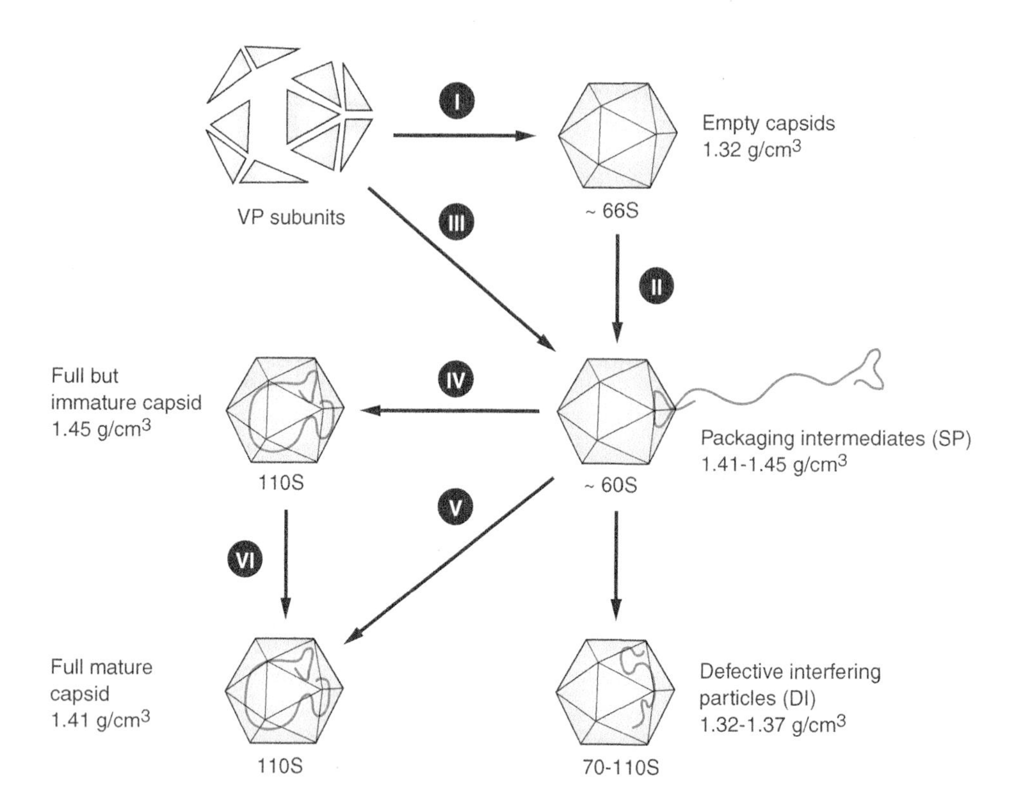

FIGURE 6.12 Possible pathways for parvovirus assembly and DNA incorporation, based on various studies of adeno-associated and autonomous viruses. Several mechanisms are possible; however, the current data propose the assembly of capsids from viral protein subunits, possibly trimers (see Fig.6.4), some of which remain as empty particles. The single-strand DNA is packaged during replication into the more or less intact capsids through the activity of the nonstructural or Rep protein. A final step involves the "maturation" of the capsids, which is seen as a small change in the buoyant density of the particle from 1.45 to 1.41 g/cm^3. (Adapted from Kleinschmidt JA, King JA. Molecular interactions involved in assembling the viral particle and packaging the genome. In: Kerr JR, Cotmore SF, Bloom ME, et al., eds. *Parvoviruses*. London: Hodder Arnold; 2006:305–319. Copyright © 2005 by Taylor & Francis Group, LLC. Reproduced by permission of Taylor and Francis Group, LLC, a division of Informa plc.)

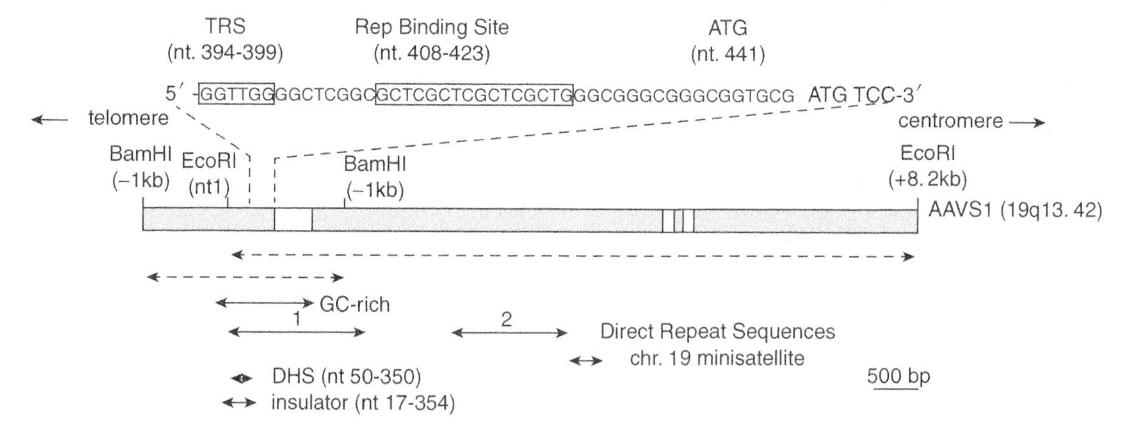

FIGURE 6.13 Schematic representation of the adeno-associated virus S1 region, the favored site of integration into the human chromosome position 19q13.42 chromosome, within the BamHI and EcoRI fragments as mapped by (REF and REF), where the EcoRI site is indicated as position 1. The sequence and position of the Rep-binding site (RBS), terminal resolution site (TRS), and the *MBS85* gene translation start sequence (ATG) are indicated, which allow Rep recognition and nicking. Locations of the GC-rich region, direct repeat sequence, chromosome 19 minisatellite sequence, DNAse I hypersensitive site (DHS), and insulator element as indicated by *arrows*. (Adapted from Dutheil N, Linden RM. Site-specific integration by adeno-associated virus. In: Kerr JR, Cotmore SF, Bloom ME, et al., eds. *Parvoviruses*. London: Hodder Arnold; 2006:213–236. Copyright © 2005 by Taylor & Francis Group, LLC. Reproduced by permission of Taylor and Francis Group, LLC, a division of Informa plc.)

TABLE 6.2 Major parvovirus pathogens of vertebrates

Virus	Disease
Human parvovirus B19 and primate erythroviruses	Erythema in children, polyarthritis and arthralgia, transient aplastic crisis, fetal hydrops
Feline parvovirus (canine parvovirus and feline panleukopenia virus, mink enteritis virus)	Enteritis; generalized neonatal disease, myocarditis, ataxia following cerebellar hypoplasia
Porcine parvovirus	Fetal infection and death, abortion, infertility
Aleutian mink disease virus	Chronic immune complexes
Canine minute virus	Mild diarrhea, fetal or neonatal death
Minute virus of mice, rat virus, H1 virus of rats	Congenital fetal malformations, persistent subclinical infections
Goose parvovirus and duck parvovirus	Hepatitis and myocarditis

organs includes enteritis in CPV-infected dogs or FPV-infected cats, hepatitis in hamsters and geese, and erythrocyte aplasia in humans (B19 and related viruses) (reviewed in Refs.[43,47,99,278,401]). Several disorders result from the host response to infection, including the chronic immune complex disease caused by persistent infection with AMDV.[1] Certain PPV isolates induce immunologically mediated vesicular skin lesions in late-gestation swine fetuses,[202] and immune responses likely cause the erythema seen in fifth disease and the polyarthropathy caused by B19 infection.[24,401]

Human Parvoviruses

There are several human parvoviruses. The B19 and the related erythroviruses are associated with primary diseases, whereas the human parvovirus 4 (Parv4) and human bocavirus appear to be associated with diseases primarily in mixed infections with other pathogens. Many parvovirus B19 infections are subclinical, and when disease occurs that is generally an acute, biphasic illness with a high viremia that peaks at days 8 and 9[17,80,295] (Fig. 6.14). Viremia is accompanied by nonspecific, influenza-like symptoms, including fever, malaise, and myalgia. Red cell aplasia coincides with viremia, leading to a drop in hemoglobin, reticulocytopenia, and modest lymphopenia and neutropenia. Specific immunoglobulin M (IgM) and IgG antibodies 10 to 14 days after inoculation results in immune complex formation and the symptoms of fifth disease (erythema infectiosum)[17,18,52,80,135] likely due to the host immune response to infection. Adults with acute B19 infection may suffer polyarthropathy that can persist for weeks or months,[387] also likely resulting from the host immune response and immune complex deposition.

Parvovirus B19 is found in the nasopharynx, and transmission is probably through the upper airway, as well as by transfer of contaminated blood products or tissues.[16,17,183,184] The major sites of viral replication are the adult bone marrow and the fetal liver.[51(p19),207] Changes in the hematopoietic tissues include giant pronormoblasts in bone marrow aspirates and fetal liver tissue, along with depletion of later erythroid precursor cells.[15,70,207,273] Temporary depression of erythropoiesis results but is not significant in most healthy people. In people with a shortened red cell life span and reduced erythropoiesis, acute B19 infection causes transient aplastic crisis (TAC) and a precipitous worsening of anemia.[16,17,51,401] Predisposing conditions include sickle cell anemia, hereditary spherocytosis, enzymopathies, thalassemias, and acquired hemolytic anemias. Resolution of the crisis begins about 7 to 10 days after onset due to antiviral antibody and viral clearance.

Fetal infection may cause nonimmune hydrops fetalis characterized by severe anemia, high-output cardiac failure, and often fetal death.[361,388,392] Erythroblasts in the fetal liver are infected, and fetal myocarditis may contribute to the pathogenesis.[70,294] The risk for a fatal outcome is greatest during the first two trimesters, and fetal infection may persist after birth as pure red cell aplasia (PRCA).[33,124,388] About 30% of maternal infections are vertically transmitted, and fetal death occurs in 2% to 10% of maternal infections.[270]

B19-related parvoviruses may be common in various primates, including rhesus monkeys, pig-tailed macaques, chimpanzees, and gorillas, but likely cause severe disease only when animals are immunosuppressed.[271,332] Acute diseases range from inapparent to very mild, and appear to lack the arthropathy seen in humans. An erythroparvovirus-like virus has been found in Manchurian chipmunks.[398]

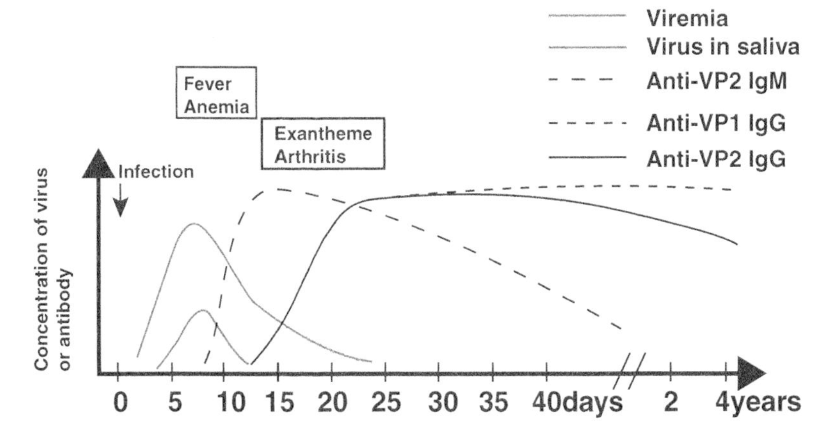

FIGURE 6.14 Pathogenesis of B19 in humans. The graph shows the changes in the amounts of the virus or the immune response to the various viral capsid components at different times in an acute human infection. (From Kerr JR, Modrow S. Human and primate erythrovirus infections and associated disease. In: Kerr JR, Cotmore SF, Bloom ME, et al., eds. *Parvoviruses*. London: Hodder Arnold; 2006:385–416. Copyright © 2005 by Taylor & Francis Group, LLC. Reproduced by permission of Taylor and Francis Group, LLC, a division of Informa plc.)

Canine and Feline Parvoviruses

CPV and FPV are very closely related strains and cause disease primarily in young animals, with a lessening of severity as the animals age.[278] The FPV-like viruses have long been found in cats, raccoons and many related hosts, while CPV is a dog-specific variant that emerged only in 1978.[12,378] CPV has since undergone variation in both antigenicity and in host range for cats and other carnivores.[14,364,375] The viruses infect through the oral–nasal route, replicate in the pharyngeal lymphoid tissues, then spread as a free or cell-associated viremia to the other lymphoid tissues.[61,62,100,235,236,248] Lymphocytes are lost from many tissues; then the virus spreads to the small intestine, infecting the rapidly dividing stem cells in the crypts of Lieberkühn, resulting in a loss of epithelial cells from the small intestine, shortened and nonabsorptive villi, and subsequent diarrhea.[60,237] Animals that survive recover normally and are protected against reinfection by the immunity they develop.

Porcine Parvovirus

A number of genotypes of PPV are now described, but fetal disease is mostly associated with the PPV type 1, while other diseases are associated with the type 2 strain.[211,247,351] Infection of older pigs by PPV-1 is mild or subclinical, but in pregnant pigs the virus takes approximately 15 days to reach the fetus, and can result in fetal death and resorption or mummification; fetuses infected prior to reaching immune competence (55 to 70 days of gestation) have an extensive infection and die.[102,182,246] After approximately 70 days of gestation, the fetuses are generally less severely infected, and the virus replicates in the lymphoid tissues.[53] PPV has also been associated with a skin vesicular disease.[202] Combined infections of PPV and porcine circovirus type 2 may cause a severe disease termed *porcine circovirus disease*.[149,155]

Aleutian Mink Disease Virus

AMDV is widespread in mink and related carnivores (skunks, ferrets, and foxes) without much associated disease. The virus mostly causes disease in farmed mink of susceptible genotypes.[43,178] In neonatal mink without maternal immunity, infection of type II pneumocytes results in pneumonitis, while older animals, or young animals with antiviral antibodies, develop a chronic infection and disease characterized by plasmocytosis, hypergammaglobulinemia, glomerulonephritis, arteritis, focal hepatitis, and death.[8–10] Lesions in chronically infected mink result from chronic viral antigen production and antibody complexes that are not efficiently cleared.[158] The Aleutian coat color mutation is linked to more severe disease because of a lysosomal storage disease similar to the human Chédiak-Higashi disease.[150] Vaccination may enhance the disease; however, control can be achieved by testing and culling of infected animals, as transmission appears relatively inefficient.

Rodent Parvovirus Diseases

Many different parvoviruses infect rodents, including experimental and wild mice and rats, as well as other rodents.[37,38,174,310,394] Rodent parvoviruses can develop persistent infections but are not usually associated with overt clinical disease.[131] They can also infect and persist in rodent and other cells in tissue culture and be introduced into animals by transfer of those cells.[37,242,394] The viruses may cause fetal abnormalities or death owing to their tropism for dividing cells. Control is most effectively by physical isolation and barriers, by serologic or DNA testing, and by culling of the infected animals or populations, followed by cesarean derivation of the young into a clean environment.[176,379]

Other Pathogenic Parvoviruses

Several goose parvoviruses have been described, and those can infect goslings, resulting in focal or diffuse hepatitis and widespread degeneration of striated, cardiac, and smooth muscles.[142,343] Duck parvovirus causes a similar disease in ducks. Bovine and rabbit parvoviruses are common, but not generally associated with clinical disease. Minute virus of canines (canine minute virus; canine bocaparvovirus) is widespread in dogs, but the infection is generally subclinical or there may be disease in association with infections by other pathogens.[64,287,326]

Dependoviruses

Natural AAV infections are assumed to occur via respiratory or gastrointestinal routes. It is not clear which tissues are the preferred sites of latency or infection in humans. The virus has not been detected in human lung samples but is recovered from a small percentage of hematopoietic cells and from the female genital tract.[129,146] AAV has been found in muscle biopsies.[360] The chromosome 19 integration site is associated with the *MBS85* gene, and integration alters that gene expression.[118] Skeletal muscle normally is not infected by adenovirus or herpesviruses, so the association with viral replication is unknown.

IMMUNE RESPONSE, KEY ANTIGENS, AND VACCINATIONS

Immunity to parvovirus infection includes both antibody and T-cell responses. Antibodies protect animals against infection by most parvoviruses and aid in recovery, as antibody therapy can resolve chronic human infections with B19 and clear canine infections by CPV.[127,206,248] The immune responses in hosts that recover protect for many years. The major antigens recognized by antibodies are the conformational epitopes of the capsids.[121,151,225,366] Antibodies to the capsids of AAV can interfere with gene therapy.[251,264,369] Other structures recognized by neutralizing antibodies include the VP1 unique region of the B19 virus[257,313] and an exposed peptide of the VP2 N-terminus of CPV.[213] Less is known about the T-cell responses to parvoviruses; however, these are likely important in recovery from infection.[173,188,308,333]

Vaccines

Modified live and inactivated or subunit vaccines have been developed against parvoviruses, and in many cases they protect against infection. A candidate recombinant vaccine has been developed against B19.[35] Modified live vaccines protect dogs and cats against CPV and FPV,[32,63] and vaccines against PPV are also successfully used.[279,280]

EPIDEMIOLOGY

Prevalence and Incidence

Many parvoviruses appear to be widespread, and most circulate readily among susceptible individuals. Parvovirus B19 infects almost all humans, and IgG antibody generally persists for life; 50% of children have anti-B19 antibodies by 15 years of age, as do more than 90% of elderly people.[50,87,136] Viremia is relatively short-lived, and although virus may be transmitted by blood, few donated blood units contain high titers of B19.[59,183] Between 10% and 60% of susceptible schoolchildren and 20% to 30% of susceptible or adult school and day care personnel can develop fifth disease in school outbreaks,[50,80,139,199] Because of the resistance of parvoviruses to heat and solvents, virus may survive the inactivation treatments employed for blood products and pass through filters; thus, the virus can be spread through pooled blood products, although infections appear uncommon.[162,197,389]

Virus is shed at very high titers in feces during CPV or FPV infections and persists in the environment.[278] Maternal antibodies protect animals against infection by CPV and FPV, but after maternal antibodies wane pups or kittens are highly susceptible.[292] Vaccination with modified live vaccines provides strong protection; however, that is also blocked when maternal antibody is present.[63,71]

Adeno-Associated Virus Infections

AAV productive infections occur in the presence of adenovirus or herpesvirus infections, and respiratory, fecal–oral, direct conjunctival, and sexual transmission have all been suggested.[40,41,138,153,325] AAVs infect a wide variety of mammals; however, cross-species transmission is not known. AAV2, AAV3, and AAV5 have been obtained from humans in the presence of numerous adenovirus serotypes.[27] AAV3 was isolated during an outbreak of adenovirus type 3 conjunctivitis among children and adults, and was found in conjunctival, throat, and fecal specimens.[325] AAV5 was isolated from a male with a flat condylomatous genital lesion.[27] AAV DNA (primarily AAV2) has been detected in peripheral blood cells, cervical biopsy samples, and tissues from spontaneous abortions, as well as tissue culture cells and adenovirus isolates.[134,146,153,324] Many humans have antibodies to various AAV serotypes, which reduce the efficiency of gene transduction.

Treatments

Few specific treatments are used for most parvovirus infections. Chronic or persistent B19 infections of naturally or therapeutically immunosuppressed individuals can be treated with immunoglobulin preparations containing antiB19 antibodies.[127,205]

ADENO-ASSOCIATED VIRUS AS A VECTOR FOR GENE THERAPY

Several AAV types has been developed as vectors for human gene therapy, and a number of treatments are now being licensed. Different AAV serotypes have varying cell receptors, tissue tropisms, and host ranges, and differ in binding to antibodies against specific serotypes.[79,144,258] Most AAV vector genomes contain the transgene(s) and regulatory sequences between two copies of the AAV ITR, and little of the AAV genome sequence remains, and their greatest capacity is approximately 4.5 kb.[143] Some approaches to expanding the capacity include packaging of different parts of a transgene in two vectors to produce a larger spliced message and a functional protein product.[115,212]

Production of AAV vectors involves helper functions, such as the adenovirus or the HSV genes required for transcription and DNA replication. Most vectors lack both Rep proteins and Rep-binding sites in the DNA and hence do not integrate into specific integration sites,[200,320] so the transduced DNA remains within the cell primarily as extrachromosomal elements, and loss by dilution occurs during cell division. Targeting site-specific integration may overcome the challenges of cell division, and providing Rep in *trans* may allow more site-specific integration.[304] Vectors may be administered to isolated cells *ex vivo* as well as after *in vivo* administration via intramuscular, intravenous, bronchial, or upper respiratory routes, and by injection into the eye, and minimal toxicity has been observed. Transgene expression may be maintained for years in experimental tests.

The list of conditions that are treated or that may be treated with AAV gene therapy is now extensive, as reviewed by[19,193,217,377]. Some conditions include hemophilia, acute macular degeneration, diabetes, parkinsonism, α1 antitrypsin deficiency, Leber congenital amaurosis, and hemophilia B. Different AAV serotypes and engineered variants show dramatically variant rates of transduction in various tissues, so that clinical trials may involve different serotypes and alternative routes of administration.

SUMMARY AND CONCLUSIONS

Parvoviruses include a wide variety of viruses that likely infect most (or even all) animals, from mammals to crustaceans. Although the long-known parvoviruses often cause various acute or chronic diseases, most of these viruses likely cause little or no disease, and those are being revealed by DNA detection or sequencing methods. The small genomes encode two large genes that are expressed in various spliced versions, as well as several small transcripts and proteins that are often less well characterized. The viral capsids are robust and survive in the environment and are assembled from 60 total copies of two or three forms of the same protein, and the overall topology and capsid forms are all similar, even when the viral sequences are very divergent. The capsids control DNA packaging, receptor binding, and cell infection. The viruses are highly dependent on host cell functions for their replication and generally complete their replication cycles in cells undergoing mitosis or that are coinfected with a helper virus. The lack of pathogenicity and efficient transduction capabilities of the AAVs has made them favored gene therapy vectors for use in humans.

REFERENCES

1. Aasted B, Alexandersen S, Christensen J. Vaccination with Aleutian mink disease parvovirus (AMDV) capsid proteins enhances disease, while vaccination with the major non-structural AMDV protein causes partial protection from disease. *Vaccine* 1998;16(11–12):1158–1165. doi: 10.1016/s0264-410x(98)80114-x.
2. Adeyemi RO, Landry S, Davis ME, et al. Parvovirus minute virus of mice induces a DNA damage response that facilitates viral replication. *PLoS Pathog* 2010;6(10):e1001141. doi: 10.1371/journal.ppat.1001141.
3. Agbandje M, McKenna R, Rossmann MG, et al. Structure determination of feline panleukopenia virus empty particles. *Proteins* 1993;16(2):155–171. doi: 10.1002/prot.340160204.
4. Agbandje-McKenna M, Kleinschmidt J. AAV capsid structure and cell interactions. *Methods Mol Biol* 2011;807:47–92. doi: 10.1007/978-1-61779-370-7_3.

5. Agbandje-McKenna M, Llamas-Saiz AL, Wang F, et al. Functional implications of the structure of the murine parvovirus, minute virus of mice. *Structure* 1998;6(11):1369–1381. doi: 10.1016/s0969-2126(98)00137-3.
6. Ahn JK, Pitluk ZW, Ward DC. The GC box and TATA transcription control elements in the P38 promoter of the minute virus of mice are necessary and sufficient for transactivation by the nonstructural protein NS1. *J Virol* 1992;66(6):3776–3783.
7. Alazard-Dany N, Nicolas A, Ploquin A, et al. Definition of herpes simplex virus type 1 helper activities for adeno-associated virus early replication events. *PLoS Pathog* 2009;5(3):e1000340. doi: 10.1371/journal.ppat.1000340.
8. Alexandersen S. Acute interstitial pneumonia in mink kits: experimental reproduction of the disease. *Vet Pathol* 1986;23(5):579–588. doi: 10.1177/030098588602300506.
9. Alexandersen S, Bloom ME, Wolfinbarger J. Evidence of restricted viral replication in adult mink infected with Aleutian disease of mink parvovirus. *J Virol* 1988;62(5):1495–1507.
10. Alexandersen S, Storgaard T, Kamstrup N, et al. Pathogenesis of Aleutian mink disease parvovirus infection: effects of suppression of antibody response on viral mRNA levels and on development of acute disease. *J Virol* 1994;68(2):738–749.
11. Allander T, Emerson SU, Engle RE, et al. A virus discovery method incorporating DNase treatment and its application to the identification of two bovine parvovirus species. *Proc Natl Acad Sci U S A* 2001;98(20):11609–11614. doi: 10.1073/pnas.211424698.
12. Allison AB, Harbison CE, Pagan I, et al. Role of multiple hosts in the cross-species transmission and emergence of a pandemic parvovirus. *J Virol* 2012;86(2):865–872. doi: 10.1128/JVI.06187-11.
13. Allison AB, Kohler DJ, Fox KA, et al. Frequent cross-species transmission of parvoviruses among diverse carnivore hosts. *J Virol* 2013;87(4):2342–2347. doi: 10.1128/JVI.02428-12.
14. Allison AB, Organtini LJ, Zhang S, et al. Single mutations in the VP2 300 loop region of the three-fold spike of the carnivore parvovirus capsid can determine host range. *J Virol* 2015;90(2):753–767. doi: 10.1128/JVI.02636-15.
15. Anand A, Gray ES, Brown T, et al. Human parvovirus infection in pregnancy and hydrops fetalis. *N Engl J Med* 1987;316(4):183–186. doi: 10.1056/NEJM198701223160403.
16. Anderson LJ. Human parvoviruses. *J Infect Dis* 1990;161(4):603–608. doi: 10.1093/infdis/161.4.603.
17. Anderson MJ, Higgins PG, Davis LR, et al. Experimental parvoviral infection in humans. *J Infect Dis* 1985;152(2):257–265. doi: 10.1093/infdis/152.2.257.
18. Anderson MJ, Lewis E, Kidd IM, et al. An outbreak of erythema infectiosum associated with human parvovirus infection. *J Hyg (Lond)* 1984;93(1):85–93. doi: 10.1017/s0022172400060964.
19. Anguela XM, High KA. Entering the modern era of gene therapy. *Annu Rev Med* 2019;70:273–288. doi: 10.1146/annurev-med-012017-043332.
20. Astell CR, Thomson M, Merchlinsky M, et al. The complete DNA sequence of minute virus of mice, an autonomous parvovirus. *Nucleic Acids Res* 1983;11(4):999–1018. doi: 10.1093/nar/11.4.999.
21. Atchison RW, Casto BC, Hammon WM. Adenovirus-associated defective virus particles. *Science* 1965;149(3685):754–756. doi: 10.1126/science.149.3685.754.
22. Badgett MR, Auer A, Carmichael LE, et al. Evolutionary dynamics of viral attenuation. *J Virol* 2002;76(20):10524–10529. doi: 10.1128/jvi.76.20.10524-10529.2002.
23. Baldauf AQ, Willwand K, Mumtsidu E, et al. Specific initiation of replication at the right-end telomere of the closed species of minute virus of mice replicative-form DNA. *J Virol* 1997;71(2):971–980.
24. Balkhy HH, Sabella C, Goldfarb J. Parvovirus: a review. *Bull Rheum Dis* 1998;47(3):4–9.
25. Ball-Goodrich LJ, Leland SE, Johnson EA, et al. Rat parvovirus type 1: the prototype for a new rodent parvovirus serogroup. *J Virol* 1998;72(4):3289–3299.
26. Ball-Goodrich LJ, Tattersall P. Two amino acid substitutions within the capsid are coordinately required for acquisition of fibrotropism by the lymphotropic strain of minute virus of mice. *J Virol* 1992;66(6):3415–3423.
27. Bantel-Schaal U, zur Hausen H. Characterization of the DNA of a defective human parvovirus isolated from a genital site. *Virology* 1984;134(1):52–63. doi: 10.1016/0042-6822(84)90271-x.
28. Bär S, Daeffler L, Rommelaere J, et al. Vesicular egress of non-enveloped lytic parvoviruses depends on gelsolin functioning. *PLoS Pathog* 2008;4(8):e1000126. doi: 10.1371/journal.ppat.1000126.
29. Bartlett JS, Wilcher R, Samulski RJ. Infectious entry pathway of adeno-associated virus and adeno-associated virus vectors. *J Virol* 2000;74(6):2777–2785. doi: 10.1128/jvi.74.6.2777-2785.2000.
30. Basak S, Turner H. Infectious entry pathway for canine parvovirus. *Virology* 1992;186(2):368–376. doi: 10.1016/0042-6822(92)90002-7.
31. Bashir T, Rommelaere J, Cziepluch C. In vivo accumulation of cyclin A and cellular replication factors in autonomous parvovirus minute virus of mice-associated replication bodies. *J Virol* 2001;75(9):4394–4398. doi: 10.1128/JVI.75.9.4394-4398.2001.
32. Bass EP, Gill MA, Beckenhauer WH. Development of a modified live, canine origin parvovirus vaccine. *J Am Vet Med Assoc* 1982;181(9):909–913.
33. Belloy M, Morinet F, Blondin G, et al. Erythroid hypoplasia due to chronic infection with parvovirus B19. *N Engl J Med* 1990;322(9):633–634. doi: 10.1056/NEJM199003013220916.
34. Belyi VA, Levine AJ, Skalka AM. Sequences from ancestral single-stranded DNA viruses in vertebrate genomes: the parvoviridae and circoviridae are more than 40 to 50 million years old. *J Virol* 2010;84(23):12458–12462. doi: 10.1128/JVI.01789-10.
35. Bernstein DI, El Sahly HM, Keitel WA, et al. Safety and immunogenicity of a candidate parvovirus B19 vaccine. *Vaccine* 2011;29(43):7357–7363. doi: 10.1016/j.vaccine.2011.07.080.
36. Berry GE, Asokan A. Chemical Modulation of Endocytic Sorting Augments Adeno-associated Viral Transduction. *J Biol Chem* 2016;291(2):939–947. doi: 10.1074/jbc.M115.687657.
37. Besselsen DG, Franklin CL, Livingston RS, et al. Lurking in the shadows: emerging rodent infectious diseases. *ILAR J* 2008;49(3):277–290. doi: 10.1093/ilar.49.3.277.
38. Besselsen DG, Romero MJ, Wagner AM, et al. Identification of novel murine parvovirus strains by epidemiological analysis of naturally infected mice. *J Gen Virol* 2006;87(Pt 6):1543–1556. doi: 10.1099/vir.0.81547-0.
39. Bieri J, Ros C. Globoside is dispensable for parvovirus B19 entry but essential at a postentry step for productive infection. *J Virol* 2019;93(20). doi: 10.1128/JVI.00972-19.
40. Blacklow NR, Hoggan MD, Kapikian AZ, et al. Epidemiology of adenovirus-associated virus infection in a nursery population. *Am J Epidemiol* 1968;88(3):368–378. doi: 10.1093/oxfordjournals.aje.a120897.
41. Blacklow NR, Hoggan MD, Sereno MS, et al. A seroepidemiologic study of adenovirus-associated virus infection in infants and children. *Am J Epidemiol* 1971;94(4):359–366. doi: 10.1093/oxfordjournals.aje.a121331.
42. Bloom ME, Kaaden OR, Huggans E, et al. Molecular comparisons of in vivo- and in vitro-derived strains of Aleutian disease of mink parvovirus. *J Virol* 1988;62(1):132–138.
43. Bloom ME, Kanno H, Mori S, et al. Aleutian mink disease: puzzles and paradigms. *Infect Agents Dis* 1994;3(6):279–301.
44. Bovo S, Mazzoni G, Ribani A, et al. A viral metagenomic approach on a non-metagenomic experiment: mining next generation sequencing datasets from pig DNA identified several porcine parvoviruses for a retrospective evaluation of viral infections. *PLoS One* 2017;12(6):e0179462. doi: 10.1371/journal.pone.0179462.
45. Brister JR, Muzyczka N. Mechanism of Rep-mediated adeno-associated virus origin nicking. *J Virol* 2000;74(17):7762–7771. doi: 10.1128/jvi.74.17.7762-7771.2000.
46. Brister JR, Muzyczka N. Rep-mediated nicking of the adeno-associated virus origin requires two biochemical activities, DNA helicase activity and transesterification. *J Virol* 1999;73(11):9325–9336.
47. Brown, Young. The simian parvoviruses. *Rev Med Virol* 1997;7(4):211–218. doi: 10.1002/(sici)1099-1654(199712)7:4<211::aid-rmv204>3.0.co;2-4.
48. Brown KE, Anderson SM, Young NS. Erythrocyte P antigen: cellular receptor for B19 parvovirus. *Science* 1993;262(5130):114–117. doi: 10.1126/science.8211117.
49. Brown KE, Hibbs JR, Gallinella G, et al. Resistance to parvovirus B19 infection due to lack of virus receptor (erythrocyte P antigen). *N Engl J Med* 1994;330(17):1192–1196. doi: 10.1056/NEJM199404283301704.
50. Brown KE, Young NS. Human parvovirus B19 infections in infants and children. *Adv Pediatr Infect Dis* 1997;13:101–126.
51. Brown KE, Young NS. Parvovirus B19 infection and hematopoiesis. *Blood Rev* 1995;9(3):176–182. doi: 10.1016/0268-960x(95)90023-3.
52. Brown KE, Young NS, Liu JM. Molecular, cellular and clinical aspects of parvovirus B19 infection. *Crit Rev Oncol Hematol* 1994;16(1):1–31. doi: 10.1016/1040-8428(94)90040-x.
53. Brownstein DG, Smith AL, Jacoby RO, et al. Pathogenesis of infection with a virulent allotropic variant of minute virus of mice and regulation by host genotype. *Lab Invest* 1991;65(3):357–364.
54. Buller RM, Janik JE, Sebring ED, et al. Herpes simplex virus types 1 and 2 completely help adenovirus-associated virus replication. *J Virol* 1981;40(1):241–247.
55. Cadar D, Lőrincz M, Kiss T, et al. Emerging novel porcine parvoviruses in Europe: origin, evolution, phylodynamics and phylogeography. *J Gen Virol* 2013;94(Pt 10):2330–2337. doi: 10.1099/vir.0.055129-0.
56. Callaway HM, Feng KH, Lee DW, et al. Parvovirus capsid structures required for infection: mutations controlling receptor recognition and protease cleavages. *J Virol* 2017;91(2). doi: 10.1128/JVI.01871-16.
57. Callaway HM, Subramanian S, Urbina CA, et al. Examination and reconstruction of three ancient endogenous parvovirus capsid protein gene remnants found in rodent genomes. *J Virol* 2019;93(6). doi: 10.1128/JVI.01542-18.
58. Canaan S, Zádori Z, Ghomashchi F, et al. Interfacial enzymology of parvovirus phospholipases A2. *J Biol Chem* 2004;279(15):14502–14508. doi: 10.1074/jbc.M312630200.
59. Candotti D, Etiz N, Parsyan A, et al. Identification and characterization of persistent human erythrovirus infection in blood donor samples. *J Virol* 2004;78(22):12169–12178. doi: 10.1128/JVI.78.22.12169-12178.2004.
60. Carlson JH, Scott FW. Feline panleukopenia. II. The relationship of intestinal mucosal cell proliferation rates to viral infection and development of lesions. *Vet Pathol* 1977;14(2):173–181. doi: 10.1177/030098587701400209.
61. Carman PS, Povey RC. Pathogenesis of canine parvovirus-2 in dogs: haematology, serology and virus recovery. *Res Vet Sci* 1985;38(2):134–140.
62. Carman PS, Povey RC. Pathogenesis of canine parvovirus-2 in dogs: histopathology and antigen identification in tissues. *Res Vet Sci* 1985;38(2):141–150.
63. Carmichael LE, Joubert JC, Pollock RV. A modified live canine parvovirus vaccine. II. Immune response. *Cornell Vet* 1983;73(1):13–29.
64. Carmichael LE, Schlafer DH, Hashimoto A. Minute virus of canines (MVC, canine parvovirus type-1): pathogenicity for pups and seroprevalence estimate. *J Vet Diagn Invest* 1994;6(2):165–174. doi: 10.1177/104063879400600206.
65. Carneiro A, Lee H, Lin L, et al. Novel lung tropic adeno-associated virus capsids for therapeutic gene delivery. *Hum Gene Ther* 2020;31(17–18):996–1009. doi: 10.1089/hum.2020.169.
66. Carter BJ, Antoni BA, Klessig DF. Adenovirus containing a deletion of the early region 2A gene allows growth of adeno-associated virus with decreased efficiency. *Virology* 1992;191(1):473–476. doi: 10.1016/0042-6822(92)90213-9.
67. Castellanos M, Pérez R, Rodríguez-Huete A, et al. A slender tract of glycine residues is required for translocation of the VP2 protein N-terminal domain through the parvovirus MVM capsid channel to initiate infection. *Biochem J* 2013;455(1):87–94. doi: 10.1042/BJ20130503.
68. Casto BC, Atchison RW, Hammon WM. Studies on the relationship between adeno-associated virus type I (AAV-1) and adenoviruses. I. Replication of AAV-1 in certain cell cultures and its effect on helper adenovirus. *Virology* 1967;32(1):52–59. doi: 10.1016/0042-6822(67)90251-6.
69. Casto BC, Goodheart CR. Inhibition of adenovirus transformation in vitro by AAV-1. *Proc Soc Exp Biol Med* 1972;140(1):72–78. doi: 10.3181/00379727-140-36397.

70. Caul EO, Usher MJ, Burton PA. Intrauterine infection with human parvovirus B19: a light and electron microscopy study. *J Med Virol.* 1988;24(1):55–66. doi: 10.1002/jmv.1890240108.
71. Cavalli A, Desario C, Marinaro M, et al. Oral administration of modified live canine parvovirus type 2b induces systemic immune response. *Vaccine* 2020;38(2):115–118 doi: 10.1016/j.vaccine.2019.10.016.
72. Chang SF, Sgro JY, Parrish CR. Multiple amino acids in the capsid structure of canine parvovirus coordinately determine the canine host range and specific antigenic and hemagglutination properties. *J Virol* 1992;66(12):6858–6867.
73. Chapman MS, Rossmann MG. Structure, sequence, and function correlations among parvoviruses. *Virology* 1993;194(2):491–508. doi: 10.1006/viro.1993.1288.
74. Chen AY, Cheng F, Lou S, et al. Characterization of the gene expression profile of human bocavirus. *Virology* 2010;403(2):145–154. doi: 10.1016/j.virol.2010.04.014.
75. Chen Z, Chen AY, Cheng F, et al. Chipmunk parvovirus is distinct from members in the genus Erythrovirus of the family Parvoviridae. *PLoS One* 2010;5(12):e15113. doi: 10.1371/journal.pone.0015113.
76. Cheung AK, Hoggan MD, Hauswirth WW, et al. Integration of the adeno-associated virus genome into cellular DNA in latently infected human Detroit 6 cells. *J Virol* 1980;33(2):739–748.
77. Chiorini JA, Wiener SM, Owens RA, et al. Sequence requirements for stable binding and function of Rep68 on the adeno-associated virus type 2 inverted terminal repeats. *J Virol* 1994;68(11):7448–7457.
78. Choi E-Y, Newman AE, Burger L, et al. Replication of minute virus of mice DNA is critically dependent on accumulated levels of NS2. *J Virol* 2005;79(19):12375–12381. doi: 10.1128/JVI.79.19.12375-12381.2005.
79. Choi VW, McCarty DM, Samulski RJ. AAV hybrid serotypes: improved vectors for gene delivery. *Curr Gene Ther* 2005;5(3):299–310. doi: 10.2174/1566523054064968.
80. Chorba T, Coccia P, Holman RC, et al. The role of parvovirus B19 in aplastic crisis and erythema infectiosum (fifth disease). *J Infect Dis* 1986;154(3):383–393. doi: 10.1093/infdis/154.3.383.
81. Christensen J, Cotmore SF, Tattersall P. A novel cellular site-specific DNA-binding protein cooperates with the viral NS1 polypeptide to initiate parvovirus DNA replication. *J Virol* 1997;71(2):1405–1416.
82. Christensen J, Cotmore SF, Tattersall P. Minute virus of mice transcriptional activator protein NS1 binds directly to the transactivation region of the viral P38 promoter in a strictly ATP-dependent manner. *J Virol* 1995;69(9):5422–5430.
83. Christensen J, Cotmore SF, Tattersall P. Parvovirus initiation factor PIF: a novel human DNA-binding factor which coordinately recognizes two ACGT motifs. *J Virol* 1997;71(8):5733–5741.
84. Christensen J, Cotmore SF, Tattersall P. Two new members of the emerging KDWK family of combinatorial transcription modulators bind as a heterodimer to flexibly spaced PuCGPy half-sites. *Mol Cell Biol* 1999;19(11):7741–7750. doi: 10.1128/mcb.19.11.7741.
85. Christensen J, Pedersen M, Aasted B, et al. Purification and characterization of the major nonstructural protein (NS-1) of Aleutian mink disease parvovirus. *J Virol* 1995;69(3):1802–1809.
86. Clemens KE, Pintel DJ. The two transcription units of the autonomous parvovirus minute virus of mice are transcribed in a temporal order. *J Virol* 1988;62(4):1448–1451.
87. Cohen BJ, Buckley MM. The prevalence of antibody to human parvovirus B19 in England and Wales. *J Med Microbiol* 1988;25(2):151–153. doi: 10.1099/00222615-25-2-151.
88. Cohen S, Panté N. Pushing the envelope: microinjection of Minute virus of mice into Xenopus oocytes causes damage to the nuclear envelope. *J Gen Virol* 2005;86(Pt 12):3243–3252. doi: 10.1099/vir.0.80967-0.
89. Corbau R, Duverger V, Rommelaere J, et al. Regulation of MVM NS1 by protein kinase C: impact of mutagenesis at consensus phosphorylation sites on replicative functions and cytopathic effects. *Virology* 2000;278(1):151–167. doi: 10.1006/viro.2000.0600.
90. Costello E, Saudan P, Winocour E, et al. High mobility group chromosomal protein 1 binds to the adeno-associated virus replication protein (Rep) and promotes Rep-mediated site-specific cleavage of DNA, ATPase activity and transcriptional repression. *EMBO J* 1997;16(19):5943–5954. doi: 10.1093/emboj/16.19.5943.
91. Cotmore SF, Agbandje-McKenna M, Canuti M, et al. ICTV virus taxonomy profile: parvoviridae. *J Gen Virol* 2019;100(3):367–368. doi: 10.1099/jgv.0.001212.
92. Cotmore SF, Christensen J, Nüesch JP, et al. The NS1 polypeptide of the murine parvovirus minute virus of mice binds to DNA sequences containing the motif [ACCA]2–3. *J Virol* 1995;69(3):1652–1660.
93. Cotmore SF, D'abramo AM, Ticknor CM, et al. Controlled conformational transitions in the MVM virion expose the VP1 N-terminus and viral genome without particle disassembly. *Virology* 1999;254(1):169–181. doi: 10.1006/viro.1998.9520.
94. Cotmore SF, Hafenstein S, Tattersall P. Depletion of virion-associated divalent cations induces parvovirus minute virus of mice to eject its genome in a 3'-to-5' direction from an otherwise intact viral particle. *J Virol* 2010;84(4):1945–1956. doi: 10.1128/JVI.01563-09.
95. Cotmore SF, Tattersall P. A genome-linked copy of the NS-1 polypeptide is located on the outside of infectious parvovirus particles. *J Virol* 1989;63(9):3902–3911.
96. Cotmore SF, Tattersall P. Encapsidation of minute virus of mice DNA: aspects of the translocation mechanism revealed by the structure of partially packaged genomes. *Virology* 2005;336(1):100–112. doi: 10.1016/j.virol.2005.03.007.
97. Cotmore SF, Tattersall P. Genome packaging sense is controlled by the efficiency of the nick site in the right-end replication origin of parvoviruses minute virus of mice and LuIII. *J Virol* 2005;79(4):2287–2300. doi: 10.1128/JVI.79.4.2287-2300.2005.
98. Cotmore SF, Tattersall P. Resolution of parvovirus dimer junctions proceeds through a novel heterocruciform intermediate. *J Virol* 2003;77(11):6245–6254. doi: 10.1128/jvi.77.11.6245-6254.2003.
99. Cotmore SF, Tattersall P. The autonomously replicating parvoviruses of vertebrates. *Adv Virus Res* 1987;33:91–174. doi: 10.1016/s0065-3527(08)60317-6.
100. Csiza CK, Scott FW, De Lahunta A, et al. Pathogenesis of feline panleukopenia virus in susceptible newborn kittens I. Clinical signs, hematology, serology, and virology. *Infect Immun* 1971;3(6):833–837.
101. Cureton DK, Harbison CE, Cocucci E, et al. Limited transferrin receptor clustering allows rapid diffusion of canine parvovirus into clathrin endocytic structures. *J Virol* 2012;86(9):5330–5340. doi: 10.1128/JVI.07194-11.
102. Cutlip RC, Mengeling WL. Pathogenesis of in utero infection: experimental infection of eight- and ten-week-old porcine fetuses with porcine parvovirus. *Am J Vet Res* 1975;36(12):1751–1754.
103. Cziepluch C, Lampel S, Grewenig A, et al. H-1 parvovirus-associated replication bodies: a distinct virus-induced nuclear structure. *J Virol* 2000;74(10):4807–4815. doi: 10.1128/jvi.74.10.4807-4815.2000.
104. D'Abramo AM, Ali AA, Wang F, et al. Host range mutants of Minute Virus of Mice with a single VP2 amino acid change require additional silent mutations that regulate NS2 accumulation. *Virology* 2005;340(1):143–154. doi: 10.1016/j.virol.2005.06.019.
105. Davis MD, Wu J, Owens RA. Mutational analysis of adeno-associated virus type 2 Rep68 protein endonuclease activity on partially single-stranded substrates. *J Virol* 2000;74(6):2936–2942. doi: 10.1128/jvi.74.6.2936-2942.2000.
106. Deleu L, Fuks F, Spitkovsky D, et al. Opposite transcriptional effects of cyclic AMP-responsive elements in confluent or p27KIP-overexpressing cells versus serum-starved or growing cells. *Mol Cell Biol* 1998;18(1):409–419. doi: 10.1128/mcb.18.1.409.
107. Deng X, Yan Z, Cheng F, et al. Replication of an autonomous human parvovirus in non-dividing human airway epithelium is facilitated through the DNA damage and repair pathways. *PLoS Pathog* 2016;12(1):e1005399. doi: 10.1371/journal.ppat.1005399.
108. Ding W, Zhang L, Yan Z, et al. Intracellular trafficking of adeno-associated viral vectors. *Gene Ther* 2005;12(11):873–880. doi: 10.1038/sj.gt.3302527.
109. Ding W, Zhang LN, Yeaman C, et al. rAAV2 traffics through both the late and the recycling endosomes in a dose-dependent fashion. *Mol Ther* 2006;13(4):671–682. doi: 10.1016/j.ymthe.2005.12.002.
110. Doerig C, Hirt B, Antonietti JP, et al. Nonstructural protein of parvoviruses B19 and minute virus of mice controls transcription. *J Virol* 1990;64(1):387–396.
111. Doerig C, Hirt B, Beard P, et al. Minute virus of mice non-structural protein NS-1 is necessary and sufficient for trans-activation of the viral P39 promoter. *J Gen Virol* 1988;69 (Pt 10):2563–2573. doi: 10.1099/0022-1317-69-10-2563.
112. Dong Y, Fasina OO, Pintel DJ. The human bocavirus 1 NP1 protein is a multifunctional regulator of viral RNA processing. *J Virol* 2018;92(22). doi: 10.1128/JVI.01187-18.
113. Dorsch S, Kaufmann B, Schaible U, et al. The VP1-unique region of parvovirus B19: amino acid variability and antigenic stability. *J Gen Virol* 2001;82(Pt 1):191–199. doi: 10.1099/0022-1317-82-1-191.
114. Dorsch S, Liebisch G, Kaufmann B, et al. The VP1 unique region of parvovirus B19 and its constituent phospholipase A2-like activity. *J Virol* 2002;76(4):2014–2018. doi: 10.1128/jvi.76.4.2014-2018.2002.
115. Duan D, Yue Y, Engelhardt JF. Expanding AAV packaging capacity with trans-splicing or overlapping vectors: a quantitative comparison. *Mol Ther* 2001;4(4):383–391. doi: 10.1006/mthe.2001.0456.
116. Dubielzig R, King JA, Weger S, et al. Adeno-associated virus type 2 protein interactions: formation of pre-encapsidation complexes. *J Virol* 1999;73(11):8989–8998.
117. Dudek AM, Pillay S, Puschnik AS, et al. An alternate route for adeno-associated virus entry independent of AAVR. *J Virol* 2018;92(7):e02213-17. doi: 10.1128/JVI.02213-17.
118. Dutheil N, Henckaerts E, Kohlbrenner E, et al. Transcriptional analysis of the adeno-associated virus integration site. *J Virol* 2009;83(23):12512–12525. doi: 10.1128/JVI.01754-09.
119. Dutheil N, Smith SC, Agúndez L, et al. Adeno-associated virus Rep represses the human integration site promoter by two pathways that are similar to those required for the regulation of the viral p5 promoter. *J Virol* 2014;88(15):8227–8241. doi: 10.1128/JVI.00412-14.
120. Eichwald V, Daeffler L, Klein M, et al. The NS2 proteins of parvovirus minute virus of mice are required for efficient nuclear egress of progeny virions in mouse cells. *J Virol* 2002;76(20):10307–10319. doi: 10.1128/jvi.76.20.10307-10319.2002.
121. Emmanuel SN, Mietzsch M, Tseng YS, et al. Parvovirus capsid-antibody complex structures reveal conservation of antigenic epitopes across the family. *Viral Immunol* 2021;34(1):3–17. doi: 10.1089/vim.2020.0022.
122. Farr GA, Tattersall P. A conserved leucine that constricts the pore through the capsid fivefold cylinder plays a central role in parvoviral infection. *Virology* 2004;323(2):243–256. doi: 10.1016/j.virol.2004.03.006.
123. Farr GA, Zhang L, Tattersall P. Parvoviral virions deploy a capsid-tethered lipolytic enzyme to breach the endosomal membrane during cell entry. *Proc Natl Acad Sci U S A* 2005;102(47):17148–17153. doi: 10.1073/pnas.0508477102.
124. Forestier F, Tissot JD, Vial Y, et al. Haematological parameters of parvovirus B19 infection in 13 fetuses with hydrops foetalis. *Br J Haematol* 1999;104(4):925–927. doi: 10.1046/j.1365-2141.1999.01241.x.
125. Fraefel C, Bittermann AG, Büeler H, et al. Spatial and temporal organization of adeno-associated virus DNA replication in live cells. *J Virol* 2004;78(1):389–398. doi: 10.1128/jvi.78.1.389-398.2004.
126. François S, Filloux D, Roumagnac P, et al. Discovery of parvovirus-related sequences in an unexpected broad range of animals. *Sci Rep* 2016;6:30880. doi: 10.1038/srep30880.
127. Frickhofen N, Abkowitz JL, Safford M, et al. Persistent B19 parvovirus infection in patients infected with human immunodeficiency virus type 1 (HIV-1): a treatable cause of anemia in AIDS. *Ann Intern Med* 1990;113(12):926–933. doi: 10.7326/0003-4819-113-12-926.
128. Frickhofen N, Young NS. Persistent parvovirus B19 infections in humans. *Microb Pathog* 1989;7(5):319–327. doi: 10.1016/0882-4010(89)90035-1.
129. Friedman-Einat M, Grossman Z, Mileguir F, et al. Detection of adeno-associated virus type 2 sequences in the human genital tract. *J Clin Microbiol* 1997;35(1):71–78.
130. Fuks F, Deleu L, Dinsart C, et al. ras oncogene-dependent activation of the P4 promoter of minute virus of mice through a proximal P4 element interacting with the Ets family of transcription factors. *J Virol* 1996;70(3):1331–1339.
131. Gaertner DJ, Smith AL, Jacoby RO. Efficient induction of persistent and prenatal parvovirus infection in rats. *Virus Res* 1996;44(1):67–78. doi: 10.1016/0168-1702(96)01351-2.

132. Gallinella G, Venturoli S, Manaresi E, et al. B19 virus genome diversity: epidemiological and clinical correlations. *J Clin Virol* 2003;28(1):1–13. doi: 10.1016/s1386-6532(03)00120-3.
133. Ganaie SS, Qiu J. Recent advances in replication and infection of human parvovirus B19. *Front Cell Infect Microbiol* 2018;8:166. doi: 10.3389/fcimb.2018.00166.
134. Gao G, Vandenberghe LH, Alvira MR, et al. Clades of adeno-associated viruses are widely disseminated in human tissues. *J Virol* 2004;78(12):6381–6388. doi: 10.1128/JVI.78.12.6381-6388.2004.
135. García-Tapia AM, Fernandez-Gutiérrez del Alamo C, Girón JA, et al. Spectrum of parvovirus B19 infection: analysis of an outbreak of 43 cases in Cadiz, Spain. *Clin Infect Dis* 1995;21(6):1424–1430. doi: 10.1093/clinids/21.6.1424.
136. Gay NJ, Hesketh LM, Cohen BJ, et al. Age specific antibody prevalence to parvovirus B19: how many women are infected in pregnancy? *Commun Dis Rep CDR Rev* 1994;4(9):R104–R107.
137. Geoffroy M-C, Epstein AL, Toublanc E, et al. Herpes simplex virus type 1 ICP0 protein mediates activation of adeno-associated virus type 2 rep gene expression from a latent integrated form. *J Virol* 2004;78(20):10977–10986. doi: 10.1128/JVI.78.20.10977-10986.2004.
138. Georg-Fries B, Biederlack S, Wolf J, et al. Analysis of proteins, helper dependence, and seroepidemiology of a new human parvovirus. *Virology* 1984;134(1):64–71. doi: 10.1016/0042-6822(84)90272-1.
139. Gillespie SM, Cartter ML, Asch S, et al. Occupational risk of human parvovirus B19 infection for school and day-care personnel during an outbreak of erythema infectiosum. *JAMA* 1990;263(15):2061–2065.
140. Giraud C, Winocour E, Berns KI. Site-specific integration by adeno-associated virus is directed by a cellular DNA sequence. *Proc Natl Acad Sci U S A* 1994;91(21):10039–10043. doi: 10.1073/pnas.91.21.10039.
141. Girod A, Wobus CE, Zádori Z, et al. The VP1 capsid protein of adeno-associated virus type 2 is carrying a phospholipase A2 domain required for virus infectivity. *J Gen Virol* 2002;83(Pt 5):973–978. doi: 10.1099/0022-1317-83-5-973.
142. Glávits R, Zolnai A, Szabó E, et al. Comparative pathological studies on domestic geese (Anser anser domestica) and Muscovy ducks (Cairina moschata) experimentally infected with parvovirus strains of goose and Muscovy duck origin. *Acta Vet Hung* 2005;53(1):73–89. doi: 10.1556/AVet.53.2005.1.8.
143. Grieger JC, Samulski RJ. Packaging capacity of adeno-associated virus serotypes: impact of larger genomes on infectivity and postentry steps. *J Virol* 2005;79(15):9933–9944. doi: 10.1128/JVI.79.15.9933-9944.2005.
144. Grimm D, Kay MA. From virus evolution to vector revolution: use of naturally occurring serotypes of adeno-associated virus (AAV) as novel vectors for human gene therapy. *Curr Gene Ther* 2003;3(4):281–304. doi: 10.2174/1566523034578285.
145. Grosse S, Penaud-Budloo M, Herrmann A-K, et al. Relevance of assembly-activating protein for adeno-associated virus vector production and capsid protein stability in mammalian and insect cells. *J Virol* 2017;91(20). doi: 10.1128/JVI.01198-17.
146. Grossman Z, Mendelson E, Brok-Simoni F, et al. Detection of adeno-associated virus type 2 in human peripheral blood cells. *J Gen Virol* 1992;73 (Pt 4):961–966. doi: 10.1099/0022-1317-73-4-961.
147. Guan W, Cheng F, Huang Q, et al. Inclusion of the central exon of parvovirus B19 precursor mRNA is determined by multiple splicing enhancers in both the exon and the downstream intron. *J Virol* 2011;85(5):2463–2468. doi: 10.1128/JVI.01708-10.
148. Guan W, Cheng F, Yoto Y, et al. Block to the production of full-length B19 virus transcripts by internal polyadenylation is overcome by replication of the viral genome. *J Virol* 2008;82(20):9951–9963. doi: 10.1128/JVI.01162-08.
149. Ha Y, Lee YH, Ahn K-K, et al. Reproduction of postweaning multisystemic wasting syndrome in pigs by prenatal porcine circovirus 2 infection and postnatal porcine parvovirus infection or immunostimulation. *Vet Pathol* 2008;45(6):842–848. doi: 10.1354/vp.45-6-842.
150. Hadlow WJ, Race RE, Kennedy RC. Comparative pathogenicity of four strains of Aleutian disease virus for pastel and sapphire mink. *Infect Immun* 1983;41(3):1016–1023.
151. Hafenstein S, Bowman VD, Sun T, et al. Structural comparison of different antibodies interacting with parvovirus capsids. *J Virol* 2009;83(11):5556–5566. doi: 10.1128/JVI.02532-08.
152. Halder S, Cotmore S, Heimburg-Molinaro J, et al. Profiling of glycan receptors for minute virus of mice in permissive cell lines towards understanding the mechanism of cell recognition. *PLoS One* 2014;9(1):e86909. doi: 10.1371/journal.pone.0086909.
153. Han L, Parmley TH, Keith S, et al. High prevalence of adeno-associated virus (AAV) type 2 rep DNA in cervical materials: AAV may be sexually transmitted. *Virus Genes* 1996;12(1):47–52. doi: 10.1007/bf00370000.
154. Harbison CE, Lyi SM, Weichert WS, et al. Early steps in cell infection by parvoviruses: host-specific differences in cell receptor binding but similar endosomal trafficking. *J Virol* 2009:83(20):10504–10514. doi: 10.1128/JVI.00295-09.
155. Hasslung F, Wallgren P, Ladekjaer-Hansen A-S, et al. Experimental reproduction of postweaning multisystemic wasting syndrome (PMWS) in pigs in Sweden and Denmark with a Swedish isolate of porcine circovirus type 2. *Vet Microbiol* 2005;106(1–2):49–60. doi: 10.1016/j.vetmic.2004.12.011.
156. Hauck B, Xiao W. Characterization of tissue tropism determinants of adeno-associated virus type 1. *J Virol* 2003;77(4):2768–2774. doi: 10.1128/jvi.77.4.2768-2774.2003.
157. Henderson KS, Pritchett-Corning KR, Perkins CL, et al. A comparison of mouse parvovirus 1 infection in BALB/c and C57BL/6 mice: susceptibility, replication, shedding, and seroconversion. *Comp Med* 2015;65(1):5–14.
158. Henson JB, Leader RW, Gorham JR, et al. The sequential development of lesions in spontaneous Aleutian disease of mink. *Pathol Vet* 1966;3(4):289–314. doi: 10.1177/030098586600300401.
159. Hermonat PL. Inhibition of bovine papillomavirus plasmid DNA replication by adeno-associated virus. *Virology* 1992;189(1):329–333. doi: 10.1016/0042-6822(92)90710-7.
160. Hickman AB, Ronning DR, Perez ZN, et al. The nuclease domain of adeno-associated virus rep coordinates replication initiation using two distinct DNA recognition interfaces. *Mol Cell* 2004;13(3):403–414. doi: 10.1016/s1097-2765(04)00023-1.
161. Hildebrandt E, Penzes JJ, Gifford RJ, et al. Evolution of dependoparvoviruses across geological timescales-implications for design of AAV-based gene therapy vectors. *Virus Evol* 2020;6(2):veaa043. doi: 10.1093/ve/veaa043.
162. van Hoeven LR, Janssen MP, Lieshout-Krikke RW, et al. An assessment of the risk, cost-effectiveness, and perceived benefits of anti-parvovirus B19 tested blood products. *Transfusion* 2019;59(7):2352–2360. doi: 10.1111/trf.15324.
163. Hoggan MD, Blacklow NR, Rowe WP. Studies of small DNA viruses found in various adenovirus preparations: physical, biological, and immunological characteristics. *Proc Natl Acad Sci U S A* 1966;55(6):1467–1474. doi: 10.1073/pnas.55.6.1467.
164. Hokynar K, Söderlund-Venermo M, Pesonen M, et al. A new parvovirus genotype persistent in human skin. *Virology* 2002;302(2):224–228. doi: 10.1006/viro.2002.1673.
165. Hoque M, Ishizu K, Matsumoto A, et al. Nuclear transport of the major capsid protein is essential for adeno-associated virus capsid formation. *J Virol* 1999;73(9):7912–7915.
166. Hörer M, Weger S, Butz K, et al. Mutational analysis of adeno-associated virus Rep protein-mediated inhibition of heterologous and homologous promoters. *J Virol* 1995;69(9):5485–5496.
167. Hueffer K, Parker JSL, Weichert WS, et al. The natural host range shift and subsequent evolution of canine parvovirus resulted from virus-specific binding to the canine transferrin receptor. *J Virol* 2003;77(3):1718–1726. doi: 10.1128/jvi.77.3.1718-1726.2003.
168. Hüser D, Gogol-Döring A, Lutter T, et al. Integration preferences of wildtype AAV-2 for consensus rep-binding sites at numerous loci in the human genome. *PLoS Pathog* 2010;6(7):e1000985. doi: 10.1371/journal.ppat.1000985.
169. Ihalainen TO, Niskanen EA, Jylhävä J, et al. Parvovirus induced alterations in nuclear architecture and dynamics. *PLoS One* 2009;4(6):e5948. doi: 10.1371/journal.pone.0005948.
170. Ilyina TV, Koonin EV. Conserved sequence motifs in the initiator proteins for rolling circle DNA replication encoded by diverse replicons from eubacteria, eucaryotes and archaebacteria. *Nucleic Acids Res* 1992;20(13):3279–3285. doi: 10.1093/nar/20.13.3279.
171. Im DS, Muzyczka N. Factors that bind to adeno-associated virus terminal repeats. *J Virol* 1989;63(7):3095–3104.
172. Im DS, Muzyczka N. The AAV origin binding protein Rep68 is an ATP-dependent site-specific endonuclease with DNA helicase activity. *Cell* 1990;61(3):447–457. doi: 10.1016/0092-8674(90)90526-k.
173. Isa A, Kasprowicz V, Norbeck O, et al. Prolonged activation of virus-specific CD8+T cells after acute B19 infection. *PLoS Med* 2005;2(12):e343. doi: 10.1371/journal.pmed.0020343.
174. Jacoby RO, Ball-Goodrich LJ, Besselsen DG, et al. Rodent parvovirus infections. *Lab Anim Sci* 1996;46(4):370–380.
175. Jang MY, Yarborough OH, Conyers GB, et al. Stable secondary structure near the nicking site for adeno-associated virus type 2 Rep proteins on human chromosome 19. *J Virol* 2005;79(6):3544–3556. doi: 10.1128/JVI.79.6.3544-3556.2005.
176. Janus LM, Bleich A. Coping with parvovirus infections in mice: health surveillance and control. *Lab Anim* 2012;46(1):14–23. doi: 10.1258/la.2011.011025.
177. Jay FT, Laughlin CA, Carter BJ. Eukaryotic translational control: adeno-associated virus protein synthesis is affected by a mutation in the adenovirus DNA-binding protein. *Proc Natl Acad Sci U S A* 1981;78(5):2927–2931. doi: 10.1073/pnas.78.5.2927.
178. Jensen TH, Chriél M, Hansen MS. Progression of experimental chronic Aleutian mink disease virus infection. *Acta Vet Scand* 2016;58(1):35. doi: 10.1186/s13028-016-0214-7.
179. Jia J, Ma Y, Zhao X, et al. Existence of various human parvovirus B19 genotypes in Chinese plasma pools: genotype 1, genotype 3, putative intergenotypic recombinant variants and new genotypes. *Virol J* 2016;13(1):155. doi: 10.1186/s12985-016-0611-6.
180. Jones MS, Kapoor A, Lukashov VV, et al. New DNA viruses identified in patients with acute viral infection syndrome. *J Virol* 2005;79(13):8230–8236. doi: 10.1128/JVI.79.13.8230-8236.2005.
181. Jongeneel CV, Sahli R, McMaster GK, et al. A precise map of splice junctions in the mRNAs of minute virus of mice, an autonomous parvovirus. *J Virol* 1986;59(3):564–573.
182. Joo HS, Donaldson-Wood CR, Johnson RH, et al. Pathogenesis of porcine parvovirus infection: pathology and immunofluorescence in the foetus. *J Comp Pathol* 1977;87(3):383–391. doi: 10.1016/0021-9975(77)90028-7.
183. Jordan J, Tiangco B, Kiss J, et al. Human parvovirus B19: prevalence of viral DNA in volunteer blood donors and clinical outcomes of transfusion recipients. *Vox Sang* 1998;75(2):97–102.
184. Juhl D, Hennig H. Parvovirus B19: what is the relevance in transfusion medicine? *Front Med (Lausanne)* 2018;5:4. doi: 10.3389/fmed.2018.00004.
185. Kailasan S, Agbandje-McKenna M, Parrish CR. Parvovirus family conundrum: what makes a killer? *Annu Rev Virol* 2015;2(1):425–450. doi: 10.1146/annurev-virology-100114-055150.
186. Kapoor A, Simmonds P, Lipkin WI. Discovery and characterization of mammalian endogenous parvoviruses. *J Virol* 2010;84(24):12628–12635. doi: 10.1128/JVI.01732-10.
187. Kapoor A, Simmonds P, Slikas E, et al. Human bocaviruses are highly diverse, dispersed, recombination prone, and prevalent in enteric infections. *J Infect Dis* 2010;201(11):1633–1643. doi: 10.1086/652416.
188. Kasprowicz V, Isa A, Tolfvenstam T, et al. Tracking of peptide-specific CD4+ T-cell responses after an acute resolving viral infection: a study of parvovirus B19. *J Virol* 2006;80(22):11209–11217. doi: 10.1128/JVI.01173-06.
189. Katzourakis A, Gifford RJ. Endogenous viral elements in animal genomes. *PLoS Genet* 2010;6(11):e1001191. doi: 10.1371/journal.pgen.1001191.
190. Kaufmann B, Baxa U, Chipman PR, et al. Parvovirus B19 does not bind to membrane-associated globoside in vitro. *Virology* 2005;332(1):189–198. doi: 10.1016/j.virol.2004.11.037.
191. Kaufmann B, Bowman VD, Li Y, et al. Structure of Penaeus stylirostris densovirus, a shrimp pathogen. *J Virol* 2010;84(21):11289–11296. doi: 10.1128/JVI.01240-10.
192. Kaufmann B, Simpson AA, Rossmann MG. The structure of human parvovirus B19. *Proc Natl Acad Sci U S A* 2004;101(32):11628–11633. doi: 10.1073/pnas.0402992101.
193. Keeler AM, Flotte TR. Recombinant adeno-associated virus gene therapy in light of luxturna (and Zolgensma and Glybera): where are we, and how did we get here? *Annu Rev Virol* 2019;6(1):601–621. doi: 10.1146/annurev-virology-092818-015530.

194. Kern A, Schmidt K, Leder C, et al. Identification of a heparin-binding motif on adeno-associated virus type 2 capsids. *J Virol* 2003;77(20):11072–11081. doi: 10.1128/jvi.77.20.11072-11081.2003.
195. Kilham L, Margolis G, Colby ED. Congenital infections of cats and ferrets by feline panleukopenia virus manifested by cerebellar hypoplasia. *Lab Invest* 1967;17(5):465–480.
196. Kilham L, Olivier LJ. A latent virus of rats isolated in tissue culture. *Virology* 1959;7(4):428–437. doi: 10.1016/0042-6822(59)90071-6.
197. Kleinman SH, Glynn SA, Lee T-H, et al. A linked donor-recipient study to evaluate parvovirus B19 transmission by blood component transfusion. *Blood* 2009;114(17):3677–3683. doi: 10.1182/blood-2009-06-225706.
198. Kleinschmidt JA, Möhler M, Weindler FW, et al. Sequence elements of the adeno-associated virus rep gene required for suppression of herpes-simplex-virus-induced DNA amplification. *Virology* 1995;206(1):254–262. doi: 10.1016/s0042-6822(95)80040-9.
199. Koch WC, Adler SP. Human parvovirus B19 infections in women of childbearing age and within families. *Pediatr Infect Dis J* 1989;8(2):83–87.
200. Kotin RM, Siniscalco M, Samulski RJ, et al. Site-specific integration by adeno-associated virus. *Proc Natl Acad Sci U S A* 1990;87(6):2211–2215. doi: 10.1073/pnas.87.6.2211.
201. Krady JK, Ward DC. Transcriptional activation by the parvoviral nonstructural protein NS-1 is mediated via a direct interaction with Sp1. *Mol Cell Biol* 1995;15(1):524–533. doi: 10.1128/mcb.15.1.524.
202. Kresse JI, Taylor WD, Stewart WW, et al. Parvovirus infection in pigs with necrotic and vesicle-like lesions. *Vet Microbiol* 1985;10(6):525–531. doi: 10.1016/0378-1135(85)90061-6.
203. Kronenberg S, Böttcher B, von der Lieth CW, et al. A conformational change in the adeno-associated virus type 2 capsid leads to the exposure of hidden VP1 N termini. *J Virol* 2005;79(9):5296–5303. doi: 10.1128/JVI.79.9.5296-5303.2005.
204. Kurian JJ, Lakshmanan R, Chmely WM, et al. Adeno-associated virus VP1u exhibits protease activity. *Viruses* 2019;11(5). doi: 10.3390/v11050399.
205. Kurtzman G, Frickhofen N, Kimball J, et al. Pure red-cell aplasia of 10 years' duration due to persistent parvovirus B19 infection and its cure with immunoglobulin therapy. *N Engl J Med* 1989;321(8):519–523. doi: 10.1056/NEJM198908243210807.
206. Kurtzman GJ, Cohen BJ, Field AM, et al. Immune response to B19 parvovirus and an antibody defect in persistent viral infection. *J Clin Invest* 1989;84(4):1114–1123. doi: 10.1172/JCI114274.
207. Kurtzman GJ, Gascon P, Caras M, et al. B19 parvovirus replicates in circulating cells of acutely infected patients. *Blood* 1988;71(5):1448–1454.
208. Kyöstiö SR, Wonderling RS, Owens RA. Negative regulation of the adeno-associated virus (AAV) P5 promoter involves both the P5 rep binding site and the consensus ATP-binding motif of the AAV Rep68 protein. *J Virol* 1995;69(11):6787–6796.
209. Labow MA, Hermonat PL, Berns KI. Positive and negative autoregulation of the adeno-associated virus type 2 genome. *J Virol* 1986;60(1):251–258.
210. Lachmann S, Rommeleare J, Nüesch JPF. Novel PKCeta is required to activate replicative functions of the major nonstructural protein NS1 of minute virus of mice. *J Virol* 2003;77(14):8048–8060. doi: 10.1128/jvi.77.14.8048-8060.2003.
211. Lagan Tregaskis P, Staines A, Gordon A, et al. Co-infection status of novel parvovirus's (PPV2 to 4) with porcine circovirus 2 in porcine respiratory disease complex and porcine circovirus-associated disease from 1997 to 2012. *Transbound Emerg Dis* 2020;00:1–16. doi: 10.1111/tbed.13846.
212. Lai Y, Yue Y, Liu M, et al. Efficient in vivo gene expression by trans-splicing adeno-associated viral vectors. *Nat Biotechnol* 2005;23(11):1435–1439. doi: 10.1038/nbt1153.
213. Langeveld JP, Casal JI, Cortés E, et al. Effective induction of neutralizing antibodies with the amino terminus of VP2 of canine parvovirus as a synthetic peptide. *Vaccine* 1994;12(15):1473–1480. doi: 10.1016/0264-410x(94)90158-9.
214. Lee H, Callaway HM, Cifuente JO, et al. Transferrin receptor binds virus capsid with dynamic motion. *Proc Natl Acad Sci U S A* 2019;116(41):20462–20471. doi: 10.1073/pnas.1904918116.
215. Lee Q, Padula MP, Pinello N, et al. Murine and related chapparvoviruses are nephrotropic and produce novel accessory proteins in infected kidneys. *PLoS Pathog* 2020;16(1):e1008262. doi: 10.1371/journal.ppat.1008262.
216. Lenghaus C, Studdert MJ. Acute and chronic viral myocarditis. Acute diffuse nonsuppurative myocarditis and residual myocardial scarring following infection with canine parvovirus. *Am J Pathol* 1984;115(2):316–319.
217. Li C, Samulski RJ. Engineering adeno-associated virus vectors for gene therapy. *Nat Rev Genet* 2020;21(4):255–272. doi: 10.1038/s41576-019-0205-4.
218. Li X, Rhode SL. Nonstructural protein NS2 of parvovirus H-1 is required for efficient viral protein synthesis and virus production in rat cells in vivo and in vitro. *Virology* 1991;184(1):117–130. doi: 10.1016/0042-6822(91)90828-y.
219. Linden RM, Winocour E, Berns KI. The recombination signals for adeno-associated virus site-specific integration. *Proc Natl Acad Sci U S A* 1996;93(15):7966–7972. doi: 10.1073/pnas.93.15.7966.
220. Linser P, Bruning H, Armentrout RW. Uptake of minute virus of mice into cultured rodent cells. *J Virol* 1979;31(2):537–545.
221. Liu H, Fu Y, Xie J, et al. Widespread endogenization of densoviruses and parvoviruses in animal and human genomes. *J Virol* 2011;85(19):9863–9876. doi: 10.1128/JVI.00828-11.
222. Liu Y, Siriwon N, Rohrs JA, et al. Generation of targeted adeno-associated virus (AAV) vectors for human gene therapy. *Curr Pharm Des* 2015;21(22):3248–3256. doi: 10.2174/1381612821666150531171653.
223. Löfling J, Lyi SM, Parrish CR, et al. Canine and feline parvoviruses preferentially recognize the non-human cell surface sialic acid N-glycolylneuraminic acid. *Virology* 2013;440(1):89–96. doi: 10.1016/j.virol.2013.02.009.
224. Lombardo E, Ramírez JC, Garcia J, et al. Complementary roles of multiple nuclear targeting signals in the capsid proteins of the parvovirus minute virus of mice during assembly and onset of infection. *J Virol* 2002;76(14):7049–7059. doi: 10.1128/jvi.76.14.7049-7059.2002.
225. López-Bueno A, Mateu MG, Almendral JM. High mutant frequency in populations of a DNA virus allows evasion from antibody therapy in an immunodeficient host. *J Virol* 2003;77(4):2701–2708. doi: 10.1128/jvi.77.4.2701-2708.2003.
226. López-Bueno A, Rubio M-P, Bryant N, et al. Host-selected amino acid changes at the sialic acid binding pocket of the parvovirus capsid modulate cell binding affinity and determine virulence. *J Virol* 2006;80(3):1563–1573. doi: 10.1128/JVI.80.3.1563-1573.2006.
227. López-Bueno A, Segovia JC, Bueren JA, et al. Evolution to pathogenicity of the parvovirus minute virus of mice in immunodeficient mice involves genetic heterogeneity at the capsid domain that determines tropism. *J Virol* 2008;82(3):1195–1203. doi: 10.1128/JVI.01692-07.
228. López-Bueno A, Valle N, Gallego JM, et al. Enhanced cytoplasmic sequestration of the nuclear export receptor CRM1 by NS2 mutations developed in the host regulates parvovirus fitness. *J Virol* 2004;78(19):10674–10684. doi: 10.1128/JVI.78.19.10674-10684.2004.
229. López-Bueno A, Villarreal LP, Almendral JM. Parvovirus variation for disease: a difference with RNA viruses? *Curr Top Microbiol Immunol* 2006;299:349–370. doi: 10.1007/3-540-26397-7_13.
230. Lorson C, Burger LR, Mouw M, et al. Efficient transactivation of the minute virus of mice P38 promoter requires upstream binding of NS1. *J Virol* 1996;70(2):834–842.
231. Lorson C, Pearson J, Burger L, et al. An Sp1-binding site and TATA element are sufficient to support full transactivation by proximally bound NS1 protein of minute virus of mice. *Virology* 1998;240(2):326–337. doi: 10.1006/viro.1997.8940.
232. Lukashov VV, Goudsmit J. Evolutionary relationships among parvoviruses: virus-host coevolution among autonomous primate parvoviruses and links between adeno-associated and avian parvoviruses. *J Virol* 2001;75(6):2729–2740. doi: 10.1128/JVI.75.6.2729-2740.2001.
233. Lusby EW, Berns KI. Mapping of the 5′ termini of two adeno-associated virus 2 RNAs in the left half of the genome. *J Virol* 1982;41(2):518–526.
234. Lyi SM, Tan MJA, Parrish CR. Parvovirus particles and movement in the cellular cytoplasm and effects of the cytoskeleton. *Virology* 2014;456–457:342–352. doi: 10.1016/j.virol.2014.04.003.
235. Macartney L, McCandlish IA, Thompson H, et al. Canine parvovirus enteritis 1: Clinical, haematological and pathological features of experimental infection. *Vet Rec* 1984;115(9):201–210. doi: 10.1136/vr.115.9.201.
236. Macartney L, McCandlish IA, Thompson H, et al. Canine parvovirus enteritis 2: Pathogenesis. *Vet Rec* 1984;115(18):453–460. doi: 10.1136/vr.115.18.453.
237. Macartney L, McCandlish IA, Thompson H, et al. Canine parvovirus enteritis 3: scanning electron microscopical features of experimental infection. *Vet Rec* 1984;115(21):533–537. doi: 10.1136/vr.115.21.533.
238. Mah C, Qing K, Khuntirat B, et al. Adeno-associated virus type 2-mediated gene transfer: role of epidermal growth factor receptor protein tyrosine kinase in transgene expression. *J Virol* 1998;72(12):9835–9843.
239. Mäntylä E, Kann M, Vihinen-Ranta M. Protoparvovirus knocking at the nuclear door. *Viruses* 2017;9(10). doi: 10.3390/v9100286.
240. Martini SV, Silva AL, Ferreira D, et al. Tyrosine mutation in AAV9 capsid improves gene transfer to the mouse lung. *Cell Physiol Biochem* 2016;39(2):544–553. doi: 10.1159/000445646.
241. McCarty DM, Pereira DJ, Zolotukhin I, et al. Identification of linear DNA sequences that specifically bind the adeno-associated virus Rep protein. *J Virol* 1994;68(8):4988–4997.
242. McKisic MD, Paturzo FX, Gaertner DJ, et al. A nonlethal rat parvovirus infection suppresses rat T lymphocyte effector functions. *J Immunol* 1995;155(8):3979–3986.
243. McLaughlin SK, Collis P, Hermonat PL, et al. Adeno-associated virus general transduction vectors: analysis of proviral structures. *J Virol* 1988;62(6):1963–1973.
244. Mendelson E, Trempe JP, Carter BJ. Identification of the trans-acting Rep proteins of adeno-associated virus by antibodies to a synthetic oligopeptide. *J Virol* 1986;60(3):823–832.
245. Meneses P, Berns KI, Winocour E. DNA sequence motifs which direct adeno-associated virus site-specific integration in a model system. *J Virol* 2000;74(13):6213–6216. doi: 10.1128/jvi.74.13.6213-6216.2000.
246. Mengeling WL, Cutlip RC. Pathogenesis of in utero infection: experimental infection of five-week-old porcine fetuses with porcine parvovirus. *Am J Vet Res* 1975;36(08):1173–1177.
247. Mészáros I, Olasz F, Cságola A, et al. Biology of porcine parvovirus (Ungulate parvovirus 1). *Viruses* 2017;9(12). doi: 10.3390/v9120393.
248. Meunier PC, Cooper BJ, Appel MJ, et al. Pathogenesis of canine parvovirus enteritis: sequential virus distribution and passive immunization studies. *Vet Pathol* 1985;22(6):617–624. doi: 10.1177/030098588502200617.
249. Mietzsch M, Pénzes JJ, Agbandje-McKenna M. Twenty-five years of structural parvovirology. *Viruses* 2019;11(4). doi: 10.3390/v11040362.
250. Miller CL, Pintel DJ. Interaction between parvovirus NS2 protein and nuclear export factor Crm1 is important for viral egress from the nucleus of murine cells. *J Virol* 2002;76(7):3257–3266. doi: 10.1128/jvi.76.7.3257-3266.2002.
251. Mingozzi F, High KA. Overcoming the host immune response to adeno-associated virus gene delivery vectors: the race between clearance, tolerance, neutralization, and escape. *Annu Rev Virol* 2017;4(1):511–534. doi: 10.1146/annurev-virology-101416-041936.
252. Mishra L, Rose JA. Adeno-associated virus DNA replication is induced by genes that are essential for HSV-1 DNA synthesis. *Virology* 1990;179(2):632–639. doi: 10.1016/0042-6822(90)90130-j.
253. Molenaar-de Backer MWA, Lukashov VV, van Binnendijk RS, et al. Global co-existence of two evolutionary lineages of parvovirus B19 1a, different in genome-wide synonymous positions. *PLoS One* 2012;7(8):e43206. doi: 10.1371/journal.pone.0043206.
254. Morgan WR, Ward DC. Three splicing patterns are used to excise the small intron common to all minute virus of mice RNAs. *J Virol* 1986;60(3):1170–1174.
255. Mühlemann B, Margaryan A, Damgaard PdB, et al. Ancient human parvovirus B19 in Eurasia reveals its long-term association with humans. *Proc Natl Acad Sci U S A* 2018;115(29):7557–7562. doi: 10.1073/pnas.1804921115.
256. Muralidhar S, Becerra SP, Rose JA. Site-directed mutagenesis of adeno-associated virus type 2 structural protein initiation codons: effects on regulation of synthesis and biological activity. *J Virol* 1994;68(1):170–176.
257. Musiani M, Manaresi E, Gallinella G, et al. Immunoreactivity against linear epitopes of parvovirus B19 structural proteins. Immunodominance of the amino-terminal half of the unique region of VP1. *J Med Virol* 2000;60(3):347–352. doi: 10.1002/(sici)1096-9071(200003)60:3<347::aid-jmv15>3.0.co;2-t.

258. Muzyczka N, Warrington KH. Custom adeno-associated virus capsids: the next generation of recombinant vectors with novel tropism. *Hum Gene Ther* 2005;16(4):408–416. doi: 10.1089/hum.2005.16.408.
259. Naeger LK, Cater J, Pintel DJ. The small nonstructural protein (NS2) of the parvovirus minute virus of mice is required for efficient DNA replication and infectious virus production in a cell-type-specific manner. *J Virol* 1990;64(12):6166–6175.
260. Nakamura M, Tohya Y, Miyazawa T, et al. A novel antigenic variant of Canine parvovirus from a Vietnamese dog. *Arch Virol* 2004;149(11):2261–2269. doi: 10.1007/s00705-004-0367-y.
261. Naumer M, Sonntag F, Schmidt K, et al. Properties of the adeno-associated virus assembly-activating protein. *J Virol* 2012;86(23):13038–13048. doi: 10.1128/JVI.01675-12.
262. Ni TH, McDonald WF, Zolotukhin I, et al. Cellular proteins required for adeno-associated virus DNA replication in the absence of adenovirus coinfection. *J Virol* 1998;72(4):2777–2787.
263. Nicolas A, Alazard-Dany N, Biollay C, et al. Identification of rep-associated factors in herpes simplex virus type 1-induced adeno-associated virus type 2 replication compartments. *J Virol* 2010;84(17):8871–8887. doi: 10.1128/JVI.00725-10.
264. Nidetz NF, McGee MC, Tse LV, et al. Adeno-associated viral vector-mediated immune responses: understanding barriers to gene delivery. *Pharmacol Ther* 2020;207:107453. doi: 10.1016/j.pharmthera.2019.107453.
265. Ning K, Liang T, Wang M, et al. Pathogenicity of a variant goose parvovirus, from short beak and dwarfism syndrome of Pekin ducks, in goose embryos and goslings. *Avian Pathol* 2018;47(4):391–399. doi: 10.1080/03079457.2018.1459040.
266. Nüesch JP, Christensen J, Rommelaere J. Initiation of minute virus of mice DNA replication is regulated at the level of origin unwinding by atypical protein kinase C phosphorylation of NS1. *J Virol* 2001;75(13):5730–5739. doi: 10.1128/JVI.75.13.5730-5739.2001.
267. Nüesch JP, Cotmore SF, Tattersall P. Sequence motifs in the replicator protein of parvovirus MVM essential for nicking and covalent attachment to the viral origin: identification of the linking tyrosine. *Virology* 1995;209(1):122–135. doi: 10.1006/viro.1995.1236.
268. Nüesch JP, Tattersall P. Nuclear targeting of the parvoviral replicator molecule NS1: evidence for self-association prior to nuclear transport. *Virology* 1993;196(2):637–651. doi: 10.1006/viro.1993.1520.
269. Olofsson A, Mittelholzer C, Treiberg Berndtsson L, et al. Unusual, high genetic diversity of Aleutian mink disease virus. *J Clin Microbiol* 1999;37(12):4145–4149.
270. Ornoy A, Ergaz Z. Parvovirus B19 infection during pregnancy and risks to the fetus. *Birth Defects Res* 2017;109(5):311–323. doi: 10.1002/bdra.23588.
271. O'Sullivan MG, Anderson DC, Fikes JD, et al. Identification of a novel simian parvovirus in cynomolgus monkeys with severe anemia. A paradigm of human B19 parvovirus infection. *J Clin Invest* 1994;93(4):1571–1576. doi: 10.1172/JCI117136.
272. Ozawa K, Ayub J, Hao YS, et al. Novel transcription map for the B19 (human) pathogenic parvovirus. *J Virol* 1987;61(8):2395–2406.
273. Ozawa K, Kurtzman G, Young N. Productive infection by B19 parvovirus of human erythroid bone marrow cells in vitro. *Blood* 1987;70(2):384–391.
274. Palermo LM, Hueffer K, Parrish CR. Residues in the apical domain of the feline and canine transferrin receptors control host-specific binding and cell infection of canine and feline parvoviruses. *J Virol* 2003;77(16):8915–8923. doi: 10.1128/jvi.77.16.8915-8923.2003.
275. Parker JS, Murphy WJ, Wang D, et al. Canine and feline parvoviruses can use human or feline transferrin receptors to bind, enter, and infect cells. *J Virol* 2001;75(8):3896–3902. doi: 10.1128/JVI.75.8.3896-3902.2001.
276. Parker JS, Parrish CR. Cellular uptake and infection by canine parvovirus involves rapid dynamin-regulated clathrin-mediated endocytosis, followed by slower intracellular trafficking. *J Virol* 2000;74(4):1919–1930. doi: 10.1128/jvi.74.4.1919-1930.2000.
277. Parks WP, Green M, Piña M, et al. Physicochemical characterization of adeno-associated satellite virus type 4 and its nucleic acid. *J Virol* 1967;1(5):980–987.
278. Parrish CR. Pathogenesis of feline panleukopenia virus and canine parvovirus. *Baillieres Clin Haematol* 1995;8(1):57–71. doi: 10.1016/s0950-3536(05)80232-x.
279. Paul PS, Mengeling WL. Oronasal and intramuscular vaccination of swine with a modified live porcine parvovirus vaccine: multiplication and transmission of the vaccine virus. *Am J Vet Res* 1984;45(12):2481–2485.
280. Paul PS, Mengeling WL, Brown TT. Effect of vaccinal and passive immunity on experimental infection of pigs with porcine parvovirus. *Am J Vet Res* 1980;41(9):1368–1371.
281. Pénzes JJ, Marsile-Medun S, Agbandje-McKenna M, et al. Endogenous amdoparvovirus-related elements reveal insights into the biology and evolution of vertebrate parvoviruses. *Virus Evol* 2018;4(2):vey026. doi: 10.1093/ve/vey026.
282. Pénzes JJ, Pham HT, Chipman P, et al. Molecular biology and structure of a novel penaeid shrimp densovirus elucidate convergent parvoviral host capsid evolution. *Proc Natl Acad Sci U S A* 2020;117(33):20211–20222. doi: 10.1073/pnas.2008191117.
283. Perabo L, Büning H, Kofler DM, et al. In vitro selection of viral vectors with modified tropism: the adeno-associated virus display. *Mol Ther* 2003;8(1):151–157. doi: 10.1016/s1525-0016(03)00123-0.
284. Pereira DJ, McCarty DM, Muzyczka N. The adeno-associated virus (AAV) Rep protein acts as both a repressor and an activator to regulate AAV transcription during a productive infection. *J Virol* 1997;71(2):1079–1088.
285. Perros M, Deleu L, Vanacker JM, et al. Upstream CREs participate in the basal activity of minute virus of mice promoter P4 and in its stimulation in ras-transformed cells. *J Virol* 1995;69(9):5506–5515.
286. Philpott NJ, Gomos J, Berns KI, et al. A p5 integration efficiency element mediates Rep-dependent integration into AAVS1 at chromosome 19. *Proc Natl Acad Sci U S A* 2002;99(19):12381–12385. doi: 10.1073/pnas.182430299.
287. Piewbang C, Jo WK, Puff C, et al. Canine bocavirus type 2 infection associated with intestinal lesions. *Vet Pathol* 2018;55(3):434–441. doi: 10.1177/0300985818755253.
288. Pillay S, Carette JE. Host determinants of adeno-associated viral vector entry. *Curr Opin Virol* 2017;24:124–131. doi: 10.1016/j.coviro.2017.06.003.
289. Pilz IH, Di Pasquale G, Rzadzinska A, et al. Mutation in the platelet-derived growth factor receptor alpha inhibits adeno-associated virus type 5 transduction. *Virology* 2012;428(1):58–63. doi: 10.1016/j.virol.2012.03.004.
290. Pittman N, Misseldine A, Geilen L, et al. Atomic resolution structure of the oncolytic parvovirus LuIII by electron microscopy and 3D image reconstruction. *Viruses* 2017;9(11). doi: 10.3390/v9110321.
291. Plevka P, Hafenstein S, Li L, et al. Structure of a packaging-defective mutant of minute virus of mice indicates that the genome is packaged via a pore at a 5-fold axis. *J Virol* 2011;85(10):4822–4827. doi: 10.1128/JVI.02598-10.
292. Pollock RV, Carmichael LE. Maternally derived immunity to canine parvovirus infection: transfer, decline, and interference with vaccination. *J Am Vet Med Assoc* 1982;180(1):37–42.
293. Porter DD. Aleutian disease: a persistent parvovirus infection of mink with a maximal but ineffective host humoral immune response. *Prog Med Virol* 1986;33:42–60.
294. Porter HJ, Quantrill AM, Fleming KA. B19 parvovirus infection of myocardial cells. *Lancet* 1988;1(8584):535–536. doi: 10.1016/s0140-6736(88)91332-3.
295. Potter CG, Potter AC, Hatton CS, et al. Variation of erythroid and myeloid precursors in the marrow and peripheral blood of volunteer subjects infected with human parvovirus (B19). *J Clin Invest* 1987;79(5):1486–1492. doi: 10.1172/JCI112978.
296. Prasad KM, Trempe JP. The adeno-associated virus Rep78 protein is covalently linked to viral DNA in a preformed virion. *Virology* 1995;214(2):360–370. doi: 10.1006/viro.1995.0045.
297. Pujol A, Deleu L, Nüesch JP, et al. Inhibition of parvovirus minute virus of mice replication by a peptide involved in the oligomerization of nonstructural protein NS1. *J Virol* 1997;71(10):7393–7403.
298. Qing K, Mah C, Hansen J, et al. Human fibroblast growth factor receptor 1 is a co-receptor for infection by adeno-associated virus 2. *Nat Med* 1999;5(1):71–77. doi: 10.1038/4758.
299. Qing K, Wang XS, Kube DM, et al. Role of tyrosine phosphorylation of a cellular protein in adeno-associated virus 2-mediated transgene expression. *Proc Natl Acad Sci U S A* 1997;94(20):10879–10884. doi: 10.1073/pnas.94.20.10879.
300. Qiu J, Cheng F, Burger LR, et al. The transcription profile of Aleutian mink disease virus in CRFK cells is generated by alternative processing of pre-mRNAs produced from a single promoter. *J Virol* 2006;80(2):654–662. doi: 10.1128/JVI.80.2.654-662.2006.
301. Qiu J, Pintel D. Processing of adeno-associated virus RNA. *Front Biosci* 2008;13:3101–3115. doi: 10.2741/2912.
302. Qiu J, Pintel DJ. The adeno-associated virus type 2 Rep protein regulates RNA processing via interaction with the transcription template. *Mol Cell Biol* 2002;22(11):3639–3652. doi: 10.1128/mcb.22.11.3639-3652.2002.
303. Ran G, Chen X, Xie Y, et al. Site-directed mutagenesis improves the transduction efficiency of capsid library-derived recombinant AAV vectors. *Mol Ther Methods Clin Dev* 2020;17:545–555. doi: 10.1016/j.omtm.2020.03.007.
304. Recchia A, Mavilio F. Site-specific integration by the adeno-associated virus rep protein. *Curr Gene Ther* 2011;11(5):399–405. doi: 10.2174/156652311797415809.
305. Résibois A, Coppens A, Poncelet L. Naturally occurring parvovirus-associated feline hypogranular cerebellar hypoplasia—a comparison to experimentally-induced lesions using immunohistology. *Vet Pathol* 2007;44(6):831–841. doi: 10.1354/vp.44-6-831.
306. Rhode SL, Paradiso PR. Parvovirus genome: nucleotide sequence of H-1 and mapping of its genes by hybrid-arrested translation. *J Virol* 1983;45(1):173–184.
307. Richardson WD, Westphal H. A cascade of adenovirus early functions is required for expression of adeno-associated virus. *Cell* 1981;27(1 Pt 2):133–141. doi: 10.1016/0092-8674(81)90367-6.
308. Rimmelzwaan GF, van der Heijden RW, Tijhaar E, et al. Establishment and characterization of canine parvovirus-specific murine CD4+ T cell clones and their use for the delineation of T cell epitopes. *J Gen Virol* 1990;71 (Pt 5):1095–1102. doi: 10.1099/0022-1317-71-5-1095.
309. Riolobos L, Reguera J, Mateu MG, et al. Nuclear transport of trimeric assembly intermediates exerts a morphogenetic control on the icosahedral parvovirus capsid. *J Mol Biol* 2006;357(3):1026–1038. doi: 10.1016/j.jmb.2006.01.019.
310. Roediger B, Lee Q, Tikoo S, et al. An atypical parvovirus drives chronic tubulointerstitial nephropathy and kidney fibrosis. *Cell* 2018;175(2):530–543.e24. doi: 10.1016/j.cell.2018.08.013.
311. Ros C, Bayat N, Wolfisberg R, et al. Protoparvovirus cell entry. *Viruses* 2017;9(11). doi: 10.3390/v9110313.
312. Ros C, Kempf C. The ubiquitin-proteasome machinery is essential for nuclear translocation of incoming minute virus of mice. *Virology* 2004;324(2):350–360. doi: 10.1016/j.virol.2004.04.016.
313. Rosenfeld SJ, Yoshimoto K, Kajigaya S, et al. Unique region of the minor capsid protein of human parvovirus B19 is exposed on the virion surface. *J Clin Invest* 1992;89(6):2023–2029. doi: 10.1172/JCI115812.
314. Rubio M-P, López-Bueno A, Almendral JM. Virulent variants emerging in mice infected with the apathogenic prototype strain of the parvovirus minute virus of mice exhibit a capsid with low avidity for a primary receptor. *J Virol* 2005;79(17):11280–11290. doi: 10.1128/JVI.79.17.11280-11290.2005.
315. Ruffing M, Zentgraf H, Kleinschmidt JA. Assembly of viruslike particles by recombinant structural proteins of adeno-associated virus type 2 in insect cells. *J Virol* 1992;66(12):6922–6930.
316. Ruiz Z, Mihaylov IS, Cotmore SF, et al. Recruitment of DNA replication and damage response proteins to viral replication centers during infection with NS2 mutants of Minute Virus of Mice (MVM). *Virology* 2011;410(2):375–384. doi: 10.1016/j.virol.2010.12.009.
317. Ryan JH, Zolotukhin S, Muzyczka N. Sequence requirements for binding of Rep68 to the adeno-associated virus terminal repeats. *J Virol* 1996;70(3):1542–1553.
318. Ryt-Hansen P, Hagberg EE, Chriél M, et al. Global phylogenetic analysis of contemporary aleutian mink disease viruses (AMDVs). *Virol J* 2017;14(1):231. doi: 10.1186/s12985-017-0898-y.
319. Saikawa T, Anderson S, Momoeda M, et al. Neutralizing linear epitopes of B19 parvovirus cluster in the VP1 unique and VP1-VP2 junction regions. *J Virol* 1993;67(6):3004–3009.
320. Samulski RJ, Zhu X, Xiao X, et al. Targeted integration of adeno-associated virus (AAV) into human chromosome 19. *EMBO J* 1991;10(12):3941–3950.
321. Sánchez-Martínez C, Grueso E, Carroll M, et al. Essential role of the unordered VP2 n-terminal domain of the parvovirus MVM capsid in nuclear assembly and endosomal enlargement of the virion fivefold channel for cell entry. *Virology* 2012;432(1):45–56. doi: 10.1016/j.virol.2012.05.025.

322. Sanlioglu S, Benson PK, Yang J, et al. Endocytosis and nuclear trafficking of adeno-associated virus type 2 are controlled by rac1 and phosphatidylinositol-3 kinase activation. *J Virol* 2000;74(19):9184–9196. doi: 10.1128/jvi.74.19.9184-9196.2000.
323. Schlehofer JR, Ehrbar M, zur Hausen H. Vaccinia virus, herpes simplex virus, and carcinogens induce DNA amplification in a human cell line and support replication of a helpervirus dependent parvovirus. *Virology* 1986;152(1):110–117. doi: 10.1016/0042-6822(86)90376-4.
324. Schmidt M, Grot E, Cervenka P, et al. Identification and characterization of novel adeno-associated virus isolates in ATCC virus stocks. *J Virol* 2006;80(10):5082–5085. doi: 10.1128/JVI.80.10.5082-5085.2006.
325. Schmidt OW, Cooney MK, Foy HM. Adeno-associated virus in adenovirus type 3 conjunctivitis. *Infect Immun* 1975;11(6):1362–1370.
326. Schwartz D, Green B, Carmichael LE, et al. The canine minute virus (minute virus of canines) is a distinct parvovirus that is most similar to bovine parvovirus. *Virology* 2002;302(2):219–223. doi: 10.1006/viro.2002.1674.
327. Schwartz RA, Carson CT, Schuberth C, et al. Adeno-associated virus replication induces a DNA damage response coordinated by DNA-dependent protein kinase. *J Virol* 2009;83(12):6269–6278. doi: 10.1128/JVI.00318-09.
328. Servant A, Laperche S, Lallemand F, et al. Genetic diversity within human erythroviruses: identification of three genotypes. *J Virol* 2002;76(18):9124–9134. doi: 10.1128/jvi.76.18.9124-9134.2002.
329. Shackelton LA, Hoelzer K, Parrish CR, et al. Comparative analysis reveals frequent recombination in the parvoviruses. *J Gen Virol* 2007;88(Pt 12):3294–3301. doi: 10.1099/vir.0.83255-0.
330. Shackelton LA, Holmes EC. Phylogenetic evidence for the rapid evolution of human B19 erythrovirus. *J Virol* 2006;80(7):3666–3669. doi: 10.1128/JVI.80.7.3666-3669.2006.
331. Shackelton LA, Parrish CR, Truyen U, et al. High rate of viral evolution associated with the emergence of carnivore parvovirus. *Proc Natl Acad Sci U S A* 2005;102(2):379–384. doi: 10.1073/pnas.0406765102.
332. Sharp CP, LeBreton M, Kantola K, et al. Widespread infection with homologues of human parvoviruses B19, PARV4, and human bocavirus of chimpanzees and gorillas in the wild. *J Virol* 2010;84(19):10289–10296. doi: 10.1128/JVI.01304-10.
333. Simmons R, Sharp C, Sims S, et al. High frequency, sustained T cell responses to PARV4 suggest viral persistence in vivo. *J Infect Dis* 2011;203(10):1378–1387. doi: 10.1093/infdis/jir036.
334. Simpson AA, Chandrasekar V, Hébert B, et al. Host range and variability of calcium binding by surface loops in the capsids of canine and feline parvoviruses. *J Mol Biol* 2000;300(3):597–610. doi: 10.1006/jmbi.2000.3868.
335. Simpson AA, Chipman PR, Baker TS, et al. The structure of an insect parvovirus (Galleria mellonella densovirus) at 3.7 A resolution. *Structure* 1998;6(11):1355–1367. doi: 10.1016/s0969-2126(98)00136-1.
336. Simpson AA, Hébert B, Sullivan GM, et al. The structure of porcine parvovirus: comparison with related viruses. *J Mol Biol* 2002;315(5):1189–1198. doi: 10.1006/jmbi.2001.5319.
337. Smith RH, Kotin RM. An adeno-associated virus (AAV) initiator protein, Rep78, catalyzes the cleavage and ligation of single-stranded AAV ori DNA. *J Virol* 2000;74(7):3122–3129. doi: 10.1128/jvi.74.7.3122-3129.2000.
338. Smith RH, Kotin RM. The Rep52 gene product of adeno-associated virus is a DNA helicase with 3'-to-5' polarity. *J Virol* 1998;72(6):4874–4881.
339. Snyder RO, Im DS, Ni T, et al. Features of the adeno-associated virus origin involved in substrate recognition by the viral Rep protein. *J Virol* 1993;67(10):6096–6104.
340. Snyder RO, Samulski RJ, Muzyczka N. In vitro resolution of covalently joined AAV chromosome ends. *Cell* 1990;60(1):105–113. doi: 10.1016/0092-8674(90)90720-y.
341. Söderlund-Venermo M. Emerging human parvoviruses: the Rocky Road to Fame. *Annu Rev Virol* 2019;6(1):71–91. doi: 10.1146/annurev-virology-092818-015803.
342. Söderlund-Venermo M, Hokynar K, Nieminen J, et al. Persistence of human parvovirus B19 in human tissues. *Pathol Biol (Paris)* 2002;50(5):307–316. doi: 10.1016/s0369-8114(02)00307-3.
343. Soliman MA, Erfan AM, Samy M, et al. Detection of novel goose parvovirus disease associated with short beak and dwarfism syndrome in commercial ducks. *Animals (Basel)* 2020;10(10). doi: 10.3390/ani10101833.
344. Song S, Lu Y, Choi Y-K, et al. DNA-dependent PK inhibits adeno-associated virus DNA integration. *Proc Natl Acad Sci U S A* 2004;101(7):2112–2116. doi: 10.1073/pnas.0307833100.
345. Sonntag F, Köther K, Schmidt K, et al. The assembly-activating protein promotes capsid assembly of different adeno-associated virus serotypes. *J Virol* 2011;85(23):12686–12697. doi: 10.1128/JVI.05359-11.
346. de Souza WM, Dennis T, Fumagalli MJ, et al. Novel parvoviruses from wild and domestic animals in Brazil provide new insights into parvovirus distribution and diversity. *Viruses* 2018;10(4). doi: 10.3390/v10040143.
347. Storgaard T, Oleksiewicz M, Bloom ME, et al. Two parvoviruses that cause different diseases in mink have different transcription patterns: transcription analysis of mink enteritis virus and Aleutian mink disease parvovirus in the same cell line. *J Virol* 1997;71(7):4990–4996.
348. Storz J, Young S, Carroll EJ, et al. Parvovirus infection of the bovine fetus: distribution of infection, antibody response, and age-related susceptibility. *Am J Vet Res* 1978; 39(7):1099–1102.
349. Strassheim ML, Gruenberg A, Veijalainen P, et al. Two dominant neutralizing antigenic determinants of canine parvovirus are found on the threefold spike of the virus capsid. *Virology* 1994;198(1):175–184. doi: 10.1006/viro.1994.1020.
350. Straus SE, Sebring ED, Rose JA. Concatemers of alternating plus and minus strands are intermediates in adenovirus-associated virus DNA synthesis. *Proc Natl Acad Sci U S A* 1976;73(3):742–746. doi: 10.1073/pnas.73.3.742.
351. Streck AF, Truyen U. Porcine parvovirus. *Curr Issues Mol Biol* 2019;37:33–46. doi: 10.21775/cimb.037.033.
352. Stutika C, Gogol-Döring A, Botschen L, et al. A comprehensive RNA sequencing analysis of the adeno-associated virus (AAV) type 2 transcriptome reveals novel AAV transcripts, splice variants, and derived proteins. *J Virol* 2016;90(3):1278–1289. doi: 10.1128/JVI.02750-15.
353. Suikkanen S, Aaltonen T, Nevalainen M, et al. Exploitation of microtubule cytoskeleton and dynein during parvoviral traffic toward the nucleus. *J Virol* 2003;77(19):10270–10279. doi: 10.1128/jvi.77.19.10270-10279.2003.
354. Suikkanen S, Antila M, Jaatinen A, et al. Release of canine parvovirus from endocytic vesicles. *Virology* 2003;316(2):267–280. doi: 10.1016/j.virol.2003.08.031.
355. Suikkanen S, Sääjärvi K, Hirsimäki J, et al. Role of recycling endosomes and lysosomes in dynein-dependent entry of canine parvovirus. *J Virol* 2002;76(9):4401–4411. doi: 10.1128/jvi.76.9.4401-4411.2002.
356. Summerford C, Bartlett JS, Samulski RJ. AlphaVbeta5 integrin: a co-receptor for adeno-associated virus type 2 infection. *Nat Med* 1999;5(1):78–82. doi: 10.1038/4768.
357. Summerford C, Samulski RJ. Membrane-associated heparan sulfate proteoglycan is a receptor for adeno-associated virus type 2 virions. *J Virol* 1998;72(2):1438–1445.
358. Tattersall P. Replication of the parvovirus MVM. I. Dependence of virus multiplication and plaque formation on cell growth. *J Virol* 1972;10(4):586–590.
359. Tattersall P, Shatkin AJ, Ward DC. Sequence homology between the structural polypeptides of minute virus of mice. *J Mol Biol* 1977;111(4):375–394. doi: 10.1016/s0022-2836(77)80060-0.
360. Tezak Z, Nagaraju K, Plotz P, et al. Adeno-associated virus in normal and myositis human skeletal muscle. *Neurology* 2000;55(12):1913–1917. doi: 10.1212/wnl.55.12.1913.
361. Tolfvenstam T, Broliden K. Parvovirus B19 infection. *Semin Fetal Neonatal Med* 2009;14(4):218–221. doi: 10.1016/j.siny.2009.01.007.
362. Toolan HW. Experimental production of mongoloid hamsters. *Science* 1960;131(3411): 1446–1448. doi: 10.1126/science.131.3411.1446.
363. Toolan HW. The parvoviruses. *Prog Exp Tumor Res* 1972;16:410–425. doi: 10.1159/000393383.
364. Truyen U, Evermann JF, Vieler E, et al. Evolution of canine parvovirus involved loss and gain of feline host range. *Virology* 1996;215(2):186–189. doi: 10.1006/viro.1996.0021.
365. Tsao J, Chapman MS, Agbandje M, et al. The three-dimensional structure of canine parvovirus and its functional implications. *Science* 1991;251(5000):1456–1464. doi: 10.1126/science.2006420.
366. Tseng Y-S, Agbandje-McKenna M. Mapping the AAV capsid host antibody response toward the development of second generation gene delivery vectors. *Front Immunol* 2014;5:9. doi: 10.3389/fimmu.2014.00009.
367. Tullis GE, Burger LR, Pintel DJ. The minor capsid protein VP1 of the autonomous parvovirus minute virus of mice is dispensable for encapsidation of progeny single-stranded DNA but is required for infectivity. *J Virol* 1993;67(1):131–141.
368. Tullis GE, Burger LR, Pintel DJ. The trypsin-sensitive RVER domain in the capsid proteins of minute virus of mice is required for efficient cell binding and viral infection but not for proteolytic processing in vivo. *Virology* 1992;191(2):846–857. doi: 10.1016/0042-6822(92)90260-v.
369. Vandenberghe LH, Wilson JM. AAV as an immunogen. *Curr Gene Ther* 2007;7(5):325–333. doi: 10.2174/156652307782151416.
370. Vibin J, Chamings A, Klaassen M, et al. Metagenomic characterisation of avian parvoviruses and picornaviruses from Australian wild ducks. *Sci Rep* 2020;10(1):12800. doi: 10.1038/s41598-020-69557-z.
371. Vihinen-Ranta M, Wang D, Weichert WS, et al. The VP1 N-terminal sequence of canine parvovirus affects nuclear transport of capsids and efficient cell infection. *J Virol* 2002;76(4):1884–1891. doi: 10.1128/jvi.76.4.1884-1891.2002.
372. Vihinen-Ranta M, Yuan W, Parrish CR. Cytoplasmic trafficking of the canine parvovirus capsid and its role in infection and nuclear transport. *J Virol* 2000;74(10):4853–4859. doi: 10.1128/jvi.74.10.4853-4859.2000.
373. Virtanen J, Smura T, Aaltonen K, et al. Co-circulation of highly diverse Aleutian mink disease virus strains in Finland. *J Gen Virol* 2019;100(2):227–236. doi: 10.1099/jgv.0.001187.
374. Viuff B, Aasted B, Alexandersen S. Role of alveolar type II cells and of surfactant-associated protein C mRNA levels in the pathogenesis of respiratory distress in mink kits infected with Aleutian mink disease parvovirus. *J Virol* 1994;68(4):2720–2725.
375. Voorhees IEH, Lee H, Allison AB, et al. Limited intrahost diversity and background evolution accompany 40 years of canine parvovirus host adaptation and spread. *J Virol* 2019;94(1). doi: 10.1128/JVI.01162-19.
376. Walters RW, Agbandje-McKenna M, Bowman VD, et al. Structure of adeno-associated virus serotype 5. *J Virol* 2004;78(7):3361–3371. doi: 10.1128/jvi.78.7.3361-3371.2004.
377. Wang D, Tai PWL, Gao G. Adeno-associated virus vector as a platform for gene therapy delivery. *Nat Rev Drug Discov* 2019;18:358–378. doi: 10.1038/s41573-019-0012-9.
378. Wasik BR, de Wit E, Munster V, et al. Onward transmission of viruses: how do viruses emerge to cause epidemics after spillover? *Philos Trans R Soc Lond B Biol Sci* 2019;374(1782):20190017. doi: 10.1098/rstb.2019.0017.
379. Watson J, Thompson KN, Feldman SH. Successful rederivation of contaminated immunocompetent mice using neonatal transfer with iodine immersion. *Comp Med* 2005;55(5):465–469.
380. Weigel-Kelley KA, Yoder MC, Srivastava A. Alpha5beta1 integrin as a cellular coreceptor for human parvovirus B19: requirement of functional activation of beta1 integrin for viral entry. *Blood* 2003;102(12):3927–3933. doi: 10.1182/blood-2003-05-1522.
381. Weindler FW, Heilbronn R. A subset of herpes simplex virus replication genes provides helper functions for productive adeno-associated virus replication. *J Virol* 1991;65(5):2476–2483.
382. Weller ML, Amornphimoltham P, Schmidt M, et al. Epidermal growth factor receptor is a co-receptor for adeno-associated virus serotype 6. *Nat Med* 2010;16(6):662–664. doi: 10.1038/nm.2145.
383. Wistuba A, Kern A, Weger S, et al. Subcellular compartmentalization of adeno-associated virus type 2 assembly. *J Virol* 1997;71(2):1341–1352.
384. Wobus CE, Hügle-Dörr B, Girod A, et al. Monoclonal antibodies against the adeno-associated virus type 2 (AAV-2) capsid: epitope mapping and identification of capsid domains involved in AAV-2-cell interaction and neutralization of AAV-2 infection. *J Virol* 2000;74(19):9281–9293. doi: 10.1128/jvi.74.19.9281-9293.2000.

385. Wolfisberg R, Kempf C, Ros C. Late maturation steps preceding selective nuclear export and egress of progeny parvovirus. *J Virol* 2016;90(11):5462–5474. doi: 10.1128/JVI.02967-15.
386. Wolter S, Richards R, Armentrout RW. Cell cycle-dependent replication of the DNA of minute virus of mice, a parvovirus. *Biochim Biophys Acta* 1980;607(3):420–431. doi: 10.1016/0005-2787(80)90152-5.
387. Woolf AD. Human parvovirus B19 and arthritis. *Behring Inst Mitt* 1990;(85):64–68.
388. Wright C, Hinchliffe SA, Taylor C. Fetal pathology in intrauterine death due to parvovirus B19 infection. *Br J Obstet Gynaecol* 1996;103(2):133–136. doi: 10.1111/j.1471-0528.1996.tb09664.x.
389. Wu C, Mason B, Jong J, et al. Parvovirus B19 transmission by a high-purity factor VIII concentrate. *Transfusion* 2005;45(6):1003–1010. doi: 10.1111/j.1537-2995.2005.04387.x.
390. Wu P, Xiao W, Conlon T, et al. Mutational analysis of the adeno-associated virus type 2 (AAV2) capsid gene and construction of AAV2 vectors with altered tropism. *J Virol* 2000;74(18):8635–8647. doi: 10.1128/jvi.74.18.8635-8647.2000.
391. Xie Q, Bu W, Bhatia S, et al. The atomic structure of adeno-associated virus (AAV-2), a vector for human gene therapy. *Proc Natl Acad Sci U S A* 2002;99(16):10405–10410. doi: 10.1073/pnas.162250899.
392. Xiong Y-Q, Tan J, Liu Y-M, et al. The risk of maternal parvovirus B19 infection during pregnancy on fetal loss and fetal hydrops: a systematic review and meta-analysis. *J Clin Virol* 2019;114:12–20. doi: 10.1016/j.jcv.2019.03.004.
393. Yakobson B, Hrynko TA, Peak MJ, et al. Replication of adeno-associated virus in cells irradiated with UV light at 254 nm. *J Virol* 1989;63(3):1023–1030.
394. Yamamoto H, Sato H, Yagami K, et al. Microbiological contamination in genetically modified animals and proposals for a microbiological test standard for national universities in Japan. *Exp Anim* 2001;50(5):397–407. doi: 10.1538/expanim.50.397.
395. Yan Z, Zak R, Zhang Y, et al. Distinct classes of proteasome-modulating agents cooperatively augment recombinant adeno-associated virus type 2 and type 5-mediated transduction from the apical surfaces of human airway epithelia. *J Virol* 2004;78(6):2863–2874. doi: 10.1128/jvi.78.6.2863-2874.2004.
396. Yang Q, Chen F, Ross J, et al. Inhibition of cellular and SV40 DNA replication by the adeno-associated virus Rep proteins. *Virology* 1995;207(1):246–250. doi: 10.1006/viro.1995.1072.
397. Ye C, Pintel DJ. The transcription strategy of bovine adeno-associated virus (B-AAV) combines features of both adeno-associated virus type 2 (AAV2) and type 5 (AAV5). *Virology* 2008;370(2):392–402. doi: 10.1016/j.virol.2007.09.007.
398. Yoo BC, Lee DH, Park SM, et al. A novel parvovirus isolated from Manchurian chipmunks. *Virology* 1999;253(2):250–258. doi: 10.1006/viro.1998.9518.
399. Yoon-Robarts M, Blouin AG, Bleker S, et al. Residues within the B' motif are critical for DNA binding by the superfamily 3 helicase Rep40 of adeno-associated virus type 2. *J Biol Chem* 2004;279(48):50472–50481. doi: 10.1074/jbc.M403900200.
400. Yoshimoto K, Rosenfeld S, Frickhofen N, et al. A second neutralizing epitope of B19 parvovirus implicates the spike region in the immune response. *J Virol* 1991;65(12):7056–7060.
401. Young NS. B19 parvovirus. *Baillieres Clin Haematol* 1995;8(1):25–56. doi: 10.1016/s0950-3536(05)80231-8.
402. Yuan W, Parrish CR. Canine parvovirus capsid assembly and differences in mammalian and insect cells. *Virology* 2001;279(2):546–557. doi: 10.1006/viro.2000.0734.
403. Zádori Z, Szelei J, Lacoste MC, et al. A viral phospholipase A2 is required for parvovirus infectivity. *Dev Cell* 2001;1(2):291–302. doi: 10.1016/s1534-5807(01)00031-4.
404. Zengel J, Carette JE. Structural and cellular biology of adeno-associated virus attachment and entry. *Adv Virus Res* 2020;106:39–84. doi: 10.1016/bs.aivir.2020.01.002.
405. Zhao Q, Gersappe A, Pintel DJ. Efficient excision of the upstream large intron from P4-generated pre-mRNA of the parvovirus minute virus of mice requires at least one donor and the 3' splice site of the small downstream intron. *J Virol* 1995;69(10):6170–6179.
406. Zhou X, Muzyczka N. In vitro packaging of adeno-associated virus DNA. *J Virol* 1998;72(4):3241–3247.

CHAPTER

7 *Circoviridae* and *Anelloviridae*

Xiang-Jin Meng • Yao-Wei Huang

The *Circoviridae* and *Anelloviridae* are two families of small, circular, single-stranded DNA viruses with nonenveloped icosahedral viruses. They are similar in that both have capsids with $T = 1$ icosahedral symmetry, exhibit a high degree of genetic diversity, replicate in nucleus of mitotically active cells, infect a large number of animal species including humans, and are ubiquitous in environments. They are distinguished by their morphology and coding strategy. The virions of anelloviruses, as revealed in chicken anemia virus (CAV), are larger with protruding pentagonal units compared to those with flat pentameric units in circoviruses. The circovirus genomes use an ambisense strategy for rolling circle replication (RCR) of the genome, whereas the anellovirus genomes employ a negative-sense strategy for replication. They are being considered in this chapter together because of their similar genome structure and ubiquity in nature.

CIRCOVIRIDAE

History

The prototype circovirus, porcine circovirus (PCV), was first reported in 1974 as papovavirus- and picornavirus-like particles in a contaminated porcine kidney cell line PK-15.[165] The name circovirus was proposed in 1982 when the viral genome was determined to be a circular single-stranded DNA molecule.[163] PCV was not known to be pathogenic[164] until 1997 when a variant strain, PCV type 2 (PCV2), was isolated from pigs with a wasting disease.[2] The PK-15 cell–derived virus was designated PCV1 to distinguish it from the pathogenic PCV2. In 2016, PCV3 was identified from pigs in the United States and subsequently from a number of other animal species.[130,135] PCV3 has been incriminated in several clinical conditions,[4] although its definitive association with a disease remains highly debatable. The avian circovirus, psittacine beak and feather disease virus (BFDV), was isolated in 1989 as a novel virus with a single-stranded circular DNA genome from cockatoos with beak and feather disease.[144]

Definitive evidence of human infections by circoviruses is lacking. Antibodies to PCV1 were reportedly detected in humans,[164] although subsequent studies could not confirm the initial report.[3,33] Evidence of productive PCV1 infection was demonstrated in human hepatocellular carcinoma cell line Huh-7,[8] and human cell lines were also reportedly infected by PCV2.[81] Contamination of PCV1 and PCV2 in live-attenuated human rotavirus vaccines prompted the FDA to temporarily suspend the use of the vaccines.[7,169]

Classification

Viruses in the family *Circoviridae* infect mainly mammalian and avian species. The genomic organization and replication strategy of circoviruses are similar to those of plant geminiviruses and nanoviruses. In fact, animal circoviruses may have evolved from a plant nanovirus through host switch followed by a recombination event with a picorna-like virus in a mammalian host.[49] Two genera of circoviruses, *Circovirus* and *Cyclovirus*, have now been recognized by the ICTV. The genus *Circovirus* consists of at least 39 species infecting a broad range of hosts such as pig, bat, bird, dog, chimpanzee, human, mink, rodent, and fish.[178] The genus *Cyclovirus*, originally discovered from stool samples of humans and chimpanzees,[76] contains at least 47 species identified from a large number of hosts including human, bat, cattle, chicken, chimpanzee, duck, cat, goat, horse, rodent, and insect.

Virion Structure

Circoviruses contain a single-strand circular DNA genome enclosed within a capsid, which is the only known structural

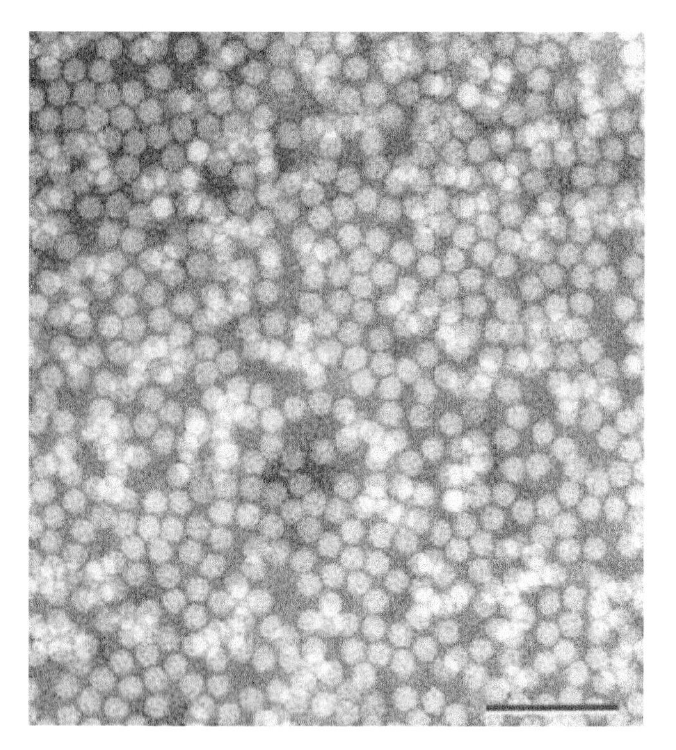

FIGURE 7.1 Transmission electron micrographs of purified PCV2 particles. Bar = 0.1 μm. (Republished with permission of Microbiology Society from Nawagitgul P, Morozov I, Bolin SR, et al. Open reading frame 2 of porcine circovirus type 2 encodes a major capsid protein. *J Gen Virol* 2000;81(Pt 9):2281–2287; permission conveyed through Copyright Clearance Center, Inc.)

protein in the virion. Morphologically, members of the genus *Circovirus* appear as small, nonenveloped, icosahedral particles of approximately 15 to 20 nm in size[28,104] (Fig. 7.1). Members of *Circoviridae* all have a $T = 1$ structure containing 60 copies of the capsid protein.[28] The capsids of genus *Circovirus* consist of 12 flat pentameric morphological units[28] (Fig. 7.2). The virion structure of genus *Cyclovirus* is currently unknown.

Genome Structure and Organization

The genome of *Circoviridae* is a single-stranded circular DNA molecule of 1.7 to 2.0 kb in size.[178] These are the smallest DNA viruses known to infect mammals and birds, and the genome size is reduced to the absolute necessities for the two basic functions of a virus, copying and packaging of viral genome.

For the genus *Circovirus*, the genome contains two major ORFs coding for the replicase protein (Rep) and capsid protein (Cap), respectively. The *rep* and *cap* genes are oriented in the opposite direction resulting in an ambisense genome organization. The Rep and Rep′ are produced from alternatively spliced RNA transcripts and contain endonuclease and helicase domains involved in rolling circle replication. An intergenic region between the 5′ ends of *rep* and *cap* genes contains the origin of viral genome replication (*Ori*), which is characterized by a stem-loop structure with a nonamer motif in its apex (Fig. 7.3). Three or four hexamer repeat motifs adjacent to the stem-loop serve as the binding sites for Rep and Rep′ to initiate rolling circle replication of viral genome.[40,94] The *rep* or *Ori* between PCV1 and PCV2 are fully exchangeable,[9–11,36–38] indicating conserved functionality of these regions among members of the genus *Circovirus*.

Like genus *Circovirus*, members of the genus *Cyclovirus* also consist of two major ORFs encoding the Cap and Rep.[76] Unlike circoviruses in which the Rep is encoded on the virion sense strand and the Cap on the complementary sense strand, the gene orientation is opposite for cycloviruses. The genes encoding the Rep and Cap of most cycloviruses overlap at their 3′ ends. The intergenic region at the 3′ end of the ORFs is relatively smaller in cyclovirus genomes than that in circovirus genomes.

Stages of Replication

Among the 39 species in the genus *Circovirus*, only PCV1 and PCV2 can be propagated *in vitro*. Currently, there is no cell culture system for members of the genus *Cyclovirus*. Thus, the knowledge of circovirus replication is derived mostly from the studies of PCV1 and PCV2.

Attachment, Entry, and Uncoating

Glycosaminoglycans (GAG), heparin, heparan sulfate, and chondroitin sulfate B are attachment receptors for PCV2.[101,177] However, the interaction between PCV2 and heparin does not follow the icosahedral symmetry of the PCV2 Cap.[31] It is not surprising that PCV2 utilizes GAG as the general attachment receptors[40] (Fig. 7.4), since the virus targets multiple organs and tissues in infected pigs.[156] The target cells for PCV2 shift from cardiomyocytes, hepatocytes, and macrophages during fetal life to only macrophages postnatally.[146] A yet to be identified specific receptor may be needed for more efficient binding and entry of PCV2 into cells.[40]

PCV2 is internalized by dendritic cells (DCs), and the internalization was observed with both mature and immature cells including blood DCs, plasmacytoid DCs, and DC precursors, and thus suggestive of a nonmacropinocytic uptake of the virus.[171,172] PCV2 virus-like particles (VLPs) quickly bound to porcine monocytic cells 3D4/31 and enter cells predominantly via clathrin-mediated endocytosis and require an acidic environment for infection.[102] PCV2 targets lymphoblasts *in vivo*, and infected pigs developed lymphocyte depletion in lymphoid tissues. PCV2 reportedly attached to 11% to 26% of the T lymphoblasts *in vitro*, and 2.6% to 12.7% of the cells showed virus internalization.[177] It is believed that PCV2 binds to T lymphoblasts via chondroitin sulfate and enters the cells via clathrin-mediated endocytosis.[177] The epithelial cells are also major targets for PCV2 *in vivo*. Although PCV2 quickly attaches to epithelial cells, virus entry is slow.[100] It appears that a dynamin- and cholesterol-independent, but actin- and small GTPase-dependent, pathway allows PCV2 entry and internalization leading to full replication in epithelial cells.[100] A nuclear localization signal (NLS) with rich positively charged residues was identified in the N terminus of the PCV2 Cap and reportedly functions as a cell-penetrating peptide (CPP), similar to the classical CPP derived from HIV TAT. In addition to entering cells via endocytic pathways, the first 17 residues of the PCV2 Cap NLS play an important role in cellular uptake of cargo molecules.[182] After entry, PCV2 is localized in the endosomes[40] (Fig. 7.4). As the endosomal vesicles move toward the nuclear membrane and become acidic, a serine protease appears to be required for PCV2 release from the endosome, suggesting that a proteolytic cleavage of Cap may be a part of the uncoating process.[99,101,102] It has been shown that the ubiquitin–proteasome system is important for early stages of PCV2

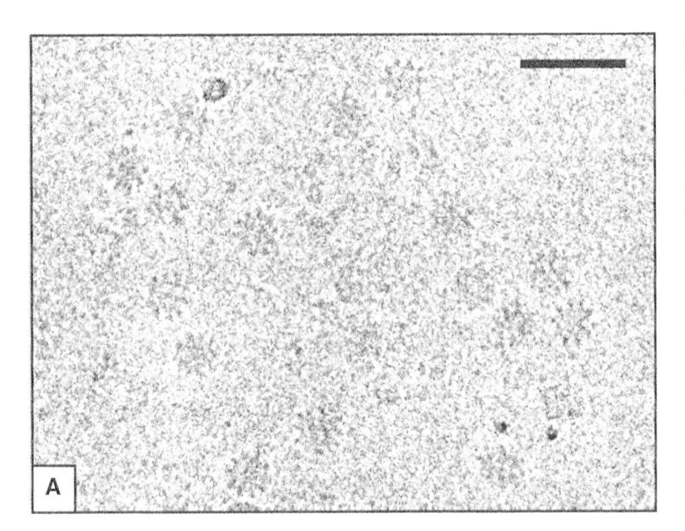

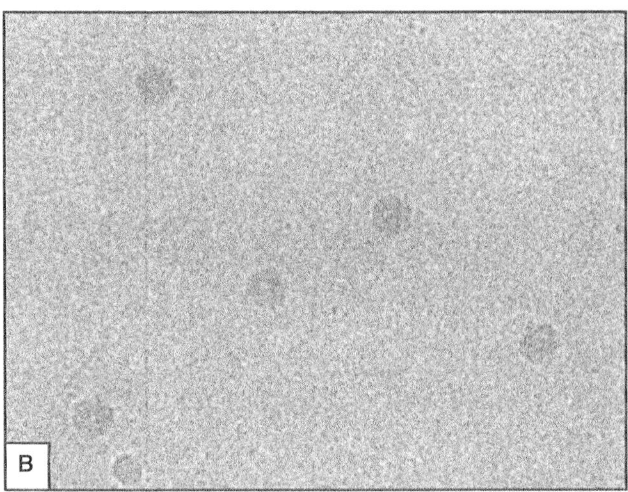

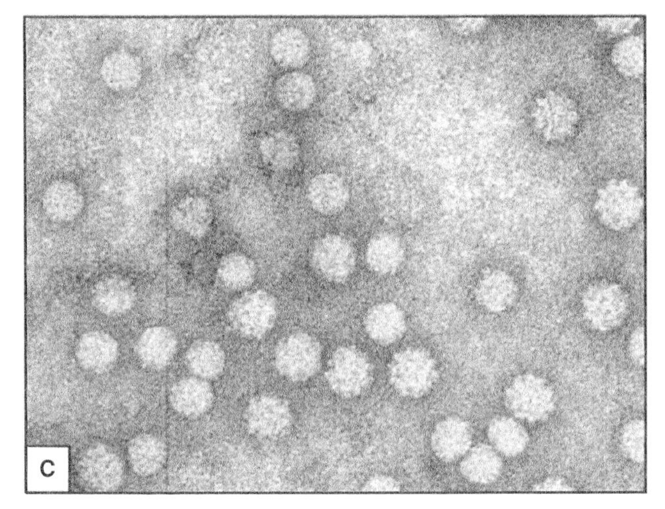

FIGURE 7.2 Micrographs of various animal circoviruses. **A:** Cryomicrograph of CAV. **B:** Cryomicrograph of PCV2. **C:** Micrograph of a negatively stained preparation of a mixture of CAV and BFDV. The larger rough particles are CAV, and the smaller smoother particles are BFDV. Scale bar = 50 nm. (From Crowther RA, Berriman JA, Curran WL, et al. Comparison of the structures of three circoviruses: chicken anemia virus, porcine circovirus type 2, and beak and feather disease virus. *J Virol* 2003;77(24):13036–13041. Copyright © 2003 American Society for Microbiology. Reproduced with permission from American Society for Microbiology.)

replication and that protein ubiquitination may play a role in PCV2 replication.[17] PCV2 infection of untreated and chloroquine diphosphate–treated porcine kidney PK-15 cells was blocked by a serine protease inhibitor, suggesting that serine protease–mediated PCV2 disassembly is enhanced in porcine epithelial cells but inhibited in monocytic cells after inhibition of endosome–lysosome system acidification.[99]

Transcription

A total of nine RNA transcripts were synthesized during productive PCV2 infection in PK-15 cells: Cap protein RNA (CR), five Rep-associated RNAs (Rep, Rep′, Rep3a, Rep3b, and Rep3c), and three NS-associated RNAs (NS515, NS672, and NS0)[18] (Fig. 7.5). Rep′, Rep3a, Rep3b, and Rep3c are produced from Rep by alternate splicing. The three NS-associated RNAs are transcribed from three different promoters inside ORF1 and share only the 3′ sequence with Rep.[18] A stop codon introduced at the 5′ end of CR did not affect Rep-associated viral antigen or DNA synthesis.[19] Altering the consensus dinucleotides at the splice junctions of the minor Rep- and NS-associated RNAs or introducing a stop codon in the abundant NS0 RNA also had no effect on viral protein or DNA synthesis. However, mutations resulting in truncated Rep or Rep′ reduced viral protein synthesis by more than 99% and abolished viral DNA replication, indicating that both Rep and Rep′ are essential for PCV2 replication.[20] In contrast to the pathogenic PCV2, a total of 12 RNAs were synthesized in PCV1-infected porcine kidney PK-15 cells[19] including the viral CR RNA, eight Rep-associated RNAs, and three NS-associated RNAs.[19] The promoter for *cap* is mapped within the ORF1 (nt 1328–1252), and the promoter for *rep* is located in the intergenic region (nt 640–796) and overlaps the *Ori* of PCV1.[91]

Several cellular gene transcripts were up-regulated in both PCV2-infected PK-15 cells and affected tissues including two transcripts with homology to an RNA splicing factor (SPF30) and a hyaluronan-mediated motility receptor. Microarray analyses of the genes in lymph nodes of PCV2-infected pigs revealed altered expression levels in genes that are involved in innate immune defense (TLR1, CD14, and CD180), immunosuppressed responses (FGL2 and GPNMB), proinflammatory signals (galectin-3), and fasting processes (ANGPTL-4), suggesting that PCV2 has developed an intricate mechanism to induce immunosuppression, inflammatory cell infiltration, and weight loss in pigs.[74] PCV2, but not PCV1, induces IL-10 secretion by monocytic cells, which led to repression of IL-12 in PBMCs.[69] The PCV2 ORF3 protein binds to a regulator of G protein signaling (RGS) and is colocalized with poRGS16 in LPS-activated porcine PBMC. The poRGS16 appeared to participate in the translocation of ORF3 protein into the nucleus.[162] NF-kB was activated concomitantly

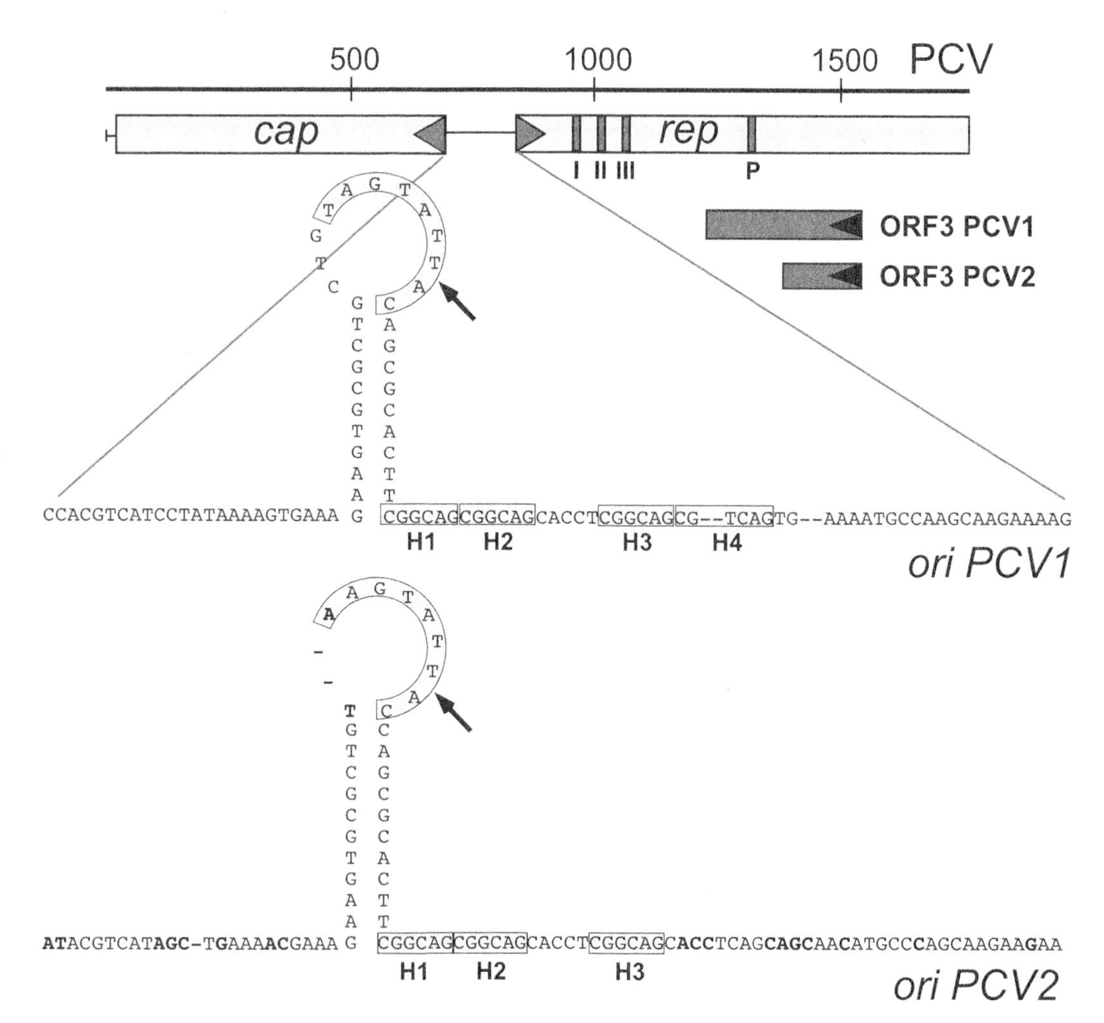

FIGURE 7.3 A linear map of the PCV genome indicates the two major ORF encoding *rep* and *cap*. Three motifs conserved in RCR enzymes (I–III) and a dNTP-binding domain (*P*) indicated within the rep gene. The ORF3 differing in length in PCV1 and PCV2 is indicated in *gray boxes*. The lower part shows a comparison of the two *Oris* of PCV1 and PCV2. Sequences have been aligned, and the hexamer repeats 1 to 4 are marked by *open boxes*. The conserved nonamer sequence within the single-stranded loop of the hairpin is indicated by a *gray box*, the nicking site by an *arrow*. (Reprinted from Finsterbusch T, Mankertz A. Porcine circoviruses—small but powerful. *Virus Res* 2009;143(2):177–183. Copyright © 2009 Elsevier. With permission.)

with PCV2 replication, and treatment of cells with an NF-kB inhibitor reduced virus protein expression and virion production, suggesting that NF-kB activation is important for PCV2 replication.[176]

Translation

The genome of genus *Circovirus* consists of two major ORFs: ORF1 encodes the Rep and Rep′, and the ORF2 encodes Cap. Rep is translated from the full-length *rep* transcript, while Rep′ is produced from a spliced transcript.[40] Both Rep and Rep′ are essential for the initiation of virus replication.[24,92,93] Mutation within motifs I-III and the GKS box of the Rep and Rep′ interfered with viral replication. Motifs I to III are essential for PCV1 *Ori* cleavage.[158] The repression of *rep* promoter is mediated by binding of Rep to H1 and H2 hexamers in the *Ori* of PCV1; however, transcription of *cap* promoter is not influenced by viral proteins.[41,93] Both Rep and Rep′ colocalize in the nucleus of infected cells and form homo- and heteromeric complexes.[41,92] Three putative NLSs are present in the N termini of Rep/Rep′: NLS1 and NSL2 mediate nuclear accumulation, whereas NSL3 enhances the nuclear transport of Rep and Rep′.[41] PCV2 Rep interacted with an intermediate filament protein, similar to human syncoilin, and with the transcriptional regulator c-myc.[161] The PCV Rep also binds three porcine cellular proteins[1,42]: ZNF265 is an alternative component of the spliceosome, whereas VG5Q and TDG were linked to transcriptional regulation.

The Cap of the genus *Circovirus* can self-assemble into VLPs[14,104] and elicits neutralizing antibodies in vaccinated animals.[13,75] At least five different but overlapping conformational epitopes were identified within residues 47 to 63 and 165 to 200 and the last four amino acids at the C terminus of PCV2 Cap.[75,90] Two amino acid mutations in the Cap, P110A and R191S, enhance the growth ability of PCV2 *in vitro* but attenuate PCV2 *in vivo*.[39] The Cap localized in the nucleoli of PCV2-infected cells[82] and in the nucleoli of cells at an early stage of PCV1 infection.[41] The PCV Cap interacts with numerous cellular proteins[42,161] including complement factor C1qB,

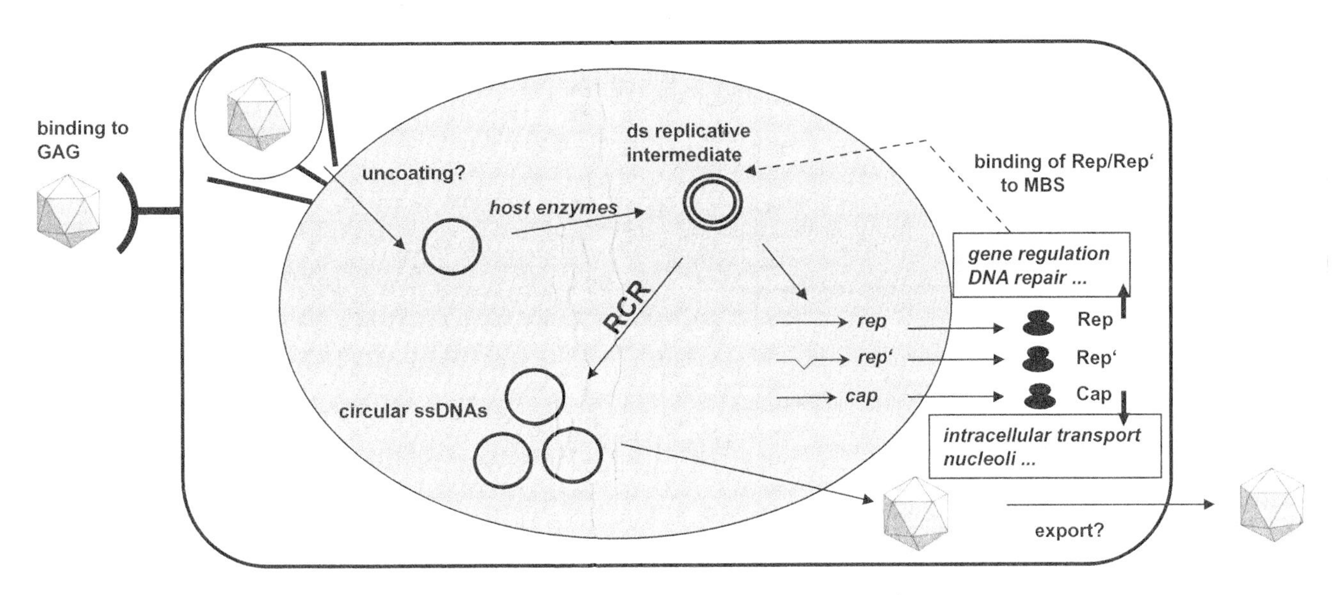

FIGURE 7.4 Life cycle of PCV. PCV uses glycosaminoglycans (GAG) as attachment receptors. After uncoating, the ssDNA genome is transported into the nucleus and converted by host enzymes into a dsDNA intermediate. The rep and cap mRNAs are transcribed, and the proteins are synthesized and imported from the cytoplasm. Rep and Rep′ bind to the dsDNA and initiate RCR by introduction of a nick that serves as primer. Elongation of the primer by host enzymes leads to replication. The Rep is covalently bound to the DNA and terminates the reaction by introduction of a second cleavage reaction via Tyr-93. Events leading to assembly and release of virions are unknown. (Reprinted from Finsterbusch T, Mankertz A. Porcine circoviruses—small but powerful. *Virus Res* 2009;143(2):177–183. Copyright © 2009 Elsevier. With permission.)

E3 ubiquitin ligase family member MKRN1, and proapoptotic gene product Par-4.[40] The exact function of these cellular factors in PCV replication remains to be elucidated.

An ORF3 has been identified in PCV1 but is truncated in PCV2. The *in vitro*–expressed ORF3 protein of PCV2 induced apoptosis through the activation of caspase 8 and caspase 3 pathways.[80] The ORF3 protein interacts with pPirh2 and competes with p53 in binding to pPirh2 and mediates the deregulation of p53 homeostasis, leading to increased p53 levels and apoptosis of the infected cells.[66,84] It was reported that abrogation of the ORF3 function attenuated PCV2 in pigs,[65] although other studies showed that PCV2 pathogenicity is not solely determined by ORF3.[15,60] In fact, whether or not PCV2 infection causes apoptosis remains controversial.[72,142,172] It has been reported that PCV2 induces ORF3-independent apoptosis, due to activation of PERK pathway, via increased cytosolic and mitochondrial Ca^{2+} levels and cellular reactive oxygen species levels.[185]

A small ORF4, which overlaps ORF3 in the same direction, was also identified in PCV2, but its function in virus replication, if any, is controversial. The ORF4 was shown to be dispensable for PCV2 replication but may play a role in inhibiting the caspase activity and regulating CD4+ and CD8+ T cells during virus infection.[51] It was suggested that ORF4 protein may play a role by restricting ORF3 transcription to prevent virus-induced apoptosis.[46] The ORF4 reportedly binds ferritin heavy chain to antagonize apoptosis by stabilizing its concentration.[85,86] By contrast, Lin et al. reported that the ORF4 actually induces apoptosis by interacting with adenine nucleotide translocase 3 (ANT3) through the mitochondrial pathway.[79]

Replication of Genomic DNA, Assembly, and Release

After uncoating, the single-strand circular viral DNA genome is converted to dsDNA intermediate by host enzymes in the nucleus. Binding of Rep and Rep′ to *Ori* unwinds the dsDNA intermediate to initiate genome replication.[21–25,40] Viral genomes with mutations on either or both arms of the inverted repeats (IR, palindrome) were still capable of synthesizing viral proteins and producing infectious viruses with restored or new palindromes, indicating that a flanking palindrome at *Ori* is not essential for initiation of viral DNA replication. A rolling circle "melting-pot" model for circovirus DNA replication was proposed[22,23] (Fig. 7.6). The Rep and Rep′ complex binds, destabilizes, and nicks the *Ori* sequence to initiate leading-strand DNA synthesis.[22] The four strands of the destabilized IRs exist in a "melted" configuration, and the minus-strand viral DNA and a palindromic strand serve as templates simultaneously during initiation or termination of viral DNA replication. The palindromic sequences flanking the *Ori* can potentially form single-stranded stem-loop cruciform structures that are essential for circovirus replication.[23] Three conserved rolling circle replication motifs (RCR-I, RCR-II, and RCR-III) and a dNTP-binding motif were identified within PCV Rep and Rep′.[40,157,168] Mutations of the conserved motifs negatively affect PCV replication.[93,158] The RCR-II motif is involved in the nicking of the viral DNA, and the Tyr-93 residue within the RCR-III motif cleaves the phosphodiester bond to produce a 3′-hydroxyl group that serves as a primer for viral genome replication and a 5′-phosphate of the cleavage product that covalently attaches to Rep and Rep′.[157,168] After a round of replication, the newly synthesized viral genome DNA is cleaved again, and the 5′-phosphate is ligated to the 3′-hydroxyl group, resulting in the release of unit-length single-strand monomer genomes.[40]

The mechanism of PCV2 assembly and release remains largely unknown. It was reported that the p32 (gC1qR) is a key regulator for PCV2 nuclear egress.[173] PCV2 Cap recruits P32 to the nucleus as an adaptor to recruit phosphorylated PKC-δ and PCV2 Cap to the nuclear membrane to phosphorylate

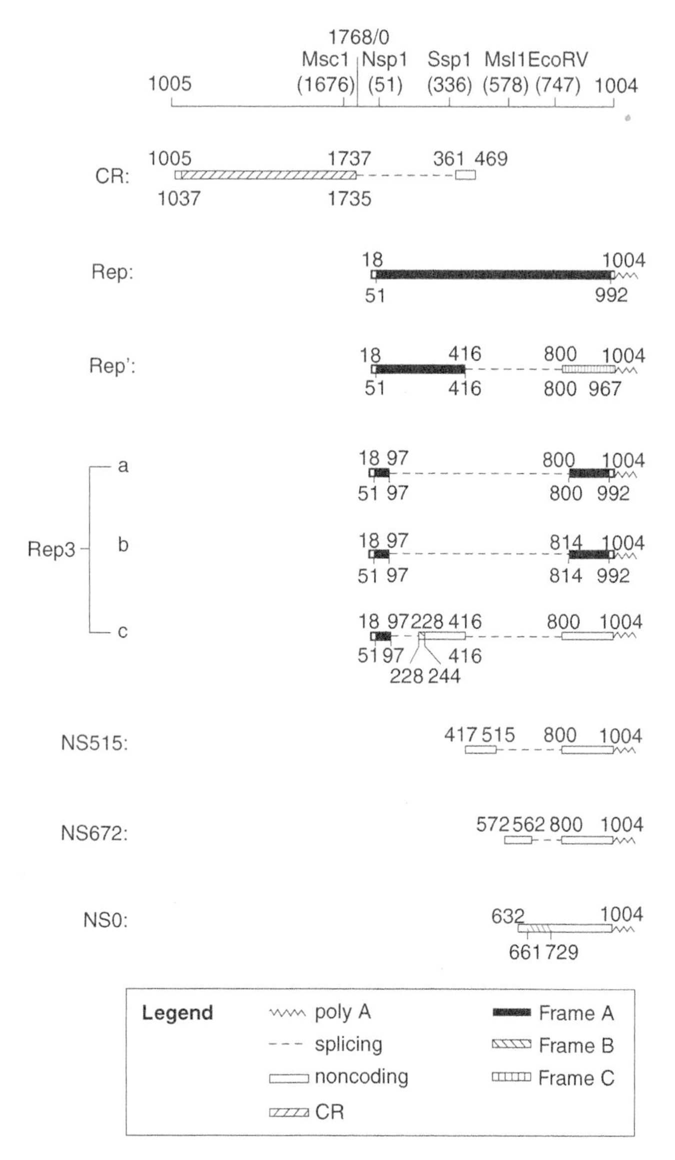

FIGURE 7.5 **Summary of the PCV2 RNA transcripts.** The schematic representation of the PCV2 genome with relevant restriction enzyme sites is shown on *top*. The RNA is annotated on *top* with nt coordinates that indicates the last nucleotide of each respective exon. The coding sequence of each transcript was shaded and their nt coordinates are indicated below each RNA. (Reprinted from Cheung AK. Transcriptional analysis of porcine circovirus type 2. *Virology* 2003;305(1):168-180. Copyright © 2003 Elsevier. With permission.)

lamin A/C, leading to the rearrangement of nuclear lamina and facilitation of PCV2 nuclear egress. It was also demonstrated that nuclear targeting of PCV2 Cap involved conformational changes, and the viral genome was released from the assembled Cap.[175]

Pathogenesis and Pathology

Porcine Circovirus–Associated Diseases

PCV2 is associated with various disease conditions in pigs including postweaning multisystemic wasting syndrome (PMWS), reproductive failures, and porcine dermatitis and nephropathy syndrome (PDNS) collectively known as porcine circovirus–associated diseases (PCVAD).[127,147] The oronasal exposure is likely the natural route of PCV2 transmission, although pigs can be experimentally infected via intramuscular, oral, oronasal, and intrauterine routes of inoculation.[88,128,129] Lymphoid depletion and histiocytic replacement are characteristic lesions in lymphoid tissues[127] (Fig. 7.7). PCV2 is likely shed through respiratory and oral secretions, urine, and feces of infected pigs.[127] The interaction of PCV2 with the host immune system is a critical factor in PCV2 pathogenesis. Immunostimulations by coinfecting agents such as porcine reproductive and respiratory syndrome virus (PRRSV) or by adjuvants such as keyhole limpet hemocyanin exacerbate PCVAD.[127] An increase in IL-10 and proinflammatory cytokines such as IL-1 and TNF-α and a decrease in IL-2, IL-4 expression were observed in PCV2-infected pigs with PCVAD. An interferon-stimulated response element (ISRE) sequence was identified in the Ori of PCV2 genome. When present in the context of intact virus but not in isolation, the ISRE influences the interferon-mediated enhancement of PCV2 replication *in vitro* and plays a potential role in viral pathogenesis *in vivo*.[140,141]

The pathogenicity of PCV3 remains debatable. PCV3 was initially identified from pigs with cardiac and multisystemic inflammation,[135] PDNS, and reproductive failure.[130] PCV3 was detected from pigs with porcine respiratory disease complex (PRDC) in Thailand,[68] and PCV3 DNA was detected by *in situ* hybridization within lesions with myocarditis, encephalitis, and PDNS.[4] PDNS-like disease, but without mortality, was reportedly reproduced in pigs experimentally inoculated with PCV3 stock derived from a PCV3 infectious DNA clone,[58] although independent confirmation of this causal relationship is still lacking. The fact that PCV3 is highly prevalent in apparently healthy pigs[48,83] suggests that the mechanism of PCV3 pathogenesis is complicated and other cofactors may be involved. Little is known regarding the ability of cross-species infection by PCV3. Replication of PCV3 in baboons was reported following transplantation of a heart from a PCV3-positive donor pig, although an attempt to infect human 293 cells with PCV3 failed.[73]

Psittacine Beak and Feather Disease

Psittacine beak and feather disease (PBFD), caused by BFDV of genus *Circovirus*, is one of the most frequently diagnosed viral diseases in psittacine birds.[144,178] BFDV is now known to infect more than 60 different species of psittacine birds, and circovirus infections are common in many other avian species. The natural routes of exposures are thought to be via aerosolized virus particles or direct ingestion of contaminated materials. BFDV has tropism for rapidly dividing cells in mitosis stage such as basal follicular epithelium, lymphoid tissues, and intestinal epithelium. Virus transmission is through virus shedding in feather dander followed by fecal shedding and feeding of chicks with regurgitated crop contents. Gross pathological lesions include feather loss and dystrophy, and beak deformities. Microscopically, necrosis and inflammation are seen in dystrophic feathers. Lymphofollicular hyperplasia with necrosis and lymphoid depletion are commonly seen in lymphoid tissues of BFDV-infected birds.[178]

Epidemiology and Clinical Features

PCVAD affects grower pigs of 5 to 18 weeks of age and rarely occurs in 1- to 3-week-old pigs presumably due to maternal antibody protection.[96] PCV2 infection is widespread worldwide

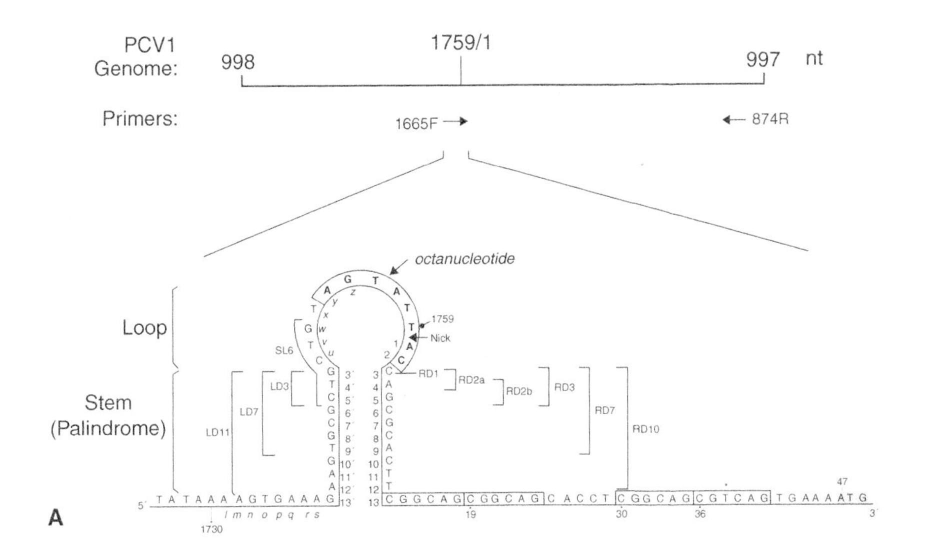

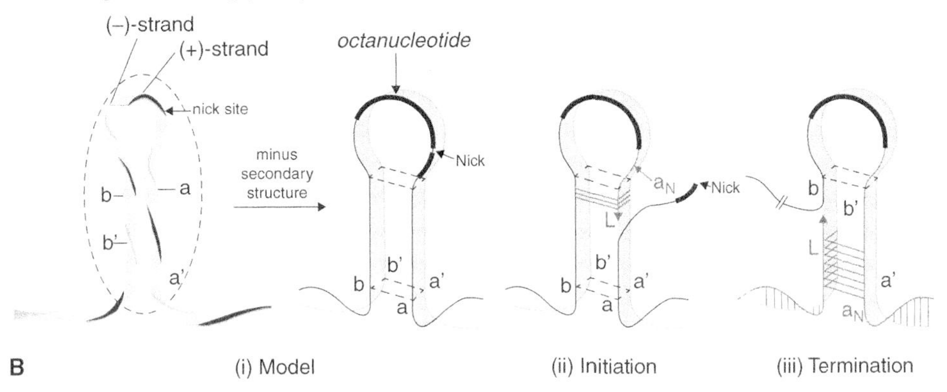

FIGURE 7.6 A: Schematic representation of the PCV1 *Ori*, indicating potential base pairing of the flanking inverted repeats. The genome sequence (1,759 nucleotides) and coordinates (1, 2, 3, etc.) are based on GenBank accession number AY184287. The nucleotide coordinates (3′, 4′, 5′, etc.) are arbitrarily assigned to show the nucleotide complementarity of the palindromic sequences. The octanucleotide containing the presumed nick site (AGTATT↓AC) is *boxed* and indicated in bold. The palindrome is divided into six regions (right arm, RD3, RD7, and RD10; left arm, LD3, LD7, and LD11). The six-nucleotide tandem repeats located at nucleotides 13, 19, 30, and 36 (not perfect at nucleotide 38 and indicated by an *asterisk*) are in *boxes*. Relevant nucleotide sequences are assigned arbitrary positions (l-m-n-o-p-q-r-s and u-v-w-x-y-z) to assist in retracing the templates used during replication. **B:** The rolling circle melting-pot replication model. (i) PCV1 *Ori* after Rep binding to the octanucleotide (prior to nicking) with the plus- and minus-strand genomes in close proximity to each other. The destabilized environment (i.e., the melting pot) is enclosed by a *dotted circle*. (ii) Schematic representation of the DNA templates available during initiation of DNA replication after removal of the secondary structure in the model. The leading strand (*L*) displaces strand a and uses strand a′ or strand b as the template. (iii) Schematic representation of the DNA templates available during termination of DNA replication after removal of the secondary structure in the model. The leading strand (*L*) displaces strand b and uses the newly synthesized strand a_N or strand b′ as the template. The plus-strand genome is indicated in *black*, the minus-strand genome is indicated in *blue*, and the potential base-pairing opportunities available for the current round of DNA replication are indicated in *red*. (From Cheung AK. Palindrome regeneration by template strand-switching mechanism at the origin of DNA replication of porcine circovirus via the rolling-circle melting-pot replication model. *J Virol* 2004;78(17):9016–9029. Copyright © 2004 American Society for Microbiology. Reproduced with permission from American Society for Microbiology.)

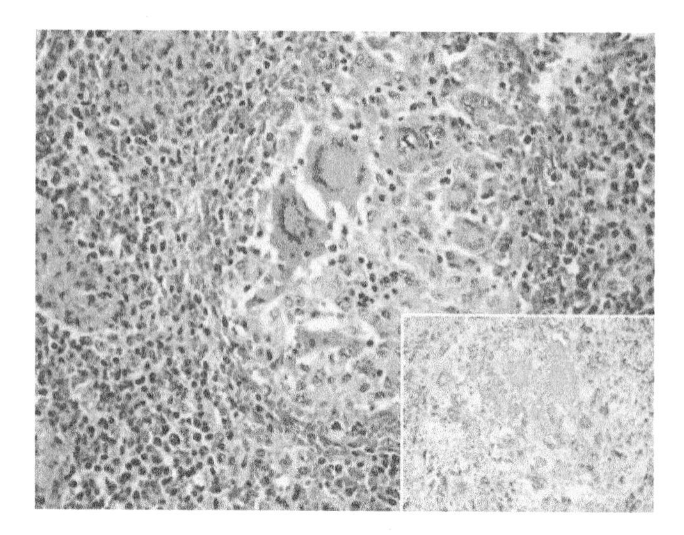

FIGURE 7.7 **PCV2-associated lymphoid depletion and histiocytic-to-granulomatous replacement of the lymphoid follicle with multinucleated giant cells in the center.** Hematoxylin and eosin staining. *Inset*, abundant PCV2 antigen (*brown color* staining) detected by immunohistochemistry. Streptavidin–biotin–peroxidase complex method, hematoxylin counterstain. (From Opriessnig T, Meng XJ, Halbur PG. Porcine circovirus type 2 associated disease: update on current terminology, clinical manifestations, pathogenesis, diagnosis, and intervention strategies. *J Vet Diagn Invest* 2007;19(6):591–615. Copyright © 2007 SAGE Publications. Reprinted by permission of SAGE Publications, Inc.)

with 100% seropositivity in some herds; however, the morbidity is low and only a small proportion of infected animals (5% to 30%) actually develop clinical PCVAD.[127] Currently, there exist at least five different PCV2 genotypes (PCV2a, 2b, 2c, 2d, 2e), and PCV2a and PCV2b differ by as much as 10% at nucleotide sequence level.[10] PCV2 continues to evolve, as evidenced by continuous genotype shifts. Since 2003, PCV2b replaced PCV2a as the predominant genotype in swine populations. Since 2012, a second major genotype shift occurred when the PCV2d genotype has essentially replaced the previously predominant PCV2b genotype worldwide.[67,126] Currently, PCV2a, 2b, and 2d are all globally prevalent and are considered of major clinical importance.[126] The main clinical signs of PCVAD include progressive weight loss or decreased rate of weight gain, paleness or icterus, and gauntness and ill thrift[127] (Fig. 7.8A). The infected pigs may also experience labored respiration with coughing and diarrhea (Fig. 7.9). PCV2 is associated with a number of diseases including pneumonia, enteritis, reproductive failure, and PDNS (Fig. 7.8B).[127]

PCV3 apparently has a broader host range than do PCV1 and PCV2. In addition to pigs, PCV3 was reportedly detected in cattle[174] and dog,[159] although the biological and clinical significance of PCV3 in nonswine species are unclear. PCV3 was thought to have originated from a bat-associated circovirus, and at least two main clades (PCV3a, 3b) have been identified thus far.[16]

BFDV infection is usually seen in young psittacine birds of less than 3 years of age and young pigeons of less than 1 year of age, although older birds can also be infected. In general, circovirus infection in birds is associated with high morbidity but low mortality. The prevalence of BFDV infection varied in wild and captive bird populations. For example, approximately 41% to 95% of the free-ranging psittacine birds in New South Wales are seropositive, whereas 5% of the captive birds in the United States are positive for BFDV.[178] Mortality and clinical signs in BFDV-infected birds varied depending on the age, species, and concurrent infection status. The most common signs in circovirus-infected pigeons include poor performance, diarrhea, and ill-thrift, whereas loss of flight and tail feathers is the main clinical sign in turtle doves.[178] The majority of the infected birds are subclinical.

Diagnosis, Prevention, and Control

The diagnosis of clinical PCVAD requires the demonstration of characteristic pathological lesions associated with the detection of PCV2 antigen or DNA in the affected tissues.[127] Prior to the availability of vaccines, good herd management practices, coinfection control, and disinfection of animal

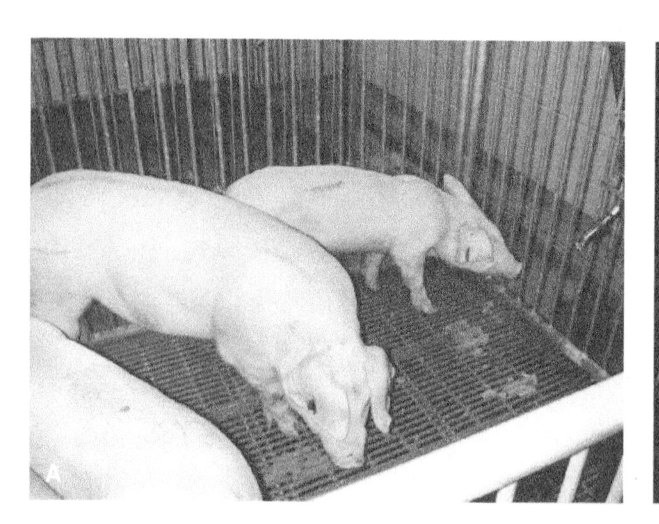

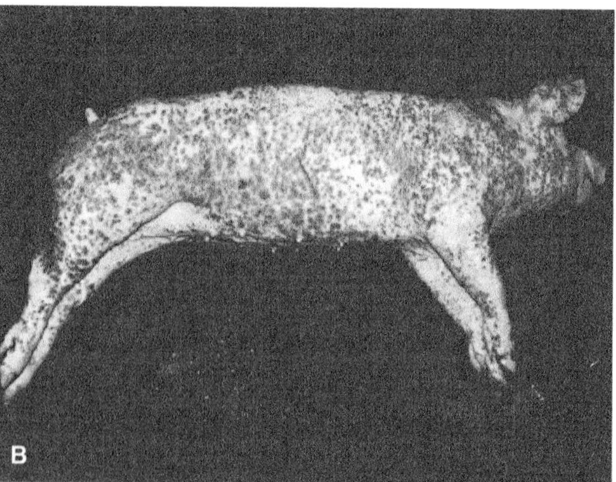

FIGURE 7.8 **A:** An 8-week-old pig experimentally coinfected with porcine circovirus type 2 (PCV2) and porcine parvovirus (PPV) showing icterus and a poor body condition typical of systemic PCVAD. **B:** A 12-week-old pig suffering from porcine dermatitis and nephropathy syndrome (PDNS). The perineal region, ventral abdomen, and legs are covered by raised coalescing *red-purple* lesions. (From Opriessnig T, Meng XJ, Halbur PG. Porcine circovirus type 2 associated disease: update on current terminology, clinical manifestations, pathogenesis, diagnosis, and intervention strategies. *J Vet Diagn Invest* 2007;19(6):591–615. Copyright © 2007 SAGE Publications. Reprinted by permission of SAGE Publications, Inc.)

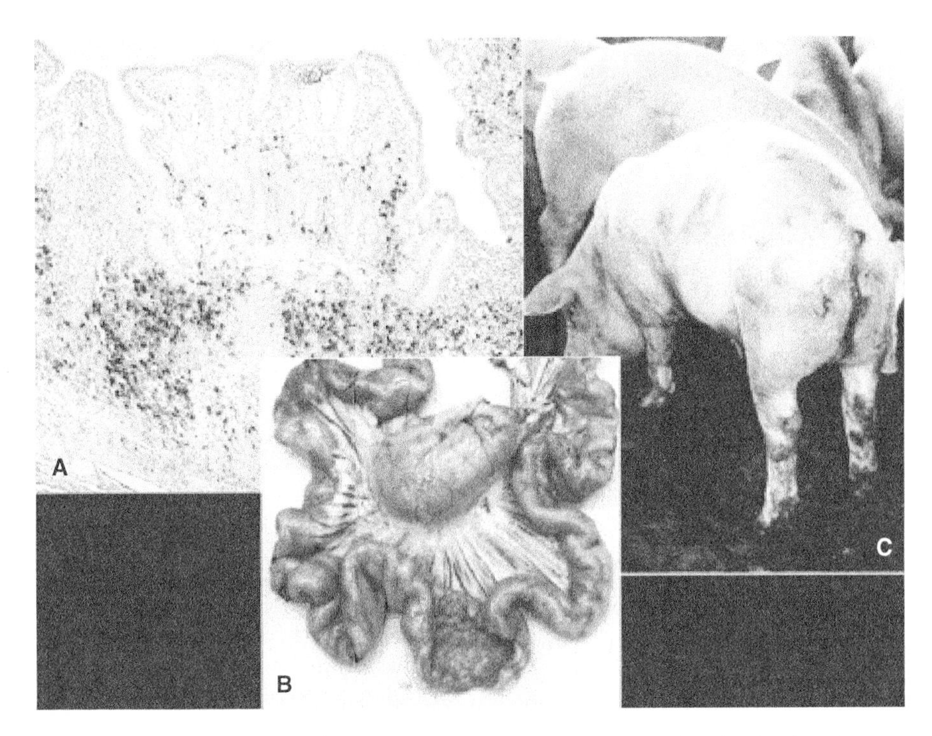

FIGURE 7.9 **PCV2-associated enteritis. A:** PCV2 antigen (*brown staining*) within lymphocytes and macrophage-like cells in the lamina propria and Peyer patches of the ileum of an infected pig. Immunohistochemistry. Streptavidin–biotin–peroxidase complex method, hematoxylin counterstain. **B:** Thickened intestinal mucosa and a markedly enlarged mesenteric lymph node. **C:** Grow-finish pig with mild diarrhea. (From Opriessnig T, Meng XJ, Halbur PG. Porcine circovirus type 2 associated disease: update on current terminology, clinical manifestations, pathogenesis, diagnosis, and intervention strategies. *J Vet Diagn Invest* 2007;19(6):591–615. Copyright © 2007 SAGE Publications. Reprinted by permission of SAGE Publications, Inc.)

facilities can minimize the impact of PCV2 infection. Several commercial vaccines are available against PCV2 infection and PCVAD,[10,11,37,38,70] and these vaccines are highly effective. Definitive diagnosis of circovirus infections in birds requires the detection of viral antigen or DNA in affected birds. Virus isolation is not possible for most circoviruses. Currently, there is no commercial vaccine against BFDV, and thus control of circovirus infection in free-ranging birds is difficult.

Perspective

Members of the *Circoviridae* are associated with important animal diseases including PCVAD in pigs and PBFD in avian species. The biological significance and pathogenic potential for members of the genus *Cyclovirus* remain unknown. Contamination of live-attenuated human rotavirus vaccines with porcine circoviruses raised a concern of vaccine safety, although definitive evidence of zoonotic human infections by animal circoviruses is still lacking. Only porcine circoviruses can be propagated *in vitro*, and a specific cellular receptor for circoviruses has not yet been identified. Many steps in the circovirus life cycle are poorly understood. Future studies are warranted to elucidate the molecular mechanism of circovirus pathogenesis, identify cellular and viral factors that determine species tropisms, assess the zoonotic potential of animal circoviruses, and determine the clinical significance of cycloviruses.

ANELLOVIRIDAE

History

Anelloviruses are single-stranded, small circular DNA viruses infecting humans and a broad range of other animal species.[120,121] The first anellovirus, torque teno virus (TTV), was discovered from a Japanese patient with posttransfusion hepatitis of unknown etiology in 1997.[109] The virus was named "TTV" after the patient's initials "T.T." but was later adopted as torque teno virus in order to preserve the original abbreviation while also implying the circular nature of the virus genome: torque (from Latin *torques*, "necklace") and teno (from Latin *tenuis*, "thin").[12]

Other related viruses such as torque teno mini virus (TTMV) and torque teno midi virus (TTMDV), with smaller genomes than TTV, were subsequently identified in humans.[63,108,160] Studies have documented anelloviruses as the most abundant component of human virome, causing lifelong viremia.[43,44] Anelloviruses have also been identified in a large number of animal species with a high degree of genetic diversity.[59,121] The porcine anelloviruses, torque teno sus viruses (TTSuV), are highly prevalent in pig population worldwide and have been studied in more detail than other TTVs.[52–55,125] Human anelloviruses are epidemiologically incriminated in a number of diseases including liver diseases, respiratory disorders, hematological disorders, and cancer; however, there is no established direct causal relationship between TTV and a disease.[43,120]

CAV was first isolated in 1979,[183] although its complete genomic sequence was not determined until 1991.[27,113,119] The virus causes bone marrow atrophy, anemia, and immunosuppression in chickens.

Classification

In the absence of a disease association or lack of knowledge on anellovirus replication, the host species and genome size are utilized as the main criteria for taxonomic classification into different genera and species within the family *Anelloviridae*. According to the ICTV 9th Report, the *Anelloviridae* family consists of at least 14 genera (*Alpha-, Beta-, Delta-, Epsilon-, Eta-, Gamma-, Iota-, Kappa-, Lambda-, Mu-, Nu-, Theta-, Zetatorquevirus,* and *Gyrovirus*) and 76 species.

The genus *Gyrovirus,* previously classified within the family *Circoviridae*, has now been reclassified into the *Anelloviridae* family.[145] CAV is the prototype species within the genus *Gyrovirus*. At least 9 other gyrovirus species have now been identified from a number of animal species including chickens, birds, humans, ferret, mice, and domestic cats.[26,34,35,77,110,143,148,180] Avian gyrovirus 2, first reported in 2011 as a distant relative of CAV,[143,148] was identified in chickens and healthy humans.[181] GyV3 and GyV4 were identified from human feces,[26,136] and GyV3 has also been identified from commercial broiler chickens with transmissible viral proventriculitis.[78] GyV5 and GyV6 were detected in diarrheic samples from Tunisian children,[137] and GyV7 was detected in chicken meats.[184] The genome of a highly divergent GyV8 was characterized in the spleen and uropygial gland tissues of a sea bird in San Francisco.[77] GyV9 was found in the feces of an adult with diarrhea,[134] and GyV10 was discovered from birds with neurologic disease and chick mortality.[50] Unfortunately, little is known regarding the biology and pathogenicity of these novel gyroviruses; no direct association with a disease has been established. The ever-expanding host range with frequent identification of novel animal anelloviruses from diverse animal species suggests that the classification of *Anelloviridae* family will continue to evolve in the future.[44,152]

Virion Structure

The virions are nonenveloped spherical particles of approximately 30 to 35 nm in size for TTVs[56] and less than 30 nm for TTMVs.[160] The virion particles of CAV in the genus *Gyrovirus* have a diameter of 25 to 26.5 nm[28,47,97] (Fig. 7.2). The capsid of CAV, encoded by ORF1, contains 12 pentagonal trumpet-shaped capsomers with a $T = 1$ icosahedral symmetry, which is different from that of *Circoviridae* that has 12 flat pentameric morphological units. Therefore, under EM, the circovirus virions have a smoother and more featureless surface than that of *Gyrovirus* CAV within the family *Anelloviridae*[28] (Fig. 7.2). Using viruses purified from sera, the virion buoyant density is 1.31 to 1.33 g cm^{-3} for TTVs[122] and 1.27 to 1.28 g cm^{-3} for TTMVs.[160] Anellovirus virion particles form immune complex with serum immunoglobulin in circulation, as visualized by immunogold electron microscopy[56] as aggregates of different sizes, while particles in feces exist as free virions.

Genome Structure and Organization

The genomes of anelloviruses are single-stranded circular DNA molecules ranging from 2.0 to 3.9 kb in size.[120,121] Members of *Anelloviridae* family contain two partially overlapping ORFs (ORF1 and ORF2),[121,125] additional ORFs with variable sizes translated from the negative strand of circular ds replicative form of viral DNA[54,55,103,139] and a short stretch of untranslated region (UTR) with high GC content (~90%).[121,122,124,125]

The genome of *gyrovirus* CAV is a negative sense with approximately 2.3 kb and contains three partially overlapping ORFs, a promoter-enhancer region, and a polyadenylation signal.[114,138] The ORF1 codes for the VP1 capsid protein, and the ORF2 and ORF3 code for VP2 and VP3 nonstructural proteins. The ORF3 completely overlaps ORF2, while ORF2 partially overlaps ORF1. The promoter-enhancer region in the 5′ NCR of CAV genome contains four or five 21-bp direct repeats (DR) and a 12-bp insert between the second and third DRs.[98,114] Host cell transcription factors bind to the DRs and the 12-bp insert, and at least two DRs and the 12-bp insert are required for efficient transcription and replication.[113–115,119]

Stages of Replication

Although CAV in the genus *Gyrovirus* can be propagated in cell cultures, other genera of the *Anelloviridae* could not be efficiently cultured *in vitro*. Therefore, knowledge of anellovirus replication especially regarding attachment, entry, and uncoating steps is very limited and derived mostly from the studies of gyrovirus CAV.

Transcription

The genome of human anelloviruses expresses at least three spliced mRNAs encoding at least six proteins: ORF1, ORF2, ORF1/1, ORF2/2, ORF1/2, and ORF2/3.[62,63,103,139] The porcine anellovirus, torque teno sus virus (TTSuV), also expresses at least three putative mRNAs encoding six proteins.[55] The transcriptional profile of human anellovirus genome has been studied by transfecting the plasmid containing the full-length viral genome in cultured cell lines.[103,139,170] Three species of TTV mRNAs (2.8 to 3.0, 1.2, and 1.0 kb) are transcribed from a single promoter located in the region −154/−76 (RNA initiation site is denoted as position +1) and are polyadenylated at the same nucleotide (nt) 2978 position.[63] Therefore, all TTV RNAs are cleaved at the same site at approximately nt 3000 and have common 5′ and 3′ ends. A small intron (~100 nt), located in approximately 70 nt from the RNA initiation site, is spliced out from all three transcripts. Among the three species of TTV mRNAs, the two short 1.2-kb and 1.0-kb mRNAs are further spliced approximately 400 nt downstream of the small intron, excising another larger intron with alternative 3′ splice sites at nt 2315 and nt 2505. The 2.8-, 1.2-, and 1.0-kb mRNAs comprise approximately 60%, 5%, and 35% of the total TTV RNAs, respectively.[103] All the splice sites utilize the conserved GT-AG donor and acceptor sequences.[63,103,139]

For CAV in the genus *Gyrovirus*, three viral proteins are derived from a single 2.0-kb mRNA species.[116,132] Several minor mRNA species of 1.6, 1.3, and 1.2 kb in size are also identified[64] (Fig. 7.10). The 1.3-kb RNA had a splice site joining nt 1222 to nt 1814 and encoded head-to-tail VP1. The 1.2-kb RNA possessed a splice site joining nt 994 to nt 1095 and encoded several putative proteins with frame-shift mutations. CAV contains a single promoter-enhancer region with 4 consensus cyclic AMP response element sequences that are similar to the estrogen response element consensus half-sites. These sequences are arranged as direct repeats, an arrangement that

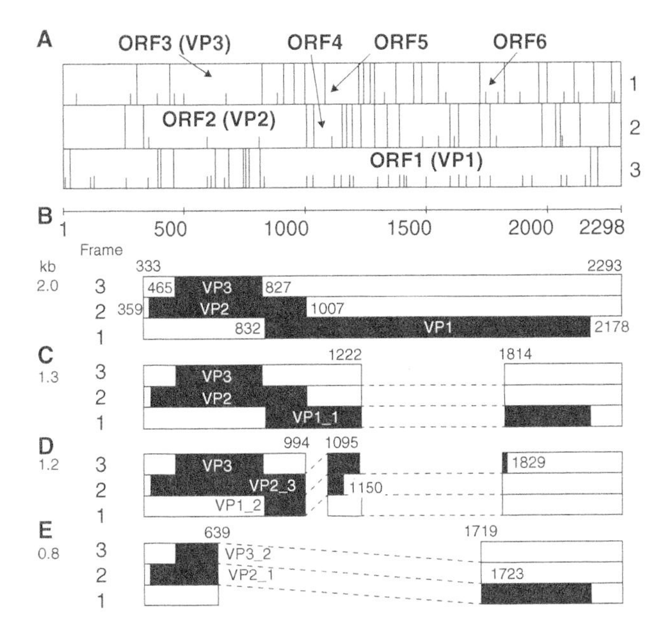

FIGURE 7.10 Schematic representation of the *Gyrovirus* CAV RNA transcripts and their candidate ORFs. A: Six ORFs of the CAV genome. *Short and long vertical lines* indicate ATG start and stop codons, respectively. Putative ORFs encoded by the RNA transcripts are indicated by *arrows*. ORFs evident in the 2.0-, 1.3-, 1.2-, and 0.8-kb transcripts are shown in panels **(B–E)**, respectively. *Dotted lines* indicate introns or deleted regions. *Black boxes* represent putative coding regions. Nucleotide numbers indicate the positions of ORF junctions or boundaries of ORFs. (Republished with permission of Microbiology Society from Kamada K, Kuroishi A, Kamahora T, et al. Spliced mRNAs detected during the life cycle of Chicken anemia virus. *J Gen Virol* 2006;87(Pt 8):2227-2233; permission conveyed through Copyright Clearance Center, Inc.)

can be recognized by members of the nuclear receptor superfamily and may provide a mechanism to regulate CAV activity in situations of low virus copy number.[98]

Translation

For human anelloviruses, the largest and most abundant 2.8-kb mRNA species expresses the ORF1 and ORF2 proteins, respectively. The smaller 1.2-kb mRNA species expresses the ORF2/2 and ORF1/1 proteins, whereas the smallest 1.0-kb mRNA species expresses the ORF2/3 and ORF1/2 proteins.[61,103,139] The ORF1, ORF1/1, and ORF1/2 expression products of human anelloviruses were localized in the nucleoli, ORF3 and ORF4 in the nucleoplasm, ORF2/2 in the nucleoli or whole nucleus, and ORF2 in the cytoplasm.[103] Similar to human TTVs, proteins encoded from ORF1 and ORF3 of TTSuV1 and TTSuV2 were also localized in the nucleoli, and ORF2 in the cytoplasm and nucleus excluding the nucleoli.[95]

The ORF1 of anelloviruses encodes a putative capsid protein containing arginine-rich, hydrophilic N-terminal sequences and replication-associated protein with the largest size relative to the other predicted viral proteins.[52,61,103] The ORF2 of TTMVs contains a highly conserved motif ($WX_7HX_3CXCX_5H$) in its N-terminal region[160] and may encode a protein with phosphatase activity. The ORF2 reportedly suppressed NF-κB pathways via interaction with IκB kinases and may involve in regulating the innate and adaptive immune responses.[186] The ORF3 of TTVs contains a serine-rich domain at the C terminus that may produce different phosphorylation sites,[5] possibly involving in maintaining persistent viral infection. The function of the other putative anellovirus proteins has not yet been demonstrated.

The gyrovirus CAV genome encodes three proteins: the VP1 Cap and the VP2 and VP3 nonstructural proteins.[150,166] The amino acid residue 394 of VP1 is a determinant of virus pathogenicity.[179] The VP2 is a multifunctional protein that also serves as a scaffold protein during virion assembly.[71,116,150] The VP2 has dual serine and tyrosine protein phosphatase activities,[132,133] and mutations in VP2 attenuated CAV.[131] Both VP1 and VP2 are required to elicit neutralizing antibodies against CAV.[32,71,115,117] The VP3 of CAV, also known as apoptin, induces apoptosis in chicken thymocytes and lymphoblastoid cells.[118] VP3 triggers the intrinsic mitochondrial death pathway resulting in loss of mitochondrial membrane and release of cytochrome c and apoptosis-inducing factors in mitochondria.[30,87] The VP3-induced apoptosis is independent of tumor suppressor p53, and Bcl-2 does not inhibit the VP3-induced apoptosis in tumor cells.[29,151] Synthesis of VP3 alone induces apoptosis in human tumor cell lines, but not in normal human diploid cells,[29] and thus VP3 is considered as an anticancer agent.[111,112]

Replication of Genomic DNA, Assembly, and Release

The viral DNA replication, assembly, and release are essentially unknown due to the lack of an efficient cell culture system for anelloviruses; however, the extensive heterogeneity among the genomes of anelloviruses suggests a poor proofreading mechanism during the viral genome replication. Anelloviruses do not encode viral polymerase and therefore rely on the host cellular DNA polymerase for its genome replication. The ORF1 possesses conserved amino acid sequence motifs, such as a RCR sequence motif, found in the Rep proteins of other circular ssDNA viruses including *Circoviridae* and *Nanoviridae*, suggesting that anelloviruses likely also use a rolling circle mechanism for virus replication.[61,62,103] A conserved sequence and structure in the UTR region are essential for the initiation of viral genome replication.[62,124] The replication-associated protein ORF1 containing the "Rep" motifs is necessary for anelloviruses to interact with host proteins during virus replication.[61–63]

The genome replication of the genus *Gyrovirus* CAV is also thought to be via a rolling circle replication mechanism.[150,167] Homologous recombination occurs in cloned head-to-tail repeat replicative form of CAV genomes.[167] The VP1 contains a 3-amino acid motif associated with rolling circle replication. The phosphatase activity of VP2 is important but not required for CAV replication.[132,133] The VP3 is essential for completion of CAV life cycle as truncated VP3 lacking the C-terminal 11 amino acid residues failed to induce apoptosis.[114,118]

Pathogenesis and Pathology

Other than CAV in the genus *Gyrovirus*, attempts to associate other anelloviruses with a specific disease have not been successful.[43,53,120] It is generally believed that anelloviruses are commensal viruses to the host, although infection of anelloviruses may play a role in the homeostatic balance of host immune system, thereby indirectly affecting the severity and outcome of diseases caused by other pathogens.[44,89,152] It has been reported that TTV DNA loads are elevated in donor lungs in allografts and that the plasma loads of TTV DNA can predict rejection in lung transplant recipients.[45,57]

Chicken Infectious Anemia (CIA)

CAV is the only known virus within the family *Anelloviridae* that causes a disease. The natural route of exposure for CAV is likely oral.[149] Feces from infected chickens are the main source of virus for horizontal transmission. Vertical transmission in commercial flocks through hatching eggs is an important means of virus dissemination. Under field condition, vertical transmission occurs for a period of 3 to 9 weeks after exposure to CAV. Gross lesions include thymic and bone marrow atrophy and less commonly bursal atrophy. Hemorrhagic-aplastic anemia syndrome characterized by intracutaneous, subcutaneous, and intramuscular hemorrhages is associated with severe anemia in CAV-infected chickens. Microscopically, CAV-infected chickens are characterized by generalized lymphoid atrophy and depletion and panmyelophthisis. Infection of hemocytoblasts in the bone marrow and lymphoblasts in the thymus cortex in the early infection stage (6 to 8 days postinfection) causes a rapid depletion of these cells by apoptosis with drastically reduced numbers of erythrocytes, white blood cells, and thrombocytes.[154]

Epidemiology and Clinical Features

Beside humans, genetically divergent anelloviruses have been identified from more than a dozen other animal species including pigs, sheep, dog, horse, elk, masked palm civet, fur seals, bats, opossums, gorillas, chimpanzees, and rodent species.[121,125,155] Whether anelloviruses infect across species remains largely unknown,[106,153] although human TTV reportedly infects chimpanzees.[123] Multiple infections of human TTV with different genotypes, as well as dual or triple infections of TTV, TTMV, and TTMDV in a single individual, have been documented and are believed to be a common event in humans.[6,107] Similarly, TTSuV infection with different genotypes or subtypes in a single pig has also been reported.[54] Antigenic cross-reactivity between two TTSuV genotypes (TTSuV1a and TTSuV1b), but not between two species (TTSuV1 and TTSuV2), has been demonstrated.[53] There appears to be antigenically distinct between human TTV and TTSuV.[53] The TTSuVs are highly prevalent in pig population worldwide, but the infection in swine is subclinical.[52,53] Human anelloviruses spread through multiple routes including blood, saliva, air, water, and contaminated food.[43,120]

Within the genus *Gyrovirus* alone, in addition to CAV, at least 9 other species of animal gyroviruses have been genetically identified through metagenomic analyses from various animals such as chickens, birds, humans, ferret, mice, and domestic cats.[26,34,35,77,110,143,148,180] CAV infection is ubiquitous in chicken flocks worldwide. CAV infection of chickens of 2 to 4 weeks of age induced anemia, which is characterized by hematocrit values ranging from 6% to 27%. The mortality is about 10% to 20% but generally does not exceed 30%. Surviving chickens completely recover from anemia by 20 to 28 days postinfection, although secondary bacterial or viral infection may slow down the recovery process. Chickens develop age resistance to CAV-induced anemia by approximately 3 weeks of age.[149]

Diagnosis, Prevention, and Control

Clinical samples such as plasma, saliva, feces, hairs, and skin biopsies can be used to detect anelloviruses by PCR, which is the most commonly used method for identification of anellovirus infection.[107,108,120,121,125] Primers specific for the highly conserved UTR region allow for PCR detection of different genotypes.[107,120,121,125] Quantitative PCR is also used for quantification of viral loads. Reagents for serological assays are very limited. TTSuV1a or TTSuV1b ELISA assays based on the respective ORF1 capsid antigen were developed to detect TTSuV antibodies in pigs.[52,53,105] With the exception of CAV, there is no cell culture system to isolate other anelloviruses. Due to ubiquitous nature and the lack of a disease association, it is rather difficult to ascertain the anellovirus-specific morbidity.

CAV can be propagated in lymphoblastoid T-cell lines (MDCC-MSB1 and MDCC-JP2) and B-cell line (LSCC-1104B1). Virus isolation in susceptible cells and detection of CAV DNA and antigen in tissues are means of diagnosis of CAV infection. Commercial live-attenuated vaccines against CAV are used to immunize chickens of 9 to 15 weeks of ages. Complete elimination of CAV from chicken flocks is not realistic and thus good management and hygiene procedures are important to minimize the impact caused by CAV infection.

Perspective

Members of the *Anelloviridae* have a very broad host range. Only *Gyrovirus* CAV is known to cause a disease in chickens, and the other anelloviruses are considered to be a part of host microbiota and not associated with a specific disease.[43] Anellovirus replication may be enhanced in infected immune-compromised individuals, and the anelloviral DNA load may be considered as a biomarker of immune suppression.[44,89] An efficient cell culture system is critically needed in order to understand the life cycle of anelloviruses. CAV can be propagated *in vitro*, although a specific cellular receptor has not been identified. TTSuV has been detected in numerous porcine tissue–derived commercial products such as meats, vaccines, enzymes for laboratory use, and human drugs, suggesting a need to better screen biomedical products for anelloviruses. The natural history, ecology, potential cross-species infection, and pathogenicity of a large number of genetically diverse anelloviruses require in-depth research.

REFERENCES

1. Adams DJ, van der Weyden L, Mayeda A, et al. ZNF265—a novel spliceosomal protein able to induce alternative splicing. *J Cell Biol* 2001;154:25–32.
2. Allan GM, McNeilly F, Kennedy S, et al. Isolation of porcine circovirus-like viruses from pigs with a wasting disease in the USA and Europe. *J Vet Diagn Invest* 1998;10:3–10.
3. Allan GM, McNeilly F, McNair I, et al. Absence of evidence for porcine circovirus type 2 in cattle and humans, and lack of seroconversion or lesions in experimentally infected sheep. *Arch Virol* 2000;145:853–857.
4. Arruda B, Pineyro P, Derscheid R, et al. PCV3-associated diseases in the United States swine herd. *Emerg Microbes Infect* 2019;8(1):684–698.
5. Asabe S, Nishizawa T, Iwanari H, et al. Phosphorylation of serine-rich protein encoded by open reading frame 3 of the TT virus genome. *Biochem Biophys Res Commun* 2001;286(2):298–304.
6. Ball JK, Curran R, Berridge S, et al. TT virus sequence heterogeneity in vivo: evidence for co-infection with multiple genetic types. *J Gen Virol* 1999;80 (Pt 7):1759–1768.
7. Baylis SA, Finsterbusch T, Bannert N, et al. Analysis of porcine circovirus type 1 detected in Rotarix vaccine. *Vaccine* 2011;29:690–697.
8. Beach NM, Córdoba L, Kenney SP, et al. Productive infection of human hepatocellular carcinoma cells by porcine circovirus type 1. *Vaccine* 2011;29(43):7303–7306.
9. Beach NM, Juhan NM, Cordoba L, et al. Replacement of the replication factors of porcine circovirus (PCV) type 2 with those of PCV type 1 greatly enhances viral replication in vitro. *J Virol* 2010;84:8986–8989.
10. Beach NM, Ramamoorthy S, Opriessnig T, et al. Novel chimeric porcine circovirus (PCV) with the capsid gene of the emerging PCV2b subtype cloned in the genomic backbone of the non-pathogenic PCV1 is attenuated in vivo and induces protective and cross-protective immunity against PCV2b and PCV2a subtypes in pigs. *Vaccine* 2010;29:221–232.
11. Beach NM, Smith SM, Ramamoorthy S, et al. Chimeric porcine circoviruses (PCV) containing amino acid epitope tags in the C-terminus of the capsid gene are infectious and elicit both anti-epitope tag antibodies and anti-PCV2 neutralizing antibodies in pigs. *J Virol* 2011;85(9):4591–4595.

12. Biagini P. Classification of TTV and related viruses (anelloviruses). *Curr Top Microbiol Immunol* 2009;331:21–33.
13. Bonne N, Shearer P, Sharp M, et al. Assessment of recombinant beak and feather disease virus capsid protein as a vaccine for psittacine beak and feather disease. *J Gen Virol* 2009;90:640–647.
14. Bucarey SA, Noriega J, Reyes P, et al. The optimized capsid gene of porcine circovirus type 2 expressed in yeast forms virus-like particles and elicits antibody responses in mice fed with recombinant yeast extracts. *Vaccine* 2009;27:5781–5790.
15. Chaiyakul M, Hsu K, Dardari R, et al. Cytotoxicity of ORF3 proteins from a nonpathogenic and a pathogenic porcine circovirus. *J Virol* 2010;84:11440–11447.
16. Chen Y, Xu Q, Chen H, et al. Evolution and genetic diversity of porcine circovirus 3 in China. *Viruses* 2019;11(9). pii: E786.
17. Cheng S, Yan W, Gu W, et al. The ubiquitin-proteasome system is required for the early stages of porcine circovirus type 2 replication. *Virology* 2014;456–457:198–204.
18. Cheung AK. Transcriptional analysis of porcine circovirus type 2. *Virology* 2003;305:168–180.
19. Cheung AK. Comparative analysis of the transcriptional patterns of pathogenic and nonpathogenic porcine circoviruses. *Virology* 2003;310:41–49.
20. Cheung AK. The essential and nonessential transcription units for viral protein synthesis and DNA replication of porcine circovirus type 2. *Virology* 2003;313:452–459.
21. Cheung AK. Identification of the essential and non-essential transcription units for protein synthesis, DNA replication and infectious virus production of Porcine circovirus type 1. *Arch Virol* 2004;149:975–988.
22. Cheung AK. Detection of template strand switching during initiation and termination of DNA replication of porcine circovirus. *J Virol* 2004;78:4268–4277.
23. Cheung AK. Palindrome regeneration by template strand-switching mechanism at the origin of DNA replication of porcine circovirus via the rolling-circle melting-pot replication model. *J Virol* 2004;78:9016–9029.
24. Cheung AK. Rolling-circle replication of an animal circovirus genome in a theta-replicating bacterial plasmid in Escherichia coli. *J Virol* 2006;80:8686–8694.
25. Cheung AK. Homologous recombination plays minor role in excision of unit-length viral genomes from head-to-tail direct tandem repeats of porcine circovirus during DNA replication in Escherichia coli. *Arch Virol* 2007;152:1531–1539.
26. Chu DKW, Poon LLM, Chiu SSS, et al. Characterization of a novel gyrovirus in human stool and chicken meat. *J Clin Virol* 2012;55:209–213.
27. Claessens JA, Schrier CC, Mockett AP, et al. Molecular cloning and sequence analysis of the genome of chicken anaemia agent. *J Gen Virol* 1991;72:2003–2006.
28. Crowther RA, Berriman JA, Curran WL, et al. Comparison of the structures of three circoviruses: chicken anemia virus, porcine circovirus type 2, and beak and feather disease virus. *J Virol* 2003;77:13036–13041.
29. Danen-Van Oorschot AA, Fischer DF, Grimbergen JM, et al. Apoptin induces apoptosis in human transformed and malignant cells but not in normal cells. *Proc Natl Acad Sci U S A* 1997;94:5843–5847.
30. Danen-van Oorschot AA, van Der Eb AJ, Noteborn MH. The chicken anemia virus-derived protein apoptin requires activation of caspases for induction of apoptosis in human tumor cells. *J Virol* 2000;74:7072–7078.
31. Dhindwal S, Avila B, Feng S, et al. Porcine circovirus 2 uses a multitude of weak binding sites to interact with heparan sulfate, and the interactions do not follow the symmetry of the capsid. *J Virol* 2019;93(6). pii: e02222-18.
32. Douglas AJ, Phenix K, Mawhinney KA, et al. Identification of a 24 kDa protein expressed by chicken anaemia virus. *J Gen Virol* 1995;76:1557–1562.
33. Ellis JA, Wiseman BM, Allan G, et al. Analysis of seroconversion to porcine circovirus 2 among veterinarians from the United States and Canada. *J Am Vet Med Assoc* 2000;217:1645–1646.
34. Fang L, Li Y, Wang Y, et al. Genetic analysis of two chicken infectious anemia virus variants-related *Gyrovirus* in stray mice and dogs: the first report in China, 2015. *Biomed Res Int* 2017;2017:6707868.
35. Fehér E, Pazár P, Kovács E, et al. Molecular detection and characterization of human gyroviruses identified in the ferret fecal virome. *Arch Virol* 2014;159:3401–3406.
36. Fenaux M, Halbur PG, Haqshenas G, et al. Cloned genomic DNA of type 2 porcine circovirus is infectious when injected directly into the liver and lymph nodes of pigs: characterization of clinical disease, virus distribution, and pathologic lesions. *J Virol* 2002;76:541–551.
37. Fenaux M, Opriessnig T, Halbur PG, et al. Immunogenicity and pathogenicity of chimeric infectious DNA clones of pathogenic porcine circovirus type 2 (PCV2) and nonpathogenic PCV1 in weanling pigs. *J Virol* 2003;77:11232–11243.
38. Fenaux M, Opriessnig T, Halbur PG, et al. A chimeric porcine circovirus (PCV) with the immunogenic capsid gene of the pathogenic PCV type 2 (PCV2) cloned into the genomic backbone of the nonpathogenic PCV1 induces protective immunity against PCV2 infection in pigs. *J Virol* 2004;78:6297–6303.
39. Fenaux M, Opriessnig T, Halbur PG, et al. Two amino acid mutations in the capsid protein of type 2 porcine circovirus (PCV2) enhanced PCV2 replication in vitro and attenuated the virus in vivo. *J Virol* 2004;78:13440–13446.
40. Finsterbusch T, Mankertz A. Porcine circoviruses—small but powerful. *Virus Res* 2009;143:177–183.
41. Finsterbusch T, Steinfeldt T, Caliskan R, et al. Analysis of the subcellular localization of the proteins Rep, Rep′ and Cap of porcine circovirus type 1. *Virology* 2005;343:36–46.
42. Finsterbusch T, Steinfeldt T, Doberstein K, et al. Interaction of the replication proteins and the capsid protein of porcine circovirus type 1 and 2 with host proteins. *Virology* 2009;386:122–131.
43. Focosi D, Antonelli G, Pistello M, et al. Torquetenovirus: the human virome from bench to bedside. *Clin Microbiol Infect* 2016;22(7):589–593.
44. Freer G, Maggi F, Pifferi M, et al. The virome and its major component, Anellovirus, a convoluted system molding human immune defenses and possibly affecting the development of asthma and respiratory diseases in childhood. *Front Microbiol* 2018;9:686.
45. Frye BC, Bierbaum S, Falcone V, et al. Kinetics of Torque Teno virus-DNA plasma load predict rejection in lung transplant recipients. *Transplantation* 2019;103(4):815–822.
46. Gao Z, Dong Q, Jiang Y, et al. ORF4-protein deficient PCV2 mutants enhance virus-induced apoptosis and show differential expression of mRNAs in vitro. *Virus Res* 2014;183:56–62.
47. Gelderblom H, Kling S, Lurz R, et al. Morphological characterization of chicken anaemia agent (CAA). *Arch Virol* 1989;109:115–120.
48. Geng S, Luo H, Liu Y, et al. Prevalence of porcine circovirus type 3 in pigs in the southeastern Chinese province of Zhejiang. *BMC Vet Res* 2019;15(1):244.
49. Gibbs MJ, Weiller GF. Evidence that a plant virus switched hosts to infect a vertebrate and then recombined with a vertebrate-infecting virus. *Proc Natl Acad Sci U S A* 1999;96:8022–8027.
50. Goldberg TL, Clyde VL, Gendron-Fitzpatrick A, et al. Severe neurologic disease and chick mortality in crested screamers (Chauna torquata) infected with a novel Gyrovirus. *Virology* 2018;520:111–115.
51. He J, Cao J, Zhou N, et al. Identification and functional analysis of the novel ORF4 protein encoded by porcine circovirus type 2. *J Virol* 2013;87(3):1420–1429.
52. Huang YW, Harrall KK, Dryman BA, et al. Expression of the putative ORF1 capsid protein of Torque teno sus virus 2 (TTSuV2) and development of Western blot and ELISA serodiagnostic assays: correlation between TTSuV2 viral load and IgG antibody level in pigs. *Virus Res* 2011;158(1–2):79–88.
53. Huang YW, Harrall KK, Dryman BA, et al. Serological profile of torque teno sus virus species 1 (TTSuV1) in pigs and antigenic relationships between two TTSuV1 genotypes (1a and 1b), between two species (TTSuV1 and −2), and between porcine and human anelloviruses. *J Virol* 2012;86(19):10628–10639.
54. Huang YW, Ni YY, Dryman BA, et al. Multiple infection of porcine Torque teno virus in a single pig and characterization of the full-length genomic sequences of four U.S. prototype PTTV strains: implication for genotyping of PTTV. *Virology* 2010;396(2):289–297.
55. Huang YW, Patterson AR, Opriessnig T, et al. Rescue of a porcine anellovirus (torque teno sus virus 2) from cloned genomic DNA in pigs. *J Virol* 2012;86(11):6042–6054.
56. Itoh Y, Takahashi M, Fukuda M, et al. Visualization of TT virus particles recovered from the sera and feces of infected humans. *Biochem Biophys Res Commun* 2000;279(2):718–724.
57. Jaksch P, Kundi M, Görzer I, et al. Torque Teno Virus as a novel biomarker targeting the efficacy of immunosuppression after lung transplantation. *J Infect Dis* 2018;218(12):1922–1928.
58. Jiang H, Wang D, Wang J, et al. Induction of porcine dermatitis and nephropathy syndrome in piglets by infection with porcine circovirus type 3. *J Virol* 2019;93(4). pii: e02045-18.
59. Jones MS, Kapoor A, Lukashov VV, et al. New DNA viruses identified in patients with acute viral infection syndrome. *J Virol* 2005;79:8230–8236.
60. Juhan NM, LeRoith T, Opriessnig T, et al. The open reading frame 3 (ORF3) of porcine circovirus type 2 (PCV2) is dispensable for virus infection but evidence of reduced pathogenicity is limited in pigs infected by an ORF3-null PCV2 mutant. *Virus Res* 2010;147:60–66.
61. Kakkola L, Bondén H, Hedman L, et al. Expression of all six human Torque teno virus (TTV) proteins in bacteria and in insect cells, and analysis of their IgG responses. *Virology* 2008;382(2):182–189.
62. Kakkola L, Hedman K, Qiu J, et al. Replication of and protein synthesis by TT viruses. *Curr Top Microbiol Immunol* 2009;331:53–64.
63. Kamada K, Kamahora T, Kabat P, et al. Transcriptional regulation of TT virus: promoter and enhancer regions in the 1.2-kb noncoding region. *Virology* 2004;321:341–348.
64. Kamada K, Kuroishi A, Kamahora T, et al. Spliced mRNAs detected during the life cycle of Chicken anemia virus. *J Gen Virol* 2006;87:2227–2233.
65. Karuppannan AK, Jong MH, Lee SH, et al. Attenuation of porcine circovirus 2 in SPF piglets by abrogation of ORF3 function. *Virology* 2009;383:338–347.
66. Karuppannan AK, Liu S, Jia Q, et al. Porcine circovirus type 2 ORF3 protein competes with p53 in binding to pPirh2 and mediates the deregulation of p53 homeostasis. *Virology* 2010;398:1–11.
67. Karuppannan AK, Opriessnig T. Porcine circovirus type 2 (PCV2) vaccines in the context of current molecular epidemiology. *Viruses*. 2017;9(5). pii: E99.
68. Kedkovid R, Woonwong Y, Arunorat J, et al. Porcine circovirus type 3 (PCV3) infection in grower pigs from a Thai farm suffering from porcine respiratory disease complex (PRDC). *Vet Microbiol* 2018;215:71–76.
69. Kekarainen T, Montoya M, Mateu E, et al. Porcine circovirus type 2-induced interleukin-10 modulates recall antigen responses. *J Gen Virol* 2008;89:760–765.
70. Kixmöller M, Ritzmann M, Eddicks M, et al. Reduction of PMWS-associated clinical signs and co-infections by vaccination against PCV2. *Vaccine* 2008;26:3443–3451.
71. Koch G, van Roozelaar DJ, Verschueren CA, et al. Immunogenic and protective properties of chicken anaemia virus proteins expressed by baculovirus. *Vaccine* 1995;13:763–770.
72. Krakowka S, Ellis J, McNeilly F, et al. Features of cell degeneration and death in hepatic failure and systemic lymphoid depletion characteristic of porcine circovirus-2-associated postweaning multisystemic wasting disease. *Vet Pathol* 2004;**41**:471–481.
73. Kruger L, Langin M, Reichart B, et al. Transmission of porcine circovirus type 3 (PCV3) by xenotransplantation of pig hearts into baboons. *Viruses* 2019;11(7). pii: E650.
74. Lee G, Han D, Song JY, et al. Genomic expression profiling in lymph nodes with lymphoid depletion from porcine circovirus 2-infected pigs. *J Gen Virol* 2010;91:2585–2591.
75. Lekcharoensuk P, Morozov I, Paul PS, et al. Epitope mapping of the major capsid protein of type 2 porcine circovirus (PCV2) by using chimeric PCV1 and PCV2. *J Virol* 2004;78:8135–8145.
76. Li L, Kapoor A, Slikas B, et al. Multiple diverse circoviruses infect farm animals and are commonly found in human and chimpanzee feces. *J Virol* 2010;84:1674–1682.
77. Li L, Pesavento PA, Gaynor AM, et al. A gyrovirus infecting a sea bird. *Arch Virol* 2015;160(8):2105–2109.
78. Li G, Yuan S, He M, et al. Emergence of gyrovirus 3 in commercial broiler chickens with transmissible viral proventriculitis. *Transbound Emerg Dis* 2018;65(5):1170–1174.
79. Lin C, Gu J, Wang H, et al. Caspase-dependent apoptosis induction via viral protein ORF4 of porcine circovirus 2 binding to mitochondrial adenine nucleotide translocase 3. *J Virol* 2018;92(10). pii: e00238-18.

80. Liu J, Chen I, Kwang J. Characterization of a previously unidentified viral protein in porcine circovirus type 2-infected cells and its role in virus-induced apoptosis. *J Virol* 2005;79:8262–8274.
81. Liu X, Ouyang T, Ouyang H, et al. Human cells are permissive for the productive infection of porcine circovirus type 2 in vitro. *Sci Rep* 2019;9(1):5638.
82. Liu Q, Tikoo SK, Babiuk LA. Nuclear localization of the ORF2 protein encoded by porcine circovirus type 2. *Virology* 2001;285:91–99.
83. Liu Y, Zhang S, Song X, et al. The prevalence of novel porcine circovirus type 3 isolates in pig farms in China. *Transbound Emerg Dis* 2019;66(5):2143–2151.
84. Liu J, Zhu Y, Chen I, et al. The ORF3 protein of porcine circovirus type 2 interacts with porcine ubiquitin E3 ligase pPirh2 and facilitates p53 expression in viral infection. *J Virol* 2007;81:9560–9567.
85. Lv Q, Guo K, Wang T, et al. Porcine circovirus type 2 ORF4 protein binds heavy chain ferritin. *J Biosci* 2015;40(3):477–485.
86. Lv Q, Guo K, Zhang G, et al. The ORF4 protein of porcine circovirus type 2 antagonizes apoptosis by stabilizing the concentration of ferritin heavy chain through physical interaction. *J Gen Virol* 2016;97(7):1636–1646.
87. Maddika S, Booy EP, Johar D, et al. Cancer-specific toxicity of apoptin is independent of death receptors but involves the loss of mitochondrial membrane potential and the release of mitochondrial cell-death mediators by a Nur77-dependent pathway. *J Cell Sci* 2005;118:4485–4493.
88. Madson DM, Patterson AR, Ramamoorthy S, et al. Reproductive failure experimentally induced in sows via artificial insemination with semen spiked with porcine circovirus type 2. *Vet Pathol* 2009;46:707–716.
89. Maggi F, Bendinelli M. Immunobiology of the Torque teno viruses and other anelloviruses. *Curr Top Microbiol Immunol* 2009;331:65–90.
90. Mahe D, Blanchard P, Truong C, et al. Differential recognition of ORF2 protein from type 1 and type 2 porcine circoviruses and identification of immunorelevant epitopes. *J Gen Virol* 2000;81:1815–1824.
91. Mankertz J, Buhk HJ, Blaess G, et al. Transcription analysis of porcine circovirus (PCV). *Virus Genes* 1998;16:267–276.
92. Mankertz A, Caliskan R, Hattermann K, et al. Molecular biology of porcine circovirus: analyses of gene expression and viral replication. *Vet Microbiol* 2004;98:81–88.
93. Mankertz A, Hillenbrand B. Replication of porcine circovirus type 1 requires two proteins encoded by the viral rep gene. *Virology* 2001;279:429–438.
94. Mankertz A, Persson F, Mankertz J, et al. Mapping and characterization of the origin of DNA replication of porcine circovirus. *J Virol* 1997;71:2562–2566.
95. Martínez-Guinó L, Ballester M, Segalés J, et al. Expression profile and subcellular localization of Torque teno sus virus proteins. *J Gen Virol* 2011;92:2446–2457.
96. McKeown NE, Opriessnig T, Thomas P, et al. Effects of porcine circovirus type 2 (PCV2) maternal antibodies on experimental infection of piglets with PCV2. *Clin Diagn Lab Immunol* 2005;12:1347–1351.
97. McNulty MS, Curran WL, Todd D, et al. Chicken anemia agent: an electron microscopic study. *Avian Dis* 1990;34:736–743.
98. Miller MM, Jarosinski KW, Schat KA. Positive and negative regulation of chicken anemia virus transcription. *J Virol* 2005;79:2859–2868.
99. Misinzo G, Delputte PL, Lefebvre DJ, et al. Increased yield of porcine circovirus-2 by a combined treatment of PK-15 cells with interferon-gamma and inhibitors of endosomal-lysosomal system acidification. *Arch Virol* 2008;153:337–342.
100. Misinzo G, Delputte PL, Lefebvre DJ, et al. Porcine circovirus 2 infection of epithelial cells is clathrin-, caveolae- and dynamin-independent, actin and Rho-GTPase-mediated, and enhanced by cholesterol depletion. *Virus Res* 2009;139:1–9.
101. Misinzo G, Delputte PL, Meerts P, et al. Porcine circovirus 2 uses heparan sulfate and chondroitin sulfate B glycosaminoglycans as receptors for its attachment to host cells. *J Virol* 2006;80:3487–3494.
102. Misinzo G, Meerts P, Bublot M, et al. Binding and entry characteristics of porcine circovirus 2 in cells of the porcine monocytic line 3D4/31. *J Gen Virol* 2005;86:2057–2068.
103. Mueller B, Maerz A, Doberstein K, et al. Gene expression of the human Torque Teno Virus isolate P/1C1. *Virology* 2008;381(1):36–45.
104. Nawagitgul P, Morozov I, Bolin SR, et al. Open reading frame 2 of porcine circovirus type 2 encodes a major capsid protein. *J Gen Virol* 2000;81:2281–2287.
105. Nieto D, Martínez-Guinó L, Jiménez-Melsió A, et al. Development of an indirect ELISA assay for the detection of IgG antibodies against the ORF1 of Torque teno sus viruses 1 and 2 in conventional pigs. *Vet Microbiol* 2015;180(1–2):22–27.
106. Ninomiya M, Takahashi M, Hoshino Y, et al. Analysis of the entire genomes of torque teno midi virus variants in chimpanzees: infrequent cross-species infection between humans and chimpanzees. *J Gen Virol* 2009;90(2):347–358.
107. Ninomiya M, Takahashi M, Nishizawa T, et al. Development of PCR assays with nested primers specific for differential detection of three human anelloviruses and early acquisition of dual or triple infection during infancy. *J Clin Microbiol* 2008;46:507–514.
108. Ninomiya M, Takahashi M, Shimosegawa T, et al. Analysis of the entire genomes of fifteen torque teno midi virus variants classifiable into a third group of genus Anellovirus. *Arch Virol* 2007;152:1961–1975.
109. Nishizawa T, Okamoto H, Konishi K, et al. A novel DNA virus (TTV) associated with elevated transaminase levels in posttransfusion hepatitis of unknown etiology. *Biochem Biophys Res Commun* 1997;241(1):92–97.
110. Niu JT, Yi SS, Dong GY, et al. Genomic characterization of diverse gyroviruses identified in the feces of domestic cats. *Sci Rep* 2019;9(1):13303.
111. Noteborn MH. Chicken anemia virus induced apoptosis: underlying molecular mechanisms. *Vet Microbiol* 2004;98:89–94.
112. Noteborn MH. Proteins selectively killing tumor cells. *Eur J Pharmacol* 2009;625:165–173.
113. Noteborn MH, de Boer GF, van Roozelaar DJ, et al. Characterization of cloned chicken anemia virus DNA that contains all elements for the infectious replication cycle. *J Virol* 1991;65:3131–3139.
114. Noteborn MH, Koch G. Chicken anaemia virus infection: molecular basis of pathogenicity. *Avian Pathol* 1995;24:11–31.
115. Noteborn MH, Kranenburg O, Zantema A, et al. Transcription of the chicken anemia virus (CAV) genome and synthesis of its 52-kDa protein. *Gene* 1992;118:267–271.
116. Noteborn MH, Todd D, Verschueren CA, et al. A single chicken anemia virus protein induces apoptosis. *J Virol* 1994;68:346–351.
117. Noteborn MH, Verschueren CA, Koch G, et al. Simultaneous expression of recombinant baculovirus-encoded chicken anaemia virus (CAV) proteins VP1 and VP2 is required for formation of the CAV-specific neutralizing epitope. *J Gen Virol* 1998;79:3073–3077.
118. Noteborn MH, Verschueren CA, van Ormondt H, et al. Chicken anemia virus strains with a mutated enhancer/promoter region share reduced virus spread and cytopathogenicity. *Gene* 1988;223:165–172.
119. Noteborn MH, Verschueren CA, Zantema A, et al. Identification of the promoter region of chicken anemia virus (CAV) containing a novel enhancer-like element. *Gene* 1994;150:313–318.
120. Okamoto H. History of discoveries and pathogenicity of TT viruses. *Curr Top Microbiol Immunol* 2009;331:1–20.
121. Okamoto H. TT viruses in animals. *Curr Top Microbiol Immunol* 2009;331:35–52.
122. Okamoto H, Akahane Y, Ukita M, et al. Fecal excretion of a nonenveloped DNA virus (TTV) associated with posttransfusion non-A-G hepatitis. *J Med Virol* 1998;56:128–132.
123. Okamoto H, Fukuda M, Tawara A, et al. Species-specific TT viruses and cross-species infection in nonhuman primates. *J Virol* 2000;74(3):1132–1139.
124. Okamoto H, Nishizawa T, Ukita M, et al. The entire nucleotide sequence of a TT virus isolate from the United States (TUS01): comparison with reported isolates and phylogenetic analysis. *Virology* 1999;259:437–448.
125. Okamoto H, Takahashi M, Nishizawa T, et al. Genomic characterization of TT viruses (TTVs) in pigs, cats and dogs and their relatedness with species-specific TTVs in primates and tupaias. *J Gen Virol* 2002;83:1291–1297.
126. Opriessnig T, Castro AMMG, Karuppanan AK, et al. A Porcine circovirus type 2b (PCV2b)-based experimental vaccine is effective in the PCV2b-Mycoplasma hyopneumoniae coinfection pig model. *Vaccine.* 2019;37(44):6688–6695.
127. Opriessnig T, Meng XJ, Halbur PG. Porcine circovirus type 2 associated disease: update on current terminology, clinical manifestations, pathogenesis, diagnosis, and intervention strategies. *J Vet Diagn Invest* 2007;19:591–615.
128. Opriessnig T, Patterson AR, Elsener J, et al. Influence of maternal antibodies on efficacy of porcine circovirus type 2 (PCV2) vaccination to protect pigs from experimental infection with PCV2. *Clin Vaccine Immunol* 2008;15:397–401.
129. Opriessnig T, Ramamoorthy S, Madson DM, et al. Differences in virulence among porcine circovirus type 2 isolates are unrelated to cluster type 2a or 2b and prior infection provides heterologous protection. *J Gen Virol* 2008;89:2482–2491.
130. Palinski R, Pineyro P, Shang P, et al. A novel porcine circovirus distantly related to known circoviruses is associated with porcine dermatitis and nephropathy syndrome and reproductive failure. *J Virol* 2016;91(1). pii: e01879-16.
131. Peters MA, Crabb BS, Tivendale KA, Browning GF. Attenuation of chicken anemia virus by site-directed mutagenesis of VP2. *J Gen Virol* 2007;88:2168–2175.
132. Peters MA, Jackson DC, Crabb BS, et al. Chicken anemia virus VP2 is a novel dual specificity protein phosphatase. *J Biol Chem* 2002;277:39566–39573.
133. Peters MA, Jackson DC, Crabb BS, et al. Mutation of chicken anemia virus VP2 differentially affects serine/threonine and tyrosine protein phosphatase activities. *J Gen Virol* 2005;86:623–630.
134. Phan TG, da Costa AC, Zhang W, et al. A new gyrovirus in human feces. *Virus Genes* 2015;51(1):132–135.
135. Phan TG, Giannitti F, Rossow S, et al. Detection of a novel circovirus PCV3 in pigs with cardiac and multi-systemic inflammation. *Virol J* 2016;13(1):184.
136. Phan TG, Li L, O'Ryan MG, et al. A third gyrovirus species in human faeces. *J Gen Virol* 2012;93(Pt 6):1356–1361.
137. Phan TG, Phung Vo N, Sdiri-Loulizi K, et al. Divergent gyroviruses in the feces of Tunisian children. *Virology* 2013;446:346–348.
138. Phenix KV, Meehan BM, Todd D, et al. Transcriptional analysis and genome expression of chicken anaemia virus. *J Gen Virol* 1994;75:905–909.
139. Qiu J, Kakkola L, Cheng F, et al. Human circovirus TT virus genotype 6 expresses six proteins following transfection of a full-length clone. *J Virol* 2005;79(10):6505–6510.
140. Ramamoorthy S, Huang FF, Huang YW, et al. Interferon-mediated enhancement of in vitro replication of porcine circovirus type 2 is influenced by an interferon-stimulated response element in the PCV2 genome. *Virus Res* 2009;145:236–243.
141. Ramamoorthy S, Opriessnig T, Pal N, et al. Effect of an interferon-stimulated response element (ISRE) mutant of porcine circovirus type 2 (PCV2) on PCV2-induced pathological lesions in a porcine reproductive and respiratory syndrome virus (PRRSV) co-infection model. *Vet Microbiol* 2011;147:49–58.
142. Resendes AR, Majo N, Segales J, et al. Apoptosis in lymphoid organs of pigs naturally infected by porcine circovirus type 2. *J Gen Virol* 2004;85:2837–2844.
143. Rijsewijk FA, Dos Santos HF, Teixeira TF, et al. Discovery of a genome of a distant relative of chicken anemia virus reveals a new member of the genus Gyrovirus. *Arch Virol* 2011;156:1097–1100.
144. Ritchie BW, Niagro FD, Lukert PD, et al. Characterization of a new virus from cockatoos with psittacine beak and feather disease. *Virology* 1989;171(1):83–88.
145. Rosario K, Breitbart M, Harrach B, et al. Revisiting the taxonomy of the family Circoviridae: establishment of the genus Cyclovirus and removal of the genus Gyrovirus. *Arch Virol* 2017;162(5):1447–1463.
146. Sanchez RE Jr, Meerts P, Nauwynck HJ, et al. Change of porcine circovirus 2 target cells in pigs during development from fetal to early postnatal life. *Vet Microbiol.* 2003;95(1–2):15–25.
147. Sanchez RE Jr, Nauwynck HJ, McNeilly F, et al. Porcine circovirus 2 infection in swine foetuses inoculated at different stages of gestation. *Vet Microbiol* 2001;83(2):169–176.
148. Sauvage V, Cheval J, Foulongne V, et al. Identification of the first human gyrovirus, a virus related to chicken anemia virus. *J Virol* 2011;85:7948–7950.
149. Schat KA, van Santen VL. Chicken infectious anemia. In: Saif YM, Fadly AM, Glisson JR, et al., eds. *Diseases of Poultry.* 12th ed. Ames, IA: Blackwell Publishing; 2008:211–235.

150. Schat KA, Woods LW. Chicken infectious anemia virus and other circovirus infections. In: Saif YM, Fadly AM, Glisson JR, et al., eds. *Diseases of Poultry*. 12th ed. Ames, IA: Blackwell Publishing; 2008:209–211.
151. Schoop RA, Kooistra K, Baatenburg De Jong RJ, et al. Bcl-xL inhibits p53- but not apoptin-induced apoptosis in head and neck squamous cell carcinoma cell line. *Int J Cancer* 2004;109:38–42.
152. Shulman LM, Davidson I. Viruses with circular single-stranded DNA genomes are everywhere! *Annu Rev Virol* 2017;4(1):159–180.
153. Singh G, Ramamoorthy S. Potential for the cross-species transmission of swine torque teno viruses. *Vet Microbiol* 2018;215:66–70.
154. Smyth JA, Moffett DA, McNulty MS, et al. A sequential histopathologic and immunocytochemical study of chicken anemia virus infection at one day of age. *Avian Dis* 1993;37:324–338.
155. de Souza WM, Fumagalli MJ, de Araujo J, et al. Discovery of novel anelloviruses in small mammals expands the host range and diversity of the Anelloviridae. *Virology* 2018;514:9–17.
156. Steiner E, Balmelli C, Herrmann B, et al. Porcine circovirus type 2 displays pluripotency in cell targeting. *Virology* 2008;378:311–322.
157. Steinfeldt T, Finsterbusch T, Mankertz A. Demonstration of nicking/joining activity at the origin of DNA replication associated with the rep and rep′ proteins of porcine circovirus type 1. *J Virol* 2006;80:6225–6234.
158. Steinfeldt T, Finsterbusch T, Mankertz A. Functional analysis of cis- and trans-acting replication factors of porcine circovirus type 1. *J Virol* 2007;81:5696–5704.
159. Sun W, Wang W, Xin J, et al. An epidemiological investigation of porcine circovirus 3 infection in dogs in the Guangxi Province from 2015 to 2017, China. *Virus Res* 2019;270:197663.
160. Takahashi K, Iwasa Y, Hijikata M, et al. Identification of a new human DNA virus (TTV-like mini virus, TLMV) intermediately related to TT virus and chicken anemia virus. *Arch Virol* 2000;145(5):979–993.
161. Timmusk S, Fossum C, Berg M. Porcine circovirus type 2 replicase binds the capsid protein and an intermediate filament-like protein. *J Gen Virol* 2006;87:3215–3223.
162. Timmusk S, Merlot E, Lövgren T, et al. Regulator of G protein signaling 16 is a target for a porcine circovirus type 2 protein. *J Gen Virol* 2009;90:2425–2436.
163. Tischer I, Gelderblom H, Vettermann W, et al. A very small porcine virus with circular single-stranded DNA. *Nature* 1982;295:64–66.
164. Tischer I, Mields W, Wolff D, et al. Studies on epidemiology and pathogenicity of porcine circovirus. *Arch Virol* 1986;91:271–276.
165. Tischer I, Rasch R, Tochtermann G. Characterization of papovavirus-and picornavirus-like particles in permanent pig kidney cell lines. *Zentralbl Bakteriol Orig A* 1974;226: 153–167.
166. Todd D, Creelan JL, Mackie DP, et al. Purification and biochemical characterization of chicken anaemia agent. *J Gen Virol* 1990;71:819–823.
167. Todd D, Creelan JL, Meehan BM, et al. Investigation of the transfection capability of cloned tandemly-repeated chicken anaemia virus DNA fragments. *Arch Virol* 1996;141:1523–1534.
168. Vega-Rocha S, Byeon IJ, Gronenborn B, et al. Solution structure, divalent metal and DNA binding of the endonuclease domain from the replication initiation protein from porcine circovirus 2. *J Mol Biol* 2007;367:473–487.
169. Victoria JG, Wang C, Jones MS, et al. Viral nucleic acids in live-attenuated vaccines: detection of minority variants and an adventitious virus. *J Virol* 2010;84:6033–6040.
170. de Villiers EM, Borkosky SS, Kimmel R, et al. The diversity of torque teno viruses: in vitro replication leads to the formation of additional replication-competent subviral molecules. *J Virol* 2011;85:7284–7295.
171. Vincent IE, Carrasco CP, Guzylack-Piriou L, et al. Subset-dependent modulation of dendritic cell activity by circovirus type 2. *Immunology* 2005;115:388–398.
172. Vincent IE, Carrasco CP, Herrmann B, et al. Dendritic cells harbor infectious porcine circovirus type 2 in the absence of apparent cell modulation or replication of the virus. *J Virol* 2003;77:13288–13300.
173. Wang T, Du Q, Niu Y, et al. Cellular p32 is a critical regulator of the porcine circovirus type 2 nuclear egress. *J Virol* 2019;93. pii: JVI.00979-19.
174. Wang W, Sun W, Cao L, et al. An epidemiological investigation of porcine circovirus 3 infection in cattle in Shandong province, China. *BMC Vet Res* 2019;15(1):60.
175. Wang H, Zhang K, Lin C, et al. Conformational changes and nuclear entry of porcine circovirus without disassembly. *J Virol* 2019;93(20). pii: e00824-19.
176. Wei L, Kwang J, Wang J, et al. Porcine circovirus type 2 induces the activation of nuclear factor kappa B by IkappaBalpha degradation. *Virology* 2008;378:177–184.
177. Wei R, Van Renne N, Nauwynck HJ. Strain-dependent porcine circovirus type 2 (PCV2) entry and replication in T-lymphoblasts. *Viruses* 2019;11(9):813.
178. Woods LW, Latimer KS. Circovirus infection of pigeons and other avian species. In: Saif YM, Fadly AM, Glisson JR, et al., eds. *Diseases of Poultry*. 12th ed. Ames, IA: Blackwell Publishing; 2008:236–249.
179. Yamaguchi S, Imada T, Kaji N, et al. Identification of a genetic determinant of pathogenicity in chicken anaemia virus. *J Gen Virol* 2001;82:1233–1238.
180. Yao S, Gao X, Tuo T, et al. Novel characteristics of the avian gyrovirus 2 genome. *Sci Rep* 2017;7:41068.
181. Ye JQ, Tian XY, Xie Q, et al. Avian gyrovirus 2 DNA in fowl from live poultry markets and in healthy humans, China. *Emerg Infect Dis* 2015;21:1486–1488.
182. Yu W, Zhan Y, Xue B, et al. Highly efficient cellular uptake of a cell-penetrating peptide (CPP) derived from the capsid protein of porcine circovirus type 2. *J Biol Chem* 2018;293(39):15221–15232.
183. Yuasa N, Taniguchi T, Yoshida I. Isolation and some characteristics of an agent inducing anemia in chicks. *Avian Dis* 1979;23:366–385.
184. Zhang W, Li L, Deng X, et al. What is for dinner? Viral metagenomics of US store bought beef, pork, and chicken. *Virology* 2014;468–470:303–310.
185. Zhang Y, Sun R, Geng S, et al. Porcine circovirus type 2 induces ORF3-independent mitochondrial apoptosis via PERK activation and elevation of cytosolic calcium. *J Virol* 2019;93(7). pii: e01784-18.
186. Zheng H, Ye L, Fang X, et al. Torque teno virus (SANBAN isolate) ORF2 protein suppresses NF-kappaB pathways via interaction with IkappaB kinases. *J Virol* 2007;81(21):11917–11924.

CHAPTER

8 The Family *Herpesviridae*: A Brief Introduction

Laurie T. Krug • Philip E. Pellett

Learn the biology.

Bernard Roizman

Herpesviruses form a taxonomic order of double-stranded DNA (dsDNA) viruses that establish lifelong infections in their animal host and cause disease that can have significant adverse effects on individuals and on host populations (e-Table 8.1). These complex biological nanomachines employ diverse mechanisms to reprogram cells to produce infectious virions, sometimes after lying dormant in a latent state for decades. Discoveries of the mechanisms by which herpesviruses subvert cellular processes and adapt to evolving host defenses will continue to have significant impacts on our understanding of molecular and cellular biology, as well as immunology and pathologies such as cancer. Development of strategies for control and prevention of societally important herpesvirus infections is dependent on appreciating and understanding the virion structure, genetic content, and biological properties of this ancient and evolving family of extraordinarily interesting pathogens.

The objectives of this chapter are to provide definitions and examples of many of the terms and concepts that define the field of herpesvirology; a glossary of terms associated with herpesvirology is provided in e-Table 8.2. Summarizing such a broad area of active research is accomplished at the cost of oversimplification and overgeneralization, with the understanding that subsequent chapters will provide deeper coverage for individual viruses. Importantly, the paradigms presented here offer opportunities for conceptual and experimental challenge.

THE FAMILY *HERPESVIRIDAE*

Herpesviruses are defined on the basis of their shared virion architecture (Fig. 8.1). A typical herpesvirion consists of a ***core*** containing a linear dsDNA genome (ranging from 109 to 241 kb among the *Herpesviridae*); an icosahedral ***capsid*** approximately 125 nm in diameter containing 161 capsomeres with a hole running down their long axis, plus one capsomeric structure that serves as the portal for packaging and release of the viral genome; the ***tegument***, which is a less-ordered and often asymmetric layer composed of proteins and RNA that surrounds the nucleocapsid; and an ***envelope*** containing viral glycoprotein spikes on its surface. Based on the morphologic criteria, highly divergent viruses with hosts that range from bivalves to humans have been identified as herpesviruses (Fig. 8.2). Originally classified as a single virus family, genome sequence data led to establishment of the order *Herpesvirales*,[110] which encompasses three virus families: the herpesviruses of mammals, birds, and reptiles (the *Herpesviridae*[111]), herpesviruses of fish and amphibians (the *Alloherpesviridae*[112]), and herpesviruses of bivalves (the *Malacoherpesviridae*[113]). This and subsequent chapters in this book are concerned primarily with viruses that have long been recognized as members of the family *Herpesviridae*, with a focus on herpesviruses of humans.

DISTRIBUTION IN NATURE

Herpesviruses are highly disseminated in nature. Most animal species examined are host to at least one, and frequently several distinct herpesviruses. Given that few herpesviruses are hosted by

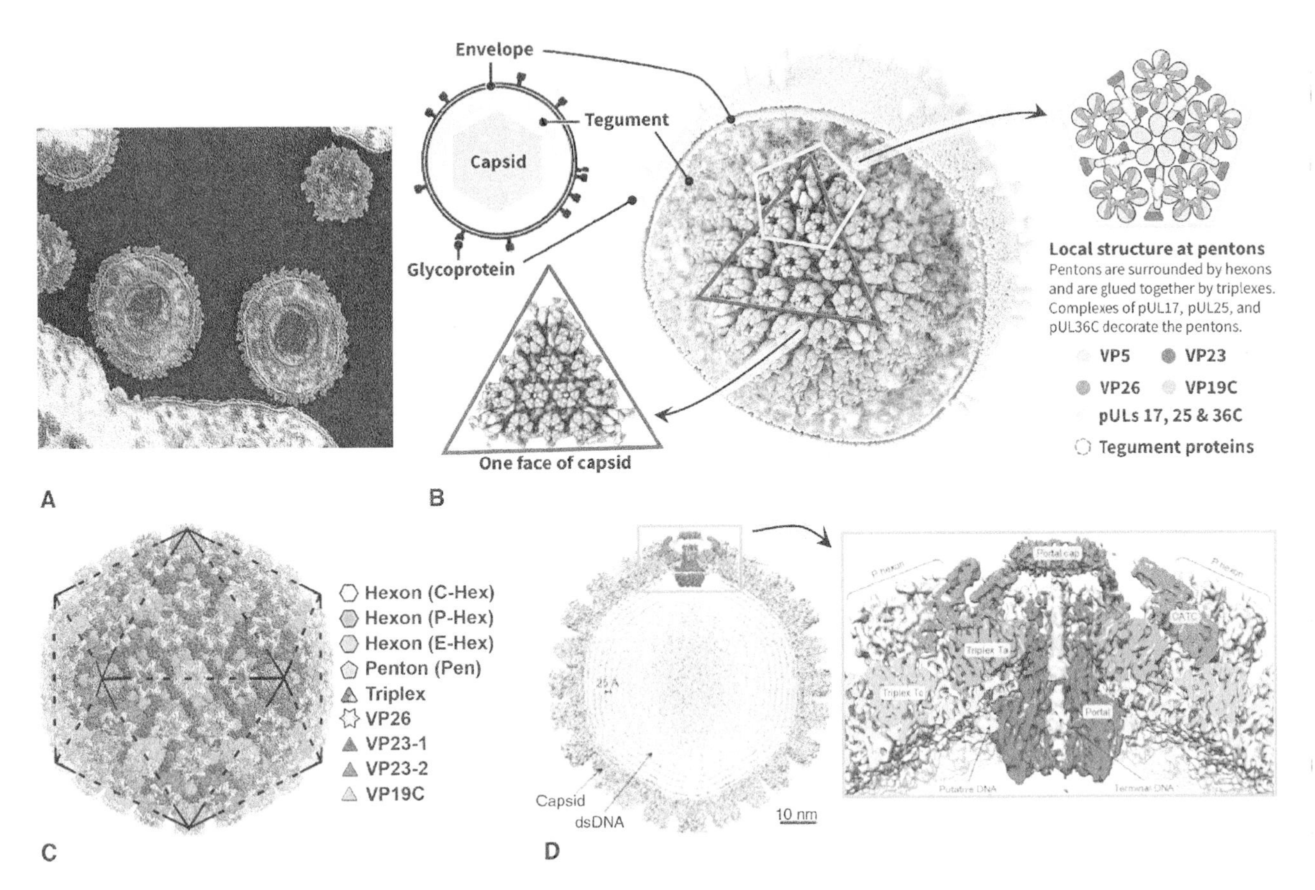

FIGURE 8.1 **Structure of herpesvirus virions. A:** False-colored electron micrograph of HSV-1 virions shows capsid (*orange*) coated with tegument (*inner-blue, outer-teal*) and surrounded by lipid envelope (*yellow*). (Image from https://www.sciencesource.com/archive/Herpes-simplex-viruses-SS2105481.html.) **B:** HSV capsid is an icosohedron with 20 faces and 12 vertices. Approximately 3,000 proteins form pentons, hexons, and triplexes. (From Heldwein EE. Up close with herpesviruses. *Science* 2018;360(6384):34–35. Reprinted with permission from AAAS. Ref.[56] Reprinted with permission from AAAS.) **C:** Surface representation 1,250 Å (angstrom)-wide capsid of HSV-2. *Black lines*, icosahedral facets. (From Yuan S, Wang J, Zhu D, et al. Cryo-EM structure of a herpesvirus capsid at 3.1 Å. *Science* 2018;360(6384):eaao7283. Reprinted with permission from AAAS.) **D:** On *left*, clipped view of KSHV capsid reconstruction, showing packaged dsDNA within the capsid and unique portal vertex. On *right*, enlarged view of the portal vertex region, showing terminal DNA (*yellow*) in the portal's translocation channel (*purple*) and encircling the lower periphery of the portal (*dark blue*). (Reprinted from Gong D, Dai X, Jih J, et al. DNA-packing portal and capsid-associated tegument complexes in the tumor herpesvirus KSHV. *Cell* 2019;178(6):1329–1343.e12. Copyright © 2019 Elsevier. With permission)

more than one species, their number in nature likely vastly exceeds the more than 300 identified to date. Nine herpesviruses have been identified that have humans as their primary host: herpes simplex viruses 1 and 2 (HSV-1 and HSV-2); human cytomegalovirus (HCMV); varicella–zoster virus (VZV); Epstein-Barr virus (EBV); human herpesviruses 6A, 6B, and 7 (HHV-6A, HHV-6B, and HHV-7); and Kaposi sarcoma herpesvirus (KSHV, also known as Kaposi's sarcoma-associated herpesvirus and HHV-8). Herpesviruses of humans and of veterinary and scientific importance are listed in Table 8.1; a more comprehensive list is provided in e-Table 8.3. We have not tabulated the many herpesviruses identified on the basis of small PCR amplimers or metagenomic sequencing data.[61,66]

BIOLOGICAL PROPERTIES

Members of family *Herpesviridae* share four significant biological properties:

1. Production of infectious progeny virus (lytic infection) is generally accompanied by destruction of the infected cell.
2. Herpesviruses examined to date employ cellular latency as a mechanism for lifelong persistence in their hosts (Fig. 8.3).
3. Virus gene transcription, replication of the dsDNA genome, and nucleocapsid assembly occur in the nucleus. Virions acquire most of their tegument and are enveloped in the cytoplasm.
4. Herpesvirus genomes encode many of the proteins needed for virus replication, as well as most of the proteins and RNAs that make up the virion; many of these genes are conserved across the family (Table 8.2). In addition, much of the genetic content of herpesvirus genomes is dedicated to production of gene products (proteins and noncoding RNAs) that play diverse roles in managing cell biology and immune responses. The array of virus genes and gene products involved in management of the host ranges widely across the family. This genetic diversity is the source of much of the biological diversity of herpesviruses—it drives and defines their pathogenesis and clinical manifestations.

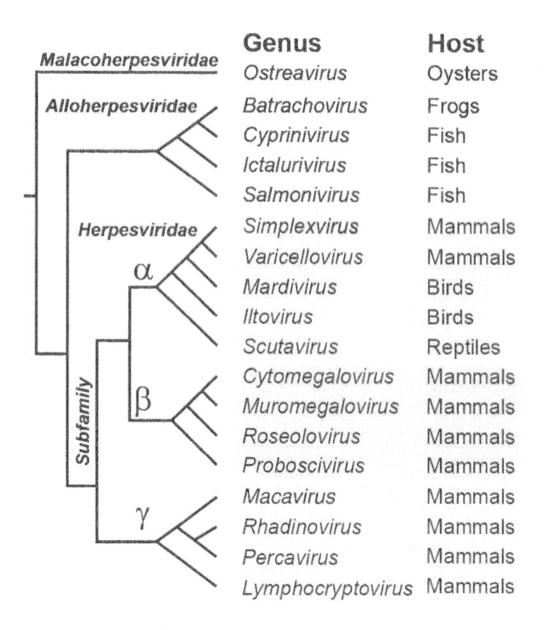

FIGURE 8.2 **Major phylogenetic relationships and taxonomic subunits within Order *Herpesvirales*.** (Adapted from Pellett PE, Davison AJ, Eberle R, et al. Order *Herpesvirales*. In: King AMQ, Adams MJ, Carstens EB, et al., eds. *Virus Taxonomy: Ninth Report of the International Committee on Taxonomy of Viruses*. Oxford: Elsevier; 2011:99–107.) The schematic shows branching patterns, not evolutionary distances.

NOMENCLATURE AND CLASSIFICATION

Classification

Before their DNA and amino acid sequences were known, herpesviruses were classified into one family (the *Herpesviridae*) and three subfamilies (the *Alphaherpesvirinae*, the *Betaherpesvirinae*, and the *Gammaherpesvirinae*) on the basis of biological properties.[126] Remarkably, this framework stands and has withstood expansion. In the current formal taxonomy,[110] herpesviruses belong to Realm *Duplodna*, Phylum *Peploviricota*, Class *Herviviricetes*, and Order *Herpesvirales*. Order *Herpesvirales* is subdivided into three Families: *Alloherpesviridae* (viruses of bony fish and amphibians), *Herpesviridae* (viruses of reptiles, birds, and mammals), and *Malacoherpesviridae* (viruses of molluscs). Species within the *Herpesviridae* subfamilies and the *Alloherpesviridae* are further classified into genera.

Herpesvirus Species

A herpesvirus may be classified as a species if it "has distinct epidemiological or biological characteristics and a distinct genome that represents an independent replicating lineage."[110] Two forms of nomenclature are employed for herpesviruses: an informal (also known as vernacular or colloquial) nomenclature that is often traced to the early days of virology, and a formal subfamily-based species nomenclature governed by the International Committee for Taxonomy of Viruses (ICTV).

TABLE 8.1 Herpesviruses of humans and select herpesviruses of veterinary, agricultural, or animal model importance[a]

Formal Name[b]	Abbreviation	Common Names and Synonyms[c]	Subfamily and Genus[d]	Genome Size (Kbp)[e]	Genome Accession No.
Family *HERPESVIRIDAE*					
Viruses of Humans					
Human αHV 1	HuAHV1	Herpes simplex virus 1, HSV-1	αS	152	NC_001806
Human αHV 2	HuAHV2	Herpes simplex virus 2, HSV-2	αS	155	NC_001798
Human αHV 3	HuAHV3	Varicella–zoster virus, VZV	αV	125	NC_001348
Human γHV 4	HuGHV4	Epstein-Barr virus, EBV	γL	172	NC_007605[f] NC_009334[f]
Human βHV 5	HuBHV5	Human cytomegalovirus, HCMV, CMV	βC	236	NC_006273[g]
				230	NC_001347[g]
Human βHV 6A	HuBHV6A	Human herpesvirus 6A, HHV-6A	βR	159/170[h]	NC_001664
Human βHV 6B	HuBHV6B	Human herpesvirus 6B, HHV-6B	βR	162/168[h]	NC_000898
Human βHV 7	HuBHV7	Human herpesvirus 7, HHV-7	βR	145	NC_001716
Human γHV 8	HuGHV8	Human herpesvirus 8, HHV-8; Kaposi sarcoma herpesvirus, KSHV; [Kaposi's sarcoma-associated herpesvirus]	γRh	170	NC_009333
Viruses of Animals					
Order *Primates*					
Cercopithecine αHV 9	CeAHV-9	Simian varicella virus, SVV	αV	124	NC_002686
Macacine αHV 1	McAHV-1	B virus, HV simiae; [*Cercopithecine HV 1*]	αS	157	NC_004812
Macacine βHV 3	McBHV-3	Rhesus monkey CMV, RhCMV; [*Cercopithecine HV 8*]	βC	221	NC_006150

TABLE 8.1 Herpesviruses of humans and select herpesviruses of veterinary, agricultural, or animal model importance[a] (Continued)

Formal Name[b]	Abbreviation	Common Names and Synonyms[c]	Subfamily and Genus[d]	Genome Size (Kbp)[e]	Genome Accession No.
Macacine γHV 4	McGHV-4	Rhesus EBV-like HV; rhesus lymphocrypto HV, RLV [*Cercopithecine HV 15*]	γL	171	NC_006146
Macacine γHV 5	McGHV-5	Rhesus Rhadinovirus, RRV; [*Cercopithecine HV 17*]	γRh	134	NC_003401
Saimiriine γHV 2	SaGHV-2	Squirrel monkey HV; HV saimiri, HVS	γRh	155	NC_001350
Order *Artiodactyla*					
Bovine αHV 1	BoAHV-1	Infectious bovine rhinotracheitis HV; bovine HV 1, BHV-1	αV	140	JX898220
Bovine αHV 5	BoAHV-5	Bovine encephalitis HV; bovine HV 5, BHV-5	αV	138	NC_005261
Suid αHV 1	SuAHV-1	Pseudorabies virus, PRV	αV	143	JF797218
Order *Carnivora*					
Felid αHV 1	FeAHV-1	Feline rhinotracheitis virus, FRV; feline HV 1	αV	136	FJ478159
Order *Rodentia*					
Murid βHV 1	MuBHV-1	Mouse CMV, MCMV	βM	235	NC_004065
Murid βHV 2	MuBHV-2	Rat CMV, RCMV	βM	230	NC_002512
Caviid βHV 2	CdBHV-2	Guinea pig cytomegalovirus, GPCMV	βU	233	NC_020231
Murid γHV 4	MuGHV-4	Murid herpesvirus 4, MuHv-4; murine gammaherpesvirus 68, γHV68, MHV68	γRh	135	NC_001826
Order *Perissodactyla*					
Equid αHV 1	EqAHV-1	Equine HV 1, EHV-1; equine abortion HV	αV	150	NC_001491
Equid αHV 4	EqAHV-4	Equine HV 4, EHV-4; equine rhinopneumonitis virus	αV	146	NC_001844
Order *Proboscidea*					
Elephantid βHV 1	ElBHV-1	Endotheliotropic elephant HV 1, EEHV	βP	180	NC_020474
Viruses of Birds					
Anatid αHV 1	AnAHV-1	Duck plague HV, DPV; duck enteritis virus, DEV	αM	161	JF999965
Gallid αHV 1	GaAHV-1	Infectious laryngotracheitis virus, ILTV	αI	165	NC_06623
Gallid αHV 2	GaAHV-2	Marek disease HV 1, MDV-1	αM	180	NC_002229
Family *ALLOHERPESVIRIDAE*					
Cyprinid HV 3	CyHV-3	Koi herpesvirus, KHV	Cy	295	NC_009127
Ictalurid HV 1	IcHV-1	Channel catfish HV, CCV	Ic	130	NC_001493
Family *MALACOHERPESVIRIDAE*					
Ostreid HV 1	OsHV-1	Pacific oyster HV, OHV	Os	207	NC_005881

[a]The table was extracted and extended from information compiled by the *Herpesvirales* Study Group of ICTV and available at ictvonline.org as ICTV Master Species List 2019.v1., plus information from the exemplar virus list provided by the Virus Metadata Resource.
[b]Formally recognized HV species are italicized. Information about hosts is in bold.
[c]Retired formal names and alternate historical names are in brackets.
[d]Genus designations: α, *Alphaherpesvirinae*: S, *Simplexvirus*; V, *Varicellovirus*; M, *Mardivirus*; I, *Iltovirus*. β, *Betaherpesvirinae*: C, *Cytomegalovirus*; M, *Muromegalovirus*; R, *Roseolovirus*; P, *Probscivirus*. γ, *Gammaherpesvirinae*: L, *Lymphocryptovirus*; Rh, *Rhadinovirus*; M, *Macavirus*; P, *Percavirus*. *Alloherpesviridae*: Ba, *Batrachovirus*, Cy, *Cyprinivirus*; Ic, *Ictalurivirus*; Sa, *Salmonivirus*. *Malacoherpesviridae*: Os, *Ostreavirus*. Species and viruses are indicated by U and the subfamily (if known).
[e]Genome sequence information is sometimes limited in the vicinity of genomic termini.
[f]Accession numbers are provided for a widely studied strain of EBV types 1 (B95-8) and 2 (AG876), respectively.
[g]Accession numbers are provided for a low-passage clinical isolate of HCMV (Merlin) and a high-passage widely studied laboratory strain (AD169), respectively.
[h]Values obtained in different laboratories may reflect differences in strains.

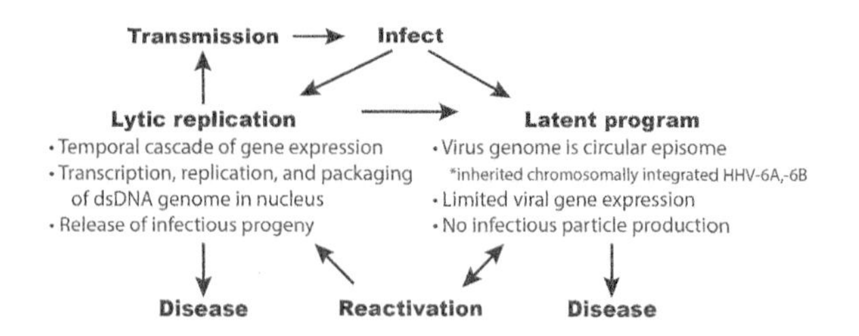

FIGURE 8.3 The complexity of herpesvirus infections. Persistence in the host organism via cellular latency is a defining property of herpesviruses. Cellular latency is different from clinical (or organismal) latency, which is the period between infection and disease, and during which extensive lytic replication might be occurring at the cellular level. Lytic replication, latent infections, and episodic reactivation at the cellular level lead to disease manifestations and transmission at the organismal level. Full-fledged reactivation from latency may be unsuccessful or may lead to productive replication, infectious particle production, and dissemination within and between hosts. Within an organism, a herpesvirus can be simultaneously latent in some cells and actively replicating in others due to periodic reactivation events. Reactivation likely plays a role in maintaining the viral load in the host and is key for transmission to new hosts upon shedding of infectious particles at mucosal tissues. (Copyright Laurie Krug and Philip Pellett.)

For example, *Human gammaherpesvirus 4* is the species name for the virus widely known as EBV. The species number enables differentiation of herpesviruses that share their host, but is not intended to imply anything about the relationship between a virus and other herpesviruses that infect the same host species (e.g., HHV-7 and HHV-8 are members of different subfamilies) or between similarly numbered viruses that infect different host species (e.g., EHV-2 and BoHV-2 are members of different subfamilies). Table 8.1 and e-Table 8.3 include informal and formal names for each virus.

Herpesvirus Phylogeny

The virus lineage that encompasses the present-day alpha-, beta-, and gammaherpesvirus subfamilies (the *Herpesviridae*) is rooted about 400 million years ago.[92] Within the major subdivisions of the three subfamilies, relationships among virus species generally mirror host phylogeny.

Alphaherpesvirinae

Alphaherpesviruses typically have relatively short reproductive cycles, spread rapidly in culture, efficiently destroy infected cells, and establish latency in sensory ganglia. Viruses of the *Simplexvirus* (HSV-1 and HSV-2), and *Varicellovirus* (VZV) genera have mammalian hosts, while *Mardiviruses* and *Iltoviruses* have avian hosts, and *Scutaviruses* have reptilian hosts.

Betaherpesvirinae

Betaherpesviruses typically have a restricted host range. The reproductive cycle can be protracted in cultured cells. Infected cells frequently become enlarged (cytomegalia), and carrier cultures are readily established. Betaherpesviruses can establish latency in secretory glands, lymphoreticular cells, kidneys, and other tissues. Betaherpesvirus genera include *Cytomegalovirus, Muromegalovirus, Proboscivirus, and Roseolovirus* (HHV-6A, HHV-6B, and HHV-7).

Gammaherpesvirinae

In vitro, all gammaherpesviruses replicate in lymphoblastoid cells, and some can lytically infect particular stromal cell types (epithelial and fibroblasts). They are usually specific for either T or B lymphocytes, and establish latency in lymphoid tissue. The subfamily contains four genera: *Lymphocryptovirus* (EBV), *Macavirus, Percavirus,* and *Rhadinovirus* (KSHV). Genus *Lymphocryptovirus* includes two major lineages that appear to have coevolved with their hosts: viruses of Old World (humans, chimpanzees) and New World (marmosets) primates.[46,93] Viruses of genus *Rhadinovirus* are mainly hosted by primates, *Macaviruses* are related to the malignant catarrhal fever viruses of ruminants, and *Percaviruses* include viruses of perissodactyls and carnivores.

VIRION ARCHITECTURE

The Virion

The virion is the vehicle for delivery of the virus genome and a set of accessory factors into newly infected cells. At the entry stage of infection, virion envelope glycoproteins bind to specific receptors on appropriate target cells to enable delivery of the cargo (nucleocapsid and tegument contents) into the cytoplasm. The tegument is an assortment, or toolbox, of proteins and RNAs that immediately upon entry begin to manage the host environment to meet the needs of the virus, for example, by shutting down host protein synthesis, inhibiting infection-triggered cell defenses, and stimulating viral gene expression. The nucleocapsid has signals that enable its transport via microtubules to a nuclear pore where it interacts with cellular machinery that facilitates injection of the genome into the nucleus. Individual herpesvirus virions are built from approximately 10,000 protein molecules, a collection of mRNAs, microRNAs, circular RNAs and other RNAs, and one molecule of the dsDNA genome. The virion thus represents the evolved solution to a significant design and manufacturing challenge: how to (a) efficiently build as many as thousands of virions in well-defended infected cells, (b) release the newly synthesized virions in a regulated manner, and (c) ensure that the mature virions are physically stable during transmission, yet able to disassemble in a regulated manner to start a new infection.

Mature herpesvirus virions vary in diameter from 120 to as much as 260 nm (reviewed in Ref.[127]). The range is due to variability in the thickness of tegument, the plane of sectioning, and the state of the envelope. The precise number of protein species contained in virions is not known and may vary from one virus to another, as well as from one virion to another of the same variety.[11] Estimates based on gel analyses of purified virions have generally been in the range of 35 to 45 major species. Proteomic analyses have identified from 24 to 71 virally encoded proteins in virions (4 to 7 in the nucleocapsid, 9 to >20 in the tegument, and 4 to 19 in the envelope, plus a number of proteins whose location within virions is unknown).[69,70,96,106,148] Numerous host proteins have been detected in virion preparations, including moderately abundant quantities of cellular structural proteins, enzymes, and chaperones; their roles and necessity are not known. The mean abundance of individual protein species varies widely, from less than one copy per virion to over 1,000.

TABLE 8.2 Genes conserved among the alpha-, beta-, and gammaherpesviruses

Function[a]	HSV Homolog	Gene Block[b]
Gene regulation		
Multifunctional regulator of expression (MRE)	UL54	3
Nucleotide metabolism		
Ribonucleotide reductase, large subunit (RR1)	UL39	1
Uracil-DNA glycosylase (UNG)	UL2	7
Deoxyuridine triphosphatase (dUTPase)	UL50	3
DNA replication		
Helicase/primase complex		
ATPase subunit (HP1)	UL5	6
RNA pol subunit (HP2)	UL52	3
Subunit C (HP3)	UL8	6
DNA polymerase (POL)	UL30	2
ssDNA binding (SSB)	UL29	2
DNA polymerase processivity subunit (PPS)	UL42	1
Virion		
Nonstructural; roles in virion maturation		
Alkaline exonuclease (NUC)	UL12	6
Capsid transport nuclear protein (CTNP)	UL32	1
Terminase binding protein (TERbp)	UL33	1
Terminase (TER)		
TER ATPase subunit (TER1)	UL15	6
TER DNA recognition subunit (TER2)	UL28	2
Assembly protease (PR)	UL26	4
Assembly protein precursor (pAP)	UL26.5	4
Capsid nuclear egress complex		1
Nuclear egress membrane protein (NEMP)	UL34	1
Nuclear egress lamina protein (NELP)	UL31	1
Capsid		
Major capsid protein (pentons and hexons; MCP)	UL19	5
Portal protein (PORT)	UL6	6
Portal capping protein (PCP)	UL25	4
Capsid triplex		
Monomer (TRI1)	UL38	1
Dimer (TRI2)	UL18	5
Small capsid protein (SCP) at hexon tips	UL35	1
Tegument		
Encapsidation and egress protein (EEP)	UL7	6
Myristoylated/palmitoylated cytoplasmic egress tegument protein (CETP)	UL11	6
Virion protein kinase (VPK)	UL13	6
Encapsidation chaperone protein (ECP)	UL14	6
CETP binding protein (CETPbp)	UL16	6
Capsid transport tegument protein (CTTP)	UL17	6
Cytoplasmic egress facilitator 2 (CEF2)	UL21	5
Cell-to-cell fusion inhibitor	UL24	4
Large tegument protein (LTP)	UL36	1
LTP binding protein (LTPbp)	UL37	1
Cytoplasmic egress facilitator 1 (CEF1)	UL51	3
Envelope		
Glycoprotein B (gB)	UL27	2
Glycoprotein H (gH)	UL22	4
Glycoprotein L (gL)	UL1	6
Glycoprotein M (gM)	UL10	6
Glycoprotein N (gN)	UL49.5	3

[a]Nomenclature and abbreviations are as described and proposed in (From Mocarski ES Jr. Comparative analysis of herpesvirus-common proteins. In: Arvin A, Campadelli-Fiume G, Mocarski E, et al., eds. *Human Herpesviruses: Biology, Therapy, and Immunoprophylaxis*. Cambridge: Cambridge University Press; 2007:44–58.).
[b]Gene blocks are as illustrated in Figure 8.4.

Most of the virus-related particles released from infected cells are not independently infectious but are nonetheless bioactive. These include particles that appear by electron microscopy to be intact and complete virions. In addition, herpesvirus-infected cells can produce large numbers of nonvirion particles of uncertain biological significance, such as the dense bodies of HCMV, which are capsid-free enveloped collections of tegument proteins. HSV-1 induces production of extracellular vesicles (exosomes) that can activate antiviral defenses in uninfected cells.[36]

Virion Components

The Core

The core of mature virions contains a single molecule of the viral genome, in the form of nonchromatinized dsDNA that is packed in the form of a left-handed spool (evident in Fig. 8.1D), with shells of progressively tighter radii.[45,89] The tight packing and the repulsive forces generated by the negatively charged phosphates along the genome backbone necessitate the abundant presence in the core of the cation spermine.[48] Packaging of the viral genome into the capsid core requires ATP and results in a pressurized system that appears to be important for injection of virus genomes through the nuclear pore complex into nuclei of newly infected cells; the pressure and bending are sufficient to denature a portion of the dsDNA genome near the center of the core.[13,81]

The Capsid

The structural features of the capsid—its approximately 130 nm diameter, 161 capsomeres (150 hexons and 11 pentons), portal complex, and capsid triangulation number

(T = 16)—are characteristic of all herpesviruses (Fig. 8.1), including the evolutionarily distant herpesviruses of fish and oysters.[59,121] Nonenveloped capsids are present in infected cells in three main forms, A-, B-, and C-capsids.[47] A-capsids have no core structure, B-capsids contain the assembly scaffold but no genome, and C-capsids are DNA-containing species that no longer house the scaffold. The four conserved capsid proteins that constitute the major structural features of the capsid include the major capsid protein (MCP), the monomer and dimer proteins of the triplex (TRI1 and TRI2, respectively), and the small capsomere-interacting protein (SCP) (Fig. 8.1; HSV homologs are listed in Table 8.2). MCP is present in six copies per hexon (6 × 150 = 900 copies per capsid) and five per penton (5 × 11 = 55 copies per capsid), for a total of 955 copies per capsid. The triplex proteins interact with $\alpha_2\beta$ stoichiometry and form complexes that are present at the 320 sites of threefold symmetry. Hexameric capsomeres are 9.5 × 12.5 nm in longitudinal section; a channel of 4 nm in diameter runs from the surface along their long axis.[155] Penton channels are generally somewhat narrower and are nearly closed at their midpoint in B-capsids.[161] The twelfth pentonal position is the portal for transit of genomic DNA into and out of the capsid; it is composed of 12 copies of the capsid portal protein (PORT) (Fig. 8.1D). The portal capping protein (PCP) is associated with mature, DNA-containing nucleocapsids. Cryoelectron microscopy has enabled determination of capsid structures for nearly all human herpesvirus to greater than 4 Å resolution.[24,50,80,82,160,162,163]

The Tegument

The tegument is the protein- and RNA-containing structure between the nucleocapsid and the envelope.[127] It has no distinctive features in thin section electron micrographs but may appear fibrous on negative staining. The tegument can be distributed asymmetrically within the virion.[11] Tegument thickness may vary, depending on the location of the virion within the infected cell, with it being thinner in virions accumulating in the perinuclear space following primary envelopment than in cytoplasmic vacuoles following secondary envelopment.[40] Teguments contain greater than 20 different virally encoded proteins, some of which are present at hundreds of copies per virion. Structural polarity across the tegument has been visualized by immunoelectron and fluorescence microscopy,[11,136] indicating that it is an ordered structure. This is further evidenced by the inner tegument proteins that associate with the capsid in the nucleus to form the capsid-associated tegument complex[24,50,80,82,160,163] and the tail-like portal vertex–associated tegument.[89] Following nuclear egress, subsequent components of the tegument are likely added in a somewhat ordered manner during its cytoplasmic maturation.[22,95]

The Envelope

Envelopes of mature virions are derived from patches of altered cellular membrane that trace to the organelle where envelopment occurs.[83] A major constituent of virion envelopes is a collection of virally encoded glycoproteins (gPs), most of which are involved in virion entry. gPs form protrusions on virion envelopes that are more numerous and shorter than those present on the surface of many other enveloped viruses.[155] The number and relative abundances of virion gPs vary among herpesviruses. HSV specifies at least 11 different virion-associated gPs; copy numbers of individual gPs can exceed 1,000 per virion. All members of the *Herpesviridae* have homologs of glycoprotein B (gB) and gH and gL, which form the gH/gL complex. These gPs are involved in virion entry, in association or concert with other gPs and gP complexes that are specific to the various herpesvirus lineages.[103,139]

HERPESVIRUS GENOMES

Herpesvirus genomes serve two major purposes: they are the stable repository of genetic information that is transmitted via the virion to newly infected cells, and they provide the instructions needed for the viruses to carry out their evolved biological programs. A curated set of reference herpesvirus genome sequences is maintained at Genbank (https://www.ncbi.nlm.nih.gov/genomes/GenomesGroup.cgi?taxid=10292).

Genomic Architecture

Herpesvirus genomes extracted from virions are predominantly linear and double stranded, but circularize immediately on release from nucleocapsids into the nuclei of infected cells. Across Order *Herpesvirales*, genome lengths range from approximately 109 to 295 kbp (Fig. 8.4, Table 8.1, and e-Table 8.2). They contain terminal and internal repeated sequences that vary in copy number, and can be oriented in the same or reverse direction relative to each other (e-Fig. 8.1). Herpesvirus genomes range from 31% to 77% in total G+C content and vary in local G+C content across the genome, with generally higher G+C composition in the terminal repeats (Table 8.1 and e-Table 8.2).

Herpesvirus genomes contain numerous *cis*-acting sequences that play critical roles in transcription regulation, function as origins of lytic (oriLyt) or latent replication, are involved in tethering latent genomes to host chromosomes during latency in dividing cells, and provide signals that direct packaging of nascent DNA into capsids and cleavage of concatemeric genomes to unit length (cleavage/packaging, or *pac* sequences).

The genetic requirements for efficient replication in cultured cells differ from *in vivo* requirements. Spontaneous deletions have been noted in HSV, EBV, and HCMV strains passaged outside the human host. A progression of changes in a small number of genes enables clinical isolates of HCMV to begin replicating efficiently in cultured cells.[25] Highly passaged strains of HCMV lack a segment encoding at least 19 genes that are present in wild-type isolates.[17]

Genetic Architecture

Herpesvirus Genes

Over the past 40 years, studies of herpesvirus gene structure, expression, and regulation defined many properties of what can be termed "canonical" genes, which are often represented in diagrams such as Figure 8.4, where the diagrammatic emphasis is on major open reading frames (ORFs) from which many well-studied proteins are expressed. In recent years, application of systems biology methods such as deep DNA sequencing, RNAseq, ribosome profiling, and temporal and spatial proteomics have greatly expanded our understanding of the

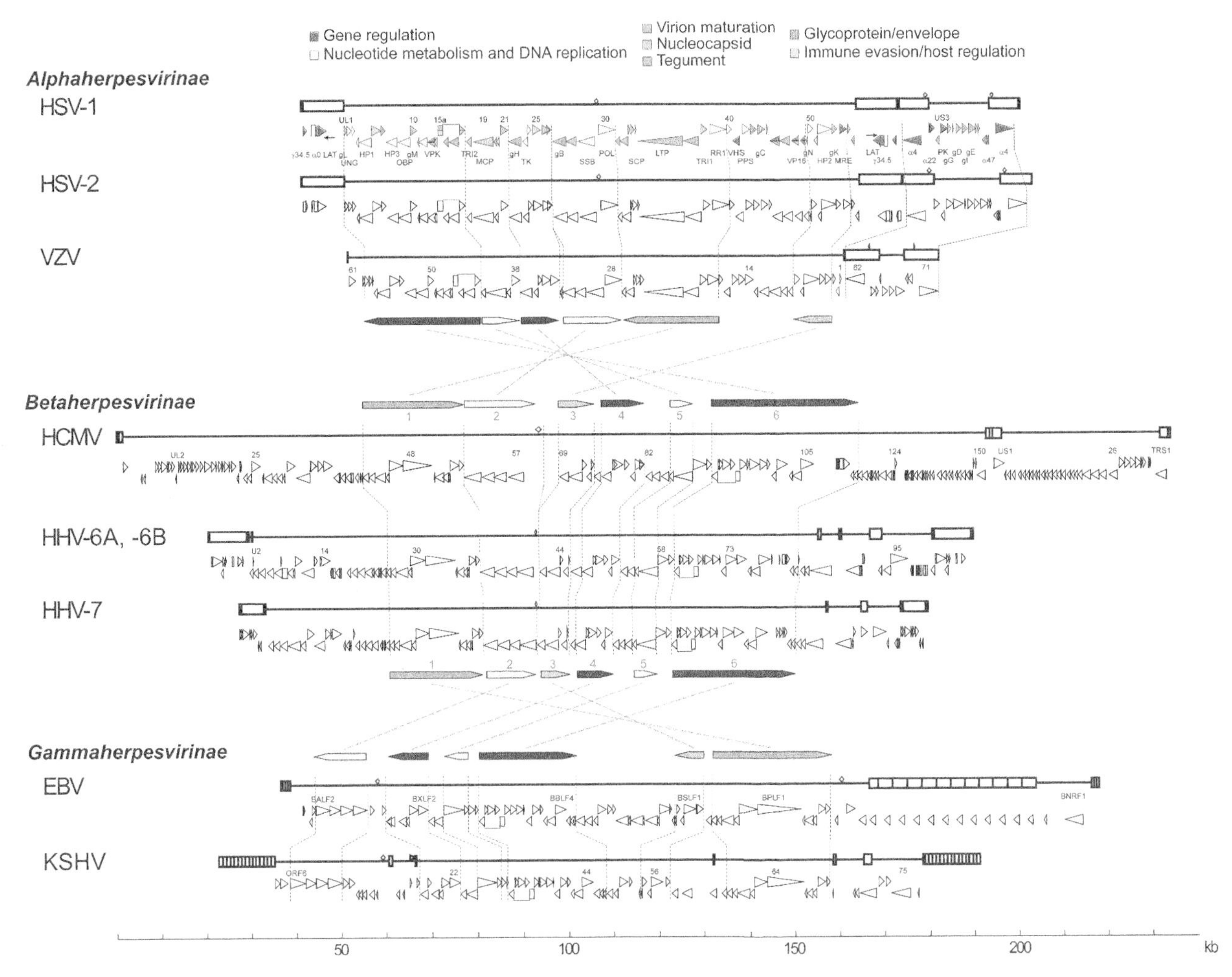

FIGURE 8.4 Genomic and genetic architectures of the human herpesviruses. Major repeat elements are indicated on each genomic schematic as boxes. Beneath each genome, open reading frames considered likely to encode expressed proteins are indicated as *triangles* that are oriented to show their direction of transcription. 5′ exons of spliced genes are indicated as boxes that are connected by bars to 3′ exons. The seven conserved herpesvirus sequence blocks (block 1 through block 6) are diagramed to show their relative locations and orientations in the three major lineages. Diagrams are based on annotations and coordinates in Genbank accession numbers X14112 (HSV-1 strain 17), Z86099 (HSV-2 strain HG52), X04370 (VZV strain Dumas), NC_006273 (HCMV strain Merlin), X83413 (HHV-6A strain U1102), AF157706 (HHV-6B strain Z29), U43400 and AF037218 (HHV-7 strains JI and RK), NC_007605 (EBV strain B95-8), and U75698 (HHV-8 BC-1). The diagram does not include details related to the complex array of RNAs expressed by the viruses (e-Fig. 8.2). Detailed descriptions are available in virus-specific chapters that follow. Abbreviations for conserved proteins are as listed in Table 8.2. (Copyright Laurie Krug and Philip Pellett.)

breadth and complexity of herpesvirus gene expression and gene function.[38,39,64,67,104,107,137,142,153] Here we summarize the new information in the context of the framework provided by our understanding of canonical genes and their expression.

Canonical herpesvirus genes have features indistinguishable from eukaryotic genes: (a) a collection of promoter/regulatory sequence elements that are located 50 to 200 bp upstream of a transcription initiation site, (b) express mRNAs with 5′-capped nontranslated leader sequences of 30 to 300 bp, (c) encode an ORF that can express a single protein of at least 100 amino acids that is initiated at a translation initiation codon that often meets the host requirements for efficient initiation, and (d) have 3′ regions that include 10 to 30 bp of nontranslated sequence followed by a canonical polyadenylation signal with standard flanking sequences (e-Fig. 8.2, panel A). Because herpesvirus genomes are dsDNA, genes can be oriented in either direction along the genome.

The predominant form of transcript for most herpesvirus genes had long been thought to be unspliced; that is, the 5′-capped primary transcript needs only to be polyadenylated to form the mature mRNA. However, recent application of deep RNA sequencing and proteomic analyses have made it clear that RNA splicing (including alternative splicing) is much more common than previously recognized, and the functional coding capacity of the viruses is greatly expanded by alternative transcription initiation and termination sites, alternative splicing, and noncanonical translation initiation signals (e-Fig. 8.2).[5,35,42,107,154] Combined transcriptional, proteomics, and genetic analyses have made it clear that the newly recognized forms of gene expression enable production of functional products that play important biological roles during infection. Such studies have also demonstrated translation of functional proteins from RNAs long thought to be noncoding.[42,64]

Gene overlaps are common in herpesvirus genomes. For head-to-tail gene arrangements, the upstream gene can overlap with the promoter-regulatory sequences of the downstream gene (e-Fig. 8.2B). Independent transcriptional units can be embedded in a protein coding sequence to yield a shorter polypeptide that is initiated at an internal methionine within the same ORF as the larger protein (e.g., HSV UL26 and UL26.5) (e-Fig. 8.2C). The resulting proteins thus share a domain of identical amino acid sequence, yet differ markedly in their function. Protein-encoding ORFs can be expressed from mRNAs that are antisense to each other (e.g., HSV-1 $\gamma_1$34.5 and ORF P and O (e-Fig. 8.2D). Common features of herpesvirus genomes are clusters of 3′ coterminal transcripts, each of which expresses a different ORF (e-Fig. 8.1B). Within these clusters, coding domains seldom overlap by more than a few codons.

Another strategy is to use splicing to enable differential regulation of a gene at different parts of the virus life cycle. In some cases, this means the same ORF is accessed from different promoters, or different ORFs can be expressed from the same primary transcript (e-Fig. 8.2E).

While they were largely ignored in many of the initial descriptions of herpesvirus genome sequences, short ORFs (sORFs) of less than 100 codons can direct translation of functional proteins.[43] Upstream open reading frames (uORFs) are sORFs that encode proteins of less than 100 amino acids, and are located in the 5′ leader sequences of mRNAs that direct translation of larger canonical proteins. Translation of uORFs is regulated via noncanonical translation initiation environments. The short translation products of uORFs can have regulatory activities, sometimes directed at the canonical ORF that is part of the same mRNA, enabling complex forms of regulation of protein expression[5,9,77] (e-Fig. 8.2, panel F).

Herpesviruses express a plethora of biologically important small noncoding RNAs (ncRNA), including microRNAs (miRNAs), long noncoding-RNAs (lncRNA; >170 nucleotides in length), and circular RNAs (circRNAs).[15,54] miRNAs are often clustered in intergenic regions and are not highly conserved across herpesvirus lineages. Highly stable circRNAs are formed via covalent linkage of a backspliced viral transcript, and can be incorporated into virions.[1,146] Although most genes are transcribed by RNA polymerase II, some small ncRNAs are transcribed by RNA polymerase III, including the EBV EBER transcripts[62] and the tRNA-miRNA molecules (TMERs) of MHV68 (MuHV-4).[15]

Naming of Genes and Their Products

There is no formalized system for naming herpesvirus genes or their products. The historical nomenclature can be particularly daunting to newcomers to the field. For example, the major HSV-1 transcriptional transactivator was first identified as a component of the virion and designated by its migration in denaturing gels relative to that of other virion proteins (VP16). Subsequently, it has been known on the basis of its migration in denaturing gels relative to other infected cell proteins (ICP25), its apparent molecular weight in denaturing polyacrylamide gels (vmw65), its best-known function (α-trans-inducing factor or α-TIF), and the gene encoding it (pUL48). EBV genes and their products are named after the restriction endonuclease-generated DNA fragment in which the gene maps; for instance, BZLF1 is BamHI, Z fragment, left frame 1. This nomenclature precludes all but the most dedicated from visualizing the position of the gene in the genome.

An additional hazard is the assumption that all functions of orthologous gene products are fully conserved from virus to virus. Most herpesvirus proteins studied in detail have multiple functions; proteins sharing a conserved block of amino acids may diverge in the functions encoded in their other domains.

Fortunately, gene name cross-references are often available in readily available compendia.[85,97,125] The nomenclature and abbreviation system proposed for genes conserved across the *Herpesviridae*[97] is used in this chapter.

Gene Functions

The cellular and organismal host ranges of herpesviruses differ enormously, from very wide (e.g., HSV) to very narrow (e.g., EBV, HHV-6B). The host range is determined only in part by the availability of receptors. Virally encoded proteins are required for entry into the cell, regulation of viral gene expression, nucleotide metabolism, synthesis of viral DNA, structural proteins, and virion assembly, as well as for management of host defenses, metabolism, and macromolecular biosynthesis and transport. Standing apart are genes expressed during latency; in the case of EBV there are multiple forms of latency differing with respect to the genes that are expressed.

Regulatory genes are specifically adapted to the requirements of the cell types inhabited by the virus *in vivo*. Some subsets of herpesviruses (e.g., the alphaherpesviruses) share clear homologs of regulatory genes such as α4, α0, and α27. Other groups of herpesviruses have important regulatory genes that have little obvious sequence similarity, although they may occupy similar genomic locations and even share splicing patterns (e.g., the immediate-early genes of the betaherpesviruses).

Viral non-coding RNAs (ncRNAs) represent a treasure trove of novel strategies evolved to promote infection and impair immune responses.[15,54,115,146] ncRNAs are highly variable in their sequence, structure, biogenesis, and the molecules with which they interact. Herpesvirus miRNAs posttrancriptionally silence mRNAs of both the virus and host; their roles in latency versus lytic infection often reflect their pattern of expression.[115] The highly expressed EBERs of EBV latency bind host proteins to protect the cell from apoptosis. The HSV latency-associated transcript (LAT) is a lncRNA that protects latently infected neurons from apoptosis. Like the lncRNAs of HCMV and KSHV, HSV LAT interacts with chromatin modifiers to regulate α/IE gene expression. Small circular RNAs bind miRNAs, functioning as molecular sponges for miRNAs to regulate viral gene expression.[146]

The functionality of herpesvirus gene products is defined by three key characteristics. ***First***, they often have multiple functions that may or may not be related. For instance, the ribonucleotide reductase, large subunit (RR1) is a key enzyme for nucleotide metabolism with additional roles in the impairment of apoptosis and necroptosis (e.g. HSV1, HSV2,) and relocalization of the host mutator APOBEC3B (e.g., HSV1, KSHV, EBV).[20,53] The decision as to which function is performed by a particular protein may be determined by the nature of posttranslational modifications, protein interactions that occur only in the context of infection, or the local environment of individual protein molecules. Full assessment of the multifunctional nature of viral proteins requires their study in the context of infection. A variety of approaches have been applied to the study of herpesvirus gene function, including cloning complete herpesvirus genomes into plasmids that can replicate in *E. coli* as bacterial artificial chromosomes. This enables rapid and precise mutagenesis of herpesvirus genomes, which can then be transfected into susceptible mammalian cells to generate virus stocks for functional studies.

The ***second*** key characteristic relates to their role(s) in virus replication. Genes necessary for replication in cultured cells are sometimes referred to as "essential," while dispensable genes can be described as "nonessential" or "accessory."[28] For HSV, more than 50% of the ORFs are dispensable for growth in cells in culture. However, most of these seemingly nonessential genes are not dispensable for virus replication or for reactivation from the latent state in experimental animal systems. Assays involving the establishment or maintenance of latency require conditional loss of function approaches to most accurately assess whether a virus gene is dispensable.

The ***third*** key characteristic is that virus proteins and RNAs mediate their activities via self-interactions or via interactions with other proteins and biomolecules of the virus or host. A conserved central intraviral protein interactome has been defined for members of the *Herpesviridae*,[60] in which clusters of protein–protein interactions enable identification of sets of viral proteins involved in critical processes such as entry, genome replication, capsid assembly, nuclear egress, cytoplasmic maturation, and egress. In addition, the interactions help to define roles of many conserved proteins in processes other than their primary function. This form of analysis has been extended to the full set of interactions between and among virus and cellular proteins during the course of infection,[105] as well to the influence of virus gene products on the properties of cellular organelles during the course of infections,[67] greatly broadening our understanding of the complex set of interactions that take place during infection.

Gene Relatedness and Arrangement

Complete genomic sequences have been determined for greater than 80 herpesviruses, and smaller segments have been obtained for many others (Table 8.1 and e-Table 8.2). From this and other information, several fundamental principles of herpesvirus genetic architecture have been deduced.

Herpesvirus gene sequences are related to each other in ways that reflect the long-standing, biology-based classification of herpesviruses into subfamilies and their respective genera. These relationships are substantial and easily detected. For viruses of the *Herpesviridae*, the nucleotide sequence of a 400-bp PCR product amplified from the viral DNA polymerase gene by the use of degenerate consensus primers is sufficient to establish the identity of a herpesvirus and place it into the appropriate subfamily. Higher resolution and more robust classification can be obtained by expanding the size of the comparison sequence and by analyzing more than one gene. A representation of herpesvirus taxonomic and phylogenetic relationships is shown in Figure 8.2.

Forty-one genes, referred to as the herpesvirus core genes, have been identified as conserved across the alpha-, beta-, and gammaherpesviruses (Table 8.2). Each gene belongs to one of six core gene blocks. Within each gene block, gene order and polarity are conserved (Fig. 8.4). Across the family, the core gene blocks are found in various permutations of order and orientation.[19,30] Block arrangement, and thus gene order, is conserved at the subfamily level. Conserved genes do not share identical sequences (e-Fig. 8.3). In some instances, homologs have readily detected sequence identity or similarity across their full lengths, while for others only a small portion is identifiably conserved. The implication is that the resulting proteins are an amalgam of conserved and diverged functions.

Some genes are conserved at the subfamily level. Thus, genes unique to alphaherpesviruses include their latency-associated genes, glycoprotein D, a tegument-associated protein that induces transcription from α-genes, and a transcriptional regulatory protein related to HSV $\alpha4$ (e-Fig. 8.3). To the left of conserved gene block 1, betaherpesviruses encode a block of 14 genes that have no counterparts elsewhere in the family (Fig. 8.4). Gammaherpesviruses uniquely encode conserved proteins needed to maintain latent genomes in dividing cells.

An interesting variation on the linkage of gene sets to subfamilies is offered by the origin-binding protein (OBP) and its binding site. OBP binds to its cognate sites in origins of lytic replication and serves to nucleate the DNA replication machinery and play a role in initiating DNA replication. Only alphaherpesviruses and members of the *Roseolovirus* genus of the betaherpesviruses encode OBP homologs and OBP binding sites[65] (e-Fig. 8.3). Other betaherpesviruses and the gammaherpesviruses initiate DNA replication by another mechanism.

Herpesviruses generally encode at least one gene of obvious host origin (reviewed in Refs.[63,118]); KSHV has acquired at least 12.[131] Examples include thymidylate synthase and *bcl*-2. These genes appear to have been acquired by retrotransposition events from cDNAs, given that they are most often encoded on the viral genome as continuous ORFs that do not require splicing. Some of these genes appear to have been acquired independently by different herpesvirus lineages (again, thymidylate synthetase and bcl-2). Host-acquired genes tend to be located toward the viral genomic termini and between core gene blocks. In some cases, the host-acquired genes retain a function similar to its cellular counterpart; expression from the viral genome allows the desired product to be produced when needed by the virus. In other cases, the host-acquired gene has been modified to alter its function. For example, the KSHV homolog of the cellular D-type cyclin is resistant to cyclin-dependent kinase inhibitors, rendering the viral version constitutively active and capable of transforming cells.[6]

BIOLOGICAL CYCLE OF HERPESVIRUSES

The herpesvirus biological cycle can be divided into four major components: initiation of infection, lytic replication, latency, and reactivation (Fig. 8.3). These components are linked by a biological decision in the infected cell to follow either the lytic or latent pathway, as well as by the ability of latently infected cells to be reactivated to a lytic state. Here we provide a general outline of the herpesvirus biological cycle; detailed descriptions of the diverse mechanisms employed by the various viruses to accomplish this are provided in subsequent chapters. It is important to bear in mind that essentially every step and stage of the herpesvirus biological cycle is dependent on the virus making use of, or adapting for its purposes, cellular systems, structures, and materials. Host interactions include modification of cellular systems for regulating gene expression, modulation of the cell cycle, reprogramming metabolic pathways for energy production and generation of biosynthetic precursors, remodeling of the secretory apparatus, using intracellular transportation systems throughout the infectious cycle, and managing host defenses.

Initiation of Infection

Initiation of infection spans the events that begin with receptor binding through the initial interactions of the virus genome with the host transcriptional machinery in the nucleus (Fig. 8.5, **Steps A1** to **A4**). The general features of this stage occur in cells destined for immediate entry into the lytic state, as well as in cells that will become latently infected.

Because they infect wide varieties of cell types, individual herpesviruses employ multiple cell surface receptors for virion entry. These interactions are mediated by individual, or combinations of, virion surface virus glycoproteins. For most, if not all herpesviruses, the initial binding of the virion to the host cell involves interactions of gB with cell surface heparan sulfate proteoglycans. After receptors are fully engaged, herpesviruses enter cells by two major pathways: fusion of the virion envelope with the plasma membrane at the cell surface (**Step A2a**), or membrane fusion after virion uptake by endocytosis (**Step A2b**). Fusion of virion and cellular membranes is mediated by gB and the gH/gL complex. gB is a class III fusion protein that has structural features in common with membrane fusion proteins encoded by viruses as diverse as vesicular stomatitis virus and baculoviruses.[57] In addition to their roles in virion entry, virion–receptor interactions activate cellular signaling pathways, some of which the virus takes advantage of, while others need to be redirected or blunted (Fig. 8.5, right side).

As part of entry, virus particles must interact with and ultimately penetrate the cytoplasm. Because of the macromolecular density and highly structured nature of the cytoplasm, objects the size of nucleocapsids are unable to migrate from the cell surface to the nucleus by diffusion alone. By way of interactions that ultimately link to microtubule motors, nucleocapsids hitch rides on microtubules for active transport to nuclear pores (**Step A3**). Next, tegument and capsid proteins mediate the docking of the nucleocapsid with the nuclear pore complex. The DNA is translocated from the capsid portal across the nuclear pore into the nucleus. Injection of the genome is powered in part by internal pressurization of the capsid during DNA packaging.[13] Almost immediately upon entry into the nucleus, the virus genome associates with histones. The organization and modification of the chromatinized genomes impacts the availability and state of particular viral and cellular transcription regulators. Thus, the epigenetic landscape is a major determinant of the biological decision to either establish a latent infection or enter the lytic replication cycle (**Steps B1a** and **B1b**).[76] Tegument proteins that are released into the cytoplasm during entry can have effector activities in the cytoplasm or nucleus. These include management of intrinsic defense responses and transcriptional activation of α genes (Fig. 8.5, right side).

Lytic Replication

The purpose of lytic replication is to manufacture infectious virions that can infect other cells and hosts. As illustrated in Figure 8.5, lytic replication includes regulated expression of virus genes, genome replication, virion assembly, egress, and transmission, all the while managing a wide range of host activities and defenses. As with any assembly line manufacturing process, virion assembly is dependent on production of appropriate levels of the various parts, plus mechanisms to ensure their presence in the proper locations when they are needed. Coordination of events during lytic infection is regulated as a function of the state of infection rather than by synchronization to a molecular clock. Lytic replication involves sophisticated use of preexisting cellular compartments such as the nucleus, cytoplasm, and cytoplasmic organelles, as well as their modification and sometimes subcompartmentalization.

As studied in detail for HSV, gene transcription, genome replication, and DNA packaging into capsids take place in subnuclear compartments. Several replication compartments, each nucleated by a single viral genome, constitute an infected cell nucleus. The compartments are dynamic, changing in size and composition as infection progresses.[73] Host chromatin is marginated to the nuclear periphery and host factors involved in gene transcription, DNA repair, and epigenetic silencing are relocalized; factors may be either recruited to, or excluded from, viral replication compartments.[18] Our understanding of the spatial–temporal changes that mediate transcription, replication, and genome packaging will continue to advance through use of super resolution microscopy and methods for purification of active transcription and replication complexes.

Expression and Activities of Lytic Genes

Herpesvirus gene expression during productive infection represents a classic regulatory cascade, the basic features of which are conserved across the family. In productively infected cells, viral genes form at least three kinetic classes that differ with respect to their order of gene expression. These are the α (immediate-early, IE) genes that require no new (cellular or viral) protein synthesis for their expression, β (early, E) genes whose transcription is totally independent of viral DNA synthesis, and γ (late, L) genes that typically follow viral DNA synthesis. In HSV, these γ genes are further categorized into γ1 (leaky-late) genes whose expression is augmented by the onset of viral DNA synthesis, and γ2 (true late) genes whose expression is absolutely dependent on viral DNA synthesis. The immediate-early, early, and late nomenclature is rooted in early phage studies; it has the virtue of instant recognition but does not fully describe the events occurring in the infected cell. Both systems are used widely and interchangeably.

Upon entry and circularization of the histone-free genome in the nucleus, the viral genome rapidly associates with nucleosomes. Epigenetic modifications of the chromatinized genome direct the availability of viral gene promoters. Regardless of whether the lytic pathway is entered directly as part of a new infection or via reactivation from latency, a key event is triggering α/IE gene transcription in a manner that drives the coordinated cascade of lytic gene infection. The activation of α/IE gene promoters is dependent on a transcriptional enhancer

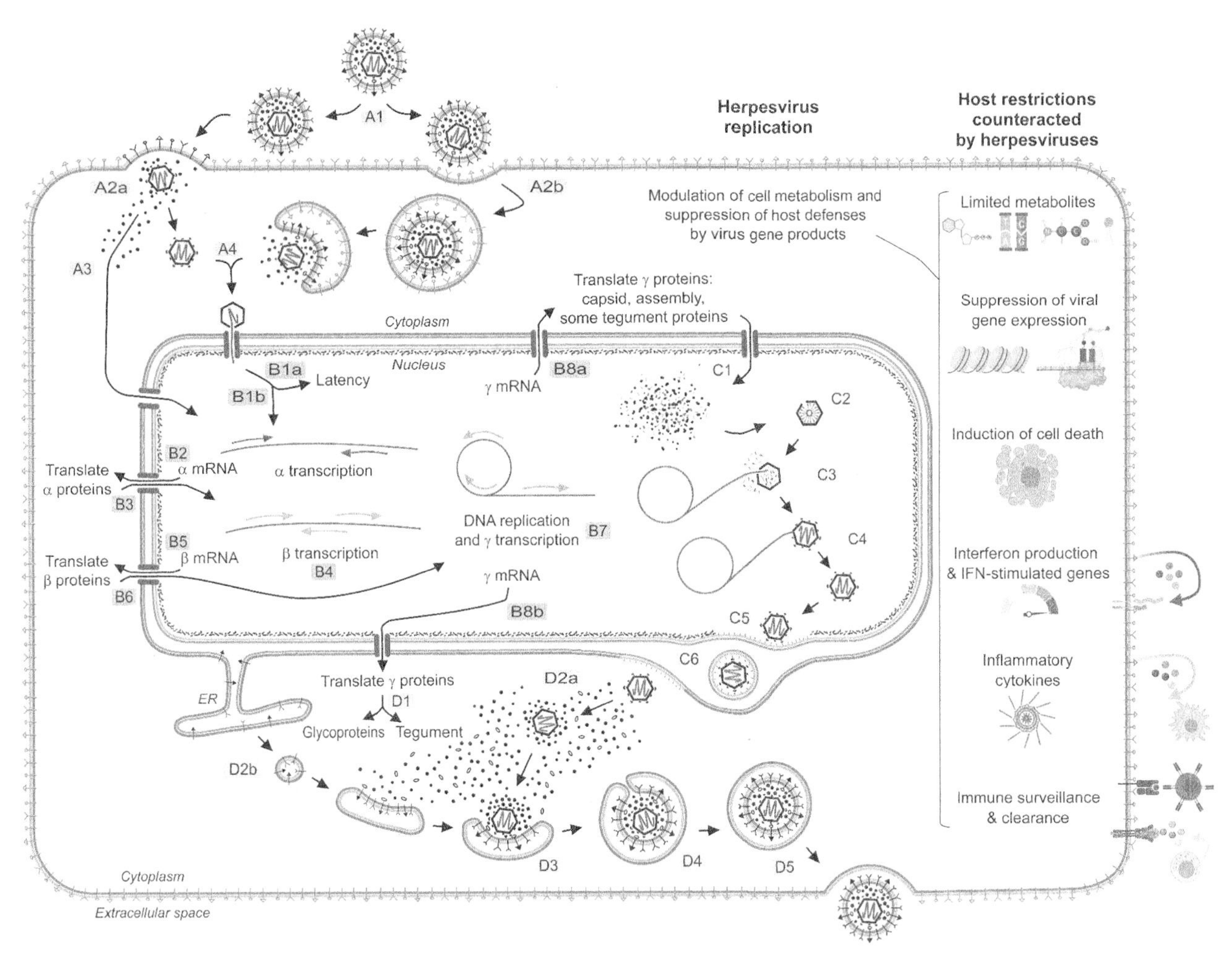

FIGURE 8.5 **Herpesvirus replication in the context of host restrictions. *Stages of lytic replication (left side).*** *Initiation of infection* (Steps **A1** to **A4**). Incoming virions engage cell surface receptors (**A1**) and then enter cells by fusion at the plasma membrane (**A2a**) or after endocytosis (**A2b**). Tegument proteins are routed to their various destinations, including the nucleus to activate α gene transcription (**A3**). Nucleocapsids are transported to nuclear pores via microtubules, and the virus genome is injected into the nucleus through a nuclear pore (**A4**). *Gene expression* (Steps **B1** to **B8**). Depending on the virus, cell type, and cell state, the virus can follow either the latent (**B1a**, details not illustrated) or lytic gene expression program, which is quickly dominated by transcription of α genes (**B1b**). α mRNAs are transported to the cytoplasm for translation (**B2**). Some α proteins are transported to the nucleus (**B3**) to initiate β gene transcription (**B4**). β mRNAs are transported to the cytoplasm (**B4**), translated, and then transported to the nucleus (**B6**) where they play various roles in replication of the virus genome (**B7**). γ genes are transcribed from replicating genomes, and the transcripts are then transported to the cytoplasm for translation (**B8a** and **B8b**). Nucleocapsid assembly and nuclear egress (Steps **C1** to **C6**). Capsid proteins and proteins required for capsid assembly and nuclear egress are transported to the nucleus (**C1**). Capsids form on a scaffold (**C2**) that is digested by a viral protease as the capsid is filled with newly replicated DNA (**C3**). Unit length virus genomes are cleaved from replicating genomes at specific sequences and the filled capsid is capped, thus forming a nucleocapsid (C4). Nuclear nucleocapsids associate with inner tegument proteins (**C4**). Nuclear egress involves modification of the nuclear lamina by viral and cellular kinases (**C5**), followed by nuclear egress complex-driven acquisition of the primary envelope by budding into the lumen of the nuclear membrane (**C6**), and then delivery into the cytoplasm after de-envelopment at the outer nuclear membrane. *Cytoplasmic virion assembly* (Steps **D1** to **D5**). The cytoplasmic steps of virion assembly begin with translation of tegument proteins and virion envelope glycoproteins (**D1**). Nonenveloped, partially tegumented nucleocapsids acquire most of their tegument during transport via microtubules (not illustrated) to their exit vesicle (**D2a**). Exit vesicles are populated with viral glycoproteins that were synthesized at the ER and then transported and processed via the Golgi apparatus and the trans-Golgi network (**D2b**). A small subset of tegument proteins associates with exit vesicles prior to nucleocapsid arrival. Nucleocapsids acquire their envelope by a budding/wrapping process (**D3**) that culminates in fully enveloped virions being contained within cytoplasmic vesicles that can be transported to the cell surface (**D4**). Virions are released to the extracellular space after fusion of the exit vesicle membrane with the plasma membrane (**D5**). While the general features of this scheme are shared by all herpesviruses, details vary from virus to virus. ***Host restrictions counteracted by herpesviruses (right side)***. Over half of the genetic content of herpesviruses is involved in counteracting the formidable array of host defenses to successfully drive a productive lytic infection. As detailed in Table 8.3 and in the text, these interactions may take place in the cytoplasm or nucleus, in subcompartments and organelles therein, or at the cell surface via receptors for extracellular factors. (Copyright Laurie Krug and Philip Pellett.)

complex of viral and host factors. For example, host transcription factors recruit the virion protein VP16 of HSV and the host coactivator HCF-1 to promote active chromatin and drive transcription from α/IE promoters.[75]

Herpesviruses typically encode a small number of α/IE genes, whose products perform a number of regulatory functions, including activation of β/E gene transcription, modulation of the cell cycle, chromatin structure, RNA transport and splicing, and blunting innate, intrinsic, and adaptive immune responses. Most β/E gene products are involved in virus genome replication. This includes enzymatic activities that ensure adequate pools of nucleotides, as well as the proteins and enzymes necessary for DNA synthesis at the replication fork. In the beta- and gammaherpesviruses, preinitiation complexes that are distinct from those that activate α/IE promoters drive transcription from γ/L promoters at a non-canonical TATT motif.[51,101] Most γ/L gene products are virion proteins.

Genome Replication

Replication of the virus genome is dependent on the presence of sufficient biosynthetic precursors, *cis*-acting signals in the virus genome that guide assembly of the replication complex and initiation of DNA replication, and *trans*-acting factors that replicate the virus genome in a manner that is sufficiently orderly to generate several thousand genomic copies from as few as one starting template and then efficiently encapsidate the nascent genomes.

Herpesvirus genomes have 1 to 3 *cis*-acting sites that can act as origins of lytic DNA replication (oriLyt). For alphaherpesviruses and a subset of betaherpesviruses (members of the *Roseolovirus* genus), assembly of the replication complex at these sites is dependent on the virally encoded OBP, which binds to specific oriLyt sequences and then triggers conformational changes in the virus genome that enable assembly of the replication complex and initiation of replication. Other herpesviruses employ virally encoded DNA-binding transcription factors for oriLyt activation. Regardless of how oriLyt is activated, a set of six proteins that are conserved across the *Herpesviridae* interact to form the enzymatic complex that replicates the genome. These proteins include the viral DNA polymerase (POL) and its associated processivity subunit (PPS), a single-stranded DNA binding protein (SSB), and the three components of the helicase–primase complex (HP1, HP2, and HP3). Some host proteins are involved, but their roles have not been fully defined. Other forms of replication might be involved, but rolling-circle replication (**Step B7**) appears to be the major source of new genomes. Because packaged genomes are not chromatinized, thus far undefined mechanisms are needed to either prevent chromatization during and after viral DNA replication or remove nucleosomes from newly replicated viral DNA prior to packaging.[102]

Virion Assembly and Egress

Biosynthesis and intracellular delivery of virion components

Dissection of the process of virion assembly needs to account for the structure of mature infectious virions and the topological constraints imposed by cellular compartmentalization. The major stages of virion assembly occur first in the nucleus and then in the cytoplasm. Extensive use is made of cellular systems for synthesis, processing, and trafficking of membrane proteins, plus nucleocytoplasmic, intracytoplasmic, and vesicular transport systems, as well as management of cellular metabolism to ensure manufacture of raw materials such as amino acids and nucleotides, in addition to lipids needed to form virion envelopes. The process is dependent on coordinated delivery of virion subcomponents to appropriate subcellular addresses at appropriate times.

Biosynthesis of most virion proteins begins with translation of mRNAs for structural genes. The mRNAs for virion glycoproteins need to be translated by ribosomes associated with the endoplasmic reticulum, to begin the trafficking through the ER, Golgi apparatus, and trans-Golgi network required for sequential maturation of nascent glycoproteins and their ultimate delivery to the organelle(s) where virions are enveloped (Fig. 8.5, **Steps D1** to **D3**). Proteins and multiprotein complexes formed in the cytoplasm are required for construction of capsids in the nucleus must associate with machinery that enables their transport to and through the nuclear pore complex. Tegument proteins that will be assembled onto nucleocapsids in the cytoplasm need to be routed to areas that will be traversed by nucleocapsids on their way to the cytoplasmic organelle where they will acquire their envelope.

Assembly and nuclear egress of the nucleocapsid

Capsids are assembled in the nucleus (**Steps C1** to **C4**).[23,59,121] In addition to its structural proteins, capsid assembly is dependent on several other viral proteins expressed from a pair of overlapping genes (*UL26* and *UL26.5* in HSV). These include the assembly protein precursor (pAP), the mature assembly protein (AP), and the assembly protease (PR), which are self-excised by PR from a precursor polyprotein (prePR) that contains PR, pAP, and AP, and proteolytic products that form the temporary scaffold during capsid assembly. Capsid assembly nucleates on the dodecameric portal complex (**Step C2**). The scaffold enables assembly of pentonal and hexagonal capsomeres and their associated proteins into closed capsids, after which the scaffold is proteolytically digested (**Steps C3** and **C4**).

The genome is packaged into the capsid by the packaging motor and site-specific endonuclease that form the terminase complex (**Step C3**), which is built from six terminase monomers that are arranged as a ring just outside the capsid portal complex at its pentonal vertex.[121,157] Each of the terminase monomers consists of three conserved subunits: the terminase binding protein (TERbp; HSV pUL33), the terminase ATPase subunit (TER1; HSV pUL15), and the TER DNA recognition subunit (TER2; pUL28). To initiate packaging, the complex recognizes and then employs its endonuclease activity to cleave the nascent genome at its packaging and cleavage sequence. With one end now precisely defined, the genome is then translocated into the capsid by the packaging motor activity of the complex.

Rather than screwing the DNA into the capsid (rotation model for packaging), which would produce torsional forces that would twist and tangle the genome, DNA is packaged via a rotational mechanism. During translocation, the DNA is passed from one terminase subunit to the next, the double helix revolving around the center of the central channel of the hexameric complex, without rotation of either the DNA or terminase complex. The DNA is advanced into the capsid at an energy cost of one ATP per terminase monomer step. The bacteriophage phi29 packaging motor, which uses a related mechanism, advances its DNA 1.75 bp per step into the capsid.[132] As packaging approaches completion, and the capsid is nearly filled, a conformational change occurs that enables the complex to cleave the genome precisely at the next packaging and cleavage sequence it encounters. The portal capping protein (PCP; HSV pUL25) is involved in securing the DNA in the highly pressurized nucleocapsid.

Filled nucleocapsids are exported from the nucleus via a process that involves primary envelopment at the inner nuclear membrane followed by deenvelopment during entry into the cytoplasm.[58,128] The viral nuclear egress complex (NEC) is made from two conserved herpesvirus proteins, nuclear egress membrane protein (NEMP; HSV pUL34) and nuclear egress lamina protein (NELP; HSV pUL31). NEC mediates a viral and cellular kinase-driven disassembly and rearrangement of the nuclear lamina that enables filled nucleocapsids to access the nuclear face of the inner nuclear membrane (**Step C5**). NEC enables generation of the inner nuclear membrane curvature needed for capsid envelopment, which is followed by NEC-driven scission of the nascent primary envelope, with no apparent requirement for ESCRT machinery. In the lumen of the nuclear membrane, nucleocapsids present in primary enveloped virions are surrounded by the NEC and a small set of capsid-associated tegument proteins (**Step C6**). The mechanism for the membrane fusion that enables primary enveloped virions to migrate from the lumen of the nuclear membrane to the cytoplasm is not well defined.

Cytoplasmic tegumentation, secondary envelopment, and egress

As delivered into the cytoplasm, nonenveloped nascent virions consist of nucleocapsids and a set of nucleocapsid-associated tegument proteins (the inner tegument) that were acquired in the nucleus (**Step D2a**). The next assembly steps involve addition of the final complement of tegument proteins and some RNAs, and then acquisition of the mature envelope while budding into a cytoplasmic organelle from which the virion can be transported to the cell surface for release[22,23,156] (**Steps D3** to **D5**). Few mechanistic details are known of the tegumentation process. Virion membrane proteins must possess trafficking signals appropriate for being routed to exit organelles (**Steps D2b** to **D3**), where they form concentrated patches. Nucleocapsids are transported from the site of nuclear egress to their exit vesicle through associations with microtubule motors. Some tegument proteins interact with each other to form subassemblies that associate with the developing virion during transport to the exit organelle. Electron micrographs make it clear that most of the tegument forms on the nucleocapsid, but some tegument proteins associate with cytoplasmic projections of virion membrane proteins. When the necessary associations and structures have formed, tegumented nucleocapsids bud into the exit organelle. The final step of envelopment is scission of the neck of the membrane that connects the tegument-containing compartment of the developing virion to liberate the mature virion into the lumen of the exit vesicle (**Steps D4** to **D5**). Topologically similar activities are important in cell biology and for other enveloped viruses (e.g., retroviruses and filoviruses), and are commonly carried out by ESCRT machinery.[8] Current evidence indicates that ESCRT machinery is employed for completion of secondary envelopment of HSV-1, but HCMV employs a different mechanism, one possibly mediated by viral proteins.[138]

Herpesviruses can differ with respect to the organelle where they acquire their mature envelope. The unifying concept is that the exit organelle is adapted from an organelle that is normally involved in vesicular transport and delivery of cargo for release at the plasma membrane. Thus, HSV uses the trans-Golgi network and early endosomes, HCMV appears to follow a secretory endosomal pathway, and HHV-6A follows a pathway used by CD63-positive multivesicular bodies.[23,156] Vesicles containing enveloped virions are transported to the plasma membrane, where vesicle membranes fuse with the plasma membrane; mature virions are then released to the extracellular space from which they can infect other cells, in the same or a different host.

Latency and Reactivation

Latency

Latency is a defining property that drives much of herpesvirus biology. Each herpesvirus establishes latency in a specific set of cells, with the cellular site of latency differing from one virus to another. In cells that harbor latent virus, viral genomes generally take the form of closed circular chromatin that is not integrated into a host chromosome (an episome), with epigenetic marks that silence transcription, enabling expression of only a small subset of viral genes (Fig. 8.3). Latently infected cells differ from chronically or persistently infected cells in that infectious progeny are not produced during latency. The limited gene expression of latency is a stealth mode that reduces potential exposure of viral antigens to the immune system. Importantly, latent genomes retain the capacity to reactivate to a lytic state during which new infectious virions are produced. The capacity to reactivate differentiates latent from abortive infections.

Epigenetic regulation to silence lytic gene expression from the viral genome is a broad strategy of latency. However, there appears to be no shared genetic component for establishment, maintenance, or termination of the latent state. Members of some genera of herpesviruses encode several proteins and ncRNAs that are expressed to facilitate latency in cells at particular states of differentiation (e.g., EBV), while others (e.g., HSV) might express ncRNAs derived from a single latency-associated transcript (LAT) to establish and maintain latency. Maintenance of the viral genome in nondividing cells, such as neurons infected by alphaherpesviruses, requires less viral activity than in cells infected by beta- and gammaherpesviruses, which typically establish latency in proliferating cells of the immune system. EBV and KSHV express latency nuclear antigens that tether the viral episome to the host chromosome and recruit the host replication machinery to the latent origin of virus replication upon host cell division.[32]

HHV-6A and HHV-6B readily integrate into the telomeres of host chromosomes in cell culture models of infection.[71] Chromosomal integration is hypothesized to provide a mechanism for maintenance and replication of the virus genome during latency. Approximately 1% of humans have germ-line integration of HHV-6A or HHV-6B, which leads to the intriguing phenomenon of inherited vertical transmission.

The molecular mechanisms that lead to establishment of, and reactivation from, the latent state are not fully understood. A central feature of latency is epigenetic regulation of transcription.

Chromatin modifications of the viral genome ensure transcription of latency-specific transcription, as well as suppression of lytic gene transcription.[32]

During the establishment of latency, host factors such as histone deacetyltransferases promote heterochromatin with repressive histone modifications to suppress lytic gene expression.[75] The host chromatin remodelers and regulatory factors vary with the type and state of the cell. Virally encoded proteins and ncRNAs modulate the activities of the host factors and directly regulate latent gene programs.[32,54,124]

Reactivation

Reactivation from latency is the reversal of suppressed lytic gene expression. In a cell type–dependent manner, cellular stress conditions and particular states of activation and differentiation serve as cues to reverse the epigenetic modifications that silence latent viral genomes. Signaling pathways culminate in the activation of transcription factors that drive α/IE lytic promoters; these vary with cell type and stimulus. Reactivation events are held in check by antiviral cytokines and the virus-specific adaptive immune response.

Defining the signals that coordinate a permissive chromatin state and the engagement of transcription enhancer complexes is a fascinating challenge. For HSV, both animal models and primary culture systems model reactivation using stress cues such as tissue explant or withdrawal of neuronal growth factors (NGFs). Molecular events during reactivation include the loss of the translational repressor 4E-BP1 that is regulated by NGF-dependent mTORC1, relocalization of host coactivator HCF-1 and its associated histone demethylases to the nucleus, and chromatin modifications that displace repressive factors.[21,72,75,76] A simple binary latent or lytic state of infection may not exist for all herpesviruses.[134] Gene expression patterns that do not fit the regulated, ordered lytic cascade is observed prior to the establishment of latency and in the early phase of reactivation. The collective molecular cues that regulate latency are likely in flux within the infected cell and its microenvironment. If the threshold to trigger the full lytic cascade is not met or if the immune system blocks this event, reactivation is aborted.

Reactivation from cellular latency can result in disease due to a combination of the cellular and tissue damage directly caused by lytic virus replication, plus the immunologic responses to the reactivated lytic replication. Within an organism, a herpesvirus can be simultaneously latent in some cells and actively replicating in others due to periodic reactivation events. Reactivation likely plays a role in maintaining the viral load in the host and is key for transmission to new hosts via infections virions shed via lesional fluid or mucosal tissues.

VIRUS–HOST INTERACTIONS

Across the herpesviruses, multiple mechanisms have evolved that accomplish the shared objective of thwarting host defenses at each step of infection, for example, the many ways they block the attempt of infected cells to undergo a form of death termed apoptosis or block the action of antiviral interferon cytokines. The diversity of approaches is a remarkable testimony both to the depth and complexity of host defenses and to the adaptive prowess of the virus (summarized in Table 8.3). That the virus wins in the infected cell but normally allows the host to survive attests to an evolutionary necessity.

Conquering the Cell

Herpesviruses are exquisite cellular parasites that transform the infected cells into a production factory for virus particles. Infection typically ramps up the acquisition and usage of fuel, in addition to the production of molecular building blocks such as nucleotides, amino acids, and lipids. Glycolysis, glutaminolysis, and the synthesis of fatty acids are common pathways boosted by infection.[140] In addition to encoding enzymes involved in nucleotide metabolism, some herpesviruses (e.g., HSV) alter the flow through metabolic pathways that result in enhanced pyrimidine biosynthesis,[149] while others (e.g., HCMV) manipulate the tricarboxylic acid cycle to ensure adequate lipids for other stages of replication.[99,149,159] Herpesvirus subversion of the metabolic microenvironment may involve increased glucose uptake, up-regulation of metabolic enzymes, and interference with cellular signaling.[84,122,140] HCMV UL38 targets the host TSC tumor suppressor to increase glycolytic and amino acid flux that promotes virus production.[123] miRNAs and proteins encoded by gammaherpesviruses subvert metabolic processes that promote cell survival.[117] The EBV latency protein EBNA2 drives one carbon metabolism via MYC up-regulation to promote transformation of primary B cells.[152]

The molecular battle with the cell occurs on many fronts. During lytic production, cell cycle progression ramps up metabolism and host factors needed to produce infectious particles. Viral proteins perturb the cell cycle by direct interaction with cyclin-dependent kinases or by the phosphorylation, degradation, and redistribution of host regulators of the cell cycle.[41,135] On the gene expression front, herpesvirus mRNAs are indistinguishable from mature host mRNAs (5′7- methylguanosine cap and 3′ polyA tails) and they rely on the transcriptional and translational machinery of the cell. How does the virus compete with the much larger host transcriptome to favor viral gene products and repress host antiviral responses? The ICP27 family of viral IE proteins exhibits a remarkable array of interactions with host factors and viral RNAs that promote the stability of viral RNAs in the nucleus. Most herpesvirus transcripts are not spliced. HSV-1 ICP27 dysregulates termination, splicing, and export of host transcripts.[145,151] KSHV ORF57 protects viral mRNAs from RNA decay in the nucleus,[130] and as reported for its HSV, HCMV, and EBV homologs, it promotes translation of intronless viral mRNAs in the cytoplasm.[49] Viral nucleases of the alphaherpesviruses (HSV-1 vhs) and gammaherpesviruses (KSHV vSox) cleave mRNAs of the host and virus to facilitate optimal viral gene expression.[49] Another broad feature of the battle at the translational front is virus-mediated stimulation of the assembly of translation initiation factor complexes. Down-regulation of stress responses to infection such as the unfolded protein response and protein kinase R activation prevents host shutdown of viral protein synthesis and cell death.[49]

Herpesvirus proteins interact with cytoskeleton components throughout the infectious cycle: retrograde virion transport to the nucleus, egress from the nucleus, and then final tegumentation and envelopment in the cytoplasm, with anterograde directional transport to release infectious particles.[100] Engagement of virion glycoproteins with surface receptors cues actin remodeling and signaling that stabilizes microtubules.[34] As exemplified by pseudorabies virus infection of neurons,

TABLE 8.3 Herpesvirus countermeasures for host restrictions

Host restriction	Virus Countermeasures	HSV-1 HSV-2	VZV	HCMV	HHV-6A HHV-6B HHV-7	EBV	KSHV
Limited metabolites	Induce nucleotide, lipid, and/or glucose metabolism	⊙	○	●	●	●	●
	Modulate host regulators of cell cycle	●	●	●	●	●	●
Suppression of viral gene expression	Impair epigenetic silencers and repressors that silence viral genomes	●	○	●	○	●	●
	Degrade host transcripts	●	○	○	○	●	●
	Alter transcription, splicing and export of transcripts to favor virus	●	○	●	⊙	●	●
	Promote translation initiation and downregulate stress responses	●	○	●	⊙	●	●
Induction of cell death	Block host sensors and signaling that activate death effectors	●	●	●	●	●	●
	Induce host survival factors or encode viral mimics	●	●	●	○	●	●
Antiviral cytokines	Block pathogen sensors and production of antiviral cytokines	●	○	●	●	●	●
	Prevent interferon signaling and interferon simulated gene expression	●	○	●	●	●	●
Immune response	Block induction of inflammatory cytokines	●	○	●	⊙	●	●
	Encode or induce immunosuppressive cytokines	○	⊙	●	●	●	●
	Pirating of chemokine, chemokine binding protein or receptor	●	●	●	●	●	●
	Alter cell surface receptors to prevent NK cell activation	●	⊙	●	●	●	●
	Interference with antigen presentation to T cells	●	●	●	●	●	●
	Latency program of restricted viral gene expression	●	●	●	●	●	●

Filled circle indicate that specific viral factors promote the indicated countermeasure.
Circles with center dot indicate viral infection impacts a particular host process, but the specific viral factor that is responsible remains undetermined.
Open circles indicate that the virus countermeasure has not been reported.

The revised version of Table 8.3 includes the following changes:

- two text changes:
  - make column heading plural to state: "Virus Countermeasures"
  - the fifth row under 'Virus Countermeasures' should have the verb "Alters" corrected to state "Alter transcription, splicing..."
- More complete virus names are used.
- The filled table fields have been replaced with filled circle symbols.
- The gray table fields have been replaced with circles that have a dot in the center.
- The white table fields have been replaced with open circles.
- The footnote has been reordered and corrected to describe the new symbols.

the inner tegument proteins bind motor proteins to facilitate transport to and from the nucleus, and virion proteins including kinases modify and dissociate nuclear lamins.[87] HCMV-infected cells form a distinct virion assembly complex in which the nucleus is bent into a kidney shape around a cylindrical organelle structure composed of virus-modified Golgi, TGN, and secretory vesicles, all radiating from a microtubule organizing center.[4]

Modulation of Host Defenses

Intrinsic Defenses

The intrinsic defense of a cell to an incoming virion in the cytoplasm or a newly deposited viral genome in the nucleus initiates with sensing by preexisting host molecules. Promyelocytic-nuclear bodies (PML-NB), also referred to as nuclear domain 10 (ND10), are nuclear hubs of host factors including the PML, Sp100, and hDaxx transcriptional regulators that restrict virus replication.[144] PML has been observed to form a cage-like lattice around the HSV-1 genome early during infection.[3] PML-NB components recruit chromatin remodelers to transcriptionally silence the promoters of immediate early genes, and they facilitate innate interferon-stimulated gene expression. Viral proteins delivered via the virion tegument (gammaherpesvirus vFGARATs and HCMV pp71) or newly synthesized during the first hours of infection (HSV-1 ICP0) neutralize these host restriction factors by ubiquitin-mediated degradation, disruption of protein–protein interactions, or relocalization of the

PML-NB components to inert subcompartments.[44,78,129] A fine balance is involved, since herpesviruses co-opt these restriction factors to facilitate their own latency. HSV-1 genomes localize to ND10 in the nuclei of neurons during latency.[37]

The interferon gamma–inducible protein IFI16 is a nuclear DNA sensor that activates host restriction factors that epigenetically silence viral genomes to prevent gene expression. Repressive histone methylation marks on KSHV lytic gene promoters that are driven by IFI16 facilitate and maintain latency in endothelial cells and B lymphocytes.[129]

Apoptosis, necroptosis, and autophagy are distinct cell death responses invoked by virus infection. Caspase-dependent apoptosis is initiated from extrinsic death receptors such as the TNFα receptor or from intrinsic pathways via the mitochondria or ER following cell stress. Herpesviruses override these death cues with glycoproteins and tegument components of the virions, in addition to newly expressed genes during lytic infection.[143] Viral strategies of subversion encompass transcriptional up-regulation or molecular mimicry of prosurvival host factors, altering the phosphorylation of host signaling intermediates or impairing the function of signaling factors and caspases through direct interactions.[7,52,158] The latency-associated transcript of HSV-1 and numerous proteins expressed in the latency programs of EBV and KSHV employ similar strategies to protect the viability of cellular reservoirs of latent infection.[7,158] Necroptosis is a fallback host defense to counter viruses that impair caspase 8. RIP kinase 3 associates with RIP1 of death receptor activated complexes to phosphorylate a host factor that disrupts plasma membranes. RIP homotypic interaction motifs found in proteins of alpha and betaherpesviruses directly impair RIPK3 interactions and protect against necroptosis.[52] The cellular recycling process of autophagy is induced in response to cell stress and can destroy virions by fusion of virion-containing endosomes with autophagolysosomes. Inhibition of autophagy increases virus yield in many systems. However, autophagy also provides an opportunity to recycle vacuolar membranes to enhance egress, increase metabolites, drive host cell survival and proliferation, and reduce inflammatory responses.[86] With each type of cell death, herpesviruses may encode gene products or employ ncRNAs that engage upstream signaling events to drive beneficial outcomes while others intervene to circumvent execution of cell death processes.

Innate Defenses

The sheer physical complexity of the virion in addition to virus-driven subversion of cellular processes triggers numerous molecular tripwires in the host. Cytoplasmic sensors of virion DNA and stress-induced release of mitochondrial DNA drive cGAS/STING activation that signals to trigger type I IFN (IFN-I) production.[164] Engagement of toll-like receptor sensors and RIG-I with double-stranded RNA produced during infection leads to a series of phosphorylation events that activate transcription factors to induce IFN-I.[147] Interferons are a potent family of cytokines that induce hundreds of interferon-stimulated genes (ISGs) that function to blunt replication in the infected cell and warn neighboring uninfected cells to bolster defenses against the imminent herpesvirus intruder. The antiviral ISGs can impair multiple stages of infection such as an early block in the delivery of the viral genome to the nucleus, a shutoff of protein translation, or the induction of apoptosis. In response to this threat, each herpesvirus employs multiple strategies to thwart host induction of, and responses to, interferons. For example, HSV-1, HCMV, and KSHV each encode over a dozen distinct proteins that block upstream events to impair key host signaling molecules STING and TBK1, interfere with the function of host transcription factors NF-kappaB and IRF3 to dampen the expression of IFN-I, directly repress the expression of key players in the IFN pathway, and block signaling downstream of IFN receptor engagement to reduce ISG expression[2,10,143,147]

Innate immune cells express high levels of pathogen recognition receptors and are responsive to chemokine-directed recruitment and cytokines produced by infected cells. As first-line responders, neutrophils and macrophage cells produce toxic moieties such as reactive oxygen species and nitric oxide. They produce soluble factors that amplify inflammation and recruit additional leukocytes of both the innate and adaptive host immune response. Herpesviruses have pirated numerous chemokine-related molecules to redirect immune cell communications. Paradoxically, some herpesviruses facilitate the recruitment of innate immune cells as a reservoir of latency or as a vehicle for dissemination. Every human herpesvirus encodes at least one chemokine homolog with distinct agonist or antagonistic relationships with host chemokine receptors.[116] Chemokine binding proteins of the alpha and beta subfamilies may enhance or inhibit their cognate chemokines while the chemokine receptors of the beta and gamma subfamilies usurp signaling pathways to drive proliferation, cell migration, and angiogenesis of the infected cell. These pirated immune modulators can profoundly influence pathogenesis. For example, the vGPCR of KSHV is a homolog of CXCR2 that constitutively drives the production of paracrine growth factors to promote endothelial cell proliferation and angiogenesis, a hallmark of the Kaposi sarcoma neoplasm.[116]

Natural killer (NK) cells survey the surface receptors of cells for signatures indicative of infection such as down-regulation of MHC I molecules or up-regulation of the activating ligand NKG2D. Potent antiviral effector functions include the production of cytokines IFNγ and TNFα, recognition of antibodies bound to infected cells, and the directed killing of target cells by perforin/granzyme B and FasL. Herpesviruses have evolved a multitude of molecular strategies to counter recognition by NK cells. Viral proteins facilitate ER retention and degradation of ligands for NK activating receptors, or they provide decoys and ligands for NK cells receptors that inhibit activation; viral miRNAs down-regulate NK activating ligands.[33] Viral glycoproteins may function as viral Fc receptors for antibodies that recognize viral antigens on a cell surface; this impairs antibody-dependent cytotoxity by NK cells.

In vivo investigations of nonhuman herpesviruses (BHV-1, MCMV, gpCMV, MHV68, RRV) in their natural hosts have proven invaluable to define critical host determinants of immune control and the role of viral genes that promote pathogenesis by evading host immune responses. For example, the biological importance of NK cell inhibition is quite apparent in mice infected with MCMV. Viral mutants that lack genes products or viral miRNAs that interfere with NK cell surveillance have reduced pathogenesis; these phenotypes are absolved when NK cells are depleted or inhibited in mice.[114]

Adaptive Defenses

B lymphocytes produce virus-reactive antibodies that either neutralize the virion particles directly or lead to the death of the infected cell when antibodies that bind viral surface antigen cue the complement cascade or innate immune cells recognition via Fc receptors. B lymphocytes also present antigen and provide help to T cells. Activation of CD4+ T cells leads to cytokine production that facilitates the expansion and activation of virus-specific CD8+ T cells. Virus-specific CD8+ T cells produce the antiviral cytokines IFNγ and TNFα, which inhibit herpesvirus replication and reactivation; most importantly, they kill infected cells via perforin/granzyme B– or Fas-mediated cytolysis.

Herpesviruses escape killing by virus-specific CD8+ T cells by preventing surface presentation of viral antigens on MHC I. Strategies to down-regulate viral antigen presentation include cleavage of MHC I transcripts, increasing MHC I turnover by viral ubiquitin ligases, retention of MHC I molecules in the ER, and blocking transport of peptides into the ER and loading onto MHC I.[109,120] The EBNA1 latency antigen contains a glycine–alanine repeat that reduces its translation and MHC I antigen presentation.[120] Many herpesviruses have either independently pirated an IL-10 homolog (vIL-10) or induce cellular IL-10 expression to suppress proinflammatory cytokine production and inhibit CD4+ and CD8+ T-cell effector responses.[108] The remarkable set of immune modulators encoded by herpesviruses coupled with the molecular program of latency bestows an invisibility cloak that is a major contributor to lifelong persistence of herpesviruses, even in immunocompetent hosts.

Animal studies provide numerous examples whereby virus-specific cells of the adaptive immune system play a critical role in acute control, prevention of latency, or long-term control of reactivation. Neutralizing antibodies suffice for sterilizing immunity for many pathogens, but antigen-specific CD8+ T cells and CD4+ helper T cells are most critical for long-term control of herpesviruses. In humans, herpesvirus pathologies that manifest upon failure of immune defenses due to genetic immunodeficiency, young or advanced age, uncontrolled HIV or pharmaceutical suppression demonstrate that chronic cycles of reactivation and reinfection that transpire must be controlled by a vigilant, armed immune system.

The success of the human VZV vaccines demonstrates that sterilizing immunity is not required for protection against herpesvirus diseases. The Oka vaccine is a live attenuated form of VZV that establishes latency and has reduced the incidence of chickenpox worldwide. For persons already infected with VZV, a glycoprotein-based subunit vaccine that is administered with a potent adjuvant markedly reduces the occurrence of shingles and the debilitating development of postherpetic neuralgia. The challenge is to understand the spatial and temporal events of the immune response required for the control of each herpesvirus and prevention of their respective diseases, and then tailor a vaccine formulation that will generate the protective determinants of humoral and/or cellular immunity to reach that end.

Pathogenesis

Human Herpesvirus Transmission and Disease

Initial infections with herpesviruses might be asymptomatic or the newly infected individual may present with disease-defining clinical manifestations (e-Table 8.1). Herpesviruses are shed at mucosal sites including the oral and genital tissues. Shedding is often asymptomatic; the periodicity and level of infectious virus in secretions is not well-characterized for most herpesviruses. Primary infection typically occurs through asexual contact in childhood and adolescence, but some viruses may be acquired through sexual contact. HCMV may be acquired by vertical transmission from the mother to the fetus *in utero* and is also shed in the urine and breast milk. Mothers who undergo primary infection with HCMV during their pregnancy are most at risk for *in utero* transmission, but reactivation and reinfection events are also sources of placental infection that contribute to more total cases of congenital HCMV disease.

Herpes is forever. Once infected, the host will perpetually harbor the virus in multiple reservoirs of the body; most reservoirs are latent with some degree of lytic replication. Reactivation or low-level persistent replication can lead to mild, even asymptomatic shedding or more severe manifestations such as cold sores and genital lesions (HSV-1 and -2), shingles (VZV), and retinitis (HCMV). As detailed below, gammaherpesviruses (EBV and KSHV) drive numerous types of cancers that manifest in the lymphoid and nonlymphoid cells in which they reside at much higher rates in individuals with weakened immune systems. Sporadic, low-level reactivation is difficult to measure. However, the increased incidence and severity of herpesvirus diseases that manifest in HIV+ patients with low CD4+ T cell counts and in individuals undergoing immunosuppressive chemotherapy are striking evidence that the immune system plays an essential role in controlling intermittent productive infection.

Oncogenesis

The gamma subfamily has a strong association with lymphomas, tumors, and neoplasms in the host, albeit most frequently in the context of immune suppression (e-Table 8.1). Rapid proliferation and a prolonged life span of newly infected lymphocytes is integral to the establishment of their latent repository. Bypass of normal checkpoints likely places the gammaherpesvirus-infected cell at risk for further genetic insults, such as the classic chromosomal translocation of the c-myc oncogene to the immunoglobulin heavy chain locus in EBV-positive Burkitt lymphoma. Few alpha- or betaherpesviruses are considered to be oncogenic. A notable exception is the alphaherpesvirus, Marek disease virus (MDV, GαAHV-2), a potent driver of T-cell lymphomas in chickens.

The exquisite and complex latency program of gammaherpesviruses in a newly infected lymphocyte contrasts sharply with the single latency-associated transcript of HSV-1/2 that is expressed in nondividing neurons. EBV latency initiates with the expression of at least ten viral proteins and dozens of ncRNAs with potent proliferative and antiapoptotic functions that drive several rounds of rapid B cell division.[68] Concomitant with the generation of an adaptive immune response that surveils and eliminates infected cells with active expression of latency antigens in the host, there is a progressive shutdown of the expression of latency genes as the cell is reprogrammed towards a more differentiated, longer-lived memory B cell. The latency program of the rhadinoviruses such as KSHV in lymphocytes appears less complex. Even so the multiple latency gene products and miRNAs expressed in newly infected cells coordinate the critical end-goal of promoting proliferation and survival while maintaining the viral genome.[16]

Kaposi sarcoma is a highly angiogenic neoplasm of endothelial cell origin that arises in the skin and numerous cutaneous sites of the body. A small population of cells in an active lytic phase of KSHV infection have paracrine effects on the majority latent population and other uninfected cell types of the tumor microenvironment. Low-level but consistent detection of KSHV lytic genes with functions that promote the hyperproliferative, inflammatory, and angiogenic characteristics of Kaposi sarcoma suggest that gammaherpesvirus pathologies are not driven solely by the latency program.[16]

Many gammaherpesvirus genes are considered to be oncogenes based on their consistent detection in cancer tissues and ability to drive transformation in cell culture and animal models. Gammaherpesviruses encode an array of proteins and noncoding RNAs with functions that can induce classical hallmarks of cancer.[15,68,94] A gammaherpesvirus arsenal may encompass surface receptors, cytokines, and chemokine receptors that engage numerous signaling pathways, potent regulators of host gene expression and epigenetic modifications to activate or silence host and viral genes of interest, and homologs of host cyclin to dysregulate the cell cycle and bcl-2 to block cell death.[68,94] Taken together, these accoutrements drive cellular proliferation while impairing host DNA damage responses and tumor suppressors that risk genome instability and bona fide transformation. Viral proteins and ncRNAs place the cell at risk for transformation, but a combination of circumstances involving immune status, infections with other pathogens (notably HIV), genetic and environmental factors, and a conducive microenvironment likely serve as contributing factors to drive neoplasms and cancers. A major challenge in the gammaherpesvirus field is to understand the mechanism and order in which viral factors drive oncogenic processes in patients that transpire many years after primary infection.

HERPESVIRUS EVOLUTION

Virus Origins

Herpesviruses and their hosts have deeply shared coevolutionary histories. As elegantly summarized by Koonin et al.[74] herpesvirus origins connect to the caudoviruses (order *Caudovirales*) of prokaryotes. Early stages of herpesvirus evolution likely involved linkage of modules of genes involved in capsid structure and assembly and genome replication, plus other genes that facilitated survival in their hosts. Consistent with this, herpesviruses have discernable structural homologs of several caudovirus proteins, including the major capsid protein (MCP; HSV pUL19), which incorporates the unique caudovirus HK97 capsid protein fold, plus capsid maturation proteases and the terminase.[26] These distantly related viruses employ similar mechanisms for capsid assembly.

Prior to the mammalian radiation,[91] the ancestral herpesviruses diverged into at least three major lineages that encompass the virus families of Order *Herpesvirales*: the Alloherpesviruses of fish and amphibians, the Malacoviruses of molluscsm and molluscs, and the α, β, and γHV of birds, reptiles, and mammals that belong to family *Herpesviridae* (Fig. 8.2, Table 8.1, and e-Table 8.3). Although there is little obvious genetic similarity between viruses from the three families, their capsid structures and genomic architectures are well conserved.[31]

The evolutionary distances between closely related herpesviruses that infect different species—such as the rhadinoviruses KSHV (humans) and Herpesvirus saimiri (squirrel monkeys)—suggest that in most instances viral and host speciation occurred at approximately the same time. Herpesviruses thus have intimate shared evolutionary history with their hosts.

Mechanisms of Evolution

A number of rational mechanisms have been used to explain the development and divergence of herpesviruses; because of their timescale and net complexity, some are essentially impossible to prove directly. Mechanisms used to assemble primordial genomes likely included recombination-based acquisition and then subsequent evolution of segments of host DNA, as well as transposition or recombination of viral or cellular DNA or cDNA.

Herpesviruses have employed diverse methods for small-scale genetic changes that have collectively had profound effects on diversification of their biological activities at relatively low cost. These include shifts in base and dinucleotide composition that can be products of viral DNA polymerase mutation rates or occur in response to concentrations of intracellular nucleotide precursors and pools. There can be positive selection for variations in sequences that regulate transcription, splicing, RNA stability, translation, and timing of signal peptidase cleavage.[98,119]

dsDNA viruses that replicate in the nucleus can take advantage of cellular recombination mechanisms to acquire new genes from the host, from unrelated viruses, or from other strains of the same virus. On an evolutionary timescale, many of the host-derived genes of herpesviruses were acquired relatively recently and are involved in modulation of host immune responses.[28] Some genes were recently introduced into limited lineages, including a glycosyltransferase (core *β*-1,6-*N*-acetylglucosaminyltransferase-mucin) acquired from an ancestor of the African buffalo that is present only in viral lineages closely related to Bovine γHV 4.[88]

Recombination between genomes of different virus strains or species is rare, because it requires their presence in the same cell at the same time.[119] Examples of intervirus gene transfers include the presence of homologs of the parvovirus *rep* gene in the genomes of some betaherpesviruses,[141,150] as well as the homolous glycoproteins encoded by members of the HCMV RL11 gene family and human adenovirus E3 genes.[27] Despite the expected rarity of the simultaneous infection step, there is abundant evidence for intraspecies recombination occurring in nature, with recombination being described as "pervasive" in HCMV genomes[133] and contributing to HSV-1 strain variability at a level comparable to mutation.[12] The frequent recombinations are dependent on coinfections of cells with dissimilar strains, which is more likely if the host is superinfected by additional strains. HCMV US2-US11 gene products encode immune suppressive genes that are not needed during primary infection, but might enable superinfections that promote emergence of recombinant strains with enhanced fitness.[79]

Recombination can lead to gene duplication and divergence that allows for neofunctionalization in one of the copies.[14] This strategy has been used across the herpesvirus family, as exemplified by the evolution of the dUTPase gene of the mammalian/avian/reptilian herpesviruses, which appears to have undergone a duplication and subsequent fusion that involved permuting the order of its subdomains.[29,90] Further duplication and divergence events led to the current family of genes that encode proteins with dUTPase function, as well as proteins that lack residues that are essential for dUTPase activity, and have diverse or unidentified functions. Some of these proteins are essential for viral replication, whereas others are not. The betaherpesviruses have exploited this duplication and divergence strategy extensively, with HCMV encoding five additional gene families that each have from 2 to 12 members.[19]

Modifying a protein that is already able to be incorporated into the virion to execute a new function is a much smaller evolutionary challenge than a *de novo* strategy that requires simultaneous or successive development of function and its incorporation into virions. Thus, the strategy of adapting functionally flexible structural scaffolds to new purposes can confer a significant selective advantage. Recent catalogs of conserved herpesvirus protein domains illuminate many of the critical steps during evolution of extant herpesviruses,[14,165] and make it clear that core replication and structural proteins are much more highly conserved than proteins involved in interactions with the host.

Some viruses have evolved to rapidly spread new genotypes through the host population, for instance, the reassortment of influenza viruses that leads to rapid global distribution of new strains by birds. This is in marked contrast to herpesviruses such as KSHV that have been relatively stable in their hosts over a time course that corresponds to the global radiation of humans from our African origins.[55] VZV is another genetically stable herpesviruses that has geographically linked genotype distributions.

In summary, herpesviruses are well adapted to their hosts. In the natural immunocompetent host, fatal infections are rare. From the point of view of virus survival, fatal infections can be counterproductive because they limit opportunities for transmission of virus. This is not always the case when herpesviruses infect a heterologous host, such as the frequently fatal outcomes of infections of cattle with pseudorabies virus of pigs, of humans with simian B virus of macaque monkeys, and the severe malignant catarrhal fever caused by infection of cattle and bison with Ovine γHV 2, a virus that is a relatively benign inhabitant of sheep, its natural host. Thus, in addition to adaptation to specific cellular niches, core lytic replication genes and accessory genes undergo positive selection for temperance properties that enable them to strike a more optimal balance between virus growth in the host and avoidance and stimulation of host responses.[98] By doing so, herpesviruses have persisted in organismal populations of over a remarkable evolutionary timescale.

THE WAY FORWARD

This chapter is intended to introduce the reader to the fascinating world of herpesvirus biology. Coevolution of multiple herpesvirus species adapted to individual species within Kingdom *Animalia* (nine distinct human herpesviruses) demonstrates their evolved success as pathogens. The herpesvirus strategy that links latency and intermittent mild reactivations to enable infection of most members of their host population makes "herpes is forever" a reality for the foreseeable future. Nonetheless, the international community of herpesvirologists is active and engaged, and on the cusp of breakthroughs on many fronts. Decades of vigorous investigation have led to development of a robust data-driven conceptual foundation regarding virion structure and morphogenesis, viral gene functions, regulation of gene expression, and virus–host interactions. The work is not finished. Unbiased and progressively deeper "-omics" approaches will enable understanding of how viral gene products reprogram host metabolism, transcriptomes, and proteomes to meet the needs of the viruses. Single cell analyses suggest that the viruses likely evolved to embrace the stochastic nature of the biology that shapes infection outcomes. Whole genome sequencing of clinical isolates has illuminated responses of the viruses to transmission bottlenecks, antiviral therapy, and immune responses, and enabled identification of nucleotide polymorphisms that influence the functions of viral gene products and ultimately disease outcomes. Understanding the large and complex datasets produced by many newer technologies requires application of quantitative systems biology approaches to enable integration of the multidisciplinary advances in structural biology, molecular biology, cell biology, cancer biology, immunobiology, epidemiology, synthetic chemistry, and computational biology. Immortalized cell lines have long offered ease of manipulation, reproducibility and permissivity for infection, but increased use of primary cells, organoids, tissues from the infected host, and animal models will be needed to develop a more physiologically relevant understanding of virus biology. Together, these approaches will enable identification of key points in latent and lytic infection processes that can be targeted by small molecule inhibitors. Advances in our understanding of virus immunobiology will hopefully enable development of vaccines that can prevent herpesvirus-associated disease, including virus-associated cancers. Subsequent chapters explore in much greater specificity and detail the unique features and strategies of the herpesviruses of humans and their close relatives that have enabled their success on an evolutionary timescale.

> "It is important to go into work you would like to do. Then it doesn't seem like work. You sometimes feel it's almost too good to be true that someone will pay you for enjoying yourself. I've been very fortunate that my work led to useful drugs for a variety of serious illnesses. The thrill of seeing people get well who might otherwise have died of diseases like leukemia, kidney failure, and herpes virus encephalitis cannot be described in words."
>
> Gertrude B. Elion
> 1988 Nobel Laureate in Physiology
> Developed the first successful antiviral drug, acyclovir, to treat herpes simplex virus infection.

REFERENCES

1. Abere B, Li J, Zhou H, et al. Kaposi's sarcoma-associated herpesvirus-encoded circRNAs are expressed in infected tumor tissues and are incorporated into virions. *MBio* 2020;11(1):e03027.
2. Alandijany T. Host intrinsic and innate intracellular immunity during herpes simplex virus type 1 (HSV-1) infection. *Front Microbiol* 2019;10:2611.
3. Alandijany T, Roberts APE, Conn KL, et al. Distinct temporal roles for the promyelocytic leukaemia (PML) protein in the sequential regulation of intracellular host immunity to HSV-1 infection. *PLoS Pathog* 2018;14(1):e1006769.
4. Alwine JC. The human cytomegalovirus assembly compartment: a masterpiece of viral manipulation of cellular processes that facilitates assembly and egress. *PLoS Pathog* 2012;8(9):e1002878.

5. Arias C, Weisburd B, Stern-Ginossar N, et al. KSHV 2.0: a comprehensive annotation of the Kaposi's sarcoma-associated herpesvirus genome using next-generation sequencing reveals novel genomic and functional features. *PLoS Pathog* 2014;10(1):e1003847.
6. Arvanitakis L, Geras-Raaka E, Varma A, et al. Human herpesvirus KSHV encodes a constitutively active G-protein-coupled receptor linked to cell proliferation. *Nature* 1997;385:347–349.
7. Banerjee S, Uppal T, Strahan R, et al. The modulation of apoptotic pathways by gammaherpesviruses. *Front Microbiol* 2016;7:585.
8. Barnes J, Wilson DW. Seeking closure: how do herpesviruses recruit the cellular ESCRT apparatus? *J Virol* 2019;93(13):e00392.
9. Bencun M, Klinke O, Hotz-Wagenblatt A, et al. Translational profiling of B cells infected with the Epstein-Barr virus reveals 5′ leader ribosome recruitment through upstream open reading frames. *Nucleic Acids Res* 2018;46(6):2802–2819.
10. Biolatti M, Gugliesi F, Dell'Oste V, et al. Modulation of the innate immune response by human cytomegalovirus. *Infect Genet Evol* 2018;64:105–114.
11. Bohannon KP, Jun Y, Gross SP, et al. Differential protein partitioning within the herpesvirus tegument and envelope underlies a complex and variable virion architecture. *Proc Natl Acad Sci U S A* 2013;110(17):E1613–E1620.
12. Bowden R, Sakaoka H, Donnelly P, et al. High recombination rate in herpes simplex virus type 1 natural populations suggests significant co-infection. *Infect Genet Evol* 2004;4(2):115–123.
13. Brandariz-Nunez A, Liu T, Du T, et al. Pressure-driven release of viral genome into a host nucleus is a mechanism leading to herpes infection. *Elife* 2019;8:e47212.
14. Brito AF, Pinney JW. The evolution of protein domain repertoires: shedding light on the origins of the *Herpesviridae* family. *Virus Evol* 2020;6(1):veaa001.
15. Bullard WL, Flemington EK, Renne R, et al. Connivance, complicity, or collusion? the role of noncoding RNAs in promoting gammaherpesvirus tumorigenesis. *Trends Cancer* 2018;4(11):729–740.
16. Cesarman E, Damania B, Krown SE, et al. Kaposi sarcoma. *Nat Rev Dis Primers* 2019;5(1):9.
17. Cha TA, Tom E, Kemble GW, et al. Human cytomegalovirus clinical isolates carry at least 19 genes not found in laboratory strains. *J Virol* 1996;70:78–83.
18. Charman M, Weitzman MD. Replication compartments of DNA viruses in the nucleus: location, location, location. *Viruses* 2020;12(2):151.
19. Chee MS, Bankier AT, Beck S, et al. Analysis of the protein-coding content of the sequence of human cytomegalovirus strain AD169. *Curr Top Microbiol Immunol* 1990;154:125–169.
20. Cheng AZ, Moraes SN, Attarian C, et al. A conserved mechanism of APOBEC3 relocalization by herpesviral ribonucleotide reductase large subunits. *J Virol* 2019;93(23):e01539.
21. Cliffe AR, Wilson AC. Restarting lytic gene transcription at the onset of herpes simplex virus reactivation. *J Virol* 2017;91(2):e01419.
22. Close WL, Anderson AN, Pellett PE. Betaherpesvirus virion assembly and egress. *Adv Exp Med Biol* 2018;1045:167–207.
23. Crump C. Virus assembly and egress of HSV. *Adv Exp Med Biol* 2018;1045:23–44.
24. Dai X, Zhou ZH. Structure of the herpes simplex virus 1 capsid with associated tegument protein complexes. *Science* 2018;360(6384):eaao7298.
25. Dargan DJ, Douglas E, Cunningham C, et al. Sequential mutations associated with adaptation of human cytomegalovirus to growth in cell culture. *J Gen Virol* 2010;91(Pt 6): 1535–1546.
26. Davison AJ. Evolution of the herpesviruses. *Vet Microbiol* 2002;86:69–88.
27. Davison AJ, Akter P, Cunningham C, et al. Homology between the human cytomegalovirus RL11 gene family and human adenovirus E3 genes. *J Gen Virol* 2003;84(Pt 3):657–663.
28. Davison AJ, Dargan DJ, Stow ND. Fundamental and accessory systems in herpesviruses. *Antiviral Res* 2002;56(1):1–11.
29. Davison AJ, Stow ND. New genes from old: redeployment of dUTPase by herpesviruses. *J Virol* 2005;79(20):12880–12892.
30. Davison AJ, Taylor P. Genetic relations between varicella-zoster virus and Epstein-Barr virus. *J Gen Virol* 1987;68:1067–1079.
31. Davison AJ, Trus BL, Cheng N, et al. A novel class of herpesvirus with bivalve hosts. *J Gen Virol* 2005;86(Pt 1):41–53.
32. De Leo A, Calderon A, Lieberman PM. Control of viral latency by episome maintenance proteins. *Trends Microbiol* 2020;28(2):150–162.
33. De Pelsmaeker S, Romero N, Vitale M, et al. Herpesvirus evasion of natural killer cells. *J Virol* 2018;92(11):e02105.
34. Denes CE, Miranda-Saksena M, Cunningham AL, et al. Cytoskeletons in the closet-subversion in alphaherpesvirus infections. *Viruses* 2018;10(2):79.
35. Depledge DP, Srinivas KP, Sadaoka T, et al. Direct RNA sequencing on nanopore arrays redefines the transcriptional complexity of a viral pathogen. *Nat Commun* 2019;10(1):754.
36. Dogrammatzis C, Deschamps T, Kalamvoki M. Biogenesis of extracellular vesicles during herpes simplex virus 1 infection: role of the CD63 tetraspanin. *J Virol* 2019;93(2):e01850.
37. Enquist LW, Leib DA. Intrinsic and innate defenses of neurons: detente with the herpesviruses. *J Virol* 2017;91(1):e01200.
38. Erhard F, Halenius A, Zimmermann C, et al. Improved Ribo-seq enables identification of cryptic translation events. *Nat Methods* 2018;15(5):363–366.
39. Ersing I, Nobre L, Wang LW, et al. A temporal proteomic map of Epstein-Barr virus lytic replication in B cells. *Cell Rep* 2017;19(7):1479–1493.
40. Falke D, Siegert R, Vogell W. [Electron microscopic findings on the problem of double membrane formation in herpes simplex virus.]. *Arch Gesamte Virusforsch* 1959;9:484–496.
41. Fan Y, Sanyal S, Bruzzone R. Breaking bad: how viruses subvert the cell cycle. *Front Cell Infect Microbiol* 2018;8:396.
42. Finkel Y, Schmiedel D, Tai-Schmiedel J, et al. Comprehensive annotations of human herpesvirus 6A and 6B genomes reveal novel and conserved genomic features. *Elife* 2020;9:e50960.
43. Finkel Y, Stern-Ginossar N, Schwartz M. Viral short ORFs and their possible functions. *Proteomics* 2018;18(10):e1700255.
44. Full F, Hahn AS, Grosskopf AK, et al. Gammaherpesviral tegument proteins, PML-nuclear bodies and the ubiquitin-proteasome system. *Viruses* 2017;9(10):308.
45. Furlong D, Swift H, Roizman B. Arrangement of herpesvirus deoxyribonucleic acid in the core. *J Virol* 1972;10(5):1071–1074.
46. Gerner CS, Dolan A, McGeoch DJ. Phylogenetic relationships in the *Lymphocryptovirus* genus of the *Gammaherpesvirinae*. *Virus Res* 2004;99(2):187–192.
47. Gibson W. Structure and assembly of the virion. *Intervirology* 1996;39(5–6):389–400.
48. Gibson W, Roizman B. Compartmentalization of spermine and spermidine in the herpes simplex virion. *Proc Natl Acad Sci U S A* 1971;68(11):2818–2821.
49. Glaunsinger BA. Modulation of the translational landscape during herpesvirus infection. *Annu Rev Virol* 2015;2(1):311–333.
50. Gong D, Dai X, Jih J, et al. DNA-packing portal and capsid-associated tegument complexes in the tumor herpesvirus KSHV. *Cell* 2019;178(6):1329–1343.e1312.
51. Gruffat H, Marchione R, Manet E. Herpesvirus late gene expression: a viral-specific preinitiation complex is key. *Front Microbiol* 2016;7:869.
52. Guo H, Kaiser WJ, Mocarski ES. Manipulation of apoptosis and necroptosis signaling by herpesviruses. *Med Microbiol Immunol* 2015;204(3):439–448.
53. Guo H, Omoto S, Harris PA, et al. Herpes simplex virus suppresses necroptosis in human cells. *Cell Host Microbe* 2015;17(2):243–251.
54. Hancock MH, Skalsky RL. Roles of non-coding RNAs during herpesvirus infection. *Curr Top Microbiol Immunol* 2018;419:243–280.
55. Hayward GS. KSHV strains: the origins and global spread of the virus. *Semin Cancer Biol* 1999;9(3):187–199.
56. Heldwein EE. Up close with herpesviruses. *Science* 2018;360(6384):34–35.
57. Heldwein EE, Lou H, Bender FC, et al. Crystal structure of glycoprotein B from herpes simplex virus 1. *Science* 2006;313(5784):217–220.
58. Hellberg T, Passvogel L, Schulz KS, et al. Nuclear egress of herpesviruses: the prototypic vesicular nucleocytoplasmic transport. *Adv Virus Res* 2016;94:81–140.
59. Heming JD, Conway JF, Homa FL. Herpesvirus capsid assembly and DNA packaging. *Adv Anat Embryol Cell Biol* 2017;223:119–142.
60. Hernandez Duran A, Grunewald K, Topf M. Conserved central intraviral protein interactome of the *Herpesviridae* family. *mSystems* 2019;4(5):e00295.
61. Houldcroft CJ, Breuer J. Tales from the crypt and coral reef: the successes and challenges of identifying new herpesviruses using metagenomics. *Front Microbiol* 2015;6:188.
62. Howe JG, Shu MD. Upstream basal promoter element important for exclusive RNA polymerase III transcription of the EBER 2 gene. *Mol Cell Biol* 1993;13(5):2655–2665.
63. Hughes AL. Origin and evolution of viral interleukin-10 and other DNA virus genes with vertebrate homologues. *J Mol Evol* 2002;54(1):90–101.
64. Ingolia NT, Brar GA, Stern-Ginossar N, et al. Ribosome profiling reveals pervasive translation outside of annotated protein-coding genes. *Cell Rep* 2014;8(5):1365–1379.
65. Inoue N, Dambaugh TR, Rapp JC, et al. Alphaherpesvirus origin-binding protein homolog encoded by human herpesvirus 6B, a betaherpesvirus, binds to nucleotide sequences that are similar to ori regions of alphaherpesviruses. *J Virol* 1994;68:4126–4136.
66. James S, Donato D, de Thoisy B, et al. Novel herpesviruses in neotropical bats and their relationship with other members of the *Herpesviridae* family. *Infect Genet Evol* 2020;84:104367.
67. Jean Beltran PM, Mathias RA, Cristea IM. A portrait of the human organelle proteome in space and time during cytomegalovirus infection. *Cell Syst* 2016;3(4):361–373.e366.
68. Jha HC, Banerjee S, Robertson ES. The role of gammaherpesviruses in cancer pathogenesis. *Pathogens* 2016;5(1):18.
69. Johannsen E, Luftig M, Chase MR, et al. Proteins of purified Epstein-Barr virus. *Proc Natl Acad Sci U S A* 2004;101(46):16286–16291.
70. Kattenhorn LM, Mills R, Wagner M, et al. Identification of proteins associated with murine cytomegalovirus virions. *J Virol* 2004;78(20):11187–11197.
71. Kaufer BB, Flamand L. Chromosomally integrated HHV-6: impact on virus, cell and organismal biology. *Curr Opin Virol* 2014;9:111–118.
72. Kobayashi M, Wilson AC, Chao MV, et al. Control of viral latency in neurons by axonal mTOR signaling and the 4E-BP translation repressor. *Genes Dev* 2012;26(14):1527–1532.
73. Kobiler O, Weitzman MD. Herpes simplex virus replication compartments: from naked release to recombining together. *PLoS Pathog* 2019;15(6):e1007714.
74. Koonin EV, Dolja VV, Krupovic M. Origins and evolution of viruses of eukaryotes: the ultimate modularity. *Virology* 2015;479–480:2–25.
75. Kristie TM. Dynamic modulation of HSV chromatin drives initiation of infection and provides targets for epigenetic therapies. *Virology* 2015;479–480:555–561.
76. Kristie TM. Chromatin modulation of herpesvirus lytic gene expression: managing nucleosome density and heterochromatic histone modifications. *mBio* 2016;7(1):e00098.
77. Kronstad LM, Brulois KF, Jung JU, et al. Reinitiation after translation of two upstream open reading frames (ORF) governs expression of the ORF35-37 Kaposi's sarcoma-associated herpesvirus polycistronic mRNA. *J Virol* 2014;88(11):6512–6518.
78. Landolfo S, De Andrea M, Dell'Oste V, et al. Intrinsic host restriction factors of human cytomegalovirus replication and mechanisms of viral escape. *World J Virol* 2016;5(3):87–96.
79. Lassalle F, Depledge DP, Reeves MB, et al. Islands of linkage in an ocean of pervasive recombination reveals two-speed evolution of human cytomegalovirus genomes. *Virus Evol* 2016;2(1):vew017.
80. Li Z, Zhang X, Dong L, et al. CryoEM structure of the tegumented capsid of Epstein-Barr virus. *Cell Res* 2020;30:873–884.
81. Liashkovich I, Hafezi W, Kuhn JM, et al. Nuclear delivery mechanism of herpes simplex virus type 1 genome. *J Mol Recognit* 2011;24(3):414–421.
82. Liu W, Cui Y, Wang C, et al. Structures of capsid and capsid-associated tegument complex inside the Epstein-Barr virus. *Nat Microbiol* 2020;5:1285–1298.
83. Liu ST, Sharon-Friling R, Ivanova P, et al. Synaptic vesicle-like lipidome of human cytomegalovirus virions reveals a role for SNARE machinery in virion egress. *Proc Natl Acad Sci U S A* 2011;108(31):12869–12874.
84. Lo AK, Dawson CW, Young LS, et al. The role of metabolic reprogramming in gammaherpesvirus-associated oncogenesis. *Int J Cancer* 2017;141(8):1512–1521.

85. Longnecker R, Neipel F. Introduction to the human gamma-herpesviruses. In: Arvin A, Campadelli-Fiume G, Mocarski E, et al., eds. *Human Herpesviruses: Biology, Therapy, and Immunoprophylaxis*. Cambridge: Cambridge University Press; 2007:341–359.
86. Lussignol M, Esclatine A. Herpesvirus and autophagy: "All right, everybody be cool, this is a robbery!". *Viruses* 2017;9(12):372.
87. Lyman MG, Enquist LW. Herpesvirus interactions with the host cytoskeleton. *J Virol* 2009;83(5):2058–2066.
88. Markine-Goriaynoff N, Georgin JP, Goltz M, et al. The core 2 beta-1,6-N-acetylglucosaminyltransferase-mucin encoded by bovine herpesvirus 4 was acquired from an ancestor of the African buffalo. *J Virol* 2003;77(3):1784–1792.
89. McElwee M, Vijayakrishnan S, Rixon F, et al. Structure of the herpes simplex virus portal-vertex. *PLoS Biol* 2018;16(6):e2006191.
90. McGeehan JE, Depledge NW, McGeoch DJ. Evolution of the dUTPase gene of mammalian and avian herpesviruses. *Curr Protein Pept Sci* 2001;2(4):325–333.
91. McGeoch DJ, Cook S, Dolan A, et al. Molecular phylogeny and evolutionary timescale for the family of mammalian herpesviruses. *J Mol Biol* 1995;247(3):443–458.
92. McGeoch DJ, Gatherer D. Integrating reptilian herpesviruses into the family *Herpesviridae*. *J Virol* 2005;79(2):725–731.
93. McGeoch DJ, Gatherer D, Dolan A. On phylogenetic relationships among major lineages of the Gammaherpesvirinae. *J Gen Virol* 2005;86(Pt 2):307–316.
94. Mesri EA, Feitelson MA, Munger K. Human viral oncogenesis: a cancer hallmarks analysis. *Cell Host Microbe* 2014;15(3):266–282.
95. Mettenleiter TC, Klupp BG, Granzow H. Herpesvirus assembly: an update. *Virus Res* 2009;143(2):222–234.
96. Michael K, Klupp BG, Mettenleiter TC, et al. Composition of pseudorabies virus particles lacking tegument protein US3, UL47, or UL49 or envelope glycoprotein E. *J Virol* 2006;80(3):1332–1339.
97. Mocarski ES Jr. Comparative analysis of herpesvirus-common proteins. In: Arvin A, Campadelli-Fiume G, Mocarski E, et al., eds. *Human Herpesviruses: Biology, Therapy, and Immunoprophylaxis*. Cambridge: Cambridge University Press; 2007:44–58.
98. Mozzi A, Biolatti M, Cagliani R, et al. Past and ongoing adaptation of human cytomegalovirus to its host. *PLoS Pathog* 2020;16(5):e1008476.
99. Munger J, Bennett BD, Parikh A, et al. Systems-level metabolic flux profiling identifies fatty acid synthesis as a target for antiviral therapy. *Nat Biotechnol* 2008;26(10):1179–1186.
100. Naghavi MH, Walsh D. Microtubule regulation and function during virus infection. *J Virol* 2017;91(16).
101. Nandakumar D, Glaunsinger B. An integrative approach identifies direct targets of the late viral transcription complex and an expanded promoter recognition motif in Kaposi's sarcoma-associated herpesvirus. *PLoS Pathog* 2019;15(5):e1007774.
102. Nevels M, Nitzsche A, Paulus C. How to control an infectious bead string: nucleosome-based regulation and targeting of herpesvirus chromatin. *Rev Med Virol* 2011;21(3):154–180.
103. Nguyen CC, Kamil JP. Pathogen at the gates: human cytomegalovirus entry and cell tropism. *Viruses* 2018;10(12):704.
104. Nightingale K, Lin KM, Ravenhill BJ, et al. High-definition analysis of host protein stability during human cytomegalovirus infection reveals antiviral factors and viral evasion mechanisms. *Cell Host Microbe* 2018;24(3):447–460.e411.
105. Nobre LV, Nightingale K, Ravenhill BJ, et al. Human cytomegalovirus interactome analysis identifies degradation hubs, domain associations and viral protein functions. *Elife* 2019;8:e49894.
106. O'Connor CM, Kedes DH. Mass spectrometric analyses of purified rhesus monkey rhadinovirus reveal 33 virion-associated proteins. *J Virol* 2006;80(3):1574–1583.
107. O'Grady T, Feswick A, Hoffman BA, et al. Genome-wide transcript structure resolution reveals abundant alternate isoform usage from murine gammaherpesvirus 68. *Cell Rep* 2019;27(13):3988–4002.e3985.
108. Ouyang P, Rakus K, van Beurden SJ, et al. IL-10 encoded by viruses: a remarkable example of independent acquisition of a cellular gene by viruses and its subsequent evolution in the viral genome. *J Gen Virol* 2014;95(Pt 2):245–262.
109. Patro ARK. Subversion of immune response by human cytomegalovirus. *Front Immunol* 2019;10:1155.
110. Pellett PE, Davison AJ, Eberle R, et al. Order *Herpesvirales*. In: King AMQ, Adams MJ, Carstens EB, et al., eds. *Virus Taxonomy: Ninth Report of the International Committee on Taxonomy of Viruses*. Oxford: Elsevier; 2011:99–107.
111. Pellett PE, Davison AJ, Eberle R, et al. Family *Herpesviridae*. In: King AMQ, Adams MJ, Carstens EB, et al., eds. *Virus Taxonomy: Ninth Report of the International Committee on Taxonomy of Viruses*. Oxford: Elsevier; 2011:81–92.
112. Pellett PE, Davison AJ, Eberle R, et al. Family *Alloherpesviridae*. In: King AMQ, Adams MJ, Carstens EB, et al., eds. *Virus Taxonomy: Ninth Report of the International Committee on Taxonomy of Viruses*. Oxford: Elsevier; 2011:78–79.
113. Pellett PE, Davison AJ, Eberle R, et al. Family *Malacoherpesviridae*. In: King AMQ, Adams MJ, Carstens EB, et al., eds. *Virus Taxonomy: Ninth Report of the International Committee on Taxonomy of Viruses*. Oxford: Elsevier; 2011:93.
114. Picarda G, Benedict CA. Cytomegalovirus: shape-shifting the immune system. *J Immunol* 2018;200(12):3881–3889.
115. Piedade D, Azevedo-Pereira JM. The role of microRNAs in the pathogenesis of herpesvirus infection. *Viruses* 2016;8(6):156.
116. Pontejo SM, Murphy PM, Pease JE. Chemokine subversion by human herpesviruses. *J Innate Immun* 2018;10(5–6):465–478.
117. Purdy JG, Luftig MA. Reprogramming of cellular metabolic pathways by human oncogenic viruses. *Curr Opin Virol* 2019;39:60–69.
118. Raftery M, Muller A, Schonrich G. Herpesvirus homologues of cellular genes. *Virus Genes* 2000;21(1–2):65–75.
119. Renner DW, Szpara ML. Impacts of genome-wide analyses on our understanding of human herpesvirus diversity and evolution. *J Virol* 2018;92(1):e00908.
120. Ressing ME, van Gent M, Gram AM, et al. Immune evasion by Epstein-Barr virus. *Curr Top Microbiol Immunol* 2015;391:355–381.
121. Rixon FJ, Schmid MF. Structural similarities in DNA packaging and delivery apparatuses in Herpesvirus and dsDNA bacteriophages. *Curr Opin Virol* 2014;5:105–110.
122. Rodriguez-Sanchez I, Munger J. Meal for two: human cytomegalovirus-induced activation of cellular metabolism. *Viruses* 2019;11(3):273.
123. Rodriguez-Sanchez I, Schafer XL, Monaghan M, et al. The human cytomegalovirus UL38 protein drives mTOR-independent metabolic flux reprogramming by inhibiting TSC2. *PLoS Pathog* 2019;15(1):e1007569.
124. Roizman B. The checkpoints of viral gene expression in productive and latent infection: the role of the HDAC/CoREST/LSD1/REST repressor complex. *J Virol* 2011;85(15):7474–7482.
125. Roizman B, Campadelli-Fiume G. Alphaherpes viral genes and their functions. In: Arvin A, Campadelli-Fiume G, Mocarski E, et al., eds. *Human Herpesviruses: Biology, Therapy, and Immunoprophylaxis*. Cambridge: Cambridge University Press; 2007:70–92.
126. Roizman B, Carmichael LE, Deinhardt F, et al. *Herpesviridae*. Definition, provisional nomenclature, and taxonomy. The Herpesvirus Study Group, the International Committee on Taxonomy of Viruses. *Intervirology* 1981;16(4):201–217.
127. Roizman B, Furlong D. The replication of herpesviruses. In: Fraenkel-Conrat H, ed. *Comprehensive Virology*. 3rd ed. New York: Plenum Press; 1974:229–403.
128. Roller RJ, Baines JD. Herpesvirus nuclear egress. *Adv Anat Embryol Cell Biol* 2017;223:143–169.
129. Roy A, Ghosh A, Kumar B, et al. IFI16, a nuclear innate immune DNA sensor, mediates epigenetic silencing of herpesvirus genomes by its association with H3K9 methyltransferases SUV39H1 and GLP. *Elife* 2019;8:e49500.
130. Ruiz JC, Hunter OV, Conrad NK. Kaposi's sarcoma-associated herpesvirus ORF57 protein protects viral transcripts from specific nuclear RNA decay pathways by preventing hMTR4 recruitment. *PLoS Pathog* 2019;15(2):e1007596.
131. Russo JJ, Bohenzky RA, Chien MC, et al. Nucleotide sequence of the Kaposi sarcoma-associated herpesvirus (HHV8). *Proc Natl Acad Sci U S A* 1996;93(25):14862–14867.
132. Schwartz C, De Donatis GM, Zhang H, et al. Revolution rather than rotation of AAA+ hexameric phi29 nanomotor for viral dsDNA packaging without coiling. *Virology* 2013;443(1):28–39.
133. Sijmons S, Thys K, Mbong Ngwese M, et al. High-throughput analysis of human cytomegalovirus genome diversity highlights the widespread occurrence of gene-disrupting mutations and pervasive recombination. *J Virol* 2015;89(15):7673–7695.
134. Singh N, Tscharke DC. Herpes simplex virus latency is noisier the closer we look. *J Virol* 2020;94(4):e01701.
135. Spector DH. Human cytomegalovirus riding the cell cycle. *Med Microbiol Immunol* 2015;204(3):409–419.
136. Stefan A, Secchiero P, Baechi T, et al. The 85-kilodalton phosphoprotein (pp85) of human herpesvirus 7 is encoded by open reading frame U14 and localizes to a tegument substructure in virion particles. *J Virol* 1997;71(8):5758–5763.
137. Stern-Ginossar N, Weisburd B, Michalski A, et al. Decoding human cytomegalovirus. *Science* 2012;338(6110):1088–1093.
138. Streck NT, Carmichael J, Buchkovich NJ. Nonenvelopment role for the ESCRT-III complex during human cytomegalovirus infection. *J Virol* 2018;92(12):e02096.
139. Tang H, Mori Y. Glycoproteins of HHV-6A and HHV-6B. *Adv Exp Med Biol* 2018;1045:145–165.
140. Thaker SK, Ch'ng J, Christofk HR. Viral hijacking of cellular metabolism. *BMC Biol* 2019;17(1):59.
141. Thomson BJ, Efstathiou S, Honess RW. Acquisition of the human adeno-associated virus type-2 rep gene by human herpesvirus type-6. *Nature* 1991;351:78–80.
142. Tirosh O, Cohen Y, Shitrit A, et al. The transcription and translation landscapes during human cytomegalovirus infection reveal novel host-pathogen interactions. *PLoS Pathog* 2015;11(11):e1005288.
143. Tognarelli EI, Palomino TF, Corrales N, et al. Herpes simplex virus evasion of early host antiviral responses. *Front Cell Infect Microbiol* 2019;9:127.
144. Tsai K, Messick TE, Lieberman PM. Disruption of host antiviral resistances by gammaherpesvirus tegument proteins with homology to the FGARAT purine biosynthesis enzyme. *Curr Opin Virol* 2015;14:30–40.
145. Tunnicliffe RB, Hu WK, Wu MY, et al. Molecular mechanism of SR Protein Kinase 1 inhibition by the herpes virus protein ICP27. *mBio* 2019;10(5):e02551.
146. Ungerleider NA, Tibbetts SA, Renne R, et al. Gammaherpesvirus RNAs come full circle. *MBio* 2019;10(2):e00071.
147. Uppal T, Sarkar R, Dhelaria R, et al. Role of pattern recognition receptors in KSHV infection. *Cancers (Basel)* 2018;10(3):85.
148. Varnum SM, Streblow DN, Monroe ME, et al. Identification of proteins in human cytomegalovirus (HCMV) particles: the HCMV proteome. *J Virol* 2004;78(20):10960–10966.
149. Vastag L, Koyuncu E, Grady SL, et al. Divergent effects of human cytomegalovirus and herpes simplex virus-1 on cellular metabolism. *PLoS Pathog* 2011;7(7):e1002124.
150. Vink C, Beuken E, Bruggeman CA. Complete DNA sequence of the rat cytomegalovirus genome. *J Virol* 2000;74:7656–7665.
151. Wang X, Hennig T, Whisnant AW, et al. Herpes simplex virus blocks host transcription termination via the bimodal activities of ICP27. *Nat Commun* 2020;11(1):293.
152. Wang LW, Shen H, Nobre L, et al. Epstein-Barr-virus-induced one-carbon metabolism drives B cell transformation. *Cell Metab* 2019;30(3):539–555.e511.
153. Weekes MP, Tomasec P, Huttlin EL, et al. Quantitative temporal viromics: an approach to investigate host-pathogen interaction. *Cell* 2014;157(6):1460–1472.
154. Whisnant AW, Jurges CS, Hennig T, et al. Integrative functional genomics decodes herpes simplex virus 1. *Nat Commun* 2020;11(1):2038.
155. Wildy P, Watson DH. Electron microscopic studies on the architecture of animal viruses. *Cold Spring Harb Symp Quant Biol* 1962;27:25–47.
156. Wofford AS, McCusker I, Green JC, et al. Betaherpesvirus assembly and egress: recent advances illuminate the path. In: Kielian M, Mettenleiter TC, Roossinck M, eds. *Advances in Virus Research* Vol. 108. 2020;108:337–392.
157. Yang K, Dang X, Baines JD. A domain of herpes simplex virus pUL33 required to release monomeric viral genomes from cleaved concatemeric DNA. *J Virol* 2017;91(20):e00854.
158. You Y, Cheng AC, Wang MS, et al. The suppression of apoptosis by alpha-herpesvirus. *Cell Death Dis* 2017;8(4):e2749.

159. Yu Y, Clippinger AJ, Pierciey FJ Jr, et al. Viruses and metabolism: alterations of glucose and glutamine metabolism mediated by human cytomegalovirus. *Adv Virus Res* 2011;80:49–67.
160. Yu X, Jih J, Jiang J, et al. Atomic structure of the human cytomegalovirus capsid with its securing tegument layer of pp150. *Science* 2017;356(6345).
161. Yu XK, O'Connor CM, Atanasov I, et al. Three-dimensional structures of the A, B, and C capsids of rhesus monkey rhadinovirus: insights into gammaherpesvirus capsid assembly, maturation, and DNA packaging. *J Virol* 2003;77(24):13182–13193.
162. Yuan S, Wang J, Zhu D, et al. Cryo-EM structure of a herpesvirus capsid at 3.1 A. *Science* 2018;360(6384):eaao7283.
163. Zhang Y, Liu W, Li Z, et al. Atomic structure of the human herpesvirus 6B capsid and capsid-associated tegument complexes. *Nat Commun* 2019;10(1):5346.
164. Zheng C. Evasion of cytosolic DNA-stimulated innate immune responses by herpes simplex virus 1. *J Virol* 2018;92(6):e00099.
165. Zmasek CM, Knipe DM, Pellett PE, et al. Classification of human *Herpesviridae* proteins using domain-architecture aware inference of orthologs (DAIO). *Virology* 2019;529:29–42.

CHAPTER 9 Herpes Simplex Viruses: Mechanisms of Lytic and Latent Infection

David M. Knipe • Ekaterina E. Heldwein • Ian J. Mohr • Catherine N. Sodroski

INTRODUCTION

The herpes simplex viruses, herpes simplex virus 1 (HSV-1) and herpes simplex virus 2 (HSV-2), are common human viruses that replicate productively in mucosal epithelium and spread to establish a latent infection in sensory neurons. HSV-1 often infects the oral mucosa and then spreads to the trigeminal ganglia where it establishes a latent infection in sensory neurons. Reactivation of the virus can lead to shedding and recurrent lesions called cold sores or fever blisters. HSV-2 often infects the genital mucosa and spreads to sensory neurons in sacral ganglia to establish a latent infection. Reactivation of the virus leads to recurrent disease and genital herpes. Importantly, HSV-1 infection can also lead to encephalitis, keratitis, and blindness as well as genital herpes, while HSV-2 infection can cause genital herpes, neonatal herpes, and meningitis and is associated with increased human immunodeficiency virus 1 acquisition and transmission (see Chapter 10).

HSV-1 and HSV-2 are two species with formal names of human herpes virus 1 (HHV-1) and human herpes virus 2 (HHV-2). They are classified within the *Simplexvirus* genus in the *Alphaherpesvirinae* subfamily in the *Herpesviridae* family in the *Herpesvirales* order (Chapter 8). These two viruses are sometimes called type 1 and type 2, but they are formally species, so the word "type" is not technically correct. Many of the genetic and phenotypic properties of HSV-1 and HSV-2 are similar, so we will describe them together as HSV where genes and mechanisms are shared by the two viruses.

They share with the other herpesviruses a common virion structure comprising a double-stranded DNA genome within a core in an icosahedral capsid surrounded by an unstructured layer, the tegument, surrounded by a lipid bilayer envelope containing glycoproteins. They also share certain replication and structural proteins with the other herpesviruses, and the ability to establish a latent infection in certain infected cells. Like the other alphaherpesviruses, the HSVs establish a latent infection in sensory neurons. Their ability to undergo lytic infection in one cell type and latent infection in another cell type is one of their most intriguing and novel biological features.

Study of the herpes simplex viruses is important to understand their mechanisms of pathogenesis and latent infection and for the design of prophylactic and therapeutic antivirals and vaccines against them. This basic knowledge is essential to understand the human biology of the virus, as described in Chapter 10. HSV-1 has been the prototype for the study of lytic infection mechanisms by herpesviruses. In addition, the study of the molecular and cellular biology of HSV-1 has illuminated many aspects of human cell and molecular biology. This legacy includes identifying the basic structure of a mammalian cell promoter—the thymidine kinase promoter, nucleoside analogs as inhibitors of DNA polymerases, structures and mechanisms of action of fusogenic proteins, mechanisms of sensing of foreign viral DNA, mechanisms of latent infection by a DNA virus, mechanisms of epigenetic regulation of DNA virus gene expression and infection, critical regulatory events in translation, and mechanisms of innate recognition and evasion.

This chapter will review the basic cellular and molecular mechanisms of HSV lytic and latent infection, their interactions with host cells, how the host cells respond to combat the virus, and the implications of this knowledge for basic cellular biology. Space limitations prevent us from comprehensively covering the large literature on HSV, and we apologize in advance for not being able to cite all of the many rigorous papers on HSV. Therefore, we have cited mostly new references since 2008 as well as selected classical references. Additional reading can be found in the Supplement in the eBook and the HSV chapter in the sixth edition of Fields Virology.[395]

VIRION STRUCTURE

The HSV virion consists of four elements: (a) an electron-opaque core containing the viral DNA, (b) an icosahedral capsid surrounding the core, (c) a largely unstructured proteinaceous layer called the tegument that surrounds the capsid, and (d) an outer lipid bilayer envelope exhibiting spikes on its surface (Fig. 9.1A). Early studies defined the structure of the HSV virion through electron microscopy and biochemical analysis of the virion components. More recent cryo-electron microscopy studies have defined the nucleocapsid structure of HSV-1 and HSV-2 to approximately 3 Angstrom resolution,[99,497,536] described in detail below. The most detailed analysis of the whole HSV-1 virions used cryo-electron tomography to define its structure to 7-nm resolution (Fig. 9.1B and C[160]). This study defined the HSV-1 virion as a spherical particle with an average diameter of approximately 225 nm, with glycoprotein spikes included in the measurement. The nucleocapsid is displaced from the virion center, however, such that it is close to the envelope at one pole, termed proximal, and is 30 to 35 nm away from the envelope at the other pole, termed distal. Single-particle fluorescence measurements of pseudorabies virus, a related alpha-herpesvirus, containing fluorescently tagged proteins confirmed the eccentric positioning of the capsid.[44] Such an asymmetric arrangement may be specific to alpha-herpesviruses because in virions of beta- or gamma-herpesviruses, capsids are positioned closer to the center.[98,534] The tegument, which lacks any regular structure, fills the space between the nucleocapsid and the envelope, forming a "cap."[160] The glycoprotein spike distribution is likewise asymmetric, with more spikes located at the tegument-rich distal pole than the tegument-poor proximal pole.[160] The pronounced asymmetry of the virions has been proposed to arise from the mechanism of tegument assembly, which appears to initiate at the distal pole. This virion asymmetry could be functionally important because during entry, the incoming virions contact the cell at the proximal pole, which is sparsely populated with glycoprotein spikes.[306]

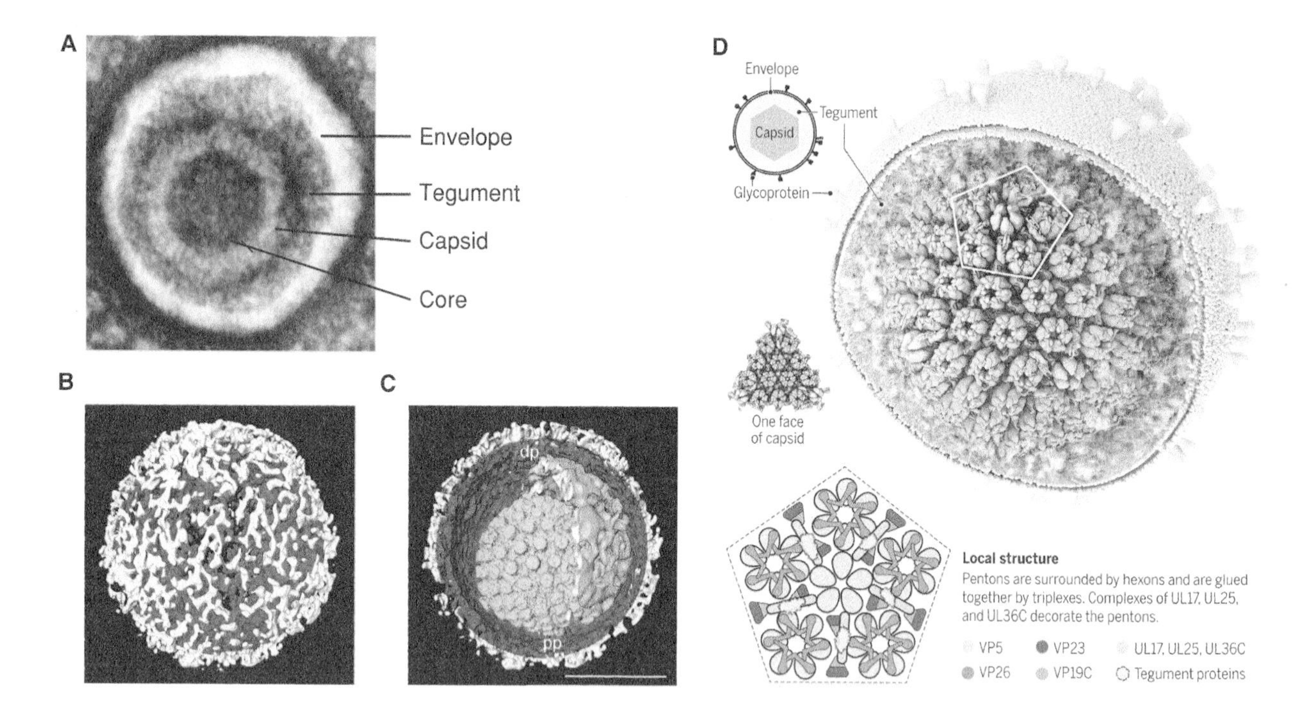

FIGURE 9.1 Structure of the herpes simplex virus (HSV) virion. A: Electron micrograph of a negative-stained HSV-1 virion. The envelope, tegument, capsid, and core are indicated. (Micrograph is provided by Travis Taylor) **B:** Surface image of HSV-1 derived from cryo-electron tomography.[160] The glycoprotein spikes are *yellow*, and the membrane is *blue*. **C:** Cutaway view of the virion interior derived from cryo-electron tomography. Capsid is shown in *light blue*, the tegument is shown in *orange*, membrane is *blue*, and the glycoprotein spikes are *yellow*. (Parts **B** and **C** are courtesy of Alasdair C. Steven) **D:** Schematic view of the HSV-1 capsid structure determined by cryogenic electron microscopy. The capsid is an icosahedron with 20 faces and 12 vertices. The outer shell is composed of four proteins that form pentons, hexons, and triplexes. Three additional proteins form complexes that decorate the vertices. (From Heldwein EE. Up close with herpesviruses. *Science* 2018;360(6384):34–35. Reprinted with permission from AAAS.)

Virion Proteins

Early studies on purified HSV-1 virions suggested that they contain more than 30 distinct proteins, which were designated as virion polypeptides (VP) and numbered sequentially from the top of the gel. HSV proteins have been named based on serial numbering of the virion proteins on a gel (e.g., VP1/2), on the open reading frame encoding them, for example, UL8, or as infected cell proteins, for example, ICP5. Mass spectrometry analysis of purified extracellular HSV-1 virions has detected 44 viral proteins and 49 host proteins.[286] Depletion of several host proteins from mature virions reduces viral replication.[444] Virions are heterogeneous both in composition[44] and structure.[44,160]

Core

The core contains the double-stranded (ds) DNA genome packaged within the capsid as a left-handed spool that is arranged in concentric shells, as revealed by cryo-EM reconstructions.[308] The viral DNA genome is tightly packaged and generates internal pressure of tens of atmospheres,[36] which is capable of driving ejection of the entire viral genome into the nucleus upon capsid docking to a nuclear pore complex.[436] The genome is tightly packaged such that it adopts a liquid crystalline state[46] with restricted mobility but becomes more fluid at physiological temperatures,[402] which should facilitate its ejection from the capsid. The viral DNA genome is described in detail below.

The core does not contain highly basic proteins, such as histones, that would neutralize the negative charges on viral DNA thereby minimizing the repulsive forces within the capsid. However, highly purified virions do contain the polyamines spermidine and spermine in a nearly constant ratio of 1.6 ± 0.2:1 or approximately 70,000 molecules of spermidine and 40,000 molecules of spermine per virion.[152] The spermine contained in the virion is sufficient to neutralize approximately 40% of the DNA phosphate.[152]

Capsid

Early cryo-EM studies have established that the HSV capsid is approximately 125 nm in diameter, with icosahedral T = 16 symmetry. The capsid is composed of 150 hexameric blocks (hexons), 11 pentameric blocks (pentons), and 1 portal. Both hexons and pentons are formed by VP5 (encoded by the U_L19 gene), the major capsid protein. Each hexon is also decorated with a hexameric ring composed of VP26 (U_L35), the small capsid protein. Instead of a 12th penton, there is a portal composed of 12 copies of the protein UL6,[282,308] through which viral DNA is packaged and, presumably, released. Linking together these hexons and pentons are 320 triplexes, heterotrimers of two copies of VP23 (U_L18) and one copy of VP19C (U_L38). Each vertex is further decorated with two additional proteins, UL25 and UL17, which are essential for reinforcing the capsid[433] so that it can withstand several atmospheres of pressure generated by the large genomes without bursting apart. UL25 and UL17 bind the C terminus of the tegument protein UL36, which anchors the tegument layer (described in detail below) to the capsid. Finally, the capsid also contains VP24 (U_L26),[286,298] the protease that cleaves the scaffold during capsid maturation and DNA encapsidation. Recent cryo-EM reconstructions of HSV-1 and HSV-2 capsids at approximately 3 Angstrom resolution (Fig. 9.1D)[99,497,536] showed extensive noncovalent and covalent interactions, particularly the disulfide bonds, that link nearly 3,000 protein copies in the capsid. These high-resolution studies have also revealed significant conformational diversity, especially in VP5, that likely ensures optimal interactions.

Tegument

The space between the capsid shell and the lipid envelope is occupied by the tegument layer unique to herpesviruses. The tegument includes up to 24 distinct virally encoded proteins (see Supplement Table 9.1 Gene List),[286,351] in addition to several host proteins.[444] The tegument has been traditionally subdivided into the inner and outer tegument.[18] The inner tegument, composed of UL36 and UL37, is directly associated with the capsid, and protein copy numbers are tightly controlled.[44,127] The outer tegument is largely unstructured and associates with the viral envelope instead of the capsid through interactions between tegument proteins and the intraviral, also referred to as cytoplasmic, tails of the envelope glycoproteins. The tegument layer is stabilized by extensive protein–protein interactions and is largely structurally maintained even if the viral membrane is removed. Some outer tegument proteins remain associated with the capsid under conditions that supposedly strip away most of the outer tegument,[44] so the boundary between inner and outer tegument may not be so clear-cut.

In addition to linking the capsid to the lipid envelope, tegument proteins play other roles during viral infection. Among the best characterized tegument proteins are UL48, also known as VP16, which activates transcription of immediate-early viral genes; the virion host shut-off (vhs) protein (encoded by the U_L41 ORF), an endonuclease that suppresses host protein expression by degrading mRNA; and UL36, the largest tegument protein (~330 kDa), also known as VP1-2, which is involved in capsid transport,[412] release of viral DNA,[2] inhibition of IFN-β–induced signaling through its ubiquitin-specific protease activity,[535] and a deubiquitinase domain essential for neuroinvasion in pseudorabies virus.[193] Other tegument proteins include UL7, UL11, UL13, UL14, UL16, UL21, UL23, UL37, VP11/12 (U_L46 gene), VP13/14 (U_L47), VP22 (U_L49), UL50, UL51, UL55, US2, US3, US10, US11, ICP0, ICP4, and ICP34.5.[286,351] Tegument proteins form an extensive network of interactions that also includes capsid and envelope proteins. Recent analysis of experimentally detected and computationally predicted protein–protein interactions in HSV-1 has expanded this interaction network.[175]

Highly purified HSV-1 virions have been reported to contain cellular and selected viral gene transcripts.[415] HSV-1 virions copurify with exosomes, which contain host and viral mRNAs and miRNAs.[219] Thus, the RNA content of HSV-1 virions needs to be re-examined.

Envelope

The envelope consists of a lipid bilayer with up to 16 distinct virion envelope proteins, of which 12 are glycosylated and 4 nonglycosylated. The virion envelope glycoproteins are gB (encoded by the U_L27 gene), gC (U_L44), gD (U_S6), gE (U_S8), gG (U_S4), gH (U_L22), gI (U_S7), gJ (U_S5), gK (U_L53), gL (U_L1), gM (U_L10), and gN ($U_L49.5$). The presence of all except gJ, gK, and gN has been demonstrated by mass spectrometry of purified extracellular virions.[286] Virion envelopes also contain at least three (U_L20, U_L56, and U_S9)[286] and possibly more (U_L24 and U_L43) nonglycosylated membrane proteins. Envelope protein composition could vary among viral strains or among virions produced in different cell types, which could explain discrepancies in the literature.

It has been assumed that HSV acquires the envelope lipids from its host. The hypothesis that the lipid composition of the viral envelope is determined by the host was supported by the observation that the buoyant density of the virus was host cell dependent on serial passage of HSV-1 alternately in HEp-2 and chick embryo cells.[440] More recent studies[479] suggest that the virion lipids are similar to those of cytoplasmic membranes and different from those of nuclear membranes of uninfected cells.

STRUCTURE AND SEQUENCE ARRANGEMENT OF VIRAL DNA

The bulk of the HSV-1 virion DNA is linear and double-stranded. Some of the ends of the genomes may be joined or in close proximity inasmuch as a small fraction of the packaged DNA appears to be circular, and the linear DNA circularizes rapidly in the absence of protein synthesis after it enters the nuclei of infected cells. DNA extracted from virions contains ribonucleotides, nicks, and gaps and thus is not super-coiled, as shown on Gardella gels.

The HSV genome can be viewed as consisting of two covalently linked components, designated as L (long) and S (short) (Fig. 9.2A). Each component consists of unique sequences bracketed by inverted repeats.[491] The repeats of the L component, R_L, have been designated as *ab* and *b'a'* (the prime symbol indicating inverted orientation), while those of the S component, R_S, are *a'c'* and *ca* (Fig. 9.2B). The inverted repeats are sometimes labeled TRL (terminal repeat of L) and IRL (internal repeat of L) or TRS (terminal repeat of S) and IRS (internal repeat of S), but these names may be misleading because due to the inversions described below, there are no differences between the terminal and internal inverted repeats. The number of "*a*" sequence repeats at the L–S junction and at the L terminus is variable; thus, the HSV genome as shown in Figure 9.2B can be represented as

$$a_L a_n \mathrm{b} - \mathrm{U_L} - b'a'_m c' - \mathrm{U_S} - \mathrm{c}a_S$$

where a_L and a_S are terminal copies of the sequences with the unique properties described below, and a_n and a_m are terminal *a* sequences directly repeated 0 or more times (n) or present in one to many copies (m).[491] The overall structure of the *a* sequence is highly conserved, but it consists of a variable number of repeat elements. As an example for one strain, the HSV-1 F strain, the structure of the *a* sequence can be represented as

$$\mathrm{DR1} - \mathrm{U_b} - \mathrm{DR2_n} - \mathrm{DR4_m} - \mathrm{U_c} - \mathrm{DR1}$$

with DR1 being a 20-bp direct repeat, U_b being a 65-bp unique sequence, DR2 being a 12-bp direct repeat present in 19 to 23 copies per "*a*" sequence, DR4 being a 37-bp direct repeat present in 2 to 3 copies, U_C being a 58-bp unique sequence, and a final copy of DR1. Adjacent "*a*" sequences share an intervening DR1. The size of the *a* sequence varies from strain to strain, reflecting in part the number of copies of DR2 and DR4.[483] Linear virion DNA contains asymmetric terminal *a* sequence ends. The terminal *a* sequence of the L component (a_L) contains a truncated DR1 with 18 bp and one 3′ nucleotide extension, whereas the terminal *a* sequence of the S component (a_S) ends with a DR1 containing only one bp and one 3′ overhanging nucleotide. The two truncated DR1 sequences form a complete DR1 upon circularization.

The L and S components of HSV are found inverted relative to one another, to yield four linear isomers (Fig. 9.2C).

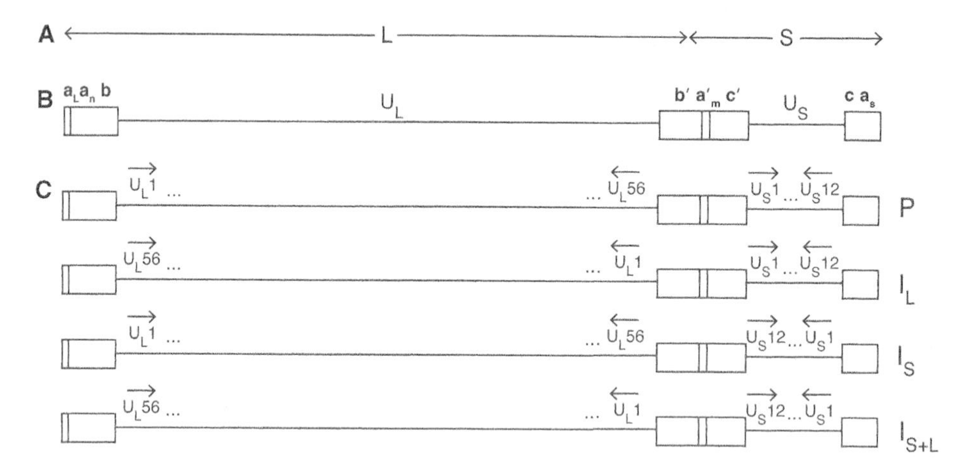

FIGURE 9.2 Schematic representation of the arrangement of DNA sequences in the HSV genome. A: The domains of the L and S components are denoted by the *arrows*. **B:** The line shows the unique sequences (*thin lines*) flanked by the inverted repeats (*boxes*). The letters above the line designate the terminal **a** sequence of the L component ($\mathbf{a}_L$), a variable (n) number of additional a sequences, the ***b*** sequence, the unique sequence of the L component (U_L), the repetitions of the ***b*** sequence and of a variable (m) number of sequences ($\mathbf{a}_m$), the inverted **c** sequence, the unique sequence of the S component (U_S), and finally the terminal **a** sequence ($\mathbf{a}_S$) of the S component. **C:** Diagram showing the orientation of the ORFs for the U_L and U_S regions of the genome for the P, I_S, I_L, and I_{SL} isomers of the DNA. The terminal genes of U_L (U_L1 and U_L56) and the terminal genes of U_S (US_1 and U_S12) are shown to denote the orientation. (Copyright, Catherine Sodroski and David Knipe.)

Populations of unit-length DNA from HSV-1–infected cells and virions consist of equimolar concentrations of the four predicted isomers. The isomers have been designated as P (prototype), I_L (inversion of the L component), I_S (inversion of the S component), and I_{S+L} (inversion of both S and L components). As a result, restriction endonucleases that cleave outside the inverted repeats yield four terminal fragments, each present in one half of the molecules (also called half molar or 0.5-M fragments), and four L–S component junction fragments that are each present in one-fourth of the molecules (also called quarter molar or 0.25-M fragments).[395]

Genetic studies showed that changes inserted into the S repeat "*b*" sequence are rapidly duplicated in the other copy of the repeat, arguing that a mechanism exists for copying one repeat into the other.[104,238,392] This was also later observed for the L component "*c*" repeats, when insertion of a deletion mutation in the *ICP0* (R_L2) gene was found in both repeats.

The internal inverted repeat sequences are not essential for growth of the virus in cell culture, as evidenced by the isolation of mutant viruses in which portions of the unique sequences and most of the internal inverted repeats have been deleted that have been obtained in all four arrangements of HSV DNA. The genomes of these mutants are frozen in one arrangement of the L and S components and do not invert, but all retain their viability in cell culture.

Biochemical studies originally estimated the genome to be approximately 150 kilobase pairs (kbp), with a G+C content of 68% for HSV-1 and 69% for HSV-2, and electron microscopic analysis demonstrated the internal inverted repeats and terminal direct repeats.[395] The first complete genomic sequence for HSV-1 was completed using conventional sequencing for the HSV-1 laboratory strain 17 genome in 1988, and this described the genome as 152,260 bp and 68.3% G+C[309] (GenBank sequence accession number NC_001806), and minor updates altered this sequence to 152,261 bp. This genomic sequence confirmed that there are inverted sequences of approximately 9 kbp bounding the unique L sequences and inverted sequences of approximately 6.2 kbp bounding the unique S sequences. The full genomic numbers were approximate, because the genomic numbers included only single copies of the *a* sequence at the ends of the L component and did not take into account the variation in the size of the *a* sequences (200 to 500 bp each) or the variable number of direct repeats present throughout the genome but especially in the inverted repeats flanking the L and S components.

Illumina high-throughput sequencing further defined the genomic sequence of two HSV-1 viruses, the F laboratory strain and the H129 clinical isolate.[454] This analysis defined the unique and single copies of the repeated sequences of the genomes and based the numbers of repeats on the strain 17 prototype genome. Comparison of the three sequences showed a limited amount of sequence diversity, less than 0.7%, between any pairs of the viruses.[454]

Next-generation sequencing of 20 additional HSV-1 genomes from around the world showed that there was limited variability between strains, the mean pairwise identity being 96.8%.[453] There was evidence of extensive recombination and evidence of as many as four geographical clusters.[453] One North American isolate, KOS, clustered with the Asian isolates[453] and seemed to be an outlier, but there has been speculation that the American source of the isolate, K.O. Smith, may have acquired this virus while serving in Asia during the Korean War.[159]

The first complete genomic sequence for HSV-2 was published for the HSV-2 HG52 laboratory strain in 1998, which defined it as 154,746 bp and 70.4% G+C[113] (GenBank sequence accession number NC_001798), and it has served as the reference genome for HSV-2. The original Sanger sequence of HSV-2 HG52 contains some errors, but these were corrected by Illumina sequencing (GenBank accession number JN561323). The complete genome of the first low-passage HSV-2 isolate, SD90e, was published in 2014.[84] Comparison of the HG52 and SD90e genomes showed only a limited number of small indels,[84] consistent with the conclusion that laboratory-passaged HSV-2 strains have not diverged substantially from primary isolates.

The HSV-1 and HSV-2 genomes are colinear and highly similar[113] with the major difference being the size of the U_S4 gene encoding glycoprotein G (gG). Based on the comparison of these initial genome sequences, the HSV-1 and HSV-2 genomes were estimated to have diverged 6.6 million years ago. However, it was later observed that the HSV-2 genome is most highly related to chimpanzee alphaherpesvirus, which suggested that HSV-2 was derived from CHV or another herpesvirus progenitor and jumped to humans in a second event.[513]

Next-generation sequencing of 34 HSV-2 low passage and lab strains showed limited diversity, less than 0.4% nucleotide diversity between any two viral genomes,[335] less than HSV-1 as described above, consistent with the hypothesized more recent divergence of HSV-2 from the chimpanzee alphaherpesvirus.[513] The limited divergence allowed only a weak geographical clustering of the HSV-2 genomes in this study,[335] but a unique sequence signature was observed in the U_S4 gene encoding glycoprotein G (gG) of certain African isolates.[259] gG is used for ELISA tests to detect HSV-1– and HSV-2–specific antibodies; therefore, this altered gG sequence in African isolates might explain the decreased sensitivity of the gG2-based ELISA test in African populations. Further sequencing studies showed no geographical clustering[210,241] or at most two lineages, one from South African isolates and one that is worldwide.[53]

Genetic Organization of HSV Genomes

HSV DNA encodes at least 84 transcriptional units that encode proteins, as well as additional noncoding RNAs. The HSV-1 and HSV-2 genomic sequences and gene maps are available through the NIAID Virus Pathogen Database and Analysis Resource (ViPR) (https://www.viprbrc.org/brc/viprStrainDetails.spg?ncbiAccession=KT899744&decorator=herpes&context=1575390364537). As described in more detail below, these genes are classified into at least four general kinetic classes, immediate-early (IE), early (E), early/late (E/L), and late (L) genes. The HSV genes are distributed largely in separate, nonoverlapping transcriptional units, although there are some in overlapping transcriptional units and antisense transcripts (Supplementary Fig. 9.1). The canonical genes, largely defined by genome sequencing definition of open reading frames and classical RNA mapping techniques, are mapped in Supplementary Figure 9.1 and listed in Supplementary Table 9.1. The genes are numbered from left to right in each region of the genome on the prototype (P) isomer of the viral genome (Fig. 9.2C). Some genes are located in the unique region of the

L component or the U_L genes. Some are in the unique region of the S component or the U_S genes, some are in the inverted repeats bounding the L component or R_L genes, and some are in the S repeats, the R_S genes. The IE genes tend to map near the termini of the L and S repeats, while the E and L genes are scattered with the U_L and U_S regions of the genome.

Recent genomic approaches have mapped additional transcripts and ORFs on the viral genome (e.g., see[45,515] and the HSV-1 genomic viewer (https://zenodo.org/record/3465873). Further studies will be needed to provide functional validation of the new transcripts and genes.

Genetic Techniques for the Manipulation of the Viral Genome

The various genetic techniques used for analysis of HSV have been described in detail previously[394]; therefore, we will review this area only briefly. Two general methods remain as the major approaches for manipulation of the HSV genomes for genetic studies, for construction of viral mutant strains for viral vectors and vaccines, and for construction of oncolytic viruses. First, genetic alterations can be introduced into the viral genome by homologous recombination following cotransfection of infectious viral DNA with a viral DNA fragment that contains a marker or mutation to be introduced into the viral genome by a double-crossover event.[238] The progeny virus can then be screened or imposed to a selection to get the correct phenotype. Although this approach can be inefficient, CRISPR/Cas9 has been used recently to promote recombination and select for the desired recombinant viruses, such that the progeny from the initial transfection can be pure recombinants.[340]

The second major technique is based on the use of bacterial artificial chromosomes (BACs) to propagate the viral genome in bacterial cells. Mutations can be introduced into the HSV sequences in the BAC, and transfection of the recombinant BAC into mammalian cells yields infectious virus.[188] The genomes cloned as bacterial accessory chromosomes are also amenable to random insertional mutagenesis by transposons.

It should be emphasized that the procedures for generating site-specific mutations, including transfection of viral DNA into mammalian cells, can introduce unintended mutations at distant sites. The obvious and necessary control is to restore the original sequence and then compare parent, mutant, and rescued virus for the predicted phenotype of the mutation. Genomic sequencing can then confirm the sequence changes between the parental wild-type virus, the recombinant mutant virus, and the rescued virus to precisely pinpoint the genetic changes responsible for the altered phenotype. Alternatively, the use of two independent isolates of a mutant that confirm the phenotype is another rigorous approach to rule out secondary mutations.

Viral mutants or recombinants are tested for the essentiality of the gene(s) that have been altered by measuring plaque formation or yields on a given cell line. The essential or nonessential nature of the HSV-1 genes is listed for each ORF in Supplementary Table 9.1. Genes dispensable for viral replication in cells in culture fall into several groups whose products are involved in entry of HSV into specific cells, regulation of gene expression in specific cells, posttranslational modification of proteins, exocytosis, inhibition of host response to infection, and spread of virus from cell to cell. Genes may also be nonessential because host functions can substitute for the viral gene function in certain cell types. For example, the viral thymidine kinase and ribonucleotide reductase can be substituted by cellular enzymes in growing cells, but the cellular enzymes are not expressed in resting neurons and other nondividing cells.

If the viral gene to be mutated is essential for growth in a cell line, stable complementing cell lines have often been used to propagate these null mutant viruses.[104] In this protocol, the gene to be mutated is transfected into and stably maintained in a cell line that serves as the complementing cell line. The complementing cell line is then transfected with intact viral DNA and the mutated DNA fragment. The progeny of transfection are screened for mutants that multiply only in the complementing cells or, if a reporter gene expression cassette has been inserted *in lieu* of the viral gene, mutants that form fluorescent or otherwise distinguishable plaques.[104] Complementing cells of this type have been used to produce replication-defective viruses for herpes vaccines[97] and for vaccine vectors and for production of adeno-associated virus gene therapy vectors.[86]

VIRAL REPLICATION

Overview of HSV Replication

We will provide an overview of the HSV lytic replication cycle (Fig. 9.3) as the foundation for the discussion of the detailed mechanisms of viral replication and interaction with host cells.

To initiate infection, HSV must attach to cell surface receptors. Fusion of the envelope with the plasma membrane or an internal membrane rapidly follows the initial attachment. The de-enveloped tegument–capsid structure is then transported to the nuclear pores where DNA is released into the nucleus.

Transcription of the viral genome, replication of viral DNA, and assembly of new capsids take place in the nucleus. Viral DNA is transcribed throughout productive infection by host RNA polymerase (pol) II, but with the participation of viral factors at all stages of infection. The synthesis of viral gene products occurs through a series of groups of viral proteins leading to the expression of the next group in a cascade fashion (Fig. 9.4). The gene products studied to date form at least four groups, immediate-early (IE), early (E), early/late (E/L), and late (L) as a result of both transcriptional and posttranscriptional regulation. These were originally called α, β, and γ,[186] but we will use IE, E, and L to conform to the more standard terminology for DNA viruses. The IE genes are expressed first and are defined as the genes that are transcribed in the absence of *de novo* viral protein synthesis. The IE gene products are involved in activating expression of the E genes. Several of the E gene products are proteins involved in viral DNA replication and localize to nuclear replication compartments (Fig. 9.5). The bulk of viral progeny DNA is synthesized as concatemers, which are cleaved into monomers during insertion into capsids in the process of nucleocapsid assembly. The L genes are then transcribed efficiently following viral DNA replication, and these gene products are largely involved in assembly of the progeny virions.

Assembly of mature, infectious virions occurs in several stages. After packaging of DNA into preassembled capsids, the nucleocapsid buds through the inner nuclear membrane to generate perinuclear enveloped vesicles that subsequently fuse with the outer nuclear membrane. This process, unique among

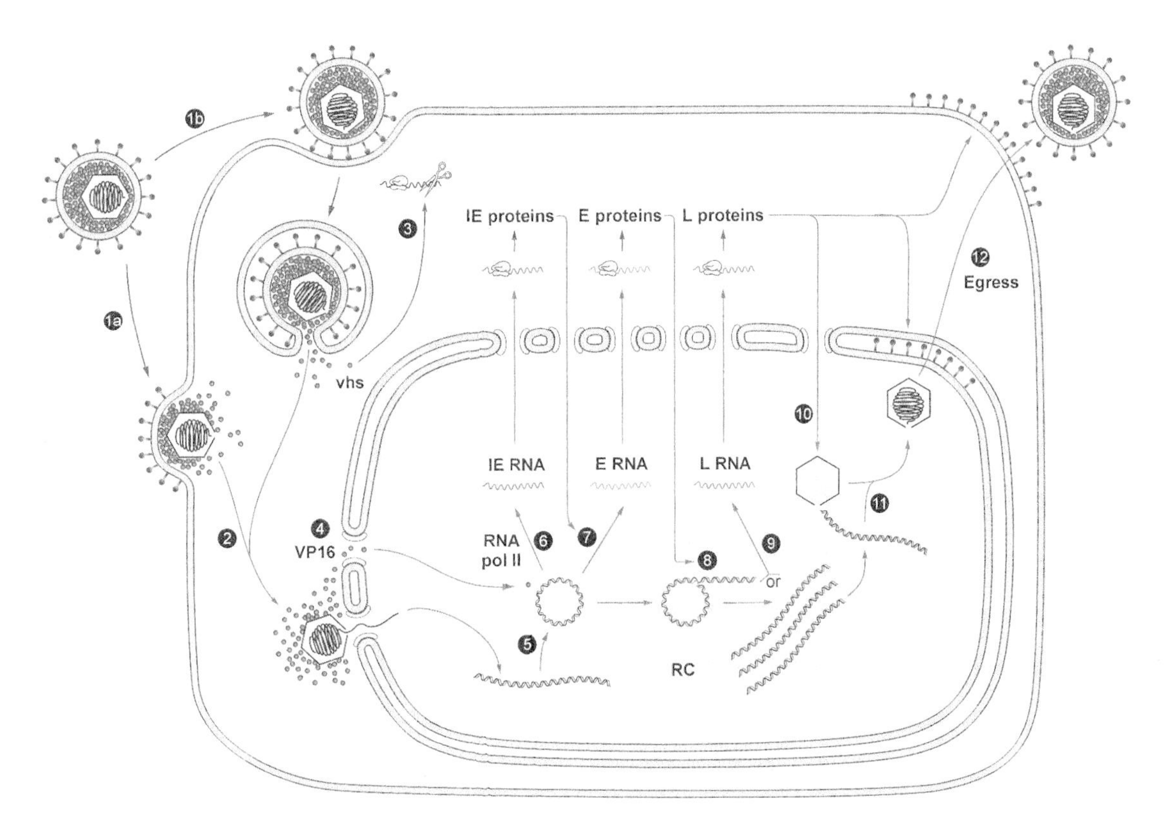

FIGURE 9.3 Diagram of the replication cycle of HSV. The virus binds to the cell plasma membrane and (*1a*) the virion envelope fuses with the plasma membrane or (*1b*) the virus enters by endocytosis, releasing the capsid and tegument proteins into the cytoplasm. (*2*) The capsid is transported to the nuclear pore where the viral DNA is released into the nucleus. (*3*) The *vhs* protein causes degradation of host mRNAs. (*4*) VP16 localizes into the nucleus. (*5*) The viral DNA circularizes and (*6*) is transcribed by host RNA pol II to give first the IE mRNAs. IE gene transcription is stimulated by the VP16 tegument protein. Five of the six IE proteins act to regulate viral gene expression in the nucleus. (*7*) IE proteins transactivate E gene transcription. (*8*) The E proteins are involved in replicating the viral DNA molecule. (*9*) Viral DNA synthesis stimulates L gene expression. (*10*) The L proteins are involved in assembling the capsid in the nucleus and modifying the membranes for virion formation. (*11*) DNA is encapsidated in the capsid. (*12*) The filled capsid buds through the inner membrane to form an enveloped virion, and the virion exits from the cell by mechanisms described below. (Copyright, Catherine Sodroski and David Knipe.)

known vertebrate viruses, allows the capsids to translocate from the nucleus into the cytoplasm. These cytoplasmic capsids next travel along microtubules to vesicles derived from the trans-Golgi network or early endosomes where a second, and final, round of envelopment takes place. There, capsids acquire their lipid envelope and most of the tegument. Cellular secretory machinery transports these mature, infectious virions out of the cell. In normal human fibroblasts, the entire process takes approximately 12 to 24 hours, depending on the multiplicity of infection.

The human host has evolved anti-HSV resistance mechanisms that are expressed constitutively or are induced by innate immunity signaling mechanisms that attempt to block these replication events. In turn, HSV has evolved viral gene products and mechanisms that neutralize these cellular resistance mechanisms. HSV has evolved for millions of years with its human host, and this has resulted in a situation where acute HSV infection is usually not life threatening unless the host is immunocompromised.

Despite the host resistance mechanisms, HSV infection reorganizes the structure of the host cell in many ways to promote its own replication. HSV causes extensive reorganization of cell structure with nuclear changes including margination of chromatin, enlargement of the cell nucleus, formation of replication compartments, disruption of the nuclear lamina and nucleoli, and cytoplasmic changes including disruption of the Golgi apparatus and microtubules.[394] Furthermore, HSV reorganizes much of the molecular machinery of the host cell to redirect transcription and translation to expression of viral RNAs and proteins, and it reorganizes the metabolic apparatus of the cell to promote its own replication. We will consider all of these virus–host interactions as we discuss the mechanisms of viral replication.

Entry of HSV

Routes of HSV Entry Into Target Cells

Early electron microscopy studies by Epstein led to the conclusion that HSV enters cells by fusing its envelope with the plasma membrane. This entry route has been well documented for Vero and HEp-2 cell lines[520] and primary neurons.[293] In contrast, entry by endocytosis only recently became accepted as a significant pathway of entry into many cell types despite the observations that date back to 1969 of enveloped virions in the cytoplasm at early times after infection. HSV enters cell types

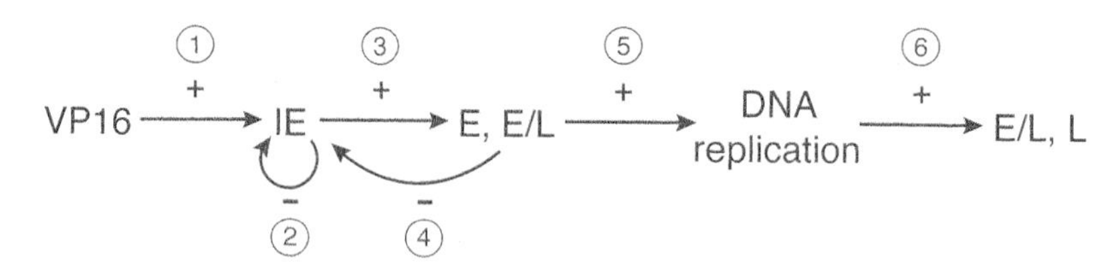

FIGURE 9.4 **Schematic representation of the regulation of HSV gene expression.** *Arrows* represent events in the reproductive cycle, which turn gene expression "on" and "off". (*1*) Turning on of IE gene transcription by VP16, an L protein packaged in the virion. (*2*) Autoregulation of IE gene expression. (*3*) Turning on of E gene transcription. (*4*) Downregulation of IE gene expression by E or L proteins. (*5*) E proteins promote viral DNA replication. (*6*) Turning on of L gene transcription by IE and E gene products through transactivation of L genes, release of L genes from repression, and replication of viral DNA. Note that E/L genes differ with respect to the stringency of the requirement for DNA synthesis. The heterogeneity is shown as a continuum in which inhibitors of viral DNA synthesis are shown to have minimal effect on E/L gene expression but totally preclude the expression of L genes.

such as Chinese hamster ovary (CHO), HeLa, corneal epithelial cells, and keratinocytes by endocytosis followed by envelope fusion with the endosomal membrane.[315,336] Furthermore, HSV appears to take different endocytic routes into different cell types as judged by differences in the sensitivity to inhibitors of endocytosis, for example, inhibitors of endosomal acidification.[336] The choice of a particular entry route, thus, depends on the target cell type.

The productive endocytic entry resulting in infection should be distinguished from the dead-end internalization by endocytosis observed under certain conditions. For example, in the absence of gD–receptor interactions, virions can be taken up by endocytosis but are then degraded by lysosomal enzymes.

A few cellular molecules that may specify entry pathways have recently come to light. For example, overexpression of paired immunoglobulin-like type 2 receptor alpha (PILRα) in CHO cells engineered to express HSV-1 receptor nectin-1 switches the HSV-1 entry route from endocytosis to fusion at the plasma membrane.[23] Another example is αν integrins. In the presence of $\alpha\nu\beta3$, $\alpha\nu\beta6$, or $\alpha\nu\beta8$ integrins, HSV-1 enters nectin-1–bearing CHO or J cells (a baby hamster kidney [BHK] cell derivative) by endocytosis that requires both dynamin and cholesterol, whereas in their absence, entry becomes independent of dynamin and cholesterol.[147,150] Nevertheless, HSV internalization routes have not yet been mapped in detail, and the available data are often contradictory, which emphasizes the need for systematic studies.

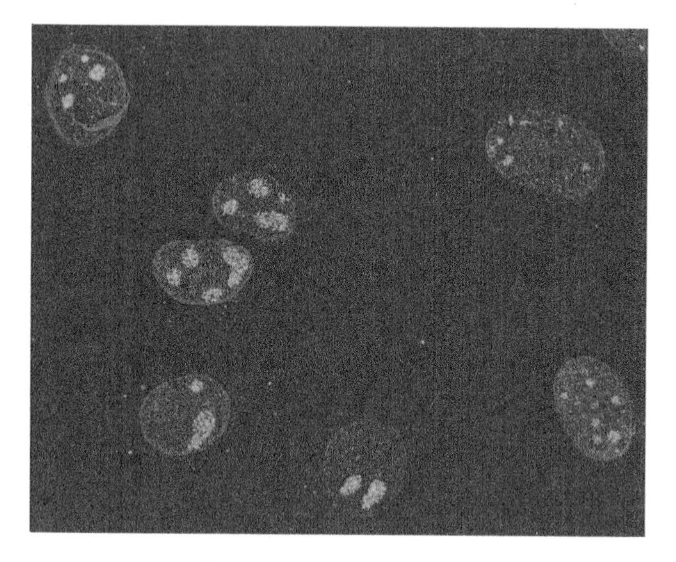

FIGURE 9.5 **Replication compartments in the nuclei of HSV-infected cells.** Shown are Vero cells infected with HSV-1 strain KOS virus and fixed at 7 hours postinfection and stained with anti-ICP8 antibody (*green*) to mark replication compartments and anti-lamin B1 antibody (*red*) to mark the nuclear lamina and define the boundaries of the nucleus. The punctate structures containing ICP8 within the larger globular replication compartments colocalize with sites of viral DNA synthesis. (Copyright, Lynne Chang and David Knipe.)

Viral contributions to the selection of a particular entry route are not well understood. In some herpesviruses, such as human cytomegalovirus (HCMV) or Epstein-Barr virus (EBV), the use of particular entry routes correlates with the involvement of specific viral glycoprotein complexes.[303] By contrast, in HSV-1, the picture is less clear,[222] because the same set of four viral glycoproteins, described in detail below, is required for entry into any cell type. Nonetheless, some nonessential glycoproteins may facilitate the selection of HSV-1 entry routes into specific cells. For example, the N terminus of gK enables HSV-1 to enter neuronal cells by fusion at the plasma membrane.[198] When the N terminus of gK was deleted, HSV-1 switched the entry route to clathrin- and dynamin-dependent endocytosis.[325]

An Overview of the Entry Mechanism

HSV entry requires multiple viral glycoproteins and diverse host receptors. HSV contains up to 16 distinct virion envelope proteins, 12 glycosylated and 4 nonglycosylated. Only 4 of the glycosylated proteins—gD, gH, gL, and gB—are essential for entry into target cells in tissue culture and in animal models, whereas the other 11 proteins are typically referred to as "nonessential" with regard to entry[126] because their deletions have mild phenotypes, if any, in cell culture.[242] Moreover, gD, gH, gL, and gB can also mediate cell–cell fusion of uninfected, receptor-bearing cells expressing these four glycoproteins.[474] gD, gH, gL, and gB are thus considered the core entry machinery of HSV.

HSV entry proceeds through three distinct steps—initial attachment, binding to one of the entry receptors, and fusion of the viral envelope with the host membrane—and requires the coordinated efforts of gD, gH, gL, and gB.[6,126,408] The prevalent model posits that the four viral glycoproteins orchestrate membrane fusion through a sequential activation process or cascade (Fig. 9.6).[27,126] First, HSV uses its receptor-binding glycoprotein, gD, to engage one of its three entry receptors.[439] Binding of gD to its receptor triggers a conformational change within gD[126,251,261] that enables it to bind the gH/gL heterodimer[58] and activate it.[26,27,146] This event, in turn, activates gB,[27,30,75] the fusogen that mediates the merger of the HSV lipid envelope with the cellular membrane.[90,126]

Attachment to the Cell Surface

Regardless of the entry route, HSV initially attaches to the surface of the host cell using gB, along with another glycoprotein, gC, to bind to heparan sulfate moieties of the cell surface proteoglycans (HSPGs). Although the attachment increases the efficiency of infection, it is not required for entry. Lack of HSPG or mutations of the putative HSPG-binding sites of gC and gB to abolish the interaction with HSPG reduces HSV yields 10- to 20-fold. HSV attachment to HSPGs is reversible and likely provides a platform from which virions can interact with entry receptors.

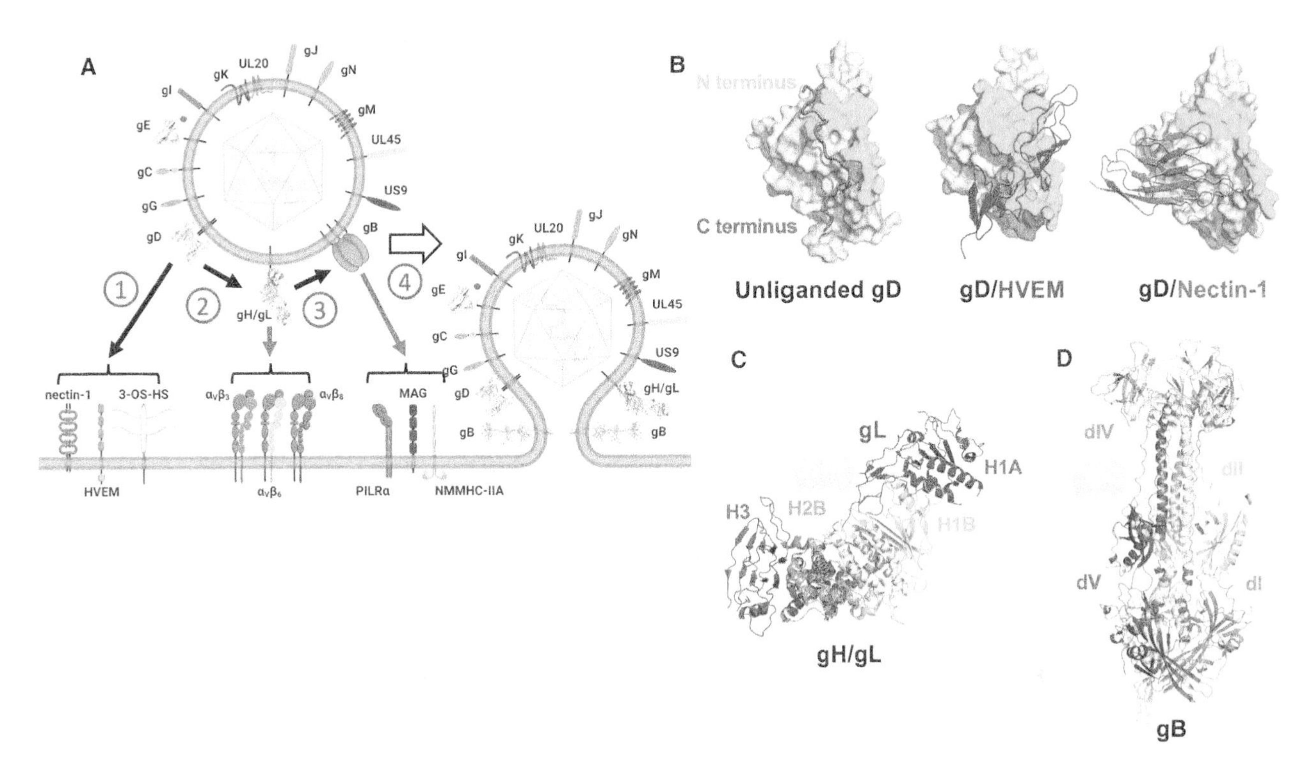

FIGURE 9.6 HSV-1 envelope proteins and their roles in entry and membrane fusion. A: HSV-1 envelope contains up to 16 proteins, 12 glycosylated [gB (RCSB PDB: 5V2S), gC, gD (RCSB PDB: 2C36), gE (RCSB PDB: 2GIY), gG, gH (RCSB PDB: 3M1C), gI, gJ, gK, gL (RCSB PDB: 3M1C), gM, gN], and 3 unglycosylated (UL20, UL45, US9). Entry into cells occurs by fusion of the envelope with the cellular membrane, plasma membrane, or the membrane of an endocytic vesicle and requires four viral glycoproteins gD, gH, gL, and gB. According to the prevalent model, the four glycoproteins orchestrate entry through a sequential activation process termed regulatory cascade. Binding of gD to one of its three cellular receptors, nectin-1, HVEM, or 3-OS-HS (*step 1*), causes conformational changes in gD that enable it to bind and activate the gH/gL heterodimer by an unknown mechanism (*step 2*). Activated gH/gL, in turn, somehow activates gB (*step 3*), the fusogen that mediates the merger of the HSV lipid envelope with the cellular membrane (*step 4*). Additionally, interactions of gH/gL and gB with cellular receptors (a_V integrins, PILRa, NMHC-IIA, and MAG) can influence entry, but how these interactions fit into the current model is unclear. Only the structure of the postfusion form of gB is known. **B:** Crystal structures of unliganded gD (RCSB PDB: 2C36), gD bound to HVEM (RCSB PDB: 1JMA), and gD bound to nectin-1 (RCSB PDB: 3SKU) shown in the same orientation. Unliganded gD is shown as a monomer, for simplicity. HVEM and nectin-1 bind to distinct sites on gD. The N terminus of gD (*green*) forms a hairpin that serves as the HVEM-binding site. Binding of nectin-1 precludes formation of the N-terminal hairpin, explaining why HVEM and nectin-1 cannot bind gD simultaneously. Binding of HVEM or nectin-1 displaces the regulatory C terminus of gD (*red*), which is thought to trigger the regulatory cascade. **C:** Crystal structure of the heterodimeric HSV-2 gH/gL ectodomain (RCSB PDB: 3M1C), colored by domain, with all domains labeled. **D:** Crystal structure of the trimeric HSV-1 gB ectodomain, in postfusion form (RCSB PDB: 2GUM). A single protomer is colored by domain. Abbreviations: HSV-1, herpes simplex virus type 1; HVEM, herpes virus entry mediator; 3-OS-HS, 3-O-sulfated-heparan sulfate; PILRα, paired immunoglobulin-like type 2 receptor alpha; NMMHC-IIA, nonmuscle myosin heavy chain IIA; MAG, myelin-associated glycoprotein. **Panel A** was generated using BioRender (https://biorender.com/). **Panels B–D** were generated using PyMOL (http://www.pymol.org/). (Copyright pending, Adam T. Hilterbrand, Ellen M. White, and Ekaterina E. Heldwein.)

gD Receptors

The interaction of gD with its receptors has been extensively studied in many laboratories. HSV entry into any cell requires the presence of one of its natural receptors that fall into three classes.[439] These various molecules bind gD independently and do not act as coreceptors during entry.

The most widely used HSV receptors are nectins, which are members of the immunoglobulin superfamily. Nectins are cellular adhesion molecules found at adherens junctions where they help maintain the integrity of cell junctions by forming homo- or heterodimers with nectins on adjacent cells. Nectins are found on the surface of many human cell types and tissues, including epithelial and neuronal cells. Nectin-1 is used by HSV-1 and HSV-2, whereas nectin-2 serves a receptor for HSV-2 and some mutant forms of HSV-1. Under selective pressure, HSV-1 can evolve to use nectin-2, -3, and -4 as entry receptors by acquiring mutations in gD and gB.[475]

The second gD receptor is a protein designated as herpes virus entry mediator (HVEM), a member of the tumor necrosis factor receptor superfamily. Both HSV-1 and HSV-2 can use HVEM as an entry receptor. HVEM is found mostly on T lymphocytes where it binds its natural ligands B and T lymphocyte attenuator (BTLA), CD160, and LIGHT and serves as a molecular switch that delivers bidirectional survival, proinflammatory and inhibitory signals to immune cells including T cells and natural killer T cells.[389]

The third gD receptor is a 3-O-sulfonated derivative of heparan sulfate (3-OS-HS) that results from modification of HS by the HS 3-O-sulfotransferase. This enzyme is present in the brain, but little is known about its role in natural HSV infection.

The presence of nectins on the surface of epithelial and neuronal cells, which are major targets of HSV, suggests that they are the primary HSV receptors. By contrast, lymphocytes are not a common target of HSV, so the importance of HVEM in HSV infection of the host is less clear. Mice with a double HVEM and nectin-1 knockout were resistant to vaginal HSV-2 infection, suggesting that these are the major receptors used during infection of epithelial cells.[465] However, single knockouts of nectin-1 or HVEM have shown that nectin-1 is more important for infection by vaginal route. For example, whereas nectin-1 knockout in mice reduced vaginal HSV-2 infection but could not prevent viral spread to enervating sensory ganglia, HVEM knockout had little effect on either parameter.[465] Likewise, in the intracranial mouse model of infection, nectin-1 knockout precluded infection and the ensuing encephalitis,[243] whereas mice lacking HVEM were indistinguishable from the wild-type mice.[243] Recent studies suggested that HVEM plays an important role during ocular infection in the context of the murine herpes keratitis model. But instead of serving as an entry receptor, HVEM appears to function as a proinflammatory factor.[124]

Both nectin-1 and HVEM are probably important in HSV infection and pathogenesis in humans because 49 tested clinical strains of HSV-1 and HSV-2 could use either nectin-1 or HVEM as entry receptors regardless of the origins of the virus (e.g., obtained from oral or genital lesions, encephalitis, or disseminated herpes of neonates). A major remaining challenge is determining the relative contributions of nectin-1 versus HVEM in human hosts because these molecules are broadly expressed and can both function as HSV entry receptors.

Structure of gD and Its Interactions With Receptors

The mature HSV-1 gD is a 369-amino acid protein, with a 316-amino acid ectodomain. Crystal structures of gD from HSV-1[251] and HSV-2[263] have revealed that the ectodomain has a V-like immunoglobulin (IgV) core, residues 56 to 184, with large N- and C-terminal extensions that are involved in receptor binding and triggering of the fusogenic cascade and undergo large conformational changes.[126] Crystal structures of several gD/receptor complexes, HSV-1 gD/HVEM, HSV-1 gD/nectin-1,[109,541] and HSV-2 gD/nectin-1,[288] along with mutational and biochemical studies,[126] have characterized gD/receptor interactions in great detail (Fig. 9.6).

The HVEM-binding site of gD is formed by the N-terminal hairpin of gD, residues 1 to 32, buttressed by the IgV core (Fig. 9.6B). Several sets of interactions at the gD/HVEM interface are critical for the stability of the complex. The N-terminal gD hairpin that composes the HVEM-binding site is conformationally flexible and only forms in the presence of HVEM. HVEM is composed of four cysteine-rich domains (CRDs), and gD binds to the most membrane distal CRD1. The gD-binding site on HVEM overlaps the binding site of one of its natural cellular ligands, BTLA, implying a possible function for gD in modulating the host immune response.

3-OS-HS likely binds gD somewhere within its N-terminal hairpin because mutations in this region have a similar effect on interactions with HVEM and 3-OST-HS. Two positively charged pockets on the surface of gD, which are occupied by sulfate ions in the crystal structure of the HSV-1 gD/HVEM complex, could potentially accommodate sulfate moieties of 3-OS-HS, and one such pocket lies in the vicinity of the HVEM-binding hairpin.

The binding site on gD for nectin-1 was mapped using mutational analysis long before the crystal structure of the gD/nectin-1 complex became available. The nectin-1–binding site is located within the IgV-like core near the HVEM-binding site but does not overlap it (Fig. 9.6B). Nevertheless, HVEM and nectin-1 cannot bind to gD simultaneously. The N-terminal hairpin of gD that forms the HVEM-binding site partially occludes the nectin-1–binding site.[109,251] Conversely, binding of nectin-1 to gD precludes the formation of the N-terminal HVEM-binding hairpin. HSV-1 gD interacts with the V domain of nectin-1[109] that mediates nectin-1 dimerization, which explains how gD can disrupt nectin/nectin interactions at cell junctions.[40]

Triggering of the Fusogenic Cascade and the Regulatory Role of the gD C Terminus

According to the prevalent model, a gD receptor triggers a cascade of events in which gD, the gH/gL heterodimer, and gB sequentially undergo conformational changes that lead to membrane fusion[27,126] (Fig. 9.6). Binding of gD to one of its receptors causes conformational changes that enable it to bind and activate the gH/gL heterodimer. The C terminus of the gD ectodomain, residues 261 to 316, plays an important role in receptor-dependent triggering of the regulatory cascade that leads to membrane fusion. The C terminus of gD, especially, a proline-rich region within the gD C terminus referred to as the profusion domain, is required for viral entry and fusion, and its truncations render gD unable to promote fusion. Moreover, antibodies targeting the gD C terminus inhibit cell–cell fusion and viral spread.[117,262]

The C terminus is disordered in the isolated, monomeric HSV-1 gD ectodomain. However, in the dimeric form stabilized by an engineered intermolecular disulfide at position 316—designed to mimic the stabilizing influence of the transmembrane domain[251]—the C terminus folds against the IgV-like core. The disulfide mutant is thought to recapitulate the native HSV-1 gD dimer on the viral envelope. The positioning of the C terminus in the unliganded HSV-1 gD occludes the nectin-1–binding site and prevents the formation of the HVEM-binding hairpin. Therefore, the C terminus must exist in a dynamic equilibrium that would enable its displacement by either nectin-1 or HVEM. Indeed, engineered disulfides that lock the C terminus in place prevent receptor binding.[251] Conversely, mutations in gD that either eliminate the C terminus or block its interactions with the IgV-like core increase the affinity of gD for both receptors.[251] A gD mutant containing a point mutation that precludes binding of the C terminus to the IgV-like core—which effectively disrupts its autoinhibitory conformation—is constitutively active in fusion even in the absence of gD receptors,[143] albeit at a reduced level. The displacement of this C terminus is thus sufficient to trigger the downstream events required for fusion. The apparent autoinhibitory nature of the C terminus of gD likely serves to couple receptor binding to the triggering of the regulatory cascade. This mechanism can also explain how binding of gD to three very different receptors produces the same triggering effect.

Additional evidence in support of the C terminus as key in downstream events comes from gD chimeras—engineered forms of gD that no longer bind its natural receptors and instead interact with heterologous receptors, used in retargeting HSV for oncolytic therapy. Surprisingly, much of gD could be substituted with heterologous sequences without any apparent defect in fusion activation. How binding of a heterologous receptor to gD chimeras can trigger subsequent fusion events is unknown, but all chimeras had the native C terminus. One possibility is that the gD chimeras may be unable to adopt the autoinhibitory conformation and are, thus, constitutively active, akin to the mutant in which the C terminus cannot bind the IgV-like core.

How the release of the C terminus activates gH/gL is unknown. It has been proposed that the C terminus binds gH/gL directly.[146] An alternative hypothesis, based on characterization of neutralizing anti-gD antibodies that do not block its receptor interactions, is that gH/gL binds the IgV-like core at a site in the vicinity of the receptor-binding site rather than the C terminus.[28,58,262] The respective interaction sites on gD and gH/gL have been mapped using antibodies that block their interactions[57,58] but await confirmation by high-resolution structures of the gD/gH/gL complexes.

gB Is the Conserved Viral Fusogen

gB is conserved across all three subfamilies of herpesviruses and is essential for viral entry, spread, and cell–cell fusion.[90,126] gB is also the target of neutralizing antibodies.[59] The first suggestion that gB was the fusogen came from the crystal structure of the postfusion form of HSV-1 gB[171] that revealed unexpected structural similarities to the fusogen of vesicular stomatitis virus (VSV), glycoprotein (G).[386] Since then, a number of structural and mutagenesis studies have firmly established gB as a viral fusogen responsible for mediating virus and host membrane fusion during viral entry.[85,126]

Viral fusogens mediate the merger of the viral envelope and host membrane during entry and cell spread by pulling the two apposed membranes together while undergoing large-scale refolding from the metastable prefusion to the stable postfusion form.[168] Three classes of viral fusogens are currently recognized.[168] gB is one of the founding members of class III, which also includes G of rhabdoviruses, for example, VSV, gp64 from baculoviruses of insects,[216] and Gp of thogotoviruses.[361] It is the newest, least well-characterized class, partly because the high-resolution structures of both the prefusion and the postfusion forms are known only for VSV G.[386] The 2.7-Angstrom crystal structure of the postfusion form of HSV-1 gB ectodomain revealed a trimeric spike composed of five distinct domains.[171] The recently determined approximately 9-Angstrom cryo-ET reconstruction of the trimeric prefusion form[490] showed a more compact conformation consistent with substantial conformational rearrangements. Therefore, despite being unusual in requiring several additional proteins for function, like other viral fusogens, gB appears to facilitate membrane fusion by undergoing large refolding.

The Fusogenic Activity of gB Is Controlled by Its Cytoplasmic Domain

In addition to the ectodomain, gB also contains the membrane-proximal (MPR), the transmembrane (TMD), and the cytoplasmic (CTD) domains that are essential for function.[90] Moreover, the CTD appears to restrain the fusogenic activity of gB because a number of point mutations, insertions, or truncations within this domain, termed hyperfusogenic or syncytial mutations, increase cell–cell fusion in the context of infected cells or uninfected cells expressing gD, gH, gL, gB,[90] presumably due to a reduced kinetic energy barrier for the fusogenic refolding of the gB ectodomain.[390] The 3.6-Angstrom crystal structure of the full-length postfusion gB from HSV-1 revealed that the MPR-TMD-CTD forms a uniquely folded trimeric pedestal underneath the ectodomain, a dynamic structure stabilized by extensive protein/protein and protein/membrane interactions.[89] Although the postfusion conformation of the ectodomain suggested that the CTD also adopted the postfusion form, the hyperfusogenic mutations target interfaces and structural motifs that stabilize the observed CTD structure, which suggests that a similar CTD structure stabilizes gB in its prefusion form. This has led to a "clamp" model whereby the CTD acts as a clamp that inhibits the fusogenic refolding of gB by somehow stabilizing the ectodomain in its prefusion conformation. Hyperfusogenic mutations would then lower the energy barrier and increase gB activity by destabilizing the inhibitory CTD structure.[89]

gB Receptors

In addition to its conserved fusogenic role, gB has been reported to bind three cellular receptors, paired immunoglobulin-like type 2 receptor-α (PILRα), nonmuscle myosin heavy chain IIA (NMMHC-IIA), and myelin-associated glycoprotein (MAG). PILRα is an inhibitory component of an immunoregulatory receptor pair, binds gB, and supports HSV-1 entry into certain cell types in the absence of gD receptors but is not required for HSV entry into all cells.[409] This receptor may contribute to infections of retinal[427] and corneal[24] epithelial cells, but the clinical significance has not yet been established. The other two receptors, NMMHC-IIA[21] and MAG,[450] have been both reported to enhance HSV entry.,

Role of gH/gL

gH and gL form a stable 1:1 complex and, in HSV, neither protein appears stable without the other. HSV-1 gH is an 838-amino acid glycoprotein that has an 802-amino acid ectodomain, a single C-terminal transmembrane anchor, and a short intraviral (or cytoplasmic) tail. HSV-1 gL is a 224-amino acid glycoprotein that lacks a transmembrane region and is retained on the viral envelope or cell surface due to its interaction with gH. The crystal structure of the extracellular portion of the HSV-2 gH/gL revealed an unusual boot-shaped complex with no structural or functional similarity to any other proteins.[75] gH is composed of individual domains H1A, H1B, H2A, H2B, and H3, sequentially arranged from N to C terminus. gL is "sandwiched" between domains H1A and H1B and interacts extensively with both, illustrating why gH and gL are always found as a complex. A similar architecture was observed in gH/gL structure from another alphaherpesvirus, varicella-zoster virus (VZV).[522]

The precise function of the gH/gL heterodimer is unclear. Initially proposed to have fusogenic properties, gH/gL does not resemble any known viral fusion proteins nor does it have a known functional counterpart in other enveloped viruses.[75] In some herpesviruses, gH/gL binds cellular receptors either directly, for example, in Kaposi's sarcoma herpesvirus (KSHV),[164] or indirectly, by forming a complex with a receptor-binding protein, for example, in HCMV.[215,303] In HSV-1, however, the evidence as to whether or not gH/gL binds integrins to enter cells is conflicting,[148,150] and the integrin-binding RGD motif in HSV-1 gH is not required for its function. Nonetheless, the requirement of gH/gL for entry and cell–cell fusion in all herpesviruses indicates a conserved function. gH/gL has been proposed to act as a unique herpesviral adaptor that transmits the triggering signals from various nonconserved receptor-binding proteins to the highly conserved fusion protein gB.[443] Specifically, HSV gH/gL is currently thought to receive a triggering signal from receptor-bound gD and transmit it to gB to activate its fusogenic function.[30,75]

To do so, gH/gL must interact with gB, but relevant complexes have not yet been detected in any herpesviruses, although a covalent gB-gH/gL complex of unknown function has been observed in HCMV.[481] Instead, gB/gH interactions have been inferred from fluorescence complementation experiments, in which two complementary segments of a split fluorescent protein were fused to the C termini of gB and gH.[29] In uninfected, receptor-bearing cells expressing gH, gL, and gB, the addition of soluble gD triggers cell–cell fusion, and in this system, fluorescence complementation was detected only in the presence of gD.[29] This observation suggested that gH/gL and gB interact only in response to a gD/receptor interaction, which implied that the gD/receptor interaction causes gH/gL to activate gB instead of relieving repression of gB by gH/gL. Several neutralizing antibodies against gB or gH/gL inhibited both fluorescence complementation and fusion, which led to the conclusion that gB and gH/gL interact through their ectodomains and that this interaction is required for membrane fusion.[27,30,75] Elucidating the role of gH/gL in promoting fusion and the mechanism by which it does so would benefit from a detailed understanding of how it interacts with gB.

Several mutational studies have shown that the 14-amino acid cytoplasmic tail of HSV-1 gH is required for fusion.[90] For example, a systematic study of HSV-1 gH C-terminal truncation mutants demonstrated a correlation between the extent of cell–cell fusion and the length of the gH cytoplasmic tail.[390] However, the mechanism is yet unclear.

Entry and Signaling

Virion attachment to cells triggers multiple signaling events inside the cell. Indeed, binding of HSV-1 to the cell surface releases intracellular Ca^{2+} stores[71] and increases intracellular levels of Cl^- ions,[544] both of which appear important for subsequent entry. One important signaling event is the activation of the cellular phosphoinositide 3-kinase (PI3K),[71,544] which induces several signaling cascades, each of which has been reported to promote virus entry, for example, Akt[70,71] and Cdc42.[343] PI3K/Akt signaling triggers calcium release from the endoplasmic reticulum.[71] PI3K/Akt signaling also leads to activation of NF-κB, which is necessary for establishing infection.

These signaling events appear to promote infection through multiple mechanisms. For example, by inhibiting actin depolymerization, HSV can promote actin polymerization underneath the cell membrane that may cluster receptors near the virion, aiding in entry.[544] Calcium release from the ER, which controls cytoskeletal dynamics, may promote capsid trafficking to the nucleus upon entry.

Translocation of Capsids to the Nucleus From the Site of De-envelopment

Upon fusion of the viral envelope with a cell membrane, the capsid—along with the tegument—is deposited into the cytoplasm. Early studies documented the accumulation of empty capsids at the nuclear membrane. The capsid must, therefore, traverse the cytoplasm, dock at a nuclear pore, and release its genome into the nucleoplasm. However, being approximately 125 nm in diameter, the capsid is too large to passively diffuse to the nucleus through the viscous, crowded cytoplasm. Instead, capsids move from the periphery to the nucleus along microtubules[436] by recruiting the microtubule motor proteins.[375,436]

This process initiates with a partial disassembly of the tegument. Most, if not all, of the outer tegument proteins dissociate from the capsid, and their destinations within the cells vary. Some stay in the cytoplasm, for example, UL41, also known as the viral host shutoff (vhs) protein, whereas others, such as VP16, travel to the nucleus independently of the capsid. The two longest known and best studied of these virion-delivered effectors are vhs, an endonuclease that rapidly shuts off host protein synthesis by degrading mRNA, and VP16, which activates transcription of viral IE genes. The roles of these and other virion-delivered tegument proteins in infection are described in detail later on in this chapter.

By contrast, the inner tegument proteins UL36, UL37, and US3 remain capsid associated as demonstrated by immunogold electron microscopy and by live-cell imaging of recombinant fluorescent viruses.[7,19] US3 is a kinase that in pseudorabies virus has been shown to activate cellular protein cofilin, which disassembles actin filaments.[197] This activity is thought to allow the capsids to breech the barrier of cortical filamentous actin, which impedes intracellular capsid trafficking.[306] UL36 facilitates capsid transport by recruiting the microtubule motor proteins dynein, dynactin, and kinesins.[375,537]

In mammalian cells, dynein and its cofactors transport cargo toward the minus-end of microtubules, whereas multiple kinesins mediate plus-end-directed transport.[381] Dynein, along with dynactin and cytoplasmic linker protein 170 (CLIP-170), is responsible for capsid trafficking toward the nucleus and their inhibition or depletion blocks long-range capsid movement postentry.[212] Dynein does not transport the capsids all the way to the nucleus, however, because the minus-ends of microtubules are bundled around the centrosome, also known as the microtubule-organizing center (MTOC). Microtubules are produced at the centrosome and radiate out from it. Indeed, capsids have been observed to transiently accumulate at the centrosome on their way to the nucleus.[436] Therefore, a plus-end-directed motor is required to transport the capsids from the centrosome to the nucleus. Kinesins have been hypothesized to fulfill this role, but this has not been formally tested yet. However, another cellular protein, dystonin/BPAG1, plays an important role during the final step of capsid transport[307] and is recruited to the capsid by binding UL37.[356] Although the precise contribution of dystonin/BPAG1 to this process is unknown, its depletion reduces transport from the centrosome to the nucleus.[307] The nuclear localization signal of UL36 also contributes to this final transport step to the nucleus.[2]

Upon reaching the nucleus, capsids bind to nuclear pore complexes (NPCs).[18] Host nuclear factor importin β as well as the nucleoporins that extend from the cytosolic surface of the NPC, Nup358/RanBP2 and Nup214/CAN, are involved in docking of capsids to nuclear pores.[91,344,355] Furthermore, *in vitro* reconstitution studies showed that capsids bind to the NPC and release viral DNA in the presence of cytosol and an energy source.[344] Interaction of the capsid with the NPC thus seems to trigger the release of the viral genome.

Both UL36[1,3] and UL25[192,369,388] are critical for the release of the viral genome from the capsid. Early studies with the temperature-sensitive HSV-1 *ts*B7 mutant, which was subsequently mapped to the U_L36 gene, showed that at the nonpermissive temperature, DNA-containing capsids accumulate at nuclear membranes.[235] The DNA is released from the capsids on temperature shift-down, and viral gene expression ensues. More recent studies have shown that UL36 must be cleaved to allow release of the viral DNA.[211] UL25, just as HSV-1 capsids, can bind to Nup214/CAN.[355,369] Mechanistic roles of either UL36 or UL25 in genome release remain unclear, however.

Capsids dock at NPCs such that a vertex points into the pore.[344] After docking, viral DNA genomes are likely released through the portal, located at one of the vertices, by a pressure-driven ejection mechanism, similar to bacteriophages.[330]

Gene Expression in HSV-Infected Cells

Classification of Viral Gene Products: General Summary

The total coding capacity of HSV includes at least 84 canonical ORFs, which encode a diversity of lytic proteins (see eBook Supplementary Fig. 9.1), a number of long noncoding RNAs, and as many as 29 microRNAs as described in the eBook Supplementary Table 9.1. Viral lytic gene products form several groups expressed coordinately in a cascade fashion defined originally in human HEp-2 cells and are grouped based on their kinetics of and requirements for expression[185,186] (Fig. 9.4). The immediate-early (IE) genes are expressed first followed by early (E), early/late (E/L) or leaky-late, and late (L) or true-late genes. The designations reflect the order of their accumulation in infected cells, and the accumulation of IE and E gene products proceeds normally in the presence of inhibitors of viral DNA synthesis. IE genes do not require prior viral protein synthesis for their expression. A common property of the six IE genes encoding the proteins ICP4, ICP0, ICP22, ICP27, US1.5, and ICP47 is the presence of a response element in their upstream sequences that is bound by a VP16-mediated complex of host proteins. At least two of the six IE proteins, ICP4 and ICP0, are required for the optimal expression of E genes, exemplified by the U_L29 gene encoding ICP8 and the U_L23 gene encoding the viral thymidine kinase. The accumulation of the products of L genes, as exemplified by the U_S11, U_L38, and U_L44 gene products, strictly requires viral DNA synthesis and the viral proteins ICP4, ICP0, ICP22, ICP27, and US1.5. A characteristic of at least some L genes is that the requirement for viral DNA synthesis is encoded within the 5′ transcribed noncoding domains.

In contrast to the E gene products, the accumulation of E/L gene products exemplified by ICP5/VP5, the major capsid protein, is affected to various degrees by inhibitors of viral DNA synthesis. Neither E nor E/L promoters share common response elements, and most likely the order and quantity of the gene product that accumulates in the infected cells reflects the cellular response elements embedded in the viral promoter and the abundance of transcriptional factors present in the infected cells.

In permissive infected cells, progeny virus accumulates at an exponential rate between 6 and 18 hours after infection and at a reduced, linear rate until at least 24 hours. In cells exposed to 10 PFU of virus per cell, IE gene products reach peak rates of synthesis between 2 and 4 hours after infection, although the actual synthesis of the proteins continues for many hours. The E gene products are expressed very soon thereafter. Overall, E gene products are readily detected by 4 hours after infection but reach highest rates of accumulation between 6 and 12 hours after infection. Viral DNA synthesis can be detected as early as 3 hours after infection and continues for at least 10 to 12 more hours.

Early Events After Entry of the DNA Into the Nucleus

After entry of viral DNA into the nucleus, as described above, several events are thought to take place, including circularization of at least part of the viral DNA, induction of a limited DNA damage repair response, and loading of heterochromatin onto the input viral DNA (Fig. 9.7).

Circularization of Viral DNA

Upon entry into the nucleus, viral DNA circularizes quickly and in the absence of viral protein synthesis, as first shown using assays that detected (a) viral DNA end joining in cells infected with recombinant viruses lacking internal repeated sequences or (b) circular viral DNA as detected in pulsed-field gels and other biochemical assays. These results also led to the development of viral DNA replication models involving theta molecule intermediates and rolling circle mechanisms, as described below. Furthermore, a later study of an HSV recombinant strain containing an insertion of the cleavage/packaging sequence within the genome confirmed the circularization

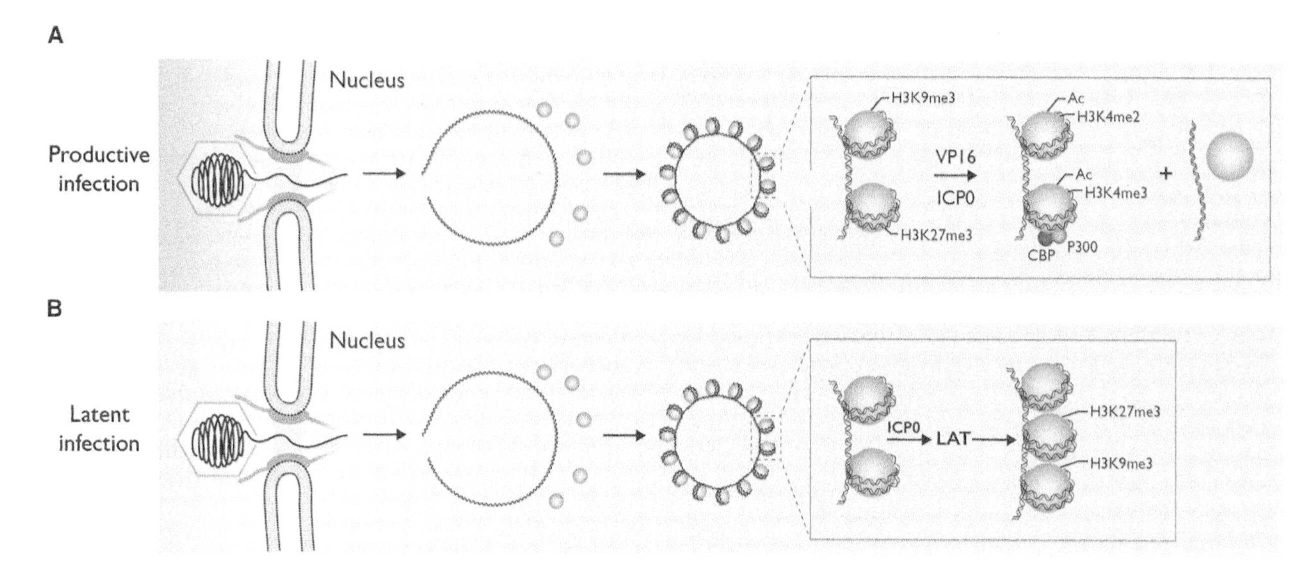

FIGURE 9.7 Epigenetic regulation of HSV-1 lytic and latent infection. A: Following infection of epithelial cells, the capsid is transported to the nuclear pore where the viral DNA is released into the nucleus where it rapidly circularizes and becomes associated with histones. VP16 from the virion tegument forms a complex with HCF-1 and Oct1 that binds to viral IE promoters and HCF-1 recruits histone modification enzymes and chromatin remodeling complexes that decrease histone association with viral IE genes and increase euchromatin marks on the remaining associated histones. ICP0 is expressed as an IE protein, and it promotes the same processes on the rest of the genome. **B:** Following infection of neuronal cells, the capsid is also transported to the nuclear pore where the viral DNA is released into the nucleus where it rapidly circularizes and becomes associated with histones. VP16 cannot be transported into the neuronal nucleus and/or HCF-1 is not localized in the nucleus, so viral IE genes are not transcribed efficiently. Instead, the latency-associated transcript is expressed, and it promotes the further association of facultative heterochromatin marks on the viral chromatin. (Copyright, Catherine Sodroski and David Knipe.)

of the HSV-1 genome during productive infection.[448] Results from the latter study also argued that the end joining reported earlier was not due to concatemer formation or recombination between terminal repeats but rather was due to circularization.[448] Circularization of viral DNA, formation of endless genomes, and efficient viral DNA synthesis and viral replication requires the cellular DNA ligase IV and its cofactor XRCC4, as shown by studies of mutant cell lines and siRNA-mediated knockdown. Knockdown of DNA ligase IV or XRCC4 causes a 100-fold reduction in viral yield, supporting the idea that early circularization of the viral DNA is part of the productive infection pathway.

Induction of the First Phase of the DNA Damage Response

HSV-1 infection causes DNA damage response (DDR) proteins to be recruited to replication compartments and to interact with viral proteins and promote viral replication.[466] HSV-1 infection activates DDR pathways,[319,511] but these could be due to input or progeny viral DNA. Various DDR proteins localize adjacent to incoming viral DNA, and ICP0 inhibits localization of at least two of these proteins: 53BP1 and BRCA1.[276] The incoming viral DNA with nicks and gaps and some linear ends as described above is an appropriate stimulus for the DNA damage response. Consistent with that, viral DNA transfected into cells induces phosphorylation of RPA, which is catalyzed by ATR and DNA-PK.[432] Infection of normal human fibroblasts with the HSV-1 *d*109 virus, which delivers its DNA to the cell nucleus but expresses little in the way of viral gene products, causes the activation of a limited DNA damage response, including the phosphorylation of Chk2 and H2AX, as well as low amounts of p53 serine 15 phosphorylation.[314] Full activation of the DNA damage response occurs after viral DNA replication and that will be discussed below in the DNA replication section. It is not apparent whether the DNA damage response to the incoming DNA in the amounts delivered by input virions is antiviral, proviral, or just a preview of things to come.

Association of Viral DNA With Histones

It was originally thought that lytic viral genomes were not associated with nucleosomes because nuclease digestion studies showed no nucleosomal-protected DNA band in lytic viral DNA.[224] However, the use of chromatin immunoprecipitation (ChIP) techniques showed that histones are associated with viral DNA during lytic infection[176,224] and that changes in the viral heterochromatin were associated with changes in viral gene expression.[176]

It then became clear that, like transfected plasmid DNAs, cells rapidly load histones on viral DNA molecules within a couple of hours (Fig. 9.7),[82,274,342] likely in an attempt to epigenetically silence the foreign, unchromatinized DNA.[234] The histones associated with viral DNA lacked euchromatin marks such as histone acetylation[82] but contained heterochromatin marks such as histone H3 lysine 9 trimethylation (H3K9me3).[264,274] However, HSV has evolved mechanisms to combat the epigenetic silencing of its lytic genes by the host cell, and to this end, VP16 organizes a complex of cellular proteins that remove histones and heterochromatin marks from IE gene promoters, ICP0 promotes the degradation of host restriction factors, leading to the reduction of histone loading on E and L gene promoters, and viral DNA replication also helps to reduce histone loading on the viral DNA molecules.[236,237]

Experiments involving pull down of labeled input viral DNA did not detect core histones associated with that DNA.[105] It is unclear why this technique gives a different result from the extensive results using ChIP, but it has been shown that nucleosomes on viral DNA are less stable in HSV-infected cells.[256,257] Therefore, the association of histones with viral DNA may not be stable enough to show association with viral DNA using pull down of labeled DNA.

Intranuclear Targeting of HSV DNA

Input viral genomic DNA is targeted to a location near the nuclear periphery and/or lamina early after entry into the nucleus. The HSV-1 genome is found initially in genome complexes and small replication compartments near the nuclear periphery.[102,428,429] The localization of the genome to the nuclear periphery may be the result of IE gene transcription rather than a cause of IE transcription, because localization of genome complexes to the periphery is reduced in cells infected with a VP16 acidic activator domain mutant virus.[429] It is noteworthy that transcriptionally active HSV genomes localize to the nuclear periphery as most of the literature considers the nuclear lamina to be silencing.[137,382] This may reflect targeting of the viral genome to specific nuclear lamina microdomains that are associated with actively transcribed chromatin.[424]

Early replication compartments, as detected by ICP8 immunofluorescence,[102,428] then form near the inner nuclear membrane. Knockout of the lamin A/C gene in mouse embryonic fibroblasts (MEFs) leads to the release of replication compartments from the nuclear periphery, increased viral heterochromatin, and reduced viral gene expression.[428] Assembly of the VP16 activator complex likely occurs on the nuclear lamina,[429] possibly because Oct-1 is believed to be associated with nuclear lamina.[299] Conceivably, this could help ensure the transcriptional activation of viral genomes immediately following nuclear entry.

Association of Viral DNA With ND10 Structures and Other Nuclear Proteins

Concurrent with the association of viral DNA with histones, histone- and chromatin-modifying enzymes, and repressors, entering viral DNA was first observed to localize in genome complexes near punctate structures within the nucleus called nuclear domain 10 (ND10) bodies or PML oncogenic domains. Later studies argued that ND10 components relocate to sites associated with the viral genome complexes.[132] While early imaging studies argued that the ND10 structures and viral DNA were adjacent, some recent studies have argued that the ND10 components are wrapped around the viral genome.[9] Thus, while we do not know the exact events taking place, we do know that at least some components of the ND10 bodies, including PML, ATRX, SP100, and SUMO2, as well as IFI16 localize to input viral genomes labeled *in situ* by click chemistry within minutes after infection.[9,55,105]

ND10 bodies have been associated with many functions including transcriptional activation and epigenetic regulation of gene expression.[470] They are dynamic structures that contain upwards of 20 proteins with PML protein acting as a scaffold. The role of ND10 body structures in viral infection is not well defined. ND10 bodies were observed to be associated with transcribing genomes and replication compartment formation and therefore were originally considered to be proviral. As described below, the protein components are antiviral under certain circumstances. Although ND10 component proteins are expressed constitutively, some are induced by interferon treatment and can act to restrict virus reproduction. In fact, interferon treatment of cells increases the number of ND10 bodies, and the effects of PML and IFI16[437] have been shown to be amplified in interferon-treated cells.

Because PML, ATRX, and IFI16 increased the steady state levels of heterochromatin under various conditions,[55,284,348] it was thought that these might be the host cell factors involved in the initial deposition of heterochromatin onto viral DNA. However, analysis of early times of infection showed that ATRX, PML, and IFI16 are not needed for loading of heterochromatin but for maintenance of heterochromatin if the genome is subjected to transcription or replication.[55,312]

Once assembled in heterochromatin, access of the viral genome to transcription factors and RNA pol II, which transcribes the HSV genome throughout infection, is restricted. The cascade of viral gene expression, while originally thought to involve transactivation of viral transcription, involves to a large part overcoming several epigenetic silencing hurdles to de-silence the viral genes, enabling the expression of the IE genes, then the expression of E and E/L genes followed by L genes.

De-Silencing and Transcription of IE Genes

IE gene promoters are loaded with histone H3 bearing heterochromatin markers by 30 minutes postinfection, but H3 levels are reduced as the infection progresses.[274] The key players in the de-silencing and transcriptional activation of IE genes are the protein complex involving the viral VP16 protein; the unique IE gene response element; the host factors recruited by the VP16 complex including Set1, LSD1, CLOCK; and a large number of epigenetic and transcriptional factors discussed below.

The IE gene promoters contain numerous cellular transcription factor binding sites, including SP1 binding sites (Fig. 9.8), but the sequence ATGCTAATGARATTCTTT,[249] sometimes shortened to TAATGARAAT, is the key sequence element defining IE gene promoters. It is present in one or several copies within several hundred base pairs upstream of the cap site (e.g., ICP4 Fig. 9.8).

The IE gene promoter element described above is targeted by a complex of host proteins organized by the tegument protein VP16. VP16, encoded by the U_L48 gene, is 1 of 18 virion tegument proteins, and upon entry into the host cell in the virion, it is a key component of the complex of proteins that de-silences and activates IE gene expression. Upon release from the tegument, VP16 binds to a cellular protein called host cell factor 1 (HCF-1). It has been reported that HCF-1 carries VP16 into the nucleus in transfected cells, but VP16 localizes normally to the cell nucleus at late times in infected cells that express a temperature-sensitive mutant HCF-1 or in cells in which HCF-1 is knocked down. Thus, at late times and conceivably at early times in infected cells, other factors, such as other viral tegument proteins, assist in nuclear localization of VP16. Within the infected cell nucleus, the VP16–HCF-1 complex binds to the cellular protein Oct-1 to form the core transcription activator complex. Oct-1 is an abundant ubiquitous transcriptional factor that, as its name indicates, binds to

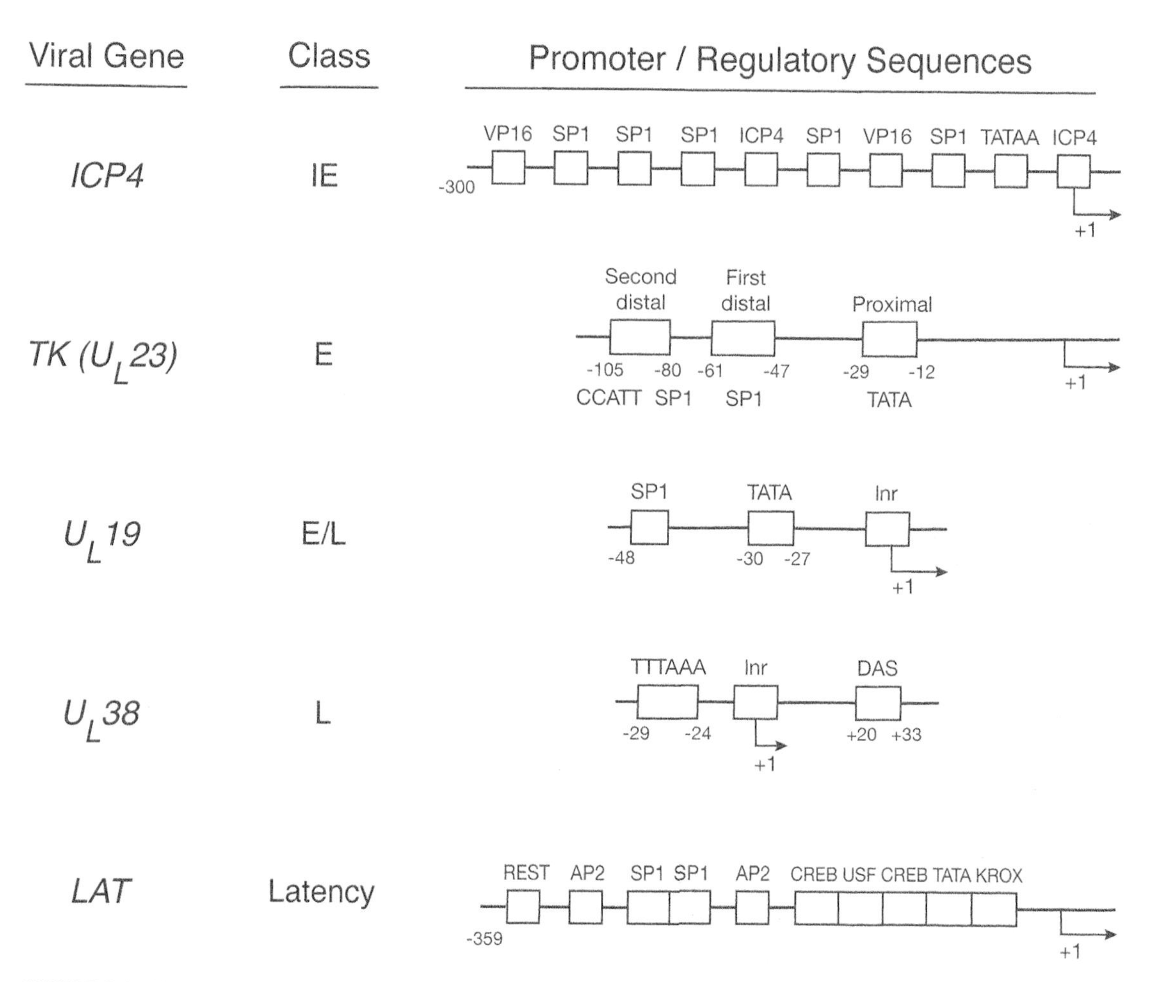

FIGURE 9.8 Diagrammatic representation of the structure of prototypic HSV gene promoters. The promoter/regulatory sequences of prototypic genes of IE, E, E/L, L lytic classes of genes and the LAT promoter of the latency gene are diagrammed. (Copyright, Catherine Sodroski and David Knipe.)

the ATGnTAAT octamer. Oct-1 binds to viral DNA at the octamer sequence found in the IE promoters and anchors the complex at the IE gene promoters. VP16 binds to adjacent DNA sequences and to HCF-1 to complete the complex.

Through the actions of this complex, VP16 acts to reduce the loading of histones and heterochromatin marks and promote the addition of euchromatin marks on viral IE gene promoters.[176] The mechanism of this has been at least partially elucidated by a variety of experiments. A key step in the expression of IE genes is the recruitment of lysine-specific demethylase 1 (LSD1), also known as lysine (K)-specific demethylase 1A (KDM1A), to the viral IE gene promoters by the HCF-1 protein in the complex. LSD1 is a flavin-dependent monoamine oxidase, which can demethylate mono- and dimethylated lysines, specifically histone 3 lysines 4 and 9 (H3K4 and H3K9). In the VP16 complex, LSD1 demethylates H3K9me2 and H3K9me moieties bound to IE promoters to shift the chromatin away from heterochromatin and enable IE gene transcription.[274] Depletion of LSD1 or pharmacologic inhibition of LSD1 increased H3K9me3 modification of histones associated with HSV IE gene promoters and decreased IE gene transcription.[274] Furthermore, HCF-1 is part of the Set1 and MLL1 histone H3 Lys4 methyltransferase complexes; therefore, the VP16 complex recruits the HCF-1-SetI or HCF-1-MLL1 histone methyltransferase (HMT) complex to IE promoters resulting in the euchromatic histone modification, trimethylation of the histone H3 lysine 4 residue (H3K4me3), which provides a euchromatic modification and binding of various factors that stimulate IE gene transcription.

The second step in IE gene expression is the activation of transcription. Part of this process involves the recruitment by the VP16 acidic C-terminal domain of transcription factors IIB (TFIIB), TFIIH, TATA-binding protein, and TBP-associated factors, which promote formation of the RNA pol II preinitiation complex on IE promoters. VP16 has also been reported to recruits chromatin-modifying coactivator proteins CBP, p300, Brg-1, or Brm onto viral promoters.[176] CBP and p300 have histone acetyltransferase (HAT) activities associated with them and promote active chromatin or euchromatin. BRM and BRG-1 are the mammalian homologs of the ATPase subunit of the yeast SWI/SNF complex, which remodels host chromatin. Interestingly, knockdown of these coactivators did not reduce HSV IE gene transcription under certain conditions, suggesting that their function is redundant with unknown host factors in some cells and/or infection conditions.[254] VP16 interacts with numerous components of the Mediator complex.[341] Because the Mediator complex plays a central role in transcriptional activation, these interactions serve to recruit the Mediator complex for transcription of the IE genes.

HCF-1 also participates in transcriptional elongation in that it recruits components of a network of transcriptional elongation components including the super elongation complex.[13] IE gene transcriptional requires the SEC-P-TEFb complex, and BET inhibitors that increase TEFb levels increase lytic reactivation and reactivation from latency.[13] Moreover, inhibitors of TEFb reduce IE gene transcription and lytic infection.[12]

Shut Off of IE Gene Expression

There is evidence for several mechanisms by which HSV controls the accumulation of at least two IE gene products, ICP4 and ICP0.

First, ICP4 can repress its own expression by binding to its own promoter. ICP4 binds to DNA in either a sequence-specific or sequence nonspecific manner. The first ICP4-specific binding sequence reported by Faber and Wilcox was ATCGTCNNNNYCGRC and is defined as the consensus binding site. The second set of sequences bears no relationship to the consensus binding sites or for that matter, to each other. Consensus binding sites that span transcription initiation sites serve as sites for repression of transcription by ICP4, as illustrated by the *ICP4* gene in Figure 9.8. Binding of ICP4 to these sites at the 5′ end of its gene leads to repression of its expression. It is less clear whether ICP4 represses the expression of the other IE genes. ICP4 binds upstream of the *ICP0* gene transcriptional initiation site, and ICP4 represses the ICP0 promoter in transfected cells. Nevertheless, the specific effect of ICP4 on *ICP0* gene expression in infected cells has not been defined by construction of a mutant virus with the binding site in the *ICP0* gene mutated. Consensus ICP4-binding sites are not evident in or near the promoters of the other IE genes. ICP4-binding sites are also found in the *ORF P* and *LAT* gene promoters and have a negative regulatory effect on their transcription. ICP4 is more generally distributed on the viral genome as the infection progresses,[116] presumably to stimulate E and L gene transcription.

Second, during productive infection, E gene products down-regulate IE gene expression.[185] One E protein identified as a candidate repressor is ICP8, the single-stranded DNA-binding protein encoded by the U_L29 gene. ICP8 has been shown to coat viral progeny DNA and to decrease the expression of all genes from those progeny genomes, in particular transcription of the *ICP4* gene,[155] which may further inhibit viral transcription. Although the mechanism of this effect of ICP8 is not known, it may involve the sequestration of viral DNA molecules in replication complexes, changes in the conformation of viral DNA, or displacement of DNA to sites of DNA synthesis away from those required for transcription.

At early times, the virion host shutoff (vhs) function has been shown to degrade both viral and cellular mRNAs. The observation that in cells infected with *vhs* mutants, the transition from IE to E and subsequently to L protein synthesis lags behind that observed in wild-type virus–infected cells led to the conclusion that one function of *vhs* is to synchronize sequential viral gene expression. The proposed model is that the rate of transcription of viral genes exceeds the ability of vhs to degrade the mRNAs and that unless destabilized, IE mRNAs would outcompete L mRNAs, and so on. Vhs is described in more detail below.

De-Silencing and Expression of E and E/L Genes

Viral E genes are associated with heterochromatin marks by 1 to 2 hpi, and this is reduced as infection progresses to allow their transcription.[82,264] Because the temporal order of expression of E and E/L genes overlap, it is convenient to lump them together. Expression of these genes requires ICP4 and is increased by ICP0, in particular at low multiplicities of infection and in normal human cells. ICP0 acts in general to make the viral genome more accessible to transcription factors and RNA pol II, and ICP4 acts to recruit the transcription factors and RNA pol II to the viral genomes. Expression of these genes also requires, to a variable extent, ICP27, ICP22, US1.5, and, in the case of E/L genes, the onset of viral DNA synthesis. We will consider the role of these viral proteins individually.

ICP0

ICP0 is an E3 ubiquitin ligase that plays a major role in the de-silencing of the post-IE genes by countering host chromatin silencing mechanisms and in countering innate immune signaling and other host responses. ICP0 is not essential for viral replication in certain cell types at high MOI. At low MOI, cells infected with *ICP0* deletion mutants yield approximately 10- to 1,000-fold less virus than cells infected with wild-type virus, with the yield reduction varying with the cell type. At greater than 5 PFU per cell or greater, the yields of ICP0 mutant virus may be similar to those of wild-type virus in tumor cells and certain cell lines. The cell line most permissive for *ICP0* mutant viruses is U20S, which is defective for restriction factors because it does not express ATRX[290] or functional IFI16 protein.[347] Thus, U20S cells serve as the standard for infectivity titrations of ICP0 mutant virus stocks for experimental studies. Even using this cell line for titrations, the particle:PFU ratio for $ICP0^-$ mutants may be higher than the $ICP0^+$ viruses[349,391]; thus, this may be a factor in differing results in certain papers. Nevertheless, ICP0 promotes HSV-1 replication by at least 10^3-fold in normal human fibroblasts,[348] consistent with the host restriction being more effective in normal human cells.[347]

The major functions of ICP0 in promoting viral replication are (a) de-silencing of the viral genome, in particular on the E and L genes and (b) inhibition of host innate immune signaling and other host responses. The former function is thought to be mainly through its E3 ubiquitin ligase-promoted degradation of restriction factors but may also occur due to disruption of inhibitory complexes.

Several lines of indirect evidence first raised the idea that ICP0 enables the expression of E genes by epigenetic de-silencing of these genes: (a) Histone deacetylase inhibitors (HDACs), such as trichostatin A and sodium butyrate, can rescue at least part of the ICP0 mutant gene expression defect, suggesting that ICP0 is overcoming epigenetic silencing in part by inhibiting HDAC activity. (b) ICP0 was reported to interact with class II histone deacetylases and to reverse repressive effects of these HDACs in transfected cells. (c) ICP0 binds to CoREST *in vitro* and dislodges HDAC1 from the HDAC1/CoREST/LSD1/REST (HCLR) complex in wild-type virus–infected cells. (d) Replacement of both copies of the *ICP0* gene with a gene encoding a dominant negative CoREST capable of binding REST but unable to bind HDAC1 led to a 100-fold increase in the yield of virus in Vero cells and an at least 10-fold increase in HEp-2 cells following low PFU/cell infection. A virus encoding an ICP0 unable to bind CoREST showed reduced ability to reactivate quiescent HSV-1, consistent with a role for REST/CoREST/HDAC1/2/LSD1 in repression of quiescent genomes.[135] Despite the weight of this evidence, knockdown of CoREST did not affect replication of an *ICP0* mutant in human HepaRG cells, a liver progenitor cell line.[130] The differences here may be due to the differences in cell types used or to the fact that CoREST both inhibits viral gene expression and stabilizes LSD1, which is needed for viral IE gene expression.[547]

Direct evidence for ICP0 promoting the de-silencing of viral chromatin came from the observation that ICP0 mutant viruses show increased total histone H3 association with viral promoters and decreased acetylation of histone H3 that is associated with viral promoters, a histone modification associated with euchromatin or active chromatin.[82] ICP0 also promotes the rapid removal of the heterochromatin H3K9 trimethylation marks from E gene chromatin in infected cells.[264] Furthermore, ICP0 promoted the removal of heterochromatin markers from viral chromatin during reactivation from quiescent infection in cell culture.[135] An unresolved issue is whether ICP0 also affects host chromatin. ICP0 increases the expression of host gene products, including p21, gadd45, and mdm2, potentially due to chromatin effects. HSV infection reduces histone H3 levels on the *GAPDH* gene promoter[166] but not on a *GAPDH* pseudogene.[82] Further studies are warranted to determine the effects of HSV infection and ICP0 specifically on host gene chromatin.

Role of the E3 Ubiquitin Ligase Activity of ICP0 in Promoting Protein Degradation

ICP0 promotes the degradation of a number of host resistance factors that can potentially restrict virus reproduction, and this is considered to be one of the major ways that ICP0 promotes the de-silencing of the viral genome. We will examine the mechanisms by which ICP0 promotes the degradation of these host proteins and then discuss the host resistance factors and their mechanism of action.

The RING domain in exon 2 of ICP0, which is a C_3HC_4 zinc-binding domain[33] from residues 106 to 149, contains a ubiquitin E3 ligase activity. The RING domain E3 ligase activity is essential for ICP0's functions in transactivation of post-IE gene expression and for promotion of viral replication at low MOI. This is likely due to ICP0's promotion of the ubiquitination of cellular restriction factors followed by their subsequent degradation. ICP0 promotes the degradation of a large number of proteins, including PML; the SUMO-modified form of Sp100; centromere proteins CENP-A, -B, and -C; the catalytic subunit of DNA-PK[354]; the ubiquitin-specific protease 7 (USP7); the RNF8 cellular RING finger ubiquitin ligase[277]; ubiquitinated histones[277]; the RNF168 cellular E3 ligase[277]; IFI16[349]; and ATRX.[214]

Mechanism of Ubiquitination

It has been puzzling that ICP0 is able to promote the degradation of so many proteins. There is evidence for some direct interactions that lead to ubiquitination. ICP0 does bind directly to a protein with ubiquitin-specific protease activity, USP7, also called herpesvirus-associated ubiquitin-specific protease or HAUSP and promotes its ubiquitination *in vitro*. ICP0 binds to the DNA repair protein RNF8 and purified ICP0 ubiquitinates RNF8 *in vitro*.[277] The interaction between ICP0 and RNF8 is believed to be due to the forkhead domain of RNF8 binding to a specific domain on ICP0 that is phosphorylated.[67] These are the only known direct substrates of the ICP0 E3 ligase activity. At least one potential contributing factor to the broad effect of ICP0 is that it contains several SUMO-interacting domains (SIMs)[47] that bind to the common peptide moiety named SUMO (small ubiquitin-like modifier), which is covalently linked as a posttranslational modification to the epsilon amino group of lysine in the tetrapeptide consensus motif Ψ-K-x-D/E where Ψ is a hydrophobic residue, K is the lysine conjugated to SUMO, x is any amino acid, and D or E is an acidic residue. Mutations in multiple SIM domains in ICP0 reduce degradation of PML isoforms in general.[47] However, the PML I isoform is also degraded in a SUMO-independent manner.[47] Therefore, the role of the SIM may be either as the primary interaction of ICP0 with proteins or to bring ICP0 into the area of proteins with which it interacts directly or indirectly for ubiquitination. Evidence for the latter was that SIM function was necessary but not sufficient for ICP0 promotion of PML isoform II degradation.[545] Proteomics analysis of ICP0 interactors showed mostly the direct binders of ICP0,[88] suggesting that the SUMO interactions may be weak interactions.

Degradation of Host Restriction Factors

A number of host cell responses to viral infection have been defined, and they have been broadly classified as intrinsic resistance and innate immune responses. Intrinsic resistance is often defined as constitutively expressed host factors that reduce viral replication, while innate immunity is considered to be factors that are induced by signaling pathways. However, this breaks down for several host factors such as PML and IFI16, which are expressed constitutively but are induced by interferons, so they could be considered to be effectors of either intrinsic resistance or innate immunity.

Host Cell Restriction Factors Affected by ICP0

Promyelocytic Leukemia (PML) Protein

The PML protein is a member of the tripartite motif (TRIM) family of proteins and contains a RING domain, two zinc-binding B-box domains, and a coiled-coil domain. As described above, PML protein localizes with and serves as a scaffold for other cellular proteins in ND10 bodies, including Sp100, DAXX, and ATRX. These proteins have all been associated with restriction of HSV gene expression.[48] PML can act independently of Sp100 and Daxx to inhibit HSV-1 replication in HepaRG cells and fibroblasts.[154] Interestingly, some studies at low multiplicity of infection show that PML can enhance HSV replication.[313,524,525] Furthermore, Ishov et al.[195] reported that PML-NBs may provide a platform for HCMV gene expression and replication, and PML-NBs have been reported to localize near incoming and early-replicating HSV-1 viral DNA (vDNA). Thus, PML is part of both a constitutive resistance mechanism and the antiviral mechanism of IFNs but may also support viral replication by other mechanisms.

PML acts to restrict HSV ICP0$^-$ mutant virus plaque formation by three- to fivefold as shown using shRNA depletion or by threefold in wild-type MEFs versus knockout MEFs. The detailed mechanism of the restriction by PML has not been defined, but PML has been shown to increase loading of heterochromatin of histone H3.3 with H3K9me3 modifications during HSV-1 quiescent infection of fibroblasts and to promote the maintenance of heterochromatin modifications including H3K9me3 and H3K27me3 on ICP0⁻ virus genomes.[55] While it is generally thought that PML promotes epigenetic silencing of the viral genome, some have reported that PML encases incoming viral DNA and sterically blocks RNA pol from transcribing the genome.[9] Thus, there are multiple mechanisms by which PML might act to epigenetically silence HSV DNA.

α-Thalassemia X-Linked Intellectual Disability (ATRX)

ATRX, a SWI/SNF chromatin remodeler protein, is a crucial epigenetic regulator of eukaryotic gene expression and silenced heterochromatin. ATRX and death domain-associated protein (Daxx) together form a histone chaperone complex that loads the noncanonical histone variant 3.3 (H3.3).[115,269] This complex is also critical for maintaining repressive heterochromatin at many repeat-rich regions, including telomeres,[287] pericentric repeats,[129] and endogenous retroviruses,[129] and mutations in the *ATRX* gene are linked to a developmental disorder and several cancer types.[287] ATRX and DAXX are also two of the core components of ND-10 structures, as described above. Depletion of ATRX increased plaque formation by an ICP0⁻ virus by sixfold, and restoration of ATRX reduced plaque formation to control levels, while ATRX depletion did not significantly affect plaque formation by an ICP0⁺ virus.[290,413,420,472] Depletion of Daxx also increased plaque formation by an ICP0⁻ virus but did not affect ICP0⁺ virus plaque formation. The Daxx interaction site on ATRX was needed for the restriction and recruitment of ATRX to genome complexes.[290,413,420,472] In total, these results argue that ATRX and Daxx act in a complex to restrict HSV-1 ICP0-deficient virus replication. HSV-1 infection reduces levels of ATRX by several mechanisms, including ICP0-promoted protein degradation, miR-H4 reduction of mRNA levels, and vhs reduction of mRNA levels.[214]

Recent studies have shown that ATRX localizes to the input HSV-1 genome within minutes after infection.[9,55] However, ATRX did not promote histone association as measured for histone H3; rather, it promoted maintenance of histone H3 and heterochromatin marks on the viral genome when the genome was transcribed or replicated to restrict transcription from parental and progeny templates.[55] Recent studies have shown that although H3 is loaded to normal levels as determined by ChIP, accessibility of the viral genome as measured by ATAC-seq is increased when ATRX is knocked out.[54]

Interferon Gamma–Inducible Protein 16 (IFI16)

IFI16 is a member of the PYHIN protein family. It contains an N-terminal pyrin domain, which mediates protein–protein interactions, and two C-terminal HIN domains, which confer sequence nonspecific double-stranded DNA (dsDNA)-binding ability.[203] IFI16 binds to dsDNA and diffuses along the DNA until it multimerizes with other IFI16 molecules to give stable binding[449]; however, positioning of a nucleosome on the DNA molecule prevents translocation and multimerization of IFI16 and inhibits stable binding of IFI16 to the DNA molecule.[449]

Depletion of IFI16 in human fibroblasts leads to an increase in replication of ICP0-null viruses and enhanced viral gene expression,[348] and overexpression of IFI16 leads to restricted replication of ICP0⁻ viruses[348] and restricted viral gene expression of ICP0⁺ viruses.[207] When IFI16 levels are increased by γ-interferon treatment of human fibroblasts, IFI16 can restrict replication and gene expression of wild-type, ICP0⁺ HSV-1 and HSV-2.[437] Thus, at baseline levels, IFI16 serves as a restriction factor for ICP0⁻ viruses and when overexpressed or when induced by interferon-γ, for wild-type viruses.

Although IFI16 has been observed to associate with ND10 proteins[110] and to colocalize with PML and ATRX at input viral genomes and genome complexes,[131,348] IFI16 restricts gene expression from both parental and progeny viral genomes by independent mechanisms.[313] It localizes to input viral genomes within 15 minutes after entry into the nucleus[55] and stabilizes histone H3 on viral chromatin.[312] In contrast, at later times after viral DNA replication in ICP0⁻ mutant–infected cells, IFI16 forms filaments decorated with PML, Sp100, and ATRX within a subset of viral replication compartments, and there is evidence that these filaments act in *trans* to reduce RNA pol II loading onto viral genomes to restrict viral transcription.[312] While the mechanism(s) of this novel structure have not been elucidated, the evidence thus far is consistent with IFI16 binding to progeny DNA molecules, multimerizing on them, and recruiting a series of restriction factors in a structure that initiates a general epigenetic restriction of viral transcription,[312] similar to supramolecular organizing centers that initiate innate signaling.[217]

Infection with viral strains expressing ICP0 causes a RING-finger–dependent, proteasome-dependent loss of IFI16, consistent with ubiquitination and degradation.[349] Some have observed no specific degradation of IFI16 due to ICP0,[94] but certain cells, especially tumor cells, were shown to encode nonfunctional IFI16.[347] The bulk of the evidence supports IFI16 functioning in normal cells and being degraded by ICP0 in those cells but that IFI16 may be defective in tumor cells,[347] due to its inhibitory effects on cell growth,[438] and thus may not be binding to viral DNA and not activated to interact with ICP0, resulting in a lack of IFI16 degradation in those cells.

DNA-Dependent Protein Kinase

The DNA-dependent protein kinase (DNA-PK) complex, consisting of the catalytic subunit (cs) and the Ku70/Ku80 heterodimer, binds to DNA breaks or ends and activates a DNA damage response (DDR) that results in repair by nonhomologous end joining. The linear ends of the incoming viral DNA may be recognized and joined together to block circle formation by DNA ligase IV/XRCC4. Consistent with this, mutant cells defective for Ku70 showed increased viral replication.[466] As described above, ICP0 promotes the degradation of DNA PKcs.

Inhibition of Activity of Host Factors

ICP0 may inhibit or sequester other host factors without promoting their degradation. ICP0 blocks the nuclear accumulation of interferon-regulatory factor 3 (IRF-3) but does not prevent its phosphorylation in the cytoplasm. There is some reduction of IRF-3 levels due to ICP0 but that shows later kinetics than the ICP0-dependent inhibition of interferon expression. At early times postinfection, ICP0 may sequester IRF-3 at nuclear sites and away from the *IFNβ* gene promoter.[350]

ICP4

ICP4 fulfills the second function needed for post-IE gene transcription, that is, recruitment of transcription factors and RNA pol II to these gene promoters. ICP4 is required for maximal levels of all post-IE gene expression,[238] and the effect of ICP4 is exerted at the transcriptional level in infected cells, as demonstrated by nuclear run-off assays.[155] ICP4 has been shown to also activate gene expression in transfected cell assays and in *in vitro* transcription systems.[395]

ICP4 is thought to function by the general mechanism of binding to the viral genome and recruiting transcription factors and RNA pol II. As discussed above, ICP4 has both sequence-specific and nonspecific DNA-binding activities. Sites bound by ICP4 with the strongest affinity are known to have their transcription repressed rather than activated by ICP4 (e.g., at the transcription initiation sites of the *ICP4* or *ORF P* genes), and destruction of the sole sequence-specific binding site of ICP4 upstream of the transcription initiation site of the *ICP4* gene attenuated repression in the context of the viral genome. With regard to the role of DNA binding in the transactivation function of ICP4, early mutational analysis studies showed that the sequence-specific binding activity of ICP4 correlated in most studies with its ability to activate E gene expression in infected cells. In addition, insertion of ICP4-binding sites was reported to render reporter genes responsive to ICP4, albeit in transfected cells. Furthermore, there was a postulated role for the DNA-binding ability of ICP4 in stabilizing the binding of cellular transcription factors to E and L gene promoters. However, one viral mutant was obtained in which the DNA-binding activity of ICP4 was greatly reduced, but the ability to activate E genes in infected cells was nearly unchanged. Originally, it was thought that most post-IE genes did not have recognizable consensus binding sites for ICP4, and mutation of consensus sites did not affect the level of expression of the surrounding genes in the viral genome. However, recent ChIP-Seq studies of ICP4 binding to the viral genome in infected cells have defined the *in vivo* consensus site as A/G/T-T-C/G/T-T/G/C-G/C/T-G/A/T/C-T/C/A-G/C/T/A-G/C/A/T-CTA-C/G-G,[116] similar to the original consensus sequence. This recent study showed that ICP4 is distributed across the viral genome, providing a potential mechanism for ICP4 to transactivate a broad range of viral genes.[116]

Second, ICP4 has been shown to interact with basal transcription factors to form complexes with TATA-binding protein, TFII-B and TAF250[268,404,492] as well as ICP27, ICP22, and the cellular CLOCK HAT.[220] ICP4 promotes the formation of transcription preinitiation complexes *in vitro* on the *gC* gene promoter, at least in part by stimulating the binding of TFIID to the promoter to form preinitiation complexes. ICP4 also interacts with the Mediator complex,[268] a large protein complex that bridges upstream activators and the preinitiation complex. ICP4 binding across the viral genome is essential for the recruitment of TBP, Mediator, and RNA pol II, and transcription of the viral genome.[116]

ICP27

ICP27 is an IE protein that is reported to have multiple regulatory functions in viral gene expression, including promoting expression of certain E proteins, L gene transcription, viral RNA export from the nucleus to cytoplasm, and translation of viral mRNAs. ICP27 comprises the following functional domains from N to C terminus: a leucine-rich region, an acidic region–nuclear localization signal, an RGG box RNA-binding domain, two predicted KLH RNA-binding domains, and a zinc finger–like region.[469] It also forms a homodimeric structure through multiple interactions in the C-terminal half of the molecule, as shown by the crystal structure of residues 241 to 512.[473]

Early studies of viral gene expression concluded that ICP27 is required only for viral DNA replication and L gene expression, but further studies showed that ICP27 is also needed for efficient expression of certain E genes, in particular the less abundant viral DNA replication proteins. Thus, ICP27 is required at least in part indirectly for viral DNA replication by increasing the mRNA levels of E gene products essential for viral DNA synthesis. These studies showed that ICP27 increases the mRNA levels for these E genes, but it has not been determined if this effect is transcriptional or posttranscriptional. ICP27 affects the cytoplasmic levels of only a subset of E mRNAs because Northern blot studies have shown that an ICP27 null mutant virus expresses levels of ICP8 mRNA at 6 hpi that are equivalent to wild-type virus. These early studies were conducted in Vero (African green monkey) cells, and similar studies in normal human cells are warranted.

HSV ICP27 mutant viruses are defective for L *gC* gene transcription as assayed by infected cell pulse labeling of RNA. ICP27 associates with the RNA pol II holoenzyme through its interaction with the C-terminal domain of the large RNA pol II subunit, consistent with an ability to enhance initiation or termination of transcription. ICP27 has been shown to bind to ICP4, to alter ICP4 phosphorylation, and to localize to replication compartments. ICP27 interacts directly with ICP8, which associates with viral progeny DNA. Therefore, ICP27, through its interactions with ICP8 and RNA pol II, is proposed to link RNA pol II to progeny viral DNA to promote late viral gene transcription. Consistent with this, some immunofluorescence studies have shown that certain *ICP27* mutant viruses are defective for recruitment of RNA pol II to replication compartments in infected cells, but others have failed to see a defect in RNA pol II recruitment with the HSV-1 *n*406 and *n*504 ICP27 mutant viruses (with nonsense mutations at the indicated codons) in human U2OS cells.[310] The difference in the latter results may be due to the fact that U2OS cells are known to have reduced restriction factor expression and activity.[290,347,532] In general, these properties are consistent with effects on transcription of late HSV genes. The ability of ICP27 to promote L viral gene expression is at least partly distinct from its ability to stimulate viral DNA synthesis because at least one mutant virus, *n*504, separates these two functions. This mutant is defective for L gene expression while maintaining normal levels of viral DNA synthesis. The *n*504 mutant virus has been used to demonstrate that ICP27 stimulates transcription of L genes independently of its role in stimulating E gene expression and viral DNA replication.[200] This study found that ICP27 promotes transcription of at least two L genes, U_L44 and U_L47, in infected cells, as assayed by *in vivo* pulse labeling of RNA, without any apparent effects on transport or stability of these transcripts. ICP27 has also been reported to affect the elongation, termination, and/or polyadenylation site selection during transcription. A recent study reported that ICP27 disrupts cellular 3′ RNA processing by binding and disrupting the cleavage and polyadenylation specific factor (CPSF) complex but preserves viral 3′ RNA processing by binding to a GC-rich sequence in viral 3′ UTRs and recruiting an alternative CPSF complex to viral transcripts.[501]

ICP27 has been shown to shuttle between the nucleus and cytoplasm and is reported to promote viral RNA export in several studies. However, in some cases, the viral mutants used may have an additional defect in late gene transcription. There are differing results on the role of ICP27 in viral mRNA export because one study found that E ICP8 mRNA is present in the cytoplasm of an *ICP27* null mutant virus–infected cell at nearly normal levels (82%) compared to that in wild-type virus–infected cells, while another study found substantially lower amounts of *ICP8* as well as other E and L transcripts in the cytoplasm of *ICP27* mutant–infected cells. Furthermore, measurement of viral transcript levels by microarray technology shows a broad spectrum of viral poly $(A)^+$ transcripts are retained in the nucleus in cells infected with *ICP27* mutant viruses,[209] while studies looking at specific viral mRNAs using Northern blot hybridization found that (a) the long U_L24 gene transcript was increased in the nucleus of *ICP27* mutant–infected cells, but the short U_L24 gene transcript was unaffected; (b) VP16 mRNA export was not altered in *ICP27* mutant–infected cells[128]; and (c) ICP27 is not required for cytoplasmic accumulation of gD and ICP5 mRNAs.[140] Therefore, these studies showed a limited number of specific transcripts that show a dependence on ICP27 for nuclear export and cytoplasmic accumulation. In total, ICP27 binds to RNA pol II, promotes late gene transcription, promotes association of RNA-binding proteins to late transcripts, may escort mRNAs to the cytoplasm, and enhances the binding of translation factors to mRNA, as discussed below.

ICP27 binds to the cellular factor Aly or REF, and this interaction promotes mRNA export out of the nucleus.[209,469] Aly/REF is an RNA export factor that functions as a molecular chaperone and export adaptor involved in nuclear export of spliced and unspliced RNAs. Aly/REF can act as a chaperone to promote dimerization of transcription factors containing basic leucine zipper (bZIP) domains and thereby promote transcription.[422,488] Aly/REF is recruited to the 5′ end of the RNA transcript by the cap-binding complex and recruits other export factors such as the TREX complex,[488] which stimulates RNA export. Thus, the interaction of ICP27 with Aly/REF could act to stimulate any of the stages of synthesis, processing, or export of viral mRNAs.

Effects of IE Gene Products on Host Transcription and RNA Splicing

HSV infection inhibits host cell transcription, including RNA pol II and RNA pol I transcription,[395] and this requires ICP4 and ICP27. Pulse labeling of nascent transcripts with 4-thiouridine (4sU), ribosomal profiling, and analysis by next-generation sequencing have confirmed the decrease in host cell transcription in infected cells. However, it was also observed that the remaining active cellular transcription units show a defect in transcriptional termination.[400] The transcriptional readthrough gives novel splice sites and an apparent inhibition of RNA splicing. ICP27 was not needed for a reduction in transcriptional termination in infected cells in an initial publication,[400] but further studies showed that ICP27 when expressed alone disrupted transcriptional termination.[501] The proposed mechanism of ICP27 action is binding to CPSF, an mRNA 3′ processing factor, and inducing the assembly of a complex that is unable to cleave 3′ ends of mRNAs.[501] Viral transcription termination continues because ICP27 binds to GC-rich regions on viral mRNA 3′ ends and activates 3′ end processing. Finally, ICP27 interacts with and leads to modification of a number of cellular splicing factors and inhibits splicing.[463,464] While most HSV mRNAs do not contain introns, some viral mRNAs (ICP0, ICP47, ICP22, UL15) are spliced; thus, viral mechanisms exist that allow these viral transcripts to be spliced in the infected cell.

Organization of E and L Gene Promoters

Unlike IE genes, E or L genes do not have unique promoter elements that predict the timing, duration, or abundance of gene expression. Rather, the overall impression is that they appear to be made up of a diversity of elements, and both the organization and the context in which these elements are placed determine the expression of the gene. Nevertheless, the E gene promoters thus far studied contain binding sites for two to three cellular transcription factors upstream of the transcriptional start site (thymidine kinase (*tk*) gene–Fig. 9.8). The mechanism of activation of E genes has also been approached in studies attempting to map the *cis*-acting sequences needed for activation by virus infection or ICP4. The most extensively studied E gene promoter is that of the U_L23 or *tk* gene. Extensive mutagenic analyses of the promoter showed that the sequences needed for basal level transcription and activated transcription were the same (Fig. 9.8): a proximal signal from bp −12 to −29 containing a TATA box and two distal signals from bp −47 to −61 and −80 to −105 containing an SP1 transcription factor binding site and an SP1 site and a CCAAT transcription factor (CTF) site, respectively. These studies also supported the hypothesis that ICP4 transactivates E gene promoters through interactions with cellular basal transcription factors.

Expression of L Genes

Once viral DNA replication (described below) has initiated, expression of L genes is increased,[185] largely as a result of increased transcription.[155] Late transcription takes place in replication compartments within the infected cell nucleus, as evidenced by (a) the localization of ICP4 and RNA pol II, to replication compartments at late times, and (b) RNA-pulse labeling of replication compartments at late times.

We know that during late gene expression: (a) transcription of late genes increases upon replication of the viral genome,[155] (b) alteration in the viral DNA template during DNA synthesis is cis-acting, (c) certain forms of heterochromatin are removed or diluted by viral DNA synthesis,[264] (d) ICP4 binding to the genome decreases to only the high affinity sites,[116] (e) ICP8 assembles on the progeny viral DNA, and (f) the ICP4, ICP22, ICP27, and ICP8 proteins are required for optimal L gene expression. The cis-acting effect on the template could be due to changes in the viral DNA molecules themselves by exposure of single-stranded regions or by conversion of the viral genome from a circular form to a linear form. Alternatively, the *cis*-acting effect could be due to proteins tightly bound to the viral parental DNA that do not exchange to other DNA molecules in the infected cell. ICP4 promotes L gene transcription by promoting the assembly of preinitiation complexes on the L *gC* gene promoter. ICP27 and ICP8 have been hypothesized to stimulate late gene transcription by recruiting RNA pol II onto progeny DNA through a direct interaction that bridges ICP27 bound to RNA pol II with ICP8 bound to viral progeny DNA.

Additional interactions of RNA pol II holoenzyme with ICP4 would lead to preinitiation complexes on late gene promoters.

As a general rule, while sequences upstream of transcriptional initiation sites are sufficient to endow a reporter gene with E gene expression kinetics both in transfected cells and in the context of the viral genome, this is not generally true of L genes. In the context of the viral genome, expression of reporter genes as L genes also requires regulatory elements present in the 5′ transcribed noncoding domains. Even then, such chimeras are expressed as E genes in cells transfected with the chimera and then superinfected with the virus.

The HSV E/L promoters have not been studied as extensively as some of the other viral promoters, but the *ICP5* (*U_L19*) gene promoter elements have been defined (Fig. 9.8). The essential elements of the minimal *ICP5* gene promoter are (a) an SP1 binding site at −48, a TATA box at −30, and an essential cis-acting element between −2 and +10 whose sequence resembles the HIV initiator element. A cellular factor that binds at the cap site has been identified. The E/L gene promoters are heterogeneous in that the minimal VP16 gene promoter from bp −90 to +6 contains an E Box (CACGTG) at −85, a CAAT box at −77, and an SP1 site at −48, and a different initiator element.

Analyses of L viral gene promoters have shown that the upstream sequences consist of a TATA box with few other upstream transcription factor binding sites and with additional sequences needed for activation within the 5′ untranslated region. For example, the L *U_L38* gene promoter (Fig. 9.8) contains three elements: (a) an unusual TATA element with the sequence TTTAAA at −29, (b) a consensus initiator element at the transcriptional start site, and (c) a downstream activation sequence (DAS) from bp +20 to +33 that is required for normal levels of gene expression. The DAS seems to increase transcriptional initiation, and several other HSV L genes, including *U_S11*, *gC* (*U_L44*), *gB* (*U_L27*), *L/ST*, and *U_L49.5*, have similar downstream control elements in their promoter. In addition, the *gC* gene DAS can partially substitute for the *U_L38* DAS, suggesting that common mechanisms may act on the different DAS sequences. The Ku70 or DNA-binding subunit of the DNA-dependent protein kinase and hTAF(II)70 have been identified as factors binding to the DAS. Given that HSV infection leads to the degradation of the catalytic subunit of DNA-PK and loss of kinase activity, this effect may free up the Ku70 subunit for interaction with viral DNA.

ICP22/US1.5

ICP22 is required in certain cell types for optimal accumulation of a subset of late (L) gene products exemplified by the US11, UL38, and UL41 proteins. This function largely maps to the C-terminal domain of ICP22 and can also be contributed by the smaller *U_S1.5* gene product.[320] In particular, in human lung fibroblasts at late stages of infection, viral transcript levels are reduced to some extent across all kinetic classes in the absence of ICP22 expression.[141] ICP0 is among the affected IE genes, and ICP22 and US1.5 have been shown in transient transfection assays in Vero cells to also limit ICP0-mediated transactivation of reporter genes.[49,320] Whether this effect is independent of ICP22-dependent effects on viral gene expression remains unclear; nor is it yet known whether the effects of ICP22 on viral transcript levels are transcriptional or posttranscriptional.

ICP22 interacts with a number of cellular proteins, and the resulting changes to the infected host cell may explain its effects on viral gene expression. First, ICP22 alters RNA pol II phosphorylation during infection, potentially affecting RNA pol II transcriptional activity. In conjunction with the UL13 protein kinase, ICP22 causes accumulation of a form of RNA pol II phosphorylated at the serine-5 position in the C-terminal domain. In addition, early in infection and independently of UL13, ICP22 causes the loss of serine 2-phosphorylated RNA pol II. ICP22 has also been found to interact with cdk9, and this complex can phosphorylate the C terminus of RNA pol II in a US3 kinase–dependent manner.[122] Second, ICP22, in conjunction with the UL13 protein kinase, mediates the activation of the cdc2 kinase and the degradation of the cdc2 binding partners, cyclins A and B. cdc2 subsequently acquires a new partner, the UL42 DNA polymerase processivity factor. The cdc2-UL42 complex recruits topoisomerase IIα in an ICP22-dependent manner to promote L gene expression. It has been proposed that the ICP22/UL42/topoisomerase complex enables transcription of newly synthesized concatemeric DNA, which in the absence of this complex could accumulate in tangles, blocking access of the transcriptional machinery. ICP22 is also required for the formation of nuclear foci that contain cellular chaperone proteins, proteasomal components, and ubiquitinated proteins.[35] These foci typically form near replication compartments and could potentially affect viral gene expression in replication compartments. Lastly, there is also evidence that ICP22 promotes the elongation of viral gene transcripts through the recruitment of cellular transcription elongation factors to viral DNA late in infection.[141] ICP22 may thus facilitate viral late gene expression through specific effects on transcription elongation.

Export of Viral RNA From the Nucleus

The export of cellular mRNA from the nucleus is coupled to RNA splicing in the nucleus. As HSV infection inhibits RNA splicing, this thus raises the question of how nascent viral transcripts are transported from their site of transcription in the nucleus to the cytoplasm for translation in HSV-infected cells. In addition to the potential role of ICP27 in nuclear export of viral RNAs as described above, HSV replication compartments move from the periphery of the nucleus of infected cells and coalesce at nuclear speckles, a movement process involving active transport using nuclear actin and myosin and ongoing transcription. This coalescence of compartments and the resulting nuclear arrangement promotes export of late viral mRNAs, the vast majority of which lack introns.[64] This argues that a new export system for viral mRNAs may be assembled in the nucleus of infected cells.

Posttranscriptional Control of Viral Gene Expression in the Cytoplasm

Subverting Host Signaling Pathways that Regulate Ribosome Loading onto mRNA

Like host cell mRNAs produced by the cellular RNA pol II, all HSV mRNAs contain a modified 5′-terminal "cap" structure composed of 7-methylguanosine (m^7G) joined via a 5′-5′ triphosphate bridge to the transcript 5′-end that is installed cotranscriptionally by cellular capping enzymes. Besides providing mRNA stability, this 5′-cap ensures recognition of viral mRNAs by host translation initiation factors that load 40S ribosomes onto mRNA.[360] While host protein synthesis is curtailed in HSV-1–infected cells, the cellular protein synthesis machinery is stimulated by multiple, independent viral functions designed to subvert host regulatory controls that normally limit mRNA translation in response to physiological stress.[199,446] Loading 40S ribosomes onto capped mRNA is tightly regulated and dependent upon eukaryotic translation initiation factors (eIFs) (Fig. 9.9). Cap recognition by the cellular cap-binding protein eIF4E is normally followed by binding to the large scaffolding component eIF4G, which associates with an ATP-dependent RNA helicase eIF4A and the eIF3-bound 40S ribosome. By binding to and sequestering the cap-recognition protein eIF4E, the eIF4E-binding protein (4E-BP) family of translational repressors regulates eIF4E availability, restricts eIF4G-binding and 40S ribosome loading, and controls cap-dependent translation.[360,446] Activation of PI-3 kinase-Akt signaling in uninfected cells stimulates mTORC1, which hyperphosphorylates 4E-BP1 and releases eIF4E from the repressor. This regulatory circuit is tightly controlled in normal primary cells and contains a negative feedback circuit to limit PI-3 kinase Akt-dependent activation of mTORC1. To prevent 4E-BP1 from restricting virus protein synthesis and enforce high-level mRNA translation in infected cells, HSV encodes the α-herpesvirus–specific ser/thr protein kinase US3 to ensure constitutive mTORC1 activation during the productive growth cycle[78] (Fig. 9.9). Even though US3 exhibits little resemblance to any specific cellular ser/thr kinase, which confounds target substrate prediction, it shares many substrates with the cellular kinase Akt, including tuberous sclerosis complex (TSC) subunit 2. By directly phosphorylating TSC2 on identical sites targeted by Akt, US3 prevents TSC from inhibiting mTORC1 and constitutively stimulates mTORC1-dependent phosphorylation and inactivation of the

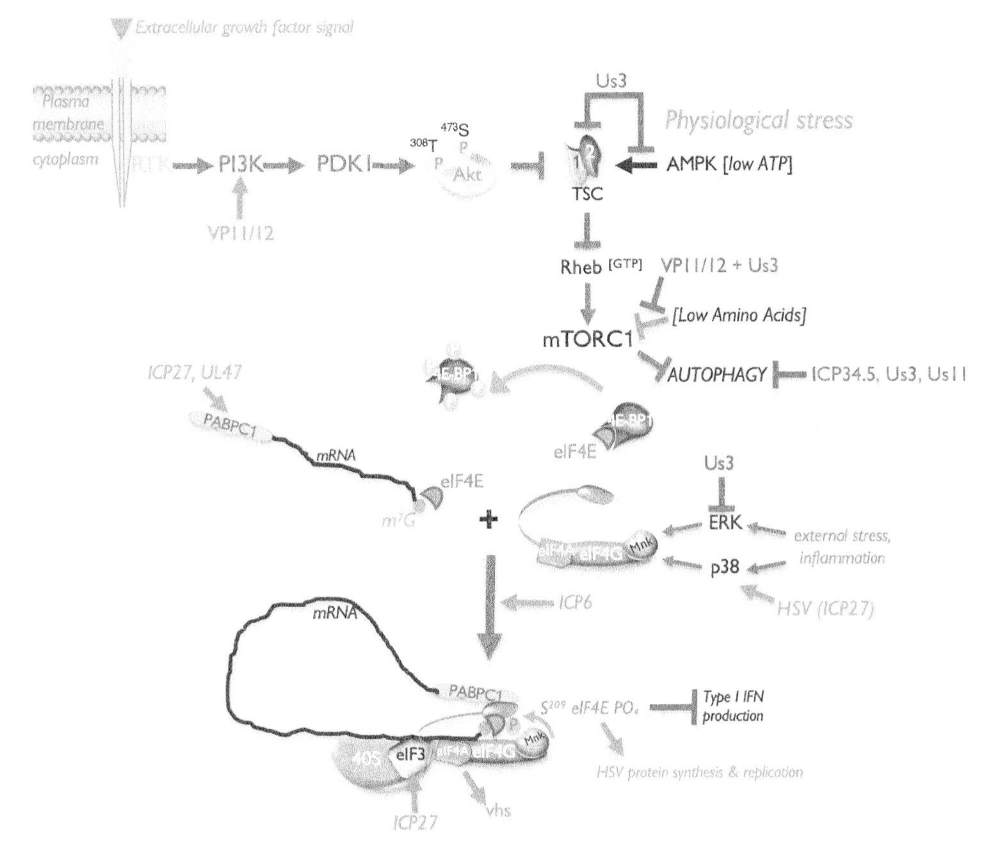

FIGURE 9.9 Regulation of the cellular cap-dependent translation initiation machinery in HSV-infected cells. Cell signaling pathways are depicted that sample extracellular and intracellular cues to regulate mTORC1 activity and allow mRNA translation to be responsive to changing environmental and physiological conditions (including infection). In uninfected cells, Akt phosphorylation (T308, S473) and activation in response to an activated growth factor receptor tyrosine kinase (RTK) represses the tuberous sclerosis complex (TSC1/2). Subsequent Rheb-GTP accumulation in response to TSC inhibition activates mTORC1. Physiological stress (energy, amino acid [aa] insufficiency) represses mTORC1 through specific effectors. Phosphorylation and inactivation of 4E-BP translational repressor family members, including 4E-BP1, by mTORC1 stimulates m^7G cap-dependent translation initiation by regulating availability of the cap-binding protein eIF4E. Once released from 4E-BP1, eIF4E physically associates with eIF4G, which interacts with the DEAD-box-containing RNA helicase eIF4A, and assembles a multisubunit protein complex called eIF4F on the m^7GTP-capped mRNA 5′-terminus (*m^7G*). Regulated assembly of eIF4E, eIF4G, and eIF4A into the eIF4F complex controls cap-dependent mRNA translation as eIF4F recruits eIF3-bound 40S subunits to the mRNA capped 5′ end. HSV-encoded factors that stimulate (*green*) and repress (*red*) the indicated cellular effectors to regulate mRNA translation in infected cells are indicated.

4E-BP1 repressor[78] (Fig. 9.9). This guarantees availability of sufficient, active eIF4E cap-binding protein pools during the viral productive replication program needed to support HSV mRNA translation.

Besides overcoming translational repression dependent upon 4E-BP1, translation initiation requires 40S ribosome recruitment onto viral mRNAs. This is stimulated by the multifunctional HSV-1 ICP6 protein, which physically interacts with eIF4G and promotes eIF4G binding to eIF4E[494] (Fig. 9.9). As eIF4G associates with eIF3-bound 40S ribosomes, this provides a molecular mechanism whereby 40S ribosome loading onto capped mRNA is stimulated in HSV-infected cells. It further represents an early role for the multifunctional ICP6 protein, originally identified as the large ribonucleotide reductase subunit, and potentially explains in part why the large subunit is expressed earlier than small subunit, the latter being required in a complex with ICP6 for ribonucleotide reductase activity.

By stimulating binding of eIF4E to eIF4G, ICP6 also stimulates eIF4E phosphorylation (Fig. 9.9) by bringing the cellular eIF4G-associated kinase Mnk1 into proximity of its substrate eIF4E.[494] Phosphorylation of eIF4E regulates selective mRNA translation and in doing so impacts innate immune responses by stimulating translation of IκBα mRNA, which in turn limits NF-κB activation and type I interferon production.[173] Thus, in addition to stimulating assembly of a translation initiation factor complex needed for viral mRNA translation, HSV functions also stimulate modification of eIF4E to selectively prevent cell intrinsic antiviral responses.

The recruitment of 40S ribosomal subunits to mRNA is also stimulated by ICP27, which associates with the host PABPC1 C-terminal domain.[431] By interacting with PABPC1, an ICP27-MS2 fusion protein tethered to a reporter gene containing 3′-MS2–binding sites enhanced translation in an eIF4G-dependent manner.[431] ICP27 is found associated with PABPC1, eIF4G, and eIF3 and stimulates translation of a subset of viral late mRNAs in infected cells.[112,128,140] Paradoxically, PABPC1 subcellular distribution is altered upon infection in an ICP27-independent manner, and the majority of the protein accumulates within nuclei late in infection.[112,403] Nuclear retention of PABP could potentially facilitate selective deposition of PABPC1 onto viral mRNAs coincident with their ICP27-dependent export, because PABPC1 nuclear export in mammalian cells predominantly reflects mRNA trafficking,[157] and ICP27 enables nuclear export of viral mRNAs.[469] PABC1, however, is not effectively retained upon isolation of cap-binding translation initiation factor complexes from HSV-1–infected

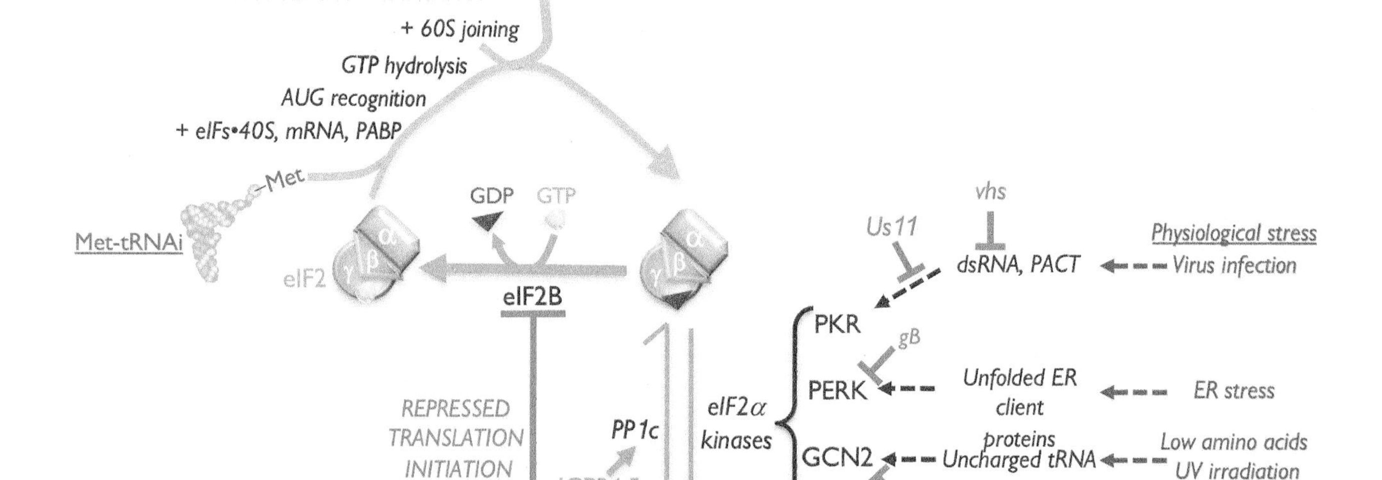

FIGURE 9.10 Multiple, independent HSV-encoded functions prevent eukaryotic initiation factor eIF2α phosphorylation and support translation initiation. Left: eIF2 is a GTP-binding, cellular translation initiation factor composed of three subunits (α, β, γ). It functions to load eIF3-bound 40S ribosomal subunits with methionyl-transfer RNA (Met-tRNAi). Following recruitment of mRNA, recognition of the AUG start codon, and GTP hydrolysis stimulated by eIF5, 60S subunit joining with 40S subunits completes 80S ribosome assembly and translation initiation commences. Inactive eIF2•GDP is released, and the guanosine nucleotide exchange factor (GEF) eIF2B is required to recycle active GTP-bound eIF2. Upon phosphorylation of eIF2α on S51 by either of four known eIF2α kinases, tight binding of eIF2B to phospho-eIF2 inhibits recycling of inactive eIF2•GDP to active eIF2•GTP thereby repressing translation initiation. **Right:** Each cellular eIF2α kinase is stimulated by specific activator molecules (*activators*) that accumulate in response to a discrete physiological stress. Partnered with the HSV-encoded regulatory subunit ICP34.5, the protein phosphatase 1 catalytic subunit (PP1c) promotes eIF2α dephosphorylation. HSV functions that activate (*green*) or repress (*red*) the indicated host effectors are shown.

cells,[493] in contrast to findings in uninfected and HCMV-infected cells. Further investigation is needed to better resolve the roles of PABPC1 in HSV-infected cells.

Finally, properties of ribosomes themselves may be altered in response to HSV-1 infection. Originally regarded as invariant, homogenous components charged exclusively with decoding mRNA, evidence now suggests that ribosome protein composition is heterogeneous and can regulate gene expression. Results from a recent siRNA screen targeting individual ribosome proteins (RPs) revealed that overall protein synthesis in uninfected cells was more sensitive to RP depletion than in HSV-1–infected cells.[485] Continued protein synthesis despite RP depletion required late viral gene expression and was specifically dependent upon the HSV-1–encoded RNA-binding protein VP22. Thus, VP22 is able to overcome RP insufficiency, which could conceivably support viral protein synthesis and replication and in response to RP variations across cell types and physiological conditions. Further work is required to decipher the underlying mechanism of how VP22 compensates for RP insufficiency.

Preserving Translation Initiation Capacity

The translation initiation factor eIF2 plays a fundamental role in uninfected and infected cell protein synthesis and is targeted by virus-encoded and host regulatory mechanisms.[446] A heterotrimeric GTP-binding protein composed of a regulatory α subunit, an RNA-binding β-subunit, and a GTP-binding γ-subunit, the GTP-bound form of eIF2, loads the 40S ribosome with initiator methionine tRNA (Fig. 9.10). Following the initiation of protein synthesis subsequent to 60S subunit joining, eIF2•GDP is released and must be recycled to the GTP-bound, active form by the guanine nucleotide exchange factor (GEF) eIF2B (Fig. 9.10). As cell intrinsic innate immune response components, several host ser/thr eIF2α kinases are activated by discrete physiological stresses and impact eIF2 activity in response to stresses including virus infection (Fig. 9.10).[446] Transcription from numerous opposing transcriptional units on opposite DNA strands in the HSV genome likely results in the accumulation of double-stranded (ds) RNA,[101] a pathogen-associated molecular pattern (PAMP) indicative of virus infection. Prior to stimulation, the cellular dsRNA-activated protein kinase PKR remains catalytically inactive until it detects and binds dsRNA in HSV-1–infected cells or is stimulated by a protein activator PACT.[446] Activated PKR phosphorylates eIF2α on residue S51 (Fig. 9.10). Phospho-eIF2 remains bound to eIF2B and inhibits the GEF from regenerating active eIF2•GTP (Fig. 9.10). Because the GEF eIF2B is limiting in most cells, modest increases in phosphorylated eIF2α can largely inhibit new protein synthesis by antagonizing eIF2B and restricting infected cell protein synthesis.[199,446] PKR itself is an interferon-stimulated gene product, emphasizing its role as an anti-HSV host defense factor.

To preserve sufficient pools of active eIF2 that are required to initiate protein synthesis, multiple independent HSV-encoded functions act to prevent phosphorylated eIF2α accumulation and/or activation of eIF2α kinases including PKR.[446] The amount of HSV genome coding capacity devoted to controlling eIF2 phosphorylation and its impact on virulence and pathogenesis emphasizes the importance of this process to virus infection biology. The viral *R_L1* gene encodes the ICP34.5 protein, which shares homology in its C terminus with the cellular GADD34 gene product. Both ICP34.5 and the host GADD34 are regulatory subunits that physically bind to the cellular ser/thr protein phosphatase 1α (PP1α) catalytic subunit and target the enzyme to specific substrates including eIF2[272] (Fig. 9.10). By functioning as a constitutively active PP1α regulatory subunit in HSV-infected cells, ICP34.5 preserves unphosphorylated eIF2α and potentially counteracts any cellular eIF2α kinase, including PKR. Significantly, ICP34.5-deficient viruses are unable to sustain infected cell protein synthesis at late times postinfection in numerous cell types, and although L mRNAs accumulate normally, late protein synthesis is arrested due to the accumulation of phosphorylated eIF2α. Not only are ICP34.5-deficient viruses hypersensitive to interferon,[62,323] they are profoundly neuroattenuated following delivery into the CNS by direct intracranial injection in mice.[74] Of all the HSV genes identified to date, removal of the gene encoding ICP34.5 results in the greatest loss of neurovirulence compared to any other single virus gene, establishing ICP34.5 as a major genetic virulence determinant.[74]

In contrast to ICP34.5, which acts broadly to counter eIF2α kinases, HSV also encodes specific effectors dedicated to inhibiting discrete eIF2α kinases (Fig. 9.10). Chief among these is the US11 gene product. The *U_S11* gene is expressed with true-late (L) kinetics and encodes an 18 Kd predicted MW protein that migrates with an apparent MW of approximately 21 Kd on SDS–polyacrylamide gels. This aberrant observed migration is likely due to a repetitive region composed of varied Arg-X-Pro motif iterations within the US11 C terminus among different HSV strains. Approximately 600 copies of the US11 protein are packaged within the tegument allowing US11 to be delivered into the host cytoplasm immediately upon infection. Although US11 has been found associated with polyribosomes at times that precede viral gene expression and accumulates within infected cell nucleoli, specific US11 functions ascribed to these discrete subcellular locales remain to be defined. Early work showed that US11 specifically binds to 60S rRNA, while later studies showed sequence and structure-specific binding of US11 to RNA.[50,228] Indeed, the repetitive R-X-P motif functions as a dsRNA-specific binding module that can physically associate with PKR in a ribonuclease-insensitive manner.[228] While US11-deficient viruses replicate to near wild-type levels in the permissive monkey kidney Vero cell line, they replicate to reduced levels and direct reduced rates of protein synthesis in primary human fibroblasts and are hypersensitive to interferon.[323] Isolation and mapping of an extragenic suppressor mutation that allowed replication of an *ICP34.5* deletion mutant in nonpermissive cells provided the first evidence that US11 and ICP34.5 were partially redundant factors that functioned in the same signaling circuit to regulate eIF2α phosphorylation. In the absence of ICP34.5, temporal deregulation of US11 allowing it to be expressed as an IE gene instead of a L gene product was sufficient to preclude both the accumulation of phosphorylated eIF2α and the premature cessation of infected cells protein synthesis prior to the completion of the viral productive growth cycle. Subsequent genetic studies confirmed that this required the C-terminal 68 RXP repeat-containing region of US11 that bound both dsRNA and PKR.[228] US11 also prevented PKR activation in response to the protein activator PACT.[366] Thus, US11 functions as a dedicated eIF2α kinase antagonist specific for PKR.

Besides PKR, three additional eIF2α kinases exist in mammals and their activities are likely countered by the ICP34.5 PP1 regulatory subunit (Fig. 9.10).[446] One of these, the ER-resident kinase PERK, is activated by ER stress resulting from accumulation of unfolded client proteins in the ER lumen.[221] HSV-1 was found to be resistant to experimentally induced ER stress, and gB was found to physically associate with the ER luminal domain of PERK. Furthermore, gB regulates viral protein accumulation in a PERK-dependent manner, defining a virus-encoded PERK-specific effector together with a new strategy by which viruses are able to maintain ER homeostasis.[322] While gB displays the hallmarks of a viral PERK-specific antagonist and US11 is a PKR-specific antagonist, gH reportedly interacts with GCN1, which is a GCN2 trans-acting positive effector, and regulates eIF2α phosphorylation in infected cells (Fig. 9.10).[179] A discrete HSV function that specifically targets the remaining cellular eIF2α kinase HRI has not been identified and may or may not exist.

Controlling Infected Cell Gene Expression by mRNA Decay

Manipulation of host gene expression begins immediately following entry when virus tegument components are released into the cytoplasm. Among them is the endoribonuclease UL41 or vhs. Early studies showed that the rapid suppression of host protein synthesis following HSV infection coincided with disruption of polyribosomes and suggested the involvement of a virion structural component. Mutant viruses unable to impair protein synthesis in the presence of actinomycin D, which prevents transcription, were isolated from mutagenized stocks and defined a single open reading frame (U_L41) encoding the virion host shutoff (vhs) function. Besides the host shut-off deficiency, vhs mutants exhibited deregulated temporal accumulation of viral IE mRNAs, consistent with a deficiency in posttranscriptional control of viral gene expression and were shown to lack a function that destabilizes viral and host mRNAs. Subsequent studies established that the vhs polypeptide is an intrinsic endoribonuclease that preferentially cleaves at single-stranded C or U residues within mRNA. Although vhs accelerates turnover of many normally stable viral and host mRNAs, its activity within infected cells principally requires a host cell translation initiation factor, eIF4H, which imparts selectivity and specificity limiting endoribonucleolytic cleavage to mRNA in polyribosomes.[407] As eIF4H stimulates the RNA helicase eIF4A that is associated with the multisubunit translation initiation factor complex assembled onto the capped mRNA 5′-end, the vhs-eIF4H association provides a mechanism to specifically load vhs onto mRNAs destined to be translationally active. Following targeting to the mRNA 5′-terminal region and primary endonucleolytic cleavage by vhs in the vicinity of translation initiation sites,[423] subsequent 5′-3′ directional degradation of the uncapped transcript body 3′-terminal fragment is dependent upon the cellular exoribonuclease Xrn1.[142] An alternate mode of vhs action has been proposed for short-lived mRNAs that contain 3′-AU–rich elements (AREs) in their 3′-UTRs, many of which encode inflammatory cytokines or stress-responsive proteins. Through a physical interaction with tristetraprolin, which recognizes AREs and promotes degradation of ARE-containing mRNAs via the exosome in uninfected cells, vhs cleavage is detected at or near AREs. While the resulting vhs-dependent 3′-cleavage products on ARE-containing mRNAs are unstable and presumed degraded by Xrn1, the remaining 5′-capped mRNA fragments reportedly have longer half-lives.

While many viral mRNAs have been shown to be sensitive to vhs-dependent turnover,[357] at least four additional virus-encoded proteins reportedly associate with vhs to regulate its endoribonuclease activity and have been proposed in part to orchestrate the accumulation of different kinetic classes of HSV-1 mRNA. Three of these proteins are tegument components (UL47, VP22, VP16) that are produced late in infection and can neutralize vhs activity.[426] This provides a mechanism to limit vhs nuclease activity while allowing quantities of vhs to accumulate for incorporation into virions. Upon delivery into the host cytoplasm following infection, vhs is released from the tegument via an unknown mechanism and accumulates in small, punctate cytoplasmic granules while it promotes selective degradation of cellular and viral mRNAs, cleaves mRNA in polyribosomes, and contributes to polyribosome disruption early in infection. Recently, vhs and cofactors including VP22 were also found to regulate nuclear export of late viral mRNAs in human fibroblasts, exposing an additional mechanism through which vhs regulates gene expression posttranscriptionally.[367]

vhs has also been found to associate with the ICP27 IE protein and the UL47 protein.[426,455] Whereas vhs is thought to load onto the mRNA 5′ end via association with cap-dependent translation initiation factors, ICP27 and UL47 interact with PABPC1, which is bound to polyA tails at the mRNA 3′-terminus.[112,403] The proximity of mRNA 5′ and 3′ ends mediated by an interaction between PABPC1 and the translation initiation factor eIF4G at the 5′ end could conceivably allow for transfer of vhs from the mRNA 5′ end to ICP27 and/or UL47 tethered via PABPC1 at the 3′ end.[426] In theory, this could provide a mechanism to regulate vhs activity and possibly spare ICP27-bound mRNAs on ribosomes from vhs-mediated destruction. Alternatively, such vhs-containing subcomplexes involving other tegument proteins could represent an early stage in virion assembly that limits unrestricted vhs activity that would otherwise suppress viral protein synthesis.[380] In addition, vhs stimulates polysome recruitment and translation of naturally occurring HSV mRNAs at late times postinfection via an unknown mechanism.[100]

While bulk host mRNA turnover is accelerated by vhs, all host mRNAs are not equivalently susceptible and mRNAs that survive vhs-induced decay have been identified. GADD45β and tristetraprolin are inducible mRNAs that did not detectably decay in productively infected cells, and their encoded polypeptide products accumulated. In addition, prior splicing or artificially tethering exon junction complex (EJC) components stabilized a reporter mRNA from virion-delivered vhs degradation and enhanced accumulation of its encoded protein late in infection.[401] While the underlying mechanism of how the splicing history of an mRNA influences its sensitivity to vhs imposed decay remains to be determined, it could impact the expression of the few spliced HSV mRNAs. Although the functional consequences of mRNAs that escape vhs-mediated turnover remain incompletely understood, accelerated mRNA decay imposed by vhs coupled with reduced transcription from cellular RNA pol II promoters and suppression of mRNA splicing by ICP27 together ensure that the vast majority of cytoplasmic mRNAs in cells productively infected with HSV are viral and effectively shut-off or severely restrict host protein synthesis.

In addition to sculpting and sharpening temporal transitions between IE, E, and L kinetic classes of viral mRNAs by promoting mRNA decay, the vhs endoribonuclease antagonizes host defenses by accelerating host mRNA decay and thereby restricting production of critical host defense components including cellular intrinsic innate immune effectors like ATRX, cytokines, IFI16, and type I interferons.[214,347,357] Notably, vhs-deficient mutants replicate to reduced levels in interferon-treated cells, more proficiently activate dendritic cells,[92] have reduced capability to down-regulate MHC class I and are severely attenuated in small animal models. Together, this underscores the critical role the HSV endoribonuclease plays in potentially modulating both innate and adaptive immunity and in pathogenesis.

Besides impacting mRNA decay, vhs also influences double-stranded RNA (dsRNA) formation in infected cells. dsRNA accumulates and concentrates at stress granules (SGs) in cells infected with vhs-deficient HSV-1.[52] SGs are dynamic aggregates comprising mRNA, translation factors, and RNA-binding proteins that accumulate in the cytoplasm in response to perturbations in protein synthesis including those associated with virus-induced shutoff of host protein synthesis.[372,446] They typically form following phosphorylation and inactivation of the translation initiation factor eIF2α, a substrate of the dsRNA-activated protein kinase PKR, and serve as hubs to potentiate PKR activation during infection. Indeed, vhs is one of several viral factors that plays a role in limiting PKR activation (Fig. 9.10),[417] interferes with SG accumulation,[138] and regulates the accumulation of viral dsRNA composed of complimentary transcripts derived from opposing DNA coding strands in infected cells.[101] Surprisingly, while innate immune activators like dsRNA and sensors including PKR are enriched at SGs in HSV-1–infected cells, this did not detectably influence IFN induction by HSV-1. Instead, the biggest effect on IFN induction was mediated by cGAS and IFI16.[52]

Viral DNA Replication

Production of progeny virus requires the amplification of the input viral DNA genomes for assembly into progeny viral particles. Many of the viral E proteins prepare the infected cell for or are directly involved in viral DNA replication through (a) targeting and assembling viral and cellular proteins into intranuclear structures where viral DNA replication initiates (prereplicative sites) and where viral DNA replication proceeds (replication compartments; Fig. 9.5), (b) enhancement of levels of nucleotide precursors for viral DNA synthesis in resting cells, and (c) catalyzing the synthesis of viral DNA. As described in the Gene Expression section above, the input viral genomes target to the nuclear periphery soon after entry into the nucleus. Following IE and E gene transcription from the viral DNA molecules, likely at these sites, the viral DNA replication proteins then localize to these genomes on the nuclear periphery to form structures called prereplicative sites.[102,374] The prereplicative sites near ND-10 bodies are the sites of initial viral DNA replication, and these structures grow into replication compartments as DNA replication proceeds.[102] The replication compartments enlarge, merge, and fill the nucleus, concomitant with peripheral margination of the host chromatin,[430] suggesting that the HSV replication compartments displace the cellular chromatin from internal sites in the nucleus. The replication compartments serve to concentrate the viral and cellular proteins needed for viral DNA replication, L gene transcription, and encapsidation of the viral DNA and exclude the cellular epigenetic silencing components and host restriction and innate sensing molecules, all of which enhance viral replication.

The full mechanism of viral DNA replication has not been elucidated, although we have significant knowledge about the viral gene products and origins of replication. Seven viral proteins are required for viral DNA replication. The seven gene products are the viral DNA polymerase catalytic subunit (UL30) and its processivity factor (UL42), an origin-binding protein (UL9), the ICP8 ssDNA-binding protein (SSB; UL29), and the helicase–primase complex of three proteins, UL5, UL8, and UL52.[63] Host cell factors are presumably also involved in viral DNA synthesis, but these have not been identified, in large part because HSV DNA replication involving origin-dependent initiation and synthesis has not been reconstituted *in vitro*. Nevertheless, it seems likely that host enzymes, including the DNA polymerase α-primase, DNA ligase, and topoisomerase II, are also required. Early immunofluorescence studies showed that cellular replication protein A (RPA), PCNA, Rb, p53, DNA ligase 1, and DNA polymerase α colocalized with ICP8. Inhibition of topoisomerase II prevents efficient replication of HSV-1 DNA, possibly by preventing decatenation of newly synthesized daughter molecules. Proteomic studies showed that a large number of cellular DNA repair, DNA damage response, and recombination proteins are associated with ICP8[466] and localize to prereplicative sites and replication compartments.[466] Mre11, Rad50, Nbs1, RPA, MSH2, BRCA1, BLM, WRN, DNA ligase 1, RAD51, and Ku86 are located in prereplicative sites and replication compartments.[158,275,466] Cells defective for WRN helicase[466] or Mre11 or ATM[275] show reduced HSV replication so these proteins promote viral replication in some way. It is not known, however, if these host proteins are directly involved in viral DNA replication.

Viral DNA Replication Proteins

The seven essential HSV DNA replication proteins are reviewed in detail elsewhere,[393,512] but brief overviews of these seven proteins and relevant accessory proteins are included below.

DNA Polymerase

The HSV DNA polymerase has been studied extensively, partly as a result of its potential as a target for antiviral drugs. A new DNA polymerase activity was detected in HSV-infected cells in the 1960s, but formal genetic proof that it was virus encoded was not provided until the late 1970s when temperature-sensitive and drug-resistant mutations affecting the properties of the polymerase were isolated and mapped to the viral genome. The HSV DNA polymerase holoenzyme is a heterodimer of the 136-kDa UL30 protein complexed with the 65-kDa UL42 protein.

UL30

The UL30 protein contains the polymerase activity, and it contains three sequence motifs that are homologous and align with sequence motifs I, II, and III of other DNA polymerases. The UL30 protein also has an intrinsic 3′-5′-exonuclease activity, which can serve as a proofreading activity during viral DNA synthesis. The crystal structure of the UL30 protein defined the following domains: pre-NH2 domain, NH2-terminal domain, 3′-5′-exonuclease domain, polymerase palm subdomain, finger subdomain, and thumb subdomain. The RNase H activity of HSV-1 DNA pol is encoded within the 3′-5′ exonuclease domain.[260] The HSV DNA polymerase interacts with a broader range of deoxynucleoside triphosphates than cellular polymerases, and this has allowed the development of drugs that specifically inhibit the viral DNA polymerase and are used clinically (Chapter 10).

UL42

The UL42 subunit increases the processivity of the UL30 DNA polymerase activity. The structure of UL42 protein bound to the C-terminal fragment of UL30 has been determined, and UL42 is unusual in binding DNA directly as a monomer rather than as a toroid wrapping around the DNA like other processivity factors. UL42 is capable of linear diffusion along DNA despite its high affinity binding to DNA. The interaction between UL30 and UL42 is essential for viral DNA replication *in vivo*, and these interaction sites are being investigated as possible targets for antiviral compounds. UL42 also interacts with cdc2 and topoisomerase IIα.

Origin-Binding Protein (UL9, OBP)

The UL9 origin-binding protein forms a homodimer and binds specifically to the sequence CGTTCGCACTT. UL9 also has ATP-binding and DNA helicase motifs that are essential for viral replication. Binding of UL9 to origin sequences induces a bend in the DNA and formation of a single-stranded stem loop structure. The addition of the HSV single-stranded DNA-binding protein, ICP8, allows UL9 to unwind Box I of *ori*S if an 18-nucleotide single-strand tail is present 3′ to Box I. Thus, ICP8 may provide a single-stranded DNA region in the AT-rich region, from which UL9 can separate the strands. As an origin-binding protein, UL9 would play a role in origin-dependent synthesis originating from circular or linear molecules, but once synthesis has converted to a rolling circle or recombination-based mode, UL9 would presumably not be needed as an origin-binding protein. Consistent with this, overexpression of UL9 inhibits viral DNA synthesis.

Single-Stranded DNA–Binding Protein (ICP8, UL29)

ICP8 is an abundant protein in HSV-infected cells and was first identified as the major DNA-binding protein in HSV-infected cells. ICP8 binds preferentially to single-stranded DNA, and this ssDNA-binding (SSB) function is essential for viral DNA replication. ICP8 exhibits a helix-destabilizing activity but can also catalyze the renaturation of complementary single strands. Probably as a consequence of the latter two activities, ICP8 can promote strand transfer and this may contribute to the high frequency of homologous recombination observed in infected cells.

In addition to its SSB function, ICP8 interacts with several other viral DNA replication proteins. ICP8 physically interacts with UL9 and stimulates UL9 helicase activity, co-immunoprecipitates with UL8, and stimulates UL5/8/52 helicase activity, and functionally interacts with the viral DNA polymerase. Consistent with these numerous interactions, ICP8 is required for localization of other viral proteins and cellular proteins to prereplicative sites in infected cell nuclei.[102] Given its size (128 kDa) and numerous protein interactions, ICP8 is likely to play a scaffold role in the assembly of HSV DNA replication complexes. The crystal structure of a 60-residue C-terminal deletion form of ICP8 showed a novel fold consisting of a large N-terminal domain (residues 9–1038) and a small C-terminal domain (residues 1049–1129). The overall structure provided a potential groove containing aromatic and basic amino acid residues that could serve as the ssDNA-binding site. ICP8 possesses strand-melting and strand-annealing activities and has been reported to mediate limited strand exchange. ICP8 can also promote strand invasion.[339] ICP8 has the molecular properties of a DDE recombinase, and mutation of this domain (E1086A/D1087A) led to a greater than 100-fold reduction in DNA replication.[51,527] HIV integrase inhibitors that reduced HSV recombination also inhibited the ICP8 strand invasion activity.[527] Mutant viruses with defective ICP8 annealing activity show reduced DNA synthesis.[509]

DNA Helicase–Primase

This complex, which contains the viral protein products of the *U_L5*, *U_L8*, and *U_L52* genes, was first identified as a helicase activity from infected cells. The complex unwinds short oligonucleotides annealed to single-stranded M13 DNA in the 5′ to 3′ direction. A complex of UL5 and UL52 has DNA-dependent ATPase and GTPase, helicase, and primase activities so this constitutes the core enzyme. UL8 promotes the nuclear localization of this complex and, in concert with ICP8, stimulates optimal activities of the core enzyme. Thus, the holoenzyme can unwind a 2.3-kbp nicked plasmid in the presence of ICP8. The primase activity produces oligoribonucleotides 6 to 13 bases in length, and the preferred template sequence is 3′AGCCCTCCCA, with synthesis initiating at the first C.

Accessory Viral Gene Products Involved in Viral DNA Synthesis

Several other HSV gene products, including the thymidine kinase, ribonucleotide reductase, deoxyuridine triphosphatase, and uracil–DNA glycosylase, are not essential for viral replication in cultured cells but are likely to be essential for nucleotide metabolism, viral DNA synthesis, and/or repair in resting cells, such as neurons. The corresponding host cell enzymes are expressed at low levels or not expressed in resting cells, and it is likely that the virus encodes these enzymes to optimize its own DNA synthesis in these cells.

Thymidine Kinase (TK)

This enzyme was first identified as a deoxythymidine kinase, which gave rise to its name. In fact, it phosphorylates pyrimidines and even purine nucleosides. In addition, it has a thymidylate activity. Its broad substrate specificity allows it to phosphorylate nucleoside analog molecules (e.g., acyclovir), which then can serve as antiviral compounds. The HSV TK consists of a homodimeric complex of the UL23 protein, the structure of which has been solved. HSV presumably encodes a TK activity to provide nucleoside triphosphate precursors for DNA synthesis in resting cells such as neurons, where the cellular enzyme is not expressed. The viral enzyme leads to an increase in dTTP pools relative to that seen in uninfected cells or early in infection. This complicates the use of radioactive thymidine for labeling of viral DNA synthesis in infected cells because the specific activity of the labeled DNA will be lower at later times of infection.

Deoxyuridine Triphosphatase (dUTPase)

The HSV dUTPase, a monomer of UL50 protein, hydrolyzes dUTP to dUMP and pyrophosphate, preventing the incorporation of uracil into DNA. HSV-1 dUTPase mutants are attenuated for neurovirulence, neuroinvasiveness, and reactivation from latency.

Ribonucleotide Reductase

Ribonucleotide reductase enzymes catalyze the reduction of ribonucleoside diphosphates to the corresponding deoxyribonucleoside diphosphate. The HSV enzyme consists of a complex of the UL39 and UL40 proteins as an $\alpha_2\beta_2$ tetramer. The HSV ribonucleotide reductase is not subject to the same allosteric controls as the cellular enzyme; thus, the HSV enzyme is not inhibited by the increased dTTP pools in HSV-infected cells. The HSV ribonucleotide reductase is required for viral replication in nondividing cells. The large subunit has an intrinsic autophosphorylating kinase activity that is separable from the ribonucleotide reductase activity.

Uracil N-Glycosylase

This enzyme removes uracil bases from DNA, bases that arise in DNA by the deamination of cytosine to form uracil, by the cleavage of the *N*-glycosidic bond linking uracil to the deoxyribose sugar. The site is then repaired so that a mutagenic event converting a G-C basepair to an A-T basepair does not occur. The HSV enzyme is encoded by the U_L2 gene.

Alkaline Nuclease

This enzyme is a phosphoprotein encoded by the U_L12 gene, has endo- and exonuclease activities, and is active at pH 9 to 10. As described below, this nuclease plays a role in viral DNA synthesis, DNA maturation, and encapsidation. The HSV nuclease may be required to resolve concatenated viral DNA for packaging. UL12 interacts with ICP8, possibly to allow the nuclease to act directly on viral replication intermediates or products. UL12 and ICP8 facilitate strand exchange *in vitro*, and ICP8 stimulates nuclease activity by increasing processivity of the enzyme.

Origins of Replication

The origins of viral DNA synthesis were identified through mapping of sequences found in defective viral genomes and sequences needed for plasmid DNA amplification in transfection studies.[489] The origins include *oriS*, a sequence located in the *c* sequences bounding the S component and therefore present in two copies in the viral genome, and *oriL*, a sequence located between the divergent transcription units of the U_L29 and U_L30 genes encoding the viral DNA replication proteins, ICP8 and DNA polymerase, respectively. Both *oriL* and *oriS* are palindromic structures, *oriL* being a 144-bp palindrome and *oriS* being a shorter palindrome of 45 bp, that center around AT-rich regions of 20 and 18 bp, respectively. Inverted repeats that contain binding sites for the UL9 protein, called Box I, are located on either side of the AT-rich region of *oriL*. *OriS* contains a Box I sequence to the 5′ side of the AT-rich region and a similar sequence with a 10-fold lower binding affinity for UL9, called Box II, located 3′ to the AT-rich region. In *oriL*, the Box I sequences are flanked by another homologous sequence, called Box III, which has greatly reduced affinity for UL9. *OriS* contains one copy of Box III flanking the 5′ Box I. *OriL* is notoriously unstable when cloned into plasmids, so little genetic analysis has been performed on this sequence. Box I is required for *oriS* function, and mutations in Box II greatly reduce DNA replication. Although Box III shows weak binding to UL9 *in vitro*, mutations in Box III reduce replication by approximately fivefold in transfection assays.

The reason(s) for three potential origins of replication in the viral genome are not apparent at this time. Neither origin is specifically required for viral replication. A mutant virus with a deletion in *oriL* is viable and showed normal burst size and latent infection. In addition, mutant viruses with both *oriS* sequences deleted showed at most a fourfold reduction in viral yields and only slightly delayed viral DNA synthesis. It has been suggested that one of these origins may represent vestigial origins from the L and S components of the viral genome and that one of these origins, *oriL*, may function in reactivation from latent infection. One study found that an *oriL* mutant virus shows reduced replication in mouse tissues and reduced reactivation from latent infection. Thus, *oriL* may be required for DNA replication in certain tissues; alternatively, the expression of the bounding U_L29 and U_L30 genes may be affected in these tissues.

Mechanisms of Viral DNA Replication

There is evidence that HSV DNA replication is a two-stage process in which an initial stage of DNA synthesis dependent on UL9 binding of viral origin sequences is followed by a switch to an origin-independent replication mechanism. The major viral DNA replicative products inside infected cells are long "head-to-tail" concatemers containing the four sequence isomers described above, and this is an important aspect of any model. There are two main basic models of HSV DNA replication as shown in Figure 9.11. The original model[37] involved binding of the HSV UL9 origin-binding protein to an origin on a circular viral DNA and subsequent formation of the HSV DNA replication complex, which replicates the molecule through an intermediate such as a Cairns circle or theta molecule (Fig. 9.11). Concatemers are then proposed to be generated following a conversion of the initial bidirectional replication to rolling circle replication. Alternatively, a replicative intermediate could undergo recombination to generate concatemeric molecules.

In the rolling circle model (Fig. 9.11), the first steps in HSV DNA replication involve the binding of UL9 protein to one or more of the origin sequences and the subsequent looping and distortion of the origin sequences by UL9. ICP8 then binds to UL9 and/or ssDNA regions, and the UL9 helicase activity unwinds the DNA. The helicase–primase complex is then recruited to the origin by interactions with UL9 and/or ICP8. Leading strand synthesis involves the unwinding of the DNA and synthesis of a primer by the HSV helicase–primase complex, from which leading strand synthesis can be accomplished by the HSV DNA polymerase UL30-UL42 holoenzyme. Alternatively, primers may be synthesized by the cellular polymerase α-primase. Lagging-strand synthesis is then accomplished by primer synthesis and UL30–UL42 extension of the DNA strand. HSV-1 progeny DNA is largely in the form of head-to-tail concatemers; thus, when viral DNA synthesis is converted to a rolling circle replicative mechanism, this would yield the concatemeric molecules observed in infected cells.

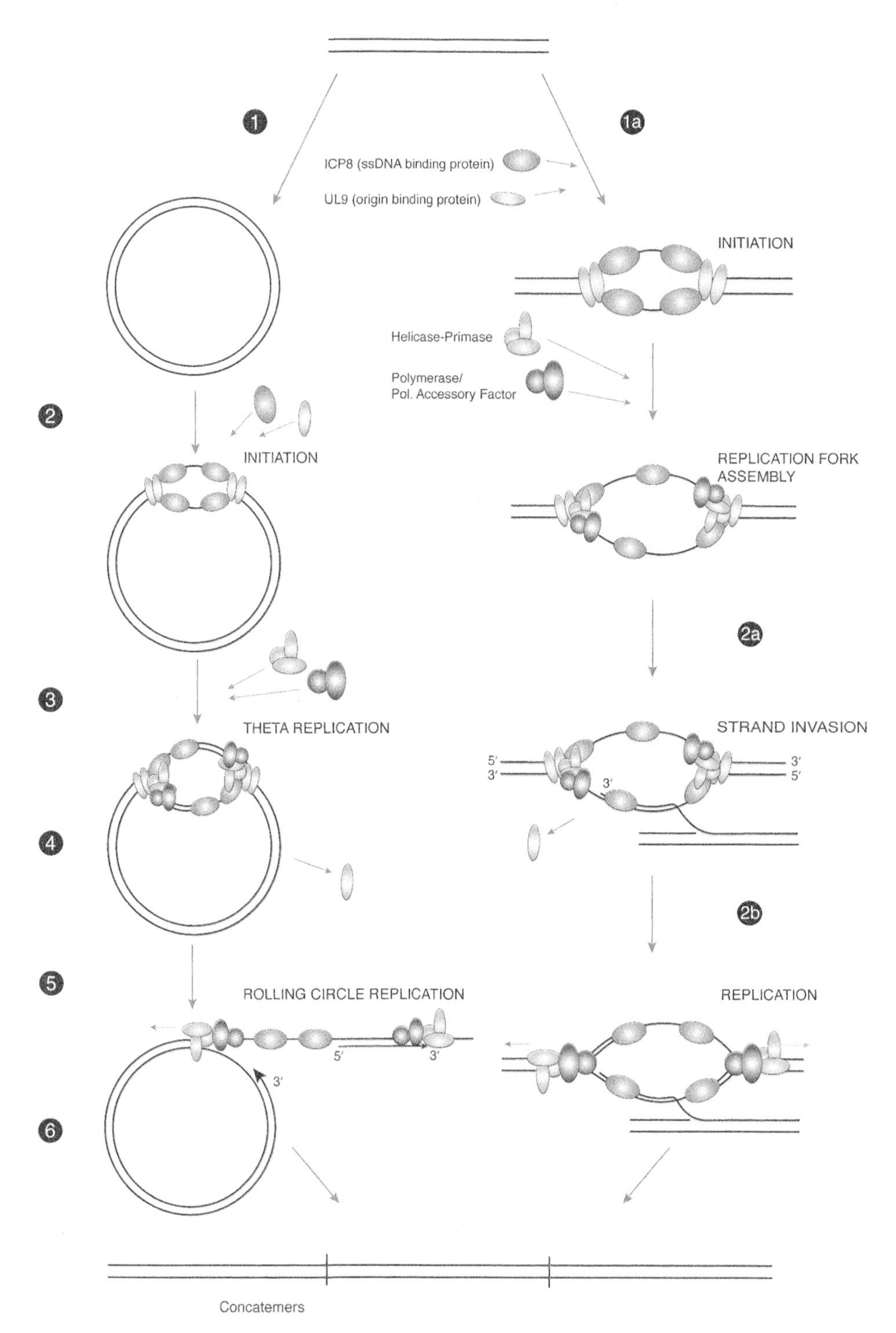

FIGURE 9.11 Diagram of models of HSV-1 DNA replication. Left: *Rolling circle replication.* (*1*) Input DNA is circularized upon entry into the nucleus. (*2*) UL9 (the origin binding protein) initially binds to specific elements in the origin (either *oriL* or *oriS*) and begins to unwind the DNA. UL9 then recruits ICP8 (the single-stranded DNA–binding protein) to the unwound single-stranded DNA. (*3*) UL9 and ICP8 recruit the five remaining viral DNA replication proteins to the replication forks. (*4*) The helicase–primase proteins and the viral polymerase complex assemble at each replication fork for initial rounds of theta form replication. (*5*) Replication switches from theta to rolling circle mode by an unknown mechanism. UL9 is not necessary for rolling circle replication, as it is not origin dependent. (*6*) Rolling circle DNA replication produces long head-to-tail concatemers of viral DNA, which are cleaved into monomeric molecules during packaging. **Right:** *Recombination-dependent replication.* (*1a*) Input DNA in linear or circular form is bound by UL9 to initiate viral DNA synthesis with subsequent recruitment of ICP8 to the unwound DNA followed by recruitment of the helicase–primase proteins and the viral polymerase complex to form an active replication fork. (*2a*) ICP8 promotes strand invasion from a separate viral genome. Strand invasion from broken strands of viral DNA or free genomic termini, resected by cellular or viral nucleases to yield single-strand templates, primes DNA synthesis. (*2b*) Recombination-dependent synthesis following priming by strand invasion enables formation of viral DNA concatemers. (Copyright, Catherine Sodroski and David Knipe.)

Replication mechanisms involving recombination have also been proposed.[339] By this model (Fig. 9.11), initiation could occur on a linear molecule or a circular molecule. ICP8 promotes strand invasion of another viral DNA molecule at a replication fork or other exposed homologous single-stranded regions of viral DNA, such as gaps in viral DNA at stalled replication forks or genomic termini, to prime viral DNA synthesis. This could then lead to the synthesis of concatemeric molecules.[509] It has been proposed that ICP8 interactions with the helicase–primase complex and the alkaline nuclease protein UL12 also contribute to recombination-mediated synthesis of viral DNA.

In support of the rolling circle model, there is evidence that viral DNA is rapidly circularized after entry.[448] In addition, DNA ligase IV and XRCC4 are required for circularization of the input viral genome for replication and knockdown of ligase IV or XRCC4-reduced viral DNA replication by 10- to 25-fold, arguing that circularization of the viral DNA leads to the majority of viral DNA synthesis. Furthermore, rolling circle replication on preformed templates has been achieved *in vitro*, and it is simpler to see how this mechanism could generate and propagate the tandem repeats of viral DNA observed in defective viral genomes.[37]

Evidence in support of recombinational mechanisms includes the need for the UL12 nuclease for optimal levels of viral DNA replication[156] and the large reduction in viral DNA replication by mutant viruses expressing ICP8 molecules that are defective for recombinase activity[51,527] or annealing activity.[509] Genomic inversions occur coincident with viral DNA synthesis[542] and are dependent upon the presence of the seven essential viral replication proteins, arguing that HSV-1 DNA synthesis and recombination are linked. Viral DNA replication intermediates include branched molecules and lariats, and this has been interpreted as evidence of recombination during replication. Alternatively, formation of these structures could be due to genomic inversions and recombination following DNA synthesis.

Rolling circle and recombinational mechanisms are not mutually exclusive, however, because models involving both rolling circle replication and recombination have been proposed.[392] Alternatively, ICP8 could play a role in strand invasion from a viral DNA molecule into the replicating circle to initiate rolling circle replication. By the latter hypothesis, both recombination and rolling circle replication would be involved in viral DNA synthesis and generation of concatemeric progeny DNA molecules. Finally, recombination could facilitate the restart of DNA synthesis at stalled replication forks. Thus, there is evidence for both recombination and a form of rolling circle replication playing roles in HSV DNA replication in separate or combined pathways.

Genomic inversions have been discussed above but do appear to occur concomitantly with viral DNA synthesis. This may be as a part of viral DNA synthesis, as proposed by Roizman et al.,[392] or by recombination following synthesis of the concatemeric molecule.

Viral DNA Recombination

Homologous recombination is very efficient in HSV-infected cells, and multiple crossover events between coinfecting viral genomes are apparent in progeny viruses, even between HSV-1 and HSV-2 genomes. Viral DNA replication is required for this high level of homologous recombination, and the time courses of DNA replication and recombination are parallel in cells transfected with viral *oriS* plasmids. As discussed above, the relationships between viral DNA replication and recombination are not well defined, but the single-stranded regions or the concatemeric molecules might be targets for cellular or viral recombination machinery. In addition, ICP8 is known to promote strand transfer, so it might play a role in recombination in infected cells. In support of this idea, HIV integrase inhibitors that inhibit the ICP8 recombinase activity reduce the generation of recombinant viruses in HSV coinfected cells.[527]

Inversion of the genomic L and S segments also involves recombination between the terminal repeats and the internal inverted repeats. As described above, HSV virion DNA contains four populations of molecules bearing the four orientations of the L and S components of the genome. This novel feature of the genome of HSV and certain other, but not all, herpesviruses (see Chapter 8) has long intrigued the field, and interest has been further piqued by the observation that viruses without internal repeats replicate well in continuous cell lines but poorly in primary human cells. These mutant viruses are nonpathogenic, suggesting that the internal inverted repeats play a key role in primary human cells and *in vivo*. The L–S junction sequences and in particular the ***a*** sequences promote high-efficiency inversion in that insertion of a copy of these sequences at other sites in the genome leads to inversion of these sequences. Duplication of certain other viral sequences at a second site in the viral genome can lead to additional inversion events, but these events appear to be less efficient than ***a*** sequence-mediated inversion. The 95bp *Uc-DR1* sequence is specifically required for inversion at the ***a*** sequence, but it remains to be determined if this event involves site-specific recombination or is a hot spot for recombination.

Activation of Host DNA Damage Response Pathways

The interactions of HSV with DNA repair pathways are complex. The presence of nicks and gaps in the incoming viral DNA is likely to result in activation of DNA repair pathways, as discussed in the Gene Expression section above. Consistent with this, HSV infection has been shown to activate the host DNA damage repair pathway.[275] Some of this host response is likely due to parental viral DNA,[314] but the peak response requires and/or coincides with viral DNA replication.[275] Phosphorylation of ATM is observed as early as 0.5 hpi but increases until 8 hpi during times of viral DNA synthesis.[275] Phosphorylation of ATM requires viral DNA replication, supporting the concept that replicating or replicated viral DNA serves as the stimulus for a more robust DDR pathway activation.[314] Thus, DNA damage sensors may recognize the input viral DNA, but the optimal response involves newly replicated DNA. HSV infection activates the ATM-dependent signaling pathway, while it inhibits the DNA-PKcs and ATR-dependent pathways.[275,318] To counter the inhibitory effects of DNA repair mechanisms on viral replication, ICP0 promotes the degradation of RNF8 and RNF168, which are mediators in the ATM pathway.[276,277] The effects of the DNA repair components on HSV replication are complex in that some components are inhibitory to viral replication while others stimulate viral replication.[275,466] It is conceivable that while HSV inhibits the DNA repair pathways, it has co-opted DNA repair mechanisms for its own genome replication, much as the host cell uses DNA repair mechanisms as part of its genomic synthesis.

In addition to maintaining genome integrity, the cellular DNA damage response (DDR) acts as an innate cell intrinsic barrier capable of limiting virus reproduction. In particular, how the repair of DNA damage associated with incoming HSV genomes and viral DNA synthesis influences virus reproduction is incompletely understood. Upon delivery of HSV-1 DNA into the host nucleus as a linear dsDNA genome containing nicks and gaps,[432] an elaborate DDR is elicited. To avoid activation of the cellular multisubunit DNA-dependent protein kinase (DNA-PK) in response to productive infection with HSV-1, the catalytic subunit is degraded in some but not all cultured cell lines in an ICP0-dependent manner.[354] Furthermore, DNA-PK–deficient murine cells support greater levels of HSV-1 productive growth.[354,466] This is consistent with proposed roles for DNA-PK as a nuclear DNA sensor that can limit virus reproductive growth.[136] While viral functions remodel facets of the host DDR to prevent viral genome silencing and suppress intrinsic antiviral defenses,[510,511] others including the cellular Fanconi anemia (FA) pathway are activated by HSV-1 infection.[223] Significantly, the FA pathway is critical for repairing interstrand DNA cross-links ensuring genome stability during DNA replication and plays a key role in the repair of endogenous dsDNA breaks (DSBs) that arise naturally during DNA synthesis through processes like replication fork stalling.[61] Cells rely on either error-prone nonhomologous end joining (NHEJ) or the more accurate homologous recombination (HR) repair pathways to repair DSBs.[66] FA pathway proteins function in part to antagonize error-prone DSB repair by NHEJ and instead stimulate more faithful DSB repair via HR. While productive HSV-1 replication was substantially impaired in FA-deficient cells, virus growth can be substantially restored by inhibiting DNA-PK to suppress NHEJ. Besides crippling the dsDNA innate immune sensor DNA-PK, FA-mediated inhibition of NHEJ via inactivating DNA-PK may represent a more physiological means to interfere with NHEJ in cells where DNA-PK is not degraded in response to HSV-1 productive growth. Although the NHEJ component DNA-PK restricts lytic virus reproduction in a cell intrinsic manner, DNA-PK activation regulates latent infections in neurons,[190] a cell type proficient in DSB repair by NHEJ compared to HR. This raises the possibility that cell type–specific, intrinsic DDR responses to DSBs play roles balancing lytic versus latent infection outcomes and will be discussed in detail in the latent infection section below.

Viral Nucleocapsid Assembly

Following their synthesis, the capsid proteins localize into the infected cell nucleus where capsid assembly occurs. Empty shells containing an internal scaffolding are assembled first and then viral DNA is inserted or encapsidated into the capsid concomitant with the loss of the scaffolding. Our knowledge of the mechanisms of assembly of the HSV capsid has come from several lines of experimentation: (a) study of infected cell complexes and structures, (b) assembly of capsid structures from extracts of insect cells infected with baculoviruses expressing HSV capsid and scaffolding proteins, (c) study of protein localization using immunofluorescence, (d) genetic analysis of the functions of capsid and scaffolding proteins, and (e) three-dimensional reconstructions obtained by cryo-EM. Each of these approaches has contributed important information to our understanding of this process.[32,87]

Immunofluorescence studies have shown that the preassembly starts in the cytoplasm where complexes involving at least some capsid proteins form prior to translocation to the nucleus. Several capsid proteins, including VP5, VP23, and VP26, cannot even enter the nucleus on their own and must bind a capsid protein partner that has a nuclear localization signal. For example, VP5, the major capsid protein, forms a 1:1 complex with pre-VP22a, a scaffold protein. Similarly, two copies of VP23 bind VP19C to form the heterotrimeric triplex. VP26, the small capsid protein, localizes into the nucleus only when it is coexpressed with VP5 and either VP19C or pre-VP22a.

Electron microscopic studies have shown that the final assembly of capsids occurs in the nucleus. Three types of capsids, called A-, B-, and C-capsids, have been identified in infected cell nuclear extracts using sucrose density gradient ultracentrifugation.[151] All three types of capsids are approximately 125 nm in diameter with an icosahedral outer shell (T = 16 symmetry) consisting of 150 hexons and 11 pentons made up of six or five copies of the major capsid protein VP5 (*U_L19*), respectively. Each hexon is additionally crowned with a hexamer of VP26 (*U_L35*), the small capsid protein. The hexons and pentons are linked by 320 triplexes, heterotrimers of two copies of VP23 (*U_L18*) and one copy of VP19C (*U_L38*). In each capsid, 1 of the 12 vertices contains a single portal composed of 12 copies of the portal protein UL6,[282,308] through which viral DNA is encapsidated during assembly[333] and ejected into the nucleus early in infection.[329] Each capsid also contains VP24 (*U_L26*),[286,298] the protease that cleaves the scaffold during capsid maturation and DNA encapsidation, described below.

C-capsids contain the viral DNA genome and go on to mature into infectious virions. Each vertex is decorated by five copies of the complex referred to as either the capsid vertex–specific complex (CVSC)[83,471] or the capsid-associated tegument complex (CATC).[99] This complex was originally thought to be specific for C-capsids but has also been observed in reconstructions of A- and B-capsids[83] albeit at, perhaps, lower amounts.[87] Each CVSC/CATC is composed of two copies of UL25, one copy of UL17 and two copies of the tegument protein UL36, or rather, its C-terminal helix.[99] UL17 and UL25, referred to as the auxiliary capsid proteins, are essential for proper DNA retention in the mature capsid and reinforce the outer shell of the capsid[433] to help it withstand the internal pressure of approximately 18 atmospheres from the encapsidated DNA genome.[36] In turn, UL36 anchors the tegument layer to the capsid.

Two additional icosahedral capsid types observed in infected cells are the empty A-capsids and the scaffold-containing B-capsids. B-capsid cavities contain VP22a and VP21, the cleaved forms of the scaffold protein, and the viral protease, VP24. A-capsids are not filled with either the DNA or the scaffold. Both capsid types are thought to be by-products of capsid assembly that result from failed attempts to package DNA.[32] Alternatively, A- and B-capsids have been proposed to represent assembly intermediates.[459]

Scaffold Proteins and Maturational Protease

HSV capsids are assembled around a protein scaffold and require proteolytic cleavage. The scaffold proteins and maturational protease are encoded by the overlapping *U_L26* and *U_L26.5* genes, which encode a complex set of gene products involved in formation of a core for capsid assembly and for capsid maturation. The U_L26 gene encodes a precursor protein with an intrinsic serine protease activity that is required for capsid assembly. The protease cleaves either in cis or in trans at two sites within the precursor molecule, the release (R) site and the maturation (M) site. Cleavage at the R site generates two products, the N-terminal VP24, a protease, and the C-terminal VP21, the large scaffold protein, which can serve as a scaffold for capsid assembly but is not the main scaffold component. Cleavage at the R site is required for viral infectivity. The $U_L26.5$ ORF initiates within the U_L26 gene and encodes a protein in the same reading frame as U_L26. This protein, pre-VP22a (or ICP35), is equivalent to the C-terminal 329 residues of VP21 and functions as the main scaffold protein for capsid assembly. The use of two overlapping genes, U_L26 and $U_L26.5$, ensures the greater than 10-fold over abundance of the scaffold proteins relative to the protease. The C termini of pre-VP22a and VP21 are recognized by VP5 during capsid assembly. Cleavage of pre-VP22a (which generates VP22a) or VP21 at the M site is thought to be involved in release of the scaffolding protein from the capsid interior. A considerable effort has been devoted to identifying specific inhibitors of the HSV protease as possible antiviral compounds, and the crystal structures of the HSV-1 and HSV-2 homologs have been determined.

Capsid Assembly

According to the currently accepted model, a spherical procapsid self-assembles in the nucleus from VP5, VP19c, VP23, and UL6, along with the scaffolding proteins, mainly, pre-VP22a. Assembly of the capsid is nucleated by the dodecameric portal around which the rest of the capsid is assembled into a sphere.[332] This strategy ensures a single portal per capsid. Assembly of the spherical structure composed of VP5–pre-VP22a complexes is driven by oligomerization of the pre-VP22a molecules, and the triplex proteins VP19c and VP23 are added subsequently. The resulting procapsid has hexons and pentons but is not angularized. Once the procapsid is assembled, the protease, triggered by an unknown mechanism, cleaves the scaffolding proteins per-VP22a and VP21 at the M site, which release them from the floor of the procapsid.[334] This causes the procapsid to undergo a structural transformation to become icosahedral. During genome encapsidation, the scaffolding proteins are expelled from the capsid interior, whereas VP24 remains inside. The icosahedral capsid then recruits outer capsid proteins, UL25, UL17, and VP26.[334]

Much of our mechanistic knowledge of the capsid assembly process comes from analyses of structures formed in insect cells infected with baculoviruses expressing HSV capsid or scaffolding proteins and in extracts from these infected cells. In these studies, a series of baculovirus recombinants were constructed that each express one capsid or scaffolding protein, and B-capsids with normal structure were formed when insect cells were coinfected with viruses encoding the VP5, VP19C, VP23, and U_L26, or $U_L26.5$ gene products. When the U_L26 and $U_L26.5$ genes were left out, no intact capsids were formed, indicating that these gene products are needed to form a scaffold structure around which VP5 and the triplex proteins could form a spherical capsid. Similar phenotypes were observed with HSV strains in which the U_L26 and $U_L26.5$ genes were mutated. In the baculovirus studies, when the U_L26 gene was omitted, B-capsids with large cores were observed because in the absence of the protease, the pre-VP22a protein was not cleaved. Thus, cleavage of the scaffolding proteins leads to condensation of the core. When the $U_L26.5$ gene was omitted, intact capsids were observed, but no core structure was apparent. Viruses mutated for $U_L26.5$ can still produce infectious virus, but progeny virus yields are reduced by 10^2- to 10^3-fold relative to wild-type virus. These data indicate that although the U_L26 gene products can serve as scaffolding proteins, they do not form a proper core necessary for assembly and maturation.

B-capsids can also assemble *in vitro* when extracts from insect cells individually infected with baculoviruses expressing VP5, VP19C, VP23, U_L26, and $U_L26.5$ gene products are mixed and incubated. However, coincubation of the purified viral components VP5, VP19C, VP23, and a scaffolding protein *in vitro* only leads to the assembly of procapsids, which suggest that while assembly of procapsids does not require the viral protease, angularization does. It has been hypothesized that the viral genomes are packaged into procapsids, similar to genome packaging into the prohead structures of bacteriophages.

Capsid assembly takes place at early times of infection within replication compartments at sites near those of viral DNA replication and at later times, perhaps, also in nuclear structures called "assemblons," in certain cell types. Genome encapsidation likely also takes place in replication compartments.

Encapsidation of Viral DNA

During encapsidation of HSV DNA, the terminal L components of concatemeric HSV progeny DNA molecules are fed into capsids in an energy-dependent process, and the concatemers are cleaved into genome-length units by a linked process, originally described for pseudorabies virus. If the L component is the first to be packaged into the capsid, then the S component would be packaged last, which is consistent with the S component being the first to exit the capsid.[330] The mechanism of the encapsidation process is not yet well defined, but the concatemeric progeny DNA molecules are likely packaged into the capsid as the scaffolding molecules, VP21 and VP22a, are displaced from it. The viral DNA concatemer is thought to be cleaved upon encapsidation of a length of DNA that fills the capsid or when a "headful" (a term that originated with bacteriophage head assembly) of DNA has been inserted. The signals for cleavage and packaging were first mapped within the U_b and U_c domains of the ***a*** sequences and later mapped precisely. The two DNA packaging elements were designated as *pac1* and *pac2*, respectively.[103]

Cleavage of the viral DNA concatemers occurs site specifically within the DR1 sequences of the ***a*** sequences and involves two site-specific breaks at defined distances from the *pac1* and *pac2* packaging signals.[103] The maturational process duplicates the sequences between these two cleavage sites so that cleavage at sites bearing only one ***a*** sequence leads to two molecules with terminal ***a*** sequences. Several models have been proposed to explain the cleavage and metabolism of viral DNA during encapsidation.[103] In general, these models propose that a packaging complex binds to the DNA and scans for a U_c sequence. Cleavage occurs at a DR1 element proximal to the U_c sequence, and then the packaging complex will scan the DNA as it is packaged until a directly repeated junction is encountered. Alternatively, two cleavages at the L and S termini will produce a monomer molecule. The amplification of the ***a*** sequence may occur by staggered nick-repair or gene conversion. The terminal ***a*** sequence generated by the cleavage may be recombinogenic in either a single-stranded or a double-stranded form and promotes inversions and/or ***a*** sequence amplification. In any event, the process must yield the proper viral genome, with an L terminus containing one or more ***a*** sequences and a 3′ single-base overhang, a unit-length genome with an L and S component, and an S terminus containing a single ***a*** sequence and a 3′ single-base overhang.

Encapsidation of viral DNA requires at least seven viral proteins, including UL6, UL15, UL17, UL25, UL28, UL32, and UL33.[87] Viral DNA is packaged into the capsid through the dodecameric portal at one capsid vertex[333] by an ATP-driven packaging motor/terminase complex of UL15, UL28, and UL33 proteins that cleaves concatemeric DNA into single-genome lengths and translocates them into the capsids. The recently 3.5-Angstrom cryo-EM structure of the HSV-1 terminase complex revealed a hexameric ring composed of UL15, UL28, and UL33.[529] The UL15 protein has an ATPase domain homologous to bacteriophage terminases. The structures of UL15 and CMV UL89, a homolog of UL15, have revealed an RNase H-like nuclease domain, which suggested that UL15 homologs also have the nuclease activity necessary for DNA cleavage.[326,418,529] The UL28 protein binds to the *pac1* cleavage-packaging sequence, a sequence needed for termination of DNA packaging, and is thus thought to provide cleavage specificity. Therefore, UL28 and UL15 provide the specific DNA-binding, nuclease, and ATPase activities needed for a terminase. Both UL28 and UL33 reinforce the terminase complex.[418,529] The cryo-EM structure of the terminase suggests a packaging mechanism in which the arginine-containing finger-like loops within UL15 that line the central pore of the terminase hexamer sequentially bind, translocate, and release the DNA, pulling it through the portal into the capsid in a manner that is coupled to the ATP hydrolysis, much like bacteriophage terminases.[418,529]

Viral Egress

Once the mature nucleocapsid is formed in the nucleus, it must traverse several membranes (the nuclear and the plasma membranes) and the cytoplasm on its route to the extracellular space while completing its maturation by acquiring the lipid envelope and the tegument layer.[205] Cell lysis typically occurs very late during HSV infection, so viral egress must occur through a specialized secretion pathway. Transit from the nucleus to the cytoplasm represents a particular obstacle because the nucleus is surrounded by a double membrane consisting of the inner nuclear membrane (INM) and the outer nuclear membrane (ONM), and most transport in and out of the nucleus occurs through nuclear pores, which are approximately 39 nm in diameter. But being approximately 125 nm in diameter, HSV capsids are too large to pass through the nuclear pores and must use a different route.

According to the prevalent model,[42,93,396] nucleocapsids first become enveloped at the inner nuclear membrane forming perinuclear enveloped virions (PEVs) in the perinuclear space (primary envelopment) (Fig. 9.12). The PEVs then fuse with the outer nuclear membrane releasing the capsid into the cytoplasm (de-envelopment). The capsid then undergoes second, final budding at cytoplasmic membranes (secondary envelopment). During this step, the capsid matures into an infectious

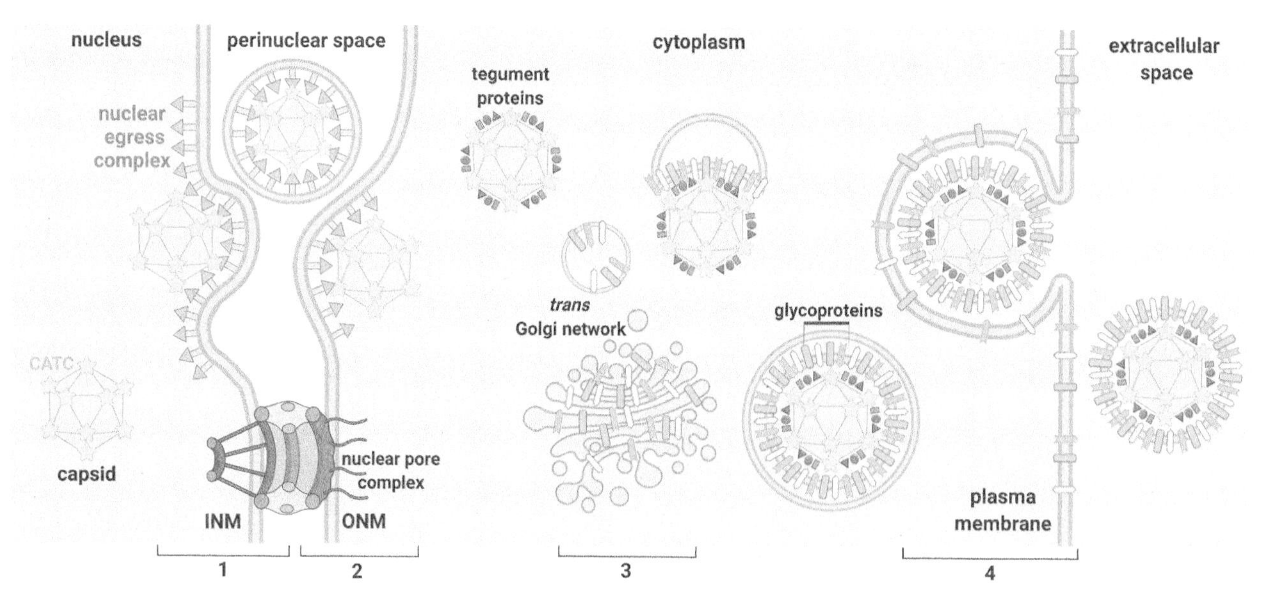

FIGURE 9.12 Overview of herpesvirus egress. Viral nucleocapsids are assembled in the nucleus and must translocate into the cytoplasm where they complete their maturation by acquiring the tegument and the envelope. Too large to fit through the nuclear pores, capsids, instead, use a different, more complex route. *Step 1*: capsids dock and bud at the inner nuclear membrane pinching off into the perinuclear space as the perinuclear enveloped virions (primary envelopment). This process is mediated by the virally encoded nuclear egress complex that, presumably, binds the CATC at the capsid vertices. *Step 2*: perinuclear enveloped virions fuse with the outer nuclear membrane and release the capsid into the cytoplasm (de-envelopment). *Step 3*: cytoplasmic capsids acquire the tegument layer and the envelope by budding at membranes derived from the trans-Golgi network or the early endosomes (secondary envelopment). *Step 4*: the mature virions inside the secretory vesicles fuse with the plasma membrane are released into the extracellular space. Abbreviations: INM, inner nuclear membrane; ONM, outer nuclear membrane; CATC, capsid-associated tegument complex. Figure generated using BioRender (https://biorender.com). (Figure generated using BioRender (https://biorender.com/). Copyright Elizabeth B. Draganova and Ekaterina E. Heldwein.)

virion by acquiring its final lipid envelope and the tegument and is released from the cell by exocytosis. While unusual, this model is the most widely accepted and is backed up by substantial data as detailed below.

Over the years, several models of egress have been proposed. According to the "luminal" egress model,[394] the PEVs instead of fusing with the ONM, acquire a second envelope and traverse the cytoplasm as double-membrane transport vesicles that fuse with the plasma membrane and release enveloped capsids into the extracellular space. Several lines of evidence argue against this model, however. First, PEVs differ from the mature, extracellular virions in their morphology and protein composition.[286,384] For example, UL31 and UL34, two viral proteins critical for nuclear egress, are found in PEVs but absent from mature HSV-1 or PRV virions.[384] Likewise, the lipid composition of extracellular virions resembles that of cytoplasmic rather than nuclear membranes.[479] Furthermore, unenveloped capsids in the cytoplasm are often found juxtaposed to curved, invaginated vesicles as evidence of envelopment at cytoplasmic membranes,[442] and deletions of particular tegument or envelope proteins, such as HSV-1 UL36 and UL37, or the glycoproteins gD and gE from either HSV-1 or PRV, result in unenveloped capsids accumulating in the cytoplasm.[106,107,133,266,385]

According to an alternative "nuclear pore" egress model, capsids escape the nucleus through enlarged pores. However, other studies have not observed enlargement or other changes in nuclear pores that would allow movement of nucleocapsids to the cytoplasm.[181] Moreover, PEVs in the perinuclear space (PNS) have been observed in many HSV-infected cells[384,442] and accumulate there as the result of some viral gene deletions,[384] which points to budding into the PNS being an intermediate stage in egress. Taken together, these observations argue strongly in favor of the envelopment–de-envelopment–re-envelopment model of egress,[42,93,205,396] in which capsids gain their initial, temporary envelope at the INM, traffic into the cytoplasm as unenveloped capsids, and then acquire their final envelope at cytoplasmic vesicles.

Primary or Nuclear Envelopment

During primary envelopment, the first step in nuclear egress, the mature nucleocapsids acquire an envelope by budding at the INM. This process requires that the capsid be recruited to and dock at the INM, the membrane be deformed around the capsid to form a nascent bud, and the bud be pinched off the INM releasing the PEV into the PNS. However, in the HSV-infected cell nucleus, the marginalized host chromatin and the nuclear lamina present barriers to capsid budding. To overcome these barriers, HSV infection causes both the dispersal of the marginalized host chromatin[430] and the disruption of the nuclear lamina.[383,430]

The nuclear lamina is a dense filamentous protein network of lamins and lamin-associated proteins (LAPs) that underlies the INM and provides shape and mechanical stability to the nuclear envelope. In uninfected cells, the nuclear lamina is completely disassembled during mitosis through phosphorylation of lamins and LAPs by cellular mitotic kinases that disrupt their interactions. However, there is no full disassembly during herpesvirus infection, presumably, to preserve the integrity of the nucleus where viral genome replication and capsid assembly occur. Instead, the lamina is disassembled locally through phosphorylation of lamins and LAPs by the HSV-1 kinase US3 and by cellular kinases that are different from the mitotic kinases,[177,292,396] notably by the protein kinase C that is recruited to the INM, along with the host protein p32 by the HSV-1 ICP34.5 protein.[504,521]

Primary envelopment requires the viral UL31 and UL34 proteins that form the heterodimeric nuclear egress complex (NEC) and are conserved across the *Herpesviridae*. In the absence of either UL31 or UL34, viral replication is reduced by three to five orders of magnitude, and capsids accumulate within the nucleus.[65,398] UL34 has a single-spanning C-terminal transmembrane region (TM) that anchors the complex to the INM. UL31 is a soluble nuclear phosphoprotein that is retained at the inner nuclear membrane through its interaction with UL34. Crystal structures of NEC homologs from HSV-1, PRV, and HCMV[41,294,495,538] have revealed an elongated cylindrical heterodimer, in which the globular core of UL31 wraps a hook-like extension around the globular UL34 pedestal.

UL31 and UL34 may promote the disruption of the nuclear lamina by binding lamins[383] and by recruitment of the viral US3 kinase and the protein kinase C to the nuclear lamina. UL31 and UL34 are also required for the dispersal of the marginalized cellular chromatin,[430] which may be an indirect effect of disruption of the nuclear lamina, to which cellular chromatin is tethered.

In addition to their roles in clearing the barriers to capsid budding at the INM, UL31 and UL34 are directly involved in the budding process. In PRV, expression of UL31 and UL34 in uninfected cells resulted in the formation of capsid-less perinuclear vesicles, which demonstrated that UL31 and UL34 are the only viral proteins necessary for nuclear budding.[233] Moreover, the NEC has an intrinsic ability to deform and bud membranes, which was established by showing that purified recombinant NEC homologs from HSV-1 or PRV can vesiculate synthetic lipid bilayers *in vitro* without any additional factors or chemical energy.[43,285]

Cryo-EM and tomography (cryo-EM/T) demonstrated that during budding *in vitro*, HSV-1 NEC oligomerizes into hexagonal "honeycomb" coats on the inner surface of lipid vesicles.[43] Coats of similar geometry have been observed on the inner surface of capsid-less perinuclear vesicles formed *in vivo* in uninfected cells expressing PRV NEC.[163] Hexagonal symmetry evident in the coats formed as the result of budding both *in vitro* and *in vivo* suggests that the hexagonal arrangement is biologically relevant. Mutations in U_L31 or U_L34 that would be predicted to disrupt the hexagonal arrangement reduce budding *in vitro*[41,43] and in infected cells,[22,397] which suggests that the hexagonal coat formation is important for the NEC budding activity.

C-capsids preferentially undergo primary envelopment at the INM,[489] implying the existence of a capsid selection mechanism that ensures that only mature, DNA-filled capsids exit the nucleus, which would increase the yield of infectious virions. The nature of this selection mechanism is yet unclear but may involve interactions between UL31 and the CVSC/CATC at the capsid vertices because CVSC/CATC components UL25 and UL17 have been shown to bind UL31[530] and because UL25 mediates interactions between purified HSV-1 nucleocapsids and recombinant NEC.[456] Furthermore, UL25 is required for nuclear egress.[252] Although CVSC/CATC is present on all three capsid types, A- and B-capsids have fewer CVSC/CATC copies on the capsid surface and may differ in the CVSC/CATC conformation.[331] Multiple NEC-binding sites on a C-capsid could thus provide the driving force for creating a PEV through avidity.

In addition to the quality control mechanism(s) that ensure budding of mature C-capsids, another mechanism appears to prevent unproductive budding in the absence of C-capsids, because during infection capsid-less perinuclear vesicles are rarely observed in infected cells. This could be achieved by down-regulating the NEC budding activity prior to the arrival of the capsid, potentially by phosphorylation of UL31 by the alphaherpesviral US3 kinase.[321]

De-envelopment

During this next step in nuclear egress, the PEVs fuse their envelopes with the ONM, which releases the capsids into the cytoplasm (Fig. 9.12). To ensure efficient nuclear egress, PEVs must preferentially fuse with the ONM rather than the INM, but how this selection is achieved is yet unknown. Defects in de-envelopment typically manifest as the accumulation of PEVs in the PNS, with a concomitant reduction in viral titer. Accumulation of PEVs in uninfected cells expressing UL31 and UL34 from HSV-1 or PRV[233] implies the involvement of viral proteins besides UL31 and UL34 in de-envelopment, and several viral proteins have been implicated in this process. Yet, proteins that mediate membrane fusion during de-envelopment have not yet been conclusively identified. The conserved viral glycoproteins gB and gH, which mediate membrane fusion during entry, have been proposed to mediate de-envelopment in HSV-1 because in a gB/gH double mutant virus,[134] PEVs accumulate in the PNS. However, the double deletion has little effect on the extracellular virions. Moreover, single deletions of gB or gH have minimal effects on de-envelopment,[134] which is at odds with both glycoproteins being essential for fusion during HSV-1 entry. Both gB and gH are dispensable for de-envelopment in the closely related PRV.[232] Therefore, other fusion mechanisms independent of these viral glycoproteins must also exist. Overexpression of another viral glycoprotein, gK from HSV-1, which localizes to the ER during infection, results in the accumulation of PEVs, but its precise role in the de-envelopment remains unclear. Elucidation of the de-envelopment mechanism requires identification of proteins on the surface of the PEVs and/or on the perinuclear surface of the ONM that would enable membrane fusion and hence de-envelopment to take place. Membrane fusion is, presumably, accompanied by disassembly of the NEC coats, to allow the naked capsids to be released into the cytoplasm, but the mechanism is yet unknown.

Secondary Envelopment

During this final step in viral morphogenesis, cytoplasmic capsids acquire their tegument and lipid envelope by budding at cytoplasmic vesicles. The identity of the cytoplasmic sites of secondary envelopment have not yet been fully elucidated. HSV has been proposed to undergo secondary envelopment at sites coincident with markers of the trans-Golgi network (TGN)[172,451] or endosomes.[184] HSV infection leads to reorganization of cytoplasmic membranes, blurring the distinction between trans-Golgi and endocytic organelles such that TGN and endosomal markers are spread throughout the cytoplasm. Regardless, both the TGN-derived secretory vesicles and the endocytic pathways contribute to secondary envelopment by mediating trafficking of viral glycoproteins required for efficient secondary envelopment of HSV-1[10,184,204] or trafficking of enveloped particles to the plasma membrane after secondary envelopment.[182,183,204]

At least 12 viral tegument proteins (UL7, UL11, UL14, UL16, UL21, UL36, UL37, UL46, UL47, UL48, UL49, UL51) form a protein interaction network that drives tegument assembly and secondary envelopment.[93,351] However, most individual tegument proteins and protein/protein or protein/membrane interactions are not essential for secondary envelopment. Therefore, this network appears to be functionally redundant.

HSV also recruits components of the cellular ESCRT (endosomal sorting complex required for transport) machinery that mediates membrane budding "away" from the cytoplasm, into either the lumenal or the extracellular space. Only ESCRT-III and Vps4, which function at late stages of the budding process, namely, the scission of the budded vesicle, are required for secondary envelopment of HSV-1 and PRV.[25,226,227,359] This suggests that the budding process during secondary envelopment utilizes a combination of viral and cellular machinery. The precise mechanism of secondary envelopment is yet to be elucidated.

In addition to infectious virions, in certain cell types, the alphaherpesviruses produce a large number of noninfectious light, or L-particles that contain only viral tegument and envelope proteins. The functions of L-particles in viral infection and pathogenesis are not entirely clear.[38,169,218]

Intracellular Transport and Exocytosis

Secondary envelopment produces an enveloped infectious virion within the lumen of a secretory vesicle. This virion-containing double-membraned vesicle then traffics to the cell periphery along the microtubules where the membrane of the secretory vesicle fuses with the plasma membrane—an SNARE-mediated process called exocytosis—to release the virion to the extracellular space.[182,183] Viral proteins may function as cargo adaptors to recruit microtubule motors to viral secretory vesicles. However, little is known about the identity of viral membrane and tegument proteins present on the cytosolic face of viral secretory vesicles or their function in virion exocytosis.

Targeting of Virus During Egress

In certain specialized cell types, HSV egress can be targeted. In polarized epithelial cells, for viruses that bud through the plasma membrane, targeting of viral glycoprotein(s) to the apical or basolateral surface defines the site of viral release from the cell. HSV glycoproteins target to the basolateral membranes of polarized epithelial cells. For HSV, with the complex pathways of release described above, targeting of viral proteins to specific plasma membrane sites does not direct virus budding to those sites. In fact, HSV egress is targeted to lateral membranes, in particular to cell–cell junctions in polarized epithelial cells, and this process requires the viral gE/gI glycoprotein complex. It is believed that the gE/gI complex accumulates in one domain of the TGN and promotes secondary envelopment there, and this domain targets the sorting of the virion vesicles to the cell–cell junctions and the basolateral membrane.[206] The ability of HSV to spread cell-to-cell is likely to occur via tight junctions in polarized epithelial cells, but the virus can also spread to other cell types in the presence of antibodies, forming the basis of plaque assays conducted in the presence of antiviral antibodies.

This allows HSV to spread *in vivo* from one epithelial cell to another without being neutralized by antiviral antibody.

INTRINSIC IMMUNITY, INNATE IMMUNITY, AND ANTI-ANTIVIRAL DEFENSES

Overview

From the initial encounters following entry into the infected cell to the release of progeny virus, the numerous events and processes required for HSV replication and their impact on cellular physiological process are subject to intense surveillance by an intricate network of host defenses. Detection of conserved viral structural components termed pathogen-associated molecular patterns or PAMPs can interfere with a cell's capacity to support virus replication by inducing a suite of proteins designed to hamper virus replication, including soluble inflammatory mediators like type I interferons that inform neighboring cells of an infectious invader and program them into an antiviral state. Furthermore, the appropriation of critical host processes vital to virus reproduction can trigger responses that restrict virus replication and spread. Included among these latter responses are those that limit viral gene expression in both nuclear and cytoplasmic compartments, result in acute physiological stress, and influence infected cell survival. While such innate, cell-intrinsic responses, if left unchecked, would inhibit virus replication and in fact may be harnessed to in part support latency in neurons, numerous HSV-encoded functions have been identified that subvert host defenses to support virus replication and effectively enable infectious virus production. The cellular factors and processes capable of detecting HSV infection and restricting virus reproduction together with viral countermeasures designed to subvert them are enumerated in the following section. These topics are reviewed in several recent review articles,[8,234,253,289,445] and the reader is referred to these for more detailed discussion.

Receptors that detect HSV infection are located throughout the cell and act to directly restrict viral replication or to initiate signaling pathways that limit viral replication. We will investigate the host cell resistance mechanisms that the virus encounters as it proceeds through the replication cycle.

Receptors at the Plasma Membrane and Endosomes

Toll-like receptor 2 (TLR2) is a cell surface receptor on various antigen-presenting cells that recognizes lipoproteins of various microbes and initiates innate signaling. TLR2 is activated by HSV infection to signal through NF-κB signaling pathways to elicit cytokine production.[149,500] Soluble forms of HSV-1 glycoprotein H and L can activate TLR2 signaling,[149] and the same events likely occur in virus-infected cells. The molecular basis for the TLR2-gH/gL interaction is not understood and could be an important model for TLR2 interaction with viruses. HSV-1 activation of TLR2 leads to MyD88-dependent induction of NF-κB signaling and expression of proinflammatory cytokines such as IL-6 and IL-8. Because of this, TLR2 activation of innate responses and cytokines is an important aspect of HSV-1 encephalitis in murine models. Other factors involved in this signaling process are αvβ3-integrin, which has been reported to act in concert with TLR2 to elicit innate signaling in response to HSV[149] and CD200R1, which increases TLR2 signing on mouse peritoneal macrophages infected with HSV-1.[435]

The HSV-1 IE ICP0 protein reduces the TLR2 signaling pathway by promoting the degradation and/or sequestration of the MyD88 adaptor protein,[480] which would limit the cytokine response in that cell. However, HSV activation of the NF-κB pathway is proviral in the infected cell,[358] and this may be due to NF-κB stimulating IE gene expression or to induction of host genes that protect from apoptosis[301] or other stress. Nevertheless, at face value, these results would seem paradoxical. HSV can activate NF-κB through other mechanisms, including by the tegument protein UL37 binding to TRAF6 and activating NF-κB signaling.[281] Therefore, proteins in incoming virions, including gH/gL and UL37, may activate a limited amount of NF-κB signaling to protect the infected cell, while the IE protein ICP0 and the L US3 protein reduce NF-κB signaling to limit innate signaling.

Toll-like receptor 9 (TLR9) is a receptor located in endosomes that recognizes unmethylated CpG-rich DNA sequences. TLR9 is important for IFN expression in HSV-1–infected dendritic cells, and TLR9 knockout mice have a reduced type I interferon response to HSV-1 infection. Nevertheless, TLR9 is not required to control HSV-1 infection in mice.[378,500] TLR9, like TLR3, TLR7, and TLR8, requires UNC93b for trafficking to endosomes.[231] Mutations in UNC93b reduce the IFN response to HSV-1 infection,[500] and patients with defects in UNC93b are highly susceptible to herpes simplex encephalitis. Although the UNC93b effect is usually associated with TLR3 deficiency, TLR9 could also play a role in the UNC93b mutation phenotype.

Toll-like receptor 3 (TLR3) is an endosomal receptor that recognizes double-stranded RNA and activates IRF-3 or NF-κB signaling. Human 293 cells expressing TLR3 did not activate NF-κB signaling, but TLR3$^{-/-}$ cells show reduced interferon induction upon HSV-1 infection. Thus, TLR3 is not sufficient for NF-κB signaling in response to HSV-1 infection but is required for optimal IFN responses to HSV-1 infection. Individuals with TLR3-related mutations are susceptible to herpes simplex virus encephalitis (HSE).[17,174,278,406] Furthermore, individuals with UNC93B mutations also show susceptibility to HSE, and as discussed above, UNC93B is involved in transport of TLRs to endosomes. Therefore, there is considerable evidence that TLR3 plays an important role in control of HSV-1 infection in neurons in the central nervous system.

Cytoplasmic Sensing of Viral PAMPS

Cyclic guanylate adenylate synthase (cGAS) is a cytoplasmic sensor that detects DNA, primarily found outside nuclear and mitochondrial subcellular compartments in the cytosol. Upon binding to DNA, cGAS undergoes a conformational change and becomes activated to synthesize cyclic guanosine monophosphate–adenosine monophosphate or cGAMP.[5,111,452] cGAMP then binds to STING to activate it and then IRF-3, which dimerizes and localizes into the nucleus to activate transcription of the *IFNB1* gene, which encodes IFN-β, and other antiviral genes. cGAS is required for induction of type 1 interferons in response to HSV-1 infection in mouse cells[271] and human fibroblasts.[346] Viral DNA is normally transported to the nucleus inside the capsid and thus should not be available for binding by cGAS. However, in macrophages, the capsid is thought to be proteolytically digested and released into the cytosol.[187] Thus, it is not clear how HSV DNA is available for binding to cytoplasmic cGAS in cells other than macrophages, and the role for cGAS in HSV induction of IFNs and its DNA ligand have not been fully defined. cGAS could be involved in sensing of HSV DNA from damaged virions or leaking out of the nucleus or in maintaining tonic or normal physiological levels of DNA sensing machinery in uninfected cells. In addition, HSV infection causes leakage of mitochondrial DNA into the cytoplasm,[514] which could be the ligand for cGAS in HSV-infected cells. Alternatively, there is evidence that some cGAS is nuclear and promotes the stability of IFI16, a nuclear sensor of HSV-1 DNA[346] or acts in cooperation with IFI16 in induction of interferons.[15] Thus, the role of cGAS in induction of interferons during HSV infection remains to be fully defined. Besides its role in controlling interferon production, interferon-independent STING functions have also been reported to promote HSV-1 resistance in mice.[526]

Absent in Melanoma 2 (AIM2). AIM2 is a cytoplasmic DNA sensor that when activated leads to a signaling pathway that activates inflammasome formation and secretion of the proinflammatory cytokines interleukin 1β (IL-1β) and IL-18. Wild-type HSV-1 does not activate AIM2 signaling,[379] but this is likely due to HSV-1 proteins blocking signaling. A recent study has shown that the HSV-1 VP22 protein blocks multimerization of AIM2 and reduces its signaling.[304]

RNA Sensors in the Cytosol

PKR and OAS. Double-stranded RNA (dsRNA) generated by transcription from primarily late genes encoded on opposing DNA strands in the viral genome is another PAMP indicative of virus infection that accumulates in HSV-infected cells.[101] Following recognition by discrete dsRNA-binding proteins that are subsequently activated by interaction with dsRNA, these host dsRNA PAMP-binding proteins interfere with key functions needed for virus reproduction including protein synthesis and global RNA stability. As discussed in the Gene Expression section above, dsRNA accumulation activates the eIF2α kinase PKR, which can block translation initiation on all mRNAs dependent upon eIF2 to load 40S ribosomes with initiator tRNA and largely inhibit infected cell protein synthesis (Fig. 9.10). Preservation of active, unphosphorylated eIF2 is achieved via the HSV-encoded PP1α-binding subunit ICP34.5 and the PKR antagonist *U_S11*. The cellular 2′-5′oligoadeylate synthetase (OAS) is another host dsRNA-activated protein that functions as an innate antiviral defense component. Upon activation by dsRNA, OAS catalyzes the *de novo* synthesis of oligoadenylate (OA) chains with a distinctive 2′-5′ linkage.[414] Three major OAS isoforms have been identified as members of a related family and while how they differ functionally is incompletely understood, each exhibits distinctive biochemical properties including their responsiveness to dsRNA concentration, the length of the 2′-5′ OA synthesized, their subcellular localization, and cell type specificity.[414] The resulting OA products bind to the inactive host ribonuclease, RNase L, and stimulate formation of active RNase L homodimers from inactive monomer subunits. By cleaving RNA at the 3′ side of UpXp sequences, activated RNase L promotes both mRNA and rRNA decay within infected cells. OAS activity is inhibited in HSV-1–infected primary human fibroblasts.[405] Furthermore, the HSV-1 *U_S11* gene product was sufficient to block OAS activation in extracts from uninfected, interferon-treated cells, and ectopically expressed US11 protein and OAS physically associated in a nuclease-sensitive manner in uninfected cells. The US11 dsRNA-binding domain was required to inhibit OAS, suggesting a mechanism that, in part, could rely on sequestering available dsRNA produced during infection.[405] Like PKR, OAS is one of hundreds of interferon-stimulated genes whose protein products accumulate in uninfected cells and in part contribute to the establishment of an "antiviral" state that is nonpermissive for virus reproduction. In addition, as dsRNA-activated host effectors, the antiviral functions of both PKR and OAS are antagonized by the HSV-encoded dsRNA-binding protein US11.

Retinoic acid–inducible gene I (RIG-I) is a cytoplasmic receptor that recognizes RNA molecules with a 5′ triphosphate or dsRNA molecules. RIG-I–dependent signaling in HSV-infected cells has been described,[72,283,543] but the RNA ligand for RIG-I had not been defined. Viral dsRNA has been reported, and it was hypothesized that small RNAs generated from HSV DNA by RNA pol III released into the cytosol could be ligands for RIG-I.[4,73] Chiang et al.[72] found that a host small RNA, 5S ribosomal RNA pseudogene 141 (RNA5SP141) RNA was the major RNA bound to RIG-I in infected cells. They found that viral inhibition of protein synthesis reduced the abundance of the proteins bound to the pseudogene RNA, exposing the 5S RNA, and releasing it to the cytoplasm where it is recognized by RIG-I.[72]

Nuclear Defenses

As described in the Gene Expression section, a variety of nuclear molecules serve as restriction factors for HSV-1 replication, including PML, Daxx, ATRX, Sp100, and IFI16. Only IFI16 has been shown to bind preferentially to unchromatinized DNA,[449] but it is believed that that many of these proteins are recruited to the entering viral DNA and promote loading and/or maintenance of heterochromatin. IFI16 has been shown to bind to viral DNA and induce IRF-3 signaling and IFN-β expression,[270,349] in addition to its epigenetic effects.

Evasion and Blunting the Interferon Response

As described above, a number of cellular receptors recognize a number of HSV PAMPs and induce interferon expression, which restricts viral replication in surrounding cells and even in the initial infected cell. However, HSV has evolved a number of viral functions that counter the induction and action of interferon. In fact, the large number of ways by which HSV counters type 1 interferon induction and action demonstrates how important interferons are as an antiviral response for protection against HSV-1. The antiviral gene functions that counter interferons include the following viral genes:

1. *ICP0* degrades IFI16[349] and inhibits and sequesters IRF3[311] to block their action in interferon induction.
2. *US3* phosphorylates a number of host proteins and thereby affects a number of host response pathways. US3 phosphorylates KIF3 (kinesin superfamily protein 3) and thereby down-regulates CD1d expression to inhibit NKT (natural killer T) cell function.[523] US3 reduces type I IFN and ISG induction in HSV-1–infected human monocytes,[362] but

the mechanism is not defined. In addition, US3 inhibits TLR2 signaling by reducing TRAF polyubiquitination through a mechanism dependent on the protein's kinase activity.[419] Furthermore, US3 is reported to hyperphosphorylate p65RelA to reduce NF-κB activation in response to TNF-α or IL-1β stimulation,[498] although this effect was not observed for other NF-κB stimuli.[419]

3. *UL37* deamidates the helicase domain of RIG-I to prevent its binding to RNA and induction of interferon expression[543] and deamidates cGAS to reduce its ability to make cGAMP.[540]
4. *ICP27* stimulates the secretion of an infected cell factor that inhibits Stat-1 nuclear accumulation by inhibiting IFN-induced Stat-1 phosphorylation at or upstream of Jak-1.[208] ICP27 also inhibits the cGAS-STING-TBK1 pathway in human macrophages by binding to TBK1 and STING.[76]
5. *ICP34.5* precludes the translational arrest imposed by activated PKR by promoting eIF2α dephosphorylation via an interaction with the PP1α host protein phosphatase. ICP34.5 also overcomes PKR-induced autophagy by binding Beclin-1 and inhibiting its autophagy function.[345] ICP34.5 was reported to reduce ISG expression by blocking the interaction of TBK1 with IRF3 through an interaction with TBK1,[484] but recent data show that this effect may be exerted more indirectly.[300]
6. *UL41/vhs* promotes degradation of host mRNAs and prevents the replenishment of host sensors and response molecules, such as TNF receptor 1, viperin,[421,539] and IFI16.[347]
7. *US11* interacts with a number of host proteins to block innate responses, including PKR to block eIF2 phosphorylation, PACT to prevent PKR activation,[366] OAS to inhibit its activity,[405] and RIG-I or MDA5 to reduce IFN induction.[225]

Catabolic Physiological Stress Responses

HSV infection results in substantial physiological stress that perturbs cellular homeostasis and evokes catabolic responses with antiviral consequences. Cell intrinsic stress responses to virus-induced disturbances, including intensive demands for amino acids and energy, can restrict virus reproduction and spread and thereby contribute to host antiviral defenses. One critical aspect of maintaining homeostasis during virus infection is balancing energy-demanding anabolic processes, including protein synthesis that is absolutely reliant upon host ribosomes, with catabolic processes poised to short circuit the virus lifecycle, prevent infectious virus production, and contain virus spread in a cell intrinsic manner. The multisubunit ser/thr kinase mTORC1 is at the nexus of information-rich cellular signaling networks that integrate physiological and environmental cues and plays essential roles in coordinating fundamental anabolic and catabolic outputs (reviewed by[229]) that profoundly influence host responses to HSV (Fig. 9.9). Moreover, mTORC1 together with virus-encoded functions that subvert mTORC1 signaling impact the proficiency with which the virus replicates during episodes of physiological stress, a defining feature of HSV infection biology.

The HSV US3 ser/thr protein kinase alters the responsiveness of mTORC1 to metabolic stress resulting from either energy or amino acid insufficiency (Fig. 9.9). In contrast to uninfected cells where energy or amino acid insufficiency inhibits mTORC1 activation to tune anabolic processes like protein synthesis to physiological stress,[229,410] mTORC1 remains activated in HSV-1–infected cells deprived of amino acids or under low energy stress. Although US3 did not detectably prevent low energy stress-induced activation of the host AMP-activated protein kinase (AMPK), it enforced mTORC1 activation despite the presence of activated AMPK, and AMPK activity in infected cells was restricted in a US3-dependent manner.[487] Similarly, synergistic action of the HSV-1 UL46 gene product, which stimulates PI 3-kinase and Akt,[123] and US3 supports virus reproduction during amino acid insufficiency.[486] Together, this defines the US3 kinase as an mTORC1 activator that subverts the host cell energy and nutrient-sensing programs to support viral productive growth and overcome cell intrinsic innate responses to metabolic physiological stress that could otherwise restrict virus protein synthesis and reproduction (Fig. 9.9). Uncoupling mTORC1 activation from energy and nutrient availability enables HSV to enforce high-level viral protein synthesis needed for replication during physiological stress and overcome what is likely an evolutionary ancient response that restricts pathogen reproduction within host cells during nutrient and energy insufficiency.

Autophagy

Besides sanctioning survival and adaptation under inauspicious conditions such as starvation and physiological stress, macroautophagy or autophagy enables cells to maintain homeostasis by recycling cytoplasmic components and is a vital innate host defense regulating infection and inflammation.[144,258,531] Cytoplasmic, double-membrane autophagosome accumulation commences in response to type 3 phosphoinositide 3-kinase (PI3KC3) activation by Beclin1. Delivery of autophagosome contents to lysosomes by fusion results in their proteolytic destruction and catabolic amino acid recycling. Autophagy is regulated in part by mTORC1, which coordinates anabolic and catabolic outcomes in response to changes in homeostasis.[229,410] While activated mTORC1 represses autophagy and stimulates anabolic responses like protein synthesis, insufficiency of nutrients, energy, or growth factors inhibits mTORC1 activation, which limits protein synthesis and promotes autophagy (Fig. 9.9). Host stress-activated eIF2α kinases that limit protein synthesis in response to virus infection, amino acid insufficiency, or ER stress also function as innate defenses and can incite autophagy.[458] By contrast, Beclin1 site–specific phosphorylation by Akt[500] restricts autophagy.

At least three independent functions encoded within the HSV genome antagonize autophagy, illustrating the importance of suppressing this catabolic process. By preventing eIF2 phosphorylation and subsequent inactivation (Fig. 9.10), both ICP34.5 and US11 curb autophagy.[291,458] While US11 also inhibits TANK-binding kinase 1 (TBK1) activation,[282] an N-terminal ICP34.5 domain interacts with and antagonizes Beclin1.[345] Significantly, HSV-1 replication was enhanced in ATG5-deficient mouse sensory neurons unable to undergo autophagy.[533] Furthermore, reduced pathogenesis in adult mice was reported following infection with HSV-1 encoding a Beclin1-binding deficient ICP34.5 mutant protein.[345,518] Greater destruction of viral proteins and/or virions following their delivery to autophagosomes likely accounts in part for this phenotype and was consistent with autophagy functioning as a neuron-specific antiviral defense.[11] In contrast to these findings in adult mice, pathogenesis was not dependent upon the ICP34.5 Beclin1-binding domain in the neonatal mouse

CNS,[518] where a greater reliance on ICP34.5 binding to PP1α to preserve unphosphorylated supplies of eIF2 was observed.[517] Thus, age-related and developmental differences in how autophagy is regulated in response to HSV-1 infection likely impact pathogenesis. Recently, however, the HSV-1 US3 ser/thr kinase was shown to be required for virus reproduction in nonneuronal cells during physiological stress, including nutrient deprivation that inhibits mTORC1 activation, and shown to inhibit autophagy.[399] By enforcing constitutive mTORC1 activation, US3 suppresses catabolic responses like autophagy while favoring anabolic responses (including protein synthesis described earlier in Gene Expression and Fig 9.9). Significantly, phosphorylation of cellular autophagy regulators ULK1 and Beclin1 in HSV-1–infected nonneuronal cells was dependent upon US3.[399] Besides preventing mTORC1-dependent autophagy by stimulating ULK1 phosphorylation, US3 was sufficient to also block autophagy in an mTORC1-independent manner and directly phosphorylated the key autophagy regulator Beclin1 on the same site targeted by the cellular kinase Akt,[399] which is known to limit autophagy.[500] Moreover, disabling autophagy by depleting ULK1 and Beclin1 partially rescued US3-deficient virus replication in primary fibroblasts.[399] Thus, autophagy generally limits HSV-1 replication in a cell intrinsic manner in nonneuronal cells, as well as neuronal cells, and is antagonized by multiple, independent virus-encoded functions that act through different mechanisms. Precisely why multiple HSV-encoded functions are needed to counter autophagy remains unknown but could conceivably either increase the probability that autophagy is inhibited in infected cells or enable different functions to predominate in different cell types encountered during the virus lifecycle.

Programmed Cell Death

By activating programmed cell death responses in response to virus infection, virus-infected cells cause their own elimination prior to the completion of the virus reproductive cycle. This cell intrinsic innate immune mechanism that results in death of the infected cell spares surrounding cells and tissues and can effectively limit virus reproduction and spread. Different programmed cell death processes have been identified with distinctive cell biological features and molecular control circuitries and likely have driven the acquisition of virus-encoded countermeasures to disarm them.

Apoptosis

Apoptosis is a developmental process that allows for cell removal via a noninflammatory cell death program characterized by a reduction in cell volume, chromatin condensation and fragmentation, phosphatidylserine exposure in the plasma membrane outer leaflet, and formation of small apoptotic cell bodies that are engulfed by phagocytes.[327] It can be triggered by an extrinsic pathway, which involves extracellular mediators such as signaling by TNF superfamily members (FasL, TNFα, TRAIL) or an intrinsic pathway activated by physiological stressors (ER, genotoxic, survival factor insufficiency, anoikis, inhibition of transcription or translation, cytoskeleton disruption). Activation of cellular pro-apoptotic BCL-2 family members (BAX, BAK, Bid) by the intrinsic pathway stimulates caspase activation, which shapes apoptotic responses by degrading numerous cellular protein substrates and results in mitochondrial outer membrane permeabilization and cytochrome c release.[327] By contrast, the extrinsic pathway requires a caspase 8-containing signaling complex that detects many pathogens including HSV.[317] Apoptosis can also result in response to perturbations in homeostasis induced by HSV-1 infection.

In the context of infection, viruses deficient in key IE regulators ICP4 or ICP27 were unable to suppress apoptosis. Subsequently, discrete HSV-1–encoded gene products whose expression was regulated by ICP4 and ICP27, including glycoproteins (gD, gJ) and the US3 protein kinase, were identified and shown to block apoptosis induced by Fas ligand, sorbitol-induced osmotic shock, virus-dependent lysosomal discharge, overexpression of proapoptotic proteins including Bcl-2 family members and caspase 3, or by viral proteins that provoke apoptotic responses.[31,546] The gD domains needed to block apoptosis induced by HSV-1 are reportedly distinct from those required for binding to the primary receptor nectin 1 or cell-to-cell fusion; however, stimulation of NF-κB activation in response to HSV infection by binding to HVEM on cells that express this TNF receptor family member has been reported.[416] Similarly, the precise mechanism underlying the inhibition of apoptosis by gJ remains unclear, although gJ is widely distributed within infected cells in the endoplasmic reticulum, *trans*-Golgi network, and early endosomes and was found to interact with FoF1 ATP synthase subunit 6.[31] By preventing cleavage of the proapoptotic BAD BCL-2 family member, the US3 ser/thr kinase blocks BAD-induced caspase 3 activation, and subsequent caspase-dependent cleavage of poly(ADP-ribose) polymerase (PARP), and fragmentation of cellular DNA.[324] While initial studies correlated this activity with US3-dependent BAD phosphorylation on Ser 112 and Ser 136, subsequent work revealed that phosphorylation on these residues was not needed for US3 antiapoptotic activity. Because the US3 ser/thr kinase activity is required to block apoptosis, it remains possible that US3 targets a caspase that cleaves BAX. US3 was also found to block apoptosis induced by overexpression of other proapoptotic BCL2 family members such as Bid and BAX, and these results suggested that US3 may in fact act to limit apoptosis both upstream and downstream of mitochondrial events. A conserved C-terminal domain within the large subunit of the ribonucleotide reductase (ICP6) encoded by both HSVs, which also is required for ribonucleotide reductase activity when physically associated with the virus-encoded R2-subunit, interacts with the caspase 8 death effector domain to suppress apoptosis induced via the extrinsic pathways.[121] Finally, a function within the latency-associated transcript (LAT) produced in latently infected neurons reportedly suppresses apoptosis and influences reactivation efficiency in the murine and rabbit models.[120,364]

Direct Activation of Programmed Necrosis/Necroptosis

As a consequence of interfering with caspase 8–dependent apoptosis, an alternative programmed cell death (PCD) pathway, necroptosis, can be triggered.[316] Characterized by intracellular organelle swelling, plasma membrane disruption, and inflammation, programmed necrosis or necroptosis is controlled by formation of the necrosome, a complex of receptor-interacting kinases (RIP1 and RIP3) via their RIP homotypic interaction motif (RHIM) domains.[77,482] Following phosphorylation of mixed lineage kinase domain like (MLKL)-protein, a kinase substrate of RIP3, MLKL oligomers trigger membrane pore formation and necrosis.[56,68,496] Besides limiting apoptosis as reviewed in the preceding section, HSV-1 also encodes effectors that disarm host necrotic cell intrinsic responses.[363] Programmed necrosis is antagonized in HSV-infected human cells through the RHIM domain within the multifunctional viral ribonucleotide reductase large subunits (ICP6), which interact with RIP1 and RIP3 to prevent MLKL-dependent necrosis.[161] Thus, the antiviral potential triggered by antagonizing caspase 8–dependent apoptosis is averted in human cells infected with HSV by enlisting the same virus-encoded ribonucleotide reductase large subunits to suppress necroptosis. In mice, however, the physical association of HSV-1 ICP6 with RIP1/3 is unable to restrain necroptosis and necrosis ensues, constraining virus propagation in this nonnatural host species and raising the possibility that necroptosis in part serves as a cross species restriction factor in infection.[191,502] This raises an additional caveat pertaining to the use of mice to model HSV infection biology.

HSV gene products also inhibit other immune responses, including adaptive responses, and these are described in the previous chapter[395] and in the Supplementary Table 9.1 Gene List.

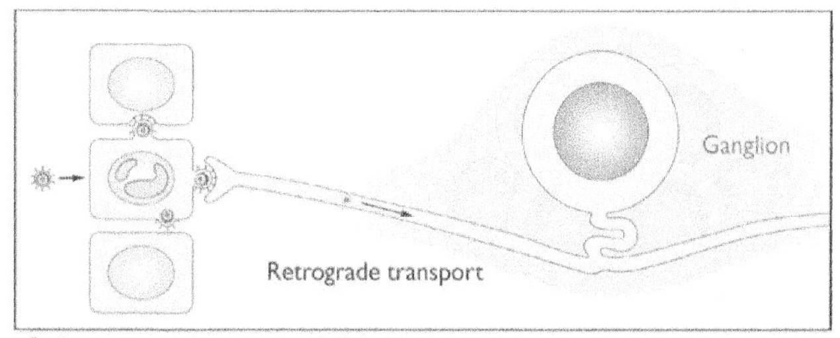

A Primary Infection and Establishment

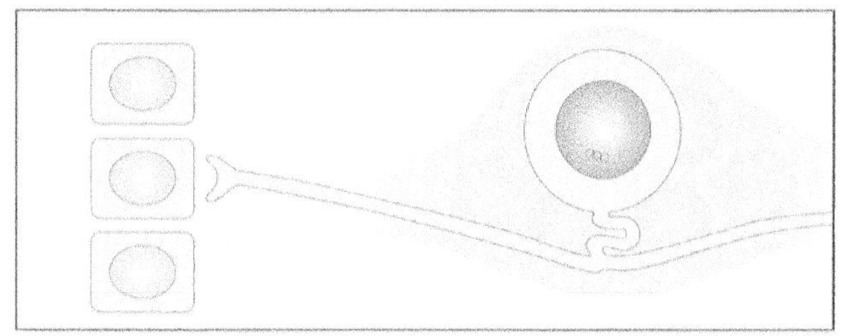

B Latent Infection

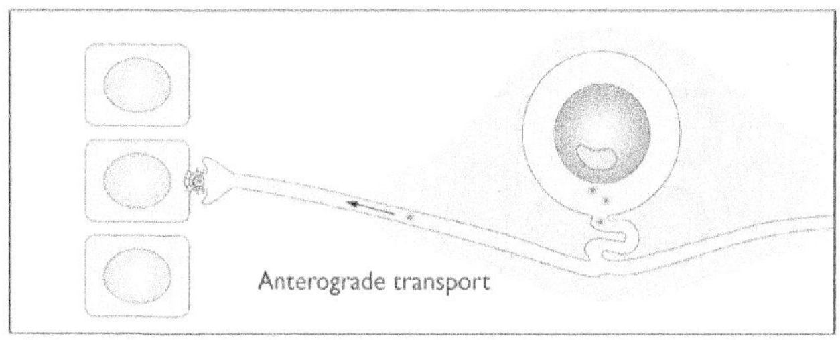

C Reactivation and Recurrent Infection

FIGURE 9.13 Stages of HSV infection of the host. A: HSV is introduced onto a mucosal surface or a break in the skin, and it replicates productively in epithelial cells at the site of inoculation and spreads through the tissue. Virus enters sensory neuron axons and is transported to the cell body in a ganglion. **B:** HSV establishes a latent infection in the neuronal cell nucleus. Viral DNA is circular and assembled in chromatin. **C:** Upon neuronal damage or activation, the virus reactivates and undergoes at least a limited productive cycle. Capsids are transported by anterograde transport to the axonal termini, and virions are released. Reactivated virus causes a recurrent infection of the mucosal tissue, causing the shedding of virus. (Copyright, Lynne Chang and David Knipe.)

LATENT INFECTION

Overview

Upon entry at oral or genital mucosal sites, HSV replicates and spreads in the tissue at the primary site of infection, and the virus enters sensory or sympathetic neurons by fusion at the axonal termini (Fig. 9.13). The nucleocapsid is carried by retrograde axonal transport to the nucleus in the neuron cell body, and the virus establishes a life-long latent infection in peripheral nervous system (PNS) neurons that innervate the infection site (Fig. 9.14). Viral DNA persists in the nucleus within neuronal cell bodies in a circular episomal form associated with nucleosomes bearing heterochromatin modifications (Fig. 9.7). In contrast to the virus lytic reproductive cycle, genes required for HSV productive replication are largely silenced through host epigenetic mechanisms during latent infection, and infectious virus may be undetectable or shed subclinically. The predominant viral gene products detected in latently infected neurons are derived from a primary latency-associated transcript (LAT), which is subsequently processed into several non–protein-coding RNA species that include a stable intron and multiple microRNAs (Fig. 9.15). Episodic emergence of the virus from latency, referred to as reactivation, commences with modifications to chromatin structure that support expression of HSV genes needed for productive virus replication. Reactivation results in virus replication within the host neuron culminating in infectious virus production. Viral latent infection is maintained by neurotrophin signaling pathways and epigenetic silencing, as evidenced by perturbations to cellular homeostasis, axonal damage, or epigenetic changes that lead to reactivation of the virus and viral gene expression. Subsequent anterograde axonal transport of virus progeny produced by reactivation to the periphery allows infection of epithelial cells innervating the axon and virus shedding at or near the anatomical site of entry. These reactivation episodes may be asymptomatic or lead to a recurrent lesion, which may vary considerably in severity from punctate lesions that are invisible to the naked eye to severe, debilitating lesions in immunosuppressed individuals. Clearance of lytically infected cells by cellular immunity resolves each recurrent episode in immune competent individuals, but the viral genome reservoir persists within the neuronal nucleus where subsequent reactivation episodes can be triggered. This lifecycle of lifelong latency within peripheral nervous system (PNS) neurons punctuated by episodic reactivation events is a defining characteristic of HSV infections and pathogenesis. While it remains incompletely understood, in part because of the challenges of modeling a human pathogen infection in other species, a powerful assortment of small animal and cell culture models have fueled our understanding of the underlying viral genetics and the cell biological and immune mechanisms that underlie latency as we know it.

Latent infection was first detected experimentally by cocultivation of explanted sensory ganglia tissue from experimentally

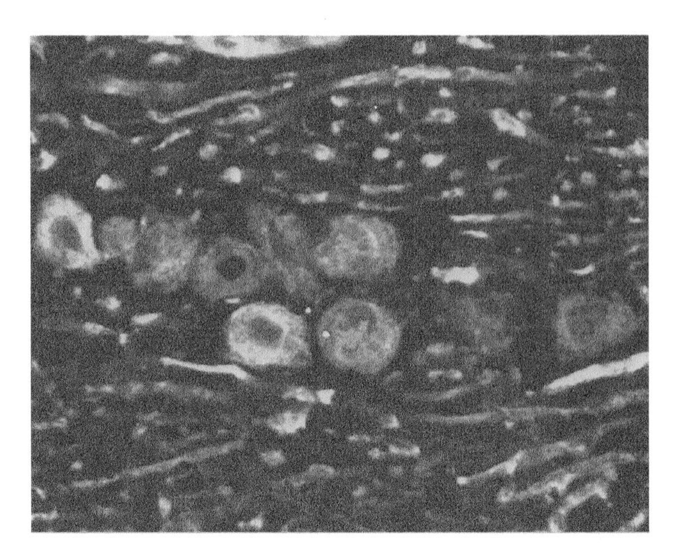

FIGURE 9.14 **Detection of HSV stable LAT RNA in latently infected murine trigeminal ganglion neurons by fluorescence *in situ* hybridization (FISH).** Mice were infected with HSV-1 following corneal scarification. At 30 days postinfection, the mice were sacrificed, and trigeminal ganglia were frozen and sectioned. The sections were hybridized with a labeled DNA probe detecting the LAT RNA (shown as *red*). Neurons were stained with antibodies detecting neurofilament proteins (*green*). (Copyright, Lynne Chang and David Knipe.)

infected mice with permissive cells and observation of cytopathic effect owing to reactivated virus. Infectious virus was not detected in homogenized ganglia tissue; therefore, the virus was considered to be latent in the tissue at the time of explant. This led to the original definition of latency: the virus must be able to reactivate from the latent state under appropriate experimental conditions. Operationally, this meant that virus could be detected after axotomy of intact ganglionic tissue and cocultivation of explanted ganglia with suitable susceptible cells in culture but not by inoculation of the susceptible cells with homogenized cell-free ganglia. The definition of latency was later extended to include viruses that can be detected in sensory ganglia several weeks after infection of experimental animals by *in situ* hybridization with probes for the latency-associated transcripts (LATs) or by assays to detect viral DNA in ganglia.[267] At the present time, the only technique for demonstrating that a virus is deficient in establishing latent infections in small animal models is the inability to detect HSV DNA by polymerase chain reaction (PCR) in total DNA isolated from whole ganglia. This more expansive definition of latent infection has enabled an assessment of the roles of specific HSV genes in the establishment and maintenance of latency, separate from their roles in reactivation. Nevertheless, it does equate the presence of viral DNA with a bona fide latent state defined biologically as capable of reactivation.

Central questions regarding the nature, control, and underlying molecular mechanisms governing HSV latency remain unanswered or incompletely understood. These include how can HSV undergo a productive infection in epithelial and other nonneuronal cells but undergo a latent infection in sensory and sympathetic PNS neurons? What intrinsic restrictive features of neurons allow the latent infection? Does the virus play an active or passive role in the latent infection? Does the host immune response control the latent infection or just the lytic infection? While our current understanding of the molecular and cellular mechanisms of HSV latency illustrates progress toward ultimately deciphering these significant gaps in knowledge, many unknowns remain.

Experimental Systems for the Study of HSV Latent Infection

Small Animal Models

The most utilized small animal model systems are laboratory mice and rabbits for HSV-1 infection and guinea pigs for genital infection by HSV-2. In all three species, inoculation of wild-type virus results in viral replication at the peripheral site and retrograde transport of virus to the nucleus of a dorsal root or trigeminal ganglion neuron, followed ultimately by establishment of latency. While the virus replicates in a fraction of sensory neurons following entry in all three animal model systems, several key features distinguish these models from each other and from infections in the natural human host. Both HSV-1 and HSV-2 reactivate spontaneously in the rabbit eye model, where the virus is readily detected in lacrimal secretions. While HSV-2 also reactivates spontaneously following genital infection of the guinea pig resulting in lesions containing small amounts of virus, the acute and recurrent phases are not always well separated. By contrast, detection of spontaneous virus reactivation in mice resulting in the appearance of infectious virus either in ganglia or at peripheral sites is exceptionally rare. Inducible reactivation has been studied in murine systems primarily following axotomy and subsequent explant of ganglia and coculture with permissive rabbit kidney cells in culture. Nevertheless, reactivation can be induced to a certain level in latently infected mice *in vivo* with peripheral tissue trauma, transient hyperthermia, UV irradiation, or epinephrine iontophoresis in the eye. Knockout mouse strains differing with respect to their susceptibility to infection have been particularly useful in studies of immune responses to acute and latent infection.

Cultured Neuron Systems

To understand molecular mechanisms underlying latency at the cell autonomous level, several cell culture models have been established to investigate virus–host interactions in the neuron itself in the absence of other cell types, including glial cells and lymphocytes that are present in ganglia. By investigating molecular interactions involving HSV-1 and the host neuron, the nuanced relationship that has evolved between the virus with this specialized host cell type can be delineated and an understanding of underlying neuronal cell intrinsic mechanisms controlling latency and reactivation at its most fundamental level can be achieved. Given that authentic, isogenic, uniform populations of human sensory or sympathetic peripheral neurons, representing archetypal host cells, are not readily available, several model systems have been developed. These include using bona fide PNS neurons harvested from rodents,[60,79,528] neuronal-like human cells differentiated from transformed, established cell lines,[125,425,467] and neurons experimentally derived from human stem cells.[96,340,368] While imperfections are associated with each of these experimental model systems, including species differences, ease of manipulation,

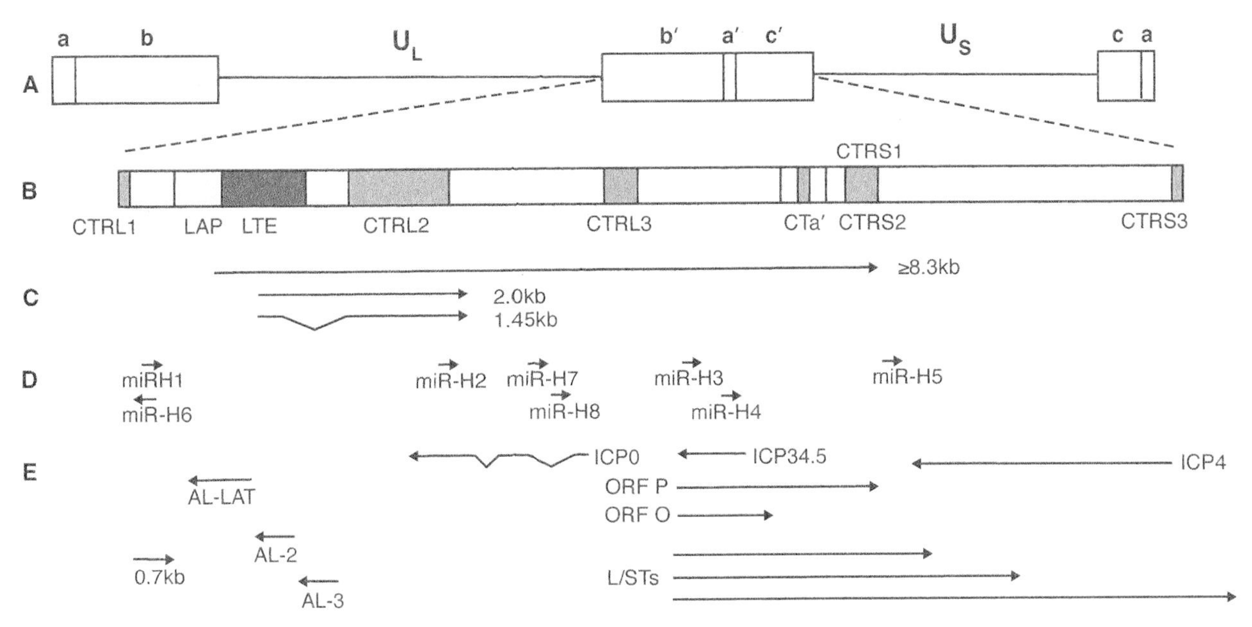

FIGURE 9.15 Map of the LAT transcriptional unit. A: HSV-1 genome in the prototype orientation; U_L and U_S denote the unique sequences of the long (L) and short (S) components of the genome, respectively. *Boxes* denote repeated sequences. **B:** Expanded view of the L–S junction of the HSV-1 genome showing the regulatory elements, including the latency-associated transcript promoter (LAP), long-term enhancer element (LTE), CTCF (CCCTC-binding factor) motifs, and putative insulator sites labeled as CTRL1, CTRL2, CTRL3, CTa′ and CTRS1, CTRS2, CTRS3. The primary LAT initiates at bp 118,802 on the HSV-1 genome based on RNase mapping of the primary transcript or at 118,803 using *in vitro* transcription. The 5′ exon extends from bp 118,803 to 119,465, and the major intron extends from bp 119,465 to 121,417. The LAT promoter is from bp 118,003 to 118,878. A second promoter, sometimes referred to as the LAP2 promoter, has been identified in transient assays and extends from bp 118,867 to 119,461. An enhancer allowing long-term expression of LAT (long-term enhancer element or LTE) extends from bp 118,077 to 119,461 and is located downstream from the LAT gene transcriptional start site. LAP2 extends from bp 118,867 to 119,461. CTCF elements containing CCTC factor (CTCF) binding sites at the U_L/c boundary (bp 120,503–120,635), and in the LAT intron (bp 117,158–117,342). **C:** LAT transcripts including the ≥ 8.3-kb LAT primary transcript; 2- and 1.5-kb LAT stable introns. **D:** Major microRNAs encoded by the LAT region: miR-H1, miR-H2, miR-H7, miR-H3, miR-H5 and miR-H4, miR-H6, miR-H8. **E:** Locations and orientations of transcripts including infected cell protein (ICP) 0, ICP4, ICP34.5,[74] open reading frame (ORF) P and ORF O, L/STs, 0.7-kb LAT (only in strain 17 and McKrae, not KOS), antisense to LAT transcripts AL-LAT, AL-2, AL-3.[196] (Copyright, Catherine Sodroski and David Knipe.)

culture purity, and the extent to which differentiated neuronal cells derived from cell lines or stem cells represent bona fide adult human sensory neurons, they continue to inform and shape our understanding of latency and reactivation despite their unavoidable strengths and weaknesses. At present, it is not possible to favor one over the other nor predict which most accurately models a natural infection in an authentic human sensory or sympathetic neuron.

To model latency in neurons, Wilcox and Johnson were among the first to utilize cultured primary sympathetic neurons isolated from the superior cervical ganglia (SCGs) of unborn rat pups and infect them with HSV-1 for latent infection.[516] Compared to sensory ganglia composed of heterogeneous neuronal types, neurons from sympathetic ganglia have an advantage in being simpler to isolate and resulted in more homogenous neuronal cultures following treatment with antimitotic agents to purge nonneuronal, dividing cells. As HSV-1 also replicates productively in neurons and cultured neurons prepared from dissociated ganglia, which are largely deficient for innate immune cells important for generating innate antiviral responses, the antiviral drug acyclovir was enlisted to uniformly suppress productive virus growth. Following removal of acyclovir, infectious virus was not detected, and a state displaying the canonical hallmarks of HSV latency defined in small animal models was reproducibly observed. Notably, productive cycle gene expression is repressed, infectious virus production is not detected, and LAT accumulation is observed in the neuronal nucleus. These pioneering studies using rat SCG sympathetic neurons latently infected with HSV-1 established that withdrawal of the neurotrophic growth factor NGF stimulated reactivation from latency[516] and first implicated NGF with a role in preserving latency in neurons. While prescient, methods for selectively manipulating host cell gene expression in neurons had not yet been developed and the molecular basis and complexity underlying NGF signaling had not yet been deciphered. Thus, these initial studies were limited to evaluating how application of varied chemical inhibitors, many of which were broadly acting, and applied physiological stresses influenced reactivation, severely limiting the utility, impact, and widespread implementation of the model.

More than 20 years later, these findings were revisited with modern methods incorporating a reporter eGFP-expressing recombinant HSV-1 enabling real-time readouts of virus reproduction in living neurons, a detailed molecular understanding of NGF-signaling, gene-specific silencing techniques capable of effectively creating hypomorphic alleles of essential host genes, and gene delivery techniques enabling ectopic expression of dominant gain of function alleles into neurons.[60,79,240]

Studies of neurons in culture have identified a defined, neuron cell autonomous relationship whereby HSV-1 persists in a nonreplicating state that is regulated by and responsive to specific cellular signaling pathways vital for neuronal homeostasis and survival. Specifically, they have revealed that (a) the virus–host neuron relationship reflects a fundamental interaction where latency can be modeled using cultured neurons and its underlying molecular circuitry dissected in the absence of an acquired immune component and (b) HSV-1 latency in cultured neurons reflects an active process maintained through continuous cell surface receptor–mediated neurotrophic factor—PI3-kinase—Akt signaling (Fig. 9.16), which maintains the viral genome in an epigenetically silenced state capable of episodic, inducible reactivation in response to defined physiological stresses.[60,79,240,305]

While neuronal latency in the natural human host and small experimental animals is established following virus infection at a peripheral nonneuronal site, available cultured neuron models are largely reliant on transient acyclovir treatment to limit virus productive growth and spread. This is not surprising, as neurons effectively support HSV productive replication and should a latently infected subpopulation stochastically form at some level following acute infection of cultured neurons, it would likely be overcome by the spread of a productive infection from neighboring cells within the culture. Nevertheless, conclusions derived from cultured neurons where latency was established using transient acyclovir administration approximate the experimental observations made without acyclovir in laboratory-infected animals. Significantly, NGF retarded whereas anti-NGF antibody accelerated the accumulation of viral mRNAs following explant-induced reactivation of sensory ganglia from experimentally infected mice.[119] Together with *in vivo* data from latently infected rabbits showing that anti-NGF administration stimulates HSV shedding,[177a] this demonstrates that HSV gene expression and reactivation are responsive to NGF in experimental latency models that do not utilize acyclovir to limit productive virus growth. Furthermore, reactivation induced by PI-3K inhibition has been reported using whole, nondissociated embryonic mouse DRG three-dimensional cultures where latency was established following *in vitro* infection without acyclovir.[305] Compartmentalized cultures that physical and fluidically separate axons from cell bodies (microfluidic or Campenot type chambers) have also been used to establish latency by infecting axons at relatively low MOI with pseudorabies virus, a related porcine α-herpesvirus, without acyclovir.[244,245] Obtaining sufficient material for biochemical analysis, however, from neurons grown in compartmentalized chambers that separate axons and soma remains a major challenge, as do studies in whole ganglia that are far from uniform and composed of varied neuronal and nonneuronal cell types. Significantly, results obtained in neuronal culture models without acyclovir are consistent with findings in models that employ acyclovir. Thus, acyclovir remains a powerful tool enabling high efficiency nonproductive infections modeling latency to be effectively established in cultured neuron models. Its use allows greater numbers of mostly homogenous populations of latently infected neurons to be made available for gene silencing, gene delivery, and biochemical analysis of neuronal cell intrinsic signaling pathways and responses.

The combination of latency studies in animal and neuron systems has yielded special insight into the mechanisms of latent infection and reactivation. Animal studies had shown the importance of epigenetic silencing of the viral genome to maintain latency,[499] and neuronal studies had shown the importance of neurotrophin signaling in maintaining latency.[60,119,240] The important connection between these two was made in neuronal studies showing that stress or signals that can arise from interruption of neurotrophin signaling leads to an epigenetic change linked to induction of viral gene expression.[79] Thus, the combination of animal studies and neuronal studies provides a powerful approach to the investigation of HSV latency, as detailed below.

Description of the Latent Infection State of HSV

The HSV-1 genome during latent infection of sensory neurons is in a covalently closed, dsDNA circle wrapped in heterochromatin. We will discuss the state of the viral latent genomes, their chromatin, and viral gene expression during latent infection. We will then describe the events of establishment, maintenance, and reactivation from latent infection.

Form and Copy Number of Viral DNA

In latently infected neurons, viral genomes are in the form of endless or circular DNA[387] assembled in nucleosomal chromatin.[108] Early studies on HSV DNA in latently infected neurons using animal models determined that there are between 0.1 and 1 viral genome equivalents per cell genome.[387] In calculations based on neurons accounting for only about 10% of the total cells in a sensory ganglion, it was obvious that each latently infected neuron must contain more than one viral genome. This was shown more directly in studies showing that approximately 20% of single purified murine trigeminal ganglion neurons contain viral DNA with an average of 20 to 30 HSV DNA molecules per cell and a range from less than 10 to greater than 1,000 molecules per cell. In studies of human neurons obtained by laser capture microdissection of trigeminal tissue, 2% to 10% of the neurons contain viral DNA with a median value of 11 genomes per cell and a range of 5 to 3,955 copies per cell. The range of DNA copy numbers raises the issue of heterogeneity of latent infection in different cells. Furthermore, only 0.2% to 1.5% of the human TG neurons express LAT, as detected by *in situ* hybridization. Thus, there are many more neurons containing DNA than expressing LAT, at least as detected by *in situ* hybridization. This extends the issue of latent infection heterogeneity by demonstrating that some latently infected neurons have all viral genes but LAT silenced, whereas other neurons have the entire viral genome silenced.

How the copy number of viral DNA molecules is established in individual neurons is not understood. High HSV genome copy numbers in latently infected cells could result in part from multiple viruses infecting each neuron. Alternatively, the viral DNA could be replicated by viral or cellular mechanisms. Studies using HSV mutant strains that do not replicate viral DNA in neurons, such as TK-negative viruses, do show lower levels of latent viral DNA per cell, supporting the idea that viral DNA replication contributes to HSV genome copy number in latently infected neurons. Nevertheless, even ganglia infected with TK-negative mutant viruses contain multiple genomes per cell, and this could be due to the slow

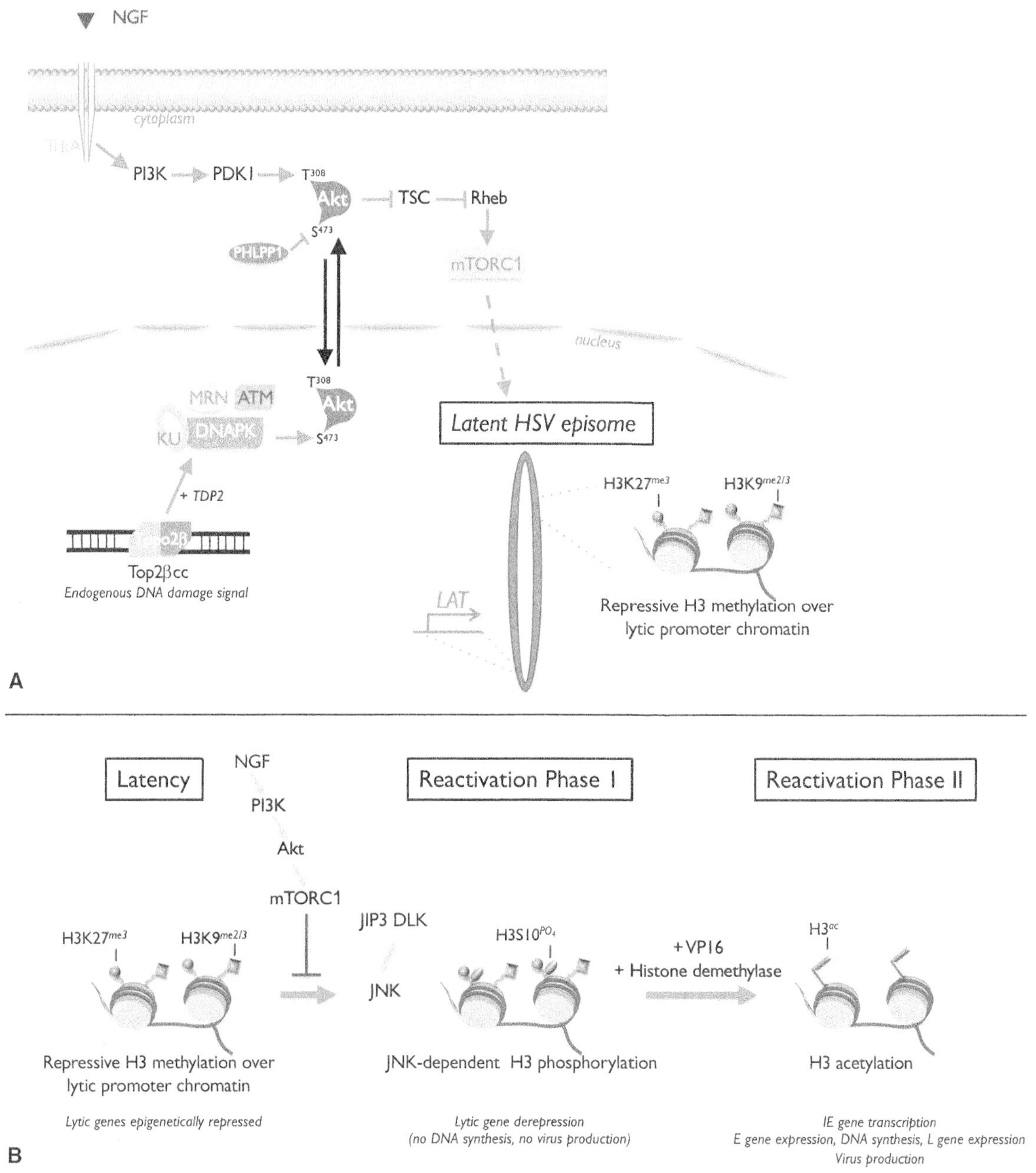

FIGURE 9.16 Regulation of HSV1 latency in cultured neurons by Akt-mTORC1 signaling and the DNA damage response. **A:** Model illustrating how activation of cellular AKT-mTORC1 signaling by extracellular NGF and cell intrinsic TOP2β-mediated nuclear DNA damage signaling maintain HSV-1 latency in cultured neurons. Binding of NGF to its high-affinity receptor TrkA stimulates PI-3 kinase (PI3K) signaling and sustained AKT Thr308 phosphorylation by PDK1. Full Akt activation in cultured sympathetic rodent neurons requires AKT to be phosphorylated on Ser473 by DNA-PK. MRN also activates ATM at DSB sites on chromatin, and ATM also promotes Akt S473 phosphorylation. DNA-PK activation results from transient DNA double-strand breaks (DSBs) generated by an endogenous DNA damage signal within the nucleus. These endogenous DSBs at promoter elements result from naturally occurring expression of host early response genes during normal neuronal activity[296] and are produced by the host topoisomerase 2β-DNA cleavage complex (TOP2βcc) intermediates acted on by TDP2. Subsequent TOP2βcc processing for both DNA repair[180] and activation of DNA-PK[190] requires the MRN complex. Presumed translocation of Akt into the nucleus allows phosphorylation by DNA-PK, and subsequent nuclear export of S473 phosphorylated Akt allows activation of cytoplasmic AKT-mTORC1 signaling. The Ser473 phosphatase PHLPP1 negatively regulates Akt activation and downstream mTORC1 signaling. Thus, sustained activation of the AKT-mTORC1 signaling axis in neurons requires consolidating at least two independent signals generated from potentially different subcellular compartments (nuclear and plasma membrane/cytoplasm). During latency, LAT is expressed from the latent genome and histones at HSV-1 lytic promoters remain in a repressed state. **B:** Neuronal stress stimuli that trigger DLK/JIP3-mediated activation of JNK contribute to a histone methyl/phospho switch[79] and subsequent replacement by euchromatin-associated marks. Interfering with continuous Akt-mTORC1 signaling results in JNK activation. The resulting histone H3 phosphorylation on residue S10 is dependent upon JNK together with JIP3/DLK and provides the trigger to initiate reactivation phase 1, which is characterized by virus genome-wide lytic gene derepression without viral DNA synthesis or infectious virus production. Subsequent expression and stochastic nuclear accumulation of VP16 in a limited cell population allows removal of repressive histone methylation marks by a histone demethylase, which coincides with the commencement of the ordered lytic gene expression program (IE genes, E genes, DNA synthesis, L genes) that culminates in infectious virus production (reactivation phase 2).

accumulation of viral DNA from the periphery or low level viral DNA replication.

Viral Chromatin

Histone modifications, particularly methylation and acetylation, play important roles in defining the type of regulation imposed on eukaryotic genes by nucleosomes, with particular modifications resulting in chromatin-mediated gene activation (active or euchromatin) or repression (inactive or heterochromatin). During latent infection, the LAT promoter and 5′ exon are associated with acetylated histones or active chromatin, whereas lytic gene promoters are not associated with acetylated histone H3. In contrast, viral lytic gene promoters are associated with heterochromatin forms of histones during latent infection.[499] The heterochromatin modifications include histone H3 lysine 9 dimethylation (H3K9me2),[499] histone H3 lysine 27 trimethylation (H3K27me3),[81,255] and H3K9 trimethylation (H3K9me3),[81] but little or none of the constitutive heterochromatin marker H3K20me3.[81] Recent studies have shown that the latent genomes in murine trigeminal ganglia[376] and in iPSC-derived sensory neurons[340] also have histones with euchromatic H3K4me3 modifications. The combination of the facultative heterochromatin mark H3K27me3 and the euchromatin mark H3K4me3 defines bivalent chromatin, a form of chromatin that is on developmentally regulated genes so they can be readily turned on at the appropriate time. Bivalent chromatin on the latent HSV genome would help it to be in a poised latency state,[265] which can reactivate with the appropriate stimulus to the latently infected neuron.

HSV DNA is not detectably methylated during latent infection in mice. The mechanism by which HSV DNA escapes methylation is a fundamental issue that remains to be defined. Current models for maintenance of HSV latent infection therefore involve the epigenetic silencing of all viral lytic genes except for the *LAT* gene and microRNAs by heterochromatin.

The three-dimensional structure of chromatin is also important for gene control. One cellular function important for higher-order structure of chromatin is CCCTC-binding factor (CTCF). CTCF promotes chromatin loop formation by two molecules of CTCF binding to separate sites and dimerization, which anchors cohesin onto the loops.[373] The loops could then define domains that are epigenetically silenced or active with the CTCF/cohesion complexes acting as chromatin insulators.

Amelio et al.[16] identified seven candidate CTCF elements containing CTCF sites, including ones at the U_L/c boundary, and in the LAT intron, and they proposed that these insulators keep the LAT enhancer activity within that boundary and heterochromatin outside of those boundaries. CTCF bound on the viral genome has also been shown to recruit polycomb repressive complex 2 (PRC2 component) Suz12,[506] which could lead to H3K27me3 modification of histones on either side of the site.

The *CTRL2*-binding site between the *ICP0* gene promoter and the *LAT* transcriptional unit (Fig. 9.15) is of particular interest because the *ICP0* gene promoter is associated with more heterochromatin and the LAT promoter is associated with more euchromatin, so *CTRL2* is a candidate insulator element between these two promoters. Comparison of an HSV-1 KOS deletion mutant virus lacking both copies of *CTRL2* with its marker rescued counterpart revealed that the *CTRL2*⁻ virus replicated normally in cultured cells and established equal viral latent DNA loads in murine trigeminal ganglia.[265] A statistically significant increase in heterochromatin on the *LAT* promoter and increased LAT expression but reduced reactivation were also observed.[265] To explain these findings, the *CTRL2* insulator was proposed to form an additional loop with a different site on the virus genome, which subsequently stimulated VP16 expression and triggered reactivation.[265] However, an independently constructed *CTRL2* deletion in the HSV-1 strain 17 genetic background resulted in a virus that replicated less well in cultured cells, and fivefold less latent DNA was detected in rabbits compared to wild-type virus. The strain 17 *CTRL2* deletion mutant also displayed reduced lytic gene transcription during latent infection and decreased H3K27me3 repressive chromatin marks over the ICP0 gene as well as other lytic genes and LAT,[507] leading the authors' to postulate that CTCF bound at the *CTRL2* site increased H3K27me3 on the viral genome. Adding to the complexity, knockdown of CTCF in rabbits latently infected with HSV-1 in the trigeminal ganglia increased ocular shedding of HSV-1.[505] Thus, at this time, we still have a complex picture with some evidence that CTCF binding to *CTRL2* serves as an insulator to prevent heterochromatin spreading,[265] while others have found that CTCF acts as an insulator to prevent spreading of chromatin from the LAT enhancer.[507]

Latent Viral Gene Expression

During latent infection, there is abundant expression of viral noncoding RNAs but very limited amounts of lytic transcripts. The major transcripts observed during latent infection are a family of noncoding RNAs known as the latency-associated transcripts (LATs)[447] and microRNAs[213,476,477] from the two copies of the R_L component of the HSV-1 genome (Fig. 9.15).

LAT

The *LAT* transcriptional unit yields a family of transcripts arising from the R_L repeat sequence (Fig. 9.15) by splicing and processing. The full-length 8.3- to 9-kb transcript accumulates at low levels in latently infected neurons, whereas the 2- and 1.5-kb introns processed from the full-length transcript are abundant and accumulate in the nucleus. These introns are highly stable as a result of unusual lariat structures. LAT was originally detected by *in situ* hybridization analysis of latently infected murine ganglia[447] and subsequently found in latently infected rabbit and human ganglia. The 2-kb LAT is the major species detected in neuronal nuclei by *in situ* hybridization[447] (Fig. 9.14).

LATs are transcribed in sensory neurons from a promoter/enhancer sequence (*LAP*; Fig. 9.15) bearing neuron-specific elements (Fig. 9.8). Although the 2-kb LAT can be detected in productively infected cells at late times postinfection, this is likely the result of splicing of read-through transcripts that are common at late times postinfection[155] or another promoter and not transcription from the true *LAT* promoter. Despite a very limited number of reports of proteins potentially encoded by LATs, most investigations have not found evidence for expression of proteins by the LATs.

A second promoter, sometimes referred to as the *LAP2* promoter, has been identified in transient assays only and is located downstream from the *in vivo LAT* gene transcriptional start site. An enhancer allowing long-term expression of LAT (long-term enhancer element or LTE) is located downstream from the *LAT* gene transcriptional start site.

Additional Transcripts

There are several additional transcripts near or overlapping the *LAT* gene or its promoter that could conceivably play a role in LAT function or contribute to the phenotypes of *LAT* gene mutant viruses (see Fig. 9.15). As a first example, a 0.7-kb transcript encoded on the same DNA strand as LAT but upstream of LAT is expressed by HSV-1 strains 17 and McKrae but not by strains KOS and F. Second, transcripts that are complementary to the *ICP4* gene transcripts, called *anti-4 transcripts*, were detected by reverse transcriptase (RT) PCR. The anti-4 transcript(s) may be expressed from a new transcriptional unit downstream of the primary LAT transcriptional unit or expressed as a read-through transcript from LAT; however, in any case, anti-4 transcription is promoted by LAT expression. Third, a transcript that is antisense to the 5′ end of LAT has been identified as encoded by HSV-1 strain McKrae and reported to express a protein in infected rabbits.

microRNAs. A number of HSV-encoded microRNAs are expressed during latent infection, as first detected in latently infected murine[476] and human ganglia.[477,478] In latently infected murine trigeminal ganglia, these include miR-H1,[248] miR-H2, miR-H3, miR-H4, miR-H5, and miR-H6,[476] as well as miR-H7, miR-H8, miR-H17, miR-H18, and miR-H24.[213] In guinea pig ganglia latently infected with HSV-2, the microRNAs shown to be expressed are miR-I (miR-H3), miR-II (miR-H4), and miR-III (miR-H2). In human trigeminal ganglia infected with HSV-1, these include miR-H1-8[477]; in human sacral ganglia infected with HSV-2, they include miR-H3, 4, 7, 9, and 10.[461,478] Of note, a subset of HSV-encoded microRNAs, while only detected at low levels during lytic infection or in latently infected samples, accumulated to higher levels upon reactivation in murine ganglia, including miR-H8, miR-H28, and miR-H29.[118,165] Many of the HSV microRNAs relevant to latency are likely to be processed from the primary LAT because their expression depends on the LAT promoter.[248,460] Interestingly, miR-H6 expression is reduced in a *LAT* promoter mutant virus,[248] despite this microRNA being encoded upstream of the *LAT* promoter, suggesting that the *LAT* promoter is bidirectional. Expression of HSV-2 miR-H3 by transfection reduced ICP34.5 expression in transfected or infected cells,[460] as did transfection of miR-H4,[462] and expression of HSV-1 miR-H2 reduced ICP0 expression.[476] Although HSV-2 miR-H6 had no effect on ICP4 expression, transfection of HSV-1 miR-H6 also reduced ICP4 expression.[476] It was thus hypothesized that these microRNAs could contribute to latent infection by down-regulating critical viral gene products needed for lytic infection.

In addition to encoding microRNAs, the HSV genome contains cis-acting elements responsive to host microRNAs that can influence latency. Two target sites for the neuron-specific microRNA, miR-138, were identified in the 3′-UTR of the mRNA encoding the HSV-1 transactivator ICP0, and one was found in the corresponding mRNA encoded by HSV-2. ICP0 and lytic gene expression in cultured cells was directly repressed by miR-138. Furthermore, disrupted miR-138–binding sites in ICP0 mRNA not only enhanced lytic gene expression in murine TGs but also enhanced virulence in mice.[352] Thus, a cell type–specific neuronal microRNA can promote latency by directly targeting ICP0 expression.

Lytic Transcripts

In murine models of HSV-1 latent infection, there is low-level expression of lytic transcripts,[246] and this may be due to abortive or nonproductive reactivation events[246] or to a limited number of cells undergoing a more complete reactivation.[170] The relatively lower levels of late viral transcripts such as *gC* gene transcripts argues that the lytic gene expression is due to abortive reactivation events in at least this murine system.[295] Single-cell RNA sequencing of dorsal root ganglia latently infected with HSV-1 showed frequent lytic gene transcription in this system.[295]

Events of Latent Infection and Reactivation

HSV latency and reactivation are complex biological processes that can be subdivided into discrete stages. Following entry into axonal termini of sensory or sympathetic neurons, HSV must reach the nucleus in the neuronal cell body to establish a permanent latent infection. Having established a latent infection by delivering its genome and effectively colonizing a postmitotic, nondividing neuron, the infection is maintained in a nonreplicating state for the life of the infected individual. Finally, in response to dynamic physiological and/or environmental cues, the virus changes its relationship with the host neuron and activates a complex gene expression program that results in the assembly and release of infectious virus particles capable of shedding at the anatomical entry portal and subsequently spreading to new hosts. In the following sections, we examine these defined stages of latency and review what is known regarding the underlying genetic and cell biological regulatory mechanisms.

Establishment of Latency

Electron microscopic studies indicate that in neurons infected in cell culture, the viral particle transported by retrograde transport along microtubules in the axon is the unenveloped nucleocapsid or nucleocapsid–tegument structure. Viral gene expression, including IE, E, L, and LAT RNAs, is observed in ganglia of infected animals over the first 24 to 72 hours. Several host immune response effectors in experimental animal models are postulated to play a role in control of early viral replication, including IFN-γ, macrophages, γδ T cells, and CD8+ T cells. CD8+ T cells infiltrate the ganglia starting around 5 to 7 days postinfection, coincident with the time at which virus starts to decrease around day 7. CD8+ T cells have been shown to play an essential role in control of HSV replication in the murine nervous system and in controlling viral replication in the ganglia during acute times of infection. Cytokine and chemokine expression increases in the acutely infected murine sensory ganglia. Silencing of HSV genes in sensory neurons in animal models appears to be a slow and multistep process.

Further evidence that entry through the axon is critical for the normal process of establishment of latent infection has come from culture systems. Studies using isolated chicken TGs cultured in a double chambered system to create an axon-only compartment showed that application of virus to distal axons resulted in nonproductive infections where LAT accumulated and lytic genes were repressed.[162] This raises the possibility that axonal entry, the natural route of virus entry from the periphery, may be a critical determinant in the lytic/latent decision in neurons.

Although the events occurring during the first few hours after entry of viral DNA into dorsal root ganglia have not been defined, a key factor is likely to be the reduced expression of IE genes. The reduced IE gene expression is likely explained by several mechanisms either as part of a common pathway or acting in a combination of pathways.

1. *Neuronal repressors.* Several neuronal repressors have been proposed to repress IE gene expression in neurons. First, the Oct-2 factor was postulated to repress IE gene expression through its interaction with TAATGARATT DNA-containing sites blocking Oct-1 activation. Oct-2 expression was not detected in sensory neurons nor was expression from a complete IE-promoter/enhancer-bearing reporter gene detectably repressed when Oct-2 was overexpressed. The neuron-specific Zhangfei/CREBZF factor has also been postulated to block activation of IE gene promoters through interaction at Oct-1–binding sites. Perhaps more significantly, expression of a dominant-negative form of the host repressor REST reduced viral replication in neurons,[119] indicating that REST could be part of the mechanism of silencing of the viral genome in neurons.
2. *Neurotrophin-regulated repression of viral gene expression.* Neurotrophins, including nerve growth factor (NGF), are host-encoded polypeptides that function in the nervous system as growth factors that promote survival, differentiation, axonal growth, and synaptic plasticity. By engaging cell surface receptors on the surface of sensory and sympathetic neurons, NGF generates signals that travel to the nucleus where they influence gene expression. NGF treatment of sensory neurons has been shown to restrict viral lytic gene expression,[516] and anti-NGF treatment of latently infected neurons increases viral lytic gene expression.[60,119] Furthermore, ocular administration of anti-NGF antibodies to latently infected rabbits resulted in virus shedding, consistent with increased reactivation *in vivo*.
3. *Lack of viral and cellular factors necessary to overcome host silencing and allow IE gene transcription.* Several studies have raised the idea that sensory neurons lack essential factors for expression of HSV IE genes, thereby explaining the latent infection in these cells. In studies using *in situ* hybridization to detect Oct-1 mRNA, Oct-1 expression was initially not detected in cells of the sensory ganglia, but more sensitive assays showed Oct-1 and GABPα/β are present but at low levels in sensory neurons. Kristie et al.[250] first showed that HCF-1, or C1, the cellular cofactor required to stimulate IE gene expression along with Oct-1 and VP16, resides in the cytoplasm in mouse trigeminal ganglion neurons and is translocated into the nucleus only under conditions of reactivation such as axotomy followed by culture of explanted ganglia. Thus, while HCF-1 is predominately nuclear in most dividing nonneuronal cells, it may not be capable of localizing to the nucleus in HSV-infected neurons, and this prevents IE gene transcription. In addition, VP16 does not contain a nuclear localization signal and is dependent upon HCF-1 for transport into the cell nucleus. VP16 in the incoming virion therefore would not accumulate in the neuronal nucleus within cell bodies and transactive IE genes. Finally, VP16 does not bind mouse Oct-1 as well as human Oct-1, potentially limiting its capacity to activate IE gene expression in neurons. The viral genome may also be localized to or near ND-10 structures, which aids in repression of the lytic gene expression.[302]
4. *Viral RNA–mediated repression of IE gene expression.* LAT-negative mutant viruses show elevated lytic gene expression in trigeminal ganglion neurons during acute infection of mice at 3 to 5 days postinfection (dpi).[145] Therefore, LAT or one of its products seems to exert some of its repressive effects at early times following infection of neurons.

Kinetics of Chromatin Silencing of Viral Lytic Genes

Chromatin assembly with incoming viral DNA is very rapid during lytic infection of cells in culture.[82] By contrast, histone H3 association with HSV DNA in murine trigeminal ganglia seems slower, possibly due to lower histone pools in resting neurons, and is apparent by 7 dpi, while the H3K9me2 modification is apparent by 15 dpi.[499] Whereas viral lytic gene promoters are associated with H3 histone by 7 dpi, further studies found that the H3K27me3 heterochromatin modification was not detected on HSV lytic gene chromatin until later, at 14 dpi,[80] arguing that the earliest chromatin effect is association of unmodified chromatin followed by the H3K27me3 modification. In this murine infection model, acute viral replication in the trigeminal ganglia has largely declined by 7 dpi; therefore, H3K27 methylation appears to occur after resolution of the infection. This is significant as it suggests that events earlier than heterochromatin modifications of histones are responsible for the initial silencing of the viral genome.

In addition to being composed of nonneuronal and neuronal cells, sensory ganglia including the trigeminal ganglia contain different neuronal subtypes. Studies on the neuronal subtype in which latent infection is established in murine model systems have shed light on the mechanisms of establishment of latent infection. In mice infected by the ocular route with HSV-1 strain KOS virus, latent infection is preferentially established in a subset of neurons identified with the A5 antibody recognizing a specific lacto-series glycoconjugate marker. Further studies showed that HSV-2 preferentially established latent infection in KH10 monoclonal antibody-reactive sensory neurons in either trigeminal or dorsal root ganglia. A recombinant HSV-2 that expresses the HSV-1 LAT showed an HSV-1 phenotype (i.e., preferential establishment of latency in A5-positive neurons), and a recombinant HSV-1 expressing the HSV-2 LAT showed an HSV-2 phenotype (i.e., preferential establishment of latency in KH10-positive neurons).[194] These studies showed that LAT influenced establishment of latent infection in discrete neuronal subtypes in mice. Furthermore, studies of infection of murine adult sensory ganglion neurons *in vitro* have shown that A5-positive sensory neurons are nonpermissive for HSV-1 strains KOS and 17 *in vitro* but are permissive for HSV-2.[39] Although the LAT recombinant viruses were not examined in the latter study, the results, in total, raise the general model of LAT controlling productive infection in specific neuronal subtypes. Therefore, these studies support the idea that both viral and host factors contribute to establishment of latent infection.

The question of whether viral infection leads directly to latent infection versus lytic infection and/or whether lytic infection can convert to latent infection has been debated extensively. Studies using viruses that express CRE recombinase from viral lytic gene promoters to activate cellular reporters and mark cells in which viral lytic gene transcription has occurred found that approximately one-third of the latently infected murine neurons have experienced IE promoter activation prior to establishment of latent infection but have not experienced TK or VP16 promoter activation.[370,371] This argues that at least some IE gene expression can precede latent infection and raises that possibility that these gene products could affect the host responses or viral chromatin and affect the type of latent infection that ensues. Furthermore, ICP0 nonsense mutant viruses show reduced H3K27me3 and LAT expression during latent infection,[377] arguing that the ICP0 protein itself increases LAT expression and indirectly increases facultative heterochromatin, during establishment and/or maintenance of latency. This raises the possibility that ICP0 could be a target for antiviral drugs during establishment and/or latency.

Maintenance Phase of Latency

The HSV-1 latent state, characterized by circular viral genomes expressing LATs and miRNAs while lytic genes are epigenetically silenced by heterochromatin, is maintained by a number of signaling pathways within the sensory neuron. Cultured neuron model systems have enabled progress toward elucidating the molecular signals that lead to viral genome repression and by extension, upon their perturbation, the earliest events resulting in inducible reactivation that are simply not possible to observe in live animal models.

By integrating numerous fundamental physiological inputs including growth factor, nutrient, energy, and oxygen sufficiency, local signaling by the mechanistic target of rapamycin complex 1 (mTORC1) in axons provides a critical signal to maintain viral genome repression and repress reactivation of HSV genomes in the nuclear compartment.[240] This defines how changes in homeostasis detected within axons can trigger genome repression or activation in spatially segregated nuclear compartments and identified how regulating neuronal gene expression posttranscriptionally at the level of mRNA translation (Fig 9.9) controls latency and reactivation (Fig. 9.16). The cellular repressor of cap-dependent translation, the eIF4E-binding protein 4E-BP1, is a key target of mTORC1 (Fig 9.9) that controls latency and reactivation, consistent with a role for differential translation of 4E-BP1–regulated neuronal mRNAs in regulating latency.[240]

Changes in genome integrity within neurons also regulate mTORC1 activation by Akt. This is significant because endogenous, cell intrinsic, double-stranded DNA (dsDNA) breaks generated by topoisomerase 2β-DNA cleavage complex (TOP2βcc) intermediates accumulate as a result of normal processes stimulating gene activation in neurons in the absence of exogenous DNA damaging agents.[297] Continued activation of the neuronal DNA damage response and DNA repair proteins is required to ensure full activation of Akt, which involves Akt S473 phosphorylation dependent upon balancing opposing activities of the cellular DNA-dependent protein kinase DNA-PK, which is required for DNA repair, and the Akt S473 phosphatase PHLPP1.[190] This provides a mechanism whereby extracellular cues in the form of neurotrophic factor signaling and nuclear genome integrity can be harnessed and integrated to control activation of neuronal Akt-mTORC1 signaling to maintain latency and repress reactivation (Fig. 9.16).

Host responses in ganglia also can contribute to the maintenance of latency. There is prolonged expression of cytokines and chemokines and $CD8^+$ T-cell infiltration[280] in the latently infected murine ganglia and prolonged expression of cytokines and chemokines in human latently infected ganglia. This indicates that there is continued antigenic stimulation of dendritic cells (DCs) and macrophages and continued T-cell activation in the ganglionic tissue both in experimental animal models and likely in the natural human host. As described elsewhere in this chapter, the ongoing immune surveillance is likely in response to the presence of viral antigens in the ganglion owing to low-level reactivation.

Latent HSV infection also leads to perturbation of neuronal host cell gene expression. Using microarrays, Kramer et al.[247] showed that numerous cellular genes were up-regulated or down-regulated in latently infected murine trigeminal ganglia. Little is known about the effects of these gene expression changes on the host neuron or whether they influence either latency or reactivation. More recent application of single-cell RNA-seq and single-molecule fluorescent *in situ* hybridization technologies using neurons prepared from rat sympathetic ganglia and latently infected with HSV-1 *in vitro* revealed that HSV-1 elicits a host gene expression signature to counteract viral reactivation in a cell type–specific manner.[189]

Reactivation of Virus From the Latent State

In humans, latent virus is reactivated after local stimuli such as injury to tissues innervated by neurons harboring latent virus or by systemic stimuli such as physical or emotional stress, hyperthermia, exposure to UV light, menstruation, and hormonal imbalance, which may reactivate virus simultaneously in neurons of various ganglia (e.g., trigeminal and sacral). Thus, injury or stimulation of cells innervated by dorsal root neurons harboring latent virus is a common trigger of recrudescence of lesions caused by reactivated virus.

The ability of sensitive PCR tests to measure HSV DNA in human genital secretions has led to the detection of frequent viral DNA shedding in the genital tract of both asymptomatic and symptomatic individuals. This raises questions about whether HSV latency is actually a low-level chronic infection producing constant virus shedding rather than a true latent infection.[411] However, the amount of virus shed by many individuals is very low, potentially representing virus DNA within desquamated epithelial cells rather than virions. Even if the limited amount of DNA detected were to result from reactivation of a small number of neurons reactivating at any one time, it seems likely that the vast majority of infected neurons are undergoing a latent infection. Nevertheless, the possibility of low-level chronic infection, especially with HSV-2, remains.

As described earlier, there are several experimental model systems for studying *in vitro* and *in vivo* reactivation of HSV. Upon induction of reactivation by *in vitro* explant of murine latently infected ganglia, LAT and microRNA transcript levels decrease, lytic gene transcripts increase,[119] and the histones associated with the *LAT* gene become deacetylated consistent with their repression. Similarly, lytic genes such as *ICP0* become associated with acetylated histones, which support epigenetic stimulation of virus gene expression and lytic gene transcripts accumulate. HSV-1 reactivates spontaneously in the rabbit ocular infection model, and HSV-2 reactivates spontaneously in the guinea pig vaginal infection model.

In cultured neuron latency models, reactivation can be induced by perturbing specific signaling pathways required to maintain latency by using chemical inhibitors, removing neuronal trophic support factors, interfering with host gene expression by RNAi, or expressing mutant alleles of signaling components. These include nerve growth factor deprivation,[60,79,516] PI-3 kinase inhibitors,[60,79,230] histone deacetylase inhibitors,[239,368] and adenyl cyclase activators.[95] Similar to reactivation induced by interfering with PI-3 kinase signaling, activation of adenyl cyclase by forskolin or cAMP mimetic treatment induced HSV reactivation in a DLK/JNK-dependent manner that involves a histone phospho/methyl switch (H3K9me3/S10p, discussed in detail later).[95] However, forskolin-induced reactivation was also dependent on neuronal activity, consistent with a role for neuronal hyperexcitability or repeated action potential firing in controlling HSV reactivation. Finally, IL-1β, a known mediator of prolonged stress inflammation and neuronal hyperexcitability, was identified as a physiological stimulus that triggers HSV reactivation in mature neurons.[95]

It was initially assumed that viral gene expression during reactivation follows the lytic gene cascade regulatory program (IE genes followed by E genes, DNA replication, and L genes) originally defined in an established, human tumor cell line,[186] and this was supported by some experimental evidence. However, Tal-Singer et al.[457] reportedly detected E gene expression prior to IE gene expression during explant-induced reactivation. While they used RT-PCR to detect viral transcripts, they did not show that the assays for each of the transcripts was equally sensitive. Thus, it remains conceivable that differences in the kinetics of observed transcript appearance reflected sensitivity of the detection assay rather than the true order of accumulation. Other *in vivo* and cell culture studies have suggested that optimal viral gene expression in neurons depends on viral DNA replication, although viral spread was not ruled out in the *in vivo* and *ex vivo* studies. However, when viral spread is prevented during ganglion explant, there is no apparent role for viral DNA synthesis in stimulation of IE and E gene expression. One study using infected rat sensory neurons in culture, however, does support the idea that viral gene expression in neurons is affected by viral DNA synthesis and found that viral DNA synthesis stimulates IE and E gene expression.

The events leading to viral gene expression during reactivation have been examined in various systems, and some understanding of the underlying mechanisms has been achieved. From studies in animal models, Thompson and Sawtell proposed defining the exit from latency as the expression of viral lytic proteins as detected by immunohistochemistry using anti-HSV antiserum, and they defined full reactivation as the production of infectious virus. Using a mouse model where reactivation is induced by transient hyperthermia, they observed an average of one cell per trigeminal ganglion in which virus has escaped latency and approximately 70% of the ganglia reactivated with an average yield of 10 pfu of virus per ganglion. An ICP0 mutant showed similar escape from latency, but infectious virus was not detected. These investigators concluded that ICP0 does not initiate reactivation from latency *in vivo*; however, the process of latency exit in this model system is of very low efficiency and could have minimized the differences between wild-type and mutant viruses.

Reactivation requires the action of LSD1, which demethylates H3Kme2 and H3Kme1 to reduce heterochromatin on viral chromatin.[273,274] LSD1 inhibitors block reactivation in explanted ganglia[273,274] or in the rabbit eye model and guinea pig infection model.[178] Thus, LSD1 inhibitors could conceivably serve as a herpes antiviral drug that prevents HSV reactivation by locking in viral latency. Antiviral targeting of a host function, however, carries toxicity risks, but this could be a useful strategy if drugs can be identified that preferentially inhibit the capacity of LSD1 to affect viral gene expression compared to gene expression in uninfected cells.

In cultured neurons, a critical role for the neuronal-specific c-Jun N-terminal kinase (JNK) stress pathway has been defined (Fig. 9.16) whereby viral genome derepression requires JNK-dependent histone H3S10 phosphorylation.[79] This comprises a histone methyl/phospho switch that allows histone H3 phosphorylation to override repressive epigenetic K9me3 methylation marks that are normally associated with gene silencing. Moreover, it defines how activation of a fundamental neuronal stress response associated with axonal damage, injury, and regeneration is subverted to overcome epigenetic repression associated with HSV genome silencing during latency. More work is required to understand how JNK activation, which is likely a near final step in modifying viral genome chromatin to overcome genome silencing, integrates with signals downstream of mTORC1 and 4E-BP1. Whether this involves the direct action of a single 4E-BP1 translationally regulated mRNA, multiple mRNAs, or a complex regulatory process with numerous molecular steps is unknown, but at least has become a tractable problem addressable with known methodologies. The molecular basis underlying how other inducers of reactivation function is also now approachable using cultured neuron models. Are other neuronal signaling pathways capable of regulating latency and reactivation? Do they all converge on a common set of downstream effectors involving PI-3K-Akt and/or mTORC1 and JNK, or are other pathways with discrete effectors involved? Can multiple pathways synergize and produce context-dependent outcomes with respect to maintaining latency and triggering reactivation? While these outcomes are presently unknown, neuronal cell culture models of HSV latency and reactivation provide a powerful opportunity to investigate these critical questions using genetic, biochemical, and cell biological methods in a quantifiable manner.

In contrast to the ordered program where IE gene products stimulate E followed by L gene expression in a cascade-like manner that characterizes acute infection and HSV productive growth, viral gene expression during reactivation is distinctively regulated. Using the mouse model, the first detectable HSV-1 gene product detected upon inducible reactivation was unexpectedly found to be VP16, a late protein. Significantly, while reactivation of the VP16 mutant virus *in*1814 was readily detected upon *in vitro* explant and coculture of ganglia with permissive cells, reactivation was not detected following induction by transient hyperthermia.[468] This suggested that VP16 was required for *in vivo* exit from latency but not for *in vitro* explant-induced reactivation. Consistent with this proposal, the

VP16 promoter, which normally is transcribed late in infection, was shown to direct VP16 expression following hyperthermia-induced reactivation in mice.[468] This led to a model where VP16 is expressed prior to IE proteins and stimulates reactivation by triggering IE gene expression to advance the lytic program much in the way that VP16 delivery by the incoming tegument functions during acute infection to initiate HSV IE gene transcription.[468] Further support for a reactivation-specific viral gene expression program was provided by experiments using *ex vivo* and *in vitro* cell culture models. Following explant of sensory ganglia from latently infected mice and incubation with NGF-neutralizing antibody in the presence or absence of cycloheximide, viral genes of IE, E, and L kinetic classes, including VP16, were found to be expressed simultaneously and not sequentially ordered.[119] A similar disordered pattern of HSV mRNA accumulation with simultaneous expression of IE, E, and L mRNAs was observed upon inducible reactivation of latently infected cultured rat and mouse SCG neurons.[79,230] These results argue that reactivation from a genome epigenetically silenced by heterochromatin occurs via cellular mechanisms affecting the entire genome uniformly and emphasize the differences in the mechanisms of reactivation versus initial acute infection of neurons and other cell types.

Two distinct reactivation-specific phases of viral gene expression were observed following inducible reactivation of rat and mouse neurons latently infected in culture. Global, simultaneous derepression of all kinetic classes of HSV-1 mRNA was observed during the initial phase, termed phase 1.[230] Neuronal JNK-dependent phosphorylation of histone H3S10, which rapidly overrides repressive methylation chromatin marks, was shown to be associated with this genome-wide burst of HSV-1 gene expression.[79] Histone demethylase inhibitors were unable to block phase 1, demonstrating that removal of repressive histone epigenetic methylation marks is not required.[79] In agreement with *in vivo* mouse models,[468] VP16 protein accumulation was detected during phase 1 as one of the earliest events following inducible reactivation.[230] However, while IE, E, and late mRNAs and proteins were readily observed in phase 1, nuclear accumulation of VP16 protein and its critical cellular cofactor HCF, viral DNA synthesis, and infectious virus were not detected.[230] Significantly, this initial widespread derepression of viral genes preceded a second phase of VP16-dependent HSV-1 gene transcription

A second discrete reactivation-specific gene expression program termed phase 2 followed the initial genome-wide phase 1 burst of HSV-1 gene expression.[79,230] The onset of phase 2 was VP16-dependent and correlated with the nuclear accumulation of VP16 and HCF-1 proteins followed by VP16-dependent viral gene transcription, HSV-1 genome amplification, and infectious virus production.[230] Thus, the production and subcellular localization of VP16 plays a critical role in enabling reactivation from latency in sympathetic neuron culture models. Unlike phase 1, cellular H3K27 demethylases (UTX/KDM6A and JMJD3/KDM6B) and the H3K9 demethylase (LSD1/KDM1) are required for full reactivation and infectious virus production in phase 2.[79] In addition, phase 2 HSV-1 gene expression more closely resembled the cascade pattern of viral gene expression during acute, productive replication.[230] The underlying mechanisms restricting virus genome amplification to phase 2 are unknown and could provide a platform to investigate and ultimately reveal unexpected nuances of viral gene expression. For example, at the single-cell level, what are the determinants of whether the genome-wide viral gene expression burst defining phase 1 will in fact progress to phase 2? Are there stochastic combinations of phase 1 gene expression more likely to progress to phase 2 or is phase 1 gene expression relatively homogenous following inducible reactivation? Does phase 1 always progress to phase 2, or are there restriction factors (perhaps including LAT products like virus microRNAs) that act as molecular hurdles that could prevent or limit the onset of phase 2 and in fact reestablish genome silencing, in effect reversing reactivation and reestablishing latency? Continued exploitation of these powerful cultured neuron models will help answer these mechanistic questions and undoubtedly raise additional new exciting questions along the way.

Role of Viral Gene Functions in Latency

Genetic analysis of mutant viruses has attempted to define the role of viral gene products in establishment of latent infection. HSV must have access to the nerve endings in order to establish latency; therefore, *in vivo* it could be expected that the greater the number of peripheral cells that become infected and support virus multiplication, the larger the number of neurons that will harbor latent virus. Indeed, replication-defective viruses show reduced levels of latent infection in animal models, although they can establish and maintain latent infections but not reactivate. In essence, no deletion mutant has totally failed to establish latent infection in mice or rabbit models, indicating an inability to identify a single viral gene product absolutely required to support latency in nonhuman animal models. Thus far, no viral gene function is essential for latent infection of neurons in culture either. Whether this reflects an intrinsic limitation of nonhuman animal models in responding to LAT function or is also true in the natural human host remains unknown.

LAT

During the establishment of latency, LAT and HSV-encoded microRNAs accumulate and contribute to silencing virus gene expression. LAT expression is detected by 26 hpi in murine trigeminal ganglia and continues to increase for at least 3 to 9 dpi.[119] Similar levels and kinetics of LAT expression are observed for a TK-negative mutant virus, which does not replicate in TG neurons, indicating that LAT expression at these times largely occurs from input viral genomes. Several studies support the possibility that LATs and HSV microRNAs could be expressed early enough to add to or synergize with the repressive effects of preexisting host repressors.[119,248]

LAT-negative mutant viruses show elevated lytic viral gene expression in murine trigeminal sensory neurons during acute infection[145] and during latent infection.[337] Consistent with these *in vivo* results, expression of LAT has been shown to reduce viral gene expression and replication in cultured cells. One study did report that LAT increases lytic gene expression during latent infection of rabbit trigeminal ganglia with the HSV-1 strain 17ΔPst mutant virus versus HSV-1 17syn+ wild-type virus.[153] However, some stocks of the HSV-1 17 ΔPst mutant used in this paper have a lytic growth defect and a rescued virus was not used.[153] Thus, the bulk of the literature documents that LAT decreases lytic gene expression with the exception of one study.

Consistent with its gene expression effects, LAT has been shown to increase H3K9me2 heterochromatin marks and decrease H3K4me2 euchromatin marks on latent HSV-1 chromatin in murine trigeminal ganglia.[499] Further analysis of the structure of the viral heterochromatin demonstrated that LAT expression shows statistically significant increases of H3K27me3 and H3K9me3 on latent viral chromatin in murine trigeminal ganglia.[81] With the exception of a single study where wild type and LAT mutants were not rigorously compared in a side-by-side experiment,[255] the bulk of the literature supports the idea that expression of LAT increases facultative heterochromatin on the latent viral genome.

LAT has been reported to have several other effects on latent infection. With regard to establishment, some studies reported that viruses deleted in various domains of *LAT* establish latency at normal levels, whereas others reported that the number of neurons harboring LAT-negative viruses is decreased by three- to fivefold.[365] It is conceivable that assaying numbers of latently infected cells is a more quantitative or accurate assay of latent infection than measurement of total viral DNA molecules. With regard to reactivation, some observed reduced explant reactivation of virus from ganglia latently infected with LAT-negative mutant viruses, although in some cases LAT-negative mutant viruses show reduced replicative ability. The region of the LATs associated with increased reactivation has been mapped to a 348-bp sequence in the 5′ end of LAT.

Consistent with increased viral gene expression, infection of mice with LAT-negative mutant viruses has been shown to result in greater cell destruction in trigeminal tissue, to cause neuronal death, and to cause higher mortality.[503] By using recombinant viruses that express reporter proteins to mark infected cells,[370] latently infected cells were shown to be lost faster with an LAT-negative mutant virus,[337] and lytic reporter gene expression during latent infection of murine decreased faster with LAT-negative mutant viruses.[338] Consistent with these findings, LATs may protect neurons from apoptosis. Thus, an LAT-deficient virus was reported to induce apoptosis in rabbit trigeminal ganglia at slightly higher levels than the wild-type virus. The effect of LAT on apoptosis in mice, however, was observed in some studies but not others. LAT expressed from a plasmid vector can protect cells of human and monkey continuous lines from cell death induced by etoposide, ceramide, or other agents.[365] Although the original hypothesis was that the LATs protected sensory neurons from apoptosis during acute infection,[365] others have argued that the effect of LATs on establishment of latent infection may be minimal and that it is more likely that the LATs play a role in blocking apoptosis during reactivation.

A role for HSV-1 LAT RNA in reactivation distinct from its function in latency establishment was recently demonstrated by depleting LAT after the establishment of HSV-1 latency in rabbits. This was accomplished by delivering an adeno-associated virus (AAV) vector to deliver a LAT-targeting hammer-head ribozyme after latency was established followed by inducible reactivation. LAT depletion in latently infected neurons with adenovirus-associated vectors expressing the ribozyme prevented reactivation in 60% of the rabbit eyes.[508] This study is also notable in that it demonstrated that AAV can be delivered to trigeminal ganglia by the corneal route.

LATs have also been reported to protect neuronal-derived cells from $CD8^+$ T-cell killing[202] and to promote $CD8^+$ T-cell exhaustion in trigeminal ganglia.[14,69] Overall, despite differences in the experimental models utilized, a common theme of LAT studies has been that LATs protect neurons from death, either by reducing viral gene expression, by protecting against apoptosis, or by other mechanisms. Studies of latent infection in human neurons, the natural host of the virus, should be very important in further defining the role of LAT in HSV-1 latent infection.

miRNAs

Although miR-H2-3p is complementary to ICP0 mRNA and could reduce ICP0 expression when coexpressed in transfected cells and miR-H6 is able to reduce ICP4 in transfected cells,[476] there have been few alterations in phenotype displayed by recombinant viruses harboring deletions of the sequences encoding these miRNAs.[248,460] Findings from studies using miR-H2 mutant viruses differ as to the impact of endogenous miR-H2 on ICP0 expression and virus replication.[139,353] While a miR-H2 mutant virus produced in a 17syn+ background displayed increased ICP0 expression in 293 cells, a miR-H2 mutant in a KOS background had no effect on ICP0 expression in Vero or Neuro2A cells or in latently infected mouse trigeminal ganglia. Furthermore, while the 17syn+ mutant virus had a reduced rate of replication following low-multiplicity infection in the Neuro2A mouse neuroblastoma cell line, there was no difference in latency establishment, maintenance, or reactivation from latency in mouse trigeminal ganglia following infection with the KOS-background miR-H2 mutant virus. The basis for this strain-specific behavior of miR-H2 mutant alleles remains unknown. Besides the miR-H2 mutant virus, miR-H3 and miR-H4 mutant viruses were produced in a 17syn+ background. Both mutant viruses had slightly increased rates of replication in Neuro2A cells following low-multiplicity infection but, while the miR-H4 mutant had increased ICP34.5 expression, there was no observed effect of miR-H3 on ICP34.5 expression in 293 cells after transfection or HSV-1 infection.[139]

Expression of a subset of these microRNAs in latently infected mouse ganglia is dependent on LAT. Because *LAT* deletion mutants can efficiently establish and maintain latency in mouse trigeminal ganglia, this indicates that LAT-encoded microRNAs are not essential for the establishment or maintenance of latency.[248] A similar dependency on LAT for expression of miR-H6 was observed in HSV-2 infection models, suggesting HSV-2 LAT-encoded microRNAs are similarly not required for latency establishment or maintenance.[460] A recent paper reported that an HSV mutant with the miR-H1 and miR-H6 sequences deleted showed slower reactivation than the wild-type parental virus.[34] The phenotype of a rescued virus remains to be explored. The limited phenotypic changes of the miRNA mutant viruses may be due to the fact that the effects of miRNAs are often subtle or human neuron specific. These miRNAs are conserved in HSV; thus, they must play a biological role, although their individual effects may be small.

ICP0

HSV-1 ICP0 increases the levels of LAT in latently infected murine ganglia and thereby increases the levels of H3K27me3 facultative heterochromatin.[377] This phenotype was observed with an *ICP0* gene nonsense mutant virus, so the effect is likely to be due to the protein itself. The mechanism could be direct or indirect but raises the possibility that viral lytic proteins could also influence latency.

Assembly of Progeny Virus in Neurons

As described earlier, reactivation leads to expression of sufficient viral proteins and viral DNA replication to produce some progeny virions. These are ultimately released at the axonal termini to initiate the recurrent infection at the site of innervation of the nerve. The mechanisms of assembly of HSV progeny virions in neurons has been controversial, as there has been evidence of intact viral particles undergoing anterograde transport ("married" model) as well as evidence of independent transport of capsids and vesicles ("separate" model) containing the viral glycoproteins.[20,519] New components of the virion move by anterograde transport to both peripheral and central branches of the neuron. Virion assembly and/or release have been reported along the axon shaft and at the axon tip.[342] The question is how virions or virion components are transported by anterograde transport to these sites of virion release. Early studies of HSV infection of human fetal neurons followed by electron microscopy, immunoelectron microscopy, and immunofluorescence analyses concluded that capsids are transported independently from vesicles containing viral glycoproteins. Immunofluorescence and live cell imaging of human neuroblastoma cells infected with HSV also showed separate sites of staining or localization for glycoproteins relative to capsid proteins.[434] A further study using high-resolution electron microscopy has shown that 75% of the capsids in the axons of rat neurons were in virion particles.[328] More recent studies of "two-color" HSV recombinants expressing fluorescent capsid proteins and a fluorescent glycoprotein have continued to find different results, in that one study found that 64% to 70% of the capsids were associated with glycoproteins while undergoing anterograde transport,[20] although another found that 80% and 67% of the capsids in two neuronal systems were independent of glycoproteins.[519] Thus, there is the potential that either of two mechanisms of transport could occur to different extents in different neuronal cells under different conditions. Genetic studies have provided some insight in this area. One study has shown a defect in transport of envelope proteins, VP22 tegument, and VP5 capsid proteins into the optic nerve in mice infected with a glycoprotein E–negative virus, implying that axonal localization of certain glycoproteins and capsid and teguments may be linked.

Role of the Host Immune Response in Latency

While the role of the host immune response in controlling acute lytic infection is clear as is the role of cellular immunity in containing reactivation events, the extent to which the host immune response is a primary component that controls latency in the neuron itself has been intensively investigated and debated. The models positing immune control as a primary regulator of latency originate with observations that immune cells are found infiltrating latently infected ganglia in naturally infected human sensory ganglia and experimentally infected mice. It has been reported that antagonizing CD8$^+$ T cells and/or IFN-γ remaining within explanted murine trigeminal ganglia at 14 days postinfection promotes viral gene expression and reactivation.[280] However, CD8$^+$ T cells remaining within TGs explanted after 34 days, a time point more consistently associated with latency in the mouse model, were unable to block reactivation. Indeed, T cells resident in infected ganglia in mice and rabbits reportedly have an exhausted phenotype and exhibit reduced function.[14,201,441] Although some studies have attempted to correlate T-cell infiltrates with LAT-positive neurons, most LAT$^+$ neurons in latently infected mice sensory ganglia are devoid of detectable associated inflammatory cells and T cells were only observed clustered around spontaneously reactivating neurons.[170] Additional studies observed that CD8$^+$ T cells nonspecifically traffic into latently infected murine sensory ganglia, although only the HSV-specific CD8$^+$ T cells are activated and specifically retained in the ganglia. Moreover, in authentic human TG, the neurons that were surrounded by T cells were not detectably positive for LAT or HSV DNA.[170] Finally, latency can be established in immunodeficient mice lacking innate and adaptive immune systems. Taken together, these studies i) imply that the role of cellular immunity is one of surveillance and control once reactivation at the molecular level has commenced within the neuron and ii) are consistent with the existence of neuronal cell-intrinsic mechanisms that are primarily responsible for controlling the lytic/latent switch in the viral lifecycle within the host neuron. This includes neuronal and viral factors including LAT and microRNAs working in concert, whereas CD8$^+$ T cells are activated and retained in the ganglia in response to low-level expression of viral antigens.

To model how latently infected neurons might respond to antiviral cytokines produced by immune cells infiltrates within ganglia, latently infected cultured rat sympathetic neurons were exposed to extrinsic interferon. Type I and type II interferon both induced neuron-specific transcriptional responses that prevented reactivation phase 1.[279] Furthermore, sensitivity to interferon action was lost once phase 1 commenced and ICP0 expression prior to phase 1 could protect neurons from type II interferon action.[279] The surprising finding that IFN acts within a limited temporal window and is antagonized by a reactivation phase 1 viral protein exemplified by ICP0 implicates the viral products produced within phase 1 in the establishment of an IFN-resistant state that allows reactivating virus to proceed into active replication during reactivation phase 2.[279] Thus, in addition to allowing immediate production of VP16,[230] the reactivation phase 1 HSV genome-wide burst of expression enables production of numerous viral functions that subvert host defenses regardless of their classification as IE, E, or L genes. Moreover, it provides a potential mechanism for reactivation events initiating from latent HSV DNA genomes to access tegument functions, which are normally expressed as late genes and delivered in the context of infecting virions where they function at times that precede viral gene expression during acute infection.

The fate of the neurons after viral reactivation has been a topic of long debate. In support of survival of the neurons is that loss of sensory perception due to virus-induced sensory neuron loss is not a common sequela in patients suffering from frequent recurrences at the same site. A formal rebuttal of this argument is that nerve endings from adjacent unaffected neurons could grow into the healed area and reestablish a network. The second and more significant observation is that women with recurrent genital lesions shed virus in the interim between clinically manifest lesions. If each local lesion arises from a reactivated neuron, there would not be enough neurons to support viral reactivation over many years if the neurons die as a consequence of this process. The fate of the infected neuron may depend on the latent viral load and the strength of the inducing signal; thus, there may be a continuum of effects of reactivation on the host neuron. A recent study evaluating reactivation in mice in response to hyperthermic stress found that fragmented viral protein–positive neurons morphologically consistent with apoptotic bodies and containing cleaved caspase-3 were detected.[114] While evidence for direct T-cell–mediated antigen recognition was not detected, inhibition of viral DNA replication with acyclovir surprisingly blocked neuronal fragmentation. Thus, at least some neurons supporting HSV-1 reactivation following hyperthermia in mice do not survive this event, and acyclovir therapy can reduce fragmentation associated with hyperthermia-induced reactivation.

PERSPECTIVES

We have considerable knowledge of the mechanisms of viral replication in cells, and future studies on the role of human host factors and how the virus interacts with those human cell factors will be important for understanding the virus and our human cells. Powerful new methods for studying the structure and function of viral and host gene products will define the molecular basis for viral pathogenesis. Exciting new applications of neuronal cell culture and human stem cell culture technology are providing us with powerful new approaches to study the interaction of HSV with human neurons and organoids in culture. These will be important for the design of new antivirals that target latent infection as well as lytic infection. HSV infections have been associated with neurodegenerative diseases,[167] and a recent study of maternal immunization of female mice with an HSV vaccine was recently shown to prevent behavioral changes due to neonatal infection.[358a] These results further raise the potential for a direct role for HSV infection on long-term neurological disease and the potential for antiviral interventions. Detailed studies of the effects of HSV infection in the neuronal systems for lytic and latent infection may provide the mechanistic basis for this and other forms of viral neuropathogenesis.

REFERENCES

1. Abaitua F, Daikoku T, Crump CM, et al. A single mutation responsible for temperature-sensitive entry and assembly defects in the VP1-2 protein of herpes simplex virus. *J Virol* 2011;85(5):2024–2036.
2. Abaitua F, Hollinshead M, Bolstad M, et al. A Nuclear localization signal in herpesvirus protein VP1-2 is essential for infection via capsid routing to the nuclear pore. *J Virol* 2012;86(17):8998–9014.
3. Abaitua F, Souto RN, Browne H, et al. Characterization of the herpes simplex virus (HSV)-1 tegument protein VP1-2 during infection with the HSV temperature-sensitive mutant tsB7. *J Gen Virol* 2009;90(Pt 10):2353–2363.
4. Ablasser A, Bauernfeind F, Hartmann G, et al. RIG-I-dependent sensing of poly(dA:dT) through the induction of an RNA polymerase III-transcribed RNA intermediate. *Nat Immunol* 2009;10(10):1065–1072.
5. Ablasser A, Schmid-Burgk JL, Hemmerling I, et al. Cell intrinsic immunity spreads to bystander cells via the intercellular transfer of cGAMP. *Nature* 2013;503(7477):530–534.
6. Agelidis AM, Shukla D. Cell entry mechanisms of HSV: what we have learned in recent years. *Future Virol* 2015;10(10):1145–1154.
7. Aggarwal A, Miranda-Saksena M, Boadle RA, et al. Ultrastructural visualization of individual tegument protein dissociation during entry of herpes simplex virus 1 into human and rat dorsal root ganglion neurons. *J Virol* 2012;86(11):6123–6137.
8. Alandijany T. Host intrinsic and innate intracellular immunity during herpes simplex virus type 1 (HSV-1) infection. *Front Microbiol* 2019;10:2611.
9. Alandijany T, Roberts APE, Conn KL, et al. Distinct temporal roles for the promyelocytic leukaemia (PML) protein in the sequential regulation of intracellular host immunity to HSV-1 infection. *PLoS Pathog* 2018;14(1):e1006769.
10. Albecka A, Laine RF, Janssen AF, et al. HSV-1 glycoproteins are delivered to virus assembly sites through dynamin-dependent endocytosis. *Traffic* 2016;17(1):21–39.
11. Alexander DE, Leib DA. Xenophagy in herpes simplex virus replication and pathogenesis. *Autophagy* 2008;4(1):101–103.
12. Alfonso-Dunn R, Arbuckle JH, Vogel JL, et al. Inhibition of the super elongation complex suppresses herpes simplex virus immediate early gene expression, lytic infection, and reactivation from latency. *mBio* 2020;11(3):e01216.
13. Alfonso-Dunn R, Turner AW, Jean Beltran PM, et al. Transcriptional elongation of HSV immediate early genes by the super elongation complex drives lytic infection and reactivation from latency. *Cell Host Microbe* 2017;21(4):507–517.e5.
14. Allen SJ, Hamrah P, Gate D, et al. The role of LAT in increased CD8+ T cell exhaustion in trigeminal ganglia of mice latently infected with herpes simplex virus 1. *J Virol* 2011;85(9):4184–4197.
15. Almine JF, O'Hare CA, Dunphy G, et al. IFI16 and cGAS cooperate in the activation of STING during DNA sensing in human keratinocytes. *Nat Commun* 2017;8:14392.
16. Amelio AL, McAnany PK, Bloom DC. A chromatin insulator-like element in the herpes simplex virus type 1 latency-associated transcript region binds CCCTC-binding factor and displays enhancer-blocking and silencing activities. *J Virol* 2006;80(5):2358–2368.
17. Andersen LL, Mork N, Reinert LS, et al. Functional IRF3 deficiency in a patient with herpes simplex encephalitis. *J Exp Med* 2015;212(9):1371–1379.
18. Anderson F, Savulescu AF, Rudolph K, et al. Targeting of viral capsids to nuclear pores in a cell-free reconstitution system. *Traffic* 2014;15(11):1266–1281.
19. Antinone SE, Smith GA. Retrograde axon transport of herpes simplex virus and pseudorabies virus: a live-cell comparative analysis. *J Virol* 2010;84(3):1504–1512.
20. Antinone SE, Zaichick SV, Smith GA. Resolving the assembly state of herpes simplex virus during axon transport by live-cell imaging. *J Virol* 2010;84(24):13019–13030.
21. Arii J, Goto H, Suenaga T, et al. Non-muscle myosin IIA is a functional entry receptor for herpes simplex virus-1. *Nature* 2010;467(7317):859–862.
22. Arii J, Takeshima K, Maruzuru Y, et al. Roles of the interhexamer contact site for hexagonal lattice formation of the herpes simplex virus 1 nuclear egress complex in viral primary envelopment and replication. *J Virol* 2019;93(14):e00498.
23. Arii J, Uema M, Morimoto T, et al. Entry of herpes simplex virus 1 and other alphaherpesviruses via the paired immunoglobulin-like type 2 receptor alpha. *J Virol* 2009;83(9):4520–4527.
24. Arii J, Wang J, Morimoto T, et al. A single-amino-acid substitution in herpes simplex virus 1 envelope glycoprotein B at a site required for binding to the paired immunoglobulin-like type 2 receptor alpha (PILRalpha) abrogates PILRalpha-dependent viral entry and reduces pathogenesis. *J Virol* 2010;84(20):10773–10783.
25. Arii J, Watanabe M, Maeda F, et al. ESCRT-III mediates budding across the inner nuclear membrane and regulates its integrity. *Nat Commun* 2018;9(1):3379.
26. Atanasiu D, Cairns TM, Whitbeck JC, et al. Regulation of herpes simplex virus gB-induced cell-cell fusion by mutant forms of gH/gL in the absence of gD and cellular receptors. *mBio* 2013;4(2).
27. Atanasiu D, Saw WT, Cohen GH, et al. Cascade of events governing cell-cell fusion induced by herpes simplex virus glycoproteins gD, gH/gL, and gB. *J Virol* 2010;84(23):12292–12299.
28. Atanasiu D, Saw WT, Lazear E, et al. Using antibodies and mutants to localize the presumptive gH/gL binding site on herpes simplex virus gD. *J Virol* 2018;92(24).
29. Atanasiu D, Whitbeck JC, Cairns TM, et al. Bimolecular complementation reveals that glycoproteins gB and gH/gL of herpes simplex virus interact with each other during cell fusion. *Proc Natl Acad Sci U S A* 2007;104(47):18718–18723.
30. Atanasiu D, Whitbeck JC, de Leon MP, et al. Bimolecular complementation defines functional regions of herpes simplex virus gB that are involved with gH/gL as a necessary step leading to cell fusion. *J Virol* 2010;84(8):3825–3834.
31. Aubert M, Chen Z, Lang R, et al. The antiapoptotic herpes simplex virus glycoprotein J localizes to multiple cellular organelles and induces reactive oxygen species formation. *J Virol* 2008;82(2):617–629.
32. Baines JD. Herpes simplex virus capsid assembly and DNA packaging: a present and future antiviral drug target. *Trends Microbiol* 2011;19(12):606–613.
33. Barlow PN, Luisi B, Milner A, et al. Structure of the C3HC4 domain by 1H-nuclear magnetic resonance spectroscopy. A new structural class of zinc-finger. *J Mol Biol* 1994;237(2):201–211.
34. Barrozo ER, Nakayama S, Singh P, et al. Deletion of herpes simplex virus 1 microRNAs miR-H1 and miR-H6 impairs reactivation. *J Virol* 2020;94(15).
35. Bastian TW, Livingston CM, Weller SK, et al. Herpes simplex virus type 1 immediate-early protein ICP22 is required for VICE domain formation during productive viral infection. *J Virol* 2010;84:2384–2394.
36. Bauer DW, Huffman JB, Homa FL, et al. Herpes virus genome, the pressure is on. *J Am Chem Soc* 2013;135(30):11216–11221.
37. Becker Y, Asher Y, Weinberg-Zahlering E, et al. Defective herpes simplex virus DNA: circular and circular-linear molecules resembling rolling circles. *J Gen Virol* 1978;40(2):319–335.
38. Bello-Morales R, Lopez-Guerrero JA. Extracellular vesicles in herpes viral spread and immune evasion. *Front Microbiol* 2018;9:2572.
39. Bertke AS, Swanson SM, Chen J, et al. A5-positive primary sensory neurons are nonpermissive for productive infection with herpes simplex virus 1 in vitro. *J Virol* 2011;85(13):6669–6677.
40. Bhargava AK, Rothlauf PW, Krummenacher C. Herpes simplex virus glycoprotein D relocates nectin-1 from intercellular contacts. *Virology* 2016;499:267–277.
41. Bigalke JM, Heldwein EE. Structural basis of membrane budding by the nuclear egress complex of herpesviruses. *EMBO J* 2015;34(23):2921–2936.
42. Bigalke JM, Heldwein EE. Nuclear exodus: herpesviruses lead the way. *Annu Rev Virol* 2016;3(1):387–409.

43. Bigalke JM, Heuser T, Nicastro D, et al. Membrane deformation and scission by the HSV-1 nuclear egress complex. *Nat Commun* 2014;5:4131.
44. Bohannon KP, Jun Y, Gross SP, et al. Differential protein partitioning within the herpesvirus tegument and envelope underlies a complex and variable virion architecture. *Proc Natl Acad Sci U S A* 2013;110(17):E1613–E1620.
45. Boldogkoi Z, Szucs A, Balazs Z, et al. Transcriptomic study of herpes simplex virus type-1 using full-length sequencing techniques. *Sci Data* 2018;5:180266.
46. Booy FP, Newcomb WW, Trus BL, et al. Liquid-crystalline, phage-like packing of encapsidated DNA in herpes simplex virus. *Cell* 1991;64(5):1007–1015.
47. Boutell C, Cuchet-Lourenco D, Vanni E, et al. A viral ubiquitin ligase has substrate preferential SUMO targeted ubiquitin ligase activity that counteracts intrinsic antiviral defence. *PLoS Pathog* 2011;7(9):e1002245.
48. Boutell C, Everett RD. Regulation of alphaherpesvirus infections by the ICP0 family of proteins. *J Gen Virol* 2013;94(Pt 3):465–481.
49. Bowman JJ, Orlando JS, Davido DJ, et al. Transient expression of herpes simplex virus type 1 ICP22 represses viral promoter activity and complements the replication of an ICP22 null virus. *J Virol* 2009;83(17):8733–8743.
50. Bryant KF, Cox JC, Wang H, et al. Binding of herpes simplex virus-1 US11 to specific RNA sequences. *Nucleic Acids Res* 2005;33(19):6090–6100.
51. Bryant KF, Yan Z, Dreyfus DH, et al. Identification of a divalent metal cation binding site in herpes simplex virus 1 (HSV-1) ICP8 required for HSV replication. *J Virol* 2012;86(12):6825–6834.
52. Burgess HM, Mohr I. Defining the role of stress granules in innate immune suppression by the herpes simplex virus 1 endoribonuclease VHS. *J Virol* 2018;92(15).
53. Burrel S, Boutolleau D, Ryu D, et al. Ancient recombination events between human herpes simplex viruses. *Mol Biol Evol* 2017;34(7):1713–1721.
54. Cabral JM, Cushman C, Sodroski CN, Knipe DM. ATRX limits the accessibility of histone H3-occupied HSV genes during lytic infection. *PLoS Pathog*, in press.
55. Cabral JM, Oh HS, Knipe DM. ATRX promotes maintenance of herpes simplex virus heterochromatin during chromatin stress. *eLife* 2018;7:e40228.
56. Cai Z, Jitkaew S, Zhao J, et al. Plasma membrane translocation of trimerized MLKL protein is required for TNF-induced necroptosis. *Nat Cell Biol* 2014;16(1):55–65.
57. Cairns TM, Atanasiu D, Saw WT, et al. Localization of the interaction site of herpes simplex virus glycoprotein D (gD) on the membrane fusion regulator, gH/gL. *J Virol* 2020;94(20).
58. Cairns TM, Ditto NT, Atanasiu D, et al. Surface plasmon resonance reveals direct binding of herpes simplex virus glycoproteins gH/gL to gD and locates a gH/gL binding site on gD. *J Virol* 2019;93(15).
59. Cairns TM, Huang ZY, Gallagher JR, et al. Patient-specific neutralizing antibody responses to herpes simplex virus are attributed to epitopes on gD, gB, or both and can be type specific. *J Virol* 2015;89(18):9213–9231.
60. Camarena V, Kobayashi M, Kim JY, et al. Nature and duration of growth factor signaling through receptor tyrosine kinases regulates HSV-1 latency in neurons. *Cell Host Microbe* 2010;8(4):320–330.
61. Ceccaldi R, Rondinelli B, D'Andrea AD. Repair pathway choices and consequences at the double-strand break. *Trends Cell Biol* 2016;26(1):52–64.
62. Cerveny M, Hessefort S, Yang K, et al. Amino acid substitutions in the effector domain of the gamma(1)34.5 protein of herpes simplex virus 1 have differential effects on viral response to interferon-alpha. *Virology* 2003;307(2):290–300.
63. Challberg MD. A method for identifying the viral genes required for herpesvirus DNA replication. *Proc Natl Acad Sci U S A* 1986;83(23):9094–9098.
64. Chang L, Godinez WJ, Kim IH, et al. Herpesviral replication compartments move and coalesce at nuclear speckles to enhance export of viral late mRNA. *Proc Natl Acad Sci U S A* 2011;108(21):E136–E144.
65. Chang YE, Van Sant C, Krug PW, et al. The null mutant of the UL31 gene of herpes simplex virus 1: construction and phenotype in infected cells. *J Virol* 1997;71:8307–8315.
66. Chapman JR, Taylor MR, Boulton SJ. Playing the end game: DNA double-strand break repair pathway choice. *Mol Cell* 2012;47(4):497–510.
67. Chaurushiya MS, Lilley CE, Aslanian A, et al. Viral E3 ubiquitin ligase-mediated degradation of a cellular E3: viral mimicry of a cellular phosphorylation mark targets the RNF8 FHA domain. *Mol Cell* 2012;46(1):79–90.
68. Chen X, Li W, Ren J, et al. Translocation of mixed lineage kinase domain-like protein to plasma membrane leads to necrotic cell death. *Cell Res* 2014;24(1):105–121.
69. Chentoufi AA, Kritzer E, Tran MV, et al. The herpes simplex virus 1 latency-associated transcript promotes functional exhaustion of virus-specific CD8+ T cells in latently infected trigeminal ganglia: a novel immune evasion mechanism. *J Virol* 2011;85(17):9127–9138.
70. Cheshenko N, Pierce C, Herold BC. Herpes simplex viruses activate phospholipid scramblase to redistribute phosphatidylserines and Akt to the outer leaflet of the plasma membrane and promote viral entry. *PLoS Pathog* 2018;14(1):e1006766.
71. Cheshenko N, Trepanier JB, Stefanidou M, et al. HSV activates Akt to trigger calcium release and promote viral entry: novel candidate target for treatment and suppression. *FASEB J* 2013;27(7):2584–2599.
72. Chiang JJ, Sparrer KMJ, van Gent M, et al. Viral unmasking of cellular 5S rRNA pseudogene transcripts induces RIG-I-mediated immunity. *Nat Immunol* 2018;19(1):53–62.
73. Chiu YH, Macmillan JB, Chen ZJ. RNA polymerase III detects cytosolic DNA and induces type I interferons through the RIG-I pathway. *Cell* 2009;138(3):576–591.
74. Chou J, Kern ER, Whitley RJ, et al. Mapping of herpes simplex virus-1 neurovirulence to gamma 134.5, a gene nonessential for growth in culture. *Science* 1990;250(4985):1262–1266.
75. Chowdary TK, Cairns TM, Atanasiu D, et al. Crystal structure of the conserved herpesvirus fusion regulator complex gH-gL. *Nat Struct Mol Biol* 2010;17(7):882–888.
76. Christensen MH, Jensen SB, Miettinen JJ, et al. HSV-1 ICP27 targets the TBK1-activated STING signalsome to inhibit virus-induced type I IFN expression. *EMBO J* 2016;35(13):1385–1399.
77. Christofferson DE, Yuan J. Necroptosis as an alternative form of programmed cell death. *Curr Opin Cell Biol* 2010;22(2):263–268.
78. Chuluunbaatar U, Roller R, Feldman ME, et al. Constitutive mTORC1 activation by a herpesvirus Akt surrogate stimulates mRNA translation and viral replication. *Genes Dev* 2010;24(23):2627–2639.
79. Cliffe AR, Arbuckle JH, Vogel JL, et al. Neuronal stress pathway mediating a histone methyl/phospho switch is required for herpes simplex virus reactivation. *Cell Host Microbe* 2015;18(6):649–658.
80. Cliffe AR, Coen DM, Knipe DM. Kinetics of facultative heterochromatin and polycomb group protein association with the herpes simplex viral genome during establishment of latent infection. *mBio* 2013;4(1):e00590.
81. Cliffe AR, Garber DA, Knipe DM. Transcription of the herpes simplex virus latency-associated transcript promotes the formation of facultative heterochromatin on lytic promoters. *J Virol* 2009;83(16):8182–8190.
82. Cliffe AR, Knipe DM. Herpes simplex virus ICP0 promotes both histone removal and acetylation on viral DNA during lytic infection. *J Virol* 2008;82(24):12030–12038.
83. Cockrell SK, Huffman JB, Toropova K, et al. Residues of the UL25 protein of herpes simplex virus that are required for its stable interaction with capsids. *J Virol* 2011;85(10):4875–4887.
84. Colgrove R, Diaz F, Newman R, et al. Genomic sequences of a low passage herpes simplex virus 2 clinical isolate and its plaque-purified derivative strain. *Virology* 2014;450–451:140–145.
85. Connolly SA, Jackson JO, Jardetzky TS, et al. Fusing structure and function: a structural view of the herpesvirus entry machinery. *Nat Rev Microbiol* 2011;9(5):369–381.
86. Conway JE, Rhys CM, Zolotukhin I, et al. High-titer recombinant adeno-associated virus production utilizing a recombinant herpes simplex virus type I vector expressing AAV-2 Rep and Cap. *Gene Ther* 1999;6(6):986–993.
87. Conway JF, Homa FL. Nucleocapsid structure, assembly and DNA packaging of herpes simplex virus. In: Weller SK, ed. *Alphaherpesviruses: Molecular Virology*. Norfolk, UK: Caister Academic Press; 2011:175–193.
88. Conwell SE, White AE, Harper JW, et al. Identification of TRIM27 as a novel degradation target of herpes simplex virus 1 ICP0. *J Virol* 2015;89(1):220–229.
89. Cooper RS, Georgieva ER, Borbat PP, et al. Structural basis for membrane anchoring and fusion regulation of the herpes simplex virus fusogen gB. *Nat Struct Mol Biol* 2018;25(5):416–424.
90. Cooper RS, Heldwein EE. Herpesvirus gB: a finely tuned fusion machine. *Viruses* 2015;7(12):6552–6569.
91. Copeland AM, Newcomb WW, Brown JC. Herpes simplex virus replication: roles of viral proteins and nucleoporins in capsid-nucleus attachment. *J Virol* 2009;83(4):1660–1668.
92. Cotter CR, Kim WK, Nguyen ML, et al. The virion host shutoff protein of herpes simplex virus 1 blocks the replication-independent activation of NF-kappaB in dendritic cells in the absence of type I interferon signaling. *J Virol* 2011;85(23):12662–12672.
93. Crump C. Virus assembly and egress of HSV. *Adv Exp Med Biol* 2018;1045:23–44.
94. Cuchet-Lourenco D, Anderson G, Sloan E, et al. The viral ubiquitin ligase ICP0 is neither sufficient nor necessary for degradation of the cellular DNA sensor IFI16 during herpes simplex virus 1 infection. *J Virol* 2013;87(24):13422–13432.
95. Cuddy SR, Schinlever AR, Dochnal S, et al. Neuronal hyperexcitability is a DLK-dependent trigger of HSV-1 reactivation that can be induced by IL-1. *eLife* 2020;9:e58037.
96. D'Aiuto L, Bloom DC, Naciri JN, et al. Modeling herpes simplex virus 1 infections in human central nervous system neuronal cells using two- and three-dimensional cultures derived from induced pluripotent stem cells. *J Virol* 2019;93(9).
97. Da Costa XJ, Jones CA, Knipe DM. Immunization against genital herpes with a vaccine virus that has defects in productive and latent infection. *Proc Natl Acad Sci U S A* 1999;96(12):6994–6998.
98. Dai W, Jia Q, Bortz E, et al. Unique structures in a tumor herpesvirus revealed by cryo-electron tomography and microscopy. *J Struct Biol* 2008;161(3):428–438.
99. Dai X, Zhou ZH. Structure of the herpes simplex virus 1 capsid with associated tegument protein complexes. *Science* 2018;360(6384).
100. Dauber B, Pelletier J, Smiley JR. The herpes simplex virus 1 vhs protein enhances translation of viral true late mRNAs and virus production in a cell type-dependent manner. *J Virol* 2011;85(11):5363–5373.
101. Dauber B, Saffran HA, Smiley JR. The herpes simplex virus host shutoff (vhs) RNase limits accumulation of double stranded RNA in infected cells: Evidence for accelerated decay of duplex RNA. *PLoS Pathog* 2019;15(10):e1008111.
102. de Bruyn Kops A, Knipe DM. Formation of DNA replication structures in herpes virus-infected cells requires a viral DNA binding protein. *Cell* 1988;55(5):857–868.
103. Deiss LP, Chou J, Frenkel N. Functional domains within the a sequence involved in the cleavage-packaging of herpes simplex virus DNA. *J Virol* 1986;59:605–618.
104. DeLuca NA, McCarthy AM, Schaffer PA. Isolation and characterization of deletion mutants of herpes simplex virus type 1 in the gene encoding immediate-early regulatory protein ICP4. *J Virol* 1985;56(2):558–570.
105. Dembowski JA, DeLuca NA. Temporal viral genome-protein interactions define distinct stages of productive herpesviral infection. *mBio* 2018;9(4).
106. Desai P, Sexton GL, McCaffery JM, et al. A null mutation in the gene encoding the herpes simplex virus type 1 UL37 polypeptide abrogates virus maturation. *J Virol* 2001;75(21):10259–10271.
107. Desai PJ. A null mutation in the UL36 gene of herpes simplex virus type 1 results in accumulation of unenveloped DNA-filled capsids in the cytoplasm of infected cells. *J Virol* 2000;74(24):11608–11618.
108. Deshmane SL, Fraser NW. During latency, herpes simplex virus type 1 DNA is associated with nucleosomes in a chromatin structure. *J Virol* 1989;63(2):943–947.
109. Di Giovine P, Settembre EC, Bhargava AK, et al. Structure of herpes simplex virus glycoprotein D bound to the human receptor nectin-1. *PLoS Pathog* 2011;7(9):e1002277.
110. Diner BA, Lum KK, Javitt A, et al. Interactions of the antiviral factor interferon gamma-inducible protein 16 (IFI16) mediate immune signaling and herpes simplex virus-1 immunosuppression. *Mol Cell Proteomics* 2015;14(9):2341–2356.

111. Diner EJ, Burdette DL, Wilson SC, et al. The innate immune DNA sensor cGAS produces a noncanonical cyclic dinucleotide that activates human STING. *Cell Rep* 2013;3(5):1355–1361.
112. Dobrikova E, Shveygert M, Walters R, et al. Herpes simplex virus proteins ICP27 and UL47 associate with polyadenylate-binding protein and control its subcellular distribution. *J Virol* 2010;84(1):270–279.
113. Dolan A, Jamieson FE, Cunningham C, et al. The genome sequence of herpes simplex virus type 2. *J Virol* 1998;72(3):2010–2021.
114. Doll JR, Hoebe K, Thompson RL, et al. Resolution of herpes simplex virus reactivation in vivo results in neuronal destruction. *PLoS Pathog* 2020;16(3):e1008296.
115. Drane P, Ouararhni K, Depaux A, et al. The death-associated protein DAXX is a novel histone chaperone involved in the replication-independent deposition of H3.3. *Genes Dev* 2010;24(12):1253–1265.
116. Dremel SE, DeLuca NA. Genome replication affects transcription factor binding mediating the cascade of herpes simplex virus transcription. *Proc Natl Acad Sci U S A* 2019;116(9):3734–3739.
117. Du R, Wang L, Xu H, et al. A novel glycoprotein D-specific monoclonal antibody neutralizes herpes simplex virus. *Antiviral Res* 2017;147:131–141.
118. Du T, Han Z, Zhou G, et al. Patterns of accumulation of miRNAs encoded by herpes simplex virus during productive infection, latency, and on reactivation. *Proc Natl Acad Sci U S A* 2015;112(1):E49–E55.
119. Du T, Zhou G, Roizman B. HSV-1 gene expression from reactivated ganglia is disordered and concurrent with suppression of latency-associated transcript and miRNAs. *Proc Natl Acad Sci U S A* 2011;108(46):18820–18824.
120. Du T, Zhou G, Roizman B. Induction of apoptosis accelerates reactivation of latent HSV-1 in ganglionic organ cultures and replication in cell cultures. *Proc Natl Acad Sci U S A* 2012;109(36):14616–14621.
121. Dufour F, Sasseville AM, Chabaud S, et al. The ribonucleotide reductase R1 subunits of herpes simplex virus types 1 and 2 protect cells against TNFalpha- and FasL-induced apoptosis by interacting with caspase-8. *Apoptosis* 2011;16(3):256–271.
122. Durand LO, Roizman B. Role of cdk9 in the optimization of expression of the genes regulated by ICP22 of herpes simplex virus 1. *J Virol* 2008;82(21):10591–10599.
123. Eaton HE, Saffran HA, Wu FW, et al. Herpes simplex virus protein kinases US3 and UL13 modulate VP11/12 phosphorylation, virion packaging, and phosphatidylinositol 3-kinase/Akt signaling activity. *J Virol* 2014;88(13):7379–7388.
124. Edwards RG, Longnecker R. Herpesvirus entry mediator and ocular herpesvirus infection: more than meets the eye. *J Virol* 2017;91(13).
125. Edwards TG, Bloom DC. Lund human mesencephalic (LUHMES) neuronal cell line supports herpes simplex virus 1 latency in vitro. *J Virol* 2019;93(6).
126. Eisenberg RJ, Atanasiu D, Cairns TM, et al. Herpes virus fusion and entry: a story with many characters. *Viruses* 2012;4(5):800–832.
127. El Bilali N, Duron J, Gingras D, et al. Quantitative evaluation of protein heterogeneity within herpes simplex virus 1 particles. *J Virol* 2017;91(10).
128. Ellison KS, Maranchuk RA, Mottet KL, et al. Control of VP16 translation by the herpes simplex virus type 1 immediate-early protein ICP27. *J Virol* 2005;79(7):4120–4131.
129. Elsasser SJ, Noh KM, Diaz N, et al. Histone H3.3 is required for endogenous retroviral element silencing in embryonic stem cells. *Nature* 2015;522(7555):240–244.
130. Everett RD. Depletion of CoREST does not improve the replication of ICP0 null mutant herpes simplex virus type 1. *J Virol* 2010;84(7):3695–3698.
131. Everett RD. Dynamic response of IFI16 and promyelocytic leukemia nuclear body components to herpes simplex virus 1 infection. *J Virol* 2016;90(1):167–179.
132. Everett RD, Murray J. ND10 components relocate to sites associated with herpes simplex virus type 1 nucleoprotein complexes during virus infection. *J Virol* 2005;79(8):5078–5089.
133. Farnsworth A, Goldsmith K, Johnson DC. Herpes simplex virus glycoproteins gD and gE/gI serve essential but redundant functions during acquisition of the virion envelope in the cytoplasm. *J Virol* 2003;77(15):8481–8494.
134. Farnsworth A, Wisner TW, Webb M, et al. Herpes simplex virus glycoproteins gB and gH function in fusion between the virion envelope and the outer nuclear membrane. *Proc Natl Acad Sci U S A* 2007;104(24):10187–10192.
135. Ferenczy MW, Ranayhossaini DJ, Deluca NA. Activities of ICP0 involved in the reversal of silencing of quiescent herpes simplex virus 1. *J Virol* 2011;85(10):4993–5002.
136. Ferguson BJ, Mansur DS, Peters NE, et al. DNA-PK is a DNA sensor for IRF-3-dependent innate immunity. *eLife* 2012;1:e00047.
137. Finlan LE, Sproul D, Thomson I, et al. Recruitment to the nuclear periphery can alter expression of genes in human cells. *PLoS Genet* 2008;4:e1000039.
138. Finnen RL, Hay TJ, Dauber B, et al. The herpes simplex virus 2 virion-associated ribonuclease vhs interferes with stress granule formation. *J Virol* 2014;88(21):12727–12739.
139. Flores O, Nakayama S, Whisnant AW, et al. Mutational inactivation of herpes simplex virus 1 microRNAs identifies viral mRNA targets and reveals phenotypic effects in culture. *J Virol* 2013;87(12):6589–6603.
140. Fontaine-Rodriguez EC, Knipe DM. Herpes simplex virus ICP27 increases translation of a subset of viral late mRNAs. *J Virol* 2008;82(7):3538–3545.
141. Fox HL, Dembowski JA, DeLuca NA. A herpesviral immediate early protein promotes transcription elongation of viral transcripts. *mBio* 2017;8(3).
142. Gaglia MM, Covarrubias S, Wong W, et al. A common strategy for host RNA degradation by divergent viruses. *J Virol* 2012;86(17):9527–9530.
143. Gallagher JR, Saw WT, Atanasiu D, et al. Displacement of the C terminus of herpes simplex virus gD is sufficient to expose the fusion-activating interfaces on gD. *J Virol* 2013;87(23):12656–12666.
144. Galluzzi L, Pietrocola F, Levine B, et al. Metabolic control of autophagy. *Cell* 2014;159(6):1263–1276.
145. Garber DA, Schaffer PA, Knipe DM. A LAT-associated function reduces productive-cycle gene expression during acute infection of murine sensory neurons with herpes simplex virus type 1. *J Virol* 1997;71(8):5885–5893.
146. Gianni T, Amasio M, Campadelli-Fiume G. Herpes simplex virus gD forms distinct complexes with fusion executors gB and gH/gL in part through the C-terminal profusion domain. *J Biol Chem* 2009;284(26):17370–17382.
147. Gianni T, Campadelli-Fiume G. αVβ3-integrin relocalizes nectin1 and routes herpes simplex virus to lipid rafts. *J Virol* 2012;86(5):2850–2855.
148. Gianni T, Cerretani A, Dubois R, et al. Herpes simplex virus glycoproteins H/L bind to cells independently of {alpha}V{beta}3 integrin and inhibit virus entry, and their constitutive expression restricts infection. *J Virol* 2010;84(8):4013–4025.
149. Gianni T, Leoni V, Campadelli-Fiume G. Type I interferon and NF-kappaB activation elicited by herpes simplex virus gH/gL via alphavbeta3 integrin in epithelial and neuronal cell lines. *J Virol* 2013;87(24):13911–13916.
150. Gianni T, Salvioli S, Chesnokova LS, et al. alphavbeta6- and alphavbeta8-integrins serve as interchangeable receptors for HSV gH/gL to promote endocytosis and activation of membrane fusion. *PLoS Pathog* 2013;9(12):e1003806.
151. Gibson W, Roizman B. Proteins specified by herpes simplex virus. VIII. Characterization and composition of multiple capsid forms of subtypes 1 and 2. *J Virol* 1972;10:1044–1052.
152. Gibson W, Roizman B. The structural and metabolic involvement of polyamines with herpes simplex virus. In: Russell DH, ed. *Polyamines in Normal and Neoplastic Growth.* New York: Raven Press; 1973:123–135.
153. Giordani NV, Neumann DM, Kwiatkowski DL, et al. During herpes simplex virus type 1 infection of rabbits, the ability to express the latency-associated transcript increases latent-phase transcription of lytic genes. *J Virol* 2008;82(12):6056–6060.
154. Glass M, Everett RD. Components of promyelocytic leukemia nuclear bodies (ND10) act cooperatively to repress herpesvirus infection. *J Virol* 2013;87(4):2174–2185.
155. Godowski PJ, Knipe DM. Transcriptional control of herpesvirus gene expression: gene functions required for positive and negative regulation. *Proc Natl Acad Sci U S A* 1986;83(2):256–260.
156. Grady LM, Szczepaniak R, Murelli RP, et al. The exonuclease activity of herpes simplex virus 1 UL12 is required for production of viral DNA that can be packaged to produce infectious virus. *J Virol* 2017;91(23).
157. Gray NK, Hrabalkova L, Scanlon JP, et al. Poly(A)-binding proteins and mRNA localization: who rules the roost? *Biochem Soc Trans* 2015;43(6):1277–1284.
158. Gregory DA, Bachenheimer SL. Characterization of mre11 loss following HSV-1 infection. *Virology* 2008;373(1):124–136.
159. Grose C. Korean war and the origin of herpes simplex virus 1 strain KOS. *J Virol* 2014;88(7):3911.
160. Grunewald K, Desai P, Winkler DC, et al. Three-dimensional structure of herpes simplex virus from cryo-electron tomography. *Science* 2003;302(5649):1396–1398.
161. Guo H, Omoto S, Harris PA, et al. Herpes simplex virus suppresses necroptosis in human cells. *Cell Host Microbe* 2015;17(2):243–251.
162. Hafezi W, Lorentzen EU, Eing BR, et al. Entry of herpes simplex virus type 1 (HSV-1) into the distal axons of trigeminal neurons favors the onset of nonproductive, silent infection. *PLoS Pathog* 2012;8:e1002679.
163. Hagen C, Dent KC, Zeev-Ben-Mordehai T, et al. Structural basis of vesicle formation at the inner nuclear membrane. *Cell* 2015;163(7):1692–1701.
164. Hahn AS, Kaufmann JK, Wies E, et al. The ephrin receptor tyrosine kinase A2 is a cellular receptor for Kaposi's sarcoma-associated herpesvirus. *Nat Med* 2012;18(6):961–966.
165. Han Z, Liu X, Chen X, et al. miR-H28 and miR-H29 expressed late in productive infection are exported and restrict HSV-1 replication and spread in recipient cells. *Proc Natl Acad Sci U S A* 2016;113(7):E894–E901.
166. Hancock MH, Cliffe AR, Knipe DM, et al. Herpes simplex virus VP16, but not ICP0, is required to reduce histone occupancy and enhance histone acetylation on viral genomes in U2OS osteosarcoma cells. *J Virol* 2010;84(3):1366–1375.
167. Harris SA, Harris EA. Herpes simplex virus type 1 and other pathogens are key causative factors in sporadic Alzheimer's disease. *J Alzheimers Dis* 2015;48(2):319–353.
168. Harrison SC. Viral membrane fusion. *Virology* 2015;479–480:498–507.
169. Heilingloh CS, Krawczyk A. Role of L-particles during herpes simplex virus infection. *Front Microbiol* 2017;8:2565.
170. Held K, Junker A, Dornmair K, et al. Expression of herpes simplex virus 1-encoded microRNAs in human trigeminal ganglia and their relation to local T-cell infiltrates. *J Virol* 2011;85(19):9680–9685.
170a. Heldwein EE. Up close with herpesviruses. *Science* 2018;360(6384):34–35.
171. Heldwein EE, Lou H, Bender FC, et al. Crystal structure of glycoprotein B from herpes simplex virus 1. *Science* 2006;313(5784):217–220.
172. Henaff D, Radtke K, Lippe R. Herpesviruses exploit several host compartments for envelopment. *Traffic* 2012;13(11):1443–1449.
173. Herdy B, Jaramillo M, Svitkin YV, et al. Translational control of the activation of transcription factor NF-kappaB and production of type I interferon by phosphorylation of the translation factor eIF4E. *Nat Immunol* 2012;13(6):543–550.
174. Herman M, Ciancanelli M, Ou YH, et al. Heterozygous TBK1 mutations impair TLR3 immunity and underlie herpes simplex encephalitis of childhood. *J Exp Med* 2012;209(9):1567–1582.
175. Hernandez Duran A, Greco TM, Vollmer B, et al. Protein interactions and consensus clustering analysis uncover insights into herpesvirus virion structure and function relationships. *PLoS Biol* 2019;17(6):e3000316.
176. Herrera FJ, Triezenberg SJ. VP16-dependent association of chromatin-modifying coactivators and underrepresentation of histones at immediate-early gene promoters during herpes simplex virus infection. *J Virol* 2004;78(18):9689–9696.
177a. Hill JM, Garza Jr., HH, Helmy MF, et al. Nerve growth factor antibody stimulates reactivation of ocular herpes simplex virus type 1 in latently infected rabbits. *J Neurovirol* 1997;3:206–211.
177. Hertel L. Herpesviruses and intermediate filaments: close encounters with the third type. *Viruses* 2011;3(7):1015–1040.
178. Hill JM, Quenelle DC, Cardin RD, et al. Inhibition of LSD1 reduces herpesvirus infection, shedding, and recurrence by promoting epigenetic suppression of viral genomes. *Sci Transl Med* 2014;6(265):265ra169.
179. Hirohata Y, Kato A, Oyama M, et al. Interactome analysis of herpes simplex virus 1 envelope glycoprotein H. *Microbiol Immunol* 2015;59(6):331–337.
180. Hoa NN, Shimizu T, Zhou ZW, et al. Mre11 is essential for the removal of lethal topoisomerase 2 covalent cleavage complexes. *Mol Cell* 2016;64(3):580–592.

181. Hofemeister H, O'Hare P. Nuclear pore composition and gating in herpes simplex virus-infected cells. *J Virol* 2008;82(17):8392–8399.
182. Hogue IB, Bosse JB, Hu JR, et al. Cellular mechanisms of alpha herpesvirus egress: live cell fluorescence microscopy of pseudorabies virus exocytosis. *PLoS Pathog* 2014;10(12):e1004535.
183. Hogue IB, Scherer J, Enquist LW. Exocytosis of alphaherpesvirus virions, light particles, and glycoproteins uses constitutive secretory mechanisms. *mBio* 2016;7(3).
184. Hollinshead M, Johns HL, Sayers CL, et al. Endocytic tubules regulated by Rab GTPases 5 and 11 are used for envelopment of herpes simplex virus. *EMBO J* 2012;31(21):4204–4220.
185. Honess RW, Roizman B. Regulation of herpesvirus macromolecular synthesis. I. Cascade regulation of the synthesis of three groups of viral proteins. *J Virol* 1974;14(1):8–19.
186. Honess RW, Roizman B. Regulation of herpesvirus macromolecular synthesis: sequential transition of polypeptide synthesis requires functional viral polypeptides. *Proc Natl Acad Sci U S A* 1975;72(4):1276–1280.
187. Horan KA, Hansen K, Jakobsen MR, et al. Proteasomal degradation of herpes simplex virus capsids in macrophages releases DNA to the cytosol for recognition by DNA sensors. *J Immunol* 2013;190(5):2311–2319.
188. Horsburgh BC, Hubinette MM, Tufaro F. Genetic manipulation of herpes simplex virus using bacterial artificial chromosomes. *Methods Enzymol* 1999:306:337–352.
189. Hu H-L, Srinivas KP, Wang S, et al. manuscript in preparation.
190. Hu HL, Shiflett LA, Kobayashi M, et al. TOP2beta-dependent nuclear DNA damage shapes extracellular growth factor responses via dynamic AKT phosphorylation to control virus latency. *Mol Cell* 2019;74(3):466–480.e4.
191. Huang Z, Wu SQ, Liang Y, et al. RIP1/RIP3 binding to HSV-1 ICP6 initiates necroptosis to restrict virus propagation in mice. *Cell Host Microbe* 2015;17(2):229–242.
192. Huffman JB, Daniel GR, Falck-Pedersen E, et al. The C terminus of the herpes simplex virus UL25 protein is required for release of viral genomes from capsids bound to nuclear pores. *J Virol* 2017;91(15).
193. Huffmaster NJ, Sollars PJ, Richards AL, et al. Dynamic ubiquitination drives herpesvirus neuroinvasion. *Proc Natl Acad Sci U S A* 2015;112(41):12818–12823.
194. Imai Y, Apakupakul K, Krause PR, et al. Investigation of the mechanism by which herpes simplex virus type 1 LAT sequences modulate preferential establishment of latent infection in mouse trigeminal ganglia. *J Virol* 2009;83(16):7873–7882.
195. Ishov AM, Stenberg RM, Maul GG. Human cytomegalovirus immediate early interaction with host nuclear structures: definition of an immediate transcript environment. *J Cell Biol* 1997;138(1):5–16.
196. Jaber T, Henderson G, Li S, et al. Identification of a novel herpes simplex virus type 1 transcript and protein (AL3) expressed during latency. *J Gen Virol* 2009;90(Pt 10):2342–2352.
197. Jacob T, Van den Broeke C, van Troys M, et al. Alphaherpesviral US3 kinase induces cofilin dephosphorylation to reorganize the actin cytoskeleton. *J Virol* 2013;87(7):4121–4126.
198. Jambunathan N, Chowdhury S, Subramanian R, et al. Site-specific proteolytic cleavage of the amino terminus of herpes simplex virus glycoprotein K on virion particles inhibits virus entry. *J Virol* 2011;85(24):12910–12918.
199. Jan E, Mohr I, Walsh D. A cap-to-tail guide to mRNA translation strategies in virus-infected cells. *Annu Rev Virol* 2016;3(1):283–307.
200. Jean S, LeVan KM, Song B, et al. Herpes simplex virus 1 ICP27 is required for transcription of two viral late (gamma 2) genes in infected cells. *Virology* 2001;283(2):273–284.
201. Jeon S, St Leger AJ, Cherpes TL, et al. PD-L1/B7-H1 regulates the survival but not the function of CD8+ T cells in herpes simplex virus type 1 latently infected trigeminal ganglia. *J Immunol* 2013;190(12):6277–6286.
202. Jiang X, Chentoufi AA, Hsiang C, et al. The herpes simplex virus type 1 latency-associated transcript can protect neuron-derived C1300 and Neuro2A cells from granzyme B-induced apoptosis and CD8 T-cell killing. *J Virol* 2011;85(5):2325–2332.
203. Jin T, Perry A, Jiang J, et al. Structures of the HIN domain:DNA complexes reveal ligand binding and activation mechanisms of the AIM2 inflammasome and IFI16 receptor. *Immunity* 2012;36(4):561–571.
204. Johns HL, Gonzalez-Lopez C, Sayers CL, et al. Rab6 dependent post-Golgi trafficking of HSV1 envelope proteins to sites of virus envelopment. *Traffic* 2014;15(2): 157–178.
205. Johnson DC, Baines JD. Herpesviruses remodel host membranes for virus egress. *Nat Rev Microbiol* 2011;9(5):382–394.
206. Johnson DC, Huber MT. Directed egress of animal viruses promotes cell-to-cell spread. *J Virol* 2002;76(1):1–8.
207. Johnson KE, Bottero V, Flaherty S, et al. IFI16 restricts HSV-1 replication by accumulating on the hsv-1 genome, repressing HSV-1 gene expression, and directly or indirectly modulating histone modifications. *PLoS Pathog* 2014;10(11):e1004503.
208. Johnson KE, Knipe DM. Herpes simplex virus-1 infection causes the secretion of a type I interferon-antagonizing protein and inhibits signaling at or before Jak-1 activation. *Virology* 2010;396(1):21–29.
209. Johnson LA, Sandri-Goldin RM. Efficient nuclear export of herpes simplex virus 1 transcripts requires both RNA binding by ICP27 and ICP27 interaction with TAP/NXF1. *J Virol* 2009;83(3):1184–1192.
210. Johnston C, Magaret A, Roychoudhury P, et al. Highly conserved intragenic HSV-2 sequences: results from next-generation sequencing of HSV-2 UL and US regions from genital swabs collected from 3 continents. *Virology* 2017;510:90–98.
211. Jovasevic V, Liang L, Roizman B. Proteolytic cleavage of VP1-2 is required for release of herpes simplex virus 1 DNA into the nucleus. *J Virol* 2008;82:3311–3319.
212. Jovasevic V, Naghavi MH, Walsh D. Microtubule plus end-associated CLIP-170 initiates HSV-1 retrograde transport in primary human cells. *J Cell Biol* 2015;211(2):323–337.
213. Jurak I, Kramer MF, Mellor JC, et al. Numerous conserved and divergent microRNAs expressed by herpes simplex viruses 1 and 2. *J Virol* 2010;84(9):4659–4672.
214. Jurak I, Silverstein LB, Sharma M, et al. Herpes simplex virus is equipped with RNA- and protein-based mechanisms to repress expression of ATRX, an effector of intrinsic immunity. *J Virol* 2012;86(18):10093–10102.
215. Kabanova A, Marcandalli J, Zhou T, et al. Platelet-derived growth factor-alpha receptor is the cellular receptor for human cytomegalovirus gHgLgO trimer. *Nat Microbiol* 2016;1(8):16082.
216. Kadlec J, Loureiro S, Abrescia NG, et al. The postfusion structure of baculovirus gp64 supports a unified view of viral fusion machines. *Nat Struct Mol Biol* 2008;15(10):1024–1030.
217. Kagan JC, Magupalli VG, Wu H. SMOCs: supramolecular organizing centres that control innate immunity. *Nat Rev Immunol* 2014;14(12):821–826.
218. Kalamvoki M, Deschamps T. Extracellular vesicles during herpes simplex virus type 1 infection: an inquire. *Virol J* 2016;13:63.
219. Kalamvoki M, Du T, Roizman B. Cells infected with herpes simplex virus 1 export to uninfected cells exosomes containing STING, viral mRNAs, and microRNAs. *Proc Natl Acad Sci U S A* 2014;111(46):E4991–E4996.
220. Kalamvoki M, Roizman B. The histone acetyltransferase CLOCK is an essential component of the herpes simplex virus 1 transcriptome that includes TFIID, ICP4, ICP27, and ICP22. *J Virol* 2011;85(18):9472–9477.
221. Karagoz GE, Acosta-Alvear D, Walter P. The unfolded protein response: detecting and responding to fluctuations in the protein-folding capacity of the endoplasmic reticulum. *Cold Spring Harb Perspect Biol* 2019;11(9).
222. Karasneh GA, Shukla D. Herpes simplex virus infects most cell types in vitro: clues to its success. *Virol J* 2011;8:481.
223. Karttunen H, Savas JN, McKinney C, et al. Co-opting the Fanconi anemia genomic stability pathway enables herpesvirus DNA synthesis and productive growth. *Mol Cell* 2014;55(1):111–122.
224. Kent JR, Zeng PY, Atanasiu D, et al. During lytic infection herpes simplex virus type 1 is associated with histones bearing modifications that correlate with active transcription. *J Virol* 2004;78(18):10178–10186.
225. Kew C, Lui PY, Chan CP, et al. Suppression of PACT-induced type I interferon production by herpes simplex virus 1 Us11 protein. *J Virol* 2013;87(24):13141–13149.
226. Kharkwal H, Smith CG, Wilson DW. Blocking ESCRT-mediated envelopment inhibits microtubule-dependent trafficking of alphaherpesviruses in vitro. *J Virol* 2014;88(24):14467–14478.
227. Kharkwal H, Smith CG, Wilson DW. Herpes simplex virus capsid localization to ESCRT-VPS4 complexes in the presence and absence of the large tegument protein UL36p. *J Virol* 2016;90(16):7257–7267.
228. Khoo D, Perez C, Mohr I. Characterization of RNA determinants recognized by the arginine- and proline-rich region of Us11, a herpes simplex virus type 1-encoded double-stranded RNA binding protein that prevents PKR activation. *J Virol* 2002;76(23):11971–11981.
229. Kim J, Guan KL. mTOR as a central hub of nutrient signalling and cell growth. *Nat Cell Biol* 2019;21(1):63–71.
230. Kim JY, Mandarino A, Chao MV, et al. Transient reversal of episome silencing precedes VP16-dependent transcription during reactivation of latent HSV-1 in neurons. *PLoS Pathog* 2012;8(2):e1002540.
231. Kim YM, Brinkmann MM, Paquet ME, et al. UNC93B1 delivers nucleotide-sensing toll-like receptors to endolysosomes. *Nature* 2008;452(7184):234–238.
232. Klupp B, Altenschmidt J, Granzow H, et al. Glycoproteins required for entry are not necessary for egress of pseudorabies virus. *J Virol* 2008;82(13):6299–6309.
233. Klupp BG, Granzow H, Fuchs W, et al. Vesicle formation from the nuclear membrane is induced by coexpression of two conserved herpesvirus proteins. *Proc Natl Acad Sci U S A* 2007;104(17):7241–7246.
234. Knipe DM. Nuclear sensing of viral DNA, epigenetic regulation of herpes simplex virus infection, and innate immunity. *Virology* 2015;479–480:153–159.
235. Knipe DM, Batterson W, Nosal C, et al. Molecular genetics of herpes simplex virus. VI. Characterization of a temperature-sensitive mutant defective in the expression of all early viral gene products. *J Virol* 1981;38(2):539–547.
236. Knipe DM, Cliffe A. Chromatin control of herpes simplex virus lytic and latent infection. *Nat Rev Microbiol* 2008;6(3):211–221.
237. Knipe DM, Lieberman PM, Jung JU, et al. Snapshots: chromatin control of viral infection. *Virology* 2013;435(1):141–156.
238. Knipe DM, Ruyechan WT, Roizman B, et al. Molecular genetics of herpes simplex virus: demonstration of regions of obligatory and nonobligatory identity within diploid regions of the genome by sequence replacement and insertion. *Proc Natl Acad Sci U S A* 1978;75(8):3896–3900.
239. Kobayashi M, Kim JY, Camarena V, et al. A primary neuron culture system for the study of herpes simplex virus latency and reactivation. *J Vis Exp* 2012(62):3823.
240. Kobayashi M, Wilson AC, Chao MV, et al. Control of viral latency in neurons by axonal mTOR signaling and the 4E-BP translation repressor. *Genes Dev* 2012;26(14):1527–1532.
241. Koelle DM, Norberg P, Fitzgibbon MP, et al. Worldwide circulation of HSV-2 x HSV-1 recombinant strains. *Sci Rep* 2017;7:44084.
242. Komala Sari T, Pritchard SM, Cunha CW, et al. Contributions of herpes simplex virus 1 envelope proteins to entry by endocytosis. *J Virol* 2013;87(24):13922–13926.
243. Kopp SJ, Banisadr G, Glajch K, et al. Infection of neurons and encephalitis after intracranial inoculation of herpes simplex virus requires the entry receptor nectin-1. *Proc Natl Acad Sci U S A* 2009;106(42):17916–17920.
244. Koyuncu OO, MacGibeny MA, Hogue IB, et al. Compartmented neuronal cultures reveal two distinct mechanisms for alpha herpesvirus escape from genome silencing. *PLoS Pathog* 2017;13(10):e1006608.
245. Koyuncu OO, Song R, Greco TM, et al. The number of alphaherpesvirus particles infecting axons and the axonal protein repertoire determines the outcome of neuronal infection. *mBio* 2015;6(2).
246. Kramer MF, Coen DM. Quantification of transcripts from the ICP4 and thymidine kinase genes in mouse ganglia latently infected with herpes simplex virus. *J Virol* 1995;69(3):1389–1399.
247. Kramer MF, Cook WJ, Roth FP, et al. Latent herpes simplex virus infection of sensory neurons alters neuronal gene expression. *J Virol* 2003;77(17):9533–9541.
248. Kramer MF, Jurak I, Pesola JM, et al. Herpes simplex virus 1 microRNAs expressed abundantly during latent infection are not essential for latency in mouse trigeminal ganglia. *Virology* 2011;417(2):239–247.
249. Kristie TM, Liang Y, Vogel JL. Control of alpha-herpesvirus IE gene expression by HCF-1 coupled chromatin modification activities. *Biochim Biophys Acta* 2010;1799(3–4):257–265.

250. Kristie TM, Vogel JL, Sears AE. Nuclear localization of the C1 factor (host cell factor) in sensory neurons correlates with reactivation of herpes simplex virus from latency. *Proc Natl Acad Sci U S A* 1999;96(4):1229–1233.
251. Krummenacher C, Supekar VM, Whitbeck JC, et al. Structure of unliganded HSV gD reveals a mechanism for receptor-mediated activation of virus entry. *EMBO J* 2005;24(23):4144–4153.
252. Kuhn J, Leege T, Klupp BG, et al. Partial functional complementation of a pseudorabies virus UL25 deletion mutant by herpes simplex virus type 1 pUL25 indicates overlapping functions of alphaherpesvirus pUL25 proteins. *J Virol* 2008;82(12):5725–5734.
253. Kurt-Jones EA, Orzalli MH, Knipe DM. Innate immune mechanisms and herpes simplex virus infection and disease. *Adv Anat Embryol Cell Biol* 2017;223:49–75.
254. Kutluay SB, DeVos SL, Klomp JE, et al. Transcriptional coactivators are not required for herpes simplex virus type 1 immediate-early gene expression in vitro. *J Virol* 2009;83(8):3436–3449.
255. Kwiatkowski DL, Thompson HW, Bloom DC. The polycomb group protein Bmi1 binds to the herpes simplex virus 1 latent genome and maintains repressive histone marks during latency. *J Virol* 2009;83(16):8173–8181.
256. Lacasse JJ, Schang LM. During lytic infections, herpes simplex virus type 1 DNA is in complexes with the properties of unstable nucleosomes. *J Virol* 2010;84(4):1920–1933.
257. Lacasse JJ, Schang LM. Herpes simplex virus 1 DNA is in unstable nucleosomes throughout the lytic infection cycle, and the instability of the nucleosomes is independent of DNA replication. *J Virol* 2012;86(20):11287–11300.
258. Lamb CA, Yoshimori T, Tooze SA. The autophagosome: origins unknown, biogenesis complex. *Nat Rev Mol Cell Biol* 2013;14(12):759–774.
259. Lamers SL, Newman RM, Laeyendecker O, et al. Global diversity within and between human herpesvirus 1 and 2 glycoproteins. *J Virol* 2015;89(16):8206–8218.
260. Lawler JL, Mukherjee P, Coen DM. Herpes simplex virus 1 DNA polymerase RNase H activity acts in a 3′-to-5′ direction and is dependent on the 3′-to-5′ exonuclease active site. *J Virol* 2018;92(5).
261. Lazear E, Carfi A, Whitbeck JC, et al. Engineered disulfide bonds in herpes simplex virus type 1 gD separate receptor binding from fusion initiation and viral entry. *J Virol* 2008;82(2):700–709.
262. Lazear E, Whitbeck JC, Ponce-de-Leon M, et al. Antibody-induced conformational changes in herpes simplex virus glycoprotein gD reveal new targets for virus neutralization. *J Virol* 2012;86(3):1563–1576.
263. Lee CC, Lin LL, Chan WE, et al. Structural basis for the antibody neutralization of herpes simplex virus. *Acta Crystallogr D Biol Crystallogr* 2013;69(Pt 10):1935–1945.
264. Lee JS, Raja P, Knipe DM. Herpesviral ICP0 protein promotes two waves of heterochromatin removal on an early viral promoter during lytic infection. *mBio* 2016;7(1):e02007.
265. Lee JS, Raja P, Pan D, et al. CCCTC-binding factor acts as a heterochromatin barrier on herpes simplex viral latent chromatin and contributes to poised latent infection. *mBio* 2018;9(1):e02372.
266. Leege T, Granzow H, Fuchs W, et al. Phenotypic similarities and differences between UL37-deleted pseudorabies virus and herpes simplex virus type 1. *J Gen Virol* 2009;90(Pt 7):1560–1568.
267. Leib DA, Coen DM, Bogard CL, et al. Immediate-early regulatory gene mutants define different stages in the establishment and reactivation of herpes simplex virus latency. *J Virol* 1989;63(2):759–768.
268. Lester JT, DeLuca NA. Herpes simplex virus 1 ICP4 forms complexes with TFIID and mediator in virus-infected cells. *J Virol* 2011;85(12):5733–5744.
269. Lewis PW, Elsaesser SJ, Noh KM, et al. Daxx is an H3.3-specific histone chaperone and cooperates with ATRX in replication-independent chromatin assembly at telomeres. *Proc Natl Acad Sci U S A* 2010;107(32):14075–14080.
270. Li T, Diner BA, Chen J, et al. Acetylation modulates cellular distribution and DNA sensing ability of interferon-inducible protein IFI16. *Proc Natl Acad Sci U S A* 2012;109(26):10558–10563.
271. Li XD, Wu J, Gao D, et al. Pivotal roles of cGAS-cGAMP signaling in antiviral defense and immune adjuvant effects. *Science* 2013;341(6152):1390–1394.
272. Li Y, Zhang C, Chen X, et al. ICP34.5 protein of herpes simplex virus facilitates the initiation of protein translation by bridging eukaryotic initiation factor 2alpha (eIF2alpha) and protein phosphatase 1. *J Biol Chem* 2011;286(28):24785–24792.
273. Liang Y, Quenelle D, Vogel JL, et al. A novel selective LSD1/KDM1A inhibitor epigenetically blocks herpes simplex virus lytic replication and reactivation from latency. *mBio* 2013;4(1):e00558.
274. Liang Y, Vogel JL, Narayanan A, et al. Inhibition of the histone demethylase LSD1 blocks alpha-herpesvirus lytic replication and reactivation from latency. *Nat Med* 2009;15(11):1312–1317.
275. Lilley CE, Carson CT, Muotri AR, et al. DNA repair proteins affect the lifecycle of herpes simplex virus 1. *Proc Natl Acad Sci U S A* 2005;102(16):5844–5849.
276. Lilley CE, Chaurushiya MS, Boutell C, et al. The intrinsic antiviral defense to incoming HSV-1 genomes includes specific DNA repair proteins and is counteracted by the viral protein ICP0. *PLoS Pathog* 2011;7(6):e1002084.
277. Lilley CE, Chaurushiya MS, Boutell C, et al. A viral E3 ligase targets RNF8 and RNF168 to control histone ubiquitination and DNA damage responses. *EMBO J* 2010;29(5):943–955.
278. Lim HK, Seppanen M, Hautala T, et al. TLR3 deficiency in herpes simplex encephalitis: high allelic heterogeneity and recurrence risk. *Neurology* 2014;83(21):1888–1897.
279. Linderman JA, Kobayashi M, Rayannavar V, et al. Immune escape via a transient gene expression program enables productive replication of a latent pathogen. *Cell Rep* 2017;18(5):1312–1323.
280. Liu T, Khanna KM, Chen X, et al. CD8(+) T cells can block herpes simplex virus type 1 (HSV-1) reactivation from latency in sensory neurons. *J Exp Med* 2000;191(9):1459–1466.
281. Liu X, Fitzgerald K, Kurt-Jones E, et al. Herpesvirus tegument protein activates NF-kappaB signaling through the TRAF6 adaptor protein. *Proc Natl Acad Sci U S A* 2008;105(32):11335–11339.
282. Liu X, Matrenec R, Gack MU, et al. Disassembly of the TRIM23-TBK1 complex by the Us11 protein of herpes simplex virus 1 impairs autophagy. *J Virol* 2019;93(17).
283. Liu Y, Goulet ML, Sze A, et al. RIG-I-mediated STING upregulation restricts herpes simplex virus 1 infection. *J Virol* 2016;90(20):9406–9419.
284. Lomonte P. The interaction between herpes simplex virus 1 genome and promyelocytic leukemia nuclear bodies (PML-NBs) as a hallmark of the entry in latency. *Microb Cell* 2016;3(11):569–572.
285. Lorenz M, Vollmer B, Unsay JD, et al. A single herpesvirus protein can mediate vesicle formation in the nuclear envelope. *J Biol Chem* 2015;290(11):6962–6974.
286. Loret S, Guay G, Lippe R. Comprehensive characterization of extracellular herpes simplex virus type 1 virions. *J Virol* 2008;82(17):8605–8618.
287. Lovejoy CA, Li W, Reisenweber S, et al. Loss of ATRX, genome instability, and an altered DNA damage response are hallmarks of the alternative lengthening of telomeres pathway. *PLoS Genet* 2012;8(7):e1002772.
288. Lu G, Zhang N, Qi J, et al. Crystal structure of herpes simplex virus 2 gD bound to nectin-1 reveals a conserved mode of receptor recognition. *J Virol* 2014;88(23):13678–13688.
289. Luecke S, Paludan SR. Innate recognition of alphaherpesvirus DNA. *Adv Virus Res* 2015;92:63–100.
290. Lukashchuk V, Everett RD. Regulation of ICP0-null mutant herpes simplex virus type 1 infection by ND10 components ATRX and hDaxx. *J Virol* 2010;84(8):4026–4040.
291. Lussignol M, Queval C, Bernet-Camard MF, et al. The herpes simplex virus 1 Us11 protein inhibits autophagy through its interaction with the protein kinase PKR. *J Virol* 2013;87(2):859–871.
292. Lv Y, Zhou S, Gao S, et al. Remodeling of host membranes during herpesvirus assembly and egress. *Protein Cell* 2019;10(5):315–326.
293. Lycke E, Hamark B, Johansson M, et al. Herpes simplex virus infection of the human sensory neuron. An electron microscopy study. *Arch Virol* 1988;101(1–2):87–104.
294. Lye MF, Sharma M, El Omari K, et al. Unexpected features and mechanism of heterodimer formation of a herpesvirus nuclear egress complex. *EMBO J* 2015;34(23):2937–2952.
295. Ma JZ, Russell TA, Spelman T, et al. Lytic gene expression is frequent in HSV-1 latent infection and correlates with the engagement of a cell-intrinsic transcriptional response. *PLoS Pathog* 2014;10(7):e1004237.
296. Madabhushi R, Gao F, Pfenning AR, et al. Activity-induced DNA breaks govern the expression of neuronal early-response genes. *Cell* 2015;161(7):1592–1605.
297. Madabhushi R, Kim TK. Emerging themes in neuronal activity-dependent gene expression. *Mol Cell Neurosci* 2018;87:27–34.
298. Maier O, Sollars PJ, Pickard GE, et al. Visualizing herpesvirus procapsids in living cells. *J Virol* 2016;90(22):10182–10192.
299. Malhas AN, Lee CF, Vaux DJ. Lamin B1 controls oxidative stress responses via Oct-1. *J Cell Biol* 2009;184(1):45–55.
300. Manivanh R, Mehrbach J, Knipe DM, et al. Role of herpes simplex virus 1 gamma34.5 in the regulation of IRF3 signaling. *J Virol* 2017;91(23).
301. Marino-Merlo F, Papaianni E, Medici MA, et al. HSV-1-induced activation of NF-kappaB protects U937 monocytic cells against both virus replication and apoptosis. *Cell Death Dis* 2016;7(9):e2354.
302. Maroui MA, Calle A, Cohen C, et al. Latency entry of herpes simplex virus 1 is determined by the interaction of its genome with the nuclear environment. *PLoS Pathog* 2016;12(9):e1005834.
303. Martinez-Martin N, Marcandalli J, Huang CS, et al. An unbiased screen for human cytomegalovirus identifies neuropilin-2 as a central viral receptor. *Cell* 2018;174(5):1158–1171.e19.
304. Maruzuru Y, Ichinohe T, Sato R, et al. Herpes simplex virus 1 VP22 inhibits AIM2-dependent inflammasome activation to enable efficient viral replication. *Cell Host Microbe* 2018;23(2):254–265.e7.
305. Mattila RK, Harila K, Kangas SM, et al. An investigation of herpes simplex virus type 1 latency in a novel mouse dorsal root ganglion model suggests a role for ICP34.5 in reactivation. *J Gen Virol* 2015;96(8):2304–2313.
306. Maurer UE, Sodeik B, Grunewald K. Native 3D intermediates of membrane fusion in herpes simplex virus 1 entry. *Proc Natl Acad Sci U S A* 2008;105(30):10559–10564.
307. McElwee M, Beilstein F, Labetoulle M, et al. Dystonin/BPAG1 promotes plus-end-directed transport of herpes simplex virus 1 capsids on microtubules during entry. *J Virol* 2013;87(20):11008–11018.
308. McElwee M, Vijayakrishnan S, Rixon F, et al. Structure of the herpes simplex virus portal-vertex. *PLoS Biol* 2018;16(6):e2006191.
309. McGeoch DJ, Dalrymple MA, Davison AJ, et al. The complete DNA sequence of the long unique region in the genome of herpes simplex virus type 1. *J Gen Virol* 1988;69:1531–1574.
310. McSwiggen DT, Hansen AS, Teves SS, et al. Evidence for DNA-mediated nuclear compartmentalization distinct from phase separation. *eLife* 2019;8:e47098.
311. Melroe GT, Silva L, Schaffer PA, et al. Recruitment of activated IRF-3 and CBP/p300 to herpes simplex virus ICP0 nuclear foci: potential role in blocking IFN-beta induction. *Virology* 2007;360(2):305–321.
312. Merkl PE, Knipe DM. Role for a filamentous nuclear assembly of IFI16, DNA, and host factors in restriction of herpesviral infection. *mBio* 2019;10(1).
313. Merkl PE, Orzalli MH, Knipe DM. Mechanisms of host IFI16, PML, and Daxx protein restriction of herpes simplex virus 1 replication. *J Virol* 2018;92(10).
314. Mertens M, Knipe DM. Herpes simplex virus 1 manipulates host cell anti-viral and pro-viral DNA damage responses. *mBio* 2021;12:e03552–20.
315. Miranda-Saksena M, Denes CE, Diefenbach RJ, et al. Infection and transport of herpes simplex virus type 1 in neurons: role of the cytoskeleton. *Viruses* 2018;10(2).
316. Mocarski ES, Guo H, Kaiser WJ. Necroptosis: the Trojan horse in cell autonomous antiviral host defense. *Virology* 2015;479–480:160–166.
317. Mocarski ES, Upton JW, Kaiser WJ. Viral infection and the evolution of caspase 8-regulated apoptotic and necrotic death pathways. *Nat Rev Immunol* 2011;12(2):79–88.

318. Mohni KN, Livingston CM, Cortez D, et al. ATR and ATRIP are recruited to herpes simplex virus type 1 replication compartments even though ATR signaling is disabled. *J Virol* 2010;84(23):12152–12164.
319. Mohni KN, Mastrocola AS, Bai P, et al. DNA mismatch repair proteins are required for efficient herpes simplex virus 1 replication. *J Virol* 2011;85(23):12241–12253.
320. Mostafa HH, Davido DJ. Herpes simplex virus 1 ICP22 but not US 1.5 is required for efficient acute replication in mice and VICE domain formation. *J Virol* 2013;87(24):13510–13519.
321. Mou F, Wills E, Baines JD. Phosphorylation of the U(L)31 protein of herpes simplex virus 1 by the U(S)3-encoded kinase regulates localization of the nuclear envelopment complex and egress of nucleocapsids. *J Virol* 2009;83(10):5181–5191.
322. Mulvey M, Arias C, Mohr I. Maintenance of endoplasmic reticulum (ER) homeostasis in herpes simplex virus type 1-infected cells through the association of a viral glycoprotein with PERK, a cellular ER stress sensor. *J Virol* 2007;81(7):3377–3390.
323. Mulvey M, Camarena V, Mohr I. Full resistance of herpes simplex virus type 1-infected primary human cells to alpha interferon requires both the Us11 and gamma(1)34.5 gene products. *J Virol* 2004;78:10193–10196.
324. Munger J, Roizman B. The US3 protein kinase of herpes simplex virus 1 mediates the posttranslational modification of BAD and prevents BAD-induced programmed cell death in the absence of other viral proteins. *Proc Natl Acad Sci U S A* 2001;98(18):10410–10415.
325. Musarrat F, Jambunathan N, Rider PJF, et al. The amino terminus of herpes simplex virus 1 Glycoprotein K (gK) is required for gB binding to Akt, release of intracellular calcium, and fusion of the viral envelope with plasma membranes. *J Virol* 2018;92(6).
326. Nadal M, Mas PJ, Blanco AG, et al. Structure and inhibition of herpesvirus DNA packaging terminase nuclease domain. *Proc Natl Acad Sci U S A* 2010;107(37):16078–16083.
327. Nagata S. Apoptosis and clearance of apoptotic cells. *Annu Rev Immunol* 2018;36:489–517.
328. Negatsch A, Granzow H, Maresch C, et al. Ultrastructural analysis of virion formation and intraaxonal transport of herpes simplex virus type 1 in primary rat neurons. *J Virol* 2010;84(24):13031–13035.
329. Newcomb WW, Booy FP, Brown JC. Uncoating the herpes simplex virus genome. *J Mol Biol* 2007;370(4):633–642.
330. Newcomb WW, Cockrell SK, Homa FL, et al. Polarized DNA ejection from the herpesvirus capsid. *J Mol Biol* 2009;392(4):885–894.
331. Newcomb WW, Fontana J, Winkler DC, et al. The primary enveloped virion of herpes simplex virus 1: its role in nuclear egress. *mBio* 2017;8(3).
332. Newcomb WW, Homa FL, Brown JC. Involvement of the portal at an early step in herpes simplex virus capsid assembly. *J Virol* 2005;79:10540–10546.
333. Newcomb WW, Juhas RM, Thomsen DR, et al. The UL6 gene product forms the portal for entry of DNA into the herpes simplex virus capsid. *J Virol* 2001;75(22):10923–10932.
334. Newcomb WW, Trus BL, Cheng N, et al. Isolation of herpes simplex virus procapsids from cells infected with a protease-deficient mutant virus. *J Virol* 2000;74(4):1663–1673.
335. Newman RM, Lamers SL, Weiner B, et al. Genome sequencing and analysis of geographically diverse clinical isolates of herpes simplex virus 2. *J Virol* 2015;89(16):8219–8232.
336. Nicola AV, Hou J, Major EO, et al. Herpes simplex virus type 1 enters human epidermal keratinocytes, but not neurons, via a pH-dependent endocytic pathway. *J Virol* 2005;79:7609–7616.
337. Nicoll MP, Hann W, Shivkumar M, et al. The HSV-1 latency-associated transcript functions to repress latent phase lytic gene expression and suppress virus reactivation from latently infected neurons. *PLoS Pathog* 2016;12(4):e1005539.
338. Nicoll MP, Proenca JT, Connor V, et al. Influence of herpes simplex virus 1 latency-associated transcripts on the establishment and maintenance of latency in the ROSA26R reporter mouse model. *J Virol* 2012;86(16):8848–8858.
339. Nimonkar AV, Boehmer PE. Reconstitution of recombination-dependent DNA synthesis in herpes simplex virus 1. *Proc Natl Acad Sci U S A* 2003;100(18):10201–10206.
340. Oh HS, Chou S-F, Raja P, Cabral JM, Knipe DM. manuscript in preparation.
341. Oh HS, Knipe DM. Proteomic analysis of the herpes simplex virus 1 virion protein 16 transactivator protein in infected Cells. *Proteomics* 15:1957–1967.
342. Oh J, Fraser NW. Temporal association of the herpes simplex virus genome with histone proteins during a lytic infection. *J Virol* 2008;82(7):3530–3537.
343. Oh MJ, Akhtar J, Desai P, et al. A role for heparan sulfate in viral surfing. *Biochem Biophys Res Commun* 2010;391(1):176–181.
344. Ojala PM, Sodeik B, Ebersold MW, et al. Herpes simplex virus type 1 entry into host cells: reconstitution of capsid binding and uncoating at the nuclear pore complex in vitro. *Mol Cell Biol* 2000;20(13):4922–4931.
345. Orvedahl A, Alexander D, Talloczy Z, et al. HSV-1 ICP34.5 confers neurovirulence by targeting the Beclin 1 autophagy protein. *Cell Host Microbe* 2007;1(1):23–35.
346. Orzalli MH, Broekema NM, Diner BA, et al. cGAS-mediated stabilization of IFI16 promotes innate signaling during herpes simplex virus infection. *Proc Natl Acad Sci U S A* 2015;112(14):E1773–E1781.
347. Orzalli MH, Broekema NM, Knipe DM. Relative contributions of herpes simplex virus 1 ICP0 and vhs to loss of cellular IFI16 vary in different human cell types. *J Virol* 2016;90(18):8351–8359.
348. Orzalli MH, Conwell SE, Berrios C, et al. Nuclear interferon-inducible protein 16 promotes silencing of herpesviral and transfected DNA. *Proc Natl Acad Sci U S A* 2013;110(47):E4492–E4501.
349. Orzalli MH, DeLuca NA, Knipe DM. Nuclear IFI16 induction of IRF-3 signaling during herpesviral infection and degradation of IFI16 by the viral ICP0 protein. *Proc Natl Acad Sci U S A* 2012;109(44):E3008–E3017.
350. Orzalli MH, Knipe DM. unpublished results.
351. Owen DJ, Crump CM, Graham SC. Tegument assembly and secondary envelopment of alphaherpesviruses. *Viruses* 2015;7(9):5084–5114.
352. Pan D, Flores O, Umbach JL, et al. A neuron-specific host microRNA targets herpes simplex virus-1 ICP0 expression and promotes latency. *Cell Host Microbe* 2014;15(4):446–456.
353. Pan D, Pesola JM, Li G, et al. Mutations inactivating herpes simplex virus 1 MicroRNA miR-H2 do not detectably increase ICP0 gene expression in infected cultured cells or mouse trigeminal ganglia. *J Virol* 2017;91(2).
354. Parkinson J, Lees-Miller SP, Everett RD. Herpes simplex virus type 1 immediate-early protein vmw110 induces the proteasome-dependent degradation of the catalytic subunit of DNA-dependent protein kinase. *J Virol* 1999;73(1):650–657.
355. Pasdeloup D, Blondel D, Isidro AL, et al. Herpesvirus capsid association with the nuclear pore complex and viral DNA release involve the nucleoporin CAN/Nup214 and the capsid protein pUL25. *J Virol* 2009;83(13):6610–6623.
356. Pasdeloup D, McElwee M, Beilstein F, et al. Herpesvirus tegument protein pUL37 interacts with dystonin/BPAG1 to promote capsid transport on microtubules during egress. *J Virol* 2013;87(5):2857–2867.
357. Pasieka TJ, Lu B, Crosby SD, et al. Herpes simplex virus virion host shutoff attenuates establishment of the antiviral state. *J Virol* 2008;82(11):5527–5535.
358. Patel CD, Backes IM, Taylor SA, et al. Maternal immunization confers protection against neonatal herpes simplex mortality and behavioral morbidity. *Sci Transl Med* 2019;11(487):eaau6039.
358a. Patel A, Hanson J, McLean TI, et al. Herpes simplex type 1 induction of persistent NF-kappa B nuclear translocation increases the efficiency of virus replication. *Virology* 1998;247(2):212–222.
359. Pawliczek T, Crump CM. Herpes simplex virus type 1 production requires a functional ESCRT-III complex but is independent of TSG101 and ALIX expression. *J Virol* 2009;83(21):11254–11264.
360. Pelletier J, Sonenberg N. The organizing principles of eukaryotic ribosome recruitment. *Annu Rev Biochem* 2019;88:307–335.
361. Peng R, Zhang S, Cui Y, et al. Structures of human-infecting Thogotovirus fusogens support a common ancestor with insect baculovirus. *Proc Natl Acad Sci U S A* 2017;114(42):E8905–E8912.
362. Peri P, Mattila RK, Kantola H, et al. Herpes simplex virus type 1 Us3 gene deletion influences toll-like receptor responses in cultured monocytic cells. *Virol J* 2008;5:140.
363. Peri P, Nuutila K, Vuorinen T, et al. Cathepsins are involved in virus-induced cell death in ICP4 and Us3 deletion mutant herpes simplex virus type 1-infected monocytic cells. *J Gen Virol* 2011;92(Pt 1):173–180.
364. Perng GC, Jones C, Ciacci-Zanella J, et al. Virus-induced neuronal apoptosis blocked by the herpes simplex virus latency-associated transcript. *Science* 2000;287(5457):1500–1503.
365. Perng GC, Slanina SM, Yukht A, et al. The latency-associated transcript gene enhances establishment of herpes simplex virus type 1 latency in rabbits. *J Virol* 2000;74(4):1885–1891.
366. Peters GA, Khoo D, Mohr I, et al. Inhibition of PACT-mediated activation of PKR by the herpes simplex virus type 1 Us11 protein. *J Virol* 2002;76(21):11054–11064.
367. Pheasant K, Moller-Levet CS, Jones J, et al. Nuclear-cytoplasmic compartmentalization of the herpes simplex virus 1 infected cell transcriptome is co-ordinated by the viral endoribonuclease vhs and cofactors to facilitate the translation of late proteins. *PLoS Pathog* 2018;14(11):e1007331.
368. Pourchet A, Modrek AS, Placantonakis DG, et al. Modeling HSV-1 latency in human embryonic stem cell-derived neurons. *Pathogens* 2017;6(2).
369. Preston VG, Murray J, Preston CM, et al. The UL25 gene product of herpes simplex virus type 1 is involved in uncoating of the viral genome. *J Virol* 2008;82(13):6654–6666.
370. Proenca JT, Coleman HM, Connor V, et al. A historical analysis of herpes simplex virus promoter activation in vivo reveals distinct populations of latently infected neurones. *J Gen Virol* 2008;89(Pt 12):2965–2974.
371. Proenca JT, Coleman HM, Nicoll MP, et al. An investigation of herpes simplex virus promoter activity compatible with latency establishment reveals VP16-independent activation of immediate-early promoters in sensory neurones. *J Gen Virol* 2011;92(Pt 11):2575–2585.
372. Protter DSW, Parker R. Principles and properties of stress granules. *Trends Cell Biol* 2016;26(9):668–679.
373. Pugacheva EM, Kubo N, Loukinov D, et al. CTCF mediates chromatin looping via N-terminal domain-dependent cohesin retention. *Proc Natl Acad Sci U S A* 2020;117(4):2020–2031.
374. Quinlan MP, Chen LB, Knipe DM. The intranuclear location of a herpes simplex virus DNA-binding protein is determined by the status of viral DNA replication. *Cell* 1984;36(4):857–868.
375. Radtke K, Kieneke D, Wolfstein A, et al. Plus- and minus-end directed microtubule motors bind simultaneously to herpes simplex virus capsids using different inner tegument structures. *PLoS Pathog* 2010;6(7):e1000991.
376. Raja P, Chou S-F, Lee JS, et al. manuscript in preparation.
377. Raja P, Lee JS, Pan D, et al. A herpesviral lytic protein regulates the structure of latent viral chromatin. *mBio* 2016;7(3):e00633.
378. Rasmussen SB, Jensen SB, Nielsen C, et al. Herpes simplex virus infection is sensed by both Toll-like receptors and retinoic acid-inducible gene- like receptors, which synergize to induce type I interferon production. *J Gen Virol* 2009;90(Pt 1):74–78.
379. Rathinam VA, Jiang Z, Waggoner SN, et al. The AIM2 inflammasome is essential for host defense against cytosolic bacteria and DNA viruses. *Nat Immunol* 2010;11(5):395–402.
380. Read GS. Virus-encoded endonucleases: expected and novel functions. *Wiley Interdiscip Rev RNA* 2013;4(6):693–708.
381. Reck-Peterson SL, Redwine WB, Vale RD, et al. The cytoplasmic dynein transport machinery and its many cargoes. *Nat Rev Mol Cell Biol* 2018;19(6):382–398.
382. Reddy KL, Zullo JM, Bertolino E, et al. Transcriptional repression mediated by repositioning of genes to the nuclear lamina. *Nature* 2008;452(7184):243–247.
383. Reynolds AE, Liang L, Baines JD. Conformational changes in the nuclear lamina induced by herpes simplex virus type 1 require genes U(L)31 and U(L)34. *J Virol* 2004;78(11):5564–5575.
384. Reynolds AE, Wills EG, Roller RJ, et al. Ultrastructural localization of the herpes simplex virus type 1 UL31, UL34, and US3 proteins suggests specific roles in primary envelopment and egress of nucleocapsids. *J Virol* 2002;76(17):8939–8952.

385. Roberts AP, Abaitua F, O'Hare P, et al. Differing roles of inner tegument proteins pUL36 and pUL37 during entry of herpes simplex virus type 1. *J Virol* 2009;83(1): 105–116.
386. Roche S, Bressanelli S, Rey FA, et al. Crystal structure of the low-pH form of the vesicular stomatitis virus glycoprotein G. *Science* 2006;313(5784):187–191.
387. Rock DL, Fraser NW. Detection of HSV-1 genome in central nervous system of latently infected mice. *Nature* 1983;302(5908):523–525.
388. Rode K, Dohner K, Binz A, et al. Uncoupling uncoating of herpes simplex virus genomes from their nuclear import and gene expression. *J Virol* 2011;85(9):4271–4283.
389. Rodriguez-Barbosa JI, Schneider P, Weigert A, et al. HVEM, a cosignaling molecular switch, and its interactions with BTLA, CD160 and LIGHT. *Cell Mol Immunol* 2019;16(7):679–682.
390. Rogalin HB, Heldwein EE. Interplay between the herpes simplex virus 1 gB cytodomain and the gH cytotail during cell-cell fusion. *J Virol* 2015;89(24):12262–12272.
391. Roizman B. The checkpoints of viral gene expression in productive and latent infection: the role of the HDAC/CoREST/LSD1/REST repressor complex. *J Virol* 2011;85(15):7474–7482.
392. Roizman B, Jacob RJ, Knipe DM, et al. On the structure, functional equivalence, and replication of the four arrangements of herpes simplex virus DNA. *Cold Spring Harb Symp Quant Biol* 1979;43 Pt 2:809–826.
393. Roizman B, Knipe DM. Herpes simplex viruses and their replication. In: Knipe DM, Howley PM, eds. *Fields Virology*. 4th ed. Philadelphia, PA: Lippincott Williams & Wilkins; 2001:2399–2460.
394. Roizman B, Knipe DM, Whitley RJ. Herpes simplex viruses. In: Knipe DM, Howley PM, eds. *Fields Virology*. Vol. 2. 5th ed. Philadelphia, PA: Lippincott Williams & Wilkins; 2007:2501–2602.
395. Roizman B, Knipe DM, Whitley RJ. Herpes simplex viruses. In: Knipe DM, Howley PM, eds. *Fields Virology*. 6th ed. Philadelphia, PA: Lippincott Williams & Wilkins; 2013:1823–1897.
396. Roller RJ, Baines JD. Herpesvirus nuclear egress. *Adv Anat Embryol Cell Biol* 2017;223: 143–169.
397. Roller RJ, Bjerke SL, Haugo AC, et al. Analysis of a charge cluster mutation of herpes simplex virus type 1 UL34 and its extragenic suppressor suggests a novel interaction between pUL34 and pUL31 that is necessary for membrane curvature around capsids. *J Virol* 2010;84(8):3921–3934.
398. Roller RJ, Zhou Y, Schnetzer R, et al. Herpes simplex virus type 1 U(L)34 gene product is required for viral envelopment. *J Virol* 2000;74:117–129.
399. Rubio RM, Mohr I. Inhibition of ULK1 and Beclin1 by an alpha-herpesvirus Akt-like Ser/Thr kinase limits autophagy to stimulate virus replication. *Proc Natl Acad Sci U S A* 2019;116:26941–26950.
400. Rutkowski AJ, Erhard F, L'Hernault A, et al. Widespread disruption of host transcription termination in HSV-1 infection. *Nat Commun* 2015;6:7126.
401. Sadek J, Read GS. The splicing history of an mRNA affects its level of translation and sensitivity to cleavage by the virion host shutoff endonuclease during herpes simplex virus infections. *J Virol* 2016;90(23):10844–10856.
402. Sae-Ueng U, Li D, Zuo X, et al. Solid-to-fluid DNA transition inside HSV-1 capsid close to the temperature of infection. *Nat Chem Biol* 2014;10(10):861–867.
403. Salaun C, MacDonald AI, Larralde O, et al. Poly(A)-binding protein 1 partially relocalizes to the nucleus during herpes simplex virus type 1 infection in an ICP27-independent manner and does not inhibit virus replication. *J Virol* 2010;84(17):8539–8548.
404. Sampath P, Deluca NA. Binding of ICP4, TATA-binding protein, and RNA polymerase II to herpes simplex virus type 1 immediate-early, early, and late promoters in virus-infected cells. *J Virol* 2008;82(5):2339–2349.
405. Sanchez R, Mohr I. Inhibition of cellular 2'-5' oligoadenylate synthetase by the herpes simplex virus type 1 Us11 protein. *J Virol* 2007;81(7):3455–3464.
406. Sancho-Shimizu V, Perez de Diego R, Lorenzo L, et al. Herpes simplex encephalitis in children with autosomal recessive and dominant TRIF deficiency. *J Clin Invest* 2011;121(12):4889–4902.
407. Sarma N, Agarwal D, Shiflett LA, et al. Small interfering RNAs that deplete the cellular translation factor eIF4H impede mRNA degradation by the virion host shutoff protein of herpes simplex virus. *J Virol* 2008;82(13):6600–6609.
408. Sathiyamoorthy K, Chen J, Longnecker R, et al. The COMPLEXity in herpesvirus entry. *Curr Opin Virol* 2017;24:97–104.
409. Satoh T, Arii J, Suenaga T, et al. PILRalpha is a herpes simplex virus-1 entry coreceptor that associates with glycoprotein B. *Cell* 2008;132(6):935–944.
410. Saxton RA, Sabatini DM. mTOR signaling in growth, metabolism, and disease. *Cell* 2017;168(6):960–976.
411. Schiffer JT, Corey L. New concepts in understanding genital herpes. *Curr Infect Dis Rep* 2009;11(6):457–464.
412. Schipke J, Pohlmann A, Diestel R, et al. The C terminus of the large tegument protein pUL36 contains multiple capsid binding sites that function differently during assembly and cell entry of herpes simplex virus. *J Virol* 2012;86(7):3682–3700.
413. Schreiner S, Burck C, Glass M, et al. Control of human adenovirus type 5 gene expression by cellular Daxx/ATRX chromatin-associated complexes. *Nucleic Acids Res* 2013;41(6):3532–3550.
414. Schwartz SL, Conn GL. RNA regulation of the antiviral protein 2'-5'-oligoadenylate synthetase. *Wiley Interdiscip Rev RNA* 2019;10(4):e1534.
415. Sciortino M-T, Suzuki M, Taddeo B, et al. RNAs extracted from herpes simplex virus 1 virions: apparent selectivity of viral but not cellular RNAs packaged in virions. *J Virol* 2001;75:8105–8116.
416. Sciortino MT, Medici MA, Marino-Merlo F, et al. Involvement of gD/HVEM interaction in NF-kB-dependent inhibition of apoptosis by HSV-1 gD. *Biochem Pharmacol* 2008;76(11):1522–1532.
417. Sciortino MT, Parisi T, Siracusano G, et al. The virion host shutoff RNase plays a key role in blocking the activation of protein kinase R in cells infected with herpes simplex virus 1. *J Virol* 2013;87(6):3271–3276.
418. Selvarajan Sigamani S, Zhao H, Kamau YN, et al. The structure of the herpes simplex virus DNA-packaging terminase pUL15 nuclease domain suggests an evolutionary lineage among eukaryotic and prokaryotic viruses. *J Virol* 2013;87(12):7140–7148.
419. Sen J, Liu X, Roller R, et al. Herpes simplex virus US3 tegument protein inhibits Toll-like receptor 2 signaling at or before TRAF6 ubiquitination. *Virology* 2013;439(2):65–73.
420. Shalginskikh N, Poleshko A, Skalka AM, et al. Retroviral DNA methylation and epigenetic repression are mediated by the antiviral host protein Daxx. *J Virol* 2013;87(4):2137–2150.
421. Shen G, Wang K, Wang S, et al. Herpes simplex virus 1 counteracts viperin via its virion host shutoff protein UL41. *J Virol* 2014;88(20):12163–12166.
422. Shi M, Hu X, Wei Y, et al. Genome-wide profiling of small RNAs and degradome revealed conserved regulations of miRNAs on auxin-responsive genes during fruit enlargement in peaches. *Int J Mol Sci* 2017;18(12).
423. Shiflett LA, Read GS. mRNA decay during herpes simplex virus (HSV) infections: mutations that affect translation of an mRNA influence the sites at which it is cleaved by the HSV virion host shutoff (Vhs) protein. *J Virol* 2013;87(1):94–109.
424. Shimi T, Pfleghaar K, Kojima S, et al. The A- and B-type nuclear lamin networks: microdomains involved in chromatin organization and transcription. *Genes Dev* 2008;22(24):3409–3421.
425. Shipley MM, Mangold CA, Kuny CV, et al. Differentiated human SH-SY5Y cells provide a reductionist model of herpes simplex virus 1 neurotropism. *J Virol* 2017;91(23).
426. Shu M, Taddeo B, Zhang W, et al. Selective degradation of mRNAs by the HSV host shutoff RNase is regulated by the UL47 tegument protein. *Proc Natl Acad Sci U S A* 2013;110(18):E1669–E1675.
427. Shukla SY, Singh YK, Shukla D. Role of nectin-1, HVEM, and PILR-alpha in HSV-2 entry into human retinal pigment epithelial cells. *Invest Ophthalmol Vis Sci* 2009;50(6):2878–2887.
428. Silva L, Cliffe A, Chang L, et al. Role for A-type lamins in herpesviral DNA targeting and heterochromatin modulation. *PLoS Pathog* 2008;4(5):e1000071.
429. Silva L, Oh HS, Chang L, et al. Roles of the nuclear lamina in stable nuclear association and assembly of a herpesviral transactivator complex on viral immediate-early genes. *mBio* 2012;3(1):e00300.
430. Simpson-Holley M, Baines J, Roller R, et al. Herpes simplex virus 1 U(L)31 and U(L)34 gene products promote the late maturation of viral replication compartments to the nuclear periphery. *J Virol* 2004;78(11):5591–5600.
431. Smith RWP, Anderson RC, Larralde O, et al. Viral and cellular mRNA-specific activators harness PABP and eIF4G to promote translation initiation downstream of cap binding. *Proc Natl Acad Sci U S A* 2017;114(24):6310–6315.
432. Smith S, Reuven N, Mohni KN, et al. Structure of the herpes simplex virus 1 genome: manipulation of nicks and gaps can abrogate infectivity and alter the cellular DNA damage response. *J Virol* 2014;88(17):10146–10156.
433. Snijder J, Radtke K, Anderson F, et al. Vertex-specific proteins pUL17 and pUL25 mechanically reinforce herpes simplex virus capsids. *J Virol* 2017;91(12).
434. Snyder A, Polcicova K, Johnson DC. Herpes simplex virus gE/gI and US9 proteins promote transport of both capsids and virion glycoproteins in neuronal axons. *J Virol* 2008;82(21):10613–10624.
435. Soberman RJ, MacKay CR, Vaine CA, et al. CD200R1 supports HSV-1 viral replication and licenses pro-inflammatory signaling functions of TLR2. *PLoS One* 2012;7(10):e47740.
436. Sodeik B, Ebersold MW, Helenius A. Microtubule-mediated transport of incoming herpes simplex virus 1 capsids to the nucleus. *J Cell Biol* 1997;136(5):1007–1021.
437. Sodroski CN, Knipe DM. manuscript in preparation.
438. Song LL, Ponomareva L, Shen H, et al. Interferon-inducible IFI16, a negative regulator of cell growth, down-regulates expression of human telomerase reverse transcriptase (hTERT) gene. *PLoS One* 2010;5(1):e8569.
439. Spear PG, Eisenberg RJ, Cohen GH. Three classes of cell surface receptors for alphaherpesvirus entry. *Virology* 2000;275(1):1–8.
440. Spear PG, Roizman B. Buoyant density of herpes simplex virus in solutions of caesium chloride. *Nature* 1967;214(5089):713–714.
441. Srivastava R, Dervillez X, Khan AA, et al. The herpes simplex virus latency-associated transcript gene is associated with a broader repertoire of virus-specific exhausted CD8+ T cells retained within the trigeminal ganglia of latently infected HLA transgenic rabbits. *J Virol* 2016;90(8):3913–3928.
442. Stackpole CW. Herpes-type virus of the frog renal adenocarcinoma. I. Virus development in tumor transplants maintained at low temperature. *J Virol* 1969;4(1):75–93.
443. Stampfer SD, Heldwein EE. Stuck in the middle: structural insights into the role of the gH/gL heterodimer in herpesvirus entry. *Curr Opin Virol* 2013;3(1):13–19.
444. Stegen C, Yakova Y, Henaff D, et al. Analysis of virion-incorporated host proteins required for herpes simplex virus type 1 infection through a RNA interference screen. *PLoS One* 2013;8(1):e53276.
445. Stempel M, Chan B, Brinkmann MM. Coevolution pays off: herpesviruses have the license to escape the DNA sensing pathway. *Med Microbiol Immunol* 2019;208(3–4):495–512.
446. Stern-Ginossar N, Thompson SR, Mathews MB, et al. Translational control in virus-infected cells. *Cold Spring Harb Perspect Biol* 2019;11(3).
447. Stevens JG, Wagner EK, Devi-Rao GB, et al. RNA complementary to a herpesvirus alpha gene mRNA is prominent in latently infected neurons. *Science* 1987;235(4792):1056–1059.
448. Strang BL, Stow ND. Circularization of the herpes simplex virus type 1 genome upon lytic infection. *J Virol* 2005;79(19):12487–12494.
449. Stratmann SA, Morrone SR, van Oijen AM, et al. The innate immune sensor IFI16 recognizes foreign DNA in the nucleus by scanning along the duplex. *eLife* 2015;4:e11721.
450. Suenaga T, Satoh T, Somboonthum P, et al. Myelin-associated glycoprotein mediates membrane fusion and entry of neurotropic herpesviruses. *Proc Natl Acad Sci U S A* 2010;107(2):866–871.
451. Sugimoto K, Uema M, Sagara H, et al. Simultaneous tracking of capsid, tegument, and envelope protein localization in living cells infected with triply fluorescent herpes simplex virus 1. *J Virol* 2008;82(11):5198–5211.
452. Sun L, Wu J, Du F, et al. Cyclic GMP-AMP synthase is a cytosolic DNA sensor that activates the type I interferon pathway. *Science* 2013;339(6121):786–791.

453. Szpara ML, Gatherer D, Ochoa A, et al. Evolution and diversity in human herpes simplex virus genomes. *J Virol* 2014;88(2):1209–1227.
454. Szpara ML, Parsons L, Enquist LW. Sequence variability in clinical and laboratory isolates of herpes simplex virus 1 reveals new mutations. *J Virol* 2010;84(10):5303–13.
455. Taddeo B, Zhang W, Roizman B. Role of herpes simplex virus ICP27 in the degradation of mRNA by virion host shutoff RNase. *J Virol* 2010;84(19):10182–10190.
456. Takeshima K, Arii J, Maruzuru Y, et al. Identification of the capsid binding site in the herpes simplex virus 1 nuclear egress complex and its role in viral primary envelopment and replication. *J Virol* 2019;93(21).
457. Tal-Singer R, Lasner TM, Podrzucki W, et al. Gene expression during reactivation of herpes simplex virus type 1 from latency in the peripheral nervous system is different from that during lytic infection of tissue cultures. *J Virol* 1997;71(7):5268–5276.
458. Talloczy Z, Jiang W, Virgin HWT, et al. Regulation of starvation- and virus-induced autophagy by the eIF2alpha kinase signaling pathway. *Proc Natl Acad Sci U S A* 2002;99(1):190–195.
459. Tandon R, Mocarski ES, Conway JF. The A, B, Cs of herpesvirus capsids. *Viruses* 2015;7(3):899–914.
460. Tang S, Bertke AS, Patel A, et al. Herpes simplex virus 2 microRNA miR-H6 is a novel latency-associated transcript-associated microRNA, but reduction of its expression does not influence the establishment of viral latency or the recurrence phenotype. *J Virol* 2011;85(9):4501–4509.
461. Tang S, Bertke AS, Patel A, et al. An acutely and latently expressed herpes simplex virus 2 viral microRNA inhibits expression of ICP34.5, a viral neurovirulence factor. *Proc Natl Acad Sci U S A* 2008;105(31):10931–10936.
462. Tang S, Patel A, Krause PR. Novel less-abundant viral microRNAs encoded by herpes simplex virus 2 latency-associated transcript and their roles in regulating ICP34.5 and ICP0 mRNAs. *J Virol* 2009;83(3):1433–1442.
463. Tang S, Patel A, Krause PR. Herpes simplex virus ICP27 regulates alternative pre-mRNA polyadenylation and splicing in a sequence-dependent manner. *Proc Natl Acad Sci U S A* 2016;113(43):12256–12261.
464. Tang S, Patel A, Krause PR. Hidden regulation of herpes simplex virus 1 pre-mRNA splicing and polyadenylation by virally encoded immediate early gene ICP27. *PLoS Pathog* 2019;15(6):e1007884.
465. Taylor JM, Lin E, Susmarski N, et al. Alternative entry receptors for herpes simplex virus and their roles in disease. *Cell Host Microbe* 2007;2(1):19–28.
466. Taylor TJ, Knipe DM. Proteomics of herpes simplex virus replication compartments: association of cellular DNA replication, repair, recombination, and chromatin remodeling proteins with ICP8. *J Virol* 2004;78(11):5856–5866.
467. Thellman NM, Botting C, Madaj Z, et al. An immortalized human dorsal root ganglion cell line provides a novel context to study herpes simplex virus 1 latency and reactivation. *J Virol* 2017;91(12).
468. Thompson RL, Preston CM, Sawtell NM. De novo synthesis of VP16 coordinates the exit from HSV latency in vivo. *PLoS Pathog* 2009;5(3):e1000352.
469. Tian X, Devi-Rao G, Golovanov AP, et al. The interaction of the cellular export adaptor protein Aly/REF with ICP27 contributes to the efficiency of herpes simplex virus 1 mRNA export. *J Virol* 2013;87(13):7210–7217.
470. Torok D, Ching RW, Bazett-Jones DP. PML nuclear bodies as sites of epigenetic regulation. *Front Biosci (Landmark Ed)* 2009;14:1325–1336.
471. Toropova K, Huffman JB, Homa FL, et al. The herpes simplex virus 1 UL17 protein is the second constituent of the capsid vertex-specific component required for DNA packaging and retention. *J Virol* 2011;85:7513–7522.
472. Tsai K, Thikmyanova N, Wojcechowskyj JA, et al. EBV tegument protein BNRF1 disrupts DAXX-ATRX to activate viral early gene transcription. *PLoS Pathog* 2011;7(11):e1002376.
473. Tunnicliffe RB, Schacht M, Levy C, et al. The structure of the folded domain from the signature multifunctional protein ICP27 from herpes simplex virus-1 reveals an intertwined dimer. *Sci Rep* 2015;5:11234.
474. Turner A, Bruun B, Minson T, et al. Glycoproteins gB, gD, and gHgL of herpes simplex virus type 1 are necessary and sufficient to mediate membrane fusion in a Cos cell transfection system. *J Virol* 1998;72(1):873–875.
475. Uchida H, Chan J, Goins WF, et al. A double mutation in glycoprotein gB compensates for ineffective gD-dependent initiation of herpes simplex virus type 1 infection. *J Virol* 2010;84(23):12200–12209.
476. Umbach JL, Kramer MF, Jurak I, et al. MicroRNAs expressed by herpes simplex virus 1 during latent infection regulate viral mRNAs. *Nature* 2008;454(7205):780–783.
477. Umbach JL, Nagel MA, Cohrs RJ, et al. Analysis of human alphaherpesvirus microRNA expression in latently infected human trigeminal ganglia. *J Virol* 2009;83(20):10677–10683.
478. Umbach JL, Wang K, Tang S, et al. Identification of viral microRNAs expressed in human sacral ganglia latently infected with herpes simplex virus 2. *J Virol* 2010;84(2):1189–1192.
479. van Genderen IL, Brandimarti R, Torrisi MR, et al. The phospholipid composition of extracellular herpes simplex virions differs from that of host cell nuclei. *Virology* 1994;200:831–836.
480. van Lint AL, Murawski MR, Goodbody RE, et al. Herpes simplex virus immediate-early ICP0 protein inhibits Toll-like receptor 2-dependent inflammatory responses and NF-kappaB signaling. *J Virol* 2010;84(20):10802–10811.
481. Vanarsdall AL, Howard PW, Wisner TW, et al. Human cytomegalovirus gH/gL forms a stable complex with the fusion protein gB in virions. *PLoS Pathog* 2016;12(4):e1005564.
482. Vandenabeele P, Galluzzi L, Vanden Berghe T, et al. Molecular mechanisms of necroptosis: an ordered cellular explosion. *Nat Rev Mol Cell Biol* 2010;11(10):700–714.
483. Varmuza SL, Smiley JR. Signals for site-specific cleavage of HSV DNA: maturation involves two separate cleavage events at sites distal to the recognition sequences. *Cell* 1985;41:793–802.
484. Verpooten D, Feng Z, Valyi-Nagy T, et al. Dephosphorylation of eIF2alpha mediated by the gamma134.5 protein of herpes simplex virus 1 facilitates viral neuroinvasion. *J Virol* 2009;83(23):12626–12630.
485. Vink EI, Andrews JC, Duffy C, et al. Productive replication during ribosomal protein insufficiency requires an HSV-1 RNA binding protein. Manuscript in revision.
486. Vink EI, Lee S, Smiley JR, et al. Remodeling mTORC1 responsiveness to amino acids by the herpes simplex virus UL46 and Us3 gene products supports replication during nutrient insufficiency. *J Virol* 2018;92(24).
487. Vink EI, Smiley JR, Mohr I. Subversion of host responses to energy insufficiency by Us3 supports herpes simplex virus 1 replication during stress. *J Virol* 2017;91(14).
488. Viphakone N, Sudbery I, Griffith L, et al. Co-transcriptional loading of RNA export factors shapes the human transcriptome. *Mol Cell* 2019;75(2):310–323.e8.
489. Vlazny DA, Kwong A, Frenkel N. Site-specific cleavage/packaging of herpes simplex virus DNA and the selective maturation of nucleocapsids containing full-length viral DNA. *Proc Natl Acad Sci U S A* 1982;79(5):1423–1427.
490. Vollmer B, Prazak V, Vasishtan D, et al. The prefusion structure of herpes simplex virus glycoprotein B. *Sci Adv* 2020;6(39).
491. Wadsworth S, Jacob RJ, Roizman B. Anatomy of herpes simplex virus DNA. II. Size, composition, and arrangement of inverted terminal repetitions. *J Virol* 1975;15(6):1487–1497.
492. Wagner LM, DeLuca NA. Temporal association of herpes simplex virus ICP4 with cellular complexes functioning at multiple steps in PolII transcription. *PLoS One* 2013;8(10):e78242.
493. Walsh D, Mohr I. Phosphorylation of eIF4E by Mnk-1 enhances HSV-1 translation and replication in quiescent cells. *Genes Dev* 2004;18(6):660–672.
494. Walsh D, Mohr I. Assembly of an active translation initiation factor complex by a viral protein. *Genes Dev* 2006;20(4):461–472.
495. Walzer SA, Egerer-Sieber C, Sticht H, et al. Crystal structure of the human cytomegalovirus pUL50-pUL53 core nuclear egress complex provides insight into a unique assembly scaffold for virus-host protein interactions. *J Biol Chem* 2015;290(46):27452–27458.
496. Wang H, Sun L, Su L, et al. Mixed lineage kinase domain-like protein MLKL causes necrotic membrane disruption upon phosphorylation by RIP3. *Mol Cell* 2014;54(1):133–146.
497. Wang J, Yuan S, Zhu D, et al. Structure of the herpes simplex virus type 2 C-capsid with capsid-vertex-specific component. *Nat Commun* 2018;9(1):3668.
498. Wang K, Ni L, Wang S, et al. Herpes simplex virus 1 protein kinase US3 hyperphosphorylates p65/RelA and dampens NF-kappaB activation. *J Virol* 2014;88(14):7941–7951.
499. Wang QY, Zhou C, Johnson KE, et al. Herpesviral latency-associated transcript gene promotes assembly of heterochromatin on viral lytic-gene promoters in latent infection. *Proc Natl Acad Sci U S A* 2005;102(44):16055–16059.
500. Wang JP, Bowen GN, Zhou S, et al. Role of specific innate immune responses in herpes simplex virus infection of the central nervous system. *J Virol* 2012;86:2273–2281.
501. Wang X, Hennig T, Whisnant AW, et al. Herpes simplex virus blocks host transcription termination via the bimodal activities of ICP27. *Nat Commun* 2020;11(1):293.
502. Wang X, Li Y, Liu S, et al. Direct activation of RIP3/MLKL-dependent necrosis by herpes simplex virus 1 (HSV-1) protein ICP6 triggers host antiviral defense. *Proc Natl Acad Sci U S A* 2014;111(43):15438–15443.
503. Wang X, Patenode C, Roizman B. US3 protein kinase of HSV-1 cycles between the cytoplasm and nucleus and interacts with programmed cell death protein 4 (PDCD4) to block apoptosis. *Proc Natl Acad Sci U S A* 2011;108(35):14632–14636.
504. Wang Y, Yang Y, Wu S, et al. p32 is a novel target for viral protein ICP34.5 of herpes simplex virus type 1 and facilitates viral nuclear egress. *J Biol Chem* 2014;289(52):35795–35805.
505. Washington SD, Edenfield SI, Lieux C, et al. Depletion of the insulator protein CTCF results in herpes simplex virus 1 reactivation in vivo. *J Virol* 2018;92(11).
506. Washington SD, Musarrat F, Ertel MK, et al. CTCF binding sites in the herpes simplex virus 1 genome display site-specific CTCF occupation, protein recruitment, and insulator function. *J Virol* 2018;92(8).
507. Washington SD, Singh P, Johns RN, et al. The CCCTC binding factor, CTRL2, modulates heterochromatin deposition and the establishment of herpes simplex virus 1 latency in vivo. *J Virol* 2019;93(13).
508. Watson ZL, Washington SD, Phelan DM, et al. In vivo knockdown of the herpes simplex virus 1 latency-associated transcript reduces reactivation from latency. *J Virol* 2018;92(16):e00812.
509. Weerasooriya S, DiScipio KA, Darwish AS, et al. Herpes simplex virus 1 ICP8 mutant lacking annealing activity is deficient for viral DNA replication. *Proc Natl Acad Sci U S A* 2019;116(3):1033–1042.
510. Weitzman MD, Lilley CE, Chaurushiya MS. Genomes in conflict: maintaining genome integrity during virus infection. *Annu Rev Microbiol* 2010;64:61–81.
511. Weller SK. Herpes simplex virus reorganizes the cellular DNA repair and protein quality control machinery. *PLoS Pathog* 2010;6(11):e1001105.
512. Weller SK, Coen DM. Herpes simplex viruses: mechanisms of DNA replication. *Cold Spring Harb Perspect Biol* 2012;4(9):a013011.
513. Wertheim JO, Smith MD, Smith DM, et al. Evolutionary origins of human herpes simplex viruses 1 and 2. *Mol Biol Evol* 2014;31(9):2356–2364.
514. West AP, Khoury-Hanold W, Staron M, et al. Mitochondrial DNA stress primes the antiviral innate immune response. *Nature* 2015;520(7548):553–557.
515. Whisnant AW, Jurges CS, Hennig T, et al. Integrative functional genomics decodes herpes simplex virus 1. *Nat Commun* 2020;11(1):2038.
516. Wilcox CL, Johnson EM Jr. Nerve growth factor deprivation results in the reactivation of latent herpes simplex virus in vitro. *J Virol* 1987;61(7):2311–2315.
517. Wilcox DR, Muller WJ, Longnecker R. HSV targeting of the host phosphatase PP1alpha is required for disseminated disease in the neonate and contributes to pathogenesis in the brain. *Proc Natl Acad Sci U S A* 2015;112(50):E6937–E6944.
518. Wilcox DR, Wadhwani NR, Longnecker R, et al. Differential reliance on autophagy for protection from HSV encephalitis between newborns and adults. *PLoS Pathog* 2015;11(1):e1004580.
519. Wisner TW, Sugimoto K, Howard PW, et al. Anterograde transport of herpes simplex virus capsids in neurons by both separate and married mechanisms. *J Virol* 2011;85(12):5919–5928.
520. Wittels M, Spear PG. Penetration of cells by herpes simplex virus does not require a low pH-dependent endocytic pathway. *Virus Res* 1991;18:271–290.
521. Wu S, Pan S, Zhang L, et al. Herpes simplex virus 1 induces phosphorylation and reorganization of lamin A/C through the gamma134.5 protein that facilitates nuclear egress. *J Virol* 2016;90(22):10414–10422.

522. Xing Y, Oliver SL, Nguyen T, et al. A site of varicella-zoster virus vulnerability identified by structural studies of neutralizing antibodies bound to the glycoprotein complex gHgL. *Proc Natl Acad Sci U S A* 2015;112(19):6056–6061.
523. Xiong R, Rao P, Kim S, Li M, Wen X, Yuan W. Herpes simplex virus 1 US3 phosphorylates cellular KIF3A to downregulate CD1d expression. *J Virol* 2015;89(13):6646–6655.
524. Xu P, Mallon S, Roizman B. PML plays both inimical and beneficial roles in HSV-1 replication. *Proc Natl Acad Sci U S A* 2016;113(21):E3022–E3028.
525. Xu P, Roizman B. The SP100 component of ND10 enhances accumulation of PML and suppresses replication and the assembly of HSV replication compartments. *Proc Natl Acad Sci U S A* 2017;114(19):E3823–E3829.
526. Yamashiro LH, Wilson SC, Morrison HM, et al. Interferon-independent STING signaling promotes resistance to HSV-1 in vivo. *Nat Commun* 2020;11(1):3382.
527. Yan Z, Bryant KF, Gregory SM, et al. HIV integrase inhibitors block replication of alpha-, beta-, and gammaherpesviruses. *mBio* 2014;5(4):e01318.
528. Yanez AA, Harrell T, Sriranganathan HJ, et al. Neurotrophic factors NGF, GDNF and NTN selectively modulate HSV1 and HSV2 lytic infection and reactivation in primary adult sensory and autonomic neurons. *Pathogens* 2017;6(1).
529. Yang B, Liu Y, Cui Y, et al. RNF90 negatively regulates cellular antiviral responses by targeting MITA for degradation. *PLoS Pathog* 2020;16(3):e1008387.
530. Yang K, Baines JD. Selection of HSV capsids for envelopment involves interaction between capsid surface components pUL31, pUL17, and pUL25. *Proc Natl Acad Sci U S A* 2011;108(34):14276–14281.
531. Yang Z, Klionsky DJ. Eaten alive: a history of macroautophagy. *Nat Cell Biol* 2010;12(9):814–822.
532. Yao F, Schaffer PA. An activity specified by the osteosarcoma line U2OS can substitute functionally for ICP0, a major regulatory protein of herpes simplex virus type 1. *J Virol* 1995;69(10):6249–6258.
533. Yordy B, Iijima N, Huttner A, et al. A neuron-specific role for autophagy in antiviral defense against herpes simplex virus. *Cell Host Microbe* 2012;12(3):334–345.
534. Yu X, Shah S, Lee M, et al. Biochemical and structural characterization of the capsid-bound tegument proteins of human cytomegalovirus. *J Struct Biol* 2011;174(3):451–460.
535. Yuan H, You J, You H, et al. Herpes simplex virus 1 UL36USP antagonizes type i interferon-mediated antiviral innate immunity. *J Virol* 2018;92(19).
536. Yuan S, Wang J, Zhu D, et al. Cryo-EM structure of a herpesvirus capsid at 3.1 A. *Science* 2018;360(6384).
537. Zaichick SV, Bohannon KP, Hughes A, et al. The herpesvirus VP1/2 protein is an effector of dynein-mediated capsid transport and neuroinvasion. *Cell Host Microbe* 2013;13(2):193–203.
538. Zeev-Ben-Mordehai T, Weberruss M, Lorenz M, et al. Crystal structure of the herpesvirus nuclear egress complex provides insights into inner nuclear membrane remodeling. *Cell Rep* 2015;13(12):2645–2652.
539. Zenner HL, Mauricio R, Banting G, et al. Herpes simplex virus 1 counteracts tethering restriction via its virion host shutoff activity. *J Virol* 2013;87(24):13115–13123.
540. Zhang J, Zhao J, Xu S, et al. Species-specific deamidation of cGAS by herpes simplex virus UL37 protein facilitates viral replication. *Cell Host Microbe* 2018;24(2):234–248.e5.
541. Zhang N, Yan J, Lu G, et al. Binding of herpes simplex virus glycoprotein D to nectin-1 exploits host cell adhesion. *Nat Commun* 2011;2:577.
542. Zhang X, Efstathiou S, Simmons A. Identification of novel herpes simplex virus replicative intermediates by field inversion gel electrophoresis: implications for viral DNA amplification strategies. *Virology* 1994;202(2):530–539.
543. Zhao J, Zeng Y, Xu S, et al. A viral deamidase targets the helicase domain of RIG-I to block RNA-induced activation. *Cell Host Microbe* 2016;20(6):770–784.
544. Zheng K, Chen M, Xiang Y, et al. Inhibition of herpes simplex virus type 1 entry by chloride channel inhibitors tamoxifen and NPPB. *Biochem Biophys Res Commun* 2014;446(4):990–996.
545. Zheng Y, Samrat SK, Gu H. A tale of two PMLs: elements regulating a differential substrate recognition by the ICP0 E3 ubiquitin ligase of herpes simplex virus 1. *J Virol* 2016;90(23):10875–10885.
546. Zhou G, Galvan V, Campadelli-Fiume G, et al. Glycoprotein D or J delivered in trans blocks apoptosis in SK-N-SH cells induced by a herpes simplex virus 1 mutant lacking intact genes expressing both glycoproteins. *J Virol* 2000;74(24):11782–11791.
547. Zhou G, Te D, Roizman B. The CoREST/REST repressor is both necessary and inimical for expression of herpes simplex virus genes. *mBio* 2010;2(1):e00313.

CHAPTER 10

Herpes Simplex Viruses: Pathogenesis and Clinical Insights

Richard J. Whitley • Christine Johnston

HISTORY

Herpes simplex viruses (HSVs) were the first of the human herpesviruses to be discovered and are among the most intensively investigated of all viruses. Attractions are their biologic properties, particularly their abilities to cause a variety of infections, to remain latent in their host for life, and to reactivate to cause lesions at or near the site of initial infection. They serve as models and tools for the study of translocation of proteins, synaptic connections in the nervous system, membrane structure, gene regulation, gene therapy, cancer therapy, and a myriad of other biological problems, both general to viruses and specific to HSV. For years, their size and complexity served as formidable obstacles to intensive research. More than 40 years passed from the time of their isolation until Schneweis demonstrated that there were two serotypes of HSV: HSV-1 and HSV-2. For a detailed history of HSV infections, the reviewer is referred to a prior edition of this chapter.

The field has grown enormously since the dawn of the molecular biology of HSV. Studies on HSV are elaborating "structure and function," and its gene products have become powerful probes for the study of cellular metabolic pathways. Host factors crucial to virus multiplication and, potentially, to latency are being identified. Notably, only a fraction of viral gene products are extensively studied and for many products their reason for existence has not been established.

PATHOGENESIS

Entry Into the Host

Transmission of HSV is dependent on intimate, personal contact between a seronegative (susceptible) individual and someone excreting HSV from skin or mucosal surfaces. Virus must come in contact with mucosal surfaces or abraded skin for infection to be initiated. Following oropharyngeal infection, usually caused by HSV-1, the trigeminal ganglion becomes infected and harbors latent virus. Although HSV-1 efficiently reactivates from the trigeminal ganglion, it can also infect the genital tract and become latent in the sacral ganglion. Acquisition of HSV-2 infection is usually the consequence of transmission by genital contact. Virus replicates in the genital, perigenital, or anal skin sites with seeding of the sacral ganglia. By comparison, HSV-2 is more pathogenic in the genital track than HSV-1, causing more frequent recurrences and reactivation from sacral ganglia than HSV-1.

Site of Primary Replication

Accumulated clinical experience suggests that after primary infection, replication of virus at the portal of entry, usually oral or genital mucosa, results in infection of sensory nerve endings; virus is transported to dorsal root ganglia.[16,17,276] The more severe the primary infection, as reflected by the size, number, and extent of lesions, the more likely it is that recurrences will ensue. This notion is attributed to the large quantity of virus present when primary disease is extensive as compared with asymptomatic infections. Primary infection can spread beyond the dorsal root ganglia, thereby becoming systemic. For example, studies of children with primary gingivostomatitis demonstrated HSV DNA in the blood by polymerase chain reaction (PCR) in about one-third of patients. Similarly, 24% of adults with primary genital herpes had viral DNA detected by PCR in the blood.[140]

Cell and Tissue Tropism

Fundamental to disease pathogenesis is the propensity of virus to replicate at mucosal surfaces, to be transported to dorsal root ganglia, and to become latent. Although replication can sometimes lead to disease and infrequently result in life-threatening central nervous system (CNS) infection, the host–virus balance between latency and reactivation predominates. With reactivation, virus travels through peripheral nerves to epithelial cells, where it replicates and is detected at mucocutaneous sites. Vesicles or pustules that coalesce into painful mucosal ulcers are classic clinical signs, but the virus can also simply be excreted in the absence of symptoms (asymptomatic shedding).

The first exposure to either HSV-1 or HSV-2 results in primary infection. Patients with primary infection may present with multiple ulcerations of the oral or genital tract, as well as systemic symptoms such as fevers, chills, or myalgias and headaches. Reactivation of HSV is known as recurrent infection and clinically results in a limited number of vesicular lesions as occurs with HSV labialis or recurrent HSV genitalis or can result in asymptomatic shedding. An individual with preexisting antibodies to one type of HSV (i.e., HSV-1) can experience a first infection with the opposite virus type (i.e., HSV-2) at a different site. Under such circumstances, the infection is known as an initial infection rather than as a primary or recurrent infection. For example, an initial infection occurs in those individuals who have preexisting HSV-1 antibodies who then acquire a genital HSV-2 infection. HSV-1 antibodies do not protect against HSV-2 infection, but those with prior HSV-1 infection may have a less severe HSV-2 initial infection.[61] While not proven, prior HSV infections may ameliorate subsequent infection with different HSV types. Because many individuals are infected with HSV and do not experience a primary infection, the first recurrence has been identified as first-episode infection. Reinfection with a different strain of HSV can occur, but it is uncommon in the normal host.[122]

Pathology

The pathologic changes induced by HSV replication are similar for both primary and recurrent infection but vary in the extent. The histopathologic characteristics of HSV skin lesions are shown in Figure 10.1,[236] representing a combination of virus-mediated cell death and associated inflammation. Viral infection induces ballooning of cells and the appearance of condensed chromatin within the nuclei, followed by subsequent degeneration of the cellular nuclei, generally within parabasal and intermediate cells of the epithelium. Cells lose intact plasma membranes and form multinucleated giant cells. With cell lysis, clear (referred to as vesicular) fluid containing virus appears between the epidermis and dermal layer. The vesicular fluid contains cell debris, inflammatory cells, and, often, multinucleated giant cells. In dermal substructures, there is an intense inflammatory response with infiltration of CD4+ and CD8+ T cells, usually in the corium of the skin. With healing, the vesicular fluid becomes pustular with the recruitment of inflammatory cells, and then it forms a wet and painful ulceration. The dry crust, or healing phase, is characterized by formation of a scab and typically occurs in the absence of viral shedding. Scarring is uncommon but has been noted in some patients with frequent recurrences. When mucous membranes are involved, vesicles are less likely to be prominent. Instead, shallow ulcers are more common because the vesicles rapidly rupture as a result of the very thin cornified epithelium.

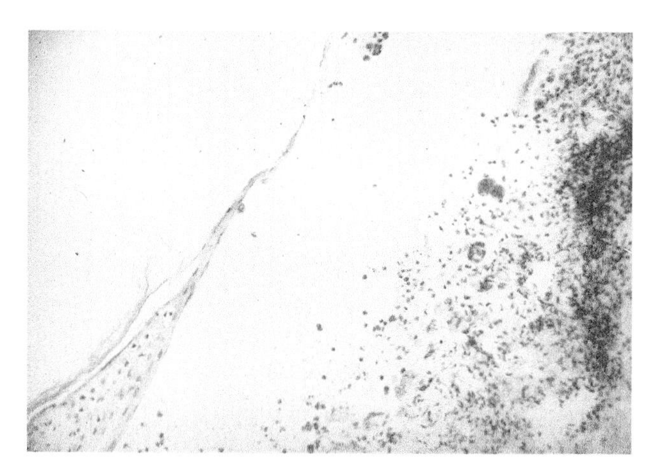

FIGURE 10.1 Histopathology of herpes simplex virus infection.

Vascular changes in infected tissue include perivascular cuffing and areas of hemorrhagic necrosis. These histopathologic findings become particularly prominent when organs other than skin are involved, for example, HSV encephalitis or disseminated neonatal HSV infection. In such cases, widespread areas of hemorrhagic necrosis, mirroring the area of infection, are prominent. With HSV encephalitis, oligodendrocytic involvement and gliosis are common, as is astrocytosis, but these changes develop late in the disease course. Local lymphatics can show evidence of infection with intrusion of inflammatory cells, draining infected secretions from the area of viral replication. The intensity of the inflammatory response is significantly less with recurrent disease. As host defenses develop, an influx of mononuclear cells is detected in infected tissue.

MODELS OF DISEASE PATHOGENESIS

Animal models allow study of the pathogenesis of infection but with fundamental problems. The animal species (indicative of susceptibility), virus type, route of infection, state of immune competence, and specific viral strain all influence disease pathogenesis. Both HSV-1 encephalitis (virulence) and latency models have been established in animals following inoculation by the eye route. However, the end points of virulence and latency do not routinely correlate with human disease. After ocular inoculation by corneal scarification, replication of virus in the eye peaks within 48 hours and declines over the next 6 days. Virus appears in the trigeminal ganglia approximately 1 day after inoculation, with peak replication occurring 4 to 6 days later. If sufficient quantities of virus and/or a virulent strain of virus are inoculated onto the eye, encephalitis follows virus replication within the trigeminal ganglia.

For HSV-1 cutaneous infections, mice (particularly the hairless mouse)[298] and rabbits or guinea pigs with abraded or punctured skin are used to study replication and disease pathogenesis as well as to evaluate antiviral therapies. The hairless mouse, guinea pig, and rabbit are all artificial models of human cutaneous infections, particularly for recurrent infections of humans.

HSV-2 mucosal infections have been studied most extensively in an intravaginal guinea pig model. Both HSV-1 and HSV-2 have been used in this model. These animals tend to experience continual recurrences of lesions, but retrieval of HSV from these lesions is variable. The guinea pig genital infection model has been used extensively in the assessment of vaccines and antiviral. The development of an intravaginal infection in rhesus macaques in which HSV-2 DNA is detected in sacral ganglia and spontaneous vaginal shedding is found up to 40 days after inoculation may also be useful to study interventions to prevent HSV-2 infection.[163]

Models of life-threatening disease include the intranasal inoculation of HSV-1 or HSV-2 in young (3-week-old) Balb/C mice, resulting in CNS and visceral (usually lung) disease (mimicking neonatal HSV infection). However, inoculation of older mice with similar quantities of either virus type may fail to cause disease, or, if it does lead to disease, it might be encephalitis but not multiorgan disease. Intracerebral inoculation of virus provides an unnatural route of infection even for the study of antiviral therapeutics; however, it is used to screen new drugs.

Accurate and predictive models of human HSV encephalitis have been described using rabbit[250,251] and mouse models. The resultant disease leads to focal localization of infection in the rabbit brain, as compared with diffuse pancortical infection of the mouse brain. Virus is inoculated directly into the olfactory bulb or upon abraded nasal epithelium of the rabbit over the nerves from the olfactory bulb.[278]

Human models of both labial and genital herpes have been reported. Induced reactivation of HSV labialis occurs by exposure of the vermilion border of the lip of seropositive individuals to UV light.[237] The resulting lesions and course of infection are similar to those that occur naturally. Lesions develop in approximately 70% of UV-exposed volunteers after approximately 3 days. This model has been exploited for the evaluation of antiviral therapies.[237,238] Similarly, UV exposure of the buttocks and thigh in HSV-2–infected individuals results in reactivation in approximately 35%, and the incubation period is longer, about 5 days.[238]

IMMUNE RESPONSE

Primary Immune Responses

The natural history of HSV infections is influenced by both innate and induced host defense mechanisms. Historically, animal models provided the majority of data that address the relationship between host defense and disease pathogenesis. Host genetic background, innate immune responses, macrophages, natural killer cells, specific T-cell subpopulations, specific antibodies, and cytokine responses are important host defenses against HSV infections. Human studies have been insightful.[273] Local control mechanisms of viral spread aim to neutralize the infectious agent and lead to viral clearance. Following primary HSV infection, the initial, local immunological responses involve both nonspecific defense mechanisms, namely interferons (IFNs) alpha and beta, activated natural killer (NK) cells, and macrophages, and HSV-specific responses, such as cytotoxic T cells (CTLs).[223] The role of T cells has attracted increasing attention, particularly as it relates to vaccine development, particularly for therapeutic, as opposed to prophylactic, vaccines.[111,116,142,156,224,241]

In response to a viral infection, the initial cellular response is synthesis and secretion of type I IFNs (α and β). IFNs induce an antiviral state in infected and surrounding cells. The antiviral activity is modulated in part by IFN-mediated activation of cellular enzymes such as 2′-5′ oligoadenylate synthetase (2′-5′ AS) and double-stranded RNA-dependent protein kinase, as well as intracellular signaling molecules through the activation of the JAK/STAT kinase pathway. More specific to HSV infection, IFN-α appears to inhibit immediate-early (IE) gene expression (see Chapter 9 for HSV cycle of replication). Thus, the antiviral mechanisms directly affect transactivation of the IE responsive element necessary for synthesis of viral proteins.

In addition to antiviral activity, IFNs are potent immunomodulators. As such, they mediate macrophage and NK cell activation, activate CTLs, induce MHC class I and MHC class II antigens, stimulate cytokine secretion, and induce local inflammation. IFN gamma may aid the control of HSV infection. Evidence that $\gamma\delta$ T cells, NK cells, CD4+ T cells, and possibly neurons produce IFN-γ and TNF in response to HSV infection in the nervous system has been reported. IFN-γ downregulates priming of CD4+ Th2 cells, which are responsible for inducing Ig isotype B cell switching from IgA to IgG, thereby exerting a major effect on humoral immune responses.[108]

NK cells lyse pathogen-infected cells before virus-specific T-cell immunity is generated and constitute first-line defense against infection. *In vitro* and *in vivo* experiments have demonstrated that NK cells protect from HSV challenge in a murine model. Severe herpetic disease has been correlated with low *in vitro* NK activity in newborns, as well as in a patient lacking NK cells.[28] Other mononuclear cells, such as macrophages, are recruited to the site of infection and, upon activation, release immune cell mediators such as TNF and interleukins. Macrophages play a major role in mediating antibody-dependent cellular cytotoxicity (ADCC) for viral clearance and antigen presentation.

Dendritic cells (DCs) travel from mucosal or skin areas of infection and prime antigen-specific, naive T cells in draining lymph nodes (DLN). Studies using HSV-1 footpad infection and fractionating DC subpopulations in the DLN show that classic, CD8α+ dermal DC, rather than specialized epidermal Langerhans cells (LCs), are able to prime naive CD8+ T cells.[19] In the case of vaginal HSV-2 infection, dermal DCs rather than LCs again seem to be the physiologically active cell population in a similar DLN investigation.[351] LCs are able to present HSV antigens to memory HSV-specific T cells and may participate in primary or recurrent immune reactions. Plasmacytoid

DCs (pDCs) react to HSV by producing IFN-α.[266] pDCs are recruited to sites of infection, participate in viral clearance, and express relevant Toll-like receptors (TLRs) including TLR 7, 8, and 9.[170,245] Low pDC number or poor pDC reactivity is associated with severe human HSV infection.[68]

As infection progresses, virus-specific immune responses are detected. On days 4 and 5 postinfection, HSV-specific CD4+ Th1 lymphocytes are detected in genital lymph nodes and in smaller numbers in peripheral blood; they can subsequently be found in the genital mucosa. CD8+ responses also occur quite quickly in the mouse.[196]

Humoral immune responses follow initial HSV infection. The predominant mucosal antibodies are of the IgA isotype, being secreted by plasma cells. Antibodies can be detected as early as day 3 following infection, peaking within the first 6 weeks after disease onset, and are followed by appearance of IgG1 and IgG3 subclasses of antibodies, which are typically found following viral infections. HSV-specific IgA antibodies are present for at least 6 weeks, gradually decreasing to undetectable levels. IgM-secreting B cells have also been detected in secretions of the female genital mucosa. Analyses of antibody responses by immunoblot and immunoprecipitation to infected cell polypeptides have been correlated with the development of neutralizing antibodies.[356] Soon after the onset of infection, antibodies to structural proteins are followed by those directed against gD, gB, ICP-4, gE, gG-1 or gG-2, and gC. Both IgM and IgG antibodies can be detected, depending on the time of assessment after infection.

Recurrent HSV Infection

Early on, cytokine production was incriminated in the pathogenesis of frequently recurrent genital and labial HSV infection. A decrease in both IFN-γ production and NK cells has been reported during the disease prodrome.[66] HSV-specific CD8 and CD4 T cells infiltrate latently infected trigeminal ganglia in mice and humans,[132,302] acting via IFN-γ. Neuronal loss is not seen clinically, and inhibitory receptor–ligand pairings can be documented in the ganglia that may modulate their cytotoxic activity.[283] HSV-2–specific CD4+ and CD8+ T cells localize to sites of recurrent HSV-2 infection and to the cervix.[144,145] Using *in situ* staining, HSV-2–specific CD8 CTLs persist at the epidermal/dermal junction adjacent to sensory nerve endings.[139,354] In human genital tissue, tissue resident memory CD8+ T cells remain at the dermal–epidermal junction in the mucosa after the resolution of lesions and are thought to play a role in immune surveillance.[355] Repeated subclinical episodes of HSV excretion may be a source of antigenic stimulation leading to long-term HSV-specific immune memory. In recurrent HSV-2 infections, NK and HSV-specific CD4+ cells are detected earlier than CD8+ cells in genital lesions.[108] CD4+ T cells and, more recently, CD8+ T cells have been highlighted as major mediators of viral clearance from mucocutaneous lesions in recurrent episodes.[144,223] Low IFN-γ titers in vesicle fluid have been associated with a shorter time to the next recurrence in patients with frequent recurrences. T-cell proliferation is decreased in these patients in comparison to patients with less-frequent recurrences. IFN-γ is associated with viral clearance from mucocutaneous sites, whereas altered cytokine production appears to correlate with recurrence.

A shorter duration of viral shedding occurs in women with recurrent genital herpes who have detectable secretory IgA in vaginal secretions. IgA, IgG1, and IgG3 antibodies develop in the sera of all patients with recurrent HSV-2 episodes, while IgM and IgG4 antibodies were detected in 70% to 80% of these patients.

Persistence of Immune Responses

The host's immune responses persist and partially control HSV disease; recurrent episodes are generally less severe and of shorter duration over the years, perhaps due to progressive enhancement of long-term immunity.[21] Differences in host immune response between episodes of symptomatic versus asymptomatic shedding have not been detected. Furthermore, some degree of cross-protection exists between HSV-1 and HSV-2, as best evidenced by partial protection of newborns by maternal antibodies.[327] HSV-specific T-cell infiltrates appear in lesions during early disease resolution.[223]

Studies indicate that persistent cell-mediated immune responses are more important than humoral immune responses in disease resolution.[26] NK cells, macrophages, and T lymphocytes as well as cytokines such as IFN-α and -γ, IL-2, and IL-12 all contribute to resolving HSV disease.[234] HSV-specific CD4+ and CD8+ cells are detected in lesions from recurrent episodes, suggesting a role in controlling HSV disease.[144,223] By contrast, agammaglobulinemic patients do not experience more severe or more frequent herpetic recurrences than the general population.[151] Several vaccine trials have demonstrated that the presence of neutralizing antibodies, albeit of varying titers, to HSV-2 glycoproteins do not provide protection against HSV-2 infection or disease.[275] However, a prophylactic vaccine study did suggest benefit for prevention of genital HSV-1 infection,[18] implying that with selection of the correct antigen and adjuvant, antibody responses may be protective against HSV infection.

Relationship Between Immune Response and Disease

Humoral immunity has been evaluated exhaustively in disease pathogenesis. In animal models, polyclonal antibodies have been used to alter disease lethality, particularly in the newborn mouse, or to limit progression of both neurologic and ocular disease. Monoclonal antibodies to selected specific infected cell polypeptides, especially the envelope glycoproteins gB and gD, confer protection from lethality.[73,232] gD2 is a known target of neutralizing antibodies, ADCC and CD4 and CD8 T-cell mediated responses[102,120,192,346]; thus, this antigen has been a prime component of subunit vaccines.

Efforts to correlate the frequency of recurrences with immune responses have failed to identify any specific humoral response to specified polypeptides.[23,126] Thus, further efforts have focused, in large part, on cell-mediated immune responses. As noted, lymphocyte blastogenic responses are demonstrable within 4 to 6 weeks after the onset of infection and sometimes as early as 2 weeks.[63,214,231,279] These responses are typically mediated by CD4 T cells. With recurrences, boosts in blastogenic responses occur; however, these responses, as after primary infection, decrease with time. Nonspecific blastogenic responses do not correlate with a history of recurrences. HSV-1 and 2 are cross-reactive in these assays at the whole virus levels, although individual T-cell clonotypic responses can be either type common or type specific.[140]

Lymphokine production has been incriminated in the pathogenesis of frequently recurrent genital and labial HSV infection. A decrease in both IFN-γ production and NK has been reported during disease prodrome.[66,208,260] No reproducible data confirm these observations. The relevance of lymphokine expression in vaccine development can be assessed only in prospective field trials.

Host response of the newborn to HSV must be defined separately from that of older individuals. Immaturity of host defense mechanisms is a cause of the increased severity of some infectious agents in the fetus and the newborn. Factors that must be considered in defining host response of the newborn include the mode of transmission of the agent (viremia vs. mucocutaneous infection without blood-borne spread) and time of acquisition of infection. Transplacentally acquired neutralizing antibodies either prevent or ameliorate infection in exposed newborns as does ADCC.[148,226,343] Preexisting antibodies, indicative of prior infection, significantly decrease the transmission of infection from pregnant women to their offspring,[32] contributing to the rationale for the development of an HSV vaccine.

Infected newborns produce IgM antibodies specific for HSV within the first 3 weeks of infection. These antibodies increase rapidly in titer during the first 2 to 3 months and may be detectable for as long as 1 year after infection. The most reactive antigens are the surface viral glycoproteins, particularly gD. Humoral antibody responses have been studied using immunoblot technology, resulting in patterns of response similar to those of adults with primary infection.[127,279] The quantity of neutralizing antibodies is lower in babies with disseminated infection.[279,343]

Cellular immunity has been considered to be important in the host response of the newborn. The T-lymphocyte proliferative responses to HSV infections are delayed in newborns compared to older individuals.[279] Most infants have no detectable T-lymphocyte responses to HSV 2 to 4 weeks after the onset of clinical symptoms.[214,230,279] The correlation between these delayed responses may be of significance in evaluating outcome to neonatal HSV infection. Specifically, if the response to T-lymphocyte antigens in children who have disease localized to the skin, eye, or mouth (SEM) at the onset of disease is significantly delayed, disease progression may occur at a much higher frequency than babies with a more appropriate response.[54,279]

Infected newborns have decreased production of IFN-α in response to HSV when compared to adults with primary HSV infection.[279] Lymphocytes from infected babies have decreased responses to IFN-γ during the first month of life.[37,279] In general, the newborn has poorer immune responses than older children and adults. Antibodies plus complement and antibodies mixed with NK, monocytes, macrophages, or polymorphonuclear leukocytes will lyse HSV-infected cells *in vitro*. ADCC is an important component of the development of host immunity to infection.[146] However, the total population of NK of the newborn seems to be lower than that found in older individuals and monocytes and macrophages of newborns are not as active as those of adults.[106,147,167,294] These findings are supported by animal model data.

Host Susceptibility

Clinically, elegant studies have identified several inborn errors involving single genes among children with HSV-1 encephalitis (HSE) and some adults. Single gene errors in the Toll-like receptor 3 (TLR3) signaling pathway have been associated with forebrain HSV-1 encephalitis (HSE), including *TLR3, TRIF, UNC93B1, TyK2, TRAF3, IRF3, and TBK1*.[194,244,349,350] Studies in two children, one with a loss of a functional mutation in nuclear factor-kB essential modulator (*NEMO*) and the other with an autosomal recessive mutation in signal transducer and activator of transcription 1 (*STAT-1*) genes, both encoding proteins essential for IFN production, developed HSE and *in vitro* studies showed that their cells had impaired interferon production upon exposure to HSV-1.[10,78] These seminal observations demonstrate the importance of the TLR3 and interferon pathways to contain HSV replication in the CNS.

Other studies of genetic susceptibility have been reported. Autosomal recessive DRB1 (an RNA lariat debranching enzyme) deficiency has been associated with brainstem HSV-1 infection.[348] Exome analysis of a cohort of patients with forebrain HSE has also revealed rare autosomal dominant variants in the small nucleolar RNA (*snoRNA*)-encoding gene, *snoRA31*, that are associated with increased HSV-1 replication in *in vitro* studies of cortical CNS neurons. The function of *snoRA31* is unknown *in vivo*, but in cortical neurons, it is a cell-intrinsic antiviral factor and is not dependent on the TLR3 pathway, suggesting a novel susceptibility mechanism for HSE.[154] In addition to identifying genetic susceptibility to HSE, these studies of rare genetic variants associated with HSE have greatly enhanced our understanding of HSV-1 pathogenesis in the CNS.[45,244,349] Such severe infections have been identified in severe combined immunodeficiency syndrome in the presence of a DOCK8 mutation.[347] Extensive studies of individuals with recurrent herpes labialis found an association with C21orf91 genotypes correlating with increased susceptibility.[152] Likely, further genetic associations will be identified.

EPIDEMIOLOGY

The development of serologic assays in the mid-1970s that reliably differentiated between HSV-1 and HSV-2 infection revolutionized the ability to understand the epidemiology of HSV infections.[200]

Orolabial HSV Infections: Primary and Recurrent

Humans are the sole reservoir for transmission of HSV to other humans. Virus is transmitted from infected to susceptible individuals during close personal contact. There is no seasonal variation in the incidence of infection. Because infection is both rarely fatal and is chronic, people have the potential to transmit HSV throughout their life span. As a result, HSV is one of the most prevalent infections worldwide. In 2012, 3.7 billion people aged 0 to 49 years were estimated to be infected with HSV-1, for a prevalence of 67% across all ages.[165] In addition, the annual incidence of HSV-1 infection is high, with an estimated 118 million new infections in 2012. Geographic location and age are primary factors that influence HSV-1 seroprevalence. For example, the worldwide prevalence of HSV-1 is estimated to increase from 27% among those aged 0 to 4, to 71% at age 15 to 19, and 79% at age 45 to 49. These estimates indicate that HSV-1 is most commonly acquired in childhood, likely through oral exposure, but acquisition can continue as people age. The prevalence of HSV-1 infection is similar

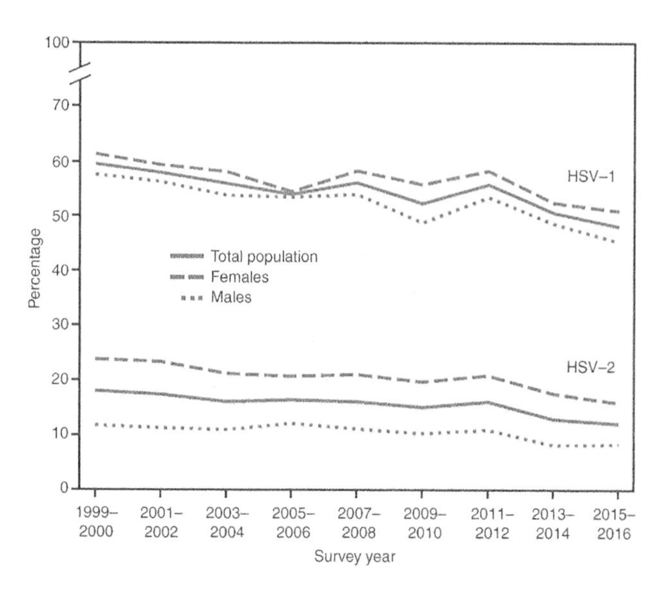

FIGURE 10.2 **QuickStats: Age-Adjusted Trends in the Prevalence of Herpes Simplex Virus Type 1 (HSV-1) and Herpes Simplex Virus Type 2 (HSV-2).** From QuickStats: Age-adjusted trends in the prevalence of Herpes Simplex Virus Type 1 (HSV-1) and Herpes Simplex Virus Type 2 (HSV-2) among adolescents and adults aged 14-49 Years - United States, 1999-2000 through 2015-2016. *MMWR Morb Mortal Wkly Rep* 2018;67(6):203. doi: http://dx.doi.org/10.15585/mmwr.mm6706a7.

among men and women. The highest HSV-1 seroprevalence rates are found in Africa (87% for both men and women), the Eastern Mediterranean (75% among men and women), and the Western Pacific (73%), with the lowest rates in the Americas (49% among women, 39% among men). Estimates are limited by small sample sizes and lack of data in some regions.

In the United States, periodic seroprevalence studies among those aged 14 to 49 have been performed in the National Health and Nutrition Examination Surveys (NHANES) since 1977,[84,200] using the same serologic assay. Between 1999–2000 and 2015–2016, the HSV-1 seroprevalence declined by over 11% to 48.1% in 2015–2016 (Fig. 10.2).[183] Between 1999 and 2010, the most substantial decline was found among those aged 14 to 19 (39% to 30%, a 23% decrease). In the United States, higher rates of HSV-1 seroprevalence are found among racial and ethnic minority groups compared to white populations. These associations are likely due to social factors such as lower household income and education and increased crowding,[31,71] rather than biologic factors. The declining HSV-1 seroprevalence is thought to be secondary to improvements in hygiene and decreased crowding, resulting in less oral HSV-1 transmission during childhood. Paradoxically, decreased HSV-1 acquisition during childhood may place adolescents at increased risk for genital HSV-1 infection when they become sexually active (see below). Similar findings have recently been observed in several European countries.[176,334]

Following the association of HSV and gingivostomatitis,[39] virologic screening was used to study the epidemiology and natural history of infection. Primary infection led to the shedding of virus in mouth and stool and from the former site for as long as 23 days (average, 7 to 10 days).[2] Neutralizing antibodies appeared between 4 and 7 days after the onset of disease and peaked in approximately 3 weeks. Virus was isolated from the saliva of asymptomatic children in approximately 20% of children 7 months to 2 years of age.[36] Virus shedding in children less than 6 months of age was uncommon. In older children, 3 to 14 years of age, asymptomatic shedding was documented in 18%. Retrieval of infectious virus decreased with advancing age, being only 2.7% in individuals over 15 years of age. These frequencies of shedding are similar to contemporary cross-sectional surveys, ranging from 2% to 5%. Application of PCR demonstrates higher frequencies of shedding and for intermittent periods.

In prospective studies of HSV-1 acquisition, evidence of oral herpetic infection was found in approximately 13% of children over a 10-year period. Children 1 to 2 years of age were most commonly infected, accounting for over half of all cases.[70,236] Most children experienced asymptomatic infection, accounting for over 65% of the seroconversions.[3,49]

In summary, these studies demonstrate that HSV-1 is acquired during childhood and adolescence, particularly in settings with greater crowding and lower socioeconomic status, and that in higher income settings there has been a significant decrease in seroprevalence over time. The frequency of direct person-to-person contact, indicative of crowding encountered with lower socioeconomic status, appears to be the major mediator of infection.

The largest human reservoir of HSV-1 is latent infection in the trigeminal ganglia, which reactivates leading to recurrent herpes labialis. Studies performed to assess the frequency and severity of recurrent infection in the immunocompetent host are limited. A positive history of recurrent herpes labialis was noted in 38% of 1,800 graduate students.[263,264] Lesions occurred at a frequency of one per month in 5% of students and at intervals of 2 to 11 months in 34% of the infected students. Recurrences of one per year or less often were found in 61%.[87,262]

Recurrent viral shedding occurs in the absence of clinical symptoms. Asymptomatic excretion of HSV in healthy children occurs in about 1% to 5%[92,318] Nearly 1% of pregnant women and nursery personnel excrete HSV at any time, providing a source of virus for transmission to the newborn. Asymptomatic shedding also occurs in nearly one-third of seropositive transplant recipients.[49,215,216]

Genital HSV Infections: Primary and Recurrent

Genital herpes can be caused by either HSV-1 or 2. Because infections with HSV-2 are usually acquired through sexual contact, antibodies to this virus are rarely found before the onset of sexual activity.[337] An increasing proportion of genital herpes is attributable to HSV-1.[79,128,335] Worldwide, there are estimated to be 140 million genital HSV-1 infections in persons aged 15 to 49.[165] Over 50% of first-episode genital herpes at some sexually transmitted disease (STD) clinics are caused by HSV-1.[67,79,337] In a recent prophylactic vaccine study enrolling sexually active HSV-1/HSV-2 seronegative women, the rate of infection for HSV-1 was more than twice that of HSV-2.[22] Modeling studies suggest that genital acquisition of HSV-1 will continue to increase over time, as oral acquisition declines.[12] The contribution of HSV-1 to overall genital infection cannot be defined by seroprevalence. Antibodies to HSV-1 do not distinguish between oral and genital infection. The distinction in virus type is not insignificant; genital HSV-1 infections are usually both less severe clinically and less prone to recur.[233]

In 2012, worldwide estimates of HSV-2 seroprevalence revealed that 11.3% of people aged 15 to 49 years were HSV-2 seropositive (an estimated 417 million people),[165] with an additional 19.2 million people with incident infection that year.

In contrast to HSV-1, HSV-2 seroprevalence is about twofold higher in women compared to men.[165] Similar to HSV-1 infection, HSV-2 seroprevalence increases with age, with an estimated 4.6% seroprevalence at age 15 to 19, increasing to 17% prevalence at age 45 to 49. The burden of HSV-2 infection is widely variable throughout the world, with an estimated 134.9 million people infected in the WHO African Region and 81.2 million in the WHO Western Pacific Region, as compared to only 24.9 and 31.4 in the WHO Eastern Mediterranean Region and WHO European Region, respectively. In the United States, the most recent NHANES survey in 2015–2016 showed an age-adjusted HSV-2 seroprevalence of 12.1% among those aged 14 to 49, a significant decrease from a high of 21.9% in 1988–1994 and from 18.0% in 1999–2000 (Tables 10.1 and 10.2 and Fig. 10.3).[183] In parallel, one study in Seattle, WA, found a significant decline in HSV-2 seroprevalence rates among pregnant women between 1989–1999 and 2000–2010, decreasing 46%, from 30.1% to 16.3%.[72] However, a NHANES study among women between 1999 and 2014 found stable HSV-2 seroprevalence among pregnant women and nonpregnant sexually active women.[84,183,219,338] Paralleling global estimates, United States seroprevalence increases with age, being 2-fold higher in women compared to men[81]. Antibodies to HSV-2 are virtually nonexistent in nuns, and HSV-2 seroprevalence increases with increasing numbers of lifetime sexual partners (Fig. 10.4),[338] indicating that sexual exposure is a significant risk factor for acquisition of HSV-2 infection. Although HSV-2 seroprevalence rates are decreasing for all racial/ethnic groups in the United States, racial disparities persist, with a 3.3-fold higher seroprevalence rate in black compared to white U.S. women in 2007–2010,[81] and worsening disparities seen in 2015–2016. Importantly, in 2007–2010, 87.4% of HSV-2 seropositive persons reported no history of an HSV-2 diagnosis.[81] NHANES last explored the association of HSV-2 seroprevalence with sexual behavior in 2001–2006. Among women who have sex exclusively with women, HSV-2 seroprevalence rates are relatively low (8.2%).[340] Men who have sex with men have a similar HSV-2 seroprevalence to men who have sex exclusively with women.[339] In 2003–2006, HSV-2 seroprevalence was significantly higher among person with HIV infection compared to the general population (59.7% vs. 19.2%).[218] HSV-2 serologic trends in the United States have been reported but require updating.[53]

Vaccine and antiviral studies have defined the risk of transmission.[64,158] First, women remain more susceptible to HSV infection than men. Second, transmission usually occurs from

TABLE 10.1 Herpes simplex virus type 2 seroprevalence[a] among persons aged 14 to 49 years, by selected characteristics—National Health and Nutrition Examination Survey, United States, 2005–2008

	Overall			Female			Male		
Characteristic	Sample Size	Sero-prevalence (%)	(95% CI[b])	Sample Size	Sero-prevalence (%)	(95% CI)	Sample Size	Sero-prevalence (%)	(95% CI)
Total	7,293	16.2	(14.6–17.9)	3,778	20.9	(18.9–23.1)	3,515	11.5	(9.8–13.3)
Age group (years)									
14–19	2,287	1.4	(1.0–2.0)	1,115	2.1	(1.4–3.0)	1,172	0.8[c]	(0.3–1.8)
20–29	1,710	10.5	(9.0–12.3)	952	14.4	(11.9–17.3)	758	6.6	(5.3–8.3)
30–39	1,657	19.6	(16.7–22.9)	861	25.2	(21.2–29.7)	796	13.9	(11.1–17.2)
40–49	1,639	26.1	(22.7–29.7)	850	32.3	(28.3–36.5)	789	19.6	(15.2–25.0)
Race/ethnicity[d]									
White, non-Hispanic	2,816	12.3	(10.7–14.2)	1,449	15.9	(13.6–18.7)	1,367	8.7	(6.9–10.9)
Black, non-Hispanic	1,742	39.2	(36.7–41.7)	893	48.0	(44.1–52.0)	849	29.0	(26.3–31.9)
Mexican American	1,822	10.1	(8.3–12.3)	944	13.2	(10.8–16.1)	878	7.5	(5.4–10.4)
Reported number of lifetime sex partners[e]									
1	879	3.9	(2.5–6.3)	587	5.4	(3.3–8.8)	292	1.7[c]	(0.7–4.2)
2–4	1,500	14.0	(12.1–16.2)	907	18.8	(16.3–21.5)	593	7.3	(5.3–9.8)
5–9	1,212	16.3	(13.4–19.6)	651	21.8	(17.6–26.7)	561	10.1	(7.6–13.4)
≥10	1,601	26.7	(23.2–30.4)	652	37.1	(33.6–40.8)	949	19.1	(15.2–23.6)

[a]All seroprevalence estimates were weighted using medical examination weights of the survey to represent the U.S. civilian, noninstitutionalized population, accounting for survey participants' unequal probabilities of selection and adjustments for nonresponse.
[b]Confidence interval.
[c]Relative standard error >30%.
[d]Data for persons of other racial/ethnic groups, including other Hispanic, Asian/Pacific Islander, American Indian/Alaska Native, and persons of multiple race/ethnicity (*n* = 913), are not presented because of small sample sizes but are included in the overall analyses.
[e]Excludes 2,101 persons who reported never having sex.
From Xu F, Sternberg MR, Gottlieb SL, Berman SM, Markowtiz LE, Division of STD Prevention, National Center for HIV/Aids, Viral Hepatitis, STD and TB Prevention, Forhan SE, Taylor LD, DrPH, EIS officers CDC. Seroprevalence of Herpes Simplex Virus Type 2 Among Persons Aged 14-49 Years - United States, 2005-2008. *MMWR Morb Mortal Wkly Rep* 2010;59(15):456-459.

TABLE 10.2 Prevalence of herpes simplex virus 2 antibodies in different populations

Site of Study	Year(s) of Study	Percent Prevalence of HSV-2 Antibodies
Different individuals		
Reykjavik, Iceland (pregnant women)	1979	4.1
	1985	23.4
Lyon, France (pregnant women)	1977–1978	10.7
	1985	17.3
Orebro, Sweden (pregnant women)	1982	11.8
	1985	16.1
Zaire	1959	21
Kinshasa	1985	60
Rural areas	1959	6
	1985	32
Same individuals		
Alabama (pregnant women)	1985	6-mo acquisition rate = 2%
South Carolina (university students)	1983	0.4 (acquisition rate = 2%/y)
San Francisco (homosexual men)	1987	7
	1978	44 (acquisition rate = 4%/y)
	1985	72

HSV-2, herpes simplex virus 2.

an asymptomatic individual and does so in over 70% of cases. Third, overall, the annual rate of transmission is approximately 4% to 5% per annum. The rate of acquisition by women is about 8% annually, whereas it is lower for men, namely 2%.

As with HSV-1 infections of the mouth, HSV-2 can be shed from the genital tract in the absence of symptoms after primary, initial, or recurrent infection.[295,312] Viral transmission most commonly occurs during episodes of asymptomatic shedding.[187] Initial studies used viral culture to detect HSV-2 from patient-collected swabs to determine rates of asymptomatic shedding.[141,312] Using HSV PCR to study HSV-2 shedding rates,[306] persons with symptomatic HSV-2 infection shed virus from the genital tract on 20% of days, while persons with asymptomatic HSV-2 shed on 10% of days.[295] Shedding rates are similar in men and women, and among those with and without HSV-1 coinfection.[295] Shedding episodes are short, lasting a

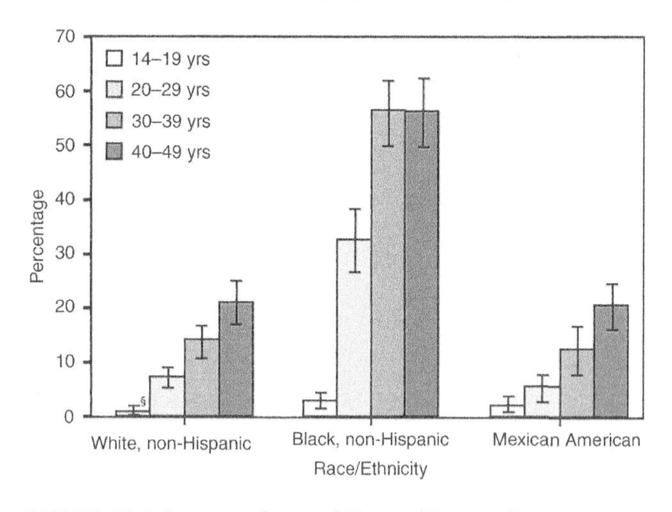

FIGURE 10.3 Seroprevalence of Herpes Simpex Virus Type 2 Among Persons Aged 14-49 years - United States 2005-2008. From Xu F, Sternberg MR, Gottlieb SL, Berman SM, Markowtiz LE, Division of STD Prevention, National Center for HIV/Aids, Viral Hepatitis, STD and TB Prevention, Forhan SE, Taylor LD, DrPH, EIS officers CDC. Seroprevalence of Herpes Simplex Virus Type 2 Among Persons Aged 14-49 Years - United States, 2005-2008. *MMWR Morb Mortal Wkly Rep* 2010;59(15):456-459.

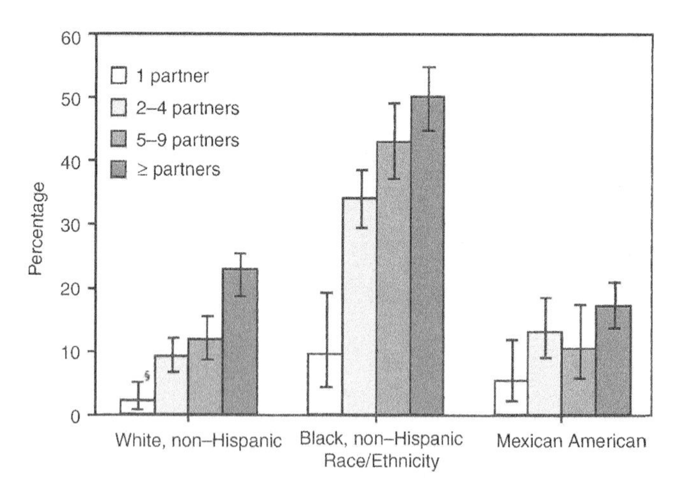

FIGURE 10.4 Seroprevalence of Herpes Simpex Virus Type 2 Among Persons Aged 14-49 years - United States 2005-2008. From Xu F, Sternberg MR, Gottlieb SL, Berman SM, Markowtiz LE, Division of STD Prevention, National Center for HIV/Aids, Viral Hepatitis, STD and TB Prevention, Forhan SE, Taylor LD, DrPH, EIS officers CDC. Seroprevalence of Herpes Simplex Virus Type 2 Among Persons Aged 14-49 Years - United States, 2005-2008. *MMWR Morb Mortal Wkly Rep* 2010;59(15):456-459.

median of 13 hours.[177] Viral shedding associated with symptomatic genital ulcer disease has higher shedding rates.[1] As a result, the viral shedding rate has been used as a marker of viral suppression in studies of novel HSV therapeutics.[1] Shedding of virus occurs more frequently in the first year following genital infection than in subsequent years,[311] but shedding persists for years or even decades after acquiring the virus.[221] Detailed anatomic surveys of genital tract shedding have also shown that shedding occurs throughout the genital tract on days with shedding, rather than being localized to a specific anatomic area.[124] These studies have helped redefine latency by demonstrating viral reactivation at the neuronal level is more permissive than realized.[121] Mathematical modeling studies suggest that HSV is frequently introduced into the genital tract in small quantities from neurons and that the immune response to infected epithelial cells is a key determinant of shedding and lesion frequency.[248,249]

The sacral ganglia contain the largest reservoir of HSV-2, and reactivation leads to recurrent HSV-2 infection. A recurrence is associated with a shorter duration of viral shedding and fewer lesions. The frequency of recurrences varies somewhat between males and females, with calculations of 2.7 and 1.9 per 100 patient-days, respectively. Detecting HSV by both culture and PCR, viral excretion was documented at 6% annually, but PCR detection of viral DNA occurred on 18% to 25% of days—a three- to fourfold increase over viral culture. Notably, there was an association between detection of virus by PCR (but not by culture) and person-to-person transmission.[295,312]

Several studies have reported a frequency of recurrence as high as 60%. Broadly, nearly 90% of HSV-2–infected patients will have one or more recurrences per year, 38% greater than 6 recurrences and 20% greater than 10 recurrences[20] HSV-1 infection recurs less frequently than does HSV-2 infection.[20,155]

HSV and HIV Interactions

HSV-2 infection, by nature of being an ulcerative disease, is associated with increased risk of acquisition of both human immunodeficiency virus type 1 (HIV-1) and human T-cell lymphotropic virus type 1 (HTLV-1) by two- to threefold,[86,309] in particular in regions where HIV and HSV-2 are both epidemic (Fig. 10.5). For example, in a prospective cohort study in Kenyan women between 1993 and 2012, prevalent HSV-2 infection was associated with 2.5-fold increased risk of acquiring HIV infection. When comparing the population attributable risk percentage (PAR%), the PAR% for prevalent HSV-2 infection was 48.3% and was stable over time, demonstrating the sustained impact of HSV-2 infection on the HIV epidemic. A systematic review and meta-analysis estimated a threefold increased risk of HIV acquisition among HSV-2 seropositive persons aged 15 to 49 in 2016, for an overall PAR% of 29.6%.[166] Not surprisingly, the PAR% was highest in settings with the highest HSV-2 seroprevalence, such as the WHO Africa region, and in women, who have a higher HSV-2 seroprevalence than men. HSV-2 infection is associated with an increased number of HIV target CCR5+CD4+ T cells in the female genital tract.[258,259] Similarly, when examining foreskin samples obtained after male medical circumcision, increased numbers of CD4+ T cells were found in the foreskin of HSV-2 seropositive men[118,119] compared to HSV-2 seronegative men, and foreskin inflammation was greatest among men with HIV and HSV-2 coinfection. At the site of a recurrent genital HSV-2 ulcer, increased numbers of CCR5+CD4+ target cells permissive for HIV infection persist[353] for weeks after the ulceration has healed. In addition, genital ulcer disease is associated with increased risk of HIV transmission to HIV seronegative partners. Unfortunately, studies of suppressive acyclovir among HSV-2 seropositive persons to prevent acquisition[47] or transmission of HIV infection did not provide evidence of effectiveness.[48] Furthermore, this study showed that acyclovir blood levels are lower in African subjects than in non-African subjects.[168]

Molecular Epidemiology

HSV molecular epidemiology has blossomed with the advent of high throughput (next-generation) sequencing. While HSV is a large (152 kB) and challenging virus to sequence given its high GC content and large repeat regions,[217] optimization of HSV sequencing has led to important insights into molecular epidemiology. Initial efforts utilized viral cultures of both laboratory strains and clinical isolates of HSV-1 for sequencing.[58,285]

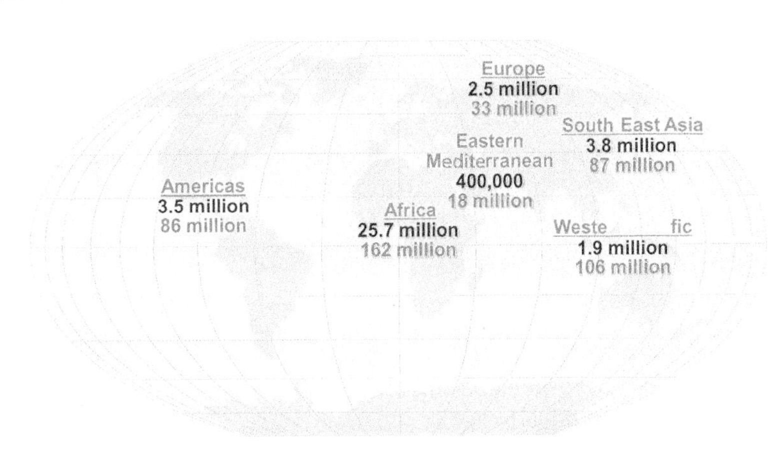

FIGURE 10.5 Persons living with HIV and persons infected with HSV-2. (Copyright David Knipe. HIV: World Health Organization; HSV-2: James et al. *Bull World Health Organ* 2020;98:315–329.)

These studies revealed both heterogeneity between laboratory and clinical strains as well as overall stability of a single strain in culture over time.[57] Twenty HSV-1 strains were sequenced from around the world, revealing both geographic clustering and a high degree of HSV-1 × HSV-1 recombination.[284] After revealing significant differences in the pathogenicity and sequence of the canonical HSV-2 laboratory strain, HG52, and a low-passage clinical isolate from South Africa, SD90e HSV-2 clinical isolates from around the world were sequenced, revealing little overall sequence variation (maximum nucleotide divergence: 0.4%) and no geographic clustering patterns.[57,203] Frequent HSV-1 × HSV-2 recombination was identified in another cohort of clinical HSV-2 samples.[143] HSV-1 sequencing in unique patient cohorts has provided insight into the exceptional stability of viral genomes over time. For instance, a father–son pair, each with 4 to 5 recurrences of oral HSV-1 infection per year had a reported transmission event nearly 20 years prior. Viral isolates collected from an oral HSV-1 recurrence were sequenced (father 43 years postinfection, son 17 years postinfection). The genomes were 98.9% identical at the consensus level, with only 2 differences that affected coding sequences.[210] These viruses had similar pathogenicity in a mouse ocular model of infection. Similarly, a woman with recurrent symptomatic genital HSV-1 infection had several samples sequenced over a 4-month period, and these were 98.5% identical overall.[265] Two participants in a prophylactic HSV-2 vaccine study had HSV-2 genomes sequenced from primary infection and with a 5th or 6th recurrence, revealing virtual identity, with fewer than 10 nonsynonymous changes between the two samples from each.[189] These studies suggest very slow evolution in the host, despite frequent recurrences. Sequencing studies have also suggested that infection with more than one strain of HSV-2 is quite rare. Only 18 (3.9%) of 459 people had dual-strain infection; HIV seropositivity was found to be a significant risk factor.[122]

Maternal Genital HSV Infections

Genital HSV infection in the pregnant woman poses a risk to fetus and newborn.[97] An uncommon problem encountered with HSV infections during pregnancy is that of widely disseminated maternal disease.[318] In a limited number of cases, dissemination after primary oropharyngeal or genital infection has led to life-threatening disease, such as necrotizing hepatitis with or without thrombocytopenia, leukopenia, disseminated intravascular coagulopathy, and encephalitis. The mortality rate among these pregnant women is reported to be greater than 50%. Fetal deaths also have occurred in more than 50% of cases, although mortality did not necessarily correlate with the death of the mother. Surviving fetuses were delivered by cesarean section and none had evidence of neonatal HSV infection. Fortunately, with the advent of safe antiviral therapy, symptomatic HSV infection can be treated in pregnant women.

From several prospective trials, the major risk to the fetus is maternal primary or initial genital HSV infection.[34,153] Thus, identification of the woman at risk for primary infection (seronegative for HSV-2 or both types) is important. Studies of the discordant serologic status of sexual partners and rates of acquisition of genital HSV-2 infection define this problem.[34] Primary or initial genital infection occurs at rates from 5.0% to 10% per year.[35] If a pregnant woman experiences initial or primary genital infection in the last trimester of gestation, the likelihood of transmission to the fetus is between 30% and 50%. On the other hand, recurrent maternal infection is associated with a rate of transmission of 3% or less.[33] These different rates of transmission have direct implications on strategies to prevent neonatal disease or at least ameliorate it if the child is inadvertently delivered through an infected birth canal. In the United States, approximately 1 in 2,000 live births (~2,000 per year) are infected with HSV.[175]

Maternal primary infection before 20 weeks of gestation in some women has been associated with spontaneous abortion. The contribution of primary maternal genital infection to spontaneous abortion must be weighed above that of a routine rate of fetal loss of approximately 20%. Infection that develops later in gestation has not been associated with the termination of pregnancy.[97,99]

Recurrent infection is the most common form of infection during gestation. Transmission of infection to the fetus is usually related to shedding of virus at the time of delivery. The actual prevalence of viral excretion at delivery is about approximately 0.5% for all women, irrespective of past history.[304]

Several prospective studies have evaluated the frequency and nature of viral shedding in pregnant women with a known history of genital herpes. In a predominantly white, middle-class population, documented recurrent infection occurred in 84% of pregnant women with a history of herpes.[304] Asymptomatic viral shedding occurred in at least 12% of the recurrent episodes. Viral shedding from the cervix occurred in 0.56% of symptomatic infections versus 0.66% of asymptomatic infections and higher in some populations (3%).[7] The frequency of recurrences has not been shown to be different from one pregnancy to the next for a given woman. The frequency of shedding does not appear to vary by trimester during gestation.[304] Most infants who develop neonatal disease are born to women who are completely asymptomatic for genital HSV infection and have neither a past history of genital herpes nor a sexual partner reporting a genital vesicular rash.[324,329,333] These women account for 60% to 80% of all women whose infected children become clinically ill.

CLINICAL MANIFESTATIONS OF DISEASE

HSV disease ranges from the usual case of mild illness or asymptomatic in the majority of individuals, to sporadic, severe, and life-threatening disease in a few infants, children, and adults. Although HSV-1 and HSV-2 are usually transmitted by different routes and can involve different areas of the body, there is a great deal of overlap between the epidemiology and clinical manifestations of these two viruses. Historically, primary HSV-1 oropharyngeal infections occurred in the young child, less than 5 years of age, and were most often asymptomatic. More recently, HSV-1 infections have become a significant cause of genital herpes as the first manifestation of disease, as is discussed below.[338] When the oropharynx is involved, the mouth and lips are the most common sites of HSV-1 infections, causing gingivostomatitis; however, any organ can become infected with this virus.

Primary/Recurrent Oropharyngeal Disease

The clinical symptoms of primary HSV-1 infections vary greatly. Infection can be totally asymptomatic or result in

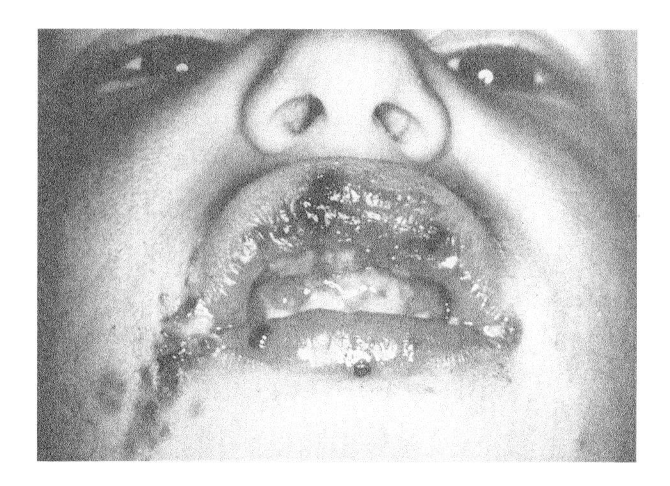

FIGURE 10.6 **Herpes simplex gingivostomatitis.**

combinations of fever, sore throat, ulcerative and vesicular lesions, gingivostomatitis, edema, localized lymphadenopathy, anorexia, and/or malaise. Asymptomatic infection is the rule rather than the exception. The incubation period ranges from 2 to 12 days, with a mean of approximately 4 days.

Symptomatic disease in children is characterized by involvement of the buccal and gingival mucosa (Fig. 10.6).[270] The duration of clinical illness may be from 2 to 3 weeks with fever of 101°F to 104°F. Children with symptomatic primary infection often are unable to swallow liquids because of the significant edema and ulcerative lesions of the mucosal membranes and the associated pain. Intraoral lesions do not scab. Submandibular lymphadenopathy is common with primary HSV gingivostomatitis but rare with recurrent infections. A clinical distinction should be drawn between intraoral gingival lesions and lip lesions indicative of presumed primary and recurrent infections, respectively. Utilizing PCR detection of viral DNA, evidence of viremia can be documented in approximately one-third of symptomatic patients with primary infection.[98]

With primary HSV infections during adulthood, HSV pharyngitis in association with a mononucleosis syndrome is common. Ulcerative tonsillar lesions on an erythematous base with associated submandibular lymphadenopathy are characteristic.[92] The differential diagnosis of both primary HSV gingivostomatitis and pharyngitis includes herpangina (caused by coxsackieviruses), *Candida albicans*, group A streptococcal infections, Epstein-Barr or cytomegalovirus-induced mononucleosis, lesions induced by chemotherapy or radiation therapy, and Stevens-Johnson syndrome.

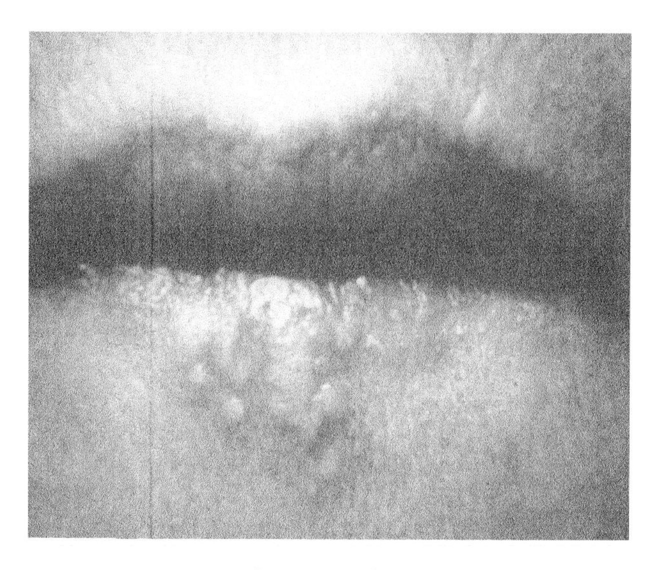

FIGURE 10.8 **Recurrent herpes simplex labialis.**

The onset of recurrent orolabial lesions is heralded by a prodrome of pain, burning, tingling, or itching, which generally lasts for less than 6 hours followed by vesicle formation.[271] The natural history of recurrent herpes labialis is illustrated in Figure 10.7.[270] Vesicles appear most commonly at the vermillion border of the lip and persist in most patients 48 hours or less (Fig. 10.8).[318] Vesicles generally number 3 to 5. The total area of involvement usually is less than 100 mm^2 and lesions progress to the pustular or ulcerative and crusting stage within 72 to 96 hours. Pain is most severe at the outset and resolves quickly over 96 to 120 hours. Similarly, the loss of

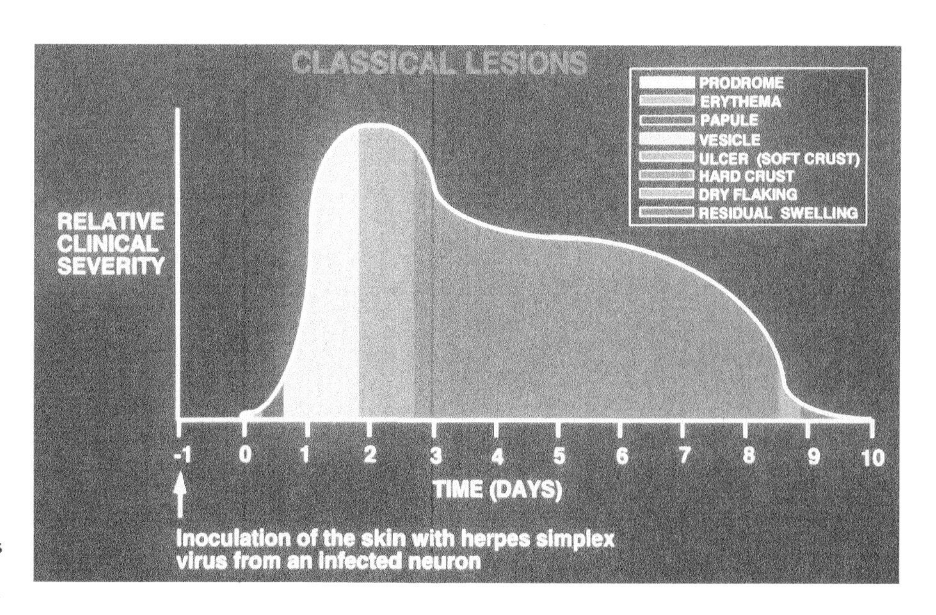

FIGURE 10.7 **Herpes simplex labialis natural history.**

virus from lesions decreases with progressive healing over 2 to 3 days.[13,271] Healing is rapid, generally being complete in 8 to 10 days. The frequency of recurrences varies among individuals.[271] Factors responsible for recurrences are highly variable but include fever, stress, immunosuppression, and exposure to UV light.[262]

Primary/Initial/Recurrent Genital Disease

Symptomatic primary genital infection is usually the most severe. After acquisition of HSV infection at a mucocutaneous site, macules and papules, followed by vesicles, pustules, and ulcers, appear. The duration of lesions averages 3 weeks. There are both similarities and differences in the clinical symptomatology between men and women with infection.[59] Furthermore, there appears to be no difference in clinical symptoms associated with primary genital HSV infection attributed to either virus type.

Primary infection is associated with (a) larger quantities of virus replicating in the genital tract (more than 10^6 viral particles per 0.2 mL of inoculum) and (b) a period of viral excretion that may persist for 3 weeks in the absence of antiviral treatment. Systemic complications in men are relatively uncommon; however, aseptic meningitis can develop. Paresthesias and dysesthesias that involve the lower extremities and perineum can result from genital herpetic infection. Primary infections can be associated with fever, dysuria, localized inguinal adenopathy, and malaise in both men and women. The severity of primary infection and its association with complications are statistically higher in women than in men, for unknown reasons. Systemic complaints are common in both sexes, approaching 70% of all cases. Extragenital lesions are common.

In women with primary infection, lesions appear on the vulva and are usually bilateral, as shown in Figure 10.9,[236] with the cervix often involved. The actual frequency of primary cervical infection in the absence of vulvar infection is unknown. Lesions usually are excruciatingly painful, associated with inguinal adenopathy and dysuria, and may involve the vulva, perineum, buttocks, cervix, and/or vagina. A urinary retention syndrome occurs in 10% to 15% of females, and as many as 25% will develop aseptic meningitis.

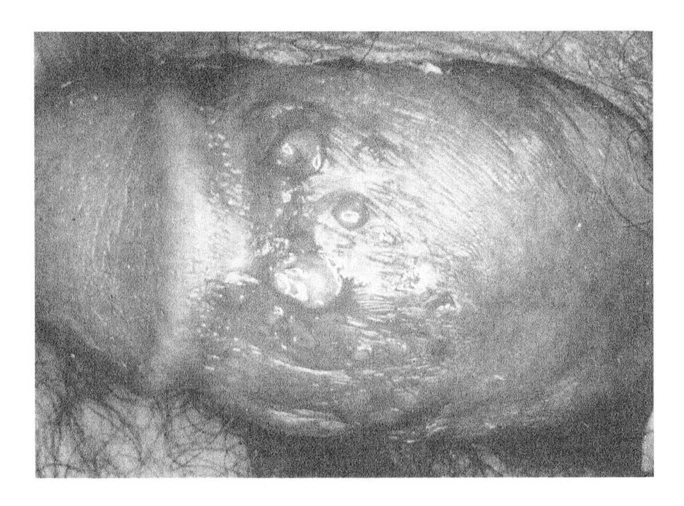

FIGURE 10.10 **Genital herpes simplex infection (male).**

In men, primary genital HSV infections are most often associated with vesicular lesions superimposed on an erythematous base, usually appearing on the glans penis or the penile shaft, as shown in Figure 10.10.[236] The total number of lesions can vary significantly. Extragenital lesions of the thigh, buttocks, and perineum can occur.

Complications of primary genital herpetic infection have included sacral radiculomyelitis, which can lead to urinary retention, neuralgias, and meningoencephalitis.[103,105,288] Primary perianal and anal HSV-2 infections, as well as associated proctitis, are common in men who have sex with men.[95] HSV-2 can be isolated from the rectum of heterosexual males and females. Many primary HSV-2 illnesses are subclinical, often involving the uterine cervix.[344]

Nonprimary but initial genital infection (i.e., occurring in an individual with preexisting antibody to the other virus type) is less severe symptomatically and heals more quickly than does primary infection. The duration of disease approximates 2 weeks. The number of lesions, severity of pain, and likelihood of complications are significantly decreased compared to primary infection. Preexisting antibodies to HSV-1 appear to

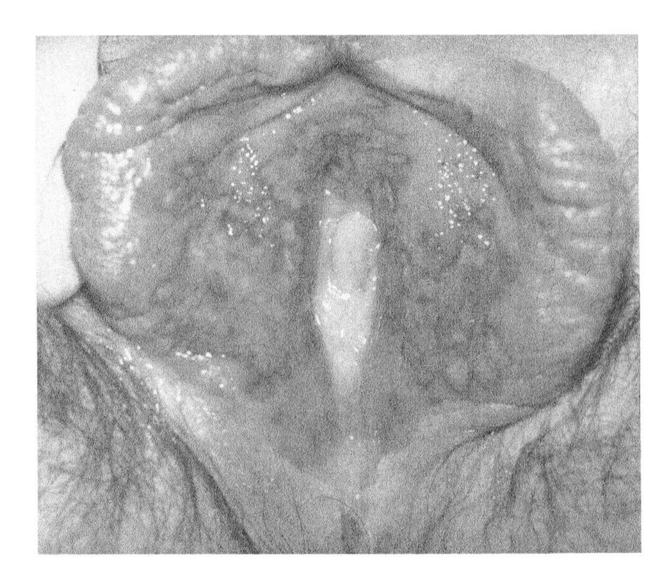

FIGURE 10.9 **Genital herpes simplex infection (female).**

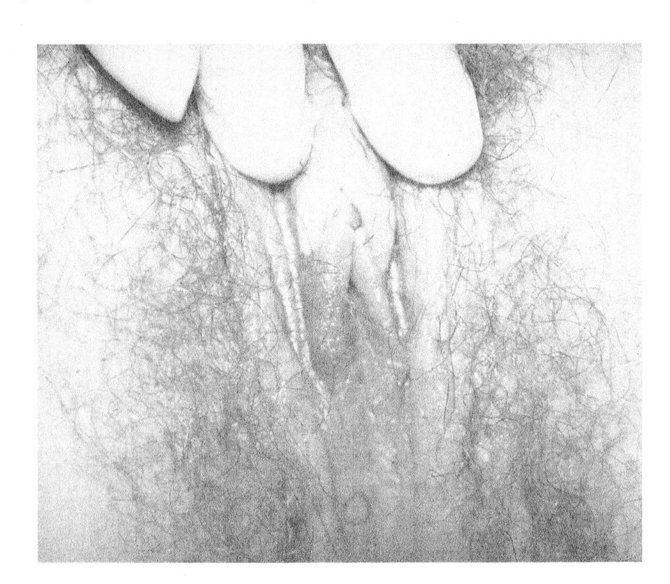

have an ameliorative effect on disease severity of HSV-2[252,312] but do not prevent infection.

Recurrent genital herpes is usually a much milder form of disease. With recurrent genital herpetic infection, a limited number of vesicles, usually 3 to 5, appear on the shaft of the penis of the male or as simply a vulvar irritation in the female. The duration of disease is approximately 7 to 10 days and parallels that encountered with recurrent HSV labialis. Neurologic or systemic complications are uncommon with recurrent disease; however, paresthesias and dysesthesias can occur.

Some individuals experience their "first-episode" genital infection years after an asymptomatic or atypical primary infection. Therefore, when antibody to the virus has already developed, it is difficult to determine when acquisition of the virus occurred.

The extent of viral replication is different for recurrent infection as compared with primary infection. Virus is shed for an average of only 2 to 5 days and at lower concentrations (~10^2 to 10^3 per 0.2 mL of inoculum in tissue culture systems). Recurrent genital infection in both men and women is characterized by prodrome consisting of tingling/itching or burning, which is thought to be caused by virus traveling down the nerves[169] and localized irritation.

A major problem with genital HSV infection is the frequency of recurrences, which varies substantially from one individual to the next. Anecdotally, the severity of primary infection correlates directly with the frequency of recurrences; that is, the more severe the primary infection, the more likely and frequent the recurrences. Notably, virtually all patients will suffer from recurrences, whether symptomatic or asymptomatic. For those individuals with genital HSV-1 infection, the probability of recurrences is significantly less and, in some patients, virtually not at all.[21] HSV-2 genital infections are prone to recur. One-third of patients are estimated to have recurrences in excess of six times per year, one-third will have two to three per year, and the remaining third will have four to six. With recurrences, either symptomatic or asymptomatic, transmission of infection to sexual partners can occur with intimate contact.

Neonatal HSV Infection

Incidence and Transmission of Newborn Infection

The estimated incidence of neonatal HSV infection is approximately 1 in 2,000 deliveries per year in the United States.[125,175] Globally, there are estimated to be 10.3 cases of neonatal herpes per 100,000 livebirths.[164] At least four factors influence transmission of infection from mother to fetus. First, maternal primary or first-episode genital infection during the third trimester results in a transmission rate of 30% to 50% as compared with 3% or less with recurrent infection.[32,34] Second, transplacental maternal neutralizing and ADCC antibodies appear to have an ameliorative effect on acquisition of infection and disease presentation.[9,226,342,343] Third, rupture of membranes more than 6 hours increases the risk of transmission. Fourth, the use of fetal scalp monitors is associated with increased risk.[130,213]

Acquisition and Presentation of Infection

Infection of the newborn can be acquired *in utero (congenital)*, intrapartum, or postnatally. The mother is the source of infection for the first two of these routes of transmission.[97,317]

Congenital Infection

In utero infection can occur as a consequence of either transplacental or ascending infection.[14,114] The incidence has been estimated to be 1 in 200,000 deliveries.[14] Intrauterine infection is characterized by the triad of skin vesicles or skin scarring, eye disease (chorioretinitis or microphthalmia), and the far more severe manifestations of microcephaly or hydranencephaly.

Intrapartum Infection

The most common route of infection is that of intrapartum contact of the fetus with infected maternal genital secretions. Likely, 80% to 90% of infected babies acquire HSV infection by this route. Babies who are infected intrapartum or postnatally with HSV infection are classified as having: (a) disease localized to the skin, eye, and mouth (SEM); (b) encephalitis with or without skin involvement; and (c) disseminated infection that involves multiple organs, including the CNS, lung, liver, adrenals, skin, eye, and/or mouth.[136,331]

Disseminated infection has the highest mortality and morbidity,[324] typically presenting for therapy at 9 to 11 days of age. The principal afflicted organs are the liver, lungs, and adrenals, but virtually all organs can be involved. Constitutional signs and symptoms include irritability, seizures, respiratory distress, jaundice, bleeding diatheses, shock, and, frequently, the characteristic vesicular exanthem, which is often considered pathognomonic for infection. Encephalitis is a common component of this form of infection, occurring in about 60% to 75%. Over 20% of these children do not develop skin vesicles during the course of their illness.[324] Mortality in the absence of therapy exceeds 80%; all but a few survivors are impaired. Death in these babies is caused either by HSV pneumonitis or by disseminated intravascular coagulopathy.

Babies with infection of the CNS alone or in combination with disseminated disease (75%) present with the findings of encephalitis. Clinical manifestations of encephalitis include seizures (both focal and generalized), lethargy, irritability, tremors, poor feeding, temperature instability, bulging fontanelle, and pyramidal tract signs. Whereas babies with disseminated infection often have skin vesicles in association with brain infection, the same is not true for the baby with encephalitis alone. This latter group of children may only have skin vesicles in approximately 60% of cases at any time during the disease.[97,280,324] Death occurs in 50% of babies with localized CNS disease who are not treated. Survivors are left with severe neurologic impairment.[319,325]

The long-term prognosis, after either disseminated infection or encephalitis, is poor in the absence of antiviral therapy. As many as 50% of surviving children have some degree of psychomotor retardation, often in association with microcephaly, hydranencephaly, porencephalic cysts, spasticity, blindness, chorioretinitis, or learning disabilities. Recent data suggest that CNS damage can be progressive after initial therapy, as predicated upon long-term antiviral suppressive data administered to babies with encephalitis. Indeed, this may represent low-grade replication of HSV in the brain.

Subclinical infection of the CNS has been detected in babies with disease apparently localized to the SEM. These children had normal cerebrospinal fluid (CSF) assessments but PCR-detectable HSV DNA at the onset of disease.[135] Subsequently, a subset of these children developed neurologic impairment.

Importantly, in as many as 40% of children with disease localized to the CNS (e.g., the 2- to 3-week-old baby with cells and protein in the CSF), skin vesicles (the classic sign of disease) are not present. For the neonate with CSF findings indicative of infection, HSV must be considered along with bacterial pathogens (e.g., group B *streptococcus*, *Escherichia coli*).

Infection localized to the SEM is associated with lower mortality, but morbidity can occur. When infection is localized to the skin, the presence of discrete vesicles remains the hallmark of disease. With time, the rash can progress to involve other areas of the body as well, particularly if viremia occurs. Vesicles occur in 90% of children with SEM infection, presenting at about 10 to 11 days of life. Skin lesions invariably will recur, regardless of whether therapy was administered. Although death is not associated with disease localized to the SEM, approximately 30% of these children eventually develop neurologic impairment.[319,325,329] The skin vesicles usually erupt from an erythematous base and are 1 to 2 mm in diameter. Other manifestations of skin lesions have included a zosteriform eruption.[198]

Infections involving the eye may manifest as keratoconjunctivitis or, later, as chorioretinitis. The eye can be the only site of HSV involvement.[325] These children present with keratoconjunctivitis or evidence of microphthalmia and retinal dysplasia.

Postnatal Acquisition

Postnatal acquisition of HSV-1 accounts for about 10% of cases.[159,160,199,281] The presentation is similar to that described above and usually is the consequence of family contact with the newborn.

Herpes Simplex Keratoconjunctivitis

Viral infections of the eye are usually caused by HSV-1 beyond the newborn age.[27,207] Approximately 300,000 cases of HSV infections of the eye are diagnosed yearly in the United States. These infections are second only to trauma as the cause of corneal blindness in the United States. Primary herpetic keratoconjunctivitis is associated with either unilateral or bilateral conjunctivitis, which can be follicular in nature, followed soon thereafter by preauricular adenopathy. HSV infection of the eye is also associated with photophobia, tearing, eyelid edema, and chemosis, accompanied by the pathognomonic findings of branching dendritic lesions (Fig. 10.11).[236] Less commonly,

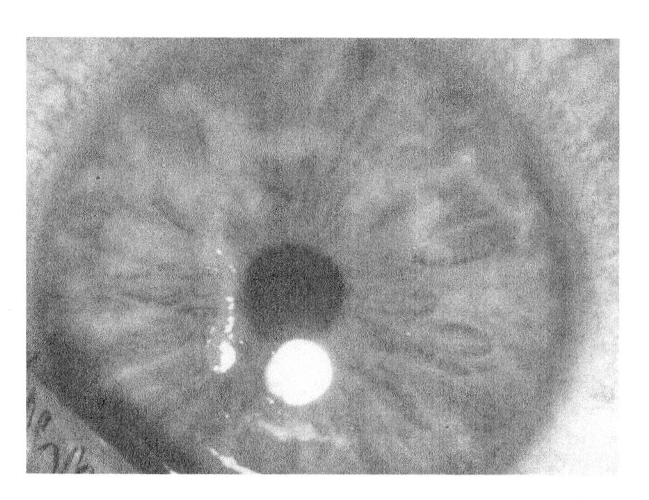

FIGURE 10.11 Dendritic lesions of herpes simplex keratoconjunctivitis.

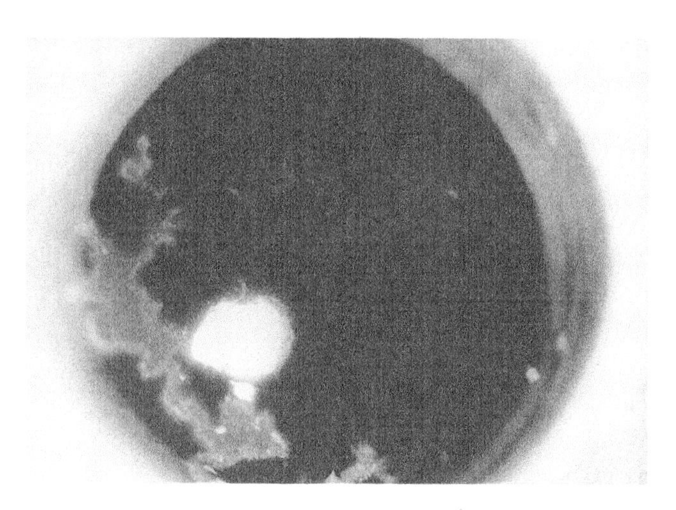

FIGURE 10.12 Geographic corneal ulcer caused by herpes simplex virus infection.

with progressive disease, the infection is associated with a geographic ulcer of the cornea (Fig. 10.12).[236] Healing of the cornea can take as long as 1 month, even with appropriate antiviral therapy.

Recurrent HSV infections of the eye are common. Most frequently, recurrences are unilateral in involvement, but a small percentage of cases involve both eyes. Characteristically, either dendritic ulceration or stromal involvement occurs. Visual acuity is decreased in the presence of the ulcers; with progressive stromal involvement, opacification of the cornea may occur. The route and pathogenesis of infection remain unknown. Progressive disease results in visual loss and even rupture of the globe.

Skin Infections

Skin infections caused by HSV generally manifest as eczema herpeticum in patients with underlying atopic dermatitis, occurring in 1% to 2%.[228,287,315] The lesions can either be localized, resembling herpes zoster with a dermatomal distribution, or disseminated. The latter occurs commonly in Kaposi's varicella-like eruption. HSV infections of the digits, known as herpetic whitlow, have been reported and are particularly common among medical and dental personnel.[239] The estimated incidence is 2.4 cases per 100,000 individuals per year, and the cause may be HSV-1 or HSV-2.[91] With the uniform use of disposable gloves by medical personnel, the incidence has decreased.

In addition to individuals with atopic disease, patients with skin abrasions or burns appear particularly susceptible to HSV-1 or HSV-2 infections and some may develop disseminated infection. Disseminated HSV infections have been also reported among wrestlers (herpes gladiatorum).[316] Other skin disorders associated with extensive cutaneous lesions include Darier disease and Sézary syndrome.[101,107] Localized recurrences followed by an episode of dissemination have been reported. HSV infections of either type can trigger erythema multiforme.[314] The presence of HSV DNA in skin lesions of erythema multiforme is as high as 80%.

Infections of the Immunocompromised Host

Patients compromised by immunosuppressive therapy, underlying disease, or malnutrition are at increased risk for

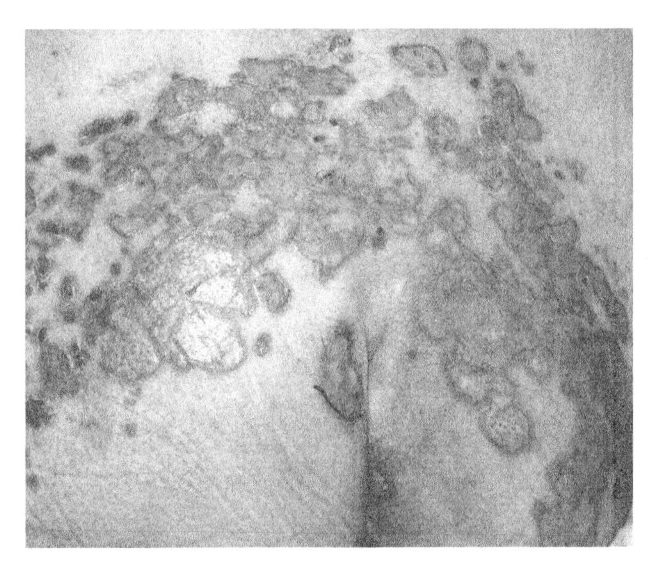
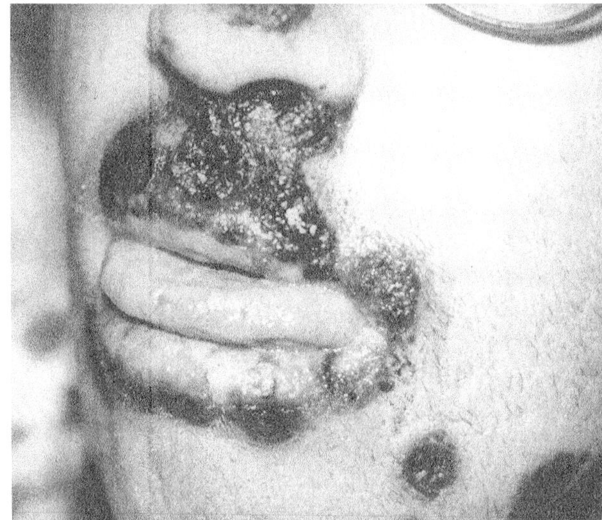

FIGURE 10.13 **Cutaneous dissemination of herpes simplex virus infection in an immunocompromised host.**

severe HSV infections. Renal, hepatic, stem cell, and cardiac recipients are all at risk for increased severity of HSV infection.[197,215,328] An example of cutaneous dissemination after shaving, in a renal transplant recipient, is shown in Figure 10.13.[236] Acquisition of HSV infection from a transplanted organ (kidney) has been reported.[77] These patients may develop progressive disease involving the respiratory tract, esophagus, or even the gastrointestinal tract.[150,193] The severe nature of progressive disease in these patients appears to be directly related to the type of immunosuppressive therapy. Esophagitis is a common occurrence in the immunocompromised host and can be caused by HSV, cytomegalovirus, or *Candida albicans*. Notably, acyclovir-resistant HSV disease can occur in the immunocompromised host and can be progressive. Reactivation of latent HSV infections in these patients can occur at multiple sites, and healing in these patients with severe progressive disease occurs over an average of 6 weeks.[332]

Since the first reports of acquired immunodeficiency syndrome (AIDS), the severity of HSV clinical disease in the absence of antiretroviral therapy was noted.[313] Disease severity correlates with CD4 count and the probability of developing resistance to antiviral therapy. Atypical, hypertrophic or "pseudotumor" lesions that mimic squamous cell carcinoma may occur in patients with HIV infection.[246] Furthermore, after starting antiretroviral therapy in persons with a low CD4 count and HSV-2 infection, genital HSV recurrences and genital ulcer disease increase, possibly as a manifestation of the immune reconstitution inflammatory syndrome.[83,225,290] Asymptomatic excretion of HSV can occur even in the immunocompromised host, as is best exemplified in HIV-infected individuals.[247,312]

Infections of the Central Nervous System

Herpes simplex encephalitis (HSE) is one of the most devastating of all HSV infections (Fig. 10.14),[236] being the most common cause of sporadic, fatal encephalitis in this country,[206,323] having an incidence of approximately 1 in 250,000 individuals per year (1,250 cases in the United States).

HSV encephalitis is primarily a focal encephalitis associated with fever, altered consciousness, bizarre behavior, disordered mentation, and localized neurologic findings.[317] These clinical signs and symptoms generally are associated with evidence of localized temporal lobe disease.[330,331] There are no pathognomonic findings of HSE; however, a progressively deteriorating level of consciousness, fever, an abnormal CSF formula with a lymphocytic predominance and/or blood, and focal neurologic findings in the absence of other causes should make this disease highly suspect. In the absence of antiviral therapy, mortality exceeds 70%, and only 2.5% of all patients return to normal neurologic function.

Neurodiagnostic procedures used in the evaluation of patients with suspected HSV encephalitis include CSF examination, electroencephalogram, and, preferably, a magnetic resonance image scan. Characteristic abnormalities of the CSF include elevated levels of cells (usually mononuclear) and protein. Red blood cells are found in most (but not all) CSF obtained from patients with HSV encephalitis. The electroencephalogram generally demonstrates localized spike and slow-wave activity in the temporal lobe. A burst suppression pattern is considered characteristic of HSV encephalitis. Imaging indicates localization of disease to the temporal lobe with evidence of edema that is followed by evidence of hemorrhage and a midline shift in the cortical structures.

PCR detection of HSV DNA in the CSF is the diagnostic modality of choice.[157] Serologic assessments of serum or CSF for HSV antibodies are not helpful early in the disease course when therapeutic decisions are mandatory.[201]

Other Neurologic Syndromes

In addition to encephalitis, HSV can involve nearly all anatomic areas of the nervous system including meningitis, myelitis, and radiculitis, among others.[65] Aseptic meningitis is a common occurrence in individuals with primary genital HSV infections. Recurrent aseptic meningitis (Mollaret syndrome) will occur in patients with genital herpes.[296] Notably, HSV DNA has been detected in the brain from all lobes at autopsy in individuals dying from other causes.[15]

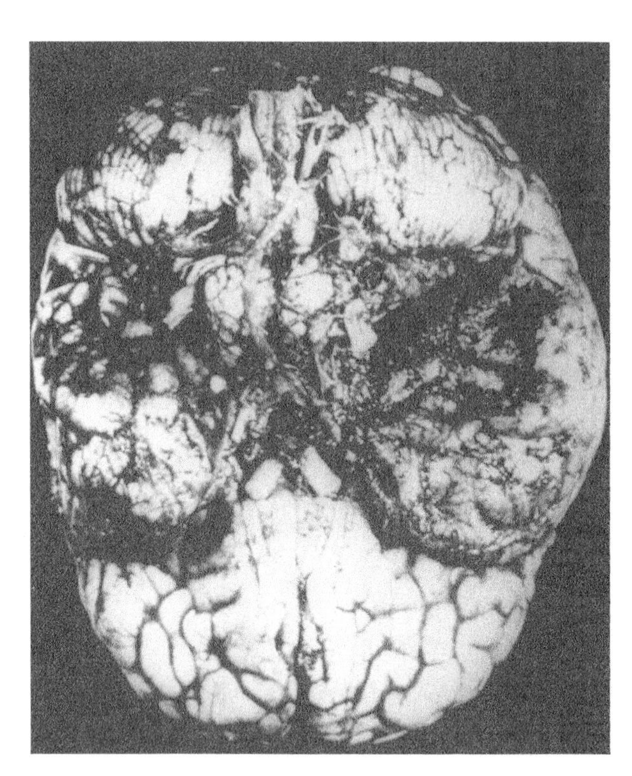

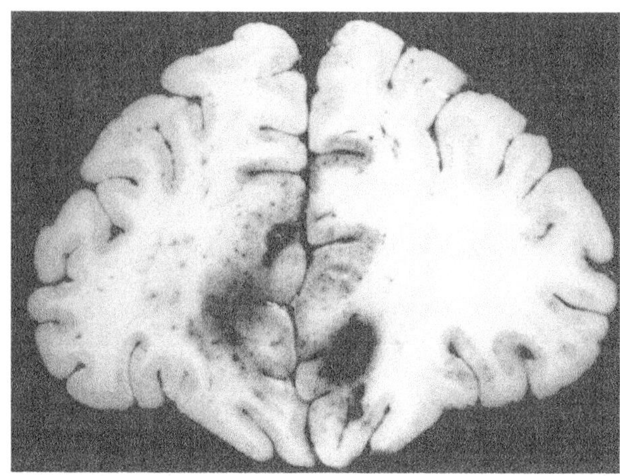

FIGURE 10.14 **Coronal section of brain from a patient with herpes simplex encephalitis.**

DIAGNOSIS

The appropriate use of laboratory tools is essential if a diagnosis of HSV infection is to be achieved.[60] Virus isolation is one definitive diagnostic method; however, PCR detection of viral DNA has replaced culture in many laboratories. If a culture is obtained, skin vesicles/lesions should be swabbed/scraped and transferred promptly in appropriate virus transport media to a diagnostic virology laboratory. In addition to skin vesicles, other sites from which virus may be isolated include the CSF (rarely), stool, urine, throat, nasopharynx, and conjunctivae. Clinical specimens should be shipped on ice for inoculation into cell culture systems (e.g., foreskin fibroblasts, Vero cells) that are appropriate for the demonstration of the cytopathic effects characteristic of HSV replication.[255] Cytopathic effect tends to develop within 24 to 48 hours after inoculation of specimens containing infectious virus. HSV is labile, and therefore the shipping and processing of specimens for viral culture should be expedited to avoid false-negative results.

The advantage of cell culture is the ability to obtain a virus isolate for further testing (e.g., resistance). Typing of an HSV isolate may be accomplished both in culture and by PCR. Differentiating between HSV-1 and HSV-2 infection in the genital tract is important for patient counseling.

Serologic diagnosis of HSV infection is clinically valuable in the counseling of patients regarding genital herpes provided that the assays are type specific (differentiate between HSV-1 and HSV-2), namely HSV-1 and HSV-2 gG-specific antibodies.[309] If a clinically apparent HSV infection is suspected, empiric therapy should be started without awaiting the commercial and FDA-approved assays that are available. IgM antibody responses do not correlate with disease activity or infection and are not recommended for diagnosis.[209,336] Screening for HSV infection by serology among persons without symptoms is not recommended by the CDC.[82]

The development of PCR has revolutionized the diagnosis of HSV infections and also allowed for detailed studies of disease pathogenesis. PCR assessment of CSF is the standard for diagnosis of HSV encephalitis[227,240,293] as well as skin lesions—either orolabial or genital. HSV DNA can be detected in the CSF of patients undergoing brain biopsies for HSV encephalitis with a sensitivity of more than 95% and a specificity that approaches 100%.[157] PCR evaluation of CSF can be used to follow therapeutic outcome in patients with HSV encephalitis. Persistence of HSV DNA in the CSF of newborns with HSV encephalitis at the completion of antiviral therapy predicts poor neurologic outcome.[138]

PREVENTION AND CONTROL OF HSV INFECTIONS

Genital HSV Infections

Because of the increased awareness of genital herpes and neonatal herpes and its association with increased risk of acquisition of HIV, every effort should be made to prevent HSV-2 infections. The use of condoms should be promoted as use moderately decreases the probability of acquiring genital HSV infection, with a 30% decreased risk of HSV-2 acquisition among people who always use condoms (compared to never users).[181] Some studies have shown that condoms are more effective in the prevention of infection of females than males.[44,174,308] Among HSV-2 heterosexual serodiscordant couples without HIV infection, use of daily suppressive valacyclovir for the HSV-2–seropositive partner is associated with a 48% decreased risk HSV-2 transmission to the seronegative partner.[64] Conflicting results have been found in studies of medical male circumcision (MMC) conducted in Africa for prevention of HIV infection.[184] Some studies have showed a significant 30% decrease in the risk of HSV-2 acquisition among men undergoing MMC,[290] and female partners of those undergoing MMC have a decreased risk of HSV-2 acquisition.[96] Disclosure of HSV serostatus to sexual partners is also associated with decreased risk of transmission.[307]

Prevention of Neonatal HSV Infection

The risk of neonatal infection is increased in the presence of genital ulcers, but HSV transmission can also occur in the absence of lesions. Surgical abdominal delivery is associated with the decreased transmission of infection when membranes are ruptured less than 4 hours, but cesarean section has not been proven efficacious when membranes are ruptured for longer periods of time.[34]

For women with a past history of genital HSV infection, some obstetricians prescribe an antiviral medication during the last 4 weeks of gestation, recognizing a decreased probability of virus excretion.[5] However, recent data indicate, that in spite of maternal compliance, maternal transmission can still occur, resulting in severe neonatal HSV disease.[222]

For babies born to mothers with known primary infection during the third trimester of gestation, the American Academy of Pediatrics Redbook Committee recommends 10 days of high-dose intravenous acyclovir therapy followed by careful serial medical assessment.[134] If a child is born through a known infected birth canal, particularly in the presence of an established genital infection, skin surface cultures and careful follow-up are in order. Should the cultures become positive or the child ill, further evaluation (i.e., CSF and blood assessment by PCR) is indicated with therapy initiated until a diagnosis is either confirmed or excluded.

At the time of presentation to the labor and delivery suite, a careful vaginal examination is of paramount importance. Although visualization of the cervix is often difficult, speculum examination for documentation of recurrent lesions is extremely important and should be attempted in all women because it will guide management of the newborn (see below).

Hospital Staff

Temporary removal of personnel who have cold sores is advocated for some clinical services. Education regarding the risk of transmission of virus and the importance of hand washing when lesions are present should be repeatedly emphasized to healthcare workers. Some infection control physicians recommend that hospital personnel should wear masks when active lesions are present.

Prevention of Other HSV Infections

At the present time, the only mechanism for prevention of mucocutaneous HSV infection is to avoid contact with infected secretions. Gloving of hospital personnel will decrease risk of hand exposure. There are no proven effective postexposure antiviral therapies or vaccines.

VACCINE DEVELOPMENT

Human HSV Vaccine Development

An important consideration for human HSV vaccines is the definition of expectations, warranting a distinction between infection and disease. From animal data, disease can be ameliorated if not prevented; however, infection still occurs and with it the potential for reactivating and transmitting infection. Similarly, the potential of altering the immune response to change the pattern of recurrences in previously infected individuals is unlikely. HSV vaccine research has focused on prevention of HSV-2 infection. Clinical trials have explored both prophylactic vaccines, which aim to prevent acquisition of HSV-2, and therapeutic vaccines, which are given to HSV-2–seropositive persons to prevent recurrences and shedding. Despite extensive research, no vaccines have elicited sufficient efficacy to gain licensure for use. Early investigations provide important insights into these expectations according to candidate vaccine: (a) wild-type virus, (b) inactivated or killed virus, (c) subunit vaccines, and (d) live vaccines.

Wild-Type Virus Vaccines

Numerous investigators have studied (a) autologous virus, (b) virus from another infected individual, or (c) virus recovered from an experimentally infected rabbit. In some cases, inoculation led to recurrences of latent infection.[29] These live viruses were subsequently abandoned because many patients failed to develop lesions at the site of inoculation; therefore, it was concluded that the virus did not produce an "adequate take," as compared to smallpox immunization.

Inactivated (or Killed) Virus Vaccines

Killed viruses were used as vaccines in a variety of animal models. The initial inactivated vaccines were made from phenol-treated tissues obtained from infected animals. Because of the potential for demyelination after the administration of animal proteins, these vaccines attracted little biomedical attention. UV light inactivation of purified virus derived from tissue culture experiments provided greater impetus for the vaccine field. Viral antigens obtained from a variety of cell cultures were inactivated by formalin, UV light, or heat and administered to thousands of patients.[320] While decreased recurrences were reported in as many as 60% to 80% of patients,[202] no controls were used.

Several important observations were made from these studies. First, despite repeated inoculations, antibody titers (as measured by neutralization or complement fixation) remained unchanged in the majority of patients or demonstrated only slight increases.[269,303] Second, although few side effects were reported, some authors noted concern that, in patients with keratitis, autoimmune phenomena might make the herpetic disease worse.[254] Lastly, placebo-controlled trial designs were not routinely employed.

Subunit Vaccines

Subunit vaccines evolved from attempts to remove viral and cellular DNA, to enhance antigenic concentration and induce stronger immune responses, and, finally, to exclude any possibility of contamination with residual live virus. The immunogenicity of envelope glycoproteins was demonstrated in animals.[42,43,188,267] The subunit vaccines elicited some protection, as evidenced by reduction of morbidity and mortality in the immunized animals. However, the predictability of these models for human studies is disappointing. Furthermore, several injections with an adjuvant were required to induce protection. Protection in a rodent model is significantly easier than that in nonhuman primates. Vaccination of primates, specifically rhesus monkeys,[41] chimpanzees,[41,42] and *Cebus* monkeys,[104] induces neutralizing antibodies, which can lead to an amnestic response after subsequent injection months later.

Subunit vaccines have failed in human experiments despite initial promising results. Both HSV-1 and HSV-2 antigens have been prepared in human diploid cells and chicken embryo fibroblasts. The first envelope subunit vaccine[8,104,345] was administered to uninfected sexual partners of patients known to have genital herpes and demonstrated that HSV infection was nearly equal for both placebo and vaccine recipients, indicating that the vaccine was not effective.

Further extensive studies have been completed with two gB and/or gD recombinant vaccines in humans, including adjuvants. Some studies demonstrated an increase in the geometric mean neutralizing antibody titer to gD-2; however, lymphocyte blastogenic responses were inconsistent.[277] Other studies afforded a high level of protection from HSV disease in animal models[243]; but with unacceptable reactogenicity. Notably, in these studies, the quantity of neutralizing antibodies elicited by immunization and the total HSV antibody titer (as measured by ELISA) were higher after vaccination than after natural infection.[274] A controlled clinical trial using gD2 and gB2 in an adjuvant of squalene oil and water emulsion failed to demonstrate efficacy for prevention of either infection or disease.[62]

A second candidate vaccine consisting of gD-2 with an alum and monophosphoryl lipid A adjuvant induced titers of HSV gD-specific antibody that were higher than those observed in patients who had sexually acquired genital HSV-2 infection. In these studies, women who were seronegative for both HSV-1 and 2 were significantly protected from disease (72% efficacy; p = 0.01 and 0.02, respectively) and there was a trend toward protection against infection (43% efficacy; p = 0.06 and 0.07). However, in individuals seropositive for HSV-1, irrespective of sex, and seronegative men, no significant clinical benefit could be demonstrated. Thus, this genital herpes vaccine (gD-Alum/MPL) was only effective in preventing HSV-1 or 2 genital herpes disease in a subset of volunteers, that is, women who were HSV-1 and 2 seronegative (HSV-1/2) prior to vaccination. However, these studies were neither designed nor powered to assess efficacy exclusively in HSV-1/2 women and therefore did not meet their primary endpoints of overall efficacy. The vaccine had no effect in women who had preexisting antibodies to HSV-1 or men regardless of their serologic status. A large placebo-controlled study to verify these results showed only 20% efficacy in preventing genital herpes disease overall (the primary endpoint) but did show 58% efficacy for preventing HSV-1 genital disease.[18] By including HSV seroconversion in the definition of genital infection, the vaccine showed only 22% protection from HSV infection overall, but 35% efficacy for preventing HSV-1 infection. A trivalent subunit vaccine appears promising in preclinical studies for prevention of genital herpes. The vaccine attempts to build on the partial successes of the prior subunit vaccine studies. The vaccine consists of HSV-2 glycoproteins C, D, and E intended to block virus entry mediated by glycoprotein D and prevent immune evasion from antibody and complement mediated by glycoproteins C and E.[11]

More recently, other approaches have either entered or are being considered for clinical trials. A therapeutic vaccine consisting of immunogenic T-cell antigens has been assessed in persons with HSV-2 infection in Phase I and II clinical studies. The vaccine decreased the frequency of shedding and recurrences by approximately 40%, demonstrating a proof of principle that stimulating T-cell responses by vaccination can alter the natural history of HSV-2 infection.[25,300] However, to date, this impact was not significant enough to pursue Phase III licensure trials.

Live Virus Vaccines

For decades, live virus vaccines have been considered most likely to provide a high level of protection as occurs with measles, mumps, and rubella. Moreover, these vaccines usually require smaller quantities of antigen and, therefore, should be more economical. Several approaches to live virus vaccines have been attempted, including HSV mutants, heterologous herpesviruses, antigens expressed in non-HSV viral vectors, and genetically engineered viruses.

Genetically Engineered HSV Vaccines

Current technology allows the construction of recombinant HSV as prototype vaccines.[185,235] These vaccines were engineered with the objectives that they should be attenuated so as not to cause primary disease or to reactivate; be able to protect against HSV-1 or HSV-2 disease; provide biomarkers that distinguish vaccine from wild-type infection; and, potentially, serve as vectors to express immunogens of other human pathogens. Notably, there is overlap between engineered vaccine candidates and HSV constructs that are used for gene therapy; see below.

The initial construction of candidate vaccines was based on the use of HSV-1. An engineered HSV was constructed that deleted the viral thymidine kinase gene and the junction region of the U_L and U_S segments in order to excise some of the genetic loci responsible for neurovirulence. An HSV-2 DNA fragment encoding the HSV-2 glycoproteins D, G, and I was inserted in place of the internal inverted repeat. The resulting recombinant, designated as R7017, was further altered by insertion of the thymidine kinase gene next to the HSV-2 DNA fragment (R7020). Because this virus expresses thymidine kinase, it is amenable to antiviral chemotherapy with acyclovir.

When evaluated in rodent models, the two constructs were considerably attenuated in pathogenicity and ability to establish latency and were capable of inducing protective immune responses. These results were corroborated by studies in owl monkeys (*Aotus trivirgatus*). Although 100 plaque-forming units of wild-type virus administered by peripheral routes were fatal to the monkeys, recombinants given by various routes in amounts at least 10^5-fold greater were innocuous or produced only mild infections, even in the presence of immunosuppression by total lymphoid irradiation.[186] When R7020 was administered to humans to determine reactogenicity, immune responses were elicited[40]; however, R7020 was not effective at the relatively low doses tested at that time.

The application of these principles to HSV-2 constructs was undertaken and assessed in animal models. The $\gamma_1 34.5$ gene of HSV-1 was proven to be a mediator of CNS replication, providing a potential vaccine construct upon deletion.[55] Furthermore, deletions of $\gamma_1 34.5$ significantly decrease the ability of this construct to establish latency.

One promising approach to an HSV vaccine is using replication-defective viruses.[75] A current construct deletes U_L5 and U_L29 in HSV-2 to generate the dl5-29 vaccine candidate.[195,204] This vaccine candidate was compared to a gD-2 subunit vaccine in Freund adjuvant. Significant protection was induced along with high titers of neutralizing antibodies and $CD8^+$ T cells.[76,109,110] This vaccine candidate has been evaluated in Phase I human trials and generated only modest immune responses.[74]

A vaccine deleted in gH was studied in a Phase II trial in the United Kingdom. This vaccine, known as the HSV-DISC vaccine, undergoes a single cycle of replication. Because gH is deleted, no further replication is possible. The results of this Phase II study failed to demonstrate effectiveness in reducing reactivation and disease in persons with recurrent HSV-2.[69] A similar approach by deleting another essential entry molecule, glycoprotein D, is under evaluation as a prophylactic vaccine for genital herpes in preclinical studies.[38]

Vectored Gene Expression and Other Approaches

Vectored approaches have utilized vaccinia virus[268] and adenoviruses[182] for expression of foreign genes, namely the gD and/or gB genes that showed varying effectiveness in animal models but have not been advanced to human trials.[352]

Other approaches being tested as therapeutic vaccines include DNA plasmid vaccines of gD2 that are optimized to generate both humoral and cell-mediated immunity (COR-1). In Phase I/II studies, this approach generated gD2-specific immune responses.[51] In addition, a "prime and pull" strategy, which uses traditional parenteral vaccination followed by application of a topical chemokine on the genital mucosa, is being studied in animal models as a therapeutic vaccine approach and generates better viral control than vaccination alone.[24,261,272]

Future vaccines must be directed against both HSV types. As noted above, one advanced at this time is a construct that deletes U_L5 and U_L29 in HSV-2 to generate the *dl5-29* vaccine candidate. One such construct will consider the utilization of immunologically dominant T-cell epitopes as a means to improve immune responses.

ONCOLYTIC HSV THERAPY

Genetically engineered HSVs have been assessed for the treatment of human glioblastoma multiforme and melanoma. These constructs have included mutations in the viral genes for thymidine kinase, DNA polymerase, ribonucleotide reductase, and $\gamma_1 34.5$[30,50,117,129,179,190] and have been identified as HF10, HSV1716, NV1020, G207, G47Δ, OncoVEX$^{GM\text{-}CSF}$, rRp450, M032, and C134.[46,80,94,161,173,185,191,205] While virtually any alteration of HSV reduces neurovirulence, only the deletions in the $\gamma_1 34.5$ gene consistently demonstrate safety and efficacy in animal models. Tumoricidal effects *in vitro* and *in vivo* in multiple glioma models (mouse, rat, and human glioma cell lines, human glioma explants) are demonstrable. Imlygic has been licensed for the treatment of melanoma.[115]

Animal Model Studies

Studies in animal models of gliomas of various constructs of HSV (engineered viruses deleted in $\gamma_1 34.5$) demonstrate the following principles: (a) the time course of infection (quantitative virology and PCR) represents impaired replication with limited spread of virus across the brain using marker genes (*lacZ* under an ICP6 promoter) with HSV antibody staining,[117,129] (b) two selected mutations appear to avoid mutations with reversion to wild-type phenotype ($\gamma_1 34.5$ and ribonucleotide reductase deletions),[341] (c) the retention of the native HSV TK allows for acyclovir susceptibility,[50] (d) the safety of these constructs was established in susceptible primates (*Aotus*),[341] and (e) HSV could be used as a vehicle to express foreign genes.[4,212,56,89]

The status of these viruses can be summarized as follows.

HF10

HF10 is derived following serial passage of the wild-type HSV-1 strain HF.[205] This virus is not neuroinvasive and was determined to have stable duplications in the U_L53, U_L54, and U_L55 genes, as well as deletion of the U_L56 gene. Notably, HF10 contains both native copies of the $\gamma_1 34.5$ neurovirulence gene, but its lack of neuroinvasiveness is presumably due to the absence of U_L56 or to *syn* alterations that may also have an effect.[299] HF10 has been evaluated in murine models of peritoneal tumor distribution as well as breast and bladder cancer.[149,286,289] Preliminary clinical studies of HF10 demonstrated the safety of HF10 following intratumoral injection into metastatic squamous cell carcinoma of the head and neck, as well as metastatic breast cancer.[88,133] A Phase I clinical trial investigating the safety of HF10 in patients with refractory head and neck cancer has been conducted.

HSV1716

HSV1716 is one of two conditionally replication-competent, engineered HSV directly injected into malignant glioma with demonstrated safety and the absence of neurovirulence. HSV1716 has been clinically studied for the treatment of malignant glioma in the United Kingdom. A series of Phase I studies of direct intratumoral and surrounding normal parenchyma administration of HSV1716 at doses ranging from 1×10^3 to 1×10^5 pfu proved safety and viral replication in the tumor.[100,211,229] HSV1716 has also been assessed as a therapy of oral squamous cell carcinoma (1×10^5 pfu of virus intratumorally) and melanoma with evidence of safety but no documentation of viral replication.[171,172]

NV1020

Engineered as a vaccine to prevent HSV-1 and -2 infections, NV1020 is deleted in only one of the two $\gamma_1 34.5$ genes.[185] NV1020 has been studied as an oncolytic HSV for hepatic colorectal adenocarcinoma metastases at doses ranging from 3×10^6 to 1×10^8 pfu followed by chemotherapy 2 to 3 days later.[131] Serious adverse events were minimal. Concomitant sampling of the hepatic vein for viral DNA by PCR detected little evidence of systemic exposure, a perceived risk of administering virus intra-arterially. Efficacy cannot be determined from these studies but the investigators concluded that NV1020 may render infected malignant cells moderately susceptible to chemotherapy regimens against which they are resistant.[85,90]

G207

G207, derived from the HSV-1 (F) strain, is deleted for both *$\gamma_1 34.5$* genes and is further attenuated by insertion of the *lacZ* gene into the *$U_L 39$* locus, preventing expression of ribonucleotide reductase. G207 was demonstrated to be safe following direct intracranial injection in both mice and in highly susceptible *Aotus nancymae* primates.[113,282]

The first Phase I safety trial with G207 evaluated direct intratumoral injection of virus in escalating doses ranging from 1×10^6 to 3×10^9 pfu. Several Phase I studies have been performed that demonstrate safety and a modicum of clinical response.[180,178]

G47Δ

G47Δ, directly derived from G207 and thus lacking both *$\gamma_1 34.5$* gene copies as well as containing a *lacZ* gene insertion within *$U_L 39$*, is additionally deleted for the *α47* gene. This latter modification prevents G47Δ from downmodulating MHC-I presentation and additionally alters the kinetics of *$U_S 11$* gene expression from late to early in infection.[292] These modifications increase the immunogenicity and replicative ability of G47Δ without affecting neurovirulence.[292] G47Δ reduces tumor mass in multiple models.[291] The *in vivo* efficacy of G207 and G47Δ has been directly compared, with G47Δ providing an equal or improved survival advantage over G207.[162,292,301] A Phase I-II clinical trial investigating the safety and efficacy of G47Δ in recurrent glioblastoma multiforme is currently recruiting patients in Japan.

OncoVEX^{GM-CSF}

OncoVEX^{GM-CSF} is derived from the pathogenic clinical isolate JS-1.[161] Attenuations in this vector include replacement of both *$\gamma_1 34.5$* genes with the gene encoding human granulocyte–macrophage stimulating factor (GM-CSF), and deletion of the *α47* coding sequence such that the *$U_S 11$* gene is expressed from the immediate-early *α47* promoter. OncoVEX^{GM-CSF} expresses a transgene hypothesized to enhance antitumor effects by complementing the lytic mechanism of tumor clearance. In the case of OncoVEX^{GM-CSF}, this additional mechanism is immune stimulation through the cytokine GM-CSF, a hematopoietic growth factor that promotes the maturation and development of dendritic cells as well as elicits the formation of Th1 skewed immune responses. OncoVEX^{GM-CSF} is the first armed oncolytic HSV vector to be evaluated in clinical trials.

OncoVEX^{GM-CSF} has been evaluated in several Phase I clinical trials enrolling patients with refractory cutaneous or subcutaneous metastases of breast, gastrointestinal adenocarcinoma, malignant melanoma, or epithelial cancer of the head and neck.[112] Direct intratumoral injection of 1 or 3 doses (1×10^6 to 1×10^8 pfu) established safety. OncoVEX^{GM-CSF} is currently being evaluated in malignant melanoma.[256] No severe events were attributable to virus administration.

rRp450

rRp450 is derived from the first-generation vector hrR3. hrR3 was engineered by replacing the *$U_L 39$* gene encoding RR of the wild-type strain KOS with *lacZ*. rRp450 followed with the replacement of the *lacZ* genes with the *CYP2B1*, the gene encoding the rat cytochrome p450 enzyme responsible for prodrug metabolism.[52] Cytochrome p450 2B1 expression is hypothesized to serve as a method of concentrating active metabolites of chemotherapeutics in malignant cells. Notably, rRp450 retains both native copies of *$\gamma_1 34.5$*. Preclinical studies with rRp450 demonstrated its selective replication in tumor cells with increased expression of mammalian ribonucleotide reductase, demonstrating a level of targeting afforded by the ICP6 deletion, as well as increased cytotoxicity of these cells when infection was combined with nitrogen mustard alkylating agents *in vitro*.[52] *In vivo* studies demonstrated synergistic efficacy of rRp450 and cyclophosphamide against a model of hepatic metastases of colon adenocarcinoma in mice.[220]

M032, C134

The engineered HSV recombinants M032 and C134 are similar in that both were originally derived from the wild-type HSV-1 (F) strain. They share identical deletions of the *$\gamma_1 34.5$* gene but differ with regard to the inserted genes replacing $\gamma_1$34.5. M032 expresses the human immunostimulatory cytokine interleukin-12 (IL-12). IL-12 promotes the activation of IFN-γ secretion and Th1 polarization of $CD8^+$ T lymphocytes and also has antiangiogenic effects. Preliminary studies of a murine IL-12–expressing virus M002 demonstrate increased survival in intracranial tumor–bearing mice treated with M002, and increased infiltration of innate and adaptive immune cells into tumors.[212]

Currently, the safety of M032, expressing human IL-12, in patients with recurrent glioblastoma is being evaluated in a Phase Ib study (NCT02062827).

C134 expresses the cytomegalovirus (CMV) PKR evasion and IFN-γ resistance molecule IRS1.[257] IRS1 has equivalent functions as the *$\gamma_1 34.5$* gene product ICP34.5 in terms of PKR evasion, but unlike ICP34.5, it does not contribute to neurovirulence. Cells infected with C134 do not undergo PKR-mediated host protein shutoff. This resistance to PKR-mediated host protein shutoff has been found to occur in neuroblastoma cell lines, prompting the submission of an IND application for a Phase I clinical trial of C134 in pediatric patients with recurrent glioblastoma.[46]

Summary

Engineered HSV constructs have been proven consistently safe when administered intracranially to humans at high doses. With some constructs, suggestions of efficacy are apparent. Likely, no one construct or approach will cure all tumors. Future work will need to focus on improving replication competence without sacrificing safety, improving delivery, and gaining a better understanding of host gene expression to optimize the oncolytic approach.

ANTIVIRAL THERAPY

Advances in the treatment of HSV infections have led the way in the development of antiviral therapeutics. The details of antiviral therapy appear elsewhere in this textbook. In the 1970s, vidarabine (adenine arabinoside) was the first licensed antiviral therapeutic for the treatment for HSE and neonatal HSV infections, as well as varicella zoster virus infections in the immunocompromised host. Vidarabine was replaced by acyclovir for the treatment of all HSV infections. Today, acyclovir and its prodrug valacyclovir as well as the prodrug of penciclovir, famciclovir, are the most useful and widely prescribed therapeutics for the treatment of HSV infections. Both valacyclovir and famciclovir have a distinct advantage over acyclovir. Specifically, the oral bioavailability of acyclovir following valacyclovir administration allows for improved pharmacokinetics. The same case is also made of plasma levels of penciclovir following famciclovir administration. The mechanism of action of acyclovir and penciclovir, as well as the details of antiherpetic therapy, is summarized elsewhere. Brief reference will be made to the use of these medications, as well as foscarnet and cidofovir, in the management of HSV infections.

Table 10.3 summarizes the use of the antiviral therapeutics in the treatment of HSV infections. A brief summary of the status of therapy is provided.

Life-threatening HSV infections, including HSE, neonatal HSV infection, and progressive or visceral disease in the immunocompromised host, are routinely treated with intravenous acyclovir. For infections involving the CNS, most notably HSE, mortality is decreased from 70% in placebo recipients to 25% in those who receive intravenous acyclovir therapy. Of the survivors, only 1 out of 3 returns to normal function. For neonatal HSV infection, multiorgan disseminated involvement, as defined above, can be treated with acyclovir with a resultant overall mortality of 25%. Neonatal HSV encephalitis is associated with a mortality of 5% following therapy. For both of these entities, survivors are left with significant neurologic impairment in the majority of cases, namely 60%. Factors that predict a poor outcome include disseminated intravascular coagulopathy and prematurity for those babies with disseminated neonatal herpes, while for those with encephalitis, seizures and prematurity predict a poor neurologic outcome.[136,321,322,326] These data indicate the requirement for improved therapies of HSV infections of the CNS.

Six months of suppressive acyclovir therapy, following 3 weeks of intravenous therapy, has been shown to improve neurologic outcome for newborns with HSV brain disease.[137] In a placebo-controlled clinical trial, the treated babies had Bailey Developmental scores that were 30 points higher on average than those for the controls. These data suggest that

TABLE 10.3 Drugs for herpes simplex virus

Infection	Drugs	Adult Dosage[a]
Orolabial	*Topical*	
	Acyclovir: ointment	5% cream 5 times/d × 4 d
	Docosanol	10% cream 5 times/d until healing
	Penciclovir	1% cream applied q2h while awake × 4
	Oral	
	Acyclovir	400 mg PO 5 times/d while awake × 4
	Famciclovir	400 mg PO bid × 7 d
	Valacyclovir	2 g PO q12h × 1 d
Genital		
First episode	Acyclovir	400 mg PO tid or 200 mg PO 5 times/d × 7–10 d[b]
	Famciclovir	250 mg PO tid × 7–10 d
	Valacyclovir	1 g PO bid × 7–10 d
Episodic treatment of recurrences	Acyclovir	800 mg tid or 400 mg PO tid × 3–5 d
	Famciclovir	125 mg PO bid × 5 d
	Valacyclovir	500 mg PO bid × 3 d
Suppression of recurrences	Acyclovir	400 mg PO bid
	Famciclovir	250 mg PO bid
	Valacyclovir	500 mg or 1 g PO 1 time/d
Mucocutaneous (immunocompromised)	Acyclovir	5 mg/kg IV q8h × 7–14 d or 400 mg PO 5 times/d ×7–10d
	Famciclovir	500 mg bid × 7–10 d
	Valacyclovir	500 mg or 1 g bid × 7–10 d
Encephalitis	Acyclovir	10–15 mg/kg IV q8h × 14–21 d
Neonatal	Acyclovir	20 mg/kg IV q8h × 14–21 d
Keratoconjunctivitis	Trifluridine	1% solution 1 drop q2h (max 9 drops/d)
Acyclovir resistant (severe infection, immunocompromised)	Foscarnet	40 mg/kg IV q8h × 14–21 d

[a]Dosage adjustment may be required for renal insufficiency.
[b]For severe initial genital herpes, IV acyclovir (5–10 mg/kg q8h for 5–7 d) can be used.
Note: Generic and trade names of drugs are as follows: acyclovir (Zovirax), docosanol (Abreva), penciclovir topical (Denavir), famciclovir (Famvir), valacyclovir (Valtrex), trifluridine (Viroptic), and foscarnet (Foscavir).

low grade continuing viral replication in the brain can be suppressed. Currently, this is the recommended standard of care.[134] Unfortunately, similar benefit was not achieved with valacyclovir suppressive therapy following HSV-1 encephalitis in adults.[93]

Ocular HSV infections are routinely treated with topical trifluorothymidine with or without concomitant oral acyclovir, valacyclovir, or famciclovir therapy. Topical idoxuridine has also been used for ocular infections. Acyclovir, and likely valacyclovir and famciclovir, can be used to suppress recurrences of HSV keratoconjunctivitis. However, it should be noted that no clinical trials of valacyclovir or famciclovir have been performed for this entity.

The most significant advances in antiviral therapy have been achieved in the management of mucocutaneous HSV infections. The prototypic treatment and suppressive regimens have been developed for the management of genital HSV infections. Acyclovir, valacyclovir, and famciclovir all are efficacious in the treatment of both primary and recurrent genital HSV infections. Valacyclovir and famciclovir[242] can be administered to patients on a suppressive basis to prevent reactivation of infection, as occurs more commonly with HSV-2 infections. While these medications significantly reduce the frequency of recurrences and, therefore, the probability of reactivation, periodic excretion of virus still occurs during suppressive therapy and can result in person-to-person transmission of infection. Indeed, even valacyclovir at approved doses does not prevent intermittent shedding of HSV.[64] In a seminal clinical trial, valacyclovir has been shown to decrease person-to-person transmission by approximately 48% when drug is administered once daily at 500 mg.[64] Suppressive therapy can be successfully achieved with valacyclovir administered once daily, whereas famciclovir requires twice daily dosing for suppression. Both valacyclovir and famciclovir[6,242] can be administered for short periods of therapy (3 days and 1 day, respectively) to treat recurrences of genital herpes with efficacy compared to longer treatment regimens.[123]

Acyclovir, valacyclovir, and famciclovir are all approved for the treatment of herpes labialis. As with genital HSV infection, short-course therapy provides excellent therapeutic results. At the present time, while acyclovir has been studied for the management of HSV gingivostomatitis, registrational trials have not been submitted to the US Food and Drug Administration.

HSV infections in the immunocompromised host pose unique challenges. Intravenous acyclovir is used routinely for progressive and/or life-threatening disease. Valacyclovir and famciclovir are useful in the management of HSV infections in individuals with HIV/AIDS. However, in some patient populations, progressive disease occurs in the presence of intravenous acyclovir therapy, implying the development of resistance. The propensity to develop resistance to these medications is greatest in patients with profound immunocompromise, such as hematopoietic stem cell transplant recipients and individuals who have advanced HIV/AIDS with low CD4 counts. When HSV isolates are mapped for resistance, the most common mutations are found in thymidine kinase.[253] Alternatively, mutations have been detected in HSV DNA polymerase rendering acyclovir triphosphate and penciclovir triphosphate ineffective. Under such circumstances, foscarnet or, rarely, cidofovir, drugs with alternative mechanisms of action have been employed.

Future Needs

The development of new antiviral agents for the management of HSV infection has been stymied by the overwhelming success of drugs like acyclovir, valacyclovir, and famciclovir. In large part, the pharmaceutical industry does not identify a niche for the development of future antiviral drugs in this area. Regardless, the persistent mortality and elevated morbidity in patients with HSV infections of the CNS define a medical need for which improved therapy should be developed. Recently, novel helicase/primase inhibitors have been effective for treatment or suppression in Phase II clinical trials, but clinical development has been stalled because of toxicity in nonhuman primates.[297,305,310]

PERSPECTIVE

HSV infections of humans are ubiquitous, being identified since ancient Greek times. Their unique biologic properties of neurovirulence and the ability to establish latency and recur create unique problems for those biomedical scientists attempting to develop either the ape tics or vaccines. Their ability to persist and cause recurrent disease despite potent host immune responses has stymied efforts to develop effective vaccines. Nevertheless, the application of genetically engineering the virus can turn a potentially lethal virus into a useful therapeutic.

REFERENCES

1. Agyemang E, Magaret AS, Selke S, et al. Herpes simplex virus shedding rate: surrogate outcome for genital herpes recurrence frequency and lesion rates, and phase 2 clinical trials end point for evaluating efficacy of antivirals. *J Infect Dis* 2018;218(11):1691–1699.
2. Amir J, Harel L, Smetana Z, et al. Treatment of herpes simplex gingivostomatitis with acyclovir in children: a randomized double blind placebo controlled study. *BMJ* 1997;314:1800–1803.
3. Anderson SG, Hamilton J. The epidemiology of primary herpes simplex infection. *Med J Aust* 1959;1:308.
4. Andreansky S, He B, van Cott J, et al. Treatment of intracranial gliomas in immunocompetent mice using herpes simplex viruses that express murine interleukins. *Gene Ther* 1998;5:121–130.
5. Andrews WW, Kimberlin DF, Whitley R, et al. Valacyclovir therapy to reduce recurrent genital herpes in pregnant women. *Am J Obstet Gynecol* 2006;194:774–781.
6. Aoki FY, Tyring S, Diaz-Mitoma F, et al. Single-day, patient-initiated famciclovir therapy for recurrent genital herpes: a randomized, double-blind, placebo-controlled trial. *Clin Infect Dis* 2006;42:8–13.
7. Arvin AM, Hensleigh PA, Prober CG, et al. Failure of antepartum maternal cultures to predict the infant's risk of exposure to herpes simplex virus at delivery. *N Engl J Med* 1986;315:796–800.
8. Ashley R, Mertz GJ, Corey L. Detection of asymptomatic herpes simplex virus infections after vaccination. *J Virol* 1987;61:264–268.
9. Ashley RL, Dalessio J, Burchett S, et al. Herpes simplex virus-2 (HSV-2) type-specific antibody correlates of protection in infants exposed to HSV-2 at birth. *J Clin Invest* 1992;90:511–514.
10. Audry M, Ciancanelli M, Yang K, et al. NEMO is a key component of NF-kappaB- and IRF-3-dependent TLR3-mediated immunity to herpes simplex virus. *J Allergy Clin Immunol* 2011;128(3):610–617 e611–e614.
11. Awasthi S, Hook LM, Pardi N, et al. Nucleoside-modified mRNA encoding HSV-2 glycoproteins C, D, and E prevents clinical and subclinical genital herpes. *Sci Immunol* 2019;4(39):eaaw7083.
12. Ayoub HH, Chemaitelly H, Abu-Raddad LJ. Characterizing the transitioning epidemiology of herpes simplex virus type 1 in the USA: model-based predictions. *BMC Med* 2019;17(1):57.
13. Bader C, Crumpacker CS, Schnipper LE, et al. The natural history of recurrent facial-oral infection with herpes simplex virus. *J Infect Dis* 1978;138:897–905.
14. Baldwin S, Whitley RJ. Intrauterine herpes simplex virus infection. *Teratology* 1989;39:1–10.
15. Baringer JR. Herpes simplex infections of the nervous system. *Neurol Clin* 2008;26(3):657–674, viii.
16. Baringer JR, Swoveland P. Recovery of herpes-simplex virus from human trigeminal ganglions. *N Engl J Med* 1973;288:648–650.
17. Bastian FO, Rabson AS, Yee CL. Herpesvirus hominis: isolation from human trigeminal ganglion. *Science* 1972;178:306.
18. Belshe RB, Leone PA, Bernstein DI, et al. Efficacy results of a trial of a herpes simplex vaccine. *N Engl J Med* 2012;366:34–43.

19. Belz GT, Behrens GM, Smith CM, et al. The CD8alpha(+) dendritic cell is responsible for inducing peripheral self-tolerance to tissue-associated antigens. *J Exp Med* 2002;196:1099–1104.
20. Benedetti J, Corey L, Ashley R. Recurrence rates in genital herpes after symptomatic first-episode infection. *Ann Intern Med* 1994;121:847–854.
21. Benedetti JK, Zeh J, Corey L. Clinical reactivation of genital herpes simplex virus infection decreases in frequency over time. *Ann Intern Med* 1999;131:14–20.
22. Bernstein DI, Bellamy AR, Hook EW III, et al. Epidemiology, clinical presentation, and antibody response to primary infection with herpes simplex virus type 1 and type 2 in young women. *Clin Infect Dis* 2013;56(3):344–351.
23. Bernstein DI, Bryson YJ, Lovett MA. Antibody response to type-common and type-unique epitopes of herpes simplex virus polypeptides. *J Med Virol* 1985;15:251–263.
24. Bernstein DI, Cardin RD, Bravo FJ, et al. Successful application of prime and pull strategy for a therapeutic HSV vaccine. *NPJ Vaccines* 2019;4:33.
25. Bernstein DI, Flechtner JB, McNeil LK, et al. Therapeutic HSV-2 vaccine decreases recurrent virus shedding and recurrent genital herpes disease. *Vaccine* 2019;37(26):3443–3450.
26. Bernstein DI, Stanberry LR. Herpes simplex virus vaccines. *Vaccine* 1999;17:1681–1689.
27. Binder PS. Herpes simplex keratitis. *Surv Ophthalmol* 1977;21:313–331.
28. Biron CA, Bryon HS, Sullivan JL. Severe herpes virus infections in an adolescent without natural killer cells. *N Engl J Med* 1989;320:1731–1735.
29. Blank H, Haines HG. Experimental human reinfection with herpes simplex virus. *J Invest Dermatol* 1973;61:223–225.
30. Boviatsis EJ, Scharf JM, Chase M, et al. Antitumor activity and reporter gene transfer into rat brain neoplasms inoculated with herpes simplex virus vectors defective in thymidine kinase or ribonucleotide reductase. *Gene Ther* 1994;1:323–331.
31. Bradley H, Markowitz LE, Gibson T, et al. Seroprevalence of herpes simplex virus types 1 and 2—United States, 1999-2010. *J Infect Dis* 2014;209(3):325–333.
32. Brown A, Benedetti J, Ashley R, et al. Neonatal herpes simplex virus infection in relation to asymptomatic maternal infection at the time of labor [see comments]. *N Engl J Med* 1991;324:1247–1252.
33. Brown ZA, Selke S, Zeh J, et al. The acquisition of herpes simplex virus during pregnancy. *N Engl J Med* 1997;337:509–515.
34. Brown ZA, Wald A, Morrow RM, et al. Effect of serologic status and cesarean delivery on transmission rates of herpes simplex virus from mother to infant. *JAMA* 2003;289:203–209.
35. Bryson Y, Dillon M, Bernstein DI, et al. Risk of acquisition of genital herpes simplex virus type 2 in sex partners of persons with genital herpes: a prospective couple study. *J Infect Dis* 1993;167:942–946.
36. Buddingh GH, Schrum DI, Lanier JC, et al. Studies of the natural history of herpes simplex infections. *Pediatrics* 1953;11:595.
37. Burchett SK, Westall J, Mohan K, et al. Ontogeny of neonatal mononuclear cell transformation and interferon gamma production after herpes simplex virus stimulation. *Clin Res* 1986;34:129.
38. Burn C, Ramsey N, Garforth SJ, et al. A herpes simplex virus (HSV)-2 single-cycle candidate vaccine deleted in glycoprotein D protects male mice from lethal skin challenge with clinical isolates of HSV-1 and HSV-2. *J Infect Dis* 2018;217(5):754–758.
39. Burnet FM, Williams SW. Herpes simplex: new point of view. *Med J Aust* 1939;1:637–640.
40. Cadoz M, Micoud M, Seigneurin JM, et al. Phase 1 trial of R7020: A live attenuated recombinant herpes simplex (HSV) candidate vaccine. Paper presented at: 32nd Interscience Conference on Antimicrobial Agents and Chemotherapy; October 11–14, 1992 October 11–14; Anaheim, CA.
41. Cappel R, de Cuyper F, Braekeler J. Antibody and cell-mediated immunity to a DNA free herpes simplex subunit vaccine. *Dev Biol Stand* 1979;43:381–385.
42. Cappel R, de Cuyper F, Rickaert F. Efficacy of a nucleic acid free herpetic subunit vaccine. *Arch Virol* 1980;65:15–23.
43. Cappel R, Sprecher S, Rickaert F, et al. Immune response to a DNA free herpes simplex vaccine in man. *Arch Virol* 1982;73:61–67.
44. Casper C, Wald A. Condom use and the prevention of genital herpes acquisition [see comment]. *Herpes* 2002;9:10–14.
45. Casrouge A, Zhang SY, Eidenschenk C, et al. Herpes simplex virus encephalitis in human UNC-93B deficiency. *Science* 2006;314:308–312.
46. Cassady KA, Parker JN. Herpesvirus vectors for therapy of brain tumors. *Open Virol J* 2010;4:103–108.
47. Celum C, Wald A, Hughes J, et al. Effect of acyclovir on HIV-1 acquisition in herpes simplex virus 2 seropositive women and men who have sex with men: a randomised, double-blind, placebo-controlled trial. *Lancet* 2008;371(9630):2109–2119.
48. Celum C, Wald A, Lingappa JR, et al. Acyclovir and transmission of HIV-1 from persons infected with HIV-1 and HSV-2. *N Engl J Med* 2010;362:427–439.
49. Cesario TC, Poland JD, Wulff H, et al. Six years experience with herpes simplex virus in a children's home. *Am J Epidemiol* 1969;90:416–422.
50. Chambers R, Gillespie GY, Soroceanu L, et al. Comparison of genetically engineered herpes simplex viruses for the treatment of brain tumors in a SCID mouse model of human malignant glioma. *Proc Natl Acad Sci U S A* 1995;92:1411–1425.
51. Chandra J, Woo WP, Dutton JL, et al. Immune responses to a HSV-2 polynucleotide immunotherapy COR-1 in HSV-2 positive subjects: a randomized double blinded phase I/IIa trial. *PLoS One* 2019;14(12):e0226320.
52. Chase M, Chung RY, Chiocca EA. An oncolytic viral mutant that delivers the CYP2B1 transgene and augments cyclophosphamide chemotherapy. *Nat Biotechnol* 1998;16:444–448.
53. Chemaitelly H, Nagelkerke N, Omori R, et al. Characterizing herpes simplex virus type 1 and type 2 seroprevalence declines and epidemiological association in the United States. *PLoS One* 2019;14(6):e0214151.
54. Chilmonczyk BA, Levin MJ, McDuffy R, et al. Characterization of the human newborn response to herpesvirus antigen. *J Immunol* 1985;134:4184–4188.
55. Chou J, Kern ER, Whitley RJ, et al. Mapping of herpes simplex virus-1 neurovirulence to gamma 134.5, a gene nonessential for growth in culture. *Science* 1990;250:1262–1266.
56. Chung S-M, Advani SJ, Bradley JD, et al. The use of a genetically engineered herpes simplex virus (R7020) with ionizing radiation for experimental hepatoma. *Gene Ther* 2002;9:75–80.
57. Colgrove R, Diaz F, Newman R, et al. Genomic sequences of a low passage herpes simplex virus 2 clinical isolate and its plaque-purified derivative strain. *Virology* 2014;450–451:140–145.
58. Colgrove RC, Liu X, Griffiths A, et al. History and genomic sequence analysis of the herpes simplex virus 1 KOS and KOS1.1 sub-strains. *Virology* 2016;487:215–221.
59. Corey L. The diagnosis and treatment of genital herpes. *JAMA* 1982;248:1041–1049.
60. Corey L. Laboratory diagnosis of herpes simplex virus infections. Principles guiding the development of rapid diagnostic tests. *Diagn Microbiol Infect Dis* 1986;4:111S–119S.
61. Corey L, Adams HG, Brown ZA, et al. Genital herpes simplex virus infections: clinical manifestations, course and complications. *Ann Intern Med* 1983;98:958–972.
62. Corey L, Langenberg AG, Ashley R, et al. Recombinant glycoprotein vaccine for the prevention of genital HSV-2 infection: two randomized controlled trials. Chiron HSV Vaccine Study Group. *JAMA* 1999;28:331–340.
63. Corey L, Reeves WC, Holmes KK. Cellular immune response in genital herpes simplex virus infection. *N Engl J Med* 1978;299:986–991.
64. Corey L, Wald A, Patel R, et al. Once-daily valacyclovir to reduce the risk of transmission of genital herpes. *N Engl J Med* 2004;350:11–20.
65. Craig CP, Nahmias AJ. Different patterns of neurologic involvement with herpes simplex virus types 1 and 2: isolation of herpes simplex virus type 2 from the buffy coat of two adults with meningitis. *J Infect Dis* 1973;127:365–372.
66. Cunningham AL, Merigan TC. Alpha interferon production appears to predict time of recurrence of herpes labialis. *J Immunol* 1983;130:2397–2400.
67. Dabestani N, Katz DA, Dombrowski J, et al. Time trends in first-episode genital herpes simplex virus infections in an urban sexually transmitted disease clinic. *Sex Transm Dis* 2019;46(12):795–800.
68. Dalloul A, Oksenhendler E, Chosidow O, et al. Severe herpes virus (HSV-2) infection in two patients with myelodysplasia and undetectable NK cells and plasmacytoid dendritic cells in the blood. *J Clin Virol* 2004;30:329–336.
69. de Bruyn G, Vargas-Cortez M, Warren T, et al. A randomized controlled trial of a replication defective (gH deletion) herpes simplex virus vaccine for the treatment of recurrent genital herpes among immunocompetent subjects. *Vaccine* 2006;24:914–920.
70. DeGiordana HM, Banza CA, Russi JC, et al. Prevalence of herpes simplex virus infection. *Arch Pediatr Urug* 1970;41:107.
71. Delaney AS, Thomas W, Balfour HH, Jr. Coprevalence of epstein-barr virus, cytomegalovirus, and herpes simplex virus type-1 antibodies among united states children and factors associated with their acquisition. *J Pediatric Infect Dis Soc* 2015;4(4):323–329.
72. Delaney S, Gardella C, Saracino M, et al. Seroprevalence of herpes simplex virus type 1 and 2 among pregnant women, 1989-2010. *JAMA* 2014;312(7):746–748.
73. Dix RD, Pereira L, Baringer JR. Use of monoclonal antibody directed against herpes simplex virus glycoproteins to protect mice against acute virus-induced neurological disease. *Infect Immun* 1981;34:192–199.
74. Dropulic LK, Oestreich MC, Pietz HL, et al. A randomized, double-blinded, placebo-controlled, phase 1 study of a replication-defective herpes simplex virus (HSV) type 2 vaccine, HSV529, in adults with or without HSV infection. *J Infect Dis* 2019;220(6):990–1000.
75. Dudek T, Knipe DM. Replication-defective viruses as vaccines and vaccine vectors. *Virology* 2006;344:230–239.
76. Dudek TE, Torres-Lopez E, Crumpacker C, et al. Evidence for differences in immunologic and pathogenesis properties of herpes simplex virus 2 strains from the United States and South Africa. *J Infect Dis* 2011;203:1434–1441.
77. Dummer JS, Armstrong J, Somers J, et al. Transmission of infection with herpes simplex virus by renal transplantation. *J Infect Dis* 1987;155:202–206.
78. Dupuis S, Jouanguy E, Al-Hajjar S, et al. Impaired response to interferon-alpha/beta and lethal viral disease in human STAT1 deficiency. *Nat Genet* 2003;33(3):388–391.
79. Durukan D, Fairley CK, Bradshaw CS, et al. Increasing proportion of herpes simplex virus type 1 among women and men diagnosed with first-episode anogenital herpes: a retrospective observational study over 14 years in Melbourne, Australia. *Sex Transm Infect* 2019;95(4):307–313.
80. Eissa IR, Bustos-Villalobos I, Ichinose T, et al. The current status and future prospects of oncolytic viruses in clinical trials against melanoma, glioma, pancreatic, and breast cancers. *Cancers (Basel)* 2018;10(10):356.
81. Fanfair RN, Zaidi A, Taylor LD, et al. Trends in seroprevalence of herpes simplex virus type 2 among non-Hispanic blacks and non-Hispanic whites aged 14 to 49 years—United States, 1988 to 2010. *Sex Transm Dis* 2013;40(11):860–864.
82. Feltner C, Grodensky C, Ebel C, et al. Serologic screening for genital herpes: an updated evidence report and systematic review for the US Preventive Services Task Force. *JAMA* 2016;316(23):2531–2543.
83. Fife KH, Mugwanya K, Thomas KK, et al. Transient increase in herpes simplex virus type 2 (HSV-2)-associated genital ulcers following initiation of antiretroviral therapy in HIV/HSV-2-coinfected individuals. *J Infect Dis* 2016;213(10):1573–1578.
84. Fleming DT, McQuillan GM, Johnson RE, et al. Herpes simplex virus type 2 in the United States, 1976 to 1994. *N Engl J Med* 1997;337:1105–1111.
85. Fong Y, Kim T, Bhargava A, et al. A herpes oncolytic virus can be delivered via the vasculature to produce biologic changes in human colorectal cancer. *Mol Ther* 2009;17:389–394.
86. Freeman EE, Weiss HA, Glynn JR, et al. Herpes simplex virus 2 infection increases HIV acquisition in men and women: systematic review and meta-analysis of longitudinal studies. *AIDS* 2006;20:73–83.
87. Friedman E, Katcher AH, Brightman VJ. Incidence of recurrent herpes labialis and upper respiratory infection: a prospective study of the influence of biologic, social, and psychologic predictors. *Oral Surg Oral Med Oral Pathol* 1977;43:873–878.
88. Fujimoto Y, Mizuno T, Sugiura S, et al. Intratumoral injection of herpes simplex virus HF10 in recurrent head and neck squamous cell carcinoma. *Acta Otolaryngol* 2006;126:1115–1117.

89. Gaston D, Whitley RJ, Parker J. Engineered herpes simplex virus vectors for antitumor therapy and vaccine delivery. *Future Virol* 2011;6:1–20.
90. Geevarghese SK, Geller DA, de Haan HA, et al. Phase I/II study of oncolytic herpes simplex virus NV1020 in patients with extensively pretreated refractory colorectal cancer metastatic to the liver. *Hum Gene Ther* 2010;21:1119–1128.
91. Gill MJ, Arlette J, Buchan K. Herpes simplex virus infection of the hand. A profile of 79 cases. *Am J Med* 1988;84:89–93.
92. Glezen WP, Fernald GW, Lohr JA. Acute respiratory disease of university students with special references to the etiologic role of herpesvirus hominis. *Am J Epidemiol* 1975;101:111–121.
93. Gnann JW Jr, Skoldenberg B, Hart J, et al. Herpes simplex encephalitis: lack of clinical benefit of long-term valacyclovir therapy. *Clin Infect Dis* 2015;61(5):683–691.
94. Goins WF, Huang S, Hall B, et al. Engineering HSV-1 vectors for gene therapy. *Methods Mol Biol* 2020;2060:73–90.
95. Goodell SE, Quinn TC, Mkritchian E, et al. Herpes simplex virus proctitis in homosexual men. *N Engl J Med* 1983;308:868.
96. Grund JM, Bryant TS, Jackson I, et al. Association between male circumcision and women's biomedical health outcomes: a systematic review. *Lancet Glob Health* 2017;5(11): e1113–e1122.
97. Gutierrez K, Whitley RJ, Arvin A. Herpes simplex virus infections. In: Remington JS, Klein JO, Wilson CB, et al., eds. *Infectious Diseases of the Fetus and Newborn Infant.* Philadelphia, PA: Elsevier; 2010.
98. Harel L, Smetana Z, Prais D, et al. Presence of viremia in patients with primary herpetic gingivostomatitis. *Clin Infect Dis* 2004;39:636–640.
99. Harger JH, Meyer MP, Amortegui AJ. Changes in the frequency of genital herpes recurrences as a function of time. *Obstet Gynecol* 1986;67:637–642.
100. Harrow S, Papanastassiou V, Harland J, et al. HSV1716 injection into the brain adjacent to tumour following surgical resection of high-grade glioma: safety data and long-term survival. *Gene Ther* 2004;11:1648–1658.
101. Hazen PG, Eppes RB. Eczema herpeticum caused by herpesvirus type 2, a case in a patient with Darier disease. *Arch Dermatol* 1977;113:1085–1086.
102. Heber-Katz E, Valentine S, Dietzchold B, et al. Overlapping T cell antigenic sites on a synthetic peptide fragment from herpes simplex virus glycoprotein D, the degenerate MHC restriction elicited, and functional evidence for antigen-Ia interaction. *J Exp Med* 1988;167:275–287.
103. Hevron JE Jr. Herpes simplex virus type 2 meningitis. *Obstet Gynecol* 1977;49(5):622–624.
104. Hilleman MR, Larson VM, Lehman ED, et al. Subunit herpes simplex virus vaccine. In: Nahmias AJ, Dowdle WR, Schinazi RF, eds. *The Human Herpesviruses: An Interdisciplinary Perspective.* North-Holland, Amsterdam, The Netherlands: Elsevier; 1982:503–506.
105. Hinthorn DR, Baker LH, Romig DA. Recurrent conjugal neuralgia caused by herpesvirus hominis type 2. *JAMA* 1976;236:587–588.
106. Hirsch MS, Zisman B, Allison AC. Macrophages and age-dependent resistance to Herpes simplex virus in mice. *J Immunol* 1970;104:1160–1165.
107. Hitselberger JF, Burns RE. Darier's disease: report of a case complicated by Kaposi's varicella-form eruption. *Arch Dermatol* 1961;83:425.
108. Holterman A-X, Rogers K, Edelmann K, et al. An important role for major histocompatibility complex class I-restricted T cells, and a limited role for gamma interferon, in protection of mice against lethal herpes simplex virus infection. *J Virol* 1999;73:2058–2063.
109. Hoshino Y, Dalai SK, Wang K, et al. Comparative efficacy and immunogenicity of replication-defective, recombinant glycoprotein, and DNA vaccines for herpes simplex virus 2 infections in mice and guinea pigs. *J Virol* 2005;79:410–418.
110. Hoshino Y, Pesnicak L, Dowdell KC, et al. Protection from herpes simplex virus (HSV)-2 infection with replication-defective HSV-2 or glycoprotein D2 vaccines in HSV-1-seropositive and HSV-1-seronegative guinea pigs. *J Infect Dis* 2009;200(7):1088–1095.
111. Hosken N, McGowan P, Meier A, et al. Diversity of the CD8+ T-cell response to herpes simplex virus type 2 proteins among persons with genital herpes. *J Virol* 2006;80:5509–5515.
112. Hu JC, Coffin RS, Davis CJ, et al. A phase I study of OncoVEXGM-CSF, a second-generation oncolytic herpes simplex virus expressing granulocyte macrophage colony-stimulating factor. *Clin Cancer Res* 2006;12:6737–6747.
113. Hunter WD, Martuza RL, Feigenbaum F, et al. Attenuated, replication-competent herpes simplex virus type 1 mutant G207: safety evaluation of intracerebral injection in nonhuman primates. *J Virol* 1999;73:6319–6326.
114. Hutto C, Arvin A, Jacobs R, et al. Intrauterine herpes simplex virus infections. *J Pediatr* 1987;110:97–101.
115. Imlygic Package Insert. 2019. https://www.pi.amgen.com/~/media/amgen/repositorysites/pi-amgen-com/imlygic/imlygic_pi.pdf. Accessed December 11, 2019.
116. Iwasaki A. Exploiting mucosal immunity for antiviral vaccines. *Annu Rev Immunol* 2016;34:575–608.
116a. James et al. *Bull World Health Organ* 2020;98:315–329.
117. Jia WW, McDermott M, Goldie J, et al. Selective destruction of gliomas in immunocompetent rats by thymidine kinase-defective herpes simplex virus type 1. *J Natl Cancer Inst* 1994;86:1209–1215.
118. Johnson KE, Redd AD, Quinn TC, et al. Effects of HIV-1 and herpes simplex virus type 2 infection on lymphocyte and dendritic cell density in adult foreskins from Rakai, Uganda. *J Infect Dis* 2011;203(5):602–609.
119. Johnson KE, Sherman ME, Ssempiija V, et al. Foreskin inflammation is associated with HIV and herpes simplex virus type-2 infections in Rakai, Uganda. *AIDS* 2009;23(14):1807–1815.
120. Johnson RM, Lancki DW, Fitch FW, et al. Herpes simplex virus glycoprotein D is recognized as antigen by CD4+ and CD8+ T lymphocytes from infected mice: characterization of T cell clones. *J Immunol* 1990;145:702–710.
121. Johnston C, Corey L. Current concepts for genital herpes simplex virus infection: diagnostics and pathogenesis of genital tract shedding. *Clin Microbiol Rev* 2016;29(1):149–161.
122. Johnston C, Magaret A, Roychoudhury P, et al. Dual-strain genital herpes simplex virus type 2 (HSV-2) infection in the US, Peru, and 8 countries in sub-Saharan Africa: a nested cross-sectional viral genotyping study. *PLoS Med* 2017;14(12):e1002475.
123. Johnston C, Saracino M, Kuntz S, et al. Standard-dose and high-dose daily antiviral therapy for short episodes of genital HSV-2 reactivation: three randomised, open-label, cross-over trials. *Lancet* 2012;379:641–647.
124. Johnston C, Zhu J, Jing L, et al. Virologic and immunologic evidence of multifocal genital herpes simplex virus 2 infection. *J Virol* 2014;88(9):4921–4931.
125. Kabani N, Kimberlin D. Neonatal herpes simplex virus infection. *NeoReviews* 2018;19(2):e89–e96.
126. Kahlon J, Lakeman FD, Ackermann M, et al. Human antibody response to herpes simplex virus-specific polypeptides after primary and recurrent infection. *J Clin Microbiol* 1986;23:725–730.
127. Kahlon J, Whitley RJ. Antibody response of the newborn after herpes simplex virus infection. *J Infect Dis* 1988;158:925–933.
128. Kalinyak JE, Fleagle G, Docherty JJ. Incidence and distribution of herpes simplex virus types 1 and 2 from genital lesions in college women. *J Med Virol* 1977;1:175–181.
129. Kaplitt MG, Tjuvajev JG, Leib DA, et al. Mutant herpes simplex virus induced regression of tumors growing in immunocompetent rats. *J Neurooncol* 1994;19:137–147.
130. Kaye EM, Dooling EC. Neonatal herpes simplex meningoencephalitis associated with fetal monitor scalp electrodes. *Neurology* 1981;31:1045–1047.
131. Kemeny N, Brown K, Covey A, et al. Phase I, open-label, dose-escalating study of a genetically engineered herpes simplex virus, NV1020, in subjects with metastatic colorectal carcinoma to the liver. *Hum Gene Ther* 2006;17:1214–1224.
132. Khanna KM, Bonneau RH, Kinchington PR, et al. Herpes simplex virus-specific memory CD8(+) T cells are selectively activated and retained in latently infected sensory ganglia. *Immunity* 2003;18:593–603.
133. Kimata H, Imai T, Kikumori T, et al. Pilot study of oncolytic viral therapy using mutant herpes simplex virus (HF10) against recurrent metastatic breast cancer. *Ann Surg Oncol* 2006;13:1078–1084.
134. Kimberlin DW, Brady MT, Jackson MA, et al., eds. *Redbook.* 31st ed. Itasca, IL: American Academy of Pediatrics; 2018.
135. Kimberlin DW, Lakeman FD, Arvin AM, et al. Application of the polymerase chain reaction to the diagnosis and management of neonatal herpes simplex virus disease. *J Infect Dis* 1996;174:1162–1167.
136. Kimberlin DW, Lin C-Y, Jacobs RF, et al. The safety and efficacy of high-dose intravenous acyclovir in the management of neonatal herpes simplex virus infections. *Pediatrics* 2001;108:230–238.
137. Kimberlin DW, Whitley RJ, Wan W, et al. Oral acyclovir suppression and neurodevelopment after neonatal herpes. *N Engl J Med* 2011;365:1284–1292.
138. Kimura H, Futamura M, Kito H, et al. Detection of viral DNA in neonatal herpes simplex virus infections: frequent and prolonged presence in serum and cerebrospinal fluid. *J Infect Dis* 1991;164:289–293.
139. Knickelbein JE, Khanna KM, Yee MB, et al. Noncytotoxic lytic granule-mediated CD8+ T cell inhibition of HSV-1 reactivation from neuronal latency. *Science* 2008;322(5899):268–271.
140. Koelle DM, Corey L, Burke RL, et al. Antigenic specificities of human CD4+ T-cell clones recovered from recurrent genital herpes simplex virus type 2 lesions. *J Virol* 1994;68:2803–2810.
141. Koelle DM, Genedetti J, Langenberg A, et al. Asymptomatic reactivation of herpes simplex virus in women after the first episode of genital herpes. *Ann Intern Med* 1992;116:433–437.
142. Koelle DM, Liu Z, McClurkan CL, et al. Immunodominance among herpes simplex virus-specific CD8 T cells expressing a tissue-specific homing receptor. *Proc Natl Acad Sci U S A* 2003;100:12899–12904.
143. Koelle DM, Norberg P, Fitzgibbon MP, et al. Worldwide circulation of HSV-2 x HSV-1 recombinant strains. *Sci Rep* 2017;7:44084.
144. Koelle DM, Posavad CM, Barnum GR, et al. Clearance of HSV-2 from recurrent genital lesions correlates with infiltration of HSV-specific cytotoxic T lymphocytes. *J Clin Invest* 1998;101:1500–1508.
145. Koelle DM, Schomogyi M, Corey L. Antigen-specific T cells localize to the uterine cervix in women with genital herpes simplex virus type 2 infection. *J Infect Dis* 2000;182: 662–670.
146. Kohl S, Frazier JP, Pickering LK, et al. Normal function of neonatal polymorphonuclear leukocytes in antibody-dependent cellular-cytotoxicity to herpes simplex virus-infected cells. *J Pediatr* 1981;98:783–785.
147. Kohl S, Shaban S, Starr S, et al. Human neonatal and maternal monocyte-macrophage and lymphocyte mediated antibody dependent cytotoxicity to herpes simplex infected cells. *J Pediatr* 1978;93:206–210.
148. Kohl S, West MS, Prober CG, et al. Neonatal antibody-dependent cellular cytotoxic antibody levels are associated with the clinical presentation of neonatal herpes simplex virus infection. *J Infect Dis* 1989;160:770–776.
149. Kohno S, Luo C, Goshima F, et al. Herpes simplex virus type 1 mutant HF10 oncolytic viral therapy for bladder cancer. *Urology* 2005;66:1116–1121.
150. Korsager B, Spencer ES, Mordhorst CH. Herpesvirus hominis infections in renal transplant recipients. *Scand J Infect Dis* 1975;7:11–19.
151. Krause PR, Straus SE. Herpesvirus vaccines: development, controversies, and applications. *Infect Dis Clin North Am* 1999;13:61–81.
152. Kriesel JD, Jones BB, Matsunami N, et al. C21orf91 genotypes correlate with herpes simplex labialis (cold sore) frequency: description of a cold sore susceptibility gene. *J Infect Dis* 2011;204(11):1654–1662.
153. Kulhanjian JA, Soroush V, Au DS, et al. Identification of women at unsuspected risk of primary infection with herpes simplex virus type 2 during pregnancy. *N Engl J Med* 1992;326:916–920.
154. Lafaille FG, Harschnitz O, Lee YS, et al. Human SNORA31 variations impair cortical neuron-intrinsic immunity to HSV-1 and underlie herpes simplex encephalitis. *Nat Med* 2019;25(12):1873–1884.
155. Lafferty WE, Coombs RW, Benedetti J, et al. Recurrences after oral and genital herpes simplex virus infection. Influence of site of infection and viral type. *N Engl J Med* 1987;316:1444–1449.

156. Laing KJ, Magaret AS, Mueller DE, et al. Diversity in CD8(+) T cell function and epitope breadth among persons with genital herpes. *J Clin Immunol* 2010;30:703–722.
157. Lakeman FD, Whitley RJ. Diagnosis of herpes simplex encephalitis: application of polymerase chain reaction to cerebrospinal fluid from brain-biopsied patients and correlation with disease. National Institute of Allergy and Infectious Diseases Collaborative Antiviral Study Group. *J Infect Dis* 1995;172:857–863.
158. Langenberg AG, Corey L, Ashley RL, et al. A prospective study of new infections with herpes simplex virus type 1 and type 2. Chiron HSV Vaccine Study Group. *N Engl J Med* 1999;341:1432–1438.
159. Light IJ. Postnatal acquisition of herpes simplex virus by the newborn infant: a review of the literature. *Pediatrics* 1979;63:480–482.
160. Linnemann CC, Jr., Buchman TG, Light IJ, et al. Transmission of herpes-simplex virus type 1 in a nursery for the newborn. Identification of viral isolates by D.N.A. "fingerprinting". *Lancet* 1978;1:964–966.
161. Liu BL, Robinson M, Han ZQ, et al. ICP34.5 deleted herpes simplex virus with enhanced oncolytic, immune stimulating, and anti-tumour properties. *Gene Ther* 2003;10:292–303.
162. Liu R, Varghese S, Rabkin SD. Oncolytic herpes simplex virus vector therapy of breast cancer in C3(1)/SV40 T-antigen transgenic mice. *Cancer Res* 2005;65:1532–1540.
163. Lo M, Zhu J, Hansen SG, et al. Acute infection and subsequent subclinical reactivation of herpes simplex virus 2 after vaginal inoculation of rhesus macaques. *J Virol* 2019;93(2):e01574-18.
164. Looker KJ, Magaret AS, May MT, et al. First estimates of the global and regional incidence of neonatal herpes infection. *Lancet Glob Health* 2017;5(3):e300–e309.
165. Looker KJ, Magaret AS, Turner KM, et al. Global estimates of prevalent and incident herpes simplex virus type 2 infections in 2012. *PLoS One* 2015;10(1):e114989.
166. Looker KJ, Welton NJ, Sabin KM, et al. Global and regional estimates of the contribution of herpes simplex virus type 2 infection to HIV incidence: a population attributable fraction analysis using published epidemiological data. *Lancet Infect Dis* 2020;20(2):240–249.
167. Lopez C, Ryshke R, Bennett M. Marrow-dependent cells depleted by 89Sr mediate genetic resistance to herpes simplex virus type 1 infection in mice. *Infect Immun* 1980;28:1028–1032.
168. Lu Y, Celum C, Wald A, et al. Acyclovir achieves a lower concentration in african HIV-seronegative, herpes simplex virus 2-seropositive women than in Non-African populations. *Antimicrob Agents Chemother* 2012(56):2777–2779.
169. Luby JP, Gnann JW Jr, Alexander WJ, et al. A collaborative study of patient-initiated treatment of recurrent genital herpes with topical acyclovir or placebo. *J Infect Dis* 1984;150:1–6.
170. Lund JM, Linehan MM, Iijima N, et al. Cutting edge: plasmacytoid dendritic cells provide innate immune protection against mucosal viral infection in situ. *J Immunol* 2006;177:7510–7514.
171. Mace AT, Ganly I, Soutar DS, et al. Potential for efficacy of the oncolytic Herpes simplex virus 1716 in patients with oral squamous cell carcinoma. *Head Neck* 2008;30:1045–1051.
172. MacKie RM, Stewart B, Brown SM. Intralesional injection of herpes simplex virus 1716 in metastatic melanoma. *Lancet* 2001;357:525–526.
173. MacLean AR, ul-Fareed M, Robertson L, et al. Herpes simplex virus type 1 deletion variants 1714 and 1716 pinpoint neurovirulence-related sequences in Glasgow strain 17+ between immediate early gene 1 and the 'a' sequence. *J Gen Virol* 1991;72:631–639.
174. Magaret AS, Mujugira A, Hughes JP, et al. Effect of condom use on per-act HSV-2 transmission risk in HIV-1, HSV-2-discordant couples. *Clin Infect Dis* 2016;62(4):456–461.
175. Mahant S, Hall M, Schondelmeyer AC, et al. Neonatal herpes simplex virus infection among medicaid-enrolled children: 2009–2015. *Pediatrics* 2019;143(4):e20183233.
176. Marchi S, Trombetta CM, Gasparini R, et al. Epidemiology of herpes simplex virus type 1 and 2 in Italy: a seroprevalence study from 2000 to 2014. *J Prev Med Hyg* 2017;58(1):E27–E33.
177. Mark KE, Wald A, Magaret AS, et al. Rapidly cleared episodes of herpes simplex virus reactivation in immunocompetent adults. *J Infect Dis* 2008;198(8):1141–1149.
178. Markert JM, Liechty PG, Wang W, et al. Phase Ib trial of mutant herpes simplex virus G207 inoculated pre-and post-tumor resection for recurrent GBM. *Mol Ther* 2009;17:199–207.
179. Markert JM, Malick A, Coen D, et al. Reduction and elimination of encephalitis in an experimental glioma therapy model with attenuated herpes simplex mutants that retain susceptibility to acyclovir. *Neurosurgery* 1993;32:597–603.
180. Markert JM, Medlock MD, Rabkin SD, et al. Conditionally replicating herpes simplex virus mutant, G207 for the treatment of malignant glioma: results of a phase I trial. *Gene Ther* 2000;7:867–874.
181. Martin ET, Krantz E, Gottlieb SL, et al. A pooled analysis of the effect of condoms in preventing HSV-2 acquisition. *Arch Intern Med* 2009;169(13):1233–1240.
182. McDermott MR, Graham FL, Hanke T, et al. Protection of mice against lethal challenge with herpes simplex virus by vaccination with an adenovirus vector expressing HSV glycoprotein B. *Virology* 1989;169:244–247.
183. McQuillan G, Kruszon-Moran D, Flagg EW, et al. Prevalence of herpes simplex virus type 1 and type 2 in persons aged 14–49: United States, 2015–2016. *NCHS Data Brief* 2018;(304):1–8.
184. Mehta SD, Moses S, Agot K, et al. Medical male circumcision and herpes simplex virus 2 acquisition: posttrial surveillance in Kisumu, Kenya. *J Infect Dis* 2013;208(11):1869–1876.
185. Meignier B, Longnecker R, Roizman B. In vivo behavior of genetically engineered herpes simplex viruses R7017 and R7020: construction and evaluation in rodents. *J Infect Dis* 1988;158:602–614.
186. Meignier B, Martin B, Whitley R, et al. In vivo behavior of genetically engineered herpes simplex viruses R7017 and R7020. II. Studies in immunocompetent and immunosuppressed owl monkeys (Aotus trivirgatus). *J Infect Dis* 1990;162:313–321.
187. Mertz GJ, Benedetti J, Ashley R, et al. Risk factors for the sexual transmission of genital herpes. *Ann Intern Med* 1992;116:197–202.
188. Mertz GJ, Peterman G, Ashley R, et al. Herpes simplex virus type-2 glycoprotein-subunit vaccine: tolerance and humoral and cellular responses in humans. *J Infect Dis* 1984;150:242–249.
189. Minaya MA, Jensen TL, Goll JB, et al. Molecular evolution of herpes simplex virus 2 complete genomes: comparison between primary and recurrent infections. *J Virol* 2017;91(23):e00942-17.
190. Mineta T, Rabkin SD, Martuza RL. Treatment of malignant gliomas using ganciclovir-hypersensitive, ribonucleotide reductase-deficient herpes simplex viral mutant. *Cancer Res* 1994;54:3963–3966.
191. Mineta T, Rabkin SD, Yazaki T, et al. Attenuated multi-mutated herpes simplex virus-1 for the treatment of malignant gliomas. *Nat Med* 1995;1:938–943.
192. Minson AC, Hodgman TC, Digar P. An analysis of the biological properties of monoclonal antibodies against glycoprotein D of herpes simplex virus and identification of amino acid substitutions that confer resistance to neutralization. *J Gen Virol* 1986;67:1001–1013.
193. Montgomerie JZ, Becroft DM, Croxson MC, et al. Herpes-simplex-virus infection after renal transplantation. *Lancet* 1969;2:867–871.
194. Mork N, Kofod-Olsen E, Sorensen KB, et al. Mutations in the TLR3 signaling pathway and beyond in adult patients with herpes simplex encephalitis. *Genes Immun* 2015;16(8):552–566.
195. Morrison LA, Knipe DM. Immunization with replication-defective mutants of herpes simplex virus type 1: sites of immune intervention in pathogenesis of challenge virus infection. *J Virol* 1994;68:689–696.
196. Mueller SN, Jones CM, Smith CM, et al. Rapid cytotoxic T lymphocyte activation occurs in the draining lymph nodes after cutaneous herpes simplex virus infection as a result of early antigen presentation and not the presence of virus. *J Exp Med* 2002;195:651–656.
197. Muller SA, Hermann FC, Winkelman RK. Herpes simplex infections in hematologic malignancies. *Am J Med* 1972;52:102–114.
198. Music SI, Fine EM, Togo Y. Zoster-like disease in the newborn due to herpes-simplex virus. *N Engl J Med* 1971;284:24–26.
199. Nahmias AJ, Keyserling HL, Kerrick GM. Herpes simplex. In: Remington JS, Klein JO, eds. *Infectious Diseases of the Fetus and Newborn Infant*. Philadelphia, PA: W. B. Saunders Company; 1983:636–678.
200. Nahmias AJ, Lee FK, Bechman-Nahmias S. Sero-epidemiological and sociological patterns of herpes simplex virus infection in the world. *Scand J Infect Dis* 1990;69:19–36.
201. Nahmias AJ, Whitley RJ, Visintine AN, et al Herpes simplex virus encephalitis: laboratory evaluations and their diagnostic significance. *J Infect Dis* 1982;145:829–836.
202. Nasemann T, Schaeg G. Herpes simplex virus. Type II: microbiology and clinical experiences with attenuated vaccine. *Hautarzt* 1973;24:133–139.
203. Newman KL, Marsh Z, Kirby AE, et al. Immunocompetent adults from human norovirus challenge studies do not exhibit norovirus viremia. *J Virol* 2015;89(13):6968–6969.
204. Nguyen LH, Knipe DM, Finberg RW. Replication-defective mutants of herpes simplex virus (HSV) induce cellular immunity and protect against lethal HSV infection. *J Virol* 1992;66:7067–7072.
205. Nishiyama Y, Kimura H, Daikoku T. Complementary lethal invasion of the central nervous system by nonneuroinvasive herpes simplex virus types 1 and 2. *J Virol* 1991;65:4520–4524.
206. Olson LC, Buescher EL, Artenstein MS, et al. Herpesvirus infections of the human central nervous system. *N Engl J Med* 1967;277:1271–1277.
207. Ostler HB. Herpes simplex: the primary infection. *Surv Ophthalmol* 1977;21:91–99.
208. Overall JCJ, Spruance SL, Green JA. Viral-induced leukocyte interferon in vesicle fluid from lesions of recurrent herpes labialis. *J Infect Dis* 1981;143:543–547.
209. Page J, Taylor J, Tideman RL, et al. Is HSV serology useful for the management of first episode genital herpes? *Sex Transm Infect* 2003;79(4):276–279.
210. Pandey U, Renner DW, Thompson RL, et al. Inferred father-to-son transmission of herpes simplex virus results in near-perfect preservation of viral genome identity and in vivo phenotypes. *Sci Rep* 2017;7(1):13666.
211. Papanastassiou V, Rampling R, Fraser M, et al. The potential for efficacy of the modified (ICP 34.5(−)) herpes simplex virus HSV1716 following intratumoural injection into human malignant glioma: a proof of principle study. *Gene Ther* 2002;9:398–406.
212. Parker J, Gillespie GY, Love CE, et al. Engineered herpes simplex virus expressing interleukin 12 in the treatment of experimental murine tumors. *Proc Natl Acad Sci U S A* 2000;97:2208–2213.
213. Parvey LS, Ch'ien LT. Neonatal herpes simplex virus infection introduced by fetal-monitor scalp electrodes. *Pediatrics* 1980;65:1150–1153.
214. Pass RF, Dworsky ME, Whitley RJ, et al Specific lymphocyte blastogenic responses in children with cytomegalovirus and herpes simplex virus infections acquired early in infancy. *Infect Immun* 1981;34:166–170.
215. Pass RF, Long WK, Whitley RJ, et al. Productive infection with cytomegalovirus and herpes simplex virus in renal transplant recipients: role of source of kidney. *J Infect Dis* 1978;137:556–563.
216. Pass RF, Whitley RJ, Whelchel JD, et al. Identification of patients with increased risk of infection with herpes simplex virus after renal transplantation. *J Infect Dis* 1979;140:487–492.
217. Patel A, Patel R. Recent insights into HSV infection and disease: results of wider genome analysis. *Curr Opin Infect Dis* 2019;32(1):51–55.
218. Patel P, Bush T, Mayer KH, et al. Prevalence and risk factors associated with herpes simplex virus-2 infection in a contemporary cohort of HIV-infected persons in the United States. *Sex Transm Dis* 2012;39(2):154–160.
219. Patton ME, Bernstein K, Liu G, et al. Seroprevalence of herpes simplex virus types 1 and 2 among pregnant women and sexually active, nonpregnant women in the United States. *Clin Infect Dis* 2018;67(10):1535–1542.
220. Pawlik TM, Nakamura H, Mullen JT, et al. Prodrug bioactivation and oncolysis of diffuse liver metastases by a herpes simplex virus 1 mutant that expresses the CYP2B1 transgene. *Cancer* 2002;95:1171–1181.
221. Phipps W, Saracino M, Magaret A, et al. Persistent genital herpes simplex virus-2 shedding years following the first clinical episode. *J Infect Dis* 2011;203(2):180–187.
222. Pinninti S, Feja K, Kimberlin D, et al. Neonatal herpes disease despite maternal antenatal antiviral suppressive therapy: a multicenter case series of the first such infants reported Paper presented at: Infectious Disease Society of America 48th Annual Meeting 2010; Vancouver, BC.
223. Posavad CM, Koelle DM, Corey L. Tipping the scales of herpes simplex virus reactivation: The important responses are local. *Nat Med* 1998;4:381–382.

224. Posavad CM, Remington M, Mueller DE, et al. Detailed characterization of T cell responses to herpes simplex virus-2 in immune seronegative persons. *J Immunol* 2010;184:3250–3259.
225. Posavad CM, Wald A, Kuntz S, et al. Frequent reactivation of herpes simplex virus among HIV-1-infected patients treated with highly active antiretroviral therapy. *J Infect Dis* 2004;190:693–696.
226. Prober CG, Sullender WM, Yasukawa LL, et al. Low risk of herpes simplex virus infections in neonates exposed to the virus at the time of vaginal delivery to mothers with recurrent genital herpes simplex virus infections. *N Engl J Med* 1987;316:240–244.
227. Puchhammer-Stockl E, Popow-Kraupp T, Heinz FX, et al. Establishment of PCR for the early diagnosis of herpes simplex encephalitis. *J Med Virol* 1990;32:77–82.
228. Pugh RCB, Dudgeon JA, Bodia M. Kaposi's varicelliform eruption (eczema herpeticum) with typical visceral necrosis. *J Pathol Bacteriol* 1955;69:67.
229. Rampling R, Cruickshang G, Papanastassiou V, et al. Toxicity evaluation of replication-competent herpes simplex virus (ICP 34.5 null mutant 1716) in patients with recurrent malignant glioma. *Gene Ther* 2000;7:859–866.
230. Rasmussen L, Merigan TC. Role of T lymphocytes in cellular immune responses during herpes simplex virus infection in humans. *Proc Natl Acad Sci U S A* 1978;75:3957–3961.
231. Rasmussen LE, Jordan GW, Stevens DA, et al. Lymphocyte interferon production and transformation after herpes simplex infections in humans. *J Immunol* 1974;112:728–736.
232. Rector JT, Lausch RN, Oakes JE. Use of monoclonal antibodies for analysis of antibody-dependent immunity to ocular herpes simplex virus type 1 infection. *Infect Immun* 1982;38:168–174.
233. Reeves WC, Corey L, Adams HG, et al. Risk of recurrence after first episodes of genital herpes: relation to HSV type and antibody response. *N Engl J Med* 1981;305:315–319.
234. Rinaldo CR Jr, Torpey DJ III. Cell-mediated immunity and immunosuppression in herpes simplex virus infection. *Immunodeficiency* 1993;5:33–90.
235. Roizman B, Jenkins FJ. Genetic engineering of novel genomes of large DNA viruses. *Science* 1985;129:1208–1214.
236. Roizman B, Knipe DM, Whitley RJ. Herpes simplex viruses. In: Knipe DM, Howley PM, eds. *Fields Virology*. 5th ed. Philadelphia, PA: Lippincott, Williams and Wilkins; 2007:2501–2602.
237. Rooney JF, Bryson Y, Mannix ML, et al. Prevention of ultraviolet-light-induced herpes labialis by sunscreen. *Lancet* 1991;338:1419–1422.
238. Rooney JF, Straus SE, Mannix ML, et al. Ultraviolet light-induced reactivation of herpes simplex virus type 2 and prevention by acyclovir. *J Infect Dis* 1992;166:500–506.
239. Rosato FE, Rosato EF, Plotkin SA. Herpetic-paronychia—an occupational hazard of medical personnel. *N Engl J Med* 1970;283:804–805.
240. Rowley A, Lakeman F, Whitley R, et al. Rapid detection of herpes simplex virus DNA in cerebrospinal fluid of patients with herpes simplex encephalitis. *Lancet* 1990;335: 440–441.
241. Roy S, Coulon PG, Srivastava R, et al. Blockade of LAG-3 immune checkpoint combined with therapeutic vaccination restore the function of tissue-resident anti-viral CD8(+) T cells and protect against recurrent ocular herpes simplex infection and disease. *Front Immunol* 2018;9:2922.
242. Sacks SL, Aoki FY, Martel AY, et al. Clinic-initiated, twice-daily oral famciclovir for treatment of recurrent genital herpes: a randomized, double-blind, controlled trial. *Clin Infect Dis* 2005;41:1097–1104.
243. Sanchez-Pescador L, Burke RL, Ott G, et al. The effect of adjuvants on the efficacy of a recombinant herpes simplex virus glycoprotein vaccine. *J Immunol* 1988;141:1720–1727.
244. Sancho-Shimizu V, Perez de Diego R, Lorenzo L, et al. Herpes simplex encephalitis in children with autosomal recessive and dominant TRIF deficiency. *J Clin Invest* 2011;121(12):4889–4902.
245. Sato A, Linehan MM, Iwasaki A. Dual recognition of herpes simplex viruses by TLR2 and TLR9 in dendritic cells. *Proc Natl Acad Sci U S A* 2006;103:17343–17348.
246. Sbidian E, Battistella M, Legoff J, et al. Recalcitrant pseudotumoral anogenital herpes simplex virus type 2 in HIV-infected patients: evidence for predominant B-lymphoplasmocytic infiltration and immunomodulators as effective therapeutic strategy. *Clin Infect Dis* 2013;57(11):1648–1655.
247. Schacker T, Zeh J, Hu HL, et al. Frequency of symptomatic and asymptomatic herpes simplex virus type 2 reactivations among human immunodeficiency virus-infected men. *J Infect Dis* 1998;178:1616–1622.
248. Schiffer JT, Abu-Raddad L, Mark KE, et al. Mucosal host immune response predicts the severity and duration of herpes simplex virus-2 genital tract shedding episodes. *Proc Natl Acad Sci U S A* 2010;107(44):18973–18978.
249. Schiffer JT, Abu-Raddad L, Mark KE, et al. Frequent release of low amounts of herpes simplex virus from neurons: results of a mathematical model. *Sci Transl Med* 2009;1(7):7ra16.
250. Schlitt M, Bucher AP, Stroop WG, et al. Mortality in an experimental focal herpes encephalitis: relationship to seizures. *Brain Res* 1988;440:293–298.
251. Schlitt M, Lakeman AD, Wilson ER, et al. A rabbit model of focal herpes simplex encephalitis. *J Infect Dis* 1986;153:732–735.
252. Schmidt OW, Fife KH, Corey L. Reinfection is an uncommon occurrence in patients with symptomatic recurrent genital herpes. *J Infect Dis* 1984;149:645–646.
253. Schmidt S, Bohn-Wippert K, Schlattmann P, et al. Sequence analysis of herpes simplex virus 1 thymidine kinase and DNA polymerase genes from over 300 clinical isolates from 1973 to 2014 finds novel mutations that may be relevant for development of antiviral resistance. *Antimicrob Agents Chemother* 2015;59(8):4938–4945.
254. Schneider J, Rohde B. Antigen therapy of recurring herpes simplex with herpes simplex vaccine LUPIDON H and G. *Z Haut Geschlechtskr* 1972;47:973–980.
255. Schneweis KE, Nahmias AJ. On the stability of three strains of herpes simplex virus at low temperatures. *Z Hyg Infektionskr* 1961;183:556.
256. Senzer NN, Kaufman HL, Amatruda T, et al. Phase II clinical trial of a granulocyte-macrophage colony-stimulating factor-encoding, second-generation oncolytic herpesvirus in patients with unresectable metastatic melanoma. *J Clin Oncol* 2009;27:5763–5771.
257. Shah AC, Parker JN, Gillespie GY, et al. Enhanced antiglioma activity of chimeric HCMV/HSV-1 oncolytic viruses. *Gene Ther* 2007;14:1045–1054.
258. Shannon B, Gajer P, Yi TJ, et al. Distinct effects of the cervicovaginal microbiota and herpes simplex type 2 infection on female genital tract immunology. *J Infect Dis* 2017;215(9):1366–1375.
259. Shannon B, Yi TJ, Thomas-Pavanel J, et al. Impact of asymptomatic herpes simplex virus type 2 infection on mucosal homing and immune cell subsets in the blood and female genital tract. *J Immunol* 2014;192(11):5074–5082.
260. Sheridan JF, Donnenberg AD, Aurelian L, et al. Immunity to herpes simplex virus type 2. IV. Impaired lymphokine production during recrudescence correlates with an imbalance in T lymphocyte subsets. *J Immunol* 1982;129:326–331.
261. Shin H, Iwasaki A. A vaccine strategy that protects against genital herpes by establishing local memory T cells. *Nature* 2012;491(7424):463–467.
262. Ship II, Miller MF, Ram C. A retrospective study of recurrent herpes labialis (RHL) in a professional population, 1958–1971. *Oral Surg Oral Med Oral Pathol* 1977;44:723–730.
263. Ship II, Morris AL, Durocher RT, et al. Recurrent aphthous ulcerations and recurrent herpes labialis in a professional school student population. I. Experience. *Oral Surg Oral Med Oral Pathol* 1960;13:1191–1202.
264. Ship II, Morris AL, Durocher RT, et al. Recurrent aphthous ulcerations and recurrent labialis in a professional school student population. IV. Twelve month study of natural disease patterns. *Oral Surg Oral Med Oral Pathol* 1961;14:39.
265. Shipley MM, Renner DW, Ott M, et al. Genome-wide surveillance of genital herpes simplex virus type 1 from multiple anatomic sites over time. *J Infect Dis* 2018;218(4):595–605.
266. Siegal FP, Kadowaki N, Shodell M, et al. The nature of the principal type 1 interferon-producing cells in human blood. *Science* 1999;284:1835–1837.
267. Skinner GR, Williams DR, Moles AW, et al. Prepubertal vaccination of mice against experimental infection of the genital tract with type 2 herpes simplex virus. *Arch Virol* 1980;64:329–338.
268. Smith GL, Mackett M, Moss B. Infectious vaccinia virus recombinants that express hepatitis B virus surface antigen. *Nature* 1983;302:490–495.
269. Soltz-Szots J. New methods of specific vaccination in recurrent herpes simplex. *Hautartz* 1960;11:465–467.
270. Spruance SL. The natural history of recurrent oral-facial herpes simplex virus infection. *Semin Dermatol* 1992;11:200–206.
271. Spruance SL, Overall JC Jr, Kern ER, et al. The natural history of recurrent herpes simplex labialis: implications for antiviral therapy. *N Engl J Med* 1977;297:69–75.
272. Srivastava R, Khan AA, Chilukuri S, et al. CXCL10/CXCR3-dependent mobilization of herpes simplex virus-specific CD8(+) TEM and CD8(+) TRM cells within infected tissues allows efficient protection against recurrent herpesvirus infection and disease. *J Virol* 2017;91(14):e00278-17.
273. Stanberry L, Koelle DM, Whitley RJ. Herpes simplex vaccines. In: Levine M, Good M, Liu M, Nabel G, Nataro J, Rappuoli R, eds. *New Generation Vaccines*. New York: Informa Healthcare; 2008.
274. Stanberry LR, Bernstein DI, Burke RL, et al. Vaccination with recombinant herpes simplex virus glycoproteins: protection against initial and recurrent genital herpes. *J Infect Dis* 1987;155:914–920.
275. Stanberry LR, Spruance SL, Bernstein DI, et al. Glycoprotein-D-adjuvant vaccine to prevent genital herpes. *N Engl J Med* 2002;347(21):1652–1661.
276. Stevens JG, Cook ML. Latent herpes simplex virus in sensory ganglia. *Perspect Virol* 1974;8:171.
277. Straus SE, Savarese B, Tigges M, et al. Induction and enhancement of immune responses to herpes simplex virus type 2 in humans by use of a recombinant glycoprotein D vaccine. *J Infect Dis* 1993;167:1045–1052.
278. Stroop WG, Schaefer DC. Production of encephalitis restricted to the temporal lobes by experimental reactivation of herpes simplex virus. *J Infect Dis* 1986;153:721–731.
279. Sullender WM, Miller JL, Yasukawa LL, et al. Humoral and cell-mediated immunity in neonates with herpes simplex virus infection. *J Infect Dis* 1987;155:28–37.
280. Sullivan-Bolyai J, Hull H, Wilson C, et al. Presentation of neonatal herpes simplex virus infections: implications for a change in therapeutic strategy. *Pediatr Infect Dis J* 1986;5:309–314.
281. Sullivan-Bolyai JZ, Fife KH, Jacobs RF, et al. Disseminated neonatal herpes simplex virus type 1 from a maternal breast lesion. *Pediatrics* 1983;71:455–457.
282. Sundaresan P, Hunter WD, Martuza RL, et al. Attenuated, replication-competent herpes simplex virus type 1 mutant G207: safety evaluation in mice. *J Virol* 2000; 74(8):3832–3841.
283. Suvas S, Azkur AK, Rouse BT. Qa-1b and CD94-NKG2a interaction regulate cytolytic activity of herpes simplex virus-specific memory CD8+ T cells in the latently infected trigeminal ganglia. *J Immunol* 2006;176:1703–1711.
284. Szpara ML, Gatherer D, Ochoa A, et al. Evolution and diversity in human herpes simplex virus genomes. *J Virol* 2014;88(2):1209–1227.
285. Szpara ML, Parsons L, Enquist LW. Sequence variability in clinical and laboratory isolates of herpes simplex virus 1 reveals new mutations. *J Virol* 2010;84(10):5303–5313.
286. Takakuwa H, Goshima F, Nozawa N, et al. Oncolytic viral therapy using a spontaneously generated herpes simplex virus type 1 variant for disseminated peritoneal tumor in immunocompetent mice. *Arch Virol* 2003;148:813–825.
287. Terezhalmy GT, Tyler MT, Ross GR. Eczema herpeticum: atopic dermatitis complicated by primary herpetic gingivostomatitis. *Oral Surg Oral Med Oral Pathol* 1979;48:513–516.
288. Terni M, Carcialanza D, Cassai E, et al. Aseptic meningitis in association with herpes progenitalis. *N Engl J Med* 1971;285:503–504.
289. Teshigahara O, Goshima F, Takao K, et al. Oncolytic viral therapy for breast cancer with herpes simplex virus type 1 mutant HF 10. *J Surg Oncol* 2004;85:42–47.
290. Tobian AA, Grabowski MK, Serwadda D, et al. Reactivation of herpes simplex virus type 2 after initiation of antiretroviral therapy. *J Infect Dis* 2013;208(5):839–846.
291. Todo T. Oncolytic virus therapy using genetically engineered herpes simplex viruses. *Front Biosci* 2008;13:2060–2064.
292. Todo T, Martuza RL, Rabkin SD, et al. Oncolytic herpes simplex virus vector with enhanced MHC class I presentation and tumor cell killing. *Proc Natl Acad Sci U S A* 2001;98:6396–6401.

293. Troendle-Atkins J, Demmler GJ, Buffone GJ. Rapid diagnosis of herpes simplex virus encephalitis by using the polymerase chain reaction. *J Pediatr* 1993;123:376–380.
294. Trofatter KF, Jr., Daniels CA, Williams RJ, Jr., et al. Growth of type 2 herpes simplex virus in newborn and adult mononuclear leukocytes. *Intervirology* 1979;11:117–123.
295. Tronstein E, Johnston C, Huang ML, et al. Genital shedding of herpes simplex virus among symptomatic and asymptomatic persons with HSV-2 infection. *JAMA* 2011;305(14):1441–1449.
296. Tyler KL. Herpes simplex virus infections of the central nervous system: encephalitis and meningitis, including Mollaret's. *Herpes* 2004;11(Suppl 2):57A–64A.
297. Tyring S, Wald A, Zadeikis N, et al. ASP2151 for the treatment of genital herpes: a randomized, double-blind, placebo- and valacyclovir-controlled, dose-finding study. *J Infect Dis* 2012;205:1100–1110.
298. Underwood GE, Weed SD. Recurrent cutaneous herpes simplex in hairless mice. *Infect Immun* 1974;10:471–474.
299. Ushijima Y, Luo C, Goshima F, et al. Determination and analysis of the DNA sequence of highly attenuated herpes simplex virus type 1 mutant HF10, a potential oncolytic virus. *Microbes Infect* 2007;9:142–149.
300. Van Wagoner N, Fife K, Leone PA, et al. Effects of different doses of GEN-003, a therapeutic vaccine for genital herpes simplex virus-2, on viral shedding and lesions: results of a randomized placebo-controlled trial. *J Infect Dis* 2018;218(12):1890–1899.
301. Varghese S, Rabkin SD, Liu R, et al. Enhanced therapeutic efficacy of IL-12, but not GM-CSF, expressing oncolytic herpes simplex virus for transgenic mouse derived prostate cancers. *Cancer Gene Ther* 2006;13:253–265.
302. Verjans GM, Hintzen RQ, van Dun JM, et al. Selective retention of herpes simplex virus-specific T cells in latently infected human trigeminal ganglia. *Proc Natl Acad Sci U S A* 2007;104:3496–3501.
303. von Rodovsky J, Dbaly V, Benda R. Preventive treatment of recurring herpes with a formaldehyde vaccine made of rabbit kidney cells. *Dermatol Monatsschr* 1971;157:701–708.
304. Vontver LA, Hickok DE, Brown Z, et al. Recurrent genital herpes simplex virus infection in pregnancy: infant outcome and frequency of asymptomatic recurrences. *Am J Obstet Gynecol* 1982;143:75–84.
305. Wald A, Corey L, Timmler B, et al. Helicase-primase inhibitor Pritelivir for HSV-2 infection. *N Engl J Med* 2014;370(3):201–210.
306. Wald A, Huang ML, Carrell D, et al. Polymerase chain reaction for detection of herpes simplex virus (HSV) DNA on mucosal surfaces: comparison with HSV isolation in cell culture. *J Infect Dis* 2003;188(9):1345–1351.
307. Wald A, Krantz E, Selke S, et al. Knowledge of partners' genital herpes protects against herpes simplex virus type 2 acquisition. *J Infect Dis* 2006;194(1):42–52.
308. Wald A, Langenberg AG, Link K, et al. Effect of condoms on reducing the transmission of herpes simplex virus type 2 from men to women. *JAMA* 2001;285:3100–3106.
309. Wald A, Link K. Risk of human immunodeficiency virus infection in herpes simplex virus type 2-seropositive persons: a meta-analysis. *J Infect Dis* 2002;185:45–52.
310. Wald A, Timmler B, Magaret A, et al. Effect of pritelivir compared with valacyclovir on genital HSV-2 shedding in patients with frequent recurrences: a randomized clinical trial. *JAMA* 2016;316(23):2495–2503.
311. Wald A, Zeh J, Barnum G, et al. Suppression of subclinical shedding of herpes simplex virus type 2 with acyclovir. *Ann Intern Med* 1996;124:8–15.
312. Wald A, Zeh J, Selke S, et al. Reactivation of genital herpes simplex virus type 2 infection in asymptomatic seropositive persons. *N Engl J Med* 2000;342:844–850.
313. Wali RK, Drachenberg C, Hirsch HH, et al. BK virus-associated nephropathy in renal allograft recipients: rescue therapy by sirolimus-based immunosuppression. *Transplantation* 2004;78:1069–1073.
314. Weston WL, Brice SL, Jester JD, et al. Herpes simplex virus in childhood erythema multiforme. *Pediatrics* 1992;89:32–34.
315. Wheeler CE, Jr., Abele DC. Eczema herpeticum, primary and recurrent. *Arch Dermatol* 1966;93:162–173.
316. Wheeler CE, Jr., Cabaniss WH, Jr. Epidemic cutaneous herpes simplex in wrestlers (herpes gladiatorum). *JAMA* 1965;194:993–997.
317. Whitley R, Roizman B. Herpes simplex virus. In: Richman D, Whitley R, Hayden F, eds. *Clinical Virology*. 4th ed. Washington, DC: ASM Press; 2017:415–445.
318. Whitley RJ. Herpes simplex virus infection. *Semin Pediatr Infect Dis* 2002;13:6–11.
319. Whitley RJ. Herpes simplex virus infections. In: Remington JS, Klein JO, eds. *Infectious Diseases of the Fetus and Newborn Infant*. 2nd ed. Philadelphia, PA: W. B. Saunders Company; 1989:282–305.
320. Whitley RJ. Herpes simplex viruses. In: Knipe DM, Howley PM, eds. *Fields Virology*. 4th ed. Philadelphia, PA: Lippincott, Williams and Wilkins; 2001:2461–2509.
321. Whitley RJ. Herpes simplex viruses. In: Fields BN, Knipe DM, eds. *Virology* Vol 2. New York: Raven Press; 1990:1844–1887.
322. Whitley RJ. Therapy of herpes simplex virus infections of the central nervous system: Neonatal herpes and herpes simplex encephalitis. In: Feigin RD, ed. *Seminars in Pediatric Infectious Diseases*. Vol 2. Philadelphia, PA: W. B. Saunders Company; 1991:263–269.
323. Whitley RJ. Viral encephalitis. *N Engl J Med* 1990;323:242–250.
324. Whitley RJ, Corey L, Arvin A, et al. Changing presentation of herpes simplex virus infection in neonates. *J Infect Dis* 1988;158:109–116.
325. Whitley RJ, Hutto C. Neonatal herpes simplex virus infections. *Pediatr Rev* 1985;7: 119–126.
326. Whitley RJ, Kimberlin DW. Herpes simplex: encephalitis children and adolescents. *Semin Pediatr Infect Dis* 2005;16:17–23.
327. Whitley RJ, Kimberlin DW, Roizman B. Herpes simplex viruses. *Clin Infect Dis* 1998;26:541–555.
328. Whitley RJ, Levin M, Barton N, et al. Infections caused by herpes simplex virus in the immunocompromised host: natural history and topical acyclovir therapy. *J Infect Dis* 1984;150:323–329.
329. Whitley RJ, Nahmias AJ, Visintine AM, et al. The natural history of herpes simplex virus infection of mother and newborn. *Pediatrics* 1980;66:489–494.
330. Whitley RJ, Soong S-J, Dolin R, et al. Adenine arabinoside therapy of biopsy-proved herpes simplex encephalitis: National Institute of Allergy and Infectious Diseases collaborative antiviral study. *N Engl J Med* 1977;297:289–294.
331. Whitley RJ, Soong S-J, Hirsch MS, et al. Herpes simplex encephalitis: vidarabine therapy and diagnostic problems. *N Engl J Med* 1981;304:313–318.
332. Whitley RJ, Spruance S, Hayden FG, et al. Vidarabine therapy for mucocutaneous herpes simplex virus infections in the immunocompromised host. *J Infect Dis* 1984;149:1–8.
333. Whitley RJ, Yeager A, Kartus P, et al. Neonatal herpes simplex virus infection: follow-up evaluation of vidarabine therapy. *Pediatrics* 1983;72:778–785.
334. Woestenberg PJ, Tjhie JH, de Melker HE, et al. Herpes simplex virus type 1 and type 2 in the Netherlands: seroprevalence, risk factors and changes during a 12-year period. *BMC Infect Dis* 2016;16:364.
335. Wolontis S, Jeansson S. Correlation of herpes simplex virus types 1 and 2 with clinical features of infection. *J Infect Dis* 1977;135:28–33.
336. Workowski KA. Centers for disease control and prevention sexually transmitted diseases treatment guidelines. *Clin Infect Dis* 2015;61(Suppl 8):S759–S762.
337. Xu F, Schillinger JA, Sternberg MR, et al. Seroprevalence and coinfection with herpes simplex virus type 1 and type 2 in the United States, 1988-1994. *J Infect Dis* 2002;185:1019–1024.
338. Xu F, Sternberg MR, Kottiri BJ, et al. Trends in herpes simplex virus type 1 and type 2 seroprevalence in the United States. *JAMA* 2006;296:964–973.
339. Xu F, Sternberg MR, Markowitz LE. Men who have sex with men in the United States: demographic and behavioral characteristics and prevalence of HIV and HSV-2 infection: results from National Health and Nutrition Examination Survey 2001–2006. *Sex Transm Dis* 2010;37(6):399–405.
340. Xu F, Sternberg MR, Markowitz LE. Women who have sex with women in the United States: prevalence, sexual behavior and prevalence of herpes simplex virus type 2 infection—results from National Health and Nutrition Examination Survey 2001–2006. *Sex Transm Dis* 2010;37(7):407–413.
341. Yazaki T, Manz HJ, Rabkin SD, et al. Treatment of human malignant meningiomas by G207, a replication-competent multimutated herpes simplex virus 1. *Cancer Res* 1995;55:4752–4756.
342. Yeager AS, Arvin AM. Reasons for the absence of a history of recurrent genital infections in mothers of neonates infected with herpes simplex virus. *Pediatrics* 1984;73:188–193.
343. Yeager AS, Arvin AM, Urbani LJ, et al, 3d. Relationship of antibody to outcome in neonatal herpes simplex virus infections. *Infect Immun* 1980;29:532–538.
344. Yen SSC, Reagan JW, Rosenthal MS. Herpes simplex infection in the female genital tract. *Obstet Gynecol* 1965;25:479–492.
345. Zarling JM, Moran PA, Brewer L, et al. Herpes simplex virus (HSV)-specific proliferative and cytotoxic T-cell responses in humans immunized with an HSV type 2 glycoprotein subunit vaccine. *J Virol* 1988;62:4481–4485.
346. Zarling JM, Moran PA, Burke RL, et al. Human cytotoxic T cells clones directed against herpes simplex virus infected cells. *J Immunol* 1986;136:4669–4673.
347. Zhang Q, Davis JC, Lamborn IT, et al. Combined immunodeficiency associated with DOCK8 mutations. *N Engl J Med* 2009;361(21):2046–2055.
348. Zhang SY, Clark NE, Freije CA, et al. Inborn errors of RNA lariat metabolism in humans with brainstem viral infection. *Cell* 2018;172(5):952–965 e918.
349. Zhang SY, Jouanguy E, Ugolini S, et al. TLR3 deficiency in patients with herpes simplex encephalitis. *Science* 2007;317:1522–1527.
350. Zhang SY, Jouanguy E, Zhang Q, et al. Human inborn errors of immunity to infection affecting cells other than leukocytes: from the immune system to the whole organism. *Curr Opin Immunol* 2019;59:88–100.
351. Zhao X, Deak E, Soderberg K, et al. Vaginal submucosal dendritic cells, but not Langerhan's cells, induce protective TH1 responses to herpes simplex virus 2. *J Exp Med* 2003;197:153–162.
352. Zheng B, Graham FL, Johnson DC, et al. Immunogenicity in mice of tandem repeats of an epitope from herpes simplex gD protein when expressed by recombinant adenovirus vectors. *Vaccine* 1993;11:1191–1198.
353. Zhu J, Hladik F, Woodward A, et al. Persistence of HIV-1 receptor-positive cells after HSV-2 reactivation is a potential mechanism for increased HIV-1 acquisition. *Nat Med* 2009;15(8):886–892.
354. Zhu J, Koelle DM, Cao J, et al. Virus-specific CD8+ T cells accumulate near sensory nerve endings in genital skin during subclinical HSV-2 reactivation. *J Exp Med* 2007;204:595–603.
355. Zhu J, Peng T, Johnston C, et al. Immune surveillance by CD8alphaalpha+ skin-resident T cells in human herpes virus infection. *Nature* 2013;497(7450):494–497.
356. Zweerink HJ, Corey L. Virus-specific antibodies in sera from patients with genital herpes simplex virus infections. *Infect Immun* 1982;37:413–421.

CHAPTER 11

Epstein-Barr Virus

Benjamin E. Gewurz • Richard M. Longnecker • Jeffrey I. Cohen

HISTORY

In 1958, Denis Burkitt described a tumor in young African children in areas where malaria was holoendemic. This tumor is now referred to as Burkitt lymphoma.[67] In 1964, Epstein, Achong, and Barr discovered a member of the herpes family in cultured Burkitt lymphoma cells using electron microscopy to detect viral particles.[172] The virus was named Epstein-Barr virus (EBV). Gertrude and Werner Henle described an immunofluorescent antibody test for EBV in 1966 finding that patients with Burkitt lymphoma as well as most American adults had antibody to EBV.[243] In 1969, a chance discovery by the Henles in serological studies investigating the prevalence of EBV found that EBV was a causative agent for mononucleosis when a control subject seroconverted and was found to have infectious mononucleosis.[245] Descriptions of patients with symptoms resembling infectious mononucleosis were first reported in the medical literature in the late 19th century and infectious mononucleosis was first named in 1920.[666] Heterophile antibodies were first used in the diagnosis of infectious mononucleosis in 1932.[530] In 1967, EBV was found to immortalize human B lymphocytes in cell culture.[242,550] In 1984, the virus was shown to replicate in human epithelial cells.[641] These discoveries allowed laboratory experimental model systems that provided a means to study the newly identified virus. Sero-epidemiologic evidence that EBV was a cause for Burkitt lymphoma came from pioneering studies of de-The and colleagues.[687] Subsequently, EBV genome positivity was discovered in nasopharyngeal carcinoma (NPC) in 1970,[766] in lymphoma/lymphoproliferative disease in posttransplant patients in late 1970, and in the analogous non-Hodgkin lymphoma in patients with AIDS in 1982,[762] in T-cell lymphoma in 1988,[301] and in some cases of Hodgkin lymphoma in 1989.[728] Since then, the virus has been detected in other malignancies, notably NK cell lymphoma and in a subset of gastric carcinoma. Its potential relationship to nonmalignant diseases such as multiple sclerosis and systemic lupus erythematosus continues to be studied and will be discussed later in this chapter.

CLASSIFICATION

EBV is a member of the gamma herpesvirus subfamily consisting of the gamma 1 or lymphocryptovirus (LCV)

genus, which includes EBV and LCVs in nonhuman primates, and the gamma 2 or rhadinovirus (RDV) genus, which includes herpesvirus saimiri (HVS) and Kaposi's sarcoma herpes virus (KSHV, also called HHV8). Many Old World and some New World primate species naturally carry their own LCVs, which are collinearly homologous to EBV. In contrast, RDVs are found not only in most primate species but also in many subprimate mammalian species. Overall, the nucleotide sequences of gamma herpesvirus genomes have substantial collinear homology and much less collinearity and homology with alpha and beta herpesvirus genomes.[145]

Among the gamma herpesvirus genomes, LCVs are likely to have evolved from RDVs. RDVs have more diverse genomes than LCVs, are naturally found in more diverse mammalian species, and characteristically have homologs of multiple cellular cDNAs in their genomes. Old World LCVs have collinear homologous genomes with a unique group of recently evolved nuclear protein-encoding genes, which lack homology to RDV or cell genes and are only partially present in New World LCV genomes. New World LCVs may therefore be intermediates in the evolution of Old World primate LCVs.

LCV genomes are very similar to each other in structure, gene organization, and have collinear homology, albeit with some exceptions in the case of New World LCVs, which as shown by the common marmoset LCV lack two EBNA3 genes, the viral interleukin-10, and EBV-encoded small RNAs (EBERs) when compared to EBV.[583] Shared features include 0.5 kbp tandem terminal direct repeats (TR), 3 kbp tandem internal direct repeats (IR1), and short tandem internal direct repeats (IR2, IR4). RDVs have longer and more highly reiterated TRs and lack long internal direct repeats. Old World primate LCV genes encode latency-associated nuclear antigen proteins EBNA1, EBNA2, EBNA3A, EBNA3B, and EBNA3C, which are expressed when EBV growth transforms primary B lymphocytes to lymphoblastoid cell lines (LCLs). LCVs also include genes that encode latent membrane proteins (LMPs) important for efficient latent infection–associated B-lymphocyte growth transformation and survival,[182] genes that encode two small nonpolyadenylated EBER RNAs,[259,372] genes that encode differentially spliced Bam A rightward transcripts (BARTs), genes that encode an IL-10 and a bcl-2 homolog,[471,531] genes that encode distinctive microRNAs (miRNAs),[542] and a large number of genes that are important for replicating and packaging the genome and infecting target cells (Table 11.1).

TABLE 11.1 EBV-encoded proteins

EBV Gene	HSV	KSHV	EBV Name	Known or Proposed Function
BNRF1		ORF75		Major tegument protein, disrupts DAXX and ATRX complex
BNLF2b				
BNLF2a				Interacts with Tap, immune evasion
EBER1,2				Small RNAs, cell survival factor, PAX5 recruitment to genome
BCRF1				IL-10 homolog—host immune modulator
BCRF2				
BCLT1				Nuclear noncoding RNA—lytic replication
BCRT2				Nuclear noncoding RNA—lytic replication
BWRF1			**EBNALP**	**Regulator of gene transcription (EBNA5)—EBV nuclear antigen**
BYRF1			**EBNA2**	**Regulator of viral gene transcription—EBV nuclear antigen**
BHRF1		ORF16		Bcl-2 homolog
BHLF1				Transcript required for OriLyt function
BFLF2	UL31	ORF69		Required for nuclear egress—binds BFRF1
BFLF1	UL32	ORF68		Virion protein—DNA cleavage/packaging
BFRF1	UL34	ORF67		Nuclear egress—binds BFLF2—ESCRT recruitment
BFRF2		ORF66		Part of vPIC with BDLF3.5, BDLF4, BGLF3, BGLF4, BVLF1
BFRF3	UL35	ORF65		Capsid protein
BPLF1	UL36	ORF64		Tegument protein—deubiquitinase
BOLF1	UL37	ORF63		Tegument protein
BORF1	UL38	ORF62		Capsid assembly
BORF2	UL39	ORF61		Ribonucleotide reductase (large subunit)—inhibits cellular APOBEC3B
BaRF1	UL40	ORF60		Ribonucleotide reductase (small subunit)
BMRF1	UL42	ORF59		Polymerase-associated processivity factor
BMRF2	UL43	ORF58		Transmembrane glycoprotein—binds integrins and BDLF2

(Continued)

TABLE 11.1 EBV-encoded proteins (Continued)

EBV Gene	HSV	KSHV	EBV Name	Known or Proposed Function
BSLF2/BMLF1	UL54	ORF57		SM, posttranscriptional regulator of viral gene expression
BSLF1	UL52	ORF56		DNA replication—helicase/primase complex
BSRF1	UL51	ORF55		Tegument protein
BLRF1		ORF53		gN, virion protein, interacts with gM
BLRF2		ORF52		Tegument protein
BLLF1a			gp350	Virion binding to CR2 (CD21), virion protein
BLLF1b			gp220	Virion binding to CR2 (CD21), virion protein
BLLF3	UL50	ORF54		dUTPase
BLRF3-BERF1			**EBNA3C**	**Regulator of gene expression (EBNA6)**
BERF2a,b			**EBNA3B**	**Regulator of gene expression (EBNA4)**
BERF3-BERF4			**EBNA3A**	**Regulator of gene expression (EBNA3)**
BZLF2			gp42	Binds HLA class II, complexes with gH/gL (gp85/gp25), virion protein
BZLF1			Zta, EB1	Lytic gene transactivator
RAZ				Z regulator
BRLF1		ORF50	Rta, EB2 LF2	Lytic gene transactivator
BRRF1		ORF49		Na—lytic gene transactivator
BRRF2		ORF48		Cytoplasmic phosphoprotein
BKRF1			**EBNA1**	**Maintenance of viral episome**
BRKF2	UL1	ORF47	gp25	gL—complexes with gp42 and gp85
BKRF3	UL2	ORF46		Uracil–DNA glycosylase
BKRF4	UL3	ORF45		Tegument phosphoprotein
BBLF4	UL5	ORF44		DNA replication—helicase/primase complex
BBRF1	UL6	ORF43		Capsid protein—portal
BBRF2	UL7	ORF42		Tegument protein
BBLF2-3	UL9	ORF40		DNA replication—helicase/primase complex
BBRF3	UL10	ORF39		gM, interacts with gN
BBLF1	UL11	ORF38		Myristoylated virion protein
BGLF5	UL12	ORF37		Exonuclease, host shutoff, immune evasion
BGLF4	UL13	ORF36		Part of vPIC with BDLF3.5, BDLF4, BFRF2, BGLF3, BVLF1
BGLF3	UL14	ORF34		Part of vPIC with BDLF3.5, BDLF4, BFRF2, BGLF4, BVLF1
BGLF3.5		ORF35		Tegument protein
BGRF1	UL15	ORF29a		Terminase—small subunit
BGLF2	UL16	ORF33		Tegument protein
BGLF1	UL17	ORF32		Capsid maturation/DNA packaging, tegument protein
BDLF4		ORF31		Part of vPIC with BDLF3.5, BFRF2, BGLF3, BGLF4, BVLF1
BDRF1	UL15	ORF29b		Terminase—small subunit
BDLF3		ORF28	gp150	Glycoprotein enhances epithelial infection
BDLF3.5		ORF30		Part of vPIC with BDLF4, BFRF2, BGLF3, BGLF4, BVLF1
BDLF2		ORF27		Gycoprotein—complexes with BMRF2
BDLF1	UL18	ORF26		Minor capsid protein
BcLF1	UL19	ORF25		Major capsid protein
BcRF1		ORF24		vTBP—viral TATA binding protein—directs vPic
BTRF1	UL21	ORF23		

TABLE 11.1 EBV-encoded proteins (Continued)

EBV Gene	HSV	KSHV	EBV Name	Known or Proposed Function
BXLF2	UL22	ORF22	gp85	gH—complexes with gp25 and gp42, virion protein
BXLF1	UL23	ORF21		Thymidine kinase
BXRF1	UL24	ORF20		
BVRF1	UL25	ORF19		Virion protein
BVRF2	UL26	ORF17		Protease, scaffold
BVLF1				Part of vPIC with BDLF3.5, BDLF4, BFRF2, BGLF3, BGLF4
BdRF1				Capsid scaffolding
BILF2			gp78/55	Virion protein
BILF1				GPCR, down-regulates MHC class I
BALF5	UL30	ORF9		DNA polymerase
BALF4	UL27	ORF8	gp110	gB—fusion protein, virion protein
BALF3	UL28	ORF7		Terminase large subunit
BALF2	UL29	ORF6		ssDNA binding protein
BALF1				Bcl-2 homolog
BARF0/ RK-BARF0				Regulator of Notch pathway
BARTS				MicroRNAs
BARF1				Soluble colony stimulating factor receptor, binds CSF1
BNLF1a,b,c			**LMP1**	**Constitutive CD40 mimic—oncoprotein**
			LMP2A	**Constitutive B-cell receptor mimic (TP1)**
			LMP2B	**Regulator of LMP2A and LMP1 function? (TP2)**
Raji LF3				
Raji LF2		ORF11		Binds BRLF1 and IRF7
RPMS1				Interacts with the CBF1-associated corepressor and negatively regulates EBNA2 and Notch
Raji LF1				Part of BILF1
BARTS				microRNAs

Genes in "EBV" column bolded are expressed in latent infection.
In the "HSV" and "KSV" columns, the homology with the proteins underlined with EBV is not significant; however, they may be positional homologs. EBV proteins and RNAs that inhibit the immune system are shown in Table 11.3. EBV, Epstein-Barr virus; HSV, herpes simplex virus; KSHV, Kaposi's sarcoma herpes virus; IL, interleukin; HLA, human leukocyte antigen; CSF-1, colony-stimulating factor-1; vPic, virus preinitiation complex; GPCR, G protein-coupled receptor; MHC, major histocompatibility complex class I.

The EBV genome and gene organization is shown in Figures 11.1 and 11.2. EBV was the first herpesvirus genome to be completely cloned in sets of overlapping fragments based in part on previously derived restriction endonuclease maps generated by Elliott Kieff's laboratory.[141,142] The EBV genome was subsequently sequenced from BamHI digested cloned DNA fragments[27] and open reading frames (ORFs) were designated by their order in a rightward or leftward direction within each BamHI fragment, which were given letters based on the size of the fragment[27] (Fig. 11.2 and Table 11.1). The majority of KSHV-predicted ORFs are collinearly homologous to ORFs of EBV[594] (Table 11.1), emphasizing the common evolutionary origin of the gamma 1 and gamma 2 herpesviruses. LCVs and RDVs also have analogous but nonhomologous DNA sequences encoding nuclear proteins that are necessary and sufficient for persistence of the genomes as episomes in dividing cells.[744]

More broadly, all alpha, beta, and gamma herpesvirus DNAs have conserved distantly homologous gene blocks with conserved gene order and collinear homology at the predicted protein level (see Chapter 8).[145] These are primarily genes that encode proteins involved in nucleotide metabolism, proteins that replicate and process viral DNA, and proteins that comprise the structural components of the virion capsid, tegument, and envelope. In addition, genes that are at least partially shared among the gamma herpesviruses and have more limited representation in the genomes of other herpesviruses include BZLF1 and BRLF1, which encode the immediate-early

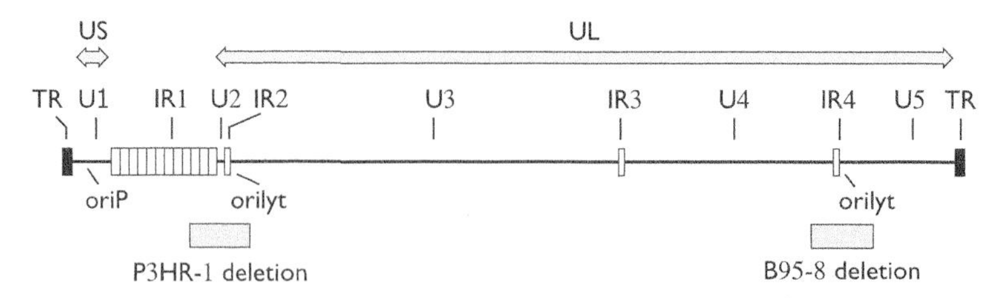

FIGURE 11.1 Schematic depiction of the linear Epstein-Barr virus (EBV) genome. Linear representation of the overall genome arrangement with the unique short (US) and unique long (UL) regions shown. Within the genome the terminal repeats (TR), internal repeats (IR1-4), and unique sequence domains (U1-U5) of the EBV genome are depicted in proportion to their overall size. The position of the cis-acting element for episome maintenance and replication in latent infection, oriP, is indicated. The origins for EBV DNA replication in lytic infection (oriLyt) are in U3 and U5 just to the right of IR2 and IR4, respectively. The deletions in B95-8 and P3HR-1 genomes are shown.[235,286,300]

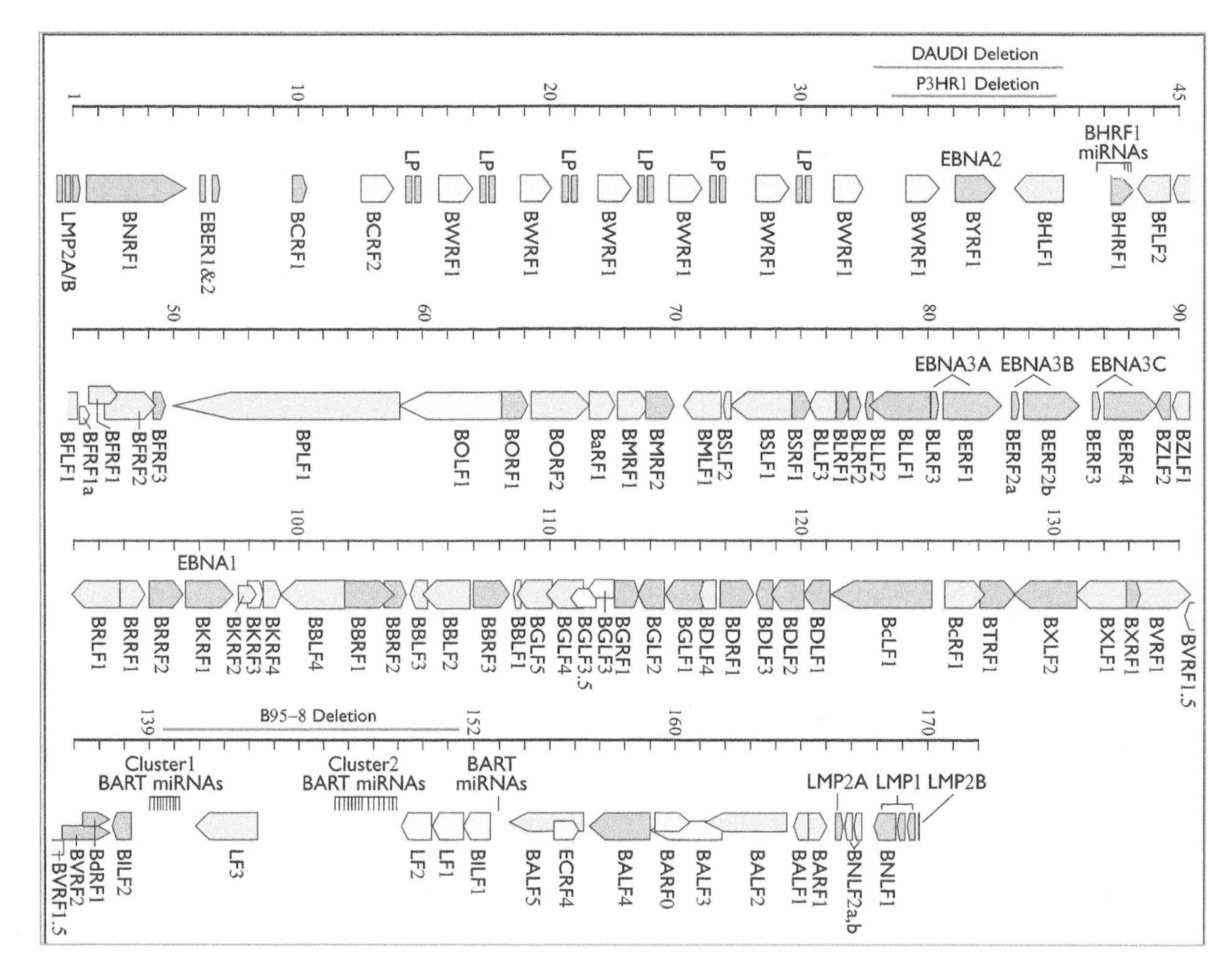

FIGURE 11.2 Schematic depiction of the linear Epstein-Barr virus (EBV) genome with encoded open reading frames (ORFs). EBV ORFs are named based on their location (first ORF, second ORF, etc.) and direction (rightward or leftward) within the Bam H1 fragment (A, B, C, and so on, in decreasing size).[27] The prototypic EBV type 1 genome DNA sequence (171,820 bp) found in the National Center for Biotechnology Information (NCBI) is actually a composite of two viral genomes (B95-8 and Raji) due to deletions within the viral genomes during passage in tissue culture.[27,526] Size and direction of the ORFs are indicated, as are the noncoding RNAs EBER1 and EBER2. The latency-associated ORFs or exons that make up these ORFs are colored purple. The early lytic ORFs are beige and late lytic ORFs are shaded with red. *Yellow arrows* depict ORFs of unknown gene class or are hypothetical. LMP2A and LMP2B are encoded across the circularized genome. The locations of microRNA (miRNAs) encoded by the genome are shown. Numbers refer to kilobase pairs. (Reprinted by permission from Springer: Sample JT, Marendy EM, Hughes DJ, et al. The Epstein-Barr virus genome. In: Damania B, Pipas JM, eds. *DNA Tumor Viruses*. New York: Springer; 2009:241–258. Copyright © 2009 Springer Science + Business Media, LLC.)

regulators of viral gene expression, BALF1, which encodes a bcl-2 homolog and LMP1 and LMP2A, which encode integral membrane proteins with 6 and 12 membrane spanning domains, respectively.

The gamma herpesvirus subfamily classification was initially established on the basis of biologic properties including oncogenic associations and restricted host range for infection in cell culture. Gamma herpesviruses also establish latent infection in lymphocytes but are not unique in this regard. Beta herpesviruses such as HHV-6, HHV-7, and CMV can also latently infect lymphocytes and other hematopoietic cells. Segregation into the gamma herpesvirus subfamily based on nucleotide and protein sequence homology and genome collinearity provides a more enduring basis for phylogenic classification.[145] Taxonomists have named EBV as human herpes virus 4 (HHV4), although EBV is typically used.

Two EBV types circulate in most populations. EBV type 1 and 2 (also named types A and B, respectively) differ largely in EBV nuclear antigen (EBNA) genes that encode leader protein (EBNA-LP), EBNA2, EBNA3A, EBNA3B, and EBNA3C, which are expressed in latency III growth transformation of B cells to LCLs.[606] The type 1 and 2 alleles for EBNA2, EBNA3A, EBNA3B, and EBNA3C differ in predicted primary amino acid sequence by 47%, 16%, 20%, and 28%, respectively. Both types are present worldwide but type 1 EBV is the more common type in most populations, particularly so in the developed world, whereas type 2 EBV reaches its highest prevalence among people in equatorial Africa and New Guinea.[159] Type 1 and 2 EBV may also be found in throat washings from immunocompromised patients, particularly HIV-infected people, who may be colonized with both EBV types and even with multiple strains of those types. Intertypic recombinants and EBNA2 deletions have been identified in the oropharynx and lymphocytes of immunocompromised people and less commonly from otherwise healthy people.[642] Aside from the EBNA differences, the genomes of EBV type 1 and 2 differ little more than that found among individual strains of either type, which mostly differ in inter- and intragenic small and large repeats. Similarities in the numbers of DNA repeats at various sites in the EBV genome among EBV isolates from a given geographic area have been used to group isolates into strains and to epidemiologically track EBV infection.

VIRUS STRUCTURE

Like other herpesviruses, EBV has a toroid-shaped DNA core in a nucleocapsid with 162 capsomeres, an outer envelope with external glycoprotein spikes, and a protein tegument between the nucleocapsid and envelope[160,297] (Fig. 11.3). EBV capsids from purified enveloped virus are composed of the 155 kD major capsid protein BcLF1, 30 kD minor capsid protein, 18 kD small capsid protein, 40 kD minor capsid protein binding protein, and 68 kD portal protein BBRF1. The EBV tegument is composed of the 350 kD large tegument protein BPLF1, 140 kD large tegument protein binding protein BOLF1, 15 kD myristoylated protein BBLF1, 32 kD Myristoylated protein binding protein BGLF2, 58 kD capsid associated protein BVRF1, 58 kD packaging protein BGLF1, 27 kD palmitylated protein BSRF1, and 47 kD serine–threonine protein kinase BGLF4, which are common components of herpesvirus teguments.[297] In addition, EBV has a 140 kD major tegument protein BNRF1, 19 kD BLRF2, 72 kD BRRF2, 54 kD BDLF2, and 42kD BKRF4, which are gamma herpesvirus specific.[297] Cellular proteins including actin, HSP70, cofilin, β-tubulin, enolase, and Hsp90 are also significant components of the EBV tegument, potentially related to cytoplasmic re-envelopment. The major glycoprotein components of the envelope are gp350 (BLLF1), gH (BXLF2), gB (BALF4), gp42 (BZLF2),

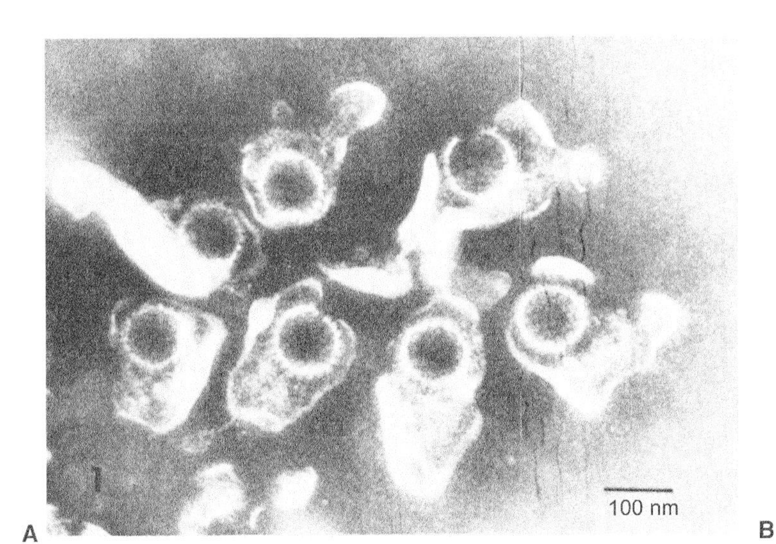

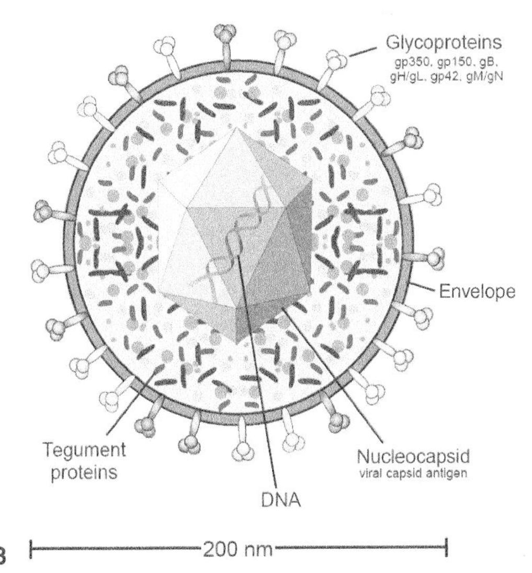

FIGURE 11.3 Electron micrograph and schematic diagram of EBV virions. A: EBV particles purified from the supernatant of B95-8 marmoset cells. Bar represents 100 nm. (Republished with permission of Rockefeller University Press from Miller G, Lipman M. Comparison of the yield of infectious virus from clones of human and simian lymphoblastoid lines transformed by Epstein-Barr virus. *J Exp Med* 1973;138(6):1398–1412; permission conveyed through Copyright Clearance Center, Inc.) **B:** Diagram of EBV virion. The major structural components of the virion are shown including the virion envelope, which is studded with glycoproteins important for binding and subsequent fusion of the virion envelope with cellular membranes, the tegument, which contains both virus-encoded proteins as well as cellular proteins, the capsid, and viral genome.

gM (BBRF3), gp78 (BILF2), gN (BLRF1), gp150 (BDLF3), and gL (BKRF2) and were also observed in virions.[297] Some EBV-encoded proteins, notably the EBNAs, LMP1, LMP2, gp64 (BILF1), BMRF2, and the homologs of HSV UL7 (BBRF2), UL14 (BGLF3), UL31, (BFLF2), and UL34 (BFRF1) were not detected in EBV virions.[297]

GENOME STRUCTURE

The EBV genome is a linear, double-stranded DNA composed of 60 mole percent guanine and cytosine as elegantly shown by Elliott Kieff prior to sequencing of the EBV genome.[27,325] As a historic first, the EBV genome was the first genome fully sequenced by a conventional subcloning and Sanger sequencing strategy.[27] The prototypic EBV type 1 genome DNA sequence (171,823 bp) found in NCBI (GI:82503188) is actually a composite of two viral genomes B95-8 and Raji, both of which carry deletions within the viral genome that may have occurred during passage in tissue culture (Fig. 11.1).[27,526] B95-8 was selected for virus production in culture and was found to be deleted for the BARTs, which is discussed in the EBV miRNAs section of this chapter.[566,648] B95-8 remains the most extensively studied EBV strain. P3HR1, another deletion virus, was important for the discovery of the essential role of EBNA2 before genetic manipulation with the EBV genome was possible (see EBNA2 section in this chapter) and the role of the Z protein in initiation of lytic replication (see lytic replication in this chapter).[135,235,286,300] Type 2 strains have been sequenced and the prototypic type 2 stain deposited in NCB1 (AG876) is 172,760 bp and as described above is highly homologous to type 1 EBV.[159] An isolate of an EBV type 1 strain (M81) has an increased ability to infect epithelial cells, reduced ability to infect B cells, and increased lytic replication, and has been proposed as a new EBV subtype.[698] The characteristic features of EBV and most other LCV genomes include (a) a single overall format and gene arrangement; (b) 2 to 5 tandem, 0.5 kbp, direct repeats of the same sequence at both termini (TR)[209]; (c) 6 to 12 tandem reiterations of a 3 kbp, internal direct repeat (IR1); (d) short and long largely unique sequence domains (US and UL) that have almost all of the genome coding capacity; (e) perfect and imperfect tandem DNA repeats, most of which are within ORFs; and (f) a duplicated region, IR2, near the left end of UL, which consists of multiple, highly conserved, G-C rich, tandem 125 bp repeats and 2 kbp of adjacent unique DNA, all of which have extensive homology to a region, IR4, near the right end of UL. IR4 is comprised of G-C rich, tandem 102 bp repeats and 1 kbp of nearby unique DNA. The IR3 and IR4 repeats are within ORFs. Because the IR3 repeat is 125 kbp and not divisible by three, sequential iterations are translated in different reading frames, resulting in an unusual protein. IR3 and IR4 also include the origins for initiation of viral DNA replication.[227]

The reiteration frequency of the EBV tandem perfect repeats becomes variable during viral DNA replication, with the average number of repeats being identical to the parent genome and most of the progeny having similar numbers of repeats as the parental genome. When EBV infects a cell, the genome becomes an episome with a characteristic number of TRs, dependent on the number of TRs in the parental genome, and the unique cleavage and joining events of the single infecting viral genome. If infection is nonpermissive for viral replication and permissive for latent infection and continued cell growth, each EBV episome in progeny infected cells will usually have the same number of TRs as the parent cell. Homogeneity or heterogeneity in the number of TRs is therefore useful in determining whether a group of latently infected cells arose from a single common progenitor infected cell or from multiple progenitors.[568] The number of 3 kbp IR1 repeats also varies among EBVs and among progeny of EBV replication but is more difficult to assess as a marker of heterogeneity because of the 18 to 30 kbp total size. Other, smaller, imperfect, or less highly reiterated repeats within ORFs are more stable during replication but differ sufficiently among different virus isolates so that the size of the encoded proteins can be used to uniquely identify each isolate.

STEPS IN REPLICATION

Attachment and Entry

EBV uses different glycoprotein combinations to infect B cells and epithelial cells (Fig. 11.4), but similar to other human herpesviruses, the core fusion complex consists of gB (originally designated gp110) and gH/gL (originally designated gp85/gp25). Antibodies directed against the core EBV fusion complex can potently neutralize fusion and infection.[613,653] EBV gB is the fusogen for viral entry, and the gB structure is composed of trimers and is similar to the structure of HSV gB.[26,239] The solved gB structure likely represents a postfusion conformation since the structure is very similar to the low-pH or postfusion form of G protein of vesicular stomatitis virus.

B Lymphocytes

B lymphocytes and epithelial cells are the major sites for EBV infection in the human host. CD21, also known as complement receptor 2 (CR2), is critical for EBV B-cell entry. Reflecting the importance of CD21 for B-cell infection, CD21 is abundantly expressed on B cells and binds the virus-encoded gp350/220.[184] gp350/220 has homologs in primate gamma herpesviruses, but there are no sequence-related proteins in the other human herpesviruses. CD21 is expressed on mature peripheral CD3+ T cells, with a higher level of expression on the naive CD4+ and CD8+ T-cell subsets and has recently been shown to be an entry receptor for the virus into T cells.[650] gp350 and gp220 are encoded by the same mRNA, but a single splice generates the gp220 reading frame.[269] No known distinct function of either gp350 or gp220 has been determined since they both contain the domain that binds CD21.[681] CD35 also binds gp350/220 and functions to allow EBV attachment to B cells.[514]

CD21 is the receptor for the C3d component of complement and is part of a large family of complement regulatory proteins. Family members have one or more extracellular structural motifs known as short consensus repeats (SCRs). As well as being expressed on B cells, CD21 is expressed on other cell types including tonsillar epithelial cells.[288] The extracellular domain of CD21 contains multiple SCRs, but only SCR-1 and SCR-2 are required for EBV and C3d binding.[86,404] Soluble CD21 binds to the EBV virion and can block B-cell infection.[499] The structure of the key gp350 binding domain on CD21 was solved[562] and the region of gp350 required for

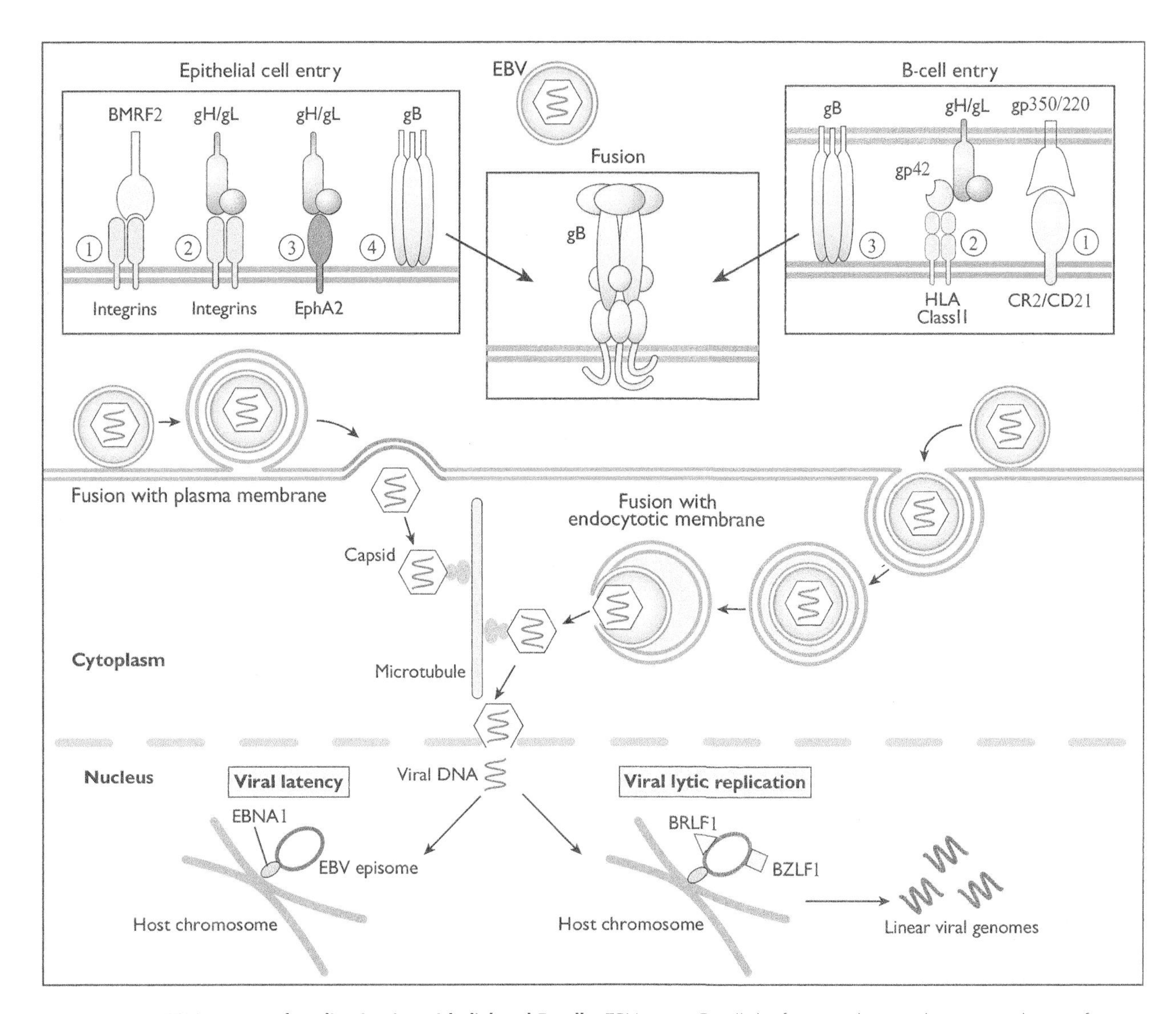

FIGURE 11.4 EBV entry and replication in epithelial and B cells. EBV enters B cells by fusion with an endocytic membrane after endocytosis. EBV enters epithelial cells by fusion at the plasma membrane. For B-cell entry, EBV virions first bind to CR2/CD21 via gp350/220 (*1*). Following this interaction, gp42 binds to HLA class II (*2*) triggering fusion mediated by gH/gL and gB (*3*). For epithelial cell entry, EBV virions may first bind via an interaction of integrins with BMRF2 (*1*). Following this binding, gH/gL binds to ephrin A2 (*2*) and triggers fusion mediated by gB (*3*). For both B and epithelial cells, following fusion, the capsid is released into the cytoplasm and is transported to the nuclear membrane by microtubule-mediated transport. The EBV genome is released into the nucleus through a nuclear pore. Latency can result, in which the genome is tethered to host chromosomes via an interaction with EBNA1. Lytic replication resulting in the production of viral genomes may also result, induced by the BRLF1 and BZLF1 EBV gene products.

binding to CD21 is contained within a portion of gp350 that is not glycosylated.[675] Compatible with this finding, deglycosylated gp350 binds to CD21 as does the fully glycosylated gp350.[675]

Binding of EBV virions or a soluble form of gp350 to CD21 results in capping of CD21 followed by endocytosis[498,681] indicating a putative role of signal transduction in EBV B-lymphocyte entry. The binding of gp350/220 to CD21 parallels the interaction of HSV gC with cell surface proteoglycans in tethering virions to target cells. This initial step is not absolutely required for infection since EBV deleted for gp350/220 or HSV-1 deleted for gC have only modest defects in virus entry *in vitro* when infections are performed with high virus titers. After binding to B cells, EBV virions are endocytosed[460] and fusion of the viral membrane is thought to occur via the interaction of gp42 with HLA class II followed by fusion mediated by gH/gL and gB.

HLA-DR was found to bind gp42 in an expression library screen for proteins that bound a soluble form of gp42.[665] Both structural and functional studies have shown that gp42 exhibits features of the C-type lectin family[480,665] and has no known sequence homologs in other human herpesviruses but is found in the EBV-related primate viruses. The gp42/HLA-DR interaction is essential for EBV infection of B cells since antibodies to gp42 and HLA-DR block infection.[380,459] In addition, virus deleted for gp42 does not infect B cells unless soluble gp42 is provided in trans or polyethylene glycol is added to promote fusion.[713] Also indicative of the important role of gp42 in B-cell infection, virosomes lacking gp42 bind B cells but are unable to fuse.[225] The binding site of gp42 on HLA class II has been extensively studied by mutagenesis[224] and by protein crystallography.[480] Specific HLA-DR alleles correlate with EBV infection and binding to gp42.[106,376] Because of the key role of antigen presentation, studies have suggested that gp42 may block HLA class II antigen presentation preventing CD4 T-cell activation.[579,665]

gp42 stably interacts with gH/gL and links receptor binding with fusion mediated by gH/gL and gB. The structure of gp42 not bound to receptor indicates that a conformational change occurs upon binding of gp42 to HLA class II, widening a hydrophobic pocket on the surface of gp42, which suggests a conformational change is important in triggering fusion by engaging other components of the EBV fusion complex.[336] The EBV gH/gL structure has also been solved,[437] revealing an elongated rod-like shape, with the middle being the widest and gL forming intimate contacts with the N-terminal residues of gH. These features are compatible with the known chaperone function of gL for gH expression, processing, and transport.[742] Of particular interest, a KGD sequence found on the gH/gL surface is implicated in integrin binding and epithelial cell entry.[437] Validating the central role of gH/gL in EBV entry, gH mutants within a gH glycosylation site, the cytoplasmic tail, or a large groove that separates domain 1 and domain 2 of gH/gL all have defects in fusion.[100,101,467]

The structure of gH/gL/gp42 complex bound to an anti-gH/gL antibody (E1D1) has been solved.[611] In these studies, it was shown that gp42 interacts with gH/gL via two domains in the gp42 amino terminus located outside the gp42 C-type lectin domain.[335,380,396] gp42 domains cross three domains on the gH surface. Both the binding of the gp42 N-terminal domain and E1D1 to gH/gL selectively inhibit epithelial cell fusion; however, they engage distinct surfaces of gH/gL. The extensive structural and mutational studies of EBV entry proteins has led to a model for the assembly of the putative B-cell entry complex comprised of gH/gL, gp42, and HLA class II (Fig. 11.5).[612] These studies provide a snapshot of an intermediate state in EBV entry and highlight the potential for the triggering complex to bring the two membrane bilayers into proximity by interactions of the constituents of the complex based on an "open" and "closed" form of the complex observed in CryoEM. These open and closed forms resemble those previous seen in Cryo-ET studies done with HSV-1.[438] Interestingly, in this assembled complex, gH/gL interacts with the gp42 hydrophobic pocket. This result suggests that following receptor engagement, binding of gp42 may drive fusion mediated by gH/gL and gB by bringing the viral and cellular membranes together. Previous studies indicated that a domain containing gL amino acids Q54 and K94[546] is important for triggering gB and may specifically interact with EBV gB to trigger fusion (Fig. 11.5).

EBV virions produced by B cells have reduced gp42 as a consequence of gp42 binding to HLA class II, which is present in infected B cells, during lytic replication.[57] EBV deficient in gp42 is defective in B-cell infectivity but is enhanced in epithelial cell infectivity.[57] The absence of gp42 enables the gH/gL complex to engage an epithelial cell receptor, which is

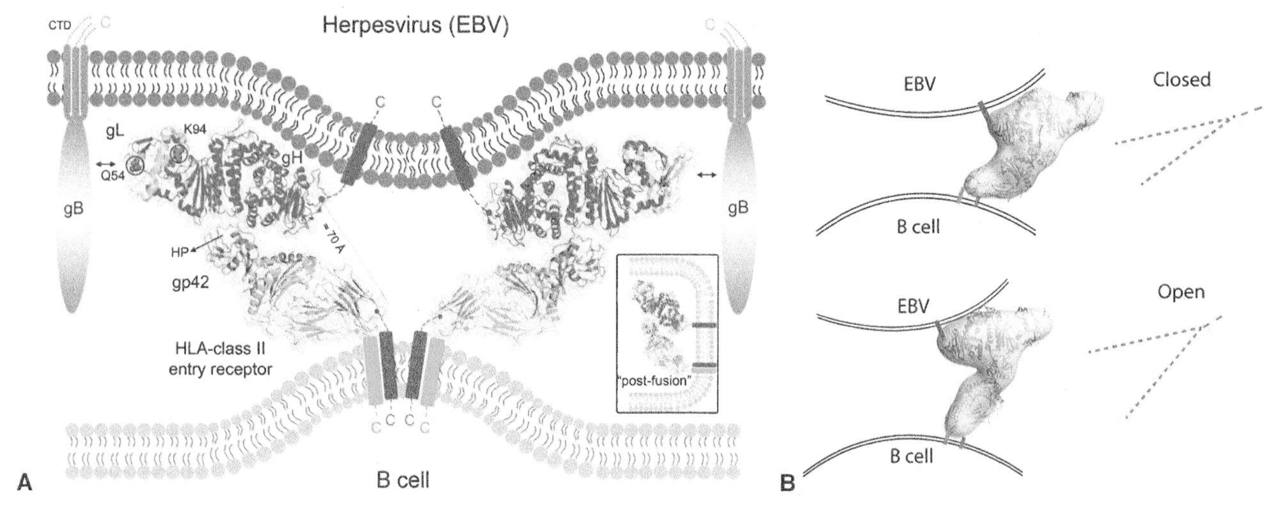

FIGURE 11.5 Proposed EBV B-cell entry complex required for B-cell fusion.[612] **A:** *Top* represents the viral membrane bilayer with prefusion gB (*purple*), gH/gL (*blue/cyan*), and gp42 (*hot pink*). The structure of gB in a prefusion form is not known. HLA class II (*green/brown*) is at the *bottom*. Locations of the transmembrane (TM) domains of gH and HLA are indicated schematically with rectangles since no structural data are available (*blue*—HLA and *green/brown*—class II). The C-termini of gH and HLA class II are also indicated. gp42 is a type II transmembrane protein and the N-terminal TM domain must be cleaved for it to be active in fusion. The location of the gp42 N-terminus is not known. The approximately 170 Å long complex shown suggests a conformation that could bridge viral–cellular membranes potentially distorting and thereby facilitating fusion between the viral and cellular membranes. This model places gL residues (Q54 and K94) involved in gB activation[546] on the opposite side of the gH and HLA membrane anchors. The external location of gB implied by this model may indicate an initial peripheral activation of gB followed by its movement to a more central position to mediate membrane fusion. The gp42 hydrophobic pocket (HP), which is critical for fusion activation and located at the gH D-II/D-III junction, is highlighted to show its location with respect to the triggering complex. A potential postfusion arrangement is shown in the **inset. B:** Representation of the V/Y shape of the respective open and closed triggering complexes highlighting their similarity to the structures observed in cryo-ET studies of HSV-1 entry described in.[612] (Reprinted from Sathiyamoorthy K, Jiang J, Hu YX, et al. Assembly and architecture of the EBV B cell entry triggering complex. *PLoS Pathog* 2014;10(8):e1004309. https://creativecommons.org/licenses/by/4.0/.)

otherwise occluded by gp42. During virus egress from epithelial cells, the absence of HLA class II results in virions containing gp42 bound to gH/gL that efficiently infect B lymphocytes.

Epithelial Cells

In contrast to B-cell entry, EBV entry into epithelial cells occurs at the cell surface in the absence of endocytosis.[460] CD21 is expressed in tonsil epithelium, but not in epithelium from buccal mucosa, uvula, soft palate, or tongue by RT-PCR suggesting that the gp350/222 interaction with CD21 may be important for epithelial cell infection.[288] BMRF2 may also have a role in epithelial cell entry. BMRF2 is a multispan membrane protein that contains an extracellular RGD motif that is a ligand for α1, α5, α3, and αv integrins.[737] This interaction is important for infection of polarized epithelial cells,[701] and antibodies to BMRF2 or to α5β1 integrin block EBV infection of polarized epithelial cells through the basolateral cell surface. Interestingly, BMRF2 is not abundant in the EBV virion[297] and appears not to have a role in fusion, so BMRF2 may function similar to gp350/220 to tether virions to target cells and to induce signal transduction pathways. Integrin signaling has been shown to be important in Kaposi's sarcoma herpesvirus (KSHV) infection.[631] Integrins αVβ5, αVβ6, and αVβ8 bind to gH,[106] but this interaction is not required for the triggering of fusion. Earlier studies had shown that a soluble form of gH/gL bound specifically to epithelial cells, but not B cells.[58] In addition, gH-null virus does not bind to epithelial cells[468,513] and a monoclonal antibody to gH/gL can reduce both gH/gL and virus binding.[58,468] In more recent studies, integrin αV knock-out HEK293 cells were generated using the CRISPR-Cas9 system. No difference between WT HEK293 and integrin αV knock-out HEK293 cells were found for viral infection or fusion activity, indicating that integrins are not essential for entry in HEK293 cells and may function as entry mediators.[104] In these same studies, a novel and more rapid approach using readily available RNA-seq databases was used to identify potential epithelial cell receptors and Ephrin A2 (EphA2) was identified as an EBV receptor for epithelial cells.[104] Another group independently identified EphA2 also as an EBV receptor in epithelial cells using microarray and RNA interference screen and CRISPR analyses.[749] EphA2 belongs to the largest receptor tyrosine kinase (RTK) family, with 14 known human members that play roles in boundary formation, cell migration, axon guidance, synapse formation, angiogenesis, proliferation, and cell differentiation. EphA2 is also a receptor for KSHV, another human gammaherpesvirus.[226]

Other modes of EBV infection may also exist for virus entry. Virus coated with IgA can bind to the polymeric IgA receptor.[643] This form of infection may be relevant in NPC, where high levels of EBV-specific IgA antibodies are found in the blood.[244] However, EBV is transcytosed in polarized epithelial cells without evidence of replication.[204] Interestingly, antibodies directed against gp350/220 can enhance EBV epithelial infection independent of Fc receptor interactions, and cell contact also enhances epithelial infection.[628,702] Cell-associated virus is very efficient in infecting epithelial cells or B cells.[278,630] Recently, a novel mechanism for EBV infection was reported for nonsusceptible epithelial cells through the formation of cell-in-cell structures.[500] Epithelial CNE-2 cells that are resistant to infection were invaded by EBV-infected Akata B cells to form cell-in-cell structures *in vitro*. Interestingly, similar unique cellular structures were observed in biopsies of NPC. How these different routes of infection impact EBV infection in humans requires further investigation.

EBV Latency Programs

An intriguing aspect of EBV is its ability to establish different types of latent B-cell infection. EBV switches between latency programs to navigate the B-cell compartment and to colonize memory B cells, the reservoir for lifelong EBV infection. Up to 9 EBV proteins are expressed in EBV latency programs (Table 11.1).[556,600] These include 6 EBNAs, 2 LMPs, and the viral BCL2 homolog BHRF1. Their key functions are shown in Table 11.1. EBV latency genes are conserved with closely related primate LCVs but not with other herpesviruses. In addition to protein products, 2 highly abundant Epstein-Barr encoded RNAs (EBERs) and up to 44 viral miRNAs are expressed.

Following primary B-cell infection, the EBV W promoter (*Wp*) drives transcription of a message that encodes EBNA-LP and EBNA2 (Fig. 11.6).[478] While this message potentially encodes all six EBNAs, at very early time points EBNA2 and EBNA-LP are preferentially expressed. BHRF1 is also expressed at low levels, and T cells can recognize BHRF1 epitopes in newly infected cells.[63,317] A *Wp* upstream element recruits YY1, Pax5, and additional transcription factors that together provide B-cell tropic expression.

EBNA-LP and EBNA2 reach levels significantly higher than those observed in LCLs by 48 hours postinfection,[478,721] contributing to major host transcriptome and proteome remodeling. At 72 hours postinfection, some infected cells rapidly proliferate.[505,543,723] Together with host factors, EBNA2 activates the EBV C promoter (*Cp*). The *Cp* CBF1 region associates with RBP-Jκ, which recruits EBNA2. The CBF2 region recruits Pax5.[693] Interestingly, *Cp* and *Wp* are mutually exclusive, and posttranscriptional mechanisms repress *Wp* upon *Cp* activation.[263,563]

Cp and *Wp* regulation is complex. RBP-Jκ/CBF1 is a host sequence specific transcription factor that associates with *Cp* and recruits EBNA2 to this and other key DNA sites. EBNA2, EBNA-LP, and EBNA1 promote *Cp*/*Wp* activity, whereas EBNA3 proteins compete with EBNA2 for binding to CBF1 to down-modulate their activity.[298,429,585,586]

Cp initially drives the viral latency IIb program, where an approximately 125 kilobase EBV transcript is alternatively spliced for expression of six EBNAs.[8,35,38,219,232,386,393,537,604,663,664] BHRF1 is also expressed, at low levels.[478] EBNA3A, EBNA3B, EBNA3C, and EBNA1 reach levels seen in LCLs at approximately 72 hours postinfection.[478,721] Pol II stalling at *Cp* promotes EBNA expression by regulating nucleosome assembly, recruiting pTEFb and maintaining Pol II C-terminal domain phosphorylation.[519] EBNA1 levels increase to assure EBV episome transmission to progeny cells and to enhance transcription from promoters around *oriP* (the origin for latent viral replication), which includes an EBNA1-dependent enhancer and an EBNA1-dependent replication origin.[28,203,576,577]

Wp and *Cp* are each important for EBV-driven B-cell transformation *in vitro*. Deletion of the control region of the upstream *Wp* copy, which also effects *Cp* activity, decreases *in vitro* B-cell transformation efficiency. Compensatory use of downstream *Wp* copies allows for a reduced level of B-cell outgrowth. *Cp* deletion reduces EBV B-cell transformation

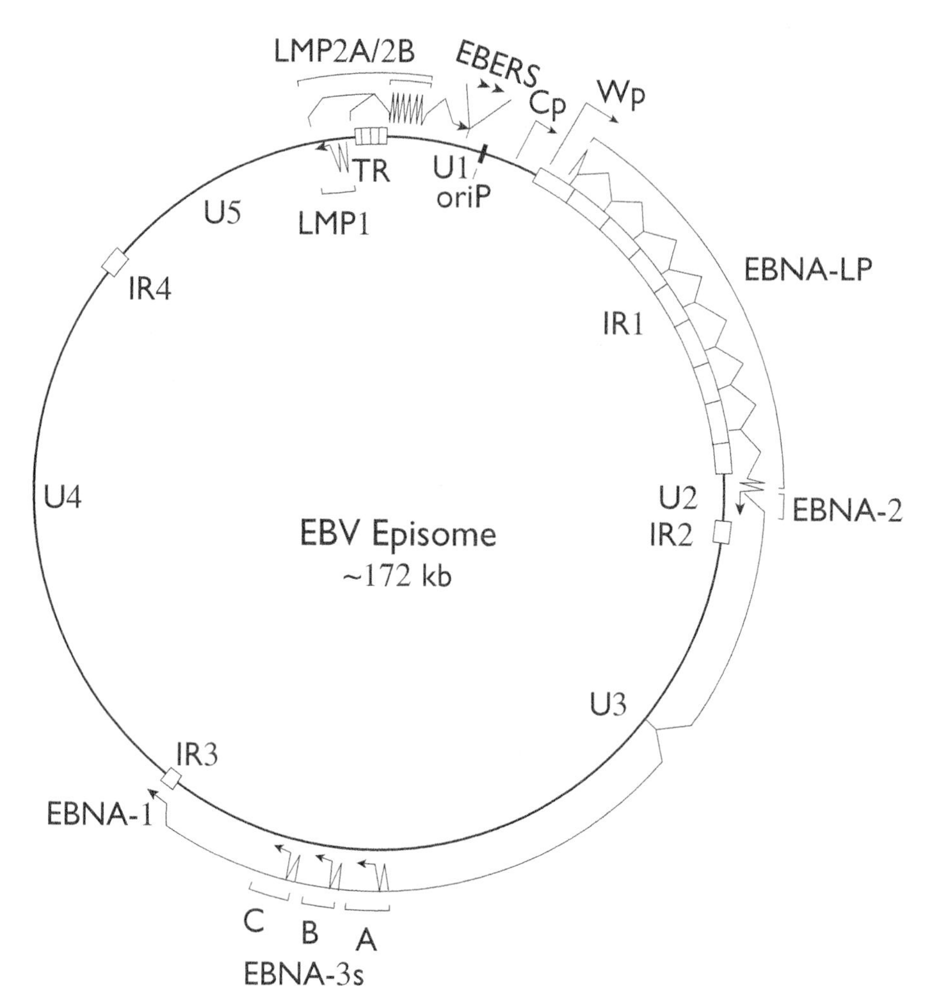

FIGURE 11.6 Schematic depiction of the EBV episome. The EBV episome is circularized through terminal repeats (TR). Shown are the transcripts, mRNAs, and major proteins in type III latent B-lymphocyte infection. Largely unique (U1-U5) and internal (IR1-4) or terminal (TR) repeat DNA segments are indicated. The origin for latent infection EBV episome replication, oriP, is also indicated. Exons encoding EBV nuclear proteins (EBNA1, EBNA2, EBNA3A, EBNA3B, EBNA3C, and EBNA-LP) or EBV integral latent membrane proteins (LMP1, LMP2A, or LMP2B) are indicated by *vertical lines* radiating from the circular episome map. EBNA transcription is shown as it is first initiated from the IR1 or Wp. In many infected lymphocytes, after expression of EBNA-LP and EBNA2, *Cp* in U1 dominates EBNA transcription. Alternative polyadenylation and splicing result in expression of the various EBNA mRNAs. EBNA-LP is encoded by repeating exons from IR1 and two short unique exons from U2. The EBERs are two small, nonpolyadenylated, RNAs. LMP1 is transcribed in direction opposite to the EBNAs, LMP2A, and LMP2B, and EBERs. LMP2A has an upstream EBNA2 response element, whereas LMP1 and LMP2B share the same EBNA2 response element.

efficiency by greater than 100-fold.[672] LCLs derived from wild-type and *Cp* deletion mutant EBV have similar EBNA levels, suggesting that *Wp* can support EBV oncoprotein expression in the absence of *Cp*.[693,746]

Latency III, also called the EBV growth program, is defined by the viral transcripts observed in LCLs with expression of six nuclear antigens (EBNAs 1, 2, LP, 3A, 3B, 3C), three membrane antigens (LMP1, LMP2A, and LMP2B), BHRF1, and noncoding RNAs.[689] BNRF1 is expressed at low levels.[4,6] EBNA2 activates the promoters that drive LMP1 and LMP2, whose levels increase over the first 2 weeks postinfection.[478,558] NF-κB, AP-2, and early B-cell factor also up-regulate LMP promoters.[150,489]

Latency III likely serves to expand the pool of EBV-infected B cells *in vivo* and drives continuous LCL proliferation in tissue culture. Latency III also up-regulates adhesion molecules and plasma membrane receptors that are thought to drive EBV-infected B cells into lymph node germinal centers, possibly for memory cell differentiation. Within the germinal center, EBV-infected cells are thought to switch to the latency II program, with EBNA1, LMP1, LMP2, and noncoding RNA expression. The viral Q promoter (*Qp*) drives EBNA1 expression, whereas LMP promoters (*LMPp*) drive LMP1/2.

Latency I is expressed in memory B cells, where EBNA1 is the only viral protein expressed (Table 11.2). Latency I is also observed in most EBV-positive Burkitt lymphomas. In latency I, EBNA1 transcription is driven by *Qp*, located more than 50 kb downstream from *Cp*.[402,483,512,615,616] However, EBNA1 negatively regulates *Qp*, allowing low EBNA1 levels for immunoevasion.[483,603] EBNA1 is not translated in resting memory cells, resulting in the latency 0 state, in which EBV evades T-cell detection in this important reservoir cell by silencing all viral encoded proteins. In up to 15% of endemic BLs, EBNA2 deleted virus is present and is associated with *Wp* activation, broadening the expression pattern seen in latency I.[317] In addition to expressing EBNAs 1 and 3, *Wp*-restricted Burkitt lymphomas express BHRF1. BHRF1 interacts with proapoptotic BH3-only family members BIM, BID, PUMA, and BAK, confers resistance to multiple apoptotic stimuli, and accelerates MYC-driven lymphomas in a mouse transgenic model.[187]

Epigenetic Regulation of EBV Programs

The viral epigenetic state resets with each lytic cycle, which produces unmethylated and unchromatinized DNA.[111,303] Linear EBV genomes are chromatinized and circularize early after infection.[110,384,402] Multiple layers of epigenetic control enable establishment of latency, control latency program selection, and ultimately support lytic reactivation.

BZLF1 preferentially activates promoters with methylated 5′-cytosine (5mC), termed meZREs,[45,303,304] limiting leaky lytic gene expression in newly infected B cells. DNA methylation levels progressively increase following EBV B-cell infection,

TABLE 11.2 EBV latency gene expression patterns

Latency	EBERs	EBNA1	EBNA2	EBNA3	EBNA-LP	LMP1	LMP2	BART miRNAs	BHRF1	Disease
0	+	−[a]	−	−	−	−	−	?	−	Blood in healthy carriers
I	+	+[b]	−	−	−	−	−	+	−	BL, gastric carcinoma
IIa[c]	+	+[b]	−	−	−	+	+	+	−	NPC, HL,TCL
IIb	+	+	+	+	+	−	−	+	+	DLBCL
III[d]	+	+[e]	+	+	+	+	+	+	+	PTLD

[a]EBNA1 is expressed only when cells divide.
[b]EBNA1 is driven by the Q promoter.
[c]A form of latency termed I/II has been proposed in which some cells do not express LMP1.
[d]BHRF1 miRNAs are also expressed along with low level expression of BHRF1.
[e]EBNA1 is driven by the C or W promoter.
BL, Burkitt lymphoma; NPC, nasopharyngeal carcinoma; HL, Hodgkin lymphoma; TCL, T-cell lymphoma; DLBCL, diffuse large B-cell lymphoma; PTLD, posttransplant lymphoproliferative disease; NPC and gastric carcinoma show variable expression of LMP1.

with higher levels achieved over the first 50 to 100 cell cycles.[304] The extent of methylation is limited by EBNA2, which induces the cytosine demethylase TET2. EBNA2 colocalizes with TET2, RBP-Jκ, and EBF1. TET2 depletion triggers lytic gene expression.[407,732] EBV also results in hypermethylation in an oral epithelial cell infection model.[49] By contrast, as detailed below, the BRLF1 immediate-early EBV transcription factor activates unmethylated sites, which facilitates induction of the lytic cycle in newly infected epithelial cells.[733]

Chromatinization has a key role in silencing EBV lytic genes in newly infected cells, and viral genomes are chromatinized by 48 hours postinfection.[69] However, over the first days postinfection, the (virion-associated) major EBV tegument protein BNRF1 supports latency gene expression by disrupting host histone chaperone ATRX/DAXX complexes, which would otherwise deposit repressive histone 3.3 complexes onto EBV genomes.[699] BNRF1 disrupts DAXX/ATRX complexes at PML bodies and is essential for EBNA2 induction.[699] Polycomb repressive complex 2 (PRC2) deposits repressive histone 3 lysine 27 trimethyl (H3K27me3) on the EBV genome, and histone 3 lysine 9 trimethyl (H3K9me3) is also deposited.[20,383,686] While BZLF1 and BRLF1 promoters are nucleosomal, open chromatin at these sites is not sufficient for lytic reactivation.[134]

DNA methylation exerts control over latency program selection and further suppress lytic gene expression. EBV also utilizes hypermethylation to silence host tumor suppressor genes.[597] As EBV-infected B cells enter lymphoid tissue germinal centers, *Cp* DNA methylation may contribute to the transition from latency III to latency II (Fig. 11.7). Initiator DNA methyltransferase DNMT3B is induced in germinal center B cells. The epigenetic enzymes UHRF1 and DNMT1, which copy methylation marks from parental to newly synthesized DNA strands, are induced in germinal center B cells and by primary B-cell infection. It is likely that UHRF1 and DNMT1 maintain methylation marks as cells differentiate into memory B cells with latency I expression. Latency III and lytic gene expression are de-repressed in latency I Burkitt B cells treated with DNA hypomethylating agents or by depletion of UHRF1.[223,435,584] Polycomb repressive complex I (PRC1) further controls LMP promoter activity in B cells and may add a layer of control over latency program switching. Depletion of PRC1 subunits de-represses LMP1 and LMP2A expression in latency I Burkitt lymphoma cells, and PRC1-mediated histone 2 lysine 119 monoubiquitination (H2Ub119Ub1) repressive marks are more abundant in Burkitt cells with latency I than latency III programs[223] (Fig. 11.7).

Higher order DNA structure also regulates EBV gene expression. The CCCTC-binding factor (CTCF) binds to multiple EBV genome sites to mediate long-range chromatin interactions or to insulate genome regions. CTCF binding to the EBV genome may anchor it to the nuclear matrix and direct specific chromatin architectures that can mediate alternative promoter targeting by the *oriP* enhancer. The *oriP* enhancer facultatively associates with either *Cp* in latency III or *Qp* in latency I.[685] Mechanistically, CTCF participates in each of these loops, and disruption of CTCF recruitment perturbs formation of either loop, highlighting how the viral genome coopts a host three-dimensional genome organizing factor for maintenance of epigenetically stable states. Furthermore, CTCF functions as a chromatin insulator at EBV genomic sites including *Qp* to block epigenetic silencing and to prevent promiscuous transcription of surrounding genes. Likewise, mutagenesis studies suggest that the CTCF site upstream of *Cp* also has roles in B-cell latency I epigenetic reprogramming.[264] CTCF activity is posttranslationally regulated by the host enzyme poly(ADP-ribose) polymerase (PARP1) and by DNA methylation. CTCF and PARP1 colocalize at specific EBV genomic sites, where PARP1 stabilizes CTCF occupancy.[410] PARP1 and CTCF suppress the *BZLF1* promoter.

EBV-induced host transcription factor MYC occupies the EBV genome origin of lytic replication (*oriLyt*) sites and prevents looping of these enhancer sites to the immediate-early BZLF1 promoter.[222] MYC depletion triggers EBV three-dimensional genome reorganization that juxtaposes *oriLyt* with the *BZLF1* promoter region. Since Blimp1 suppresses MYC expression, EBV may have evolved this mechanism to sense MYC abundance and link lytic reactivation to plasma cell differentiation. Elevated MYC levels present in newly infected B cells suppress LMP1 expression,[557] further highlighting the intimate relationship between MYC and EBV epigenetic regulation. Latent EBV genomes preferentially associate with human genome heterochromatin regions characterized by lower densities of coding genes and the repressive H3K9me3 mark. Upon lytic reactivation or EBNA1 depletion, EBV genomes move toward active chromatin.[328,473]

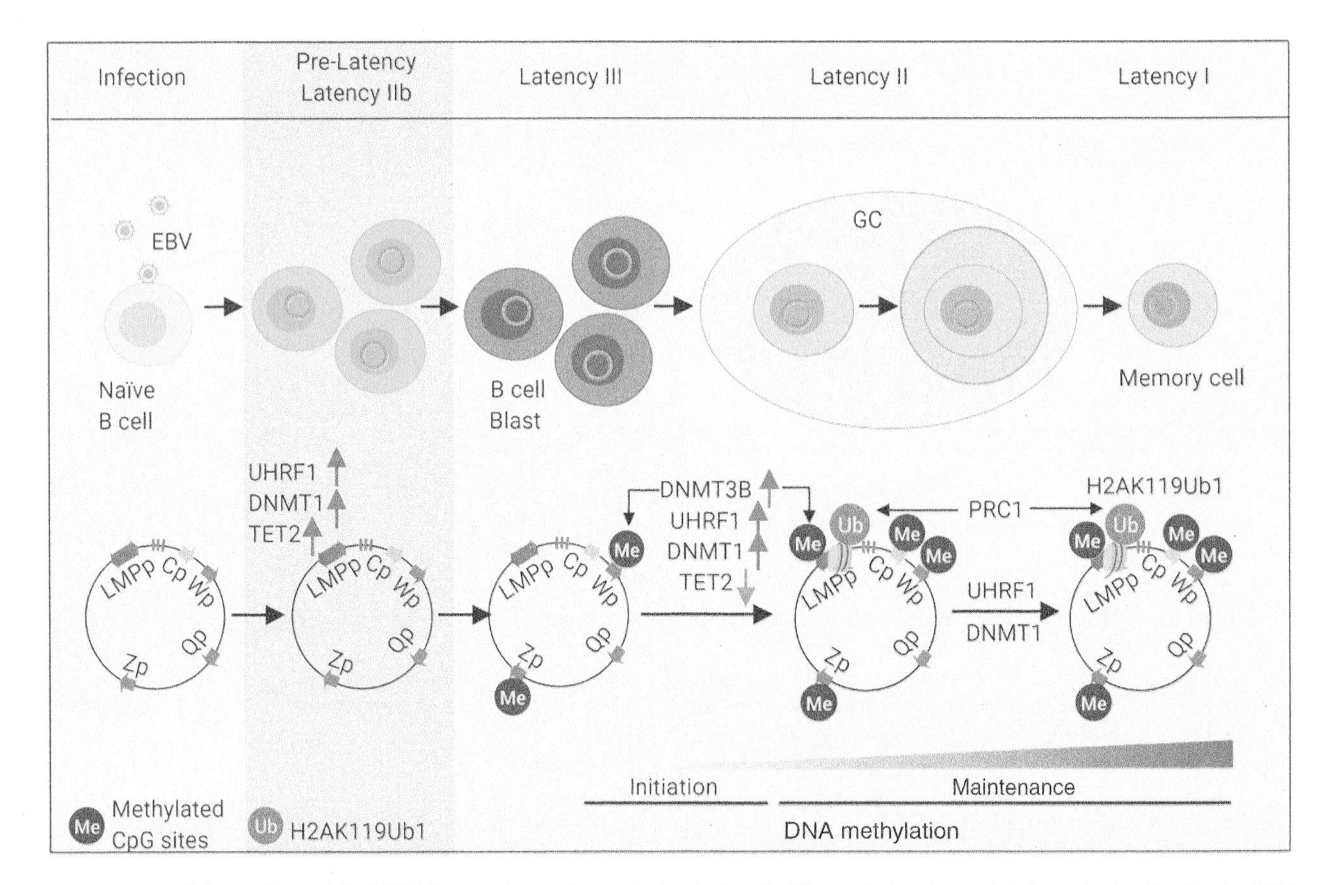

FIGURE 11.7 Schematic model of EBV/host epigenetic regulation in B-cell differentiation. In newly infected naïve B cells, the EBV genome circularizes and is chromatinized. EBNA2 expression in the prelatency and latency IIb phases induces the host DNA demethylase TET2, as well as the maintenance of methylation enzymes UHRF1 and DNMT1. EBNA2 induces the LMP promoter, driving LMP1 and LMP2A expression and causing methylation of *Wp*. The initiator DNA methyltransferase DNMT3B is induced in germinal centers (GC), where *Cp* is methylated and inactivated. Loss of EBNA2 expression diminishes TET2 abundance, potentiating EBV genome methylation. As B cells further differentiate, polycomb repressive complex 1 (PRC1) marks the LMP promoter with histone 2 lysine 199 monoubiquitin (H2AK119Ub1), which together with LMP promoter methylation silences LMP1 and LMP2A expression and allowing *Qp* activation. UHRF1 and DNMT1 propagate DNA methylation marks across cell cycles to maintain latency I.

Latency Gene Functions

EBNA1

EBNA1 (Fig. 11.8A) is the only EBNA that directly binds DNA. To ensure replication and stable maintenance of EBV genomes, EBNA1 binds both to the viral episome and serves to tether the viral genome to host chromosomes in mitosis. EBNA1 binds to *oriP*, which is the viral genome origin of DNA replication in latency.[577,743] Remarkably, it was subsequently discovered that *oriP* and EBNA1 are sufficient for partitioning of EBV genomes, or plasmids containing *oriP*, to progeny cells.[455,496] EBNA1 and *oriP* maintain the EBV genome as a replicon that is copied by host machinery once per cell cycle in S-phase. Catenation of newly replicated viral genomes appears to lead to their pairing on sister chromatids, which serves to mediate equal partitioning of episomes to daughter cells.[228]

The *oriP* family of repeats (FR), dyad symmetry (DS) element, and two cis-acting elements are critical for maintenance of EBV episomes. FR serves as a approximately 650 bp maintenance element and an EBNA1-dependent enhancer important for *Cp* activity.[28,203,228,321,402,540,547] FR is located approximately 1 kb upstream of DS and contains multiple 18 bp copies of an EBNA1 recognition sequence[412,573,577] (Fig. 11.8B). The EBNA1 N-terminus binds to perichromatic regions enriched for histone methylation marks that are hallmarks of transcriptionally active regions.[151] In this manner, EBNA1 tethers FR-bound episomes to condensed mitotic chromosomes. DS serves as the latency origin for episome DNA synthesis. It contains 4 EBNA1 recognition sites and a 65 bp region of dyad symmetry.[719] DS is necessary for EBNA1-dependent plasmid replication.[228]

EBNA1 binds DNA as a homodimer (Fig. 11.8B–D). The EBNA1 dimerization domain extends from residues 504 to 604. Amino acids 470 to 503 include a helix that projects into the DNA major groove and an extended chain that moves along the minor groove and makes all the DNA sequence specific contacts. Smooth DNA bending stabilizes interactions between EBNA1 dimers.[422] An extensive hydrogen bonding network connects the dimer–dimer interface, disruption of which compromises *oriP*-dependent plasmid replication and MCM3 complex recruitment to *oriP*. The EBNA1 DNA-binding domain itself forms a hexameric ring, highlighting that EBNA1 dimers assemble into higher-order structures. Point mutations at the oligomeric interface destabilize higher-order complex formation, alter cooperative DNA binding, and

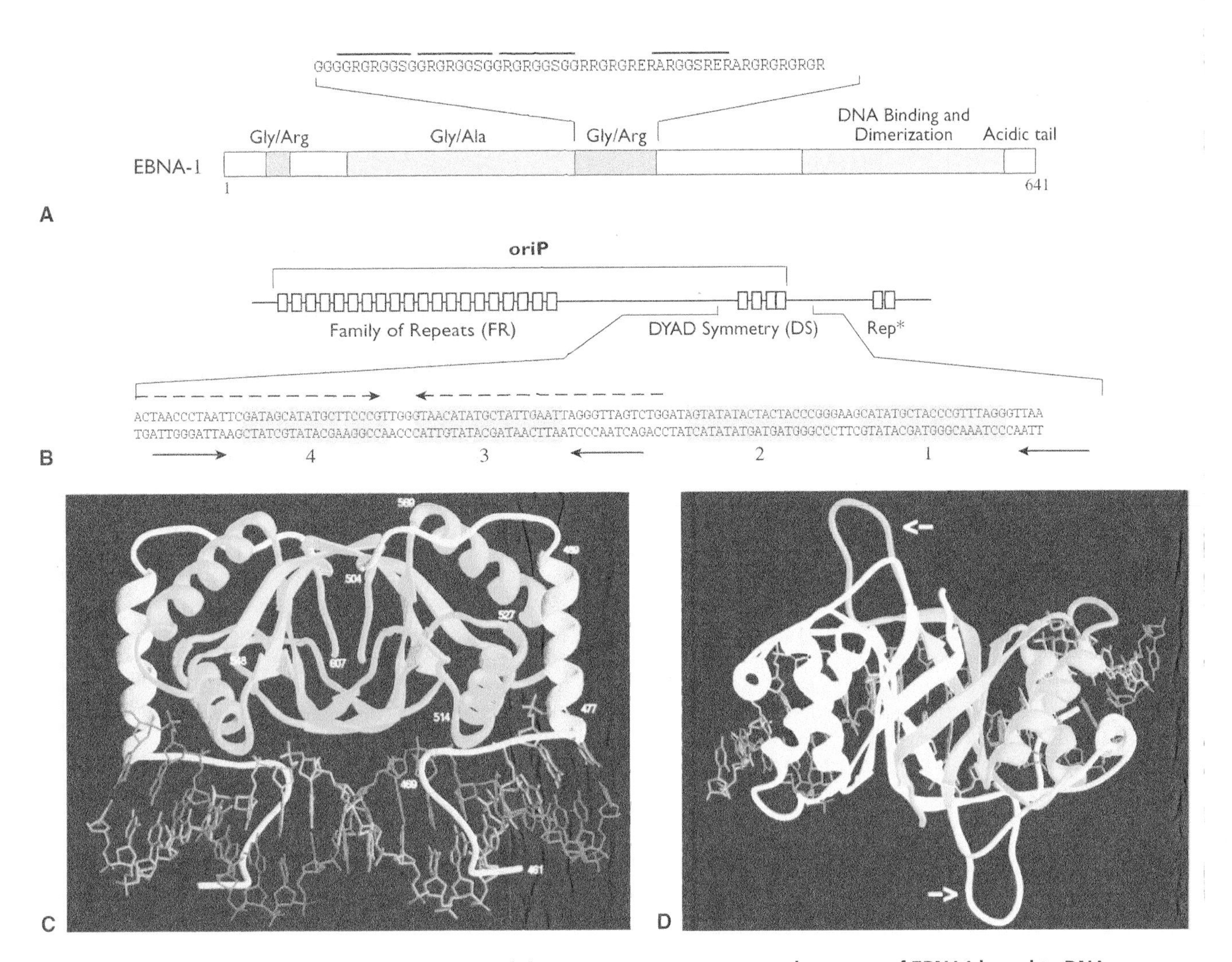

FIGURE 11.8 EBNA1 functional domains, schematic of the *oriP* DNA arrangement, and structure of EBNA1 bound to DNA. **A:** Important EBNA1 functional domains. The amino terminal Gly/Arg domain is important for replication, segregation, and transcription and has been shown to bind P32/TAP. The central Gly/Arg sequence is also important for replication, segregation, and transcription. This domain has been shown to bind a variety of cell proteins including EBP2, Nap1, p32/TAP, MDF1, PRMT1, and PRMT5. The DNA binding and dimerization domain at the C-terminus of EBNA1 is essential for all known functions of EBNA1 including replication, segregation, and transcription. Regions outside these domains of EBNA1 are generally thought to be nonessential but have been shown to bind cellular proteins including tankyrase and USP7. **B:** The *oriP* family of repeats (FRs) and dyad symmetry (DS) elements are shown with an expanded view of the nucleotide sequence of DS with the EBNA1 binding sites 1 to 4. The nonamer repeats (*solid arrows*) and the 65 base-pair dyad symmetry (*broken arrows*) are also shown. EBNA1-binding sites are shown as *open boxes* with the dyad present in DS denoted by the *head-to-head arrows*. The Rep* element is located 240 bp downstream of DS. **C:** EBNA1 bound to DNA with a ribbon diagram showing the core domain, which contains residues 504 to 607 from each monomer, in *blue*. The flanking domains from each monomer are shown in *yellow*. The amino acids are numbered according to their position in the full-length EBNA1 protein derived from B95-8. **D:** A view down the noncrystallographic axis that shows one monomer in white and the other monomer in the same color scheme as used in **(C)**. The proline loops are indicated by the *arrows*. (Reprinted from Bochkarev A, Barwell JA, Pfuetzner RA, et al. Crystal structure of the DNA-binding domain of the Epstein-Barr virus origin-binding protein, EBNA1, bound to DNA. *Cell* 1996;84(5):791–800. Copyright © 1996 Elsevier. With permission. Ref.[52])

can either positively or negatively affect EBNA1-dependent functions.[148] Using a structure and fragment-based approach, small molecule inhibitors of EBNA1 DNA binding activity were identified. Remarkably, EBNA1 inhibitors impair LCL and EBV-infected NPC cell survival *in vitro* and xenograft models *in vivo*.[453] Similarly, a small molecule that blocks the ability of the N-terminal EBNA1 AT-hooks to bind host chromosomes causes EBV genome loss in tissue culture.[94]

The repeat unit of *oriP* acts as an enhancer in the presence of EBNA1, which is important for latent gene transcription from *Cp*.[197,228] Host cell factor 1 (HCF1) and octamer-binding transcription factor 2 (OCT2) cooperatively bind *oriP* with EBNA1 and are each important for *oriP* H3K4 trimethylation, *Cp* and *Qp* activity.[154] HCF1 knockdown causes EBV episome loss from Burkitt lymphoma cells, suggesting a potential HCF1 episome maintenance role. EBP2 is important for interactions between EBNA1 and chromosomes in metaphase and association with metaphase chromosomes. The MCM complex associates with DS and may have roles in initiation and licensing of EBV genome replication. EBNA1 may facilitate

ORC recruitment to DS by disrupting nucleosomes to provide ORC with DNA access.[197] Timeless and timeless interacting proteins, which have roles in stabilizing replication forks, are also recruited to *oriP*.[153] Timeless depletion from Burkitt cells causes loss of closed circular EBV episomes, accumulation of linear EBV DNA and double-strand breaks at *oriP*, suggesting an important role in replication fork stabilization in episome maintenance.[153]

USP7, which is a key regulator of p53 and Mdm2, stimulates EBNA1 DNA binding activity. USP7 forms a ternary complex with DNA-bound EBNA1[609] and is part of a histone deubiquitylating complex. USP7 depletion increases monoubiquitylated histone H2B at EBV FR and decreases its transcriptional activation activity.[255] Crystallographic studies reveal that EBNA1 and p53 bind the same USP7 pocket, but that EBNA1 makes more extensive contacts with USP7. Association between EBNA1 and USP7 protects cells from apoptotic challenge by p53 depletion. EBNA1 partially protects them from p53 overexpression-driven apoptosis.[608] Conversely, depletion of EBNA1 in EBV-positive Burkitt cells induces apoptosis.[320] USP7 and EBNA1 also have joint roles in disruption of PML nuclear bodies.[197]

EBNA1 deletion does not prevent EBV-driven B-cell outgrowth or establishment of LCLs,[268,543] likely since episome integration into host chromosomes enables DNA maintenance in the absence of EBNA1. This is apparently rare, as LCLs emerge nearly 1,000-fold less frequently from EBNA1-deficient virus.[268] LCLs established from wild-type versus EBNA1 deletion mutant virus grow at comparable rates and each can form xenografts in SCID mice. Thus, the contribution of EBNA1 to B-cell immortalization outside of activation of EBV latent genes[12] and maintaining the EBV genomes in infected cells may be limited in comparison with roles of other EBV latency oncoproteins.

A large number of putative EBNA1 host genome targets have been identified. EBNA1 ChIP-seq was used together with RNA-seq analysis following EBNA1 depletion from LCLs, Burkitt, and NPC cells.[684] Interestingly, approximately 1,000 host genome EBNA1 binding sites are mostly conserved across cell types, share a consensus DNA motif, and are frequently located proximal to transcription start sites, particularly at highly expressed genes.[408] EBNA1 binding sites are also enriched for LINE 1 retrotransposons. The antiapoptotic host factor survivin is up-regulated by EBNA1.[42]

EBNA2

Early studies by Elliott Kieff's group identified a B-cell transformation incompetent, but lytic replication competent EBV strain derived from Jijoye Burkitt cells called P3HR-1.[126,141,143,144,246,325,334,559,570] The search for the biochemical basis of the nontransforming phenotype led to the discovery and characterization of EBNA2, which is the principal ORF deleted in P3HR-1.[126,141,143,144,246,325,334,559,570] While EBNA-LP is also truncated in P3HR-1, it was found that restoring type 1 EBV EBNA2 expression rescued P3HR-1 B-cell growth transformation.[28,124,126,402] Transfection with cloned EBV DNA fragments deleted for part of the EBNA2 ORF or containing a stop codon one-third of the way into the EBNA2 ORF failed to restore transforming ability. Recombinant EBVs with a nontransforming EBNA2 mutation could also be recovered by infection of EBV negative BL cells.[403] More recently, the role of EBNA2 in EBV-driven primary B-cell transformation was again highlighted, where EBNA2 was the only latency gene found to be essential for newly infected B-cell outgrowth over the first 8 days.[543]

EBNA2 typically functions as an activator of B-cell viral and host gene transcription.[126,319,722] EBNA2 is the major viral transactivator of the C and LMP promoters.[722] Genetic analysis identified three essential EBNA2 domains critical for LMP and C promoter up-regulation (Fig. 11.9). These correspond to EBNA2 residues 1 to 58 or 97 to 210, which mediate

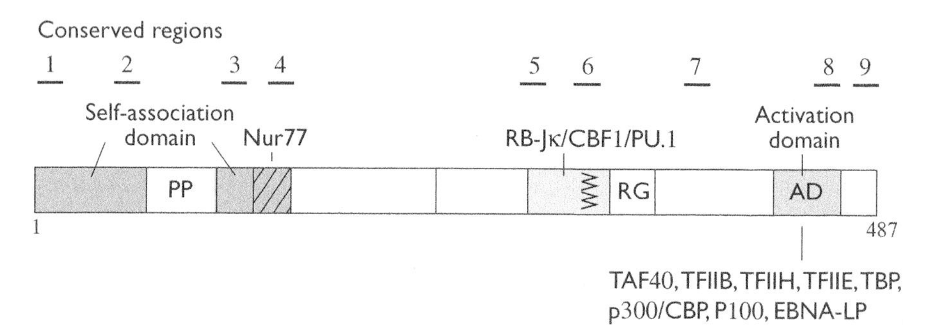

FIGURE 11.9 Schematic depiction of Epstein-Barr virus nuclear antigen (EBNA)-2 domains. EBNA2 contains a domain that interacts with the cellular sequence-specific DNA binding proteins RBP-Jκ and PU.1 to bring it to specific promoters, including the LMP1 promoter. The EBNA2 N-terminus has two domains that can mediate homotypic association with other EBNA2 molecules. Within this region, there is an interactive domain for Nur77. The poly-proline (PP) and poly-arginine-glycine (RG) as well as the activation domain (AD) are shown. The tryptophan-tryptophan-proline (WW) sequence in EBNA2, which is similar to a sequence in the Notch receptor intracellular domain, that normally mediates tight association with RBP-Jκ in up-regulating HES-1 in tissue development is shown. Mutation of this sequence in ablates EBNA2 transactivation.[219] The EBNA2 acidic domain (AD) interacts with TAF40, TFIIB, TFIIH, TFIIE, TBP, P300/CBP, p100, and EBNA-LP in stimulating transcription. The EBNA2 acidic domain is extensively associated with p100, which is a scaffolding protein for c-myb and PIM-1. Nine conserved regions of EBNA2 (bars above the protein) have been identified by comparing type 1 and type 2 EBNA2 with those from related LCVs that infect nonhuman primates.

homotypic association, amino acids 280 to 337, which mediate interaction with RBP-Jκ, and C-transactivation domain (TAD) residues 420 to 464.[118,124,126,219,229,233,241,313,319,758] In B lymphocytes, the EBNA2 C-terminal transactivation domain (TAD) is nearly as strong in activation of basal reporter constructs as the core herpes simplex VP16 activation domain.[124] The VP16 core 14 amino acids can substitute for the corresponding EBNA2 C-terminal transactivation domain residues in primary B-lymphocyte conversion to LCLs in recombinant EBV.[118] The EBNA2 C-terminal TAD recruits basal and activation associated transcription factors including TFB1/p62, TFIIB, TAF40, RPA70, TFIIH, and the histone acetyltransferases CBP/P300 and PCAF[319] (Fig. 11.9). An intrinsically unstructured EBNA2 region folds into a 9 amino acid alpha helix upon complex formation.[92]

EBNA2 is recruited to DNA through association with host transcription factors, particularly the Notch pathway sequence-specific DNA binding protein RBP-Jκ/CBF1.[38,219,241,296] Whereas RBP-Jκ assembles corepressor complexes in B cells in the absence of EBNA2, EBNA2 often converts RBP-Jκ into an activator by competing for corepressor binding, through EBNA2 TADs, and through recruitment of coactivators, including EBNA-LP. RBP-Jκ is critical for LCL growth and survival.[416] EBNA2 is at least partially dependent on Jκ DNA sites for transactivation of *Cp*,[293] LMP1, and LMP2.[207,296,362] The *Cp* and *LMPp* sites contain EBNA2 response elements that carry Jκ DNA motifs.

EBNA2 mimics key aspects of activated Notch signalling. The EBNA2 WWP motif (Fig. 11.9) resembles a Notch intracellular domain "WFP" sequence that tightly associates with RBP-Jκ,[679] and EBNA2 and Notch binding to RBP-Jκ are mutually exclusive.[260] EBNA2 residues 318 to 327 mediate RBP-Jκ association.[393] EBNA2 induces formation of new RBP-Jκ occupied sites.[405] Yet, constitutive Notch signaling cannot replace EBNA2 to maintain EBV-transformed lymphoblastoid B-cell proliferation.[211,253]

Microarray profiling of EBV-uninfected Burkitt cell lines with conditional EBNA2 expression identified 311 significantly EBNA2-induced genes, including CD21, CD23, CCR7, RUNX3, and CD83. Likewise, conditional EBNA2 expression identified key EBNA2 down-regulated targets, including CD79B, TCL-1, and MEF2B.[420,753] ChIP-seq identified a much larger number of host genomic sites occupied by EBNA2[405,420,441,751,755] and suggested that EBNA2 subverts intrinsic B-cell transcriptional programs. Thousands of host genome sites are co-occupied by RBP-Jκ and EBNA2 in LCLs. EBNA2 and RBP-Jκ predominantly co-occupy intergene and intron sites, with only a small proportion proximal to transcription start sites.[221,441,755] Jκ DNA motifs are highly enriched at EBNA2/RBP-Jκ co-occupied sites, whereas EBF1 DNA motifs are enriched at sites occupied by EBNA2 but not RBP-Jκ. EBNA2 reorganizes genomic binding sites of RBP-Jκ and EBF1, and EBNA2-EBF1-RBP-Jκ co-occupancy appears to transcriptionally activate target genes.[210,405]

EBNA2 alleles differ significantly in amino acid sequence between type 1 and 2 EBV strains.[126,143,581] Reconstitution of the type 2 P3HR-1 EBV strain with a type 1, but not a type 2 EBNA2 gene, yields virus that transforms B cells as efficiently as type 1 EBV strains.[126] A single EBNA2 transactivating domain amino acid at residue 442 appears to underlie this phenotype. Substitution of type 2 serine 442 with type 1 aspartic acid confer enhanced LMP1 up-regulation and type 1 transforming activity on a type 2 EBV strain.[705] In contrast, recombination of cloned type 2 EBNA2 DNA in place of the P3HR-1 deletion results in deficient transformation characteristic of type 2 EBV. EBNA2 encoded by type 1 EBV more strongly induces LMP1 and a small number of host cell genes than EBNA2 encodes by type 2 EBV.[409] Similarly, type 2 EBNA2 associates more strongly with the BS69 repressor protein.[549]

Super-enhancers (SEs) are particularly strong enhancers that drive expression of genes critical for cell identity and oncogenic states. EBNA2 occupied 888 SE in LCLs.[221,292,735,759] Often located far from transcriptional start sites, these SE loop to targets, including *RBPJ*, *EBF1*, *BATF*, and *RUNX3*. A subset of EBNA2 SEs, termed EBV SEs, are co-occupied by EBNAs LP, 3A, 3C, and LMP1-activated NF-κB transcription factors.[292,759] EBV SEs often loop to more than one target gene, enabling them to target 1992 sites. EBV SE targets were enriched for host genes essential for LCL growth and survival,[292,416] including *MYC*, *IRF4*, and *CFLAR*. Two EBV SEs loop to the *MYC* promoter from 525 and 428 kbp upstream,[292,735,759] and EBNA2 is important for formation of these loops in newly infected B cells.[292] EBNA2 recruits the SWI/SNF chromatin remodeler complex to *MYC* enhancers to promote interactions with the *MYC* promoter.[735] The pioneer transcription factor MEF2C was also found to be important for MYC-targeting EBV SE activity.[715] Deletion of either *MYC*-targeting EBV SE by CRISPR genome editing diminished MYC expression and LCL proliferation.[292]

EBNA2 also has key roles in host metabolism pathway remodeling in newly infected B cells, both by strongly inducing MYC and also by EBNA2 target gene regulation.[721] EBNA2 has important roles in up-regulation of aerobic glycolysis (the Warburg effect) within the first days of infection.[442,478,721] EBV-mediated NF-κB and PI3K activity are each important for up-regulation of the glucose transporter GLUT1 in transformed cells at later timepoints,[656] though interestingly GLUT1 is up-regulated even before LMP1 and 2A reach significant levels in newly infected cells.[721] EBV infection also markedly remodels mitochondria, most of whose components are encoded by nuclear genes that can be regulated by EBNA and LMP signaling. Consequently, oxidative phosphorylation is also strongly up-regulated in the first week postinfection and plays similarly important roles in B-cell growth transformation.

Maximal EBNA2 RNA and protein abundance is observed by 48 hours postinfection.[478,717,721] Proteomic analysis highlighted that EBV strongly induces the mitochondrial one-carbon (1C) pathway within the first days of infection, reaching maximal expression levels during the period of hyperproliferation[721] to convert serine into glycine, carbon units, ATP, and NAD(P)H for use in anabolic reactions. Lipid metabolism pathways are also highly induced by EBNA2, which functions with host transcription factors such as SREBP and MYC to remodel mevalonate and fatty acid synthesis pathways. EBV-induced lipid metabolism enables cross-talk between EBNA and LMP oncoproteins.[723]

EBNA-LP

EBNA-LP is a major coactivator of EBNA2 host and viral target genes.[8,200,232,509,636] EBNA-LP targets include the C and LMP1 promoters as well as a large number of host genomic sites. EBNA-LP coactivation with EBNA2 is evident in

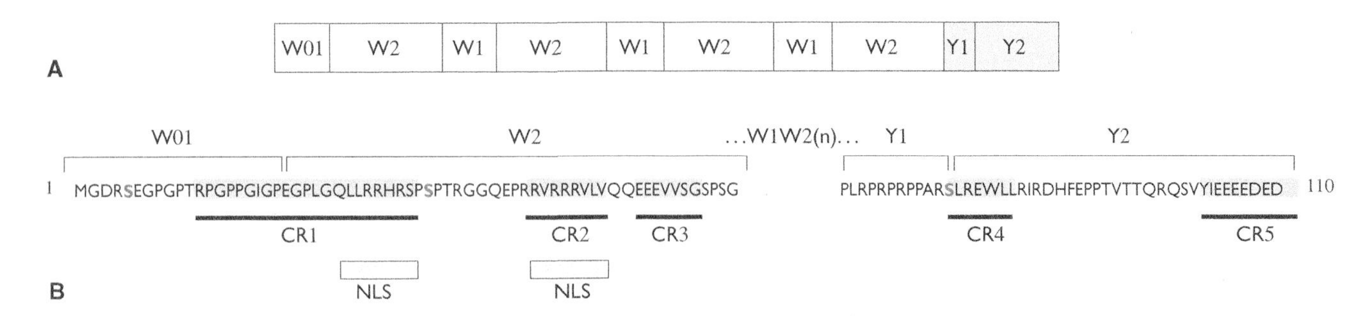

FIGURE 11.10 Schematic diagram of the repeat and unique exon and domain structure of Epstein-Barr virus nuclear antigen leader protein (EBNA-LP). The exons of EBNA-LP are derived from the BamHI W and Y fragments with initiation of transcription from *Wp* or *Cp*. **A:** The EBNA-LP AUG is generated by a unique alternative 5′ splicing event. The W1 and W2 regions are repeats of 22 and 44 amino acids, respectively. This EBNA-LP repeat domain coactivates transcription mediated by the EBNA2 acidic domain. The unique C-terminus of EBNA-LP consists of Y1 and Y2, which is dispensable for EBNA2 coactivation and modulates EBNA-LP function. **B:** Amino acid sequence of the unique W01 exon and the W2, Y1, and Y2 exons. A single W1/W2 repeat is shown. Also shown are serines that are phosphorylated and conserved regions (CRs) in EBNA-LP proteins encoded in EBV and the nonhuman primate LCVs.

transient expression assays with artificial LMP1 promoter constructs, and in inducing the latency III program in Burkitt cells when coexpressed by gene transfer together with EBNA2. Yet, EBNA-LP does not globally coactivate EBNA2 targets.[319,402]

EBNA-LP is comprised of 22 and 44 amino acid regions of variable copy number, fused to 11 and 34 residue carboxy-terminal regions. These are encoded by the W1, W2, Y1, and Y2 exons, respectively (Fig. 11.10A and B). The W1 and W2 encoded regions enable homodimerization and association with the EBNA2 acidic activating domain.[232,537] In newly infected B cells, *Wp* drives expression of a 5′ W0 exon, which is alternatively spliced either to the W1 or to a W1' exon and then to W2. Since W0, W1, and W2 reside within the EBV genome internal repeat 1 (IR1) region, EBNA-LP size varies between viral strains with differing IR1 copy number. Likewise, transcripts can initiate from distinct W0 exons, giving rise to EBNA-LP products of variable length early in B-cell infection. Upon the switch to *Cp* driven transcription, EBNA-LP mRNAs are instead comprised of 5′ C1 and C2 exons that are joined with W and Y exons.[319] At least 5 W repeats are required for optimal B-cell outgrowth, at least two of which are necessary for B-cell transformation in culture.[692] This requirement results from the optimization of *Wp*-driven transcriptional activity. Clinical EBV strains typically have at least 5 to 8 W copies.[692]

EBNA2 and EBNA-LP interact in yeast two-hybrid assays[77] and as recombinant proteins *in vitro*. However, association between wild-type EBNA-LP and EBNA2 is difficult to detect in LCL extracts. EBNA-LP can bind to and coactivate transcription through the EBNA2 acidic activating domain or through an EBNA2 N-terminal 58 amino acid domain.[537] EBNA-LP potentiates EBNA2-mediated transcription from the C and LMP1 promoters in transient transfection assays with reporter constructs and also coactivates EBNA2 up-regulation of LMP1 expression in type 1 EBV-infected BL cells.

EBNA-LP localizes predominantly to promyelocytic leukemia (PML) nuclear bodies and to a lesser extent in the cytosol.[319] An EBNA-LP region conserved in nonhuman primate LCVs interacts with and displaces Sp100 from PML nuclear bodies.[394] Sp100A mutants deleted for the PML targeting domain, which also interacts with EBNA-LP, can coactivate EBNA2 independently of EBNA-LP, suggesting that displacement of Sp100A from PML nuclear bodies is an important EBNA-LP function.[394] Deletion of a Sp100A domain that interacts with the transcriptional repressor heterochromatin protein 1 (HP1) prevents Sp100A coactivation function, suggesting that EBNA-LP function may in part involve chromatin modification.[394] Together with HA95, EBNA-LP also activates transcription by displacing NCoR and histone deacetylases (HDACs) from matrix-associated deacetylase (MAD) bodies.[551] EBNA-LP can also coactivate host target genes with the host histone acetyltransferase EP300/P300, apparently independently of EBNA2.[725] ChIP-Seq identified nearly 20,000 EBNA-LP occupied host genomic regions.[552] Only 29% were co-occupied by EBNA2, in large part because approximately 50% of EBNA-LP sites were within 2 kb of transcriptional start sites. Long-range DNA interactions may increase contact between EBNA2-bound enhancer and EBNA-LP occupied promoter sites.

Recombinant EBV studies suggest that EBNA-LP is important for B-cell transformation. Complete repair of the P3HR1-1 deletion encoding EBNA2 and the Y1/Y2 EBNA-LP exons restores B-cell immortalization, whereas repair of only EBNA2 reduces immortalization efficiency by approximately 10-fold.[28,425] EBNA-LP knockout (KO) virus exhibited reduced naive B-cell transformation efficiency. Deletion of just the Y1 and Y2 exons also substantially decreased the rate of EBV-driven B-cell outgrowth.[676] EBNA-LP KO EBV likewise slows outgrowth of tonsil B cells.[543] By contrast, EBNA-LP KO virus failed to establish LCLs from umbilical cord B cells, which underwent cell death by 2 weeks postinfection. Absence of EBNA-LP significantly diminished recruitment of EBNA2, EBF1, and RBP-Jκ to the viral genome, but not to the EBNA2 target *IL7* host target gene.[676]

EBNA3A, EBNA3B, and EBNA3C

EBNA3 proteins have important roles in host and viral gene regulation. EBNA3s share an N-terminal homology domain, a proline-rich region and repeat sequences. EBNA3C also has a putative leucine zipper that mediates association with the host transcription factor PU.1/SP1.[754] EBNA3s target DNA sites through interactions with host factors, in particular RBP-Jκ.[585,586] Each EBNA3 has transcription repression activity when tethered to DNA by a heterologous GAL4 DNA binding domain.

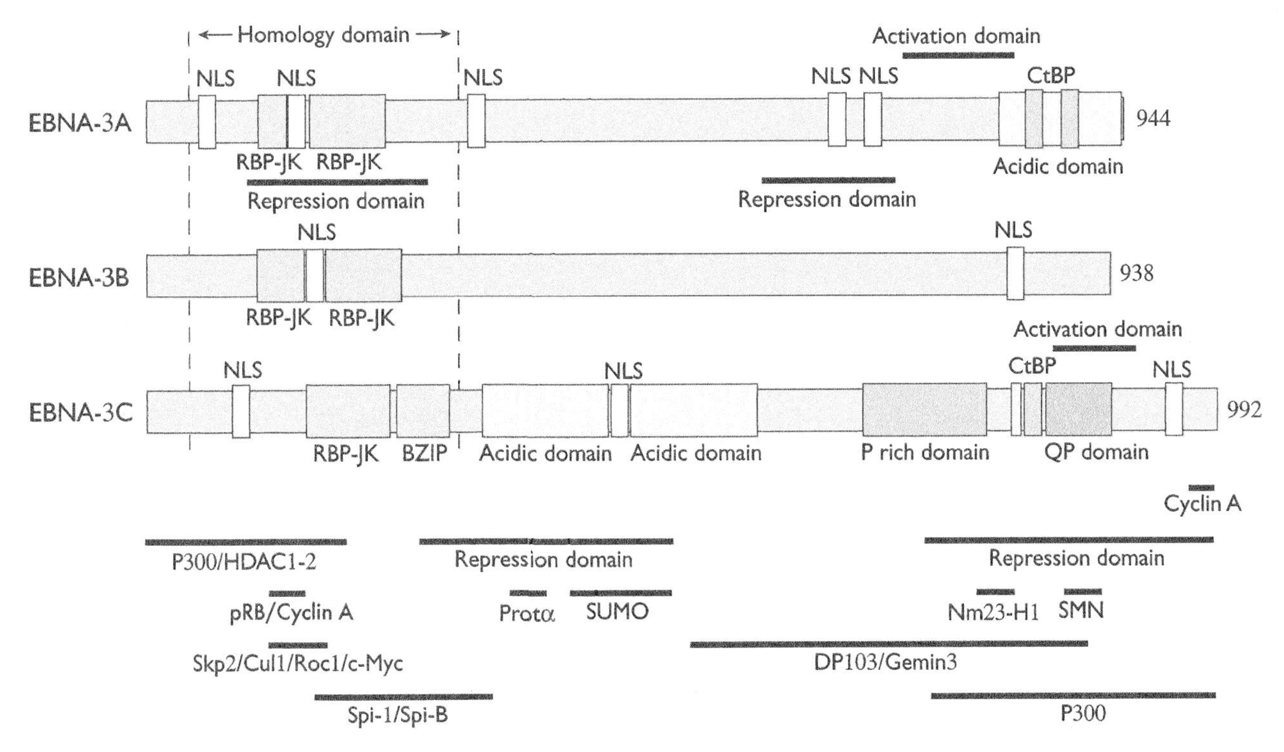

FIGURE 11.11 Schematic diagram of the Epstein-Barr virus nuclear antigen (EBNA)3A, EBNA3B, and EBNA3C and their functional domains. EBNA3A, EBNA3B, and EBNA3C proteins are shown with the number of their amino acids and with a common domain that contains the RBP-Jκ interaction domain. Also indicated are domains that have activating or repressive effects in addition to a variety of domains that associate with cellular proteins including CtBP, p300/HDAC1-2, pRB/cyclin A, prothymosin-α (Protα), Skp2/Cull/Rocl/c-Myc, Spi-1/Spi-B, SUMO, Nm23-H1. SMN, DP103/Gemin3, and p300. Nuclear localization signals (NLS), a leucine zipper (BZIP), acidic domains, proline (P)-rich region, and a glutamine (Q) and proline region are shown. (Reprinted with permission from Sims K, Saha A, Robertson ES. Regulation of Cellular Processes by the Epstein-Barr Virus Nuclear Antigen 3 Family of Proteins. In: Robertson ES, ed. *Epstein-Barr Virus—Latency and Transformation.* Norfolk, UK: Caister Academic Press; 2010:81–100. Ref.[635])

EBNA3A, 3B, and *3C* genes are arranged in tandem (Fig. 11.11) and are conserved with primate LCVs, but do not have homology with host proteins. EBNA3 proteins are expressed from a polycistronic transcript that encodes all 6 EBNAs, that is alternatively spliced, and that is present at low abundance in LCLs.[9] *Wp* or *Cp* drive expression of EBNA3 transcripts in the latency IIb and III programs, respectively. EBNA3 messages share a U exon with EBNA1 and have individual splice acceptor sites that compete with EBNA1. EBNA3 transcripts have individual downstream polyA sites. EBNA3s are expressed within 48 hours of primary B-cell infection, reaching maximal levels between 4 and 7 days postinfection cell culture.[478,717,721] EBNA3s inhibit EBNA2 activation of *Cp*, which may account for the significant drop in EBNA2 expression by 96 hours postprimary B-cell infection.

EBNA3s compete with EBNA2 for the same RBP-Jκ binding surface.[585,586,752] However, EBNA3s bind more tightly to RBP-Jκ,[690] reminiscent of the *Drosophila* Notch antagonist Hairless. Deletion of the EBNA3A or EBNA3C RBP-Jκ association region abrogates their EBNA2 antagonism.[431,729] Interaction between EBNA3A or 3C and RBP-Jκ is essential for LCL growth and survival.[116,368,433]

EBNA3s also repress target genes through assembly of corepressor complexes. EBNA3s associate with host corepressors C-terminal binding protein (CtBP), Sin3A, NCoR, and HDACs HDAC-1 and 2.[9,600] The EBNA3A and EBNA3C region that associates with CtBP1 is required for LCL growth.[368,644] CtBP1 is important for LCL, but not Burkitt growth and survival.[416] EBNA3A and EBNA3C recruit CtBP by mimicking "PLDLS" domains that mediate association between CtBP and transcription corepressors. EBNA3s association with CtBP is important for the assembly of polycomb repressive complex 2 (PRC2) at target gene sites, where the histone methyl transferase subunit EZH2 deposits histone 3 lysine 27 trimethyl (H3K27me3) repressive chromatin marks.[9] H3K27me3 have been identified at EBNA3A and EBNA3C occupied sites proximal to transcriptional start sites of major tumor suppressor genes, including *BCL2L11*.[527,735]

ChIP-Seq has identified a wide range of EBNA3 host and viral target gene sites. Greater than 13,000 EBNA3C sites were identified in LCLs, 64% of which were at chromatin sites with activating H3K4me1 and H3K27ac enhancer marks. DNA motifs for RUNX3, BATF, IRF4, and ATF2 are enriched at these sites.[291] EBNA3C ChIP-seq signals were strongest at sites with either composite BATF/IRF4 elements (also known as ATF–interferon composite elements, or AICE) or composite SPI1/IRF4 elements (also known as ETS–interferon composite elements, or EICE). Similarly, ChIP-seq identified 10,000 EBNA3A host genome binding sites in LCLs, 55% of which were active enhancers and 11% of which were at active or weakly active promoters.[617] AICE and EICE motifs were enriched at EBNA3A occupied sites. A total of 25% of host genomic binding sites were shared between EBNA2 and EBNA3 proteins in Burkitt lymphoma cells with latency III expression.[441]

EBNA3s can also serve as transcriptional activators, alone or in concert with EBNA2. EBNA3C associates with PU.1/SPI1[754] and with the histone acetyltransferase p300.[133] The EBNA3C leucine zipper interacts *in vitro* with the PU.1-Ets domain and appears to up-regulate transcription through the LMP1 promoter PU.1 binding site.[754] The EBNA3C effect is independent of the RBP-Jκ binding site in the LMP1 promoter and of the RBP-Jκ interaction domain in EBNA3C.[754] Furthermore, EBNA3C fully coactivates with an EBNA2 mutant that does not interact with RBP-Jκ.[389]

Using EBV-negative Burkitt lymphoma cells infected by wild-type versus EBNA3 knockout EBV, microarray analysis identified greater than 1,000 host genes whose expression significantly changed with EBNA3 deficiency.[730] More than one EBNA3 protein regulated a third of these, with EBNA3C apparently cooperating with EBNA3A, EBNA3B, or both. Expression profiling identified 167 up-regulated and 129 down-regulated host genes in LCLs established from EBNA3A-deficient versus wild-type virus.[247] EBNA3A-regulated genes were enriched for targets previously identified as being regulated by EBNA2. Likewise, 550 host genes were at least 1.5-fold differentially regulated in LCLs with conditional EBNA3C inactivation, and these significantly overlapped with genes regulated by EBNA2 and EBNA3A.[751]

EBNA3A and EBNA3C, but not EBNA3B, are each important for B-cell transformation into LCLs.[9,600,695] EBNA3A KO virus is attenuated for B-cell transformation and gives rise to LCLs with increased apoptosis and reduced proliferation rates.[247] Conditional EBNA3C inactivation results in the accumulation of cell cycle inhibitors p16(INK4A), p14(ARF), p53, and hypophosphorylation of Rb.[432,751] Similarly, EBNA3A or 3C inactivation results in active chromatin marks at the p14 and p16 encoding *CDKN2A* locus.[291] Knockdown of p14 or p16 partially rescues LCL growth in the absence of either EBNA3A or EBNA3C.[434] B cells obtained from an individual with a homozygous *CDKN2A* locus deletion that causes p16 deficiency are transformed equally well by wild-type and EBNA3C-deficient virus, highlighting an EBNA3C role in overcoming a p16-dependent block to B-cell proliferation 2 to 4 weeks postinfection.[645]

EBNA3A and EBNA3C have key roles in regulation of B-cell differentiation.[670] B cells infected by EBNA3A and EBNA3C conditionally inactivated virus, or virus deficient for EBNA3s altogether, initially proliferate. However, they subsequently undergo plasmablast differentiation at 20 days postinfection. This phenotype may result from EBNA3C suppression of *BCL6*[535] and BLIMP1. Once committed to plasmablast differentiation, re-expression of EBNA3A and EBNA3C does not rescue LCL differentiation.[670] EBNA3A or 3C have key roles in repressing the *BCL2L11* encoded tumor suppressor BIM. EBNA3A and 3C co-occupy assemble a PRC2 repressive complex upstream of the *BCL2L11* promoter.[441,527,735] Inhibition of EZH2 up-regulates BIM expression,[735] as does KO of BATF or IRF4, suggesting that they may play roles in EBNA3 recruitment to this site.[416] The H3K4me3 chromatin mark, which can be found at activated promoters, does not change with H3K27me3 deposition, suggesting that bivalent chromatin is formed.[645] EBNA3A also has key roles in up-regulation of the antiapoptotic *MCL-1* gene to promote infected B-cell survival at early timepoints postinfection.[555]

The onset of EBV-induced hyperproliferation at 3 days postinfection induces DNA replication stress and the DNA damage response (DDR) pathway.[113,505] EBNA3C suppresses the ATM/Chk2-mediated DNA damage responsive signaling pathway in newly EBV-infected cells.[113,505] The DNA damage response has an important tumor suppression role in limiting EBV-induced B-cell transformation *in vitro*, as inhibition of the DNA damage response pathway kinases ATM or CHK2 increased B-cell transformation efficiency.[505]

Functionally important EBNA3C interactions have been defined, many of which regulate cell cycle progression, the G1/S checkpoint, and cell survival. EBNA3C binds p53 and represses its functions by interacting with the inhibitor of growth family proteins ING4 and ING5.[595,599] EBNA3C recruits the ubiquitin ligase Skp1/Cul1/F-box complex resulting in ubiquitination of the cell cycle regulators Rb and p27.[340,341] EBNA3C also interacts with and modulates the activity of cyclins A, D1, and E.[338,339,596] EBNA3C associates with the transcription repressor E2F6 to reduce E2F1 activity.[534] Furthermore, the EBNA3C N- and C-terminal domains associate with E2F1 to block its induction of apoptosis stimulated by the DNA damage response.[598] EBNA3C up-regulates and associates with PIM-1 kinase to down-modulate activity of the cell cycle inhibitor p21/WAF1.[32] EBNA3C also recruits Skp2 ubiquitin ligase complexes to cyclin A to target degradation of the kinase inhibitor p27 and further promote cell proliferation.[341] The EBNA3C N-terminal domain associates with IRF4 and IRF8 and stabilizes IRF4. IRF4 depletion causes decreased MYC and CDK6 expression and causes LCL death.[33,416] EBNA3C induces and associates with the WTAP N6-methyladenosine transferase, which in turn regulates EBV transcript stability and promotes EBV-transformed cell growth.[360]

In cord blood humanized mouse models, EBNA3C-deficient EBV induced lymphomas at decreased frequency and with delayed onset in comparison to wild-type virus. P16 levels were increased in tumors that arose from EBNA3C knockout virus in comparison to wild-type virus-infected tumors.[589] EBNA3C-deficient tumors had increased T-cell infiltration and up-regulation of the type 1 interferon response, suggesting additional EBNA3C immunomodulation roles *in vivo*. EBV deficient for either EBNA3A or 3C establishes persistent infection but fails to induce tumors in humanized NOD-SCID mouse models.[491] EBNA3B is not critical for EBV-driven primary B-cell conversion to LCLs.[11,141,694] EBNA3B epitopes are frequently recognized by cytotoxic T lymphocytes. Interestingly, humanized mouse infection by EBNA3B-deficient EBV causes aggressive monomorphic lymphomas, which are not infiltrated by EBV-reactive T cells despite their expansion in this model.[731] EBNA3B knockout deficient B cells secreted less CXCL10, a chemokine that attracts T cells, a phenotype that was also observed in EBNA3B-deficient LCLs. Thus, EBNA3B can be considered to have tumor suppressor roles *in vivo*, perhaps safeguarding against malignancy during the establishment of latency.

LMP1

LMP1 was identified by Elliott Kieff's group as the most abundant viral mRNA in lymphoblastoid B cells.[182] LMP1 mimicks CD40 signaling to subvert a major B/T-cell communication pathway[476] and is essential for *in vitro* B-cell conversion into

LCLs.[156,314,316,327] LMP1 also promotes differentiation-induced lytic replication.[88] As described in detail below, LMP1 constitutively activates NF-κB, mitogen-activated protein kinase (MAPK), phosphatidylinositol 3-kinase (PI3K), JAK/STAT, interferon regulatory factor (IRF), and SUMOylation pathways in a ligand-independent manner. In single gene transfer experiments using heterologous promoters, LMP1 has transforming or "oncogene" effects in continuous rodent fibroblast cell lines.[718] LMP1 alters Rat-1 or NIH 3T3 cell morphology, enables growth in medium supplemented with low serum, causes loss of contact inhibition, and enhances growth as tumors in nude mice. Rat-1 or Balb/c 3T3 cells also lose anchorage dependence and grow in soft agar after LMP1 expression.[541,718] The growth of Balb/c 3T3 cells in soft agar correlates quantitatively with the extent of LMP1 expression up to the levels ordinarily expressed in LCLs.[29,472,541]

LMP1 is transcribed from one of two viral promoters separated by approximately 600 bp. In B cells, LMP1 is encoded by a 2.8-kb mRNA, which initiates from the ED-L1 promoter that is dependent on EBNA2.[296] ED-L1 can also be activated independently of EBNA2 by cellular factors, such as the STATs, IRF7, NF-κB, ATF4, PAX5, AP-2, and EBF1.[102,150,369,489,507,720] The p38 signaling pathway also up-regulates LMP1 expression.[299] Enhancement of LMP1 expression up to 200-fold can be mediated by the EBNA1-dependent transcriptional enhancer FR in *oriP* acting across the fused TRs.[203] Looping of the *oriP* enhancer to the LMP1 promoter also contributes to LMP1 expression.[685] LMP1 transcripts are detectable within 48 hours of B-cell infection and steadily increase over the first 2 weeks postinfection.[558] LMP1 also activates the unfolded protein response to drive its own synthesis, and LMP1 levels in individual cells vary by over 100-fold in clonal LCL cultures.[369] Highly elevated MYC levels early after EBV infection dampen B-cell LMP1 expression.[557]

In epithelial cells, LMP1 transcription is mediated by the upstream L1-TR promoter that initiates transcription from multiple TATA-less sites in the nearest copy of TR, resulting in a 3.5-kb transcript with a long untranslated 5′ exon.[208,529] Transcription is in part dependent on the cellular factors Sp1 and STAT3.[208,529] LMP2A can negatively regulate the expression of LMP1 from this promoter,[667] whereas TR copy number varies inversely to LMP1 expression.[578] The LMP1 ORF has two short introns.[35,182] Epithelial cell differentiation regulates LMP1 expression, where the host transcription factors KLF4 and BLIMP1 jointly up-regulate LMP1 through coactivation of the two LMP1 promoters.[497] L1-TR is active in NPC and interestingly also in Hodgkin lymphoma.[102,578]

LMP1 induces many of the changes usually associated with EBV infection of primary B cells or with antigen activation of primary B cells, including homotypic adhesion, villous projections, increased vimentin expression, increased cell surface expression of CD23, CD39, CD40, CD44, and class II MHC, increased IL-10 expression, decreased expression of CD10, and increased expression of the cell adhesion molecules LFA-1, ICAM-1, and LFA-3.[2] LMP1 is not required for EBV-induced B-cell outgrowth over the first week of infection.[543,558] EBV-infected cells become dependent on LMP1 and NF-κB approximately 1 to 2 weeks postinfection *in vitro*,[558] and conditional LMP1 inactivation or NF-κB blockade triggers LCL growth arrest and apoptosis.[70-73,327]

Reverse genetic experiments defined key LMP1 domains important for B-cell transformation (Fig. 11.12). Deletion of the 24 residue N-terminal cytoplasmic tail reduces transforming efficiency, possibly because of effects on trafficking or stability.[281] The LMP1 six transmembrane domains induce intra- and intermolecular association that drive LMP1 signaling. The 200 residue LMP1 C-terminal tail contains three signaling regions and is critical for B-cell transformation. Of these, CTAR/transformation effector site (TES) 1 and 2 are critical for EBV-mediated B-cell transformation into LCLs.[282,314-316] An EBV recombinant lacking CTAR1 residues 185 to 211 is unable to transform primary human cells into LCLs *in vitro*, suggesting obligatory CTAR1 role(s).[282,314-316] Interestingly, recombinant EBV that expresses only the first 231 LMP1 residues and therefore lacks CTAR2/TES2 and CTAR3 transforms primary B cells into LCLs, so long as they are either grown on fibroblast feeder layers or high-titers of EBV are used.[282,314-316] While deletion of LMP1 residues encompassing CTAR3 does not abrogate B-cell growth transformation,[280,282] *in vivo* roles remain possible. Indeed, CTAR3 alters cell migration and promotes the establishment of latency.[40,42,279] CTAR3 associates with the SUMO ligase Ubc9, which itself is induced by LMP1 CTAR1/2.[42,199,601]

LMP1 activates two NF-κB pathways, termed canonical and noncanonical. CTAR2/TES2 associates with TRADD and TNIK and activates the ubiquitin ligase TRAF6 to initiate canonical NF-κB signaling.[280,619,621,634] In turn, TRAF6 activates the kinase TAK1, which phosphorylates the IκB kinase (IKK) IKKβ[724] (Fig. 11.12). The linear ubiquitin assembly complex (LUBAC) also plays a key role in IKK activation.[206] IKK phosphorylates IκBα, promoting its ubiquitination by β-TRCP and proteasomal turnover. IκBα degradation releases dimeric NF-κB transcription factors, typically RelA:p50 or cRel:p50 for nuclear translocation and to target gene activation. CRISPR loss-of-function analysis identified TRAF6, TAK1, LUBAC, IKKβ, RelA, and cRel as important for LCL growth and survival.[416]

CTAR1 induces a complex NF-κB response, as determined by electrophoretic mobility shift assays.[313,457] Recombinant LMP1 lacking CTAR2 efficiently induces NF-κB target genes including ICAM-1 at levels similar to wild-type virus.[282,314-316] LMP1 CTAR1/TES1 uses a PXQXT motif to recruit TRAFs 1, 2, 3, and 5.[152,476,745] PxQxT motifs were subsequently found to also be used by immune receptors including CD40. CTAR1 sequesters TRAF3, which likely prevents it from suppressing levels of the NF-κB inducing kinase (NIK).[34] NIK then likely autophosphorylates to activate the IKKα kinase, which triggers production of the active p52 NF-κB subunit. p52 homodimers or heterodimers then regulate target genes. p52 is necessary for LCL growth and survival, though interestingly RelB is not, perhaps because of redundancy.[416] Association with TRAF1 enhances CTAR1/TES1 activation of the canonical NF-κB pathway, where TRAF1:TRAF2 heterotrimers recruit LUBAC and lysine-63 ubiquitin ligases to activate TAK1.[216]

In epithelial cells, a key LMP1 target is the epithelial growth factor receptor (EGFR), which is induced by CTAR1 signaling through NF-κB, BCL3, and STAT3. LMP1-activated STAT3 induces BCL3, which co-occupies the EGFR promoter together with p50 homodimers.[349,691] Similarly, LMP1 suppression of the junctional protein plakoglobin influences a cadherin switch, with effects on cell migration relevant to

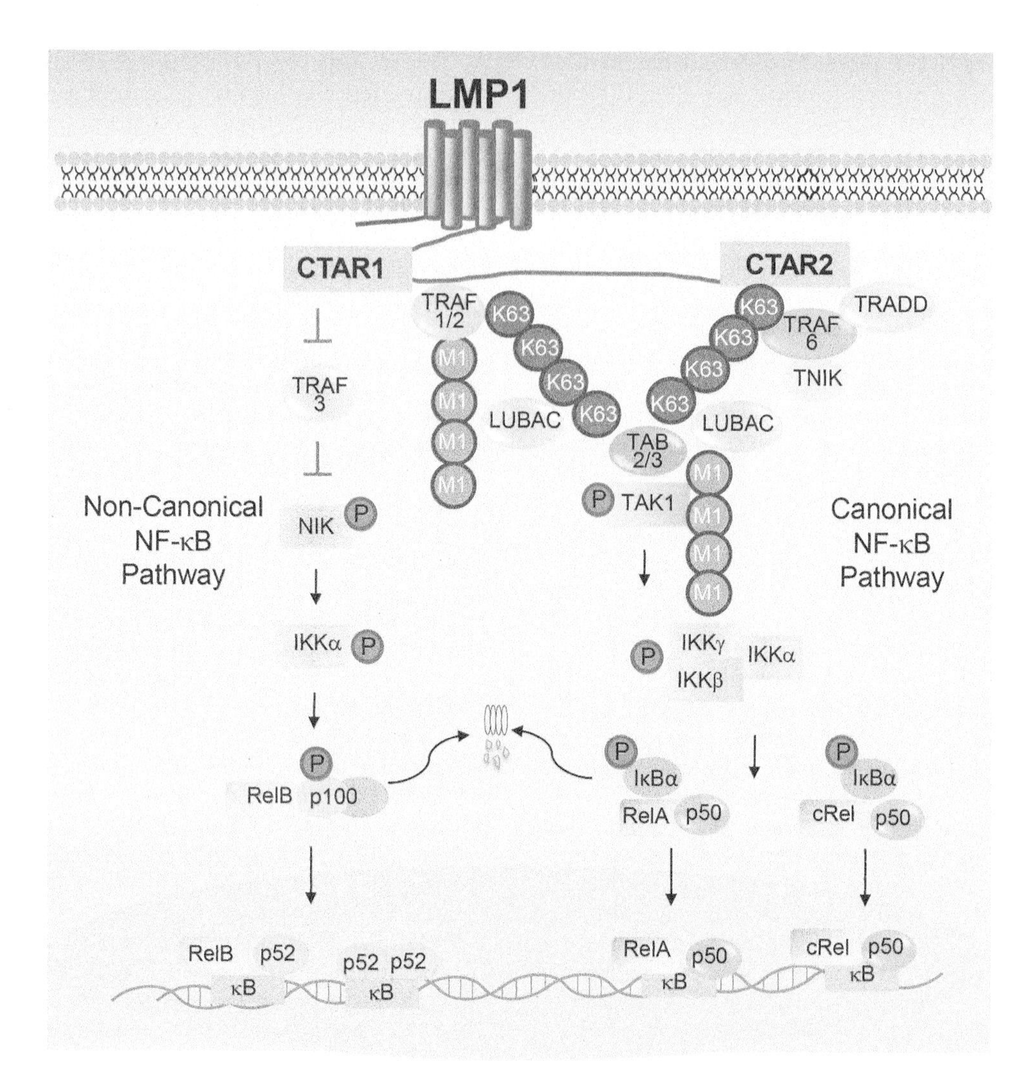

FIGURE 11.12 Schematic diagram of biochemical mechanisms by which latent membrane protein 1 (LMP1) activates NF-κB pathways. The six LMP1 transmembrane domains enable LMP1 aggregation and activation of signaling. The LMP1 C-terminal tail has two regions that activate NF-κB pathways, termed CTAR1/TES1 and CTAR2/TES2. CTAR1/TES1 sequesters TRAF3 to de-repress its negative regulation of the kinase NIK. In the absence of suppression by TRAF3, NIK activates the non-canonical NF-κB pathway by phosphorylating the kinase IKKα. IKKα triggers processing of p100 to p52, which translocates to the nucleus as homodimers or as heterodimers with RelB. LMP1 CTAR2/TES2 associates with the TNFR1-associated death domain (TRADD) and activates the canonical pathway. CTAR2/TES2 activates TRAF6 and the linear ubiquitin assembly complex (LUBAC), which synthesize lysine 63-linked (K63) and linear (M1 Ub) polyubiquitin chains, respectively, culminating in activation of the kinases TAK1 and IKKβ. IKKβ phosphorylates IκBα, causing its proteasomal degradation and nuclear translocation of RelA/p50 and cRel/p50 complexes. TRAF1 enables CTAR1 to cross-talk with the canonical NF-κB pathway through polyubiquitin signaling. Not shown here, LMP1 CTAR1/2 also activates p38, JNK, ERK, and IRF7 pathways, and the linker region between CTAR1/2 contains the LMP1 CTAR3 region that activates UBC9, but which is not required for B-cell transformation.

NPC metastasis.[627] LMP1 also blocks p53-mediated apoptosis through induction of the NF-κB target gene A20.[198]

Constitutive LMP1 activation of canonical and noncanonical pathways gives rise to a complex genomic NF-κB binding landscape. Indeed, as many as 13 NF-κB dimeric transcription factors may form in LCL nuclei.[750] NF-κB occupies 73% of LCL active enhancers but does not readily reflect the two NF-κB pathway paradigm. Rather, 11 distinct NF-κB profiles were present at enhancers and 10 at promoters, suggesting that there is significant cross-talk between the canonical and noncanonical NF-κB pathways at the level of the host genome.[750] NF-κB targets critical for LCL survival include c-FLIP[416] and BCL2 family members.[240,555] Proteomic analysis found that greater than 80% of LMP1 gene targets were encoded by genes identified to be targeted by NF-κB.[149] LMP1 further influences host target gene regulation through effects on PARylation.[430]

LMP1 strongly activates the JNK, p38, and ERK MAP and PI3 kinase pathways.[326,714] Experiments with dominant negative JNK or with JNK chemical inhibitors indicate that JNK activation is critical for LMP1 effects on transformed cell growth. TAK1 plays multiple roles in MAPK activation, including a kinase-independent role in LMP1 signaling complex formation that contributes to downstream TPL2 and JNK kinase activation. This does not appear to be shared with CD40.[712] TRAF1 enables LMP1 TES1 to also strongly activate MAPK pathways.[216] Also differing from CD40, LMP1 activates IRF7.[739] LMP1 CTAR2 binds to IRF7 and induces K63-linked ubiquitination in a RIP1- and TRAF6-dependent fashion.[506,508,657] LMP1 induces IRF7 sumoylation,[41] which limits IRF7 DNA binding and transcriptional activation and thereby potentially limits innate immune responses. LMP1 associates with PI3 kinase through CTAR1.[146,358] CTAR1 but not CTAR2 is necessary for LMP1-mediated rodent and human fibroblast transformation through the activation of the PI3K and AKT kinases.[421] The cytoskeleton protein vimentin, which associates with LMP1, is important for LMP1-mediated PI3K/AKT pathway activation.[445]

LMP1 oligomers form patches at the plasma membrane and endosomal membrane sites.[388] LMP1 signals from cholesterol-rich membrane microdomains termed lipid rafts,[311] and egress from the endoplasmic reticulum is necessary for LMP1 signaling.[357] The Rab family protein Rab13 is induced by EBV within the first days of B-cell infection, colocalizes with LMP1 and LMP2A, and has key roles in their intracellular trafficking to signaling sites.[723] LMP1 is released from infected cells in extracellular vesicles, which regulate LMP1 levels and affect the nearby microenvironment.[447,511,567,711]

Mouse models have highlighted LMP1 oncogenicity. Transgenic LMP1 expression causes B-cell lymphoproliferative disease in mice.[348,748] Mice expressing an LMP1/CD40 chimera, in which the LMP1 transmembrane domains (TMs) drive constitutive signaling from the CD40 cytoplasmic tail develop B-cell lymphomas as result of hyperactive CD40 signaling.[236,256,572] By contrast, transgenic mice expressing a chimeric CD40 extracellular and transmembrane domain fused to the LMP1 C-terminal tail are relatively normal. Immunoglobulin heavy chain promoter and enhancer driven LMP1 expression results in B-cell hyperplasia and lymphomas in aged mice.[348] By contrast, when expressed from a CD19 promoter, LMP1-positive cells are recognized and destroyed by T and NK cell responses.[748] T-cell depletion causes fatal lymphoproliferative disease, which was also seen in mice with conditional LMP1 and LMP2A coexpression following T and NK cell suppression.[463,734] LMP1 is not absolutely necessary for EBV-driven lymphomagenesis in a cord blood humanized mouse model, apparently because CD40 signaling may compensate to some degree.[417] Likewise, EBV deficient for LMP1 and LMP2A could cause lymphoma in a cord blood-humanized mouse model, albeit at reduced frequency from wild-type EBV.[415]

LMP1 remodels host metabolic pathways, in part through effects on PARP1-mediated posttranslational modification of target genes, including hypoxia-inducible factor 1-alpha (HIF-1a). This potentiates glycolytic Warburg metabolism.[267] PARP1 inhibition causes accumulation of repressive histone methylation marks and results in EBV lytic reactivation, likely through effects on the BZLF1 promoter.[411] EBV similarly up-regulates glycolysis in transformed epithelial cells, and EBV-driven cell metabolism remodeling likely has key roles in NPC pathogenesis.[747]

LMP2A and LMP2B

LMP2A acts as a broad inducer of cellular signal transducers in part by acting as a B-cell receptor mimic but also by rewiring B-cell signal transduction resulting in differential phosphorylation of kinases, phosphatases, adaptor proteins, transcription factors such as NF-κB and TCF3, as well as widespread changes in the transcriptional output of LMP2A-expressing B cells[91,185] (Fig. 11.13). As a result, the two EBV latent membrane proteins provide two signals that are essential for normal B-cell development and function—LMP1 providing a CD40-like signal and LMP2A a BCR-like signal. Together, LMP1 and LMP2A direct EBV-infected B cells to the memory B-cell compartment where EBV establishes a latent infection. LMP2B is related to LMP2A but lacks the amino terminal domain required for LMP2A signaling function (Fig. 11.13). LMP2A and LMP2B in latency III are expressed from unique EBNA2 responsive promoters with RBP-Jκ and PU.1 binding sites.[448,605,763]

In latency IIa, in which EBNA2 is not expressed, LMP2A may autoactivate its own expression through Notch providing a mechanism for expression independent of EBNA2.[15] The LMP2A first exon encodes 119 N-terminal cytosolic amino acids that precede a methionine, which is the translational start site for the LMP2B mRNA. LMP2A and 2B mRNAs share the remaining exons, which encode 12 transmembrane (TM) spanning domains separated by short reverse turns and a 27 amino acid C-terminal cytosolic domain[363,605] (Fig. 11.13). Several studies have suggested that LMP2B can augment LMP1 signaling and negatively regulate the function of LMP2A.[574,575,591] LMP2A colocalizes with LMP1 in patches in membranes of latently infected B lymphocytes.[401] LMP2A is palmitylated[250,312,436] and associates with lipid rafts, which is likely important for initial contact with Src family tyrosine kinases such as Lyn. Along with lipid raft association, Lyn is likely recruited to LMP2A by the amino acids DQSL in the LMP2A C-terminal cytoplasmic domain, which is similar to the amino acids DCSM in the BCR-associated protein Ig-α. This interaction is required for the phosphorylation of LMP2A tyrosines found within the LMP2A amino terminal domain, including an ITAM motif, which binds the Syk tyrosine kinase via two Syk SH2 domains.[66,456,592] This results in the activation of a variety of cellular signal transducers, including RAS, PI3K, Btk, BLNK, Akt, mTor, and MAPK[91,171,451,452,456,470,674] (Fig. 11.13).

Antiphosphotyrosine antibodies localize to LMP2A sites of constitutive tyrosine phosphorylation in the plasma membrane of infected cells.[400] LMP2A is also serine/threonine phosphorylated. LMP2A S15 and S102 bind MAPK *in vitro* and are substrates for MAPK phosphorylation.[523] The LMP2A N-terminus has two PPPPY motifs, which bind WW domains of Nedd4 family ubiquitin ligases, such as AIP4/Itchy, WWP2, Nedd4, or Nedd4-2.[273,274] This interaction results in the ubiquitination and degradation of LMP2A and LMP2A-associated proteins.

LMP2A and 2B have been extensively mutated within the EBV genome indicating that LMP2A and LMP2B are not absolutely essential for transforming primary B lymphocytes in culture, but in some cases can provide a growth advantage.[60,423,424,543,587,662] Compatible with this observation,

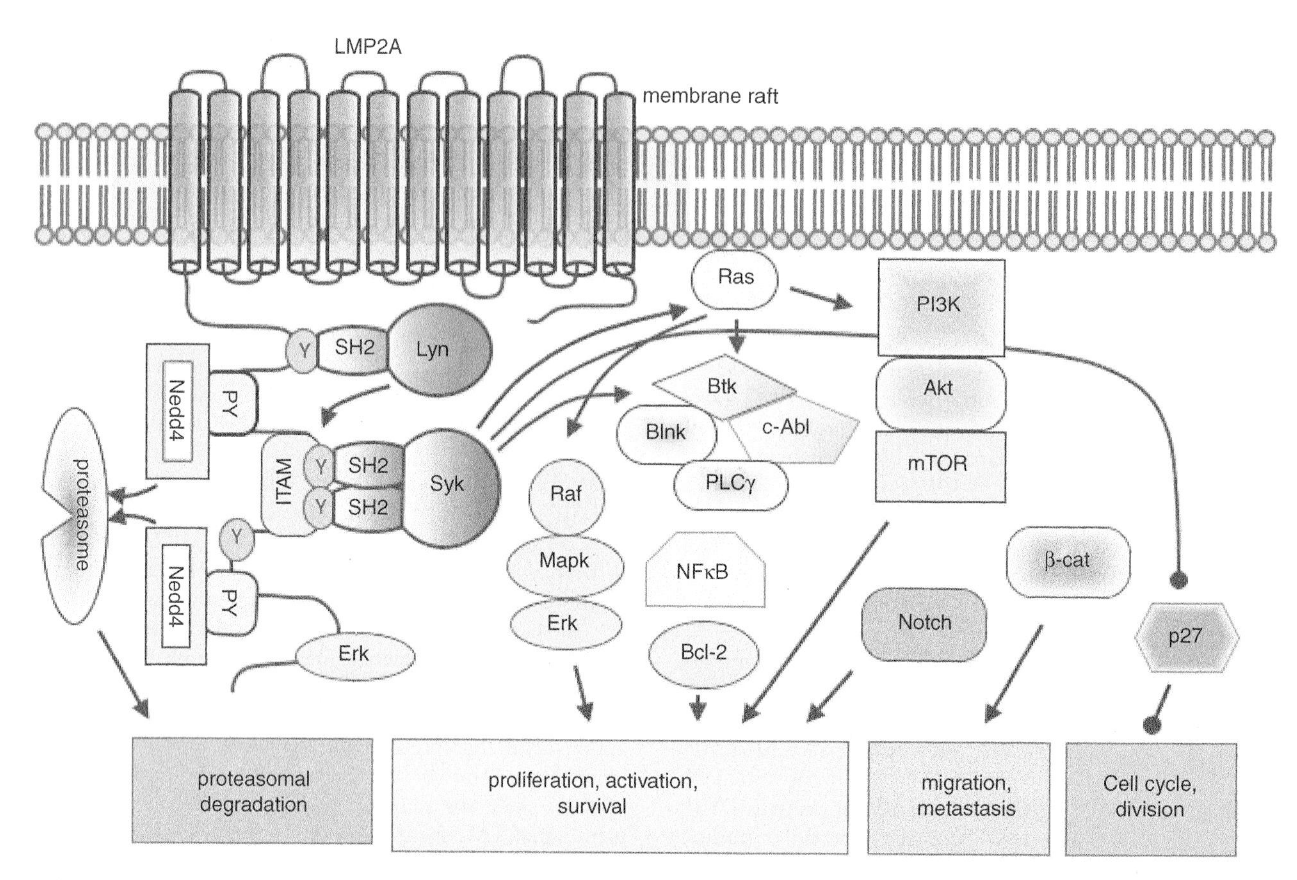

FIGURE 11.13 **Latent membrane protein 2A (LMP2A) activates B-cell signaling pathways by constitutively mimicking an activated BCR.** LMP2A is constitutively localized to lipid rafts and binds Src family tyrosine kinases such as Lyn leading to constitutive phosphorylation of LMP2A at multiple tyrosine residues. Syk is recruited to LMP2A by the phosphorylated ITAM in the amino-terminal domain of LMP2A and becomes activated. LMP2A also binds E3 ubiquitin ligases in the Nedd4 family and MAPK. LMP2A blocks BCR entry into lipid rafts. PI-3K is constitutively phosphorylated in cells expressing LMP2A, as is BLNK, and Btk. The antiapoptotic serine/threonine kinase Akt is constitutively phosphorylated in cells expressing LMP2A, representing one mechanism, by which LMP2A inhibits apoptosis. MAPK and Ca2+ dependent signal transduction may result from activation of PI-3K, BLNK, and Btk. LMP2A also activates β-catenin that is important in LMP2A effects in epithelial cells. (Reprinted by permission from Springer: Cen O, Longnecker R. Latent Membrane Protein 2 (LMP2). In: Münz C, ed. Epstein Barr Virus Volume 2. *Current topics in microbiology and immunology,* Vol 391. Cham: Springer; 2015:151-180. Copyright © 2015 Springer International Publishing Switzerland.)

CRISPR/Cas9 dependency screens have shown that LMP2A targets such as Syk, Btk, BLNK, PI3Kinase, and cell cycle regulators are important for LCL growth in culture.[416] LMP2A, like LMP1, provides survival and differentiation signals to B cells *in vivo*. This was first shown using transgenic mice where LMP2A expression in transgenic mice was directed to B cells, which allowed BCR negative B cells to escape from the bone marrow and colonize peripheral lymphoid organs, bypassing normal B-cell developmental checkpoints by constitutive activation of BCR signal transducers.[16,78] The LMP2A effect is also evident in RAG1 KO mice and a number of proteins important for BCR signaling, such as Syk, Btk, and BLNK. The LMP2A ITAM is important for this effect.[171,451,452] Thus, LMP2A has a role in latency type II infected lymphocytes in enhancing B-cell survival through activation of B-cell signal transducers.

In transgenic mice, high level LMP2A expression results in B-1 cells in bone marrow, spleen, and the periphery, whereas low level expression results in spontaneous germinal centers.[87,276] More recent studies using engineered mice confirm the role of LMP2A and LMP1 to mimic signals B cells receive in a germinal center reaction. LMP2A provides an antigen-independent signal, and a T-cell help signal mediated by LMP1 allows antigen-independent proliferation.[463,757]

The level of LMP2 expression is regulated by N-terminal monoubiquitination, which is mediated by Nedd4 ubiquitin ligases that bind to the PY motifs found in the LMP2A amino terminus.[273,275] In murine models of Burkitt lymphoma using a *myc* transgene expressed in B cells, LMP2A has been shown to dramatically accelerate tumor development, by bypassing the requirement of mutation of the p53 pathway[46] and by activating the cell cycle through increasing p27kip1 degradation.[658] Remarkably, tumors derived from LMP2A/MYC mice share a similar pattern of gene expression with MYC tumors derived from transgenic mice, despite the absence of p53 pathway mutations in LMP2A/MYC mice.[47] LMP2A expression is detected as mRNA transcripts and protein in Burkitt and Hodgkin lymphoma biopsies. Like Burkitt lymphoma, Hodgkin lymphoma exhibits latency II, which includes EBNA1, LMP1, and LMP2A. EBV-associated diffuse large B-cell lymphoma shows latency II or III, including LMP1 and LMP2A. In HIV/AIDS-related lymphomas, EBV latent gene expression is heterogeneous, and LMP1 and LMP2A, in addition to EBNA2 and EBNA3A/B/C, are variably expressed.

Constitutive activation of important cellular signal transducers by LMP2A is likely important in the pathogenesis of EBV-associated malignancies. An important role for LMP2A in classical Hodgkin lymphoma can be surmised, since crippling mutations in the immunoglobulin genes are found, which would normally result in the death of these cells. LMP2A and LMP1 are uniformly expressed, providing a role for LMP2A and LMP1 in classical Hodgkin lymphoma, by allowing bypass of apoptotic signals that should normally result in cell death due to the absence of the expression of the BCR. Also in support of a role of LMP2A in classical Hodgkin lymphoma, LMP2A expression during B-cell development in mice results in decreased expression of E2A, EBF, and Pax-5, which are important for normal B-cell development.[553,554] Furthermore, LMP2A activates Notch, which alters B-cell identity.[17] Similar changes and loss of B-cell identity are observed in classical Hodgkin lymphoma.

Studies have shown that LMP2A is an important factor in NPC and gastric carcinoma. LMP2A expression in epithelial cells line results in hyperproliferation in raft cultures, alterations in differentiation, increased cloning efficiency in soft agar, and promotes epithelial cell spreading and migration.[10,194,345,406,620] AKT activation increases β-catenin and cell growth through the LMP2A ITAM and PY motif.[474,475,533] LMP2A inhibits TGF-β associated apoptosis.[202] In summary, LMP2A, like LMP1, delivers a potent cell survival signal to B lymphocytes and may provide a therapeutic target in EBV-associated cancers.

EBERs

EBERs 1 and 2 are transcribed by RNA pol III in a manner enhanced by EBNA1 as nonpolyadenylated transcripts of 167 and 172 nucleotides, respectively. The EBERs have intragenic A and B box transcriptional control regions common to pol III transcripts.[647] At steady state levels in latently infected B lymphocytes, the EBERs are the most abundant viral RNAs, reaching 1 to 5 million copies per cell. Since EBERs are expressed in all B-cell latency states, they are widely used to identify EBV-infected cells in histological samples. EBERs localize to the nucleus, where they are complexed with the cellular La and L22 proteins. Despite their high expression levels, the role of the EBERs in EBV pathogenesis remain incompletely defined.

EBER2 associates with the EBV genomic terminal repeats, where it has a role in recruiting the transcription factor PAX5 to down-modulate LMP expression.[366] In support, LCLs established from EBV deficient for EBERs express elevated LMP2 RNA levels, though protein levels were unaffected.[218] Several overexpression studies suggest that EBERs have a role in EBV oncogenicity. However, the effects of EBER expression can be opposed by concomitant L22 expression, suggesting that the interaction between EBERs and L22 is functionally significant. Indeed, overexpression of an EBER1 mutant deficient for binding L22 in EBV-negative Akata cells failed to enhance soft agar colony formation.

EBERs are similar in size and structure to adenovirus VA1 and VAII RNAs, which block PKR phosphorylation and translation inhibition and are important for adenovirus replication. EBER1 and EBER2 can partially substitute for VA1 in adenovirus replication and can inhibit PKR *in vitro*, at levels similar to VA1 RNA. In contrast, PKR activation *in vivo* is unaffected by EBER expression. This may reflect the distinct subcellular compartmentalization, of the EBERs being exclusively nuclear, while PKR is predominately found in the cytoplasm. Both EBERs can activate the cytosolic double-stranded RNA sensor RIG-I and stimulate type I interferon production when overexpressed,[602] but like PKR, RIG-I is thought to be a cytosolic protein, calling into question the physiological significance of this interaction.

Studies of the effects of EBER deletion on primary human B-cell outgrowth have yielded conflicting results. EBER-deleted EBV generated by homologous recombination into the P3HR-1 genome was equivalent to wild-type EBV in efficiency of primary B-cell conversion to LCLs, in time to LCL outgrowth, and in lytic reactivation.[673] No significant change in B-cell outgrowth was observed between wild-type and EBER-deficient recombinant B95-8 virus over 8 days of infection.[543] Yet, the 50% transforming dose was 100-fold less for wild-type than recombinant Akata EBER deletion mutants. Restoration of EBER expression resulted rescued transformation efficiency. LCLs established from EBER-deleted Akata virus had reduced growth rates.[741] Differences in methodology or in virus strains utilized may explain discrepancies between these studies. EBER-deficient recombinant EBV established infection of humanized mice with similar efficiency as wild-type mice, with similar spleen and blood viral loads at 4 weeks postinfection.[218] Nonetheless, EBER functions are likely to be important *in vivo*, as recent experiments with the closely related murine gammaherpesvirus 68 found that the noncoding RNA TMER4 promotes infected B-cell egress from lymph nodes into the peripheral circulation. Interestingly, this TMER4 function could be replaced by EBER1.[254]

EBV miRNAs

EBV was the first human virus identified to encode miRNAs.[542] miRNAs are 20 to 22 basepair noncoding single-stranded RNAs that broadly regulate virus and host gene expression through repression of translation or through mRNA degradation. miRNAs usually fine-tune target gene expression by less than 50%, but summed activities of miRNAs on a given transcript can strengthen phenotypes. EBV miRNAs are incorporated into the RNA-induced silencing complex (RISC), which then associates with viral and host mRNA 3′ untranslated regions. Around 25 viral pre-miRNAs encoded by two viral genome clusters give rise to at least 44 miRNAs, which are expressed in LCLs and in tonsils.[485] The majority of EBV miRNAs are encoded in the BART cluster, with several also encoded in the BHRF1 cluster. Both clusters are expressed within 48 hours of EBV B-cell infection and increase over the first week.[647] A total of 21 EBV miRNAs are conserved with rhesus LCV.[647] EBV miRNAs can be expressed as abundantly as cellular miRNAs.

The BART cluster encodes 22 miRNA precursors (ebv-miR-BART1-22), from which 44 miRNAs are produced.[177] Two clusters of BART miRNAs are separated by an intron. BART miRNAs are expressed at highest levels in latently infected epithelial cells, including nasopharyngeal and gastric epithelial cells.[569] BART miRNAs are also highly expressed in EBV-infected primary effusion lymphoma. By contrast, BART miRNAs are expressed at low levels in all stages of B-cell infection, with the lowest expression found in latency I.[74] Two TATA-less promoter regions, P1 at nucleotide 150641 and

P2 at nt 150357 in the B95 sequence, likely transcribe the BARTs.[11,27,287,651] P1 is active in epithelial cells, is the initial B-cell promoter, and is down-regulated by IRF7 and IRF5, whereas P2 is more active in epithelial cells and is up-regulated by c-MYC and C/EBP.[11] Other studies have suggested that the EBV-encoded miRNA profile in infected cells may differ when normal infected tissues are compared to neoplastic tissues.[564] Interestingly, BART miRNAs promote tumor growth in murine xenograft gastric carcinoma models, suggesting epithelial transforming properties *in vivo*.[565]

The commonly used B95-8 laboratory strain lacks most BART miRNAs.[566,648] Consistent with this observation, studies with BART locus miRNAs did not uncover any gross defect in regard to EBV transformation as monitored in cell culture.[626] However, BART miRNAs may have important *in vivo* roles in immunoevasion, for example suppressing transcripts encoding RIG-I and Toll-like receptors, the NK cell ligand MICA, the IL-1 and IL-6 receptors, the NLRP3 inflammasome, the cytokine IL-12, and the NK and T-cell chemoattractant CXCL11. EBV miRNAs also suppress class I and II major histocompatibility complex antigen presentation at the levels of the TAP transporter and lysosomal proteases, respectively.[7,677] This may explain why EBV miRNA KO decreases titers and diminishes B-cell proliferation in humanized models.[492] T-cell depletion allowed miRNA-deficient EBV to achieve similar viral loads as wild-type EBV and to induce tumors. In epithelial cells, high level BART expression contributes to immunoevasion.[271]

BART miRNAs target tumor suppressor gene mRNAs, including those encoding BIM, PUMA, and PTEN.[427] BART miRNAs inhibit etoposide-triggered apoptosis in epithelial cells through effects on the BIM 3′UTR.[427] BART miRNAs enhance gastric carcinoma tumorigenicity in a murine xenograft model and block apoptosis responses in EBV-infected Burkitt cells through effects on caspase 3.[709] Burkitt cells with induced EBV-genome loss could be propagated so long as BART miRNAs were ectopically expressed.[709] EBV re-infection of these EBV-negative Burkitt cells restores their growth on soft agar and tumorigenicity in SCID mice.[344]

BART miRNA viral targets include mRNAs encoding LMP1, LMP2A, the immediate-early BZLF1, and the viral polymerase BALF5. BART9 miRNA alters LMP1 levels and affects the growth rate of NK T-cell lymphomas.[571] Interestingly, editing of BART6 miRNA results in suppression of EBNA2.[272] Induction of lytic replication enhances expression of many EBV miRNAs, even though miR-BART20-5p targets BZLF1 and BRFL1.[302] Recombinant EBV lacking BART miRNAs cause increased lytic replication, likely given increased BZLF1 expression.[391] EBV genomic deletions observed in NK and T-cell lymphomas affect the BART miRNAs, perhaps increasing lytic gene expression.[517] Indeed, the BART miRNAs most frequently deleted were mir-BART6-5p and mir-BART6-p, which target BZLF1 and BRFL1. Alternatively, multiple EBV miRNAs target B-cell receptor signaling mediators to promote EBV B-cell latency by desensitizing infected cells to antigen receptor stimuli.[99]

Alternatively spliced BART transcripts are the most abundant viral-encoded polyadenylated RNAs in EBV-infected epithelial cancers.[426] Highly spliced, nuclear polyadenylated exons, from which the primary BART miRNA intronic sequences are removed, do not appear to be translated. Rather, they function as nuclear long-noncoding RNAs (lncRNAs). In gastric carcinoma cells, these target thousands of cellular genes, with approximately equal numbers of up-regulated and down-regulated targets. Targets include components of the unfolded protein response. Interestingly, many of the BART lncRNA target genes have also been identified as being regulated upon EBV infection.[426]

miR-BHRF1-3 are encoded within EBNA transcripts and are strongly expressed in B cells with latency III expression but are nearly undetectable in B cells or epithelial cells with latency I or II infection.[74] Two BHRF1 miRNAs accumulate with lytic replication.[13] BHRF1 miRNAs promote cell cycle progression and block apoptosis. BHRF1 miRNAs target the tumor suppressors PTEN and p27.[548] miR-BHRF1-2 reduces NF-κB activation in response to IL-1.[649] BHRF1 miRNAs also down-modulate expression of *EBNA2, LMP1,* and *LMP2* and up-regulate SUMO-conjugation via down-regulation of the SUMO-targeted ubiquitin ligase RNF4 SUMO to promote secretion of infectious virus.[377] miR-BHRF1-2-5p targets the 3′ UTR of the mRNAs encoding immune checkpoint PD-L1 and PD-L2.[137]

EBV miRNAs predominantly target host gene products, many of which are evolutionarily conserved RISC-accessible sites.[647] LMP1 and NF-κB up-regulate the oncogenic miR-155, whose overexpression induces lymphomas in mice and is required for LCL proliferation.[395] EBNA3A/C induce host miR-221 and 222, which targeted the mRNA of the p57KIP2 cyclin-dependent kinase inhibitor.[37] Even in LCLs established with B95-8 EBV, PAR-CLIP identified nearly 8,000 miRNA interaction sites in approximately 3,500 transcript UTRs.[646]

Extracellular vesicles (exosomes) can transfer EBV miRNAs to cells in the microenvironment, including on neighboring dendritic cells.[446,532] Viral miRNAs, which are stable within exosomes, therefore have potential for serving as biomarkers for EBV-associated diseases.

Gammaherpesviruses encode circular RNAs (circRNAs), which are small noncoding RNAs that are produced by back-splicing of a 3′ donor to a 5′ acceptor.[706] EBV circRNAs are expressed from *Cp*, the EBNA U exon, *LMP2, BHLF1,* and from the *RPMS1* locus. CircRNA roles remain to be defined but may include functions in sequestration of miRNAs or interactions with *oriLyt* in lytic DNA replication, as lytic circRNA clusters are located in the vicinity of lytic replication origins in multiple gamma-herpesviruses.

EBV Lytic Replication

Lytic replication is necessary for transmission of EBV between hosts and for cell-to-cell spread. Lytic genes are increasingly recognized to also have oncogenic roles, in particular for NPC, where elevated antibody titers against EBV lytic proteins are disease biomarkers.[443] EBV gene expression follows a temporal and sequential order as with other herpesviruses. Nearly all EBV genes are expressed in the viral lytic cycle, where by late timepoints most of the viral genome is transcribed in both directions.[515] The majority of genes required for EBV lytic DNA replication, cleavage, assembly, and packaging of the viral genome are conserved across the three herpesvirus families. Table 11.1 lists EBV protein-coding genes and their HSV and KSHV homologs. EBV lytic reactivation remodels the B-cell proteome, with multiple effects on cell cycle proteins and immune pathways, including up-regulation of complement and depletion of the B-cell receptor complex.[174]

Lytic replication may contribute to EBV-associated cancers by at least three mechanisms: (a) expansion and replenishment of the population of infected cells; (b) conditioning of the microenvironment, including induction of angiogenesis, genomic instability, and secretion of proinflammatory cytokines and growth factors[322,485]; and (c) abortive lytic expression of oncogenic noncoding RNA and proteins.[518] Immediate-early and early gene expression contributes to B-cell lymphomagenesis in humanized mouse models.[418]

Immediate-Early Genes

The EBV immediate-early viral genes *BZLF1* and *BRLF1* are transactivators of virus replication. BZLF1 was originally identified in studies using variants of the EBV-positive HR1 cell line. A rare variant spontaneously released virus that could induce early lytic antigens in Raji cells. These early studies identified that a 2.7-kb DNA rearranged in the rare P3HR-1 variant cells was sufficient to trigger lytic replication in latently infected cells.[48,136,462,678] Subsequent studies showed that rearranged BZLF1, contained in this fragment, was sufficient to disrupt latency in HR-1 cells.[135] BZLF1 and BRLF1 are expressed shortly after induction of lytic replication by immunoglobulin cross-linking and are essential for lytic replication.[180] BZLF1 and BRLF1 cross-regulate one another and synergistically induce EBV early genes. Studies comparing BZLF1 and BRLF1 deletion viruses, and analyzing the temporal order of BZLF1 and BRLF1 expression following induction of EBV lytic replication, indicate that BZLF1 is critical in the initial stages of B-cell induction of lytic replication.

BZLF1 is encoded by a three exon transcript initiating from the *BZLF1* promoter (*Zp*). The first exon encodes a TAD.[382,385,387] The second exon encodes a strongly basic domain with homology to AP1 that interacts with DNA sites. BZLF1 and AP-1 bind to similar DNA motifs, although BZLF1 preferentially binds to methylated Z-responsive elements (meZRE). Underscoring their close relationship, several alanine-to-serine point mutants enable AP-1 to phenocopy key BZLF1 functions, including binding to meZREs and inducing BRLF1 and early gene expression.[414] The third exon encodes a coiled-coil leucine/isoleucine heptad repeat.[191]

Phosphorylation by host and viral kinases regulate BZLF1 activity, including casein kinase II (CKII) and protein kinases A and C (PKA and PKC). PKC phosphorylates BZLF1 DNA binding domain serine 186, and this residue is absolutely required for lytic reactivation.[196] CKII phosphorylates BZLF1 serines 167 and 173, the latter of which is required for lytic DNA replication but not for early gene activation.[443] The EBV serine/threonine kinase BGLF4 further regulates BZLF1 activity and supports its expression.[21,22,379]

BZLF1 activates transcription of BRLF1 (also known as RTA or R), which is a DNA sequence specific transcription activator with distant amino acid sequence similarity to the host transcription factor c-MYB. RTA binds to RTA-response elements (RREs) and to viral promoters through association with host transcription factors.[443] BRLF1 and BZLF1 activate their own as well as each others' promoters.[322] BRFL1 has an N-terminal DNA recognition domain, a dimerization domain, and a C-terminal transcription activation domain that is a potent acidic activator similar to VP16. BZLF1 and BRLF1 synergistically induce transcription from viral early gene promoters, which frequently contain DNA elements for both. BRLF1 binds to unmethylated DNA motifs and preferentially induces activating H3K9 histone acetyl marks at unmethylated promoters, which is important for epithelial cell lytic induction.[733]

The *BZLF1* promoter is tightly repressed to maintain latency. Seven *cis*-acting, BZLF1-bound DNA elements, termed ZIA-D, ZII, ZIIIA, and ZIIIB regulate Z promoter (Zp) activity (Fig. 11.14).[191] Multiple host transcription factors also bind to Zp elements, including Sp1/Sp3 and the myocyte enhancer factor 2D (MEF2D). Depending on cell type, the host repressors ZEB1 and/or ZEB2 bind to the Z promoter ZV/ZV' element to suppress induction of lytic replication.[169,346,347] Mutations that disrupt these silencing elements result in hyperlytic viruses that are deficient in B-cell transformation. The host miRNAs 200b and 429 can induce EBV latently infected cells to undergo lytic replication, in part by reducing expression of ZEB1/ZEB2.[170] STAT3 and PARP1 exert additional repressive effects on EBV lytic reactivation.[342,411] As mentioned above, MYC represses EBV lytic reactivation.[222]

Variants of the Z promoter alter the extent of lytic protein expression in B cells. The Zp-V3 variant, found in type 2 EBV strains and in some type 1 strains, contains a binding motif for NFAT. While type 2 EBV causes higher levels of lytic protein expression in cord blood-humanized mouse infection models as well as in LCLs,[588] Zp-V3 is not sufficient for this phenotype. Elevated NFATc1 and NFATc2 abundance may also contribute lytic replication levels in type 2 EBV infected cells. The M81 EBV strain, isolated from a patient with NPC, has high spontaneous lytic replication, linked to lower BART miRNAs levels[391] and to higher expression of the EBV DNA polymerase BALF5.[115] Sumoylation also regulates BZLF1 and BRLF1 activities.[322] EBV lytic factor LF2 induces BRLF1 sumoylation and relocalizes it to the extranuclear cytoskeleton, resulting in repression of BRLF1 activity.[76,238]

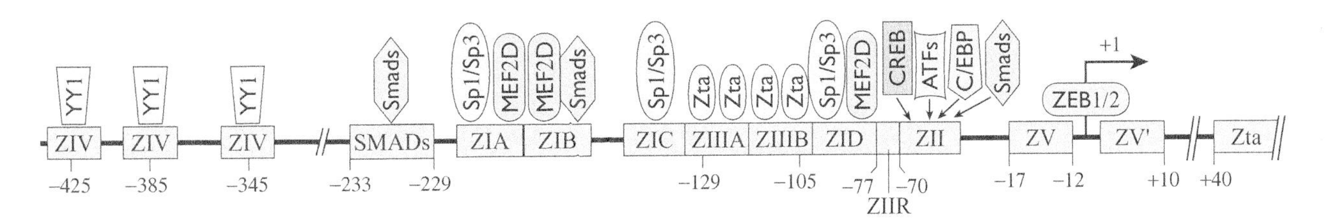

FIGURE 11.14 Schematic representation of EBV BZLF1 promoter elements. The BZLF1 promoter has a large number of binding sites for regulators of gene expression. Shown in the diagram are the cis-acting regulatory elements present within nucleotides −221 through +40 of the BZLF1 promoter relative to the transcription initiation site. *Shaded rectangles* along the BZLF1 promoter indicate approximate locations of identified regulatory elements with the relevant transacting factors indicated above.

Cellular differentiation is increasingly linked to EBV reactivation. B-cell differentiation into plasma cells is a major trigger for EBV lytic replication.[355] Likewise, studies of oral hairy leukoplakia found that EBV lytic replication occurred in the outer most differentiated layers of the epithelium[503] and in raft culture models EBV lytic replication is dependent on epithelial cell differentiation.[89,166] Mechanistically, the plasma cell differentiation master regulators BLIMP1 and XBP-1 are essential for B-cell lytic induction.[44,580] In epithelial cells, differentiation-dependent expression of BLIMP1 and KLF4 synergistically support EBV lytic reactivation. KLF4 and BLIMP1 induce LMP1 in epithelial cells in an immediate-early gene independent manner, and LMP1 in turn supports BZLF1 and BRLF1 expression.[497] Hypoxia, transforming growth factor beta, and B-cell receptor stimulation also trigger lytic gene expression.[322]

Early Genes

The 38 EBV early genes are operationally differentiated from late genes by their transcription in the absence of viral DNA synthesis. Early genes are transcribed from nucleosome-bound DNA templates, with promoters often initiating nested transcripts that terminate at the same polyadenylation site. Lytic replication leads to amplification of EBV DNA by the BALF5 polymerase by 100 to 1,000-fold within 1 to 2 days, likely by a mixture of semiconservative and rolling circle DNA amplification. EBV lytic replication produces long head-to-tail concatemers that are cleaved and packaged as linear, unchromatinized genomes.[228] Considerable progress has been made in constituting an *in vivo* minimal DNA replication system similar to the Challberg HSV system.[188,189] The components include BALF5, which encodes the core DNA polymerase, BALF2 the single strand DNA binding protein, BMRF1 the processivity factor, BSLF1 and BBLF4 the primase and helicase complex, BBLF2/3 a spliced primase helicase complex component, and BKRF3 the uracil DNA glycosylase.

Lytic DNA amplification is accompanied by extensive nuclear reorganization, with the appearance of large regions termed replication compartments in which EBV DNA is replicated. These occupy approximately 30% of the nuclear volume and result in the margination of host DNA, causing a honeycombing nuclear appearance.[111,494] Host DNA and histones are excluded from these regions. Lytic DNA replication begins synchronously from EBV episomes within a given cell that serve as templates, but is delayed until cells reach S-phase, at which point single EBV genomes seed individual replication compartments. Only approximately 30% of EBV episomal DNA serves as templates for DNA synthesis. Within the replication compartments, the DNA processivity factor BMRF1 forms core structures surrounding newly replicated DNA and late gene mRNAs.[671]

The viral lytic origin *oriLyt* is an approximately 8 kb, cis-acting element with multiple lytic cycle roles.[228] Nearly all EBV strains have two copies of *oriLyt*, located approximately 100 kbp apart. *Orilyt* is comprised of a approximately 1 kb core region with 7 ZREs flanked by upstream and downstream auxiliary regions. BZLF1 occupancy converts *oriLyt* into a strong enhancer and mediates interactions with viral replication proteins.[458,490] Recombinant EBV deficient for all oriLyt ZREs could only support low-level lytic replication.[179] *OriLyt* interacts with multiple viral factors, which assemble into a replication complex, including BALF5 polymerase, BMRF1 polymerase processivity factor, BBLF4 helicase, and BSLF1 primase. *OriLyt* also has key roles in late gene expression and must be present in *cis* for late gene transcription.[157]

The small, nuclear RNA-binding protein BSMLF1 (SM) is essential for lytic replication.[710] SM is the functional homolog of HSV US11/ICP27. SM increases the export and levels of most intronless RNAs, binds to and inhibits PKR, and binds EBV transcripts to enhance their stability, nuclear export, splicing, and translation efficiency. SM is important for the expression of 15 late lytic genes.[688,710] SM also recruits the xeroderma pigmentosum group B-complementing protein (XBV), a component of the transcription factor II H (TFIIH) complex, to EBV lytic promoters to induce lytic genes. The hypertension medication, spironolactone, which triggers XBP degradation, inhibits SM-dependent late gene transcription.[710]

The BGLF4 serine threonine protein kinase, which is homologous to the HSV UL13 and KSHV ORF36, is necessary for most late gene expression, even following lytic DNA replication.[167] BGLF4 dissociates from the virion and phosphorylates several viral proteins, including BZLF1 and BMRF1. BGLF4 activates topoisomerase II, contributes to changes in nuclear morphology and modification of the DNA damage response. BGLF4 rather than the EBV thymidine kinase encoded by BXLF1 is the viral kinase that activates ganciclovir or acyclovir for inhibition of EBV lytic replication.[450]

Late Genes

EBV encodes approximately 36 late mRNAs, whose expression requires lytic DNA replication. However, a subset of EBV "leaky late" genes are expressed with both early and late kinetics. CAGE-seq analysis identified 16 true-late and 16 leaky-late genes.[158] Late genes include proteins necessary for DNA packing into capsids, virion assembly, virion structure, and glycoproteins. Viral IL-10 is also expressed with late kinetics.[487] Expression of nearly all true late genes is dependent on the viral pre-initiation complex (vPIC), which is assembled by six EBV proteins with orthologs in β and γ, but not in α-herpesviruses. vPIC recruits RNA polymerase II to late gene promoter TATTWAA elements, where W represents either A or T,[158] which drives transcription of late genes. Since vPIC functions in the context of a *cis*-acting *oriLyt*, it is likely that vPIC drives transcription from newly replicated viral DNA, perhaps explaining why late gene mRNAs are found in replication compartments. Therefore, late gene expression is dependent on three factors: viral DNA replication proteins, *oriLyt* in *cis*, and the vPIC.

Precisely why these genes are only expressed from lytic DNA remains an open question, but hypotheses include that these require the absence of histones and/or epigenetic marks or a host repressor that requires these marks, that replication may recruit factors necessary for transcription from late promoters, that topological changes resulting from linear EBV genomes are required, or that replication compartments allow sufficient concentration of viral components important for late gene expression.[115]

Head-to-tail EBV DNA concatemers produced by lytic replication must be cleaved for packaging of unit length genomes into procapsids. EBV BALF3 is homologous to the HSV terminase UL28 and is a component of the viral terminase that cleaves EBV concatemers, together with BGRF1/BDRF1 and BFRF1A.[112] The EBV terminal repeats, comprised of 538 base pair sequences that are located at the ends of the linear EBV genome, are packaging signals. Sequence alignments of EBV and other herpesvirus genomic termini suggest that conserved packaging signals are present within the EBV TRs.[112] The EBV GCATGGGGG motif, referred to as DR1, brackets the multiple copies of TR. In HSV-1, DR1 is the site of cleavage of headful length DNA for packaging into virions. The sequence $C(G)_5TGT(T)_2CCT(G)_5CC$ occurs 25 base pairs before the EBV DR1, is similar to sequences in HSV and CMV, and is also the key cleavage packaging recognition sequence for EBV. The EBV rightmost TR acquires a short unique sequence from the leftmost TR during cleavage and packaging and that sequence becomes the left end of the DNA.[764] Interestingly, lytic replication of recombinant EBV lacking terminal repeats results in the production of empty capsids and viral particles, demonstrating that DNA packaging is not necessary for virion formation and egress.[181]

Herpesvirus nucleocapsids are greater than 100 nM in size, whereas nuclear pores are 40 nM.[140] Nonetheless, nucleocapsids are observed in the cytoplasm in cells with lytic replication. In common with other herpesviruses, encapsidated EBV genomes exit the nucleus by budding through the inner and outer nuclear membranes for further maturation in the cytosol and secretory pathways. The EBV nuclear egress complex (NEC) is comprised of BFRF1 and BFLF2, which are orthologs of UL31 and UL34 of HSV. The BFRF1 NEC core and BFLF2 hook segments are highly structurally conserved with other herpesvirus NEC complexes.[481]

Tegumentation and maturation occurs in the cytosol. EBV then buds into compartments with cis and trans-Golgi markers. Viral particles subvert cellular secretion pathway machinery to travel through secretory vesicles in a manner dependent on Rab GTPases, including Rabs8, 10, and 11. As in other herpesviruses, EBV gM and gN are important for egress of EBV virions from infected cells. These two proteins form a stable complex in infected cells, and EBV that lacks gN is deficient in envelopment and de-envelopment. Matured EBV particles are released as enveloped virions via fusion with the plasma membrane.[495]

ENTRY INTO HOST—PORTAL OF ENTRY, SITE OF PRIMARY REPLICATION, CELL TYPES INFECTED

Most EBV infections occur through contact with infected saliva from persons infected in the past. Saliva contains virus that is high in EBV gp42. This suggests that the virus is derived predominantly from MHC class II negative cells (i.e., epithelial cells rather than B cells)[290] and will therefore be more efficient in binding B cells than epithelial cells. During primary infection, EBV either infects epithelial cells in Waldeyer's ring in the oropharynx where it replicates[641] and then can infect resting naïve B cells that traffic through the oropharynx, or the virus may infect resting, naïve B cells in the tonsilar crypts directly (Fig. 11.15). In addition to its high gp42 content, the presence of EBV in the blood 3 weeks before the onset of IM and in throat washings only 1 week before the disease suggests that B cells are the first cell type infected.[164] Virus replication has been reported in orally shed epithelial cells during IM,[371] but subsequent studies on tissue sections have found replication only in B cells in the tonsils. While some oropharyngeal B cells undergo lytic infection, most become latently infected. Initially the cells are lymphoblasts with a type III pattern of latency and express each of the EBV latency genes[352] (Table 11.2). Up to 10% of the B cells in the blood are EBV-positive early in infection but it appears that, even by this stage, most of these cells have the phenotype of resting memory B cells and have escaped immune surveillance by down-regulating the latency III program.

These early events remain poorly understood, in particular how an initial growth-transforming infection, potentially involving all infectable B-cell subsets in the oropharynx, results in selective colonization of just the memory B-cell compartment. Thorley-Lawson and colleagues have postulated that EBV preferentially infects and activates only naïve B cells, which then enter germinal centers and differentiate into resting memory B cells, similar to the physiologic process through which naïve B cells are activated by cognate antigen to become B-cell blasts, enter the germinal center of lymphoid follicles, undergo class switch recombination, somatic hypermutation, and, if positively selected, differentiate into resting memory B cells[252] (Fig. 11.16). Physiologically, only B cells whose surface immunoglobulin (B-cell receptor) has a high affinity for antigen are selected, thereby avoiding apoptosis and becoming $CD27^+$ memory B cells. Accordingly, it is postulated that naïve B cells infected with EBV express EBV type III latency genes resulting in B-cell proliferation and blast formation. These cells then migrate to a lymphoid follicle to begin the germinal center reaction. EBV-infected cells then switch to express only EBV latency II genes. Of these, EBV LMP1 up-regulates activation-induced cytidine deaminase (AID) to induce somatic hypermutation or immunoglobulin class switching. EBV LMP2 stimulates antigen receptor signaling.[78] This allows the infected cell to survive its transit through the germinal center. Upon exiting the germinal center into the blood, the virus-infected cells are thought to differentiate into memory B cells and express the EBV latency 0 pattern of gene expression with no viral proteins expressed.[252] Subsequently, some of these cells may undergo differentiation to plasma cells with EBV lytic replication. The resulting virus may then infect nearby naïve B cells, or if differentiation and virus replication occurs after the B cells traffic back to the oropharnyx, the resultant virus may be shed into the saliva directly, or may infect permissive epithelial cells, which can also shed EBV into the saliva.

While the above model has its attractions, it is worth noting several lines of evidence that remain difficult to reconcile with the model as proposed. First, EBV can infect both naïve and memory B cells not only *in vitro* but also *in vivo*; thus, within the tonsils of persons with IM, Ig gene sequencing of single cells picked from tissue sections reveals clonal expansions of both naïve and fully mature memory B cells, with various patterns of latency displayed even within individual clones.[352] Importantly, however, these expansions are occurring in extrafollicular areas of the tonsil and not in germinal centers; indeed Ig sequencing of the few infected cells that are localized within germinal center areas shows that they are infiltrating B cells and not part of the germinal center reaction.[352,502] Second, in healthy carriers EBV is present in both the non–isotype-switched as well as isotype-switched memory B-cell subset; however, the non–isotype-switched subset is thought by many to be independent of the germinal center. Third, patients with

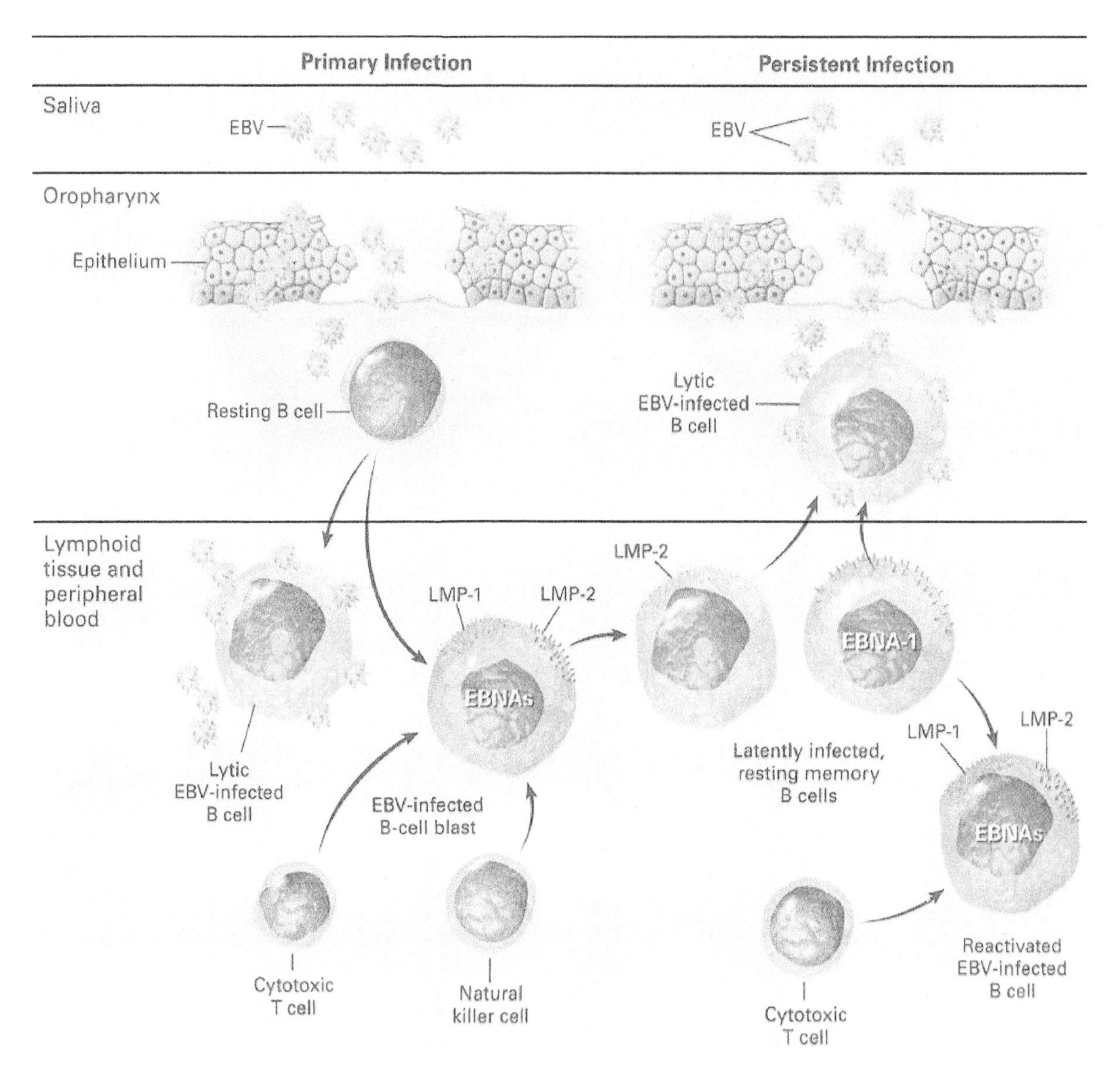

FIGURE 11.15 EBV life cycle. EBV infects resting B cells either directly or by virus released from epithelial cells in the oropharynx. EBV-infected B cells in the lymphoid tissues and blood undergo lytic infection or become B-cell blasts, which are controlled by NK cells and cytotoxic T cells. Latently infected resting memory B cells express no viral proteins unless they divide; if they reactivate, they are controlled by cytotoxic T cells. Some latently infected cells traffic to the oropharynx where they undergo lytic replication and release virus. (Adapted from Cohen JI. Epstein-Barr virus infection. *N Engl J Med* 2000:343(7):481-492. Copyright © 2000 Massachusetts Medical Society. Reprinted with permission from Massachusetts Medical Society.)

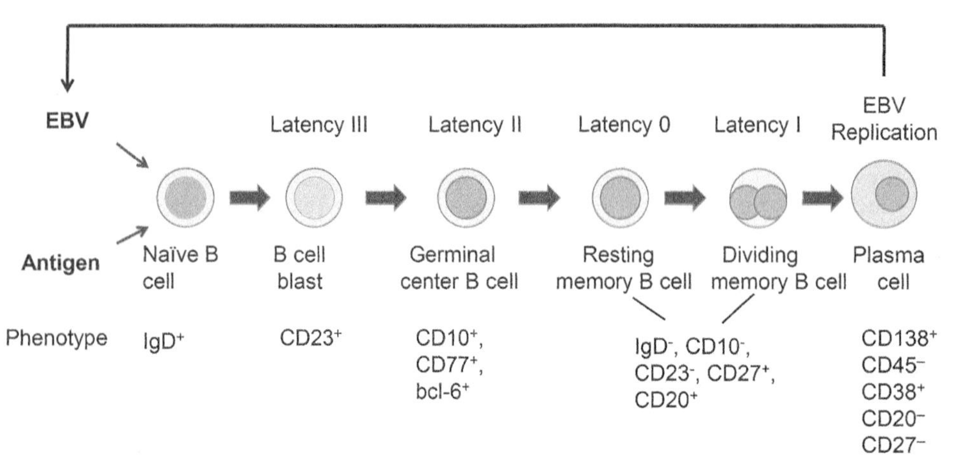

FIGURE 11.16 EBV infection of B cells parallels the response of B cell to antigenic stimulation. EBV infects naïve B cells, which become B-cell blasts with type III EBV latency. The cells undergo a germinal center reaction with type II EBV latency and exit the germinal center with type 0 EBV latency. EBV-infected resting memory B cells can differentiate in plasma cells whereby EBV undergoes lytic replication and can infect new naïve B cells.

X-linked lymproliferative disease have absent or poorly formed germinal centers, but they clearly become infected with EBV (see below). Likewise patients with X-linked hyperimmunoglobulin M syndrome cannot form germinal centers and lack class switched (IgD⁻, CD27⁺) classical memory B cells; however, these patients can be infected with EBV and the virus is found in nonclassical memory B cells (IgD⁺, CD27⁺).[130] Thus, EBV infection of the B cells can occur in the absence of germinal centers and a conventional memory B-cell population. Indeed much of the above evidence suggests that, even in the normal course of events, the virus populates the memory B-cell compartment without involving passage through a germinal center.[59]

While EBV infects naïve and memory B cells from tonsils *ex vivo*, EBV is less efficient in infecting memory B cells from the blood.[162] IgA-positive or IgG-positive memory B cells from the tonsils are infected more efficiently with EBV than IgM memory B cells from the tonsils. EBV infects memory B cells in nasal-associated lymphoid tissue more efficiently than memory B cells in other lymphatic tissues. EBV has been detected in plasmacytoid B cells.[14]

B cells are essential for EBV latency. Persons with X-linked agammaglobulinemia who lack mature B cells are not infected with EBV and have no cellular immunity to EBV.[178] Hematopoietic stem cell transplantation, which eliminates host B cells, but not epithelial cells, can eliminate EBV from the body.[215] EBV replication is detected in epithelial cells of the tongue, but not in epithelial cells of the salivary glands. EBV also infects human umbilical cord-derived endothelial cells.

While EBV is present in B cells in the blood of healthy individuals, in some patients with elevated EBV levels in the blood (e.g., patients with HIV, transplant recipients), EBV has been detected in other cell types, usually at a lower frequency than in B cells. EBV has been detected in the blood in cells other than B cells including CD4+ and CD8+ T cells in patients with HIV, γ/δ T cells, and NK cells in patients with chronic active EBV disease, plasmablasts/plasma cells and monocytes in patients with lymphoproliferative diseases and HIV,[75] and pre-Langerhans cells in the blood of persons with HIV as well as healthy individuals. Detection of EBV in cells other than B cells by cell sorting using flow cytometry must be carefully verified by additional techniques due to possibility of contamination with small numbers of B cells during the sort.[195]

IMMUNE RESPONSE

Innate Immune Response

The innate immune response is comprised of rapidly mobilized humoral and cellular processes that limit the replication and spread of pathogens prior to the development of antigen-specific adaptive responses, but that by themselves do not result in the generation of immunological memory. Key components of the innate immune response to EBV include natural killer (NK) cells, **γ/δ**, and invariant natural-killer (iNKT) T cells.

NK cell expansion is observed with acute infection and the levels of proliferating NK cells correlate with the EBV load.[30,486,683] Cytokines that regulate NK cell activation (IFN-α, IFN-β, IFN-γ, and IL-12) are significantly increased in persons with IM compared with healthy controls. In the peripheral blood of patients with IM, the CD56^{dim} CD16⁻ NK subset preferentially expands. These NK cells recognize and lyse cells undergoing EBV replication *in vitro*.[683] The expansion of early differentiated NK cells persists for at least 6 months. However, in the months after acute infection, these cells up-regulate senescence markers and cease to proliferate. The CD56^{dim}/KIR⁻/CD57⁻ NK cell frequency is higher in early childhood than later in adulthood, raising the possibility that more robust CD8+ T-cell responses may be required to control EBV when acquired at later ages, and that this may in turn drive IM.[486]

Differentiated CD56^{dim} CD16⁺ cells are primed for cytotoxic activity against EBV-infected cells and are also found in the peripheral blood. Less mature CD56^{bright}/CD16⁻ NK cells predominate in secondary lymphoid organs, including the tonsils. These early differentiated NK cells do not appear to exert cytotoxic effects against EBV-transformed B cells, and instead limit EBV-driven B-cell growth transformation *in vitro*, likely due to IFN-γ secretion.[683]

Humanized mouse models highlight roles for NK cells in control of B-cell EBV infection. Early differentiated NK cells expand by 3 weeks post-EBV infection, the timepoint at which lytic replication is also first seen in this model. NK cell depletion results in elevated EBV genome copy numbers in humanized mice infected with wild-type virus, but not in mice infected by BZLF1 KO virus, underscoring a key role for NK cells in control of B-cell EBV lytic replication.[109] NK cell depletion also results in CD8+ T-cell expansion, splenomegaly, and monoclonal B-cell lymphoproliferation, reminiscent of IM. Indeed, impairment in NK cell differentiation by loss-of-function *IRF8* mutation is associated with severe EBV disease, including fulminant infectious mononucleosis.

Invariant NK T (iNKT) cells are innate-like T cells with α/β receptors that may also exert an important layer of control over newly EBV-infected B cells. iNKT cells express a semi-invariant T-cell receptor that recognizes glycolipid antigens presented by the MHC class-1 related CD1d molecule. Activated iNKT cells secrete large quantities of cytokines, including IFN-γ, have cytotoxic activity, and limit EBV-driven B-cell growth transformation *in vitro*. However, iNKT cells may preferentially control newly EBV-infected B cells, because CD1d is down-modulated early during EBV-driven B-cell transformation *in vitro*.[114] Notably, patients with X-linked lymphoproliferative disease lack iNKT cells, and this may be linked to their susceptibility to EBV.

γ/δ T cells may also exert important anti-EBV responses.[399] Activated **γ/δ** T cells exert cytotoxicity toward EBV-transformed B cells in cell culture and in a murine LCL xenograft model.[736] Interestingly, Vg9Vd2 T cells could be expanded *in vitro* by administration of bisphosphonate pamidronate and then adoptively transferred to humanized mice, where they inhibited xenograft LCLs.

Antibody Response

Acute EBV infection induces polyclonal B-cell activation with elevated levels of IgG, IgM, and IgA. Humoral responses to many EBV lytic and latent antigens are observed in IM. Heterophile antibodies are produced, which are not EBV-specific, and instead are largely IgM antibodies directed toward glycoplipid antigens on red blood cells.[454] One type of heterophile antibody used for diagnosis of acute infection measures the

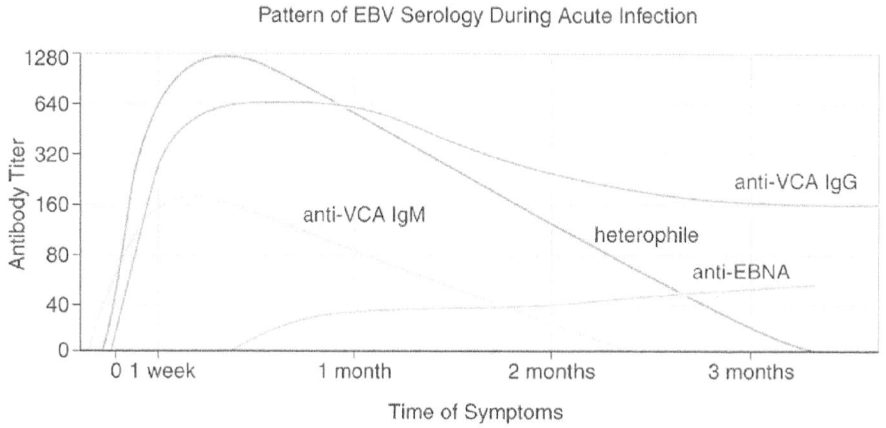

FIGURE 11.17 Pattern of antibodies to EBV during acute infection. (Reprinted from Cohen JI. Epstein-Barrr virus. In: Young NS, Gerson SL, High KA, eds. *Clinical Hematology.* Philadelpha, PA: Elsevier; 2006:956–966. Copyright © 2006 Elsevier. With permission.)

dilution of serum that agglutinates sheep, horse, or cow erythrocytes after absorption with guinea pig kidney. Heterophile antibodies persist for up to 1 year after IM and are often absent in children less than 5 years old or in the elderly. IgM and IgG antibodies to VCA are usually present at the onset of symptoms of IM (Fig. 11.17).[454] Later in infection, antibody to EBNA is detected and IgM to VCA disappears. IgG antibody to VCA and EBNA persists for life.[683] Antibodies to EBV early antigens (EAs) are classified as either diffuse (EA-D, diffusely in the nucleus and cytoplasm, methanol resistant) or restricted (EA-R, restricted to the cytoplasm, methanol sensitive). EA-D antibodies are often present 3 to 4 weeks after the onset of IM, especially in patients with severe illness, and are frequently detected in patients with NPC or CAEBV. EA-R antibodies are often detected in CAEBV or African BL. IgA antibody to EBV is often elevated in patients with NPC and IgA antibody to EBV EA is present in patients with IM.[43]

There has been growing interest in the identification of anti-EBV glycoprotein antibodies that block EBV entry into epithelial and/or B cells. Neutralizing anti-gp350 antibodies reached their highest levels at approximately 6 months postinfection, and these were not found to be more abundant in individuals with symptomatic disease. Anti-gH/gL and gp42 antibodies contribute to neutralization of B-cell infection,[65] and anti-gH/gL antibodies also neutralize EBV epithelial cell infection.[65] Monoclonal antibodies targeting gH/gL potently neutralize both epithelial and B-cell infection.[65,653] Interestingly, elevated levels of antibodies that bind gp350 and neutralize B-cell infection are associated with a lower risk of NPC in certain populations.[117]

T-Cell Immune Response

The importance of T-cell immunity toward EBV is highlighted by the high frequency of EBV-associated malignancies in patients with congenital immunodeficiency syndromes that restrain T-cell responses, in patients with HIV/AIDS, or who receive T-cell immunosuppression posttransplant. Nearly eighty EBV-encoded polypeptides are a potentially rich source of epitopes for CD4+ and CD8+ T-cell activation. CD8+ T cells, which recognize infected cells through viral peptides presented by MHC I molecules on the cell surface, play key roles in control of both acute and persistent EBV infection, and the CD8+ T-cell response in infectious mononucleosis (IM) is one of the strongest human T-cell responses described.[220] These are the "atypical lymphocytes" whose presence is used clinically to help establish the diagnosis of IM. The increase in anti-EBV CD8+ T-cell abundance correlates with the onset of IM symptoms (Fig. 11.18), consistent with the hypothesis that antiviral and proinflammatory cytokines secreted by this population of cells drives IM symptoms. Anti-EBV responses can exceed 50% of the CD8+ T-cell population.[683] Anti-EBV CD8+ T cells proliferate and have activated/memory phenotypes.

Primary CD8+ T-cell responses to EBV, as seen in acute IM patients, are most robust against immediate-early and to a lesser extent to certain early antigens, including BMRF1 and BMLF1[683] (Fig. 11.19). This hierarchy appears to follow the abundance of viral peptides presented by MHC I molecules on the infected cell surface prior to the induction of EBV immunoevasins that perturb antigen presentation.[193] While responses to immediate-early and particular early antigens dominate the primary response, a recent study has shown that the response broadens over time to reveal new late antigen responses in the blood of long-term carriers.[4] Although T-cell responses to EBV contract after resolution of IM, even in chronic carriers, EBV-specific memory cells can account for up to 3% of the circulating CD8+ T-cell pool.[399] In humans, a virus-driven memory response of this magnitude in the blood is only exceeded by memory to another herpesvirus, CMV.

Plasmacytoid dendritic cells (pDCs) detect EBV, produce interferons, and prime CD8+ T-cell responses but may not be required for control of EBV infection.[220] Expression of programmed death receptor 1 (PD1), a marker of T-cell exhaustion, is elevated on EBV-specific CD8+ T cells during IM, correlates with the EBV viral load, and returns to low levels during convalescence. PD-1+ T cells expand in IM and in humanized mice infected by EBV, where they and other expanded T-cell subsets are important for control of EBV.[97] EBV-specific CD8+ T cells persist and have cytotoxic

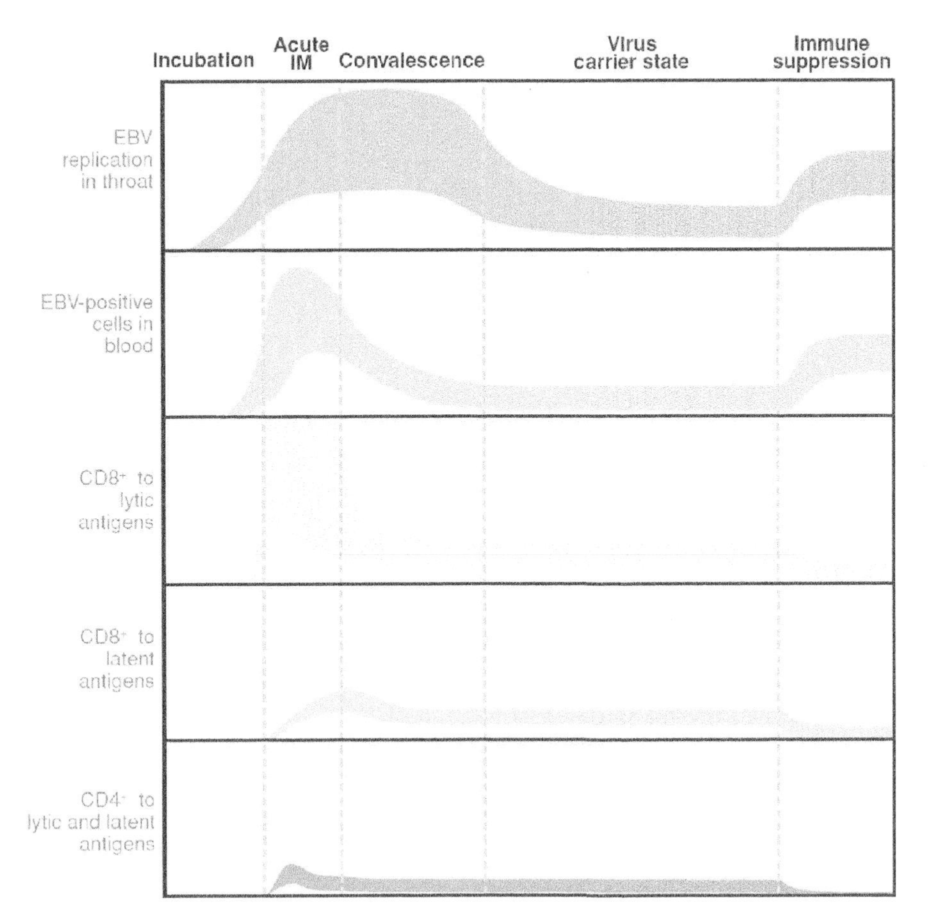

FIGURE 11.18 Levels of EBV in the throat and blood and cellular immunity during the course of infection. (Republished with permission of Annual Reviews, Inc. from Hislop AD, Taylor GS, Sauce D, et al. Cellular responses to viral infection in humans: lessons from Epstein-Barr virus. *Annu Rev Immunol* 2007;25:587–617; permission conveyed through Copyright Clearance Center, Inc.)

activity. In healthy carriers, the frequency of EBV-specific CD8+ T cells is about 0.2% to 2% for viral lytic proteins and 0.05% to 1% for latent proteins and remains stable over time. A large proportion of these responses are directed at EBNA3A, EBNA3B, and EBNA3C antigens. BZLF1, BRLF1, BMRF1, and BMLF1 antigens are also prominent targets (Fig. 11.19).[165,683] A smaller number of CD8+ T cells are specific for EBNA2, EBNA-LP, LMP1, or LMP2. However, CD8+ T cells responsive to EBNA2 and EBNA-LP peptides can recognize newly infected B cells *in vitro* and inhibit outgrowth of

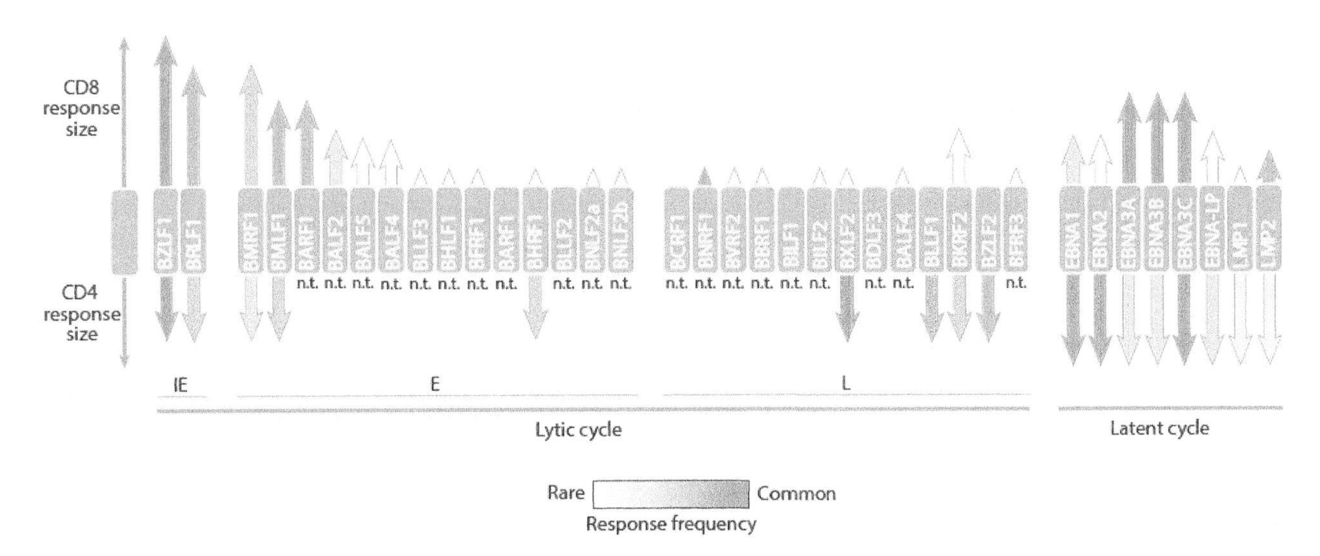

FIGURE 11.19 CD8+ and CD4+ T-cell responses to EBV immediate-early (IE), early (E), late (L), and latent proteins. (Republished with permission of Annual Reviews, Inc. from Taylor GS, Long HM, Brooks JM, et al. The immunology of Epstein-Barr virus-induced disease. *Annu Rev Immunol* 2015;33:787–821; permission conveyed through Copyright Clearance Center, Inc.)

these cells in culture, suggesting a possible role for these cells in adoptive or vaccine approaches.[63] During chronic infection, T cells specific for EBV epitopes are typically antigen-experienced, resting cells that do not express activation markers. However, these T cells secrete cytokines and exhibit potent cytotoxicity upon re-challenge.[399]

T-cell responses may be different during asymptomatic infection in early childhood, but the differences appear to be quantitative rather than qualitative. Thus, studies of newly infected African children show that, although they have high IM-like EBV genome copy numbers in the blood, they do not show a gross expansion of the CD8+ compartment; there is a detectable EBV-specific CD8+ T-cell response against the known immunodominant antigens but the response does not amplify to the unusually high level seen in IM.[285,399] Despite these differences, once the long-term virus carrier state is established, anti-EBV CD8+ T-cell frequencies are similar in individuals who experienced asymptomatic or symptomatic primary infection.[683] There is growing interest in the use of adoptive CD8+ T-cell therapy to augment anti-EBV responses in patients with primary or secondary immunodeficiency.

CD4+ T cells recognize peptide antigens presented by major histocompatibility class (MHC) II molecules on the surface of professional antigen presenting cells such as dendritic cells and macrophages. Such cells engulf virion particles or viral antigens released from infected cells and then present them to CD4+ T cells.[398] However, B cells also naturally express MHC class II molecules and have antigen-processing capacity, as do certain other cell types when induced to express MHC II by IFN-γ. Though classically seen as providing help for CD8+ T-cell responses, CD4+ T cells can themselves become cytotoxic after activation, as recently shown for the EBV-specific T-cell response.[399] The CD4+ T-cell response to EBV is different in several respects from that shown by CD8+ T cells; the response is numerically smaller, latent cycle reactivities tend to be dominant, and lytic cycle responses are more evenly spread across IE, E, and L antigens, both in primary and persistent infection (Fig. 11.19).[30,683] The breadth of the CD4+ T-cell response presumably reflects the large array of antigens released from infected cells and available for processing by professional antigen-presenting cells. In addition, cross-presentation of intracellular EBV antigens between infected B cells themselves, as has been observed *in vitro*, may also play a role both in priming the response and in rendering infected cells susceptible to direct CD4+ T-cell recognition.

In children, CD4+ T-cell responses emerge within the first year of infection and are directed at multiple viral latent and lytic antigens.[356] Anti-EBV CD4+ responses are amplified with primary infection and individual epitope restricted T-cell frequencies can reach 1% to 2% of the peripheral blood CD4+ T-cell compartment (Fig. 11.18).[399,683] In chronic infection, similar numbers of CD4+ T-cell CCR7+ central memory and CCR7-effector memory are detectable.[399] CD4+ T cells in IM have a Th1-like profile, with expression of the transcription factor T-Bet and robust IFN-γ expression upon *ex vivo* stimulation. Particular CD4+ T cells responding to EBV antigens also express perforin and granzyme B and exert cytotoxic activity. Most of these cells have a very short half-life and undergo apoptosis when the level of EBV antigen declines. For incompletely understood reasons, CD4+ T-cell responses to EBNA1 epitopes are delayed, which likely connects to the similar delay in appearance of anti-EBNA1 IgG. Ultimately, anti-EBNA1 responses are a major component of anti-EBV CD4+ T-cell responses in healthy EBV carriers. To a lesser extent, EBNA2 and EBNA3C peptide-restricted T cells are also present in the peripheral blood.[399]

Despite the exaggerated size of the T-cell response, particularly the CD8 response, seen in the blood of IM patients, virus replication and shedding in the oropharynx continues at high levels after disease symptoms and the atypical blood picture have resolved.[399] This may reflect the fact that relatively few of the activated EBV-specific T cells in the blood seem able to traffic to the tonsils, perhaps because the necessary lymphoid homing receptors CCR7 and CD632L are down-modulated by activation. Anti-EBV T-cell frequency increases over time in the tonsils, perhaps reflecting the recovery of the T cells' homing markers and/or antigen drive from the persistent EBV infection in oropharyngeal tissues. Remarkably, in long-term carriers, the tonsils show a 10- to 20-fold enrichment of CD8+ T cells that recognize latent epitopes and a 2- to 5-fold enrichment of CD8+ T cells that recognize lytic epitopes compared with the peripheral blood.

EBV Evasion of the Immune Response

EBV has evolved multiple mechanisms to down-modulate presentation (Table 11.3). BNLF2A blocks the transporter associated with antigen processing (TAP) to prevent translocation of peptides from the cytoplasm to the endoplasmic reticulum.[294] Furthermore, the large tegument protein BPLF1 is a deubiquitylating (DUB) enzyme that blocks the proteasomal degradation of cytosolic proteins by removing polyubiquitin tags.[173] The EBV late gene *BDLF3* encodes a 150 kDa protein that inhibits MHC class I and II as well as lipid antigen presentation by CD1 molecules. Abundant glycosylation of gp150 shields surface presentation of the antigen to the immune system. Similarly, the EBV lytic protein BILF1, which is a constitutively active G protein-coupled receptor, targets HLA-A and HLA-B molecules for destruction, but spares HLA-C, presumably because this allele can activate NK inhibitor receptors. EBV also targets the MHC class II pathways via gp42 (BZLF2), which binds the HLA-DR β chain and soluble gp42 inhibits antigen presentation. gp42 binds to class II peptide complexes and inhibits MHC class II antigen presentation to T cells.

The dominant role of the EBNA1 Gly-Ala repeats is to reduce the translation efficiency of EBNA1, resulting in fewer EBNA1 peptides and less efficient recognition by EBV-specific CD8+ T cells.[399] Defective ribosome EBNA1 products are the major source of EBNA1 epitopes presented to CD8+ T cells.

LMP1 inhibits its presentation to MHC class I by self-aggregation and possible destruction of LMP1 epitopes in proteasomes. LMP1 levels in EBV-infected cells vary over time, and this may allow cells expressing low levels of the protein to avoid killing by CD8 T cells.[62] LMP1 peptides suppress T-cell activation, inhibit T-cell proliferation, and reduce NK cell cytotoxicity; however, it is not clear if such peptides are present and at levels required to have immunosuppressive activity. LMP1, secreted in exosomes from virus-infected cells, inhibits T-cell

TABLE 11.3 EBV proteins and RNAs that inhibit the immune system

EBV Protein	Effect
EBNA1	Inhibits its own proteasome processing Reduces translational efficiency and initiation of translation
LMP1	Up-regulates galectin promoter to induce apoptosis of CTLs Up-regulates IL-10, up-regulates A20 and bcl-2 to inhibit apoptosis
LMP2	Increases degradation of IFN receptors Up-regulates galectin promoter to induce apoptosis of CTLs
BARF1	Soluble colony stimulating factor receptor, inhibits IFN-α secretion
BCRF1	IL-10 homolog, inhibits synthesis of IFN-γ by T cells, reduces MHC class II expression, reduces IL-1α, IL-1β, TNF-α, and IL-6 production in monocytes, reduces levels of MHC class I, ICAM1, CD80, and CD86 on monocytes, reduces mRNA levels of TAP1 and proteasome protein LMP2
BDLF3	Inhibits presentation of MHC class I and II
BGLF2	Binds TYK-2 and inhibits type I IFN
BGLF5	Blocks synthesis of MHC I and II molecules Down-regulates TLR9
BHRF1	Bcl-2 homolog, blocks apoptosis
BILF1	Binds MHC class I molecules and removes MHC class I from cell surface Reduces rate of newly synthesized class I molecules on the cell surface by diverting them from the exocytic pathway Forms heterodimers with CXCR4 and impairs binding to CXCL12
BLLF3 (dUTPase)	Up-regulates IL-10, TNF-α, IL-1β, IL-8, and IL-6
BNLF2a	Interacts with TAP, inhibits its ATP and peptide binding functions, reduces MHC class I at the cell surface
BORF2	Inhibits APOBEC3B to evade innate immunity
BPLF1	Blocks proteasomal degradation of cytosolic proteins by removing polyubiquitin tags
BZLF1	Up-regulates IL-10, inhibits IRF7 (and type I IFN), inhibits IFN-γ-induced MHC class II expression, inhibits activation of IRF1, CIITA, and p48, nuclear translocation of STAT1, decreases levels of IFN-γ receptor-α mRNA and level of TNF receptor 1
BZLF2 (gp42)	Binds the HLA-DRβ chain of class II and inhibits antigen presentation, inhibits generation of CTLs in mixed lymphocyte reactions
LF2	Inhibits dimerization of IRF7, inhibits IFN-α production
EBV RNA	
EBER	Up-regulates IL-10, induces resistance to IFN-α-mediated apoptosis
miR-BART2-5P	Reduces expression of MICB, a stress-induced NK cell ligand to reduce killing by NK cells
miR-146a	Inhibits expression of IFN-responsive genes

proliferation.[190,324] LMP2A and LMP2B increase the degradation of IFN receptors in epithelial cells, which may limit the antiviral response in virus-infected cells. LMP1 and LMP2A up-regulate the galectin-1 promoter; galectin-1 triggers apoptosis of EBV-specific cytotoxic T cells.

The EBV late gene *BCRF1* encodes a viral homolog of the cytokine IL-10, which protects newly infected B cells from killing by NK cells and has inhibitory effects on CD4+ T-cell cytokine secretion.[294] BCRF1 shares 70% amino acid identity with human IL-10 and inhibits T-cell IFN-γ synthesis. EBV BLLF3 (dUTPase) up-regulates IL-10, as well as TNF-α, IL-1β, IL-8, and IL-6 in resting PBMCs. The EBV-encoded alkaline exonuclease BGLF5 exerts host shut-off activity. However, host-shutoff unmasks a 5S ribosomal RNA pseudogene, *RNA5SP141*, which then binds to and activates RIG-I, resulting in TNF-α but not type I IFN secretion.[107] EBV lytic genes further perturb interferon pathways. The EBV tegument protein BGLF2 binds to Tyk-2 and inhibits type I, but not type II IFN signaling.[397] Similarly, the LF2 tegument protein interacts with IRF7, inhibiting its dimerization, and reducing production of IFN-α.

Monocytes and plasmacytoid dendritic cells sense EBV, in part through recognition of EBV virion-associated unmethylated DNA or through release of EBERs.[683] EBV-encoded BARF1 inhibits monocyte-colony stimulating factor, and BARF1 knockout recombinant rhesus LCV had lower EBV viral loads in acute and chronic infection.[516]

EBV perturbs inflammasome pathways on multiple levels. Lytic replication in Burkitt cells causes depletion of AIM2, a component of a double-stranded DNA sensing inflammasome.[174] Interestingly, EBV subverts caspase pathways to regulate the lytic switch.[68,413] EBV targets JAK-STAT signaling pathways, where BZLF1 inhibits JAK1/2 tyrosine phosphorylation and together with BGLF4 inhibits STAT1 phosphorylation. Lytic replication also results in depletion of IRF1 and STAT2.[174]

The EBV ribonucleotide reductase large subunit BORF2 inhibits the host DNA cytosine deaminase APOBEC3B to evade this important innate antiviral pathway.[105] Interestingly, BORF2 stoichiometrically inhibits APOBEC3B DNA cytosine deaminase activity and sequesters APOBEC3B to perinuclear bodies. In the absence of BORF2, APOBEC deaminates EBV genomes in cells with lytic reactivation, resulting in diminished EBV titers and lower infectivity of target cells.

Several EBV gene products inhibit apoptosis. EBV BHRF1 is a viral BCL2 homolog that binds to proapoptotic BIM, BID, PUMA, and BAK.[187] BHRF1 is expressed in newly infected B cells as well as upon lytic reactivation, and has pro-survival roles in *Wp*-restricted Burkitt cells. The role of a second putative EBV-encoded BCL2 homolog, BALF1, remains less well characterized. EBV also induces multiple BCL2 family members at different stages of growth transformation. LMP1 also inhibits apoptosis. EBV-encoded and up-regulated host miRNAs also perturb apoptosis pathways.

EPIDEMIOLOGY

Over 90% of adults in all human populations are infected with EBV. In many developing countries, primary infection typically occurs between the ages of 2 and 4 and is usually asymptomatic or results in nonspecific symptoms.[501] Infection may occur even earlier, with 50% of children in areas of Africa where Burkitt lymphoma is common acquiring the virus before 1 year of age. In the developed world, especially in more affluent populations, infection is often delayed until the second decade or later. In the United States, for example, white children tend to acquire the virus later than their black, Asian or Hispanic counterparts.[131] Overall the proportion of seronegatives among 6 to 19 year olds in United States increased in the period from 2003–2004 to 2009–2010, mostly in whites.[31] Accordingly, the incidence of IM is increasing.[351] How many delayed infections become symptomatic has long been of interest. A recent detailed prospective study of EBV seronegative freshman college students showed that 46% became infected during the next 3 years and 77% of infections resulted in 2 or more symptoms of IM.[30] Increased numbers of CD8+ and NK cells were observed, and the severity of disease correlated both with EBV viral load and with CD8+ T-cell numbers.

EBV is usually spread by infected saliva. Parents or siblings are likely the source of EBV transmission to young children.[90] Transmission among sexually active young adults may be due to kissing with sharing of oral secretions, but some observations suggest that the virus may be spread by sexual intercourse. Thus the risk of IM was lower in students who always used condoms,[249] was higher in women than men in sexually active persons, and in those with a higher number of sexual partners. In addition, EBV has been detected in both male and female genital secretions, albeit at lower levels than in saliva. EBV has also been transmitted iatrogenically, notably by latently infected B cells through blood transfusion or bone marrow transplantation from seropositive donors.

EBV is classified into two types, 1 and 2, based on sequence polymorphisms in EBNA2, EBNA3A, EBNA3B, and EBNA3C. Type 1 EBV isolates are more efficient in B-cell transformation *in vitro* than type 2 isolates, although to date differences in EBV type have not correlated with disease potential. Both EBV types coexist in all populations that have been studied. While type 1 strains are believed to be more common in most populations, type 2 isolates are nearly equal in prevalence to type 1 isolates in New Guinea and equatorial Africa. Coinfections with both virus types have been observed, often in immunocompromised individuals, and indeed intertypic recombinants containing portions of type I and type II EBV strains have been found. Type 2 viruses are reported to have a predilection for infection of T cells *in vitro*, with production of numerous cytokines.[128] Type 2 infection of T cells has also been seen in Kenyan children,[127] but adults in Kenya and patients with EBV T-cell CAEBV are usually infected with type 1 virus.

EBV is further classified into strains based on sequence differences. Strain differences are generally segregated with different ethnicities (African, Southeast Asia, and Caucasian), presumably reflecting many thousands of years of virus–host coevolution within geographically separate host populations. This has complicated work investigating the possible existence of "more oncogenic" EBV strains. For example, particular polymorphisms in EBNA1 and LMP1 sequences have been linked to endemic Burkitt lymphoma and NPC respectively, but it is likely that they were in fact a reflection of naturally prevalent strains in the risk populations. Asymptomatic carriers have multiple strains of EBV that are often different in the blood and in the throat and the balance between individual strains may change over time.[638] Patients with IM have multiple strains of EBV in the oropharynx, plasma, and PBMCs, suggesting simultaneous acquisition; indeed, multiple strains have been shown to be transmitted from a carrier resulting in primary infection.[639]

PRIMARY INFECTION

Healthy Carriers

In healthy carriers in developed countries, EBV is reported to be present in about 1 to 50 per million B cells in the peripheral blood.[465] While the number of latent EBV genomes various between healthy individuals up to 100-fold, within an individual the latent viral load is relatively constant both in healthy persons and in asymptomatic HIV carriers.[465] In Africa, particularly in areas where malaria is endemic, EBV is present in the blood of children at unusually high levels, approaching those seen in acute IM.[510] The latently infected cells in the blood are classic antigen-selected resting memory B cells (IgD$^-$, CD27$^+$, sIg$^+$, CD20$^+$) and are isotype-switched and somatically mutated.[24,25,659] All EBV-infected persons shed infectious virus into the saliva, reflecting on-going virus replication in the oropharynx, but levels of virus shedding vary considerably even following the same individual over time.

While transcripts for LMP2 and EBNA1 have been detected in cells of the blood of carriers, more recent studies suggest that virus-infected cells in the blood have a latency 0 phenotype and express no viral genes with the exception of the EBERs[23] and selected BART miRNAs.[564] EBV-infected memory B cells in the tonsils are IgD$^-$ and express a type 2 latency phenotype.[24,25] EBV-infected B cells are present at similar levels in the tonsils, adenoids, and the peripheral blood, but at 20-fold lower levels in the spleen and the mesenteric lymph nodes, suggesting preferential trafficking of circulating infected cells back to oropharyngeal sites.[354] EBV gene expression is similar in the spleen and tonsil (latency II), unlike that of the blood (latency 0). When B cells in the tonsils differentiate into plasma cells, the EBV BZLF1 promoter is activated and viral replication initiates.

While the EBV viral load is similar in the peripheral blood and the bone marrow, there is a 3-fold higher number of EBV lytic antigen-specific T cells in the bone marrow compared with the blood, although the numbers of latent antigen-specific T cells are similar at both sites.

Infectious Mononucleosis

The incubation period for IM is about 4 to 6 weeks. IM presents with fever, lymphadenopathy, and pharyngitis in more than half of patients.[119] Posterior cervical lymphadenopathy and a tonsillar exudate are common. Other signs and symptoms include splenomegaly, hepatomegaly, rash, periorbital edema, and fatigue. Rarely EBV-positive genital ulcers can occur. Serious complications include upper airway obstruction due to enlarged tonsils, aplastic anemia, severe thrombocytopenia, granulocytopenia, autoimmune hemolytic anemia, hemophagocytic syndrome, hepatitis, jaundice, myocarditis, splenic rupture, encephalitis, meningitis, and Guillain-Barré syndrome. Most patients with EBV encephalitis do not present with IM. While most patient's symptoms resolve in 2 to 4 weeks, up to 10% will have fatigue persisting for 6 months or more. Patients with persistent symptoms do not have higher EBV DNA levels or obvious differences in immune responses to the virus.[80]

The peripheral blood in persons with IM shows leukocytosis, an increase in T cells but not B cells, and atypical lymphocytes. These latter cells have large amounts of cytoplasm often with vacuoles (Fig. 11.20) and are predominantly activated T cells (HLA-DR$^+$), but also include NK cells. There is an increase in CD8+ T cells and a relative decrease in CD4+ T cells. T cells from patients with IM have reduced responses to mitogens *in vitro*. Pathology of lymph nodes and tonsils show reactive follicles with proliferation of immunoblasts with reactive T cells; binuclear immunoblasts that resemble Reed-Sternberg cells are often present, which can confuse the diagnosis of IM with B-cell lymphoma. Polyclonal B-cell activation results in elevated levels of immunoglobulins, production of heterophile antibody (see Diagnosis below) and in some cases antinuclear antibodies, cold agglutinins, rheumatoid factor, or antiplatelet antibodies. Tissues have elevated levels of IL-1β. IL-6, IL-10, TNF-α, lymphotoxin, and IFN-γ-induced chemokines (MIG, IP10). The serum shows elevated levels of liver enzymes including serum transaminases and alkaline phosphatase. Symptoms of IM are due to the large expansion of CD8+ T cells and the cytokines they produce (IL-6, IL-10, IL-12, IFN-γ, TNF-α, TGF-β), rather than to lytic infection of B cells. In contrast, asymptomatic EBV infection is associated with a high level of EBV in the blood, but not the large expansion of CD8+ T cells, which occurs in IM.[3] Therefore. the large expansion of CD8+ T cells in IM that are associated with symptoms might not be required for control of virus infection.

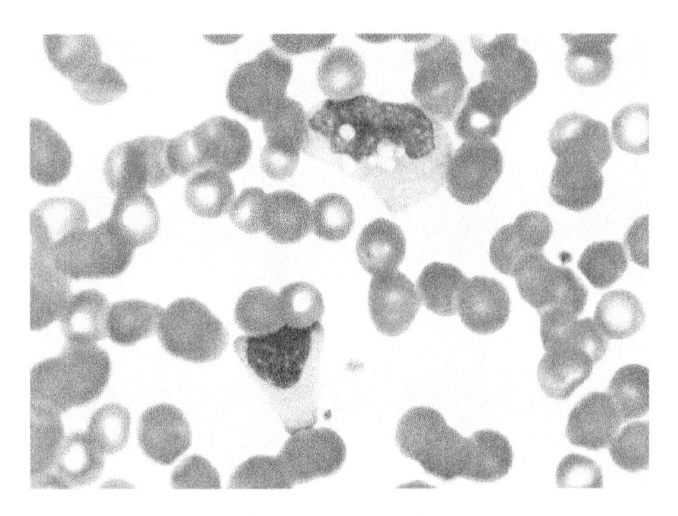

FIGURE 11.20 Atypical lymphocytes with prominent cytoplasm and vacuoles. (Reprinted from Cohen JI. Epstein-Barrr virus. In: Young NS, Gerson SL, High KA, eds. *Clinical Hematology*. Philadelpha, PA: Elsevier; 2006:956–966. Copyright © 2006 Elsevier. With permission.)

MHC class I polymorphisms in HLA-A01 correlate with development of IM, severity of symptoms, and viral load in persons with primary EBV infection.[439] HLA DR polymorphisms also correlated with development of IM. Persons with certain polymorphisms in IL-10 have more severe disease with acute infection.

Patients with IM have high levels of EBV in the peripheral blood and shed high titers of virus from the throat (Fig. 11.18). Virus may be produced in lytically infected B cells[310] as well as in epithelial cells. The level of EBV-infected B cells in the blood drops rapidly ($t_{1/2}$ = 7.5 days) after infection, followed by a slow decline during the first year. During the latter slow decline, the half-life of the viral load is 39 days.[258] High levels of virus shedding persist in the throat for prolonged periods (>180 days) of time after IM. After recovery, the number of infected B cells falls to within the same range as seen in healthy carriers with no history of IM.[24] The half-life of EBV-specific T cells during the first 2 weeks of IM is 2.9 days.[258]

Viral replication in the blood is rare during IM, and nearly all the cells are latently infected. EBV-positive cells in the blood have more somatic hypermutation than EBV-negative cells.[660] Patients in the acute phase of IM have reduced memory B cells in the blood, reduced plasmacytoid dendritic cells, and undetectable antibody-secreting cells and EBV neutralizing antibody.[164,521,522] Neutralizing antibody, gp350 binding antibody, and ADCC increase over time after IM and these peak only during convalescence.[64,726] The frequency of regulatory T cells (CD4+, CD25^{hi}) in the blood is significantly lower in persons with IM than in seropositive blood bank donors; however, a similar frequency of regulatory T cells was observed in the tonsils of patients with IM and controls. B cells in tonsils from persons with IM show EBV latency III gene expression along with other forms of latency including type I and type II with variable expression of LMP1.[352]

EBV-ASSOCIATED DISEASES

X-Linked Lymphoproliferative Disease

X-Linked lymphoproliferative disease type 1 (XLP1), first described as "fatal IM," is a complex immunodeficiency with various sequelae, but best characterized by an extreme susceptibility to symptomatic EBV infection. Patients can present with hemophagocytic syndrome (32% of cases), dysgammaglobulinemia (22%), a family history of XLP1 (17%), lymphoma (14%), fulminant IM (8%), or other symptoms.[56] Acute infection with EBV usually results in a fulminant infection with organs infiltrated by proliferating B and T cells; hemophagocytic lymphohistiocytosis (HLH), bone marrow failure with lymphocytopenia, and hepatic failure often occur.[623] Other patients have aplastic anemia, lymphomatoid granulomatosis, or vasculitis. Patients have an excessive Th1 response with elevation of IFN-γ levels and large numbers of activated T cells and NK cells in the blood. Survivors of acute EBV infection often have low levels of IgG and high levels of IgM and IgA; about 20% subsequently develop B-cell lymphomas. Some patients with XLP1 develop B-cell lymphomas, vasculitis, or hypogammaglobulinemia even in the absence of EBV infection, reflecting a broader immune impairment. These patients do not have more severe infections with other viruses. Patients with XLP1 have reduced IgG responses to vaccines, reduced IL-10 production in T cells[5] and absent NKT cells.[528] SAP knock-out mice have impaired B-cell memory.

XLP1 is due to a mutation in SAP (SLAM-associated protein) encoded by the *SH2D1A* gene on the X chromosome[614] (Fig. 11.21A). SAP, an adapter protein containing a single SH2 domain, is expressed in T, NK, NKT, and in some B cells and interacts with SLAM on T, B, and dendritic cells.[82] This interaction negatively regulates the production of IFN-γ, which is normally induced by T-cell activation. This is thought to occur either by (a) impairment of SLAM binding to SHIP[614] or (b) recruitment of FynT, SHIP, Dok1, and Dok2 with activation of Ras-GTPase-activating protein. SAP also interacts with other members of the SLAM family.[82] These include 2B4 and NTB-A, which mediate CD8+ T-cell and NK cell killing, Ly9, and CD84. The interaction of SAP with 2B4 results in recruitment of FynT, SHIP, and Vav-1 that result in increased NK cell cytotoxicity. Impaired SAP interactions with SLAM, 2B4, and NTB-A may reduce CD8+T and NK cell killing of EBV-infected B cells and result in excessive production of IFN-γ, which can contribute to uncontrolled T-cell proliferation and HLH. SAP also has proapoptotic activity and promotes reactivation-induced cell death, which is important for T-cell homeostasis.[654] T cells from patients with XLP1 are resistant to apoptosis mediated by T-cell receptor stimulation, which may contribute to the massive lymphoproliferative disease with the disease.

Patients with XLP1 who survive infection with EBV have quantitatively normal EBV-specific CD8+ T-cell responses, but their T cells are impaired for recognition of SLAM ligand-positive (but not SLAM-negative) EBV-infected B cells. Patients with XLP1 lack $IgD^{-}CD27^{+}$ class-switched memory B cells, and those who survive carry EBV in nonswitched memory cells (IgM+, IgD+, CD27+).[93] Patients with other family members with XLP1 nearly always have mutations in SAP, whereas sporadic cases are less likely to have mutations. CD4+ T cells from patients with XLP1 do not provide optimal B-cell help, efficiently differentiate into IL-10-positive effector cells, or efficiently up-regulate inducible costimulator (ICOS), a potent inducer of IL-10. Adoptive transfer experiments in mice lacking SAP show that the animals have normal B cells, but defective CD4+ T cells. This results in markedly reduced numbers of virus-specific long-lived plasma cells and memory B cells with impaired long-term antibody responses, but normal or increased levels of virus-specific memory CD4+ T cells. Mice and humans lacking SAP have markedly reduced germinal center B cells; germinal center responses require early and sustained interactions between B and T cells, and SAP is essential for these interactions. SAP expression in T cells, but not B cells, is required for normal antibody production and formation of germinal centers.[708]

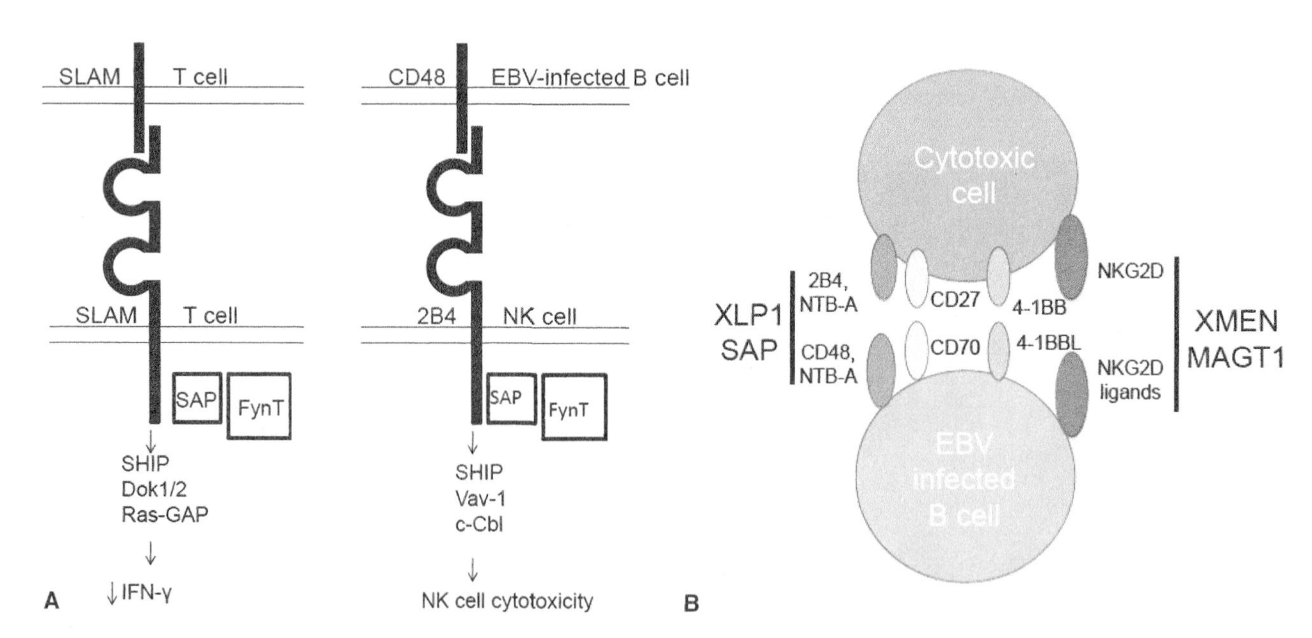

FIGURE 11.21 Interaction of SAP with SLAM and 2B4 and proteins important for B- and T- or NK cell interactions. A: SAP binds to SLAM on T cells and initiates a cascade resulting in decreased IFN-γ. SAP binds to 2B4 on NK cells, which results in increased NK cell cytotoxicity. **B:** Mutations in SAP (which impair 2B4-CD48 and NTB-A self interactions), CD27, CD70, 4-1BB (CD137), or MAGT1 (which up-regulates NKG2D) impair the interaction of EBV-infected B cells with cytotoxic T or NK cells.

Intravenous immunoglobulin has been used to prevent EBV infection in boys with mutations in SAP; fatal breakthroughs have occurred. While antiviral therapy and cytotoxic chemotherapy have not been successful, rituximab (anti-CD20 monoclonal antibody) has been reported to be life-saving in several patients with XLP1 and fulminant IM. Hematopoietic stem cell transplantation (HSCT) cures the disease and survival rates of 80% have been reported with good immune reconstitution. Patients with active HLH have a lower rate (50%) of survival.

Patients with mutations in X-linked inhibitor of apoptosis (XIAP, encoded by *BIRC4*) have many features of XLP1, and this disease is referred to as XLP2.[582] These patients often present with HLH, recurrent splenomegaly, fever, and cytopenia. The disease is usually triggered by primary infection with EBV. XLP2 is usually less severe than XLP1. HLH is more common with XLP2 than XLP1, while hypogammaglobulinemia and low NKT cell numbers are more common in XLP1. The high incidence of HLH and the lack of lymphomas in patients with XLP2 have caused some authors to reconsider its classification as a form of X-linked familial HLH rather than XLP2.[183] Lymphocytes from patients deficient in XIAP have increased apoptosis in response to Fas and the TRAIL receptor.[582] HSCT is recommended for XLP2.[183]

Several other mutations have been associated with poorly controlled EBV and risk of B-cell lymphoma or lymphoproliferative disease. These include mutations in genes important for (a) T-cell interactions with EBV-infected B cells *CD27, CD70, 4-1BB* (CD137), *MAGT1,* which up-regulates NKG2D (Fig. 11.21B); (b) T-cell signaling including *ITK*; (c) nucleotide metabolism (*CTPS1*); and (d) NK or T-cell degranulation (*PRF1, UNC13D, STXBP2*). Other genes are important for protection against EBV and other infections including *GATA2, STK4, CORO1A, RAG1, RAG2, LIG4, MCM4, FCGR3, PIK3CD, PIK3R1, RASGRP1, DOCK8, WAS,* and *NFKB1*.[120,361,680]

Chronic Active EBV and Related Disorders

Chronic active EBV (CAEBV) disease is a rare disease more common in Asia and natives of Mexico, Central and South America. Patients present with IM-like symptoms with fever, lymphadenopathy, hepatosplenomegaly, and develop lymphoproliferative disease involving the liver, lungs, nervous system, or other organs.[123,329] HLH is common with fever and pancytopenia. Asian patients may have severe mosquito bite allergy. The disease often presents after primary EBV infection and patients have high viral loads and/or extremely high antibody titers to EBV VCA and EA, and infiltration of tissues with EBV-positive T, NK, or much less commonly B cells. Many patients have absent antibody to EBNA1. In Japanese patients with CAEBV, EBV is often clonal in T or NK cells, while in the United States, the virus has been reported in T, NK, or B cells. Patients with CAEBV have dysregulation of cytokines and often have elevations in both Th1 and Th2 cytokines. Patients often have low levels of EBV-specific CD8+ T cells implying a failure to control infection. Some patients with NK or T-cell CAEBV have somatic mutations in DDX3X and other cancer driver genes in NK cells, or more rarely in T cells; the EBV genome frequently has deletions especially in BART miRNAs, which can otherwise inhibit lytic activation.[518] In contrast, in patients with B-cell CAEBV, some patients have been found to have germline mutations.[120] Patients with EBV in T cells have a poorer prognosis than those with virus in NK cells, while patients with EBV in NK cells often have severe mosquito bite allergy, high IgE, and large granular lymphocytes in the blood. If untreated, most patients die from hepatic failure, refractory T or NK cell lymphomas, or opportunistic infections due to a progressive loss of immune cell function. EBV latency II gene expression is present in the peripheral blood of many patients with CAEBV. While a number of therapies, including antiviral agents, immunosuppressive agents, cytotoxic chemotherapy, and autologous EBV-specific cytotoxic T cells (CTLs) have been tried, only hematopoietic stem cell transplantation (HSCT) has been curative.[54,212]

Hydroa vacciniforme-like lymphoproliferative disorder is associated with chronic active EBV and is more common in Asians and natives of Central and South America. Patients have high levels of EBV in T or NK cells in the blood. The disease presents with papules and vesicles on sun-exposed areas of the skin (e.g., face) that heal with scarring. In Asia and Latin America, the disease can remain localized to the skin or become systemic similar to CAEBV and require HSCT. In the United States and Europe, Caucasians with the disease usually only have cutaneous disease and the prognosis is often good; some cases resolve spontaneously.[125] EBV-positive cells are usually clonal and can have different forms of EBV latency. Expression of BZLF1 in tissue and age greater than 9 years are indicative of a poor prgnsosis.[464]

Severe mosquito bite allergy presents with deep ulcerations and scarring after mosquito bites. Patients have high levels of EBV in NK cells.[122] While some patients have disease limited to the skin, others develop systemic disease with CAEBV.

Hemophagocytic lymphohistiocytosis (HLH) is associated with immune deficiencies, with CAEBV, or as a rare manifestation of primary EBV infection.[428] Patients with HLH present with fever, pancytopenia, and liver dysfunction. Many patients presenting with HLH and primary EBV infection have virus in T cells and if supported with immunosuppressive therapy, using the HLH 2004 protocol, undergo long-term remissions.[343] In contrast, patients with HLH and immunodeficiencies or CAEBV typically require HSCT. Infection of T cells *in vitro* with EBV results in up-regulation of TNF-α and IFN-γ, which activates macrophages and may drive HLH.[364] Elevated levels of IFN-γ, MIP-1α, MIG, and IP10 are present in tissues

Systemic EBV-positive T-cell lymphoma of childhood is a disease of EBV-positive clonal activated CTLs.[122] While it can present after primary EBV infection, it can also be associated with CAEBV. Patients typically have HLH with fulminant disease.

EBV Lymphoproliferative Disease: Congenital, Iatrogenic, and Posttransplant

Patients with congenital (e.g., genetic disorders described above), acquired (e.g., HIV), or iatrogenic (e.g., methotrexate therapy) T-cell immunodeficiencies often have elevated EBV DNA levels in the peripheral blood and throat and are at risk for EBV lymphoproliferative disease and lymphoma (Table 11.4). The underlying defect in these patients is impaired T-cell function and inability to control EBV-infected B cells. Pathology ranges from polymorphic lymphoproliferative disease to diffuse large B-cell lymphoma.

Patients with rheumatoid arthritis or polymyositis who receive methotrexate may develop EBV lymphoproliferative

TABLE 11.4 EBV-associated malignancies in immunocompromised persons

Disease	EBV Frequency	EBV Gene Expression	EBV Latency	Genetic Mutations	Cell of Origin	Latency Period After EBV Infection	Comments
Lymphoproliferative disease in immune deficiency	100%	EBNA1,2,3,LP; LMP1,2	3		B cell, GC or post-GC	<3 mo	Reduced T-cell immunity
Posttransplant lymphoproliferative disease	Early: <1 year after transplant >90%; late: EBV less common	EBNA1,2,3,LP; LMP1,2	3	Early: none; late: bcl-6 +/− ras, p53, c-myc	B-cell, GC or post-GC	Early: <1 year; late: >1 year	Reduced T-cell immunity
HIV malignancies							
Burkitt lymphoma	30%–70%	EBNA1	1	c-myc, bcl-6, +/−p53	B-cell, GC	Early in HIV	35% of HIV lymphomas
Hodgkin lymphoma	>95%	EBNA1, LMP1, LMP2	2		B cell, post-GC	Early in HIV	5% of HIV lymphomas
DLBCL-centroblast	30%	EBNA1	1	+/−bcl-6	B cell, GC	Early in HIV	25% of HIV lymphomas
DLBCL-immunoblastic	>90%	EBNA1,2,3,LP; LMP1,2	3		B cell, GC or post-GC	Late in HIV	15% of HIV lymphomas, low CD4+ cell numbers
Primary CNS lymphoma	>95%	EBNA1, 2, 3, LP; LMP1,2	3		B cell, GC or post-GC	Late in HIV	Low CD4+ cell numbers
Primary effusion lymphoma	>90%	EBNA1, +/− LMP1, LMP2	1 or 1/2	bcl-6	B cell, GC or post-GC	Late in HIV	HIV lymphomas HHV-8+
Plasmablastic lymphoma	50%–80%	EBNA1 +/− LMP1	1 or 1/2		B cell, post-GC	Late in HIV	Very rare; CD20−
Smooth muscle tumors	>95%	EBNA2, +/− LMP1	?		Smooth muscle cell	Late in HIV	Rare

GC, germinal center; DLBCL, diffuse large B-cell lymphoma; CNS, central nervous system.

disease that often resolves when methotrexate is discontinued.[466] In this case, methotrexate may increase the risk of virus reactivation as well as impair T-cell function. Patients receiving TNF-α inhibitors for rheumatoid arthritis have also developed EBV lymphoproliferative disease; some cases resolve after stopping the drug.

EBV posttransplant lymphoproliferative disease (PTLD) occurs in 1% of kidney transplant recipients, 1% to 2% of liver transplant recipients, 1% to 3% of heart transplant patients, 2% to 5% of lung transplants recipients, and 20% of small intestine transplant patients. Early-stage PTLD lesions do not necessarily meet the true definition of EBV lymphoma. The risk of EBV PTLD is increased in persons who have a primary EBV infection posttransplant, graft versus host disease, cytomegalovirus infection, or who receive second transplants or anti–T-cell antibodies.[359] Certain immunosuppressive drugs, including tacrolimus and IL-2 receptor antagonists, are associated with an increased risk of disease; other immunosuppressive drugs such as alemtuzumab are associated with a high viral load but a low risk of PTLD.

Patients with PTLD often have elevated levels of IL-6, a B-cell growth factor, in the peripheral blood.[697] Polymorphisms in the TNF-α promoter, the TNF receptor I promoter, Nramp, IFN-γ, IL-10, or TGF-β are more frequent in transplant patients with PTLD. Patients with EBV PTLD have a significantly higher frequency of an HLA B51 allele than transplant patients without the allele. HLA-B18 and HLA-B21 are associated with a higher risk of developing PTLD, while HLA-A03 and HLA-DR7 are associated with a lower risk. EBV PTLD is higher in persons homozygous for HLA-A1 and lower in those homozygous for HLA-A2.[333]

About 55% of patients (especially early after transplant) present with an IM-like illness with fever, enlargement of tonsils and adenoids, and lymphadenopathy; biopsies show plasmacytic hyperplasia and lesions are polyclonal or oligoclonal. PTLD may involve the lymph nodes, but lesions are often extranodal and present in the gastrointestinal tract, liver, lungs, kidney, or central nervous system. In organ transplant recipients, the lesions are often in the transplanted organ, probably due to antigenic stimulation with production of cytokines and B-cell growth factors. Tumors are usually of donor origin in bone marrow transplant recipients and of recipient origin in solid organ transplant recipients. About 30% of patients have polymorphic PTLD with monoclonal or oligoclonal lesions (Fig. 11.22). About 15% of patients have monomorphic PTLD with monoclonal disease, which include diffuse large B cell lymphoma, Burkitt lymphoma, classical Hodgkin lymphoma-like PTLD, and plasma cell myeloma. Distinct EBV-positive

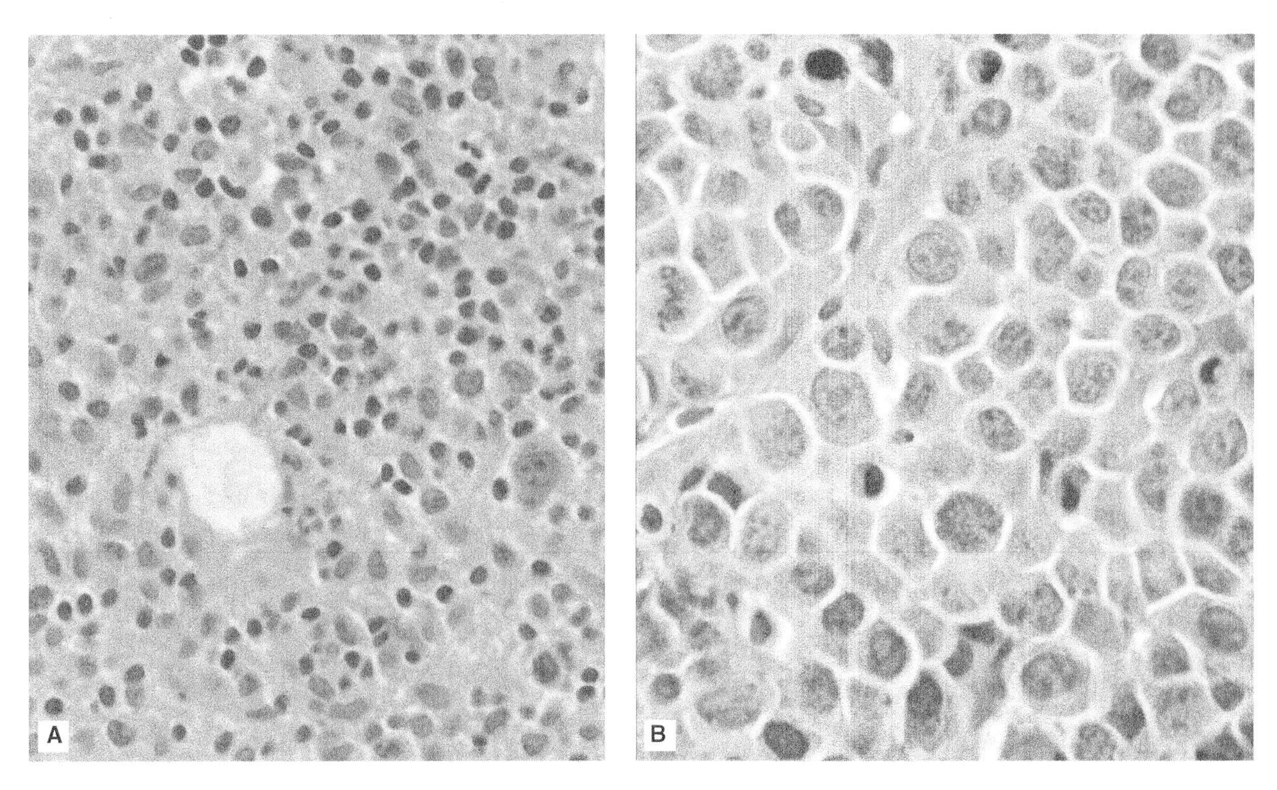

FIGURE 11.22 Biopsy from a patient with (A) polymorphic or (B) monomorphic posttransplant lymphoproliferative disease. (Courtesy of Dr. Elaine Jaffe.)

clones can arise at one or more sites. In contrast, T-cell lymphomas after transplant are rarely EBV positive. The polyclonal and polymorphic PTLD lesions that occur during the first year after transplant are almost always EBV positive and have a type 3 pattern of latency. In contrast, the later monomorphic lesions are often, but not always EBV positive, and may have different patterns of latency with variable expression of EBNA2 and LMP1. Early plasmacytic hyperplastic or polymorphic PTLD lesions usually do not have chromosomal abnormalities, providing further evidence that these tumors are driven by EBV. In contrast, monomorphic PTLD lesions that occur later after transplant that are centroblastic diffuse large B-cell lymphomas may have mutations in *bcl-6*.[83] Monomorphic lesions may also have mutations in *p53, N-ras,* and *c-myc*. Unlike many Burkitt lymphoma cell lines that have *c-myc* translocations and often do not require EBV for survival, cells from PTLD patients require EBV to inhibit apoptosis and to drive the cells out of the G1/G0 phase of the cell cycle. Sequencing of immunoglobulin heavy chain (IgH) genes from PTLD lesions show that some (especially early after transplant) have germline IgH sequences indicative of naïve B cells, while others have IgH somatic mutations that arise from antigen-selected memory B cells; in contrast, others (usually late after transplant) have mutated IgH genes (lacking a functional B-cell receptor) that is often not compatible with B-cell survival, but more commonly seen with Hodgkin lymphoma.[493]

Detection of elevated levels of viral DNA in the blood or CSF may provide a clue to the diagnosis of PTLD and also may be useful for follow-up after treatment.[213] In general, very high levels of EBV DNA in the blood are predictive of PTLD. Detection of EBV DNA in the plasma is more predictive of PTLD than detection in whole blood.[332] Patients at risk for EBV PTLD have lower levels of EBV-specific CD8+ T cells in the blood and combined viral load measurements and EBV-specific T cells may be more predictive of PTLD than either alone. Staging of the extent of disease is performed with CT and PET scans. Diagnosis of EBV PTLD requires demonstration of EBV and appropriate histopathology in tissue biopsies. Biopsies of PTLD lesions usually show type III EBV latency; the peripheral blood often shows type 0 EBV latency, while in some cases additional genes (*LMP1, LMP2, BZLF1*) may be expressed. PTLD biopsies overexpress galectin-1, which tolerizes dendritic cells and induces apoptosis of cytotoxic T cells.

Burkitt Lymphoma

Endemic Burkitt lymphoma (BL) is usually an EBV-positive tumor that occurs in equatorial Africa and New Guinea where *Plasmodium falciparum* malaria is also endemic[469] (Table 11.5). The disease occurs at 5-10 cases per 100,000 children and is the most common childhood tumor in these areas. Endemic BL usually presents as a tumor in the jaw.

Sporadic BL occurs in the United States and Europe at a rate of 0.2 to 0.3 cases per 100,000 persons and only 10% to 20% of tumors are EBV positive. The disease is more common in South America and North Africa with rates of 1 to 2 per 100,000 persons where up to 85% of BL is EBV positive. Sporadic BL usually presents in children with abdominal tumors. AIDS-related BL represents yet another form of the tumor, seen at high incidence in AIDS patients; about 35% of these tumors are EBV positive. The disease occurs early in the course of HIV when immune function is relatively intact

TABLE 11.5 EBV-associated malignancies in nonimmunocompromised persons

Disease	EBV Frequency	EBV Gene Expression	EBV Latency	Genetic Mutations	Cell of Origin	Latency Period After EBV Infection
Burkitt lymphoma	Endemic 95%–100%; sporadic 15%–85%	EBNA1	I	*c-myc, +/-p53, RB2*	B-cell GC centroblast	3–8 y
Hodgkin lymphoma	MC, LD 60%–80%; NS 20%–40%	EBNA1, LMP1, LMP2	II		B-cell post-GC	1 y or more
Nasopharyngeal carcinoma	Anaplastic 100%; keratinizing; 30%–100%	EBNA1, LMP2, +/–LMP1	II	Various tumor suppressor genes	Undifferentiated epithelial cell	>30 y
Gastric carcinoma	Lymphoepithelioma 100%; adenocarcinoma 5%–15%	EBNA1, LMP2 +/–LMP1	I or I/II		Gastric epithelial cell	>30 y
Diffuse large B-cell lymphoma of the elderly	Up to 25%	EBNA1, LMP1,2 +/–EBNA2	II or III		B cell, GC or post-GC	>30 y
Peripheral T-cell lymphoma-associated with CAEBV or acute EBV infection	100%	EBNA1, LMP2, +/–LMP1	2		Mature CD4+ T cell	None or several months
Angioimmunoblastic T-cell lymphoma	>90%	EBNA1, LMP1,2	2	Trisomy 3 or 5	Lymphoma in CD4+ T cells; EBV in B cells, GC	>30 y
Pyothorax lymphoma	100%	EBNA1, 2, +/–LMP1	3	p53	B cell, GC or post-GC	>30 y
Extranodal NK/T Nasal	100%	EBNA1, LMP2, +/–LMP1	2		$CD3^-$, $CD56^+$	>30 y

MC, mixed cellularity; LD, lymphocyte depleted; NS, nodular sclerosis; GC, germinal center; RB2, retinoblastoma-like 2.

and, unlike the EBV-positive PTLD-like lesions that were often seen in late stage HIV infection, AIDS-BL incidence has not fallen with the advent of effective antiretroviral therapy. HIV, like malaria, also induces B-cell proliferation and impairs EBV-specific CTL activity. Pathology of BL shows atypical B cells with basophilic, vacuolated cytoplasm and irregular nuclei with prominent nucleoli in a background of phagocytic histiocytes resulting in a "starry sky" pattern (Fig. 11.23). The lymphoid tumor cells often show mitotic figures and evidence of apoptosis.

BL cells shows dysregulation of the *c-myc* oncogene due to an 8:14, 8:2, or 8:22 chromosomal translocation in which a portion of the immunoglobulin heavy chain (on chromosome 14) or light chain (on chromosome 2 or 22) is fused to *c-myc* (on chromosome 8). Analysis of the structure of the chromosome breakpoints suggest that the *c-myc*/immunoglobulin gene translocations occur during the germinal center reaction either due to somatic hypermutation or to an error during class-switch recombination.[350] Increased expression of *c-myc,* due to its proximity to the immunoglobulin enhancer sequence, is a major determinant of the tumor phenotype, affecting the expression of greater than 15% of genes in BL cells. In particular, c-myc reduces the immunogenicity of EBV-positive cells by inhibiting expression of TAPs, reducing expression of MHC class I, and inhibiting expression of proteasome subunits that are important for antigen presentation. Expression of c-myc also impairs NF-κB and interferon responses in BL cells. Transgenic mice expressing c-myc driven by immunoglobulin light chain sequences develop tumors resembling BL. Expression of c-myc is not compatible with expression of EBNA2 which, if transcriptionally active, is functionally mutated. In addition, EBNA2 down-regulates expression of c-myc. Therefore, high levels of MYC expression limit EBV latency gene expression in B cells and appear to substitute for many of the growth transforming functions of LMP1 and EBNA2.

Infection with malaria not only increases the EBV load but also increases germinal center B-cell numbers and the expression of activation-induced cytidine deaminase (AID) and, thereby, the rate of mutations, including c-myc translocations.[696] EBV-positive BL has a high rate of somatic mutations, which may be associated with activation of AID or defective mismatch DNA repair in the cell.[214] EBV-positive BL has fewer mutations in driver genes that promote lymphoma, particularly those associated with protection from apoptosis including *TP53* than EBV-negative disease. In contrast, EBV-positive endemic BL and AIDS-related BL have high IgH mutation rates with signs of antigen selection, while EBV-negative sporadic BL have low mutation rates without signs of antigen selection.

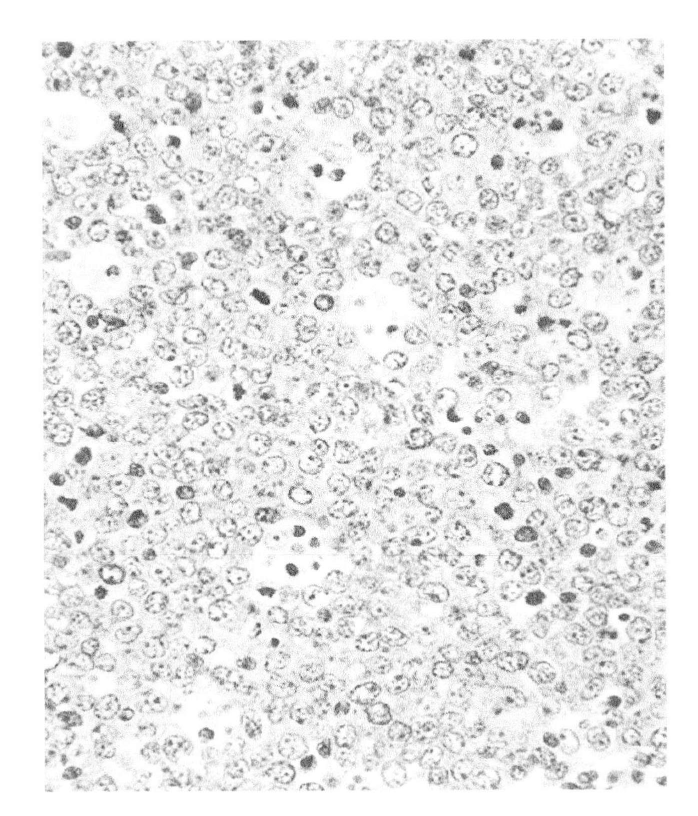

FIGURE 11.23 Biopsy from a patient with Burkitt lymphoma. The intensely stained B cells in a background of lightly stained histiocytes give a "starry sky" appearance. (Courtesy of Dr. Elaine Jaffe.)

This indicates that endemic and AIDS-associated EBV-positive BL evolve from late germinal center B cells (or memory B cells), while sporadic EBV-negative BL evolve from early centroblasts. Sequencing of immunoglobulin genes from endemic BL cells showed that multiple mutations evolve *in vivo*. BL cells express cell surface markers present on germinal center cells with CD77 (BL antigen), CD10, BCL6, CD38, and PAX5, but not adhesion molecules (e.g., LFA-1, ICAM1), B-cell activation antigens (e.g., CD23, CD70), costimulatory molecules (e.g., CD80, CD86), or BCL2. EBV inhibits expression of the apototic genes *BIM* and *PUMA* to increase survival of BL cells.[186] Endemic EBV-positive BL differs from sporadic disease in having fewer mutations in *CCND3* (a cyclin that regulates the cell cycle in germinal center B cells), *TCF3* (which activates PI3K), and *ID3* (which inhibits *TCF3*).[618] EBV-positive BL has a higher frequency of somatic mutations in the genome; type 1 EBV-positive BL had more somatic mutations than type 2.[520]

EBV endemic BL contains clonal viral genomes and usually has a type I EBV latency pattern in tissues and *in vitro*. The cells express EBNA1 driven by the *Qp* promoter and grow as single cells *in vitro*. EBNA1 expression is critical for survival of BL cells; inhibition of EBNA1 induces apoptosis and reduces survival of EBV-positive BL cells.[320] More sensitive assays indicate that some BL cells express LMP2[39] and some lytic genes, especially BHRF1 and LF3 at high levels. Other endemic BLs have high c-myc expression and grow as single cells *in vitro* but have a different pattern of virus latency called "*Wp*-restricted."[318] Such tumors carry an EBNA2-deleted EBV genome, placing the downstream BHRF1 gene under the control of the latent *Wp* promoter. These cells express EBNA1, EBNA3A, EBNA3B, EBNA3C, a truncated EBNA-LP, BHRF1 from *Wp*, and low level LMP2, but not LMP1.

While some EBV BL cells lose their EBV genome during passage *in vitro*, this has not been observed *in vivo*, indicating that the EBV genome has an important role in maintaining the tumor even with limited viral gene expression. In addition, BL cells that lost their EBV genomes *in vitro* had a less malignant phenotype with reduced tumorigenicity in mice. Much of the available evidence suggests that the main role of EBV in BL pathogenesis is not to promote cell growth but rather to counteract the high susceptibility to apoptosis as a consequence of high level c-myc expression. In *Wp*-restricted BLs, cell survival is greatly enhanced through expression of BHRF1, due at least in part to antagonizing Bim-mediated apoptosis.[317] With increasing passage in cell culture, some BL cell lines switch from a latency I to a latency III pattern of EBV expression and the EBNAs are driven by *Cp* or *Wp*. These cells now become LCL-like, grow in clumps, express adhesion molecules (ICAM1, LFA3), B-cell activation markers (CD23, CD70), costimulatory molecules (e.g., CD80, CD86), and bcl-2. Though they still carry the myc/Ig chromosomal translocation identifying their malignant origin, these phenotypically switched BL lines express lower levels of c-myc and are no longer representative of the tumor *in vivo*.

Epidemiologic evidence has implied that a high EBV load is a risk factor for endemic BL; high levels of EBV are common in children with chronic malaria. Accordingly, children in Africa with increased antibody titers to EBV VCA were found to be at increased risk of BL.[687] Patients with endemic BL also often have elevated antibody titers to EBV VCA as well as EA-R. Elevated serum antibody titers to EBV lytic and latent proteins were observed in children in areas where malaria was holoendemic and the levels remained elevated, while antibody titers were lower and declined in persons from areas where malaria was sporadic.[545] Children in Africa from an area with a high prevalence of endemic BL were infected with EBV at a younger age and had higher viral loads than those in another area of Africa.[544] Persons in regions with malaria transmission had higher numbers of EBV-specific T cells, especially targeting latent antigens, than those living in areas without transmission.[98] Children aged 5 to 9 years old who lived in an area holoendemic for malaria had lower EBV-specific IFN-γ responses than those in a nonholoendemic area; this coincided with the peak age incidence of endemic BL in this area. A domain in the *P. falciparum* membrane protein 1 is a polyclonal B-cell activator and incubation of this protein domain with PBMCs increases the EBV DNA copy number. This suggests that chronic exposure to malaria may promote B-cell proliferation and BL.

Hodgkin Lymphoma

Classical Hodgkin lymphoma (HL) consists of 4 histologic subtypes. The frequency of EBV positivity, as defined by detection of the viral genome and certain latency proteins in the malignant Reed-Sternberg cells, is 80% to 90% for lymphocyte depleted, 60% to 75% for mixed cellularity, 20% to 40% for nodular sclerosis, and less than 10% for lymphocyte rich.[270] Reed-Sternberg cells (large multinucleated cells of B-cell lineage) have clonal immunoglobulin gene rearrangements and

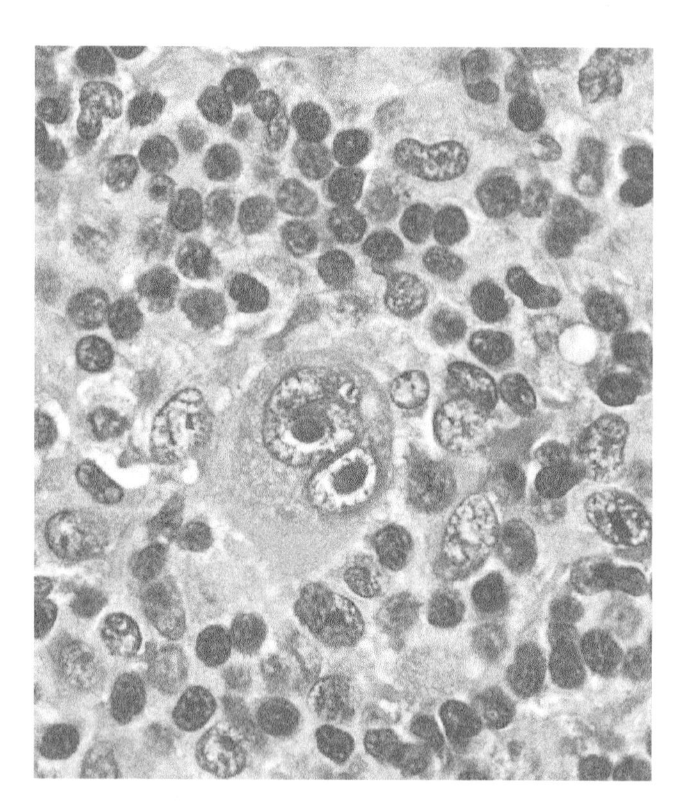

FIGURE 11.24 Biopsy from a patient with Hodgkin lymphoma, mixed cellularity. The large binucleate cell in the center is a Reed-Sternberg cell. (Courtesy of Dr. Elaine Jaffe.)

express B-cell activation antigens CD25 and CD70, although they usually do not express conventional B-cell markers such as CD19 or CD20. Patients present with lymphadenopathy and often have involvement of the bone marrow, liver, and spleen. Pathology shows small numbers of Reed-Sternberg cells in a background of nonmalignant lymphocytes, granulocytes, histiocytes, and plasma cells (Fig. 11.24).

EBV-positive HL is more common than EBV-negative disease in patients in developing countries including Central and South America (80% to 90% EBV positive) compared with affluent countries (30% to 40% EBV positive) in some, but not all studies. HL is more commonly EBV positive in childhood and older adults than in young adults. HL is nearly always EBV positive in immunosuppressed patients.

Elevations in IgG antibody to EBV VCA, EBNA2, and EA-D are present at a mean of 4 years before diagnosis of HL.[479] Increases in each of these antibodies carries a 3- to 4-fold relative risk of subsequent development of HL. Patients with EBV-positive HL have detectable EBV DNA in the plasma before therapy. EBV DNA in the plasma declines in response to therapy and increases before disease recurs.[661] The level of EBV is higher in the blood of persons with EBV-positive HL compared with EBV-negative disease and higher in patients with advanced stage disease. Overall there is a 2.6- to 3.4-fold increased risk of EBV-positive HL after IM, reaching 4-fold in younger adults.[251] The risk is highest within the first year and decreases to normal after 10 years; the median time for HL presentation post-IM is 2.9 years. In contrast, there is no increase in other lymphoid tumors after EBV IM, including EBV-negative HL or non-Hodgkin lymphoma.

Sequencing of immunoglobulin genes from HL indicates that the tumor cells have mutated immunoglobulin genes and in some cases are derived from crippled germinal center B cells.[309] Such crippling mutations, which result in loss of functional immunoglobulin, would normally lead to counter-selection and B-cell death. About 90% of EBV-positive HL had crippling mutations compared to about 40% of EBV-negative HL. This is consistent with the hypothesis that two of the EBV proteins expressed in HL cells, LMP1, which inhibits apoptosis by stimulating NF-κB, and LMP2A, which provides a B-cell growth stimulus mimicking the Ig receptor, may help the crippled B cells to survive.

Biopsies from EBV-positive HL have type II EBV latency with expression of LMP1, LMP2A and LMP2B, EBNA1 driven by the *Qp* promoter, EBERs, and BARTs.[147] Expression of LMP1 in germinal center B cells results in reduced expression of genes that are commonly down-regulated in HL such as CD79A, CD19, CD20, and CD22. EBNA1 down-regulates expression of Smad2, which in turn down-regulates expression of the protein tyrosine phosphatase receptor κ, which enhances proliferation and viability of HL cells. LMP1 up-regulates Bim-1 in HL cells, which may increase survival of these cells. EBV infection of HL cells induces expression of autotoxin, which increases lysophosphatidic acid and increases growth and survival of HL cells. EBV-positive HL shows higher levels of CCL20, which can induce trafficking of regulatory T cells into the tumors.

Polymorphisms in the HLA class I region associate with EBV-positive HL, while those in HLA class III correlate with EBV-negative disease.[155] The class I association suggests that the strength of immune surveillance by EBV-specific CD8+ T cells could influence disease development. Further studies showed that Caucasian patients with an HLA-A*0201 allele have a reduced risk of developing EBV-positive HL; conversely those with an HLA-A*0101 allele have an increased risk.[504] In addition, a polymorphism in the IL-10 promoter is more common in persons with EBV-positive HL than in EBV-negative disease. Biopsies from patients with EBV-positive, but not EBV-negative, classical HL show down-regulation of miR-96, miR-128a, and miR-128b.

EBV-specific T-cell function is partially impaired in HL. Galectin-1, an immunomodulatory protein, was expressed in the majority of classical HL tissues examined (and in Reed-Sternberg cell lines from HL) and expression was associated with reduced LMP1- and LMP2-CD8+ T-cell responses and reduced CD8+ T-cell infiltrates in tumor tissues.[205] CD8+ T cells specific for LMP1 and LMP2, but not EBNA or lytic proteins, from patients with HL have impaired function. Galectin-1 reduces degranulation and recognition of epitopes by LMP-specific T cells. Regulatory T cells are increased in the blood of patients with HL with active disease, compared with those in remission. Expression of LAG-3, which is a marker of regulatory T cells, is increased in infiltrating lymphocytes in EBV-positive HL tissue and is associated with impaired EBV LMP1- and LMP2-specific CD8+ T-cell responses. Many patients with EBV-associated HL lack detectable CD4+ specific T-cell responses to EBNA1. Overall survival is higher in patients with EBV-positive HL than EBV-negative disease, independent of gender, stage of disease, and B symptoms.[284]

Nasopharyngeal Carcinoma

NPC is classified as keratinizing (WHO type I) or nonkeratinizing with differentiated (WHO type II) or undifferentiated (WHO type III) subtypes. Virtually all nonkeratinizing undifferentiated (WHO type III) NPC is EBV positive.[700] Undifferentiated NPC is more prevalent in Southeast Asia (especially Southern China), Northern Africa, and Eskimos in the Arctic. In Southern China, the rate of NPC is 50 per 100,000 in men over 50 years old. The disease has a 2- to 3-fold higher rate in men than in women. The incidence of NPC peaks at ages 50 to 59, with a smaller peak in adolescents and young adults. The rates are also elevated in Chinese persons who migrate from China. Environmental factors, especially dietary habits (use of salted fish and preserved foods), as well as genetic factors, may play a role in development of the disease. The rate of NPC has been declining in developed areas of Southeast Asia, perhaps due to changes in dietary habits. NPC occurs less commonly in the United States and Europe with rates of 0.5 to 2 per 100,000. In the United States, 63% of NPC is undifferentiated.

EBV is clonal in high grade preinvasive lesions (carcinoma *in situ* or dysplasia) as well as in NPC,[529] but not in low grade preinvasive lesions. Thus, the virus likely infects epithelial cells that already have a genetic abnormality. Undifferentiated NPC shows uniform malignant epithelial cells with prominent nuclei in a dense background of lymphocytes (Fig. 11.25). EBV DNA is present in the transformed epithelial cells, but not in the infiltrating lymphocytes. The tumors are sometimes referred to as lymphoepitheliomas. About 30% of NPCs have mutations in the MHC locus that may allow escape from virus-specific CTLs.[378]

Development of NPC is believed to be a multistep process initially with overexpression of *p53* and loss of expression of the tumor suppressor genes *p16* and *p27* (and in some cases increased *p21Ras*) resulting in a hyperplastic lesion. This is followed by EBV infection and increased expression of *bcl-2* resulting in a dysplastic lesion and then overexpression of *p53* and invasive NPC (Fig. 11.26). A large number of tumor suppressor genes are hypermethylated resulting in reduced expression in NPC including *TFPI-2, DLEC1, BLU, and E-cadherin.* Twist and Snail, which are repressors of E-cadherin and regulators of epithelial–mesenchymal transition, are induced by LMP1 and correlate with the metastatic behavior of NPC. Whole exome sequencing and genome-wide association studies identified genetic variants in numerous genes including cancer driver genes (*PIK3CA, TP53, ERBB2, ERBB3, KRAS*), chromatin modifier genes (*ARID1A, MLL2, BAP1, MLL3, TET2, TSHZ3*), and autophagy genes (*ATG13, ATG7*).[390] In addition, mutations resulting in loss of function in NF-κB regulators (*CYLD, TRAF3, NFKBIA, NLRC5, TNFAIP3*) are also common in NPC.[378,756] Interesting, the loss of function in NF-κB regulators were only observed in LMP1-negative NPC.

The risk for NPC is much higher (hazard ratio 6.8) for family members (when one member has the disease) compared with others in the same community.[261] The risk of NPC is higher for those with elevated anti-EBV DNAase antibody or

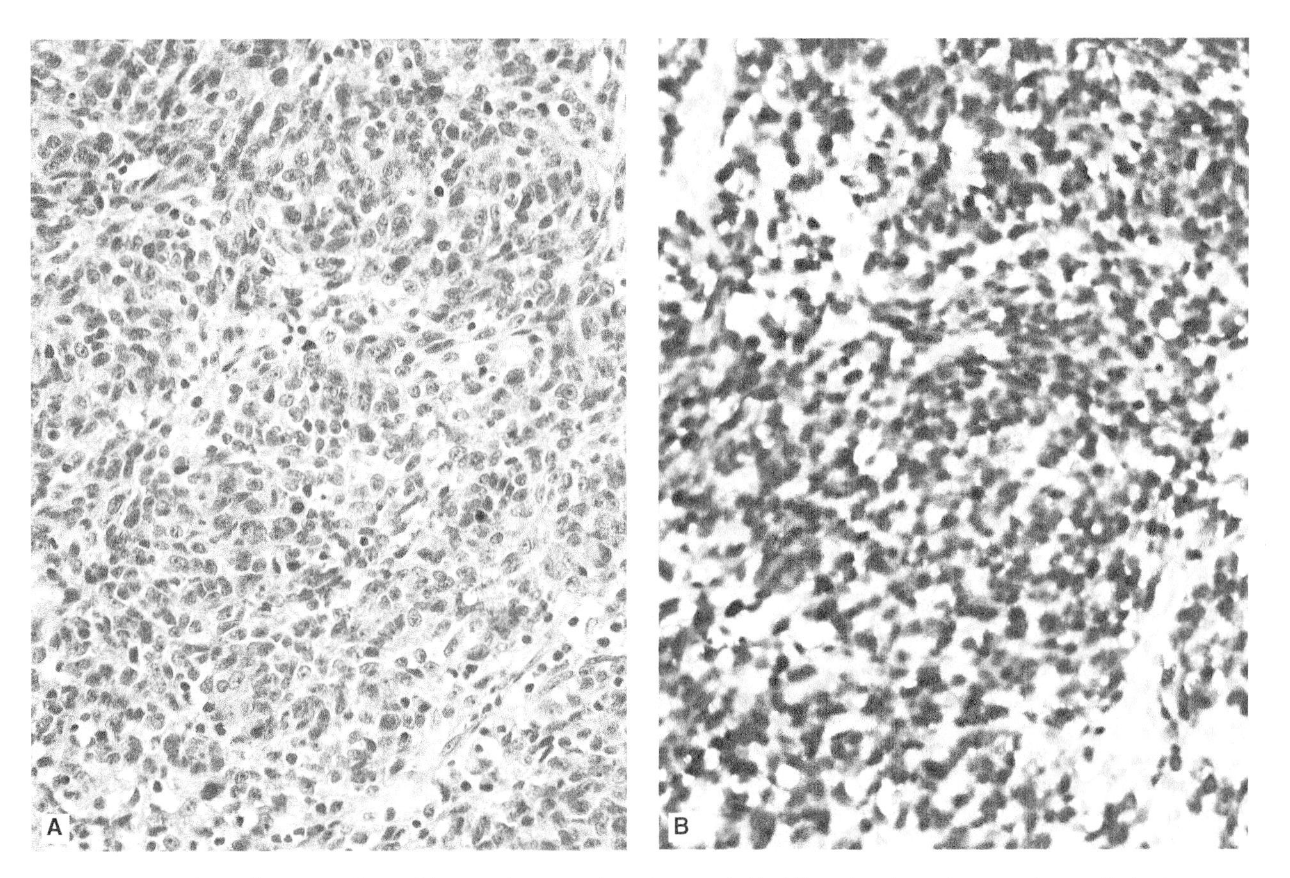

FIGURE 11.25 Biopsy from a patient with nasopharyngeal carcinoma. A: Undifferentiated anaplastic carcinoma. **B:** *In situ* hybridization shows EBV-encoded RNA (EBER)-positive carcinoma cells. (Courtesy of Dr. Paul A. VanderLaan.)

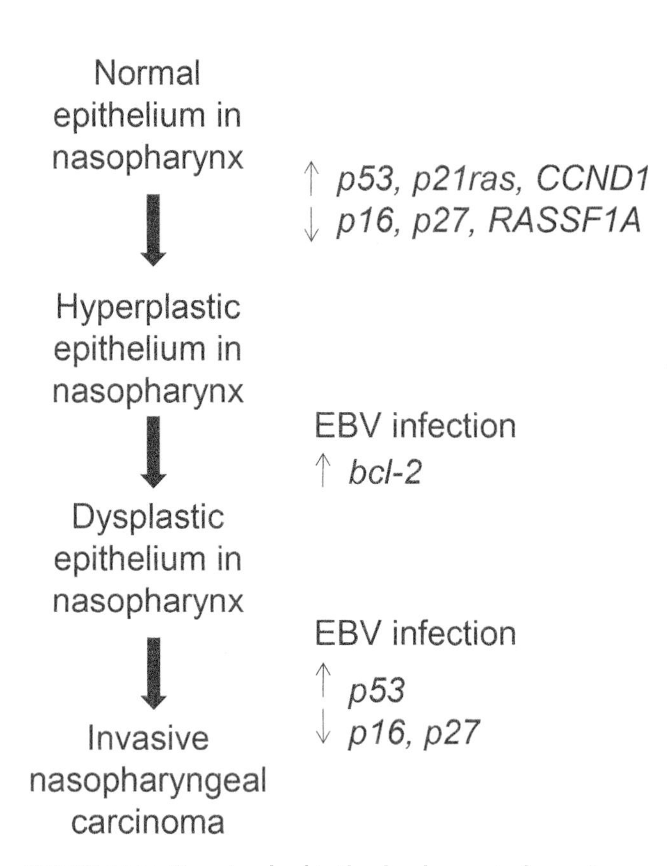

FIGURE 11.26 **Steps involved in the development of nasopharyngeal carcinoma.** EBV infection occurs after the cells have undergone initial genetic changes and have a hyperplastic or dysplastic phenotype. (Modified from Fan SQ, Ma J, Zhou J, et al. Differential expression of Epstein-Barr virus-encoded RNA and several tumor-related genes in various types of nasopharyngeal epithelial lesions and nasopharyngeal carcinoma using tissue microarray analysis. *Hum Pathol* 2006;37(5):593–605. Copyright © 2006 Elsevier. With permission.)

anti-EBV VCA IgA (hazard ratio 2.8) and even higher when both antibodies are elevated (adjusted hazard ratio 15.1). Persons with a family history of NPC and elevated EBV serologies had a higher risk of NPC (hazard ratio was 31) than those without a family history and negative serology for DNAse and VCA IgA. A prospective study found a 21-fold increased risk of NPC in persons with rising titers of IgA antibody to EBV VCA. Elevated levels of anti-EBV EBNA1 IgA were associated with a 5-fold risk of NPC.

Patients with NPC usually have high titers of antibody to EBV VCA, EBNA, and EA-D IgA; unlike other EBV tumors, elevated antibodies to EBV occur in NPC regardless of the geographical location. IgA to EBV VCA or EBV DNAse in serum or saliva has been used for screening in endemic areas[108]; persons with a four fold increase in IgA VCA have an 18% risk of developing NPC within 3 years in China; some patients have loss of antibody and loss of risk. EBV IgA antibody levels are elevated up to 10 years before the diagnosis of NPC with a mean duration of 37 months before diagnosis.

NPC patients often have elevated levels of EBV DNA in the plasma[392]; this viral DNA is due to apoptosis of tumor cells with EBV DNA released into the blood, not to increased numbers of EBV-infected B cells. The sensitivity of EBV DNA, VCA IgA antibody, and combined EBV DNA and VCA IgA for diagnosis of NPC was 95%, 81%, and 99%, respectively. The specificity of EBV DNA and VCA IgA was 98% and 96%, respectively.[373] Higher EBV plasma levels at the time of diagnosis and rising levels of EBV VCA or EA IgA antibody, or EBV DNA after therapy is associated with a poorer prognosis. After therapy, the serum level of EBV DNA often declines. Another noninvasive test for NPC involves brushing suspicious areas of the nasopharynx and performing PCR for EBV DNA and detecting EBV DNA and RNA. High levels of EBV DNA in brushings had a specificity of 98% and sensitivity of 90% for NPC. EBNA1 and BARF1 mRNA were found in 86% and 74% of brushings, respectively, from NPC-positive patients. A prospective study of over 1,000 persons showed that detection of EBV DNA in plasma is helpful for detecting asymptomatic NPC at an early stage.[96]

Patients with NPC have lower levels of EBNA1-specific CD8+ T cells and lower levels of LMP1- and LMP2-specific T cells than controls.[192] Patients with NPC have lower levels of naïve CD3+CD45+RA+ and CD4+CD25− cells in the blood, and higher levels of activated CD4+CD25+ T cells and CD3⁻CD16+ NK cells than controls. EBV-specific cytotoxic T-cell (CTL) activity could be reactivated in peripheral blood mononuclear cells by incubation with autologous lymphoblastoid cells lines, while tumor infiltrating lymphocytes from NPC biopsies lacked cytotoxic activity and did not produce IFN-γ when incubated with autologous lymphoblastoid cells lines. NPC tumors have high levels of regulatory T cells (CD4+CD25^{hi}, Foxp3).

NPC usually has type II EBV latency with EBNA1 driven by the *Qp* promoter, expression of EBER, BARTs, and variable expression of LMP1; in many cases, LMP1 is undetectable. In contrast, LMP1 is routinely expressed in preinvasive lesions.[529] LMP2A is usually expressed in NPC biopsies, and its expression may be important for NPC, since LMP2A expression in epithelial cells increases expression of integrin α6 proteins, which increases their migration and invasiveness. Higher mutation rates in the sequence of LMP2 were seen in NPC tumors than in isolates from the oropharynx of healthy persons. While BARF1 and BZLF1 were present in some tumor cells, other lytic proteins were generally not expressed. miRNAs from BART, but not BHRF1, are expressed in NPC.[1,132,761] BART miRNAs interact with the 3′ NTR of LMP1 and reduce its expression. miR-218 suppresses NPC progression by down-regulating survivin. A polymorphism in one the EBV EBERs was associated with an increased risk of NPC.[265] Two variants in the BALF2 gene resulted in an 8.7-fold and 6.1-fold increased risk of NPC in Southern China, and these variants contributed to 83% of the risk of NPC in the area.[738] A variant in the EBV BZLF1 promoter is increased in patients with NPC.[61]

NPC cells release exosomes that contain galectin-9, which can induce apoptosis of EBV-specific CD4+ T cells; galectin-9 is also present in exosomes from plasma of patients with NPC.[337] Exosomes from NPC cells also contain LMP1, viral miRNAs, and signal transduction molecules, which activate signaling pathways in recipient cells.[447] Lesions from patients with NPC often show down-regulation of TAP1, tapasin, and MHC class I, and up-regulation of IL-10.

EBV is also present in other epithelial cell tumors (known as lymphoepitheliomas or undifferentiated carcinomas of the nasopharyngeal type) including the tonsils, salivary glands, thymus, larynx, lungs, skin, and cervix. Like NPC, these tumors are more common in certain areas of the world, especially Southeast Asia and Eskimos in the Arctic. Also similar to NPC, pathology shows malignant EBV-positive epithelial cells with a dense infiltrate of lymphocytes. When a family member is diagnosed with NPC, there is an 8.4-fold risk to other members for carcinoma of the salivary gland.

Gastric Carcinoma

EBV is present in about 9% to 10% of gastric carcinomas including over 90% of gastric lymphoepithelioma-like carcinomas, 7% of moderately to well-differentiated gastric adenocarcinomas, and 6% of poorly differentiated gastric adenocarcinomas.[201,277] Since the vast majority of gastric carcinomas are adenocarcinomas, most EBV-positive gastric cancers are adenocarcinomas. Worldwide, gastric carcinomas are the most common EBV-associated malignancy. The prevalence of EBV-positive gastric carcinoma is similar in the United States, Europe, and Asia. Lymphoepithelioma-like carcinomas have a similar pathology to NPC with EBV DNA in malignant epithelial cells and a dense infiltrate of EBV-negative lymphocytes and macrophages surrounding the tumor cells. EBV-positive gastric carcinomas often involve the upper third of the stomach. Meta-analyses found that the prevalence of EBV-positivity in gastric carcinoma was 2-fold higher in men than in women, more common in younger persons, more frequent in the gastric cardia or corpus than the antrum, and more common in post-surgical gastric remnants.

EBV-positive gastric carcinoma has a higher frequency of mutations in *PIK3CA, ARID1A, BCOR*, amplification of *JAK2, ERBB2, PD-L1*, and *PD-L2*, DNA hypermethylation (resulting in silencing of many genes), and a lower frequency of mutations in TP53 compared with EBV-negative gastric carcinoma.[81,161,716] Expression of p16, p27, E-cadherin, and p73 is reduced in EBV-positive gastric cancer, while expression of cyclin D1 and NF-κB are increased compared with EBV-negative cancer. Somatic mutations in EBV-positive gastric carcinoma have been associated with up-regulation of APOBEC in the tumors.[51] DNA methylation of CpG sequences in the promoters of tumor suppressor genes such as *PTEN* is induced by LMP2 by up-regulation of de novo methyltransferase 1. MHC class I is down-regulated in EBV-positive gastric carcinoma cells.

Gastric carcinoma cells are clonal or oligoclonal for EBV DNA. EBV-positive gastric carcinomas have an EBV type I latency pattern, with EBNA1 driven by the *Qp* promoter, expression of EBERs, BARTs, and variable expression of LMP2A.[201] EBNA1 expression in gastric carcinoma cells is associated with loss of PML bodies, impaired response to DNA damage, and reduced apoptosis.[640] BARF1 is also expressed in the tumors and like NPC, BART miRNAs, but not BHRF1 miRNAs, are expressed in tissues from patients with EBV-positive gastric carcinoma.

EBV was not detected in preneoplastic (dysplasia and intestinal metaplasia) lesions in patients with EBV-positive gastric carcinomas, but only in the carcinomas.[767] This suggests that like NPC, EBV infection is a late event in the development of gastric carcinoma. EBV gastric carcinoma is associated with atrophic gastritis and lymphocytic infiltration.

Like NPC, levels of anti-EBV VCA IgA are higher in persons who subsequently develop EBV-positive gastric carcinoma than controls. Levels of anti-EBV VCA IgG and anti-EA IgG antibodies are higher in patients with EBV-positive gastric carcinoma than those with EBV-negative cancer.[277] EBV anti-VCA and anti-EBNA antibodies titers are higher in persons with dysplasia on gastric biopsy, suggesting that EBV reactivation could be related to an early phase of gastric carcinoma.

EBV-positive gastric carcinomas with a lymphoepithelial-like histology and large numbers of tumor infiltrating lymphocytes generally have a better prognosis than EBV-positive carcinomas with an adenocarcinoma histology and a patchy lymphocytic infiltrate. Patients with EBV-positive gastric carcinomas have a better survival rate than those with EBV-negative carcinomas.

Non-Hodgkin Lymphomas and Other Malignancies in Nonimmunocompromised Persons

EBV is present in about 6% of cases of non-Hodgkin lymphoma (NHL) in Europe.[629] This includes diffuse large B-cell lymphoma, lymphomatoid granulomatosis, pyothorax-associated lymphoma, peripheral T-cell lymphoma, and angioimmunoblastic T-cell lymphoma. In Asia, EBV is associated with NK/T-cell lymphoma and aggressive NK cell leukemia/lymphoma.[122]

Diffuse large B-cell lymphomas are EBV positive in 10% of nonimmunosuppressed persons; the rate of EBV positivity is higher in immunocompromised persons. EBV-positive diffuse large B-cell lymphomas have a poorer prognosis than EBV-negative lymphomas and are associated with increased age, extranodal disease, fever, and a poorer response to therapy. The most frequently mutated genes in EBV-positive DLBCL were *MYC, RHOA, PIM1, MEF2B, MYD88*, and *CD79B*.[760] About 40% of CD30+ anaplastic large B-cell lymphomas are EBV positive and express LMP1 with variable expression of EBNA2.[353] About 15% of large B-cell lymphomas in the oral cavity are EBV positive, while approximately 20% of T-cell-rich B-cell NHL is EBV positive.

Lymphomatoid granulomatosis usually presents with fever and masses in the lungs but also can involve the kidneys, skin, liver, and central nervous system.[449] Many patients with lymphomatoid granulomatosis have reduced numbers of CD8+ and CD4+ T cells; some patients have HIV, XLP1, or have received organ transplants. Pathology shows EBV in rare B cells, an exuberant T-cell response, and destruction of small blood vessels. Separate clonal lesions can arise at different sites. Lesions express EBV EBNA2 and LMP1, and EBV DNA levels in the blood are often not elevated. IFN-α is often effective in early stage disease, while late stage disease requires cytotoxic chemotherapy.

Pyothorax-associated lymphoma is an EBV-positive diffuse large B-cell lymphoma that originates in the pleural cavity after a history of pyothorax. Tumors usually express EBNA1, EBNA2, and/or LMP.[19] The disease is probably due to chronic inflammation, persistent cytokine production, and reduced host immunosurveillance. Similar localized EBV-positive lymphomas, termed diffuse large B-cell lymphoma associated with chronic inflammation, can occur at sites of chronic osteomyelitis, cardiac myxomas, splenic cysts, skin ulcers, and near metallic prostheses.

EBV-positive mucocutaneous ulcers are more common in the elderly and they respond to reduction in immunosuppression or may spontaneously regress.

Peripheral T-cell lymphomas usually present with fever and lymphadenopathy and are often associated with HLH.

The disease is more common in Asians and persons from South America. Macrophage activation is often present with elevated serum levels of TNF-α, IFN-γ, and other cytokines. Elevated levels of TNF-α in the serum are associated with a poorer prognosis. T-cell lymphomas have clonal EBV DNA and usually have type II EBV latency, although expression of LMP1 can be variable.[103] The lymphoma can involve α/β or γ/δ T cells.

Angioimmunoblastic T-cell lymphoma is a peripheral T-cell lymphoma that presents with fever, night sweats, weight loss, hepatosplenomegaly, lymphadenopathy, and hypergammaglobulinemia. The malignant T cells are usually clonal and patients may develop EBV-positive diffuse large B-cell lymphoma. Autoantibodies including immune complexes, cold agglutinins, rheumatoid factor, and antismooth muscle antibodies may be present. EBV is present in over 90% of cases, and the virus is present in the proliferating B cells that accompany the malignant T cells.[727] EBV-infected B cells can be polyclonal, oligoclonal, or clonal and are deficient in the immunoglobulin receptor. EBV DNA is elevated in the serum and parallels the clinical course.

Extranodal NK/T-cell lymphoma—nasal type (formally lethal midline granuloma) usually presents in nose, but can also involve the sinuses and palate. Other portions of the upper airway may be involved; much less commonly the gastrointestinal tract and skin are infected. Pathology shows invasion of blood vessels with necrosis. Most tumor cells are CD56+ and surface CD3− and express granzyme and perforin; however, in some cases, cells are CD56−, CD3+. These tumors are more common in Southeast Asia and Central and South America, especially in men. The disease may be associated with HLH. The tumors are nearly always EBV positive, clonal for EBV, and have type II EBV latency with variable expression of LMP1. Extranodal NK/T-cell lymphomas often have mutations in *STAT3, BCOR,* and *MLL2,* and *DDX3X.*[289,367] Some tumors have mutations in PD-L1/PD-L2. Tumor cells often show NF-κB and Akt activation and express TNF-α with dysregulation of STATs and Rel A. High levels of EBV DNA in the blood correlate with a poorer prognosis.

Aggressive NK leukemia/lymphoma presents with fever, night sweats, weight loss, pancytopenia, hepatosplenomegaly, and large granular lymphocytes in the blood and bone marrow. About 50% of cases are EBV positive and the disease is more common in Asians; some patients initially present with CAEBV. The level of EBV DNA in the plasma is elevated at onset of disease and parallels the course of the disease. Mutations in *STAT3, DDX3X, RAS-MAPK,* and histone modifier genes are often present.[163]

Inflammatory pseudotumor-like follicular dendritic cell sarcoma presents with fever and usually involves the spleen and liver. The tumors contain clonal EBV DNA with a type II pattern of EBV latency.

Breast cancer has been associated with EBV based on earlier reports, using PCR and antibodies to EBV proteins that detected EBV in a small fraction of the tumor cells; however, more recent studies using *in situ* hybridization and immunochemistry have generally not supported an association of EBV with the disease.

EBV and HIV

Patients with late stage HIV often have higher levels of EBV-specific antibodies, lower levels of virus-specific CTLs, shed higher levels of virus from the throat, and have 10-fold higher levels of EBV in the peripheral blood than healthy persons.[50,84] Detectable EBV DNA in the blood was predictive of EBV lymphoma in patients with HIV.[482] In patients begun on highly active antiretroviral therapy, the EBV DNA load did not change, and there was a decline in BZLF-1-specific CD4+ and CD8+ T cells suggestive of less EBV reactivation. In contrast, there was an increase in EBNA1-specific CD4+ and CD8+ T cells to levels similar to those seen in healthy persons. A variant in the EBV BZLF1 promoter was increased in patients with HIV-associated lymphomas.[61]

A longitudinal study of EBV DNA loads and cellular immunity in HIV patients showed that patients who did not develop NHL had stable levels of EBV DNA and EBV-specific CTL precursors, while patients who developed NHL had increasing EBV loads and decreasing EBV-specific CTLs before the onset of lymphoma.[323] In another study, HIV patients who developed NHL had increasing EBV DNA levels in the blood and although they did not have a decline in the number of EBV-specific T cells, these cells lost their ability to produce IFN-γ in response to EBV peptides. Primary infection with EBV does not alter the HIV viral load or progression to AIDS.

The overall rate of EBV-positive lymphomas has declined with highly active antiretroviral therapy. However, this is highly dependent upon tumor type. Lymphomas that occur early in the course of HIV infection—BL and HL—have not declined in incidence with highly active antiretroviral therapy, while lymphomas that occur later when patients are very immunocompromised—immunoblastic and primary CNS lymphomas—have decreased.

Oral hairy leukoplakia is a nonmalignant disease that occurs in patients with late-stage AIDS and in some transplant recipients.[217] The disease presents with white corrugated "hairy" lesions on lateral aspect of the tongue or occasionally on the palate or buccal mucosa and is due to lytic EBV replication in the outer layer of epithelial cells, without evidence of latent infection in the basal layers. Pathology shows hyperkeratosis of the squamous epithelium with acanthosis and intranuclear inclusions, but no inflammatory cells. Biopsies show linear (replicating) EBV DNA and herpesvirus particles on EM. EBV lytic antigens BZLF1, EA, VCA, as well as EBNA1, EBNA2, and LMP1 are expressed in lytically infected epithelial cells. Multiple EBV strains have been detected in single lesions with EBV variants due to recombination in and adjacent to the EBNA2 gene between viruses. The disease responds to acyclovir, which inhibits EBV replication; however, relapses are common when acyclovir is stopped. Highly active antiretroviral therapy can resolve lesions.

Lymphoid interstitial pneumonitis is characterized by diffuse interstitial pulmonary infiltrates. The alveoli are infiltrated with EBV-positive B cells, immunoblasts, and plasma cells. The disease is more common in children with HIV, although it can occur in adults with autoimmune disease.

Burkitt lymphomas account for about 35% of cases of AIDS-associated lymphoma (Table 11.4). About 30% of BL in HIV are EBV positive. The disease occurs in patients with HIV usually before they develop severe immunodeficiency. These tumors usually have a type I EBV latency pattern, or less commonly a type II pattern, and have *c-myc* translocations.

Hodgkin lymphoma occurs early in the course of HIV and like patients without HIV, EBV is more often present in tumors of the lymphocyte depleted or mixed cellularity subtypes.

Non-Hodgkin lymphomas in patients with HIV are EBV positive in 50% of cases and are clonal for the viral genome.[85] EBV was detected more often in benign lymph nodes of HIV patients who subsequently or concurrently had NHL than in those without lymphoma. Patients with HIV progressing to NHL had loss of EBV-specific CD8+ T and CD4+ T cells, including EBNA1-specific CD4+ and CD8+ T-cell responses.

Diffuse large B-cell lymphomas include centroblastic and immunoblastic lymphomas. Centroblastic lymphoma involves the lymph nodes, accounts for 25% to 30% of HIV lymphomas, and 30% of the tumors are EBV positive. Immunoblastic lymphomas account for 10% of HIV lymphomas, 90% are EBV positive, and the tumors are extranodal. Diffuse large B-cell lymphomas often have type II or type III EBV latency, although variable expression of latent EBV genes has been reported.

CNS lymphomas in patients with AIDS are nearly always EBV positive, are immunoblastic lymphomas with type III EBV latency, and occur late in the course of AIDS when CD4+ T-cell counts are low[419] (Fig. 11.27). The cerebrospinal fluid is usually EBV positive. While studies before the era of highly active antiretroviral therapy found that detection of EBV in the cerebrospinal fluid of patients with mass lesions was highly predictive of CNS lymphoma, more recent studies suggest that the positive predictive value may be 30% or less. Increased metabolic activity on a PET scan along with EBV DNA in the CSF increases the likelihood of CNS lymphoma in these patients. HIV patients who subsequently developed CNS lymphomas lacked EBV-specific CD4+ T cells. Other immunoblastic lymphomas in patients with AIDS occur in the late stages of the disease and are usually EBV positive.

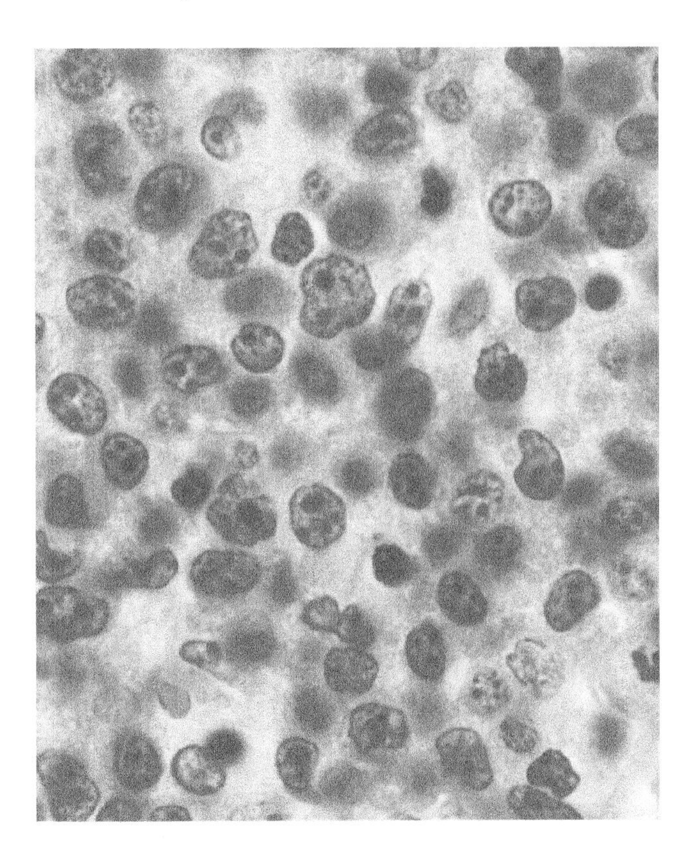

FIGURE 11.27 Biopsy from a patient with immunoblastic lymphoma of the central nervous system (Courtesy of Dr. Elaine Jaffe.)

Plasmablastic lymphomas are usually EBV positive and occur in the mouth or jaw of patients with HIV; less often they present in the sinus, gastrointestinal tract, or soft tissues. These tumors are EBER positive, have a type I latency pattern, and do not express CD20. They generally occur late in the course of HIV and have a poor prognosis.

Primary effusion lymphomas are located in the pleural, pericardial, or peritoneal cavity. The cells are positive for HHV-8 DNA and ≥90% of tumors contain EBV DNA. When positive for EBV, the EBV genome is required for cell proliferation. EBV inhibits HHV-8 lytic replication in primary effusion lymphoma cells. The tumor cells express EBNA1 and may express LMP1 and LMP2.

EBV-positive smooth muscle tumors, leiomyosarcomas, and leiomyomas occur in patients with AIDS,[440] transplant recipients,[365] and in patients with congenital immunodeficiencies. These tumors usually present in the lungs or gastrointestinal tract but also can involve the liver, kidney, lymph nodes, central nervous system, and adrenal glands. The smooth muscle cells contain clonal or oligoclonal EBV DNA. Multiple tumors in the same patient may be from distinct EBV clones, indicating that they can arise independently. The disease usually occurs in the late stage of AIDS or at a mean of 3 years after organ transplant. Persons with primary EBV infection after transplant are at high risk.[669] Tumors can be either of donor or recipient origin in transplant patients. EBV gene expression varies; some tumors show type III EBV latency, while others express EBNA2, but not LMP1. In contrast, leiomyomas and leiomyosarcomas from immunocompetent persons do not contain EBV DNA.

Model for EBV Oncogenesis

While a large number of malignancies are associated with EBV, and new associations continue to be made, certain criteria have proved important for linking EBV to tumors. First, EBV should be in virtually every tumor cell. Second, the viral DNA should be clonal (or oligoclonal), indicating that the malignancy arose from an EBV-infected cell(s). Third, in the case of epithelial cell malignancies, viral DNA should be in dysplastic lesions, indicating that EBV infection occurred during oncogenesis. Fourth, at least one EBV-associated latency gene should be expressed, indicating that the virus has an active role in maintaining the tumor.

Some EBV-associated malignancies are strongly linked with the virus, which clearly is required for development of the tumor (Fig. 11.28). These malignancies have a short latency period between EBV infection or virus reactivation and development of malignancy and occur in highly immunosuppressed persons with little or no EBV-specific T-cell immunity. The tumor cells express most or all of the EBV-associated latency proteins and have few if any host gene mutations. Examples include EBV lymphoproliferative disease occurring early after transplantation or in patients with congenital immunodeficiencies. The low level of cellular immunity to EBV allows expression of the EBV transforming proteins, which rapidly results in transformation without the need for secondary cellular genetic changes.

In contrast, other malignances (e.g., HL) occur in otherwise healthy persons, have longer latency periods, and express an intermediate number of EBV latency genes. These patients

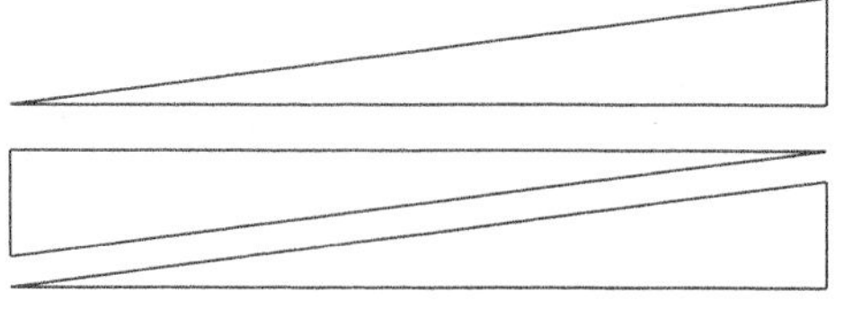

FIGURE 11.28 Model of EBV oncogenesis. EBV-associated malignancies in immunocompromised patients show full expression of EBV latency genes and few or no mutations or changes in cellular gene expression (left), while EBV-associated malignancies in persons with otherwise normal immunity have limited expression of EBV latency genes and more mutations or changes in cellular gene expression (right).

have a degree of impaired T-cell immunity, but to much less an extent than those with EBV PTLD. Viral gene products can substitute for mutations in host cell genes that occur in the analogous EBV-negative tumors (e.g., crippled germinal center cells in HL).

A third class of EBV-associated malignancies (e.g., BL, NPC, gastric carcinoma) arise in patients who seem to be fully immunocompetent or challenged by another infection (e.g., malaria in the case of endemic BL) that may interfere with control of EBV infection. These tumors have mutations in cellular genes and more limited EBV latent gene expression. In EBV-associated epithelial cell malignancies (e.g., NPC, gastric carcinoma), genetic mutations are associated with inactivation of tumor suppressor genes and hyperplastic changes occur before EBV infection of the cells. In BL, EBV may initially drive proliferation of B cells resulting in chromosomal translocation and oncogene activation (e.g., *c-myc* in BL). In these diseases, EBV is clearly a cofactor and virus infection is one of several steps in development of the fully malignant phenotype. However, the presence of clonal EBV in every tumor cell, without loss of viral DNA after tumors are established, indicates that the fully malignant phenotype is dependent on EBV.

Other Diseases Associated With EBV

Chronic lymphocytic leukemia may have a subpopulation of cells infected with EBV and these cells express LMP1 and EBERs. EBV has been associated with transformation of chronic lymphocytic leukemia to diffuse large B-cell lymphoma. EBV has also been detected in T-cell prolymphocytic leukemia cells.

Rheumatoid arthritis patients often have elevated EBV DNA loads in the blood.[79] These patients have an increased risk of lymphomas (HL and diffuse large B-cell lymphoma), even in the absence of immunosuppressive therapy, and 24% of the lymphomas are EBV positive.

Multiple sclerosis (MS) has been associated with EBV in several studies.[36] Unlike the association of EBV with lymphoid and epithelial cell malignancies, the association of EBV with MS (and systemic lupus erythematosis) is primarily epidemiologic and EBV is likely to be a cofactor in these diseases. Primary infection with EBV is associated with an increased risk of MS[374]; persons who are EBV seronegative have a very low risk of MS. A meta-analysis showed a 2.2-fold increased risk of MS after IM. A case–control study showed that 83% of children with MS had evidence of EBV infection, compared with 43% of controls. A study of the prevalence of EBV-specific antibodies prior to the onset of MS found that serum antibodies to the EBNA complex in persons ≥25 years old were 2- to 3-fold higher in those who subsequently developed MS compared to those who did not.[375] The risk of MS was 36-fold higher in persons with high titers of anti-EBNA complex IgG antibodies and 8-fold higher in those with high EBNA1 titers than those with low titers titers.[484] Women in the highest quintile of EBNA1 IgG levels had a 3-fold higher risk of MS than the lowest quintile[483] Children of mothers with high VCA IgG during pregnancy had a 2.4-fold relative risk of MS.[483] A meta-analysis of several studies found an association between MS and anti-EBV VCA IgG, anti-EBNA IgG, and anti-EBNA1 antibody, but not anti-EBV EA IgG, viral DNA in the serum, or DNA in CSF or brain.

Patients with MS have increased numbers and broadened specificity of CD4+ T cells to EBNA1. Patients with active MS have increased CD8+ T-cell responses to lytic EBV antigens.[18] CD107a+ CD8+ T cells recognizing lytic and latent EBV antigens were detected in the meninges or MS lesions of 11 of 12 patients.[625] Elevated levels of both antibodies and T cells to EBNA1 were associated with development of MS. EBNA1-specific T cells cross-reacted with myelin more frequently than autoantigens not associated with MS, and the myelin cross-reactive T cells produced IFN-γ and IL-2.

While most studies have not found EBV DNA or RNA in the brain, one study reported that nearly all postmortem brains from patients with MS showed EBV RNA (EBER) and BFRF1 protein in B-cell follicles, and LMP1 and EBNA2 in perivascular areas in white matter lesions. In contrast, EBV RNA was generally not detected in active plaques or in B cells in the CSF in another study. One study reported higher levels of antibodies to peptide sequences from EBV BRRF2 and EBNA1 in the serum and CSF from patients with MS compared with controls; antibodies to the viral proteins were present in oligoclonal CSF IgG. Increased levels of EBV antibody were detected in the serum and CSF of patients with MS; however, intrathecal synthesis of EBV antibody was uncommon, absent, or nonspecific in other studies. Of 10 patients with MS, treated with autologous EBNA1, LMP1, and LMP2A-specific T cells, 6 had both symptomatic and neurologic improvement and those who improved had T cells with high EBV reactivity.[536]

Systemic lupus erythematosus (SLE) is associated with elevated antibody titers to EBV; however, a prior history of IM is not associated with increased risk of SLE. In one study, 99% of children with SLE had evidence of prior infection with EBV compared with 70% of age matched controls.[283] EBV DNA was detected in the blood of 100% of patients with SLE, compared with 72% of controls. Patients with SLE often have higher EBV loads, increased numbers of latently infected B cells, and have certain EBV-specific antibodies that cross-react with SLE autoantigens. Patients with SLE more often have antibody to EBNA1 and produce antibody to more regions of EBNA1 than healthy persons. Antibody to 60 kDa Ro, which cross-reacts with EBNA1, was detected in some patients with SLE prior to the onset of disease; rabbits immunized with either a 60 kDa Ro or a cross-reacting EBNA1 peptide developed autoantibodies and SLE-like autoimmune disease. Increased levels of EBV VCA IgG and EA IgG were associated with a 1.3-fold or 1.4-fold risk of relatives of patients with SLE transitioning to SLE.[295] Meta-analyses showed a 2-fold higher risk of SLE for persons seropositivity to VCA IgG, a 8-fold higher risk for those who were EA IgG positive, and a 4-fold high risk for persons EBV DNA positive in blood.[381] Evaluation of transcription factors binding sites showed that almost half of GWAS loci associated with SLE are occupied by EBV EBNA2; similar GWAS loci for multiple sclerosis were also shared with EBNA2 sites.[234]

DIAGNOSIS

The diagnosis of IM in patients with typical symptoms is made by a positive heterophile antibody. In patients with atypical symptoms, or in those with typical symptoms and a negative heterophile test, titers of EBV-specific antibodies are measured. Antibody to EBV VCA IgM antibody is the most useful test since the antibody is present only during the first 2 to 3 months of the illness (Fig. 11.17). EBV VCA IgG antibody is often elevated at the time of diagnosis, but since it persists for life, it is not useful for diagnosis of acute infection. Seroconversion to EBV EBNA positivity can be useful since antibodies take 3 to 6 weeks after the onset of illness to become positive and they persist for life. Antibody to EBNA2 is present early in IM, while antibody to EBNA1 is present later during convalescence.

Measurement of plasma EBV DNA is helpful when monitoring for EBV-associated tumors, which release DNA from apoptotic cells into the blood. Detection of EBV DNA in the blood can be useful for diagnosis of IM if serologic results are equivocal. Measurement of EBV DNA is also used to follow patients after transplant to predict the development of EBV PTLD or to follow patients with EBV PTLD, Hodgkin lymphoma, or NK/T-cell lymphoma after therapy.[212,330] Measurement of EBV DNA in whole blood (combined plasma and cells) is helpful for monitoring patients with EBV lymphoproliferative diseases associated with immune deficiencies and with CAEBV. The World Health Organization international standard for EBV has reduced the variability of whole-blood EBV DNA PCR results between laboratories.[624] Elevated levels of plasma EBV DNA is more specific than whole-blood EBV DNA for diagnosis of EBV diseases, but the latter is more sensitive to detect EBV in blood of immunocompromised persons.[306] Detection of cell-free EBV DNA in blood has been a useful marker to follow patients with NPC, NK/T-cell lymphoma, and Hodgkin lymphoma.[305]

Detection of EBV DNA in the cerebrospinal fluid of AIDS patients with lesions in the brain can be helpful for prediction of lymphoma. Culture of throat washings for EBV is not useful for diagnosis of IM since the virus persists for life in the throat of infected persons. PCR for the terminal repeats is used to determine if EBV is clonal in tissues, since individual clones have a fixed number of terminal repeats.

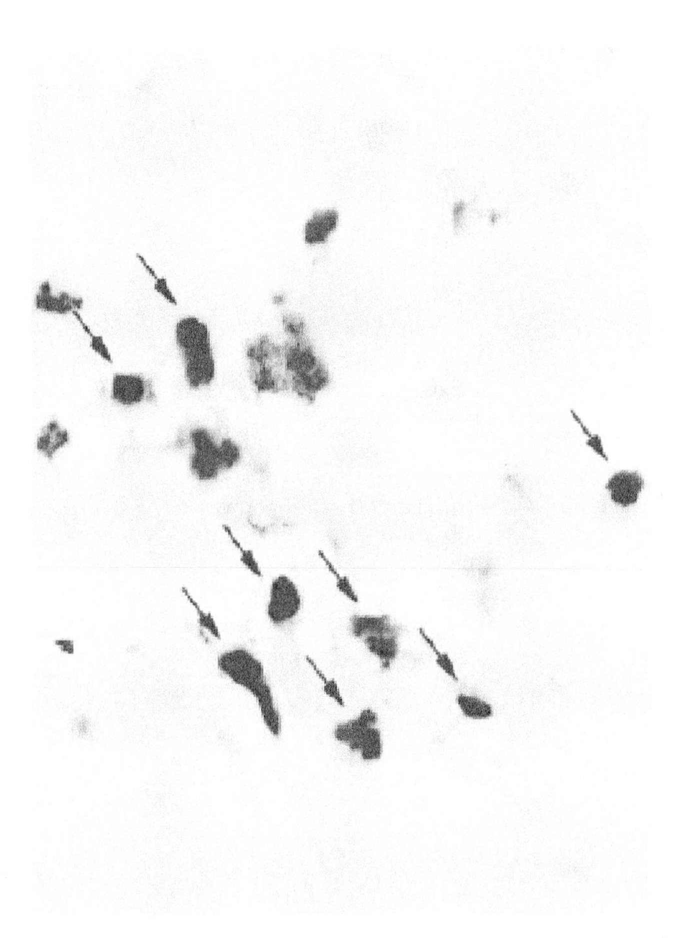

FIGURE 11.29 **EBER staining from a biopsy showing EBV lymphoma.** *Arrows* show cells that hybridize with the EBER probe. (From Cohen JI. Epstein-Barr virus infection. *N Engl J Med* 2000:343(7): 481–492. Copyright © 2000 Massachusetts Medical Society. Reprinted with permission from Massachusetts Medical Society.)

EBV is usually detected in tissue by *in situ* hybridization using a probe for EBER (Fig. 11.29) since this RNA is present at thousands of copies per cell. EBV latency proteins, including EBNA1, EBNA2, or LMP1, can also be detected in tissues. The characteristics of cells that EBV infects in blood can be determined by combined fluorescence *in situ* hybridrization and cell surface staining, or by staining for EBER and cell markers followed by flow cytometry.[129,195,331]

INHIBITORS OF REPLICATION

Acyclovir and ganciclovir inhibit the viral DNA polymerase but do not inhibit latent infection. Phosphorylation of acyclovir and ganciclovir is mediated by the EBV BGLF4 protein kinase, not the viral thymidine kinase (encoded by BXLF1). While treatment of chronic EBV carriers with acyclovir stops EBV shedding from the oropharynx, 1 month of therapy has no effect on the EBV viral load in the blood.[740] However, 1 year of antiviral therapy resulted in a modest reduction in the EBV viral load in the blood but did not affect the EBV DNA copy number per B cell.[257] Brincidofovir, a hexadecyloxypropyl ester of cidofovir, is greater than 100 times more potent as an inhibitor of EBV replication than acyclovir. Maribavir, an

L-ribofuranoside benzimidazole, blocks phosphorylation of viral proteins by the EBV protein kinase and inhibits viral transcription, which results in reduced EBV replication.

TREATMENT

Infectious Mononucleosis

Treatment of IM is supportive. Contact sports should be avoided during the acute phase of the disease due to the risk of splenic rupture. While antiviral therapy reduces or eliminates virus replication and shedding from the oropharynx, it has no effect on symptoms. Corticosteroids reduce the duration of fever and sore throat; however, they may inhibit the development of cellular immunity to the virus and are not recommended for most cases of IM. The combination of corticosteroids and antiviral therapy did not reduce time off from work or school or the duration of the disease.[703] Corticosteroids are used for life-threatening complications such as upper airway obstruction due to tonsil enlargement, severe hemolytic anemia, and some cases of cardiac or central nervous system EBV disease.

EBV Posttransplant Lymphoproliferative Disease

Reduction in immunosuppression can allow an increase in EBV-specific T-cell activity against virus-infected B cells and in some cases, especially disease that occurs early after organ transplant, can cause tumor regression.[213] Rituximab, which depletes CD20-positive B cells, can be effective, especially in combination with chemotherapy. Surgery can be effective when PTLD lesions are confined to a single site. Cytotoxic chemotherapy (e.g., CHOP) is often effective early after transplant or in cases of rituximab failure. Radiation as well as high-dose methotrexate is often used for disease involving the central nervous system. Antiviral therapy has no effect once PTLD is established, since the EBV genome replicates in latently infected cells using the host, not viral, DNA polymerase.

Most tumors are of donor origin in hematopoietic stem transplant (HSCT) recipients. Thus, in these patients, infusion of donor lymphocytes has been successful although GVHD can occur.[524] EBV-specific T cells, either from stem cell donors[525] or HLA-matched donors from a donor bank,[561,704] have been used to treat EBV PTLD. Functional gene-marked CTLs persisted for up to 9 years. Immune escape from EBV-specific CTLs was reported in one bone marrow transplant recipient whose tumor cells mutated, deleting two EBNA3B epitopes, which resulted in a fatal outcome.

Most EBV PTLD in organ transplant patients is recipient in origin. In these patients, reduction of immunosuppressive therapy can increase the level of EBV-specific T cells and may cure the disease. In some cases, EBV-specific CTLs have been expanded from organ transplant recipients and successfully treated the disease. Partially HLA-matched allogeneic T cells from a donor bank that covered 95% of common HLA haplotypes resulted in a complete remission in 42% of patients with PTLD (most of whom had undergone organ transplant) who had progressive disease despite conventional therapy.[231,561]

CTLs that recognize adenovirus, CMV, and EBV have been developed by incubating PBMCs with autologous EBV LCLs transducted with an adenovirus vector expressing a CMV gene; infusions of the CTLs into transplant recipients and their subsequent expansion in the blood were associated with lower levels of EBV DNA in the blood and resolution of EBV PTLD.[370] A rapid method of producing EBV-specific T cells involves stimulation of donor cells with EBV-specific peptides and antibody-mediated capture of cells expressing surface IFN-γ; this technique allowed isolation of EBV-specific T cells from donor blood in 36 hours and resulted in remissions in patients with early-stage PTLD.

While most EBV-specific T-cell therapies have focused on CD8+ T cells that recognize EBV antigen, some CD4+ T cells recognize EBV-transformed B cells not through viral antigens, but likely by cellular antigens that are induced by the virus. The latter may provide additional targets for T-cell therapy. Lymphokine-activated autologous killer cells have been effective in small numbers of organ transplant recipients with disease.

Hodgkin Lymphoma

Infusion of allogeneic EBV-specific CTLs into patients with refractory HL resulted in reduction in disease in some patients; however, the donor cells could not be detected in the recipients. CTLs were made to EBV-transformed B cells and infused into patients with EBV-positive HL; of 11 patients with measurable tumors, 2 had a complete response, 5 had stable disease, 1 had a partial response, and 3 had no response.[53] However, CTLs produced using dendritic cells transduced with LMP2 resulted in a higher frequency of LMP2-specific CTLs and induced a complete response in 4 of 6 patients with HL or NHL and relapsed disease, and maintained remissions in 9 of 10 patients. Infusion of EBV LMP1- and LMP2-specific CTLs into 21 patients with resistant or relapsed EBV-positive lymphomas resulted in 11 complete responses.[55]

Nasopharyngeal Carcinoma

A phase I trial showed that vaccination with a poxvirus (MVA) expressing the carboxyl terminal half of EBNA1 fused to LMP2 showed that the vaccine induced EBV-specific T-cell responses *in vivo*.[682] Dendritic cells from patients with NPC were pulsed with LMP2 peptides *in vitro*, and when injected into patients, they resulted in epitope-specific T-cell responses in the blood coincident with tumor regression in some patients.

Infusion of autologous EBV-specific T cells in patients with late-stage NPC resulted in control of disease in 6 of 10 patients; 3 of 4 patients with LMP2-specific immune responses after infusion had a clinical benefit. A second study by the same authors used higher doses of EBV-specific T cells after lymphodepletion by chemotherapy and reported control of disease in 6 of 11 patients.[622] In another trial, 10 patients with advanced NPC were treated with autologous EBV-specific CTLs; 4 patients who had been in remission remained disease free, and of 6 with refractory disease before treatment, 2 had complete responses, 1 had a partial remission, 1 had stable disease, and 2 had no response.[668] A phase I/II study of 23 patients (including 10 patients reported previously[668] with recurrent or refractory NPC showed that infusion of autologous EBV-specific T cells resulted in disease-free outcomes in 62% of patients who had been in remission at the time of infusions, while 49% who had active disease at the time of the infusions had a complete or partial response. Patients with metastatic disease had a worse outcome than those with locoregional disease. A phase 1/2 trial of autologous EBV-specific CTLs in 21 patients with recurrent metastatic NPC yielded a median progression-free survival of only 2.2 months.[262] EBNA1-, LMP1-, and LMP2-specific

T cells from patients with NPC were expanded ex vivo and infused into the patients resulting in an increased median overall survival compared with patients who did not receive the cells.[652]

Other Therapies

Other therapies to treat EBV diseases include the use of combined cytotoxic chemotherapeutic agents and ganciclovir to induce virus replication, express the viral protein kinase to phosphorylate ganciclovir (which is toxic to cells), and kill EBV-infected cells. Combined administration of ganciclovir and arginine butyrate (a HDAC inhibitor) resulted in EBV-positive tumor responses in 10 of 15 patients.[539] Romidepsin is the most effective of the FDA-approved HDAC inhibitors to induce lytic replication of EBV *in vitro*.[266]

HDAC inhibitors also increase the effectiveness of chemotherapeutic agents by inducing lytic replication in animal models of EBV lymphoma. Adenovirus expressing EBV IE genes reduced EBV tumor growth in mice. Demethylating agents such as 5-azacytadine also activate viral gene expression. Other approaches include low-dose hydroxyurea to reduce EBV episome copy number and rapamycin, which induces cell cycle arrest at the G1 phase in EBV-transformed B cells and inhibits growth of EBV lymphomas in SCID mice. Ritonavir, an HIV protease inhibitor, down-regulates survivin and cyclin D2, inhibits activation of NF-κB, and induces apoptosis in EBV-transformed B cells and inhibits growth of lymphoma cells in immunocompromised mice. Hsp90 inhibitors reduce EBNA1 expression and inhibit the growth EBV-transformed B cells in SCID mice. Ganetespib, an HSP90 inhibitor, improved survival in mice inoculated with transformed B cells and reduced the percentage of EBV-infected cells in the blood of a patient.[632] An HSP90 inhibitor reduced tumor formation with NPC cell xenografts in mice.[95] An HSP90 inhibitor reduced the growth of EBV-positive NK cell xenografts in mice.[488]

Bortezomib, a proteasome inhibitor, and Bay 11-7082 block NF-κB, induce apoptosis of EBV-transformed B cells, and enhance survival of mice injected with LCLs.[765] SAHA and bortezomib inhibit EBV lymphomas in a mouse model. Combined inhibitor of mTOR and PI3K/Akt inhibited EBV tumor growth in immunocompromised mice.[607] JQ1, an inhibitor of bromodomain and extra-terminal (BET) proteins, inhibited tumor growth in a mouse xenograft model.[237] Monoclonal antibody to CCR4 (mogamulizumab) inhibited the growth of EBV-positive NK cell lymphoma in mice.[307]

Based on the structure of EBNA1, benzoic acid–based inhibitors were designed that inhibit EBNA1 binding to DNA, block EBV transcription, and reduce growth of patient-derived tumors in mice[453]; one of these inhibitors has been tested in patients with EBV-positive nasopharyngeal carcinoma. A computational designed inhibitor of the apoptosis inhibitor EBV BHRF1 induced apoptosis in tumor cells and prolonged survival of EBV-positive lymphomas in mice.[560] GAP31, a plant-derived protein, inhibited EBNA1 dimerization and EBV transformation of B cells and reduced growth of EBV-positive tumors in mice.[633]

PREVENTION AND VACCINES

Preemptive therapy for EBV lymphoproliferative disease has included antiviral therapy with acyclovir or ganciclovir. Results have been mixed, with more recent studies reporting a reduction in disease, while other studies showing no effect. Depletion of B cells from bone marrow used for transplantation reduces the risk of EBV PTLD, presumably due to removal of virus-infected cells. A single dose of rituximab (anti-CD20 antibody) given to allogeneic HSCT patients at high risk for EBV PTLD with rising viral loads reduced the rate of disease from 49% based on an historical cohort to 18% in the treated group and prevented death at 6 months.[176] However, relapses due to CD20-negative EBV-infected B cells have occurred that require other therapy. An alternative approach is to monitor patients with rising viral loads and to give rituximab or EBV-specific CTLs only when systemic symptoms occur. Infusion of EBV-specific T cells (directed again EBV latency-associated proteins) has been effective in reducing the EBV load in the blood and preventing EBV-associated PTLD in HSCT recipients.[213,248,590] A study of EBV-specific CTLs for prevention of EBV PTLD found that none of 101 patients who received CTLs developed the disease. Donor-derived EBV-specific CTLs have prevented disease in matched unrelated and haploidentical stem cell transplants. Prophylactic treatment with rituximab markedly reduced the risk of PTLD in haplo-cord blood transplant recipients.[707]

Reduction of immunosuppression is often effective early after transplantation when viral loads increase. In a study of 73 liver transplant recipients in which immunosuppression was tapered when EBV viral loads were elevated, one patient developed allograft rejection, but the incidence of PTLD declined from 16% to 2%. EBV-specific T cells prevented development of EBV-positive lymphomas when they were given as prophylaxis to T-cell depleted bone marrow transplant recipients with high EBV loads after transplant and at high risk of the disease; the cells can persist for at least 18 months.[248] Autologous EBV-specific T cells have also been used to prevent EBV lymphomas in solid organ transplants with high viral loads. Donor-derived LMP1-specific T cells reduced the rate of relapse after transplant for B-cell or T-cell EBV lymphoma or lymphoproliferative disease.[444]

Vaccination to prevent EBV infection or disease will be important in certain high-risk groups including transplant recipients, boys with mutations in SAP or XIAP, and areas where the frequency of NPC and BL are high.[121] Vaccination that reduces the rate of IM might reduce the frequency of EBV-positive HL, which is increased during the first 5 years after IM.

gp350 has been the major immunogen in vaccine studies; it is the major target for neutralizing antibody[65] and it is a target of CTLs. Infusion of immunodeficient mice, reconstituted with PBMCs from EBV negative persons, with monoclonal antibody to gp350 prevented development of EBV lymphomas after challenge with virus[230] and a monoclonal antibody to gH/gL reduced viremia in humanized mice challenged with EBV and monkeys challenged with rhesus LCV.[637] Vaccination with soluble gp350 protected cottontop tamarins from lymphoma when challenged with EBV. While immunization of marmosets with gp350 reduced infection, protection did not always correlate with development of neutralizing antibody. Rhesus LCV is the homolog of EBV in rhesus macaques. Immunization of rhesus macaques with soluble rhesus LCV gp350 resulted in better protection from infection and reduced viral loads 2 years after infection in animals that became infected after challenge, when compared with virus-like replicon particles expressing rhesus LCV gp350, EBNA3A, and EBNA3B.[610]

A study of 19 seronegative children (1 to 3 years old) in China randomized to vaccination with vaccinia virus expressing gp350 or control found that at 16 months all 10 unvaccinated children were infected with EBV, while only 3 of 9 vaccinated children were infected. A study of 181 EBV-seronegative adults randomized to receive three doses of soluble gp350 in monophosphoryl lipid A/alum adjuvant or placebo showed that the vaccine reduced the rate of EBV IM by 78% but did not affect the rate of virus infection.[477,655] A phase I trial of children with chronic kidney disease using three injections of a lower dose of gp350 in alum showed that the vaccine induced neutralizing antibody in 33% of subjects receiving the highest dose of gp350 and immune responses declined rapidly; the authors concluded that a more prolonged vaccine schedule or an improved adjuvant was needed for these patients.

Vaccination of mice with a tetrameric form of gp350[139] or rabbits with trimeric gH/gL or trimeric gB[138] induced higher levels of antibody than the monomeric gp350. Vaccination of mice with gH/gL-EBNA1 and gB-LMP2 virus-like particles also induced high titer neutralizing antibody as well as virus-specific T-cell responses.[538] Vaccination of rabbits with gp350, gB, gp42, gH, and gL virus-like particles induced antibodies that protected B cells and epithelial cells from infection *in vitro*.[175] Presentation of gp350 on nanoparticles enhanced the levels of neutralizing antibody in monkeys compared with soluble gp350 and focused the immune response on the CR2 (receptor) binding site on gp350 in monkeys.[308] Vaccination of mice and nonhuman primates with nanoparticles displaying EBV glycoproteins (gH/gL/gp42) induced potent neutralizing antibody that protected B cells and epithelial cells from infection and blocked EBV glycoprotein-mediated cell fusion.[65]

An alternative or complementary strategy is to induce potent T-cell responses to control primary infection so as to reduce the viral load after infection and potentially reduce the risk of EBV-associated malignancy. A study of 14 HLA B*0801 EBV-seronegative adults randomized to receive an HLA B*0801 EBV EBNA3A peptide (FLRGRAYGL) and tetanus toxoid in a water in oil adjuvant showed that 8 of the 9 volunteers developed epitope-specific T-cell responses.[168] At 2 to 12 years after follow-up, 1 of 2 placebo recipients developed IM, while 4/4 vaccinees that became infected with EBV did not develop IM. Virus-like particles expressing nearly all the EBV genes except for BZLF1, EBNA2, 3A, 3B, 3C, and LMP1 and the terminal repeats induced neutralizing antibody and T-cell responses in mice. Vaccination of mice with virus-like and light particles that contain lytic and latent EBV antigens resulted in virus-specific T cells that controlled outgrowth of EBV, and particles containing EBNA1 protected mice from wild-type EBV in humanized mice.[768] Vaccination of transgenic mice with adenovirus expressing EBNA1, following by boosting with MVA expressing EBNA1, resulted in protection both as a prophylactic and therapeutic vaccine to prevent or treat EBV lymphoma.[593]

PERSPECTIVE

While we have learned much about EBV, many important questions remain. The precise mechanisms by which EBV is associated with malignancies, and how these relate to the establishment and reactivation from latency, are still being uncovered. Much remains to be learned about EBV gene regulation in newly infected and latently infected cells, including how long-range DNA interactions and epigenetic pathways control EBV programs. Knowledge remains incomplete of how EBV causes these cells to differentiate into memory B cells, and whether these reservoir cells differ from uninfected memory B cells. Many EBV lytic gene products remain poorly studied, and roles for miRNAs and circular RNAs remain to be fully characterized. It is not fully apparent why EBV IM is primarily a disease of adolescents and young adults, though humanized mouse models and human studies will continue to provide new insights. The types of immune responses needed to prevent EBV infection, EBV mononucleosis, or virus-associated malignancies are uncertain. The role of EBV in multiple sclerosis and other autoimmune diseases is still unclear. While EBV-specific CTLs have often been effective in the treatment of EBV posttransplant lymphoma, these cells have been less effective in the treatment of NPC and EBV-associated lymphomas, and improved virus-specific therapies are needed. Newer therapies to block EBV immune evasion mechanisms or to alter EBV genome programs to allow latently infected cells to be better recognized and killed by the immune system are needed. Finally, while small scale trials have shown that an EBV vaccine can reduce the incidence of IM but not the rate of infection, larger trials with more effective vaccines are needed to prevent EBV infection and/or disease. EBV continues to teach us about B-cell biology, and studies of immune deficiencies that predispose to severe EBV infections inform us about how the immune system controls virus infections. Thus, the study of EBV continues to enrich our knowledge of human biology and virology and further progress should help to reduce the burden of EBV-associated cancer.

ACKNOWLEDGMENTS

The authors acknowledge the mentorship of Elliott Kieff, with whom all of us trained and who has greatly influenced our understanding of EBV. We also acknowledge Alan Rickinson, who along with Elliott Kieff wrote earlier versions of this chapter, and who have shaped our knowledge about EBV. We thank Nancy Raab-Traub and Alan Rickinson for reviewing this chapter and for valuable suggestions. We acknowledge the assistance of our colleagues, in particular Dr. Rui Guo. J.I.C. is supported by the Intramural Research Program of NIAID. R.L. is the Dan and Bertha Spear Research Professor and is supported by grants from the NIAID and NINDS. B.E.G. is supported by grants from NIAID, NCI, and a Burroughs Wellcome Career Award in Medical Sciences. Additional references can be found in the prior edition of this chapter in Fields Virology.

REFERENCES

1. Aalto SM, Juvonen E, Tarkkanen J, et al. Epstein-Barr viral load and disease prediction in a large cohort of allogeneic stem cell transplant recipients. *Clin Infect Dis* 2007;45(10):1305–1309.
2. Abbot SD, Rowe M, Cadwallader K, et al. Epstein-Barr virus nuclear antigen 2 induces expression of the virus- encoded latent membrane protein. *J Virol* 1990;64(5):2126–2134.
3. Abbott RJ, Pachnio A, Pedroza-Pacheco I, et al. Asymptomatic primary infection with Epstein-Barr virus: observations on young adult cases. *J Virol* 2017;91(21).
4. Abbott RJ, Quinn LL, Leese AM, et al. CD8+ T cell responses to lytic EBV infection: late antigen specificities as subdominant components of the total response. *J Immunol* 2013;191(11):5398–5409.
5. Adamson AL. Effects of SUMO-1 upon Epstein-Barr virus BZLF1 function and BMRF1 expression. *Biochem Biophys Res Commun* 2005;336(1):22–28.

6. Adhikary D, Damaschke J, Mautner J, et al. The Epstein-Barr virus major tegument protein BNRF1 is a common target of cytotoxic CD4+ T cells. *J Virol* 2020;94:e00284.
7. Albanese M, Tagawa T, Bouvet M, et al. Epstein-Barr virus microRNAs reduce immune surveillance by virus-specific CD8+ T cells. *Proc Natl Acad Sci U S A* 2016;113(42): E6467–E6475.
8. Alfieri C, Birkenbach M, Kieff E. Early events in Epstein-Barr virus infection of human B lymphocytes [published erratum appears in Virology 1991 Dec;185(2):946]. *Virology* 1991;181(2):595–608.
9. Allday MJ, Bazot Q, White RE. The EBNA3 family: two oncoproteins and a tumour suppressor that are central to the biology of EBV in B cells. *Curr Top Microbiol Immunol* 2015;391:61–117.
10. Allen MD, Young LS, Dawson CW. The Epstein-Barr virus-encoded LMP2A and LMP2B proteins promote epithelial cell spreading and motility. *J Virol* 2005;79(3):1789–1802.
11. Altmann M, Hammerschmidt W. Epstein-Barr virus provides a new paradigm: a requirement for the immediate inhibition of apoptosis. *PLoS Biol* 2005;3(12):e404.
12. Altmann M, Pich D, Ruiss R, et al. Transcriptional activation by EBV nuclear antigen 1 is essential for the expression of EBV's transforming genes. *Proc Natl Acad Sci U S A* 2006;103(38):14188–14193.
13. Amoroso R, Fitzsimmons L, Thomas WA, et al. Quantitative studies of Epstein-Barr virus-encoded microRNAs provide novel insights into their regulation. *J Virol* 2011;85(2):996–1010.
14. Anagnostopoulos I, Hummel M, Kreschel C, et al. Morphology, immunophenotype, and distribution of latently and/or productively Epstein-Barr virus-infected cells in acute infectious mononucleosis: implications for the interindividual infection route of Epstein-Barr virus. *Blood* 1995;85(3):744–750.
15. Anderson LJ, Longnecker R. An auto-regulatory loop for EBV LMP2A involves activation of Notch. *Virology* 2008;371(2):257–266.
16. Anderson LJ, Longnecker R. EBV LMP2A provides a surrogate pre-B cell receptor signal through constitutive activation of the ERK/MAPK pathway. *J Gen Virol* 2008;89(Pt 7): 1563–1568.
17. Anderson LJ, Longnecker R. Epstein-Barr virus latent membrane protein 2A exploits Notch1 to alter B-cell identity in vivo. *Blood* 2009;113(1):108–116.
18. Angelini DF, Serafini B, Piras E, et al. Increased CD8+ T cell response to Epstein-Barr virus lytic antigens in the active phase of multiple sclerosis. *PLoS Pathog* 2013;9(4):e1003220.
19. Aozasa K, Takakuwa T, Nakatsuka S. Pyothorax-associated lymphoma: a lymphoma developing in chronic inflammation. *Adv Anat Pathol* 2005;12(6):324–331.
20. Arvey A, Tempera I, Lieberman PM. Interpreting the Epstein-Barr Virus (EBV) epigenome using high-throughput data. *Viruses* 2013;5(4):1042–1054.
21. Asai R, Kato A, Kato K, et al. Epstein-Barr virus protein kinase BGLF4 is a virion tegument protein that dissociates from virions in a phosphorylation-dependent process and phosphorylates the viral immediate-early protein BZLF1. *J Virol* 2006;80(11):5125–5134.
22. Asai R, Kato A, Kawaguchi Y. Epstein-Barr virus protein kinase BGLF4 interacts with viral transactivator BZLF1 and regulates its transactivation activity. *J Gen Virol* 2009;90(Pt 7): 1575–1581.
23. Babcock GJ, Decker LL, Freeman RB, et al. Epstein-barr virus-infected resting memory B cells, not proliferating lymphoblasts, accumulate in the peripheral blood of immunosuppressed patients. *J Exp Med* 1999;190(4):567–576.
24. Babcock GJ, Decker LL, Volk M, et al. EBV persistence in memory B cells in vivo. *Immunity* 1998;9(3):395–404.
25. Babcock GJ, Thorley-Lawson DA. Tonsillar memory B cells, latently infected with Epstein-Barr virus, express the restricted pattern of latent genes previously found only in Epstein-Barr virus-associated tumors. *Proc Natl Acad Sci U S A* 2000;97(22):12250–12255.
26. Backovic M, Longnecker R, Jardetzky TS. Structure of a trimeric variant of the Epstein-Barr virus glycoprotein B. *Proc Natl Acad Sci U S A* 2009;106(8):2880–2885.
27. Baer R, Bankier AT, Biggin MD, et al. DNA sequence and expression of the B95-8 Epstein-Barr virus genome. *Nature* 1984;310(5974):207–211.
28. Baichwal VR, Hammerschmidt W, Sugden B. Characterization of the BNLF-1 oncogene of Epstein-Barr virus. *Curr Top Microbiol Immunol* 1989;144:233–239.
29. Baichwal VR, Sugden B. Transformation of Balb 3T3 cells by the BNLF-1 gene of Epstein-Barr virus. *Oncogene* 1988;2(5):461–467.
30. Balfour HH, Jr., Odumade OA, Schmeling DO, et al. Behavioral, virologic, and immunologic factors associated with acquisition and severity of primary Epstein-Barr virus infection in university students. *J Infect Dis* 2013;207(1):80–88.
31. Balfour HH Jr, Sifakis F, Sliman JA, et al. Age-specific prevalence of Epstein-Barr virus infection among individuals aged 6-19 years in the United States and factors affecting its acquisition. *J Infect Dis* 2013;208(8):1286–1293.
32. Banerjee S, Lu J, Cai Q, et al. EBNA3C augments Pim-1 mediated phosphorylation and degradation of p21 to promote B-cell proliferation. *PLoS Pathog* 2014;10(8):e1004304.
33. Banerjee S, Lu J, Cai Q, et al. The EBV latent antigen 3C inhibits apoptosis through targeted regulation of interferon regulatory factors 4 and 8. *PLoS Pathog* 2013;9(5):e1003314.
34. Bangalore-Prakash P, Stunz LL, Mambetsariev N, et al. The oncogenic membrane protein LMP1 sequesters TRAF3 in B-cell lymphoma cells to produce functional TRAF3 deficiency. *Blood Adv* 2017;1(27):2712–2723.
35. Bankier AT, Deininger PL, Farrell PJ, et al. Sequence analysis of the 17,166 base-pair EcoRI fragment C of B95-8 Epstein-Barr virus. *Mol Biol Med* 1983;1(1):21–45.
36. Bar-Or A, Pender MP, Khanna R, et al. Epstein-Barr virus in multiple sclerosis: theory and emerging immunotherapies. *Trends Mol Med* 2020;26(3):296–310.
37. Bazot Q, Paschos K, Skalska L, et al. Epstein-Barr virus proteins EBNA3A and EBNA3C together induce expression of the oncogenic MicroRNA cluster miR-221/miR-222 and ablate expression of its target p57KIP2. *PLoS Pathog* 2015;11(7):e1005031.
38. Beaufils P, Choquet D, Mamoun RZ, et al. The (YXXL/I)2 signalling motif found in the cytoplasmic segments of the bovine leukaemia virus envelope protein and Epstein-Barr virus latent membrane protein 2A can elicit early and late lymphocyte activation events. *EMBO J* 1993;12(13):5105–5112.
39. Bell AI, Groves K, Kelly GL, et al. Analysis of Epstein-Barr virus latent gene expression in endemic Burkitt's lymphoma and nasopharyngeal carcinoma tumour cells by using quantitative real-time PCR assays. *J Gen Virol* 2006;87(Pt 10):2885–2890.
40. Bentz GL, Moss CR II, Whitehurst CB, et al. LMP1-induced sumoylation influences the maintenance of Epstein-Barr virus latency through KAP1. *J Virol* 2015;89(15):7465–7477.
41. Bentz GL, Shackelford J, Pagano JS. Epstein-Barr virus latent membrane protein 1 regulates the function of interferon regulatory factor 7 by inducing its sumoylation. *J Virol* 2012;86(22):12251–12261.
42. Bentz GL, Whitehurst CB, Pagano JS. Epstein-Barr virus latent membrane protein 1 (LMP1) C-terminal-activating region 3 contributes to LMP1-mediated cellular migration via its interaction with Ubc9. *J Virol* 2011;85(19):10144–10153.
43. Bhaduri-McIntosh S, Landry ML, Nikiforow S, et al. Serum IgA antibodies to Epstein-Barr virus (EBV) early lytic antigens are present in primary EBV infection. *J Infect Dis* 2007;195(4):483–492.
44. Bhende PM, Dickerson SJ, Sun X, et al. X-box-binding protein 1 activates lytic Epstein-Barr virus gene expression in combination with protein kinase D. *J Virol* 2007;81(14):7363–7370.
45. Bhende PM, Seaman WT, Delecluse HJ, et al. The EBV lytic switch protein, Z, preferentially binds to and activates the methylated viral genome. *Nat Genet* 2004;36(10):1099–1104.
46. Bieging KT, Amick AC, Longnecker R. Epstein-Barr virus LMP2A bypasses p53 inactivation in a MYC model of lymphomagenesis. *Proc Natl Acad Sci U S A* 2009;106(42): 17945–17950.
47. Bieging KT, Fish K, Bondada S, et al. A shared gene expression signature in mouse models of EBV-associated and non-EBV-associated Burkitt lymphoma. *Blood* 2011;118(26): 6849–6859.
48. Biggin M, Bodescot M, Perricaudet M, et al. Epstein-Barr virus gene expression in P3HR1-superinfected Raji cells. *J Virol* 1987;61(10):3120–3132.
49. Birdwell CE, Queen KJ, Kilgore PC, et al. Genome-wide DNA methylation as an epigenetic consequence of Epstein-Barr virus infection of immortalized keratinocytes. *J Virol* 2014;88(19):11442–11458.
50. Birx DL, Redfield RR, Tosato G. Defective regulation of Epstein-Barr virus infection in patients with acquired immunodeficiency syndrome (AIDS) or AIDS-related disorders. *N Engl J Med* 1986;314(14):874–879.
51. Bobrovnitchaia I, Valieris R, Drummond RD, et al. APOBEC-mediated DNA alterations: a possible new mechanism of carcinogenesis in EBV-positive gastric cancer. *Int J Cancer* 2020;146:181–191.
52. Bochkarev A, Barwell JA, Pfuetzner RA, et al. Crystal structure of the DNA-binding domain of the Epstein-Barr virus origin-binding protein, EBNA1, bound to DNA. *Cell* 1996;84(5):791–800.
53. Bollard CM, Aguilar L, Straathof KC, et al. Cytotoxic T lymphocyte therapy for Epstein-Barr virus+ Hodgkin's disease. *J Exp Med* 2004;200(12):1623–1633.
54. Bollard CM, Cohen JI. How I treat T-cell chronic active Epstein-Barr virus disease. *Blood* 2018;131(26):2899–2905.
55. Bollard CM, Gottschalk S, Torrano V, et al. Sustained complete responses in patients with lymphoma receiving autologous cytotoxic T lymphocytes targeting Epstein-Barr virus latent membrane proteins. *J Clin Oncol* 2014;32(8):798–808.
56. Booth C, Gilmour KC, Veys P, et al. X-linked lymphoproliferative disease due to SAP/SH2D1A deficiency: a multicenter study on the manifestations, management, and outcome of the disease. *Blood* 2011;117:53–63.
57. Borza CM, Hutt-Fletcher LM. Alternate replication in B cells and epithelial cells switches tropism of Epstein-Barr virus. *Nat Med* 2002;8(6):594–599.
58. Borza CM, Morgan AJ, Turk SM, et al. Use of gHgL for attachment of Epstein-Barr virus to epithelial cells compromises infection. *J Virol* 2004;78(10):5007–5014.
59. Brauninger A, Spieker T, Mottok A, et al. Epstein-Barr virus (EBV)-positive lymphoproliferations in post-transplant patients show immunoglobulin V gene mutation patterns suggesting interference of EBV with normal B cell differentiation processes. *Eur J Immunol* 2003;33(6):1593–1602.
60. Brielmeier M, Mautner J, Laux G, et al. The latent membrane protein 2 gene of Epstein-Barr virus is important for efficient B cell immortalization. *J Gen Virol* 1996;77(Pt 11): 2807–2818.
61. Bristol JA, Djavadian R, Albright ER, et al. A cancer-associated Epstein-Barr virus BZLF1 promoter variant enhances lytic infection. *PLoS Pathog* 2018;14(7):e1007179.
62. Brooks JM, Lee SP, Leese AM, et al. Cyclical expression of EBV latent membrane protein 1 in EBV-transformed B cells underpins heterogeneity of epitope presentation and CD8+ T cell recognition. *J Immunol* 2009;182(4):1919–1928.
63. Brooks JM, Long HM, Tierney RJ, et al. Early T cell recognition of B cells following Epstein-Barr virus infection: identifying potential targets for prophylactic vaccination. *PLoS Pathog* 2016;12(4):e1005549.
64. Bu W, Hayes GM, Liu H, et al. Kinetics of Epstein-Barr Virus (EBV) neutralizing and virus-specific antibodies after primary infection with EBV. *Clin Vaccine Immunol* 2016;23(4):363–369.
65. Bu W, Joyce MG, Nguyen H, et al. Immunization with components of the viral fusion apparatus elicits antibodies that neutralize Epstein-Barr Virus in B cells and epithelial cells. *Immunity* 2019;50(5):1305–1316.e1306.
66. Burkhardt AL, Bolen JB, Kieff E, et al. An Epstein-Barr virus transformation-associated membrane protein interacts with src family tyrosine kinases. *J Virol* 1992;66(8): 5161–5167.
67. Burkitt D. A sarcoma involving the jaws in African children. *Br J Surg* 1958;46(197): 218–223.
68. Burton EM, Goldbach-Mansky R, Bhaduri-McIntosh S. A promiscuous inflammasome sparks replication of a common tumor virus. *Proc Natl Acad Sci U S A* 2020;117(3):1722–1730.
69. Buschle A, Hammerschmidt W. Epigenetic lifestyle of Epstein-Barr virus. *Semin Immunopathol* 2020;42(2):131–142.
70. Cahir McFarland ED, Izumi KM, Mosialos G. Epstein-Barr virus transformation: involvement of latent membrane protein 1-mediated activation of NF-kappaB. *Oncogene* 1999;18(49):6959–6964.
71. Cahir-McFarland ED, Carter K, Rosenwald A, et al. Role of NF-kappa B in cell survival and transcription of latent membrane protein 1-expressing or Epstein-Barr virus latency III-infected cells. *J Virol* 2004;78(8):4108–4119.

72. Cahir-McFarland ED, Davidson DM, Schauer SL, et al. NF-kappa B inhibition causes spontaneous apoptosis in Epstein-Barr virus-transformed lymphoblastoid cells. *Proc Natl Acad Sci U S A* 2000;97(11):6055–6060.
73. Cahir-McFarland E, Kieff E. NF-kappaB inhibition in EBV-transformed lymphoblastoid cell lines. *Recent Results Cancer Res* 2002;159:44–48.
74. Cai X, Schafer A, Lu S, et al. Epstein-Barr virus microRNAs are evolutionarily conserved and differentially expressed. *PLoS Pathog* 2006;2(3):e23.
75. Calattini S, Sereti I, Scheinberg P, et al. Detection of EBV genomes in plasmablasts/plasma cells and non-B cells in the blood of most patients with EBV lymphoproliferative disorders by using Immuno-FISH. *Blood* 2010;116(22):4546–4559.
76. Calderwood MA, Holthaus AM, Johannsen E. The Epstein-Barr virus LF2 protein inhibits viral replication. *J Virol* 2008;82(17):8509–8519.
77. Calderwood MA, Venkatesan K, Xing L, et al. Epstein-Barr virus and virus human protein interaction maps. *Proc Natl Acad Sci U S A* 2007;104(18):7606–7611.
78. Caldwell RG, Wilson JB, Anderson SJ, et al. Epstein-Barr virus LMP2A drives B cell development and survival in the absence of normal B cell receptor signals. *Immunity* 1998;9(3):405–411.
79. Callan MF. Epstein-Barr virus, arthritis, and the development of lymphoma in arthritis patients. *Curr Opin Rheumatol* 2004;16(4):399–405.
80. Cameron B, Bharadwaj M, Burrows J, et al. Prolonged illness after infectious mononucleosis is associated with altered immunity but not with increased viral load. *J Infect Dis* 2006;193(5):664–671.
81. Cancer Genome Atlas Research Network. Comprehensive molecular characterization of gastric adenocarcinoma. *Nature* 2014:513(7517):202–209.
82. Cannons JL, Tangye SG, Schwartzberg PL. SLAM family receptors and SAP adaptors in immunity. *Annu Rev Immunol* 2011;29:665–705.
83. Capello D, Cerri M, Muti G, et al. Molecular histogenesis of posttransplantation lymphoproliferative disorders. *Blood* 2003;102(10):3775–3785.
84. Carbone A. Emerging pathways in the development of AIDS-related lymphomas. *Lancet Oncol* 2003;4(1):22–29.
85. Carbone A, Cesarman E, Spina M, et al. HIV-associated lymphomas and gamma-herpesviruses. *Blood* 2009;113(6):1213–1224.
86. Carel JC, Myones BL, Frazier B, et al. Structural requirements for C3d,g/Epstein-Barr virus receptor (CR2/CD21) ligand binding, internalization, and viral infection. *J Biol Chem* 1990;265(21):12293–12299.
87. Casola S, Otipoby KL, Alimzhanov M, et al. B cell receptor signal strength determines B cell fate. *Nat Immunol* 2004;5(3):317–327.
88. Caves EA, Butch RM, Cook SA, et al. Latent membrane protein 1 is a novel determinant of Epstein-Barr virus genome persistence and reactivation. *mSphere* 2017;2(6).
89. Caves EA, Cook SA, Lee N, et al. Erratum for Caves et al., "Air-Liquid interface method to study Epstein-Barr virus pathogenesis in nasopharyngeal epithelial cells". *mSphere* 2019;4(2).
90. Cederberg LE, Rabinovitch MD, Grimm-Geris JM, et al. Epstein-Barr virus DNA in parental oral secretions: a potential source of infection for their young children. *Clin Infect Dis* 2019;68(2):306–312.
91. Cen O, Longnecker R. Latent membrane protein 2 (LMP2). *Curr Top Microbiol Immunol* 2015;391:151–180.
92. Chabot PR, Raiola L, Lussier-Price M, et al. Structural and functional characterization of a complex between the acidic transactivation domain of EBNA2 and the Tfb1/p62 subunit of TFIIH. *PLoS Pathog* 2014;10(3):e1004042.
93. Chaganti S, Ma CS, Bell AI, et al. Epstein-Barr virus persistence in the absence of conventional memory B cells: IgM+IgD+CD27+ B cells harbor the virus in X-linked lymphoproliferative disease patients. *Blood* 2008;112(3):672–679.
94. Chakravorty A, Sugden B. The AT-hook DNA binding ability of the Epstein Barr virus EBNA1 protein is necessary for the maintenance of viral genomes in latently infected cells. *Virology* 2015;484:251–258.
95. Chan KC, Ting CM, Chan PS, et al. A novel Hsp90 inhibitor AT13387 induces senescence in EBV-positive nasopharyngeal carcinoma cells and suppresses tumor formation. *Mol Cancer* 2013;12(1):128.
96. Chan KCA, Woo JKS, King A, et al. Analysis of plasma Epstein-Barr virus DNA to screen for nasopharyngeal cancer. *N Engl J Med* 2017;377(6):513–522.
97. Chatterjee B, Deng Y, Holler A, et al. CD8+ T cells retain protective functions despite sustained inhibitory receptor expression during Epstein-Barr virus infection in vivo. *PLoS Pathog* 2019;15(5):e1007748.
98. Chattopadhyay PK, Chelimo K, Embury PB, et al. Holoendemic malaria exposure is associated with altered Epstein-Barr virus-specific CD8(+) T-cell differentiation. *J Virol* 2013;87(3):1779–1788.
99. Chen Y, Fachko D, Ivanov NS, et al. Epstein-Barr virus microRNAs regulate B cell receptor signal transduction and lytic reactivation. *PLoS Pathog* 2019;15(1):e1007535.
100. Chen J, Jardetzky TS, Longnecker R. The large groove found in the gH/gL structure is an important functional domain for Epstein-Barr virus fusion. *J Virol* 2013;87(7):3620–3627.
101. Chen J, Jardetzky TS, Longnecker R. The cytoplasmic tail domain of Epstein-Barr virus gH regulates membrane fusion activity through altering gH binding to gp42 and epithelial cell attachment. *MBio* 2016;7(6).
102. Chen H, Lee JM, Zong Y, et al. Linkage between STAT regulation and Epstein-Barr virus gene expression in tumors. *J Virol* 2001;75(6):2929–2937.
103. Chen CL, Sadler RH, Walling DM, et al. Epstein-Barr virus (EBV) gene expression in EBV-positive peripheral T-cell lymphomas. *J Virol* 1993;67(10):6303–6308.
104. Chen J, Sathiyamoorthy K, Zhang X, et al. Ephrin receptor A2 is a functional entry receptor for Epstein-Barr virus. *Nat Microbiol* 2018;3(2):172–180.
105. Cheng AZ, Yockteng-Melgar J, Jarvis MC, et al. Epstein-Barr virus BORF2 inhibits cellular APOBEC3B to preserve viral genome integrity. *Nat Microbiol* 2019;4(1):78–88.
106. Chesnokova LS, Nishimura SL, Hutt-Fletcher LM. Fusion of epithelial cells by Epstein-Barr virus proteins is triggered by binding of viral glycoproteins gHgL to integrins alphavbeta6 or alphavbeta8. *Proc Natl Acad Sci U S A* 2009;106(48):20464–20469.
107. Chiang JJ, Sparrer KMJ, van Gent M, et al. Viral unmasking of cellular 5S rRNA pseudogene transcripts induces RIG-I-mediated immunity. *Nat Immunol* 2018;19(1):53–62.
108. Chien YC, Chen JY, Liu MY, et al. Serologic markers of Epstein-Barr virus infection and nasopharyngeal carcinoma in Taiwanese men. *N Engl J Med* 2001;345(26):1877–1882.
109. Chijioke O, Muller A, Feederle R, et al. Human natural killer cells prevent infectious mononucleosis features by targeting lytic Epstein-Barr virus infection. *Cell Rep* 2013;5(6):1489–1498.
110. Chiu YF, Sugden B. Epstein-Barr virus: the path from latent to productive infection. *Ann Rev Virol* 2016;3(1):359–372.
111. Chiu YF, Sugden AU, Sugden B. Epstein-Barr viral productive amplification reprograms nuclear architecture, DNA replication, and histone deposition. *Cell Host Microbe* 2013;14(6):607–618.
112. Chiu SH, Wu MC, Wu CC, et al. Epstein-Barr virus BALF3 has nuclease activity and mediates mature virion production during the lytic cycle. *J Virol* 2014;88(9):4962–4975.
113. Choudhuri T, Verma SC, Lan K, et al. The ATM/ATR signaling effector Chk2 is targeted by Epstein-Barr virus nuclear antigen 3C to release the G2/M cell cycle block. *J Virol* 2007;81(12):6718–6730.
114. Chung BK, Tsai K, Allan LL, et al. Innate immune control of EBV-infected B cells by invariant natural killer T cells. *Blood* 2013;122(15):2600–2608.
115. Church TM, Verma D, Thompson J, et al. Efficient translation of Epstein-Barr virus (EBV) DNA polymerase contributes to the enhanced lytic replication phenotype of M81 EBV. *J Virol* 2018;92(6).
116. Cludts I, Farrell PJ. Multiple functions within the Epstein-Barr virus EBNA-3A protein. *J Virol* 1998;72(3):1862–1869.
117. Coghill AE, Bu W, Nguyen H, et al. High levels of antibody that neutralize B-cell infection of Epstein-Barr virus and that bind EBV gp350 are associated with a lower risk of nasopharyngeal carcinoma. *Clin Cancer Res* 2016;22(14):3451–3457.
118. Cohen JI. A region of herpes simplex virus VP16 can substitute for a transforming domain of Epstein-Barr virus nuclear protein 2. *Proc Natl Acad Sci U S A* 1992;89(17):8030–8034.
119. Cohen JI. Epstein-Barr virus infection. *N Engl J Med* 2000;343(7):481–492.
120. Cohen JI. Primary immunodeficiencies associated with EBV disease. *Curr Top Microbiol Immunol* 2015;390(Pt 1):241–265.
121. Cohen JI, Fauci AS, Varmus H, et al. Epstein-Barr virus: an important vaccine target for cancer prevention. *Sci Transl Med* 2011;3(107):107fs7.
122. Cohen JI, Iwatsuki K, Ko YH, et al. Epstein-Barr virus NK and T cell lymphoproliferative disease: report of a 2018 international meeting. *Leuk Lymphoma* 2020;61(4):808–819.
123. Cohen JI, Jaffe ES, Dale JK, et al. Characterization and treatment of chronic active Epstein-Barr virus disease: a 28-year experience in the United States. *Blood* 2011;117(22):5835–5849.
124. Cohen JI, Kieff E. An Epstein-Barr virus nuclear protein 2 domain essential for transformation is a direct transcriptional activator. *J Virol* 1991;65(11):5880–5885.
125. Cohen JI, Manoli I, Dowdell K, et al. Hydroa vacciniforme-like lymphoproliferative disorder: an EBV disease with a low risk of systemic illness in whites. *Blood* 2019;133(26):2753–2764.
126. Cohen JI, Wang F, Mannick J, et al. Epstein-Barr virus nuclear protein 2 is a key determinant of lymphocyte transformation. *Proc Natl Acad Sci U S A* 1989;86(23):9558–9562.
127. Coleman CB, Daud II, Ogolla SO, et al. Epstein-Barr virus type 2 infects T cells in healthy kenyan children. *J Infect Dis* 2017;216(6):670–677.
128. Coleman CB, Lang J, Sweet LA, et al. Epstein-Barr virus type 2 infects T cells and induces B cell lymphomagenesis in humanized mice. *J Virol* 2018;92(21).
129. Collins P, Fox CP, George LC, et al. Characterising EBV-associated lymphoproliferative diseases and the role of myeloid-derived suppressor cells. *Blood* 2020.
130. Conacher M, Callard R, McAulay K, et al. Epstein-Barr virus can establish infection in the absence of a classical memory B-cell population. *J Virol* 2005;79(17):11128–11134.
131. Condon LM, Cederberg LE, Rabinovitch MD, et al. Age-specific prevalence of Epstein-Barr virus infection among Minnesota children: effects of race/ethnicity and family environment. *Clin Infect Dis* 2014;59(4):501–508.
132. Cosmopoulos K, Pegtel M, Hawkins J, et al. Comprehensive profiling of Epstein-Barr virus microRNAs in nasopharyngeal carcinoma. *J Virol* 2009;83(5):2357–2367.
133. Cotter MA II, Robertson ES. Modulation of histone acetyltransferase activity through interaction of epstein-barr nuclear antigen 3C with prothymosin alpha. *Mol Cell Biol* 2000;20(15):5722–5735.
134. Countryman JK, Gradoville L, Miller G. Histone hyperacetylation occurs on promoters of lytic cycle regulatory genes in Epstein-Barr virus-infected cell lines which are refractory to disruption of latency by histone deacetylase inhibitors. *J Virol* 2008;82(10):4706–4719.
135. Countryman J, Jenson H, Seibl R, et al. Polymorphic proteins encoded within BZLF1 of defective and standard Epstein-Barr viruses disrupt latency. *J Virol* 1987;61(12):3672–3679.
136. Countryman J, Miller G. Activation of expression of latent Epstein-Barr herpesvirus after gene transfer with a small cloned subfragment of heterogeneous viral DNA. *Proc Natl Acad Sci U S A* 1985;82(12):4085–4089.
137. Cristino AS, Nourse J, West RA, et al. EBV microRNA-BHRF1-2-5p targets the 3′UTR of immune checkpoint ligands PD-L1 and PD-L2. *Blood* 2019;134(25):2261–2270.
138. Cui X, Cao Z, Chen Q, et al. Rabbits immunized with Epstein-Barr virus gH/gL or gB recombinant proteins elicit higher serum virus neutralizing activity than gp350. *Vaccine* 2016;34(34):4050–4055.
139. Cui X, Cao Z, Sen G, et al. A novel tetrameric gp350 1-470 as a potential Epstein-Barr virus vaccine. *Vaccine* 2013;31(30):3039–3045.
140. Dai YC, Liao YT, Juan YT, et al. The novel nuclear targeting and BFRF1-interacting domains of BFLF2 are essential for efficient Epstein-Barr virus virion release. *J Virol* 2020;94(3).
141. Dambaugh T, Beisel C, Hummel M, et al. Epstein-Barr virus (B95-8) DNA VII: molecular cloning and detailed mapping. *Proc Natl Acad Sci U S A* 1980;77(5):2999–3003.
142. Dambaugh T, Heller M, Raab-Traub N, et al. DNAs of Epstein-Barr virus and herpes virus Papio. In: Nahmias AJ, Dowdles WR, Schinazi RF, eds., *The Human Herpes Viruses.* New York: Elsevier; 1981:85–90.
143. Dambaugh T, Hennessy K, Chamnankit L, et al. U2 region of Epstein-Barr virus DNA may encode Epstein-Barr nuclear antigen 2. *Proc Natl Acad Sci U S A* 1984;81(23):7632–7636.
144. Dambaugh T, Wang F, Hennessy K, et al. Expression of the Epstein-Barr virus nuclear protein 2 in rodent cells. *J Virol* 1986;59(2):453–462.
145. Davison AJ. Evolution of the herpesviruses. *Vet Microbiol* 2002;86(1-2):69–88.

146. Dawson CW, Tramountanis G, Eliopoulos AG, et al. Epstein-Barr virus latent membrane protein 1 (LMP1) activates the phosphatidylinositol 3-kinase/Akt pathway to promote cell survival and induce actin filament remodeling. *J Biol Chem* 2003;278(6):3694–3704.
147. Deacon EM, Pallesen G, Niedobitek G, et al. Epstein-Barr virus and Hodgkin's disease: transcriptional analysis of virus latency in the malignant cells. *J Exp Med* 1993;177(2):339–349.
148. Deakyne JS, Malecka KA, Messick TE, et al. Structural and functional basis for an EBNA1 hexameric ring in Epstein-Barr virus episome maintenance. *J Virol* 2017;91(19).
149. DeKroon RM, Gunawardena HP, Edwards R, et al. Global proteomic changes induced by the Epstein-Barr virus oncoproteins latent membrane protein 1 and 2A. *MBio* 2018;9(3).
150. Demetriades C, Mosialos G. The LMP1 promoter can be transactivated directly by NF-kappaB. *J Virol* 2009;83(10):5269–5277.
151. Deutsch MJ, Ott E, Papior P, et al. The latent origin of replication of Epstein-Barr virus directs viral genomes to active regions of the nucleus. *J Virol* 2010;84(5):2533–2546.
152. Devergne O, Hatzivassiliou E, Izumi KM, et al. Association of TRAF1, TRAF2, and TRAF3 with an Epstein-Barr virus LMP1 domain important for B-lymphocyte transformation: role in NF-kappaB activation. *Mol Cell Biol* 1996;16(12):7098–7108.
153. Dheekollu J, Lieberman PM. The replisome pausing factor Timeless is required for episomal maintenance of latent Epstein-Barr virus. *J Virol* 2011;85(12):5853–5863.
154. Dheekollu J, Wiedmer A, Sentana-Lledo D, et al. HCF1 and OCT2 cooperate with EBNA1 to enhance orip-dependent transcription and episome maintenance of latent Epstein-Barr virus. *J Virol* 2016;90(11):5353–5367.
155. Diepstra A, Niens M, Vellenga E, et al. Association with HLA class I in Epstein-Barr-virus-positive and with HLA class III in Epstein-Barr-virus-negative Hodgkin's lymphoma. *Lancet* 2005;365(9478):2216–2224.
156. Dirmeier U, Hoffmann R, Kilger E, et al. Latent membrane protein 1 of Epstein-Barr virus coordinately regulates proliferation with control of apoptosis. *Oncogene* 2005;24(10):1711–1717.
157. Djavadian R, Chiu YF, Johannsen E. An Epstein-Barr virus-encoded protein complex requires an origin of lytic replication in cis to mediate late gene transcription. *PLoS Pathog* 2016;12(6):e1005718.
158. Djavadian R, Hayes M, Johannsen E. CAGE-seq analysis of Epstein-Barr virus lytic gene transcription: 3 kinetic classes from 2 mechanisms. *PLoS Pathog* 2018;14(6):e1007114.
159. Dolan A, Addison C, Gatherer D, et al. The genome of Epstein-Barr virus type 2 strain AG876. *Virology* 2006;350(1):164–170.
160. Dolyniuk M, Pritchett R, Kieff E. Proteins of Epstein-Barr virus. I. Analysis of the polypeptides of purified enveloped Epstein-Barr virus. *J Virol* 1976;17(3):935–949.
161. Dong M, Wang HY, Zhao XX, et al. Expression and prognostic roles of PIK3CA, JAK2, PD-L1, and PD-L2 in Epstein-Barr virus-associated gastric carcinoma. *Hum Pathol* 2016;53:25–34.
162. Dorner M, Zucol F, Alessi D, et al. beta1 integrin expression increases susceptibility of memory B cells to Epstein-Barr virus infection. *J Virol* 2010;84(13):6667–6677.
163. Dufva O, Kankainen M, Kelkka T, et al. Aggressive natural killer-cell leukemia mutational landscape and drug profiling highlight JAK-STAT signaling as therapeutic target. *Nat Commun* 2018;9(1):1567.
164. Dunmire SK, Grimm JM, Schmeling DO, et al. The incubation period of primary Epstein-Barr virus infection: viral dynamics and immunologic events. *PLoS Pathog* 2015;11(12):e1005286.
165. Dunne PJ, Faint JM, Gudgeon NH, et al. Epstein-Barr virus-specific CD8(+) T cells that re-express CD45RA are apoptosis-resistant memory cells that retain replicative potential. *Blood* 2002;100(3):933–940.
166. Eichelberg MR, Welch R, Guidry JT, et al. Epstein-Barr virus infection promotes epithelial cell growth by attenuating differentiation-dependent exit from the cell cycle. *MBio* 2019;10(4).
167. El-Guindy A, Lopez-Giraldez F, Delecluse HJ, et al. A locus encompassing the Epstein-Barr virus bglf4 kinase regulates expression of genes encoding viral structural proteins. *PLoS Pathog* 2014;10(8):e1004307.
168. Elliott SL, Suhrbier A, Miles JJ, et al. Phase I trial of a CD8+ T-cell peptide epitope-based vaccine for infectious mononucleosis. *J Virol* 2008;82(3):1448–1457.
169. Ellis AL, Wang Z, Yu X, et al. Either ZEB1 or ZEB2/SIP1 can play a central role in regulating the Epstein-Barr virus latent-lytic switch in a cell-type-specific manner. *J Virol* 2010;84(12):6139–6152.
170. Ellis-Connell AL, Iempridee T, Xu I, et al. Cellular microRNAs 200b and 429 regulate the Epstein-Barr virus switch between latency and lytic replication. *J Virol* 2010;84(19):10329–10343.
171. Engels N, Merchant M, Pappu R, et al. Epstein-Barr virus latent membrane protein 2A (LMP2A) employs the SLP-65 signaling module. *J Exp Med* 2001;194(3):255–264.
172. Epstein MA, Achong BG, Barr YM. Virus particles in cultured lymphoblasts from burkitt's lymphoma. *Lancet* 1964;1(7335):702–703.
173. Ernst R, Claessen JH, Mueller B, et al. Enzymatic blockade of the ubiquitin-proteasome pathway. *PLoS Biol* 2011;8(3):e1000605.
174. Ersing I, Nobre L, Wang LW, et al. A temporal proteomic map of Epstein-Barr virus lytic replication in B cells. *Cell Rep* 2017;19(7):1479–1493.
175. Escalante GM, Foley J, Mutsvunguma LZ, et al. A pentavalent Epstein-Barr virus-like particle vaccine elicits high titers of neutralizing antibodies against Epstein-Barr virus infection in immunized rabbits. *Vaccines (Basel)* 2020;8(2).
176. van Esser JW, Niesters HG, van der Holt B, et al. Prevention of Epstein-Barr virus-lymphoproliferative disease by molecular monitoring and preemptive rituximab in high-risk patients after allogeneic stem cell transplantation. *Blood* 2002;99(12):4364–4369.
177. Farrell PJ. Epstein-Barr virus and cancer. *Annu Rev Pathol* 2019;14:29–53.
178. Faulkner GC, Burrows SR, Khanna R, et al. X-Linked agammaglobulinemia patients are not infected with Epstein-Barr virus: implications for the biology of the virus. *J Virol* 1999;73(2):1555–1564.
179. Feederle R, Delecluse HJ. Low level of lytic replication in a recombinant Epstein-Barr virus carrying an origin of replication devoid of BZLF1-binding sites. *J Virol* 2004;78(21):12082–12084.
180. Feederle R, Kost M, Baumann M, et al. The Epstein-Barr virus lytic program is controlled by the co-operative functions of two transactivators. *EMBO J* 2000;19(12):3080–3089.
181. Feederle R, Shannon-Lowe C, Baldwin G, et al. Defective infectious particles and rare packaged genomes produced by cells carrying terminal-repeat-negative epstein-barr virus. *J Virol* 2005;79(12):7641–7647.
182. Fennewald S, van Santen V, Kieff E. Nucleotide sequence of an mRNA transcribed in latent growth- transforming virus infection indicates that it may encode a membrane protein. *J Virol* 1984;51(2):411–419.
183. Filipovich AH, Zhang K, Snow AL, et al. X-linked lymphoproliferative syndromes: brothers or distant cousins? *Blood* 2010;116(18):3398–3408.
184. Fingeroth JD, Weis JJ, Tedder TF, et al. Epstein-Barr virus receptor of human B lymphocytes is the C3d receptor CR2. *Proc Natl Acad Sci U S A* 1984;81(14):4510–4514.
185. Fish K, Comoglio F, Shaffer V III, et al. Rewiring of B cell receptor signaling by Epstein-Barr virus LMP2A. *Proc Natl Acad Sci U S A* 2020;117:26318–26327.
186. Fitzsimmons L, Boyce AJ, Wei W, et al. Coordinated repression of BIM and PUMA by Epstein-Barr virus latent genes maintains the survival of Burkitt lymphoma cells. *Cell Death Differ* 2018;25(2):241–254.
187. Fitzsimmons L, Cartlidge R, Chang C, et al. EBV BCL-2 homologue BHRF1 drives chemoresistance and lymphomagenesis by inhibiting multiple cellular pro-apoptotic proteins. *Cell Death Differ* 2020;27:1554–1568.
188. Fixman ED, Hayward GS, Hayward SD. trans-acting requirements for replication of Epstein-Barr virus ori-Lyt. *J Virol* 1992;66(8):5030–5039.
189. Fixman ED, Hayward GS, Hayward SD. Replication of Epstein-Barr virus oriLyt: lack of a dedicated virally encoded origin-binding protein and dependence on Zta in cotransfection assays. *J Virol* 1995;69(5):2998–3006.
190. Flanagan J, Middeldorp J, Sculley T. Localization of the Epstein-Barr virus protein LMP 1 to exosomes. *J Gen Virol* 2003;84(Pt 7):1871–1879.
191. Flemington E, Speck SH. Identification of phorbol ester response elements in the promoter of Epstein-Barr virus putative lytic switch gene BZLF1. *J Virol* 1990;64(3):1217–1226.
192. Fogg MH, Wirth LJ, Posner M, et al. Decreased EBNA-1-specific CD8+ T cells in patients with Epstein-Barr virus-associated nasopharyngeal carcinoma. *Proc Natl Acad Sci U S A* 2009;106(9):3318–3323.
193. Forrest C, Hislop AD, Rickinson AB, et al. Proteome-wide analysis of CD8+ T cell responses to EBV reveals differences between primary and persistent infection. *PLoS Pathog* 2018;14(9):e1007110.
194. Fotheringham JA, Mazzucca S, Raab-Traub N. Epstein-Barr virus latent membrane protein-2A-induced DeltaNp63alpha expression is associated with impaired epithelial-cell differentiation. *Oncogene* 2010;29(30):4287–4296.
195. Fournier B, Boutboul D, Bruneau J, et al. Rapid identification and characterization of infected cells in blood during chronic active Epstein-Barr virus infection. *J Exp Med* 2020;217(11).
196. Francis AL, Gradoville L, Miller G. Alteration of a single serine in the basic domain of the Epstein-Barr virus ZEBRA protein separates its functions of transcriptional activation and disruption of latency. *J Virol* 1997;71(4):3054–3061.
197. Frappier L. Ebna1. *Curr Top Microbiol Immunol* 2015;391:3–34.
198. Fries KL, Miller WE, Raab-Traub N. Epstein-Barr virus latent membrane protein 1 blocks p53-mediated apoptosis through the induction of the A20 gene. *J Virol* 1996;70(12):8653–8659.
199. Fries KL, Miller WE, Raab-Traub N. The A20 protein interacts with the Epstein-Barr virus latent membrane protein 1 (LMP1) and alters the LMP1/TRAF1/TRADD complex. *Virology* 1999;264(1):159–166.
200. Fuentes-Panana EM, Peng R, Brewer G, et al. Regulation of the Epstein-Barr virus C promoter by AUF1 and the cyclic AMP/protein kinase A signaling pathway. *J Virol* 2000;74(17):8166–8175.
201. Fukayama M. Epstein-Barr virus and gastric carcinoma. *Pathol Int* 2010;60(5):337–350.
202. Fukuda M, Longnecker R. Latent membrane protein 2A inhibits transforming growth factor-beta 1-induced apoptosis through the phosphatidylinositol 3-kinase/Akt pathway. *J Virol* 2004;78(4):1697–1705.
203. Gahn TA, Sugden B. An EBNA-1-dependent enhancer acts from a distance of 10 kilobase pairs to increase expression of the Epstein-Barr virus LMP gene. *J Virol* 1995;69(4):2633–2636.
204. Gan YJ, Chodosh J, Morgan A, et al. Epithelial cell polarization is a determinant in the infectious outcome of immunoglobulin A-mediated entry by Epstein-Barr virus. *J Virol* 1997;71(1):519–526.
205. Gandhi MK, Moll G, Smith C, et al. Galectin-1 mediated suppression of Epstein-Barr virus specific T-cell immunity in classic Hodgkin lymphoma. *Blood* 2007;110(4):1326–1329.
206. Gewurz BE, Towfic F, Mar JC, et al. Genome-wide siRNA screen for mediators of NF-kappaB activation. *Proc Natl Acad Sci U S A* 2012;109(7):2467–2472.
207. Ghosh D, Kieff E. cis-acting regulatory elements near the Epstein-Barr virus latent-infection membrane protein transcriptional start site. *J Virol* 1990;64(4):1855–1858.
208. Gilligan K, Rajadurai P, Resnick L, et al. Epstein-Barr virus small nuclear RNAs are not expressed in permissively infected cells in AIDS-associated leukoplakia. *Proc Natl Acad Sci U S A* 1990;87(22):8790–8794.
209. Given D, Yee D, Griem K, et al. DNA of Epstein-Barr virus. V. Direct repeats of the ends of Epstein-Barr virus DNA. *J Virol* 1979;30(3):852–862.
210. Glaser LV, Rieger S, Thumann S, et al. EBF1 binds to EBNA2 and promotes the assembly of EBNA2 chromatin complexes in B cells. *PLoS Pathog* 2017;13(10):e1006664.
211. Gordadze AV, Peng R, Tan J, et al. Notch1IC partially replaces EBNA2 function in B cells immortalized by Epstein-Barr virus. *J Virol* 2001;75(13):5899–5912.
212. Gotoh K, Ito Y, Shibata-Watanabe Y, et al. Clinical and virological characteristics of 15 patients with chronic active Epstein-Barr virus infection treated with hematopoietic stem cell transplantation. *Clin Infect Dis* 2008;46(10):1525–1534.
213. Gottschalk S, Rooney CM, Heslop HE. Post-transplant lymphoproliferative disorders. *Annu Rev Med* 2005;56:29–44.
214. Grande BM, Gerhard DS, Jiang A, et al. Genome-wide discovery of somatic coding and noncoding mutations in pediatric endemic and sporadic Burkitt lymphoma. *Blood* 2019;133(12):1313–1324.

215. Gratama JW, Oosterveer MA, Lepoutre JM, et al. Serological and molecular studies of Epstein-Barr virus infection in allogeneic marrow graft recipients. *Transplantation* 1990;49(4):725–730.
216. Greenfeld H, Takasaki K, Walsh MJ, et al. TRAF1 coordinates polyubiquitin signaling to enhance Epstein-Barr virus LMP1-mediated growth and survival pathway activation. *PLoS Pathog* 2015;11(5):e1004890.
217. Greenspan JS, Greenspan D, Lennette ET, et al. Replication of Epstein-Barr virus within the epithelial cells of oral "hairy" leukoplakia, an AIDS-associated lesion. *N Engl J Med* 1985;313(25):1564–1571.
218. Gregorovic G, Boulden EA, Bosshard R, et al. Epstein-Barr viruses (EBVs) deficient in EBV-encoded RNAs have higher levels of latent membrane protein 2 RNA expression in lymphoblastoid cell lines and efficiently establish persistent infections in humanized mice. *J Virol* 2015;89(22):11711–11714.
219. Grossman SR, Johannsen E, Tong X, et al. The Epstein-Barr virus nuclear antigen 2 transactivator is directed to response elements by the J kappa recombination signal binding protein. *Proc Natl Acad Sci U S A* 1994;91(16):7568–7572.
220. Gujer C, Murer A, Muller A, et al. Plasmacytoid dendritic cells respond to Epstein-Barr virus infection with a distinct type I interferon subtype profile. *Blood Adv* 2019;3(7):1129–1144.
221. Gunnell A, Webb HM, Wood CD, et al. RUNX super-enhancer control through the Notch pathway by Epstein-Barr virus transcription factors regulates B cell growth. *Nucleic Acids Res* 2016;44(10):4636–4650.
222. Guo R, Jiang C, Zhang Y, et al. MYC controls the Epstein-Barr virus lytic switch. *Mol Cell* 2020;78(4):653–669.e658.
223. Guo R, Zhang Y, Teng M, et al. DNA methylation enzymes and PRC1 restrict B-cell Epstein-Barr virus oncoprotein expression. *Nat Microbiol* 2020;5:1051–1063.
224. Haan KM, Longnecker R. Coreceptor restriction within the HLA-DQ locus for Epstein-Barr virus infection. *Proc Natl Acad Sci U S A* 2000;97(16):9252–9257.
225. Haddad RS, Hutt-Fletcher LM. Depletion of glycoprotein gp85 from virosomes made with Epstein-Barr virus proteins abolishes their ability to fuse with virus receptor- bearing cells. *J Virol* 1989;63(12):4998–5005.
226. Hahn AS, Kaufmann JK, Wies E, et al. The ephrin receptor tyrosine kinase A2 is a cellular receptor for Kaposi's sarcoma-associated herpesvirus. *Nat Med* 2012;18(6):961–966.
227. Hammerschmidt W, Sugden B. Identification and characterization of oriLyt, a lytic origin of DNA replication of Epstein-Barr virus. *Cell* 1988;55(3):427–433.
228. Hammerschmidt W, Sugden B. Replication of Epstein-Barr viral DNA. *Cold Spring Harb Perspect Biol* 2013;5(1):a013029.
229. Han I, Harada S, Weaver D, et al. EBNA-LP associates with cellular proteins including DNA-PK and HA95. *J Virol* 2001;75:2475–2481.
230. Haque T, Johannessen I, Dombagoda D, et al. A mouse monoclonal antibody against Epstein-Barr virus envelope glycoprotein 350 prevents infection both in vitro and in vivo. *J Infect Dis* 2006;194(5):584–587.
231. Haque T, Wilkie GM, Jones MM, et al. Allogeneic cytotoxic T-cell therapy for EBV-positive posttransplantation lymphoproliferative disease: results of a phase 2 multicenter clinical trial. *Blood* 2007;110(4):1123–1131.
232. Harada S, Kieff E. Epstein-Barr virus nuclear protein LP stimulates EBNA-2 acidic domain- mediated transcriptional activation. *J Virol* 1997;71(9):6611–6618.
233. Harada S, Yalamanchili R, Kieff E. Residues 231 to 280 of the Epstein-Barr virus nuclear protein 2 are not essential for primary B-lymphocyte growth transformation. *J Virol* 1998;72(12):9948–9954.
234. Harley JB, Chen X, Pujato M, et al. Transcription factors operate across disease loci, with EBNA2 implicated in autoimmunity. *Nat Genet* 2018;50(5):699–707.
235. Hatfull G, Bankier AT, Barrell BG, et al. Sequence analysis of Raji Epstein-Barr virus DNA. *Virology* 1988;164(2):334–340.
236. Hatzivassiliou EG, Kieff E, Mosialos G. Constitutive CD40 signaling phenocopies the transforming function of the Epstein-Barr virus oncoprotein LMP1 in vitro. *Leuk Res* 2007;31(3):315–320.
237. He A, Miranda JL. JQ1 reduces Epstein-Barr virus-associated lymphoproliferative disease in mice without sustained oncogene repression. *Leuk Lymphoma* 2018;59(5):1248–1251.
238. Heilmann AM, Calderwood MA, Johannsen E. Epstein-Barr virus LF2 protein regulates viral replication by altering Rta subcellular localization. *J Virol* 2010;84(19):9920–9931.
239. Heldwein EE, Lou H, Bender FC, et al. Crystal structure of glycoprotein B from herpes simplex virus 1. *Science* 2006;313(5784):217–220.
240. Henderson S, Rowe M, Gregory C, et al. Induction of bcl-2 expression by Epstein-Barr virus latent membrane protein 1 protects infected B cells from programmed cell death. *Cell* 1991;65(7):1107–1115.
241. Henkel T, Ling PD, Hayward SD, et al. Mediation of Epstein-Barr virus EBNA2 transactivation by recombination signal-binding protein J kappa. *Science* 1994;265(5168):92–95.
242. Henle W, Diehl V, Kohn G, et al. Herpes-type virus and chromosome marker in normal leukocytes after growth with irradiated Burkitt cells. *Science* 1967;157(3792):1064–1065.
243. Henle G, Henle W. Immunofluorescence in cells derived from Burkitt's lymphoma. *J Bacteriol* 1966;91(3):1248–1256.
244. Henle G, Henle W. Serum IgA antibodies of Epstein-Barr virus (EBV)-related antigens. A new feature of nasopharyngeal carcinoma. *Bibl Haematol* 1975;(43):322–325.
245. Henle G, Henle W, Diehl V. Relation of Burkitt's tumor-associated herpes-type virus to infectious mononucleosis. *Proc Natl Acad Sci U S A* 1968;59(1):94–101.
246. Hennessy K, Fennewald S, Kieff E. A third viral nuclear protein in lymphoblasts immortalized by Epstein-Barr virus. *Proc Natl Acad Sci U S A* 1985;82(17):5944–5948.
247. Hertle ML, Popp C, Petermann S, et al. Differential gene expression patterns of EBV infected EBNA-3A positive and negative human B lymphocytes. *PLoS Pathog* 2009;5(7):e1000506.
248. Heslop HE, Ng CY, Li C, et al. Long-term restoration of immunity against Epstein-Barr virus infection by adoptive transfer of gene-modified virus-specific T lymphocytes. *Nat Med* 1996;2(5):551–555.
249. Higgins CD, Swerdlow AJ, Macsween KF, et al. A study of risk factors for acquisition of Epstein-Barr virus and its subtypes. *J Infect Dis* 2007;195(4):474–482.
250. Higuchi M, Izumi KM, Kieff E. Epstein-Barr virus latent-infection membrane proteins are palmitoylated and raft-associated: protein 1 binds to the cytoskeleton through TNF receptor cytoplasmic factors. *Proc Natl Acad Sci U S A* 2001;98(8):4675–4680.
251. Hjalgrim H, Askling J, Rostgaard K, et al. Characteristics of Hodgkin's lymphoma after infectious mononucleosis. *N Engl J Med* 2003;349(14):1324–1332.
252. Hochberg D, Middeldorp JM, Catalina M, et al. Demonstration of the Burkitt's lymphoma Epstein-Barr virus phenotype in dividing latently infected memory cells in vivo. *Proc Natl Acad Sci U S A* 2004;101(1):239–244.
253. Hofelmayr H, Strobl LJ, Marschall G, et al. Activated Notch1 can transiently substitute for EBNA2 in the maintenance of proliferation of LMP1-expressing immortalized B cells. *J Virol* 2001;75(5):2033–2040.
254. Hoffman BA, Wang Y, Feldman ER, et al. Epstein-Barr virus EBER1 and murine gammaherpesvirus TMER4 share conserved in vivo function to promote B cell egress and dissemination. *Proc Natl Acad Sci U S A* 2019;116(51):25392–25394.
255. Holowaty MN, Zeghouf M, Wu H, et al. Protein profiling with Epstein-Barr nuclear antigen-1 reveals an interaction with the herpesvirus-associated ubiquitin-specific protease HAUSP/USP7. *J Biol Chem* 2003;278(32):29987–29994.
256. Homig-Holzel C, Hojer C, Rastelli J, et al. Constitutive CD40 signaling in B cells selectively activates the noncanonical NF-kappaB pathway and promotes lymphomagenesis. *J Exp Med* 2008;205(6):1317–1329.
257. Hoshino Y, Katano H, Zou P, et al. Long-term administration of valacyclovir reduces the number of Epstein-Barr virus (EBV)-infected B cells but not the number of EBV DNA copies per B cell in healthy volunteers. *J Virol* 2009;83(22):11857–11861.
258. Hoshino Y, Nishikawa K, Ito Y, et al. Kinetics of Epstein-Barr virus load and virus-specific CD8(+) T cells in acute infectious mononucleosis. *J Clin Virol* 2010.
259. Howe JG, Shu MD. Epstein-Barr virus small RNA (EBER) genes: unique transcription units that combine RNA polymerase II and III promoter elements. *Cell* 1989;57(5):825–834.
260. Hsieh JJ, Hayward SD. Masking of the CBF1/RBPJ kappa transcriptional repression domain by Epstein-Barr virus EBNA2. *Science* 1995;268(5210):560–563.
261. Hsu WL, Yu KJ, Chien YC, et al. Familial tendency and risk of nasopharyngeal carcinoma in Taiwan: effects of covariates on risk. *Am J Epidemiol* 2011;173:292–299.
262. Huang J, Fogg M, Wirth LJ, et al. Epstein-Barr virus-specific adoptive immunotherapy for recurrent, metastatic nasopharyngeal carcinoma. *Cancer* 2017;123(14):2642–2650.
263. Hughes DJ, Dickerson CA, Shaner MS, et al. Trans-repression of protein expression dependent on the Epstein-Barr virus promoter Wp during latency. *J Virol* 2011;85:11435–11447.
264. Hughes DJ, Marendy EM, Dickerson CA, et al. Contributions of CTCF and DNA methyltransferases DNMT1 and DNMT3B to Epstein-Barr virus restricted latency. *J Virol* 2012;86(2):1034–1045.
265. Hui KF, Chan TF, Yang W, et al. High risk Epstein-Barr virus variants characterized by distinct polymorphisms in the EBER locus are strongly associated with nasopharyngeal carcinoma. *Int J Cancer* 2019;144(12):3031–3042.
266. Hui KF, Cheung AK, Choi CK, et al. Inhibition of class I histone deacetylases by romidepsin potently induces Epstein-Barr virus lytic cycle and mediates enhanced cell death with ganciclovir. *Int J Cancer* 2016;138(1):125–136.
267. Hulse M, Caruso LB, Madzo J, et al. Poly(ADP-ribose) polymerase 1 is necessary for coactivating hypoxia-inducible factor-1-dependent gene expression by Epstein-Barr virus latent membrane protein 1. *PLoS Pathog* 2018;14(11):e1007394.
268. Humme S, Reisbach G, Feederle R, et al. The EBV nuclear antigen 1 (EBNA1) enhances B cell immortalization several thousandfold. *Proc Natl Acad Sci U S A* 2003;100(19):10989–10994.
269. Hummel M, Thorley-Lawson D, Kieff E. An Epstein-Barr virus DNA fragment encodes messages for the two major envelope glycoproteins (gp350/300 and gp220/200). *J Virol* 1984;49(2):413–417.
270. Huppmann AR, Nicolae A, Slack GW, et al. EBV may be expressed in the LP cells of nodular lymphocyte-predominant Hodgkin lymphoma (NLPHL) in both children and adults. *Am J Surg Pathol* 2014;38(3):316–324.
271. Iizasa H, Kim H, Kartika AV, et al. Role of viral and host microRNAs in immune regulation of Epstein-Barr virus-associated diseases. *Front Immunol* 2020;11:367.
272. Iizasa H, Wulff BE, Alla NR, et al. Editing of Epstein-Barr virus-encoded BART6 microRNAs controls their dicer targeting and consequently affects viral latency. *J Biol Chem* 2010;285(43):33358–33370.
273. Ikeda A, Caldwell RG, Longnecker R, et al. Itchy, a Nedd4 ubiquitin ligase, downregulates latent membrane protein 2A activity in B-cell signaling. *J Virol* 2003;77(9):5529–5534.
274. Ikeda M, Ikeda A, Longan LC, et al. The Epstein-Barr virus latent membrane protein 2A PY motif recruits WW domain-containing ubiquitin-protein ligases. *Virology* 2000;268(1):178–191.
275. Ikeda M, Ikeda A, Longnecker R. Lysine-independent ubiquitination of Epstein-Barr virus LMP2A. *Virology* 2002;300(1):153–159.
276. Ikeda A, Merchant M, Lev L, et al. Latent membrane protein 2A, a viral B cell receptor homologue, induces CD5+ B-1 cell development. *J Immunol* 2004;172(9):5329–5337.
277. Imai S, Koizumi S, Sugiura M, et al. Gastric carcinoma: monoclonal epithelial malignant cells expressing Epstein-Barr virus latent infection protein. *Proc Natl Acad Sci U S A* 1994;91(19):9131–9135.
278. Imai S, Nishikawa J, Takada K. Cell-to-cell contact as an efficient mode of Epstein-Barr virus infection of diverse human epithelial cells. *J Virol* 1998;72(5):4371–4378.
279. Izumi KM, Cahir McFarland ED, Riley EA, et al. The residues between the two transformation effector sites of Epstein-Barr virus latent membrane protein 1 are not critical for B-lymphocyte growth transformation. *J Virol* 1999;73(12):9908–9916.
280. Izumi KM, Cahir McFarland ED, Ting AT, et al. The Epstein-Barr virus oncoprotein latent membrane protein 1 engages the tumor necrosis factor receptor-associated proteins TRADD and receptor-interacting protein (RIP) but does not induce apoptosis or require RIP for NF-kappaB activation. *Mol Cell Biol* 1999;19(8):5759–5767.
281. Izumi KM, Kaye KM, Kieff ED. Epstein-Barr virus recombinant molecular genetic analysis of the LMP1 amino-terminal cytoplasmic domain reveals a probable structural role, with no component essential for primary B-lymphocyte growth transformation. *J Virol* 1994;68(7):4369–4376.

282. Izumi KM, Kaye KM, Kieff ED. The Epstein-Barr virus LMP1 amino acid sequence that engages tumor necrosis factor receptor associated factors is critical for primary B lymphocyte growth transformation. *Proc Natl Acad Sci U S A* 1997;94(4):1447–1452.
283. James JA, Kaufman KM, Farris AD, et al. An increased prevalence of Epstein-Barr virus infection in young patients suggests a possible etiology for systemic lupus erythematosus. *J Clin Invest* 1997;100(12):3019–3026.
284. Jarrett RF, Stark GL, White J, et al. Impact of tumor Epstein-Barr virus status on presenting features and outcome in age-defined subgroups of patients with classic Hodgkin lymphoma: a population-based study. *Blood* 2005;106(7):2444–2451.
285. Jayasooriya S, de Silva TI, Njie-jobe J, et al. Early virological and immunological events in asymptomatic Epstein-Barr virus infection in African children. *PLoS Pathog* 2015;11(3):e1004746.
286. Jeang KT, Hayward SD. Organization of the Epstein-Barr virus DNA molecule. III. Location of the P3HR-1 deletion junction and characterization of the NotI repeat units that form part of the template for an abundant 12-O-tetradecanoylphorbol-13-acetate-induced mRNA transcript. *J Virol* 1983;48(1):135–148.
287. de Jesus O, Smith PR, Spender LC, et al. Updated Epstein-Barr virus (EBV) DNA sequence and analysis of a promoter for the BART (CST, BARF0) RNAs of EBV. *J Gen Virol* 2003;84(Pt 6):1443–1450.
288. Jiang R, Gu X, Nathan CO, et al. Laser-capture microdissection of oropharyngeal epithelium indicates restriction of Epstein-Barr virus receptor/CD21 mRNA to tonsil epithelial cells. *J Oral Pathol Med* 2008;37(10):626–633.
289. Jiang L, Gu ZH, Yan ZX, et al. Exome sequencing identifies somatic mutations of DDX3X in natural killer/T-cell lymphoma. *Nat Genet* 2015;47(9):1061–1066.
290. Jiang J, Lee EJ, Schmittgen TD. Increased expression of microRNA-155 in Epstein-Barr virus transformed lymphoblastoid cell lines. *Genes Chromosomes Cancer* 2006;45(1):103–106.
291. Jiang S, Willox B, Zhou H, et al. Epstein-Barr virus nuclear antigen 3C binds to BATF/IRF4 or SPI1/IRF4 composite sites and recruits Sin3A to repress CDKN2A. *Proc Natl Acad Sci U S A* 2014;111(1):421–426.
292. Jiang S, Zhou H, Liang J, et al. The Epstein-Barr virus regulome in lymphoblastoid cells. *Cell Host Microbe* 2017;22(4):561–573.e564.
293. Jin XW, Speck SH. Identification of critical cis elements involved in mediating Epstein-Barr virus nuclear antigen 2-dependent activity of an enhancer located upstream of the viral BamHI C promoter. *J Virol* 1992;66(5):2846–2852.
294. Jochum S, Moosmann A, Lang S, et al. The EBV immunoevasins vIL-10 and BNLF2a protect newly infected B cells from immune recognition and elimination. *PLoS Pathog* 2012;8(5):e1002704.
295. Jog NR, Young KA, Munroe ME, et al. Association of Epstein-Barr virus serological reactivation with transitioning to systemic lupus erythematosus in at-risk individuals. *Ann Rheum Dis* 2019;78(9):1235–1241.
296. Johannsen E, Koh E, Mosialos G, et al. Epstein-Barr virus nuclear protein 2 transactivation of the latent membrane protein 1 promoter is mediated by J kappa and PU.1. *J Virol* 1995;69(1):253–262.
297. Johannsen E, Luftig M, Chase MR, et al. Proteins of purified Epstein-Barr virus. *Proc Natl Acad Sci U S A* 2004;101(46):16286–16291.
298. Johannsen E, Miller CL, Grossman SR, et al. EBNA-2 and EBNA-3C extensively and mutually exclusively associate with RBPJkappa in Epstein-Barr virus-transformed B lymphocytes. *J Virol* 1996;70(6):4179–4183.
299. Johansson P, Jansson A, Ruetschi U, et al. The p38 signaling pathway upregulates expression of the Epstein-Barr virus LMP1 oncogene. *J Virol* 2010;84(6):2787–2797.
300. Jones MD, Foster L, Sheedy T, et al. The EB virus genome in Daudi Burkitt's lymphoma cells has a deletion similar to that observed in a non-transforming strain (P3HR-1) of the virus. *EMBO J* 1984;3(4):813–821.
301. Jones JF, Shurin S, Abramowsky C, et al. T-cell lymphomas containing Epstein-Barr viral DNA in patients with chronic Epstein-Barr virus infections. *N Engl J Med* 1988;318(12):733–741.
302. Jung YJ, Choi H, Kim H, et al. MicroRNA miR-BART20-5p stabilizes Epstein-Barr virus latency by directly targeting BZLF1 and BRLF1. *J Virol* 2014;88(16):9027–9037.
303. Kalla M, Gobel C, Hammerschmidt W. The lytic phase of epstein-barr virus requires a viral genome with 5-methylcytosine residues in CpG sites. *J Virol* 2012;86(1):447–458.
304. Kalla M, Schmeinck A, Bergbauer M, et al. AP-1 homolog BZLF1 of Epstein-Barr virus has two essential functions dependent on the epigenetic state of the viral genome. *Proc Natl Acad Sci U S A* 2010;107(2):850–855.
305. Kanakry J, Ambinder R. The biology and clinical utility of EBV monitoring in blood. *Curr Top Microbiol Immunol* 2015;391:475–499.
306. Kanakry JA, Hegde AM, Durand CM, et al. The clinical significance of EBV DNA in the plasma and peripheral blood mononuclear cells of patients with or without EBV diseases. *Blood* 2016;127(16):2007–2017.
307. Kanazawa T, Hiramatsu Y, Iwata S, et al. Anti-CCR4 monoclonal antibody mogamulizumab for the treatment of EBV-associated T- and NK-cell lymphoproliferative diseases. *Clin Cancer Res* 2014;20(19):5075–5084.
308. Kanekiyo M, Bu W, Joyce MG, et al. Rational design of an Epstein-Barr virus vaccine targeting the receptor-binding site. *Cell* 2015;162(5):1090–1100.
309. Kanzler H, Kuppers R, Hansmann ML, et al. Hodgkin and Reed-Sternberg cells in Hodgkin's disease represent the outgrowth of a dominant tumor clone derived from (crippled) germinal center B cells. *J Exp Med* 1996;184(4):1495–1505.
310. Karajannis MA, Hummel M, Anagnostopoulos I, et al. Strict lymphotropism of Epstein-Barr virus during acute infectious mononucleosis in nonimmunocompromised individuals. *Blood* 1997;89(8):2856–2862.
311. Katano H, Pesnicak L, Cohen JI. Simvastatin induces apoptosis of Epstein-Barr virus (EBV)-transformed lymphoblastoid cell lines and delays development of EBV lymphomas. *Proc Natl Acad Sci U S A* 2004;101(14):4960–4965.
312. Katzman RB, Longnecker R. LMP2A does not require palmitoylation to localize to buoyant complexes or for function. *J Virol* 2004;78(20):10878–10887.
313. Kaye KM, Devergne O, Harada JN, et al. Tumor necrosis factor receptor associated factor 2 is a mediator of NF- kappa B activation by latent infection membrane protein 1, the Epstein- Barr virus transforming protein. *Proc Natl Acad Sci U S A* 1996;93(20):11085–11090.
314. Kaye KM, Izumi KM, Kieff E. Epstein-Barr virus latent membrane protein 1 is essential for B-lymphocyte growth transformation. *Proc Natl Acad Sci U S A* 1993;90(19):9150–9154.
315. Kaye KM, Izumi KM, Li H, et al. An Epstein-Barr virus that expresses only the first 231 LMP1 amino acids efficiently initiates primary B-lymphocyte growth transformation. *J Virol* 1999;73(12):10525–10530.
316. Kaye KM, Izumi KM, Mosialos G, et al. The Epstein-Barr virus LMP1 cytoplasmic carboxy terminus is essential for B-lymphocyte transformation; fibroblast cocultivation complements a critical function within the terminal 155 residues. *J Virol* 1995;69(2):675–683.
317. Kelly GL, Long HM, Stylianou J, et al. An Epstein-Barr virus anti-apoptotic protein constitutively expressed in transformed cells and implicated in burkitt lymphomagenesis: the Wp/BHRF1 link. *PLoS Pathog* 2009;5(3):e1000341.
318. Kelly GL, Milner AE, Tierney RJ, et al. Epstein-Barr virus nuclear antigen 2 (EBNA2) gene deletion is consistently linked with EBNA3A, -3B, and -3C expression in Burkitt's lymphoma cells and with increased resistance to apoptosis. *J Virol* 2005;79(16):10709–10717.
319. Kempkes B, Ling PD. EBNA2 and its coactivator EBNA-LP. *Curr Top Microbiol Immunol* 2015;391:35–59.
320. Kennedy G, Komano J, Sugden B. Epstein-Barr virus provides a survival factor to Burkitt's lymphomas. *Proc Natl Acad Sci U S A* 2003;100(24):14269–14274.
321. Kennedy G, Sugden B. EBNA-1, a bifunctional transcriptional activator. *Mol Cell Biol* 2003;23(19):6901–6908.
322. Kenney SC, Mertz JE. Regulation of the latent-lytic switch in Epstein-Barr virus. *Semin Cancer Biol* 2014;26:60–68.
323. Kersten MJ, Klein MR, Holwerda AM, et al. Epstein-Barr virus-specific cytotoxic T cell responses in HIV-1 infection: different kinetics in patients progressing to opportunistic infection or non-Hodgkin's lymphoma. *J Clin Invest* 1997;99(7):1525–1533.
324. Keryer-Bibens C, Pioche-Durieu C, Villemant C, et al. Exosomes released by EBV-infected nasopharyngeal carcinoma cells convey the viral latent membrane protein 1 and the immunomodulatory protein galectin 9. *BMC Cancer* 2006;6:283.
325. Kieff E, Levine J. Homology between Burkitt herpes viral DNA and DNA in continuous lymphoblastoid cells from patients with infectious mononucleosis. *Proc Natl Acad Sci U S A* 1974;71(2):355–358.
326. Kieser A, Sterz KR. The latent membrane protein 1 (LMP1). *Curr Top Microbiol Immunol* 2015;391:119–149.
327. Kilger E, Kieser A, Baumann M, et al. Epstein-Barr virus-mediated B-cell proliferation is dependent upon latent membrane protein 1, which simulates an activated CD40 receptor. *EMBO J* 1998;17(6):1700–1709.
328. Kim KD, Tanizawa H, De Leo A, et al. Epigenetic specifications of host chromosome docking sites for latent Epstein-Barr virus. *Nat Commun* 2020;11(1):877.
329. Kimura H, Ito Y, Kawabe S, et al. Epstein-Barr virus (EBV)-associated T/NK lymphoproliferative diseases in non-immunocompromised hosts: prospective analysis of 108 cases. *Blood* 2012;119:673–686.
330. Kimura H, Kwong YL. EBV Viral loads in diagnosis, monitoring, and response assessment. *Front Oncol* 2019;9:62.
331. Kimura H, Miyake K, Yamauchi Y, et al. Identification of Epstein-Barr virus (EBV)-infected lymphocyte subtypes by flow cytometric in situ hybridization in EBV-associated lymphoproliferative diseases. *J Infect Dis* 2009;200(7):1078–1087.
332. Kinch A, Oberg G, Arvidson J, et al. Post-transplant lymphoproliferative disease and other Epstein-Barr virus diseases in allogeneic haematopoietic stem cell transplantation after introduction of monitoring of viral load by polymerase chain reaction. *Scand J Infect Dis* 2007;39(3):235–244.
333. Kinch A, Sundstrom C, Tufveson G, et al. Association between HLA-A1 and -A2 types and Epstein-Barr virus status of post-transplant lymphoproliferative disorder. *Leuk Lymphoma* 2016;57(10):2351–2358.
334. King W, Dambaugh T, Heller M, et al. Epstein-Barr virus DNA XII. A variable region of the Epstein-Barr virus genome is included in the P3HR-1 deletion. *J Virol* 1982;43(3):979–986.
335. Kirschner AN, Lowrey AS, Longnecker R, et al. Binding-site interactions between Epstein-Barr virus fusion proteins gp42 and gH/gL reveal a peptide that inhibits both epithelial and B-cell membrane fusion. *J Virol* 2007;81(17):9216–9229.
336. Kirschner AN, Sorem J, Longnecker R, et al. Structure of Epstein-Barr virus glycoprotein 42 suggests a mechanism for triggering receptor-activated virus entry. *Structure* 2009;17(2):223–233.
337. Klibi J, Niki T, Riedel A, et al. Blood diffusion and Th1-suppressive effects of galectin-9-containing exosomes released by Epstein-Barr virus-infected nasopharyngeal carcinoma cells. *Blood* 2009;113(9):1957–1966.
338. Knight JS, Robertson ES. Epstein-Barr virus nuclear antigen 3C regulates cyclin A/p27 complexes and enhances cyclin A-dependent kinase activity. *J Virol* 2004;78(4):1981–1991.
339. Knight JS, Sharma N, Kalman DE, et al. A cyclin-binding motif within the amino-terminal homology domain of EBNA3C binds cyclin A and modulates cyclin A-dependent kinase activity in Epstein-Barr virus-infected cells. *J Virol* 2004;78(23):12857–12867.
340. Knight JS, Sharma N, Robertson ES. Epstein-Barr virus latent antigen 3C can mediate the degradation of the retinoblastoma protein through an SCF cellular ubiquitin ligase. *Proc Natl Acad Sci U S A* 2005;102(51):18562–18566.
341. Knight JS, Sharma N, Robertson ES. SCFSkp2 complex targeted by Epstein-Barr virus essential nuclear antigen. *Mol Cell Biol* 2005;25(5):1749–1763.
342. Koganti S, Clark C, Zhi J, et al. Cellular STAT3 functions via PCBP2 to restrain Epstein-Barr Virus lytic activation in B lymphocytes. *J Virol* 2015;89(9):5002–5011.
343. Kogawa K, Sato H, Asano T, et al. Prognostic factors of Epstein-Barr virus-associated hemophagocytic lymphohistiocytosis in children: report of the Japan Histiocytosis Study Group. *Pediatr Blood Cancer* 2014;61(7):1257–1262.

344. Komano J, Sugiura M, Takada K. Epstein-Barr virus contributes to the malignant phenotype and to apoptosis resistance in Burkitt's lymphoma cell line Akata. *J Virol* 1998;72(11):9150–9156.
345. Kong QL, Hu LJ, Cao JY, et al. Epstein-Barr virus-encoded LMP2A induces an epithelial-mesenchymal transition and increases the number of side population stem-like cancer cells in nasopharyngeal carcinoma. *PLoS Pathog* 2010;6(6):e1000940.
346. Kraus RJ, Mirocha SJ, Stephany HM, et al. Identification of a novel element involved in regulation of the lytic switch BZLF1 gene promoter of Epstein-Barr virus. *J Virol* 2001;75(2):867–877.
347. Kraus RJ, Perrigoue JG, Mertz JE. ZEB negatively regulates the lytic-switch BZLF1 gene promoter of Epstein-Barr virus. *J Virol* 2003;77(1):199–207.
348. Kulwichit W, Edwards RH, Davenport EM, et al. Expression of the Epstein-Barr virus latent membrane protein 1 induces B cell lymphoma in transgenic mice. *Proc Natl Acad Sci U S A* 1998;95(20):11963–11968.
349. Kung CP, Raab-Traub N. Epstein-Barr virus latent membrane protein 1 induces expression of the epidermal growth factor receptor through effects on Bcl-3 and STAT3. *J Virol* 2008;82(11):5486–5493.
350. Kuppers R. B cells under influence: transformation of B cells by Epstein-Barr virus. *Nat Rev Immunol* 2003;3(10):801–812.
351. Kuri A, Jacobs BM, Vickaryous N, et al. Epidemiology of Epstein-Barr virus infection and infectious mononucleosis in the United Kingdom. *BMC Public Health* 2020;20(1):912.
352. Kurth J, Spieker T, Wustrow J, et al. EBV-infected B cells in infectious mononucleosis: viral strategies for spreading in the B cell compartment and establishing latency. *Immunity* 2000;13(4):485–495.
353. Kuze T, Nakamura N, Hashimoto Y, et al. Clinicopathological, immunological and genetic studies of CD30+ anaplastic large cell lymphoma of B-cell type; association with Epstein-Barr virus in a Japanese population. *J Pathol* 1996;180(3):236–242.
354. Laichalk LL, Hochberg D, Babcock GJ, et al. The dispersal of mucosal memory B cells: evidence from persistent EBV infection. *Immunity* 2002;16(5):745–754.
355. Laichalk LL, Thorley-Lawson DA. Terminal differentiation into plasma cells initiates the replicative cycle of Epstein-Barr virus in vivo. *J Virol* 2005;79(2):1296–1307.
356. Lam JKP, Hui KF, Ning RJ, et al. Emergence of CD4+ and CD8+ polyfunctional T cell responses against immunodominant lytic and latent EBV antigens in children with primary EBV infection. *Front Microbiol* 2018;9:416.
357. Lam N, Sugden B. LMP1, a viral relative of the TNF receptor family, signals principally from intracellular compartments. *EMBO J* 2003;22(12):3027–3038.
358. Lambert SL, Martinez OM. Latent membrane protein 1 of EBV activates phosphatidylinositol 3-kinase to induce production of IL-10. *J Immunol* 2007;179(12):8225–8234.
359. Landgren O, Gilbert ES, Rizzo JD, et al. Risk factors for lymphoproliferative disorders after allogeneic hematopoietic cell transplantation. *Blood* 2009;113(20):4992–5001.
360. Lang F, Singh RK, Pei Y, et al. EBV epitranscriptome reprogramming by METTL14 is critical for viral-associated tumorigenesis. *PLoS Pathog* 2019;15(6):e1007796.
361. Latour S, Fischer A. Signaling pathways involved in the T-cell-mediated immunity against Epstein-Barr virus: lessons from genetic diseases. *Immunol Rev* 2019;291(1):174–189.
362. Laux G, Adam B, Strobl LJ, et al. The Spi-1/PU.1 and Spi-B ets family transcription factors and the recombination signal binding protein RBP-J kappa interact with an Epstein-Barr virus nuclear antigen 2 responsive cis-element. *EMBO J* 1994;13(23):5624–5632.
363. Laux G, Economou A, Farrell PJ. The terminal protein gene 2 of Epstein-Barr virus is transcribed from a bidirectional latent promoter region. *J Gen Virol* 1989;70(Pt 11):3079–3084.
364. Lay JD, Tsao CJ, Chen JY, et al. Upregulation of tumor necrosis factor-alpha gene by Epstein-Barr virus and activation of macrophages in Epstein-Barr virus-infected T cells in the pathogenesis of hemophagocytic syndrome. *J Clin Invest* 1997;100(8):1969–1979.
365. Lee ES, Locker J, Nalesnik M, et al. The association of Epstein-Barr virus with smooth-muscle tumors occurring after organ transplantation. *N Engl J Med* 1995;332(1):19–25.
366. Lee N, Moss WN, Yario TA, et al. EBV noncoding RNA binds nascent RNA to drive host PAX5 to viral DNA. *Cell* 2015;160(4):607–618.
367. Lee S, Park HY, Kang SY, et al. Genetic alterations of JAK/STAT cascade and histone modification in extranodal NK/T-cell lymphoma nasal type. *Oncotarget* 2015;6(19):17764–17776.
368. Lee S, Sakakibara S, Maruo S, et al. Epstein-Barr virus nuclear protein 3C domains necessary for lymphoblastoid cell growth: interaction with RBP-Jkappa regulates TCL1. *J Virol* 2009;83(23):12368–12377.
369. Lee DY, Sugden B. The LMP1 oncogene of EBV activates PERK and the unfolded protein response to drive its own synthesis. *Blood* 2008;111(4):2280–2289.
370. Leen AM, Myers GD, Sili U, et al. Monoculture-derived T lymphocytes specific for multiple viruses expand and produce clinically relevant effects in immunocompromised individuals. *Nat Med* 2006;12(10):1160–1166.
371. Lemon SM, Hutt LM, Shaw JE, et al. Replication of EBV in epithelial cells during infectious mononucleosis. *Nature* 1977;268(5617):268–270.
372. Lerner MR, Andrews NC, Miller G, et al. Two small RNAs encoded by Epstein-Barr virus and complexed with protein are precipitated by antibodies from patients with systemic lupus erythematosus. *Proc Natl Acad Sci U S A* 1981;78(2):805–809.
373. Leung SF, Tam JS, Chan AT, et al. Improved accuracy of detection of nasopharyngeal carcinoma by combined application of circulating Epstein-Barr virus DNA and anti-Epstein-Barr viral capsid antigen IgA antibody. *Clin Chem* 2004;50(2):339–345.
374. Levin LI, Munger KL, O'Reilly EJ, et al. Primary infection with the Epstein-Barr virus and risk of multiple sclerosis. *Ann Neurol* 2010;67(6):824–830.
375. Levin LI, Munger KL, Rubertone MV, et al. Temporal relationship between elevation of epstein-barr virus antibody titers and initial onset of neurological symptoms in multiple sclerosis. *JAMA* 2005;293(20):2496–2500.
376. Li Q, Bu W, Gabriel E, et al. HLA-DQ beta1 alleles associated with Epstein-Barr virus (EBV) infectivity and EBV gp42 binding to cells. *JCI Insight* 2017;2(4):e85687.
377. Li J, Callegari S, Masucci MG. The Epstein-Barr virus miR-BHRF1-1 targets RNF4 during productive infection to promote the accumulation of SUMO conjugates and the release of infectious virus. *PLoS Pathog* 2017;13(4):e1006338.
378. Li YY, Chung GT, Lui VW, et al. Exome and genome sequencing of nasopharynx cancer identifies NF-kappaB pathway activating mutations. *Nat Commun* 2017;8:14121.
379. Li X, Kozlov SV, El-Guindy A, Bhaduri-McIntosh S. Retrograde regulation by the viral protein kinase epigenetically sustains the Epstein-Barr virus latency-to-lytic switch to augment virus production. *J Virol* 2019;93(17).
380. Li Q, Turk SM, Hutt-Fletcher LM. The Epstein-Barr virus (EBV) BZLF2 gene product associates with the gH and gL homologs of EBV and carries an epitope critical to infection of B cells but not of epithelial cells. *J Virol* 1995;69(7):3987–3994.
381. Li ZX, Zeng S, Wu HX, et al. The risk of systemic lupus erythematosus associated with Epstein-Barr virus infection: a systematic review and meta-analysis. *Clin Exp Med* 2019;19(1):23–36.
382. Lieberman P. Identification of functional targets of the Zta transcriptional activator by formation of stable preinitiation complex intermediates. *Mol Cell Biol* 1994;14(12):8365–8375.
383. Lieberman PM. Chromatin structure of Epstein-Barr virus latent episomes. *Curr Top Microbiol Immunol* 2015;390(Pt 1):71–102.
384. Lieberman PM. Epigenetics and genetics of viral latency. *Cell Host Microbe* 2016;19(5):619–628.
385. Lieberman PM, Berk AJ. The Zta trans-activator protein stabilizes TFIID association with promoter DNA by direct protein-protein interaction. *Genes Dev* 1991;5(12B):2441–2454.
386. Lieberman PM, Hardwick JM, Sample J, et al. The zta transactivator involved in induction of lytic cycle gene expression in Epstein-Barr virus-infected lymphocytes binds to both AP-1 and ZRE sites in target promoter and enhancer regions. *J Virol* 1990;64(3):1143–1155.
387. Lieberman PM, Ozer J, Gursel DB. Requirement for transcription factor IIA (TFIIA)-TFIID recruitment by an activator depends on promoter structure and template competition. *Mol Cell Biol* 1997;17(11):6624–6632.
388. Liebowitz D, Wang D, Kieff E. Orientation and patching of the latent infection membrane protein encoded by Epstein-Barr virus. *J Virol* 1986;58(1):233–237.
389. Lin J, Johannsen E, Robertson E, et al. Epstein-Barr virus nuclear antigen 3C putative repression domain mediates coactivation of the LMP1 promoter with EBNA-2. *J Virol* 2002;76(1):232–242.
390. Lin DC, Meng X, Hazawa M, et al. The genomic landscape of nasopharyngeal carcinoma. *Nat Genet* 2014;46(8):866–871.
391. Lin X, Tsai MH, Shumilov A, et al. The Epstein-Barr virus BART miRNA cluster of the M81 strain modulates multiple functions in primary B cells. *PLoS Pathog* 2015;11(12):e1005344.
392. Lin JC, Wang WY, Chen KY, et al. Quantification of plasma Epstein-Barr virus DNA in patients with advanced nasopharyngeal carcinoma. *N Engl J Med* 2004;350(24):2461–2470.
393. Ling PD, Hayward SD. Contribution of conserved amino acids in mediating the interaction between EBNA2 and CBF1/RBPJk. *J Virol* 1995;69(3):1944–1950.
394. Ling PD, Peng RS, Nakajima A, et al. Mediation of Epstein-Barr virus EBNA-LP transcriptional coactivation by Sp100. *EMBO J* 2005;24(20):3565–3575.
395. Linnstaedt SD, Gottwein E, Skalsky RL, et al. Virally induced cellular microRNA miR-155 plays a key role in B-cell immortalization by Epstein-Barr virus. *J Virol* 2010;84(22):11670–11678.
396. Liu F, Marquardt G, Kirschner AN, et al. Mapping the N-terminal residues of Epstein-Barr virus gp42 that bind gH/gL by using fluorescence polarization and cell-based fusion assays. *J Virol* 2010;84(19):10375–10385.
397. Liu X, Sadaoka T, Krogmann T, et al. Epstein-Barr virus (EBV) tegument protein BGLF2 suppresses type I interferon signaling to promote EBV reactivation. *J Virol* 2020;94(11).
398. Long HM, Leese AM, Chagoury OL, et al. Cytotoxic CD4+ T cell responses to EBV contrast with CD8 responses in breadth of lytic cycle antigen choice and in lytic cycle recognition. *J Immunol* 2011;187(1):92–101.
399. Long HM, Meckiff BJ, Taylor GS. The T-cell response to Epstein-Barr virus-new tricks from an old dog. *Front Immunol* 2019;10:2193.
400. Longnecker R, Druker B, Roberts TM, et al. An Epstein-Barr virus protein associated with cell growth transformation interacts with a tyrosine kinase. *J Virol* 1991;65(7):3681–3692.
401. Longnecker R, Kieff E. A second Epstein-Barr virus membrane protein (LMP2) is expressed in latent infection and colocalizes with LMP1. *J Virol* 1990;64(5):2319–2326.
402. Longnecker RM, Kieff E, Cohen JI. Epstein-barr virus. In: Knipe DM, Howley PM, eds. *Fields Virology*. Vol. 1. 6th ed. Philadelphia, PA: Wolters Kluwer, Lippincott Williams & Wilkins; 2013:1898–1959.
403. Longnecker R, Miller CL, Miao XQ, et al. The only domain which distinguishes Epstein-Barr virus latent membrane protein 2A (LMP2A) from LMP2B is dispensable for lymphocyte infection and growth transformation in vitro; LMP2A is therefore nonessential. *J Virol* 1992;66(11):6461–6469.
404. Lowell CA, Klickstein LB, Carter RH, et al. Mapping of the Epstein-Barr virus and C3dg binding sites to a common domain on complement receptor type 2. *J Exp Med* 1989;170(6):1931–1946.
405. Lu F, Chen HS, Kossenkov AV, et al. EBNA2 drives formation of new chromosome binding sites and target genes for B-cell master regulatory transcription factors RBP-jkappa and EBF1. *PLoS Pathog* 2016;12(1):e1005339.
406. Lu J, Lin WH, Chen SY, et al. Syk tyrosine kinase mediates Epstein-Barr virus latent membrane protein 2A-induced cell migration in epithelial cells. *J Biol Chem* 2006;281(13):8806–8814.
407. Lu F, Wiedmer A, Martin KA, et al. Coordinate regulation of TET2 and EBNA2 control DNA methylation state of latent Epstein-Barr virus. *J Virol* 2017;91:e00804.
408. Lu F, Wikramasinghe P, Norseen J, et al. Genome-wide analysis of host-chromosome binding sites for Epstein-Barr Virus Nuclear Antigen 1 (EBNA1). *Virol J* 2010;7:262.
409. Lucchesi W, Brady G, Dittrich-Breiholz O, et al. Differential gene regulation by Epstein-Barr virus type 1 and type 2 EBNA2. *J Virol* 2008;82(15):7456–7466.
410. Lupey-Green LN, Caruso LB, Madzo J, et al. PARP1 stabilizes CTCF binding and chromatin structure to maintain Epstein Barr virus latency type. *J Virol* 2018;92:e00755.
411. Lupey-Green LN, Moquin SA, Martin KA, et al. PARP1 restricts Epstein Barr Virus lytic reactivation by binding the BZLF1 promoter. *Virology* 2017;507:220–230.
412. Lupton S, Levine AJ. Mapping genetic elements of Epstein-Barr virus that facilitate extrachromosomal persistence of Epstein-Barr virus-derived plasmids in human cells. *Mol Cell Biol* 1985;5(10):2533–2542.

413. Lv DW, Zhang K, Li R. Interferon regulatory factor 8 regulates caspase-1 expression to facilitate Epstein-Barr virus reactivation in response to B cell receptor stimulation and chemical induction. *PLoS Pathog* 2018;14(1):e1006868.
414. Lyons DE, Yu KP, Vander Heiden JA, et al. Mutant cellular AP-1 proteins promote expression of a subset of Epstein-Barr virus late genes in the absence of lytic viral DNA replication. *J Virol* 2018;92(19).
415. Ma SD, Tsai MH, Romero-Masters JC, et al. Latent membrane protein 1 (LMP1) and LMP2A collaborate to promote Epstein-Barr virus-induced B cell lymphomas in a cord blood-humanized mouse model but are not essential. *J Virol* 2017;91(7).
416. Ma Y, Walsh MJ, Bernhardt K, et al. CRISPR/Cas9 screens reveal Epstein-Barr virus-transformed B cell host dependency factors. *Cell Host Microbe* 2017;21(5):580–591.e587.
417. Ma SD, Xu X, Plowshay J, et al. LMP1-deficient Epstein-Barr virus mutant requires T cells for lymphomagenesis. *J Clin Invest* 2015;125(1):304–315.
418. Ma SD, Yu X, Mertz JE, et al. An Epstein-Barr Virus (EBV) mutant with enhanced BZLF1 expression causes lymphomas with abortive lytic EBV infection in a humanized mouse model. *J Virol* 2012;86(15):7976–7987.
419. MacMahon EM, Glass JD, Hayward SD, et al. Epstein-Barr virus in AIDS-related primary central nervous system lymphoma. *Lancet* 1991;338(8773):969–973.
420. Maier S, Staffler G, Hartmann A, et al. Cellular target genes of Epstein-Barr virus nuclear antigen 2. *J Virol* 2006;80(19):9761–9771.
421. Mainou BA, Everly DN Jr, Raab-Traub N. Epstein-Barr virus latent membrane protein 1 CTAR1 mediates rodent and human fibroblast transformation through activation of PI3K. *Oncogene* 2005;24(46):6917–6924.
422. Malecka KA, Dheekollu J, Deakyne JS, et al. Structural basis for cooperative binding of EBNA1 to the Epstein-Barr virus dyad symmetry minimal origin of replication. *J Virol* 2019;93(20).
423. Mancao C, Altmann M, Jungnickel B, et al. Rescue of "crippled" germinal center B cells from apoptosis by Epstein-Barr virus. *Blood* 2005;106(13):4339–4344.
424. Mancao C, Hammerschmidt W. Epstein-Barr virus latent membrane protein 2A is a B-cell receptor mimic and essential for B-cell survival. *Blood* 2007;110(10):3715–3721.
425. Mannick JB, Cohen JI, Birkenbach M, et al. The Epstein-Barr virus nuclear protein encoded by the leader of the EBNA RNAs is important in B-lymphocyte transformation. *J Virol* 1991;65(12):6826–6837.
426. Marquitz AR, Mathur A, Edwards RH, et al. Host gene expression is regulated by two types of noncoding RNAs transcribed from the Epstein-Barr virus BamHI A rightward transcript region. *J Virol* 2015;89(22):11256–11268.
427. Marquitz AR, Mathur A, Nam CS, et al. The Epstein-Barr virus BART microRNAs target the pro-apoptotic protein Bim. *Virology* 2011;412(2):392–400.
428. Marsh RA. Epstein-Barr virus and hemophagocytic lymphohistiocytosis. *Front Immunol* 2017;8:1902.
429. Marshall D, Sample C. Epstein-Barr virus nuclear antigen 3C is a transcriptional regulator. *J Virol* 1995;69(6):3624–3630.
430. Martin KA, Lupey LN, Tempera I. Epstein-Barr virus oncoprotein LMP1 mediates epigenetic changes in host gene expression through PARP1. *J Virol* 2016;90(19):8520–8530.
431. Maruo S, Johannsen E, Illanes D, et al. Epstein-Barr virus nuclear protein 3A domains essential for growth of lymphoblasts: transcriptional regulation through RBP-Jkappa/CBF1 is critical. *J Virol* 2005;79(16):10171–10179.
432. Maruo S, Wu Y, Ishikawa S, et al. Epstein-Barr virus nuclear protein EBNA3C is required for cell cycle progression and growth maintenance of lymphoblastoid cells. *Proc Natl Acad Sci U S A* 2006;103(51):19500–19505.
433. Maruo S, Wu Y, Ito T, et al. Epstein-Barr virus nuclear protein EBNA3C residues critical for maintaining lymphoblastoid cell growth. *Proc Natl Acad Sci U S A* 2009;106(11):4419–4424.
434. Maruo S, Zhao B, Johannsen E, et al. Epstein-Barr virus nuclear antigens 3C and 3A maintain lymphoblastoid cell growth by repressing p16INK4A and p14ARF expression. *Proc Natl Acad Sci U S A* 2011;108(5):1919–1924.
435. Masucci MG, Contreras-Salazar B, Ragnar E, et al. 5-Azacytidine up regulates the expression of Epstein-Barr virus nuclear antigen 2 (EBNA-2) through EBNA-6 and latent membrane protein in the Burkitt's lymphoma line rael. *J Virol* 1989;63(7):3135–3141.
436. Matskova L, Ernberg I, Pawson T, et al. C-terminal domain of the Epstein-Barr virus LMP2A membrane protein contains a clustering signal. *J Virol* 2001;75(22):10941–10949.
437. Matsuura H, Kirschner AN, Longnecker R, et al. Crystal structure of the Epstein-Barr virus (EBV) glycoprotein H/glycoprotein L (gH/gL) complex. *Proc Natl Acad Sci U S A* 2010;107(52):22641–22646.
438. Maurer UE, Sodeik B, Grunewald K. Native 3D intermediates of membrane fusion in herpes simplex virus 1 entry. *Proc Natl Acad Sci U S A* 2008;105(30):10559–10564.
439. McAulay KA, Higgins CD, Macsween KF, et al. HLA class I polymorphisms are associated with development of infectious mononucleosis upon primary EBV infection. *J Clin Invest* 2007;117(10):3042–3048.
440. McClain KL, Leach CT, Jenson HB, et al. Association of Epstein-Barr virus with leiomyosarcomas in children with AIDS. *N Engl J Med* 1995;332(1):12–18.
441. McClellan MJ, Wood CD, Ojeniyi O, et al. Modulation of enhancer looping and differential gene targeting by Epstein-Barr virus transcription factors directs cellular reprogramming. *PLoS Pathog* 2013;9(9):e1003636.
442. McFadden K, Hafez AY, Kishton R, et al. Metabolic stress is a barrier to Epstein-Barr virus-mediated B-cell immortalization. *Proc Natl Acad Sci U S A* 2016;113(6):E782–E790.
443. McKenzie J, El-Guindy A. Epstein-Barr virus lytic cycle reactivation. *Curr Top Microbiol Immunol* 2015;391:237–261.
444. McLaughlin LP, Rouce R, Gottschalk S, et al. EBV/LMP-specific T cells maintain remissions of T- and B-cell EBV lymphomas after allogeneic bone marrow transplantation. *Blood* 2018;132(22):2351–2361.
445. Meckes DG Jr, Menaker NF, Raab-Traub N. Epstein-Barr virus LMP1 modulates lipid raft microdomains and the vimentin cytoskeleton for signal transduction and transformation. *J Virol* 2013;87(3):1301–1311.
446. Meckes DG Jr, Raab-Traub N. Microvesicles and viral infection. *J Virol* 2011;85(24):12844–12854.
447. Meckes DG Jr, Shair KH, Marquitz AR, et al. Human tumor virus utilizes exosomes for intercellular communication. *Proc Natl Acad Sci U S A* 2010;107(47):20370–20375.
448. Meitinger C, Strobl LJ, Marschall G, et al. Crucial sequences within the Epstein-Barr virus TP1 promoter for EBNA2- mediated transactivation and interaction of EBNA2 with its responsive element. *J Virol* 1994;68(11):7497–7506.
449. Melani C, Jaffe ES, Wilson WH. Pathobiology and treatment of lymphomatoid granulomatosis, a rare EBV-driven disorder. *Blood* 2020;135(16):1344–1352.
450. Meng Q, Hagemeier SR, Fingeroth JD, et al. The Epstein-Barr virus (EBV)-encoded protein kinase, EBV-PK, but not the thymidine kinase (EBV-TK), is required for ganciclovir and acyclovir inhibition of lytic viral production. *J Virol* 2010;84(9):4534–4542.
451. Merchant M, Caldwell RG, Longnecker R. The LMP2A ITAM is essential for providing B cells with development and survival signals in vivo. *J Virol* 2000;74(19):9115–9124.
452. Merchant M, Longnecker R. LMP2A survival and developmental signals are transmitted through Btk-dependent and Btk-independent pathways. *Virology* 2001;291(1):46–54.
453. Messick TE, Smith GR, Soldan SS, et al. Structure-based design of small-molecule inhibitors of EBNA1 DNA binding blocks Epstein-Barr virus latent infection and tumor growth. *Sci Transl Med* 2019;11(482).
454. Middeldorp JM. Epstein-Barr virus-specific humoral immune responses in health and disease. *Curr Top Microbiol Immunol* 2015;391:289–323.
455. Middleton T, Sugden B. Retention of plasmid DNA in mammalian cells is enhanced by binding of the Epstein-Barr virus replication protein EBNA1. *J Virol* 1994;68(6):4067–4071.
456. Miller CL, Burkhardt AL, Lee JH, et al. Integral membrane protein 2 of Epstein-Barr virus regulates reactivation from latency through dominant negative effects on protein- tyrosine kinases. *Immunity* 1995;2(2):155–166.
457. Miller WE, Cheshire JL, Raab-Traub N. Interaction of tumor necrosis factor receptor-associated factor signaling proteins with the latent membrane protein 1 PXQXT motif is essential for induction of epidermal growth factor receptor expression. *Mol Cell Biol* 1998;18(5):2835–2844.
458. Miller G, El-Guindy A, Countryman J, et al. Lytic cycle switches of oncogenic human gammaherpesviruses. *Adv Cancer Res* 2007;97:81–109.
459. Miller N, Hutt-Fletcher LM. A monoclonal antibody to glycoprotein gp85 inhibits fusion but not attachment of Epstein-Barr virus. *J Virol* 1988;62(7):2366–2372.
460. Miller N, Hutt-Fletcher LM. Epstein-Barr virus enters B cells and epithelial cells by different routes. *J Virol* 1992;66(6):3409–3414.
461. Miller G, Lipman M. Comparison of the yield of infectious virus from clones of human and simian lymphoblastoid lines transformed by Epstein-Barr virus. *J Exp Med* 1973;138(6):1398–1412.
462. Miller G, Rabson M, Heston L. Epstein-Barr virus with heterogeneous DNA disrupts latency. *J Virol* 1984;50(1):174–182.
463. Minamitani T, Ma Y, Zhou H, et al. Mouse model of Epstein-Barr virus LMP1- and LMP2A-driven germinal center B-cell lymphoproliferative disease. *Proc Natl Acad Sci U S A* 2017;114(18):4751–4756.
464. Miyake T, Yamamoto T, Hirai Y, et al. Survival rates and prognostic factors of Epstein-Barr virus-associated hydroa vacciniforme and hypersensitivity to mosquito bites. *Br J Dermatol* 2015;172(1):56–63.
465. Miyashita EM, Yang B, Lam KM, et al. A novel form of Epstein-Barr virus latency in normal B cells in vivo. *Cell* 1995;80(4):593–601.
466. Miyazaki T, Fujimaki K, Shirasugi Y, et al. Remission of lymphoma after withdrawal of methotrexate in rheumatoid arthritis: relationship with type of latent Epstein-Barr virus infection. *Am J Hematol* 2007;82(12):1106–1109.
467. Mohl BS, Chen J, Park SJ, et al. Epstein-Barr virus fusion with epithelial cells triggered by gB is restricted by a gL glycosylation site. *J Virol* 2017;91(23).
468. Molesworth SJ, Lake CM, Borza CM, et al. Epstein-Barr virus gH is essential for penetration of B cells but also plays a role in attachment of virus to epithelial cells. *J Virol* 2000;74(14):6324–6332.
469. Molyneux EM, Rochford R, Griffin B, et al. Burkitt's lymphoma. *Lancet* 2012;379(9822):1234–1244.
470. Moody CA, Scott RS, Amirghahari N, et al. Modulation of the cell growth regulator mTOR by Epstein-Barr virus-encoded LMP2A. *J Virol* 2005;79(9):5499–5506.
471. Moore KW, O'Garra A, de Waal Malefyt R, et al. Interleukin-10. *Annu Rev Immunol* 1993;11:165–190.
472. Moorthy RK, Thorley-Lawson DA. Biochemical, genetic, and functional analyses of the phosphorylation sites on the Epstein-Barr virus-encoded oncogenic latent membrane protein LMP-1. *J Virol* 1993;67(5):2637–2645.
473. Moquin SA, Thomas S, Whalen S, et al. The Epstein-Barr virus episome maneuvers between nuclear chromatin compartments during reactivation. *J Virol* 2018;92(3).
474. Morrison JA, Gulley ML, Pathmanathan R, et al. Differential signaling pathways are activated in the Epstein-Barr virus-associated malignancies nasopharyngeal carcinoma and Hodgkin lymphoma. *Cancer Res* 2004;64(15):5251–5260.
475. Morrison JA, Klingelhutz AJ, Raab-Traub N. Epstein-Barr virus latent membrane protein 2A activates beta-catenin signaling in epithelial cells. *J Virol* 2003;77(22):12276–12284.
476. Mosialos G, Birkenbach M, Yalamanchili R, et al. The Epstein-Barr virus transforming protein LMP1 engages signaling proteins for the tumor necrosis factor receptor family. *Cell* 1995;80(3):389–399.
477. Moutschen M, Leonard P, Sokal EM, et al. Phase I/II studies to evaluate safety and immunogenicity of a recombinant gp350 Epstein-Barr virus vaccine in healthy adults. *Vaccine* 2007;25(24):4697–4705.
478. Mrozek-Gorska P, Buschle A, Pich D, et al. Epstein-Barr virus reprograms human B lymphocytes immediately in the prelatent phase of infection. *Proc Natl Acad Sci U S A* 2019;116(32):16046–16055.
479. Mueller N, Evans A, Harris NL, et al. Hodgkin's disease and Epstein-Barr virus. Altered antibody pattern before diagnosis. *N Engl J Med* 1989;320(11):689–695.
480. Mullen MM, Haan KM, Longnecker R, et al. Structure of the Epstein-Barr virus gp42 protein bound to the MHC class II receptor HLA-DR1. *Mol Cell* 2002;9(2):375–385.

481. Muller YA, Hage S, Alkhashrom S, et al. High-resolution crystal structures of two prototypical beta- and gamma-herpesviral nuclear egress complexes unravel the determinants of subfamily specificity. *J Biol Chem* 2020;295(10):3189–3201.
482. Muncunill J, Baptista MJ, Hernandez-Rodriguez A, et al. Plasma Epstein-Barr virus load as an early biomarker and prognostic factor of human immunodeficiency virus-related lymphomas. *Clin Infect Dis* 2019;68(5):834–843.
483. Munger KL, Hongell K, Cortese M, et al. Epstein-barr virus and multiple sclerosis risk in the finnish maternity cohort. *Ann Neurol* 2019;86(3):436–442.
484. Munger KL, Levin LI, O'Reilly EJ, et al. Anti-Epstein-Barr virus antibodies as serological markers of multiple sclerosis: a prospective study among United States military personnel. *Mult Scler* 2011;17(10):1185–1193.
485. Munz C. Latency and lytic replication in Epstein-Barr virus-associated oncogenesis. *Nat Rev Microbiol* 2019;17(11):691–700.
486. Munz C, Chijioke O. Natural killer cells in herpesvirus infections. *F1000Res* 2017;6:F1000.
487. Murata T. Encyclopedia of EBV-encoded lytic genes: an update. *Adv Exp Med Biol* 2018;1045:395–412.
488. Murata T, Iwata S, Siddiquey MN, et al. Heat shock protein 90 inhibitors repress latent membrane protein 1 (LMP1) expression and proliferation of Epstein-Barr virus-positive natural killer cell lymphoma. *PLoS One* 2013;8(5):e63566.
489. Murata T, Noda C, Narita Y, et al. Induction of Epstein-Barr virus oncoprotein LMP1 by transcription factors AP-2 and early B cell factor. *J Virol* 2016;90(8):3873–3889.
490. Murata T, Tsurumi T. Switching of EBV cycles between latent and lytic states. *Rev Med Virol* 2014;24(3):142–153.
491. Murer A, McHugh D, Caduff N, et al. EBV persistence without its EBNA3A and 3C oncogenes in vivo. *PLoS Pathog* 2018;14(4):e1007039.
492. Murer A, Ruhl J, Zbinden A, et al. MicroRNAs of Epstein-Barr virus attenuate T-cell-mediated immune control in vivo. *MBio* 2019;10(1).
493. Murray PG, Lissauer D, Junying J, et al. Reactivity with A monoclonal antibody to Epstein-Barr virus (EBV) nuclear antigen 1 defines a subset of aggressive breast cancers in the absence of the EBV genome. *Cancer Res* 2003;63(9):2338–2343.
494. Nagaraju T, Sugden AU, Sugden B. Four-dimensional analyses show that replication compartments are clonal factories in which Epstein-Barr viral DNA amplification is coordinated. *Proc Natl Acad Sci U S A* 2019;116(49):24630–24638.
495. Nanbo A. Epstein-Barr virus exploits the secretory pathway to release virions. *Microorganisms* 2020;8(5).
496. Nanbo A, Sugden A, Sugden B. The coupling of synthesis and partitioning of EBV's plasmid replicon is revealed in live cells. *EMBO J* 2007;26(19):4252–4262.
497. Nawandar DM, Ohashi M, Djavadian R, et al. Differentiation-dependent LMP1 expression is required for efficient lytic epstein-barr virus reactivation in epithelial cells. *J Virol* 2017;91(8).
498. Nemerow GR, Cooper NR. Early events in the infection of human B lymphocytes by Epstein-Barr virus: the internalization process. *Virology* 1984;132(1):186–198.
499. Nemerow GR, Mullen JJD, Dickson PW, et al. Soluble recombinant CR2 (CD21) inhibits Epstein-Barr virus infection. *J Virol* 1990;64(3):1348–1352.
500. Ni C, Chen Y, Zeng M, et al. In-cell infection: a novel pathway for Epstein-Barr virus infection mediated by cell-in-cell structures. *Cell Res* 2015;25(7):785–800.
501. Niederman JC, Evans AS. Epstein-Barr virus. In: Evans AS, Kaslow RA, eds. *Viral Infections of Humans: Epidemiology and Control*. 4th ed. New York: Plenum Medical Book Co.; 1997:253–283.
502. Niedobitek G, Herbst H, Young LS, et al. Patterns of Epstein-Barr virus infection in non-neoplastic lymphoid tissue. *Blood* 1992;79(10):2520–2526.
503. Niedobitek G, Young LS, Lau R, et al. Epstein-Barr virus infection in oral hairy leukoplakia: virus replication in the absence of a detectable latent phase. *J Gen Virol* 1991;72(Pt 12):3035–3046.
504. Niens M, Jarrett RF, Hepkema B, et al. HLA-A*02 is associated with a reduced risk and HLA-A*01 with an increased risk of developing EBV+ Hodgkin lymphoma. *Blood* 2007;110(9):3310–3315.
505. Nikitin PA, Yan CM, Forte E, et al. An ATM/Chk2-mediated DNA damage-responsive signaling pathway suppresses Epstein-Barr virus transformation of primary human B cells. *Cell Host Microbe* 2010;8(6):510–522.
506. Ning S, Campos AD, Darnay BG, et al. TRAF6 and the three C-terminal lysine sites on IRF7 are required for its ubiquitination-mediated activation by the tumor necrosis factor receptor family member latent membrane protein 1. *Mol Cell Biol* 2008;28(20):6536–6546.
507. Ning S, Hahn AM, Huye LE, et al. Interferon regulatory factor 7 regulates expression of Epstein-Barr virus latent membrane protein 1: a regulatory circuit. *J Virol* 2003;77(17):9359–9368.
508. Ning S, Pagano JS. The A20 deubiquitinase activity negatively regulates LMP1 activation of IRF7. *J Virol* 2010;84(12):6130–6138.
509. Nitsche F, Bell A, Rickinson A. Epstein-Barr virus leader protein enhances EBNA-2-mediated transactivation of latent membrane protein 1 expression: a role for the W1W2 repeat domain. *J Virol* 1997;71(9):6619–6628.
510. Njie R, Bell AI, Jia H, et al. The effects of acute malaria on Epstein-Barr virus (EBV) load and EBV-specific T cell immunity in Gambian children. *J Infect Dis* 2009;199(1):31–38.
511. Nkosi D, Howell LA, Cheerathodi MR, et al. Transmembrane domains mediate intra- and extracellular trafficking of Epstein-Barr virus latent membrane protein 1. *J Virol* 2018;92(17).
512. Nonkwelo C, Skinner J, Bell A, et al. Transcription start sites downstream of the Epstein-Barr virus (EBV) Fp promoter in early-passage Burkitt lymphoma cells define a fourth promoter for expression of the EBV EBNA-1 protein. *J Virol* 1996;70(1):623–627.
513. Oda T, Imai S, Chiba S, et al. Epstein-barr virus lacking glycoprotein gp85 cannot infect B cells and epithelial cells [In Process Citation]. *Virology* 2000;276(1):52–58.
514. Ogembo JG, Kannan L, Ghiran I, et al. Human complement receptor type 1/CD35 is an Epstein-Barr Virus receptor. *Cell Rep* 2013;3(2):371–385.
515. O'Grady T, Cao S, Strong MJ, et al. Global bidirectional transcription of the Epstein-Barr virus genome during reactivation. *J Virol* 2014;88(3):1604–1616.
516. Ohashi M, Fogg MH, Orlova N, et al. An Epstein-Barr virus encoded inhibitor of Colony Stimulating Factor-1 signaling is an important determinant for acute and persistent EBV infection. *PLoS Pathog* 2012;8(12):e1003095.
517. Okuno Y, Murata T, Sato Y, et al. Publisher correction: defective Epstein-Barr virus in chronic active infection and haematological malignancy. *Nat Microbiol* 2019;4(3):544.
518. Okuno Y, Murata T, Sato Y, et al. Defective Epstein-Barr virus in chronic active infection and haematological malignancy. *Nat Microbiol* 2019;4(3):404–413.
519. Palermo RD, Webb HM, West MJ. RNA polymerase II stalling promotes nucleosome occlusion and pTEFb recruitment to drive immortalization by Epstein-Barr virus. *PLoS Pathog* 2011;7(10):e1002334.
520. Panea RI, Love CL, Shingleton JR, et al. The whole genome landscape of Burkitt lymphoma subtypes. *Blood* 2019;134:1598–1607.
521. Panikkar A, Smith C, Hislop A, et al. Impaired Epstein-Barr virus-specific neutralizing antibody response during acute infectious mononucleosis is coincident with global B-cell dysfunction. *J Virol* 2015;89(17):9137–9141.
522. Panikkar A, Smith C, Hislop A, et al. Cytokine-mediated loss of blood dendritic cells during Epstein-Barr virus-associated acute infectious mononucleosis: implication for immune dysregulation. *J Infect Dis* 2015;212(12):1957–1961.
523. Panousis CG, Rowe DT. Epstein-Barr virus latent membrane protein 2 associates with and is a substrate for mitogen-activated protein kinase. *J Virol* 1997;71(6):4752–4760.
524. Papadopoulos EB, Ladanyi M, Emanuel D, et al. Infusions of donor leukocytes to treat Epstein-Barr virus-associated lymphoproliferative disorders after allogeneic bone marrow transplantation. *N Engl J Med* 1994;330(17):1185–1191.
525. Papadopoulou A, Gerdemann U, Katari UL, et al. Activity of broad-spectrum T cells as treatment for AdV, EBV, CMV, BKV, and HHV6 infections after HSCT. *Sci Transl Med* 2014;6(242):242ra83.
526. Parker BD, Bankier A, Satchwell S, et al. Sequence and transcription of Raji Epstein-Barr virus DNA spanning the B95-8 deletion region. *Virology* 1990;179(1):339–346.
527. Paschos K, Parker GA, Watanatanasup E, et al. BIM promoter directly targeted by EBNA3C in polycomb-mediated repression by EBV. *Nucleic Acids Res* 2012;40(15):7233–7246.
528. Pasquier B, Yin L, Fondaneche MC, et al. Defective NKT cell development in mice and humans lacking the adapter SAP, the X-linked lymphoproliferative syndrome gene product. *J Exp Med* 2005;201(5):695–701.
529. Pathmanathan R, Prasad U, Sadler R, et al. Clonal proliferations of cells infected with Epstein-Barr virus in preinvasive lesions related to nasopharyngeal carcinoma. *N Engl J Med* 1995;333(11):693–698.
530. Paul JR, Bunnell BW. The presence of heterophile antibodies in infectious mononucleosis. *Am J Med Sci* 1932;183:90–104.
531. Pearson GR, Luka J, Petti L, et al. Identification of an Epstein-Barr virus early gene encoding a second component of the restricted early antigen complex. *Virology* 1987;160(1):151–161.
532. Pegtel DM, Cosmopoulos K, Thorley-Lawson DA, et al. Functional delivery of viral miRNAs via exosomes. *Proc Natl Acad Sci U S A* 2010;107(14):6328–6333.
533. Pegtel DM, Subramanian A, Sheen TS, et al. Epstein-Barr-virus-encoded LMP2A induces primary epithelial cell migration and invasion: possible role in nasopharyngeal carcinoma metastasis. *J Virol* 2005;79(24):15430–15442.
534. Pei Y, Banerjee S, Sun Z, et al. EBV nuclear antigen 3C mediates regulation of E2F6 to inhibit E2F1 transcription and promote cell proliferation. *PLoS Pathog* 2016;12(8):e1005844.
535. Pei Y, Singh RK, Shukla SK, et al. Epstein-Barr virus nuclear antigen 3C facilitates cell proliferation by regulating cyclin D2. *J Virol* 2018;92(18).
536. Pender MP, Csurhes PA, Smith C, et al. Epstein-Barr virus-specific T cell therapy for progressive multiple sclerosis. *JCI Insight* 2018;3(22).
537. Peng CW, Xue Y, Zhao B, et al. Direct interactions between Epstein-Barr virus leader protein LP and the EBNA2 acidic domain underlie coordinate transcriptional regulation. *Proc Natl Acad Sci U S A* 2004;101(4):1033–1038.
538. Perez EM, Foley J, Tison T, et al. Novel Epstein-Barr virus-like particles incorporating gH/gL-EBNA1 or gB-LMP2 induce high neutralizing antibody titers and EBV-specific T-cell responses in immunized mice. *Oncotarget* 2017;8(12):19255–19273.
539. Perrine SP, Hermine O, Small T, et al. A phase 1/2 trial of arginine butyrate and ganciclovir in patients with Epstein-Barr virus-associated lymphoid malignancies. *Blood* 2007;109(6):2571–2578.
540. Pesano RL, Pagano JS. Herpesvirus papio contains a plasmid origin of replication that acts in cis interspecies with an Epstein-Barr virus trans-acting function. *J Virol* 1986;60(3):1159–1162.
541. Petti L, Sample J, Wang F, et al. A fifth Epstein-Barr virus nuclear protein (EBNA3C) is expressed in latently infected growth-transformed lymphocytes. *J Virol* 1988;62(4):1330–1338.
542. Pfeffer S, Zavolan M, Grasser FA, et al. Identification of virus-encoded microRNAs. *Science* 2004;304(5671):734–736.
543. Pich D, Mrozek-Gorska P, Bouvet M, et al. First days in the life of naive human B lymphocytes infected with Epstein-Barr virus. *MBio* 2019;10(5).
544. Piriou E, Asito AS, Sumba PO, et al. Early age at time of primary Epstein-Barr virus infection results in poorly controlled viral infection in infants from Western Kenya: clues to the etiology of endemic Burkitt lymphoma. *J Infect Dis* 2012;205(6):906–913.
545. Piriou E, Kimmel R, Chelimo K, et al. Serological evidence for long-term Epstein-Barr virus reactivation in children living in a holoendemic malaria region of Kenya. *J Med Virol* 2009;81(6):1088–1093.
546. Plate AE, Smajlovic J, Jardetzky TS, et al. Functional analysis of glycoprotein L (gL) from rhesus lymphocryptovirus in Epstein-Barr virus-mediated cell fusion indicates a direct role of gL in gB-induced membrane fusion. *J Virol* 2009;83(15):7678–7689.
547. Platt TH, Tcherepanova IY, Schildkraut CL. Effect of number and position of EBNA-1 binding sites in Epstein-Barr virus oriP on the sites of initiation, barrier formation, and termination of replication. *J Virol* 1993;67(3):1739–1745.
548. Poling BC, Price AM, Luftig MA, et al. The Epstein-Barr virus miR-BHRF1 microRNAs regulate viral gene expression in cis. *Virology* 2017;512:113–123.

549. Ponnusamy R, Khatri R, Correia PB, et al. Increased association between Epstein-Barr virus EBNA2 from type 2 strains and the transcriptional repressor BS69 restricts EBNA2 activity. *PLoS Pathog* 2019;15(7):e1007458.
550. Pope JH. Establishment of cell lines from peripheral leucocytes in infectious mononucleosis. *Nature* 1967;216(5117):810–811.
551. Portal D, Zhao B, Calderwood MA, et al. EBV nuclear antigen EBNALP dismisses transcription repressors NCoR and RBPJ from enhancers and EBNA2 increases NCoR-deficient RBPJ DNA binding. *Proc Natl Acad Sci U S A* 2011;108(19):7808–7813.
552. Portal D, Zhou H, Zhao B, et al. Epstein-Barr virus nuclear antigen leader protein localizes to promoters and enhancers with cell transcription factors and EBNA2. *Proc Natl Acad Sci U S A* 2013;110(46):18537–18542.
553. Portis T, Dyck P, Longnecker R. Epstein-Barr Virus (EBV) LMP2A induces alterations in gene transcription similar to those observed in Reed-Sternberg cells of Hodgkin lymphoma. *Blood* 2003;102(12):4166–4178.
554. Portis T, Longnecker R. Epstein-Barr virus (EBV) LMP2A mediates B-lymphocyte survival through constitutive activation of the Ras/PI3K/Akt pathway. *Oncogene* 2004;23(53):8619–8628.
555. Price AM, Dai J, Bazot Q, et al. Epstein-Barr virus ensures B cell survival by uniquely modulating apoptosis at early and late times after infection. *Elife* 2017;6:e22509.
556. Price AM, Luftig MA. To be or not IIb: a multi-step process for Epstein-Barr virus latency establishment and consequences for B cell tumorigenesis. *PLoS Pathog* 2015;11(3):e1004656.
557. Price AM, Messinger JE, Luftig MA. c-Myc represses transcription of Epstein-Barr virus latent membrane protein 1 early after primary B cell infection. *J Virol* 2018;92(2).
558. Price AM, Tourigny JP, Forte E, et al. Analysis of Epstein-Barr virus-regulated host gene expression changes through primary B-cell outgrowth reveals delayed kinetics of latent membrane protein 1-mediated NF-kappaB activation. *J Virol* 2012;86(20):11096–11106.
559. Pritchett RF, Hayward SD, Kieff ED. DNA of Epstein-Barr virus. I. Comparative studies of the DNA of Epstein-Barr virus from HR-1 and B95-8 cells: size, structure, and relatedness. *J Virol* 1975;15(3):556–559.
560. Procko E, Berguig GY, Shen BW, et al. A computationally designed inhibitor of an Epstein-Barr viral Bcl-2 protein induces apoptosis in infected cells. *Cell* 2014;157(7):1644–1656.
561. Prockop S, Doubrovina E, Suser S, et al. Off-the-shelf EBV-specific T cell immunotherapy for rituximab-refractory EBV-associated lymphoma following transplantation. *J Clin Invest* 2020;130(2):733–747.
562. Prota AE, Sage DR, Stehle T, et al. The crystal structure of human CD21: implications for Epstein-Barr virus and C3d binding. *Proc Natl Acad Sci U S A* 2002;99(16):10641–10646.
563. Puglielli MT, Desai N, Speck SH. Regulation of EBNA gene transcription in lymphoblastoid cell lines: characterization of sequences downstream of BCR2 (Cp). *J Virol* 1997;71(1):120–128.
564. Qiu J, Cosmopoulos K, Pegtel M, et al. A novel persistence associated EBV miRNA expression profile is disrupted in neoplasia. *PLoS Pathog* 2011;7(8):e1002193.
565. Qiu J, Smith P, Leahy L, et al. The Epstein-Barr virus encoded BART miRNAs potentiate tumor growth in vivo. *PLoS Pathog* 2015;11(1):e1004561.
566. Raab-Traub N, Dambaugh T, Kieff E. DNA of Epstein-Barr virus VIII: B95-8, the previous prototype, is an unusual deletion derivative. *Cell* 1980;22(1 Pt 1):257–267.
567. Raab-Traub N, Dittmer DP. Viral effects on the content and function of extracellular vesicles. *Nat Rev Microbiol* 2017;15(9):559–572.
568. Raab-Traub N, Flynn K. The structure of the termini of the Epstein-Barr virus as a marker of clonal cellular proliferation. *Cell* 1986;47(6):883–889.
569. Raab-Traub N, Hood R, Yang CS, et al. Epstein-Barr virus transcription in nasopharyngeal carcinoma. *J Virol* 1983;48(3):580–590.
570. Raab-Traub N, Pritchett R, Kieff E. DNA of Epstein-Barr virus. III. Identification of restriction enzyme fragments that contain DNA sequences which differ among strains of Epstein-Barr virus. *J Virol* 1978;27(2):388–398.
571. Ramakrishnan R, Donahue H, Garcia D, et al. Epstein-Barr virus BART9 miRNA modulates LMP1 levels and affects growth rate of nasal NK T cell lymphomas. *PLoS One* 2011;6(11):e27271.
572. Rastelli J, Homig-Holzel C, Seagal J, et al. LMP1 signaling can replace CD40 signaling in B cells in vivo and has unique features of inducing class-switch recombination to IgG1. *Blood* 2008;111(3):1448–1455.
573. Rawlins DR, Milman G, Hayward SD, et al. Sequence-specific DNA binding of the Epstein-Barr virus nuclear antigen (EBNA-1) to clustered sites in the plasmid maintenance region. *Cell* 1985;42(3):859–868.
574. Rechsteiner MP, Berger C, Weber M, et al. Silencing of latent membrane protein 2B reduces susceptibility to activation of lytic Epstein-Barr virus in Burkitt's lymphoma Akata cells. *J Gen Virol* 2007;88(Pt 5):1454–1459.
575. Rechsteiner MP, Berger C, Zauner L, et al. Latent membrane protein 2B regulates susceptibility to induction of lytic Epstein-Barr virus infection. *J Virol* 2008;82(4):1739–1747.
576. Reisman D, Sugden B. trans activation of an Epstein-Barr viral transcriptional enhancer by the Epstein-Barr viral nuclear antigen 1. *Mol Cell Biol* 1986;6(11):3838–3846.
577. Reisman D, Yates J, Sugden B. A putative origin of replication of plasmids derived from Epstein-Barr virus is composed of two cis-acting components. *Mol Cell Biol* 1985;5(8):1822–1832.
578. Repic AM, Shi M, Scott RS, et al. Augmented latent membrane protein 1 expression from Epstein-Barr virus episomes with minimal terminal repeats. *J Virol* 2010;84(5):2236–2244.
579. Ressing ME, van Leeuwen D, Verreck FA, et al. Interference with T cell receptor-HLA-DR interactions by Epstein-Barr virus gp42 results in reduced T helper cell recognition. *Proc Natl Acad Sci U S A* 2003;100(20):11583–11588.
580. Reusch JA, Nawandar DM, Wright KL, et al. Cellular differentiation regulator BLIMP1 induces Epstein-Barr virus lytic reactivation in epithelial and B cells by activating transcription from both the R and Z promoters. *J Virol* 2015;89(3):1731–1743.
581. Rickinson AB, Young LS, Rowe M. Influence of the Epstein-Barr virus nuclear antigen EBNA 2 on the growth phenotype of virus-transformed B cells. *J Virol* 1987;61(5):1310–1317.
582. Rigaud S, Fondaneche MC, Lambert N, et al. XIAP deficiency in humans causes an X-linked lymphoproliferative syndrome. *Nature* 2006;444(7115):110–114.
583. Rivailler P, Cho YG, Wang F. Complete genomic sequence of an Epstein-Barr virus-related herpesvirus naturally infecting a new world primate: a defining point in the evolution of oncogenic lymphocryptoviruses. *J Virol* 2002;76(23):12055–12068.
584. Robertson KD, Ambinder RF. Methylation of the Epstein-Barr virus genome in normal lymphocytes. *Blood* 1997;90(11):4480–4484.
585. Robertson ES, Grossman S, Johannsen E, et al. Epstein-Barr virus nuclear protein 3C modulates transcription through interaction with the sequence-specific DNA-binding protein J kappa. *J Virol* 1995;69(5):3108–3116.
586. Robertson ES, Lin J, Kieff E. The amino-terminal domains of Epstein-Barr virus nuclear proteins 3A, 3B, and 3C interact with RBPJ(kappa). *J Virol* 1996;70(5):3068–3074.
587. Rochford R, Miller CL, Cannon MJ, et al. In vivo growth of Epstein-Barr virus transformed B cells with mutations in latent membrane protein 2 (LMP2). *Arch Virol* 1997;142(4):707–720.
588. Romero-Masters JC, Huebner SM, Ohashi M, et al. B cells infected with Type 2 Epstein-Barr virus (EBV) have increased NFATc1/NFATc2 activity and enhanced lytic gene expression in comparison to Type 1 EBV infection. *PLoS Pathog* 2020;16(2):e1008365.
589. Romero-Masters JC, Ohashi M, Djavadian R, et al. An EBNA3C-deleted Epstein-Barr virus (EBV) mutant causes B-cell lymphomas with delayed onset in a cord blood-humanized mouse model. *PLoS Pathog* 2018;14(8):e1007221.
590. Rooney CM, Smith CA, Ng CY, et al. Use of gene-modified virus-specific T lymphocytes to control Epstein-Barr-virus-related lymphoproliferation. *Lancet* 1995;345(8941):9–13.
591. Rovedo M, Longnecker R. Epstein-barr virus latent membrane protein 2B (LMP2B) modulates LMP2A activity. *J Virol* 2007;81(1):84–94.
592. Rovedo M, Longnecker R. Epstein-Barr virus latent membrane protein 2A preferentially signals through the Src family kinase Lyn. *J Virol* 2008;82(17):8520–8528.
593. Ruhl J, Citterio C, Engelmann C, et al. Heterologous prime-boost vaccination protects against EBV antigen-expressing lymphomas. *J Clin Invest* 2019;129(5):2071–2087.
594. Russo JJ, Bohenzky RA, Chien MC, et al. Nucleotide sequence of the Kaposi sarcoma-associated herpesvirus (HHV8). *Proc Natl Acad Sci U S A* 1996;93(25):14862–14867.
595. Saha A, Bamidele A, Murakami M, et al. EBNA3C attenuates the function of p53 through interaction with inhibitor of growth family proteins 4 and 5. *J Virol* 2011;85(5):2079–2088.
596. Saha A, Halder S, Upadhyay SK, et al. Epstein-Barr virus nuclear antigen 3C facilitates G1-S transition by stabilizing and enhancing the function of cyclin D1. *PLoS Pathog* 2011;7(2):e1001275.
597. Saha A, Jha HC, Upadhyay SK, et al. Epigenetic silencing of tumor suppressor genes during in vitro Epstein-Barr virus infection. *Proc Natl Acad Sci U S A* 2015;112(37):E5199–E5207.
598. Saha A, Lu J, Morizur L, et al. E2F1 mediated apoptosis induced by the DNA damage response is blocked by EBV nuclear antigen 3C in lymphoblastoid cells. *PLoS Pathog* 2012;8(3):e1002573.
599. Saha A, Murakami M, Kumar P, et al. Epstein-Barr virus nuclear antigen 3C augments Mdm2-mediated p53 ubiquitination and degradation by deubiquitinating Mdm2. *J Virol* 2009;83(9):4652–4669.
600. Saha A, Robertson ES. Mechanisms of B-Cell oncogenesis induced by Epstein-Barr virus. *J Virol* 2019;93(13).
601. Salahuddin S, Fath EK, Biel N, et al. Epstein-Barr virus latent membrane protein-1 induces the expression of SUMO-1 and SUMO-2/3 in LMP1-positive lymphomas and cells. *Sci Rep* 2019;9(1):208.
602. Samanta M, Iwakiri D, Kanda T, et al. EB virus-encoded RNAs are recognized by RIG-I and activate signaling to induce type I IFN. *EMBO J* 2006;25(18):4207–4214.
603. Sample J, Henson EB, Sample C. The Epstein-Barr virus nuclear protein 1 promoter active in type I latency is autoregulated. *J Virol* 1992;66(8):4654–4661.
604. Sample J, Hummel M, Braun D, et al. Nucleotide sequences of mRNAs encoding Epstein-Barr virus nuclear proteins: a probable transcriptional initiation site. *Proc Natl Acad Sci U S A* 1986;83(14):5096–5100.
605. Sample J, Liebowitz D, Kieff E. Two related Epstein-Barr virus membrane proteins are encoded by separate genes. *J Virol* 1989;63(2):933–937.
606. Sample J, Young L, Martin B, et al. Epstein-Barr virus types 1 and 2 differ in their EBNA-3A, EBNA-3B, and EBNA-3C genes. *J Virol* 1990;64(9):4084–4092.
607. Sang AX, McPherson MC, Ivison GT, et al. Dual blockade of the PI3K/Akt/mTOR pathway inhibits posttransplant Epstein-Barr virus B cell lymphomas and promotes allograft survival. *Am J Transplant* 2019;19(5):1305–1314.
608. Saridakis V, Sheng Y, Sarkari F, et al. Structure of the p53 binding domain of HAUSP/USP7 bound to Epstein-Barr nuclear antigen 1 implications for EBV-mediated immortalization. *Mol Cell* 2005;18(1):25–36.
609. Sarkari F, Sanchez-Alcaraz T, Wang S, et al. EBNA1-mediated recruitment of a histone H2B deubiquitylating complex to the Epstein-Barr virus latent origin of DNA replication. *PLoS Pathog* 2009;5(10):e1000624.
610. Sashihara J, Hoshino Y, Bowman JJ, et al. Soluble rhesus lymphocryptovirus gp350 protects against infection and reduces viral loads in animals that become infected with virus after challenge. *PLoS Pathog* 2011;7(10):e1002308.
611. Sathiyamoorthy K, Hu YX, Mohl BS, et al. Structural basis for Epstein-Barr virus host cell tropism mediated by gp42 and gHgL entry glycoproteins. *Nat Commun* 2016;7:13557.
612. Sathiyamoorthy K, Jiang J, Hu YX, et al. Assembly and architecture of the EBV B cell entry triggering complex. *PLoS Pathog* 2014;10(8):e1004309.
613. Sathiyamoorthy K, Jiang J, Mohl BS, et al. Inhibition of EBV-mediated membrane fusion by anti-gHgL antibodies. *Proc Natl Acad Sci U S A* 2017;114(41):E8703–E8710.
614. Sayos J, Wu C, Morra M, et al. The X-linked lymphoproliferative-disease gene product SAP regulates signals induced through the co-receptor SLAM. *Nature* 1998;395(6701):462–469.
615. Schaefer BC, Strominger JL, Speck SH. Redefining the Epstein-Barr virus-encoded nuclear antigen EBNA-1 gene promoter and transcription initiation site in group I Burkitt lymphoma cell lines. *Proc Natl Acad Sci U S A* 1995;92(23):10565–10569.
616. Schaefer BC, Woisetschlaeger M, Strominger JL, et al. Exclusive expression of Epstein-Barr virus nuclear antigen 1 in Burkitt lymphoma arises from a third promoter, distinct from the promoters used in latently infected lymphocytes. *Proc Natl Acad Sci U S A* 1991;88(15):6550–6554.

617. Schmidt SC, Jiang S, Zhou H, et al. Epstein-Barr virus nuclear antigen 3A partially coincides with EBNA3C genome-wide and is tethered to DNA through BATF complexes. *Proc Natl Acad Sci U S A* 2015;112(2):554–559.
618. Schmitz R, Young RM, Ceribelli M, et al. Burkitt lymphoma pathogenesis and therapeutic targets from structural and functional genomics. *Nature* 2012;490(7418):116–120.
619. Schneider F, Neugebauer J, Griese J, et al. The viral oncoprotein LMP1 exploits TRADD for signaling by masking its apoptotic activity. *PLoS Biol* 2008;6(1):e8.
620. Scholle F, Bendt KM, Raab-Traub N. Epstein-Barr virus LMP2A transforms epithelial cells, inhibits cell differentiation, and activates Akt. *J Virol* 2000;74(22):10681–10689.
621. Schultheiss U, Puschner S, Kremmer E, et al. TRAF6 is a critical mediator of signal transduction by the viral oncogene latent membrane protein 1. *EMBO J* 2001;20(20):5678–5691.
622. Secondino S, Zecca M, Licitra L, et al. T-cell therapy for EBV-associated nasopharyngeal carcinoma: preparative lymphodepleting chemotherapy does not improve clinical results. *Ann Oncol* 2012;23:435–441.
623. Seemayer TA, Gross TG, Egeler RM, et al. X-linked lymphoproliferative disease: twenty-five years after the discovery. *Pediatr Res* 1995;38(4):471–478.
624. Semenova T, Lupo J, Alain S, et al. Multicenter evaluation of whole-blood Epstein-Barr viral load standardization using the WHO International standard. *J Clin Microbiol* 2016;54(7):1746–1750.
625. Serafini B, Rosicarelli B, Veroni C, et al. Epstein-Barr virus-specific CD8 T cells selectively infiltrate the multiple sclerosis brain and interact locally with virus infected cells: clue for a virus-driven immunopathological mechanism. *J Virol* 2019;93:e00980.
626. Seto E, Moosmann A, Gromminger S, et al. Micro RNAs of Epstein-Barr virus promote cell cycle progression and prevent apoptosis of primary human B cells. *PLoS Pathog* 2010;6(8).
627. Shair KH, Schnegg CI, Raab-Traub N. Epstein-Barr virus latent membrane protein-1 effects on junctional plakoglobin and induction of a cadherin switch. *Cancer Res* 2009;69(14):5734–5742.
628. Shannon-Lowe CD, Neuhierl B, Baldwin G, et al. Resting B cells as a transfer vehicle for Epstein-Barr virus infection of epithelial cells. *Proc Natl Acad Sci U S A* 2006;103(18):7065–7070.
629. Shannon-Lowe C, Rickinson A. The global landscape of EBV-associated tumors. *Front Oncol* 2019;9:713.
630. Shannon-Lowe C, Rowe M. Epstein-Barr virus infection of polarized epithelial cells via the basolateral surface by memory B cell-mediated transfer infection. *PLoS Pathog* 2011;7(5):e1001338.
631. Sharma-Walia N, Naranatt PP, Krishnan HH, et al. Kaposi's sarcoma-associated herpesvirus/human herpesvirus 8 envelope glycoprotein gB induces the integrin-dependent focal adhesion kinase-Src-phosphatidylinositol 3-kinase-rho GTPase signal pathways and cytoskeletal rearrangements. *J Virol* 2004;78(8):4207–4223.
632. Shatzer A, Ali MA, Chavez M, et al. Ganetespib, an HSP90 inhibitor, kills Epstein-Barr virus (EBV)-infected B and T cells and reduces the percentage of EBV-infected cells in the blood. *Leuk Lymphoma* 2017;58(4):923–931.
633. Shen CL, Huang WH, Hsu HJ, et al. GAP31 from an ancient medicinal plant exhibits anti-viral activity through targeting to Epstein-Barr virus nuclear antigen 1. *Antiviral Res* 2019;164:123–130.
634. Shkoda A, Town JA, Griese J, et al. The germinal center kinase TNIK is required for canonical NF-kappaB and JNK signaling in B-cells by the EBV oncoprotein LMP1 and the CD40 receptor. *PLoS Biol* 2012;10(8):e1001376.
635. Sims K, Saha A, Robertson ES. Regulation of cellular processes by the Epstein-Barr virus nuclear antigen 3 family of proteins. In: Robertson ES, ed. *Epstein-Barr Virus—Latency and Transformation.* Philadelphia, PA: Caister Academic Press; 2010:81–100.
636. Sinclair AJ, Palmero I, Peters G, et al. EBNA-2 and EBNA-LP cooperate to cause G0 to G1 transition during immortalization of resting human B lymphocytes by Epstein-Barr virus. *EMBO J* 1994;13(14):3321–3328.
637. Singh S, Homad LJ, Akins NR, et al. Neutralizing antibodies protect against oral transmission of lymphocryptovirus. *Cell Rep Med* 2020;1(3).
638. Sitki-Green D, Covington M, Raab-Traub N. Compartmentalization and transmission of multiple epstein-barr virus strains in asymptomatic carriers. *J Virol* 2003;77(3):1840–1847.
639. Sitki-Green DL, Edwards RH, Covington MM, et al. Biology of Epstein-Barr virus during infectious mononucleosis. *J Infect Dis* 2004;189(3):483–492.
640. Sivachandran N, Dawson CW, Young LS, et al. Contributions of the Epstein-Barr virus EBNA1 protein to gastric carcinoma. *J Virol* 2012;86(1):60–68.
641. Sixbey JW, Nedrud JG, Raab-Traub N, et al. Epstein-Barr virus replication in oropharyngeal epithelial cells. *N Engl J Med* 1984;310(19):1225–1230.
642. Sixbey JW, Shirley P, Sloas M, et al. A transformation-incompetent, nuclear antigen 2-deleted Epstein-Barr virus associated with replicative infection. *J Infect Dis* 1991;163(5):1008–1015.
643. Sixbey JW, Yao QY. Immunoglobulin A-induced shift of Epstein-Barr virus tissue tropism. *Science* 1992;255(5051):1578–1580.
644. Skalska L, White RE, Franz M, et al. Epigenetic repression of p16(INK4A) by latent Epstein-Barr virus requires the interaction of EBNA3A and EBNA3C with CtBP. *PLoS Pathog* 2010;6(6):e1000951.
645. Skalska L, White RE, Parker GA, et al. Induction of p16(INK4a) is the major barrier to proliferation when Epstein-Barr virus (EBV) transforms primary B cells into lymphoblastoid cell lines. *PLoS Pathog* 2013;9(2):e1003187.
646. Skalsky RL, Corcoran DL, Gottwein E, et al. The viral and cellular MicroRNA targetome in lymphoblastoid cell lines. *PLoS Pathog* 2012;8(1):e1002484.
647. Skalsky RL, Cullen BR. EBV noncoding RNAs. *Curr Top Microbiol Immunol* 2015;391:181–217.
648. Skare J, Edson C, Farley J, et al. The B95-8 isolate of Epstein-Barr virus arose from an isolate with a standard genome. *J Virol* 1982;44(3):1088–1091.
649. Skinner CM, Ivanov NS, Barr SA, et al. An Epstein-Barr virus MicroRNA blocks interleukin-1 (IL-1) signaling by targeting IL-1 receptor 1. *J Virol* 2017;91(21).
650. Smith NA, Coleman CB, Gewurz BE, et al. CD21 (Complement Receptor 2) is the receptor for Epstein-Barr virus entry into T cells. *J Virol* 2020;94(11).
651. Smith PR, de Jesus O, Turner D, et al. Structure and coding content of CST (BART) family RNAs of Epstein-Barr virus. *J Virol* 2000;74(7):3082–3092.
652. Smith C, Tsang J, Beagley L, et al. Effective treatment of metastatic forms of Epstein-Barr virus-associated nasopharyngeal carcinoma with a novel adenovirus-based adoptive immunotherapy. *Cancer Res* 2012;72(5):1116–1125.
653. Snijder J, Ortego MS, Weidle C, et al. An antibody targeting the fusion machinery neutralizes dual-tropic infection and defines a site of vulnerability on Epstein-Barr virus. *Immunity* 2018;48(4):799–811.e799.
654. Snow AL, Marsh RA, Krummey SM, et al. Restimulation-induced apoptosis of T cells is impaired in patients with X-linked lymphoproliferative disease caused by SAP deficiency. *J Clin Invest* 2009;119(10):2976–2989.
655. Sokal EM, Hoppenbrouwers K, Vandermeulen C, et al. Recombinant gp350 vaccine for infectious mononucleosis: a phase 2, randomized, double-blind, placebo-controlled trial to evaluate the safety, immunogenicity, and efficacy of an Epstein-Barr virus vaccine in healthy young adults. *J Infect Dis* 2007;196(12):1749–1753.
656. Sommermann TG, O'Neill K, Plas DR, et al. IKKbeta and NF-kappaB transcription govern lymphoma cell survival through AKT-induced plasma membrane trafficking of GLUT1. *Cancer Res* 2011;71(23):7291–7300.
657. Song YJ, Izumi KM, Shinners NP, et al. IRF7 activation by Epstein-Barr virus latent membrane protein 1 requires localization at activation sites and TRAF6, but not TRAF2 or TRAF3. *Proc Natl Acad Sci U S A* 2008;105(47):18448–18453.
658. Sora RP, Ikeda M, Longnecker R. Two pathways of p27(Kip1) degradation are required for murine lymphoma driven by Myc and EBV latent membrane protein 2A. *MBio* 2019;10(2).
659. Souza TA, Stollar BD, Sullivan JL, et al. Peripheral B cells latently infected with Epstein-Barr virus display molecular hallmarks of classical antigen-selected memory B cells. *Proc Natl Acad Sci U S A* 2005;102(50):18093–18098.
660. Souza TA, Stollar BD, Sullivan JL, et al. Influence of EBV on the peripheral blood memory B cell compartment. *J Immunol* 2007;179(5):3153–3160.
661. Spacek M, Hubacek P, Markova J, et al. Plasma EBV-DNA monitoring in Epstein-Barr virus-positive Hodgkin lymphoma patients. *APMIS* 2010;119(1):10–16.
662. Speck P, Kline KA, Cheresh P, et al. Epstein-Barr virus lacking latent membrane protein 2 immortalizes B cells with efficiency indistinguishable from that of wild-type virus [In Process Citation]. *J Gen Virol* 1999;80(Pt 8):2193–2203.
663. Speck SH, Pfitzner A, Strominger JL. An Epstein-Barr virus transcript from a latently infected, growth- transformed B-cell line encodes a highly repetitive polypeptide. *Proc Natl Acad Sci U S A* 1986;83(24):9298–9302.
664. Speck SH, Strominger JL. Epstein-Barr virus transformation. *Prog Nucleic Acid Res Mol Biol* 1987;34:189–207.
665. Spriggs MK, Armitage RJ, Comeau MR, et al. The extracellular domain of the Epstein-Barr virus BZLF2 protein binds the HLA-DR beta chain and inhibits antigen presentation. *J Virol* 1996;70(8):5557–5563.
666. Sprunt TP EF. Mononuclear leukocytosis in reaction to acute infections ("infectious mononucleosis"). *Johns Hopkins Hosp Bull* 1920;31:410–417.
667. Stewart S, Dawson CW, Takada K, et al. Epstein-Barr virus-encoded LMP2A regulates viral and cellular gene expression by modulation of the NF-kappaB transcription factor pathway. *Proc Natl Acad Sci U S A* 2004;101(44):15730–15735.
668. Straathof KC, Bollard CM, Popat U, et al. Treatment of nasopharyngeal carcinoma with Epstein-Barr virus--specific T lymphocytes. *Blood* 2005;105(5):1898–1904.
669. Stubbins RJ, Alami Laroussi N, Peters AC, et al. Epstein-Barr virus associated smooth muscle tumors in solid organ transplant recipients: incidence over 31 years at a single institution and review of the literature. *Transpl Infect Dis* 2019;21(1):e13010.
670. Styles CT, Bazot Q, Parker GA, et al. EBV epigenetically suppresses the B cell-to-plasma cell differentiation pathway while establishing long-term latency. *PLoS Biol* 2017;15(8):e2001992.
671. Sugimoto A, Kanda T, Yamashita Y, et al. Spatiotemporally different DNA repair systems participate in Epstein-Barr virus genome maturation. *J Virol* 2011;85(13):6127–6135.
672. Swaminathan S. Characterization of Epstein-Barr virus recombinants with deletions of the BamHI C promoter. *Virology* 1996;217(2):532–541.
673. Swaminathan S, Tomkinson B, Kieff E. Recombinant Epstein-Barr virus with small RNA (EBER) genes deleted transforms lymphocytes and replicates in vitro. *Proc Natl Acad Sci U S A* 1991;88(4):1546–1550.
674. Swart R, Ruf IK, Sample J, et al. Latent membrane protein 2A-mediated effects on the phosphatidylinositol 3-Kinase/Akt pathway. *J Virol* 2000;74(22):10838–10845.
675. Szakonyi G, Klein MG, Hannan JP, et al. Structure of the Epstein-Barr virus major envelope glycoprotein. *Nat Struct Mol Biol* 2006;13(11):996–1001.
676. Szymula A, Palermo RD, Bayoumy A, et al. Epstein-Barr virus nuclear antigen EBNA-LP is essential for transforming naive B cells, and facilitates recruitment of transcription factors to the viral genome. *PLoS Pathog* 2018;14(2):e1006890.
677. Tagawa T, Albanese M, Bouvet M, et al. Epstein-Barr viral miRNAs inhibit antiviral CD4+ T cell responses targeting IL-12 and peptide processing. *J Exp Med* 2016;213(10):2065–2080.
678. Takada K, Ono Y. Synchronous and sequential activation of latently infected Epstein-Barr virus genomes. *J Virol* 1989;63(1):445–449.
679. Tamura K, Taniguchi Y, Minoguchi S, et al. Physical interaction between a novel domain of the receptor Notch and the transcription factor RBP-J kappa/Su(H). *Curr Biol* 1995;5(12):1416–1423.
680. Tangye SG, Latour S. Primary immunodeficiencies reveal the molecular requirements for effective host defense against EBV infection. *Blood* 2020;135(9):644–655.
681. Tanner J, Weis J, Fearon D, et al. Epstein-Barr virus gp350/220 binding to the B lymphocyte C3d receptor mediates adsorption, capping, and endocytosis. *Cell* 1987;50(2):203–213.
682. Taylor GS, Jia H, Harrington K, et al. A recombinant modified vaccinia ankara vaccine encoding Epstein-Barr Virus (EBV) target antigens: a phase I trial in UK patients with EBV-positive cancer. *Clin Cancer Res* 2014;20(19):5009–5022.
683. Taylor GS, Long HM, Brooks JM, et al. The immunology of Epstein-Barr virus-induced disease. *Annu Rev Immunol* 2015;33:787–821.

684. Tempera I, De Leo A, Kossenkov AV, et al. Identification of MEF2B, EBF1, and IL6R as direct gene targets of Epstein-Barr virus (EBV) nuclear antigen 1 critical for EBV-infected B-lymphocyte survival. *J Virol* 2016;90(1):345–355.
685. Tempera I, Klichinsky M, Lieberman PM. EBV Latency types adopt alternative chromatin conformations. *PLoS Pathog* 2011;7(7):e1002180.
686. Tempera I, Wiedmer A, Dheekollu J, et al. CTCF prevents the epigenetic drift of EBV latency promoter Qp. *PLoS Pathog* 2010;6(8):e1001048.
687. de-The G, Geser A, Day NE, et al. Epidemiological evidence for causal relationship between Epstein-Barr virus and Burkitt's lymphoma from Ugandan prospective study. *Nature* 1978;274(5673):756–761.
688. Thompson J, Verma D, Li D, et al. Identification and characterization of the physiological gene targets of the essential lytic replicative Epstein-Barr virus SM protein. *J Virol* 2016;90(3):1206–1221.
689. Thorley-Lawson DA. EBV persistence—introducing the virus. *Curr Top Microbiol Immunol* 2015;390(Pt 1):151–209.
690. Thorley-Lawson DA, Allday MJ. The curious case of the tumour virus: 50 years of Burkitt's lymphoma. *Nat Rev Microbiol* 2008;6(12):913–924.
691. Thornburg NJ, Raab-Traub N. Induction of epidermal growth factor receptor expression by Epstein-Barr virus latent membrane protein 1 C-terminal-activating region 1 is mediated by NF-kappaB p50 homodimer/Bcl-3 complexes. *J Virol* 2007;81(23):12954–12961.
692. Tierney RJ, Kao KY, Nagra JK, et al. Epstein-Barr virus BamHI W repeat number limits EBNA2/EBNA-LP coexpression in newly infected B cells and the efficiency of B-cell transformation: a rationale for the multiple W repeats in wild-type virus strains. *J Virol* 2011;85(23):12362–12375.
693. Tierney RJ, Nagra J, Rowe M, et al. The Epstein-Barr virus BamHI C promoter is not essential for B cell immortalization in vitro, but it greatly enhances B cell growth transformation. *J Virol* 2015;89(5):2483–2493.
694. Tomkinson B, Kieff E. Second-site homologous recombination in Epstein-Barr virus: insertion of type 1 EBNA 3 genes in place of type 2 has no effect on in vitro infection. *J Virol* 1992;66(2):780–789.
695. Tomkinson B, Robertson E, Kieff E. Epstein-Barr virus nuclear proteins EBNA-3A and EBNA-3C are essential for B-lymphocyte growth transformation. *J Virol* 1993;67(4):2014–2025.
696. Torgbor C, Awuah P, Deitsch K, et al. A multifactorial role for P. falciparum malaria in endemic Burkitt's lymphoma pathogenesis. *PLoS Pathog* 2014;10(5):e1004170.
697. Tosato G, Jones K, Breinig MK, et al. Interleukin-6 production in posttransplant lymphoproliferative disease. *J Clin Invest* 1993;91(6):2806–2814.
698. Tsai MH, Raykova A, Klinke O, et al. Spontaneous lytic replication and epitheliotropism define an Epstein-Barr virus strain found in carcinomas. *Cell Rep* 2013;5(2):458–470.
699. Tsai K, Thikmyanova N, Wojcechowskyj JA, et al. EBV tegument protein BNRF1 disrupts DAXX-ATRX to activate viral early gene transcription. *PLoS Pathog* 2011;7(11):e1002376.
700. Tsao SW, Tsang CM, Lo KW. Epstein-Barr virus infection and nasopharyngeal carcinoma. *Philos Trans R Soc Lond B Biol Sci* 2017;372(1732).
701. Tugizov SM, Berline JW, Palefsky JM. Epstein-Barr virus infection of polarized tongue and nasopharyngeal epithelial cells. *Nat Med* 2003;9(3):307–314.
702. Turk SM, Jiang R, Chesnokova LS, et al. Antibodies to gp350/220 enhance the ability of Epstein-Barr virus to infect epithelial cells. *J Virol* 2006;80(19):9628–9633.
703. Tynell E, Aurelius E, Brandell A, et al. Acyclovir and prednisolone treatment of acute infectious mononucleosis: a multicenter, double-blind, placebo-controlled study. *J Infect Dis* 1996;174(2):324–331.
704. Tzannou I, Papadopoulou A, Naik S, et al. Off-the-shelf virus-specific T cells to treat BK virus, human herpesvirus 6, cytomegalovirus, Epstein-Barr virus, and adenovirus infections after allogeneic hematopoietic stem-cell transplantation. *J Clin Oncol* 2017;35(31):3547–3557.
705. Tzellos S, Correia PB, Karstegl CE, et al. A single amino acid in EBNA-2 determines superior B lymphoblastoid cell line growth maintenance by Epstein-Barr virus type 1 EBNA-2. *J Virol* 2014;88(16):8743–8753.
706. Ungerleider N, Concha M, Lin Z, et al. The Epstein Barr virus circRNAome. *PLoS Pathog* 2018;14(8):e1007206.
707. Van Besien K, Bachier-Rodriguez L, Satlin M, et al. Prophylactic rituximab prevents EBV PTLD in haplo-cord transplant recipients at high risk. *Leuk Lymphoma* 2019;60(7):1693–1696.
708. Veillette A, Zhang S, Shi X, et al. SAP expression in T cells, not in B cells, is required for humoral immunity. *Proc Natl Acad Sci U S A* 2008;105(4):1273–1278.
709. Vereide DT, Seto E, Chiu YF, et al. Epstein-Barr virus maintains lymphomas via its miRNAs. *Oncogene* 2014;33(10):1258–1264.
710. Verma D, Church TM, Swaminathan S. Epstein-Barr virus co-opts TFIIH component XPB to specifically activate essential viral lytic promoters. *Proc Natl Acad Sci U S A* 2020;117(23):13044–13055.
711. Verweij FJ, van Eijndhoven MA, Hopmans ES, et al. LMP1 association with CD63 in endosomes and secretion via exosomes limits constitutive NF-kappaB activation. *EMBO J* 2011;30(11):2115–2129.
712. Voigt S, Sterz KR, Giehler F, et al. A central role of IKK2 and TPL2 in JNK activation and viral B-cell transformation. *Nat Commun* 2020;11(1):685.
713. Wang X, Hutt-Fletcher LM. Epstein-Barr virus lacking glycoprotein gp42 can bind to B cells but is not able to infect. *J Virol* 1998;72(1):158–163.
714. Wang LW, Jiang S, Gewurz BE. Epstein-Barr virus LMP1-mediated oncogenicity. *J Virol* 2017;91(21).
715. Wang C, Jiang S, Zhang L, et al. TAF family proteins and MEF2C are essential for Epstein-Barr virus super-enhancer activity. *J Virol* 2019;93(16).
716. Wang K, Kan J, Yuen ST, et al. Exome sequencing identifies frequent mutation of ARID1A in molecular subtypes of gastric cancer. *Nat Genet* 2011;43(12):1219–1223.
717. Wang C, Li D, Zhang L, et al. RNA sequencing analyses of gene expression during Epstein-Barr virus infection of primary B lymphocytes. *J Virol* 2019;93(13).
718. Wang D, Liebowitz D, Kieff E. An EBV membrane protein expressed in immortalized lymphocytes transforms established rodent cells. *Cell* 1985;43(3 Pt 2):831–840.
719. Wang J, Lindner SE, Leight ER, et al. Essential elements of a licensed, mammalian plasmid origin of DNA synthesis. *Mol Cell Biol* 2006;26(3):1124–1134.
720. Wang Q, Lingel A, Geiser V, et al. Tumor suppressor p53 stimulates the expression of Epstein-Barr virus latent membrane protein 1. *J Virol* 2017;91(20).
721. Wang LW, Shen H, Nobre L, et al. Epstein-Barr-virus-induced one-carbon metabolism drives B cell transformation. *Cell Metab* 2019;30:539–555.e11.
722. Wang F, Tsang SF, Kurilla MG, et al. Epstein-Barr virus nuclear antigen 2 transactivates latent membrane protein LMP1. *J Virol* 1990;64(7):3407–3416.
723. Wang LW, Wang Z, Ersing I, et al. Epstein-Barr virus subverts mevalonate and fatty acid pathways to promote infected B-cell proliferation and survival. *PLoS Pathog* 2019;15(9):e1008030.
724. Wang L, Wang Y, Zhao J, et al. The linear ubiquitin assembly complex modulates latent membrane protein 1 activation of NF-kappaB and interferon regulatory factor 7. *J Virol* 2017;91(4).
725. Wang C, Zhou H, Xue Y, et al. Epstein-Barr virus nuclear antigen leader protein coactivates EP300. *J Virol* 2018;92(9).
726. Weiss ER, Alter G, Ogembo JG, et al. High Epstein-Barr virus load and genomic diversity are associated with generation of gp350-specific neutralizing antibodies following acute infectious mononucleosis. *J Virol* 2017;91(1).
727. Weiss LM, Jaffe ES, Liu XF, et al. Detection and localization of Epstein-Barr viral genomes in angioimmunoblastic lymphadenopathy and angioimmunoblastic lymphadenopathy-like lymphoma. *Blood* 1992;79(7):1789–1795.
728. Weiss LM, Movahed LA, Warnke RA, et al. Detection of Epstein-Barr viral genomes in Reed-Sternberg cells of Hodgkin's disease. *N Engl J Med* 1989;320(8):502–506.
729. West MJ, Webb HM, Sinclair AJ, et al. Biophysical and mutational analysis of the putative bZIP domain of Epstein-Barr virus EBNA 3C. *J Virol* 2004;78(17):9431–9445.
730. White RE, Groves IJ, Turro E, et al. Extensive co-operation between the Epstein-Barr virus EBNA3 proteins in the manipulation of host gene expression and epigenetic chromatin modification. *PLoS One* 2010;5(11):e13979.
731. White RE, Ramer PC, Naresh KN, et al. EBNA3B-deficient EBV promotes B cell lymphomagenesis in humanized mice and is found in human tumors. *J Clin Invest* 2012;122(4):1487–1502.
732. Wille CK, Li Y, Rui L, et al. Restricted TET2 expression in germinal center type B cells promotes stringent Epstein-Barr virus latency. *J Virol* 2017;91(5).
733. Wille CK, Nawandar DM, Panfil AR, et al. Viral genome methylation differentially affects the ability of BZLF1 versus BRLF1 to activate Epstein-Barr virus lytic gene expression and viral replication. *J Virol* 2013;87(2):935–950.
734. Wirtz T, Weber T, Kracker S, et al. Mouse model for acute Epstein-Barr virus infection. *Proc Natl Acad Sci U S A* 2016;113(48):13821–13826.
735. Wood CD, Veenstra H, Khasnis S, et al. MYC activation and BCL2L11 silencing by a tumour virus through the large-scale reconfiguration of enhancer-promoter hubs. *Elife* 2016;5.
736. Xiang Z, Liu Y, Zheng J, et al. Targeted activation of human Vgamma9Vdelta2-T cells controls epstein-barr virus-induced B cell lymphoproliferative disease. *Cancer Cell* 2014;26(4):565–576.
737. Xiao J, Palefsky JM, Herrera R, et al. Characterization of the Epstein-Barr virus glycoprotein BMRF-2. *Virology* 2007;359(2):382–396.
738. Xu M, Yao Y, Chen H, et al. Genome sequencing analysis identifies Epstein-Barr virus subtypes associated with high risk of nasopharyngeal carcinoma. *Nat Genet* 2019;51(7):1131–1136.
739. Xu D, Zhang Y, Zhao L, et al. Interferon regulatory factor 7 is involved in the growth of Epstein-Barr virus-transformed human B lymphocytes. *Virus Res* 2015;195:112–118.
740. Yager JE, Magaret AS, Kuntz SR, et al. Valganciclovir for the suppression of Epstein-Barr virus replication. *J Infect Dis* 2017;216(2):198–202.
741. Yajima M, Kanda T, Takada K. Critical role of Epstein-Barr Virus (EBV)-encoded RNA in efficient EBV-induced B-lymphocyte growth transformation. *J Virol* 2005;79(7):4298–4307.
742. Yaswen LR, Stephens EB, Davenport LC, et al. Epstein-Barr virus glycoprotein gp85 associates with the BKRF2 gene product and is incompletely processed as a recombinant protein. *Virology* 1993;195(2):387–396.
743. Yates J, Warren N, Reisman D, et al. A cis-acting element from the Epstein-Barr viral genome that permits stable replication of recombinant plasmids in latently infected cells. *Proc Natl Acad Sci U S A* 1984;81(12):3806–3810.
744. Yates JL, Warren N, Sugden B. Stable replication of plasmids derived from Epstein-Barr virus in various mammalian cells. *Nature* 1985;313(6005):812–815.
745. Ye H, Park YC, Kreishman M, et al. The structural basis for the recognition of diverse receptor sequences by TRAF2. *Mol Cell* 1999;4(3):321–330.
746. Yoo L, Speck SH. Determining the role of the epstein-barr virus Cp EBNA2-dependent enhancer during the establishment of latency by using mutant and wild-type viruses recovered from cottontop marmoset lymphoblastoid cell lines [In Process Citation]. *J Virol* 2000;74(23):11115–11120.
747. Zhang J, Jia L, Tsang CM, et al. EBV infection and glucose metabolism in nasopharyngeal carcinoma. *Adv Exp Med Biol* 2017;1018:75–90.
748. Zhang B, Kracker S, Yasuda T, et al. Immune surveillance and therapy of lymphomas driven by Epstein-Barr virus protein LMP1 in a mouse model. *Cell* 2012;148(4):739–751.
749. Zhang H, Li Y, Wang HB, et al. Ephrin receptor A2 is an epithelial cell receptor for Epstein-Barr virus entry. *Nat Microbiol* 2018;3(2):1–8.
750. Zhao B, Barrera LA, Ersing I, et al. The NF-kappaB genomic landscape in lymphoblastoid B cells. *Cell Rep* 2014;8(5):1595–1606.
751. Zhao B, Mar JC, Maruo S, et al. Epstein-Barr virus nuclear antigen 3C regulated genes in lymphoblastoid cell lines. *Proc Natl Acad Sci U S A* 2011;108(1):337–342.
752. Zhao B, Marshall DR, Sample CE. A conserved domain of the Epstein-Barr virus nuclear antigens 3A and 3C binds to a discrete domain of Jkappa. *J Virol* 1996;70(7):4228–4236.
753. Zhao B, Maruo S, Cooper A, et al. RNAs induced by Epstein-Barr virus nuclear antigen 2 in lymphoblastoid cell lines. *Proc Natl Acad Sci U S A* 2006;103(6):1900–1905.

754. Zhao B, Sample CE. Epstein-barr virus nuclear antigen 3C activates the latent membrane protein 1 promoter in the presence of Epstein-Barr virus nuclear antigen 2 through sequences encompassing an spi-1/Spi-B binding site. *J Virol* 2000;74(11):5151–5160.
755. Zhao B, Zou J, Wang H, et al. Epstein-Barr virus exploits intrinsic B-lymphocyte transcription programs to achieve immortal cell growth. *Proc Natl Acad Sci U S A* 2011;108(36):14902–14907.
756. Zheng H, Dai W, Cheung AK, et al. Whole-exome sequencing identifies multiple loss-of-function mutations of NF-kappaB pathway regulators in nasopharyngeal carcinoma. *Proc Natl Acad Sci U S A* 2016;113(40):11283–11288.
757. Zhong L, Wang W, Ma M, et al. Chronic active Epstein-Barr virus infection as the initial symptom in a Janus kinase 3 deficiency child: Case report and literature review. *Medicine (Baltimore)* 2017;96(42):e7989.
758. Zhou S, Fujimuro M, Hsieh JJ, et al. A role for SKIP in EBNA2 activation of CBF1-repressed promoters. *J Virol* 2000;74(4):1939–1947.
759. Zhou H, Schmidt SC, Jiang S, et al. Epstein-Barr virus oncoprotein super-enhancers control B cell growth. *Cell Host Microbe* 2015;17(2):205–216.
760. Zhou Y, Xu Z, Lin W, et al. Comprehensive genomic profiling of EBV-positive diffuse large B-cell lymphoma and the expression and clinicopathological correlations of some related genes. *Front Oncol* 2019;9:683.
761. Zhu JY, Pfuhl T, Motsch N, et al. Identification of novel Epstein-Barr virus microRNA genes from nasopharyngeal carcinomas. *J Virol* 2009;83(7):3333–3341.
762. Ziegler JL, Drew WL, Miner RC, et al. Outbreak of Burkitt's-like lymphoma in homosexual men. *Lancet* 1982;2(8299):631–633.
763. Zimber-Strobl U, Kremmer E, Grasser F, et al. The Epstein-Barr virus nuclear antigen 2 interacts with an EBNA2 responsive cis-element of the terminal protein 1 gene promoter. *Embo J* 1993;12(1):167–175.
764. Zimmermann J, Hammerschmidt W. Structure and role of the terminal repeats of Epstein-Barr virus in processing and packaging of virion DNA. *J Virol* 1995;69(5):3147–3155.
765. Zou P, Kawada J, Pesnicak L, et al. Bortezomib induces apoptosis of Epstein-Barr virus (EBV)-transformed B cells and prolongs survival of mice inoculated with EBV-transformed B cells. *J Virol* 2007;81(18):10029–10036.
766. zur Hausen H, Schulte-Holthausen H, Klein G, et al. EBV DNA in biopsies of Burkitt tumours and anaplastic carcinomas of the nasopharynx. *Nature* 1970;228(5276):1056–1058.
767. Zur Hausen A, van Rees BP, van Beek J, et al. Epstein-Barr virus in gastric carcinomas and gastric stump carcinomas: a late event in gastric carcinogenesis. *J Clin Pathol* 2004;57(5):487–491.
768. van Zyl DG, Tsai MH, Shumilov A, et al. Immunogenic particles with a broad antigenic spectrum stimulate cytolytic T cells and offer increased protection against EBV infection ex vivo and in mice. *PLoS Pathog* 2018;14(12):e1007464.

CHAPTER

12 Cytomegalovirus

Felicia Goodrum • William Britt • Edward S. Mocarski

CYTOMEGALOVIRUS

Cytomegalovirus (CMV) is a genus of herpesvirus in the subfamily of β-*Herpesvirinae*. CMV is the prototypical β-herpesvirus and has a protracted replication cycle characteristic of its subfamily. The name CMV (from the Greek cyto-, "cell," and megalo-, "large") comes from the fact that this virus causes enlargement of the infected cell with nuclear and cytoplasmic inclusions. Humans, monkeys, and other mammals serve as natural hosts. CMVs co-speciated with their host at least 90 million years ago. Co-speciation resulted in these viruses being highly restricted to their natural host species.

Human CMV (HCMV) infects between 40% and 99% of the population worldwide depending on geographical region and socioeconomic factors. Primary infection with CMV most commonly results in subclinical infection and long-term (months to years) virus shedding. Like all herpesviruses, HCMV infection is never completely cleared. The virus persists in the host indefinitely by establishing a latent infection—the maintenance of viral genomes in the absence of virus replication—punctuated by sporadic, frequent, and, in healthy hosts, asymptomatic reactivation events that result in subclinical virus shedding.

While reactivation of CMV in healthy individuals is typically asymptomatic, HCMV is an important opportunistic pathogen in immunocompromised individuals, such as following solid organ transplantation (SOT) and hematopoietic cell transplantation (HCT), patients undergoing immunosuppressive therapies, and persons affected by genetic or acquired immunodeficiency. Despite available antiviral therapies that can provide benefit in the control of CMV disease, the virus remains a significant cause of morbidity and mortality in individuals with inadequate cellular immunity. There are currently no approved vaccines, and more effective, safe and orally bioavailable antiviral drugs are needed.

HCMV is the most significant infectious cause of intrauterine infection and a leading cause of disease in the new born. Transplacental transmission of CMV to the fetus during pregnancy, which occurs rarely with other herpesviruses, leads to a congenital (present at birth) infection in approximately 1% of pregnancies worldwide regardless of the maternal CMV serostatus prior to conception. Congenital cCMV infection results in clinically significant neurodevelopmental abnormalities in 10% to 15% of congenitally infected newborns, the most common being sensorineural hearing loss. The frequency of congenital infections caused by CMV and the associated damage to the developing nervous system further underscores the importance of CMV as a human pathogen.

The virion of HCMV (~200 nm) is composed of an enveloped icosahedral capsid encasing a 236-kilobase pair double-stranded DNA genome (Fig. 12.1). CMV genomes have exceptionally large protein-coding capacities, much greater than other herpesviruses (>170 proteins). HCMV proteins with known functions are summarized in Supplementary e-Table 12.1. The viral genome also encodes microRNAs (miRNAs, Supplementary e-Table 12.2) and long RNAs thought to be noncoding (lncRNAs), although there is some evidence for coding potential discussed in later sections. The protein content of CMV particles is large and complex due to the tegument (viral and host proteins and RNAs packaged between the envelope and the capsid). Despite the restricted species host range, within the host HCMV causes systemic infection and replicates in diverse cell types, including but not limited to epithelial cells, endothelial cells, fibroblasts, and hematopoietic cells. HCMV may also enter and remain quiescent such that outcomes of infection are dictated by cell type and differentiation status, and include productive, chronic/persistent, and latent patterns. In the following sections, we review the biology and pathogenesis of HCMV infection. While a historical perspective is provided, older editions of this chapter should be consulted for the literature supporting findings that predate the year 2000 due to space constraints.

HISTORY

HCMV has been recognized as an opportunistic pathogen and an important infectious cause of birth defects for well over half a century. Nearly 100 years ago, histopathology provided the first evidence of this filterable infectious disease agent associated with congenital disease together with type A intranuclear inclusions typical of herpesvirus-infected cells. Infected cells present in tissues of immunocompromised adults or congenitally infected newborns have unmistakable large cell, "owl's eye" cytopathology, or cytomegaly.[246] By the early 1950's, diagnosis of HCMV disease was facilitated by the identification of inclusion-bearing cells in urine along with the demonstration of virus-like particles by electron microscopy. Human salivary gland virus was isolated from the urine of newborns with characteristic clinical and histopathological findings that was termed cytomegalic inclusion disease (CID), now known to be caused by HCMV. By the early 1970s, diagnosis of CMV infection in newborns and transplant recipients by virus isolation was established as a gold standard.

Surrogate animal models using related viruses infecting mice, rats, and guinea pigs play important roles defining the pathogenesis. Rat CMV (RCMV) and murine CMV (MCMV) (classified as *Muromegaloviruses*) replicate and produce a similar cytopathology to HCMV but only on fibroblasts from the homologous species. More recent studies using rhesus CMV (RhCMV) have been possible due to isolation of specific pathogen-free rhesus macaques.[492] Species specificity is recognized as a key characteristic of all CMVs.

Given the low frequency of the clinically apparent or symptomatic congenital CMV infection, the high, worldwide seroprevalence of CMV was unexpected. CMV is recognized as a common asymptomatic virus infection. In 1975 it was reported that transplantation of kidneys from seropositive individual results in a seroconversion in 83% previously seronegative recipients. This finding was confirmed for any transplanted organ—indicating the existence of a latent infection given the lack of detectable virus.

The CMV genome was first sequenced in 1990, revealing the largest human viral genome sequence known. The genome was originally annotated as open reading frames (ORFs) of 100 or more contiguous codons and that did not overlap other ORFs by more than 60%. This led to the identification of 189 putative unique genes. Since this seminal work, our appreciation of the HCMV coding potential has expanded with the identification of additional sequences, many smaller ORFs, noncanonical initiation codons and products from spliced genes. The first HCMV isolate (Toledo strain) to be sequenced prior to extensive passage in cultured fibroblasts revealed a 15-kilobase sequence in the unique long (U_L) region of the genome, referred to as the *b'* region that happened to be inverted but naturally present in all clinical isolates (Fig. 12.2). This region is often lost during serial passage in cultured fibroblasts. The *b'* region encodes 19 to 22 genes with functions related to the broad cellular tropism of HCMV, immune modulation, and latency (Fig. 12.3).[96] Further, reevaluation of the coding potential and RNAs associated with ribosomes during infection has also expanded HCMVs actual potential well beyond 200 unique genes.[161,425,427,597]

Genetic variation within the DNA genome of HCMV strains was first appreciated around the turn of 21st century.[142,213,495] The genetic instability of HCMV genomes propagated in fibroblasts led to cloning a number of low-passage clinical strains as bacterial artificial chromosomes.[410,690] This not only resulted in genomes that could be stably propagated but permitted the use of techniques in prokaryotic molecular biology to introduce mutations to target genes and define gene function.

Beyond congenitally infected infants, the most severe manifestations of uncontrolled HCMV replication have occurred in AIDS patients. During the emergence of the HIV epidemic and before the introduction of highly active antiretroviral therapies, CMV disease occurred in 21% to 44% of AIDS patients late in their disease when CMV retinitis was prevalent. Currently, the most significant setting for CMV disease is associated with immunosuppressive therapy and allograft rejection following SOT and HCT, particularly evident in developed countries. CMV is the single most important cause of infectious disease after organ transplantation and affects 75% of transplant recipients with high morbidity and mortality within the first year following transplantation.

The most important antiviral with clinically demonstrable activity against HCMV, ganciclovir and its oral form, valganciclovir, are derivatives of an aciclovir nucleoside that targets the viral DNA polymerase. These antivirals were initially used to treat end-organ disease associated with CMV infection in AIDS. It is now common practice to use these antivirals for prophylaxis or for preemptive therapy in the setting of SOT or HCT. Although typically beneficial, treatment with these antiviral drugs is sometimes ineffective in controlling virus levels or altering the clinical outcomes in the settings of transplantation

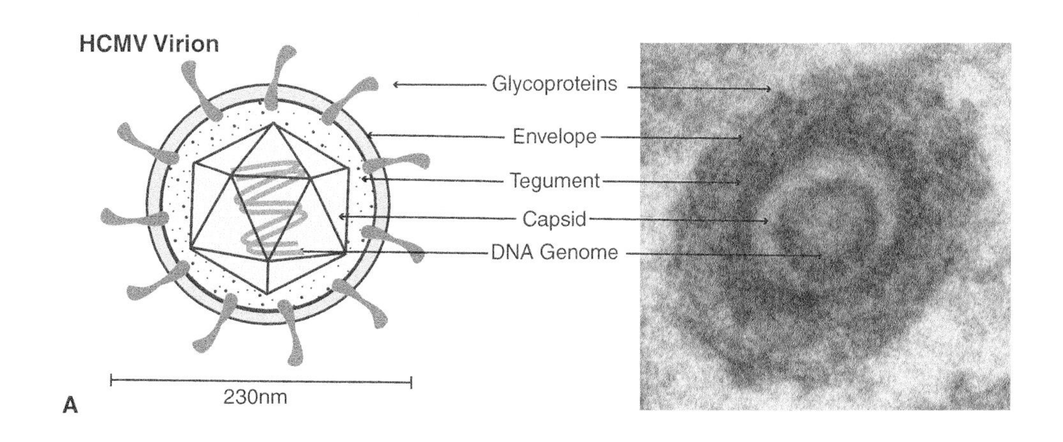

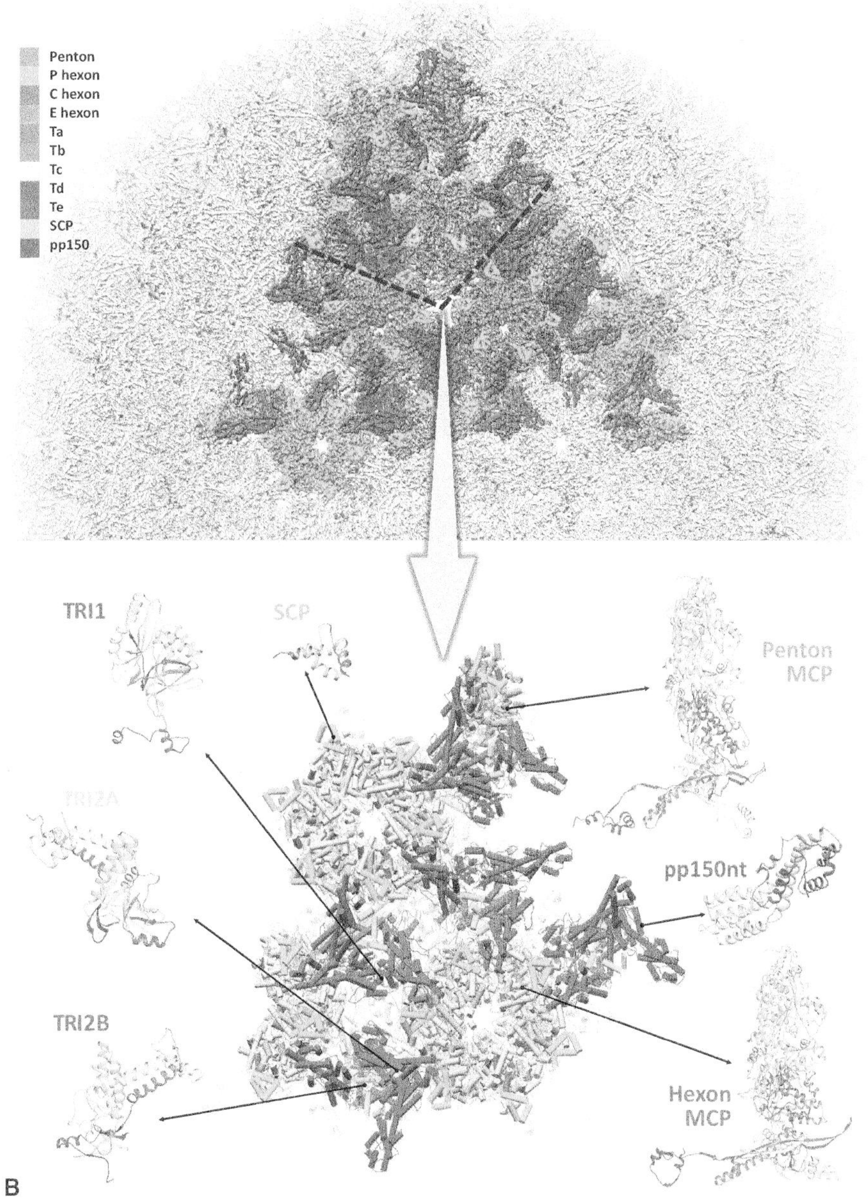

FIGURE 12.1 Virus structure. **A:** Schematic and electron micrograph of HCMV virion. The double-stranded DNA genome core, capsid, tegument, envelope (cell-derived lipid bilayer) and glycoproteins are indicated. There are numerous glycoprotein complexes on the surface of the virion and these are represented in Figure 12.6. **B:** Cryo-EM showing nucleocapsid structure from within a virion (strain AD169) showing capsomeres. The capsid proteins smallest capsid protein (SCP), pentons and hexons of major capsid protein (MCP) and Triplex (TRI2A, TRI2B, and TRI1) and the pp150 tegument protein are indicated. Peripentonal (P), center (C) and edge (E) hexons are also shown. Each asymmetric unit contains a C hexon, P hexon, one-half of an E hexon, and one-fifth of a penton plus 16 copies of SCP that sit atop each MCP, five and one-third heterotrimeric triplexes (indicated with different colors). (Panel B—courtesy of Dr. Hong Zhou, University of California, Los Angeles, California.)

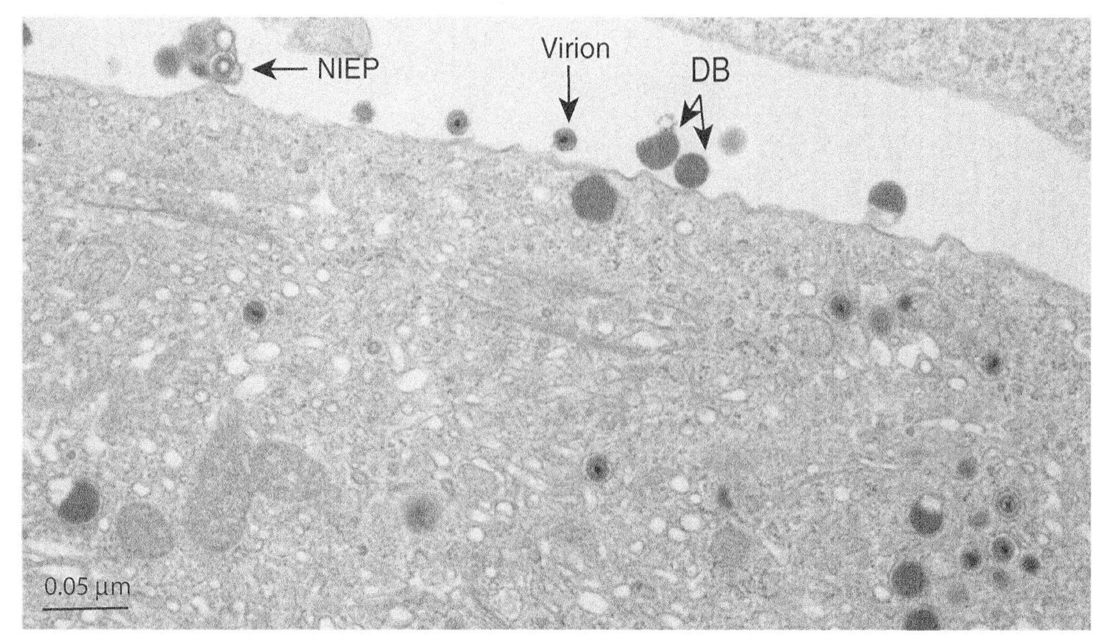

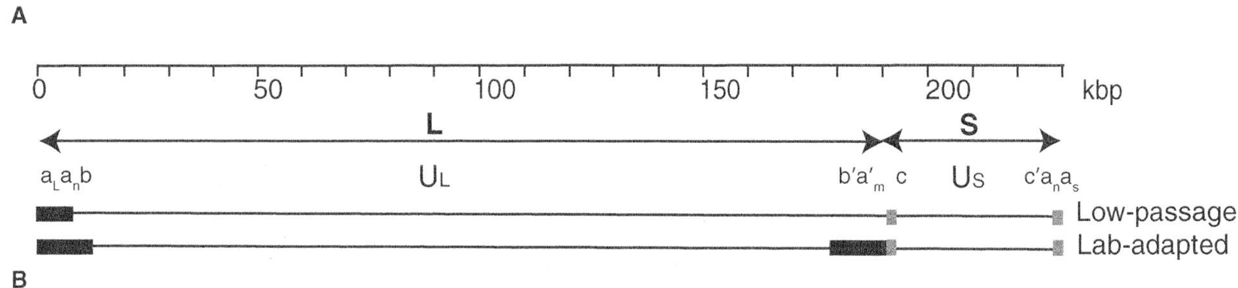

FIGURE 12.2 **HCMV infection and genome structure. A:** Electron micrograph of infected human fibroblasts with intracellular and extracellular HCMV virions, noninfectious enveloped particles (NIEP) and dense bodies (DB). Scale bar, 5 mM. **B:** HCMV genome structure. The size scale (*top line*) is in kilobase pairs (1 kbp = 1,000 base pairs). The long (L) and short (S) segments of the genome are shown with arrows. Schematics for common lab-adapted (e.g., AD169) and low-passage (e.g., TB40/E, Merlin, Toledo, etc.) strains are shown. The L-terminus is composed of the *a* sequence repeat (a_L) where zero to several copies of the *a* sequence may exist (a_n). The *b* sequence repeats at the opposite end of the U_L region near the L–S junction of the unique long (U_L) coding region in AD169. However, the *b* sequence inverted repeat is replaced by additional U_L sequence in the low-passage strains, referred to as U_Lb'. This is followed by one to several additional copies of the *a* sequence inverted repeats (a_m') at the L–S junction. The S segment of coding sequences is bordered by the c′ inverted repeat at the L–S junction and the c sequence inverted repeat and an *a* sequence repeat (a_S) with a variable number of additional copies of the *a* sequence (a_n).

as well as congenital disease. Antiviral prophylaxis with a recently available drug, letermovir, targeting the viral terminase can prevent CMV disease particularly in the HCT setting. Importantly, no existing antiviral therapies target the latent virus reservoir.

CMV was declared a priority for vaccine development byt the US Academy of Medicine in 2004. While CMV vaccines reached Phase I or II trials, there currently is no approved vaccine against CMV. A number of challenges exist to development of an effective vaccine against CMV due to its exquisite ability to evade clearance by a natural immune response and the inability of the natural immune response to prevent superinfection by additional CMV strains. Comprehensively defining the complex immune response to CMV is key to understanding viral persistence and pathology and critical to CMV vaccine development. Major advances in the 21st century have provided insights into the strikingly unique immune response associated with CMV persistence and viral genes required for reactivation, which hold exciting promise for future development of tailored vaccine vectors to target historically intractable pathogens and cancers.[90,235–238]

CLASSIFICATION

CMV is a genus of viruses in the order *Herpesvirales*, in the family *Herpesviridae*, and in the β-*Herpesvirinae* subfamily. HCMV carries the official ICTV designation as human herpesvirus 5. The betaherpesvirus subfamily exhibits a greater level of evolutionarily and genetic divergence than either the α- or γ-herpesvirus subfamilies. Higher order primate CMV species including chimpanzee CMV (ChCMV), which infects chimpanzees and orangutans; simian (SCMV); and RhCMV that infect macaques resemble HCMV and serve as promising animal models. One hundred sixty-three of the predicted 168 ChCMV genes are homologous and colinear with HCMV.[150]

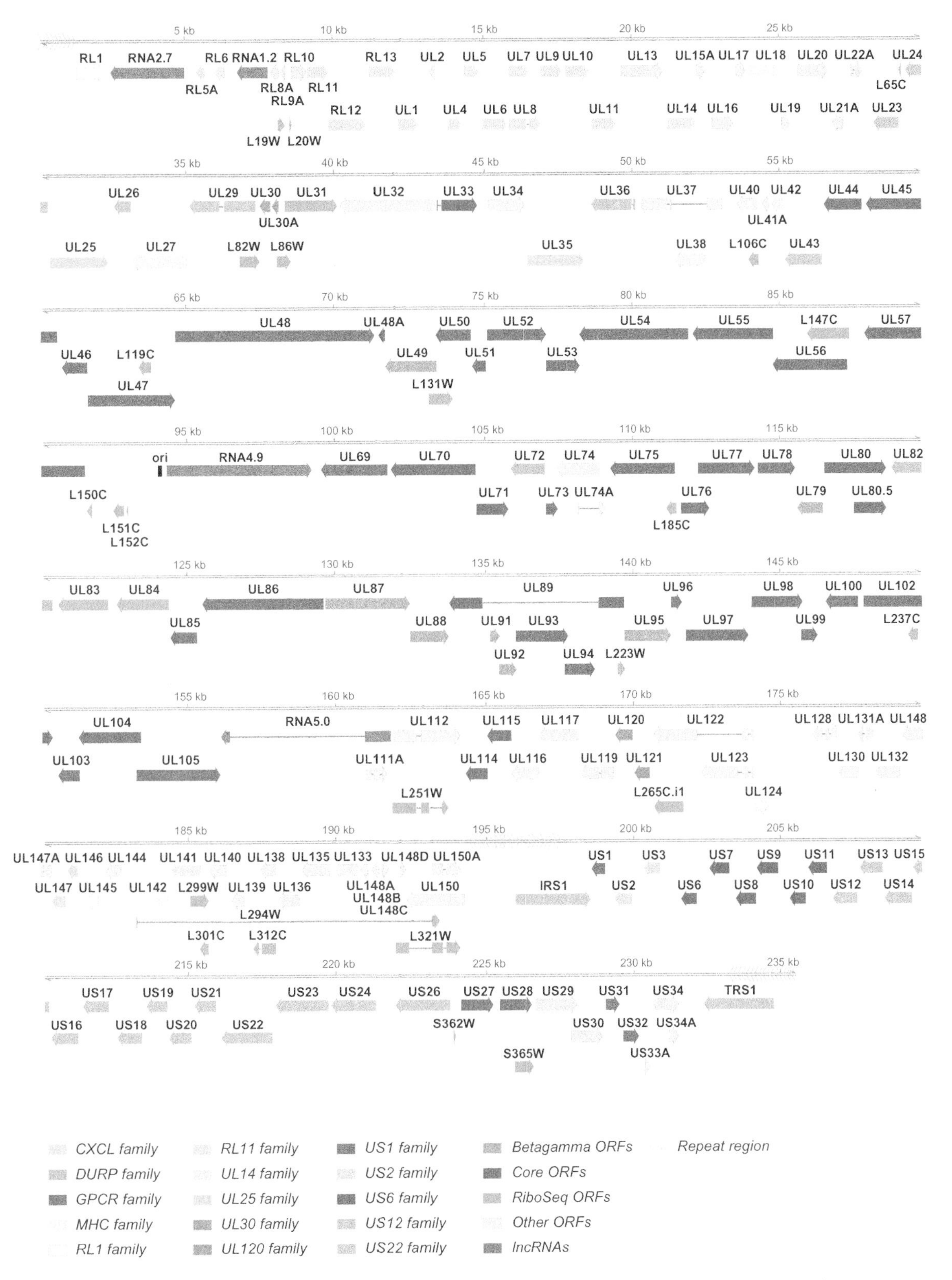

FIGURE 12.3 Genome schematic. Genome map of HCMV based on low-passage strain Merlin. The inverted repeats (RL, IRS, and TRS) are shown by the arrow fletching bordering the unique regions (U_L and U_S). Protein-coding ORFs (previously annotated or validated from ribosome profiling) and lncRNAs are indicated by colored arrows grouped according to the key shown at the foot, with gene nomenclature. Introns connecting protein-coding regions or exons in noncoding RNA5.0 are shown as a line. The colors of ORFs indicate conservation among members of the family *Herpesviridae* (core ORFs) or the subfamilies *β-herpesvirinae* and *δ-herpesvirinae* (betagamma ORFs), with subsets of the remaining noncore ORFs grouped into gene families. UL72 is both a core ORF and a member of the DURP gene family. (Courtesy of Noam Stern-Ginossar and Yaara Finkel, Weizmann Institute, Israel.)

While RhCMV is a more tractable model than ChCMV, only 111 genes share homology with HCMV.[527] The relatedness between HCMV and *muromegaloviruses* (MCMV and RCMV) that were previously classified as CMVs, falls off dramatically such that less than 80 genes exhibiting sequence homology. Nonetheless, MCMV and HCMV exhibit many common biological attributes in infection, pathogenesis, immune modulation, and latency. CMVs achieve these ends via divergent mechanisms and distinct gene products. For the purposes of this chapter, CMV is used to collectively refer to the entire genus or when referencing clinical disease (e.g., CMV disease in the immunocompromised host or congenital CMV). The chapter is focused on HCMV, and research findings that rely on other species of CMV are specified. Due to constraints inherent in studying CMV pathogenesis in humans, many key observations are referenced from the study of animal models.

VIRION STRUCTURE

Capsid

The HCMV virion ranges from 200 to 300 nM in diameter and consists of three structurally definable regions, the innermost DNA containing capsid, a structurally less well-defined tegument layer, and the outermost lipid-containing envelope (Fig. 12.1A). Of these, the capsid of HCMV shows relatedness to capsids of other herpesviruses, including the most well studied herpesvirus, herpes simplex virus-1 (HSV-1). The HCMV capsid is approximately 130 nM in diameter. Due to the size of the HCMV genome, viral DNA within the HCMV nucleocapsid is likely near the limit of viral DNA that can be packaged.[692] Because of a predicted high internal pressure of the HCMV nucleocapsid secondary to the charged and tightly packed genomic DNA, several unique structural properties of the capsid have been proposed to facilitate packaging of the viral genome and subsequent stabilization of the nucleocapsid. Major capsid protein (MCP, encoded by UL86), minor capsid protein (MnCP or Triplex 1, TRI1, encoded by UL85), minor capsid binding protein (MnCBP or Triplex 2, TRI2, encoded by UL46), smalllest capsid protein (SCP, encoded by UL48.5), and the portal proteinn (encoded by UL104). Assemblin, encoded by UL80.5, is cleared from the mature capsid prior to genome packaging, significant quantities it its cleavage product is associated with the mature particle.[526,640] In addition to mature nucleocapsids associated with infectious virions, capsids lacking genomes may be enveloped producing noninfectious enveloped particles (NIEPs) (Fig. 12.2A). Furthermore, infection results in noninfectious particles that lack both viral DNA and capsids that are termed dense bodies (DB), based on their appearance in electron micrographs. Characteristically, DB are larger than virions and more heterogeneous in their protein composition than virions, and their relative abundance is viral strain dependent. Both NIEPs and DBs are produced and released from infected cells, particularly in culture. The mature capsid of the infectious virion contains five virus-encoded proteins.

Using cryo-electron microscopy, the structure of the HCMV capsid was solved at an average resolution of 3.9 Å[692] (Fig. 12.1B). Several key protein structures and protein–protein interactions have been defined that, in turn, have provided explanations for the stability of DNA containing nucleocapsid.[692] The icosahedral structure of the HCMV capsid consists of 12 pentons, 150 hexons, and 320 triplexes with a triangulation number of 16.[144,692] A single SCP molecule associates with each MCP and a single pp150 (*UL32*) tegument protein is present on each MCP/SCP heterodimer.[692] Unique to the structure of the MCP is the presence of a Johnson-fold, a motif homologous to a structural feature in all herpesviruses and some bacteriophages that stabilizes the capsid.[692] In addition, favorable charge interactions between the HCMV DNA and hexons provide a mechanism for packing of the viral DNA as well as stabilizing the nucleocapsid.[692] These features support remarkable stability of the capsid structure. Lastly, the tegument protein pp150 interaction with MCP/SCP heterodimers as well as with triplexes creates a net or a skein-like structure to further maintain the structural integrity of the nucleocapsid, a feature unique to primate CMVs.[692,693] For more detailed discussion of capsid assembly, see section *Capsid assembly, DNA encapsidation, and nuclear egress.*

Tegument

The virion tegument layer resides between the envelope and the capsid and remains the least well-characterized region of the virion both in terms of composition and organization. The tegument consists of dozens of proteins, many of which carry out critical functions in the replicative cycle and in the modification of host responses to infection. Over 50% of the total number of virus-encoded proteins are located in the tegument[526,640]; however, only a small fraction contribute directly to the structural integrity of the virion. A majority of tegument proteins contribute to HCMV genome replication, efficient cytoplasmic assembly of infectious progeny, and modulation of host innate and adaptive immune responses. Most tegument proteins are phosphorylated, and phosphorylation may regulate tegument protein function.[214] Ultrastructural studies of the HCMV capsid have localized pp150 to the innermost layer of the tegument through its interaction with the SCP.[144] Beyond pp150, our understanding of the order of tegument protein remains rudimentary.

Although there is little evidence that individual virus-encoded proteins are required to maintain the structural integrity of tegument, deletion of individual tegument proteins can dramatically impact the assembly of infectious virions.[111] It is difficult to discern whether the loss of an single tegument protein has a direct impact on virion instability or alternatively, impacts stability by altering the incorporation of other tegument proteins important for early steps in infection, as has been described for the role of pp65 (*UL83*) in the incorporation of UL69 and UL97 proteins into the virion.[111] Tegument proteins also impact CMV replication by contributing to viral modulation of host intrinsic and innate immune responses. Functions that have been assigned to individual tegument proteins in the replication of HCMV do not provide clues to their location in the tegument. As an example, tegument proteins such as pp150 that function in both stabilization of the nucleocapsid and potentially in the transport of the nucleocapsid to sites of virion assembly presumably must belocalized to the inner tegument layer.[144,263,612,692] Finally, proteomic studies have also identified a substantial number of host cell proteins as well as virus-encoded RNAs within the tegument of extracellular virions,[526,620,640] even though these do not play any obvious a role in infection.

Envelope

The tegumented nucleocapsid is surrounded by a lipid bilayer envelope derived from the endoplasmic reticulum–Golgi intermediate compartment and contains a large number of virus-encoded proteins. The envelope exhibits a unique lipid content including very long chain fatty acids and cholesterol that distinguishes it from membranes of uninfected cells.[222,319] The lipid composition of the HCMV virion envelope is similar to that of synaptic vesicles and exocytic vesicles produced by exocrine cells.[367] It is perhaps not surprising that the lipid composition of the HCMV virion envelope differs from that of intracellular membranes in uninfected cells given the major alterations in host cell lipid metabolism and extensive spatial reorganization of intracellular membranes that accompanies generation of the membranous virus assembly compartment in the late phase of virus replication.[201,330,545] Interestingly, the cholesterol content of the infected cell increases significantly during infection and may contribute to the fusogenic activity of the envelope.[222,474] The membrane lipids incorporated into the virion envelope may also be derived from inhibition of lipid transport from the infected cells.[544,694,695] Thus, the characteristic spatial reorganization of host cell membranes in virus infected cells is accompanied by increased lipid production as well as inhibition of fatty acid oxidation and changes in intermediary metabolism to support increased lipogenesis required for virus membrane production and additional sources of carbon for ATP production.[563,647,694]

The HCMV envelope contains orthologs of core herpesvirus glycoproteins, glycoprotein B (gB), gH, gL, gM, and gN. In addition, glycoproteins unique to HCMV, including gO together with UL128, UL130, and UL131A proteins, contribute to early events of virus infection including virion attachment, fusion, and penetration of the target cell, contributing to the broad cellular tropism.[224,385,671,702] Each of these proteins is present within functional glycoprotein complexes in the virion. For more detailed discussion of glycoprotein complexes and function, see section *Attachment and Entry*. HCMV envelope protein complexes likely provide a level of regulation of the entry process into the host cell. Complex formation may also ensure functional activity of individual glycoproteins regardless of the overall stoichiometry of individual glycoproteins in the virion envelope. This possibility is consistent with findings that the composition of the envelope, including the relative amounts of individual core envelope protein complexes, can vary depending on the level of expression of nonenvelope viral proteins as well as the cell type in which the virus is propagated.[336,350,353,557] Most of the core envelope glycoproteins are involved in entry, with the exception of gM, which has been implicated in assembly and release of virions and noninfectious viral particles.[224,247,267,325] Beyond gB, gH, gL, gM, gN, gO and the UL128, UL130, and UL131A gene products, as many as 50 to 70 glycoproteins are encoded by HCMV. Many of these glycoproteins traffic to sites of virion assembly and can be incorporated into the envelope of HCMV; however, none of these has been shown to be required for virion envelopment, attachment, entry, or maturation and release arguing that they likely do not play a direct role in assembly or function of the virion envelope. Yet these viral proteins are likely required for efficient *in vivo* replication, immune modulation, and persistence of HCMV. Examples of these functions include incorporation of the viral G protein–coupled receptor (GPCR), US28, which modifies the cellular responses to HCMV infection.[47,395]

GENOME STRUCTURE AND ORGANIZATION

Genome Organization

The HCMV genome is one of the largest and most complex of any characterized herpesvirus. Initial DNA sequence analysis and conventional annotation of the 236 kb strain AD169 genome, together with follow-up investigation[142,161] established the presence of 40 conserved core protein-coding genes common to all subfamilies of mammalian herpesviruses along with a larger subset (~70) conserved across the β-herpesviruses with some of these encoding late transcription machinery that is also preserved in γ-herpesviruses (Supplementary e-Table 12.1 and Figs. 12.2 and 12.3). Taxonomy of herpesviruses is based on common virion structure together with the level of conservation of predicted protein coding genes.[148,149] β-herpesviruses are the most diverse herpesvirus subfamily such that even primate relatives show remarkable differences in genetic content. Despite this, HCMV and nonhuman primate β-herpesviruses exhibit a colinear genome organization where genes encoding different HCMV temporal classes of protein-coding and noncoding RNAs are interspersed as with other herpesvirus subfamilies. In addition, betaherpesviruses have characteristic gene families that are not observed in either alphaherpesviruses or gammaherpesviruses.

The genomes of HCMV and closely related chimpanzee CMV share high identity,[150] and both retain a class E genome arrangement with unique long (U_L) and unique short (U_S) regions flanked by terminal and internal repeats in an arrangement first described for HSV-1 (*ab*-U_L-*b'a'c'*-U_S-*ca*), shown in Figure 12.2 and summarized.[147,148] This arrangement of terminal and internal inverted *a* sequences, which contain the genome cleavage/packaging signals, promotes intramolecular recombination (genome inversion) during replication such that virus stocks are composed of four equimolar and independently infectious isomers with regard to the orientation of the short (S) and long (L) genome components. As with HSV1, genome inversion is dispensable for replication in cell culture[551] although likely provides some fitness advantage. The *c'* and *c* repeats (also called IRS and TRS) flanking the S genome component have a partially duplicated IE gene set (IRS1 and TRS1). In contrast, the large *b* and *b'* repeats (also called TRL and IRL) flanking the L genome component in viral strains that underwent extensive propagation are absent low-passage strains.[149] The RhCMV and cynomolgus monkey CMV genomes show a simpler structure with direct terminal repeats without internal repeats or genome isomerization. Directly repeated *a* sequences of variable length and copy number are found at genome termini and include two herpesvirus-conserved DNA cleavage and encapsidation (packaging) signals, called *pac1* and *pac2* near the cleavage site that dictate the position of the genome termini.[656] These elements are recognized by the machinery that is conserved in herpesviruses to cleave and feed the DNA into a capsid as well as to cut a second time once a genome length is packaged, leaving single overhanging 3′-nucleotides.

The viral genome origin of DNA synthesis (*ori*Lyt) controls genome replication during productive infection from a location between the divergent *UL57* and *UL69* genes in the middle of the U_L region. This position of *ori*Lyt is conserved in all characterized betaherpesviruses, apparently along with a lncRNA (RNA4.9 in HCMV) that is transcribed from the *ori*-Lyt region and localizes to the nuclear replication compartment (RC) where it is required for efficient expression of *UL57* and DNA replication.[611] The *ori*Lyt in CMVs is large (~1,500 bp) and structurally complex, and in HCMV, includes a pyrimidine-rich sequence, reiterated elements, direct and inverted repeat sequences, and transcription factor–binding sites.

Early on, AD169 and Towne strains were selected for research purposes. Both were readily propagated in fibroblasts owing to adaptation through serial passage that had also attenuated virulence and supported testing as live attenuated vaccines. Both were overattenuated, leading to alternative, ongoing live attenuated vaccine strategies.[6,7] Both of these so-called laboratory-adapted strains are available from ATCC as a mixture of variants with varying degrees of gene loss.[59,140,161,225] The substantial gene loss in clonal derivatives of common strains first came to light through comparison to cosmid cloned DNA of strain Toledo,[96] a low-passage strain that exhibited virulence compared to Towne[495] and because Towne-Toledo chimeras were being evaluated as vaccine candidates.[7,605] Toledo carried a larger number of genes than higher passage strains, but its genome carries substantial mutations and alterations compared to clinical isolates,[495] most markedly lacking a functional gH/gL pentamer complex[224,641] that is critical for epithelial and endothelial cell attachment and other clinically relevant activities.[536,600,653,654]

It is now very clear that HCMV rapidly develops a pattern of specific as well as more random mutations that generally subvert restrictions on cell-to-cell spread and/or cell-free release during propagation on susceptible cell substrates, including fibroblasts and epithelial cells, as well as endothelial cells and myeloid cells.[669] Although several low-passage virus strains, such as TB40/E, VR1814 and TR and their respective bacmid cloned derivatives (TB40E-BAC4, FIX-BAC, and TR-BAC) have been employed as more representative of HCMV clinical virus because they support entry and replication in all known susceptible cell types as well as human tissue explants or tissue implants (in mice), these strains represent mixtures of variants with accumulated mutations in a variety of genes and, once converted to a bacmid allows only a single clonal derivative to be the focus of study. Even though HCMV strains are most readily isolated on fibroblasts, propagation on epithelial cells or endothelial cells preserves gH/gL pentamer function, at least for the Merlin strain, for entry and the ability to infect a broader range of cell types in culture than strains propagated on fibroblast.[432]

Most recently, the Merlin strain has been presented as a potential prototype strain for detailed evaluation of HCMV biology.[198,587,669] Genome sequence analysis starting with non-propagated clinical material provided exemplary information on genome changes that accompany propagation of HCMV strains in cell culture.[145] Such alterations are known to be relevant to other HCMV strains.[336,430–432,460,556,644,669] HCMV in clinical material remains highly cell associated, revealing remarkable levels of instability when propagated in cell culture, indicating strong selective pressure for accumulation of both cell type–common and cell type–specific mutations during passage. Based on evaluation of Merlin[145] and information from other cultured strains, RL13, encoding a virus-encoded IgG Fc receptor, appears to be a very unstable viral gene independent of cell type. In fibroblasts, gH/gL pentamer components (UL128, UL130, and UL131A proteins, also known as the *UL128* locus) show dramatic instability. Merlin strain was harnessed to conditionally express the principal viral genes (RL13 and the UL128 locus) otherwise lost upon passage, allowing studies with a fully competent strain with a full complement of viral genes approximating prototypic HCMV[587]. Resulting observations help address broad concerns about unrecognized chance mutations accumulating in cultured viral stocks.[336,431,432,669] While some strains have been propagated with either intact RL13 or intact UL128 locus, these studies brought to light how RL13 and pentamer function together contribute to restriction of cell-free virus production during infection. It is becoming clear that characteristic cell-to-cell spread possibly proceeds independent of the gH/gL/gO glycoprotein complex,[556] but dependent on long-suspected and recently described gH/gL/gB complexes that predominate on virions.[635] The presence of an apparently intact RL13 in low-passage strains (e.g., TR) where gH/gL pentamer levels are distinctly low, but not absent, suggests that reduced expression may also occur during propagation.[431,556] Thus, strong selective pressure drives genomic modification to overcome restriction and facilitate efficient replication, production of cell-free virus and improved spread from cell to cell. Curiously, this selective pressure to mutate RL13 and UL128 locus may be negated by clinical strain isolation in the presence of pooled human gammaglobulin, presumably owing to the effects of anti-CMV antibodies that themselves limit cell-free spread of this virus in fibroblasts.[460] There are a wide range of additional unstable genes that have been noted but where the mechanism of restriction is less well established.

In addition to the variation observed upon propagation in cell culture, recent deep DNA sequence evaluation of HCMV genomes directly in clinical materials has revealed an apparent abundance of variation in natural infections that have been ascribed to error-prone replication, substantial recombination, and/or mixed infections with multiple strains.[139,518–520,606,607] As this area matures with more incisive methods of analysis, it is likely to have tremendous impact on many aspects of HCMV biology, immunology, therapy, and immune prophylaxis.

Coding Potential and Variation

Remarkable efforts in sequence analysis, comparative genomics, annotation of predicted protein-coding regions and study of both strain variants and additional primate CMVs has since revealed remarkable levels of genome evolution, recombination, and diversity as a variety of HCMV strains have been dissected.[84] HCMV genome annotation continues to be provisional with canonical protein-coding regions shorter than about 80 codons, use of unusual translation initiation codons and overlap with larger ORFs not included without substantial verification of their biological significance. The refinement of HCMV annotation has included many methods, including comparisons to HCMV that have not been propagated, as well as comparison to chimpanzee CMV. In addition, alternative bioinformatic algorithms and relating protein composition continues to be applied to the challenge of estimating coding capacity. Initial genome annotation methods gave a reasonable estimate of 170

TABLE 12.1 Clinical and laboratory findings in infants with symptomatic congenital HCMV infections[a]

Clinical Findings	Frequency
Hepatosplenomegaly	17%
Petechiae	55%
Jaundice	40%
Microcephaly	35%
Seizures	1%
Intrauterine growth restriction	27%
Laboratory Findings	
Elevated transaminases (liver)	55%
Decreased platelets	38%
Elevated bilirubin (direct)	46%
Cranial imaging abnormalities	71%

[a]Finding in 78 infants with symptomatic congenital HCMV infection identified by screening enrollment in natural history study of cCMV infections.[162]

protein-coding genes that formed a foundation for purposes of functional dissection of genome organization. Except for a few outliers, the order of ORFs has been depicted as RL1-to-RL13-UL1-to-150-IRS1-US1-to-US34-TRS1 (Table 12.1 and Figs. 12.2 and 12.3). Emphasis has therefore been on a uniform nomenclature where genes are numbered in sequential order and the gene product is either identified by the same name or includes a prefix. In addition to these genes, HCMV encodes four lncRNAs, two short embedded oriLyt RNAs and as many as 26 miRNA genes.[482] Recent transcript mapping,[198] ribosomal profiling,[265,595,597] mass spectrometry,[443,660] and further characterization of abundantly expressed lncRNAs[595] have revealed a growing complexity associated with HCMV genome annotation and functional organization. HCMV benefitted from being selected for evaluation in the first application of ribosomal profiling to a mammalian system.[597] Ribosomal profiling identified many previously unidentified ORFs, internal ORFs lying within known ORFs, ORFs in alternative reading frames, upstream ORFs, and ORFs encoded antisense to canonical ORFs.[597] Strikingly, these studies also identified a number of polypeptides initiating at nonconical codons and eight novel ORFs within the β2.7 RNA that has been designated as a lncRNA; two of these proteins were identified in infected fibroblasts and are recognized by CD4+ and CD8+ T cells.[265,597] When transcribed lncRNAs, miRNAs and mRNAs are considered,[265,482,597] HCMV may encode as many as 800 gene products, a complexity that is supported by remarkable parallels in roseolaviruses HHV6A and HHV6B.[183]

Accurately estimating the true functional organization of the HCMV genome has been compromised by shortcomings in annotation methods that have overlooked the existence of multi-cistronic transcripts, as well as small, multiple and overlapping ORFs that employ translation initiation codons other than canonical AUG. RNA polymerase II initiation of viral transcription is promiscuous with transcriptional start sites clustering within a 20-basepair interval,[468,597] indicating that HCMV may have regions to initiate transcription, rather than precise transcriptional start sites.[468] The over 7,000 transcriptional start sites detected during lytic replication are in vast excess of the number of ORFs that have been predicted. Alternative transcriptional starts generate overlapping or nested ORFs that produce multiple variants of a protein.[94,501,502,586] Well characterized examples in HCMV include *UL44* and *UL136*, which each give rise to overlapping transcripts with unique 5′ ends and co-terminal 3′ ends. Alternative *UL44* transcripts arise from a noncanonical TATA element.[271] At least five nested UL136 proteins with distinct localization and roles in replication are synthesized from alternative transcriptional starts.[93,94] *UL93-UL99* is also well appreciated to be a complex transcriptional unit encoding several polycistronic transcripts and overlapping 3′ coterminal transcripts that encode the UL99/pp28 protein. Some of alternative transcription start sites may result in alternative 5′ untranslated regions for differential regulation of translation, affecting ribosome initiation and progression.[418] As an example, the 5′ UTR of major immediate early transcripts is inhibitory to translation in transient reporter assays, but critical for IE protein accumulation in the context of infection, suggesting the existence of important translation regulatory sequences in the UTR.[25]

HCMV-encoded genes (~70) that contribute to productive replication in cultured fibroblasts are more likely to have more accurate functional assignments than viral genes that modulate the cellular or organismal immune environment, particularly when the species specificity of HCMV is factored in. The challenges to investigators seeking biological function of viral gene products that modulate infected cells or the host response to infection is to choose an appropriate strain variant and cell type that maximizes the expectation that accurate insights will emerge. This issue remains daunting as, for example, the *UL36*-encoded viral inhibitor of caspase-8 activation (vICA), originally characterized as a suppressor of extrinsic cell death, is commonly mutated in laboratory strain variants,[572] including a single amino acid substitution (C131R) that ablates cell death suppression. This unnoticed mutation is carried by widely studied variants of strain AD169 distributed by the ATCC (AD169*var*ATCC), as well as clonal derivatives (e.g., AD169-BAC or BADwt) used for experimental mutagenesis[691] and vaccine development.[194] This loss-of-function mutation is found in by other AD169 variants (e.g., AD169*var*UC and AD169*var*UK) as well as other viral strains (e.g., Towne*var*RIT); however, gene function has been preserved in other variants (e.g., AD169*var*DE and Towne*var*ATCC) in use around the world.[60,161,572] This diversity allowed initial characterization of mutant phenotype in monocyte lineage cells.[405] Such a pattern implied vICA function, though not obvious, was deleterious in fibroblasts dependent on additional factors as virus was passaged. Any phenotypic evaluation of *UL36*-mutant viruses requires a *UL36* competent strain for comparison.[163,405,572] The consequences of inapparent mutations is broad as a great many single gene mutants, including many implicated in cell death, have been studies in an UL36-deficient parental background without acknowledging the potential impact of caspase-8 activity, one of the most aggressive signaling systems present in all mammalian cells[419] but one that is normally completely suppressed by vICA during infection.[572] This issue has also impacted characterization of nonhuman primate CMVs. The *UL36* homolog is nonfunctional in RhCMV strain 68-1 and fails to suppress apoptosis unless repaired.[406] Unexpectedly, this defect does not undermine the ability of RhCMV 68-1 to replicate in fetal macaques.[102] Somewhat mysteriously, the repair of UL36 function had no impact on replication or vaccine vector efficacy in macaques but unveiled a significant contribution of this cell death suppressor to replication and immunogenicity in adult cynomolgus monkeys.[81] These examples illustrate the substantial challenges to fully account for underlying inapparent or unnoticed mutations that are likely to accumulate with cell culture passage of CMV variants chosen for study.

The analysis of HCMV gene function has generally followed one of two strategies. Viral genes may yield insights into biological activity when studied in isolation, when mutated in the virus or through a combination of both. This applies to studies in cultured cells, organoid cultures or human tissue–implanted mice because humans are the only available host for HCMV. A wider variety of viral gene products have been studied in isolation than have been studied in the context of viral infection, particularly in the context of engineered fully competent strains of virus,[336,431,432,587] leaving opportunities to investigate viral gene products that modulate the host response to infection. Some viral genes have revealed aspects of their function through specific phenotypes affecting replication, cell function, immune parameters, and latency. Directed or random mutagenesis of viral genomes has yielded phenotypes that help define biological function. The virus strain, host cell type, precision of the mutagenesis, and approaches for evaluation may all impact the physiological relevance of the data that are generated by these approaches. The genome complexity of HCMV, together with the range of settings where this virus interfaces with host cell and host defense pathways for replication, persistence, pathogenesis, and latency provides opportunities for investigation and discovery.

STAGES OF REPLICATION

CMV is a slow replicating virus that produces low viral yields in comparison to other viruses (10- to 100-fold less compared to HSV-1). While CMV infects and replicates in a wide variety of cells in the host organism, the replicative cycle has largely been studied in fibroblasts. Fibroblasts, a stromal cell present in all tissues, has been the model of choice because of their relative ease of isolation from a variety of discarded tissues and ready propagation in culture, as well as their capacity to support viral gene expression and progeny virus production. Figure 12.4 summarizes the replicative cycle and compares it to the latent state.

Attachment and Entry

Entry occurs in seven distinct steps (1): viral glycoprotein attachment to heparan sulfate glycosaminoglycans, (2) viral glycoprotein-mediated binding to specific cell surface receptors, (3) entry via (3a) endocytosis/micropinocytosis or (3b) gB-mediated fusion at the plasma membrane, (4) release of the capsid into the cytoplasm following fusion with the (4a) endosomal membrane or (3b) the plasma membrane, (5) microtubule (MT)-mediated transport of the capsid towards the nucleus, (6) likely docking at the nuclear pore, and (7) extrusion of the viral genome through the portal and into the nucleus (Fig. 12.5).

As in all herpesviruses, virion envelope glycoproteins are essential for virus attachment and entry and are also important targets of the host humoral immune response.[116,682] A number of different glycoprotein complexes support attachment and entry into different cells types, underlying, in part, the broad tropism of HCMV for many cell types.[440,550] Initial contact with cells is mediated by gB and the gM/gN complex binding

FIGURE 12.4 **Overview of infection: replicative and latent states. A: The HCMV replicative cycle** has been most thoroughly characterized in primary human fibroblasts. (*1*) HCMV attaches to the cell surface and binds cellular receptors to trigger (*2*) entry by endocytosis or fusion at the plasma membrane (detailed in Fig. 12.5). (*3*) The virion has been proposed to translocate along microtubules to the nuclear pore and following docking, extrudes the viral genome into the nucleus. (*4*) The genome is circularized and chromatinized by cellular histones. Viral tegument proteins (*yellow stipples*) are also translocated to the nucleus where they function to block cellular restrictions to viral gene expression and replication, including genome silencing. (*5*) Immediate early gene expression (*green*) begins and does not require, although maybe enhanced by, other viral factors, such as tegument proteins. (*6*) IE proteins are synthesized in the cytoplasm and then transported back into the nucleus where they stimulate early gene expression. (*7–8*) Early transcripts (*blue*) will be synthesized and translated and the early proteins stimulate viral genome synthesis. (*9*) Following the onset of viral DNA synthesis, late transcripts accumulate (*red*), and late proteins are synthesized. (10) Late structural proteins will be transported into the nucleus for assembly of capsids (detailed in Figs. 12.9 and 12.10). (*11*) Concatemeric genomes will be resolved and encapsidated. (*12*) Nucleocapsids receive the first layer of tegument and then egress by budding through the nuclear envelope, where they become enveloped and then de-enveloped. (*13*) Capsids will be further tegumented and enveloped within the viral assembly compartment (detailed in Figs. 12.12 and 12.13). (*14*) Mature virus particles and dense bodies (vesicles of viral tegument protein) egress via exocytic mechanisms that remain poorly characterized. **B: Latency** is studied in primary and cell line hematopoietic progenitor and myeloid lineage systems. (*1*) The virus enters through pentamer–cellular receptor interactions and endocytosis. (*2*) The capsid is translocated to the nucleus with delayed kinetics relative to fibroblasts and tegument proteins are retained in the cytoplasm. (*3*) The genome is extruded into the nucleus where it is circularized. (*4*) Broad, low-level viral gene expression from across the genome is detected and (*5*) viral proteins are synthesized. (*6*) The viral genome is further silenced, as indicated by limited viral gene expression (e.g., IE and *UL135* among others). Some genes such as *UL138* and Luna remain detectable by assays for RNA or protein expression. It is not known how the genome is maintained in latently infected cells, but viral proteins and miRNAs have been shown to be important for latency, maintenance of the genome and reactivation. (*7*) Cellular triggers such as differentiation or inflammation will trigger reexpression of viral genes and reactivation of replication. (*8*) The cascade of events from reexpression of genes to egress of virions following reactivation are poorly characterized.

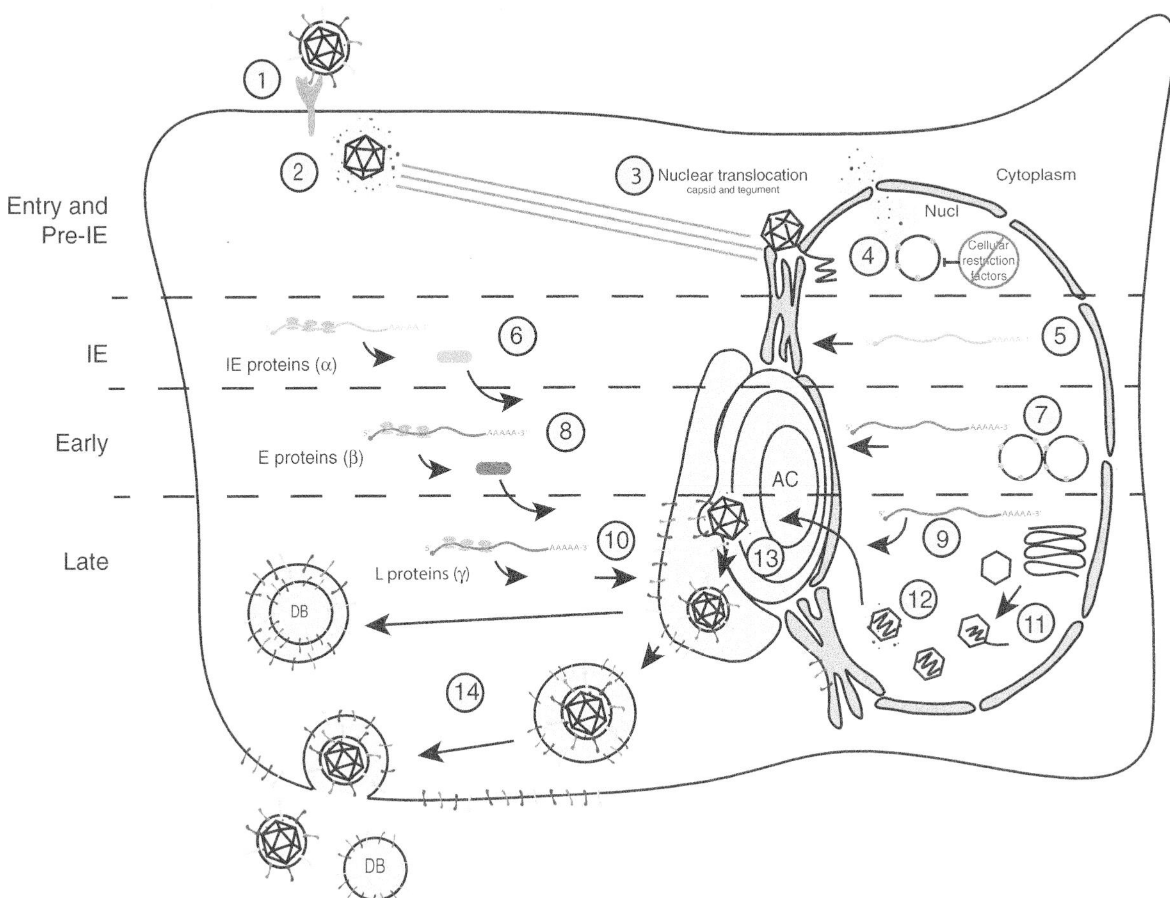
Replicative Cycle
1
2
3 Nuclear translocation
capsid and tegument
Cytoplasm
Nucl
4
Cellular restriction factors
Entry and Pre-IE
IE
IE proteins (α)
6
5
Early
E proteins (β)
8
7
AC
Late
L proteins (γ)
10
9
13
12
11
DB
14
DB
A

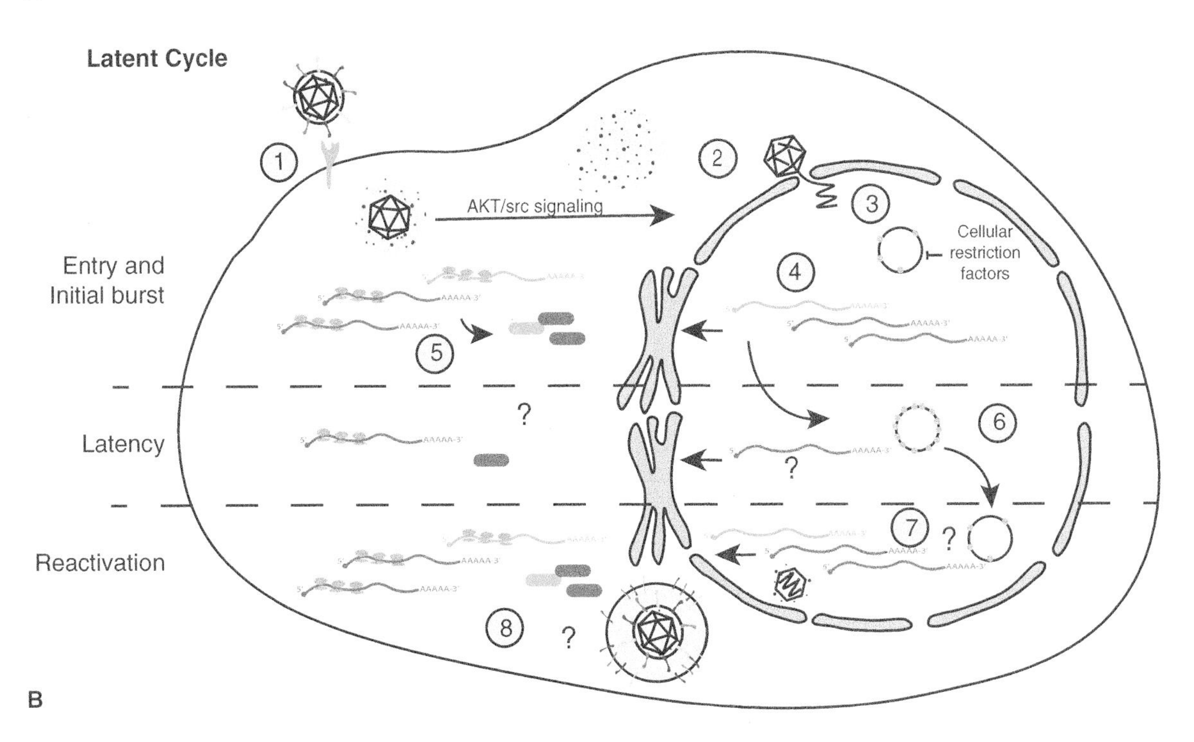
Latent Cycle
1
2
AKT/src signaling
3
Cellular restriction factors
Entry and Initial burst
4
5
Latency
?
6
?
Reactivation
7
?
8
?
B

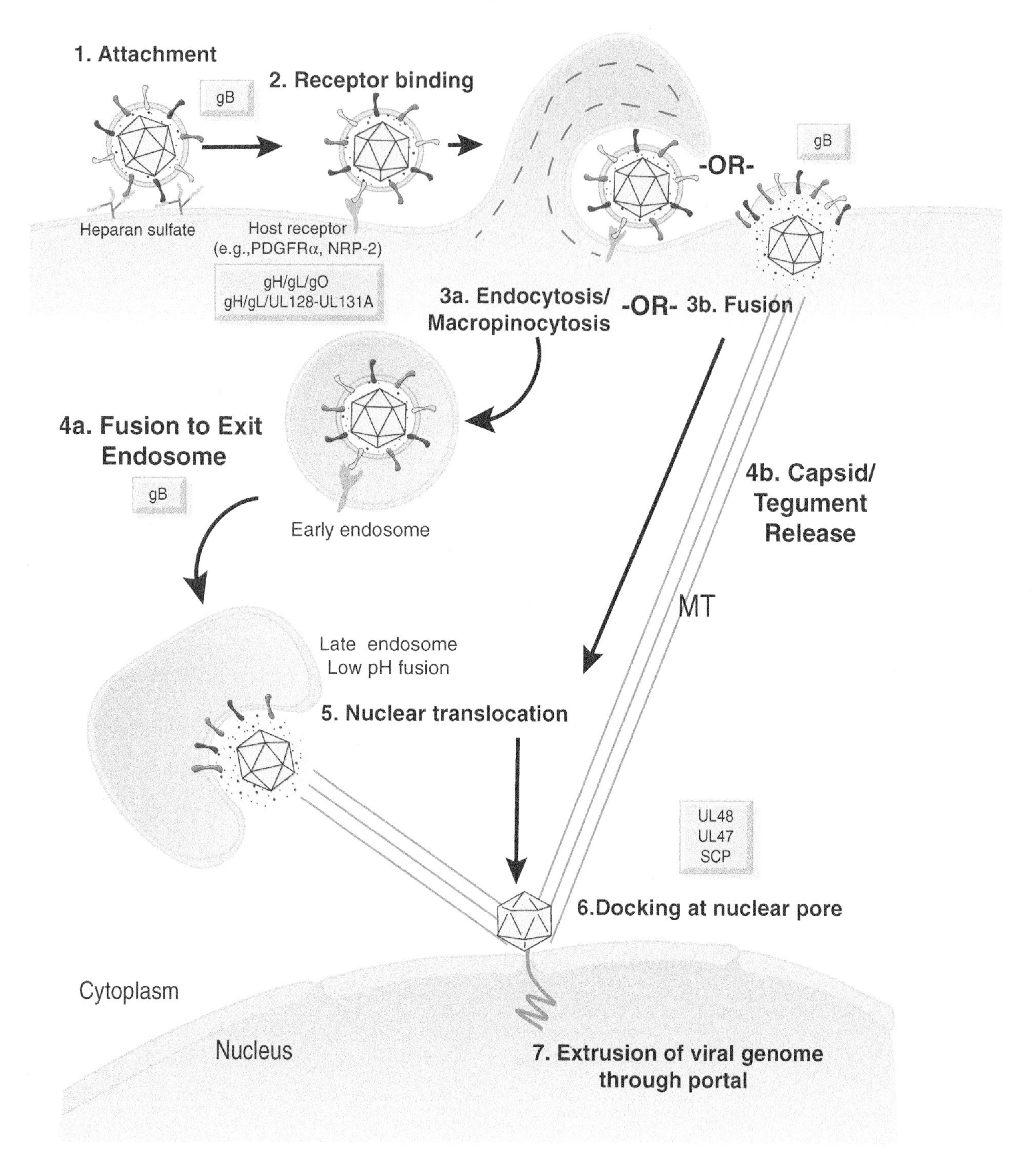

FIGURE 12.5 **HCMV entry and translocation to the nucleus.** (*1*) HCMV attaches to cells through an interaction of gB with heparan sulfate. (*2*) CMV trimer (gH/gL/gO) and pentamer (gH/gL/UL128/UL130/UL131A) will engage receptors on the cell surface, including PDGFRα and NRP-2, respectively. (*3a*) HCMV will enter the cells by endocytosis/macropinocytosis or (*3b*) through direct fusion with the plasma membrane. (*4a*) The endocytosed capsid and tegument (stippled) enters the cytoplasm by gB-mediated fusion of between the viral envelope and the endocytic membrane, possibly requiring low pH for gB-mediated fusion or (*4b*) tegument and capsid are released into the cytoplasm following fusion at the plasma membrane. (*5*) The capsid is translocated by microtubules to the nuclear membrane. (*6*) The capsid interacts with the nuclear pore. (*7*) The genome is translocated into the nucleus where it will associate with ND10. The UL47 and UL48 tegument proteins and SCP facilitate this process. Viral transcription and genome synthesis will begin at ND10s, forming viral replication compartments (detailed in Fig. 12.9). (Adapted from David Johnson, Oregon Health and Science University, Portland, Oregon.)

to heparan sulfate glycosaminoglycans, as is common to many herpesviruses. Heparan sulfate proteoglycans are diverse in structure and expressed on the surface of all cells. gB is synthesized as a 160-kDa precursor that is cleaved by furin in the Golgi body to produce 116-kDa and 55-kDa fragments that remain disulfide linked, and both full-length and cleaved forms are present on infected cells.[67] Soluble gB binds cells with or without heparan sulfate and high concentration of soluble gB blocks HCMV entry. gM/gN is the most abundant glycoprotein complex on virions,[324,640] although with the exception of heparan sulfate binding, a role for this glycoprotein complex during entry has not been observed.[386]

Critical to HCMV entry is the specific binding between cell surface receptors and gH/gL complexes on the virus particle (Fig. 12.6). gH/gL on the virion surface forms complexes with either gO to form the "trimer" or UL128-UL131 to form the "pentamer" entry complexes.[5,115,224,653,654] There is little evidence for the presence of free gH/gL complexes on the virion.[703] gO functions to incorporate gH/gL into the virion envelope[671] and the gH/gL/gO trimer and the gH/gL/UL128-UL131 pentamer form mutually exclusive complexes for entry mediated by disulfide bonds between gL Cys[144] and gO Cys[351] or UL128 Cys[162], respectively.[101,115] The trimer is required for entry into all cell types but is not required for cell-to-cell spread.[671] A approximately 2.8 Å cryo-EM structure of the trimer reveals that gH, gL, and gO interact in a linear orientation to assemble into a boot-like structure.[329] gH/gL has been recently shown to form a complex with gB, although a role for this complex in entry has not been defined.[635] Given the evidence that gH/gL complexes with only a small proportion of gB and only in the pre-fusion conformation, gH/gL may stabilize the pre-fusion conformation of gB until receptor binding triggers fusion.[567]

The gH/gL pentamer contributes to HCMV tropism for epithelial, endothelial, and hematopoietic cells, but is dispensable for entry into fibroblasts.[536,600,653,654] The *UL128-UL131* locus is unstable during passage in fibroblasts and accumulates mutations that restricts viral tropism for endothelial, epithelial, and myeloid cells,[224,431,432,536,654] largely explaining the reticence of these cells to infection by laboratory-adapted virus strains. Additionally, the loss of any one of the these components (UL128, UL130, and UL131A) results in failure to assemble pentamer and compromises replication in epithelial and endothelial cells.[523,535,537,653] 3.0 and 5.9 Å X-ray crystal structures of the pentamer bound to neutralizing antibodies demonstrate that gL forms a three-helix bundle and beta hairpin that acts as a docking site for UL128/UL130/UL131A.[101] Beyond its importance to tropism, the pentamer increases the cell

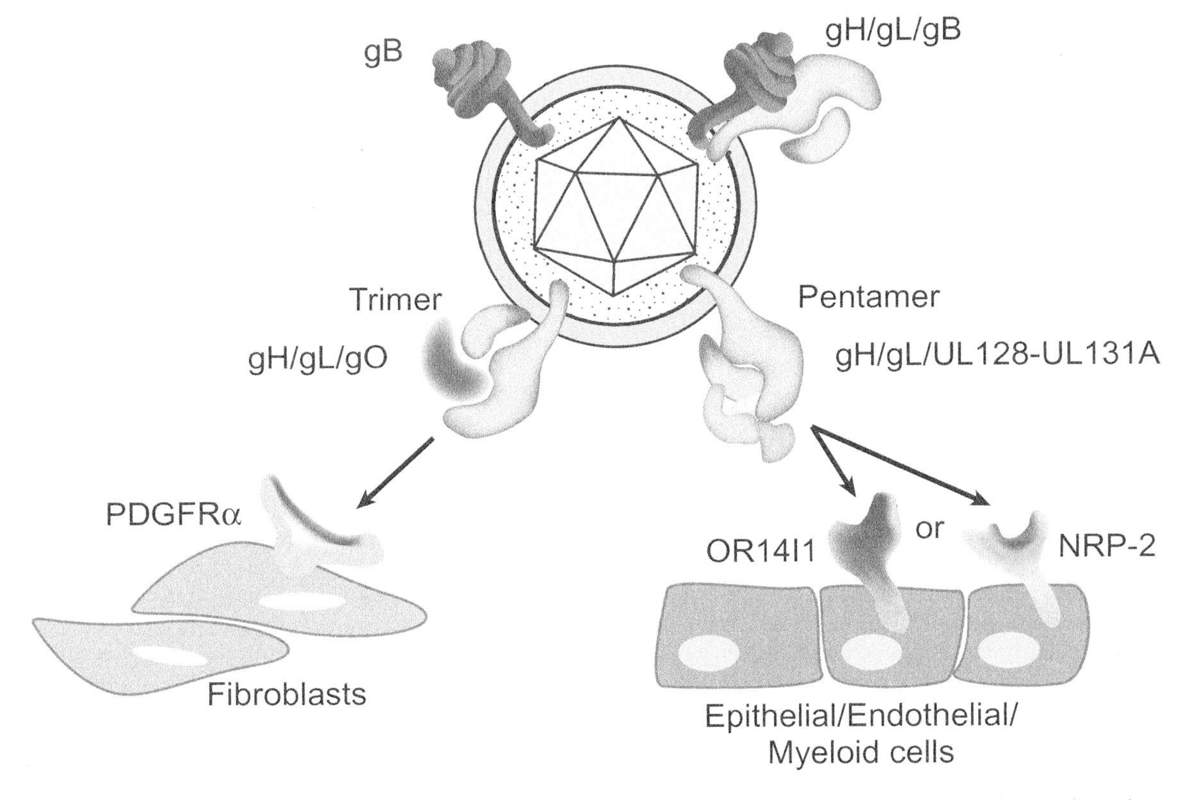

FIGURE 12.6 HCMV glycoproteins and cellular receptors/coreceptors. Glycoprotein B (gB) mediates the initial attachment to cells by binding heparan sulfate. gH and gL form a number of additional complexes that interact with specific receptors to mediate entry into a variety of cell types. gH/gL/gO forms the trimer to mediate entry into fibroblasts through its interaction with PDGFRα. Additional unknown trimer receptors likely exist for entry into epithelial and endothelial cells. gH/gL/UL128/UL130/UL131A forms the pentamer to mediate entry into epithelial, endothelial and hematopoietic cells and interacts with neuropilin-2 (NRP-2) or the OR14I1 coreceptor to mediate entry. Both the trimer and the pentamer likely bind other cellular coreceptors or mediators for entry, perhaps depending on the cell type. A complex gH/gL/gB has recently been discovered, but its role in entry has not been defined. [Courtesy of David Johnson, Oregon Health and Science University, Portland, Oregon.]

association of progeny virus and facilitates cell-to-cell spread.[5] Recent evidence indicates that entry into fibroblasts is mediated via trimer–host receptor interaction and occurs through a rapid form of clathrin-independent, pH-independent macropinocytosis.[243,638] However, entry into epithelial cells, requires the pentamer in addition to the trimer and entry occurs through an abnormal macropinocytosis followed by low pH-dependent fusion at the endosome.[638,654]

The majority of BAC clones of low-passage HCMV strains (the exception being the Merlin strain[703]) express high levels of gH/gL/gO trimer and lower levels of gH/gL/pUL128-UL131A pentamer. The *UL148* gene, encoded within the UL*b*' region typically absent in fibroblast-adapted strains, increases levels of trimer complexes on virions, while not affecting levels of pentamer.[353] UL148 protein dampens ER-associated degradation (ERAD) of gO, possibly through an interaction with SEL1L or other elements of the ER quality control machinery.[441,447] US16 interacts with and facilitates incorporation of pentamer into the virion by unknown mechanisms and its deletion results in a defect in entry into epithelial and endothelial cells.[379]

The ability of the various glycoprotein complexes formed on the HCMV virion to engage with multiple host surface receptors and coreceptors underlies the broad cellular tropism of HCMV. The criteria for establishing a cellular protein as a receptor for CMV entry relies on (a) defining an interaction between the receptor and a virion protein, (b) the ability of antibodies or peptides that interfere with the interaction to block infection, and (c) correlating cellular permissivity to infection with receptor expression. Cellular receptors, coreceptors, or mediators for HCMV entry include platelet-derived growth factors alpha (PDGFRα),[287,399,581,591,679,681] transforming growth factor beta receptor 3 (TGFβR3),[329,398] epidermal growth factor receptor (EGFR),[657,658] integrins,[180,181,657] paxillin,[448] neuropilin-2,[399] and OR14I1.[683] PDGFRα was identified as the cellular receptor for the gH/gL/gO trimer, interacting with gO, to directly mediate entry into fibroblasts,[287,581,591,681] but not epithelial and endothelial cells.[287,591,638] While the ectodomain of PDGFRα is required, its signaling activity is dispensable for entry and spread in fibroblast cultures.[679,681] Indeed, trimer engagement with PDGFRa competes directly with PDGF binding and interferes with PDGFRα signaling.[329] Neuropilin-2 (NRP-2) was identified as a receptor for the HCMV pentamer using a high-throughput avidity-based extracellular interaction screen to define interactions between single pass transmembrane proteins and trimer or pentamer.[399] NRP-2 binds soluble pentamer and silencing of NRP-2 or soluble NRP-2 reduces entry into cells. This study identified a number of other candidates, including TGFβR3, which interacts with the trimer independently of PDGFRα.[329] A CRISPR/cas9 screen identified the multi-pass membrane-associated, olfactory receptor, OR14I1, as a receptor for the pentamer (in addition to NRP-2 and a coreceptor, CD147). OR14I1 and its induction of AC/PK/AKT signaling is required for endocytic entry into epithelial cells; silencing OR14I1 or synthetic N-terminal peptides of OR14I1 reduces entry[683]; however, interaction with the pentameric complex has not been observed.

While strong structural data support PDGFRα/TGFβR3 and NRP-2 as bona fide cellular receptors required for HCMV entry, many other cellular proteins function as coreceptors or mediators of entry. Mediators of HCMV entry promote or enhance entry by a variety of mechanisms, including the clustering or processing of other proteins important to attachment or entry. EGFR facilitates entry,[657,658] and EGFR signaling is important to entry and virus trafficking to the nucleus,[98,303,657] but its role as a receptor remains controversial.[268,638] There is yet no evidence for an interaction between EGFR and HCMV glycoprotein complexes, and no direct interaction with the pentamer has been detected.[287] Integrins α2β, α6β1, and αvβ3 interact with a highly conserved disintegrin domain on gB to mediate entry.[180,181,657] Pentamer-mediated stimulation of EGFR and integrin signaling and their downstream stimulation of paxillin, a regulator of actin rearrangement, is important for entry into monocytes, as well as virus-stimulated motility.[448,449] CD90/Thy-1 interacts with gB and αvβ3 integrins and recruits paxillin, which act as gH-dependent coreceptors.[356,657] CD90/Thy-1 stimulates EGFR and PI3K signaling important for entry, suggesting the EGFR, integrins, paxillin, and CD90/Thy-1 form a signalosome necessary for HCMV entry.[356,657] CD147 is another important mediator of entry that specifically increases pentamer-mediated entry and cell–cell fusion in epithelial and endothelial cells, although soluble CD147 does not block entry and it does not bind pentamer directly.[636] Other factors mediating entry include US16, which mediates efficient viral infection of endothelial and epithelial cells when the pentamer complex is absent.[70] More recently, a novel complex between gH and gpUL116 (gH/UL116) has been reported in the virion that forms independently of gL and does not appear to form a complex with other gH containing complexes (gH/gL/gO; pentamer).[85] From this collective work, it is clear that HCMV enters cells through interactions between viral glycoproteins and constituents of the plasma membrane; however, much remains to be understood about the details of the processes involved in entry.[440,550]

gB functions as a membrane fusogen and is critical for cell-to-cell spread in addition to virus entry.[267,672] gB associates with gH/gL complexes following its synthesis and gH/gL regulates gB-mediated cell–cell fusion.[567,635,637] In the prefusion form, the gB fusion loops are thought to be tucked close to the viral envelope and out of reach of the target membrane. A 3.6 Å resolution crystal structure of gB in its prefusion form reveals a tripod structure where the fusion loops are sequestered In the prefusion form, the gB fusion loops are sequestered by interactions with internal domains of the protein closer to the viral envelope.[372] Two 3.6 Å resolution crystal structures of the postfusion form of the gB ectodomain establish it as a class III viral fusogen, resembling that of HSV-1 and EBV.[80,100] gB is thought to mediate entry by rapid, low pH–independent fusion of the virus at the plasma membrane, at least in fibroblasts. While gB is reported to interact with cellular receptors such as PDGFRα,[581] EGFR,[658] and integrins,[180,181] it is not clear what role, if any, these interactions play in entry given the fusogenic nature of gB.[672] gB may also mediate low pH–dependent fusion events in the endosome for entry of low-passage strains into epithelial and endothelial cells.[536] Most recently, gB-mediated fusion at the plasma membrane of fibroblasts has been shown to be associated with a single amino acid substitution (D275Y), resulting in a highly fusogenic gB variant in the AD169 laboratory strain and activation of caspase 2 and aberrant mitosis.[613] This finding suggests that highly fusogenic properties of laboratory-adapted virus strains may represent an adaptation that arose during passage in cell culture, although this has yet to be investigated.

Intracellular Trafficking and Genome Release

Tegument proteins are released upon entry into the cytoplasm and traffic to sites where they function in modulating the initial host response to infection and modulate transcription of IE genes[34,61] to either initiate or delay virus gene expression to ensure successful infection. As one well-characterized example, pp71 tegument protein targets the host factors that otherwise silence gene expression from the viral genome, including hDaxx[539] and BclAF1.[349] Exogenously expressed pp71 is used experimentally to enhance the infectivity of and replication from transfected viral genomes.[34] This theme is discussed further in section *Pre-IE events and Intrinsic Responses to Infection.*

Cytoplasmic microtubules facilitate translocation of the capsid to the nucleus where viral DNA is released[457] (Fig. 12.5). While genome uncoating and nuclear translocation are poorly defined in CMV infection, the capsid is thought to release viral DNA at the nuclear pore by extrusion of the genome through the same portal composed of UL104 proteins that was employed for packaging.[158] Although few viral proteins have been defined as required for this process, UL47 and UL48 tegument proteins are required for steps following entry at the plasma membrane but preceding IE gene expression.[38] The deubiquitinase activity of UL48 (cleaves K11, K48, and K63 linkages) is autocatalytic regulating its own stability and is important for virion stability such that disruption of *UL48* reduces levels of intracellular genomes following infection.[301,309,655] While the HCMV genome traffics to the nucleus and expresses IE proteins within 30 minutes in infected fibroblasts, the process of nuclear translocation is delayed in hematopoietic cells (≥4 hours in CD34+ progenitor cells and ≥3 days in CD14+ monocytes). In these settings of delayed expression, a distinct early endosome to trans-Golgi network route requires pentamer-induced integrin-Src signaling.[303,304] Upon entry into the nucleus, the linear genome is predicted to circularize by mechanisms that are yet to be investigated for any herpesvirus.

Replicative Program

During a replicative infection *in vitro*, viral genes are expressed in a temporal cascade of three phases: immediate-early, early, and late genes. These phases of gene expression have been classically defined through the use of metabolic inhibitors. Immediate early RNAs can be detected new protein synthesis is inhibited (e.g., cycloheximide) because their expression does not require *de novo* synthesis of viral proteins, whereas all early and late viral gene expression is restricted under such conditions due to the requirement for IE proteins to control activation. Further, late gene expression is blocked by inhibitors of viral DNA synthesis (e.g., phosphonoacetate or phosphonoformate) whereas early gene expression is unaffected. A fourth class of genes includes early-late genes, which accumulate to low levels in the early phase and more robustly at late times, and are partially reduced by inhibitors of viral DNA synthesis. Global analysis of viral protein accumulation indicates greater complexity in the accumulation of viral proteins, with five distinct temporal protein clusters.[660] This analysis reveals HCMV proteins that accumulate with delayed early kinetics (beginning at 24 hpi and peaking at 48 to 72 hpi) and that are either sustained or reduced at later times (72 to 96 hpi), indicating greater complexity in the regulation of viral gene expression than previously characterized.

Pre-IE Events and Intrinsic Responses to Infection

Upon delivery of the viral genome to the nucleus, viral genomes reside at the periphery of the nucleus and colocalize with RNA polymerase II transcription factors, TATA-binding protein, and transcription factor IIB.[270] The viral genome localizes to promyelocytic leukemia (PML) nuclear domains (ND10 or PML bodies), which sequester growth promoting or pathogen restricting factors. ND10-associated proteins serve to cooperatively repress viral transcription[203] and contribute to the silencing of viral gene expression for latency.[143,648] Yet, ND10s serve as sites where nuclear viral RCs initiate.[12,13] Therefore, viruses, including HCMV, target ND10-associated restriction factors, as well as others not associated with ND10, for dispersion or destruction to promote viral gene expression.[616] Host factors restrictive to IE gene expression and the replicative cycle include histone deacetylase 1 (HDAC1),[43] Daxx,[539,540,676] ATRX,[380] IFI16,[136] SPOC1,[514] and SAMHD1.[82,151,302] Tegument protein pp71 (encoded by *UL82*) is a virion transactivator that traffics to the nucleus where it targets the host transcriptional repressor Daxx for proteasomal degradation[89,136,248,539,540,676] and redistributes ATRX,[380] leading to the activation of IE genes. *UL82*-mutant viruses are growth defective at low multiplicities of infection, and this defect is overcome by Daxx knockdown.[61] The importance of pp71 in preventing silencing of viral gene expression is further reflected in that overexpression of *UL82* enhances infectivity of HCMV genomes.[34] In addition to targeting Daxx, pp71 promotes HCMV replication by enhancing transcription from cellular promoters alone or in cooperation with cellular transcription factors.[104,251,366] Another tegument protein, pp65 (encoded by *UL83*) interacts with and targets IFI16 to the major immediate early promoter (MIEP), where it drives IE2 gene expression and limits interferon (IFN) responses.[136] The UL97 serine/threonine-specific kinase is delivered to infected cells as part of the tegument and is expressed *de novo* at approximately 5 hpi.[633] It functions to support replication and maturation and is the kinase that activates ganciclovir.[364] Unique phosphorylation of HDAC1 by UL97 decreases its association with Daxx and the HCMV MIEP sequences to maintain the chromatin around the MIEP in an active conformation for MIE gene expression.[43] Infection with UV-inactivated HCMV, which enters but cannot express viral genes, retains the ability to stimulate SAMHD1 phosphorylation, indicating a role for either UL97 in the viral tegument or a host kinase.[82,302] The UL97 HCMV kinase, as well as other conserved β- and γ-herpesvirus kinases, phosphorylate and inactivate SAMHD1 in primary human fibroblasts and macrophages to unarm this host defense,[82,155,302,698] although cyclin dependent kinase 2 (CDK2) also regulates the phosphorylation of SAMHD1 in HCMV infection.[151] SAMHD1 also is targeted for proteasomal degradation during HCMV infection by a mechanism dependent on Cullin-RING-E3 ligases.[82,262] While some studies have shown an NFκB-dependent, dNTPase-independent SAMHD1-mediated down-regulation of MIE gene expression that may contribute to the establishment of quiescence,[302] other studies find no effects on MIE gene expression[151] and others have shown effects on late gene expression.[262] Taken together, tegument proteins function, at least in part, to reduce cellular restrictions, priming the cell for replication, effectively kickstarting viral gene expression and the productive replication cycle. As viral gene expression begins, the IE proteins, IE1-86 kDa and IE2-72 kDa proteins, both localize to ND10s and

IE1 disrupts ND10 by stimulating proteasome-independent loss of SUMOylated PML.[11,317,685] Other CMV proteins that contribute to ND10 remodeling include US25, UL29/UL30, UL69, UL76, UL98, and TLR9.[543]

HCMV-mediated alteration of cell cycle progression is also important for initiation of productive replication. pp71 and UL69 drives cells infected in G0 or G1 to the G1/S boundary and pp71 blocks their further progression into S phase by targeting the retinoblastoma growth suppressor (pRb) for degradation.[160,291] The UL97 kinase also acts as a viral cyclin-dependent kinase and phosphorylates and inactivates pRb, thereby inducing E2F transactivation.[258] IE2-86 kDa restricts progression into S phase.[668] When HCMV infects cells in S phase, initiation of the replication cycle is delayed until the cell enters G1/G0[187] whereas infection in mitosis results in mitotic catastrophe and an abortive infection.[242,661] A chromatin-tethering domain in a minor variant of IE1, IE1-19 kDa, tethers viral genomes to chromatin either directly or indirectly and is important for maintaining genomes during mitosis when cells are infected during S phase.[384]

The pp150 tegument protein is a substrate of cyclin A2/CDK and its phosphorylation in cyclin A2 expressing cells restricts IE gene expression, representing a mechanism by which the virus has evolved to control the timing of its gene expression.[49] Viral gene expression will initiate as cyclin A2 is degraded when cells enter G1. Much remains to be understood about how tegument proteins and their host interactions control the initial events of infection to impact the commitment to productive replication or alternatively, the establishment of latency.

The HCMV genome associates with host histones upon its translocation to the nucleus. Chromatinization occurs in a nonrandom and predictable manner based on intrinsic DNA sequence, but as infection progresses, nucleosome occupancy drops precipitously in a manner dependent on IE1 gene function.[697] One mechanism by which the IE1-72 kDa protein facilitates virus replication is by antagonizing deacetylation of histones associated with the viral genome and histone deacetylase inhibitors rescue IE-mutant virus replication defects.[439] IE1 was shown to interact with HDAC3, presumably to inhibit its activity.

Regulation of Major Immediate Early Gene Expression

Immediate early genes are expressed in the first few hours of infection, and although they may be enhanced by other viral factors, IE gene expression does not require them. IE gene expression arises from five loci across the HCMV genome: *UL123* (IE1) and *UL122* (IE2), *UL36* and *UL37*, TRS1/IRS1, and *US3*. The MIEP is located between *UL124* and *UL128* and drives the expression of *UL123* and *UL122*. The MIEP is a complex promoter, consisting of an enhancer (−520 to −65 nucleotides, nt), a unique region (−780 to −610 nt), and a modulator (−1,145 to −750 nt) in addition to the core promoter (−65 to +3 nt) (Fig. 12.7). While the promoter is sufficient for transcription of IE genes, the enhancer element increases the rate of transcription. The modulator has context dependent roles, repressive to MIEP activity in undifferentiated cells, but actively drives the MIEP in permissive fibroblasts. The MIEP is initially activated by host transcription factors and gives rise to a common RNA precursor that is alternatively spliced,[125,366,592] which encodes two major phosphoproteins known as IE1-72 kDa and IE2-86 kDa and several minor proteins (Fig. 12.8). IE1-72 kDa is encoded by exons 1 to 4, and IE2-86 kDa is produced by an exon skipping event and is encoded by exons 1 to 3 and 5. Preferential splicing results in early accumulation of IE1, which switches at later times to favor IE2.[362,456,546] The host cyclin A2 and ubiquitin-dependent segregase VCP/p97 differentially regulates alternative splicing of IE2.[362,456] Other splice variants including portions of

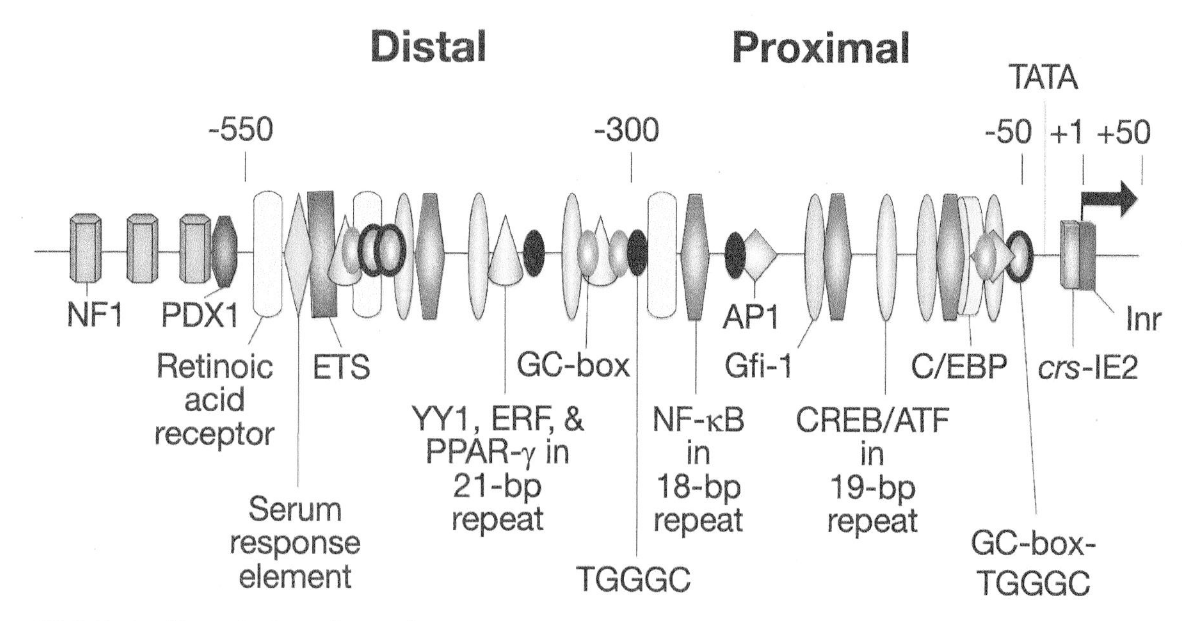

FIGURE 12.7 **The major immediate early promoter.** The major immediate early promoter (MIEP) consists of the core promoter (−65 to +3 nt), enhancer (−520 to −65 nt), unique region (−780 to −610 nt), and modulator (−1,145 to −750). The schematic diagrams the distal and proximal promoter/enhancer and the relative locations of binging sites for both activating and repressing transcription factors. (Courtesy of Jeffery Meier, University of Iowa, Iowa City, Iowa.)

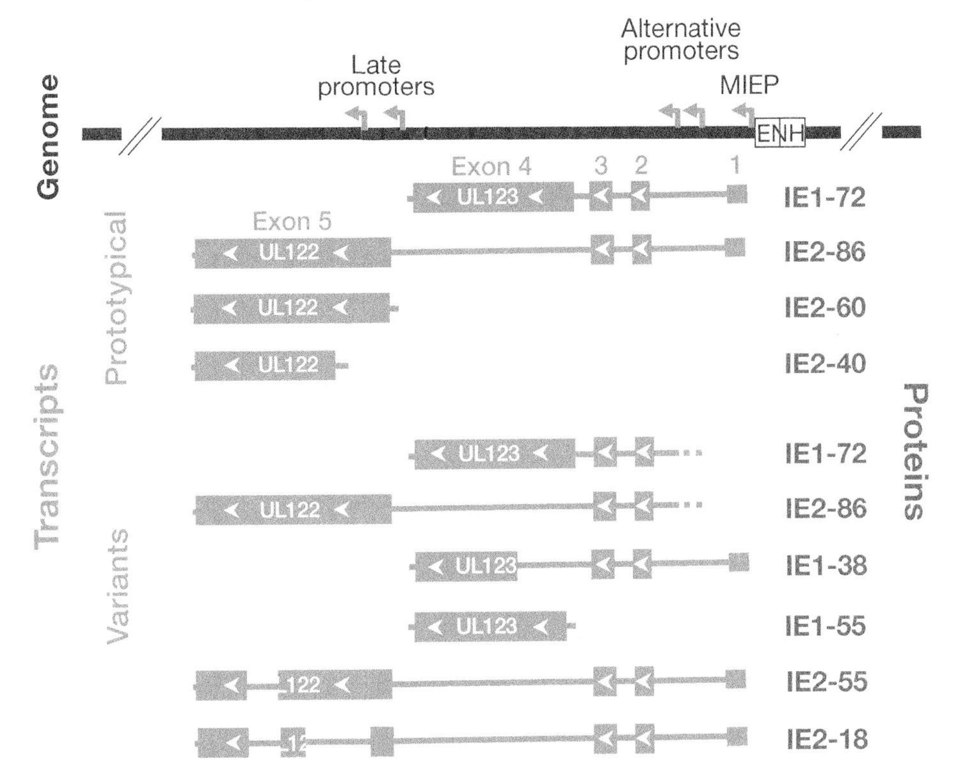

FIGURE 12.8 Transcripts and proteins originating from the major immediate early transcription unit. The major immediate transcription unit gives rise to ten distinct transcripts through alternative splicing and alternative transcription initiation site usage. The primary transactivators for virus replication and most well studied are the IE1-72 kDa and IE2-86 kDa proteins. Roles for other IE gene products have yet to be fully defined. (Courtesy of Jeffery Meier, University of Iowa, Iowa City, Iowa.)

exon 4 (IE1) or exon 5 (IE2) identified include: IE1-9 kDa, IE1-17.5 kDa, IE1-19 kDa, IE2-18 kDa, and IE2-55 kDa.[30,564,592] The MIEP is negatively regulated by the 14-basepair palindromic cis repression site at −13 to −1 relative to the MIEP transcriptional start site.[110] The strength of the MIEP in driving gene expression is best demonstrated by its broad use in driving transgene expression in viral and plasmid vectors.

The MIEP-enhancer regulatory region is composed of a dense assembly of transcription factor binding sites (Fig. 12.7), indicative of its complex landscape of regulation. The regulatory region extends beyond the region required to regulate IE gene expression, suggesting an additional role in persistence or latency. MIEP-driven transcription is strongly regulated by host factors that bind to the modulator (e.g., ETS-1 repressive factor, ERF, and YY1), unique (e.g., nuclear factor 1), and enhancer regions (e.g., NFκB/rel, CREB/ATF, Sp-1, retinoic acid, AP1, serum response factor (SRF)/Elk, and γ-IFN activating sequence (GAS) as reviewed.[125] The enhancer region also contains sequences for binding repressive YY1 and methylated DNA-binding protein (MDBP). Further, SPOC1 (also known as PHF13) is a regulator of chromatin structure induced by infection that binds to the MIEP, that recruits heterochromatin promoting factors, such as KAP1 and histone 3 lysine 9 methyltransferases to suppress expression and replication.[514] The MIEP is also regulated by viral proteins, including TRS1, UL83, pp71, IE1-72 kDa, and IE2-86 kDa.[61,89]

At late times in infection (coincident with or following viral genome synthesis), IE2-86 kDA along with intermediate and late IE2 gene products bind to a cis repression site (crs) within the MIEP and represses its activity through a self-cooperative transcriptional negative-feedback loop.[110,365,387,483,618] While this autoregulation does not prevent basal transcription factors from binding the MIEP, RNA polymerase II recruitment to the MIEP is reduced. Repression of the MIEP at late times is also mediated by recruitment of deacetylases and methyltransferases that silence the promoter.[348,507] Following DNA synthesis and cis-repression of the MIEP, transcripts driven from alternative promoters within intron A of the MIE locus accumulate to support a second phase of IE1-72 kDa and IE2-86 kDa protein synthesis.[26,129] Transcripts initiating from these intronic promoters differ in their 5′ untranslated region but support the synthesis of full length IE1-72 kDa and IE2-86 kDa proteins because exon 1 of the MIE locus is noncoding. CTCF binding within intron A of the MIE locus negatively regulates MIE gene expression.[398] The 5′ UTR of MIE transcripts have been shown to be a critical determinant of IE protein accumulation and may allow for context-dependent regulation of IE protein translation.[25]

Immediate Early Proteins

IE1-72 kDa activates transcription and regulates intrinsic and innate responses to infection. IE1-72 kDa is required for replication at lower multiplicities of infection and its role as a transcriptional activator was first appreciated through its ability to stimulate its own promoter, through its association with host transcription factors, and its sequestration of histone deacetylases.[127,439] IE1-72 kDa also indirectly affects gene expression as IE1-72 kDa stimulates expression of LUNA latency antigen not through direct interaction with the LUNA promoter, but rather through blocking Daxx-mediated suppression of LUNA.[509] Further, IE1-72 kDa binds condensed chromatin through a chromatin tethering domain and interacts with histones H2A and H2B,[175] inhibiting the deposition of histones onto the viral genome,[439,697] although this role is dispensable during replication in fibroblasts. Related to its ability to maintain active chromatin, IE1-72 kDa disrupts ND10s to antagonize intrinsic antiviral defenses and genome silencing.[10,346,670] PML-mediated sumoylation of IE1-72 kDa[522,585] functions to sustain accumulation of IE2-86 kDa to promote viral gene expression and replication.[438,639] While IE1 does not stimulate the turnover of PML like HSV-1 ICP0, it inhibits the sumoylation of PML to inhibit a type I IFN response, and induces the ubiquitination of Sp100, another ND10 component.[308,371] In addition to SP100, the ubiquitination of HES1, a neural progenitor cell regulator of Notch signaling, is stimulated by IE1-72 kDa.[371] The acidic domain of IE1 is required to down-regulate the IFN response to viral infection.[320,475] While IE1 does not disrupt the transcription of IFN, it associates with STAT1 and 2 transcription factors to inhibit the IFN-stimulated gene factor 3 complex (ISGF3: STAT1, STAT2, and IRF9) from binding DNA and inducing a JAK/STAT-mediated IFN response.[256,320] IE1-72 kDa also binds to and traps STAT3 in the nucleus and represses IL6-induced/STAT3-responsive gene expression, which rewires IL6 signaling to downstream proinflammatory IFNγ-like signaling (repressing STAT3 and activating STAT1) and tempers HCMV replication.[239,313,516]

IE2-86 kDa is a potent transcription factor that stimulates activation of viral and host promoters. IE2-86 kDa regulates viral gene expression and productive infection.[163,393,690] In addition to its role in directly transactivating the MIEP, the IE2-86 kDa protein interacts with p300/CBP associated factor (P/CAF),[72] HDAC1, and some methyltransferase,[507] suggesting a mechanism by which HCMV differentially regulates acetylation of histone tails associated with the MIEP depending on the timing in infection. Further, IE2 may indirectly facilitate E2F-mediated activation of the MIEP through its interaction with and inhibition of the retinoblastoma protein (pRB).[223] By contrast to its role as a transactivator, IE2-86 kDa represses the transcription and induces the degradation of immature interleukin 1β (IL-1β) following activation of the AIM2 inflammasome.[56] Importantly, at later points in infection, homomultimers (6 to 8 monomers) of IE2-86 kDa bind to the cis-repression element in the MIEP to repress its own expression, and this negative feedback contributes to localization of incoming viral genomes to ND10s, transcriptional strength, and viral fitness.[199,618] During early and late phases of infection, IE2 p60 and p40 variants are expressed and repress IE gene expression.[30]

The complexity of MIE locus structure and transcription through the MIE region is just one example of the complexity of transcription across the genome that includes differential transcriptional starts, exon skipping, alternative splicing, and differential polyadenylation. Despite decades of intense work on the MIEP and MIE gene products, more remains to be learned about how IE proteins impact early gene expression and the role of IE1 and IE2 protein variants and context-dependent regulation of transcription and translation.

US3, *UL36-38*, and *TRS1/IRS1*, expressed with IE kinetics, are critical for viral gene expression and regulate key host responses to infection. Similar to IE2, *US3* expression is regulated by *crs* upstream of its transcriptional start.[99,339] US3 post-ranslationally impedes the trafficking and peptide loading of MHCI to evade cytotoxic T-cell activation.[14,285,469] While CMV encodes a number of related proteins to disrupt MHC–peptide presentation, *US3* is the first expressed. UL37 exon 1 (UL37x1, also known as vMIA) potently inhibits mitochondrial-mediated cell death by sequestering Bax and Bak in the outer mitochondrial membrane to prevent cytochrome *c* release.[204] *UL36* is a *US22* family member and also inhibits cell death by blocking caspase 8 activation initially observed in macrophages.[405] IRS1 and TRS1 are highly homologous *US22* family members with identical amino termini and unique carboxy termini that share 50% identity. Both TRS1 and IRS1 inhibit the IFN-based induction of protein kinase R (PKR), and both are required for virus replication.[112,397,405] The proteins encoded by IRS1 and TRS1 both contain RNA binding domains in their amino termini and PKR binding domains in their carboxy termini.[226,227] TRS1 stimulates translation of transcripts, particularly those with HCMV 5′ UTRs, prevents stress granule formation resulting from PKR-mediated phosphorylation of eIF2α.[705] Independent of its role in inhibiting PKR-mediated phosphorylation of eIF2α, TRS1 blocks macroautophagy through an interaction with Beclin1 with the amino terminal end of TRS1.[105] Without the modulation of these host responses during IE times, infection would be terminated.

Early/Delayed Early Genes

Following peak expression of IE genes between 8 and 12 hpi, delayed early or early genes are transcriptionally activated. Most of the 65 early phase proteins and miRNAs (Supplementary e-Tables 12.1 and 12.2) accumulate gradually until the onset of viral DNA synthesis. Early genes have important roles in the regulation of IE and late transcription, the synthesis of viral genomes, encapsidation of viral genomes, the regulation of the cell cycle, and the evasion of adaptive immune responses. Many early proteins, as well as IE proteins, localize to nuclear RCs where viral DNA and RNA accumulates as both are synthesized. Disruption of early genes typically results significant defects DNA synthesis, late gene expression, and virus production.[163,690]

The promoter region of three early genes, *UL112-113*, *UL54* (DNA polymerase), and *UL4* illustrate the complexity of HCMV transcriptional control and provide insight into the dependence of early gene expression on IE gene expression as well as the differential regulation of gene expression by host and viral functions as infection proceeds. *UL112-113* transcripts[666] are detected beginning at 8 hpi and remain constant through late times. The transcripts are differentially spliced to yield four unique proteins (pp34, pp43, pp50, pp84). At late times, the transcriptional start sites are altered but the mRNA splicing pattern and polyadenylation remain the same throughout infection. The UL112-113 pp84 isoform is proposed to interact with and target the UL44 DNA processivity factor to RCs and the oriLyt for viral DNA synthesis.[307,310,470,555] Promoter-proximal ATF/CREB and IE2-86 kDa binding sites are important for sustained transcription of *UL112-113*, but most important during late times of infection.[337,529] The HCMV DNA polymerase, UL54, is also detected by 8 hpi and continues through late times of infection, relying on a single transcriptional start but two polyadenylation sites. Host transcription factors regulated by IE2-86 kDa control expression of *UL54*. *UL4* encodes a minor virion glycoprotein (gp48) that is transcribed early and continues late and is dependent on Elk1 and IE2-86 kDa binding to its promoter and the TATA element is stimulated by MAPK signaling.[107,108] *UL4* expression is regulated at the translational level by a short 22 amino acid upstream ORF, uORF2, within the *UL4* leader sequence[16] that induces ribosome stalling.[41,538,673] Much remains to be understood about the cellular and viral factors controlling early gene activation, transcriptional start site selection and switching, and protein isoforms.

Early gene products regulate viral gene expression broadly. *UL34* is encoded by transcripts with alternate transcriptional start sites that result in two proteins that differ by 21 amino terminal amino acids. The UL34 proteins localize to RCs, bind multiple sites across the HCMV genome, and are required broadly for viral gene expression and viral replication.[503] UL34 represses some genes, including *US3* and *US9* expression, acting on a novel cis repression site.[352,373] UL21A enhances viral genome synthesis and the expression of IE genes in the later phases of infection necessary for maximal virus replication.[179] The UL21A protein interacts with the multiple subunits of the anaphase promoting complex (APC) E3 ubiquitin ligase and with cyclin A2, resulting in its proteasomal degradation.[83,117,170] This may function to relieve the early restrictions imposed on viral gene expression by cyclin A2 in S/G2 cells.[49] Targeting cyclin A2 and APC neutralizes the cyclin A2 restriction to virus replication and halts cell cycle progression in infected cells into or through mitosis. UL21a–cyclin A2 interaction is important for viral genome synthesis and maintaining chromosome stability in infected cells.[170] Further, UL38 and UL28-29 proteins interact with protein complexes containing histone deacetylate 1 (HDAC1) and recruit the nucleosome remodeling and deacetylase complex (NuRD) to maintain derepression of MIE gene expression throughout infection.[417,619] These examples highlight examples of early genes targeting host pathways to ensure viral gene expression and successful viral genome synthesis.

UL97, a serine/threonine kinase, is the only conventional protein kinase encoded by HCMV. Defining a kinase and its physiologically relevant substrates requires demonstrating that the purified kinase is sufficient to phosphorylate the substrate *in vitro* on specific residues and that the phosphorylation matters by mutation of phosphorylation sites or phenotype due to loss of the kinase. It is important at all stages of viral gene expression and replication and, as such, is a major target for antiviral drug development. Depending on the state of the cells, mutational or pharmacological inactivation of the kinase results in a minimal or as much as a tenfold reduction in viral genome accumulation and an approximately 10- to 1,000-fold reduction in virus progeny yield, with defects beginning prior to viral genome synthesis and extending through late phase virion maturation.[46,326,498,515,675] The loss of UL97 results in a more severe replication defect during infection with low-passage strains that contain the ULb' region of the genome, and specifically *UL135*, compared to laboratory-adapted strains.[354,652] UL97 has a number of cellular substrates including histone deacetylate 1 (HDAC1), the retinoblastoma tumor suppressor (pRb), elongation factor delta, and lamin A/C.[43,229,258,296,414,497] Tegument-derived UL97-mediated phosphorylation of HDAC1 is important to maintain the MIEP in a de-repressed state for optimal IE gene expression.[43] UL97 phosphorylation of viral proteins inhibits the aggregation of PML nuclear bodies.[326,333,493,497,625] UL97 is a functional orthologue of human cyclin dependent kinases (CDKs) with overlapping contributions to infection.[242] Like CDK1, UL97 phosphorylation and inactivation of growth suppressor, pRB, and the related proteins, p107 and p130, activates E2F-responsive genes to stimulate the cell cycle. However, unlike CDK1, UL97 is not susceptible to p21 inhibition.[258,273] The role of UL97 in activating E2F transcription of cellular genes, late viral genes, and in viral genome synthesis can be complemented by the human papilloma virus E7 oncoprotein,[293] indicating conservation in the importance of modulating these host pathways for DNA virus infection. UL97 promotes KAT5/Tip60 histone acetyltransferase (HAT) phosphorylation to increase expression, while UL27 inhibits KAT5/Tip60 HAT to decrease expression of CDKs.[517] This dual pronged regulation indicates to importance of regulating CDK activity during infection. Further, the putative processivity factor, UL44, is heavily phosphorylated by UL97 and cellular kinases (candidates include CDK1 and CK2).[327] The role of UL97 phosphorylation of UL44 is not clear, but phosphorylation by host kinases near its nuclear localization signal is critical for viral DNA synthesis and replication.[568] Finally, UL97 phosphorylation of the nuclear lamina component, lamin A/C, promotes disassembly of the nuclear lamina and thus nuclear egress of newly formed capsids. How this happens is a subject of debate where one group finds the viral nuclear egress complex (NEC) recruits UL97 for this purpose and that dominant negative laminA/C can complement the loss of UL97,[561,562] while another group reports that lamin-associated protein p32 recruits UL97.[229] UL97 is also important for formation of the cytoplasmic viral assembly compartment and infectious virus particle maturation.[31]

HCMV encodes polyadenylated long RNAs, RNA2.7, RNA1.2, RNA4.9, and RNA5.0 (number indicating length in kilobases) transcripts that are expressed early and dominate the HCMV transcriptome, but have poorly ascribed functions. While these have been thought to be noncoding, RNA2.7, RNA1.2, and RNA4.9 are detected on polyribosomes, protein products from these RNAs have been confirmed and are proteins are recognized as antigens in humans based on CD4 and CD8 responses.[265,597] The β2.7 RNA stabilizes mitochondrial membrane potential through its interaction with mitochondrial enzyme complex 1 to prevent apoptosis.[512] The 4.9-kb RNA localizes to nuclear RCs, forming an RNA–DNA hybrid at the origin of lytic replication (*oriLyt*). RNA4.9 transcription or the RNA–DNA hybrid formation stimulate viral genome synthesis, perhaps by stimulating *oriLyt* unwinding.[611] RNA4.9 has also been shown to interact with the viral genome and the polycomb repressive complex 2 (PRC2),[533] and may regulate gene expression for latency.

DNA Synthesis

HCMV DNA synthesis occurs in the nucleus of infected fibroblasts, starting at 14 to 16 hours post infection *in vitro*. Upon delivery to the nucleus, the linear double-stranded genome circularizes and localizes to PML bodies or ND10s by unknown mechanisms.[12,13] These sites constitute prereplication foci where viral transcription and genome synthesis are initiated to form RCs. The formation of RCs depends on polarization of the inner nuclear membrane SUN1 proteins to reorganize actin filaments to spatially segregate viral DNA from inactive histones and host DNA.[500] As discussed further below, the compartmentalization and the concentration of viral and cellular DNA synthesis, transcription, and RNA processing factors at RCs are important for efficient *de novo* synthesis of viral genomes.

Initiation of HCMV genome replication occurs from a complex, bidirectional *oriLyt* encompassing at least 1,500 bp between *UL57* and *UL69* genes, an origin of replication considerably larger and more complex than other beta-herpesviruses and other herpesviruses.[466] In contrast to α- and β-herpesvirus genomes, HCMV contains only one *oriLyt* since deletion of minimal or complete *oriLyt* sequences abolishes virus replication.[55] The *oriLyt* can be divided into essential region I containing a bidirectional UL84-IE2-86 kDa-responsive promoter and a pyridine-rich Y block and essential region II containing a RNA-DNA hybrid (R loop) formed via G-C rich DNA. When R loops interact with UL84, IE2 and/or UL112-113 gene products, initiation of DNA replication proceeds.[122,290,305] UL34 protein binds to the *oriLyt* to facilitate replication protentially through interactions with IE2-86 kDa, UL44, and UL84.[574]

The core replication fork is composed of six proteins conserved among herpesviruses, the DNA polymerase (UL54), the DNA processivity factor (UL44), a single stranded DNA binding protein (UL57), and the heterotrimeric helicase–primase complex (UL105, UL102, UL70) (Fig. 12.9). Additional proteins, including UL36-38, IRS1/TRS1, and IE1/2, UL84, and UL112-113 regulate *oriLyt* activity.[467,549] CMV lacks an origin-binding protein with enzymatic activity such as found in α-herpesviruses or in γ-herpevirsues (latent origin), and likely initiates productive DAN replication in a manner similar to gammaherpesvirus oriLyt. UL84 is expressed early and multimers of the UL84 protein binds IE2-86 kDa protein through leucine zipper motifs.[123] The UL84-IE2 interaction is only important for *oriLyt*-dependent DNA replication in certain viral strains[123] and antagonizes IE2 transactivating activity, but not *crs* functions.[199] However, UL84 is not essential in all HCMV strains, and differences in IE2 or other viral functions compensate and function in its place.[583] The UL112-113 gene expresses four phosphoproteins p34, p43, p50, and p84, which are all expressed early and accumulate at nuclear RCs. While p34 and p50 are dispensable for replication, p43 and p84 isoforms are required for replication[555] and the interaction between p84 and UL54 and UL44 proteins is specifically required for genome replication.[307] UL114 interacts with UL54–UL44 complex and is important for maintaining genome integrity, excising uracil that is misincorporated into the genome or that results from spontaneous deamination of cytosine,[494] and it is important for late phase amplification of viral genomes.[132]

A growing list of host transcription factors, DNA damage factors, and other regulators are known to be relocalized to viral RCs during virus replication to regulate genome synthesis and gene expression. The C-EBPα transcription factor localizes to RCs through its interaction with UL84.[289] The nucleolar host protein nucleolin associates with UL44, and this interaction is required for the localization of UL84 and UL44 within nuclear RCs.[39,599] Some DNA damage factors, including γH2AX and ATM, are recruited to RCs where they may contribute to replication.[381,684] The altered localization of p53 and DNA damage response factors may facilitate replication, recombination or repair of viral genomes at the expense of the host genome.[188,454,684] While much remains to be understood about the presence of these host factors in RCs, virus replication is compromised in ataxia telangiectasia-mutated (ATM) protein kinase–deficient cells due to the failure to up-regulate γH2AX-mediated stabilization of the MRE11–RAD50–NSB1 (MRN) complex.[684]

Components of the ubiquitin proteasome systems assemble into domains at the periphery of HCMV RCs and ongoing proteasome activity is required for viral gene expression, particularly in early and late phases of infection.[188] Further, UL35 associates with the ubiquitin-specific protease (USP) 7 and components of the Cullin 4A (DCAF1, DDB1, and DDA1) E3 ubiquitin ligase complex, localizing these proteins to nuclear foci.[542] Together, with tegument-derived pp71 (UL82), UL35 directs the degradation of BclAF1, which restricts HCMV gene expression and replication. UL35 also induces γH2AX and p53 binding protein 1 (53BP1) foci, suggesting activation of a DNA damage response, and activates a G2 cell cycle checkpoint.[542] UL76 recruits and concentrates the polyubiquitinated protein receptor S5a by binding its von Willebrand factory type A domain and K48- and K63-linked polyubiquitinated proteins in nuclear foci juxtaposed with RCs, which is important for the formation of the RCs and the ubiquitin proteasomal factor aggresome.[361] Together these findings indicate the importance of host processes in viral genome synthesis and RNA processing that have yet to be fully understood.

UL44 stably associates with the C-terminus of the viral DNA polymerase UL54 and stimulates its activity in a DNA-dependent, sequence-independent manner, similar to the role of cellular processivity factor PCNA or the processivity factors encoded by other herpesviruses.[22,376,377] UL44 forms a C clamp–shaped dimer that binds DNA and is important for *oriLyt*-dependent replication, which represents a mechanism distinct from both the trimeric PCNA ring and the monomeric HSV UL42 processivity factor.[23,314,570] UL44 is phosphorylated by UL97, CDK1/cyclin B, CK1, and CK2 to generate a number of phosphorylated isoforms.[17,18,568] Substitution of UL97-phosphorylation sites on UL44, remarkably, does not reduce the efficiency of viral DNA synthesis in fibroblasts. C-terminal sequences containing a nuclear localization signal and CK2 phosphorylation sites are critical for UL44 interaction with importin α/β and nuclear import of UL44.[17] Intriguingly, a role for UL44 in suppressing IRF3 and NF-κB transcription suggests links between DNA replication and repair and the innate immune response.[195]

Herpesvirus DNA synthesis is thought to start as a theta form before switching to rolling circle. The mode of HCMV genome replication is largely inferred because the structure is consistent with head-to-tail concatemeric genomes thought to be produced by rolling circle during HSV replication. Genomes will accumulate to several thousand genome copies per cell by the time progeny is released from fibroblasts.[466,626] In epithelial and astrocytoma cells, replication is more subdued and viral genome levels do not exceed 1,000 copies per cell. In cells supporting high levels of replication, the accumulation of

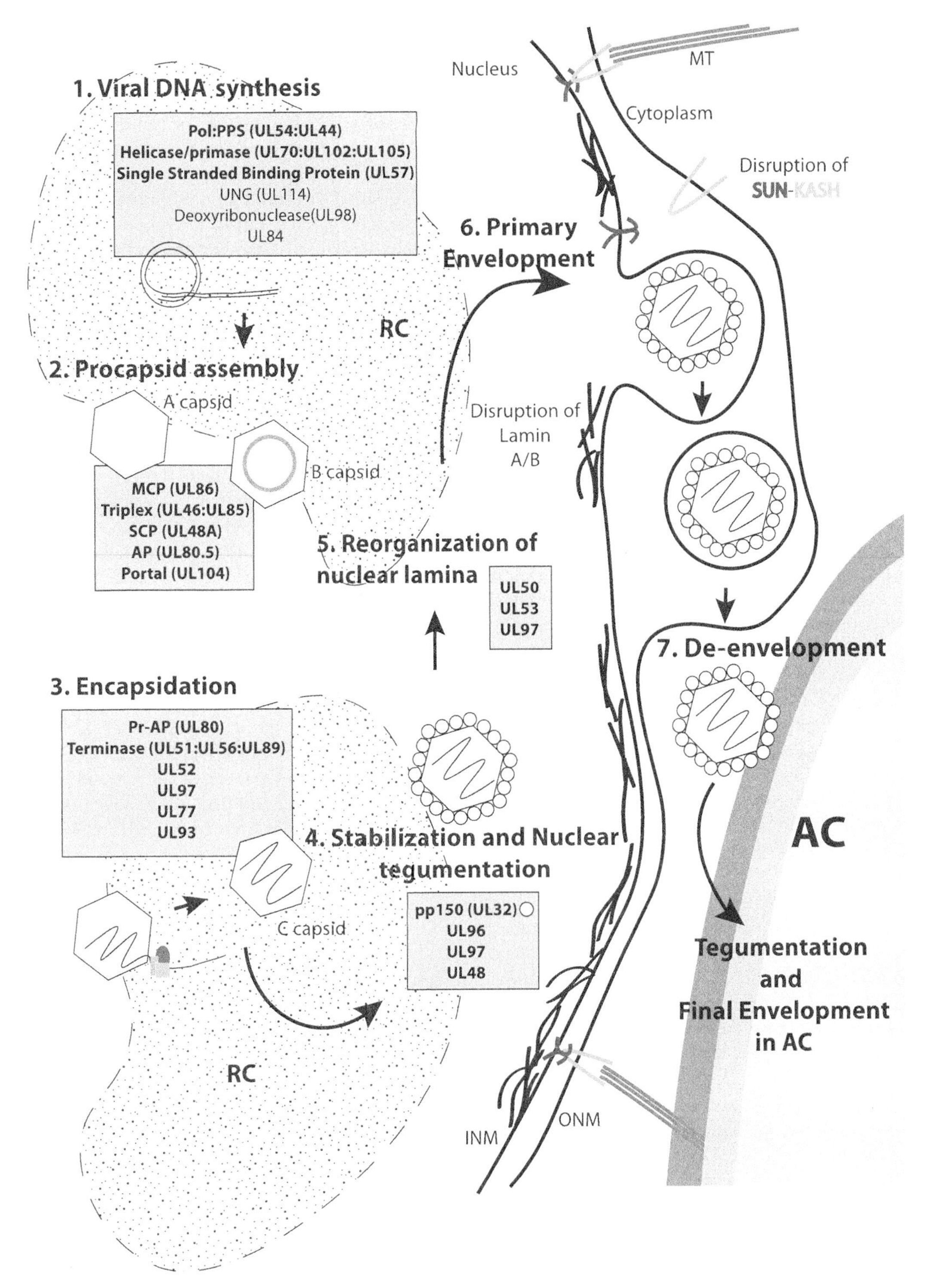

FIGURE 12.9 **Schematic of viral genome replication to nucleocapsid nuclear egress.** (*1*) The 230-kb ds-DNA genome is synthesized in viral replication compartments (RC, *stippled areas*) by a rolling circle mechanism. Six proteins make up the core replication machinery, including the DNA polymerase (Pol, UL54), the putative DNA processivity factor (PPS, UL44), the helicase/primase complex (UL70, UL102, UL105), and the single stranded DNA-binding protein (UL57). Other proteins important to genome synthesis includes the uracil–DNA deglycosylase (UNG, UL114), the deoxyribonuclease (UL98), and pUL84 (function unknown). (*2*) Procapsid assembly requires the MCP, the Triplex, SCP (UL48A), pAP (UL80.5), and the portal protein (UL104). From these proteins, A and B type capsids are formed. (*3*) Encapsidation of genome length viral DNA results in the formation of C type capsids and requires the maturational protease (Pr-AP), the terminase complex (UL51, UL56, and UL89) and UL52 (supports the terminase, required for concatemer cleavage). Other proteins important to encapsidation include UL97 (viral protein kinase) and UL77 and UL93 (links capsid triplex and terminase). (*4*) Nucleocapsids acquire pp150 tegument in the nucleus, which functions to stabilize the nucleocapsid with UL96 and UL48 (*5*) The nuclear egress complex composed of UL50 and UL53 proteins, which recruit the UL97 viral kinase to activate UL50 and UL53 and phosphorylate lamin A/B for breakdown. (*6*) Capsids egress out of the nucleus by budding through the inner nuclear membrane (INM) into the perinuclear space and then (*7*) de-envelop and enter the cytoplasm through fusion with the outer nuclear membrane (ONM). Egress of nucleocapsids into the perinuclear space requires the dissociation of SUN and KASH proteins, which tether the INM and ONM to the cytoskeleton/microtubules (MT). Once in the cytoplasm, virion maturation will continue through the viral assembly compartment (detailed in Fig. 12.12).

viral genomes may ultimately result in several compartments coalescing to a single compartment that fills the nucleus.[598,599]

Late Genes

Late gene expression is maximal after the onset of viral DNA replication, and this class of genes is largely comprised of genes with structural roles in virion assembly and maturation. For example, all capsid proteins are encoded by late genes, and their expression is inhibited if viral DNA synthesis is blocked. By contrast, while many tegument proteins are encoded by genes expressed with late kinetics, about half of the tegument-encoding genes are expressed with immediate-early, early, or early-late kinetics, suggesting nonstructural roles.[660] Expression of early-late or leaky late subsets of late genes are those that are expressed prior to the onset or without requirement for the onset of viral DNA synthesis, but that may not achieve maximal expression until after the onset of viral DNA synthesis. Late genes are controlled by simple promoters defined by regions surrounding the TATA or TATT motif, although some have multiple transcriptional start sites. Late mRNAs conserved among β- and γ-herpesviruses are spliced and arise from symmetric transcription from both DNA strands.[198]

HCMV encodes six viral transcription factors, *UL49, UL79, UL87* (viral TATA-binding protein, preferring TATT), *UL91, UL92*, and *UL95*, that are essential for late phase expression of *UL44* and other true late genes.[272,458,459,480] For example, transcription of true late genes requires UL92 function, which is conserved with γ-herpesviruses, but strikingly different from that of α-herpesviruses.[459] UL79 interacts with host RNA polymerase II, UL87, and UL95, as well as components of the DNA replication complex and stimulates RNA pol II processivity and prevents stalling on the viral genomes.[479] Further, IE2 strengthens the expression of 16 early-late or late genes, including *UL83* and *UL146*, by increasing RNA polymerase II initiation of transcription independent of TATT sequences or the late viral transcription factors.[355]

The late viral transcription factors also stimulate expression of separate promoters controlling IE2-60 kDa and IE2-40 kDa at late times in infection. IE2-40 kDa synergizes with IE2-86 kDa in transactivation of early and late promoters, and both recognize the cis repression signal (crs) of the MIEP.[548,665] The roles of MIE variants (Fig. 12.8) in contexts beyond productive infection in fibroblasts have been less thoroughly investigated.

Capsid Assembly, DNA Encapsidation, and Nuclear Egress

The process of capsid formation, encapsidation of DNA and virus maturation is conserved across herpesviruses.[202] As an overview, three HCMV capsid forms accumulate in the nucleus, denoted as A, B, and C capsids (Figs. 12.9 and 12.11). A-type capsids lack scaffold and viral DNA. B-type capsids contain the scaffold of UL80 proteins but lack viral DNA. Both A and B capsids are thought to be terminal structures, although B capsids may be enveloped as NIEPs. C capsids have both scaffold and DNA and represent true nucleocapsids assumed to be in the process of maturing. The capsid is composed of MCP, MnCP/TRI1, MnCBP/TRI2, SCP, and the portal protein. Proteins of the capsid are organized into 162 capsomers (150 hexamers plus 12 pentamers) and 320 triplexes located between capsomers (discussed in detail, see Virion Structure). Capsomers are composed of six copies of the MCP per hexon and five copies of the MnCP per penton. Hexons and pentons associate in the cytoplasm before being transported into the nucleus to assemble into capsids (Fig. 12.10). One of the 12 pentons in each capsid is composed of entirely of portal protein, which self-assembles into a homododecamer complex for controlling viral DNA encapsidation.[249] SCP is present as 1 molecule attached to the tip of each MCP of the hexon and penton.[144,692]

UL80 encodes four in-frame, carboxy co-terminal proteins: the UL80a encodes the protease precursor (pPR, 74-kDa), UL80.5, the assembly protein precursor (pAP, 38-kDa), as well as two additional proteins. The process of capsid maturation begins when the MCP associates with protease precursor complex (pPR-pAP:pAP) and is transported into the nucleus where proteolytic processing results in assembly of procapsid shells (Fig. 12.10).[202,378,442] SCP interacts with MCP and presumably translocates to the nucleus with MCP/pPR/pAP.[335,692] Heterotrimeric complexes between the two dimer-forming TRI2 conformers of the MnCP and one TRI1 protein assemble in the cytoplasm and are translocated to the nucleus (Fig. 12.10).[202] Where the triplex stabilizes hexons and pentons, completing the capsid floor between capsomers.[692]

Capsid assembly is coordinated by the pAP, and the pPR, PR, self-cleaves to produce pAP (Fig. 12.9). Precise protease cleavage steps releases MCP, inactivates the protease, and orchestrates the replacement of the scaffold in procapsids with viral DNA. PR, AP, and pAP are removed from nucleocapsids into which DNA has been packaged. Properly formed capsids (C capsids) mature more efficiently than defective nucleocapsids, such as the NIEPs lacking DNA.

Encapsidation of unit length genomes depends on the terminase proteins, encoded by UL51, UL56 (encoding TER2), and UL89 (encoding TER1) and interactions with the portal protein complex.[622,623] The terminase is a target for the antiviral drug letermovir.[206,357] The portal protein forms a multimeric ring thought to consist of a self-generated dodecameric oligomer for entry of the DNA into the capsid.[249] Terminase machinery (the ATPase encoded by UL56 and the nuclease encoded by UL89) recognizes free genomic ends, cleaves viral genomes at the portal leaving a single-base 3′ extensions at both genomic ends, and powers a single genome length of DNA through the portal and into the capsid by ATP hydrolysis.[260,623] A 129-bp region contains both cis-acting, AT-rich *pac* elements, which are sufficient for cleavage and packaging.[656] UL89 encodes a curvilinear monomer with single amino acids known to be important for DNA binding (R544) and nuclease (D463) activity through mutagenesis.[621] The portal protein interacts with the UL56 protein subunit of the terminase complex, linking the production of unit-length genomes with packaging.[159] The terminase complex dissociates after cleavage and is not part of the mature virion. UL93 and UL77 proteins associate with capsids and have roles in retaining viral DNA in the nucleocapsid.[54,316]

Tegumentation begins with association of SCP on hexons and pentons with pp150 in the nucleus.[692] As intact C capsids cannot be isolated from the nuclei of infected cells, the net-like pp150 tegument is thought to stabilize DNA-containing capsids against the high pressure exerted by encapsidation of the large genome.[144,692] Although the CMV and HSV-1 capsids are similar in size, the CMV packages about 50%

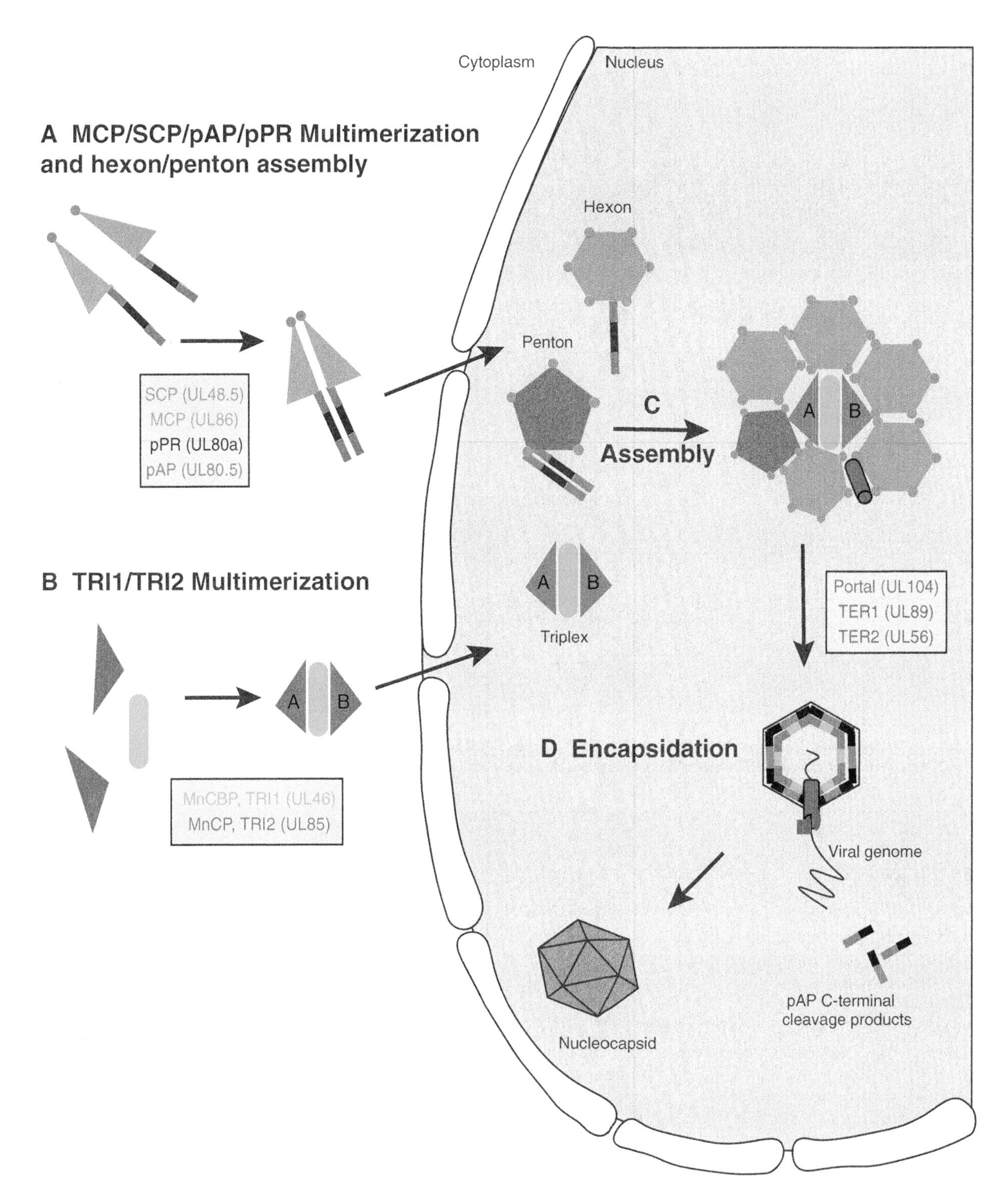

FIGURE 12.10 **HCMV nucleocapsid assembly. A:** Initial interactions between MCP protein and SCP, the assembly protein pAP and the protease precursor pPR take place in the cytoplasm resulting in the formation of multimers following interactions between conserved domains in the amino and carboxyl domains of pAP and pPR depicted as red boxes. The expression of a nuclear localization signal (NLS) by pAP and pPR permits translocation of MCP-containing multimers into the nucleus. **B:** Similarly, a triplex consisting of two molecules of MnCP/TRI2 and one molecule of MnCBP/TRI1 takes place in the cytoplasm prior to translocation into the nucleus secondary to an NLS present in MnCBP. **C:** Once in the nucleus, multimerization leads to self-assembly of hexons and pentons followed by assembly of the procapsid that also incorporates a dodecamer of the portal protein UL104 in an asymmetric vertex. **D:** Packaging of the concatemeric viral DNA is accompanied by cleavage of the pAP and pPR by the protease activity present in pPR, thus allowing sufficient volume within the procapsid for packaging of full length HCMV DNA.

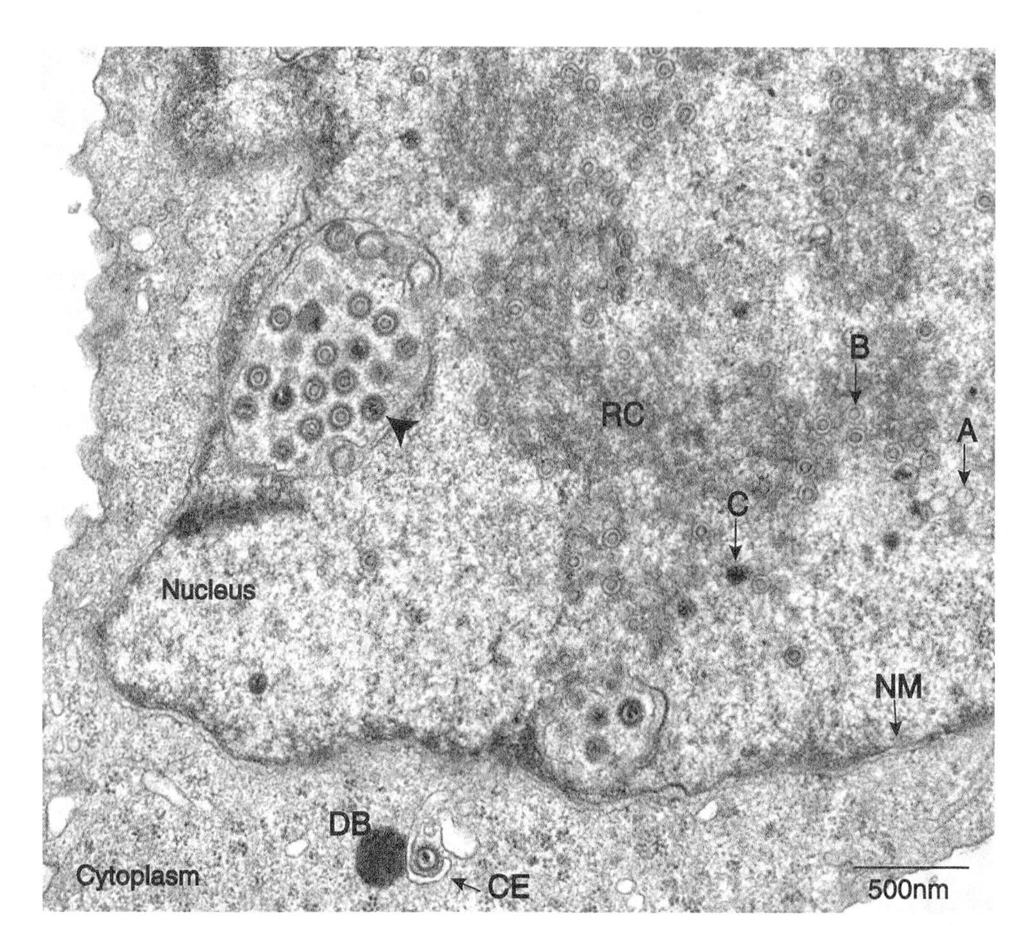

FIGURE 12.11 Nucleocapsids and nuclear egress in infected fibroblast. Transmission electron micrograph of HCMV-infected fibroblast. Replication compartments (RC) marked by accumulation of viral nucleic acids mark the site of genome encapsidation. Type A (lack scaffold and DNA), B (contain scaffold, but not DNA) and C (viral genome containing) capsids are marked with arrows. Nucleocapsid with initial layer of tegument is marked by an arrowhead. CE, capsid undergoing cytoplasmic envelopment; DB, dense body; NM, nuclear membrane.

more viral DNA, providing an explanation for the significant differences in the structure of the capsids between the two herpesviruses.[692] Tegumentation continues in the cytoplasm in conjunction with envelopment within the viral assembly compartment.[91,144,693]

The passage of the approximately 100 nm CMV nucleocapsid from the nucleus to the cytoplasm for continued maturation requires the capsids to move through the nuclear lamina and inner and outer nuclear membranes (Fig.12.9, UL80). In HCMV, the viral UL50- and UL53-encoded proteins form the core of the NEC, and structures of truncated forms of the NEC and subunits have been solved.[383,650] Heterodimers recruit the UL97-encoded viral kinase and thin and disperse nuclear lamina.[562] Nucleocapsids dock at lamina-depleted areas on the inner nuclear membrane and interact with NEC components at budding sites.[413,643] The viral protein kinase phosphorylates both NEC components, UL50 (Ser 216) and UL53 (Ser 19)[561] and phosphorylates the lamina A/C (Ser 22) on th same site that is targeted by the cellular Cdc2/cyclin-dependent kinase (CDK)1 for breakdown of the nuclear lamina during mitosis.[229] Acetylation of lamin B1 impedes disruption of lamin structure and the nuclear egress of virions.[429] Host proteins, including the inner nuclear membrane protein emerin, also associate with the NEC and emerin knockdown results in defects in all classes of viral gene expression, virus maturation, and infectious progeny production.[412] UL97 is important for viral genome synthesis and accumulation of capsids in the cytoplasm (nuclear egress).[326]

Nucleocapsids reach the cytoplasm by acquiring a temporary envelope from the inner nuclear membrane as the nucleocapsid buds into the perinuclear space (Figs. 12.9 and 12.11). To accommodate this process, the nuclear periphery juxtaposed to the virus-induced, membranous cytoplasmic AC is altered, indicated by enlargement of the perinuclear space as the result of decreased SUN domain proteins, which tether inner and outer nuclear membranes through their interaction with KASH domain proteins in the outer nuclear membrane.[73] This envelope is lost by a process of de-envelopment that involves fusion with the outer nuclear membrane as the capsid enters the cytoplasm. Once in the cytoplasm, pp150pAP associated with the nucleocapsid interacts with the ER chaperone, BiP/GRP78, and the dynein-associated motor protein, bicaudal D1, resulting in translocation to the AC for further tegumentation and final envelopment.[73,263] UL47, UL48, and UL88 are required for accumulation and tegumentation of virions within the AC.[91,332]

Envelopment and Egress

Envelopment of HCMV is proposed to occur following budding of tegumented particles into viral glycoprotein studded membrane bound vacuoles, a process that is believed to occur within the AC.[19,146,545] The AC was initially described as an isolable membranous compartment that contained virion envelope and tegument proteins.[545] The AC represents an extensive, sequential remodeling of secretory membranes, including the Golgi and trans-Golgi, endocytic membranes, and is surrounded in what appeared to be concentric layers of membranes from the ER-Golgi intermediate compartment (ERGIC) and ER (Fig. 12.12A and B).[19,146,252,506,545] Components of the late endocytic compartment are also associated with the AC, including SNARE family members[95,328] and the ER chaperone, BiP.[74,75] BiP depletion results in disintegration of the AC and diminishes infectious progeny production, suggesting the importance of host proteins in maintaining the AC and for virus production.[74] A number of activated signaling proteins are relocalized and sequestered in the AC, including mTOR and EGFR, although their role in the function of the AC is less clear.[77,118] Transferrin, β-catenin, and components of ESCRT also localize to the AC[21,146,328] (Fig. 12.13A–D).

The inhibition of AC morphogenesis has been shown to both decrease the yield of infectious virus and increase the number of defective particles released from the infected cell arguing that a major role of the AC is to facilitate virion maturation: the acquisition of tegument and envelope through the budding into or envelopment of tegumented particles by cytoplasmic vesicles containing essential virion envelope proteins (Fig. 12.13E).[253,264,506] The accumulation of membrane-bound viral glycoproteins in the AC (Fig. 12.13C and D) results from a combination of viral miRNA-mediated inhibition of vesicular trafficking from the secretory pathway and the endocytic recycling pathway while sustaining anterograde traffic in the

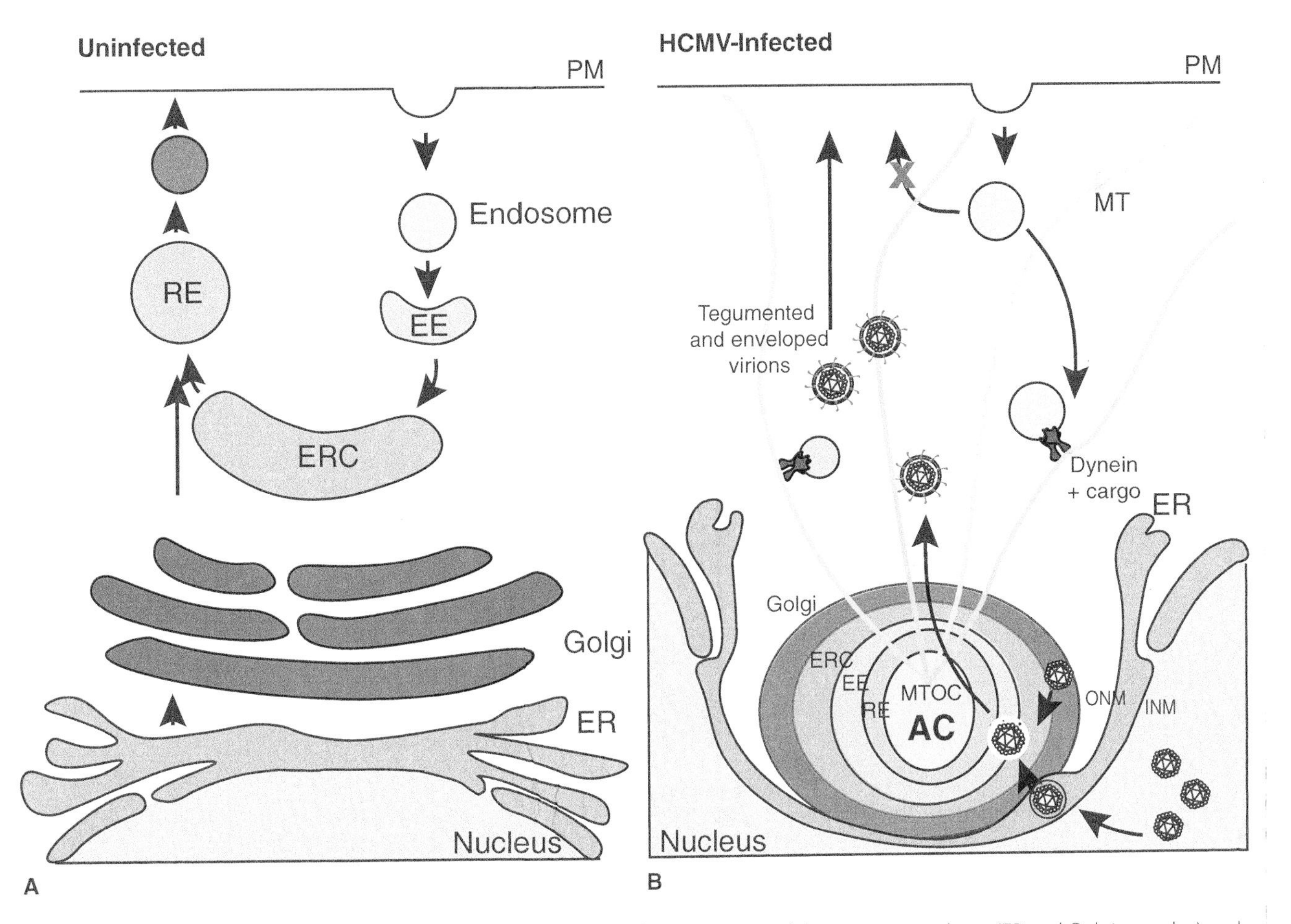

FIGURE 12.12 Cytoplasmic virus maturation. A: Uninfected cell with components of the secretory pathway (ER and Golgi complex) and endocytic pathway (early endosomes [EE]; endocytic recycling compartment [ERC]; recycling endosome [RE]). **B:** Productively infected cell with concentration of components of secretory (Golgi) and endocytic pathway (ERC, RE, EE) into a juxtanuclear compartment designated the virion assembly compartment (AC). The AC colocalizes and is formed from a Golgi-derived microtubule organizing center (MTOC) in the infected cells. Dynein motor proteins traffic endocytic vesicles and cell surface cargo to the AC, but recycling to the plasma membrane is largely blocked late in infection. The topology of the assembly compartment has been depicted as concentric rings or spheres of the different components of the secretory pathway on the outside and components of the endocytic pathway inside of AC. Virion structural proteins are concentrated in the AC by virus-induced trafficking of proteins in the secretory pathway to the AC and by the inhibition of recycling of endocytosed proteins by viral microRNAs. The tegumented capsids are enveloped by budding of particles into virion glycoprotein–containing membranous vesicles in the AC. (Adapted from Andrew Townsend, Oregon Health and Science University, Portland, Oregon.)

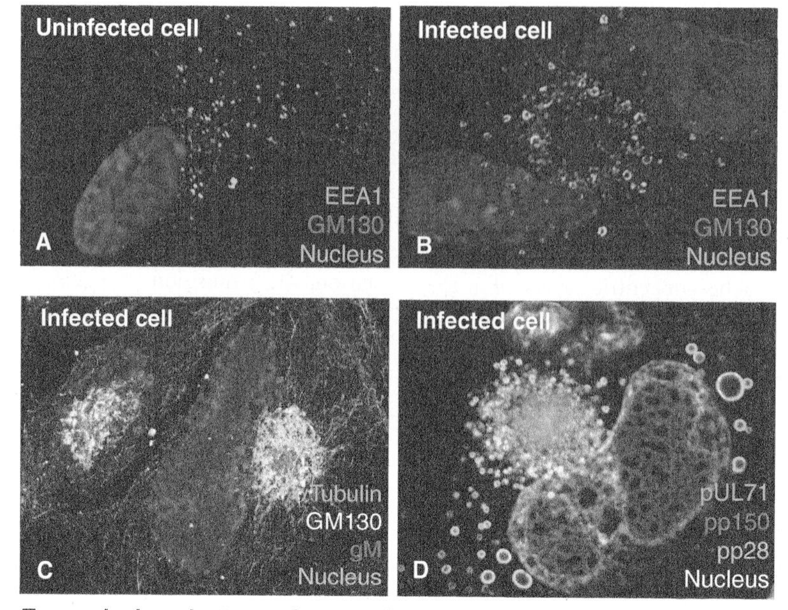

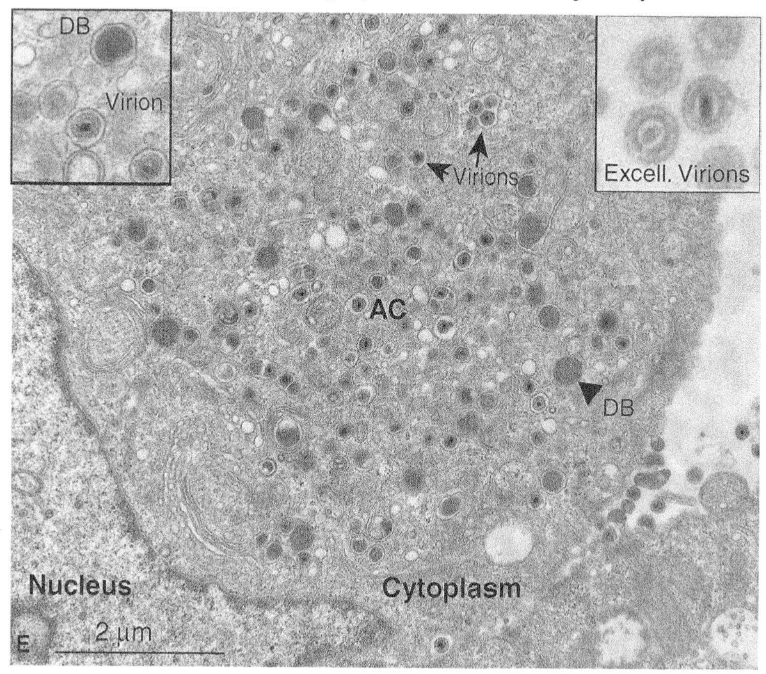

FIGURE 12.13 **Viral assembly compartment.** Immunofluorescent microscopy image of an **(A)** uninfected or **(B)** HCMV-TB40/E-infected primary human fibroblast (MOI = 1) at 72 hours. Rearrangement of Golgi (GM130 cis-Golgi marker, *Red*) and early endosomes (EEA1, *green*) and are shown. Enlarged distorted nuclei from syncytia and AC formation are evident in infected cells (DAPI, *blue*). **C:** AD169-infected cells showing tubulin (*green*), Golgi (GM130, *white*), glycoprotein M (gM, *red*) forming AC and DNA/nuclei (DAPI, *blue*). **D:** AD169-infected cell showing UL71 (*green*), pp150 (*red*), pp28 (*blue*) staining AC and DNA/nuclei (DAPI, *white*). **E:** Transmission electron micrograph of TB40/E-infected fibroblast at 96 hpi showing the viral AC, intracellular and extracellular virions, and dense bodies (DB). Insets contain enlargements of intracellular virions (left) and extracellular virions (right). (Courtesy of Felicia Goodrum and Sebastian Zeltzer (panel A-B) and William Day (panel E), University of Arizona, Tucson, Arizona; William Britt (panel C-D), University of Alabama, Birmingham.)

secretory pathway and endocytosis[253] (Fig. 12.12). HCMV-induced membrane reorganization in infected cells is not seen in other herpesviruses and allows concentration of the large number of virus-encoded glycoproteins, providing coordinated genesis of the HCMV envelope at a single cellular location and the maturation infectious progeny. Transport of the tegumented particle to sites of envelopment is thought to be microtubule dependent as inhibition of microtubule nucleation and function decreases the assembly of infectious virus.[263,499] Further, the formation of the AC depends on the motor protein, dynein, and a dynein-interacting protein, bicaudal D1.[73,263] Forces exerted by dynein contribute to the deformation of the nucleus into the kidney bean shape characteristic of cells in the late stages of CMV infection (Fig. 12.13D).[73,499] The AC acts as a Golgi-based microtubule organizing center (MTOC) by enhancing Golgi-based microtubule nucleation, a process requiring microtubule acetylation driven specifically by plus end binding protein EB3 (or MAPRE3) and resulting in nuclear rotation.[499] These microtubule-mediated changes also serve to create polarity in the nucleus for virus-induced compartmentalization.[500] Microtubules have long been appreciated to emanate from the AC (Fig. 12.13C)[545] and likely direct the transport of glycoprotein containing vesicles and possibly tegumented virus particles to the AC. Although specific protein interactions that direct the tegumented particle to sites of envelopment in the AC are not well defined, tegument proteins including UL47 and pp150 have been implicated.[91,264] The interaction between the cellular protein bicaudal D1 and pp150 has been shown to be essential for efficient infectious virus production as well as trafficking of pp150 to the AC.[263] Interestingly, a small GTPase Rab6a plays a key role in vesicular trafficking in the Golgi body and also targets bicaudal D1 and pp150 to the AC, suggesting a linkage between microtubule transport of tegumented particles to the AC and AC formation.[264] Viral gpUL132 is required for reorganizing of viral and cellular proteins to form the AC and is required for efficient replication.[678]

Subsequent budding of tegumented particles into viral glycoprotein containing vacuoles presumably requires some specificity that can be inferred by interactions between the cytoplasmic tail of a viral glycoprotein(s) and tegument proteins on the maturing particle, or alternatively between tegument proteins on the particle and the membrane bound viral tegument pp28 (*UL99*) or possibly pUL71.[156,547] These mechanisms of particle envelopment are similar to those described for RNA viruses that acquire their envelope through interactions between viral glycoproteins and viral matrix proteins. Alternatively, in the case of HCMV envelopment, budding into an envelope protein–studded vacuole and assembly of an infectious virion could be entirely random and perhaps account for the large numbers of enveloped but noninfectious particles that are released from HCMV infected cells maintained in culture. Evidence consistent with such a random process of envelopment was provided by quantitative analyses of different types of virion associated vacuoles in the AC using EM.[553] Results from this study indicated that tegumented particles were enveloped in all regions of the AC and not in a specific location within the AC. Finally, it is important to note that most of the current understanding of envelopment and in particular, the morphogenesis of the AC, has been derived from studies of laboratory adapted strains of HCMV utilizing productive infections in human fibroblast cells. Studies using clinical isolates and nonfibroblast cells have demonstrated the formation of the AC and cytoplasmic envelopment of tegumented particles. However, studies to align findings from human fibroblasts with results obtained in cells such as endothelial cells are limited as illustrated by the importance of UL135 and UL136 proteins for the formation of cytoplasmic structures required for assembly in endothelial cells but not fibroblasts.[78]

Once enveloped, mechanisms leading to the release of the infectious HCMV virions from infected cells remain undefined, particularly mechanisms that could account for the cell-to-cell spread of clinical strains of HCMV. Observations from *in vitro* studies of productive infections in human fibroblasts infected with laboratory strains of HCMV suggested that extensive cell lysis could be the major source of cell-free virus. Yet even under productive infection in permissive human fibroblasts, only about 50% of total infectious virus is released into the supernatant with the remaining infectivity associated with the infected cell. Moreover, in many low-passage clinical isolates almost all infectious virus is retained intracellularly and spread within cell monolayers.[430] Relevant to any mechanism that can account for cell-to-cell virus spread are observations from studies of viral mutants with deletions in virion structural proteins that nearly eliminate the release of cell-free infectious virus, yet appear to spread equally as well as wild type virus in assays of cell-to-cell spread.[569] In contrast, deletion of essential envelope glycoproteins including gB, gO, and gM can limit both the production of infectious extracellular virions and cell-to-cell spread.[267,282,386] Utilizing high-throughput siRNA screens, two groups have identified host cell proteins that appear to interfere with release of HCMV into the supernatant of infected cells.[407,486] Although findings from at least one of these studies provided insight into possible mechanisms virus release including exocytosis, definitive evidence of this pathway is lacking.[486]

LATENCY

A unifying characteristic of herpesviruses is that they persist for the lifetime of their host by way of a latent infection. Latency at the cellular level is the maintenance of viral genomes in a reversibly quiescent state such that the virus does not replicatein the absence of a reactivation stimulus. Within the host organism, true latency is elusive as sporadic and localized reactivation events are thought to occur frequently and subclinically in immune competent individuals. The universal risk of transplanting stem cells or an organ from a CMV-seropositive individual into a CMV-seronegative individual provides the most striking evidence of lifelong infection and the propensity for virus reactivation. Reactivation from latency in the context of immune deficiency and during pregnancy remain is central to CMV disease pathogenesis.[593] The disease implications of CMV in transplant recipients highlight the importance of understanding the mechanisms governing latency and reactivation and in designing antiviral strategies to target latent reservoirs.

The first evidence of HCMV latency came from the observation that infectious virus-free leukocytes could transmit HCMV infection. While CMV infects a diverse array of cells in the human host, the latent reservoir for HCMV is primarily considered to be hematopoietic, including CD34+ hematopoietic progenitor cells and cells of the myeloid lineage, including monocytes. The evidence for a hematopoietic reservoir consists of the detection of viral genomes in these cells in seropositive individuals in the absence of disease and the ability to stimulate reactivation from latently infected hematopoietic cells. The HCMV genome is estimated to persist episomally at a frequency of 10^{-4} to 10^{-5} with 2 to 15 genome equivalents per infected cell in myeloid progenitors.[50,576] While multiple hematopoietic cell subtypes may support latent infection, there are undoubtedly important differences that remain to be systematically understood.

Latent persistence of the virus poses a number of molecular and cellular challenges for the virus, including maintaining viral genomes through cellular division, reversibly repressing viral gene expression, and sensing host cues for reactivation. Defining natural latency beyond the identification of cell lineages that carry the HCMV genome has been challenging to understand at the molecular level in hematopoietic cells because of the heterogeneity of primary hematopoietic subpopulations cells and the scarcity of primary human progenitor cells. In an attempt to circumvent this issue, a number of cell line models have been developed that recapitulate varying degrees of the latent infection. These include acute monocytic leukemia THP-1 cells,[129,688] acute myeloblastic leukemia Kasumi 3 cells,[451] embryonal carcinoma NTera2,[208] and inducible pluripotent stem cells (iPSC)[488] and human embryonic stem cell (hESC)-derived CD34+ HPCs.[134] Cell line models offer key advantages in their homogeneity and synchronous reexpression of viral gene expression following a reactivation stimulus, and the absence of donor variability—all limitations inherent to primary cell systems. While cell line models recapitulate key aspects of CMV latency (e.g., MIEP silencing, genome maintenance), some have blocks in later steps associated with reactivation, such as amplification of the viral genome or progeny virus production. hESC-derived CD34+ HPCs offer a strong alternative to primary cells as a model that supports multi-lineage hematopoietic differentiation, HCMV-mediated myelosuppression, and recapitulate quantifiable phenotypes associated with viral genes important to latency or reactivation.[134] A key advantage is that reactivation in hESC-derived CD34+ HPCs occurs at a frequency approximately 30 times greater than that of primary cells. It is important to recognize that none of these experimental models factor contribution of the antiviral T cell immune response that dictates outcomes in immunocomppromised hosts.

Establishment and Maintenance

HCMV latency is established through a complex network of virus–host interactions that remain ill defined (Fig. 12.14). Even more ill defined are the means by which the HCMV genome and its latent state are maintained. HCMV binding to the cell surface stimulates EGFR signaling in CD14+ monocytes[98] and CD34+ progenitor cells[303] and results in downstream activation of AKT. EGFR and integrin signaling up-regulates the cytoskeletal regulators N-WASP and paxillin, which drives trafficking of the internalized virion to the nucleus and increases infected monocyte motility. These initial signaling events are also important for the establishment of latency.[303] Trafficking of the viral genome in primary monocytes is delayed relative to fibroblasts permissive for virus replication and takes a retrograde route through the trans-Golgi network and recycling endosomes that requires Src signaling.[304] Similar to monocytes, trafficking of the HCMV genome to the nucleus requires 4 to 8 hours in CD34+ cells.[303]

A prerequisite for latency is the maintenance of the viral genome, although these mechanisms have not been defined for HCMV. This is particularly important because latency is established in cells capable of division. The γ-herpesviruses EBV and KSHV encode proteins that tether the viral genome to host chromosomes. HCMV IE1-72 kDa associates with mitotic chromatin and binds histones H2A-H2B and H3-H4 and these interactions may serve to tether chromatin in the context of the latent infection,[423] although such a role has been elusive. Further, a smaller IE1 protein composed only of exon 4 is reported to interact with topoisomerase IIb for maintenance of the viral genome.[615] In the absence of a fully defined mechanism for genome maintenance, it remains possible that frequent subclinical reactivation events serve to constantly reseed the population of infected hematopoietic cells.

Critical to latency is the ability of infected hematopoietic cells to avoid programmed cell death pathways, including apoptosis. While the virus encodes a number of anti-apoptosis and anti-necroptosis factors (e.g., UL36, UL37, UL38, TRS1, and β2.7RNA, see section *Regulation of Host Cell Death*), it is not clear if these are expressed or functioning in the context of latency.[97] Infection up-regulates cellular survival signals, including ERK/MAPK[298] and Mcl-1[510] in CD34+ cells and Mcl-1[97] and Bcl-2[128] in monocytes. Mcl-1 and Bcl-2 block the formation of proapoptotic complexes, such as Bax and Bak, in mitochondrial membranes. In the case of monocytes, activated cell survival pathways dramatically extends the life span of otherwise short-lived monocytes (1 to 3 days in circulation). Mcl-1 is induced through EGFR and integrin activation during virus entry via PI3K signaling and an atypical AKT pathway.[97,121] However, Mcl-1 is down-regulated to allow basal activation of caspase-3 as a requirement for differentiation and integrin-dependent Bcl-2 increases concomitantly to continue to ensure survival. This Mcl-1-to-Bcl-2 switch is an example of the intricacy of viral manipulation of the host cell underlying HCMV persistence. Sustained PI3K/AKT signaling downstream of EGFR is important for the establishment and maintenance of HCMV latency in CD34+ HPCs, as well as that of other herpesviruses. Inhibition of the EGFR, PI3K/AKT or MEK/ERK pathways in CD34+ cells stimulate reactivation.[76,77]

In monocyte-derived dendritic cells, the signaling changes associated with reactivation are distinct. IL-6-stimulated reactivation requires MEK/ERK signaling[299,511] and the concomitant activation of src family kinase, hematopoietic cell kinase (HCK), which is up-regulated upon DC differentiation.[164] The activation of these pathways results in increased acetylation of histones and CREB binding to the MIEP.[299] Importantly, contact with infected cells stimulates uninfected monocyte-derived DCs to secrete soluble, non-IFN factors that suppress expression of viral genes and inhibit CMV spread.[294] However, direct infection of monocyte-derived DCs and macrophages stimulates cGAS/STING-dependent type-I IFN (IFN) production,[462] and type I and type II IFNs reversibly suppress viral gene expression or reactivation in mice infected with MCMV.[143,250] Direct infection of monocytes in culture or monocytes from patient samples induces up-regulation of IFN-stimulated genes, contributing to an inflammatory response in the hematopoietic niche.[559] Together these studies suggest that the establishment and maintenance of latency are driven by both infected cell–extrinsic as well as infected cell–intrinsic factors.

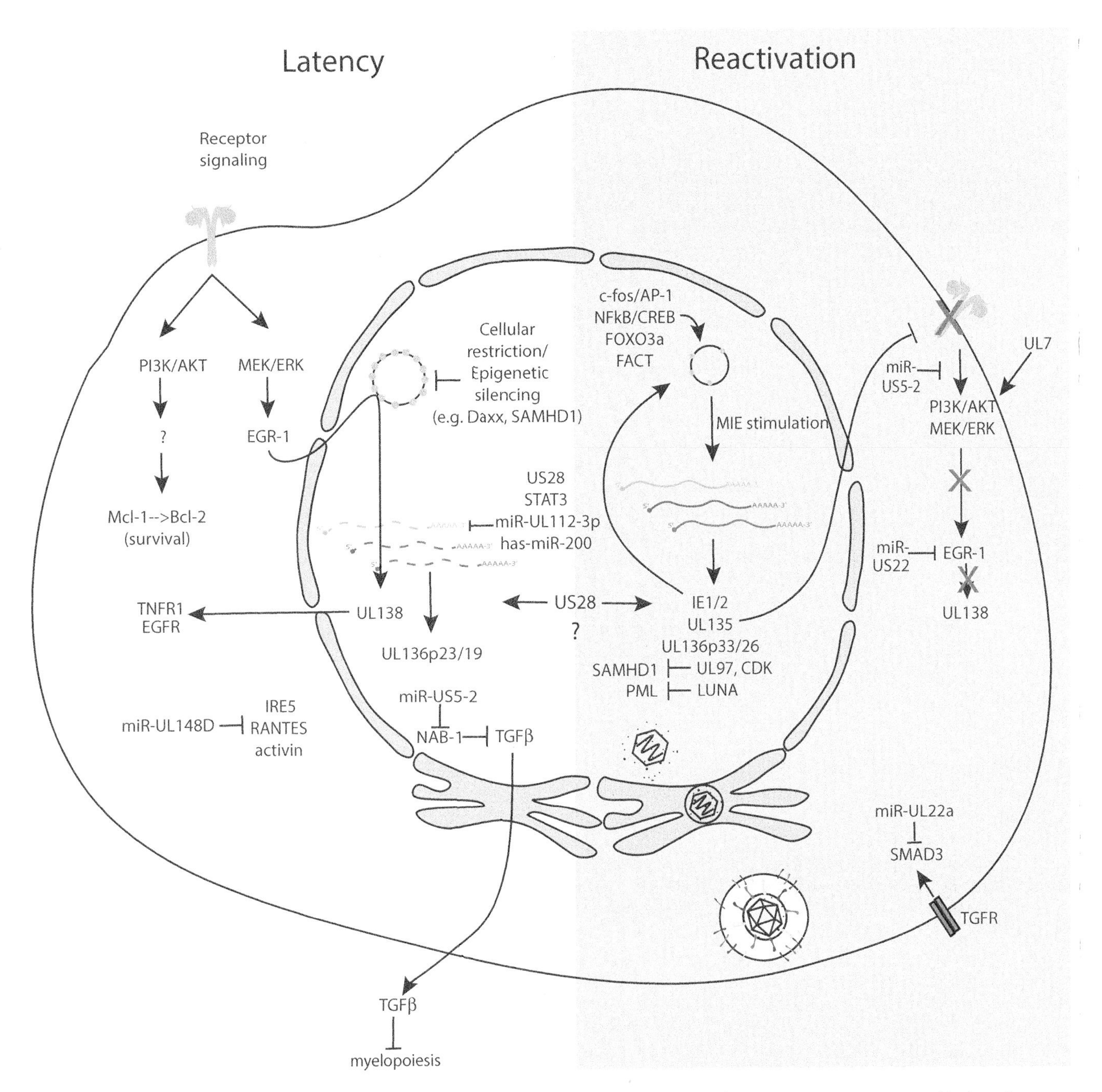

FIGURE 12.14 Latency and reactivation. During latency, viral genome is chromatinized and gene expression is restricted by host factors, including, but not limited to, PML, SAMHD1, PRC2, and FACT. Viral genes appear to be broadly expressed but at very low levels, in part due to viral and host miRNAs. miRNAs also regulate cellular responses to infection. Sustained PI3K/AKT signaling is important for cell survival and HCMV latency, as it is for all herpesviruses. MEK/ERK signaling stimulates the transcription factor, EGR-1, which drives the expression of the UL138 latency determinant. Viral proteins and miRNAs contributing to the establishment of latency are indicated. miRNAs regulate the signaling and secretion of TGFb, which is responsible for HCMV inhibition of myelopoiesis in uninfected bystander cells. During reactivation, host signaling changes induce reexpression of viral gene expression and viral replication ensues. Viral proteins and miRNAs target host cell signaling to facilitate reactivation. UL135 and viral miRNAs attenuate PI3K/AKT and MEK/ERK signaling, while UL7 is activated later and stimulates. miR-UL22a blocks TGFb signaling in infected cells to maintain myelopoiesis. US28 has been described to play roles in both latency and reactivation, likely depending on mode of signaling and context.

Control of Gene Expression for Latency

The latent program of gene expression has been an area of intense focus and controversy. Classically, herpesvirus latency is characterized by a transcriptionally silent state where gene expression is limited to a small number of genes that play important roles in establishing or maintaining latency. However, sensitive transcriptomic evaluation reveals broader patterns of gene expression associated with latency. As has been observed for other α- and γ-herpesviruses, HCMV infection of cells destined to support a latent infection results in a low-level, but promiscuous burst of gene expression from across the HCMV genome.[109,129,533,565] While this initial burst of gene expression eventually subsides,[129] low-level, broad gene expression may persist.[109,565] Although defining the latent transcriptome is complicated by the heterogeneous nature of bulk hematopoietic cell populations, the observation of broad low level gene expression is mirrored in studies of cells from latently infected healthy carriers.[109] Further, single-cell RNA sequencing has revealed heterogeneity in patterns of expression and also support low level gene expression from across the genome.[565] Therefore, while gene expression is restricted, it is likely not entirely silenced nor limited to a small number of latency genes.

In cell types that support latency, viral gene expression is restricted by chromatinization and epigenetic regulation of the viral chromosome. Many host factors with the potential to suppress viral gene expression are components of PML or ND10 bodies, including PML, Daxx, and Sp100[539,540,676] (see sections *Pre-IE Events and Intrinsic Responses to Infection* and *Regulation of Major Immediate Early Gene Expression* for further discussion). Type 1 IFN up-regulates these host factors and reversibly blocks IE gene expression for latency in MCMV-infected endothelial cells.[143] While knockdown of Daxx increases IE gene expression in THP-1 or CD34+ cells infected with the AD169 laboratory strain,[540] it fails to rescue IE expression in cells infected with a low-passage strain[541] or in undifferentiated THP-1[648] or NTera2[221] cells. These findings indicate that the repression of gene expression for latency is multifactorial. Despite the ability of the pp71 tegument protein to stimulate viral gene expression by antagonizing Daxx, pp71 fails to traffic to the nucleus and degrade Daxx in cells that support latency,[541] although high intravirion pp71 may be able to overcome this restriction and enhance replicative fitness and impede the establishment of latency.[103]

A number of other restriction factors are emerging that contribute to the establishment of latency. SAMHD1, a host factor that depletes the pool of available dNTPs to suppress DNA polymerase processivity, has been shown to restrict MIE gene expression and replication by impeding NFκB activation in myeloid cells.[302] In primary human macrophages, HCMV counteracts this restriction by inducing SAMHD1 phosphorylation (T592) through the activation of CDKs and/or through UL97 kinase-mediated phosphorylation, in addition to transcriptional down-regulation and increased proteasomal degradation.[82,155,302,698] This viral strategy is conserved in MCMV where the M97 kinase phosphorylates SAMHD1.[155] These findings suggest that SAMHD1 suppresses replication for latency and SAMHD1 inactivation is required for reactivation. Further, the phosphatases CDC25B and CDK1 are repressive to viral gene expression, and inhibition of CDK1 stimulates viral gene expression in the Kasumi-3 model of latency.[463] Finally, cellular miRNAs have also been shown to down-regulate *UL122* and *UL123* transcripts encoding IE2 and IE1, respectively.[216,453] The human miR-200 cluster is more highly expressed in undifferentiated hematopoietic progenitors or early myeloid lineage-committed cells than more differentiated cells and targets *UL122* transcripts encoding IE2 to reduce viral gene expression.[453]

Genome chromatinization is an important control point in regulating programs of gene expression that ultimately dictate replicative or latent states.[1,15,428,513] The histone tails to nucleosomes associating with viral genomes are regulated by posttranslational modifications, such as acetylation and methylation, which regulate chromatin structure and gene expression. Studies of chromatin changes associated with latency and reactivation have primarily focused on chromatinization and regulation of the MIEP as control of IE gene expression is critical for productive replication or the establishment of latency.[220,676] In cell line models for quiescent infection, histone deacetylase activity reduces viral gene expression, corresponding to increased association of heterochromatin protein 1 (HP1)[428] and the corepressor KAP1[504] with the MIEP to contribute silencing the viral genome. Heterochromatinization of the HCMV genome has not been defined as facultative or constitutive, which is an important determinant in HSV-1 latency. However, PRC2 increases trimethylation of histone 3 at lysine 27 (H3K27me3), a promiscuous chromatin mark indicative of facultative heterochromatin, on the HCMV genome in undifferentiated THP-1 cells,[1] which correlates with reduced viral gene expression. Despite an apparent role for PRC2 in chromatinization and repression of the viral genome for latency, PRC1 and 2 have also been shown to promote replication in fibroblasts as inhibition of the histone H3K27 methylase EZH2 component of PRC2 impairs HCMV gene expression[24,582] and promotes viral genome synthesis and replication in a catalytically independent manner.[609]

Viral Determinants Associated With Latency and Reactivation

In the past decade, viral genes and miRNAs have been identified that impact infection outcomes in hematopoietic cells. A polycistronic locus within the UL*b′* region of the viral genome that spans *UL133-UL138* encoding, UL133, UL135, UL136, and UL138 encode genes that are repressive to viral replication in contexts of latency and contribute to the establishment of latency or are required for reactivation.[165,210] These genes are largely dispensable for replication in fibroblasts, but they have been genetically defined to promote or suppress virus replication in hematopoietic cells; however, much remains to be understood about their mechanisms of action. Recombinant viruses lacking *UL138* exhibit a loss of latency and replicate in CD34+ HPCs without a reactivation stimulus.[210,481,631] UL138 prevents the association of lysine-specific demethylases with the viral genome to limit IE gene expression.[348] By contrast, *UL135* is important for virus replication when *UL138* is expressed; disruption of *UL135* results in a severe defect for reactivation.[632] UL138 and UL135 functionally antagonize one another by differentially regulating the trafficking and signaling activity of EGFR.[77] Interactions between UL135 and the host adapter proteins, Abelson interacting protein 1 (Abi-1) and CIN85/CD2AP are requisite for UL135-mediated turnover of EGFR and mutant viruses where these interactions are disrupted or that fail to regulate EGFR are defective for reactivation in CD34+ HPCs.[502] Inhibition of EGFR or downstream PI3K/AKT signaling potently induces reactivation when coupled with stimuli for reactivation in CD34+ HPCs,[76,77,303] suggesting a role for sustained EGFR/PI3K/AKT signaling in maintaining HCMV latency, as has been shown for other herpesvirus family members. UL138-mediated stimulation of EGFR induces the early growth response-1 (EGR1) cellular transcription factor, which in turn binds to the viral genome to drive *UL138* gene expression.[76] EGR1 is highly expressed in hematopoietic stem cells and is important for maintenance of stemness. Disruption of EGR1 binding to the viral genome reduces *UL138* expression relative to *UL135* and increases virus replication in CD34+ HPCs.

UL138 also increases TNFR1 on the surface of infected cells,[344,421] which potentiates NFκB signaling in the context of infection[421] but does not drive apoptosis due to the function of UL36.[391] TNFα signaling is a signal for reactivation *in vitro*,[186] in mice, and in the context of transplantation,[130,169] and can stimulate reexpression of viral gene expression independently of differentiation.[186] Therefore, UL138-mediated up-regulation of TNFR1 on the surface of infected cells may provide a means by which the cell can sense cues for reactivation; however, role of UL138 modulation of TNFR1 on latency and reactivation remains to be evaluated.

In contrast to EGFR and TNFR1, UL138 decreases the cell surface levels of multidrug resistance-associated protein-1 (MRP1/ABC transporter multidrug resistance protein ABCC1).[659] In hematopoietic cells, UL138 down-regulation of MRP-1 results in increased sensitivity to killing by Vincristine, but it is not known why the virus targets MRP-1. It is not clear how UL138 differentially modulates levels of host receptors at the cell surface; however, mutation of dileucine or Golgi sorting motifs within UL138 that are important for the down-regulation of MRP1 do not impact Golgi localization or the maintenance of latency in embryonic stem cells.[200]

UL136 is expressed with later kinetics than UL135 and UL138 as maximal expression requires viral DNA synthesisor entry into late phase in the context of productive infection. *UL136* is expressed as multiple protein isoforms (p33, p26, p25, p23, and p19), differing only in their amino terminal end, that differentially suppress replication for latency or contribute to reactivation in both CD34+ HPCs *in vitro* and humanized mouse models.[93,94] The mechanism by which UL136 isoforms regulate the transition between latency and reactivation is unknown.

US28 has been reported to be important for both maintaining latency and for reactivation, making its precise role in latency controversial and possibly dependent on context (e.g., cell type and culture conditions, ligand binding). HCMV encodes four GPCR homologs (UL33, UL78, US27, and US28) where US28 is the best characterized.[190] US28 is constitutively active and promiscuously activated by host chemokines CCL2 (monocyte chemoattractant protein 1, MCP-1), CCL3 (macrophage inflammatory protein 1-alpha, MIP-1α), CCL4 (macrophage inflammatory protein 1-beta, MIP-1β), CCL5 (regulated on activation, normal T cell expressed and secreted, RANTES) and CXC3CL1 (fractalkine), inducing numerous ligand- and G protein–dependent signaling pathways. US28 induces chemotactic migration, chemokine scavenging, cellular adherence and tumor promotion through its binding to CC (e.g., CCL5/RANTES) and CX3C (e.g., CX3CL1/Fractalkine) families of chemokines.[403,646] Constitutive signaling (independent of ligand binding) drives induction of NFκB/PLCβ, NFAT, p38-MAPK, and CREB signaling. A 2.9 Å structure of US28 in complex with CX3CL1/Fractalkine shows that the unique structure of the C-terminus may underlie its ligand-independent (constitutive) activity through the generation of inositol phosphates in productive infection.[79,92,416] US28 signaling drives MAPK, NFκB, and Wnt signaling in productive infection,[92,338,415,575] which likely contributes to pathogenesis of HCMV infection and spread in the host, despite being dispensable for virus replication in cultured fibroblasts.[450,642] US28 has also been shown to transcriptionally down-regulate IFN-responsive genes for latency.[171] US28 binding to RANTES stimulates smooth muscle cell migration, which can be blocked by binding to Fractalkine to stimulate migration of macrophages.[603,645] The complexity of US28 is further exemplified by its context-dependent signaling and differential functions are dictated by association with different G proteins.[420,645]

US28 is packaged within the virion tegument and is expressed during latency (prior to differentiation) and following reactivation in cell lines and primary cell models.[257,680] US28 modulates a number of signaling pathways, attenuating mitogen activated protein (MAP) kinase, NFκB, c-foscarnet, and activating STAT3.[321,322,704] US28-mediated induction of STAT3 in infected HPCs reprograms differentiation to generate a rare immunosuppressive monocyte subset that expresses high levels of IL-10 and inducible nitric oxide synthase (iNOS) and STAT3 activation is important to suppressing IE gene expression.[704] STAT3 is an important target of regulation for many contexts of HCMV infection.[239,388,516,575,628,677,699,704] In Kasumi-3 or CD34+ cells, recombinant viruses lacking US28 expresses higher levels of the MIE genes and produce infectious progeny, indicating that US28 suppresses viral gene expression and replication for latency.[257] A number of mechanistic studies have provided insights into how US28 may contribute to establishing latency. Ectopic expression of US28 in THP-1 cells attenuates MAP kinase and NFκB signaling for the establishment of latency in undifferentiated cells, which correlates with increased levels of *UL138* gene expression relative to IE gene expression.[322] However, in the same system, constitutive US28 signaling also activates MIE gene expression in TPA-differentiated cells. It was further shown that US28 decreases binding of c-foscarnet, a subunit of the AP-1 cellular transcription factor, to the MIEP, which correlates with reduced MIE gene expression.[321]

In contrast to these studies, US28 mutant viruses (nonsense and destabilized variants) maintained genomes but failed to reactivate in both CD34+ primary cells and in a humanized mouse model of latency.[133] In these studies, nonsense mutation of *US28* results in a virus that failed to reactivate, but a mutation that blocks CC- and CX3C-chemokine binding (Y16F) results in a failure to establish latency and persistent replication in the absence of a reactivation stimulus. A mutation disrupting constitutive US28 signaling through the DRY box (R129A mutation) had no effect on latency and reactivation. US28 was further shown to stimulate hematopoietic cell differentiation, driving cells toward a CD14+ lineage. Constitutive US28 signaling activity stimulates PLCβ and PKC in THP-1 monocytes, an activity that stimulates monocyte-to-endothelial cell adhesion.[680] The interactions between US28 and other signaling complexes in the membrane, the resulting conformational changes, differential association with G proteins, and regulation by GPCRs that phosphorylate C-terminal residues in a tissue-specific manner may contribute to differences in US28 function in different contexts of infection or experimental systems. Resolving the complexity in US28 function will require the use of precise mutations and highly controlled contexts to assign specific functions to distinct ligand binding and constitutive signaling activities in regulating decisions to enter into or exit latency.

HCMV miRNAs represent a powerful mechanism to fine-tune expression of viral or cellular gene expression to regulate latency since they are nonimmunogenic (Supplementary e-Table 12.2). miRNA expression patterns have been shown to be distinct in the THP-1 monocytic cell line or CD34+ HPCs relative to that measured during productive infection in fibroblasts.[193,341,409] In CD34+ HPCs, all miRNAs are detected at 4 dpi[341] and decrease over time to 10 dpi with the exception of miR-UL22A-5p, miR-UL112-3p, and miR-UL148D.[463] miR-UL112-3p targets HCMV UL123 (IE1-72 kDa),[216,426] UL112/UL113 (viral DNA synthesis),[216] UL114 (viral DNA glycosylase),[596] UL17/18 (MHC-I homologue), and UL120/UL121 (MIE region exons)[216] to inhibit IE gene expression and DNA replication. miR-UL112-1-3p is reported to down-regulate IE gene expression during latency, although disruption of miR-UL112-1-3p alone did not result in reactivation.[342] miRUL112-1-3p works in conjunction with miR-US5-1 and the UL7 protein to control FOXO3a activity and preventing cell death in CD34+ HPCs,[232] indicating a role for this miRNA in reactivation other than regulating viral gene expression. As HSV, KSHV, and EBV also encode miRNAs that can down-regulate their own IE gene expression, this may be a common strategy evolved to fine-tune viral gene expression for the establishment of latency. In addition to these viral targets, miR-UL112-1-3p targets a number of cellular genes that may also contribute to latency, although this has yet to be demonstrated. These include immune activators (MICB, an NK cell activating receptor ligand),[594] IL-32,[255] vesicular trafficking proteins that modulate cytokine secretion (e.g., VAMP3, Rab5C, Rab11A, SNAP23),[253] and host restriction factors that suppress IE gene expression (e.g., BclAF1).[349]

miR-UL148D accumulates late during the latent infection *in vitro* and regulates cytokine secretion, targeting the RANTES proinflammatory cytokine,[306] which may serve to reduce recruitment of mononuclear cells to infected cells. Further, miR-UL148D targets the activin ACVR1B receptor, which promotes monocyte to dendritic cell differentiation. miR-UL148D also limits IL-6 secretion from infected monocytes,[341] which may dampen the inflammatory response during latency. However, disruption of miR-UL148D did not alter viral gene expression or the ability of the TB40/E strain to establish or reactivate from latency. miR-UL148D was also shown to target immediate early response gene 5 (IER5), which suppresses the CDC25B phosphatase that positively regulates CDK1.[463] In this study, miR-UL148D silencing of IER5 rescued CDC25B levels, resulting in CDK1-mediated silencing of the MIE gene expression in the Kasumi 3 cell line. It should also be noted that two groups independently characterized the phenotypes of miR-UL148D-mutant viruses with differing results in terms of the regulation of IE gene expression, possibly due to differences in the model systems (CD14+ monocytes vs. Kasumi-3 cell line) and virus strains (TB40/E vs. NR1).[341,463]

The reactivation of CMV from latency is intimately linked to hematopoietic differentiation. Differentiation of latently infected cells along the myeloid lineage or allogenic stimulation results in the reexpression of viral genes and reactivation.[508,578,579] Given the extent of chromatinization and repression of the viral genome that accompanies the establishment of latency, a primary objective in changes accompanying reactivation is to de-repress the restriction of viral gene expression imposed by host factors, such as Daxx, SAMHD1, IFN, or histone methylation. Chromatin remodeling is a critical part of reactivation associated with hematopoietic differentiation,[164,513] but not fully understood. The FACT (facilitates chromatin transcription) complex functions to reposition histones and to increase accessibility to RNA polymerase. FACT is bound to the MIEP both prior to and following reactivation events in Kasumi 3 cells and is important for the reexpression of IE genes.[452]

The MIE locus contains a high density of binding sites for host transcription factors with roles in inflammation and differentiation (Fig. 12.7). Differentiation-associated changes in levels or binding of host transcriptional activators or repressors to the MIE region regulates MIE gene expression to maintain latency.[33,299,321,370,452] Because the MIEP is repressed during latency, it has been presumed that de-repression of the MIEP is a prerequisite to reexpression of IE genes upon reactivation. The CREB host transcription factor binds to CRE sites within the MIEP resulting in increased IE gene expression in infected monocytes.[299] CREB in cooperation with NF-κB also stimulates MIE expression in NTera2 cells stimulated to differentiate.[368,696] Recent studies demonstrate that additional MIE promoter elements within intron A of the MIE locus predominantly drive IE1-72 kDa and IE2-86 kDa accumulation in both in primary and cell line latency models in response to cues for reactivation.[129] FOXO3a, a member of the forkhead family of transcription factors, is induced upon differentiation and stimulates reexpression of IE gene expression from intronic promoters.[228] Host transcription factor binding in the MIE promoter or enhancer may influence 3D chromatin structure and the activity of other regions of the MIE locus, such as the intronic promoters, to drive MIE reexpression. The presence and differential use of multiple promoter elements for MIE expression in contexts of productive infection versus reactivation provides versatility to strongly repress MIE gene expression for latency, while preserving responsiveness to specific host cues for reactivation.

The identification of viral genes required for reactivation remains as elusive as those required for latency. While viral IE gene expression is sometimes observed in the context of latency, it is clear that IE gene expression alone is not sufficient for reactivation.[688] UL135 is required for reactivation[632] with functions in targeting EGFR for degradation and rearrangement of the host cytoskeleton for immune evasion.[76,502,588] The attenuation of signaling pathways downstream of EGFR, including PI3K/AKT and MEK/ERK, stimulates reactivation indicating the importance of host signaling to the maintenance of and reactivation from latency.[76,77,502] HCMV miRNA, miR-US5-2 targets the EGFR adapter protein, GAB-1, to attenuate EGFR signaling through the PI3K/AKT and MEK/ERK pathways.[234] Further, miR-US22-1 (or miR-US22a) down-regulates the EGF-responsive EGR1 host transcription factor and is required for reactivation.[411] Targeting of GAB1 and EGR1 by miR-US5-2 and miR-US22-1, respectively, indirectly decreases *UL138* expression and increases replication in CD34+ HPCs.[76,234] HCMV miR-UL22A is also required for reactivation and targets SMAD3 to negatively regulate myelo-suppressive TGF-β signaling in infected cells.[233]

By contrast to the role of MEK/ERK signaling in latency, other studies have shown an important role for MEK/ERK signaling in reactivation to ensure cell survival. ERK up-regulates the cellular pro-survival factors, Mcl-1 and Elk-1, to counter proapoptotic pathway stimulation during reactivation.[298,510] Further, UL7 is a secreted protein and a ligand for the cellular Fms-like tyrosine kinase 3 receptor (Flt-3R).[135] UL7 is expressed and secreted following a stimulus that induces reactivation. UL7 binding to Flt-3 activates the PI3K/AKT and MAPK signaling cascades to prevent cell death in CD34+ HPCs and stimulate differentiation and reactivation in CD34+ HPCs, monocytes and humanized mice.[135,232] Contrasting but clear roles for PI3K/AKT and MAPK signaling in both latency and reactivation illustrate the complexity of latency and reactivation and may indicate roles dependent on timing and context of infection.

The LUNA latency-associated nuclear antigen is encoded antisense to *UL81-82* and is important for reactivation in monocytes.[300] LUNA possesses deSUMOylase activity and its overexpression induces desumoylation and dispersal of PML domains or ND10s.[490] The desumoylase activity of LUNA is required for reexpression of MIE genes, further suggesting that PML provides an important restriction contributing to viral latency.

HCMV and Hematopoietic Differentiation

The outcome of HCMV infection in hematopoietic cells depends on the lineage of cells infected within heterogeneous populations of HPCs.[134,209,315,369] This complicates understanding latency and reactivation in bulk, multilineage hematopoietic populations. In either primary or hESC-derived CD34+ HPCs, the most immature cells (CD34+/CD38-/CD90+ or lin-) support a persistent infection, whereas CD34+/CD38+/CD90+ or CD34+/CD38lo/CD90- cells support latency.[134,209] Other lineages that become infected presumably undergo abortive infection since they fail to reactivate or require a different stimulus for reactivation. Inhibition of signaling pathways (e.g., PI3K/AKT) can increase the frequency of infectious centers indicative of reactivation, but it not known if this represents an increased frequency of reactivation from CD34+/CD38+ subpopulations or if reactivation is induced in additional subpopulations.

While hematopoietic differentiation triggers reactivation of HCMV from latency, HCMV also has profound effects on hematopoietic differentiation and fate. HCMV has long been appreciated to be myelosuppressive in the context of hematopoietic stem cell transplantation.[375] The problem of myelosuppression is further complicated in the context of transplantation by the use of the antivirals, ganciclovir, foscarnet, and cidofovir, which have myelosuppressive affects. While the mechanisms by which HCMV inhibits hematopoietic differentiation are not fully mapped, there are both direct effects on the infected cell, as well as indirect effects on bystander cells or on the stroma supporting hematopoiesis. *In vitro*, direct infection reduces the formation of hematopoietic colonies, particularly multilineage colony formation by ≥50%.[233] The indirect effects on hematopoiesis are of central importance given that very few cells are infected in the host (an estimated 1 in 10,000 to 100,000 cells).[576]

Recent studies have defined HCMV gene products that induce or suppress myelopoiesis. miRUS5-2 blocks myelopoiesis by down-regulating the TGF-β transcriptional repressor, NGFI-A-binding protein (NAB1).[233] The resulting increase in TGF-β secretion is inhibitory to myelopoiesis of uninfected cells. Importantly, miR-UL22A down-regulates SMAD3 to block intracellular TGF-β signaling in infected CD34+ HPCs. These findings suggesting an intriguing model whereby HCMV miRNAs stimulate TGF-β secretion to block myelopoiesis of uninfected cells while maintaining proliferation and differentiation of infected cells. In contrast to miR-US5-2, the UL7 HCMV Flt-3R ligand stimulates myeloid differentiation *in vitro* and *in vivo*, increasing HCMV genome-positive CD14+ monocytes in the tissues of humanized mice.[135] Further, miR-US22-1 targeting of EGR1 is required for differentiation of infected CD34+ HPCs, in addition to reactivation.[411]

VIRUS CONTROL OF CELL BIOLOGY

HCMV is exquisite in its ability to manipulate cell biology for virus objectives, to replicate or establish or reactivate from latency. Virus-induced manipulation of signaling and stress pathways though virus entry and synthesis of viral genomes and proteins or through the action of specific viral proteins or miRNAs can have broad consequences for the outcome of infection and the infected cell. HCMV has been a fertile area of research for understanding the complexity of virus–host interactions—how the virus manipulates pathways for replication that might result in cell death or termination of infection unless further manipulated to precisely regulate the response. Due to space limitations, we provide online access to examples of host pathways manipulated by the virus to affect the outcome of infection. Most of these examples are best defined in the context of replicative infection in fibroblasts, and implications for latency, while likely important, are less clear.

Regulation of Cell Death

Cell death is an ancient host defense strategy that eliminates stressed or infected cells to limit viral spread. As cell death represents an immediate dead end for infection, all viruses have evolved mechanisms to control cell death. HCMV expresses cell death suppressor proteins and lncRNA early during infection of many cell types. A number of virus-encoded IE proteins were initially found to individually block apoptosis.[404] IE proteins play diverse roles impacting different regulated cell death pathways.[71,126,404] For in-depth discussion of HCMV proteins and lncRNAs that control cell death, please refer to supplementary online content: *Cell Biology of HCMV Infection 1: Regulation of Cell Death*

Regulation of the Infected Cell Proteome

As obligate intracellular parasites, viruses have evolved an array of mechanisms to ensure the synthesis of their own proteins and to shape the proteome of the infected cells for successful infection. Viruses are ultimately parasites of the host translation machinery as no virus encodes complete translation machinery. While many viruses all but eliminate host protein synthesis, cellular protein synthesis continues largely unabated or even increases in HCMV-infected cells.[649] HCMV impacts the global proteome by specifically recruiting or excluding mRNAs from polyribosomes. mRNAs encoding proteins involved in the DNA damage response, proliferation, ribosomal biogenesis, chromatin remodeling, organelle function, and vesicular transport are increased, whereas those involved in cellular differentiation and acquired immunity are decreased.[408]

HCMV regulates more than 10,000 host proteins and their transcripts during virus replication by a variety of mechanisms to shape the infected cell proteome.[443] Global proteome analysis has revealed that 89% of the 927 host proteins detected on the plasma membrane of fibroblasts change by at least twofold during HCMV infection[660] and 131 host proteins are targeted during HCMV infection for proteasomal or lysosomal degradation,[443] indicating a dramatic redesign of the host proteome. Only 1% to 5% of these have a corresponding change in mRNA, indicating a high level of regulation at the protein level. HCMV is understood to regulate the proteome by targeted proteasomal and lysosomal degradation and by miRNAs that target host RNAs for suppression. For more in-depth discussion, please refer to supplementary online content: *Cell Biology of HCMV Infection 2: Regulation of the infected cell proteome.*

Regulation of Host Cell Metabolism

Viruses depend on the host cell's metabolic resources for their replication, and cellular metabolic regulation has increasingly emerged as central to a wide range of cell fate outcomes, including oncogenesis, immune cell activation, proliferation, and cell death. Given the extent of HCMV's interactions with host cell biology, it is not surprising that it extensively modulates cellular metabolism. HCMV induces central carbon metabolism, including glycolysis, glutaminolysis, tricarboxylic acid cycle, fatty acid biosynthesis, and pyrimidine synthesis, all of which have been found to support productive virus replication.[530,563] While many questions remain, HCMV-mediated modulation of cellular stress, nutrient sensing, and proliferative pathways appears to be critical for instituting a metabolic state conducive to productive viral replication.[530,563] As an obligate parasite, it can be assumed that HCMV depends on the host cell for energy and biomolecular building blocks, yet it also appears that HCMV modulates metabolic activities for the production of specific virion components.[530,563] Many questions remain regarding the impact of HCMV-induced metabolic remodeling of host metabolism beyond virus maturation. For more in-depth discussion, please refer to supplementary online content: *Cell Biology of HCMV Infection 3: Regulation of host metabolism.*

PATHOGENESIS AND PATHOLOGY

HCMV infection and transmission in most people proceeds without symptoms or disease. Clinically apparent manifestations of HCMV infection are expressed almost exclusively in the context of congenital infection and in the immunocompromised host, including transplant recipients and HIV/AIDS and cancer patients undergoing immunosuppressive chemotherapy. This virus is also an occasional cause of infectious mononucleosis. Characteristics of CMV disease are discussed in section *Clinical Features.* Numerous books, reviews, and chapters have described person-to-person transmission, dissemination, and host control characteristics that place individuals at risk for HCMV disease.[63,66] From initial infection at the mucosal epithelium, HCMV infects diverse cell types and tissues, causing a systemic infection with persistent and sporadic shedding for life, as discussed in section *Latency.*

Entry and Transmission

Community acquisition of HCMV follows mucosal exposure to virus that is shed into oral and genital fluids, urine, and breast milk. Thus, repeated exposures to infectious virus in saliva or urine leads to virus transmission in adults and young children. Individuals exposed to infants shedding virus and infants exposed to HCMV through breast-feeding are high-risk settings for infection. Approximately 50% of breast-fed infants born to HCMV seropositive women will acquire the virus in the first few months of life and subsequently shed virus in saliva and urine for prolonged periods of time during infancy, exposing others. The high incidence of transmission in these settings makes these important routes of community acquired infections worldwide.[231] Rates of transmission between children less than 2 years of age are also elevated, likely the result of frequent exchange of saliva between young children.[88] In adults, sexual transmission has been documented with virus shed into both cervical secretions and semen.[124] Mucous membrane epithelial cells are a portal of entry and produce progeny virus that spreads to microvascular endothelial and myelomonocytic leukocytes provide the means of dissemination throughout the body. In immunocompetent adults, these infected leukocytes likely seed the secretory organs such as salivary glands and kidneys and likely carry the virus to the placenta during pregnancy[476] as well as to bone marrow where this virus establishes lifelong residence.[566,576] Myeloid cell–mediated dissemination to distant tissues has been well described in MCMV models of virus dissemination.[176,177] The variety of cell types and organs that become involved depends on many poorly studied factors, including the size of the inoculum, the intensity of initial infection, innate immune clearance and, particularly, the adaptive immune response that generates antiviral antibodies and T cells.

Hospital-acquired (nosocomial) infections with HCMV can result from mucosal exposure but more often follows exposure to infected blood products or from allografts after transplantation. Transfusion of blood products from HCMV infected donors has long been known to represent a significant risk for the acquisition of HCMV and as a result, blood products from noninfected donors or that are leukocyte depleted[706] are now commonly employed for transfusion of at risk individuals such as premature infants and pediatric transplant recipients. In contrast to the success of strategies to limit HCMV infection from blood products, transmission of HCMV with any solid organ from infected donors remains a major route of HCMV infection in transplant recipients. Although HCMV is latent in myeloid progenitors, HCMV immunity is conferred along with bone marrow–derived cells in hematopoietic stem cell transplantation. The most risky setting for serious HCMV disease in HCT remains a HCMV seropositive recipient (R+) who receives a transplant from an HCMV seronegative donor (D-) because the donor cells lack immune experience with HCMV.

Intrauterine HCMV transmission from mother to the developing fetus results in cCMV infection. HCMV is transmitted *in utero* relatively frequently with congenital infection being present 0.2% to 1.0% of all live births.[297] Rates of cCMV are higher in maternal populations with increased rates of HIV infections, a finding that has been argued as evidence for the role of CD4 T cell–mediated immunity in limiting maternal to fetal HCMV transmission.[2,435] Interestingly, the increased transmission in pregnant women with poorly control HIV infection has been modeled in pregnant rhesus macaques which have been depleted of CD4+ T lymphocytes and challenged with rhesus CMV.[42] Unique to the epidemiology of cCMV infection is the observation that rates of cCMV infection are directly related to the seroprevalence of maternal population. There are examples of populations with high seroprevalence rates associated with high prevalence of cCMV in offspring.[65] Accordingly, cCMV can follow infection in both nonimmune women (primary maternal infection) as well as in women with preexisting immunity (nonprimary maternal infection).[65]

Intrauterine HCMV transmission has been proposed to follow maternal viremia that seeds the intervillous space of the placenta leading to infection of the villous, resulting in a villitis and loss of the cellular barrier that separates maternal and fetal blood. Because the human placenta is a hemochorial, only a single layer of cells, the placental syncytiotrophoblasts, separates the fetal circulation from the maternal circulation. Thus, focal loss of the barrier function provided by the syncytiotrophoblast layer is believed to lead to infection of underlying villous cytotrophoblasts and cells within the villous stroma containing fetal capillaries. Interestingly, HCMV DNA and HCMV-infected cells have been detected frequently in the decidua and from several sites in the placentas from seropositive pregnant women who did not transmit HCMV to their fetuses.[477] Given that infection of the placenta is not sufficient for intrauterine transmission, there are likely to be host determinants of transmission to the fetal circulation. Finally, infection of the decidua has been shown to be associated with the infiltration of inflammatory cells, prompting suggestions that these cells serve as a reservoir for infection of the placenta and transmission to the fetus.[184,477,662] Once HCMV enters the fetal circulation, HCMV disseminates hematogenously within the systemic circulation of the fetus.

Although there have been many studies seeking to understand immune correlates in pregnant women that may guide strategies to prevent congenital infection[358,525] as well as to prevent or treat transplacental transmission,[444] the overarching picture remains complex. Mechanisms through which antiviral antibodies, T cells, or other immune mechanisms act at the maternal–fetal interface remain to be determined.[66,476] On one hand, HCMV is able to transmit in the face of natural levels of antiviral immunity during either reacquisition or reactivation from latency even though the frequency of transplacental transmission and congenital infection is dramatically lower than during primary maternal infection. On the other hand, there has been little progress in understanding differences in virus transmission occurring in primary or recurrent infection.

Even though antiviral immunity develops following acquisition of HCMV and systemic infection is brought under control, virus continues to be shed from secretory epithelium in body fluids for weeks, months or even years. The reasons for such prolonged shedding despite evidence of antiviral immunity has not been resolved, but immune mechanisms are certainly central given that the extended pattern of shedding in young children has been related to weaker CD4 T-cell response patterns.[218,359] During asymptomatic infection, epithelial, vascular endothelial and myelomonocytic cells that support HCMV replication are also likely targets of immune modulation by viral gene functions.

Immune Response and Immune Modulation

CMVs persist for life in the face of robust antiviral immunity that reduces risk of disease and sustains lifelong latency. Antiviral immune defenses are important from the initial encounter with this virus, acting within the infected cells (cell-autonomous response) as well as locally and systemically in the host. Host defense mechanisms are counterbalanced by virus-encoded immune modulators that mold response patterns to suit viral persistence and contribute to the status of HCMV as an opportunistic pathogen. Shortly after infection, nonspecific (innate) immune mechanisms restrict virus spread, handing off to antigen-specific (adaptive) immune mechanisms that generate lifelong immune memory. Natural killer (NK) cells, together with adaptive immunity mediated via B cells (antibody) and, in particular, T cells contribute to protection from reinfection and suppression of viral reactivation. Cytotoxic CD8+ T cells in particular, maintain control over this virus; although, host control is counterbalanced by viral functions that counteract T-cell effector mechanisms.[279,390,473] Evidence supporting this key immune control includes HCMV disease susceptibility of individuals with defects in T-cell function or undergoing T cell–suppressive immunotherapy.[275,277] Antiviral CD4+ T-cell immunity correlates with control over CMV shedding during childhood[491,629] and CD8+ T-cell transfer has long been recognized for conferring a benefit in settings of severe HCMV disease risk such as HCT.[560] HCMV infection has a unique relationship with the immune system, inducing virus-specific T-cell memory that expands over time (a pattern called memory inflation), with decrease in CD4+ naïve T cells, and may reduce the ability to respond to other pathogens in old age.[276,630,664] HCMV infection shows a positive correlation with immune response parameters to other infectious agents and vaccines in small studies of young individuals, including identical twins,[68,69,196] although direct vaccination responses and host susceptibility to tuberculosis both show a negative correlation with HCMV infection.[58,424] Efforts to tie down health impacts of coinfection with HCMV in HIV-exposed newborns and children have suggested poorer outcomes[207] without any obvious impact on immune parameters.[577] Such correlations may reflect demographic or environmental factors unrelated to this particular virus,[87] such as comorbidities and other lifestyle issues, including the total number of lifelong infections.

Despite systemic HCMV-specific immunity, reinfection episodes[57] and infection with multiple strains of virus occurs relatively frequently.[139] Sporadic shedding may be high in children and young adults, but prevalence decreases with age.[20] Host immune control over HCMV is often incomplete[66] as observed in younger individuals as well as HIV-infected adults on antiretroviral therapy.[554] The extent to which host defenses are sidestepped by this virus may be ascribed to the arsenal of gene products elaborated during productive infection, persistence, and latency that act in a concerted fashion to mold cell-intrinsic, innate, and adaptive immune response parameters (see Supplementary e-Table 12.1). Because CMVs are species restricted and only infect their natural host, animal surrogates, primarily MCMV, RCMV, GPCMV, and RhCMV, have been studied in mice, rats, guinea pigs, and rhesus macaques, respectively. Information is imprecise owing to the fact that each of these surrogate models shows distinct genetic and environmental features, not the least of which is the high level of evolutionary divergence across the β-herpesvirus subgroup despite a common biology. Nevertheless, the study of such surrogates, particularly in mice and macaques has reinforced immune mechanisms that are most important in control of HCMV.[277,359] The unusual ability of CMV to superinfect, to maintain high frequencies of effector memory T cells and the ability of Rh CMV vectors lacking homologs of *UL128* and *UL130* to elicit unconventionally MHC-II-restricted and nonpolymorphic MHC-E-restricted CD8+ T-cell responses in lieu of conventionally MHC-I-restricted T cells has inspired the evaluation of HCMV vectors against immune evasive pathogens, such as HIV or TB.[191]

Immunity

Immunocompetent individuals generally retain an upper hand in the lifelong control over herpesviruses, including HCMV. Cellular immunity, both innate natural killer (NK) and adaptive T lymphocyte–mediated mechanisms, enable the host to maintain control, suppress replication, and sustain latency. Certain viral proteins, including m157-encoded NK cell activator in MCMV and the major viral tegument protein in RhCMV appear to promote host immune control over the virus. The importance of cellular immune surveillance to lifelong control over HCMV is revealed by the impact of this pathogen in immunocompromised host, supporting the importance of NK cells, helper T cells, and cytotoxic T cells in the control overactive viral infection. Sporadic virus replication in secretory epithelial cells and shedding in body fluids occurs independently of cellular immunity, but this immunity impacts systemic levels of virus. HCMV is rarely detected in the bloodstream in the immunocompetent host. Immunosuppressive therapies such as those used to prevent T cell–dependent allograft rejection following SOT suppress cellular immunity and allow active systemic virus replication detected in the bloodstream that, depending on levels, promotes the progression to disease.

NK cells are the most prominent contributors to the innate antiviral immune response. As the major subset of group 1 innate lymphoid cells (ILCs), NK cells patrol systemically for abnormal cells, such as virus-infected and transformed cells. NK cells recognize reduced levels of natural MHC class I in the face of elevated levels of infection-induced stress ligands that trigger cytotoxic clearance.[455] These innate lymphocytes, first characterized during MCMV infection, mediate early control over HCMV as well as RhCMV.[37,185,472,604] Studies of the antiviral response to HCMV and MCMV suggest that clonal expansion of NK cells following their activation upon encounter with virus-infected cells leads to lifelong memory and readiness to respond to reinfection.[3,455] In mice that carry the NK-activating Ly49H receptor (an MHC I allele characteristic of C57BL/6 mice), MCMV-encoded m157 directly engages this receptor to trigger massive proliferation of NK cells that, despite contraction, remain elevated for life. Such memory NK cells respond to restimulation in a pattern reminiscent of memory T cells, giving this innate response at least some of the characteristics of adaptive immunity.[3] In humans, NK cells capable of an adaptive response are marked by expression of heterodimeric CD94/NKG2C receptor. Cells bearing this receptor increase dramatically over time in HCMV seropositive healthy donors, although the viral function responsible for triggering such behavior remains unknown. The inflammatory and regulatory cytokines that control NK cell expansion are better understood in MCMV-infected mice than in HCMV-infected humans. Overall the cytokine requirements for selection, expansion, contraction, and maintenance appear similar to T-cell expansion in response to viral antigen,[3] although this may be a consequence of MCMV m157 as a virus-specific activating ligand.[37,185] Much less is known about response and memory of NK cells that are activated independently of the m157–Ly49H axis, though m157-independent NK responses have been characterized.[197,436]

There is such an overwhelming and sustained expansion of antiviral T cells to CMVs that studies have sought to determine whether lifelong HCMV infection influences life span and other aspects of healthy aging.[217] Although a clear picture is yet to emerge, the commitment that most individuals make to control of HCMV is exceptionally robust. This may be important because individuals without adequate cellular immunity are at increased risk of disease, as occurs in seropositive recipients of allogenic HCT transplants from HCMV-naïve donors as compared to allogeneic transplants from MHC-matched HCMV immune donors.[560] In such settings, despite sustained serum antibody levels, host control is highly dependent on levels of memory T cells that are absent in HCMV naïve donors. Control over HCMV may be enhanced by direct transfer of MHC-matched CMV-specific CD8+ T-cell therapy. There are also specific settings where antiviral antibody contributes to host control over infection, through neutralization as well as other antibody-dependent mechanisms. Anti-HCMV antibody makes a contribution to host resistance, best illustrated by the long-standing observation that transferred maternal antibody prevents transfusion-acquired HCMV in low birth weight infants. In addition, an envelope gB subunit vaccine candidate reduces rates of infection in HCMV naive women, possibly through antibody-mediated mechanisms.[280] Protection conferred by other viral envelope glycoproteins such as the gH/gL pentamer has not yet been evaluated.[552,634] In line with the expectation that antibody directed against viral glycoproteins would protect, there is growing interest in the potential for intravenous gammaglobulin enrichs for HCMV-specific antibodies to provide prophylactic benefit by limiting intrauterine HCMV transmission or even therapeutic benefit by limiting the congenital disease.[444]

MHC class I restricted cytotoxic CD8 T effector cells are the single most important host defense pathway responsible for controlling lifelong HCMV infection,[275,277,571] as first recognized in studies with MCMV.[487] Further insights have emerged from observational studies on clinically relevant HCMV reactivation in immunocompromised patients receiving immunosuppressive therapies that reduce cell-mediated immune surveillance, particularly in the context of SOT or HCT.[560] The appearance of active systemic infection in transplant recipients begins with triggering events that involve inflammatory cytokines, potentially acting to stimulate activation or differentiation of myeloid cells in which latent virus resides. These events compromise cell intrinsic host control mechanisms favoring reactivation (see section *Latency*). In the natural infection setting, major histocompatibility antigen mismatch triggers tissue rejection that is also associated with the production of inflammatory cytokines such as TNF.[534] These contributions are supported by studies in MCMV[130,259] in addition to direct evaluation of HCMV.[186] Most recently, SOT studies in MCMV-infected mice have brought to light a potential role of organ ischemia–reperfusion independently of MHC class I mismatch[700] that deserves additional investigation. Disease results when viral levels, as assessed by measuring viral DNA in whole blood or plasma, rise above a threshold that informs preemptive approaches for therapeutic intervention.[66]

Although viral infection is systemic, HCMV disease generally affects a particular tissue, particular organs, such as lungs, gastrointestinal tract or liver, or specific sites such as the retinal neuroepithelium or vascular endothelium. The pattern of disease suggests that immune/inflammatory signals act in concert with viral replication levels despite the immunocompromised state of the individual.[66] Analogous events likely occur in other settings where HCMV reactivation contributes to disease, such as during pregnancy in seropositive women, where reactivation and amplification precede transplacental transmission to the fetus. The cellular arm of the immune response is responsible for protection in transplant settings based on three considerations: (a) when cellular immunity is compromised, virus reactivation risk increases and classic opportunistic disease consequences follow, (b) therapies that disrupt cellular immunity, particular CD8-dependent cytotoxic T effector cells, pose the greatest threat, and (c) adoptive T-cell therapy prevents disease. Virus-specific antibody is likely to contribute to protection from exogenous infection and transplacental transmission but appears to be less critical overall for control of HCMV. Importantly, these host defense mechanisms operate despite the arsenal of immune modulators encoded by this virus.

Immune Modulation

HCMV commits the majority of its genome coding capacity to altering host defense against infection (Supplementary e-Tables 12.1 and 12.2). All classes of viral gene products expressed during productive replication (IE, E, and L) as well as latency-associated proteins and noncoding RNAs make major contributions to modulation of the host response to infection. Notably, viral genes committed to immune modulation are themselves typically dispensable for replication within cultured fibroblasts. These are sometimes lost spontaneously from laboratory strains over the course of passage in cell culture. Modulatory activity has typically been revealed experimentally by expressing an isolated viral gene product and characterized as sufficient to suppress some specific immune pathway. The necessity for particular virus-encoded modulators to have an impact on a particular pathway can only be established using infected cells, typically comparing mutant viruses to a parental strain. Human host specificity limits full evaluation of individual HCMV-encoded modulatory gene products, driving interest in use of surrogate animal betaherpesvirus models. There are three major categories of modulatory functions: (a) gene products acting within the infected cell (intrinsic or autonomous) to restrict infection, including those that impact gene regulation, pathogen sensing, cellular metabolism, cell cycle, and cell death pathways; (b) gene products acting within the host organism in concert with innate immune mechanisms, including those that affect inflammatory cytokine and NK cell responses; and, (c) gene products acting within the host organism at the adaptive immune level, modulating either elicitation or execution of antigen-specific T- and B-lymphocyte responses. Many viral functions target immune effector mechanisms that are dependent on lymphocytes. In addition to modulatory functions that evade host clearance mechanisms, virus-encoded proteins and RNAs also exploit host response pathways. The arsenal of virus-encoded modulators ensures the success of viral infection, supporting systemic dissemination, sporadic shedding, and persistence. As with other herpesviruses, major viral regulatory and replication functions often carry secondary roles in modulating the host cell response.[4] These functions make a substantial commitment to suppressing pathogen sensing, IRF3 and NF-κB activation, type I IFN induction, and the antiviral consequences of IFN-dependent host defense pathways as well as INF-independent host-encoded restriction factors,[28,45,153,211] as overviewed in earlier sections.

Each HCMV-encoded immune modulator targets one or more steps in a host defense pathway, most often dampening the impact of the pathway. Despite elaboration of many such modulators, the host defense mechanisms against which they are deployed have proved important in the control of infection. Thus, HCMV commits substantial coding potential towards functions that modulate innate NK- and adaptive T-cell immune mechanisms that are also recognized to control infection. CMVs that infect different, even closely related animal species typically encode modulatory functions that target different points in otherwise conserved host defense pathways. Remarkably, each species of CMV appears to have coevolved within the mammalian species with which it is associated today. CMVs do not appear to jump from species to species. This species-specific evolution produced different solutions to the general problem of how to evade a common set of host immune effector mechanisms.

Although many host pathways have been shown to be suppressed by HCMV gene products, this virus also enhances specific immune pathways, including the production of certain cytokines and chemokines that recruit and activate immune cells as well as deployment of virus-encoded chemokine receptors to modulate myeloid cell behavior. These functions exploit cytokine-dependent signaling to benefit the virus.[28,76,212,279,345,422,472,473] On balance, there are more virus-encoded inhibitors than there are functions that exploit immune stimulation. Stimulated pathways are nevertheless likely to provide the signature features of HCMV infection, persistence, and disease. Virus-encoded functions that either modulate or mimic cytokine and chemokine pathways serve important roles in infection, orchestrating immune cell development, homeostasis, and trafficking in the interests of the virus. Important examples of exploitation include HCMV-encoded *UL138* enhancement of TNFR1[344,421] and EGFR,[77] conferring increased sensitivity to cytokine (TNF) and growth factor (EGF) stimulation, viral US28-encoded chemokine receptor acting constitutively as well as following stimulation by host CC and CX3C chemokines, and viral *UL146*-encoded vCXCL1 recruitment of leukocytes bearing hCXCR1 and hCXCR2. These positive-acting modulators potentially shape the antiviral immune response as much as those that suppress immune pathways. Furthermore, UL138 and US28 have an impact on latency, but it is important to recognize that these potent positive-acting immune modulators are expressed at all times of infection.

Modulation of Cell Autonomous Response to Infection

CMVs encode many gene products that alter the cell-intrinsic response of infected cells and production of cytokines, particularly type I IFN.[28,153,212,345] HCMV counteracts host cell sensing and restriction metered out via cGAS-STING, IFI16, ZBP1, ND10-Sp100-hDaxx complex, SPOC1 and GAL-9, and MxB together with the effectors controlled by pathogen sensors and the IFN response.[153] Impacts on epigenetic regulation via LUNA, IE72, and pp71/UL35 affects replication, latency, and reactivation. NF-κB, IRF3, and IFN are all targeted by viral proteins as well as by lncRNA1.2.[340] Other IE proteins assure that viral and cellular transcriptional regulators remain balanced as described in section *Pre-IE Events and Intrinsic Responses to Infection* and ensure survival of the infected cells by inhibiting cell death. *UL36*-encoded vICA and UL37x1-encoded viral mitochondrial inhibitor of apoptosis (vMIA) are cell death suppressors whose mechanisms are well understood and whose functions are evolutionarily conserved in MCMV and HCMV.[71] In addition, studies of MCMV M45-encoded viral inhibitor of RIP activation (vIRA) brought the unique host defense value of necroptosis to light. Cell death suppressor vMIA has a direct impact on the timing and death pathways elaborated during infection of cultured cells, and the function of vICA provides broad protection from the death consequences of TNF signaling[391] as described in *Cell Biology of HCMV Infection 1: Regulation of Cell Death*.

Modulation of the Innate Immune Response to Infection

HCMV modulates cytokine signaling and encodes cytokine, chemokines, and chemokine receptors. The *UL22A* gene product is a secreted CC chemokine sponge, suggesting that attraction of certain leukocytes to sites of infection is discouraged. US28 responds to some of the same CC chemokines targeted by UL22A but in addition is a receptor for CX3CR1/fractalkine, a chemokine system that supports leukocyte patrolling the bloodstream. The balance of constitutive US28 activity and chemokine-induced activation has many effected on infected cells and viral dissemination (see section *Latency*). Virus-encoded UL146 is a potent CXCL8/IL-8–like chemokine (vCXCL1) that recruits cells expressing CXCR1 or CXCR2, including granulocytes (neutrophils) and monocytes.[274] The recruitment of these populations alters the inflammatory environment and likely facilitates viral dissemination.[241]

NK cells eliminate virus-infected cells, produce antiviral cytokines, and recruit and activate T cells. They are crucial for control over herpesviruses based on the susceptibility of individuals with NK-cell primary immunodeficiencies.[153] HCMV encodes a remarkably expansive set of gene products aimed at disarming the innate NK-cell response.[153,472] In humans, where the NKG2C receptor–positive NK cells become a long-lived memory population[3,153,185] the initial expansion appears to be mediated by a long-recognized UL40 leader peptide presented in HLA-E, a ligand for the activating CD94/NKG2C receptor[230] that may influence CD8+ T cells as well.[286] HCMV manipulates the availability of ligands for the NKG2D receptor, all stress-induced ligands rarely displayed on healthy cells that, when present, trigger NK-mediated destruction. These MHC class I–like family proteins (MICA, MICB and ULBP1 to ULBP6) contain alpha domains but do not bind β2-microglobulin-like conventional MHC class I and are targeted for degradation by viral modulators. MICA is targeted by UL142, UL148A, US9, US18, and US20, possibly because there are many allelic variants of this stress signal. MICB is targeted by noncoding RNA miR-UL112 as well as UL16, a promiscuous modulator that also targets ULBP1, ULBP2, and ULBP6. UL142 targets ULBP3 and US18 and US20 target B7-H6, a ligand for NKp30, in addition to MICA. Other adhesion molecules that are ligands for NK CD226/DNAM-1 are targeted by UL141, which also inhibits TRAIL-dependent NK activity, and US2, most well known as an MHC class I inhibitor. Finally, MHC class I–like UL18 on the infected cell surface engages NK inhibitory receptor LIR1/ILT2. Other adhesion proteins on infected cells are impacted by UL148. This multitude of functions supports viral evasion of NK cell killing although they do not prevent control via this host defense pathway.

Modulation of Adaptive Immune Response to Infection

Natural HCMV infection is highly immunogenic, resulting in broad humoral antibody as well as cellular T-lymphocyte responses that persist for life and maintain control over the virus. Nevertheless, HCMV encodes a wide range of functions that disarm both the elicitation and the execution of the adaptive immune response. Classical DCs carry out antigen presentation. Both Langerhans cells and myeloid DCs are susceptible to HCMV infection and are likely to be impacted by viral modulation of MHC class I antigen presentation, particularly by US2, US11, and major viral tegument proteins pp65 and pp71. The elaboration of cmvIL-10 results in the activation of DC-SIGN, potentially increasing susceptibility to infection, altering the behavior of lymphocytes, and inhibiting DC functions to aid viral escape from the full brunt of adaptive immunity.

T-cell immune surveillance provides crucial control preventing amplification of virus throughout life. Some of the first HCMV-encoded immunomodulatory functions discovered downmodulate the ability of T cells to recognize HCMV-infected cells.[473] Thus, classical and nonclassical MHC class I antigen presentation is targeted by US2, US3, US6, and US11, as well as US8 and US10. UL144 triggers coinhibitory receptors on infected cells, and UL11 drives cellular IL-10 production to dovetail with viral *UL111A*-encoded cmvIL-10,[29] altogether impeding T-cell activation and effector function to the benefit of the viral persistence.[489] Importantly, cmvIL-10 is detected in the bloodstream of healthy HCMV-seropositive individuals consistent with experimental studies showing its impact on the host immune environment.[689] The ability of viral IL-10 to tag-team with host regulatory cytokines is shared with RhCMV.[168] Although each of these modulatory functions is sufficient to have an impact, it is important to note that host antiviral CD8+ T cells remain essential in lifelong immune control over systemic levels of HCMV, although specific modulation of CD4+ T cells potentially relates to patterns of viral shedding. Deletion mutant unable to reactivate from latent infection retain the ability to induce effector memory T-cell responses, providing a potential live attenuated HCMV vaccine or vector.[90] The qualities of the human immune response directed against HCMV represent the consequences of an ancient evolutionary relationship between a multitude of viral modulators and mechanisms of host defense.

EPIDEMIOLOGY

Prevalence and Epidemiology in Populations

HCMV is ubiquitous in all populations in the world with rates of infection as determined by serological evidence of infection (seroprevalence) ranging from 45% to 100% worldwide.[87] There are nearly universal rates of infection in South America, Africa, and Asia, and lower seroprevalence is reported in the United States and in some countries in northern Europe. In populations with high rates of HCMV seroprevalence, HCMV is acquired early in childhood such that by late adolescence, most individuals are infected. In the United States and in some countries in northern Europe, HCMV seroprevalence has been shown to vary between different racial and ethnic groups and is dependent on socioeconomic status resulting in the epidemiology of HCMV in some urban populations in the United States and Europe being more similar to populations in South America and Asia.[173,189,351] Sources of virus that are associated with increased rates of virus acquisition in community settings include breast-feeding, exposure to young children, crowded living conditions, group child care, and poverty.[231,261,589,701] HCMV is considered a sexually transmitted infection (STI); thus the seroprevalence in sexually active populations is increased and risk factors for acquisition of other STIs are also linked to HCMV infection.[590]

As with other human pathogens, the average age of initial acquisition depends on frequency of contacts as well as hygiene. Although breast-feeding in areas of high seroprevalence contributes substantially to early acquisition, most transmission in the world occurs early in life in direct correlation with crowding and contact frequency, features that were first established by observing transmission patterns in day care centers.[63]

Reacquisition of HCMV throughout life apparently occurs frequently in certain populations[36] despite the apparent benefit of adaptive antiviral immunity, with the consequence of that lifelong mixed infection appears more prevalent in some populations. The ability of HCMV to overcome levels of natural antiviral immunity remains a recognized concern for vaccine development. Women, as well as men, under the age of 50 who carry HCMV from childhood represent a reservoir where sporadic reactivation and shedding in urine (as well as saliva, vaginal secretions, seminal fluid, and breast milk) contribute to spread. The U.S. population sheds virus in urine between 3% and 10% of the time, decreasing with age.[20]

Genetic Diversity

Studies utilizing next generation sequencing NGS have described considerable genetic sequence diversity in virus populations even within a single individual and have provided evidence that HCMV infection is usually associated with transmission of a population of viruses with diverse genotypes.[139,465,485,521] Although there is debate about the extent of genetic diversity in viral populations from different patient populations, there is agreement that population of viruses can replace existing populations of viruses in patients who are reinfected (superinfected) by an exogenous source of virus.[139,485] The source of the genetic diversity of HCMV likely involves recombination events between viruses with different viral genotypes.[139] In addition, genetic diversity is believed to follow selection of viral mutants secondary to exposure to different pressures during virus replication such as host antiviral immune responses, antiviral therapies, or the presence of genetic bottlenecks secondary to restricted replication in different host compartments following virus dissemination.[485] Lastly, it has been argued that the generation of genetic diversity by recombination between different viral genotypes is a relatively slow process that can explain HCMV evolution but is inconsistent with divergence of viral populations within a single individual over a short period of time.[607] Thus, the increased genetic diversity that has been observed in some individuals is believed to reflect the acquisition of new populations of viruses and potentially, the *de novo* expansion of genetic variants.

Mechanisms that contribute to the observed genetic diversity in HCMV isolates have considerable relevance to the natural history of perinatal HCMV infections. Maternal nonprimary HCMV infections during pregnancy account for most cases of congenital HCMV infection, yet the source of these infections remains poorly defined in most maternal populations.[434,651] Two mechanisms have been suggested: (a) reactivation of virus during pregnancy in a previously infected women and spread to the developing fetus, and (b) exogenous infection with a new and genetically diverse populations of HCMV.[64] Even though virus reactivation leading to a recurrent infection represents a decades-old paradigm, evidence supporting this mechanism cannot be considered definitive because of limitations in methodologies used to establish this paradigm in these early studies. Exogenous reinfection of previously infected women as a mechanism for nonprimary maternal infection is supported by several findings including (a) early studies that demonstrated sequential infection by new viral genotypes in normal infants and children in group care settings, (b) epidemiological associations between nonprimary infections and known exposures risks for virus acquisition, (c) sequential recovery of genetically divergent viruses from women attending an STI clinic, and (d) evidence of serological conversion to a new "serotype" of HCMV in women undergoing nonprimary infection during pregnancy with subsequent transmission their fetus.[36,52,531,687] Although ongoing studies will more definitively address the importance of genetic diversity of HCMV in maternal nonprimary infections, defining the source of HCMV infection in previously infected women is of considerable importance to current strategies to induce protective immunity through vaccination of women of childbearing age.

CLINICAL FEATURES

Immunocompetent Host

Community acquisition of HCMV is sometimes associated with mild influenza-like symptoms or infectious mononucleosis, but disease is typically self-limiting. Although HCMV infections are common in all age groups, clinically apparent infection is infrequent in every age group. Early studies described an infectious mononucleosis syndrome similar to that described in EBV infection and estimated that HCMV could account for 20% of cases of heterophile negative infectious mononucleosis. Although clinical and laboratory findings in cases of HCMV mononucleosis are nonspecific, individuals with HCMV mononucleosis and those with asymptomatic infection can shed infectious virus in the saliva, urine, and genital secretions for prolonged periods of time. In young children and in particular, infants infected in the postnatal period, high levels of virus shedding can persist for months and, in some cases, years after infection and thus, likely represent a major source of community exposure to HCMV.[86]

Perinatal Infections

Perinatal HCMV infections include infants infected *in utero* (congenital infection, cCMV), during birth, and following exposure to virus containing breast milk. Of these, cCMV infections are the most important. cCMV infection is the most frequent viral infection acquired *in utero* with a prevalence of 2 to 10 per 1,000 live births. More than one million new congenital infections are predicted to occur each year worldwide with 20% of these babies showing damage either present at birth or developing over the first few years of life. About 30% of women undergoing a primary HCMV infection during pregnancy transmit virus to their offspring with virus transmission to the fetus being highest in the late 2nd and 3rd trimester, but reported in all trimesters of pregnancy.[172,297] Intrauterine transmission in the late 1st trimester and early 2nd trimester is associated with a greater likelihood of clinical abnormalities at birth (symptomatic infection), central nervous system (CNS) damage, and long-term neurodevelopmental abnormalities.[172,178] Transmission rates following nonprimary maternal infections remain undefined, and definitive data demonstrating that maternal immunity prior to pregnancy can limit intrauterine transmission are limited.[65] Notably, the incidence of symptomatic infection and neurodevelopmental sequelae in infants infected *in utero* following a nonprimary maternal infection is strikingly similar to that in infants infected *in utero* after primary maternal infection.[62,614,627] Lastly, the incidence of hearing loss, the most frequent long-term sequelae in infants with cCMV infection, appears similar in infected infants regardless if born to women with primary or nonprimary infections during pregnancy.[532,686] Thus, the role of preexisting maternal adaptive immunity in the natural history of cCMV infection, in modifying both intrauterine transmission and the consequences of intrauterine infection, remains incompletely defined and impacts strategies to limit disease by prophylactic vaccines.

Overall, about 90% of infants with cCMV have asymptomatic infections with 10% having clinical findings associated with intrauterine infection. Clinical and laboratory findings in infants with symptomatic infections are described in Table 12.1. Nearly 50% of infants with symptomatic infection will have long-term neurodevelopmental sequelae while about 10% to 15% of infants with asymptomatic infection will have long-term neurodevelopmental abnormalities. Long-term sequelae of cCMV are limited almost exclusively to the CNS and can include severe neurodevelopmental findings in infants with microcephaly and structural brain damage, findings present in about 35% of infants with symptomatic infection and overall, less than 5% of all infants with cCMV infections.[162] More frequently, infants with symptomatic infection exhibit delayed neurodevelopment, hearing loss, disorders in balance, and, rarely, visual disturbances. Sequelae in infants with asymptomatic infections are most often limited to hearing loss and balance disturbances. While viral burden appears to be related to the severity of cCMV infection,[51] recent results from animal models of CNS disease in infants with cCMV suggest that the pathogenesis of the CNS infection in infants with cCMV cannot be attributed solely to virus replication and that other mechanisms of disease including virus-induced neuroinflammation could contribute to CNS damage.[558] Lastly, infants with cCMV, regardless whether with symptomatic or asymptomatic infections, shed large amounts of virus, sometimes on the order of 10^6 genomes/mL of urine or saliva for years and thus serve as a reservoir for spread of HCMV to other infants and adult caretakers.[86]

HCMV infection acquired during birth or early in the perinatal period rarely result in clinical symptoms and long-term sequelae in term infants. In contrast, premature infants infected in the postnatal period can develop severe infections with multiorgan disease. More recently, the importance of HCMV infection in premature infants exposed to HCMV containing breast milk from seropositive women has been well documented as a cause of clinically significant infections, including hepatitis, pneumonitis, and sepsis-like syndromes; however, quantifying the importance of HCMV infection to long-term neurodevelopmental outcomes in these infants has been confounded by the impact of prematurity on neurodevelopment.

Opportunistic Infections in Immunocompromised Hosts

Serious HCMV disease generally follows when virus levels rise above a threshold, such as in immunocompromised people with genetic or acquired immunodeficiency or when subjected to immunosuppressive therapy, after transplantation or during cancer chemotherapy.[66,217] HCMV pathogenesis in the immunocompromised first came to attention in solid organ transplant recipients[663] but rose to prominence with the AIDS epidemic.[245]

HIV/AIDS

Prior to remarkable success achieved by antiretroviral therapies (ART) for HIV/AIDS, HCMV was one of the most common opportunistic infection in patients with HIV/AIDS. Not only was HCMV a major cause of end organ disease, but HCMV DNAemia was strongly associated with more rapid progression to AIDS defining illnesses and mortality in individuals with HIV.[584] Common clinical manifestations of end-organ disease associated with HCMV infections included esophagitis, colitis, hepatitis, and, unique to HIV-infected hosts, retinitis. Although HCMV retinitis has been rarely reported even in the most immunocompromised transplant recipients, prior to the availability of ART HCMV retinitis was commonly diagnosed in patients with AIDS.[608] Currently, HCMV end-organ disease is relatively infrequent and is observed only in untreated HIV/AIDS patients or those with poorly controlled HIV infection.

Solid Organ Transplantation

Herpesvirus infections in allograft recipients are frequent in the posttransplant period secondary to transplant protocols and immunosuppressive agents that limit both adaptive and innate responses. Infections with HCMV are perhaps the most common and occur in a significant number of SOT recipients, depending on specific risk factors. Although a risk stratification based on the HCMV immune status of the SOT recipient was established decades ago, it remains relevant for all but the most immunosuppressed SOT recipients. The highest risk category is an allograft from a seropositive donor transplanted into a seronegative recipient (D+/R−), whereas the lowest risk is an allograft from a seronegative donor transplanted in a seronegative recipient (D−/R−). The transplantation of an allograft from a seropositive (or seronegative) donor into a seropositive recipient (D+/R+ or D−/R+) represents an intermediate risk. In addition to these risk stratifications, the selection of T lymphocyte–depleting agents used to prevent early graft rejection are also major determinants of the risk for HCMV infections. The use of a polyvalent rabbit antithymocyte globulin (ATG) may result in a higher risk of severe infection than treatment with monoclonal antibodies against CD25 or CD52.[244,624,667] These and other data argue strongly for the critical role HCMV-specific T-cell immunity plays in the control of HCMV in SOT recipients, a finding that was first described in the 1980s and that now has been translated into quantitative assays of HCMV-specific T-cell reactivity to refine estimates of the risk for HCMV infection and disease in SOT recipients.[331]

The clinical spectrum of HCMV infection in the early posttransplant period of SOT recipients ranges from a collection of clinical findings and symptoms described as the CMV syndrome to organ- and life-threatening end organ disease. The CMV syndrome is perhaps the most common presentation of HCMV infection in SOT recipients and includes fever, fatigue, low white blood counts, reactive lymphocytes, elevated hepatic transaminases, and HCMV DNAemia.[374] Other manifestations of HCMV infection in the early posttransplant period are described in Table 12.2. In contrast to a direct role for HCMV in end organ disease in the early posttransplant period that is likely related to virus replication, the contribution of HCMV to chronic rejection and graft loss in the late posttransplant period is well appreciated but poorly defined mechanistically. HCMV infection has been associated with loss of cardiac allografts secondary to graft rejection and the development of characteristic histopathological findings associated with narrowing of the lumen of coronary arteries of the allograft termed cardiac allograft vasculopathy (CAV).[152,283] Although mechanisms leading to CAV remain undefined, the combination of ongoing allograft rejection and HCMV replication appears to hasten the loss of the allograft.[278] Similarly, HCMV has been linked to chronic rejection and loss of renal allografts with characteristic histopathological findings of tubulointerstitial nephritis and tubular atrophy.[166,461,580] Animal models of both CAV and chronic renal allograft rejection have provided evidence consistent with the contribution of HCMV to chronic allograft rejection, including a direct role for HCMV infection of relevant cell types in the allograft.[266,601,602]

Hematopoietic Cell Transplantation

HCMV infection or reactivation in HCT recipients has been associated with decreased survival, including decreased survival unrelated to relapse of the underlying malignancy.[215,617] HCMV infection can be demonstrated in about 50% of HCT recipients and depends on several risk factors for HCMV acquisition and/or reactivation. A significant risk for HCMV in HCT is previous HCMV infection in the recipient such that the highest risk category is donor seronegative and recipient seropositive (D−/R+) while the combination of donor seropositive and recipient seronegative (D+/R−) represents an intermediate risk category. This risk stratification is in contrast to donor/risk stratification in SOT presumably because the risk for HCMV transmission from a seropositive donor is dependent on the number of nucleated cells in the graft and the efficiency of transmission relative to that of an infected allograft in SOT is reduced.[464,478] Other risk factors for HCMV infection that have been identified are related to the level of suppression of adaptive immune responses and include specific T lymphocyte–depleting strategies, MHC (HLA) mismatches between donor and recipient, umbilical cord stem cell transplantation into seropositive recipients, and graft versus host disease requiring steroid therapy.[394,573] The clinical findings in HCT transplant recipients with HCMV infection range from virus shedding to life-threatening end organ disease, such as HCMV pneumonia (Table 12.2). In these severely immunocompromised populations, differentiating patients with asymptomatic virus shedding from those who will progress to end-organ disease and thus benefit from aggressive interventions with antiviral agents remains a significant challenge. Lastly, an issue that continues to complicate HCT in a small but significant number of recipients is the development of late-onset HCMV disease after discontinuation of antiviral prophylaxis.[27,48] Clinically, late-onset disease can have mortality rates as high as 50%.[174] Analogous to the role of adaptive immune response in the control of HCMV in the early transplant period, individuals with late-onset disease appear to have persistent deficits in HCMV-specific T-lymphocyte responses.[48,141,182]

Associations With Other Diseases Including Chronic Disease

HCMV infections have been associated with a spectrum of human diseases for which specific etiologies remain undefined. In some cases, HCMV has been proposed to exacerbate the underlying mechanism of disease such as the proposed role of HCMV in vasculature disease including coronary artery disease

TABLE 12.2 Clinical manifestations of HCMV infections in solid organ transplant recipients

Clinical Findings	Laboratory Findings
CMV syndrome • Fever • Fatigue • Nonspecific clinical findings	• Decreased white blood cells • Decreased platelets • Reactive lymphocytes • Elevation of hepatic transaminases • HCMV DNAemia
End organ disease • Gastrointestinal disease, including esophagitis, colitis, and hepatitis • Pulmonary disease with increasing oxygen requirements • Central nervous system findings consistent with encephalitis	• HCMV DNAemia • Elevation of hepatic transaminases • Biopsy evidence of HCMV infection • Abnormal lung imaging findings • HCMV positive bronchoalveolar lavage fluid • CSF pleocytosis • Abnormal CNS imaging findings
Allograft dysfunction	• Declining graft function • Evidence of graft rejection

through its contribution to both local and systemic inflammation.[138,528] HCMV has also been associated with human cancers, including glioblastoma.[119,343] Studies from a number of laboratories have consistently demonstrated the presence of HCMV-encoded proteins or viral nucleic acids in tissues from human glioblastoma and animal models have provided evidence for a contribution of HCMV to malignant phenotype of these tumors, yet a mechanistic role for HCMV in this human cancer remains to be defined.[167] Diseases commonly associated with lifelong HCMV infection include other cancers, inflammatory syndromes, chronic periodontal disease, neurodegenerative diseases, and immune deterioration as individuals age.[281]

In contrast to these associations, HCMV infections have been more convincingly argued to contribute to the immune dysfunction observed in older individuals.[446] The immune dysfunction associated with HCMV has been attributed to the large proportion of the adaptive immune response directed against this persistent virus.[312] Studies have demonstrated that in normal individuals persistently infected with HCMV, up to 15% of circulating T lymphocytes will have reactivity specifically for HCMV.[610] The commitment of significant proportion of the normal T-cell repertoire to HCMV is thought to contribute to immune dysfunction described in older individuals, although recent studies have argued against restriction of the T-cell repertoire by HCMV infection or loss of function of T cells as explanations for the immune dysfunction in the elderly.[363] HCMV infections have also been proposed to increase the severity of the clinical course of patients with bacterial sepsis through mechanisms that do not appear directly related to virus replication.[360,392] Lastly, HCMV infection as defined by the presence of HCMV DNAemia or HCMV in biopsy specimens has been considered to be a cofactor in the exacerbations of inflammatory bowel disease (IBD), particularly ulcerative colitis.[120,157,347] The role of HCMV in exacerbations of intestinal inflammation in patients with IBD remains to be defined, but recent studies have suggested that HCMV infection could induce a proinflammatory phenotype in lamina propria macrophages.[154] In summary, these examples of interactions between HCMV and the adaptive and innate immune systems argue that persistence of this virus and its capacity to induce a variety of proinflammatory responses that could, in turn, negatively impact human health, at least in later years. Curiously, the overall elevation of immune markers in matched HCMV-seropositive and -naive twins together with a direct correlation of long-term HCMV infection with better vaccine responses in young adults has suggested this infection comes with benefits to the host.[68]

DIAGNOSIS

Characteristic cytomegalic cells are present in the epithelium lining the secretory ducts of the salivary glands, kidney, lactating breast, vaginal tract, seminal vesicles, and placenta of both immunocompromised adults or congenitally infected newborns and asymptomatic immunocompetent individuals, consistent with ubiquitous patterns of persistent shedding and transmission across the general population[20] as well as across the placenta.[63,66] Within the host HCMV remains cell associated such that common patterns of shedding in saliva and urine originates from infected epithelial cells in secretory organs. In other secretions such as semen and breast milk, both cell-free and cell-associated viruses have been observed. Whether present in healthy or diseased tissues, or in cultured cells, HCMV cytopathology coincides with late-phase productive infection (Fig. 12.13) in which enlarged cells take on a kidney-shaped nucleus distorted by a distinct cytoplasmic inclusion formed by the viral assembly compartment (Fig. 12.12).

Viral nucleic acid amplification technologies (NAATs) and viral antigen detection represent contemporary approaches for the laboratory diagnosis of HCMV infections. Virus-specific serology, including IgM testing and IgG avidity assays, remains an important tool for detection of both recent and previous HCMV infection (Table 12.3). The detection of HCMV DNA by quantitative PCR is the most frequently employed approach for the diagnosis of HCMV infection, and serial measurements of viral DNA has largely replaced other assays for virological monitoring patients at risk for invasive HCMV infection. Harmonization of the results from NAAT assays reported from laboratories in different centers has been attempted because center-specific methodologies have often confounded the interpretation of viral loads that have been reported in clinical studies.[192,240,505] In contrast to the experience in monitoring of transplant patients, successful application of qPCR assays to large-scale screening of newborn infants for HCMV shedding was accomplished in a multi-institutional study (CHIMES) using a saliva-based qPCR assay.[53] Detection of HCMV nucleic acids in tissues from biopsy by *in situ* DNA hybridization represents a sensitive approach to identify invasive HCMV infections by providing definitive evidence of HCMV in tissues from infected individuals. Viral antigen detection by immunohistochemistry remains a standard approach to complement routine histopathology of tissue specimens from patients suspected of having invasive HCMV disease and often provides evidence of HCMV infection with a greater sensitivity than that achieved with routine histologic stains.

The demonstration of HCMV-specific antibody reactivity has been long recognized as a reliable approach for the detection of HCMV infection and remains a standard laboratory approach for identification of infected individuals, for seroprevalence studies, and in stratifying risk for HCMV infection in allograft donors and recipients. Although the detection of HCMV-specific anti-IgM antibodies in immunocompetent individual has been used to estimate recent infection with HCMV, results from this assay can be confounded by the persistence of anti-HCMV IgM antibodies for months following primary infection in some individuals and limited sensitivity secondary to low titers of HCMV-specific anti-IgM antibodies. Modification of standard assays for anti-HCMV IgG antibodies by the inclusion of chaotropes such as urea to disrupt IgG antibody binding to HCMV antigens have been used to classify anti-HCMV IgG binding antibody responses into high and low avidity as an estimate of the duration of the IgG responses following primary HCMV infection. This assay has been used to identify pregnant women undergoing primary infection with only IgG anti-HCMV reactivity and without evidence of IgG seroconversion during pregnancy. The IgG avidity assay as well as most standard serological assays have limited use in monitoring transplant populations in the posttransplant period because of the confounder of immunosuppressive therapies.

TABLE 12.3 Diagnostic approaches for detection of HCMV infection

Assay	Application	Characteristics
Traditional assays		
Virus Isolation	Recovery infectious virus from clinical specimens	Dependent on quality of clinical material; prolonged culture periods; low sensitivity
Histopathology	Identification of HCMV infected with typical inclusions (owl-eyes)	Routine tissue processing; low sensitivity
Contemporary assays		
Nucleic acid amplification (NAT)	Quantitation of HCMV DNA in variety of specimens	Rapid, sensitive, and quantitative; can be used to define viral genotypes
DNA *in-situ* hybridization	Semiquantitative, sensitive detection of HCMV DNA in tissue	Technically challenging; long turnaround times
Viral antigen detection (Immunohistochemistry)	Sensitive detection of HCMV in tissue, blood cells, and infected cells in tissue culture	Rapid; technically straightforward; semiquantitative
HCMV-specific IgM serology	Identification of recent infections	Limited by variability in duration of response and low titers of IgM antibodies
HCMV-specific IgG serology	Detection of past infection with HCMV; seroprevalence studies; risk stratification for allograft recipients	Rapid; technically straightforward; quantitative
HCMV-specific IgG avidity	Useful to estimate duration of HCMV infection when only IgG serological reactivity present	Interpretation limited to high and low values of avidity; not of value in allograft recipients

PREVENTION AND CONTROL

Treatment/Antivirals and Antiviral Resistance

Antiviral agents have been used to control HCMV infections in allograft recipients, individuals with HIV/AIDS, and, more recently, infants with cCMV infections. With the advent of ART, the number of HIV/AIDS patients with invasive HCMV infections has fallen significantly, and currently, HCMV infections in allograft recipients represent the most frequent indication for HCMV antiviral therapy. Approaches for antiviral treatment of HCMV infections in transplant recipients include (a) prophylaxis in which antiviral drugs are given immediately after transplantation and continued for the period of most significant immunosuppression and (b) preemptive therapy in which transplant recipients are monitored intensively during the posttransplant period and treatment initiated when quantitative assays indicate increasing virus replication. It should be noted that current antiviral therapies have provided clear clinical benefit but overall, there remains an unmet for more effective antiviral agents and treatment strategies. The superiority of one strategy for improving outcomes of allograft recipients remains to be determined. Lastly, treatment of infants with cCMV infections with antiviral agents has been reported to improve short-term outcomes in infants with symptomatic infections.[311]

Currently approved antiviral agents for the treatment of HCMV infection include four agents that target viral genome replication either by inhibition of the activity of the UL54 DNA polymerase or by preventing viral DNA packaging through inhibition of the virus-encoded terminase complex (UL51:UL56:UL89). The agents include ganciclovir (and its oral formulation valganciclovir), cidofovir, foscarnet, and the terminase inhibitor, letermovir. Other agents include an antisense phosphorothioate oligonucleotide, fomivirsen, that has specific indications for local therapy of HCMV retinitis. There are a number of newer agents that have been tested in clinical trials, but with the exception of the UL97 inhibitor, maribavir (Maribavir), interest in further development of these agents is limited. Ganciclovir remains the widely used agent, and treatment with this drug has been shown to provide clinical benefit in immunocompromised patients and infants with cCMV infections.[311,318] Ganciclovir is an analog of deoxyguanosine and is a nonobligate DNA chain terminator that must be phosphorylated by UL97 and cellular kinases to a triphosphate metabolite to inhibit the viral DNA polymerase. Once fully active, the drug inhibits DNA chain elongation.[106] Because of the dependence on phosphorylation by UL97, resistance to ganciclovir can develop following mutations in UL97, the UL54 viral DNA polymerase, or both with mutations leading to resistance under clinical settings more commonly mapping to UL97.[113,382] Resistance to ganciclovir develops at different rates depending on the clinical setting and duration of therapy with ganciclovir such that resistance can develop in up to 10% in high-risk SOT recipients.[113]

A recently approved antiviral agent, letermovir, has been shown to be of considerable value in HCMV prophylaxis in HCT recipients secondary to both its antiviral activity and, importantly, a lack of myelosuppression that is associated with ganciclovir therapy. Letermovir is a small molecule inhibitor that specifically inhibits the packaging of HCMV DNA but not rodent CMVs or other herpesviruses.[396] Letermovir inhibits the activity of the terminase complex and resistance to the drug has been mapped to UL56, UL89, and more recently, UL51.[114,205] Letermovir is currently licensed for HCMV prophylaxis in HCT recipients, and clinical studies are currently under way in the SOT. Two less commonly used agents, cidofovir and foscarnet, both target viral DNA replication. Cidofovir is an analog of deoxycytidine monophosphate and has activity against a broad spectrum of DNA viruses. Activity of cidofovir requires only host cell kinases for conversion to a deoxycytidine triphosphate analog that is incorporated into viral DNA and inhibits viral DNA elongation secondary to chain termination. Cidofovir resistance mutations in HCMV map to UL54 and can map to the same region of the enzyme that confers resistance to ganciclovir, thus conferring cross resistance.[382] Although a potent and effective antiviral agent, it also has significant toxicity including irreversible renal toxicity that often precludes its use in some patients. Foscarnet is a broad spectrum inhibitor of viral DNA polymerases that acts as a noncompetitive inhibitor of polymerase activity that interferes with incorporation of nucleoside triphosphates into viral DNA.[137] Resistance maps to UL54, and although infrequent, cross-resistance between ganciclovir and cidofovir and foscarnet has been reported.[382] As in the case of cidofovir, foscarnet can have dose-limiting toxicity and is utilized primarily to treat HCMV infections associated with the development of ganciclovir resistance.

A number of newer agents in varying stages of testing and/or development, of which two have been tested in human transplant populations. Brincidofovir (CMX001), a derivative of cidofovir with improved bioavailability has demonstrated potent activity in preclinical animal models of HCMV infections.[254] Although early clinical trials were encouraging, a Phase III trial in HCT failed to reach the primary endpoint of the trial.[401] Maribavir was shown to be a specific inhibitor of the kinase activity of UL97.[46] Because UL97 has pleiotropic effects in the infected cell, maribavir has been shown to inhibit phosphorylation of viral targets of UL97 including UL44, UL83, UL27, and its own autophosphorylation.[44,292,493] In addition, phosphorylation of a number of cellular targets by UL97 kinase activity are also inhibited by maribavir including Rb, RNA pol II, eF1, and components of the nuclear lamina.[32,258,295,414] There remains continued interest in this agent for treatment of HCMV infections in transplant population even though in Phase III study in HCT recipients, treatment with maribivir failed to meet the primary endpoint of the trial.[402] More recently, maribivir was shown to have efficacy similar to that of valganciclovir in the clearance of HCMV viremia when used in a preemptive treatment protocol but adverse effects were more frequent in the maribivir-treated patients.[389] Resistance to maribivir maps to UL97 and interestingly to UL27 secondary to the role of UL97 in the inhibition of the activity of UL27 on Tip60, a host acetyltransferase that induces expression of the host cell cyclin-dependent kinase inhibitor P21.[44] Of note, a mutant virus containing a deletion of UL27 exhibits a less than one-log decrease in virus production, suggesting that this mechanism of resistance could be of uncertain clinical importance *in vivo*.[496]

Vaccines to Prevent or Modify Infection

The decreased risk of invasive HCMV infection in seropositive as compared to seronegative SOT recipients (D+/R+ vs. D+/R−) and an extensive literature suggesting that HCMV seroimmunity can limit transmission and severity of fetal infection in pregnant women have resulted in considerable effort directed towards the development of prophylactic HCMV vaccines. Notably, the Institute of Medicine has identified the development of a HCMV vaccine as a high priority. Vaccine trials in seronegative SOT recipients using an attenuated replication-competent HCMV (Towne strain) suggested that protection from symptoms consistent with what is now termed the CMV syndrome could be achieved with this vaccine and that vaccine recipients could be protected from low titers of HCMV in challenge studies.[484] Subsequent studies have provided conflicting data on the protection induced by this vaccine, including clinical trials in seronegative women of childbearing age.[8] This vaccine has not been licensed for use in any human population.

Interest in subunit vaccines increased following the identification of antigenic virion proteins and targets of functional antiviral antibodies, primarily virus neutralizing antibodies. An adjuvanted recombinant glycoprotein B vaccine has been tested in women of childbearing age and in SOT recipients.[219,471] Although not controlled for the effect of the adjuvant, the results from the trial in women of childbearing age suggested a modest efficacy in prevention of virus infection.[471] A subsequent trial with the same gB vaccine in adolescent women failed to demonstrate a difference in HCMV infection between vaccine recipients and placebo recipients.[40] Although discordant, these studies raised that possibility that immunity induced by this recombinant gB vaccine could provide some degree of protection. Similarly, immunization of SOT recipients with this vaccine demonstrated some benefit as reflected by a decrease in the duration of antiviral treatment and longer intervals without detectable DNAemia in vaccinated SOT recipients.[219] The correlates of protective immunological responses induced by this vaccine in both SOT recipients and women of childbearing age have been difficult to deconvolute because the vaccine induced both HCMV-specific T-lymphocyte reactivity and a broad spectrum of antiviral antibody activities. Attempts to identify specific antiviral antibody responses that correlated with outcomes in vaccine recipients have provided inconclusive and discrepant results.[35,437] The development of prophylactic HCMV vaccines remains a high priority with several candidate vaccines progressing through early clinical trials in humans including an adjuvanted replication defective HCMV, a mRNA-based candidate vaccine, a replication competent attenuated virus consisting of a chimeric genomes derived from multiple virus isolates, and a vectored peptide-based vaccine.[6,7,284,334]

The enthusiasm for vaccine development to limit HCMV disease in transplant recipient and intrauterine HCMV transmission and fetal damage in pregnant women has been tempered by the recognition of potential hurdles including the lack of an understanding of qualitative and quantitative correlates of protective immune responses in transplant recipients and in pregnant women. As an example, deficits in HCMV-specific T-lymphocyte immunity in the posttransplant period appear to be the best predictor for the development of invasive HCMV infections with a less convincing role for antiviral antibodies. Yet this interpretation of existing data must be tempered by the results from studies in animal models of HCMV infections in the posttransplant period that have repeatedly demonstrated a protective role for antiviral antibodies.[323,400] In addition, early trials with intravenous immunoglobulins in SOT recipients indicated that antibody preparations could modify HCMV infections in these patients. Finally, the design of clinical trials to define HCMV vaccine efficacy in limiting the impact of HCMV infection in graft loss during the late posttransplant period will represent a significant challenge.

In addition to hurdles for vaccine development that are shared with transplant recipients, several unanswered questions continue to surround the potential efficacy of HCMV vaccines to modify the natural history of cCMV infections, including identification of the end point such vaccines, that is, prevention of maternal infection, prevention of fetal infection, and/or prevention of sequelae associated with fetal infection. A second conundrum relevant to HCMV vaccine development is the large number of infants with cCMV born to women with preexisting HCMV immunity derived from natural infections. In some populations, over 90% of infected infants are born to women with immunity prior to conception and antiviral antibody responses are similar between women who transmitted virus *in utero* and those who did not.[433,634] Furthermore, because in most populations 3 to 4 times as many infants with cCMV are born to women with preexisting HCMV immunity as compared to women with primary infections during pregnancy, clinical trials of HCMV vaccines must also define the impact of such vaccines in women with preexisting HCMV immunity.[433,651]

Biologics

Biologics, such as intravenous immune globulins (IVIG), have been used as prophylactic and therapeutic agents for control of HCMV infections and for the prophylaxis of SOT recipients. However, with the exception of their continued use in heart–lung allograft transplantation, the routine use of these products diminished rapidly with the introduction of effective antiviral agents. Although studies also suggested that HCMV IVIG products could also provide some benefit in HCT recipients, careful analysis of the results from these trials suggested that the benefit was secondary to immunomodulatory effects and not an antiviral activity.[9,131,674] Finally, there has been considerable interest in the use of human anti-HCMV monoclonal antibodies as prophylaxis for HCMV infections in SOT. Specific monoclonal antibodies have been selected primarily based on their functional capacity in *in vitro* neutralization assays. Recent clinical trials using a cocktail of anti-gH and antipentamer (gH/gL UL128-131) monoclonal antibodies have provided evidence that such preparations could modify HCMV infections in high-risk SOT.[269]

The success of HCMV IVIG preparations in prophylaxis in SOT prompted interest in the potential use of these biologics to modify HCMV infections in pregnant women and in infants infected *in utero*. Results from a controversial study suggested that treatment of pregnant women with primary HCMV infection could dramatically reduce transmission as well as the severity of infection in infants infected *in utero*.[445] This study was uncontrolled and contaminated by selection bias and thus, was not viewed as definitive. Subsequently, a controlled trial using the same IVIG preparation failed to demonstrate any benefit of IVIG in the prevention of intrauterine transmission.[524] Most recently, an expansive clinical trial sponsored by the NIH in the United States to determine the impact of IVIG on intrauterine HCMV transmission in women with primary HCMV infections in pregnancy was discontinued secondary to lack of statistically differences between outcomes in the treatment and control groups. In contrast to results from these large clinical studies, a smaller study carried out in Germany using more frequent infusions of IVIG provided some evidence of protection from intrauterine transmission by HIG.[288] Thus, the potential value of antibodies present in IVIG in prevention of intrauterine transmission and modification of fetal infection in HCMV infected pregnant women remains to be defined.

PERSPECTIVES

HCMV is one of the most complex viruses infecting humans. HCMV infection and its inevitable persistence in the host has been fine-tuned over millions of years of coevolution. The study of HCMV has revealed tremendous depth in our understanding of the biology of virus infection and replication. In addition, the complexity of interactions with the host cell and its biology makes HCMV a master teacher of cell biology, providing a remarkable path towards discerning pivotal control points for cellular pathways and responses to infection. The advent and application of advanced genetic, molecular, and global omics approaches to HCMV infection has permitted unprecedented advancement in understanding the intricate biology of CMV infection. However, much work remains to achieve successful control of HCMV disease and congenital infection. The large HCMV genome has yet to be fully annotated, yet it is clear that it has greater potential for protein coding capacity than we currently understand. Many viral genes have yet to have functions fully ascribed. Further, functions of the lncRNAs and miRNAs encoded by HCMV are just beginning to emerge. While much is understood about the biology of infection in fibroblasts, the important differences in the biology of infection in other cell types that undoubtedly contribute to persistence and pathogenesis in the host is far from complete. HCMV offers a powerful model to understand the coup d'etat resulting in persistence of the virus at the level of latency in infected cells. It is important to continue to understand the unique immune response to HCMV infection and to define how this immune response impacts persistence and the host. Understanding virus–host interactions important to viral persistence, viral immunology, and multipathogen infection is an important future goal, as is defining the costs or benefits of CMV persistence. CMV is currently investigated as a cofactor or driver in the development of pathologies associated with aging and cancer. Long-term, low-level virus shedding and the corresponding inflammatory response, in addition to CMV-induced alterations to metabolic, signaling, and stress pathways may contribute to chronic pathologies that are not currently attributed to CMV infection.

ACKNOWLEDGMENTS

The authors gratefully acknowledge the assistance of their colleagues in helpful discussions and art for the chapter. FG, WB, and EM are supported by grants from the NIH. We apologize to those investigators whose contributions could not be included due to space constraints. This chapter focuses largely on work since the year 2000, and previous editions should be consulted for earlier work.

REFERENCES

1. Abraham CG, Kulesza CA. Polycomb repressive complex 2 silences human cytomegalovirus transcription in quiescent infection models. *J Virol* 2013;87(24):13193–13205.
2. Adachi K, Xu J, Ank B, et al. Cytomegalovirus urinary shedding in HIV-infected pregnant women and congenital cytomegalovirus infection. *Clin Infect Dis* 2017;65(3):405–413.
3. Adams NM, Grassmann S, Sun JC. Clonal expansion of innate and adaptive lymphocytes. *Nat Rev Immunol* 2020;20(11):694–707.
4. Adamson CS, Nevels MM. Bright and early: inhibiting human cytomegalovirus by targeting major immediate-early gene expression or protein function. *Viruses* 2020;12(1):110.
5. Adler B, Scrivano L, Ruzcics Z, et al. Role of human cytomegalovirus UL131A in cell type-specific virus entry and release. *J Gen Virol* 2006;87(Pt 9):2451–2460.
6. Adler SP, Lewis N, Conlon A, et al. Phase 1 clinical trial of a conditionally replication-defective human cytomegalovirus (CMV) vaccine in CMV-seronegative subjects. *J Infect Dis* 2019;220(3):411–419.
7. Adler SP, Manganello AM, Lee R, et al. A phase 1 study of 4 live, recombinant human cytomegalovirus towne/toledo chimera vaccines in cytomegalovirus-seronegative men. *J Infect Dis* 2016;214(9):1341–1348.
8. Adler SP, Starr SE, Plotkin SA, et al. Immunity induced by primary human cytomegalovirus infection protects against secondary infection among women of childbearing age. *J Infect Dis* 1995;171:26–32.
9. Ahn H, Tay J, Shea B, et al. Effectiveness of immunoglobulin prophylaxis in reducing clinical complications of hematopoietic stem cell transplantation: a systematic review and meta-analysis. *Transfusion* 2018;58(10):2437–2452.
10. Ahn JH, Brignole EJ, 3rd, Hayward GS. Disruption of PML subnuclear domains by the acidic IE1 protein of human cytomegalovirus is mediated through interaction with PML and may modulate a RING finger-dependent cryptic transactivator function of PML. *Mol Cell Biol* 1998;18(8):4899–4913.
11. Ahn JH, Hayward GS. The major immediate-early proteins IE1 and IE2 of human cytomegalovirus colocalize with and disrupt PML-associated nuclear bodies at very early times in infected permissive cells. *J Virol* 1997;71(6):4599–4613.
12. Ahn JH, Hayward GS. Disruption of PML-associated nuclear bodies by IE1 correlates with efficient early stages of viral gene expression and DNA replication in human cytomegalovirus infection. *Virology* 2000;274(1):39–55.
13. Ahn JH, Jang WJ, Hayward GS. The human cytomegalovirus IE2 and UL112-113 proteins accumulate in viral DNA replication compartments that initiate from the periphery of promyelocytic leukemia protein-associated nuclear bodies (PODs or ND10). *J Virol* 1999;73(12):10458–10471.
14. Ahn K, Angulo A, Ghazal P, et al. Human cytomegalovirus inhibits antigen presentation by a sequential multistep process. *Proc Natl Acad Sci U S A* 1996;93(20):10990–10995.
15. Albright ER, Kalejta RF. Canonical and variant forms of histone H3 are deposited onto the human cytomegalovirus genome during lytic and latent infections. *J Virol* 2016;90(22):10309–10320.
16. Alderete JP, Child SJ, Geballe AP. Abundant early expression of gpUL4 from a human cytomegalovirus mutant lacking a repressive upstream open reading frame. *J Virol* 2001;75(15):7188–7192.
17. Alvisi G, Jans DA, Guo J, et al. A protein kinase CK2 site flanking the nuclear targeting signal enhances nuclear transport of human cytomegalovirus ppUL44. *Traffic* 2005;6(11):1002–1013.
18. Alvisi G, Marin O, Pari G, et al. Multiple phosphorylation sites at the C-terminus regulate nuclear import of HCMV DNA polymerase processivity factor ppUL44. *Virology* 2011;417(2):259–267.
19. Alwine JC. The human cytomegalovirus assembly compartment: a masterpiece of viral manipulation of cellular processes that facilitates assembly and egress. *PLoS Pathog* 2012;8(9):e1002878.
20. Amin MM, Bialek SR, Dollard SC, et al. Urinary cytomegalovirus shedding in the united states: the National Health and Nutrition Examination Surveys, 1999-2004. *Clin Infect Dis* 2018;67(4):587–592.
21. Angelova M, Zwezdaryk K, Ferris M, et al. Human cytomegalovirus infection dysregulates the canonical Wnt/beta-catenin signaling pathway. *PLoS Pathog* 2012;8(10):e1002959.
22. Appleton BA, Brooks J, Loregian A, et al. Crystal structure of the cytomegalovirus DNA polymerase subunit UL44 in complex with the C terminus from the catalytic subunit. Differences in structure and function relative to unliganded UL44. *J Biol Chem* 2006;281(8):5224–5232.
23. Appleton BA, Loregian A, Filman DJ, et al. The cytomegalovirus DNA polymerase subunit UL44 forms a C clamp-shaped dimer. *Mol Cell* 2004;15(2):233–244.
24. Arbuckle JH, Gardina PJ, Gordon DN, et al. Inhibitors of the histone methyltransferases EZH2/1 induce a potent antiviral state and suppress infection by diverse viral pathogens. *mBio* 2017;8(4).
25. Arend KC, Lenarcic EM, Moorman NJ. The 5' untranslated region of the major immediate early mRNA is necessary for efficient human cytomegalovirus replication. *J Virol* 2018;92(7):e02128-17.
26. Arend KC, Ziehr B, Vincent HA, et al. Multiple transcripts encode full-length human cytomegalovirus IE1 and IE2 proteins during lytic infection. *J Virol* 2016;90(19):8855–8865.
27. Asano-Mori Y, Kanda Y, Oshima K, et al. Clinical features of late cytomegalovirus infection after hematopoietic stem cell transplantation. *Int J Hematol* 2008;87(3):310–318.
28. Ashley CL, Abendroth A, McSharry BP, et al. Interferon-independent innate responses to cytomegalovirus. *Front Immunol* 2019;10:2751.
29. Avdic S, McSharry BP, Slobedman B. Modulation of dendritic cell functions by viral IL-10 encoded by human cytomegalovirus. *Front Microbiol* 2014;5:337.
30. Awasthi S, Isler JA, Alwine JC. Analysis of splice variants of the immediate-early 1 region of human cytomegalovirus. *J Virol* 2004;78(15):8191–8200.
31. Azzeh M, Honigman A, Taraboulos A, et al. Structural changes in human cytomegalovirus cytoplasmic assembly sites in the absence of UL97 kinase activity. *Virology* 2006;354(1):69–79.
32. Baek MC, Krosky PM, Pearson A, et al. Phosphorylation of the RNA polymerase II carboxyl-terminal domain in human cytomegalovirus-infected cells and in vitro by the viral UL97 protein kinase. *Virology* 2004;324(1):184–193.
33. Bain M, Mendelson M, Sinclair J. Ets-2 Repressor Factor (ERF) mediates repression of the human cytomegalovirus major immediate-early promoter in undifferentiated non-permissive cells. *J Gen Virol* 2003;84(Pt 1):41–49.
34. Baldick CJ, Jr., Marchini A, Patterson CE, et al. Human cytomegalovirus tegument protein pp71 (ppUL82) enhances the infectivity of viral DNA and accelerates the infectious cycle. *J Virol* 1997;71(6):4400–4408.
35. Baraniak I, Kropff B, Ambrose L, et al. Protection from cytomegalovirus viremia following glycoprotein B vaccination is not dependent on neutralizing antibodies. *Proc Natl Acad Sci U S A* 2018;115(24):6273–6278.
36. Barbosa NG, Yamamoto AY, Duarte G, et al. Cytomegalovirus shedding in seropositive pregnant women from a high-seroprevalence population: the Brazilian Cytomegalovirus Hearing and Maternal Secondary Infection Study. *Clin Infect Dis* 2018;67(5):743–750.
37. Barnes S, Schilizzi O, Audsley KM, et al. Deciphering the immunological phenomenon of adaptive natural killer (NK) cells and cytomegalovirus (CMV). *Int J Mol Sci* 2020;21(22):8864.
38. Bechtel JT, Shenk T. Human cytomegalovirus UL47 tegument protein functions after entry and before immediate-early gene expression. *J Virol* 2002;76(3):1043–1050.
39. Bender BJ, Coen DM, Strang BL. Dynamic and nucleolin-dependent localization of human cytomegalovirus UL84 to the periphery of viral replication compartments and nucleoli. *J Virol* 2014;88(20):11738–11747.
40. Bernstein DI, Munoz FM, Callahan ST, et al. Safety and efficacy of a cytomegalovirus glycoprotein B (gB) vaccine in adolescent girls: a randomized clinical trial. *Vaccine* 2016;34(3):313–319.
41. Bhushan S, Meyer H, Starosta AL, et al. Structural basis for translational stalling by human cytomegalovirus and fungal arginine attenuator peptide. *Mol Cell* 2010;40(1):138–146.
42. Bialas KM, Tanaka T, Tran D, et al. Maternal CD4+ T cells protect against severe congenital cytomegalovirus disease in a novel nonhuman primate model of placental cytomegalovirus transmission. *Proc Natl Acad Sci U S A* 2015;112(44):13645–13650.
43. Bigley TM, Reitsma JM, Mirza SP, et al. Human cytomegalovirus pUL97 regulates the viral major immediate early promoter by phosphorylation-mediated disruption of histone deacetylase 1 binding. *J Virol* 2013;87(13):7393–7408.
44. Bigley TM, Reitsma JM, Terhune SS. Antagonistic relationship between human cytomegalovirus pUL27 and pUL97 activities during infection. *J Virol* 2015;89(20):10230–10246.
45. Biolatti M, Gugliesi F, Dell'Oste V, et al. Modulation of the innate immune response by human cytomegalovirus. *Infect Genet Evol* 2018;64:105–114.
46. Biron KK, Harvey RJ, Chamberlain SC, et al. Potent and selective inhibition of human cytomegalovirus replication by 1263W94, a benzimidazole L-riboside with a unique mode of action. *Antimicrob Agents Chemother* 2002;46(8):2365–2372.
47. Boeck JM, Stowell GA, O'Connor CM, et al. The human cytomegalovirus US27 gene product constitutively activates antioxidant response element-mediated transcription through gbetagamma, phosphoinositide 3-kinase, and nuclear respiratory factor 1. *J Virol* 2018;92(23):e00644-18.
48. Boeckh M, Leisenring W, Riddell SR, et al. Late cytomegalovirus disease and mortality in recipients of allogeneic hematopoietic stem cell transplants: importance of viral load and T-cell immunity. *Blood* 2003;101(2):407–414.
49. Bogdanow B, Weisbach H, von Einem J, et al. Human cytomegalovirus tegument protein pp150 acts as a cyclin A2-CDK-dependent sensor of the host cell cycle and differentiation state. *Proc Natl Acad Sci U S A* 2013;110(43):17510–17515.
50. Bolovan-Fritts CA, Mocarski ES, Wiedeman JA. Peripheral blood CD14(+) cells from healthy subjects carry a circular conformation of latent cytomegalovirus genome. *Blood* 1999;93(1):394–398.
51. Boppana SB, Fowler KB, Pass RF, et al. Congenital cytomegalovirus infection: association between virus burden in infancy and hearing loss. *J Pediatr* 2005;146(6):817–823.
52. Boppana SB, Rivera LB, Fowler KB, et al. Intrauterine transmission of cytomegalovirus to infants of women with preconceptional immunity. *N Engl J Med* 2001;344(18):1366–1371.
53. Boppana SB, Ross SA, Shimamura M, et al. Saliva polymerase-chain-reaction assay for cytomegalovirus screening in newborns. *N Engl J Med* 2011;364(22):2111–2118.
54. Borst EM, Bauerfeind R, Binz A, et al. The essential human cytomegalovirus proteins pUL77 and pUL93 are structural components necessary for viral genome encapsidation. *J Virol* 2016;90(13):5860–5875.
55. Borst EM, Messerle M. Analysis of human cytomegalovirus oriLyt sequence requirements in the context of the viral genome. *J Virol* 2005;79(6):3615–3626.
56. Botto S, Abraham J, Mizuno N, et al. Human cytomegalovirus immediate early 86-kDa protein blocks transcription and induces degradation of the immature interleukin-1beta protein during virion-mediated activation of the AIM2 inflammasome. *mBio* 2019;10(1):e02510-18.
57. Boucoiran I, Mayer BT, Krantz EM, et al. Nonprimary maternal cytomegalovirus infection after viral shedding in infants. *Pediatr Infect Dis J* 2018;37(7):627–631.
58. Bowyer G, Sharpe H, Venkatraman N, et al. Reduced Ebola vaccine responses in CMV+ young adults is associated with expansion of CD57+KLRG1+ T cells. *J Exp Med* 2020;217(7):e20200004.
59. Bradley AJ, Kovacs IJ, Gatherer D, et al. Genotypic analysis of two hypervariable human cytomegalovirus genes. *J Med Virol* 2008;80(9):1615–1623.
60. Bradley AJ, Lurain NS, Ghazal P, et al. High-throughput sequence analysis of variants of human cytomegalovirus strains Towne and AD169. *J Gen Virol* 2009;90(Pt 10):2375–2380.
61. Bresnahan WA, Shenk TE. UL82 virion protein activates expression of immediate early viral genes in human cytomegalovirus-infected cells. *Proc Natl Acad Sci U S A* 2000;97(26):14506–14511.
62. Britt W. Controversies in the natural history of congenital human cytomegalovirus infection: the paradox of infection and disease in offspring of women with immunity prior to pregnancy. *Med Microbiol Immunol* 2015;204(3):263–271.

63. Britt W. Cytomegalovirus. In: Wilson CB, Nizet V, Maldonado Y, Remington JS, Klein JO, eds. *Remington and Klein's Infectious Diseases of the Fetus and Newborn Infant*. 8th ed. Philadelphia, PA: Saunders; 2016.
64. Britt W. Human cytomegalovirus infection in women with preexisting immunity: sources of infection and mechanisms of infection in the presence of antiviral immunity (In Press). *J Infect Dis* 2020;221(Suppl 1):S1–S8.
65. Britt WJ. Congenital human cytomegalovirus infection and the enigma of maternal immunity. *J Virol* 2017;91(15):e02392-16.
66. Britt WJ. Cytomegalovirus. In: Bennett JE, Dolin R, Blaser MJ, eds. *Mandell Douglas and Bennett's Principles and Practice of Infectious Diseases*. 9th ed. Vol 1. New York: Elsevier; 2020.
67. Britt WJ, Auger D. Synthesis and processing of the envelope gp55-116 complex of human cytomegalovirus. *J Virol* 1986;58(1):185–191.
68. Brodin P, Davis MM. Human immune system variation. *Nat Rev Immunol* 2017;17(1):21–29.
69. Brodin P, Jojic V, Gao T, et al. Variation in the human immune system is largely driven by non-heritable influences. *Cell* 2015;160(1–2):37–47.
70. Bronzini M, Luganini A, Dell'Oste V, et al. The US16 gene of human cytomegalovirus is required for efficient viral infection of endothelial and epithelial cells. *J Virol* 2012;86:6875–6888.
71. Brune W, Andoniou CE. Die another day: inhibition of cell death pathways by cytomegalovirus. *Viruses* 2017;9(9):249.
72. Bryant LA, Mixon P, Davidson M, et al. The human cytomegalovirus 86-kilodalton major immediate-early protein interacts physically and functionally with histone acetyltransferase P/CAF. *J Virol* 2000;74(16):7230–7237.
73. Buchkovich NJ, Maguire TG, Alwine JC. Role of the endoplasmic reticulum chaperone BiP, SUN domain proteins, and dynein in altering nuclear morphology during human cytomegalovirus infection. *J Virol* 2010;84(14):7005–7017.
74. Buchkovich NJ, Maguire TG, Paton AW, et al. The endoplasmic reticulum chaperone BiP/GRP78 is important in the structure and function of the human cytomegalovirus assembly compartment. *J Virol* 2009;83(22):11421–11428.
75. Buchkovich NJ, Maguire TG, Yu Y, et al. Human cytomegalovirus specifically controls the levels of the endoplasmic reticulum chaperone BiP/GRP78, which is required for virion assembly. *J Virol* 2008;82(1):31–39.
76. Buehler J, Carpenter E, Zeltzer S, et al. Host signaling and EGR1 transcriptional control of human cytomegalovirus replication and latency. *PLoS Pathog* 2019;15(11):e1008037.
77. Buehler J, Zeltzer S, Reitsma J, et al. Opposing regulation of the EGF receptor: a molecular switch controlling cytomegalovirus latency and replication. *PLoS Pathog* 2016;12(5):e1005655.
78. Bughio F, Umashankar M, Wilson J, et al. Human cytomegalovirus UL135 and UL136 genes are required for postentry tropism in endothelial cells. *J Virol* 2015;89(13):6536–6550.
79. Burg JS, Ingram JR, Venkatakrishnan AJ, et al. Structural biology. Structural basis for chemokine recognition and activation of a viral G protein-coupled receptor. *Science* 2015;347(6226):1113–1117.
80. Burke HG, Heldwein EE. Crystal structure of the human cytomegalovirus glycoprotein B. *PLoS Pathog* 2015;11(10):e1005227.
81. Burwitz BJ, Malouli D, Bimber BN, et al. Cross-species rhesus cytomegalovirus infection of Cynomolgus Macaques. *PLoS Pathog* 2016;12(11):e1006014.
82. Businger R, Deutschmann J, Gruska I, et al. Human cytomegalovirus overcomes SAMHD1 restriction in macrophages via pUL97. *Nat Microbiol* 2019;4(12):2260–2272.
83. Caffarelli N, Fehr AR, Yu D. Cyclin A degradation by primate cytomegalovirus protein pUL21a counters its innate restriction of virus replication. *PLoS Pathog* 2013;9(12):e1003825.
84. Cagliani R, Forni D, Mozzi A, et al. Evolution and genetic diversity of primate cytomegaloviruses. *Microorganisms* 2020;8(5):624.
85. Calo S, Cortese M, Ciferri C, et al. The human cytomegalovirus UL116 gene encodes an envelope glycoprotein forming a complex with gH independently from gL. *J Virol* 2016;90(10):4926–4938.
86. Cannon MJ, Hyde TB, Schmid DS. Review of cytomegalovirus shedding in bodily fluids and relevance to congenital cytomegalovirus infection. *Rev Med Virol* 2011;21(4):240–255.
87. Cannon MJ, Schmid DS, Hyde TB. Review of cytomegalovirus seroprevalence and demographic characteristics associated with infection. *Rev Med Virol* 2010;20(4):202–213.
88. Cannon MJ, Stowell JD, Clark R, et al. Repeated measures study of weekly and daily cytomegalovirus shedding patterns in saliva and urine of healthy cytomegalovirus-seropositive children. *BMC Infect Dis* 2014;14:569.
89. Cantrell SR, Bresnahan WA. Interaction between the human cytomegalovirus UL82 gene product (pp71) and hDaxx regulates immediate-early gene expression and viral replication. *J Virol* 2005;79(12):7792–7802.
90. Caposio P, van den Worm S, Crawford L, et al. Characterization of a live-attenuated HCMV-based vaccine platform. *Sci Rep* 2019;9(1):19236.
91. Cappadona I, Villinger C, Schutzius G, et al. Human cytomegalovirus pUL47 modulates tegumentation and capsid accumulation at the viral assembly complex. *J Virol* 2015;89(14):7314–7328.
92. Casarosa P, Bakker RA, Verzijl D, et al. Constitutive signaling of the human cytomegalovirus-encoded chemokine receptor US28. *J Biol Chem* 2001;276(2):1133–1137.
93. Caviness K, Bughio F, Crawford LB, et al. Complex interplay of the UL136 isoforms balances cytomegalovirus replication and latency. *mBio* 2016;7(2):e01986.
94. Caviness K, Cicchini L, Rak M, et al. Complex expression of the UL136 gene of human cytomegalovirus results in multiple protein isoforms with unique roles in replication. *J Virol* 2014;88(24):14412–14425.
95. Cepeda V, Esteban M, Fraile-Ramos A. Human cytomegalovirus final envelopment on membranes containing both trans-Golgi network and endosomal markers. *Cell Microbiol* 2010;12(3):386–404.
96. Cha TA, Tom E, Kemble GW, et al. Human cytomegalovirus clinical isolates carry at least 19 genes not found in laboratory strains. *J Virol* 1996;70(1):78–83.
97. Chan G, Nogalski MT, Bentz GL, et al. PI3K-dependent upregulation of Mcl-1 by human cytomegalovirus is mediated by epidermal growth factor receptor and inhibits apoptosis in short-lived monocytes. *J Immunol* 2010;184(6):3213–3222.
98. Chan G, Nogalski MT, Yurochko AD. Activation of EGFR on monocytes is required for human cytomegalovirus entry and mediates cellular motility. *Proc Natl Acad Sci U S A* 2009;106(52):22369–22374.
99. Chan YJ, Tseng WP, Hayward GS. Two distinct upstream regulatory domains containing multicopy cellular transcription factor binding sites provide basal repression and inducible enhancer characteristics to the immediate-early IES (US3) promoter from human cytomegalovirus. *J Virol* 1996;70(8):5312–5328.
100. Chandramouli S, Ciferri C, Nikitin PA, et al. Structure of HCMV glycoprotein B in the postfusion conformation bound to a neutralizing human antibody. *Nat Commun* 2015;6(1):8176.
101. Chandramouli S, Malito E, Nguyen T, et al. Structural basis for potent antibody-mediated neutralization of human cytomegalovirus. *Sci Immunol* 2017;2(12):eaan1457.
102. Chang WL, Tarantal AF, Zhou SS, et al. A recombinant rhesus cytomegalovirus expressing enhanced green fluorescent protein retains the wild-type phenotype and pathogenicity in fetal macaques. *J Virol* 2002;76(18):9493–9504.
103. Chaturvedi S, Klein J, Vardi N, et al. A molecular mechanism for probabilistic bet hedging and its role in viral latency. *Proc Natl Acad Sci U S A* 2020;117(29):17240–17248.
104. Chau NH, Vanson CD, Kerry JA. Transcriptional regulation of the human cytomegalovirus US11 early gene. *J Virol* 1999;73(2):863–870.
105. Chaumorcel M, Lussignol M, Mouna L, et al. The human cytomegalovirus protein TRS1 inhibits autophagy via its interaction with Beclin 1. *J Virol* 2012;86(5):2571–2584.
106. Chen H, Beardsley GP, Coen DM. Mechanism of ganciclovir-induced chain termination revealed by resistant viral polymerase mutants with reduced exonuclease activity. *Proc Natl Acad Sci U S A* 2014;111(49):17462–17467.
107. Chen J, Stinski MF. Activation of transcription of the human cytomegalovirus early UL4 promoter by the Ets transcription factor binding element. *J Virol* 2000;74(21):9845–9857.
108. Chen J, Stinski MF. Role of regulatory elements and the MAPK/ERK or p38 MAPK pathways for activation of human cytomegalovirus gene expression. *J Virol* 2002;76(10):4873–4885.
109. Cheng S, Caviness K, Buehler J, et al. Transcriptome-wide characterization of human cytomegalovirus in natural infection and experimental latency. *Proc Natl Acad Sci U S A* 2017;114(49):E10586–E10595.
110. Cherrington JM, Khoury EL, Mocarski ES. Human cytomegalovirus ie2 negatively regulates alpha gene expression via a short target sequence near the transcription start site. *J Virol* 1991;65(2):887–896.
111. Chevillotte M, Landwehr S, Linta L, et al. Major tegument protein pp65 of human cytomegalovirus is required for the incorporation of pUL69 and pUL97 into the virus particle and for viral growth in macrophages. *J Virol* 2009;83(6):2480–2490.
112. Child SJ, Hakki M, De Niro KL, et al. Evasion of cellular antiviral responses by human cytomegalovirus TRS1 and IRS1. *J Virol* 2004;78(1):197–205.
113. Chou S. Approach to drug-resistant cytomegalovirus in transplant recipients. *Curr Opin Infect Dis* 2015;28(4):293–299.
114. Chou S. A third component of the human cytomegalovirus terminase complex is involved in letermovir resistance. *Antiviral Res* 2017;148:1–4.
115. Ciferri C, Chandramouli S, Donnarumma D, et al. Structural and biochemical studies of HCMV gH/gL/gO and Pentamer reveal mutually exclusive cell entry complexes. *Proc Natl Acad Sci U S A* 2015;112(6):1767–1772.
116. Ciferri C, Chandramouli S, Leitner A, et al. Antigenic characterization of the HCMV gH/gL/gO and pentamer cell entry complexes reveals binding sites for potently neutralizing human antibodies. *PLoS Pathog* 2015;11(10):e1005230.
117. Clark E, Spector DH. Studies on the contribution of human cytomegalovirus UL21a and UL97 to viral growth and inactivation of the anaphase-promoting complex/cyclosome (APC/C) E3 ubiquitin ligase reveal a unique cellular mechanism for downmodulation of the APC/C subunits APC1, APC4, and APC5. *J Virol* 2015;89(13):6928–6939.
118. Clippinger AJ, Maguire TG, Alwine JC. Human cytomegalovirus infection maintains mTOR activity and its perinuclear localization during amino acid deprivation. *J Virol* 2011;85(18):9369–9376.
119. Cobbs CS, Harkins L, Samanta M, et al. Human cytomegalovirus infection and expression in human malignant glioma. *Cancer Res* 2002;62(12):3347–3350.
120. Cohen S, Martinez-Vinson C, Aloi M, et al. Cytomegalovirus infection in pediatric severe ulcerative colitis—a Multicenter Study from the Pediatric Inflammatory Bowel Disease Porto Group of the European Society of Pediatric Gastroenterology, Hepatology and Nutrition. *Pediatr Infect Dis J* 2018;37(3):197–201.
121. Cojohari O, Peppenelli MA, Chan GC. Human cytomegalovirus induces an atypical activation of Akt to stimulate the survival of short-lived monocytes. *J Virol* 2016;90(14):6443–6452.
122. Colletti KS, Smallenburg KE, Xu Y, et al. Human cytomegalovirus UL84 interacts with an RNA stem-loop sequence found within the RNA/DNA hybrid region of oriLyt. *J Virol* 2007;81(13):7077–7085.
123. Colletti KS, Xu Y, Cei SA, et al. Human cytomegalovirus UL84 oligomerization and heterodimerization domains act as transdominant inhibitors of oriLyt-dependent DNA replication: evidence that IE2-UL84 and UL84-UL84 interactions are required for lytic DNA replication. *J Virol* 2004;78(17):9203–9214.
124. Collier AC, Handsfield HH, Ashley R, et al. Cervical but not urinary excretion of cytomegalovirus is related to sexual activity and contraceptive practices in sexually active women. *J Infect Dis* 1995;171:33–38.
125. Collins-McMillen D, Buehler J, Peppenelli M, et al. Molecular determinants and the regulation of human cytomegalovirus latency and reactivation. *Viruses* 2018;10(8):444.
126. Collins-McMillen D, Chesnokova L, Lee BJ, et al. HCMV infection and apoptosis: how do monocytes survive HCMV infection? *Viruses* 2018;10(10):533.
127. Collins-McMillen D, Kamil J, Moorman N, et al. Control of immediate early gene expression for human cytomegalovirus reactivation. *Front Cell Infect Microbiol* 2020;10:476.

128. Collins-McMillen D, Kim JH, Nogalski MT, et al. Human cytomegalovirus promotes survival of infected monocytes via a distinct temporal regulation of cellular Bcl-2 family proteins. *J Virol* 2015;90(5):2356–2371.
129. Collins-McMillen D, Rak M, Buehler JC, et al. Alternative promoters drive human cytomegalovirus reactivation from latency. *Proc Natl Acad Sci U S A* 2019;116(35):17492–17497.
130. Cook CH, Trgovcich J, Zimmerman PD, et al. Lipopolysaccharide, tumor necrosis factor alpha, or interleukin-1beta triggers reactivation of latent cytomegalovirus in immunocompetent mice. *J Virol* 2006;80(18):9151–9158.
131. Cordonnier C, Chevret S, Legrand M, et al. Should immunoglobulin therapy be used in allogeneic stem-cell transplantation? A randomized, double-blind, dose effect, placebo-controlled, multicenter trial. *Ann Intern Med* 2003;139(1):8–18.
132. Courcelle CT, Courcelle J, Prichard MN, et al. Requirement for uracil-DNA glycosylase during the transition to late-phase cytomegalovirus DNA replication. *J Virol* 2001;75(16):7592–7601.
133. Crawford LB, Caposio P, Kreklywich C, et al. Human cytomegalovirus US28 ligand binding activity is required for latency in CD34(+) hematopoietic progenitor cells and humanized NSG mice. *mBio* 2019;10(4):e01889-19.
134. Crawford LB, Hancock MH, Struthers HM, et al. CD34+ hematopoietic progenitor cell subsets exhibit differential ability to maintain HCMV latency and persistence. *J Virol* 2021;95(3):e02105-20.
135. Crawford LB, Kim JH, Collins-McMillen D, et al. Human cytomegalovirus encodes a novel FLT3 receptor ligand necessary for hematopoietic cell differentiation and viral reactivation. *mBio* 2018;9(2).
136. Cristea IM, Moorman NJ, Terhune SS, et al. Human cytomegalovirus pUL83 stimulates activity of the viral immediate-early promoter through its interaction with the cellular IFI16 protein. *J Virol* 2010;84(15):7803–7814.
137. Crumpacker CS. Mechanism of action of foscarnet against viral polymerases. *Am J Med* 1992;92(2a):3s–7s.
138. Crumpacker CS. Invited commentary: human cytomegalovirus, inflammation, cardiovascular disease, and mortality. *Am J Epidemiol* 2010;172(4):372–374.
139. Cudini J, Roy S, Houldcroft CJ, et al. Human cytomegalovirus haplotype reconstruction reveals high diversity due to superinfection and evidence of within-host recombination. *Proc Natl Acad Sci U S A* 2019;116(12):5693–5698.
140. Cui X, Adler SP, Davison AJ, et al, Habib el SE, McVoy MA. Bacterial artificial chromosome clones of viruses comprising the Towne cytomegalovirus vaccine. *J Biomed Biotechnol* 2012;2012:428498.
141. Cummins NW, Deziel PJ, Abraham RS, et al. Deficiency of cytomegalovirus (CMV)-specific CD8+ T cells in patients presenting with late-onset CMV disease several years after transplantation. *Transpl Infect Dis* 2009;11(1):20–27.
142. Cunningham C, Gatherer D, Hilfrich B, et al. Sequences of complete human cytomegalovirus genomes from infected cell cultures and clinical specimens. *J Gen Virol* 2010;91(Pt 3):605–615.
143. Dag F, Dolken L, Holzki J, et al. Reversible silencing of cytomegalovirus genomes by type I interferon governs virus latency. *PLoS Pathog* 2014;10(2):e1003962.
144. Dai X, Yu X, Gong H, et al. The smallest capsid protein mediates binding of the essential tegument protein pp150 to stabilize DNA-containing capsids in human cytomegalovirus. *PLoS Pathog* 2013;9(8):e1003525.
145. Dargan DJ, Douglas E, Cunningham C, et al. Sequential mutations associated with adaptation of human cytomegalovirus to growth in cell culture. *J Gen Virol* 2010;91(Pt 6): 1535–1546.
146. Das S, Pellett PE. Spatial relationships between markers for secretory and endosomal machinery in human cytomegalovirus-infected cells versus those in uninfected cells. *J Virol* 2011;85(12):5864–5879.
147. Davison AJ. Comparative analysis of the genomes. In: Arvin A, Campadelli-Fiume G, Mocarski E, et al., eds. *Human Herpesviruses: Biology, Therapy, and Immunoprophylaxis.* 2011/02/25 ed. Cambridge: Cambridge Press; 2007:10–26.
148. Davison AJ. Overview of classification. In: Arvin A, Campadelli-Fiume G, Mocarski E, et al., eds. *Human Herpesviruses: Biology, Therapy, and Immunoprophylaxis.* 2011/02/25 ed. Cambridge: Cambridge Press; 2007:3–9.
149. Davison AJ, Bhella D. Comparative genome and virion structure. In: Arvin A, Campadelli-Fiume G, Mocarski E, et al., eds. *Human Herpesviruses: Biology, Therapy, and Immunoprophylaxis.* 2011/02/25 ed. Cambridge: Cambridge Press; 2007:177–203.
150. Davison AJ, Dolan A, Akter P, et al. The human cytomegalovirus genome revisited: comparison with the chimpanzee cytomegalovirus genome. *J Gen Virol* 2003;84(Pt 1): 17–28.
151. De Meo S, Dell'Oste V, Molfetta R, et al. SAMHD1 phosphorylation and cytoplasmic relocalization after human cytomegalovirus infection limits its antiviral activity. *PLoS Pathog* 2020;16(9):e1008855.
152. Delgado JF, Reyne AG, de Dios S, et al. Influence of cytomegalovirus infection in the development of cardiac allograft vasculopathy after heart transplantation. *J Heart Lung Transplant* 2015;34(8):1112–1119.
153. Dell'Oste V, Biolatti M, Galitska G, et al. Tuning the Orchestra: HCMV vs. Innate Immunity. *Front Microbiol* 2020;11:661.
154. Dennis EA, Smythies LE, Grabski R, et al. Cytomegalovirus promotes intestinal macrophage-mediated mucosal inflammation through induction of Smad7. *Mucosal Immunol* 2018;11(6):1694–1704.
155. Deutschmann J, Schneider A, Gruska I, et al. A viral kinase counteracts in vivo restriction of murine cytomegalovirus by SAMHD1. *Nat Microbiol* 2019;4(12):2273–2284.
156. Dietz AN, Villinger C, Becker S, et al. A tyrosine-based trafficking motif of the tegument protein pUL71 is crucial for human cytomegalovirus secondary envelopment. *J Virol* 2018;92(1):e00907-17.
157. Dimitroulia E, Spanakis N, Konstantinidou AE, et al. Frequent detection of cytomegalovirus in the intestine of patients with inflammatory bowel disease. *Inflamm Bowel Dis* 2006;12(9):879–884.
158. Dittmer A, Bogner E. Analysis of the quaternary structure of the putative HCMV portal protein PUL104. *Biochemistry* 2005;44(2):759–765.
159. Dittmer A, Drach JC, Townsend LB, et al. Interaction of the putative human cytomegalovirus portal protein pUL104 with the large terminase subunit pUL56 and its inhibition by benzimidazole-D-ribonucleosides. *J Virol* 2005;79(23):14660–14667.
160. Dittmer D, Mocarski ES. Human cytomegalovirus infection inhibits G1/S transition. *J Virol* 1997;71(2):1629–1634.
161. Dolan A, Cunningham C, Hector RD, et al. Genetic content of wild-type human cytomegalovirus. *J Gen Virol* 2004;85(Pt 5):1301–1312.
162. Dreher AM, Arora N, Fowler KB, et al. Spectrum of disease and outcome in children with symptomatic congenital cytomegalovirus infection. *J Pediatr* 2014;164(4):855–859.
163. Dunn W, Chou C, Li H, et al. Functional profiling of a human cytomegalovirus genome. *Proc Natl Acad Sci U S A* 2003;100(24):14223–14228.
164. Dupont L, Du L, Poulter M, et al. Src family kinase activity drives cytomegalovirus reactivation by recruiting MOZ histone acetyltransferase activity to the viral promoter. *J Biol Chem* 2019;294(35):12901–12910.
165. Dutta N, Lashmit P, Yuan J, et al. The human cytomegalovirus UL133–138 gene locus attenuates the lytic viral cycle in fibroblasts. *PLoS One* 2015;10(3):e0120946.
166. Dzabic M, Rahbar A, Yaiw KC, et al. Intragraft cytomegalovirus protein expression is associated with reduced renal allograft survival. *Clin Infect Dis* 2011;53(10):969–976.
167. Dziurzynski K, Chang SM, Heimberger AB, et al. Consensus on the role of human cytomegalovirus in glioblastoma. *Neuro Oncol* 2012;14(3):246–255.
168. Eberhardt MK, Deshpande A, Fike J, et al. Exploitation of interleukin-10 (IL-10) signaling pathways: alternate roles of viral and cellular IL-10 in rhesus cytomegalovirus infection. *J Virol* 2016;90(21):9920–9930.
169. Eid AJ, Razonable RR. New developments in the management of cytomegalovirus infection after solid organ transplantation. *Drugs* 2010;70(8):965–981.
170. Eifler M, Uecker R, Weisbach H, et al. PUL21a-Cyclin A2 interaction is required to protect human cytomegalovirus-infected cells from the deleterious consequences of mitotic entry. *PLoS Pathog* 2014;10(10):e1004514.
171. Elder EG, Krishna BA, Williamson J, et al. Interferon-responsive genes are targeted during the establishment of human cytomegalovirus latency. *mBio* 2019;10(6).
172. Enders G, Daiminger A, Bader U, et al. Intrauterine transmission and clinical outcome of 248 pregnancies with primary cytomegalovirus infection in relation to gestational age. *J Clin Virol* 2011;52(3):244–246.
173. Enders G, Daiminger A, Lindemann L, et al. Cytomegalovirus (CMV) seroprevalence in pregnant women, bone marrow donors and adolescents in Germany, 1996-2010. *Med Microbiol Immunol* 2012;201(3):303–309.
174. Erard V, Guthrie KA, Seo S, et al. Reduced mortality of cytomegalovirus pneumonia after hematopoietic cell transplantation due to antiviral therapy and changes in transplantation practices. *Clin Infect Dis* 2015;61(1):31–39.
175. Fang Q, Chen P, Wang M, et al. Human cytomegalovirus IE1 protein alters the higher-order chromatin structure by targeting the acidic patch of the nucleosome. *Elife* 2016;5:e11911.
176. Farrell HE, Bruce K, Lawler C, et al. Murine cytomegalovirus spreads by dendritic cell recirculation. *mBio* 2017;8(5):e01264-17.
177. Farrell HE, Bruce K, Lawler C, et al. Murine cytomegalovirus spread depends on the infected myeloid cell type. *J Virol* 2019;93(15):e00540-19.
178. Faure-Bardon V, Magny JF, Parodi M, et al. Sequelae of congenital cytomegalovirus following maternal primary infections are limited to those acquired in the first trimester of pregnancy. *Clin Infect Dis* 2019;69(9):1526–1532.
179. Fehr AR, Yu D. Human cytomegalovirus early protein pUL21a promotes efficient viral DNA synthesis and the late accumulation of immediate-early transcripts. *J Virol* 2011;85(2):663–674.
180. Feire AL, Koss H, Compton T. Cellular integrins function as entry receptors for human cytomegalovirus via a highly conserved disintegrin-like domain. *Proc Natl Acad Sci U S A* 2004;101(43):15470–15475.
181. Feire AL, Roy RM, Manley K, et al. The glycoprotein B disintegrin-like domain binds beta 1 integrin to mediate cytomegalovirus entry. *J Virol* 2010;84(19):10026–10037.
182. Fernandez-Ruiz M, Gimenez E, Vinuesa V, et al. Regular monitoring of cytomegalovirus-specific cell-mediated immunity in intermediate-risk kidney transplant recipients: predictive value of the immediate post-transplant assessment. *Clin Microbiol Infect* 2019;25(3):381.e381–381.e310.
183. Finkel Y, Schmiedel D, Tai-Schmiedel J, et al. Comprehensive annotations of human herpesvirus 6A and 6B genomes reveal novel and conserved genomic features. *Elife* 2020;9:e50960.
184. Fisher S, Genbacev O, Maidji E, et al. Human cytomegalovirus infection of placental cytotrophoblasts in vitro and in utero: implications for transmission and pathogenesis. *J Virol* 2000;74(15):6808–6820.
185. Forrest C, Gomes A, Reeves M, et al. NK cell memory to cytomegalovirus: implications for vaccine development. *Vaccines (Basel)* 2020;8(3):394.
186. Forte E, Swaminathan S, Schroeder MW, et al. Tumor necrosis factor alpha induces reactivation of human cytomegalovirus independently of myeloid cell differentiation following posttranscriptional establishment of latency. *mBio* 2018;9(5):e01560-18.
187. Fortunato EA, Sanchez V, Yen JY, et al. Infection of cells with human cytomegalovirus during S phase results in a blockade to immediate-early gene expression that can be overcome by inhibition of the proteasome. *J Virol* 2002;76(11):5369–5379.
188. Fortunato EA, Spector DH. p53 and RPA are sequestered in viral replication centers in the nuclei of cells infected with human cytomegalovirus. *J Virol* 1998;72(3):2033–2039.
189. Fowler KB, Ross SA, Shimamura M, et al. Racial and ethnic differences in the prevalence of congenital cytomegalovirus infection. *J Pediatr* 2018;200:196–201.e1.
190. Frank T, Niemann I, Reichel A, et al. Emerging roles of cytomegalovirus-encoded G protein-coupled receptors during lytic and latent infection. *Med Microbiol Immunol* 2019;208(3–4):447–456.
191. Fruh K, Picker L. CD8+ T cell programming by cytomegalovirus vectors: applications in prophylactic and therapeutic vaccination. *Curr Opin Immunol* 2017;47:52–56.
192. Fryer JF, Heath AB, Minor PD. A collaborative study to establish the 1st WHO International Standard for human cytomegalovirus for nucleic acid amplification technology. *Biologicals* 2016;44(4):242–251.

193. Fu M, Gao Y, Zhou Q, et al. Human cytomegalovirus latent infection alters the expression of cellular and viral microRNA. *Gene* 2014;536(2):272–278.
194. Fu TM, Wang D, Freed DC, et al. Restoration of viral epithelial tropism improves immunogenicity in rabbits and rhesus macaques for a whole virion vaccine of human cytomegalovirus. *Vaccine* 2012;30(52):7469–7474.
195. Fu YZ, Su S, Zou HM, et al. Human cytomegalovirus DNA polymerase subunit UL44 antagonizes antiviral immune responses by suppressing IRF3- and NF-kappaB-mediated transcription. *J Virol* 2019;93(11):e00181-19.
196. Furman D, Jojic V, Sharma S, et al. Cytomegalovirus infection enhances the immune response to influenza. *Sci Transl Med* 2015;7(281):281ra243.
197. Gamache A, Cronk JM, Nash WT, et al. Ly49R activation receptor drives self-MHC-educated NK cell immunity against cytomegalovirus infection. *Proc Natl Acad Sci U S A* 2019;116(52):26768–26778.
198. Gatherer D, Seirafian S, Cunningham C, et al. High-resolution human cytomegalovirus transcriptome. *Proc Natl Acad Sci U S A* 2011;108(49):19755–19760.
199. Gebert S, Schmolke S, Sorg G, et al. The UL84 protein of human cytomegalovirus acts as a transdominant inhibitor of immediate-early-mediated transactivation that is able to prevent viral replication. *J Virol* 1997;71(9):7048–7060.
200. Gelbmann CB, Kalejta RF. The membrane-spanning peptide and acidic cluster dileucine sorting motif of UL138 are required to downregulate MRP1 drug transporter function in human cytomegalovirus-infected cells. *J Virol* 2019;93(11):e00430-19.
201. Gentile G, Picardi A, Capobianchi A, et al. A prospective study comparing quantitative Cytomegalovirus (CMV) polymerase chain reaction in plasma and pp65 antigenemia assay in monitoring patients after allogeneic stem cell transplantation. *BMC Infect Dis* 2006;6:167.
202. Gibson W. Structure and formation of the cytomegalovirus virion. *Curr Top Microbiol Immunol* 2008;325:187–204.
203. Glass M, Everett RD. Components of promyelocytic leukemia nuclear bodies (ND10) act cooperatively to repress herpesvirus infection. *J Virol* 2013;87(4):2174–2185.
204. Goldmacher VS, Bartle LM, Skaletskaya A, et al. A cytomegalovirus-encoded mitochondria-localized inhibitor of apoptosis structurally unrelated to Bcl-2. *Proc Natl Acad Sci U S A* 1999;96(22):12536–12541.
205. Goldner T, Hempel C, Ruebsamen-Schaeff H, et al. Geno- and phenotypic characterization of human cytomegalovirus mutants selected in vitro after letermovir (AIC246) exposure. *Antimicrob Agents Chemother* 2014;58(1):610–613.
206. Goldner T, Hewlett G, Ettischer N, et al. The novel anticytomegalovirus compound AIC246 (Letermovir) inhibits human cytomegalovirus replication through a specific antiviral mechanism that involves the viral terminase. *J Virol* 2011;85(20):10884–10893.
207. Gompels UA, Larke N, Sanz-Ramos M, et al. Human cytomegalovirus infant infection adversely affects growth and development in maternally HIV-exposed and unexposed infants in Zambia. *Clin Infect Dis* 2012;54(3):434–442.
208. Gonczol E, Andrews PW, Plotkin SA. Cytomegalovirus infection of human teratocarcinoma cells in culture. *J Gen Virol* 1985;66 (Pt 3):509–515.
209. Goodrum F, Jordan CT, Terhune SS, et al. Differential outcomes of human cytomegalovirus infection in primitive hematopoietic cell subpopulations. *Blood* 2004;104(3):687–695.
210. Goodrum F, Reeves M, Sinclair J, et al. Human cytomegalovirus sequences expressed in latently infected individuals promote a latent infection in vitro. *Blood* 2007;110(3):937–945.
211. Goodwin CM, Ciesla JH, Munger J. Who's driving? Human cytomegalovirus, interferon, and NFkappaB signaling. *Viruses* 2018;10(9):447.
212. Goodwin CM, Munger J. The IkappaB kinases restrict human cytomegalovirus infection. *J Virol* 2019;93(9):e02030-18.
213. Gorzer I, Guelly C, Trajanoski S, et al. Deep sequencing reveals highly complex dynamics of human cytomegalovirus genotypes in transplant patients over time. *J Virol* 2010;84(14):7195–7203.
214. Graf L, Feichtinger S, Naing Z, et al. New insight into the phosphorylation-regulated intranuclear localization of human cytomegalovirus pUL69 mediated by cyclin-dependent kinases (CDKs) and viral CDK orthologue pUL97. *J Gen Virol* 2016;97(1):144–151.
215. Green ML, Leisenring W, Xie H, et al. Cytomegalovirus viral load and mortality after haemopoietic stem cell transplantation in the era of pre-emptive therapy: a retrospective cohort study. *Lancet Haematol* 2016;3(3):e119–e127.
216. Grey F, Meyers H, White EA, et al. A human cytomegalovirus-encoded microRNA regulates expression of multiple viral genes involved in replication. *PLoS Pathog* 2007;3(11):e163.
217. Griffiths P. The direct and indirect consequences of cytomegalovirus infection and potential benefits of vaccination. *Antiviral Res* 2020;176:104732.
218. Griffiths P, Baraniak I, Reeves M. The pathogenesis of human cytomegalovirus. *J Pathol* 2015;235(2):288–297.
219. Griffiths PD, Stanton A, McCarrell E, et al. Cytomegalovirus glycoprotein-B vaccine with MF59 adjuvant in transplant recipients: a phase 2 randomised placebo-controlled trial. *Lancet* 2011;377(9773):1256–1263.
220. Groves IJ, Reeves MB, Sinclair JH. Lytic infection of permissive cells with human cytomegalovirus is regulated by an intrinsic 'pre-immediate-early' repression of viral gene expression mediated by histone post-translational modification. *J Gen Virol* 2009;90(Pt 10):2364–2374.
221. Groves IJ, Sinclair JH. Knockdown of hDaxx in normally non-permissive undifferentiated cells does not permit human cytomegalovirus immediate-early gene expression. *J Gen Virol* 2007;88(Pt 11):2935–2940.
222. Gudleski-O'Regan N, Greco TM, Cristea IM, et al. Increased expression of LDL receptor-related protein 1 during human cytomegalovirus infection reduces virion cholesterol and infectivity. *Cell Host Microbe* 2012;12(1):86–96.
223. Hagemeier C, Caswell R, Hayhurst G, et al. Functional interaction between the HCMV IE2 transactivator and the retinoblastoma protein. *EMBO J* 1994;13(12):2897–2903.
224. Hahn G, Revello MG, Patrone M, et al. Human cytomegalovirus UL131-128 genes are indispensable for virus growth in endothelial cells and virus transfer to leukocytes. *J Virol* 2004;78(18):10023–10033.
225. Hahn G, Rose D, Wagner M, et al. Cloning of the genomes of human cytomegalovirus strains Toledo, TownevarRIT3, and Towne long as BACs and site-directed mutagenesis using a PCR-based technique. *Virology* 2003;307(1):164–177.
226. Hakki M, Geballe AP. Double-stranded RNA binding by human cytomegalovirus pTRS1. *J Virol* 2005;79(12):7311–7318.
227. Hakki M, Marshall EE, De Niro KL, et al. Binding and nuclear relocalization of protein kinase R by human cytomegalovirus TRS1. *J Virol* 2006;80(23):11817–11826.
228. Hale AE, Collins-McMillen D, Lenarcic EM, et al. FOXO transcription factors activate alternative major immediate early promoters to induce human cytomegalovirus reactivation. *Proc Natl Acad Sci U S A* 2020;117(31):18764–18770.
229. Hamirally S, Kamil JP, Ndassa-Colday YM, et al. Viral mimicry of Cdc2/cyclin-dependent kinase 1 mediates disruption of nuclear lamina during human cytomegalovirus nuclear egress. *PLoS Pathog* 2009;5(1):e1000275.
230. Hammer Q, Ruckert T, Borst EM, et al. Peptide-specific recognition of human cytomegalovirus strains controls adaptive natural killer cells. *Nat Immunol* 2018;19(5):453–463.
231. Hamprecht K, Goelz R. Postnatal cytomegalovirus infection through human milk in preterm infants: transmission, clinical presentation, and prevention. *Clin Perinatol* 2017;44(1):121–130.
232. Hancock MH, Crawford LB, Perez W, et al. Human cytomegalovirus UL7, miR-US5-1, and miR-UL112-3p inactivation of FOXO3a protects CD34(+) hematopoietic progenitor cells from apoptosis. *mSphere* 2021;6(1):e00986-20.
233. Hancock MH, Crawford LB, Pham AH, et al. Human cytomegalovirus miRNAs regulate TGF-beta to mediate myelosuppression while maintaining viral latency in CD34(+) hematopoietic progenitor cells. *Cell Host Microbe* 2020;27(1):104–114.e4.
234. Hancock MH, Mitchell J, Goodrum FD, et al. Human cytomegalovirus miR-US5-2 downregulation of GAB1 regulates cellular proliferation and UL138 expression through modulation of epidermal growth factor receptor signaling pathways. *mSphere* 2020;5(4).
235. Hansen SG, Powers CJ, Richards R, et al. Evasion of CD8+ T cells is critical for superinfection by cytomegalovirus. *Science* 2010;328(5974):102–106.
236. Hansen SG, Sacha JB, Hughes CM, et al. Cytomegalovirus vectors violate CD8+ T cell epitope recognition paradigms. *Science* 2013;340(6135):1237874.
237. Hansen SG, Wu HL, Burwitz BJ, et al. Broadly targeted CD8(+) T cell responses restricted by major histocompatibility complex E. *Science* 2016;351(6274):714–720.
238. Hansen SG, Zak DE, Xu G, et al. Prevention of tuberculosis in rhesus macaques by a cytomegalovirus-based vaccine. *Nat Med* 2018;24(2):130–143.
239. Harwardt T, Lukas S, Zenger M, et al. Human cytomegalovirus immediate-early 1 protein rewires upstream STAT3 to downstream STAT1 signaling switching an IL6-Type to an IFNgamma-like response. *PLoS Pathog* 2016;12(7):e1005748.
240. Hayden RT, Sun Y, Tang L, et al. Progress in quantitative viral load testing: variability and impact of the WHO quantitative international standards. *J Clin Microbiol* 2017;55(2):423–430.
241. Heo J, Dogra P, Masi TJ, et al. Novel human cytomegalovirus viral chemokines, vCXCL-1s, display functional selectivity for neutrophil signaling and function. *J Immunol* 2015;195(1):227–236.
242. Hertel L, Chou S, Mocarski ES. Viral and cell cycle-regulated kinases in cytomegalovirus-induced pseudomitosis and replication. *PLoS Pathog* 2007;3(1):e6.
243. Hetzenecker S, Helenius A, Krzyzaniak MA. HCMV induces macropinocytosis for host cell entry in fibroblasts. *Traffic* 2016;17(4):351–368.
244. Hill P, Cross NB, Barnett AN, et al. Polyclonal and monoclonal antibodies for induction therapy in kidney transplant recipients. *Cochrane Database Syst Rev* 2017;1:CD004759.
245. Ho M. *Cytomegalovirus: Biology and Infection.* 2nd ed. New York: Plenum Publishing; 1991.
246. Ho M. The history of cytomegalovirus and its diseases. *Med Microbiol Immunol* 2008;197(2):65–73.
247. Hobom U, Brune W, Messerle M, et al. Fast screening procedures for random transposon libraries of cloned herpesvirus genomes: mutational analysis of human cytomegalovirus envelope glycoprotein genes. *J Virol* 2000;74(17):7720–7729.
248. Hofmann H, Sindre H, Stamminger T. Functional interaction between the pp71 protein of human cytomegalovirus and the PML-interacting protein human Daxx. *J Virol* 2002;76(11):5769–5783.
249. Holzenburg A, Dittmer A, Bogner E. Assembly of monomeric human cytomegalovirus pUL104 into portal structures. *J Gen Virol* 2009;90(Pt 10):2381–2385.
250. Holzki JK, Dag F, Dekhtiarenko I, et al. Type I interferon released by myeloid dendritic cells reversibly impairs cytomegalovirus replication by inhibiting immediate early gene expression. *J Virol* 2015;89(19):9886–9895.
251. Homer EG, Rinaldi A, Nicholl MJ, et al. Activation of herpesvirus gene expression by the human cytomegalovirus protein pp71. *J Virol* 1999;73(10):8512–8518.
252. Homman-Loudiyi M, Hultenby K, Britt W, et al. Envelopment of human cytomegalovirus occurs by budding into Golgi-derived vacuole compartments positive for gB, Rab 3, trans-golgi network 46, and mannosidase II.[erratum appears in J Virol. Arch 2003 Jul;77(14):8179]. *J Virol* 2003;77(5):3191–3203.
253. Hook LM, Grey F, Grabski R, et al. Cytomegalovirus miRNAs target secretory pathway genes to facilitate formation of the virion assembly compartment and reduce cytokine secretion. *Cell Host Microbe* 2014;15(3):363–373.
254. Hostetler KY. Alkoxyalkyl prodrugs of acyclic nucleoside phosphonates enhance oral antiviral activity and reduce toxicity: current state of the art. *Antiviral Res* 2009;82(2):A84–A98.
255. Huang Y, Qi Y, Ma Y, et al. The expression of interleukin-32 is activated by human cytomegalovirus infection and down regulated by hcmv-miR-UL112-1. *Virol J* 2013;10:51.
256. Huh YH, Kim YE, Kim ET, et al. Binding STAT2 by the acidic domain of human cytomegalovirus IE1 promotes viral growth and is negatively regulated by SUMO. *J Virol* 2008;82(21):10444–10454.
257. Humby MS, O'Connor CM. Human cytomegalovirus US28 is important for latent infection of hematopoietic progenitor cells. *J Virol* 2015;90(6):2959–2970.
258. Hume AJ, Finkel JS, Kamil JP, et al. Phosphorylation of retinoblastoma protein by viral protein with cyclin-dependent kinase function. *Science* 2008;320(5877):797–799.
259. Hummel M, Abecassis MM. A model for reactivation of CMV from latency. *J Clin Virol* 2002;25(Suppl 2):S123–S136.
260. Hwang JS, Bogner E. ATPase activity of the terminase subunit pUL56 of human cytomegalovirus. *J Biol Chem* 2002;277(9):6943–6948.

261. Hyde TB, Schmid DS, Cannon MJ. Cytomegalovirus seroconversion rates and risk factors: implications for congenital CMV. *Rev Med Virol* 2010;20(5):311–326.
262. Hyeon S, Lee MK, Kim YE, et al. Degradation of SAMHD1 restriction factor through Cullin-ring E3 ligase complexes during human cytomegalovirus infection. *Front Cell Infect Microbiol* 2020;10:391.
263. Indran SV, Ballestas ME, Britt WJ. Bicaudal D1-dependent trafficking of human cytomegalovirus tegument protein pp150 in virus-infected cells. *J Virol* 2010;84(7):3162–3177.
264. Indran SV, Britt WJ. A role for the small GTPase Rab6 in assembly of human cytomegalovirus. *J Virol* 2011;85(10):5213–5219.
265. Ingolia NT, Brar GA, Stern-Ginossar N, et al. Ribosome profiling reveals pervasive translation outside of annotated protein-coding genes. *Cell Rep* 2014;8(5):1365–1379.
266. Inkinen K, Soots A, Krogerus L, et al. Cytomegalovirus enhance expression of growth factors during the development of chronic allograft nephropathy in rats. *Transpl Int* 2005;18(6):743–749.
267. Isaacson MK, Compton T. Human cytomegalovirus glycoprotein B is required for virus entry and cell-to-cell spread but not for virion attachment, assembly, or egress. *J Virol* 2009;83(8):3891–3903.
268. Isaacson MK, Feire AL, Compton T. Epidermal growth factor receptor is not required for human cytomegalovirus entry or signaling. *J Virol* 2007;81(12):6241–6247.
269. Ishida JH, Patel A, Mehta AK, et al. Phase 2 randomized, double-blind, placebo-controlled trial of RG7667, a combination monoclonal antibody, for prevention of cytomegalovirus infection in high-risk kidney transplant recipients. *Antimicrob Agents Chemother* 2017;61(2):e01794-16.
270. Ishov AM, Stenberg RM, Maul GG. Human cytomegalovirus immediate early interaction with host nuclear structures: definition of an immediate transcript environment. *J Cell Biol* 1997;138(1):5–16.
271. Isomura H, Stinski MF, Kudoh A, et al. Noncanonical TATA sequence in the UL44 late promoter of human cytomegalovirus is required for the accumulation of late viral transcripts. *J Virol* 2008;82(4):1638–1646.
272. Isomura H, Stinski MF, Murata T, et al. The human cytomegalovirus gene products essential for late viral gene expression assemble into prereplication complexes before viral DNA replication. *J Virol* 2011;85(13):6629–6644.
273. Iwahori S, Umana AC, VanDeusen HR, et al. Human cytomegalovirus-encoded viral cyclin-dependent kinase (v-CDK) UL97 phosphorylates and inactivates the retinoblastoma protein-related p107 and p130 proteins. *J Biol Chem* 2017;292(16):6583–6599.
274. Jackson JW, Sparer T. There is always another way! Cytomegalovirus' multifaceted dissemination schemes. *Viruses* 2018;10(7):383.
275. Jackson SE, Mason GM, Wills MR. Human cytomegalovirus immunity and immune evasion. *Virus Res* 2011;157(2):151–160.
276. Jackson SE, Redeker A, Arens R, et al. CMV immune evasion and manipulation of the immune system with aging. *Geroscience* 2017;39(3):273–291.
277. Jackson SE, Sedikides GX, Okecha G, et al. Generation, maintenance and tissue distribution of T cell responses to human cytomegalovirus in lytic and latent infection. *Med Microbiol Immunol* 2019;208(3–4):375–389.
278. Jansen MA, Otten HG, de Weger RA, et al. Immunological and fibrotic mechanisms in cardiac allograft vasculopathy. *Transplantation* 2015;99(12):2467–2475.
279. Jasinski-Bergner S, Mandelboim O, Seliger B. Molecular mechanisms of human herpes viruses inferring with host immune surveillance. *J Immunother Cancer* 2020;8(2):e000841.
280. Jenks JA, Nelson CS, Roark HK, et al. Antibody binding to native cytomegalovirus glycoprotein B predicts efficacy of the gB/MF59 vaccine in humans. *Sci Transl Med* 2020;12(568):eabb3611.
281. Jergovic M, Contreras NA, Nikolich-Zugich J. Impact of CMV upon immune aging: facts and fiction. *Med Microbiol Immunol* 2019;208(3–4):263–269.
282. Jiang XJ, Adler B, Sampaio KL, et al. UL74 of human cytomegalovirus contributes to virus release by promoting secondary envelopment of virions. *J Virol* 2008;82(6): 2802–2812.
283. Johansson I, Andersson R, Friman V, et al. Cytomegalovirus infection and disease reduce 10-year cardiac allograft vasculopathy-free survival in heart transplant recipients. *BMC Infect Dis* 2015;15:582.
284. John S, Yuzhakov O, Woods A, et al. Multi-antigenic human cytomegalovirus mRNA vaccines that elicit potent humoral and cell-mediated immunity. *Vaccine* 2018;36(12):1689–1699.
285. Jones TR, Wiertz EJ, Sun L, et al. Human cytomegalovirus US3 impairs transport and maturation of major histocompatibility complex class I heavy chains. *Proc Natl Acad Sci U S A* 1996;93(21):11327–11333.
286. Jouand N, Bressollette-Bodin C, Gerard N, et al. HCMV triggers frequent and persistent UL40-specific unconventional HLA-E-restricted CD8 T-cell responses with potential autologous and allogeneic peptide recognition. *PLoS Pathog* 2018;14(4):e1007041.
287. Kabanova A, Marcandalli J, Zhou T, et al. Platelet-derived growth factor-alpha receptor is the cellular receptor for human cytomegalovirus gHgLgO trimer. *Nat Microbiol* 2016;1(8):16082.
288. Kagan KO, Enders M, Schampera MS, et al. Prevention of maternal-fetal transmission of cytomegalovirus after primary maternal infection in the first trimester by biweekly hyperimmunoglobulin administration. *Ultrasound Obstet Gynecol* 2019;53(3):383–389.
289. Kagele D, Gao Y, Smallenburg K, et al. Interaction of HCMV UL84 with C/EBPalpha transcription factor binding sites within oriLyt is essential for lytic DNA replication. *Virology* 2009;392(1):16–23.
290. Kagele D, Rossetto CC, Tarrant MT, et al. Analysis of the interactions of viral and cellular factors with human cytomegalovirus lytic origin of replication, oriLyt. *Virology* 2012;424(2):106–114.
291. Kalejta RF, Bechtel JT, Shenk T. Human cytomegalovirus pp71 stimulates cell cycle progression by inducing the proteasome-dependent degradation of the retinoblastoma family of tumor suppressors. *Mol Cell Biol* 2003;23(6):1885–1895.
292. Kamil JP, Coen DM. Human cytomegalovirus protein kinase UL97 forms a complex with the tegument phosphoprotein pp65. *J Virol* 2007;81(19):10659–10668.
293. Kamil JP, Hume AJ, Jurak I, et al. Human papillomavirus 16 E7 inactivator of retinoblastoma family proteins complements human cytomegalovirus lacking UL97 protein kinase. *Proc Natl Acad Sci U S A* 2009;106(39):16823–16828.
294. Kasmapour B, Kubsch T, Rand U, et al. Myeloid dendritic cells repress human cytomegalovirus gene expression and spread by releasing interferon-unrelated soluble antiviral factors. *J Virol* 2018;92(1):e01138-17.
295. Kawaguchi Y, Kato K, Tanaka M, et al. Conserved protein kinases encoded by herpesviruses and cellular protein kinase cdc2 target the same phosphorylation site in eukaryotic elongation factor 1delta. *J Virol* 2003;77(4):2359–2368.
296. Kawaguchi Y, Matsumura T, Roizman B, et al. Cellular elongation factor 1delta is modified in cells infected with representative alpha-, beta-, or gammaherpesviruses. *J Virol* 1999;73(5):4456–4460.
297. Kenneson A, Cannon MJ. Review and meta-analysis of the epidemiology of congenital cytomegalovirus (CMV) infection. *Rev Med Virol* 2007;17(4):253–276.
298. Kew V, Wills M, Reeves M. HCMV activation of ERK-MAPK drives a multi-factorial response promoting the survival of infected myeloid progenitors. *J Mol Biochem* 2017;6(1):13–25.
299. Kew VG, Yuan J, Meier J, et al. Mitogen and stress activated kinases act co-operatively with CREB during the induction of human cytomegalovirus immediate-early gene expression from latency. *PLoS Pathog* 2014;10(6):e1004195.
300. Keyes LR, Hargett D, Soland M, et al. HCMV protein LUNA is required for viral reactivation from latently infected primary CD14(+) cells. *PLoS One* 2012;7(12):e52827.
301. Kim ET, Oh SE, Lee YO, et al. Cleavage specificity of the UL48 deubiquitinating protease activity of human cytomegalovirus and the growth of an active-site mutant virus in cultured cells. *J Virol* 2009;83(23):12046–12056.
302. Kim ET, Roche KL, Kulej K, et al. SAMHD1 modulates early steps during human cytomegalovirus infection by limiting NF-kappaB activation. *Cell Rep* 2019;28(2):434–448 e436.
303. Kim JH, Collins-McMillen D, Buehler JC, et al. Human cytomegalovirus requires epidermal growth factor receptor signaling to enter and initiate the early steps in the establishment of latency in CD34(+) human progenitor cells. *J Virol* 2017;91(5):e01206-16.
304. Kim JH, Collins-McMillen D, Caposio P, et al. Viral binding-induced signaling drives a unique and extended intracellular trafficking pattern during infection of primary monocytes. *Proc Natl Acad Sci U S A* 2016;113(31):8819–8824.
305. Kim S, Seo D, Kim D, et al. Temporal landscape of MicroRNA-mediated host-virus crosstalk during productive human cytomegalovirus infection. *Cell Host Microbe* 2015;17(6):838–851.
306. Kim Y, Lee S, Kim S, et al. Human cytomegalovirus clinical strain-specific microRNA miR-UL148D targets the human chemokine RANTES during infection. *PLoS Pathog* 2012;8(3):e1002577.
307. Kim YE, Ahn JH. Role of the specific interaction of UL112-113 p84 with UL44 DNA polymerase processivity factor in promoting DNA replication of human cytomegalovirus. *J Virol* 2010;84(17):8409–8421.
308. Kim YE, Ahn JH. Positive role of promyelocytic leukemia protein in type I interferon response and its regulation by human cytomegalovirus. *PLoS Pathog* 2015;11(3):e1004785.
309. Kim YE, Oh SE, Kwon KM, et al. Involvement of the N-terminal deubiquitinating protease domain of human cytomegalovirus UL48 tegument protein in autoubiquitination, virion stability, and virus entry. *J Virol* 2016;90(6):3229–3242.
310. Kim YE, Park MY, Kang KJ, et al. Requirement of the N-terminal residues of human cytomegalovirus UL112-113 proteins for viral growth and oriLyt-dependent DNA replication. *J Microbiol* 2015;53(8):561–569.
311. Kimberlin DW, Jester PM, Sanchez PJ, et al. Valganciclovir for symptomatic congenital cytomegalovirus disease. *N Engl J Med* 2015;372(10):933–943.
312. Klenerman P, Oxenius A. T cell responses to cytomegalovirus. *Nat Rev Immunol* 2016;16(6):367–377.
313. Knoblach T, Grandel B, Seiler J, et al. Human cytomegalovirus IE1 protein elicits a type II interferon-like host cell response that depends on activated STAT1 but not interferon-gamma. *PLoS Pathog* 2011;7(4):e1002016.
314. Komazin-Meredith G, Petrella RJ, Santos WL, et al. The human cytomegalovirus UL44 C clamp wraps around DNA. *Structure* 2008;16(8):1214–1225.
315. Kondo K, Kaneshima H, Mocarski ES. Human cytomegalovirus latent infection of granulocyte-macrophage progenitors. *Proc Natl Acad Sci U S A* 1994;91(25):11879–11883.
316. Koppen-Rung P, Dittmer A, Bogner E. Intracellular distribution of capsid-associated pUL77 of human cytomegalovirus and interactions with packaging proteins and pUL93. *J Virol* 2016;90(13):5876–5885.
317. Korioth F, Maul GG, Plachter B, et al. The nuclear domain 10 (ND10) is disrupted by the human cytomegalovirus gene product IE1. *Exp Cell Res* 1996;229(1):155–158.
318. Kotton CN, Kumar D, Caliendo AM, et al. International consensus guidelines on the management of cytomegalovirus in solid organ transplantation. *Transplantation* 2010;89(7):779–795.
319. Koyuncu E, Purdy JG, Rabinowitz JD, et al. Saturated very long chain fatty acids are required for the production of infectious human cytomegalovirus progeny. *PLoS Pathog* 2013;9(5):e1003333.
320. Krauss S, Kaps J, Czech N, et al. Physical requirements and functional consequences of complex formation between the cytomegalovirus IE1 protein and human STAT2. *J Virol* 2009;83(24):12854–12870.
321. Krishna BA, Humby MS, Miller WE, et al. Human cytomegalovirus G protein-coupled receptor US28 promotes latency by attenuating c-fos. *Proc Natl Acad Sci U S A* 2019;116(5):1755–1764.
322. Krishna BA, Poole EL, Jackson SE, et al. Latency-associated expression of human cytomegalovirus US28 attenuates cell signaling pathways to maintain latent infection. *mBio* 2017;8(6):e01754-17.
323. Krmpotic A, Podlech J, Reddehase MJ, et al. Role of antibodies in confining cytomegalovirus after reactivation from latency: three decades' resume. *Med Microbiol Immunol* 2019;208(3–4):415–429.

324. Kropff B, Burkhardt C, Schott J, et al. Glycoprotein N of human cytomegalovirus protects the virus from neutralizing antibodies. *PLoS Pathog* 2012;8(10):e1002999.
325. Kropff B, Koedel Y, Britt W, et al. Optimal replication of human cytomegalovirus correlates with endocytosis of glycoprotein gpUL132. *J Virol* 2010;84(14):7039–7052.
326. Krosky PM, Baek MC, Coen DM. The human cytomegalovirus UL97 protein kinase, an antiviral drug target, is required at the stage of nuclear egress. *J Virol* 2003;77(2):905–914.
327. Krosky PM, Baek MC, Jahng WJ, et al. The human cytomegalovirus UL44 protein is a substrate for the UL97 protein kinase. *J Virol* 2003;77(14):7720–7727.
328. Krzyzaniak MA, Mach M, Britt WJ. HCMV-encoded glycoprotein M (UL100) interacts with Rab11 effector protein FIP4. *Traffic* 2009;10(10):1439–1457.
329. Kschonsak M, Rouge L, Arthur CP, et al. Structures of HCMV Trimer reveal the basis for receptor recognition and cell entry. *Cell* 2021;184(5):1232-1244 e1216.
330. Kudchodkar SB, Yu Y, Maguire TG, et al. Human cytomegalovirus infection alters the substrate specificities and rapamycin sensitivities of raptor- and rictor-containing complexes. *Proc Natl Acad Sci U S A* 2006;103(38):14182–14187.
331. Kumar D, Mian M, Singer L, et al. An interventional study using cell-mediated immunity to personalize therapy for cytomegalovirus infection after transplantation. *Am J Transplant* 2017;17(9):2468–2473.
332. Kumar R, Cruz L, Sandhu PK, et al. UL88 mediates the incorporation of a subset of proteins into the virion tegument. *J Virol* 2020;94(14):e00474-20.
333. Kuny CV, Chinchilla K, Culbertson MR, et al. Cyclin-dependent kinase-like function is shared by the beta- and gamma- subset of the conserved herpesvirus protein kinases. *PLoS Pathog* 2010;6(9):e1001092.
334. La Rosa C, Longmate J, Martinez J, et al. MVA vaccine encoding CMV antigens safely induces durable expansion of CMV-specific T cells in healthy adults. *Blood* 2017;129(1):114–125.
335. Lai L, Britt WJ. The interaction between the major capsid protein and the smallest capsid protein of human cytomegalovirus is dependent on two linear sequences in the smallest capsid protein. *J Virol* 2003;77(4):2730–2735.
336. Laib Sampaio K, Stegmann C, Brizic I, et al. The contribution of pUL74 to growth of human cytomegalovirus is masked in the presence of RL13 and UL128 expression. *J Gen Virol* 2016;97(8):1917–1927.
337. Lang D, Gebert S, Arlt H, et al. Functional interaction between the human cytomegalovirus 86-kilodalton IE2 protein and the cellular transcription factor CREB. *J Virol* 1995;69(10):6030–6037.
338. Langemeijer EV, Slinger E, de Munnik S, et al. Constitutive beta-catenin signaling by the viral chemokine receptor US28. *PLoS One* 2012;7(11):e48935.
339. Lashmit PE, Stinski MF, Murphy EA, et al. A cis repression sequence adjacent to the transcription start site of the human cytomegalovirus US3 gene is required to down regulate gene expression at early and late times after infection. *J Virol* 1998;72(12):9575–9584.
340. Lau B, Kerr K, Gu Q, et al. Human cytomegalovirus long non-coding RNA1.2 suppresses extracellular release of the pro-inflammatory cytokine IL-6 by blocking NF-κB activation. *Front Cell Infect Microbiol* 2020;10:361.
341. Lau B, Poole E, Krishna B, et al. The Expression of Human Cytomegalovirus MicroRNA MiR-UL148D during Latent Infection in Primary Myeloid Cells Inhibits Activin A-triggered Secretion of IL-6. *Sci Rep* 2016;6:31205.
342. Lau B, Poole E, Van Damme E, et al. Human cytomegalovirus miR-UL112-1 promotes the down-regulation of viral immediate early-gene expression during latency to prevent T-cell recognition of latently infected cells. *J Gen Virol* 2016;97(9):2387–2398.
343. Lawler SE. Cytomegalovirus and glioblastoma; controversies and opportunities. *J Neurooncol* 2015;123(3):465–471.
344. Le VT, Trilling M, Hengel H. The cytomegaloviral protein pUL138 acts as potentiator of tumor necrosis factor (TNF) receptor 1 surface density to enhance ULb'-encoded modulation of TNF-alpha signaling. *J Virol* 2011;85(24):13260–13270.
345. Le-Trilling VTK, Wohlgemuth K, Ruckborn MU, et al. STAT2-dependent immune responses ensure host survival despite the presence of a potent viral antagonist. *J Virol* 2018;92(14):e00296-18.
346. Lee HR, Kim DJ, Lee JM, et al. Ability of the human cytomegalovirus IE1 protein to modulate sumoylation of PML correlates with its functional activities in transcriptional regulation and infectivity in cultured fibroblast cells. *J Virol* 2004;78(12):6527–6542.
347. Lee HS, Park SH, Kim SH, et al. Risk factors and clinical outcomes associated with cytomegalovirus colitis in patients with acute severe ulcerative colitis. *Inflamm Bowel Dis* 2016;22(4):912–918.
348. Lee SH, Albright ER, Lee JH, et al. Cellular defense against latent colonization foiled by human cytomegalovirus UL138 protein. *Sci Adv* 2015;1(10):e1501164.
349. Lee SH, Kalejta RF, Kerry J, et al. BclAF1 restriction factor is neutralized by proteasomal degradation and microRNA repression during human cytomegalovirus infection. *Proc Natl Acad Sci U S A* 2012;109(24):9575–9580.
350. Lemmermann NA, Krmpotic A, Podlech J, et al. Non-redundant and redundant roles of cytomegalovirus gH/gL complexes in host organ entry and intra-tissue spread. *PLoS Pathog* 2015;11(2):e1004640.
351. Leruez-Ville M, Magny JF, Couderc S, et al. Risk factors for congenital cytomegalovirus infection following primary and nonprimary maternal infection: a prospective neonatal screening study using polymerase chain reaction in saliva. *Clin Infect Dis* 2017;65(3):398–404.
352. Lester E, Rana R, Liu Z, et al. Identification of the functional domains of the essential human cytomegalovirus UL34 proteins. *Virology* 2006;353(1):27–34.
353. Li G, Nguyen CC, Ryckman BJ, et al. A viral regulator of glycoprotein complexes contributes to human cytomegalovirus cell tropism. *Proc Natl Acad Sci U S A* 2015;112(14):4471–4476.
354. Li G, Rak M, Nguyen CC, et al. An epistatic relationship between the viral protein kinase UL97 and the UL133-UL138 latency locus during the human cytomegalovirus lytic cycle. *J Virol* 2014;88(11):6047–6060.
355. Li M, Ball CB, Collins G, et al. Human cytomegalovirus IE2 drives transcription initiation from a select subset of late infection viral promoters by host RNA polymerase II. *PLoS Pathog* 2020;16(4):e1008402.
356. Li Q, Wilkie AR, Weller M, et al. THY-1 cell surface antigen (CD90) has an important role in the initial stage of human cytomegalovirus infection. *PLoS Pathog* 2015;11(7):e1004999.
357. Ligat G, Cazal R, Hantz S, et al. The human cytomegalovirus terminase complex as an antiviral target: a close-up view. *FEMS Microbiol Rev* 2018;42(2):137–145.
358. Lilleri D, Gerna G. Maternal immune correlates of protection from human cytomegalovirus transmission to the fetus after primary infection in pregnancy. *Rev Med Virol* 2017;27(2).
359. Lim EY, Jackson SE, Wills MR. The CD4+ T cell response to human cytomegalovirus in healthy and immunocompromised people. *Front Cell Infect Microbiol* 2020;10:202.
360. Limaye AP, Stapleton RD, Peng L, et al. Effect of ganciclovir on IL-6 levels among cytomegalovirus-seropositive adults with critical illness: a randomized clinical trial. *JAMA* 2017;318(8):731–740.
361. Lin SR, Jiang MJ, Wang HH, et al. Human cytomegalovirus UL76 elicits novel aggresome formation via interaction with S5a of the ubiquitin proteasome system. *J Virol* 2013;87(21):11562–11578.
362. Lin YT, Prendergast J, Grey F. The host ubiquitin-dependent segregase VCP/p97 is required for the onset of human cytomegalovirus replication. *PLoS Pathog* 2017;13(5):e1006329.
363. Lindau P, Mukherjee R, Gutschow MV, et al. Cytomegalovirus exposure in the elderly does not reduce CD8 T cell repertoire diversity. *J Immunol* 2019;202(2):476–483.
364. Littler E, Stuart AD, Chee MS. Human cytomegalovirus UL97 open reading frame encodes a protein that phosphorylates the antiviral nucleoside analogue ganciclovir. *Nature* 1992;358(6382):160–162.
365. Liu B, Hermiston TW, Stinski MF. A cis-acting element in the major immediate early (IE) promoter of human cytomegalovirus is required for negative regulation by IE2. *J Virol* 1991;65:897–903.
366. Liu B, Stinski MF. Human cytomegalovirus contains a tegument protein that enhances transcription from promoters with upstream ATF and AP-1 cis-acting elements. *J Virol* 1992;66(7):4434–4444.
367. Liu ST, Sharon-Friling R, Ivanova P, et al. Synaptic vesicle-like lipidome of human cytomegalovirus virions reveals a role for SNARE machinery in virion egress. *Proc Natl Acad Sci U S A* 2011;108(31):12869–12874.
368. Liu X, Yuan J, Wu AW, et al. Phorbol ester-induced human cytomegalovirus major immediate-early (MIE) enhancer activation through PKC-delta, CREB, and NF-kappaB desilences MIE gene expression in quiescently infected human pluripotent NTera2 cells. *J Virol* 2010;84(17):8495–8508.
369. Liu XF, Swaminathan S, Yan S, et al. A novel murine model of differentiation-mediated cytomegalovirus reactivation from latently infected bone marrow haematopoietic cells. *J Gen Virol* 2019;100(12):1680–1694.
370. Liu XF, Yan S, Abecassis M, et al. Establishment of murine cytomegalovirus latency in vivo is associated with changes in histone modifications and recruitment of transcriptional repressors to the major immediate-early promoter. *J Virol* 2008;82(21):10922–10931.
371. Liu XJ, Yang B, Huang SN, et al. Human cytomegalovirus IE1 downregulates Hes1 in neural progenitor cells as a potential E3 ubiquitin ligase. *PLoS Pathog* 2017;13(7):e1006542.
372. Liu Y, Heim KP, Che Y, et al. Prefusion structure of human cytomegalovirus glycoprotein B and structural basis for membrane fusion. *Sci Adv* 2021;7(10):eabf3178.
373. Liu Z, Biegalke BJ. Human cytomegalovirus UL34 binds to multiple sites within the viral genome. *J Virol* 2013;87(6):3587–3591.
374. Ljungman P, Boeckh M, Hirsch HH, et al. Definitions of cytomegalovirus infection and disease in transplant patients for use in clinical trials. *Clin Infect Dis* 2017;64(1):87–91.
375. Ljungman P, Hakki M, Boeckh M. Cytomegalovirus in hematopoietic stem cell transplant recipients. *Hematol Oncol Clin North Am* 2011;25(1):151–169.
376. Loregian A, Appleton BA, Hogle JM, et al. Residues of human cytomegalovirus DNA polymerase catalytic subunit UL54 that are necessary and sufficient for interaction with the accessory protein UL44. *J Virol* 2004;78(1):158–167.
377. Loregian A, Appleton BA, Hogle JM, et al. Specific residues in the connector loop of the human cytomegalovirus DNA polymerase accessory protein UL44 are crucial for interaction with the UL54 catalytic subunit. *J Virol* 2004;78(17):9084–9092.
378. Loveland AN, Nguyen NL, Brignole EJ, et al. The amino-conserved domain of human cytomegalovirus UL80a proteins is required for key interactions during early stages of capsid formation and virus production. *J Virol* 2007;81(2):620–628.
379. Luganini A, Cavaletto N, Raimondo S, et al. Loss of the human cytomegalovirus US16 protein abrogates virus entry into endothelial and epithelial cells by reducing the virion content of the pentamer. *J Virol* 2017;91(11).
380. Lukashchuk V, McFarlane S, Everett RD, et al. Human cytomegalovirus protein pp71 displaces the chromatin-associated factor ATRX from nuclear domain 10 at early stages of infection. *J Virol* 2008;82(24):12543–12554.
381. Luo MH, Rosenke K, Czornak K, et al. Human cytomegalovirus disrupts both ataxia telangiectasia mutated protein (ATM)- and ATM-Rad3-related kinase-mediated DNA damage responses during lytic infection. *J Virol* 2007;81(4):1934–1950.
382. Lurain NS, Chou S. Antiviral drug resistance of human cytomegalovirus. *Clin Microbiol Rev* 2010;23(4):689–712.
383. Lye MF, Sharma M, El Omari K, et al. Unexpected features and mechanism of heterodimer formation of a herpesvirus nuclear egress complex. *EMBO J* 2015;34(23):2937–2952.
384. Lyon SM, Yetming KD, Paulus C, et al. Human cytomegalovirus genomes survive mitosis via the IE19 chromatin-tethering domain. *mBio* 2020;11(5):e02410-20.
385. Mach M, Kropff B, Dal Monte P, et al. Complex formation by human cytomegalovirus glycoproteins M (gpUL100) and N (gpUL73). *J Virol* 2000;74(24):11881–11892.
386. Mach M, Osinski K, Kropff B, et al. The carboxy-terminal domain of glycoprotein N of human cytomegalovirus is required for virion morphogenesis. *J Virol* 2007;81(10):5212–5224.
387. Macias MP, Stinski MF. An in vitro system for human cytomegalovirus immediate early 2 protein (IE2)-mediated site-dependent repression of transcription and direct binding of IE2 to the major immediate early promoter. *Proc Natl Acad Sci U S A* 1993;90(2):707–711.
388. MacManiman JD, Meuser A, Botto S, et al. Human cytomegalovirus-encoded pUL7 is a novel CEACAM1-like molecule responsible for promotion of angiogenesis. *mBio* 2014;5(6):e02035.

389. Maertens J, Cordonnier C, Jaksch P, et al. Maribavir for preemptive treatment of cytomegalovirus reactivation. *N Engl J Med* 2019;381(12):1136–1147.
390. Manandhar T, Hò GT, Pump WC, et al. Battle between host immune cellular responses and HCMV immune evasion. *Int J Mol Sci* 2019;20(15):3626.
391. Mandal P, McCormick AL, Mocarski ES. TNF signaling dictates myeloid and non-myeloid cell crosstalk to execute MCMV-induced extrinsic apoptosis. *Viruses* 2020;12(11):1221.
392. Mansfield S, Griessl M, Gutknecht M, et al. Sepsis and cytomegalovirus: foes or conspirators? *Med Microbiol Immunol* 2015;204(3):431–437.
393. Marchini A, Liu H, Zhu H. Human cytomegalovirus with IE-2 (UL122) deleted fails to express early lytic genes. *J Virol* 2001;75(4):1870–1878.
394. Marek A, Stern M, Chalandon Y, et al. The impact of T-cell depletion techniques on the outcome after haploidentical hematopoietic SCT. *Bone Marrow Transplant* 2014;49(1):55–61.
395. Margulies BJ, Gibson W. The chemokine receptor homologue encoded by US27 of human cytomegalovirus is heavily glycosylated and is present in infected human foreskin fibroblasts and enveloped virus particles. *Virus Res* 2007;123(1):57–71.
396. Marschall M, Stamminger T, Urban A, et al. In vitro evaluation of the activities of the novel anticytomegalovirus compound AIC246 (letermovir) against herpesviruses and other human pathogenic viruses. *Antimicrob Agents Chemother* 2012;56(2):1135–1137.
397. Marshall EE, Bierle CJ, Brune W, et al. Essential role for either TRS1 or IRS1 in human cytomegalovirus replication. *J Virol* 2009;83(9):4112–4120.
398. Martinez FP, Cruz R, Lu F, et al. CTCF binding to the first intron of the major immediate early (MIE) gene of human cytomegalovirus (HCMV) negatively regulates MIE gene expression and HCMV replication. *J Virol* 2014;88(13):7389–7401.
399. Martinez-Martin N, Marcandalli J, Huang CS, et al. An unbiased screen for human cytomegalovirus identifies neuropilin-2 as a central viral receptor. *Cell* 2018;174(5):1158–1171 e1119.
400. Martins JP, Andoniou CE, Fleming P, et al. Strain-specific antibody therapy prevents cytomegalovirus reactivation after transplantation. *Science* 2019;363(6424):288–293.
401. Marty FM, Ljungman P, Chemaly RF, et al. Letermovir prophylaxis for cytomegalovirus in hematopoietic-cell transplantation. *N Engl J Med* 2017;377(25):2433–2444.
402. Marty FM, Ljungman P, Papanicolaou GA, et al. Maribavir prophylaxis for prevention of cytomegalovirus disease in recipients of allogeneic stem-cell transplants: a phase 3, double-blind, placebo-controlled, randomised trial. *Lancet Infect Dis* 2011;11(4):284–292.
403. Maussang D, Verzijl D, van Walsum M, et al. Human cytomegalovirus-encoded chemokine receptor US28 promotes tumorigenesis. *Proc Natl Acad Sci U S A* 2006;103(35):13068–13073.
404. McCormick AL, Mocarski ES. Cell death pathways controlled by cytomegaloviruses. In: Reddehase MJ, ed. *Cytomegaloviruses: From Molecular Pathogenesis to Intervention*. Vol I. Norfolk, United Kingdom: Caister Scientific Press; 2013:263–276.
405. McCormick AL, Roback L, Livingston-Rosanoff D, et al. The human cytomegalovirus UL36 gene controls caspase-dependent and -independent cell death programs activated by infection of monocytes differentiating to macrophages. *J Virol* 2010;84(10):5108–5123.
406. McCormick AL, Skaletskaya A, Barry PA, et al. Differential function and expression of the viral inhibitor of caspase 8-induced apoptosis (vICA) and the viral mitochondria-localized inhibitor of apoptosis (vMIA) cell death suppressors conserved in primate and rodent cytomegaloviruses. *Virology* 2003;316(2):221–233.
407. McCormick D, Lin YT, Grey F. Identification of host factors involved in human cytomegalovirus replication, assembly, and egress using a two-step small interfering RNA screen. *mBio* 2018;9(3):e00716-18.
408. McKinney C, Zavadil J, Bianco C, et al. Global reprogramming of the cellular translational landscape facilitates cytomegalovirus replication. *Cell Rep* 2014;6(1):9–17.
409. Meshesha MK, Bentwich Z, Solomon SA, et al. In vivo expression of human cytomegalovirus (HCMV) microRNAs during latency. *Gene* 2016;575(1):101–107.
410. Messerle M, Crnkovic I, Hammerschmidt W, et al. Cloning and mutagenesis of a herpesvirus genome as an infectious bacterial artificial chromosome. *Proc Natl Acad Sci U S A* 1997;94(26):14759–14763.
411. Mikell I, Crawford LB, Hancock MH, et al. HCMV miR-US22 down-regulation of EGR-1 regulates CD34+ hematopoietic progenitor cell proliferation and viral reactivation. *PLoS Pathog* 2019;15(11):e1007854.
412. Milbradt J, Kraut A, Hutterer C, et al. Proteomic analysis of the multimeric nuclear egress complex of human cytomegalovirus. *Mol Cell Proteomics* 2014;13(8):2132–2146.
413. Milbradt J, Sonntag E, Wagner S, et al. Human cytomegalovirus nuclear capsids associate with the core nuclear egress complex and the viral protein kinase pUL97. *Viruses* 2018;10(1):35.
414. Milbradt J, Webel R, Auerochs S, et al. Novel mode of phosphorylation-triggered reorganization of the nuclear lamina during nuclear egress of human cytomegalovirus. *J Biol Chem* 2010;285(18):13979–13989.
415. Miller WE, Zagorski WA, Brenneman JD, et al. US28 is a potent activator of phospholipase C during HCMV infection of clinically relevant target cells. *PLoS One* 2012;7(11):e50524.
416. Minisini R, Tulone C, Luske A, et al. Constitutive inositol phosphate formation in cytomegalovirus-infected human fibroblasts is due to expression of the chemokine receptor homologue pUS28. *J Virol* 2003;77(8):4489–4501.
417. Mitchell DP, Savaryn JP, Moorman NJ, et al. Human cytomegalovirus UL28 and UL29 open reading frames encode a spliced mRNA and stimulate accumulation of immediate-early RNAs. *J Virol* 2009;83(19):10187–10197.
418. Mizrahi O, Nachshon A, Shitrit A, et al. Virus-induced changes in mRNA secondary structure uncover cis-regulatory elements that directly control gene expression. *Mol Cell* 2018;72(5):862–874 e865.
419. Mocarski ES, Upton JW, Kaiser WJ. Viral infection and the evolution of caspase 8-regulated apoptotic and necrotic death pathways. *Nat Rev Immunol* 2011;12(2):79–88.
420. Moepps B, Tulone C, Kern C, et al. Constitutive serum response factor activation by the viral chemokine receptor homologue pUS28 is differentially regulated by Galpha(q/11) and Galpha(16). *Cell Signal* 2008;20(8):1528–1537.
421. Montag C, Wagner JA, Gruska I, et al. The latency-associated UL138 gene product of human cytomegalovirus sensitizes cells to tumor necrosis factor alpha (TNF-alpha) signaling by upregulating TNF-alpha receptor 1 cell surface expression. *J Virol* 2011;85(21):11409–11421.
422. Moss P. 'From immunosenescence to immune modulation': a re-appraisal of the role of cytomegalovirus as major regulator of human immune function. *Med Microbiol Immunol* 2019;208(3–4):271–280.
423. Mucke K, Paulus C, Bernhardt K, et al. Human cytomegalovirus major immediate early 1 protein targets host chromosomes by docking to the acidic pocket on the nucleosome surface. *J Virol* 2014;88(2):1228–1248.
424. Müller J, Tanner R, Matsumiya M, et al. Cytomegalovirus infection is a risk factor for tuberculosis disease in infants. *JCI Insight* 2019;4(23):e130090.
425. Murphy E, Rigoutsos I, Shibuya T, et al. Reevaluation of human cytomegalovirus coding potential. *Proc Natl Acad Sci U S A* 2003;100(23):13585–13590.
426. Murphy E, Vanicek J, Robins H, et al. Suppression of immediate-early viral gene expression by herpesvirus-coded microRNAs: implications for latency. *Proc Natl Acad Sci U S A* 2008;105(14):5453–5458.
427. Murphy E, Yu D, Grimwood J, et al. Coding potential of laboratory and clinical strains of human cytomegalovirus. *Proc Natl Acad Sci U S A* 2003;100(25):14976–14981.
428. Murphy JC, Fischle W, Verdin E, et al. Control of cytomegalovirus lytic gene expression by histone acetylation. *EMBO J* 2002;21(5):1112–1120.
429. Murray LA, Sheng X, Cristea IM. Orchestration of protein acetylation as a toggle for cellular defense and virus replication. *Nat Commun* 2018;9(1):4967.
430. Murrell I, Bedford C, Ladell K, et al. The pentameric complex drives immunologically covert cell-cell transmission of wild-type human cytomegalovirus. *Proc Natl Acad Sci U S A* 2017;114(23):6104–6109.
431. Murrell I, Tomasec P, Wilkie GS, et al. Impact of sequence variation in the UL128 locus on production of human cytomegalovirus in fibroblast and epithelial cells. *J Virol* 2013;87(19):10489–10500.
432. Murrell I, Wilkie GS, Davison AJ, et al. Genetic stability of bacterial artificial chromosome-derived human cytomegalovirus during culture in vitro. *J Virol* 2016;90(8):3929–3943.
433. Mussi-Pinhata M, Yamamoto A. Natural history of congenital cytomegalovirus infection in highly seropositive populations (In Press). *J Infect Dis* 2020;221(Suppl 1):S15–S22.
434. Mussi-Pinhata MM, Yamamoto AY, Aragon DC, et al. Seroconversion for Cytomegalovirus infection during pregnancy and fetal infection in a highly seropositive population: "The BraCHS Study". *J Infect Dis* 2018;218(8):1200–1204.
435. Mwaanza N, Chilukutu L, Tembo J, et al. High rates of congenital cytomegalovirus infection linked with maternal HIV infection among neonatal admissions at a large referral center in sub-Saharan Africa. *Clin Infect Dis* 2014;58(5):728–735.
436. Nabekura T, Lanier LL. Tracking the fate of antigen-specific versus cytokine-activated natural killer cells after cytomegalovirus infection. *J Exp Med* 2016;213(12):2745–2758.
437. Nelson CS, Huffman T, Jenks JA, et al. HCMV glycoprotein B subunit vaccine efficacy mediated by nonneutralizing antibody effector functions. *Proc Natl Acad Sci U S A* 2018;115(24):6267–6272.
438. Nevels M, Brune W, Shenk T. SUMOylation of the human cytomegalovirus 72-kilodalton IE1 protein facilitates expression of the 86-kilodalton IE2 protein and promotes viral replication. *J Virol* 2004;78(14):7803–7812.
439. Nevels M, Paulus C, Shenk T. Human cytomegalovirus immediate-early 1 protein facilitates viral replication by antagonizing histone deacetylation. *Proc Natl Acad Sci U S A* 2004;101(49):17234–17239.
440. Nguyen CC, Kamil JP. Pathogen at the gates: human cytomegalovirus entry and cell tropism. *Viruses* 2018;10(12):704.
441. Nguyen CC, Siddiquey MNA, Zhang H, et al. Human cytomegalovirus tropism modulator UL148 interacts with SEL1L, a cellular factor that governs endoplasmic reticulum-associated degradation of the viral envelope glycoprotein gO. *J Virol* 2018;92(18):e00688-18.
442. Nguyen NL, Loveland AN, Gibson W. Nuclear localization sequences in cytomegalovirus capsid assembly proteins (UL80 proteins) are required for virus production: inactivating NLS1, NLS2, or both affects replication to strikingly different extents. *J Virol* 2008;82(11):5381–5389.
443. Nightingale K, Lin KM, Ravenhill BJ, et al. High-definition analysis of host protein stability during human cytomegalovirus infection reveals antiviral factors and viral evasion mechanisms. *Cell Host Microbe* 2018;24(3):447–460 e411.
444. Nigro G. Hyperimmune globulin in pregnancy for the prevention of congenital cytomegalovirus disease. *Expert Rev Anti Infect Ther* 2017;15(11):977–986.
445. Nigro G, Adler SP, La Torre R, et al, Congenital Cytomegalovirus Collaborating Group. Passive immunization during pregnancy for congenital cytomegalovirus infection. *N Engl J Med* 2005;353(13):1350–1362.
446. Nikolich-Zugich J, van Lier RAW. Cytomegalovirus (CMV) research in immune senescence comes of age: overview of the 6th International Workshop on CMV and Immunosenescence. *Geroscience* 2017;39(3):245–249.
447. Nobre LV, Nightingale K, Ravenhill BJ, et al. Human cytomegalovirus interactome analysis identifies degradation hubs, domain associations and viral protein functions. *Elife* 2019;8:e49894.
448. Nogalski MT, Chan G, Stevenson EV, et al. Human cytomegalovirus-regulated paxillin in monocytes links cellular pathogenic motility to the process of viral entry. *J Virol* 2011;85(3):1360–1369.
449. Nogalski MT, Chan GC, Stevenson EV, et al. The HCMV gH/gL/UL128-131 complex triggers the specific cellular activation required for efficient viral internalization into target monocytes. *PLoS Pathog* 2013;9(7):e1003463.
450. Noriega VM, Gardner TJ, Redmann V, et al. Human cytomegalovirus US28 facilitates cell-to-cell viral dissemination. *Viruses* 2014;6(3):1202–1218.
451. O'Connor CM, Murphy EA. A myeloid progenitor cell line capable of supporting human cytomegalovirus latency and reactivation, resulting in infectious progeny. *J Virol* 2012;86(18):9854–9865.
452. O'Connor CM, Nukui M, Gurova KV, et al. Inhibition of the FACT complex reduces transcription from the human cytomegalovirus major immediate early promoter in models of lytic and latent replication. *J Virol* 2016;90(8):4249–4253.
453. O'Connor CM, Vanicek J, Murphy EA. Host microRNA regulation of human cytomegalovirus immediate early protein translation promotes viral latency. *J Virol* 2014;88(10):5524–5532.

454. O'Dowd JM, Zavala AG, Brown CJ, et al. HCMV-infected cells maintain efficient nucleotide excision repair of the viral genome while abrogating repair of the host genome. *PLoS Pathog* 2012;8(11):e1003038.
455. O'Sullivan TE, Sun JC, Lanier LL. Natural killer cell memory. *Immunity* 2015;43(4):634–645.
456. Oduro JD, Uecker R, Hagemeier C, et al. Inhibition of human cytomegalovirus immediate-early gene expression by cyclin A2-dependent kinase activity. *J Virol* 2012;86(17):9369–9383.
457. Ogawa-Goto K, Tanaka K, Gibson W, et al. Microtubule network facilitates nuclear targeting of human cytomegalovirus capsid. *J Virol* 2003;77(15):8541–8547.
458. Omoto S, Mocarski ES. Cytomegalovirus UL91 is essential for transcription of viral true late (gamma2) genes. *J Virol* 2013;87(15):8651–8664.
459. Omoto S, Mocarski ES. Transcription of true late (gamma2) cytomegalovirus genes requires UL92 function that is conserved among beta- and gammaherpesviruses. *J Virol* 2014;88(1):120–130.
460. Ourahmane A, Cui X, He L, et al. Inclusion of antibodies to cell culture media preserves the integrity of genes encoding RL13 and the pentameric complex components during fibroblast passage of human cytomegalovirus. *Viruses* 2019;11(3):221.
461. Ozdemir BH, Sar A, Uyar P, et al. Posttransplant tubulointerstitial nephritis: clinicopathological correlation. *Transplant Proc* 2006;38(2):466–469.
462. Paijo J, Doring M, Spanier J, et al. cGAS senses human cytomegalovirus and induces type I interferon responses in human monocyte-derived cells. *PLoS Pathog* 2016;12(4):e1005546.
463. Pan C, Zhu D, Wang Y, et al. Human cytomegalovirus miR-UL148D facilitates latent viral infection by targeting host cell immediate early response gene 5. *PLoS Pathog* 2016;12(11):e1006007.
464. Panagou E, Zakout G, Keshani J, et al. Cytomegalovirus pre-emptive therapy after hematopoietic stem cell transplantation in the era of real-time quantitative PCR: comparison with recipients of solid organ transplants. *Transpl Infect Dis* 2016;18(3):405–414.
465. Pang J, Slyker JA, Roy S, et al. Mixed cytomegalovirus genotypes in HIV-positive mothers show compartmentalization and distinct patterns of transmission to infants. *Elife* 2020;9:e63199.
466. Pari GS. Nuts and bolts of human cytomegalovirus lytic DNA replication. *Curr Top Microbiol Immunol* 2008;325:153–166.
467. Pari GS, Anders DG. Eleven loci encoding trans-acting factors are required for transient complementation of human cytomegalovirus oriLyt-dependent DNA replication. *J Virol* 1993;67(12):6979–6988.
468. Parida M, Nilson KA, Li M, et al. Nucleotide resolution comparison of transcription of human cytomegalovirus and host genomes reveals universal use of RNA polymerase II elongation control driven by dissimilar core promoter elements. *mBio* 2019;10(1):e02047-18.
469. Park B, Kim Y, Shin J, et al. Human cytomegalovirus inhibits tapasin-dependent peptide loading and optimization of the MHC class I peptide cargo for immune evasion. *Immunity* 2004;20(1):71–85.
470. Park MY, Kim YE, Seo MR, et al. Interactions among four proteins encoded by the human cytomegalovirus UL112-113 region regulate their intranuclear targeting and the recruitment of UL44 to prereplication foci. *J Virol* 2006;80(6):2718–2727.
471. Pass RF, Zhang C, Evans A, et al. Vaccine prevention of maternal cytomegalovirus infection. *N Engl J Med* 2009;360(12):1191–1199.
472. Patel M, Vlahava VM, Forbes SK, et al. HCMV-encoded NK modulators: lessons from in vitro and in vivo genetic variation. *Front Immunol* 2018;9:2214.
473. Patro ARK. Subversion of immune response by human cytomegalovirus. *Front Immunol* 2019;10:1155.
474. Patrone M, Coroadinha AS, Teixeira AP, et al. Palmitoylation strengthens cholesterol-dependent multimerization and fusion activity of human cytomegalovirus glycoprotein B (gB). *J Biol Chem* 2016;291(9):4711–4722.
475. Paulus C, Krauss S, Nevels M. A human cytomegalovirus antagonist of type I IFN-dependent signal transducer and activator of transcription signaling. *Proc Natl Acad Sci U S A* 2006;103(10):3840–3845.
476. Pereira L. Congenital viral infection: traversing the uterine-placental interface. *Annu Rev Virol* 2018;5(1):273–299.
477. Pereira L, Maidji E, McDonagh S, et al. Human cytomegalovirus transmission from the uterus to the placenta correlates with the presence of pathogenic bacteria and maternal immunity. *J Virol* 2003;77(24):13301–13314.
478. Pergam SA, Xie H, Sandhu R, et al. Efficiency and risk factors for CMV transmission in seronegative hematopoietic stem cell recipients. *Biol Blood Marrow Transplant* 2012;18(9):1391–1400.
479. Perng YC, Campbell JA, Lenschow DJ, et al. Human cytomegalovirus pUL79 is an elongation factor of RNA polymerase II for viral gene transcription. *PLoS Pathog* 2014;10(8):e1004350.
480. Perng YC, Qian Z, Fehr AR, et al. The human cytomegalovirus gene UL79 is required for the accumulation of late viral transcripts. *J Virol* 2011;85(10):4841–4852.
481. Petrucelli A, Rak M, Grainger L, et al. Characterization of a novel Golgi apparatus-localized latency determinant encoded by human cytomegalovirus. *J Virol* 2009;83(11):5615–5629.
482. Pfeffer S, Sewer A, Lagos-Quintana M, et al. Identification of microRNAs of the herpesvirus family. *Nat Methods* 2005;2(4):269–276.
483. Pizzorno MC, Hayward GS. The IE2 gene products of human cytomegalovirus specifically down-regulate expression from the major immediate-early promoter through a target located near the cap site. *J Virol* 1990;64:6154–6165.
484. Plotkin SA, Starr SE, Friedman HM, et al. Protective effects of Towne cytomegalovirus vaccine against low-passage cytomegalovirus administered as a challenge. *J Infect Dis* 1989;159:860–865.
485. Pokalyuk C, Renzette N, Irwin KK, et al. Characterizing human cytomegalovirus reinfection in congenitally infected infants: an evolutionary perspective. *Mol Ecol* 2017;26(7):1980–1990.
486. Polachek WS, Moshrif HF, Franti M, et al. High-throughput small interfering RNA screening identifies phosphatidylinositol 3-kinase class II alpha as important for production of human cytomegalovirus virions. *J Virol* 2016;90(18):8360–8371.
487. Polic B, Hengel H, Krmpotic A, et al. Hierarchical and redundant lymphocyte subset control precludes cytomegalovirus replication during latent infection. *J Exp Med* 1998;188(6):1047–1054.
488. Poole E, Huang CJZ, Forbester J, et al. An iPSC-derived myeloid lineage model of herpes virus latency and reactivation. *Front Microbiol* 2019;10:2233.
489. Poole E, Sinclair J. Sleepless latency of human cytomegalovirus. *Med Microbiol Immunol* 2015;204(3):421–429.
490. Poole EL, Kew VG, Lau JCH, et al. A virally encoded DeSUMOylase activity is required for cytomegalovirus reactivation from latency. *Cell Rep* 2018;24(3):594–606.
491. Popescu I, Pipeling MR, Mannem H, et al. IL-12-dependent cytomegalovirus-specific CD4+ T cell proliferation, T-bet induction, and effector multifunction during primary infection are key determinants for early immune control. *J Immunol* 2016;196(2):877–890.
492. Powers C, Fruh K. Rhesus CMV: an emerging animal model for human CMV. *Med Microbiol Immunol* 2008;197(2):109–115.
493. Prichard MN, Britt WJ, Daily SL, et al. Human cytomegalovirus UL97 Kinase is required for the normal intranuclear distribution of pp65 and virion morphogenesis. *J Virol* 2005;79(24):15494–15502.
494. Prichard MN, Duke GM, Mocarski ES. Human cytomegalovirus uracil DNA glycosylase is required for the normal temporal regulation of both DNA synthesis and viral replication. *J Virol* 1996;70(5):3018–3025.
495. Prichard MN, Penfold ME, Duke GM, et al. A review of genetic differences between limited and extensively passaged human cytomegalovirus strains. *Rev Med Virol* 2001;11(3):191–200.
496. Prichard MN, Quenelle DC, Bidanset DJ, et al. Human cytomegalovirus UL27 is not required for viral replication in human tissue implanted in SCID mice. *Virol J* 2006;3:18.
497. Prichard MN, Sztul E, Daily SL, et al. Human cytomegalovirus UL97 kinase activity is required for the hyperphosphorylation of retinoblastoma protein and inhibits the formation of nuclear aggresomes. *J Virol* 2008;82(10):5054–5067.
498. Prichard MN, Williams JD, Komazin-Meredith G, et al. Synthesis and antiviral activities of methylenecyclopropane analogs with 6-alkoxy and 6-alkylthio substitutions that exhibit broad-spectrum antiviral activity against human herpesviruses. *Antimicrob Agents Chemother* 2013;57(8):3518–3527.
499. Procter DJ, Banerjee A, Nukui M, et al. The HCMV assembly compartment is a dynamic golgi-derived MTOC that controls nuclear rotation and virus spread. *Dev Cell* 2018;45(1):83–100 e107.
500. Procter DJ, Furey C, Garza-Gongora AG, et al. Cytoplasmic control of intranuclear polarity by human cytomegalovirus. *Nature* 2020;587(7832):109–114.
501. Qian Z, Xuan B, Hong TT, et al. The full-length protein encoded by human cytomegalovirus gene UL117 is required for the proper maturation of viral replication compartments. *J Virol* 2008;82(7):3452–3465.
502. Rak MA, Buehler J, Zeltzer S, et al. Human cytomegalovirus UL135 interacts with host adaptor proteins to regulate epidermal growth factor receptor and reactivation from latency. *J Virol* 2018;92(20):e00919-18.
503. Rana R, Biegalke BJ. Human cytomegalovirus UL34 early and late proteins are essential for viral replication. *Viruses* 2014;6(2):476–488.
504. Rauwel B, Jang SM, Cassano M, et al. Release of human cytomegalovirus from latency by a KAP1/TRIM28 phosphorylation switch. *Elife* 2015;4:e06068.
505. Razonable RR, Humar A. Cytomegalovirus in solid organ transplant recipients-Guidelines of the American Society of Transplantation Infectious Diseases Community of Practice. *Clin Transplant* 2019;33(9):e13512.
506. Rebmann GM, Grabski R, Sanchez V, et al. Phosphorylation of golgi peripheral membrane protein Grasp65 is an integral step in the formation of the human cytomegalovirus cytoplasmic assembly compartment. *mBio* 2016;7(5):e01554-16.
507. Reeves M, Murphy J, Greaves R, et al. Autorepression of the human cytomegalovirus major immediate-early promoter/enhancer at late times of infection is mediated by the recruitment of chromatin remodeling enzymes by IE86. *J Virol* 2006;80(20):9998–10009.
508. Reeves M, Sinclair J. Regulation of human cytomegalovirus transcription in latency: beyond the major immediate-early promoter. *Viruses* 2013;5(6):1395–1413.
509. Reeves M, Woodhall D, Compton T, et al. Human cytomegalovirus IE72 protein interacts with the transcriptional repressor hDaxx to regulate LUNA gene expression during lytic infection. *J Virol* 2010;84(14):7185–7194.
510. Reeves MB, Breidenstein A, Compton T. Human cytomegalovirus activation of ERK and myeloid cell leukemia-1 protein correlates with survival of latently infected cells. *Proc Natl Acad Sci U S A* 2012;109(2):588–593.
511. Reeves MB, Compton T. Inhibition of inflammatory interleukin-6 activity via extracellular signal-regulated kinase-mitogen-activated protein kinase signaling antagonizes human cytomegalovirus reactivation from dendritic cells. *J Virol* 2011;85(23):12750–12758.
512. Reeves MB, Davies AA, McSharry BP, et al. Complex I binding by a virally encoded RNA regulates mitochondria-induced cell death. *Science* 2007;316(5829):1345–1348.
513. Reeves MB, MacAry PA, Lehner PJ, et al. Latency, chromatin remodeling, and reactivation of human cytomegalovirus in the dendritic cells of healthy carriers. *Proc Natl Acad Sci U S A* 2005;102(11):4140–4145.
514. Reichel A, Stilp AC, Scherer M, et al. Chromatin-remodeling factor SPOC1 acts as a cellular restriction factor against human cytomegalovirus by repressing the major immediate early promoter. *J Virol* 2018;92(14):e00342-18.
515. Reim NI, Kamil JP, Wang D, et al. Inactivation of retinoblastoma protein does not overcome the requirement for human cytomegalovirus UL97 in lamina disruption and nuclear egress. *J Virol* 2013;87(9):5019–5027.
516. Reitsma JM, Sato H, Nevels M, et al. Human cytomegalovirus IE1 protein disrupts interleukin-6 signaling by sequestering STAT3 in the nucleus. *J Virol* 2013;87(19):10763–10776.
517. Reitsma JM, Savaryn JP, Faust K, et al. Antiviral inhibition targeting the HCMV kinase pUL97 requires pUL27-dependent degradation of Tip60 acetyltransferase and cell-cycle arrest. *Cell Host Microbe* 2011;9(2):103–114.
518. Renzette N, Bhattacharjee B, Jensen JD, et al. Extensive genome-wide variability of human cytomegalovirus in congenitally infected infants. *PLoS Pathog* 2011;7(5):e1001344.

519. Renzette N, Gibson L, Jensen JD, et al. Human cytomegalovirus intrahost evolution-a new avenue for understanding and controlling herpesvirus infections. *Curr Opin Virol* 2014;8:109–115.
520. Renzette N, Pfeifer SP, Matuszewski S, et al. On the analysis of intrahost and interhost viral populations: human cytomegalovirus as a case study of pitfalls and expectations. *J Virol* 2017;91(5).
521. Renzette N, Pokalyuk C, Gibson L, et al. Limits and patterns of cytomegalovirus genomic diversity in humans. *Proc Natl Acad Sci U S A* 2015;112(30):E4120–E4128.
522. Reuter N, Schilling EM, Scherer M, et al. The ND10 component promyelocytic leukemia protein acts as an E3 ligase for SUMOylation of the major immediate early protein IE1 of human cytomegalovirus. *J Virol* 2017;91(10):e02335-16.
523. Revello MG, Genini E, Gorini G, et al. Comparative evaluation of eight commercial human cytomegalovirus IgG avidity assays. *J Clin Virol* 2010;48(4):255–259.
524. Revello MG, Lazzarotto T, Guerra B, et al. A randomized trial of hyperimmune globulin to prevent congenital cytomegalovirus. *N Engl J Med* 2014;370(14):1316–1326.
525. Revello MG, Tibaldi C, Masuelli G, et al. Prevention of Primary Cytomegalovirus Infection in Pregnancy. *EBioMedicine* 2015;2(9):1205–1210.
526. Reyda S, Buscher N, Tenzer S, et al. Proteomic analyses of human cytomegalovirus strain AD169 derivatives reveal highly conserved patterns of viral and cellular proteins in infected fibroblasts. *Viruses* 2014;6(1):172–188.
527. Rivailler P, Kaur A, Johnson RP, et al. Genomic sequence of rhesus cytomegalovirus 180.92: insights into the coding potential of rhesus cytomegalovirus. *J Virol* 2006;80(8):4179–4182.
528. Roberts ET, Haan MN, Dowd JB, et al. Cytomegalovirus antibody levels, inflammation, and mortality among elderly Latinos over 9 years of follow-up. *Am J Epidemiol* 2010;172(4):363–371.
529. Rodems SM, Clark CL, Spector DH. Separate DNA elements containing ATF/CREB and IE86 binding sites differentially regulate the human cytomegalovirus UL112-113 promoter at early and late times in the infection. *J Virol* 1998;72(4):2697–2707.
530. Rodriguez-Sanchez I, Munger J. Meal for two: human cytomegalovirus-induced activation of cellular metabolism. *Viruses* 2019;11(3):273.
531. Ross SA, Arora N, Novak Z, et al. Cytomegalovirus reinfections in healthy seroimmune women. *J Infect Dis* 2010;201(3):386–389.
532. Ross SA, Fowler KB, Ashrith G, et al. Hearing loss in children with congenital cytomegalovirus infection born to mothers with preexisting immunity. *J Pediatr* 2006;148(3):332–336.
533. Rossetto CC, Tarrant-Elorza M, Pari GS. Cis and trans acting factors involved in human cytomegalovirus experimental and natural latent infection of CD14 (+) monocytes and CD34 (+) cells. *PLoS Pathog* 2013;9(5):e1003366.
534. Rubin RH. The pathogenesis and clinical management of cytomegalovirus infection in the organ transplant recipient: the end of the 'silo hypothesis'. *Curr Opin Infect Dis* 2007;20(4):399–407.
535. Ryckman BJ, Chase MC, Johnson DC. HCMV gH/gL/UL128-131 interferes with virus entry into epithelial cells: evidence for cell type-specific receptors. *Proc Natl Acad Sci U S A* 2008;105(37):14118–14123.
536. Ryckman BJ, Jarvis MA, Drummond DD, et al. Human cytomegalovirus entry into epithelial and endothelial cells depends on genes UL128 to UL150 and occurs by endocytosis and low-pH fusion. *J Virol* 2006;80(2):710–722.
537. Ryckman BJ, Rainish BL, Chase MC, et al. Characterization of the human cytomegalovirus gH/gL/UL128-131 complex that mediates entry into epithelial and endothelial cells. *J Virol* 2008;82(1):60–70.
538. Sachs MS, Geballe AP. Downstream control of upstream open reading frames. *Genes Dev* 2006;20(8):915–921.
539. Saffert RT, Kalejta RF. Inactivating a cellular intrinsic immune defense mediated by Daxx is the mechanism through which the human cytomegalovirus pp71 protein stimulates viral immediate-early gene expression. *J Virol* 2006;80(8):3863–3871.
540. Saffert RT, Kalejta RF. Human cytomegalovirus gene expression is silenced by Daxx-mediated intrinsic immune defense in model latent infections established in vitro. *J Virol* 2007;81(17):9109–9120.
541. Saffert RT, Penkert RR, Kalejta RF. Cellular and viral control over the initial events of human cytomegalovirus experimental latency in CD34+ cells. *J Virol* 2010;84(11): 5594–5604.
542. Salsman J, Jagannathan M, Paladino P, et al. Proteomic profiling of the human cytomegalovirus UL35 gene products reveals a role for UL35 in the DNA repair response. *J Virol* 2012;86(2):806–820.
543. Salsman J, Zimmerman N, Chen T, et al. Genome-wide screen of three herpesviruses for protein subcellular localization and alteration of PML nuclear bodies. *PLoS Pathog* 2008;4(7):e1000100.
544. Sanchez V, Dong JJ. Alteration of lipid metabolism in cells infected with human cytomegalovirus. *Virology* 2010;404(1):71–77.
545. Sanchez V, Greis KD, Sztul E, et al. Accumulation of virion tegument and envelope proteins in a stable cytoplasmic compartment during human cytomegalovirus replication: characterization of a potential site of virus assembly. *J Virol* 2000;74(2):975–986.
546. Sanchez V, McElroy AK, Yen J, et al. Cyclin-dependent kinase activity is required at early times for accurate processing and accumulation of the human cytomegalovirus UL122-123 and UL37 immediate-early transcripts and at later times for virus production. *J Virol* 2004;78(20):11219–11232.
547. Sanchez V, Sztul E, Britt WJ. Human cytomegalovirus pp28 (UL99) localizes to a cytoplasmic compartment which overlaps the endoplasmic reticulum-golgi-intermediate compartment. *J Virol* 2000;74(8):3842–3851.
548. Sanders RL, Clark CL, Morello CS, et al. Development of cell lines that provide tightly controlled temporal translation of the human cytomegalovirus IE2 proteins for complementation and functional analyses of growth-impaired and nonviable IE2 mutant viruses. *J Virol* 2008;82(14):7059–7077.
549. Sarisky RT, Hayward GS. Evidence that the UL84 gene product of human cytomegalovirus is essential for promoting oriLyt-dependent DNA replication and formation of replication compartments in cotransfection assays. *J Virol* 1996;70(11):7398–7413.
550. Sathiyamoorthy K, Chen J, Longnecker R, et al. The COMPLEXity in herpesvirus entry. *Curr Opin Virol* 2017;24:97–104.
551. Sauer A, Wang JB, Hahn G, et al. A human cytomegalovirus deleted of internal repeats replicates with near wild type efficiency but fails to undergo genome isomerization. *Virology* 2010;401(1):90–95.
552. Schampera MS, Arellano-Galindo J, Kagan KO, et al. Role of pentamer complex-specific and IgG subclass 3 antibodies in HCMV hyperimmunoglobulin and standard intravenous IgG preparations. *Med Microbiol Immunol* 2019;208(1):69–80.
553. Schauflinger M, Villinger C, Mertens T, et al. Analysis of human cytomegalovirus secondary envelopment by advanced electron microscopy. *Cell Microbiol* 2013;15(2):305–314.
554. Schoenfisch AL, Dollard SC, Amin M, et al. Cytomegalovirus (CMV) shedding is highly correlated with markers of immunosuppression in CMV-seropositive women. *J Med Microbiol* 2011;60(Pt 6):768–774.
555. Schommartz T, Tang J, Brost R, et al. Differential requirement of human cytomegalovirus UL112-113 protein isoforms for viral replication. *J Virol* 2017;91(17):e00254-17.
556. Schultz EP, Lanchy JM, Day LZ, et al. Specialization for cell-free or cell-to-cell spread of BAC-cloned human cytomegalovirus strains is determined by factors beyond the UL128-131 and RL13 loci. *J Virol* 2020;94(13):e00034-20.
557. Scrivano L, Esterlechner J, Muhlbach H, et al. The m74 gene product of murine cytomegalovirus (MCMV) is a functional homolog of human CMV gO and determines the entry pathway of MCMV. *J Virol* 2010;84(9):4469–4480.
558. Seleme MC, Kosmac K, Jonjic S, et al. Tumor necrosis factor alpha-induced recruitment of inflammatory mononuclear cells leads to inflammation and altered brain development in murine cytomegalovirus-infected newborn mice. *J Virol* 2017;91(8):e01983-16.
559. Sen P, Wilkie AR, Ji F, et al. Linking indirect effects of cytomegalovirus in transplantation to modulation of monocyte innate immune function. *Sci Adv* 2020;6(17):eaax9856.
560. Shafat MS, Mehra V, Peggs KS, et al. Cellular therapeutic approaches to cytomegalovirus infection following allogeneic stem cell transplantation. *Front Immunol* 2020;11:1694.
561. Sharma M, Bender BJ, Kamil JP, et al. Human cytomegalovirus UL97 phosphorylates the viral nuclear egress complex. *J Virol* 2015;89(1):523–534.
562. Sharma M, Kamil JP, Coughlin M, et al. Human cytomegalovirus UL50 and UL53 recruit viral protein kinase UL97, not protein kinase C, for disruption of nuclear lamina and nuclear egress in infected cells. *J Virol* 2014;88(1):249–262.
563. Shenk T, Alwine JC. Human cytomegalovirus: coordinating cellular stress, signaling, and metabolic pathways. *Annu Rev Virol* 2014;1(1):355–374.
564. Shirakata M, Terauchi M, Ablikim M, et al. Novel immediate-early protein IE19 of human cytomegalovirus activates the origin recognition complex I promoter in a cooperative manner with IE72. *J Virol* 2002;76(7):3158–3167.
565. Shnayder M, Nachshon A, Krishna B, et al. Defining the transcriptional landscape during cytomegalovirus latency with single-cell RNA sequencing. *mBio* 2018;9(2):e00013-18.
566. Shnayder M, Nachshon A, Rozman B, et al. Single cell analysis reveals human cytomegalovirus drives latently infected cells towards an anergic-like monocyte state. *Elife* 2020;9:e52168.
567. Si Z, Zhang J, Shivakoti S, et al. Different functional states of fusion protein gB revealed on human cytomegalovirus by cryo electron tomography with Volta phase plate. *PLoS Pathog* 2018;14(12):e1007452.
568. Silva LA, Strang BL, Lin EW, et al. Sites and roles of phosphorylation of the human cytomegalovirus DNA polymerase subunit UL44. *Virology* 2011;417(2):268–280.
569. Silva MC, Schroer J, Shenk T. Human cytomegalovirus cell-to-cell spread in the absence of an essential assembly protein. *Proc Natl Acad Sci U S A* 2005;102(6):2081–2086.
570. Sinigalia E, Alvisi G, Mercorelli B, et al. Role of homodimerization of human cytomegalovirus DNA polymerase accessory protein UL44 in origin-dependent DNA replication in cells. *J Virol* 2008;82(24):12574–12579.
571. Sissons JG, Wills MR. How understanding immunology contributes to managing CMV disease in immunosuppressed patients: now and in future. *Med Microbiol Immunol* 2015;204(3):307–316.
572. Skaletskaya A, Bartle LM, Chittenden T, et al. A cytomegalovirus-encoded inhibitor of apoptosis that suppresses caspase-8 activation. *Proc Natl Acad Sci U S A* 2001;98(14):7829–7834.
573. Slade M, Goldsmith S, Romee R, et al. Epidemiology of infections following haploidentical peripheral blood hematopoietic cell transplantation. *Transpl Infect Dis* 2017;19(1):e12629.
574. Slayton M, Hossain T, Biegalke BJ. pUL34 binding near the human cytomegalovirus origin of lytic replication enhances DNA replication and viral growth. *Virology* 2018;518:414–422.
575. Slinger E, Maussang D, Schreiber A, et al. HCMV-encoded chemokine receptor US28 mediates proliferative signaling through the IL-6-STAT3 axis. *Sci Signal* 2010;3(133):ra58.
576. Slobedman B, Mocarski ES. Quantitative analysis of latent human cytomegalovirus. *J Virol* 1999;73(6):4806–4812.
577. Smith C, Moraka NO, Ibrahim M, et al. Human immunodeficiency virus exposure but not early cytomegalovirus infection is associated with increased hospitalization and decreased memory T-cell responses to tetanus vaccine. *J Infect Dis* 2020;221(7):1167–1175.
578. Soderberg-Naucler C, Fish KN, Nelson JA. Reactivation of latent human cytomegalovirus by allogeneic stimulation of blood cells from healthy donors. *Cell* 1997;91(1):119–126.
579. Soderberg-Naucler C, Streblow DN, Fish KN, et al. Reactivation of latent human cytomegalovirus in CD14(+) monocytes is differentiation dependent. *J Virol* 2001;75(16):7543–7554.
580. Solez K, Colvin RB, Racusen LC, et al. Banff 07 classification of renal allograft pathology: updates and future directions. *Am J Transplant* 2008;8(4):753–760.
581. Soroceanu L, Akhavan A, Cobbs CS. Platelet-derived growth factor-alpha receptor activation is required for human cytomegalovirus infection. *Nature* 2008;455(7211):391–395.
582. Sourvinos G, Morou A, Sanidas I, et al. The downregulation of GFI1 by the EZH2-NDY1/KDM2B-JARID2 axis and by human cytomegalovirus (HCMV) associated factors allows the activation of the HCMV major IE promoter and the transition to productive infection. *PLoS Pathog* 2014;10(5):e1004136.
583. Spector DJ. UL84-independent replication of human cytomegalovirus strains conferred by a single codon change in UL122. *Virology* 2015;476:345–354.

584. Spector SA, Wong R, Hsia K, et al. Plasma cytomegalovirus (CMV) DNA load predicts CMV disease and survival in AIDS patients. *J Clin Invest* 1998;101(2):497–502.
585. Spengler ML, Kurapatwinski K, Black AR, et al. SUMO-1 modification of human cytomegalovirus IE1/IE72. *J Virol* 2002;76(6):2990–2996.
586. Stamminger T, Gstaiger M, Weinzierl K, et al. Open reading frame UL26 of human cytomegalovirus encodes a novel tegument protein that contains a strong transcriptional activation domain. *J Virol* 2002;76(10):4836–4847.
587. Stanton RJ, Baluchova K, Dargan DJ, et al. Reconstruction of the complete human cytomegalovirus genome in a BAC reveals RL13 to be a potent inhibitor of replication. *J Clin Invest* 2010;120(9):3191–3208.
588. Stanton RJ, Prod'homme V, Purbhoo MA, et al. HCMV pUL135 remodels the actin cytoskeleton to impair immune recognition of infected cells. *Cell Host Microbe* 2014;16(2):201–214.
589. Staras SA, Flanders WD, Dollard SC, et al. Cytomegalovirus seroprevalence and childhood sources of infection: a population-based study among pre-adolescents in the United States. *J Clin Virol* 2008;43(3):266–271.
590. Staras SA, Flanders WD, Dollard SC, et al. Influence of sexual activity on cytomegalovirus seroprevalence in the United States, 1988-1994. *Sex Transm Dis* 2008;35(5):472–479.
591. Stegmann C, Hochdorfer D, Lieber D, et al. A derivative of platelet-derived growth factor receptor alpha binds to the trimer of human cytomegalovirus and inhibits entry into fibroblasts and endothelial cells. *PLoS Pathog* 2017;13(4):e1006273.
592. Stenberg RM, Witte PR, Stinski MF. Multiple spliced and unspliced transcripts from human cytomegalovirus immediate-early region 2 and evidence for a common initiation site within immediate-early region 1. *J Virol* 1985;56(3):665–675.
593. Stern L, Withers B, Avdic S, et al. Human cytomegalovirus latency and reactivation in allogeneic hematopoietic stem cell transplant recipients. *Front Microbiol* 2019;10:1186.
594. Stern-Ginossar N, Elefant N, Zimmermann A, et al. Host immune system gene targeting by a viral miRNA. *Science* 2007;317(5836):376–381.
595. Stern-Ginossar N, Ingolia NT. Ribosome profiling as a tool to decipher viral complexity. *Annu Rev Virol* 2015;2(1):335–349.
596. Stern-Ginossar N, Saleh N, Goldberg MD, et al. Analysis of human cytomegalovirus-encoded microRNA activity during infection. *J Virol* 2009;83(20):10684–10693.
597. Stern-Ginossar N, Weisburd B, Michalski A, et al. Decoding human cytomegalovirus. *Science* 2012;338(6110):1088–1093.
598. Strang BL, Boulant S, Chang L, et al. Human cytomegalovirus UL44 concentrates at the periphery of replication compartments, the site of viral DNA synthesis. *J Virol* 2012;86(4):2089–2095.
599. Strang BL, Boulant S, Kirchhausen T, et al. Host cell nucleolin is required to maintain the architecture of human cytomegalovirus replication compartments. *mBio* 2012;3(1):e00301-11.
600. Straschewski S, Patrone M, Walther P, et al. Protein pUL128 of human cytomegalovirus is necessary for monocyte infection and blocking of migration. *J Virol* 2011;85(10):5150–5158.
601. Streblow DN, Hwee YK, Kreklywich CN, et al. Rat cytomegalovirus vaccine prevents accelerated chronic rejection in CMV-naive recipients of infected donor allograft hearts. *Am J Transplant* 2015;15(7):1805–1816.
602. Streblow DN, Orloff SL, Nelson JA. Acceleration of allograft failure by cytomegalovirus. *Curr Opin Immunol* 2007;19(5):577–582.
603. Streblow DN, Soderberg-Naucler C, Vieira J, et al. The human cytomegalovirus chemokine receptor US28 mediates vascular smooth muscle cell migration. *Cell* 1999;99(5):511–520.
604. Sturgill ER, Malouli D, Hansen SG, et al. Natural killer cell evasion is essential for infection by rhesus cytomegalovirus. *PLoS Pathog* 2016;12(8):e1005868.
605. Suarez NM, Lau B, Kemble GM, et al. Genomic analysis of chimeric human cytomegalovirus vaccine candidates derived from strains Towne and Toledo. *Virus Genes* 2017;53(4):650–655.
606. Suarez NM, Musonda KG, Escriva E, et al. Multiple-strain infections of human cytomegalovirus with high genomic diversity are common in breast milk from HIV-positive women in Zambia. *J Infect Dis* 2019;220(5):792–801.
607. Suarez NM, Wilkie GS, Hage E, et al. Human cytomegalovirus genomes sequenced directly from clinical material: variation, multiple-strain infection, recombination, and gene loss. *J Infect Dis* 2019;220(5):781–791.
608. Sugar EA, Jabs DA, Ahuja A, et al. Incidence of cytomegalovirus retinitis in the era of highly active antiretroviral therapy. *Am J Ophthalmol* 2012;153(6):1016–1024.e1015.
609. Svrlanska A, Reichel A, Schilling EM, et al. A noncanonical function of polycomb repressive complexes promotes human cytomegalovirus lytic DNA replication and serves as a novel cellular target for antiviral intervention. *J Virol* 2019;93(9):e02143-18.
610. Sylwester AW, Mitchell BL, Edgar JB, et al. Broadly targeted human cytomegalovirus-specific CD4+ and CD8+ T cells dominate the memory compartments of exposed subjects. *J Exp Med* 2005;202(5):673–685.
611. Tai-Schmiedel J, Karniely S, Lau B, et al. Human cytomegalovirus long noncoding RNA4.9 regulates viral DNA replication. *PLoS Pathog* 2020;16(4):e1008390.
612. Tandon R, Mocarski ES. Control of cytoplasmic maturation events by cytomegalovirus tegument protein pp150. *J Virol* 2008;82(19):9433–9444.
613. Tang J, Brixel R, Brune W. Copy-paste mutagenesis: a method for large-scale alteration of viral genomes. *Int J Mol Sci* 2019;20(4):913.
614. Tanimura K, Tairaku S, Morioka I, et al. Universal screening with use of immunoglobulin G avidity for congenital cytomegalovirus infection. *Clin Infect Dis* 2017;65(10):1652–1658.
615. Tarrant-Elorza M, Rossetto CC, Pari GS. Maintenance and replication of the human cytomegalovirus genome during latency. *Cell Host Microbe* 2014;16(1):43–54.
616. Tavalai N, Papior P, Rechter S, et al. Evidence for a role of the cellular ND10 protein PML in mediating intrinsic immunity against human cytomegalovirus infections. *J Virol* 2006;80(16):8006–8018.
617. Teira P, Battiwalla M, Ramanathan M, et al. Early cytomegalovirus reactivation remains associated with increased transplant-related mortality in the current era: a CIBMTR analysis. *Blood* 2016;127(20):2427–2438.
618. Teng MW, Bolovan-Fritts C, Dar RD, et al. An endogenous accelerator for viral gene expression confers a fitness advantage. *Cell* 2012;151(7):1569–1580.
619. Terhune SS, Moorman NJ, Cristea IM, et al. Human cytomegalovirus UL29/28 protein interacts with components of the NuRD complex which promote accumulation of immediate-early RNA. *PLoS Pathog* 2010;6(6):e1000965.
620. Terhune SS, Schroer J, Shenk T. RNAs are packaged into human cytomegalovirus virions in proportion to their intracellular concentration. *J Virol* 2004;78(19):10390–10398.
621. Theiss J, Sung MW, Holzenburg A, et al. Full-length human cytomegalovirus terminase pUL89 adopts a two-domain structure specific for DNA packaging. *PLoS Pathog* 2019;15(12):e1008175.
622. Thoma C, Bogner E. Short hairpin RNAs specific to human cytomegalovirus terminase subunit pUL89 prevent viral maturation. *Antivir Ther* 2010;15(3):391–400.
623. Thoma C, Borst E, Messerle M, et al. Identification of the interaction domain of the small terminase subunit pUL89 with the large subunit pUL56 of human cytomegalovirus. *Biochemistry* 2006;45(29):8855–8863.
624. Thomusch O, Wiesener M, Opgenoorth M, et al. Rabbit-ATG or basiliximab induction for rapid steroid withdrawal after renal transplantation (Harmony): an open-label, multicentre, randomised controlled trial. *Lancet* 2016;388(10063):3006–3016.
625. Tower C, Fu L, Gill R, et al. Human cytomegalovirus UL97 kinase prevents the deposition of mutant protein aggregates in cellular models of Huntington's disease and ataxia. *Neurobiol Dis* 2011;41(1):11–22.
626. Towler JC, Ebrahimi B, Lane B, et al. Human cytomegalovirus transcriptome activity differs during replication in human fibroblast, epithelial and astrocyte cell lines. *J Gen Virol* 2012;93(Pt 5):1046–1058.
627. Townsend CL, Forsgren M, Ahlfors K, et al. Long-term outcomes of congenital cytomegalovirus infection in Sweden and the United Kingdom. *Clin Infect Dis* 2013;56(9):1232–1239.
628. Tu CC, Arnolds KL, O'Connor CM, et al. Human cytomegalovirus UL111A and US27 gene products enhance the CXCL12/CXCR4 signaling axis via distinct mechanisms. *J Virol* 2018;92(5):e01981-17.
629. Tu W, Chen S, Sharp M, et al. Persistent and selective deficiency of CD4+ T cell immunity to cytomegalovirus in immunocompetent young children. *J Immunol* 2004;172(5):3260–3267.
630. Tu W, Rao S. Mechanisms underlying T cell immunosenescence: aging and cytomegalovirus infection. *Front Microbiol* 2016;7:2111.
631. Umashankar M, Petrucelli A, Cicchini L, et al. A novel human cytomegalovirus locus modulates cell type-specific outcomes of infection. *PLoS Pathog* 2011;7(12):e1002444.
632. Umashankar M, Rak M, Bughio F, et al. Antagonistic determinants controlling replicative and latent states of human cytomegalovirus infection. *J Virol* 2014;88(11):5987–6002.
633. van Zeijl M, Fairhurst J, Baum EZ, et al. The human cytomegalovirus UL97 protein is phosphorylated and a component of virions. *Virology* 1997;231(1):72–80.
634. Vanarsdall AL, Chin AL, Liu J, et al. HCMV trimer- and pentamer-specific antibodies synergize for virus neutralization but do not correlate with congenital transmission. *Proc Natl Acad Sci U S A* 2019;116(9):3728–3733.
635. Vanarsdall AL, Howard PW, Wisner TW, et al. Human cytomegalovirus gH/gL forms a stable complex with the fusion protein gB in virions. *PLoS Pathog* 2016;12(4):e1005564.
636. Vanarsdall AL, Pritchard SR, Wisner TW, et al. CD147 promotes entry of pentamer-expressing human cytomegalovirus into epithelial and endothelial cells. *mBio* 2018;9(3):e00781-18.
637. Vanarsdall AL, Ryckman BJ, Chase MC, et al. Human cytomegalovirus glycoproteins gB and gH/gL mediate epithelial cell-cell fusion when expressed either in cis or in trans. *J Virol* 2008;82(23):11837–11850.
638. Vanarsdall AL, Wisner TW, Lei H, et al. PDGF receptor-alpha does not promote HCMV entry into epithelial and endothelial cells but increased quantities stimulate entry by an abnormal pathway. *PLoS Pathog* 2012;8(9):e1002905.
639. Vardi N, Chaturvedi S, Weinberger LS. Feedback-mediated signal conversion promotes viral fitness. *Proc Natl Acad Sci U S A* 2018;115(37):E8803–E8810.
640. Varnum SM, Streblow DN, Monroe ME, et al. Identification of proteins in human cytomegalovirus (HCMV) particles: the HCMV proteome. *J Virol* 2004;78(20):10960–10966.
641. Vashee S, Stockwell TB, Alperovich N, et al. Cloning, assembly, and modification of the primary human cytomegalovirus isolate toledo by yeast-based transformation-associated recombination. *mSphere* 2017;2(5):e00331-17.
642. Vieira J, Schall TJ, Corey L, et al. Functional analysis of the human cytomegalovirus US28 gene by insertion mutagenesis with the green fluorescent protein gene. *J Virol* 1998;72(10):8158–8165.
643. Villinger C, Neusser G, Kranz C, et al. 3D analysis of HCMV induced-nuclear membrane structures by FIB/SEM tomography: insight into an unprecedented membrane morphology. *Viruses* 2015;7(11):5686–5704.
644. Vo M, Aguiar A, McVoy MA, et al. Cytomegalovirus strain TB40/E restrictions and adaptations to growth in ARPE-19 epithelial cells. *Microorganisms* 2020;8(4):615.
645. Vomaske J, Melnychuk RM, Smith PP, et al. Differential ligand binding to a human cytomegalovirus chemokine receptor determines cell type-specific motility. *PLoS Pathog* 2009;5(2):e1000304.
646. Vomaske J, Nelson JA, Streblow DN. Human cytomegalovirus US28: a functionally selective chemokine binding receptor. *Infect Disord Drug Targets* 2009;9(5):548–556.
647. Vysochan A, Sengupta A, Weljie AM, et al. ACSS2-mediated acetyl-CoA synthesis from acetate is necessary for human cytomegalovirus infection. *Proc Natl Acad Sci U S A* 2017;114(8):E1528–E1535.
648. Wagenknecht N, Reuter N, Scherer M, et al. Contribution of the major ND10 proteins PML, hDaxx and Sp100 to the regulation of human cytomegalovirus latency and lytic replication in the monocytic cell line THP-1. *Viruses* 2015;7(6):2884–2907.
649. Walsh D, Perez C, Notary J, et al. Regulation of the translation initiation factor eIF4F by multiple mechanisms in human cytomegalovirus-infected cells. *J Virol* 2005;79(13):8057–8064.

650. Walzer SA, Egerer-Sieber C, Sticht H, et al. Crystal structure of the human cytomegalovirus pUL50-pUL53 core nuclear egress complex provides insight into a unique assembly scaffold for virus-host protein interactions. *J Biol Chem* 2015;290(46):27452–27458.
651. Wang C, Zhang X, Bialek S, et al. Attribution of congenital cytomegalovirus infection to primary versus non-primary maternal infection. *Clin Infect Dis* 2011;52(2):e11–e13.
652. Wang D, Li G, Schauflinger M, et al. The ULb' region of the human cytomegalovirus genome confers an increased requirement for the viral protein kinase UL97. *J Virol* 2013;87(11):6359–6376.
653. Wang D, Shenk T. Human cytomegalovirus UL131 open reading frame is required for epithelial cell tropism. *J Virol* 2005;79(16):10330–10338.
654. Wang D, Shenk T. Human cytomegalovirus virion protein complex required for epithelial and endothelial cell tropism. *Proc Natl Acad Sci U S A* 2005;102(50):18153–18158.
655. Wang J, Loveland AN, Kattenhorn LM, et al. High-molecular-weight protein (pUL48) of human cytomegalovirus is a competent deubiquitinating protease: mutant viruses altered in its active-site cysteine or histidine are viable. *J Virol* 2006;80(12):6003–6012.
656. Wang JB, McVoy MA. A 128-base-pair sequence containing the pac1 and a presumed cryptic pac2 sequence includes cis elements sufficient to mediate efficient genome maturation of human cytomegalovirus. *J Virol* 2011;85(9):4432–4439.
657. Wang X, Huang DY, Huong SM, et al. Integrin alphavbeta3 is a coreceptor for human cytomegalovirus. *Nat Med* 2005;11(5):515–521.
658. Wang X, Huong SM, Chiu ML, et al. Epidermal growth factor receptor is a cellular receptor for human cytomegalovirus. *Nature* 2003;424(6947):456–461.
659. Weekes MP, Tan SY, Poole E, et al. Latency-associated degradation of the MRP1 drug transporter during latent human cytomegalovirus infection. *Science* 2013;340(6129):199–202.
660. Weekes MP, Tomasec P, Huttlin EL, et al. Quantitative temporal viromics: an approach to investigate host-pathogen interaction. *Cell* 2014;157(6):1460–1472.
661. Weisbach H, Schablowsky C, Vetter B, et al. Synthetic lethal mutations in the cyclin A interface of human cytomegalovirus. *PLoS Pathog* 2017;13(1):e1006193.
662. Weisblum Y, Panet A, Zakay-Rones Z, et al. Modeling of human cytomegalovirus maternal-fetal transmission in a novel decidual organ culture. *J Virol* 2011;85(24):13204–13213.
663. Weller TH. The cytomegaloviruses: ubiquitous agents with protean clinical manifestations I. *N Engl J Med* 1971;285(4):203–214.
664. Wertheimer AM, Bennett MS, Park B, et al. Aging and cytomegalovirus infection differentially and jointly affect distinct circulating T cell subsets in humans. *J Immunol* 2014;192(5):2143–2155.
665. White EA, Del Rosario CJ, Sanders RL, et al. The IE2 60-kilodalton and 40-kilodalton proteins are dispensable for human cytomegalovirus replication but are required for efficient delayed early and late gene expression and production of infectious virus. *J Virol* 2007;81(6):2573–2583.
666. White EA, Spector DH. Early viral gene expression and function. In: Arvin A, Campadelli-Fiume G, Mocarski E, et al., eds. *Human Herpesviruses: Biology, Therapy, and Immunoprophylaxis*. 2011/02/25 ed. Cambridge: Cambridge Press; 2007:264–294.
667. Whited LK, Latran MJ, Hashmi ZA, et al. Evaluation of alemtuzumab versus basiliximab induction: a retrospective cohort study in lung transplant recipients. *Transplantation* 2015;99(10):2190–2195.
668. Wiebusch L, Hagemeier C. Human cytomegalovirus 86-kilodalton IE2 protein blocks cell cycle progression in G(1). *J Virol* 1999;73(11):9274–9283.
669. Wilkinson GW, Davison AJ, Tomasec P, et al. Human cytomegalovirus: taking the strain. *Med Microbiol Immunol* 2015;204(3):273–284.
670. Wilkinson GW, Kelly C, Sinclair JH, et al. Disruption of PML-associated nuclear bodies mediated by the human cytomegalovirus major immediate early gene product. *J Gen Virol* 1998;79(Pt 5):1233–1245.
671. Wille PT, Knoche AJ, Nelson JA, et al. A human cytomegalovirus gO-null mutant fails to incorporate gH/gL into the virion envelope and is unable to enter fibroblasts and epithelial and endothelial cells. *J Virol* 2010;84(5):2585–2596.
672. Wille PT, Wisner TW, Ryckman B, et al. Human cytomegalovirus (HCMV) glycoprotein gB promotes virus entry in trans acting as the viral fusion protein rather than as a receptor-binding protein. *mBio* 2013;4(3):e00332-13.
673. Wilson DN, Arenz S, Beckmann R. Translation regulation via nascent polypeptide-mediated ribosome stalling. *Curr Opin Struct Biol* 2016;37:123–133.
674. Winston DJ, Antin JH, Wolff SN, et al. A multicenter, randomized, double-blind comparison of different doses of intravenous immunoglobulin for prevention of graft-versus-host disease and infection after allogeneic bone marrow transplantation. *Bone Marrow Transplant* 2001;28(2):187–196.
675. Wolf DG, Courcelle CT, Prichard MN, et al. Distinct and separate roles for herpesvirus-conserved UL97 kinase in cytomegalovirus DNA synthesis and encapsidation. *Proc Natl Acad Sci U S A* 2001;98(4):1895–1900.
676. Woodhall DL, Groves IJ, Reeves MB, et al. Human Daxx-mediated repression of human cytomegalovirus gene expression correlates with a repressive chromatin structure around the major immediate early promoter. *J Biol Chem* 2006;281(49):37652–37660.
677. Wu CC, Jiang X, Wang XZ, et al. Human cytomegalovirus immediate early 1 protein causes loss of SOX2 from neural progenitor cells by trapping unphosphorylated STAT3 in the nucleus. *J Virol* 2018;92(17):e00340-18.
678. Wu H, Kropff B, Mach M, et al. Human cytomegalovirus envelope protein gpUL132 regulates infectious virus production through formation of the viral assembly compartment. *mBio* 2020;11(5).
679. Wu K, Oberstein A, Wang W, et al. Role of PDGF receptor-alpha during human cytomegalovirus entry into fibroblasts. *Proc Natl Acad Sci U S A* 2018;115(42):E9889–E9898.
680. Wu SE, Miller WE. The HCMV US28 vGPCR induces potent Galphaq/PLC-beta signaling in monocytes leading to increased adhesion to endothelial cells. *Virology* 2016;497:233–243.
681. Wu Y, Prager A, Boos S, et al. Human cytomegalovirus glycoprotein complex gH/gL/gO uses PDGFR-alpha as a key for entry. *PLoS Pathog* 2017;13(4):e1006281.
682. Wussow F, Chiuppesi F, Contreras H, et al. Neutralization of human cytomegalovirus entry into fibroblasts and epithelial cells. *Vaccines (Basel)* 2017;5(4):39.
683. Xiaofei E, Meraner P, Lu P, et al. OR14I1 is a receptor for the human cytomegalovirus pentameric complex and defines viral epithelial cell tropism. *Proc Natl Acad Sci U S A* 2019;116(14):7043–7052.
684. Xiaofei E, Pickering MT, Debatis M, et al. An E2F1-mediated DNA damage response contributes to the replication of human cytomegalovirus. *PLoS Pathog* 2011;7(5):e1001342.
685. Xu Y, Ahn JH, Cheng M, et al. Proteasome-independent disruption of PML oncogenic domains (PODs), but not covalent modification by SUMO-1, is required for human cytomegalovirus immediate-early protein IE1 to inhibit PML-mediated transcriptional repression. *J Virol* 2001;75(22):10683–10695.
686. Yamamoto AY, Anastasio ART, Massuda ET, et al. Contribution of congenital cytomegalovirus (cCMV) to permanent hearing loss in a highly seropositive population: "The BraCHS study". *Clin Infect Dis* 2019;70(7):1379–1384.
687. Yamamoto AY, Mussi-Pinhata MM, Boppana SB, et al. Human cytomegalovirus reinfection is associated with intrauterine transmission in a highly cytomegalovirus-immune maternal population. *Am J Obstet Gynecol* 2010;202(3):297.e291–297.e298.
688. Yee LF, Lin PL, Stinski MF. Ectopic expression of HCMV IE72 and IE86 proteins is sufficient to induce early gene expression but not production of infectious virus in undifferentiated promonocytic THP-1 cells. *Virology* 2007;363(1):174–188.
689. Young VP, Mariano MC, Tu CC, et al. Modulation of the host environment by human cytomegalovirus with viral interleukin 10 in peripheral blood. *J Infect Dis* 2017;215(6):874–882.
690. Yu D, Silva MC, Shenk T. Functional map of human cytomegalovirus AD169 defined by global mutational analysis. *Proc Natl Acad Sci U S A* 2003;100(21):12396–12401.
691. Yu D, Smith GA, Enquist LW, et al. Construction of a self-excisable bacterial artificial chromosome containing the human cytomegalovirus genome and mutagenesis of the diploid TRL/IRL13 gene. *J Virol* 2002;76(5):2316–2328.
692. Yu X, Jih J, Jiang J, et al. Atomic structure of the human cytomegalovirus capsid with its securing tegument layer of pp150. *Science* 2017;356(6345):eaam6892.
693. Yu X, Shah S, Lee M, et al. Biochemical and structural characterization of the capsid-bound tegument proteins of human cytomegalovirus. *J Struct Biol* 2011;174(3):451–460.
694. Yu Y, Clippinger AJ, Alwine JC. Viral effects on metabolism: changes in glucose and glutamine utilization during human cytomegalovirus infection. *Trends Microbiol* 2011;19(7):360–367.
695. Yu Y, Maguire TG, Alwine JC. Human cytomegalovirus infection induces adipocyte-like lipogenesis through activation of sterol regulatory element binding protein 1. *J Virol* 2012;86(6):2942–2949.
696. Yuan J, Liu X, Wu AW, et al. Breaking human cytomegalovirus major immediate-early gene silence by vasoactive intestinal peptide stimulation of the protein kinase A-CREB-TORC2 signaling cascade in human pluripotent embryonal NTera2 cells. *J Virol* 2009;83(13):6391–6403.
697. Zalckvar E, Paulus C, Tillo D, et al. Nucleosome maps of the human cytomegalovirus genome reveal a temporal switch in chromatin organization linked to a major IE protein. *Proc Natl Acad Sci U S A* 2013;110(32):13126–13131.
698. Zhang K, Lv DW, Li R. Conserved herpesvirus protein kinases target SAMHD1 to facilitate virus replication. *Cell Rep* 2019;28(2):449–459 e445.
699. Zhang S, Liu L, Wang R, et al. miR-138 promotes migration and tube formation of human cytomegalovirus-infected endothelial cells through the SIRT1/p-STAT3 pathway. *Arch Virol* 2017;162(9):2695–2704.
700. Zhang Z, Qiu L, Yan S, et al. A clinically relevant murine model unmasks a "two-hit" mechanism for reactivation and dissemination of cytomegalovirus after kidney transplant. *Am J Transplant* 2019;19(9):2421–2433.
701. Zheng QY, Huynh KT, van Zuylen WJ, et al. Cytomegalovirus infection in day care centres: A systematic review and meta-analysis of prevalence of infection in children. *Rev Med Virol* 2019;29(1):e2011.
702. Zhou M, Lanchy JM, Ryckman BJ. Human cytomegalovirus gH/gL/gO promotes the fusion step of entry into all cell types, whereas gH/gL/UL128-131 broadens virus tropism through a distinct mechanism. *J Virol* 2015;89(17):8999–9009.
703. Zhou M, Yu Q, Wechsler A, et al. Comparative analysis of gO isoforms reveals that strains of human cytomegalovirus differ in the ratio of gH/gL/gO and gH/gL/UL128-131 in the virion envelope. *J Virol* 2013;87(17):9680–9690.
704. Zhu D, Pan C, Sheng J, et al. Human cytomegalovirus reprogrammes haematopoietic progenitor cells into immunosuppressive monocytes to achieve latency. *Nat Microbiol* 2018;3(4):503–513.
705. Ziehr B, Vincent HA, Moorman NJ. Human cytomegalovirus pTRS1 and pIRS1 antagonize protein kinase R to facilitate virus replication. *J Virol* 2016;90(8):3839–3848.
706. Ziemann M, Thiele T. Transfusion-transmitted CMV infection—current knowledge and future perspectives. *Transfus Med* 2017;27(4):238–248.

CHAPTER

13 Varicella–Zoster Virus

Ann M. Arvin • Allison Abendroth

INTRODUCTION AND HISTORY

Varicella–zoster virus (VZV) belongs to the alphaherpesvirus subfamily of the *Herpesviridae.* Primary VZV infection usually occurs in childhood and causes varicella (chickenpox), characterized by a pruritic vesicular rash. VZV tropism for T lymphocytes allows viral dissemination from mucosal sites of inoculation to skin (Fig. 13.1). VZV then becomes latent in ganglionic neurons and may reactivate to cause zoster (shingles), characterized by pain and a dermatomal rash due to anterograde axonal transport of the virus. VZV persists in the human population by transmission to susceptible individuals from contacts with either varicella or zoster.

Milestones in understanding VZV include the distinction between varicella and smallpox by Herberden (1768), the association of ganglion inflammation with the dermatomal distribution of the zoster rash by Von Barensprung (1863) and Head and Campbell (1900),[158] and confirmation of a proposed common infectious etiology for varicella and zoster (1892)[37] by the observation of varicella in children inoculated with zoster lesion fluid.[393] The suggestion by Garland[119] and Hope-Simpson[166] that zoster resulted from reactivation was documented by Weller et al. who showed that inoculation of varicella and zoster lesion fluid produced identical virions and cytopathic effects in cultured cells.[461,462] VZV latency in neurons was proved by Gilden et al. using VZV DNA probes[129] and Hyman et al. with VZV RNA.[171] Straus et al. compared restriction endonuclease patterns of VZV DNA from episodes of varicella and zoster in an immunocompromised patient to show that reactivation was caused by the original infecting virus.[402] Breuer et al. documented VZV reinfection using genotyping of viruses from two episodes of zoster in an immunocompetent person.[42]

VZV was the first herpesvirus genome to be fully sequenced, done by Davison and Scott,[90] and genome sequencing has since revealed several geographically distributed clades.[41,181,307,376] The

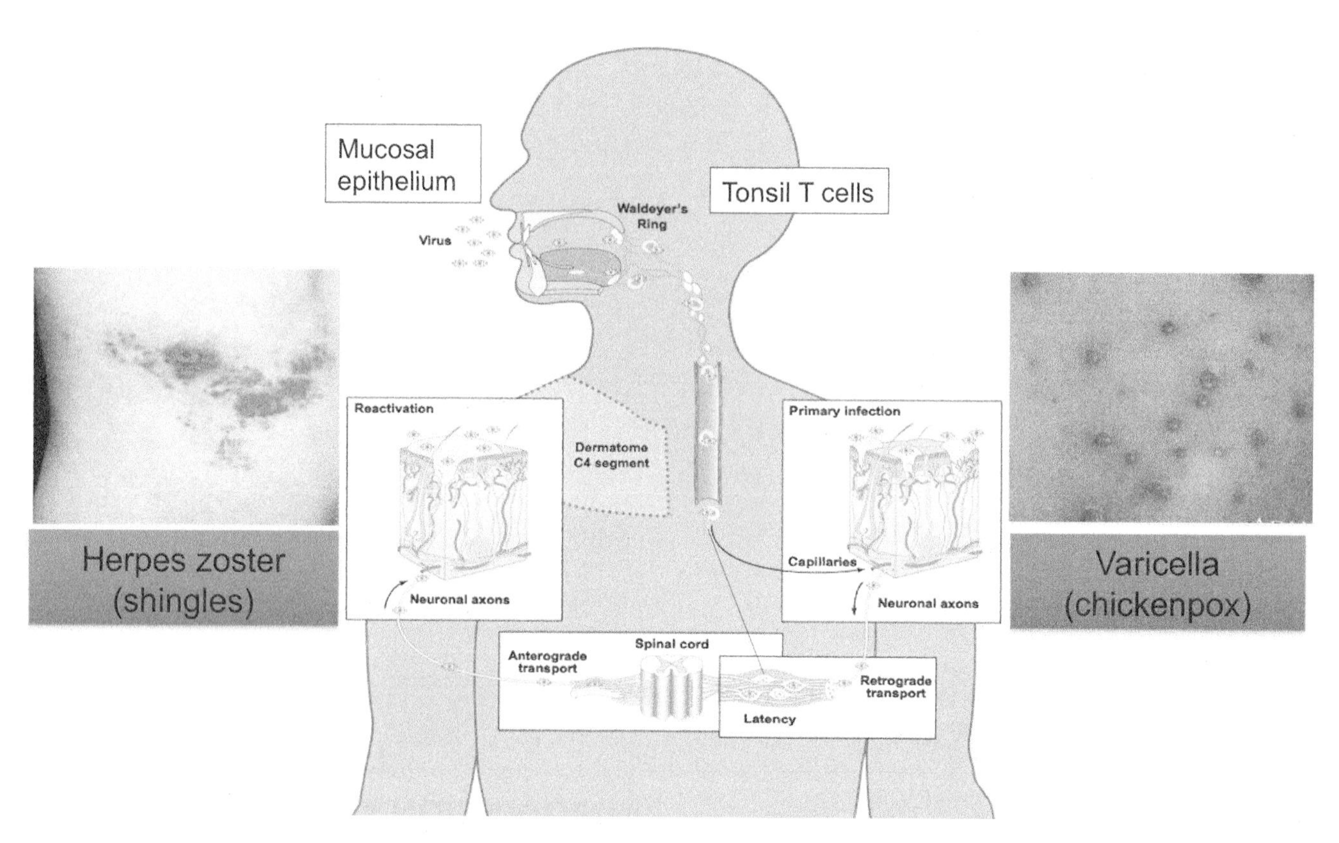

FIGURE 13.1 **Model of the pathogenesis of varicella–zoster virus (VZV) infection**. Primary VZV infection is acquired by inoculation of mucosal epithelial cells of the upper respiratory tract. Replication at the site of entry allows VZV transfer into tonsils and other local lymphoid tissues, where T cells become infected. Infection of dendritic cells in the mucosal epithelium may support virus transfer to regional lymph nodes. VZV-infected T cells transport the virus to skin sites of replication via a cell-associated viremia. After a 10- to 21-day interval, skin infection produces the vesicular rash associated with varicella (chickenpox). In the course of primary infection, VZ virions gain access to the sensory nerve cell body by retrograde axonal transport or via T-cell viremia to establish latent infection within neurons of the sensory ganglia. Episodes of reactivation, during which VZV gains access to skin via anterograde axonal transport, can cause symptoms of zoster (shingles).

construction of recombinant viruses with targeted mutations using cosmids or bacterial artificial chromosomes (BAC) has established the functions of many VZV genes and promoter elements *in vitro*[30,261,413,496] and for VZV pathogenesis *in vivo* by Arvin et al. using human tissue xenografts in a severe combined immunodeficiency (SCID) mouse model.[281,282,486,488,489] Major clinical advances were achieved with the development of effective antiviral drugs,[24,102,465] the live attenuated Oka vaccine derived from a clinical isolate by Takahashi (1974),[323,408] and the recombinant glycoprotein E vaccine.[87,235] VZV remains the only vaccine-preventable human herpesvirus infection.

CLASSIFICATION

The genus *Varicellovirus* of the alphaherpesvirus subfamily includes VZV, simian varicella virus (SVV) (cercopithecrine herpesvirus 9), pseudorabies virus (PRV) (suid herpesvirus 1), and equine herpesvirus 1 (equid herpesvirus 1). VZV is most closely related to SVV.[140] These viruses infect the skin, mucous membranes, and visceral and nervous system tissues and share a genomic arrangement encoding many orthologous genes. Of the three human alphaherpesviruses, VZV is a highly human-restricted pathogen, whereas the other human alphaherpesviruses, herpes simplex viruses HSV-1 and HSV-2 can infect many species.

VIRION STRUCTURE

Morphology

The four major components of VZV particles are the core, nucleocapsid, tegument, and envelope (Fig. 13.2). One copy of the linear, double-stranded (ds) DNA VZV genome is presumed to be incorporated into each virion forming the core. Particles imaged by electron microscopy (EM) have a loose fibrillar cage of strands surrounding a dense cylindrical core of DNA fibers.

Like other herpesviruses, the VZV nucleocapsid consists of 162 capsomere proteins with a 5:3:2 axial symmetry, in which pentameric proteins form the vertices of an 80 to 120 nm icosahedron, while hexameric elements constitute its facets. VZV nucleocapsids recovered from cell culture often lack genomes, consistent with the low infectivity of VZV particles produced *in vitro*. The VZV gene products that constitute the nucleocapsid have not all been verified but are expected to include the products of VZV open reading frames (ORFs) *20, 21, 23, 33, 40*, and *41*, by analogy with their herpesvirus orthologs.

The VZV tegument includes three immediate early (IE) proteins encoded by *ORFs 4, 62*, and *63*.[213,216] In addition, the *ORF9* to *ORF12* gene cluster, conserved in alphaherpesviruses, encodes three tegument proteins, ORF9 to ORF11, and

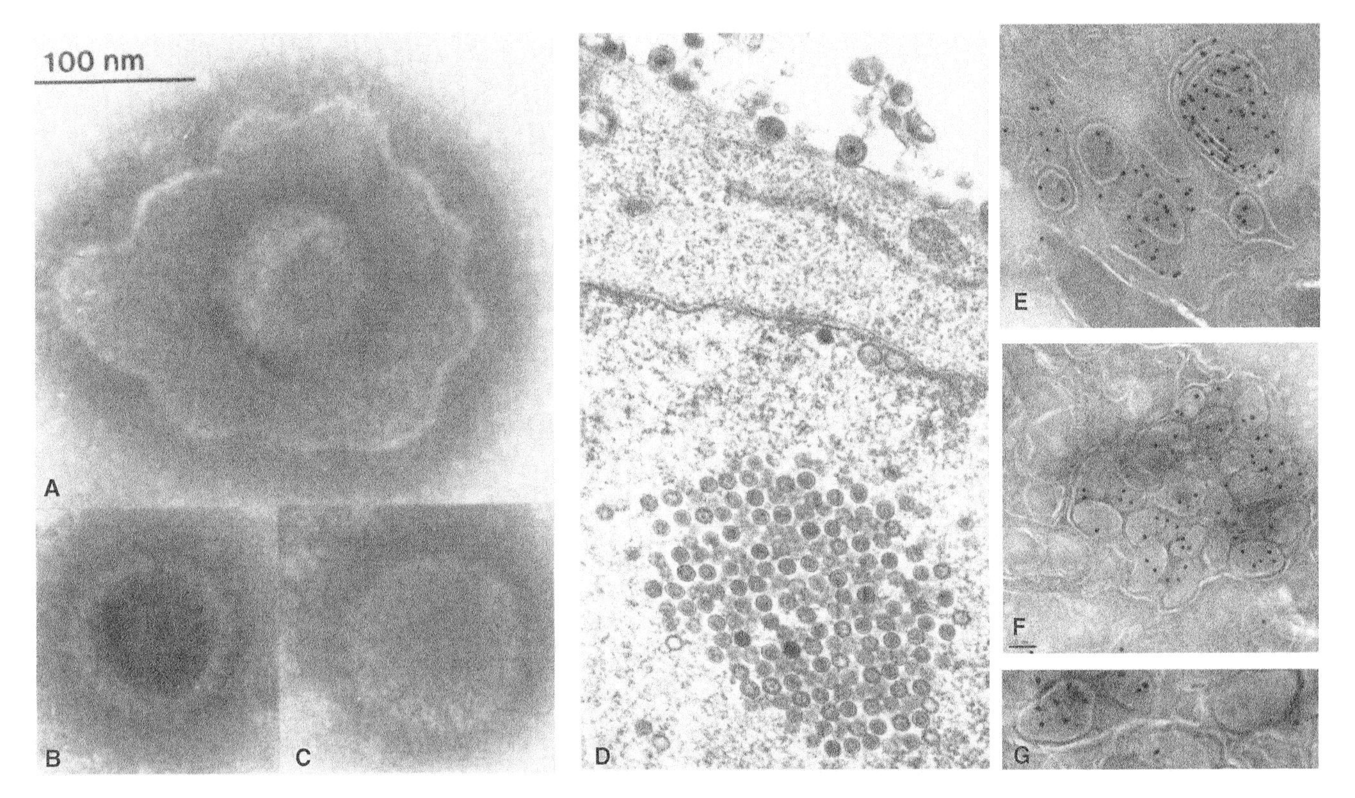

FIGURE 13.2 Electron microscopic appearance of the varicella–zoster virus particle, infected cells, and a representative tegument protein. A: Enveloped particle. **B:** Purified nucleocapsid. **C:** Negatively stained nucleocapsid preparation. **D:** Infected melanoma cell. **E–G:** Localization of the ORF9 tegument protein in Golgi **(E)**, intracellular vacuole **(F)**, and extracellular virions **(G)** shown in 100-nm Tokuyasu cryosections with immunogold staining using rabbit anti-ORF9 (**A, C** adapted from Straus SE, Ostrove JM, Inchauspé G, et al. Varicella-zoster virus infections: biology, natural history, treatment, and prevention. *Ann Intern Med* 1988;108(2):221–237. Courtesy of Dr. William Ruyechan.)

the putative tegument protein, ORF12.[61,248] The viral kinases, encoded by *ORF47* and *ORF66*, are also tegument proteins. ORFs 22, 38, 53, 57, and 64/69 are putative tegument proteins.[496] Nucleocapsids and associated tegument proteins are enveloped within patches of host cellular membranes that display virally encoded glycoproteins. Since particles can capture membranous elements of the endoplasmic reticulum (ER), cytoplasmic vesicles, and the cell surface, the VZV envelope does not appear to have a single source. The mature VZV particle, consisting of the nucleocapsid, tegument, and lipid membrane envelope, is pleomorphic to spherical and 180 to 200 nm in diameter.

Physical and Chemical Properties

The lipid envelope renders VZV susceptible to loss of infectivity by organic solvents, detergents, or proteases; heating to 60°C; prolonged storage at temperatures of −70°C or above; extremes of pH; or ultrasonic disruption. In cesium chloride gradients, enveloped VZV particles band at a buoyant density of 1.274 g/cm^3, while VZV DNA exhibits a buoyant density in cesium chloride of 1.705 g/cm^3.

GENOMIC STRUCTURE AND ORGANIZATION

The VZV dsDNA genome is approximately 125,000 bp,[90] consists of a unique long region (UL) of about 105,000 bp flanked by inverted repeat regions, the terminal repeat long (TRL) and internal repeat long (IRL) sequences (88.5 bp), and a unique short region (US) (5,232 bp) flanked by the terminal repeat short (TRS) and inverted repeat short (IRS) (7,319.5 bp) (Fig. 13.3). Overall, 46% of VZV bases are G + C, whereas the G + C content of its repeat elements is approximately 60% to 68%.[401] Unlike SVV and other varicelloviruses, VZV lacks a terminal region with flanking inverted repeats at the left end of the genome.[140]

VZ virions usually contain the viral genome as a linear molecule; a circular, supercoiled conformation is rarely detected.[219] The genome has two predominant isoforms,[105] with 50% having the US and 95% having the UL region directed in a single orientation.[89,219] An unpaired cytosine at its left end and a guanine at the right end allow the genome to form a circular molecule[89]; the termini are covalently joined in latency.[69] ORFS/L (or ORF 0), located at the end of the UL, encodes a protein essential for replication[194,197,495] and the sequence at the 5′ terminus of ORFS/L is required for DNA cleavage.[194] This UL sequence is not duplicated at the opposite end of the UL, which may explain the single orientation of UL in 95% of VZV genomes.

The VZV genome encodes at least 71 ORFs, 3 of which are present in two copies in the IRS and TRS regions, 63 are in the UL, 4 are in the US and the ORF-S/L gene (Fig. 13.3; Table 13.1). Mutagenesis studies indicate that about 44 ORFs are required for replication *in vitro*, with some variations depending on conditions. Twelve of twenty-six dispensable genes are in the *ORFS/L* to *ORF15* region.[66,496] Gene duplications are

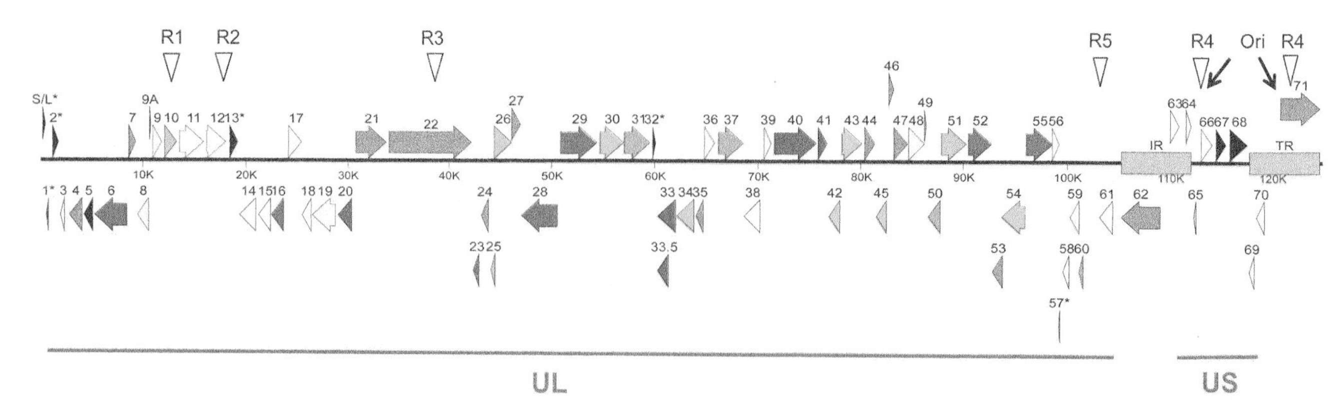

FIGURE 13.3 Organization of the varicella–zoster virus (VZV) genome and known or predicted open reading frames encoding viral proteins. The VZV genome has unique long (UL) and unique short (US) regions flanked by internal repeat (IR) and terminal repeat (TR) regions. VZV has 40 core genes that are conserved among α-, β-, and γ-herpesviruses; these gene products participate in DNA replication (*blue*), DNA cleavage and packaging (*green*), nucleic acid metabolism (*yellow*), and capsid protein assembly (*red*); or envelope glycoproteins (*orange*); or have other functions (*pink*). The genes that are not conserved among the other herpesviruses may be nonessential for VZV replication in cultured cells (*white*) or may be essential (*gray*), three of which are envelope glycoproteins (*black*). Six VZV genes have no HSV-1 ortholog (*). *Open arrows* and *black arrows* indicate repeats (R1–R5) and the origins of DNA replication (ori_S), respectively. When the genome is circularized, ORF S/L (ORF 0) begins at the right end and extends across the terminal repeat into the UL region at the left end.

TABLE 13.1 VZV genes and proteins with known or predicted functions

ORF	Virion Location	Protein Characteristics and/or Functions[a]	Requirement for Growth in Cell Culture[b]	Infection of Skin and T-Cell Xenografts in the SCID Mouse Model		HSV-1 Homolog
				Skin	T cells	
0 (S/L)		RNA transport	Essential/ impaired[b]			None
1		Membrane protein	Dispensable			None
2			Dispensable			None
3			Impaired			UL55
4	Tegument	Transactivator	Essential			UL54 (ICP 27)
5		gK[a]	Essential			UL53
6		Helicase/primase complex[a]	Essential			UL52
7			Dispensable			UL51
8		Deoxyuridine triphosphatase	Impaired			UL50
9	Tegument	Complex with gE	Essential			UL49
9A		gN[a]; syncytia formation	Essential[b]			UL49A
10	Tegument	Transactivator; efficient virion assembly	Dispensable	Impaired	NL	UL4 (VP16)
11	Tegument	RNA binding	Dispensable	Δ10:impaired (−) RNA binding: NL		UL47 (VP13-14)
12		Predicted tegument protein	Dispensable	NL		UL46 (VP11/12)
13		Thymidylate synthetase	Dispensable			None
14	Envelope	gC	Impaired			UL44
15		Integral membrane protein	Dispensable			UL43
16		DNA Polymerase processivity factor[a]	Essential			UL42
17		RNA cleavage	Essential[b]			UL41 (VHS)
18		Ribonucleotide reductase, small subunit	Impaired			UL40

TABLE 13.1 VZV genes and proteins with known or predicted functions (*Continued*)

ORF	Virion Location	Protein Characteristics and/or Functions[a]	Requirement for Growth in Cell Culture[b]	Infection of Skin and T-Cell Xenografts in the SCID Mouse Model		HSV-1 Homolog
				Skin	T cells	
19		Ribonucleotide reductase, large subunit	Impaired			UL39
20	Capsid[c]	Intercapsomeric triplex component[a]	Essential			UL38 (VP19C)
21	Capsid[c]	Nucleocapsid protein	Essential			UL37
22	Tegument[c]		Essential			UL36
23	Capsid	Small capsid surface protein	Impaired	Required		UL35 (VP26)
24			Essential			UL34
25		DNA packaging[a]	Essential			UL33
26		DNA packaging[a]	Essential			UL32
27		Nuclear matrix protein[a]	Essential			UL31
28		DNA polymerase	Essential			UL30
29		ssDNA-binding protein	Essential			UL29 (ICP8)
30		DNA packaging[a]	Essential			UL28
31	Envelope	gB	Essential	(–) furin cleavage: impaired		UL27
32		ORF47 kinase substrate	Dispensable			None
33		Major capsid scaffold protein; protease[a]	Essential			UL26 (VP24)
33.5		Minor capsid scaffold protein[a]	Essential			UL26.5 (VP22)
34		DNA packaging[a]	Essential			UL25
35		Cell–cell fusion	Impaired	Impaired	Impaired	UL24
36		Deoxypyrimidine (thymidine) kinase	Dispensable			UL23
37	Envelope	gH; three domains DI–DIII	Essential	(–) DI extreme N terminus: impaired (–) DIII fusion loop residues: impaired		UL22
38	Tegument[c]		Essential			UL21
39		Integral membrane protein[a]	Essential			UL20
40	Capsid	Major nucleocapsid protein; hexon/penton component[a]	Essential			UL19 (VP5)
41		Minor capsid protein[a]	Essential			UL18 (VP23)
42/45		DNA packaging[a]	Essential			UL15
43		DNA packaging[a]	Essential			UL17
44	Tegument[c]		Essential			UL16
46	Tegument[c]		Essential			UL14
47	Tegument	Serine/threonine kinase (conserved)	Dispensable (defective virion assembly)	Δ47: No growth (–) kinase: impaired	No growth No growth	UL13
48		Deoxyribonuclease[a]	Essential			UL12
49			Impaired			UL1
50		gM	Impaired[b]			UL10
51		Origin-binding protein	Essential			UL9
52		Helicase/primase complex (presumed)	Essential			UL8

(*Continued*)

TABLE 13.1 VZV genes and proteins with known or predicted functions (*Continued*)

ORF	Virion Location	Protein Characteristics and/or Functions[a]	Requirement for Growth in Cell Culture[b]	Infection of Skin and T-Cell Xenografts in the SCID Mouse Model		HSV-1 Homolog
				Skin	T cells	
53			Essential			UL7
54			Essential			UL6
55		Helicase/primase complex[a]	Essential			UL5
56			Essential			UL4
57	Tegument[c]	Virion egress[a]	Dispensable			None
58			Dispensable			UL3
59		Uracil–DNA glycosylase	Dispensable			UL2
60	Envelope	gL, chaperone for gH	Essential			UL1
61		Transactivator/repressor; PML dispersal by SUMO binding motifs (SIMs); E3 ligase	Essential[b]	ΔSIM: impaired Δ250–320 hydrophobic domain: impaired		ICP0
62/71	Tegument	Transactivator; IFN inhibition	Essential	Single copy: no growth		ICP4
63/70	Tegument	Phosphoprotein	Essential[b]	Single copy: NL (–) S/T residues: impaired	NL NL	US1.5 (colinear ICP22)
64/69			Dispensable (large plaques)	NL	NL	US10
65		Virion protein	Dispensable	NL	NL	US9
66		Serine/threonine kinase (α herpesviruses only)	Dispensable	Δ66: Sl. impaired (–) kinase: Sl. impaired	Impaired Impaired	US3
67	Envelope	gI; binds gE	Impaired	ΔgI: no growth (–) gE binding: impaired Δ105-125: no growth	No growth	US7
68	Envelope	gE; large unique N terminus (aa 1–187); binds gI, IDE; natural variant: MSP-gE	Essential	(–) gI binding: impaired (–) IDE binding: impaired Δ51-187: no growth (–) TGN targeting: impaired MSP gE: enhanced	T-cell entry NL NL No growth Impaired	US8

NL: normal as compared to wild-type VZV.
[a]Defined by mutagenesis of the VZV genome (pOka or vaccine Oka) using cosmids or BACs to delete, insert stop codon or introduce targeted changes in the coding sequence.
[b]Indicates differences among published observations about whether the gene is essential or dispensable, including variations in mutations tested and/or experimental conditions used to assess growth requirement.
[c]Indicates predicted function based on conserved sequence.
Abbreviations: TGN-trans Golgi Network; IDE-insulin degrading enzyme

highly preserved since removal of one copy of the gene pairs *ORF62/71, ORF63/70,* or *ORF64/69* is corrected after a few replication cycles.[316,387] Many VZV ORFs are arranged in unidirectional groups of up to four genes with a single putative polyadenylation signal at the 3′ end of the group. Eleven VZV ORFs have overlapping coding sequences. *ORFs 42* and *45* are thought to be spliced segments of the same gene.[90] *ORFS/L* is spliced in the 3′ noncoding region[197] in VZV strains including parent Oka but not vaccine Oka.[226] Small noncoding RNAs, including potential micro-RNAs, have also been identified in VZV-infected cells, which may contribute to the regulation of VZV gene expression and viral replication.[268]

The VZV genome has five small regions of unknown function, R1 through R5, which vary in length and contain different numbers of identically oriented short tandemly repeating elements,[90,180,400] which are relatively few compared to PRV and HSV-1.[407] R1, located within *ORF11*, consists of four separate 15- or 18-bp repeats. R2, located within *ORF14*, which encodes glycoprotein C (gC), consists of 42-bp repeats in multiples that differ among VZV isolates. The largest, R3 (1,000 bp), is in *ORF22*.[90] R4 has multiple 27-bp elements located in both IRS and TRS regions between *ORF62* and *ORF63* (and *ORF70* and *ORF71*). R5 is A-T instead of G-C rich and consists of 88-bp and 24-bp repeats located between *ORF60* and *ORF61*. The Dumas strain of VZV has only one copy of the R5 repeat.

The VZV genome exhibits limited geographic diversity.[41,181,307,376] The classification of geographically distinct VZV isolates into seven phylogenetic clades using single nucleotide polymorphisms (SNP) has been modified based on whole VZV genome sequences, which has identified six clades (1 to 6) and three provisional clades (VII-IX) (Fig. 13.4).[181,307] Their predominant distributions are Europe, clades 1 and 3 with some clade 6; Japan and East Asia, clade 2 with some clade 4; and Africa, clade 5.[337] Clades 1 and 2 are the most divergent but are still 99.83% identical. Comparison of the sequence of the Oka vaccine virus (clade 2) with that of the parent Oka virus revealed 63 sites that differ[81]; however, the analysis was limited because the Oka vaccine stock is a mixture of genomes reflecting its derivation by tissue culture passage. Deep sequencing demonstrates at least 224 SNP differences between vaccine and the parent Oka virus[95] and also that despite the presence of multiple genome populations, the genetic composition of these vaccines remains stable. VZV has been calculated to undergo about 20 replicative cycles in the human host before latency is established, suggesting limited opportunity for the accumulation of genetic mutations. Whole genome sequencing has also revealed that circulating VZV strains exhibit markers of homologous recombination, including both intraclade and interclade events,[307] which is evidence of both reinfection of an individual host and simultaneous replication of different VZV strains within a single host cell.

Comparison of the VZV genome with those of the seven other human herpesviruses indicates that VZV shares at least 40 conserved genes, all of which are among the 62 genes located in the UL region. These conserved genes encode an IE protein (*ORF4*); the DNA polymerase; helicase–primase complex proteins; other viral enzymes; the ORF47 kinase and structural proteins, including the major nucleocapsid and related proteins for assembly; and the glycoproteins gB, gH, gL, gM, and gN.

The predicted amino acid sequences of many VZV and HSV-1 gene products have similarities (Table 13.1). Of the 62 genes in the VZV UL region, 56 have HSV orthologs, as do all 4 of the genes encoded in the VZV US region. Nevertheless, while functions may be conserved even with limited sequence similarities,[116] they must be confirmed experimentally, as illustrated by differences in the roles of VZV ORF61 and HSV-1–infected cell protein (ICP) 0,[443] and of ORF10 and HSV-1 VP16 (UL48).[62] Each of the six VZV ORFs (*ORFs 1, 2, 13, 32, 57,* and *S/L*) that lack HSV-1 orthologs is dispensable for VZV replication in cell culture.[78,80,86,197,227,349,370] *ORFs 1, 32,* and *57* have orthologs in SVV and the equine herpesviruses.[140] *ORF13* has no related gene in the other alphaherpesviruses but has an ortholog in human herpesvirus 8, a gammaherpesvirus. The VZV genome can be engineered to express genes from other viruses.

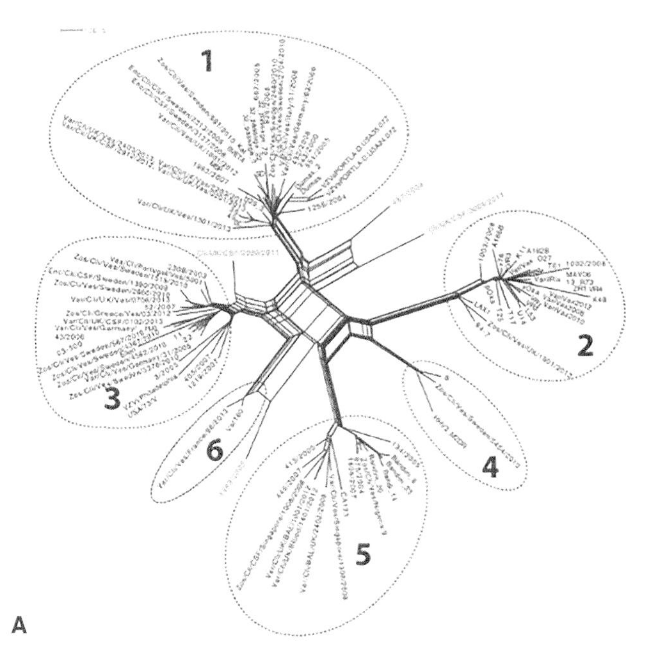

B

Position	33725	37902	38055	52365	69424	98437	114639
ORF	21	22	22	29	38	55	67
Clade 1	T	A	T	C	G	T	T
Clade 2	C	G	C	C	G	C	T
Clade 3	C	A	T	C	A	T	T
Clade 4	C	A	C	T	G	C	T
Clade 5	C	A	T	T	G	T	T
Clade 6	C	A	T	C	A	C	C
Clade VIII	C	A	T	C	G	C	T
Clade 9	C	A	C	C	A	C	T

FIGURE 13.4 **Phylogenetic network based on complete genomes of VZV strains and VZV single nucleotide polymorphisms SNP-based genotyping**. **A:** Full VZV genomes recovered from 115 zoster cases cluster in clades *1* to *5* and a novel sixth clade; four outliers are classified as putative interclade recombinants or novel clades (in *red*). Clades *1*, *3*, and *5* include isolates of European origin; clade *2* has Asian isolates, including the parent Oka virus used to derive VZV vaccines; and clade *4* has isolates from tropical Africa. (From Norberg P, Depledge DP, Kundu S, et al. Recombination of globally circulating varicella zoster virus. *J Virol* 2015;89(14):7133–7146. Copyright © 2015 American Society for Microbiology. Reproduced with permission from American Society for Microbiology.) **B:** Genotyping of 89 full VZV genomes identified single nucleotide SNP at positions based on the reference strain Dumas (Clade 1, GenBank accession #NC 001348). (Republished with permission of Microbiology Society Jensen NJ, Rivailler P, Tseng HF, et al. Revisiting the genotyping scheme for varicella-zoster viruses based on whole-genome comparisons. *J Gen Virol* 2017;98(6):1434–1438.)

STAGES OF REPLICATION

Overall Pattern of Replication

VZV is presumed to attach to cells by fusion of the viral envelope with the cytoplasmic membrane followed by endocytosis (Fig. 13.5). On entry, VZV tegument proteins encoded by *ORFs 4, 10,* and *62*[213,216] are likely transported with the nucleocapsid to the nucleus to initiate transcription. ORF61 is expressed along with IE62 shortly after virus entry[351] but is not a tegument protein. IE63 and the viral kinases ORF 47 and 66 are also likely to be important early in infection. Replication

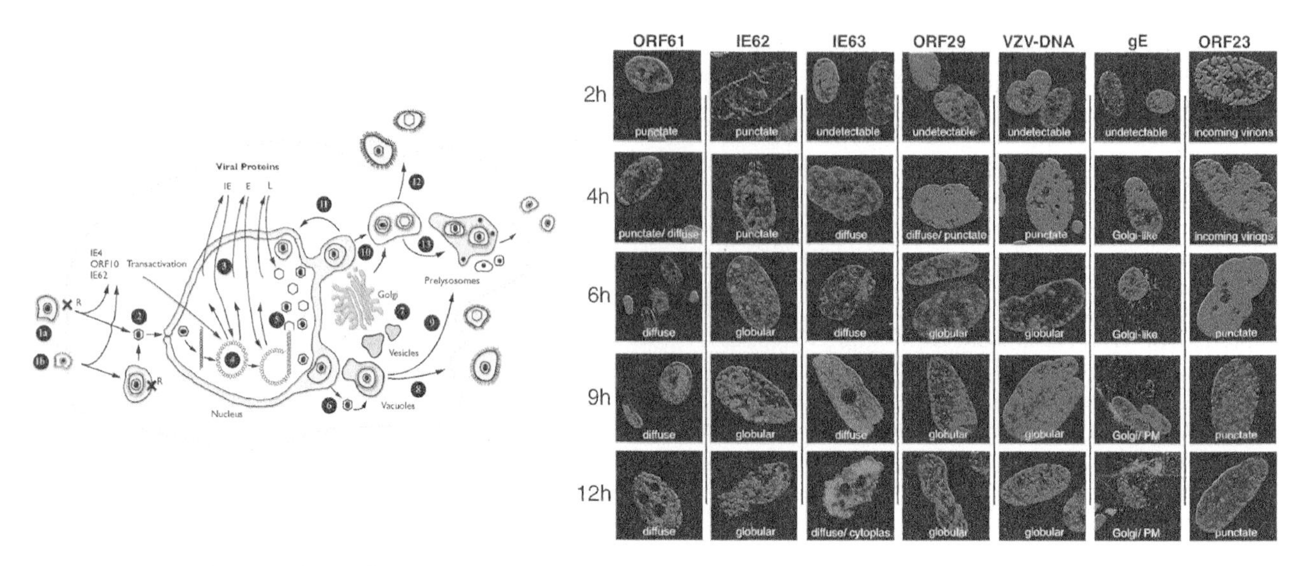

FIGURE 13.5 Replication of varicella–zoster virus (VZV). Left panel: The schema shown accommodates observations from multiple sources and relies on analogies drawn from studies of herpes simplex virus (HSV) replication. VZV may enter cells by attaching to cell surface glycosaminoglycans followed by binding to receptor(s) (*R*) on the plasma membrane (*1a*), or by endocytosis followed by interaction with a receptor(s) in the endosome (*1b*). The nucleocapsids penetrate the cell (*2*) and enter the nucleus where, with the aid of regulatory tegument proteins encoded by IE4, ORF10, and IE62, a cascade of viral immediate-early (*IE*), early (*E*), and late (*L*) transcripts and proteins is synthesized (*3*). Viral DNA replication follows a rolling-circle model (*4*). Nucleocapsids are assembled and package newly synthesized DNA (*5*). Nucleocapsids appear to be transiently enveloped as they bud through the inner nuclear lamellae (*6*). These nucleocapsids lose their envelopes upon fusion with the rough endoplasmic reticulum, resulting in the release of naked nucleocapsids into the cytoplasm (*7*). Virion glycoproteins are synthesized in the rough endoplasmic reticulum, mature in the Golgi apparatus, and line the inner surfaces of cytoplasmic vesicles. Viral tegument proteins are synthesized by free ribosomes and line the outer surfaces of the cytoplasmic vesicles. Nascent particles are drawn into these vesicles, where intact, enveloped virions coalesce (*8*). (From Gershon AA, Sherman DL, Zhu Z, et al. Intracellular transport of newly synthesized varicella-zoster virus: final envelopment in the trans-Golgi network. *J Virol* 1994;68:6372–6390.) These vacuoles may fuse with the cell membrane to release infectious progeny (*9*), although some fuse with prelysosomes in which the particle is partially degraded before release. Alternatively, nucleocapsids may retain their envelopes as they egress the nucleus. (*10*) Their envelopes are glycosylated by fusion with Golgi-derived vesicles. Late in infection, some particles may reenter the nucleus (*11*), although most are transported to the cell surface for release (*12*) or to prelysosomes (*13*). **Right panel:** The spatiotemporal pattern of expression of selected varicella–zoster virus (VZV) immediate-early, early, and late proteins and viral genomic DNA. Cells were fixed and imaged at 0 (not shown), 2, 4, 6, 9, and 12 hours after inoculation of unlabeled human fibroblasts with input cells labeled with green CellTracker. Cells were then stained with specific antibodies for VZV proteins ORF61, IE62, IE63, ORF29, gE, and ORF23 (*from left to right*) followed by Texas red–conjugated secondary antibodies to detect proteins (*red*). VZV DNA was detected by *in situ* hybridization (*red*). Cell nuclei were counterstained with Hoechst 22358. Ten fields of 30 to 50 output cells were scanned to determine the representative staining patterns in newly infected cells at each time point. Single representative cells or nuclei are shown. PM, plasma membrane; cytoplas, cytoplasm. (Reprinted from Reichelt M, Brady J, Arvin AM. The replication cycle of varicella-zoster virus: analysis of the kinetics of viral protein expression, genome synthesis, and virion assembly at the single-cell level. *J Virol* 2009;83(8):3904–3918.)

compartments containing IE62, the single-stranded DNA (ssDNA)-binding protein, ORF29, and nascent VZV DNA are formed within 4 hours after infection[351] (Fig. 13.5). Thereafter, proteins encoded by late mRNAs enter the nucleus for assembly into nascent capsids and VZV DNA is encapsidated by mechanisms that are not well defined[426]; ORF25 protein interacts with several encapsidation proteins.[427] The life cycle from entry to formation of mature enveloped VZ virions is completed in about 9 hours *in vitro*. By 12 hours, enveloped viruses are abundant in the cytoplasm and extracellularly along plasma membranes where they are presumed to bind surface receptors, fuse with membranes of adjacent cells, and begin synthesis of progeny virions. While syncytia formation is a hallmark of VZV infection, cell–cell fusion is not required to initiate the infectious process; however, the uninfected cell must be in close proximity to an infected cell, suggesting that virions attached to cell surfaces are transferred into neighboring cells.[351]

The basic events in VZV replication have been defined in cell culture using intact virus and VZV recombinants with targeted mutations in viral genes and promoter regions to map protein and promoter functions (Table 13.1).[30,206,208] However, many important characteristics of the regulation of gene expression and the essential or important functions of viral gene products during the viral life cycle are not identifiable *in vitro* but are evident when human tissue explants or differentiated human cells are infected *in vitro* or in their tissue microenvironments in human xenografts in the SCID mouse model *in vivo* (Table 13.1).

Attachment, Entry, and Uncoating

The initial attachment of alphaherpesvirus particles to the cell surface appears to entail nonspecific electrostatic interactions between viral envelope glycoproteins and cell surface glycosaminoglycans such as heparan sulfate. Whereas HSV gD and its orthologs in other alphaherpesviruses bind to cell surface receptor molecules known as herpesvirus entry mediators, VZV lacks a gD ortholog and may not use any of these receptors. The αV integrin subunit contributes to VZV-mediated fusion and infection,[477] and the cation-independent mannose-6-phosphate receptor may facilitate VZV entry by interacting with viral glycoproteins that contain phosphorylated N-linked complex oligosaccharides.[67,498]

After attachment, the herpesvirus glycoproteins gB, gH, and gL are required for fusion of the viral envelope with the cell membrane. In VZV, these glycoproteins also form the core fusion complex required for cell–cell fusion. High-resolution structures of VZV gB and gH show similarities and differences from their orthologs in other herpesviruses[315,472] (Fig. 13.6). VZV gB residues in the primary loop are essential for VZV replication[312] and gB domain IV is important for triggering fusion.[315] VZV gH appears to facilitate fusion of the VZV envelope with the cell membrane since antibodies to gH block VZV entry in cultured cells; however, anti-gH antibody is also internalized by infected cells,[429] inhibiting syncytia formation and virion egress. The gH C terminus has a loop structure essential for gB/gH/gL-mediated fusion.[428] The extreme N terminus of VZV gH is important for replication *in vitro* and in skin and may bind the αV subunit since this region of gH in other herpesviruses interacts with αβ integrins.[428,477] Interactions of gB with the myelin-associated glycoprotein (MAG) contribute to cell–cell fusion mediated by gB and gH/gL in neural cells.[404]

VZV gE is an abundant glycoprotein that forms heterodimers with gI and binds to insulin-degrading enzyme (IDE) in VZV-infected cells.[5,244,245] Inhibition of IDE reduces VZV infectivity, while IDE expression enhances infection of nonhuman cell lines, suggesting a contribution to entry.[54] However, since gE mutants with disrupted IDE binding can infect cells in culture and are not impaired in their ability to enter T cells *in vitro* or *in vivo*, gE does not appear to be a primary entry mediator.[29]

Once virus entry has occurred, herpesvirus nucleocapsids are transported to the nuclear membrane and the viral genome is delivered into the nucleus. Neither the role of specific viral proteins and cellular cytoskeletal elements in facilitating the movement of VZ virions to the nucleus nor the composition of the virion reaching the nuclear membrane has been determined, although dynamic changes in the cytoskeleton appear upon infection.[314]

Transcription and Translation

The transcription and translation of VZV genes in infected cells depends on viral transactivating proteins that act in conjunction with host cell RNA polymerase II and the cellular transcription and translation machinery (Fig. 13.5). VZV proteins with transactivating capacity are encoded by *ORFs 4, 10, 61, 62,* and *63*; IE62 is the predominant viral transcription factor. Infection in the presence of cycloheximide followed by actinomycin-D indicates that VZV *ORF4*,[91] as well as *ORF62* and *ORF63*, encodes IE proteins. Although each of the

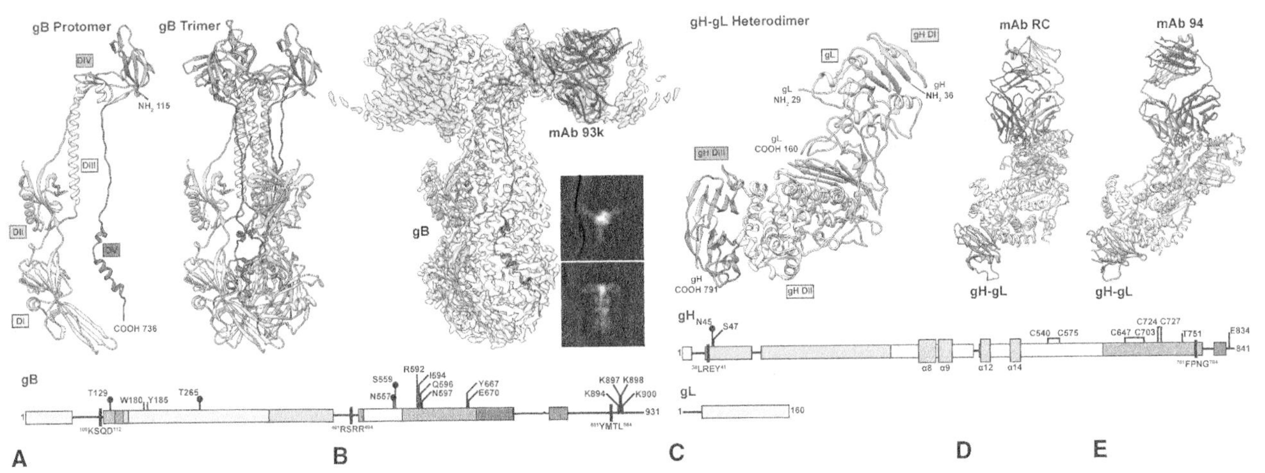

FIGURE 13.6 VZV gB and gH–gL structures and disruption of VZV gB/gH–gL fusion function by human neutralizing antibodies and site-directed mutagenesis. A and B: X-ray crystallography structure of the VZV gB trimer (A; 2.4Å) and a cryo-EM structure (B; 2.8Å) of native VZV gB (*gray*) in complex with Fab fragments from human neutralizing mAb 93k. A single gB protomer along with the VH and VL chains of mAb 93k are represented as ribbons. The two inset panels show examples of 2D class averages used to generate the cryo-EM structure of the gB-93k complex. **C–E:** X-ray crystallography structures of the VZV gH–gL heterodimer (**C**; 3.2 Å) and gH–gL in complex with Fab fragments from human neutralizing mAbs RC (**D**; 3.1Å) and 94 (**E**; 3.6Å). The gH–gL heterodimer and either mAb RC or mAb 94 are represented as ribbons. Each domain of the VZV gB, gH–gL, and the mAb structures are colored accordingly: gB structures DI (*cyan*), DII (*green*), DIII (*yellow*), DIV (*orange*), DV (*red*), linker regions (*hot pink*); gH–gL structures DI (*green*), DII (*yellow*), DIII (*orange*), and gL (*cyan*); mAb VH (*blue*) and VL (*light blue*) chains. Sites of mutagenesis that effect gB/gH–gL fusion function are mapped on the linear diagrams below the structures. All domains are colored as for the X-ray crystallography structures in **(A)** and **(C)**. Other features include the signal sequence (*light gray box*), the transmembrane domain (*dark gray box*), and sites of mutagenesis. Mutations that affect fusion function are either shown above (single) or below (motifs) the diagrams. Glycosylation sites are indicated by *black bars* with *black circles*. For gH, the disrupted α-helices (8, 9, 12, and 14) that abolished fusion are depicted as *plum-colored boxes*. The disulfide bonds in gH that were mutated are shown with connecting *lines*. (**A, B** adapted from Oliver SL, Xing Y, Chen DH, et al. A glycoprotein B-neutralizing antibody structure at 2.8 Å uncovers a critical domain for herpesvirus fusion initiation. *Nat Commun* 2020;11(1):4141. https://creativecommons.org/licenses/by/4.0/. **C, D, and E** based on Xing Y, Oliver SL, Nguyen T, et al. A site of varicella-zoster virus vulnerability identified by structural studies of neutralizing antibodies bound to the glycoprotein complex gHgL. *Proc Natl Acad Sci U S A* 2015;112:6056–6061.)

HSV-1 orthologs of *ORF 4, 62,* and *63* contains an upstream TAATGARAT sequence element, only the VZV *ORF62* promoter region has TAATGARAT-like promoter elements.[220] The transcriptional cascade of VZV gene expression has remained undefined because synchronous infection cannot be established due to low titers of cell-free VZV recoverable from cultured cells. However, the kinetics of expression of six representative VZV proteins, ORF61, IE62, IE63, ORF29 (ssDNA-binding protein), ORF23 (small capsid protein), and gE was established using markers differentiating inoculum from newly infected cells[351] (Fig. 13.5). IE62 and ORF61 are synthesized first (within 1 hour); IE63 is expressed at 4 hours. The localization of IE62 to small nuclear puncta is a marker of the earliest stage of replication.

Transcriptional arrays from VZV-infected melanoma cells showed highest expression of *ORFs 9, 48, 49, 57, 58,* and *64.*[198] VZV transcription mapping revealed 78 abundant transcripts of 6.8 kb or smaller, many of which were located in regions corresponding to ORFs predicted by Davison and Scott.[90] Long-read sequencing reveals that lytic infection is associated with novel mRNAs, suggesting that VZV encodes viral proteins not yet identified, together with start- and end-site isoforms and splicing for many viral transcripts, and noncoding RNAs of undefined function.[338]

As is observed in other herpesviruses, multiple colinear and coterminal transcripts can encode a single VZV protein. VZV uses TATA elements and polyadenylation signals whose sequences may differ from consensus sequences.[90,246,330] VZV, like HSV-1, contains GU-rich sequences GTCTGTGT and TGGTGGTA downstream of polyadenylation sites that may be important for termination of transcription.[246] *ORF14* (gC)[246] and *ORF61*[76,446] appear to be expressed from unspliced transcripts, in contrast to their HSV-1 orthologs. VZV strain differences may also affect the level of transcription of a given gene. For example, VZV strain Scott expresses about 20 times more gC mRNA than does VZV strain Oka.[246] Another feature of VZV transcription is the regulation of VZV polymerase (ORF28) and the major DNA-binding protein (ORF29) by a single bidirectional promoter with shared promoter elements. Both this *ORF28–29* bidirectional promoter[270,348,360] and the *ORF4* promoter are activated by the interaction of IE62 with the transcription factor upstream stimulatory factor (USF). A binding site for the nuclear regulatory protein Sp1 modulates the activity of both of these promoters, whereas one TATA box controls expression from the *ORF28* promoter and two other TATA elements regulate expression from the *ORF29* promoter.[478] Transcription of *ORFs 62* and *63* is also mediated from a bidirectional promoter.[190]

VZV Proteins That Regulate Viral Gene Transcription

Five VZV proteins, encoded by *ORFs 4, 10, 61, 62,* and *63*, can regulate viral gene expression. Most promoters of VZV genes also have binding motifs for cellular transcription factors, such as Sp1, USF, and activating transcription factor (ATF), that contribute to viral gene expression. These cellular transactivators can be critical for VZV replication *in vitro* and in human skin and T-cell xenografts *in vivo.*[360] ORF61 and IE62 also have important functions in counteracting intrinsic antiviral cellular responses (see **VZV Effects on Host Cell Functions**).

IE62

ORF62 (at least one copy) is essential for VZV replication.[369] This gene encodes IE62, a 1310-amino acid protein that is the most potent and promiscuous viral transactivating factor.[216] IE62 has an acidic transcriptional activation domain (TAD) and a DNA-binding domain.[417] IE62 binds directly to the cellular transcription factors Sp1 and USF and to the cellular TATA-binding protein and general transcription factor (TFIIB).[360] The serine-rich tract of IE62 interacts with the nuclear ribosomal protein EAP and is important for *ORF61* transcription.[212] IE62 binding to the viral proteins IE4 and IE63 modulates its transactivating functions. IE62 has a nuclear localization signal (NLS)[27] and is localized primarily in the nuclei of infected cells (Fig. 13.5). IE62 is phosphorylated and requires the kinase activity of ORF47 protein for cytoplasmic versus nuclear localization.[32,302] Coexpression of the ORF66 kinase with IE62 results in cytoplasmic accumulation of IE62[215] (although not in T cells),[375] and ORF66 is required for IE62 incorporation into virions in cultured cells. Mutations of the IE62 NLS and the S686A/S722A phosphorylation sites in recombinant viruses are not lethal but delay VZV growth.[206]

A single amino acid change in the DNA-binding domain of IE62 results in loss of its transactivating function[478] and is lethal for VZV replication, as is disrupting the IE62 dimerization domain.[206] IE62 is the ortholog of HSV-1 ICP4 and can complement ICP4 mutants. However, the DNA-binding domain of IE62 is less sequence specific and, unlike ICP4, does not induce DNA binding on binding its own promoter.[417] The TAD at the IE62 amino terminus is not conserved in HSV-1 ICP4 or HSV-1 viral protein (VP)16.[72] This IE62 TAD interacts with the mammalian Mediator complex involved in RNA polymerase II–mediated transcription,[479] an interaction that appears to be required for IE62 TAD–mediated activation, specifically through the MED25 subunit (e-Fig. 13.1).

IE62 transactivates expression of putative IE (*ORF4, ORF61*), early, and late gene promoters in transient expression assays[172,333] and activates its own promoter in a lymphocyte-derived cell line but not in simian cells.[100,332] The differential activation of promoters by IE62 reflects its capacity to interact with cellular transcription factors and depends on the sequence of the TATA motif in the targeted promoter.[330]

Recruitment of IE62 is enhanced by the presence of an Sp1 site within the gI promoter.[329] Interaction with Sp1 and other Sp family members is an important aspect of IE62 activation and can also reduce effects of IE62 on a promoter-specific basis, as shown for the *ORF28/29* promoter; Sp proteins may have differential effects on the same promoter, illustrated by reduced IE62-mediated activation of gI by Sp2.[207] Several other Sp1 sites within VZV promoters have been validated as important for IE62-mediated activation, including gE[30] and ORF61.[446] Bioinformatics analysis of the VZV genome has identified Sp1 sites within almost all predicted promoter elements.[360] The YY1 cellular transcription factor also facilitates IE62 function, shown by impaired transactivation when YY1 binding sites in the promoters of ORF10, ORF28/29, and gI are mutated.[209]

The mechanism of activation of the *ORF62* promoter is important because of the central role of IE62 in VZV gene transcription. The upstream region of *ORF62* contains three

TAATGARAT-like elements that contribute to the ability of VZV ORF10 protein to transactivate expression of IE62. The *ORF62* promoter also contains cAMP-responsive and GA-rich elements that are important for its transactivation. The ORF10 protein forms a complex with two of the TAATGARAT-like elements in the *ORF62* promoter that lack an overlapping octamer-binding motif, but not with the TAATGARAT-like element that possesses an octamer motif. Two cellular proteins, Oct1 and host cell factor (HCF), form a complex with ORF10 and at least one of the TAATGARAT-like elements on the *ORF62* promoter. HCF-1 is critical for activation of immediate–early gene expression by ORF10.[301] The Oct2 cellular protein binds to the TAATGARAT-like elements on the *ORF62* promoter and inhibits ORF10-mediated transactivation. However, ORF10 is dispensable for VZV replication *in vitro* and *in vivo*. Thus, self-regulation of the *ORF62* promoter by IE62 that enters the cell with the infecting virion may be the mechanism that initiates expression of additional IE62 and other IE regulatory proteins.[360,464] The NF-Y CCAAT box-binding protein and the activating transcription factor/adaptor protein 1 (ATF/AP-1) family also bind to the *ORF62* promoter.[286]

ORF61 Protein

ORF61 encodes a 467-amino acid protein that is expressed shortly after VZV entry and localizes to the nuclei of infected cells[351,396](Fig. 13.5); ORF61 is not detected in the virion tegument. ORF61 protein transactivates putative IE, early, and late promoters in transient expression assays,[291] although not in a T-cell line.[332] When ORF61 is truncated or mutations of *ORF61* promoter elements restrict its expression, VZV replication is severely compromised.[76,446,496] Limiting ORF61 expression by promoter mutations also shows that ORF61 is most important for gE expression. ORF61 dimerization through a domain located at residues 250 to 320 is required for ORF61 regulatory functions and normal replication *in vitro* and in skin xenografts *in vivo*.[444,445]

ORF61 can either repress or enhance activation of other VZV genes by IE4 and IE62, depending on the cell line and transfection conditions.[291,332,446] The ORF61 N terminus contains a RING-finger domain that is required for the transactivating activity of the full-length protein.[437] Carboxyl-terminal truncation mutants of ORF61 that retain the RING-finger domain act as dominant-negative transrepressors and reduce the infectivity of viral DNA. Transient expression of ORF61 enhances the infectivity of VZV DNA,[291] which can be explained by its critical role in dispersing promyelocytic leukemia (PML) nuclear bodies through sumoylating motifs.[443] ORF61 is related to HSV ICP0 and can functionally complement an HSV-1 ICP0 deletion mutant.[289]

IE4

ORF4 encodes the 52-kd essential immediate–early protein IE4,[320,371] which requires coexpression with *ORF62* for its nuclear localization.[91] IE4 must dimerize for gene activation, and several regions of the protein are required for its transactivation function.[26,287] Mutation of the KYFKC residues that mediate IE4 dimerization is lethal.[371] In transient expression assays, IE4 transactivates some, but not all, putative IE, early or late promoters, and also synergizes with IE62 to transactivate promoters of genes from all three kinetic classes. IE4 activation of target genes occurs at both transcriptional[331] and posttranscriptional levels.[91] IE4 interacts directly with TFIIB and the nuclear factor-κB (NF-κB) p50 and p65 subunits and also binds to an underphosphorylated form of IE62.[320,389] IE4 may function as a viral mRNA export factor through its RNA-binding capacity.[319]

IE4 is the ortholog of HSV-1 ICP27 but the proteins do not complement each other.[74] The IE4 carboxyl portion contains putative zinc-finger domains; several cysteine residues in IE4 are not required for its regulatory activity,[331] and, unlike ICP27, IE4 does not appear to have transrepressing activity.[91,172,332]

IE63

ORF63 encodes a 287-amino acid protein and additional smaller products of 38- and 28-kd.[213] IE63 is phosphorylated predominantly in the carboxy-terminal region by casein kinases I and II, CDK1, and CDK5.[147] Deletion of greater than 90% of both *ORF63* and its duplicate *ORF70* was compatible with very limited VZV replication in melanoma cells, providing IE62 allows an *ORF63* deletion mutant to replicate in U2OS cells.[73,182,387] The carboxy-terminal 70 amino acids of IE63 are dispensable, but further deletion of the carboxy-terminus or replacement of some of the serine or threonine phosphorylation sites of the protein with alanine impairs VZV replication[21,73] and skin infection.[21] IE63 is located primarily in nuclei of infected cells (Fig. 13.5). Phosphorylation of certain amino acids of IE63 is important for its cellular localization when expressed alone[38,73,397] and IE63 nuclear import requires ORF61 in neurons.[438] IE63 binds to IE62 and the two proteins exhibit some colocalization in infected cells; IE63 also binds to the cellular RNA polymerase II[252] and to antisilencing protein 1, interfering with its histone-binding capacity.[6] IE63 is reported to repress expression of VZV promoters in some transient transfection assays,[176,228,252] but IE62 is the only viral gene product that is significantly reduced in cells infected with an IE63-null mutant.[165] IE63 also transactivates the EF-1α promoter in the absence of other viral proteins.[501] IE63 is the ortholog of the HSV-1 $U_S1.5$ protein, which is expressed colinearly with HSV-1 ICP22 (U_S1).[21] IE63 was identified as important for latency in a rodent model.[70,71]

Replication of Viral DNA

Replication Proteins

The minimal repertoire of genes needed for VZV DNA replication is not known although VZV encodes orthologs of each of the seven HSV-1 genes required for origin-of-replication (ori)-dependent replication of viral DNA (Table 13.1).

DNA polymerase

ORF28 encodes the large subunit of the VZV DNA polymerase.[90] Unlike the cellular polymerase, the VZV enzyme is sensitive to phosphonoacetic acid and its activity is enhanced in the presence of ammonium sulfate. *ORF16* is predicted to encode the small subunit processivity factor of the VZV polymerase.

DNA-binding proteins

ORF29 encodes a 130-kd protein that localizes to nuclei of infected cells via a noncanonical NLS[390] (Fig. 13.5). ORF29 binds ssDNA, although the VZV protein binds with lower efficiency and cannot substitute for its HSV-1 ortholog, ICP8.[217] ORF29 binds to the gI promoter[39] and increases or decreases IE62 transactivation of a reporter gene, depending on the cell line.[39] ORF29 protein is secreted from VZV-infected cells and can be endocytosed by neurons.[9] ORF29 is also part of a complex that binds to a sequence in Ori-s, which functions as a negative regulator of VZV DNA replication.[205]

ORF51 encodes the ori-binding protein.[399] The carboxyl portion of ORF51 protein binds *in vitro* to three DNA sequence motifs in the VZV ori with similar affinities. As in the HSV-1 ortholog, UL9, a CGC triplet in the VZV ori, is required for ORF51 binding. ORF51 can substitute for HSV-1 UL9 in an origin-dependent HSV DNA replication assay and can partially complement growth of an HSV-1 UL9-null mutant.[66] VZV DNA binds five other proteins of unknown identity or function, ranging from 21- to 175-kd in size.

Genome Replication

By analogy with HSV, VZV DNA replication is presumed to occur in four stages.[89] First, the linear DNA molecule circularizes shortly after virion entry via the complementary unpaired nucleotides at each 3′ end of the genome, demonstrated by the presence of a fused U_L-U_S joint. The second stage involves replication of the circular genomic template. Isomerization of progeny genomes is thought to occur by homologous recombination between the inverted repeats. Third, replication of the circular molecule generates head-to-tail concatemers, probably by a rolling-circle mechanism (Fig. 13.5). Fourth, these concatemers are cleaved by sequence-specific nucleases to generate linear DNA for packaging into virions. Processing of VZV genomic DNA for encapsidation requires the ORF54 portal protein.[426]

The VZV genome contains AT-rich and GC-rich sequences near the left and right termini, respectively, also found in HSV-1 and implicated in cleavage and packaging of HSV-1 DNA. Because VZV exists predominantly as two isomers, 95% of cleavage appears to occur at one U_L-U_S junction, with cleavage at the other U_L-U_S joint yielding the two minor isomers.[219]

The VZV genome contains duplicate ori_S between ORFs *62* and *63* in the IRS and between ORFs *70* and *71* in the TR_S,[90,398] which are A-T rich and contain three origin-binding protein sites, two of which are important for *ORF62* and *ORF63* expression (Fig. 13.3). Transfection of cells with plasmids containing the VZV ori_S followed by VZV infection results in replication of these plasmids. The VZV genome does not have an ortholog of the HSV-1 ori_L sequence. However, VZV may have another origin of replication since a recombinant with mutations of the ori_S core sequences retained infectivity in melanoma cells.[210]

The VZV ori_S contains a near-perfect 45-bp palindrome with the sequence $(TA)_{17}$ at its center. Mutations of the palindrome impair replicative activity. The VZV ori_S also includes a GA-rich region and three binding sites for the VZV origin-binding protein, ORF51. These sequences are CGTTCGCACTT (also found in both the ori_S and the ori_L of HSV-1)[399] and CATTCGCACTT. Unlike the HSV ori_S and the ori_L, all three VZV ori-binding protein sites are upstream of the palindrome on the same strand and are oriented in the same direction.[65] Dpn1 DNA replication assays indicate that the 45-bp palindrome and the sequence CGTTCGCACTT closest to the palindrome are essential for replication, whereas the sequence CATTCGCACTT contributes additional activity but is not essential.

Viral Enzymes

Thymidine Kinase

ORF36 encodes a viral thymidine kinase (TK) dispensable for VZV replication. Since the VZV enzyme has more deoxycytidine than does TK activity, it is more accurately a deoxypyrimidine kinase. The enzyme is a 70-kd homodimer composed of two 35-kd subunits. It is most active *in vitro* at a higher pH and has broader substrate specificity than its cellular ortholog. VZV TK is more thermostable and more susceptible to inhibition by deoxythymidine triphosphate than is HSV-1 TK. TK phosphorylates and thereby activates acyclovir and its analogs. Most acyclovir-resistant VZV isolates have point mutations in the TK gene near the adenosine triphosphate (ATP) or thymidine-binding sites or have mutations that result in a truncated protein.[373] Differences between the structures of VZV and HSV TK may explain some differences in their substrate activities.[34]

Ribonucleotide reductase

ORFs *18* and *19* encode proteins orthologous to the small and large subunits of HSV-1 ribonucleotide reductase, respectively,[90] and their enzymatic activities are similar. Unlike cellular ribonucleotide reductase, the VZV and HSV-1 enzymes are not inhibited by increased intracellular levels of deoxyribonucleotides.[388] Inhibition of VZV ribonucleotide reductase with small molecules enhances the antiviral activity of acyclovir, presumably by decreasing the intracellular pool of deoxyribonucleoside triphosphates and increasing the concentration of acyclovir triphosphate. Deletion of *ORF19* from the viral genome abolishes viral ribonucleotide reductase activity, impairs the growth of the virus *in vitro*, and potentiates inhibition of replication by acyclovir.[159]

ORF47 and ORF66 protein kinases

As components of the virion tegument, ORF47 and ORF66 are likely to be important for activation of regulatory proteins in the newly infected cell. *ORF47* encodes a 54-kd serine–threonine protein kinase that phosphorylates both acidic and basic proteins, but with a marked preference for acidic amino acids, using both ATP and guanosine triphosphate (GTP) as phosphate donors; it also phosphorylates casein kinase II.[203] The HSV ortholog, UL13, has a similar catalytic domain.[395] ORF47 protein autophosphorylates and also phosphorylates viral proteins ORF32,[349] IE62,[204,302] IE63,[204] gI,[203] and gE[202] but is not required for phosphorylation of gE, IE62, or IE63 in VZV-infected cells.[160,204] ORF47 binds to IE62 through an N-terminal domain.[32] The N-terminal DYS motif is required for ORF47 kinase activity that, if disrupted, results in nuclear retention of ORF47 and IE62. Deletion of ORF47 does not alter plaque formation[160] but does lead to accelerated gE expression on membranes and cell–cell spread.[203] However, even though plaques appear normal in the absence of ORF47, the protein and its kinase activity are required for efficient VZ virion assembly and transport to cell surfaces.[32] ORF47 is important for T cell and dendritic cell infection *in vitro,*[168] is important for skin infection, and is essential for T-cell tropism *in vivo.*[31,32]

ORF66 encodes a 393-amino acid phosphoprotein expressed in the nucleus, in puncta surrounding nucleoli, and in cytoplasm of infected cells.[395,375] ORF66 is a serine–threonine protein kinase that autophosphorylates[374] and phosphorylates IE62.[214] The ORF66 catalytic domain (residues 93–378) is orthologous to the HSV-1 US3 and other members of this protein kinase superfamily.[106] IE62 phosphorylation by ORF66 determines its late accumulation in the cytoplasm of infected cells, where packaging into virions occurs. Mutagenesis of the glycine 102 residue in a highly conserved, glycine-rich ATP-binding motif in this domain blocks ORF66 kinase function.[375] ORF66 also phosphorylates the cellular nuclear matrix protein, matrin 3, which may modulate RNA processing[109,110] and targets histone deacetylases to promote transcription.[435,436] ORF66 is dispensable for replication *in vitro*[163] and in human skin xenografts in the SCID mouse model; however, the absence of ORF66 or disruption of its kinase activity leads to impaired growth and production of virions in human T cells in xenografts.[282,374,375] VZV infection of primary corneal fibroblasts also requires ORF66 functions.

Other viral enzymes

ORF8 encodes a deoxyuridine 5′-triphosphate nucleotidohydrolase (dUTPase), which hydrolyzes deoxyuridine 5′-triphosphate (dUTP) to deoxyuridine 5′-monophosphate (dUMP) and pyrophosphate.[358] *ORF8* is not required for growth *in vitro* nor is *ORF13*, which encodes the viral thymidylate synthetase.[78,412] *ORF59* encodes the VZV uracil DNA glycosylase that removes uracil residues incorporated into newly synthesized DNA strands. This protein is not necessary for replication in cell culture. VZV-infected cells express a DNase activity encoded by ORF48, the ortholog of HSV-1 UL12.[293]

ORF33 encodes the precursor of the VZV serine protease, which is cleaved autocatalytically at two sites.[118] The mature 31-kd protease is the amino-terminal cleavage product. The active form of the protease is predicted to be a homodimer. The VZV protease crystal structure is similar to that of the cytomegalovirus (CMV) protease.[343] A serine and two histidines constitute the catalytic site of the VZV protease; mutation of either one of these histidines in the protease precursor protein prevents self-cleavage.

ORF17 encodes the ortholog of the virion host shutoff (VHS) protein encoded by HSV-1 UL41. *ORF17* is dispensable for replication, but deletion of this gene yields a temperature-sensitive mutant. ORF17 protein induces RNA cleavage much less effectively than does its HSV-1 ortholog,[368] and the host shutoff function in VZV-infected cells is correspondingly less efficient.

The *ORF9-12* Gene Cluster

ORF9 encodes an essential protein present in the virion tegument that interacts with IE62 and is phosphorylated by ORF47, which supports virion egress.[46,61,237,355,356,413] The ORF9 protein functions in secondary envelopment through interactions with the cellular protein, AP-1, involved in clathrin-coated vesicle transport of proteins from endosomes to the trans-Golgi network (TGN).[237] *ORF9A* encodes the putative 7-kd gN protein located in the membranes of infected cells.[358] Although this protein is not required for replication, blocking ORF9A expression impairs syncytia formation.

ORF10 encodes a 50-kd protein that is incorporated into the viral tegument[216] and localizes to the TGN in infected cells. ORF10 is the ortholog of HSV-1 VP16, but unlike its HSV-1 counterpart, it is dispensable for replication.[62,79] ORF10 complements an HSV VP16 mutant and enhances the infectivity of transfected VZV virion DNA.[290] ORF10 transactivates the *ORF62* promoter, but not the *ORF4* or *ORF61* promoter. ORF10 forms a complex with TAATGARAT-like sequences and Oct1 and HCF to transactivate the ORF62 promoter.[288] ORF10 is important for replication in human skin, but not in T-cell xenografts in SCID mice.[62]

ORF11 is expressed as a 118-kd polypeptide present in the virion tegument and in the nucleus and cytoplasm of infected cells; ORF11 binds to the ORF9 protein.[59] ORF11 alone has little effect on VZV gene transcription, but levels of IE4, IE62, IE63, and gE proteins are reduced if ORF11 is deleted from the viral genome.[60,61] ORF11 functions as an RNA-binding protein with the binding region in the first 22 residues of the protein. RNA binding is conserved among the UL47 alphaherpesvirus orthologs. ORF11 is critical for VZV infection of human skin xenografts, but its RNA-binding function is not required.[60]

ORF12 encodes a predicted tegument protein that affects cell cycle progression by activation of the P13 kinase/Akt pathway.[248] It is dispensable for replication *in vitro;* a spontaneous deletion mutant associated with tissue culture passage has been reported[83] and ORF12 protein is not required for skin tropism.[61]

Nucleocapsid Proteins

Three forms of nucleocapsids are found in VZV-infected cells.[154] Immature B capsids lack viral DNA and contain 32- and 36-kd proteins, presumed to be the mature viral protease and assembly proteins, respectively, present in the nuclear matrix of VZV-infected cells.[132] Mature C capsids contain viral DNA but lack the 32- and 36-kd proteins. Intermediate B/C capsids are thought to contain the VZV genome and the 32- and 36-kd proteins.

ORF40

ORF40 encodes the 155-kd major nucleocapsid protein that localizes to the nuclei of infected cells.

ORF33

ORF33.5, located in the 3′ portion of the *ORF33* gene, encodes the 40-kd precursor of the VZV assembly protein. The mature 37-kd assembly protein is released after cleavage from its precursor by the VZV protease.[339] The assembly protein is presumed to provide a scaffold for nucleocapsid assembly. When expressed *in vitro*, ORF33.5 forms long, hollow rods that accumulate predominantly in the nuclei of cells.[339]

ORF23

ORF23 encodes a conserved capsid protein, called VP26 (UL35) in other alphaherpesviruses, which is expressed as a late protein[58,351] (Fig. 13.5). Unlike VP26, ORF23 localizes to nuclei through an SRSRVV motif in the carboxy-terminus and mediates nuclear import of ORF40, the major capsid protein. ORF40 is also translocated by ORF33.5. ORF23 is not essential for VZV replication, but deletion disrupts capsid assembly *in vitro*. ORF23-mediated nuclear transport of the major capsid protein is necessary in skin xenografts *in vivo*, and the ORF33.5 interaction with ORF40 does not provide a redundant capacity for this function.

ORF21

ORF21 encodes a 115-kd protein located in the nucleocapsid.[257] The protein localizes to both the nucleus and the cytoplasm of infected cells. ORF21 is essential for VZV replication, and its HSV-1 ortholog, UL37, cannot complement its absence *in vitro*.[471]

Other Putative Late Proteins

ORF35 encodes a protein that localizes to the nuclei of infected cells. A mutant deleted for this gene is impaired for cell–cell spread and for infection of human skin and T-cell xenografts in SCID mice.[175] *ORF44* encodes a nonessential tegument protein that interacts with the ORF49 gene product to support efficient infection.[363] ORF58 is nonessential, but functions have not been defined.[482] Deletion of *ORF64* results in virions that induce extensive cell fusion with large syncytia.[387] *ORF65* encodes a 16-kd virion protein that localizes to the Golgi apparatus of virus-infected cells[77]; it is dispensable for VZV infection of human T cells and skin xenografts in SCID mice.[304]

Glycoproteins

VZV glycoproteins are major constituents of the viral envelope that are also expressed on intracellular membranes and have critical interactions with other viral and cellular proteins during VZV entry, replication, cell–cell spread, and cell–cell fusion.

Glycoprotein B

gB, encoded by *ORF31*, is the most highly conserved of the herpesvirus glycoproteins. In addition to its presumed role in attachment and entry, gB expression along with gH/gL is sufficient to induce cell fusion.[178,310,314,315,404,428,476]

VZV gB has a furin recognition motif at residues 491 to 494 and is cleaved into two polypeptides that are bound together by disulfide residues. Thus, under nonreducing conditions, gB migrates in gels as a 140-kd protein, whereas under reducing conditions, gB resolves as two proteins of 60 and 70 kd. Virion morphology, protein localization, plaque size, and replication kinetics are not altered by mutations eliminating gB furin cleavage, but furin cleavage is necessary for normal VZV replication in human skin xenografts *in vivo*.[312] gB contains two tyrosine-based motifs in its cytoplasmic domain that are required for endocytosis to the Golgi network[161]; gB associates with clathrin during endocytosis. Sialic acids on gB are implicated in gB-mediated fusion by interaction with MAG.[403] The carboxy-terminal 36 amino acids of gB are required for normal trafficking to the cell surface.[162] gB has both N- and O-linked sugars and is sialylated, sulfated, and palmitylated.[141]

The 2.8Å near atomic resolution of the gB structure in complex with a human neutralizing monoclonal antibody (mAb) identified the critical role of domain IV (DIV) residues for initiation of fusion, based on using structure-guided mutagenesis of gB to define effects on gB/gH-gL fusion and VZV infection in the presence of other viral proteins.[315] (Fig. 13.6) These findings indicate that these DIV residues are accessible in prefusion conformations of gB. The gB N-terminus is also important for fusion.[313] An immunoreceptor tyrosine-based inhibition motif in the gB cytoplasmic domain regulates fusion, which when mutated causes exaggerated cell–cell fusion and severely impaired skin pathogenesis[310] and disrupts the typical transcription of VZV and host cell genes and modifications of the host cell actin cytoskeleton associated with efficient replication.[314] Regulation of cell–cell fusion by the lysine cluster in the gB cytoplasmic domain is also critical for VZV skin infection.[476]

Glycoprotein C

gC, encoded by *ORF14*, is dispensable for growth in cell culture. Because the number of R2 repeats in the gC coding sequence differs, gC varies from 80- to 170-kd. The gC endodomain consists of only six amino acids. gC is heavily glycosylated, with about one-third of its molecular weight resulting from N- and O-linked glycosylation.[141] gC transcription and translation is delayed compared to other VZV glycoproteins, with little VZV gC detected until 72 hours after infection.[142] The quantity of gC transcripts and protein produced also varies depending on the VZV isolate.[218,246] In contrast to cultured cells, skin lesions show abundant gC in a pattern consistent with virion envelope expression (e-Fig. 13.2). VZV gC also enhances the leukocyte inflammatory response.[136]

Glycoprotein E

gE, encoded by *ORF68*, is an 85- to 100-kd protein. Unlike its orthologs, VZV gE is an essential protein[284] and has a unique N terminus of 188 residues necessary for VZV replication.[29] Although gE has been considered to be a late gene product, it is detectable in a Golgi-like cytoplasmic distribution by 4 hours and is expressed extensively on plasma membranes by 9 hours[351] (Fig. 13.5). While gE orthologs are encoded within the US, *ORF68* extends into the repeat regions. gE contains both N- and O-linked sugars, is heavily sialylated, and is modified by myristoylation, palmitoylation, and sulfation.[284] Its monomeric form is phosphorylated at serine and threonine residues by casein kinase II, whereas the homodimeric form of gE is phosphorylated by a tyrosine kinase.[480] gE binds the Fc receptor of human immunoglobulin.[247,367] Expression of gE in epithelial cells induces formation of tight junctions.[277]

After synthesis and maturation in the Golgi apparatus, gE is transported to the cell membrane. The short gE cytoplasmic domain (62 amino acids) has an endocytosis motif, YAGL, a TGN-targeting AYRV tyrosine motif, and an acidic amino acid–rich phosphorylation motif.[202,280] The AYRV motif and the acid patch are required for gE transport.[499] Endocytosis to the TGN requires the YAGL motif, which allows recycling of gE through endosomes back to the cell membrane.[317] Phosphorylation of gE by the ORF47 protein kinase is necessary for endocytosed gE to traffic to the TGN. In cells infected with a mutant unable to express ORF47, gE accumulates on cell membranes.[202,203] gE endocytosis from the plasma membrane is necessary for incorporation into virions.[263] The YAGL endocytosis motif is required for virus replication; the AYRV motif is important for VZV replication in human skin and T-cell xenografts in SCID mice.[280]

Residues in the unique gE N terminus are important for normal gE expression, secondary envelopment and cell-cell spread, and are essential for skin infection.[29] Residues within amino acids 27 to 90 are necessary for gE binding to IDE, normal cell–cell spread *in vitro*,[5,28,29] and virulence in skin xenografts, but not for virus entry into T cells.[28] Nonglycosylated immature gE binds to IDE in the ER. The unique gE residues 51 to 187 are necessary for VZV infection of skin as well as T cells. VZV-MSP is a naturally occurring mutation in the unique gE N terminus, changing the amino acid of codon 150 from aspartic acid to asparagine. The mutant shows altered cellular egress and enhanced cell–cell spread *in vitro* and in skin xenografts.[366]

Correct gE trafficking and maturation requires heterodimerization of gE with gI.[247,276] gE/gI heterodimer formation depends on the cysteine-rich region (amino acids 208–236) also present in gE encoded by other alphaherpesviruses. The capacity of gE to bind to gI is a major determinant of VZV virulence in skin xenografts, indicating that cell–cell fusion and polykaryocyte formation depends on this interaction.[28] Disrupting gE/gI heterodimer formation also results in aberrant VZV infection of dorsal root ganglion (DRG) xenografts, causing severe tissue damage despite impaired cell–cell spread. By contrast, mutations of the gE AYRV *trans*-Golgi localization motif and blocking gE/IDE binding did not alter VZV neurovirulence in DRG xenografts.[484] VZV gE has essential functions in neuropathogenesis.[484]

Glycoprotein I

gI, encoded by *ORF67*, is a 58- to 62-kd glycoprotein that contains N- and O-linked sugars.[284] gI heterodimer formation with gE requires residues 105 to 125 and four highly conserved cysteine residues that are also necessary for gI structure and virion incorporation.[311] gI is not required for VZV replication in cultured human cells but is required in Vero cells. Deleting gI impairs efficient cell–cell spread of virus, adsorption to cells, and syncytia formation *in vitro*. gI is essential for infection of human skin and T-cell xenografts in SCID mice.[75,261,279] Mutations that alter Sp1- or USF-binding sites in the gI promoter reduce gI expression and impair infection of human T-cell and skin xenografts in SCID mice, but not in cultured cells.[174]

The gI cytoplasmic tail is phosphorylated but the phosphorylation sites are not required for VZV skin infection. A threonine residue in the gI endodomain targets gI to the TGN when expressed alone in cultured cells, although gI is more rapidly localized to the TGN in the presence of gE.[4] The carboxy-terminal domain of gI is required for envelopment of VZ virions in the TGN.[439] While gI is also endocytosed from the cell surface and has a methionine–leucine internalization motif in its cytoplasmic tail, the gE–gI complex undergoes endocytosis more efficiently than does gE or gI alone.[4,318] VZV gI is required for normal maturation of gE and for efficient distribution of gE to the cell surface.

Glycoprotein H

gH, the product of *ORF37*, is a 118-kd glycoprotein that contains N-linked but not O-linked sugars and is sialylated and sulfated.[141,196,283,472] The structure of gH–gL has been resolved to show gH–gL heterodimer formation (Fig. 13.6).[472] This interaction is required for entry, based on the binding of neutralizing antibodies to a site formed by residues of both gH and gL. The gH binding to gL is required for its processing in the Golgi network and transport to the cell surface.[262] Endocytosis of gH results in reduced cell surface expression and decreased cell–cell fusion. gH forms a complex with gE in virus-infected cells and during incorporation into virions.[263,327] Coexpression of gH with either gE or gI allows transport of an immature form of gH to the cell surface, but this form is not fusogenic.[103] The short cytoplasmic tail of gH contains a tyrosine-based motif (YNKI) that mediates clathrin-dependent endocytosis of gH in infected cells.[326] The gH cytoplasmic domain regulates gB/gH–gL mediated cell–cell fusion, which depends on its length rather than sequence, and is necessary for skin infection.[475]

The gH ectodomain has three functional subdomains, DI–DIII, that were defined by site-directed mutagenesis and shown to have specific functions in cell fusion and VZV pathogenesis.[428] The extreme N-terminal residues in DI are important for skin tropism, T-cell entry, and fusion. DII helices and a conserved disulfide bond are essential for gH structure and VZV replication. Disulfide bonds and a bridging strand in DIII are required for the structural stability of this domain and are critical for membrane fusion. The biologic importance of gH DIII function during VZV replication is evident since a naturally occurring compensatory mutation was acquired during VZV replication when the ^{724}CXXC^{727} motif was mutated; this DIII mutation stabilized the bridging strand and rescued both a replication-deficient virus and a lethal cysteine mutation that disrupted the fusion function of gH.[428]

Glycoprotein L

gL, encoded by *ORF60*, is a 20-kd glycoprotein that forms a complex with gH, acting as a chaperone that associates with the immature but not the mature form of gH. gL is thought to be glycosylated with an N-linked oligosaccharide. Whereas gH requires gL for its maturation, gL is fully processed in the absence of gH. When expressed alone or with gH, gL accumulates only in the cytoplasm.[103] gL contains an ER-targeting sequence and is recycled between the ER and the Golgi network.[103] Coexpression of gH and gL supports syncytia formation, whereas expression of either protein alone does not.[103]

Glycoprotein K

gK, encoded by *ORF5*, is a 40-kd glycoprotein containing N-linked sugars and is required for VZV replication.[148,278] Overexpression of gK in a cell line inhibited syncytia formation by wild-type virus. HSV gK cannot complement growth of gK-deleted VZV.

Glycoprotein M and Glycoprotein N

gM, encoded by *ORF50*, is a 435-amino acid membrane glycoprotein.[364,473] *ORF50* has one full-length transcript that produces gM and three alternatively spliced transcripts that are rarely translated *in vitro*.[285] gM is predicted to contain eight transmembrane domains, an N-glycosylation site, and a cysteine residue in the first ectodomain. gM is 42- to 48-kd in infected cells and virus particles; a 37-kd precursor, not yet modified by N-linked oligosaccharides, is present in infected cells. gM localizes to the Golgi and endosomes, where it may be incorporated into the virion envelope. The functions of gM are not defined, although its presence in virus particles suggests a role in viral entry and virion maturation[285] and its trafficking motifs are required for VZV skin tropism.[493] As observed in other herpesviruses, gM forms a complex with gN through a disulfide bond; the interaction with gN is necessary for gM maturation, transport, and virion incorporation. *ORF50* is dispensable, but gM deletion mutants have impaired plaque formation and spread, with vacuoles containing electron-dense material appearing in the cytoplasm.[364] An *ORF50* deletion mutant did not replicate in melanoma cells.[496]

Assembly and Release

Infectious VZV progeny are synthesized as large numbers of cell-free virions and released efficiently from cells infected *in vivo* (see **Pathogenesis and Pathology**), whereas VZV is highly cell associated in cultured cells. Infectious cell-free virus can be recovered by sonicating VZV-infected cells, but yields are low, the particle-to-infectivity ratio is very high (40,000:1),[51] and virions remain attached to cell membrane fragments. VZ virions are usually enclosed in membrane-lined cytoplasmic vacuoles and some may be degraded during transit through the cytoplasm.

Because VZV replication in cultured cells is expected to differ from that in differentiated cells in the human host, any model of assembly and egress derived from *in vitro* observations will be incomplete. However, the current model is that nucleocapsids assemble in the nucleus and transit the inner and outer nuclear membranes for delivery into the cytoplasm in a process that involves envelopment, fusion, and de-envelopment.[125] VZV capsid assembly within the infected cell nucleus has not been well defined but procapsids, partial capsids, and complete capsids accumulate at sites adjacent to replication compartments early in infection.[238] VZV ORF24 and ORF27 are likely to have functions in nuclear egress similar to those of their respective HSV orthologs, UL31 and UL34. The nucleocapsids are thought to undergo secondary envelopment by budding through TGN membranes where the cisternae have been decorated with VZV-encoded glycoproteins with their cytoplasmic tails extending into the cytosol. Tegument proteins adhere to the remodeled cytosolic faces of TGN membranes (Fig. 13.5). The naked nucleocapsids attach to the tegument and invaginate into the cisternae. In cultured cells, these vesicles are usually diverted to prelysosomes, where they are subjected to degrading enzymes (Fig. 13.5). Mannose-6-phosphate side chains render the evolving particles susceptible to binding and uptake by lysosomes bearing the cation-independent mannose-6-phosphate receptor (MPR^{ci}).[67] Cell lines deficient in MPR^{ci} release cell-free VZV more efficiently than other cultured cells, implying that an alternative secretory pathway is operative in some cell types *in vivo* to allow virus egress without lysosomal degradation (Fig. 13.5). Superficial epidermal skin cells, which lack MPR^{ci}, show a pattern of VZV maturation resembling that seen in cells deficient in this receptor.[67]

Syncytia Formation

Cell–cell fusion with formation of large syncytia is a hallmark of VZV replication in cell culture (Fig. 13.7), becoming detectable at about 9 hours after infection of melanoma cells,[351] and involves about 75% of the monolayer by 48 hours, with detachment of fused cells from the surface at about 60 hours. These multinucleated giant cells have enlarged nuclei, abnormal nucleoli, and marginated chromatin. Fusion between nuclear membranes also occurs within syncytia.[448] Syncytia formation is important for VZV pathogenesis in skin, where polykaryocytes are prominent. VZV also induces the fusion of neurons and satellite cells in DRG.[112,354] By contrast, VZV does not cause fusion of T cells; instead, spread in T-cell xenografts is associated with the release of infectious cell-free virions.[281,282] VZV also induces the formation of "viral highways" in which viral particles decorate the surface of infected cells, especially within the syncytia and on filopodia[52] (Fig. 13.7), and an increase in cell surface virions is associated with more rapid cell–cell spread.[366]

The formation of the core fusion complex, consisting of gB, gH, and gL, which is presumed to function in fusion of the viral envelope with the cell surface membrane during entry, is essential for cell fusion and syncytia formation.[315,428,472] The regulation of syncytia formation is required for VZV skin infection, shown by severely impaired pathogenesis and reduced progeny virions when fusion is exaggerated; this regulatory function is mediated by the C-terminal domains of gB and gH (see **Glycoprotein B** and **Glycoprotein H**). This effect was associated with up-regulation of Ras GTPase genes associated with membrane remodeling.[314] The calcineurin pathway contributes to the regulation of gB/gH–gL dependent fusion, as shown by enhanced cell fusion when calcineurin phosphatase activation is blocked.[497] Residues in gH domain III are necessary for cell-cell fusion and virulence in skin xenografts. Formation of typical VZV syncytia also requires gE/gI heterodimerization and functions that depend on the unique gE N terminus.[28,29] Deleting gI (*ORF67*) or reducing its expression by promoter mutations results in a small-plaque phenotype with distorted polykaryocyte formation.[75,261] Syncytial formation is also reduced in the absence of ORF8 and ORF9A proteins.[358] Conversely, typical syncytial formation can be retained *in vitro* even with mutations that severely disrupt VZ virion formation, such as those blocking ORF47 expression or eliminating its kinase activity; the deficiency is evident only by markedly impaired skin infection.[29,31,310]

Replication in Specialized Cells in Culture

VZV replication and gene requirements have been studied *in vitro* using primary human cells and organ cultures that reflect the tropisms of the virus for T cells, skin, and neural cells *in vivo*. Human tonsil T cells are highly permissive for VZV replication[230] (Fig. 13.8), whereas VZV infects T cells at low frequencies in peripheral blood mononuclear cell (PBMC) cultures; infection can be increased by T-cell activation.[225] VZV infection remodels tonsil T cells dramatically to promote their trafficking to skin (see **Pathogenesis and Pathology**) (Fig. 13.9).[380] VZV has only limited capacity to replicate in transformed human B cells.[225] Human natural killer (NK) cells, in particular the $CD56^{dim}$ subset that predominates in peripheral blood, are highly permissive to productive VZV infection and were more permissive to infection when compared to T cells, NKT cells, and $CD3^{-}CD56^{-}$ lymphocytes[47,48] (Fig. 13.8). VZV infection alters the NK cell surface landscape and functionality[47,48] (see **Modulation of Surface Expression of Cellular Proteins Involved in the Host Response** and **Interference**

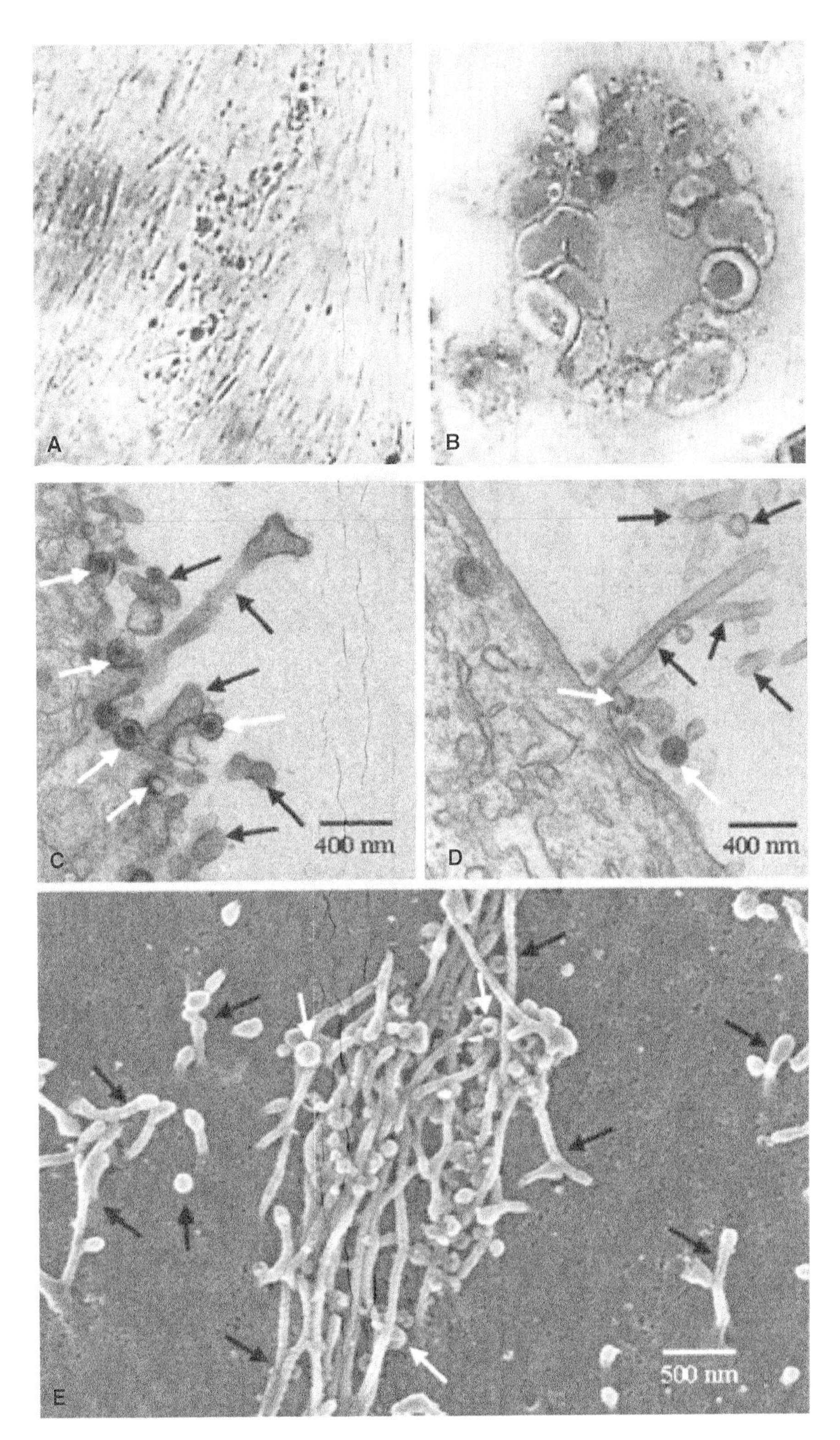

FIGURE 13.7 **Varicella–zoster virus (VZV) infection of human cells *in vitro*. A:** An early focus of VZV infection in a monolayer of human fibroblasts stained with hematoxylin and eosin (H&E, × 240). **B:** A multinucleated cell containing intranuclear inclusion bodies from a monolayer of VZV-infected human fibroblasts (H&E, × 2,600). **C–E:** Microstructural composition of "viral highways," the distinctive linear patterns from which VZV emerges as complete and aberrant viral particles (*white arrows*) and cellular projections (*black arrows*) of 70- to 100-nm diameter (by transmission electron microscopy): **C:** five viral particles and several projections; **D:** one elongated projection surrounded by portions of other projections; **E:** viral highway covered by cellular projections with viral particles in between (by scanning electron microscopy). (**A,B** from Garcia-Valcarcel M, Fowler WJ, Harper DR, et al. Cloning, expression, and immunogenicity of the assembly protein of varicella-zoster virus and detection of the products of open reading frame 33. *J Med Virol* 1997;53(4):332-339. Copyright © 1997 Wiley-Liss, Inc. Reprinted by permission of John Wiley & Sons, Inc. **C–E** from Carpenter JE, Hutchinson JA, Jackson W, et al. Egress of light particles among filopodia on the surface of varicella-zoster virus-infected cells. *J Virol* 2008;82(6):2821-2835. Copyright © 2008 American Society for Microbiology. Reproduced with permission from American Society for Microbiology.)

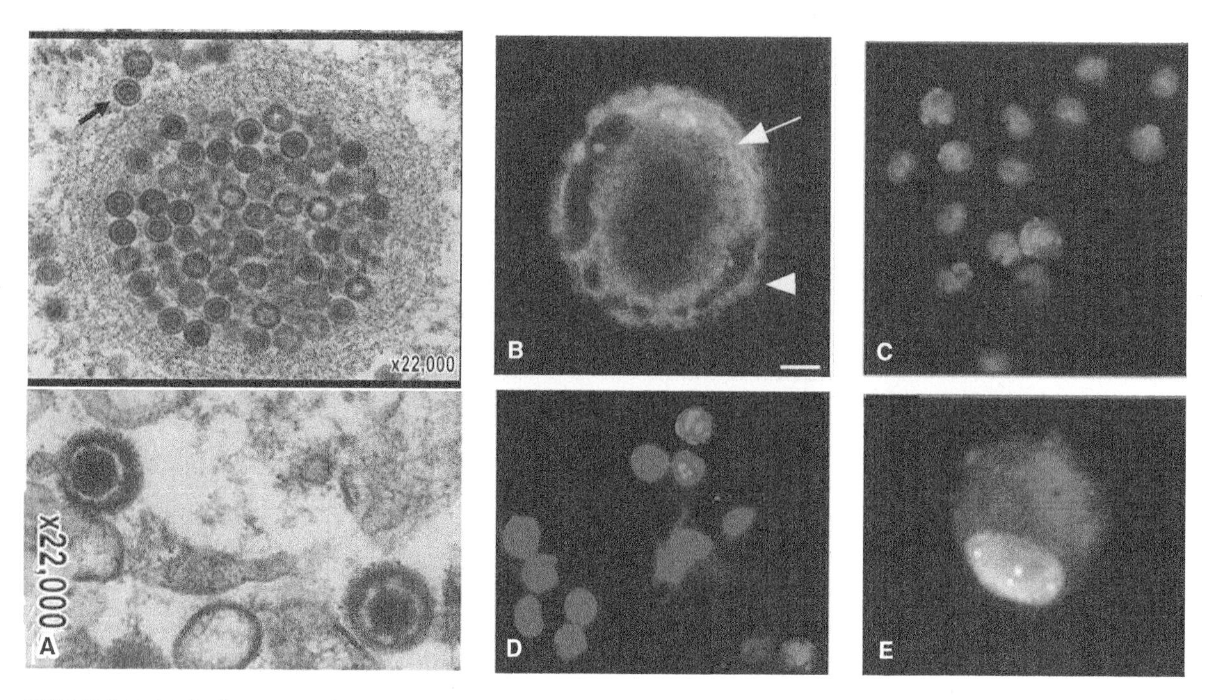

FIGURE 13.8 **Varicella–zoster virus (VZV) infection of immune cells. A:** VZ virions in T cells infected with pOka at 14 days postinoculation, showing intranuclear capsids (*upper; arrow*) and complete virions within a large cytoplasmic vesicle (*lower*). **B:** Dendritic cells 2 days after infection and stained with monoclonal antibody to CD1a (*arrowhead*) and rabbit antibody to IE4 (*arrow*). **C:** Monocytes 2 days after infection and stained with monoclonal antibody to VZV gE (*red staining*) and DAPI (*blue staining*).**D:** NK cells 1 day after infection with VZV and stained with monoclonal antibody to IE63 (*red staining*) and DAPI (*blue staining*). **E:** Merged image of monocyte-derived macrophages 2 days after VZV infection and stained with monoclonal antibody to HLA-DR (*purple staining*), rabbit antibody to VZV pORF29 (*red staining*), and DAPI (*blue staining*). (**A** adapted from Schaap A, Fortin JF, Sommer M, et al. T-cell tropism and the role of ORF66 protein in pathogenesis of varicella-zoster virus infection. *J Virol* 2005;79(20):12921-12933. **B:** adapted from Abendroth A, Morrow G, Cunningham AL, et al. Varicella-zoster virus infection of human dendritic cells and transmission to T cells: implications for virus dissemination in the host. *J Virol* 2001;75(13):6183–6192. **C and E:** adapted from Kennedy JJ, Steain M, Slobedman B, et al. Infection and functional modulation of human monocytes and macrophages by varicella-zoster virus. *J Virol* 2019;93(3):e01887-18. **D:** adapted from Campbell TM, McSharry BP, Steain M, et al. Varicella zoster virus productively infects human natural killer cells and manipulates phenotype. *PLoS Pathog* 2018;14(4):e1006999. https://creativecommons.org/licenses/by/4.0/.)

with Intrinsic Antiviral Responses). Other immune cells that can be productively infected with VZV include immature and mature dendritic cells,[2,168,169,292] plasmacytoid dendritic cells (pDCs), NKT cells, $CD3^-CD56^-$ lymphocytes, monocytes, macrophages, and B cells[47,169,188,201] (Fig. 13.8).

In skin organ cultures, deleting *ORF 7, 10, 14*, and *47* disrupts VZV infection, whereas deletion of *ORFs 0, 18, 19, 23, 32, 35, 49*, or *68* affects replication in fibroblasts as well.[496] Infected keratinocytes release cell-free virus *in vitro* but infectious virus yields are low, whereas *in vivo* infection yields high titers. VZV modifies host cell gene transcription in differentiated keratinocytes by increasing the expression of the cytokeratin gene encoding *KRT15*, a stem cell marker found at the hair follicle isthmus, and inhibiting the cytokeratin genes *KRT1* and *KRT10*, associated with keratinocyte differentiation.[189]

VZV infects dissociated cells cultured from nervous system tissues, including both neuronal and nonneuronal cells (Schwann cells and astrocytes).[164] VZV also infects neurons and supporting cells in explanted intact ganglia,[138] neurons derived from human embryonic stem cells,[362] and tissue assemblies derived from neural progenitors.[137] A model of latency and reactivation has been developed using neuronal stem cells[269] with detection of small noncoding RNAs during lytic infection.[135] Infection of differentiated neurons in culture with cell-free VZV did not produce cytopathic effects or infectious virus, although VZV DNA, virus-specific transcripts, and protein, including gE, were found several weeks later,[340] and VZV gI is required for spread and virion localization to axons in DRG explants.[68] Virion assembly in neurons requires gC,[142] and in addition to its role in skin, ORF7 functions in virion envelopment in differentiated neurons.[182] While the capacity of vaccine Oka to establish latency was maintained, reactivation was reduced in a neuronal cell model *in vitro*.[361]

VZV Effects on Host Cell Functions

Cell Protein Synthesis, Cell Cycle Changes, and Other Effects

Although *ORF17* encodes an ortholog of the HSV VHS protein, ORF17 is not present in the tegument and has little impact on host protein synthesis.[368] However, VZV infection dysregulates and arrests the cell cycle in fibroblasts (e-Fig. 13.3), an effect characterized by high levels of expression of cyclins A, B1, and D3 without extensive synthesis of cellular DNA.[239,240] Cyclin-dependent kinase (CDK) activity is essential for VZV replication; CDK1 phosphorylates IE62 and is present in viri-

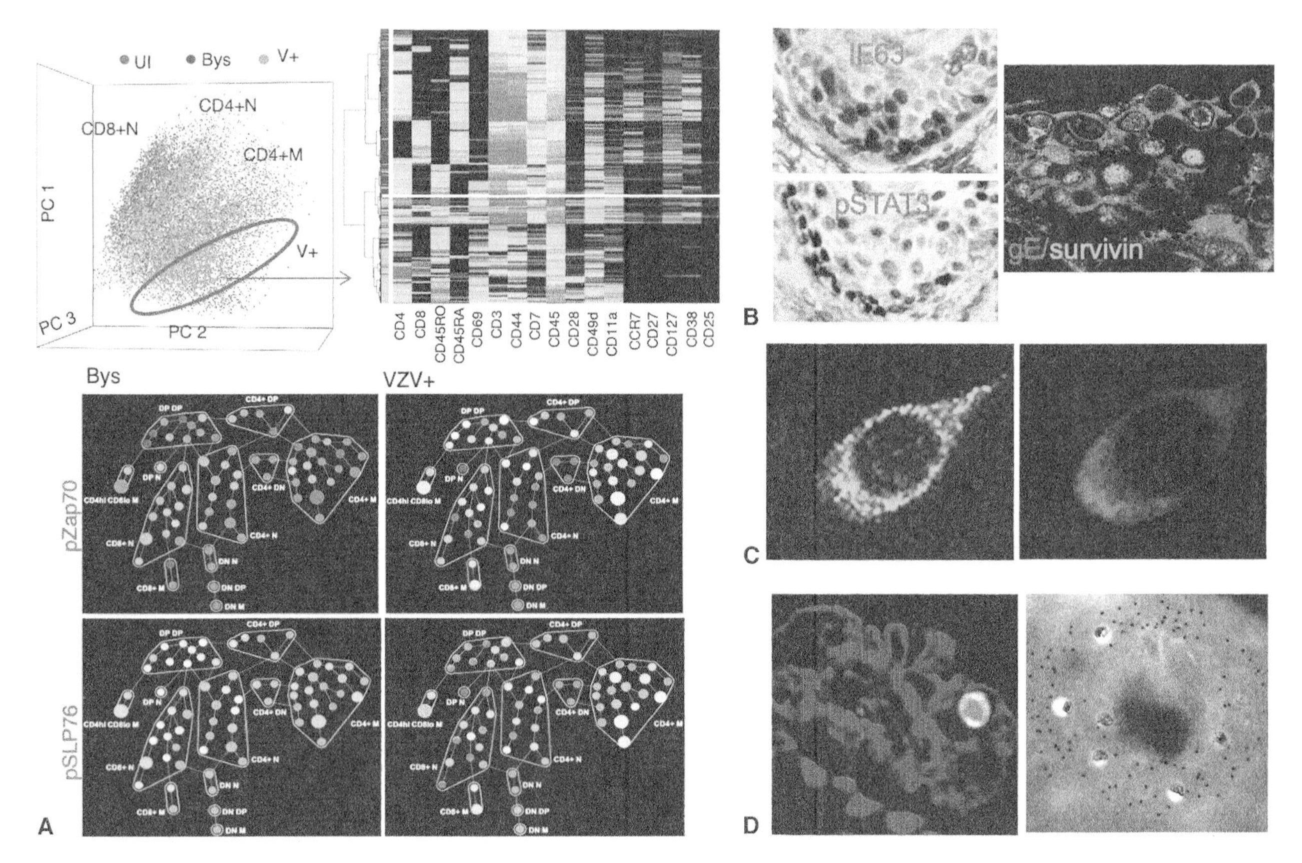

FIGURE 13.9 Varicella–zoster virus (VZV) and host cell interactions. A: Remodeling of T cells by takeover of host cell signaling pathways. *Upper*: Hierarchical relationship of pooled uninfected (UI), bystander (Bys), and VZV-infected (V+) T cells based on surface phenotypes by PCA (*left*) and agglomerative clustering (*right*) of equal numbers of cells from each population. V+ T cells were iteratively compared with a randomly selected equal number of UI and Bys T cells. *Lower*: Activation of T-cell signaling pathways shown in Bys or VZV+ T cells (each node represents a T-cell subpopulation) as the fold change in expression of pZap70 and pSLP76 at 48 hpi (*blue*: minimum; *red*: maximum) using Spanning Tree Progression Analysis of Density Normalization Events (SPADE).**B:** STAT3 activation and induction of survivin in VZV-infected skin sections obtained 21 days after infection and analyzed by immunohistochemistry. *Left two panels:* Sections were probed with antibodies to VZV IE63 to identify foci of infected cells and pSTAT3; expression was detected with DAB (*brown*) chromogen and hematoxylin counterstain. *Right panel:* VZV-infected skin sections were stained with antibodies to gE (*red*) and survivin (*green*) and examined by confocal microscopy.**C:** Autophagosomes in a varicella lesion. A keratinocyte exhibited LC3B puncta characteristic of LC3B-II in autophagosomes (*green*) in a VZV-infected cell identified by expression of IE62 (*red*). **D:** PML entrapment of nucleocapsids in neurons in human DRG xenografts in SCID mice. *Left panel:* Neural cell with large ring-like PML cage (*yellow*) that sequesters ORF23 protein (*red*) in infected human DRG xenograft. *Right panel:* a large, ring-like PML cage that sequesters numerous VZV NCs in infected neural cells shown by PML-specific immunogold-labeling of ultrathin (80-nm) cryosection. (**A:** adapted from Sen N, Mukherjee G, Sen A, et al. Single-cell mass cytometry analysis of human tonsil T cell remodeling by varicella zoster virus. *Cell Rep* 2014; 8(2):633–645. Copyright © 2014 Elsevier. With permission. **B:** adapted with permission from Sen N, Che X, Rajamani J, et al. Signal transducer and activator of transcription 3 (STAT3) and survivin induction by varicella-zoster virus promote replication and skin pathogenesis. *Proc Natl Acad Sci* U S A 2012;109(2):600–605. **C:** adapted from Carpenter JE, Jackson W, Benetti L, et al. Autophagosome formation during varicella-zoster virus infection following endoplasmic reticulum stress and the unfolded protein response. *J Virol* 2011;85(18):9414–9424. Copyright © 2011 American Society for Microbiology. Amended with permission from American Society for Microbiology. **D:** adapted from Reichelt M, Wang L, Sommer M, et al. Entrapment of viral capsids in nuclear PML cages is an intrinsic antiviral host defense against varicella-zoster virus. *PLoS Pathog* 2011;7(2):e1001266. https://creativecommons.org/licenses/by/3.0/.)

ons.[239] VZV replication may be associated with activation of the DNA damage response, leading to cell cycle arrest.[474] VZV may also activate transcription factors and increase cell cycle regulatory proteins through the mitogen-activated protein kinase pathways, extracellular-regulated kinase (ERK), c-Jun N-terminal kinase (JNK), and PI3 kinase.[347] JNK activation by VZV contributes to both replication and reactivation in the neuronal model.[231] VZV induces the phosphorylation of CREB in T cells and fibroblasts, which has multifactorial effects on host cell gene expression by binding the coactivator, p300/CBP, and is needed for cell–cell spread *in vitro* and in skin xenografts.[117] p27, p53, and ATM kinase are other examples of host regulatory proteins induced in infected cells. VZV infection also alters the organization of actin in the cell, with dramatic effects observed when gB-mediated regulation of cell fusion is disrupted.[314]

Inflammasome formation

In response to VZV infection, host cells mount an innate response through pattern recognition receptors and the formation of the nucleotide-binding domain and leucine-rich repeat-containing/pyrin domain–containing 3 (NLRP3) inflammasome. NLRP3 protein recruits the adaptor apoptosis-associated speck-like protein (ASC) and caspase-1, resulting in processing of the proinflammatory cytokine interleukin (IL)-1β by activated caspase-1 and NLRP3 is also up-regulated in VZV-infected skin xenografts *in vivo*.[308]

Interference With Intrinsic Antiviral Responses

Cell signaling

VZV targets the activation of several cellular pathways that support antiviral responses for inhibition. ORF66 interferes with the induction of phosphorylated signal transducer and activator of transcription 1 (STAT1) after exposure to interferon gamma (IFN-γ) in VZV-infected T cells and fibroblasts.[374] VZV also interferes with nuclear factor (NF)-κB activation in cultured fibroblasts and in epidermal cells in skin xenografts *in vivo* by rapidly sequestering p50 and p65 in the cytoplasm and by inhibiting degradation of the NF-κB inhibitor, IκBα.[186] However, VZV infection of human monocytes induces NF-κB and IL-6 through the Toll-like receptor 2 pathway.[440] VZV also inhibits the expression of STAT 1-α and Janus kinase 2 (JAK2) proteins as well as the transcription of IFN regulatory factor I and the major histocompatibility complex (MHC) class II transactivator, mediating IFN-γ signal transduction.[3]

In contrast to its inhibition of STAT1, VZV induces STAT3 activation in T cells and fibroblasts, as is also observed in cells infected with the oncogenic herpesviruses Kaposi Sarcoma herpesvirus (KSHV) and Epstein-Barr virus (EBV).[379] STAT3 phosphorylation requires infectious VZV and is a direct rather than a cytokine-mediated effect. STAT3 phosphorylation leads to the induction of the cell protein survivin *in vitro* and in infected skin cells (Fig. 13.9). Inhibition of STAT3 phosphorylation diminishes VZV virulence in skin xenografts and survivin inhibition reduces VZV replication, indicating that constitutive survivin expression in epithelial stem cells that line hair follicles, is important for initiating skin infection. Since STAT1 and STAT3 activation are inversely activated signaling events, VZV-mediated STAT3 activation may enhance replication indirectly by blocking STAT1-mediated innate responses and directly by promoting survival of infected cells through enhanced survivin expression (Fig. 13.9).

Interferon and interferon-regulated responses

As is true of other viruses, IFNs significantly inhibit VZV. The induction of the type I IFN pathway is initiated by IFN-β primarily through activation of IFN regulatory factor (IRF)-3, leading to IFN-α production. VZV blocks IFN-β production efficiently and down-regulates transcription of IRF3-dependent genes, as shown by comparing VZV-infected and uninfected cells from the same culture.[381] IE62 alone prevents TANK-binding kinase (TBK1)-mediated IRF3 function and IFN-β secretion through a novel mechanism in which IRF3 phosphorylation is blocked. This antiviral activity of IE62 is independent of its function as a transactivating protein. IFN-α triggers production of cell proteins that phosphorylate the alpha subunit of eukaryotic initiation factor 2 (eIF-2α), which blocks translation. VZV can block eIF-2α phosphorylation through an IE63-dependent process, preventing this IFN-α effect,[7] possibly as a redundant mechanism if IE62 interference with IFN-β is incomplete. ORF47 kinase contributes to inhibition of IRF3 activation by altering its phosphorylation and blocking homodimer formation, and ORF61 degrades phosphorylated IRF3 in HEK293 cells[500]; however, these cells do not support productive infection. While IFN-α is an important initial inhibitory response, IFN-γ induces a different pattern of host cell gene expression that is associated with blocking VZV replication in fibroblasts.[382] The downstream mechanisms by which IFN-α and IFN-γ inhibit VZV, which are the IRF-9 and IRF-1 pathways, respectively, account for their differential effects, and again, IE62 functions as a VZV countermeasure by inhibiting IRF-9 transcription. When epithelial cells and fibroblasts are treated with IFN-γ before infection, the transactivating capacity of IE62 is inhibited and the effect is reversed by interfering with JAK/STAT-1 signaling.[383]

VZV can productively infect pDCs and inhibit their ability to produce IFN-α, even when stimulated with a TLR9 agonist.[169] Since VZV infects pDCs in skin, IFN-α production may be impaired *in vivo*. IFN-γ could promote survival of VZV-infected human neurons *in vitro,* which might ensure the efficient establishment of latency *in vivo*[23] and type I IFNs had an inhibitory effect on VZV replication in human induced pluripotent stem cell (iPSC)-derived neurons *in vitro*.[85] VZV infection of DRG in SCID mice resulted in increased production of IFN-α, IFN-γ, and other proinflammatory cytokines.[483]

Promyelocytic leukemia protein nuclear bodies (PML-NBs)

PML-NBs, also known as ND10 bodies, restrict herpesvirus gene expression in newly infected cells and are up-regulated by IFNs. Whereas HSV ICP0 degrades PML protein and PML-NBs, VZV-infected cells do not exhibit PML degradation.[233] Instead, the architecture of PML-NBs is disrupted in VZV-infected cells *in vitro* and in human skin xenografts through an ORF61-mediated effect that depends on small ubiquitin-like modifier (SUMO)-interacting motifs (SIMs) in ORF61.[443] In the absence of SIMs, ORF61 association with PML-NBs is reduced, most PML-NBs remain intact, and VZV skin infection is severely impaired. The ORF61 SUMO-binding capacity is necessary to counteract the intrinsic barrier created when the IFN response in VZV-infected skin induces even higher numbers of PML-NBs in dermal and epidermal cells. Furthermore, incomplete dispersal of PML-NBs by VZV inhibits egress of VZV capsids from the infected-cell nucleus, impairing the synthesis of infectious virus progeny[352,353] This antiviral mechanism has biologic significance, since neurons and satellite cells in human DRG and skin cells infected with VZV *in vivo* contain large PML-NBs that sequester newly assembled nucleocapsids (Fig. 13.9).[353] This function is mediated by the unique carboxy-terminus of PML IV (a splice variant of PML), which interacts with the ORF23 capsid surface protein to trap capsids and inhibit VZV replication. PML-dependent sequestration of nucleocapsids appears to be a common cytoprotective function of these PML-NBs, in which aberrant proteins are sensed and aggregated in neuronal cell nuclei.

Modulation of Surface Expression of Cellular Proteins Involved in the Host Response

VZV down-regulates expression of MHC class I proteins on the surface of infected fibroblasts and T cells, through their retention in the Golgi compartment,[1] although the total amount and rate of synthesis of class I molecules is unchanged in VZV-infected cells. Most of this effect, which blocks CD8+ T cell responses is mediated by ORF66.[1,107] VZV also inhibits IFN-γ induction of MHC class II molecules on the infected cell surface,[3] preventing recognition by VZV-specific CD4+ T cells. Infection of mature dendritic cells (DCs) with VZV results in down-regulation of surface MHC class I, CD80, CD83, and CD86, and inhibits their ability to stimulate proliferation of allogeneic T cells.[292] VZV also down-regulates Fas expression on the surface of DCs.[168] VZV infection of immature DCs fails to up-regulate CD80, CD83, CD86, MHC I and CCR7 which are important for DC maturation and antiviral responses,[2] and is most likely due to VZV regulation of the NF-κB pathway[186,385] that controls the expression of these immune molecules.

Down-regulation of surface MHC class I by VZV renders infected cells a target for NK cell–mediated killing. Further alteration of the infected cell surface is needed for VZV to prevent recognition and clearance by both cytotoxic T cells and NK cells. Analysis of viral regulation of cell surface ligands for NKG2D, a potent activating receptor expressed ubiquitously on NK cells, revealed that VZV selectively down-regulates expression of ULBP2 and ULBP3 and up-regulates MICA on the surface of infected cells.[49] Furthermore, NK cell activity is not enhanced when NK cells are cocultured with VZV-infected target cells *in vitro*, indicating VZV modulates NK cell–mediated detection and activation.[49]

Profiling of the VZV-infected NK cell surface receptor phenotype by flow cytometry revealed increased expression of the skin homing chemokine receptors, cutaneous lymphocyte–associated antigen (CLA), and chemokine receptor (CCR)4.[47] This remodeling to induce a skin homing phenotype is similar to effects observed on VZV-infected T cells.[380] VZV may use a pan lymphocyte mechanism to hijack lymphocyte trafficking to promote virus spread to the skin. Interestingly, VZV infection of NK cells down-regulates surface expression of CD16, an FcγRIII receptor that enables their function in antibody-dependent cell-mediated cytotoxicity (ADCC).[47] NK cells infiltrating the site of VZV antigen challenge also had significantly reduced CD16 expression,[306] suggesting that the virus may inhibit ADCC function *in vivo*. NK cells also produce proinflammatory cytokines such as tumor necrosis factor (TNF) and IFN-γ that have potent inhibitory effects on VZV replication.[97,382] VZV reduces NK cell secretion of both of these cytokines and VZV infection of NK cells paralyzes their cytotoxic function.[48] Thus, VZV has multiple mechanisms to disarm NK cells.

VZV infection of human monocytes and macrophages *in vitro* down-regulates surface expression of CD14, MHC class II, CD11b, and macrophage colony-stimulating factor (MCSF) receptor expression.[201] In addition, infection impairs dextran-mediated endocytosis by monocytes, suggesting VZV has evolved strategies to modulate the ability of monocytes to take up and present antigen in the context of surface MHC class II. VZV-infected monocytes are also unable to differentiate into macrophages, whereas macrophages were shown to be highly permissive to infection.[201] Thus, VZV encodes an immune evasion strategy to prevent CD4+ T-cell activation.

VZV infection of human PBMCs including NK cells, T cells, NKT cells, B cells, and monocytes has been reported to up-regulate surface programmed cell death ligand 1 (PD-L1) expression,[188] potentially disrupting effective immune responses via the inhibitory signal that is transmitted to PD1. By contrast, VZV down-regulates PD-L1 in infected human brain vascular adventitial fibroblasts, perineural cells, and fetal lung fibroblasts, which may promote persistent vessel inflammation observed in patients with VZV vasculopathy and persistent inflammation in infected lungs.[187]

VZV can up-regulate surface CD59 (a host regulator of complement activation) in infected T cells and DRG, but not skin.[447] This tissue-specific regulation of surface CD59 may provide a mechanism of complement evasion.

Regulation of Apoptosis and Autophagy

VZV regulates apoptosis in a cell type–specific manner. VZV induces apoptosis with chromatin condensation and DNA fragmentation in Vero cells, B cells, T cells, and human fibroblasts, but not in primary human DRG neurons. Conversely, expression of IE63 in sensory neurons inhibits apoptosis induced by withdrawal of nerve growth factor.[164] IE63 interferes with apoptosis in keratinocytes as well as neurons, in association with cytoplasmic accumulation of IE63.[122] Transcriptome profiles indicate a propensity for VZV to up-regulate antiapoptotic genes in neurons and proapoptotic genes in fibroblasts.[267] In VZV-infected T cells, caspase-8 transcripts are reduced, whereas two IRF gene transcripts (ADAR and MxA) are increased. By contrast, caspase-8 transcripts are not reduced in virus-infected fibroblasts or skin cells.[185] VZV ORF66 expression inhibits apoptosis induced by VZV in T cells[374] and is required for efficient growth in corneal epithelial cells, although interference with apoptosis is not the only ORF66 function required in these cells.[111] STAT3 activation by VZV results in up-regulation of survivin in skin, exerting a proviral effect by inhibiting apoptosis.[379] The proapoptotic activity of Bcl-2 interacting mediator of cell death (BIM) was inhibited by its phosphorylation in VZV-infected cells, mediated through the MEK/ERK pathway, which is enhanced by ORF12, whereas without phosphorylation, Bim reduced plaque formation.[249]

Activated cytotoxic T lymphocytes (CTLs) and NK cells secrete granzyme B, which cleaves multiple apoptotic pathway components, resulting in apoptosis of the target cell. VZV ORFs 4 and 62 were identified to contain granzyme B cleavage sites and could be cleaved by granzyme B. However, only ORF4 conferred protection in a NK cell–mediated cytotoxicity assay. Mutation of the ORF4 granzyme B cleavage site did not alter the ability of ORF4 to modulate NK cell cytotoxicity, suggesting a novel ORF4 immunoevasion function independent from the granzyme B cleavage site.[121]

Whereas the HSV-1 neurovirulence protein ICP34.5 inhibits autophagy, VZV lacks an ICP34.5 ortholog. By contrast, VZV induces autophagy-associated proteins and formation of autophagosomes in cultured cells as well as in human keratinocytes that express IE62 in skin lesions (Fig. 13.9).[53,409] Autophagy appears to be a stress response of cells to VZV and the subsequent abundant synthesis of viral glycoproteins.[43] VZV titers are reduced when completion of autophagic flux is inhibited by siRNA against ATG5, and bafilomycin A1 inhibition of autophagy impairs secondary envelopment and trafficking of VZ virions.[132] While engulfment of viral particles within lysosomes (xenophagy) has not been observed, many VZV particles are transported to the outer cell membrane after secondary envelopment in single-walled vacuoles with properties of late endosomes or amphisomes.[44] Based on the effects of its inhibition, the autophagy pathway is likely to be involved in the initial stress response to VZV and the transport of some progeny virions to the cell surface.

PATHOGENESIS AND PATHOLOGY

In the usual course of VZV infection, the virus exhibits tropism for T cells, cutaneous epithelial cells, and cells of sensory nerve ganglia (Fig. 13.1). VZV can also infect other tissues when cell-associated viremia and viral replication are not controlled by intrinsic or adaptive host immune responses. Under these circumstances, disseminated infection may involve the lungs, liver, central nervous system (CNS), and many other organs. Pathologic changes in these tissues may be caused by replicating virus and, in some instances, by inflammatory or immune-mediated injury. VZV and SVV pathogenesis have similarities consistent with the genetic relatedness of these two primate *Varicelloviruses.*[105,140,170,199,224,256,258] In some cases, the SVV model permits investigations, such as the host cell transcriptome profile triggered by acute lung infection, that are difficult in human infection.[10,11,322] The clinical manifestations of varicella and zoster that are associated with events in VZV pathogenesis and the pathologic changes associated with VZV syndromes are described in **Clinical Features**.

Entry Into the Host

Initial VZV replication is likely to occur in respiratory mucosal epithelial cells (Fig. 13.1). Primary VZV infection (varicella) is presumed to be initiated by inhalation of respiratory droplets containing virus particles or by inoculation of mucosal epithelium with infectious vesicular fluid from an individual with varicella or zoster. Following an incubation period of 10 to 21 days, primary VZV infection results in varicella. The potential for aerosol transmission is suggested by epidemiologic reports, and VZV DNA is detected in air samples from rooms occupied by patients with varicella or disseminated zoster.[372]

T-cell Tropism

Although T-cell tropism appears to be a necessary component of primary VZV infection, the site and mechanisms whereby T cells become infected cannot be defined in the human host. Tonsillar T cells are most permissive for VZV infection, suggesting that spread of VZV from infected mucosal epithelial cells to these T cells initiates cell-associated viremia.[229] Respiratory mucosal epithelial cells line tonsil crypts, penetrating deep into tonsillar tissues that contain many T cells, and migrating T cells traffic across this epithelial cell layer into tonsils. Dendritic cells are also present in mucosal epithelium and may transfer the virus to T cells in regional lymph nodes.[2] Viremia may be amplified during infection as T cells traffic through infected skin and visceral organs, such as the liver. VZV is detected in PBMCs from individuals just before or after the onset of the rash.[17,324] Infected cells are present at low frequency (0.01% to 0.001% of PBMCs)[225] and are usually cleared within 24 to 72 hours after the appearance of the rash. SVV causes a robust cell-associated viremia that precedes the cutaneous exanthem.[272]

The unexpected capacity of VZV to dramatically remodel the cell surface proteins of T cells and to promote the skin trafficking potential of VZV-infected T cells has been documented using multiparameter single-cell mass cytometry (CYTOF) with 25 surface markers and 16 cell signaling phosphoproteins[380] (Fig. 13.9). VZV increased CD69, PD-1, and CD45RO, creating an effector phenotype, and increased integrins, CD11a and CD28, along with CCR4 and CLA, and decreased CCR7 and CD7, which promotes skin homing. VZV remodeled purified naïve T cells similarly. VZV triggered the cell signaling pathways that result in T-cell responses to cognate antigens, including Zap70 (TCR stimulation via the MHC) and Akt (ligand binding to costimulatory molecules, such as CD28). Thus, reprogramming occurs from within VZV-infected T cells, not by antigen stimulation or cytokine-mediated effects. Instead of selectively infecting tonsil T cells with skin homing properties, VZV takes over the T-cell signaling pathways that normally regulate cell surface proteins during differentiation from naïve to adaptive, antigen-specific memory T cells.[380]

VZV proteins that are required for or contribute to T-cell tropism *in vivo* as identified in T cell–containing xenografts in the SCID mouse model include gI, ORFs 66, 35, and 47 as well as residues 51 to 187 in the unique gE N terminus, the residues required for gE binding to gI and, to a lesser extent, the gE AYRV TGN-targeting motif (Table 13.1). VZV T cell–associated viremia is likely to be facilitated by down-regulation of MHC class I protein, inhibition of apoptosis by ORF66, and STAT3 activation with survivin induction.

Experiments in the SCID mouse model indicate that VZV is transported by infected human T cells to skin xenografts soon after they enter the circulation. However, the spread of VZV in skin is countered by a potent innate immune barrier resulting from constitutive IFN expression and up-regulation of the cellular transactivators STAT1 and NF-κB in epidermal cells, along with the high frequency of PML nuclear bodies in basement membrane cells of the dermis[186,230,443] (Fig. 13.9). Blocking IFN responses accelerates VZV infection in skin dramatically. The long interval between VZV exposure and the appearance of varicella skin lesions appears to reflect the time required for VZV to overcome these robust intrinsic obstacles.

Skin Tropism

During varicella, skin cells become major sites of virus replication (Fig. 13.10). The virus may gain access to cutaneous epithelial cells by migration of intact, infected T cells out of the capillaries into cutaneous tissue, followed by release of virions. Alternatively, infectious virus may move from T cells into capillary endothelial cells. Inclusions and VZV proteins have been observed in capillary endothelial cells and adjacent epithelial cells in VZV lesions.[305] Cells lining the lymphatics of the superficial dermis become dilated and contain intranuclear inclusions, suggesting VZV infection. Cutaneous DCs and Langerhans cells are susceptible to VZV and may contribute to local replication and spread.[2,169]

Classic studies of varicella lesions by Tyzzer in 1906[419] showed that the earliest changes consist of vasculitis involving the endothelium of small blood vessels, whereas the emergence of enlarged, multinucleated epithelial cells with intranuclear eosinophilic inclusions is typical of the second, maculopapular stage of the lesions. Progressive degeneration of epithelial cells, coalescence of fluid-filled vacuoles between cells, and destruction of the basement membrane occur as maculopapular lesions evolve into vesicles (Fig. 13.10).

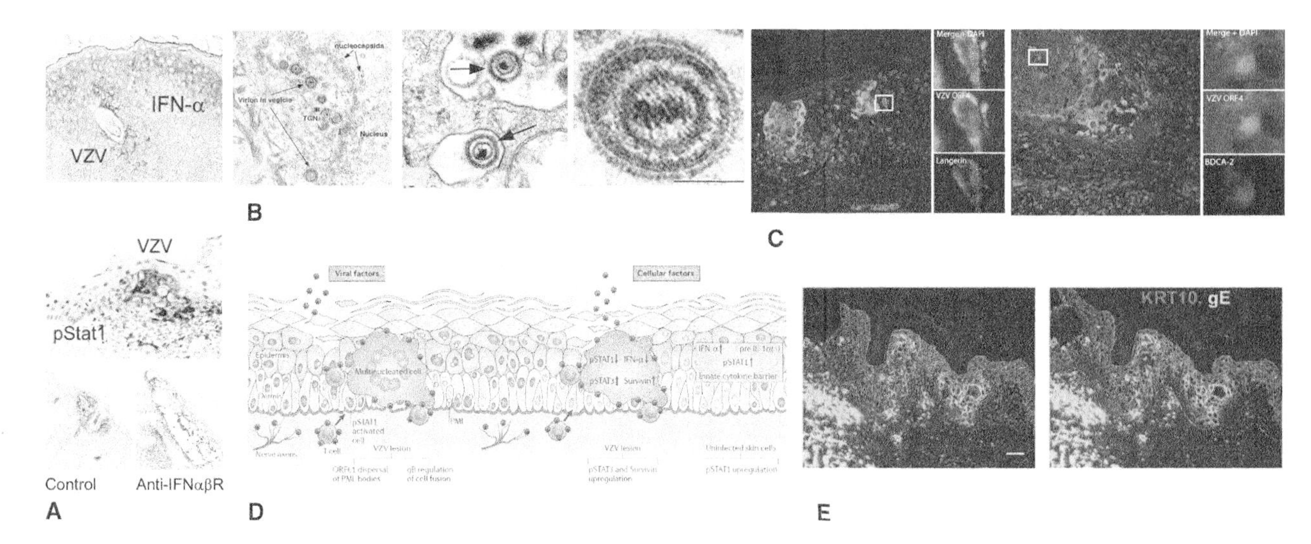

FIGURE 13.10 Varicella–zoster virus (VZV) infection of skin. Formation of epidermal lesions that penetrate the skin surfaces requires 10 to 21 days because of potent innate antiviral responses of epidermal cells. **A:** VZV lesions are formed by cell–cell spread overcoming the interferon barrier (IFN-α and pSTAT) in surrounding uninfected cells; interference with the innate IFN response by treatment of SCID mice with antibody against the IFNα/β receptor results in formation of large skin lesions. **B:** Electron micrograph of the suprabasal epidermis of a varicella skin lesion showing all stages of viral envelopment in infected keratinocytes. Unenveloped nucleocapsids are seen in the nucleus while nucleocapsids are being enveloped (*) by specialized cisternae of the TGN transport vesicles (*arrows*), each containing a single enveloped virion (*left panel*). Accumulating cytokeratin filaments are visible in the cytoplasm of the keratinocytes (*lower left of center panel*). Keratinocytes of the suprabasal layers of the VZV-infected epidermis secrete intact virions to the extracellular space (*arrows in middle panel* indicate two extracellular virions). A virion from a varicella vesicle is illustrated at high magnification and imaged in brightfield; note the spikes on the viral envelope, the complexity of the underlying tegument, and the apparent connections between the nucleocapsid and the tegument (scale bar = 100 nm) (*right panel*). **C:** Sections of varicella and herpes zoster skin lesions were immunofluorescently stained for combinations of DC markers and VZV antigens. Langerhans cell marker langerin (*red staining*) and VZV antigen ORF 4 (*green staining*) (*left panel*) and plasmacytoid dendritic cells with BDCA-2 marker (*red staining*) and VZV ORF4 (*green staining*) (*right panel*) are shown with 4′,6-diamidino-2-phenylindole (DAPI) (*blue staining*). Examples of dual positive cells are boxed and shown at higher magnification as insets. **D:** Schema of skin infection during primary VZV infection. Activation of innate responses (IFN, pStat1, and NF-κB) in uninfected cells is triggered by VZV replication. Within infected cells, VZV activates STAT3 and the antiapoptotic protein survivin. Uninfected T cells that traffic through sites of VZV lesion formation may amplify VZV viremia, and infected dendritic cells may transfer the virus to regional lymph nodes, enhancing T cell–mediated viremia. **E:** Immunofluorescent staining of a human varicella skin biopsy, showing *KRT10* (*red*) expression in the spinous layer; the loss of *KRT10* is seen in VZV-positive areas, shown by gE expression (*green*), scale bars 50 μm. (**A** adapted with permission from Ku CC, Zerboni L, Ito H, et al. Varicella-zoster virus transfer to skin by T cells and modulation of viral replication by epidermal cell interferon-α. Originally published in *Journal of Experimental Medicine*. doi: https://doi.org/10.1084/jem.20040634. Copyright © 2004 Rockefeller University Press. **B:** adapted by permission from Springer: Gershon MD, Gershon AA. VZV infection of keratinocytes: production of cell-free infectious virions in vivo. In: Abendroth A, Arvin A, Moffat J, eds. *Varicella-zoster virus. Current topics in microbiology and immunology*, Vol 342. Berlin, Heidelberg: Springer; 2010:173-188. Copyright © 2010 Springer-Verlag Berlin Heidelberg. **C:** adapted from Huch JH, Cunningham AL, Arvin AM, et al. Impact of varicella-zoster virus on dendritic cell subsets in human skin during natural infection. *J Virol* 2010;84(8):4060–4072. **D:** adapted with permission from Ku CC, Zerboni L, Ito H, et al. Varicella-zoster virus transfer to skin by T cells and modulation of viral replication by epidermal cell interferon-α. Originally published in *Journal of Experimental Medicine*. doi: https://doi.org/10.1084/jem.20040634. Copyright © 2004 Rockefeller University Press. **E:** adapted from Jones M, Dry IR, Frampton D, et al. RNA-seq analysis of host and viral gene expression highlights interaction between varicella zoster virus and keratinocyte differentiation. *PLoS Pathog* 2014;10(1):e1003896. https://creativecommons.org/licenses/by/4.0/.)

VZ virions are abundant in keratinocytes and in vesicular fluid (Fig. 13.10). Epithelial stem cells lining the hair follicles become infected first, allowing rapid delivery of the virus to the surface as these cells differentiate into keratinocytes. In skin biopsy specimens, early lesions show IE63 in keratinocytes; later, gE, gB, and IE63 are detected in keratinocytes, sebocytes, Langerhans cells, dermal dendrocytes, monocyte–macrophages, and endothelial cells. Viral proteins are also expressed in dermal nerves.[9] Cytokeratin and desmosomal proteins that preserve the epidermal structure are reduced substantially within skin lesions in a pattern associated with skin-blistering disorders.[189] Infiltration of the involved skin sites by inflammatory cells is minimal in the early vesicular phase, whereas later, up-regulation of adhesion molecules on capillary endothelial cells is associated with extensive mononuclear cell migration into the skin lesions. In the final phase, cutaneous lesions progress to ulceration and necrosis.

VZV proteins that are required for skin tropism, as assessed in skin xenografts in the SCID mouse model, include ORFs 10, 11, 31, 35, 47, 61, and 66; gI and particular residues in gI; and specific motifs within gE (Table 13.1). The passage of the Oka virus in tissue culture alters its capacity to infect skin, and analysis using vaccine/parental Oka chimeric viruses indicates that multiple VZV genes are involved in skin tropism.[485]

In addition to viral proteins, VZV skin tropism depends upon the capacity of the virus to up-regulate host cell signaling pathways, including STAT3 and pCREB, and down-regulate IFN-mediated innate defenses[117,379] (Fig. 13.10). Age-related differences have been identified that permit more VZV replication in aging skin.[492] Like VZV, SVV produces a cutaneous rash within 10 to 12 days after close contact with infected animals or following intratracheal inoculation.[272]

Release From the Host

Many cell-free VZ virions are released into vesicular fluid of skin lesions, which facilitates transmission by direct contact. VZV differs from other human herpesviruses in that infectious virus can be released into respiratory secretions and spread to susceptible persons by airborne transmission.[372] Viral DNA can be detected by PCR in specimens obtained from respiratory sites in the late stage of the incubation period and during the first few days of rash.[17,123] VZV DNA can also be detected in saliva during and after zoster, but it is not known whether infectious particles are present.[298] Compared to HSV-1, VZV DNA is rarely found in oral secretions in the absence of symptoms even in patients with HIV infection.[424]

Virulence

Naturally circulating strains of VZV do not exhibit intrinsic differences in virulence, as judged by the clinical consequences of primary VZV infection. Nonetheless, circulating strains of VZV do differ in their genome sequences, allowing assignment to clades (Fig. 13.4). The enhanced growth of the naturally occurring VZV–MSP variant in skin xenografts in SCID mice suggests that a single amino acid change in gE can alter pathogenesis.[366] VZV TK-negative viruses have been isolated from patients given prolonged acyclovir therapy, but altered pathogenicity has not been described. VZV isolates from three patients with encephalitis did not have distinctive genetic characteristics.[41] A study of Oka vaccine viruses isolated from skin revealed the same DNA sequence (a clonal isolate), whereas virus isolated from lungs contained mixed DNA sequences but with no identifiable changes related to tropism.[346] In addition, viruses isolated from skin lesions after vaccination have been found to have *ORF62* genes that encode amino acids characteristic of the parent strain rather than the substitutions identified in the vaccine, suggesting that a natural selection for these residues occurs during replication in the human host.[345] As demonstrated in the SCID mouse model, many VZV genes and promoter regulatory elements contribute to VZV cell tropism and virulence (Table 13.1).

Latency

VZV gains access to sensory ganglia, either hematogenously or by retrograde neural transport from mucocutaneous lesions during primary infection, where it establishes latency. The importance of cell-associated viremia in the delivery of the varicelloviruses to sensory ganglia is supported by VZV detection at these sites before rash has appeared and in nonhuman primates infected with SVV, and the occurrence of two episodes of zoster due to distinct strains in one individual[42,258] Alphaherpesvirus latency is characterized by the presence of viral DNA in ganglionic neurons (Fig. 13.11), limited viral gene transcription, and the potential for reactivation. VZV becomes latent in neurons in cranial nerve, dorsal root, and autonomic ganglia along the human neuraxis.[171,200,260,441] Based on autopsy studies, the prevalence of VZV latency in the population varies from 63% to 100%[84,335]; in the largest study, VZV DNA was found in 94% of 414 trigeminal ganglia.[173] Use of precise laser capture microdissection and PCR revealed VZV DNA in 4.1% of neurons and in less than 0.1% of satellite cells.[441]

Latent VZV DNA assumes a circular or concatemeric form[69] and is present at a frequency of 2 to 9 genome copies in 1% to 7% of neurons, which corresponds to a virus burden of 30 to 3,500 copies per 100 ng of ganglionic DNA.[84,165,200,335,441] The wide range of genome copy number in latently infected ganglia may reflect variability in the extent of cell-associated viremia and that the number of cutaneous lesions in primary VZV infection can range from a few to many hundreds.[357] Episodes of VZV reactivation or possibly reinfection may also increase the virus burden in latently infected ganglia.

The use of deep sequencing to evaluate trigeminal ganglia obtained less than 9 hours postmortem demonstrates that VZV gene expression is highly restricted during latency[94,321] in contrast to earlier reports of transcripts mapping to many *ORFs* when only less precise methods were available, including *in situ* hybridization, PCR amplification of cDNA libraries,[82,84] and multiplex PCR of mRNA.[299] By deep sequencing, gene expression was limited to *ORF63* and a transcript antisense to *ORF61* in trigeminal ganglia. Notably, the antisense transcript suppressed *ORF61* expression in cotransfection; isoforms of this latency-associated transcript that expressed a viral protein were identified in lytic infection and in zoster lesions. By contrast, a different isoform is expressed in latency, designated the VZV latency-associated transcript (VLT), that does not encode a protein.[94] VZV transcripts are also detected in enteric neurons that may indicate persistent gene expression or its triggering by surgical removal of intestinal tissues.[124]

Whereas the VLT was detected in 90% of early postmortem ganglia, ORF63 was also present in 63%. In earlier studies, *ORF63* transcripts in individual ganglia were found to vary more than 2,000-fold, ranging from 1 to 2,785 copies per 10,000 copies of GAPDH transcript,[84] and *ORF63* transcripts were detected in 17 of 28 ganglia, with as many as 29,000 copies per 1 μg of input mRNA. The consistent detection of *ORF63* transcripts in high abundance is not understood. Deep sequencing of RNA extracted from human trigeminal ganglia positive for VZV and HSV-1 DNA revealed microRNAs (miRNAs), the small noncoding RNA molecules that can alter transcript stability and translation, mapping to the HSV-1 genome but not the VZV genome.[420] Some of the small noncoding RNAs in VZV-infected neurons may be consistent with miRNA structures.[135]

Chromatin remodeling appears to contribute to the restricted pattern of latent VZV gene transcription based on chromatin immunoprecipitation (ChIP) assays.[120] Like HSV-1 DNA, histones are associated with VZV DNA at all stages of the viral life cycle, but the histone composition differs during productive infection and latency. Acetylated histone H3K9(Ac), indicative of a euchromatic (transcriptionally active) state, is associated with the *ORF62* and *ORF63* promoters during both latent infection in human ganglia and lytic infection of human melanoma (MeWo) cells. Neither *ORF14* (glycoprotein C) nor *ORF36* (thymidine kinase) is transcribed or associated with H3K9(Ac) during latent infection. An IE63 interaction with human antisilencing function 1 protein interferes with its capacity to bind histones h3.1 and h3.3.[6]

Some VZV protein expression may be detected in autopsy ganglia from patients with no evidence of zoster. IE63 was first identified in rare ganglion neurons by Mahalingam et al.[259]

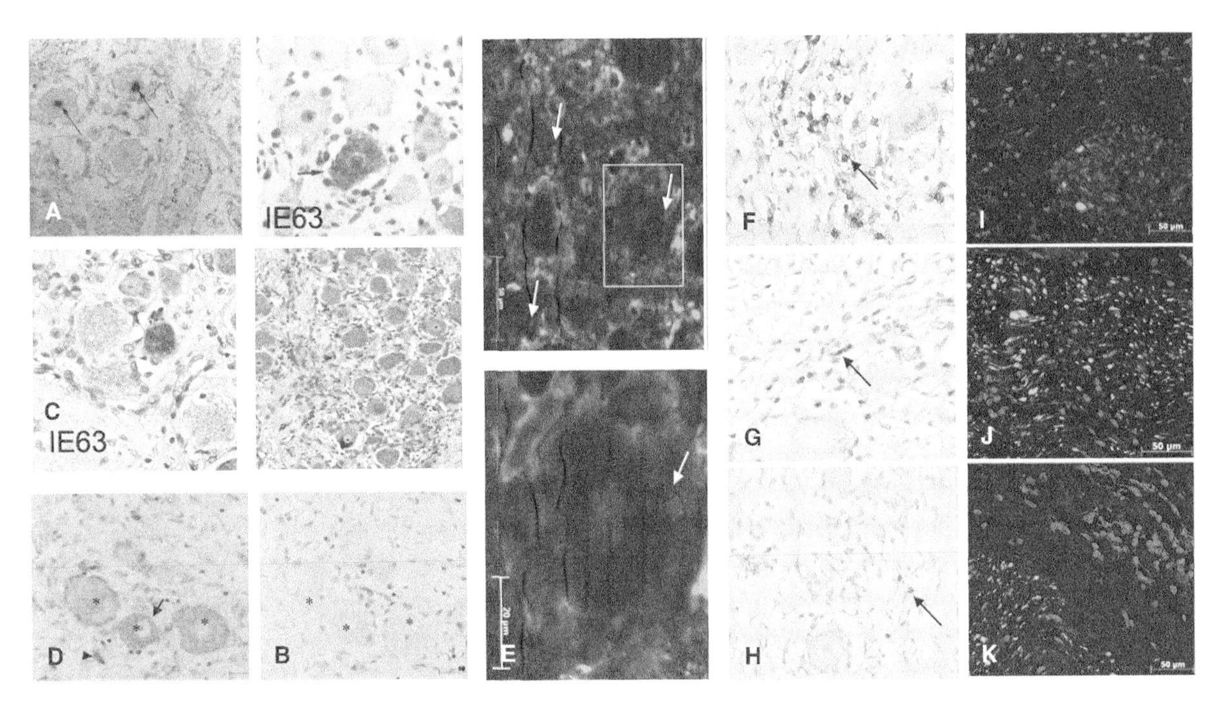

FIGURE 13.11 Varicella–zoster virus infection of human sensory ganglia. A: Detection of VZV DNA by *in situ* hybridization in the nucleus of a neuron (*arrow*) in sensory ganglion section obtained postmortem from a patient without signs of zoster. **B:** Immunohistochemical detection of IE63 protein in neuron cytoplasm (*arrow*) in a thoracic ganglion section using rabbit anti-VZV ORF63. **C:** Immunohistochemical detection of IE63 protein in dorsal root ganglion sequential sections using rabbit preimmune IgG antibody (*left panel*) and matched high-titer rabbit anti-IE63 IgG at magnifications ×100 (*right panel*) and ×200 (*lower panel*).**D:** Immunohistochemical detection of CXCL10 in dorsal root ganglia from a patient with zoster rash at time of death. The ganglion innervating the site of the rash contained CXCL10-positive neurons (*arrow*) and infiltrating cells (*arrowhead, left panel*). *Right panel* shows isotype control staining of the consecutive section. Stars indicate the same cells. **E:** Immunofluorescence detection of CXCR3 (*red*) and S100b (*green*) and counterstained with DAPI (*blue*) in the same ganglia as in **(F).** Nonneuronal CXCR3-positive cells were observed throughout the reactivated lumbar DRG (*arrows*), with some CXCR3-positive cells juxtaposed to neurons (*boxed region, upper panel*); higher-power magnification of the inset box (*lower panel*). **F-H:** Immunohistochemical detection of immune cell subsets: CD8-positive T cells, (*arrow*) **(F)** T-cell intracellular antigen (TIA)-positive cells, (*arrow*) **(G)** and granzyme B positive (*arrow*) **(H)** in DRG from a patient with zoster rash at time of death. **I–K:** Immunofluorescence detection of immune cell subsets (*red*) and S100b (*green*) and counterstained with DAPI (*blue*) in ganglia from a postherpetic neuralgia–affected patient years following zoster rash resolution. **I:** shows CD4-positive staining (red), **J:** CD8-positive staining (red), and **K:** CD20-positive staining. (**A** adapted by permission from Springer: Mahalingam R, Kennedy PGE, Gilden D. The problems of latent varicella zoster virus in human ganglia: precise cell location and viral content. *J Neurovirol* 1999;5:445–448. Copyright © 1999 Springer Nature. **C** adapted from Zerboni L, Sobel RA, Ramachandran V, et al. Expression of varicella-zoster virus immediate-early regulatory protein IE63 in neurons of latently infected human sensory ganglia. *J Virol* 2010;84(7):3421–3430. **E** adapted from Steain M, Gowrishankar K, Rodriguez M, et al. Up-regulation of CXCL10 in human dorsal root ganglia during experimental and natural varicella-zoster virus infection. *J Virol* 2011;85(1):626–631. **F-H** adapted from Gowrishankar K, Steain M, Cunningham AL, et al. Characterization of the host immune response in human ganglia after herpes zoster. *J Virol* 2010;84(17):8861–8870. **I-K** adapted from Sutherland JP, Steain M, Buckland ME, et al. Persistence of a T cell infiltrate in human ganglia years after herpes zoster and during post-herpetic neuralgia. *Front Microbiol* 2019;10:2117. https://creativecommons.org/licenses/by/4.0.)

(Fig. 13.11). Detection of IE62, IE63,[251] ORF66,[82] and proteins encoded by *ORFs 4, 21,* and *29* was also described in early studies and restriction of IE62 and IE63 to the cytoplasm of neurons was proposed as a mechanism by which latency is maintained. However, ascites-derived monoclonal antibodies and rabbit antisera may contain endogenous antibodies to human blood group A determinants, including antibodies to VZV IE62, gE, and ORF40 capsid protein that produce a cytoplasmic Golgi-like pattern of staining in neurons of blood group A subjects (~30% to 40% prevalence).[490] IE63 expression was confirmed as being rare when ganglion sections were stained with anti-IE63 rabbit antiserum and with preimmune serum to control for blood group A reactivity[259,491] (Fig. 13.11). Detection of VZV proteins in a few neurons from autopsy ganglia is likely to reflect early or abortive reactivation.

Investigations of VZV tropism for human neural cells *in vivo* have used the SCID mouse model, in which human DRG is xenografted under the mouse kidney capsule and maintained ≥20 weeks until neuronal subtype heterogeneity is established before infection. In this model, a limited lytic infection of DRG occurs in the first 14 days (Fig. 13.12). VZ virions are detected in neurons and satellite cells, and infectious virus is produced[354,486,488] and is accompanied by both proinflammatory host factors and IFNs and neuroprotective responses. Peripherin+ nociceptive and RT97+ mechanoreceptive neurons are infected by VZV via axonal transport and contiguous

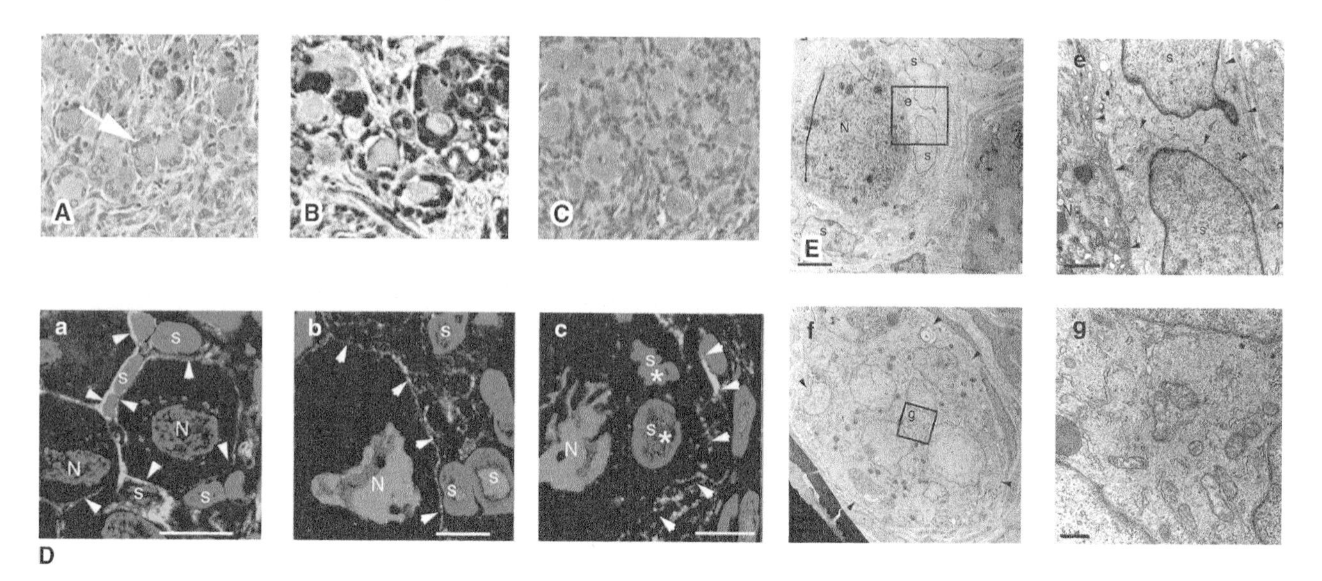

FIGURE 13.12 Varicella–zoster virus (VZV) infection of dorsal root ganglia xenografts and neuron-satellite cell fusion in the SCID mouse model. A: DRG xenograft 14 days after infection; *arrow* indicates cytopathology in neurons (H&E stain; ×200). **B:** DRG xenograft 14 days after infection stained with rabbit polyclonal antibody to VZV IE63 (*brown,* DAB signal) and counterstained with hematoxylin (×200). **C.** DRG xenograft 56 days after VZV infection, showing no evidence of productive infection (H&E stain;x200). **D**: *a–c*. Immunofluorescence analysis of acutely infected DRG. Cryosections of VZV-infected DRG were stained with mouse monoclonal anti-NCAM antibody (*a–c; green*), rabbit polyclonal antisynaptophysin antibody (*a; red*), rabbit polyclonal anti-IE62 antibody (*b; red*) and Hoechst stain (*blue*). Texas red-labeled goat antirabbit or FITC-labeled goat antimouse antibodies were used for secondary detection. Satellite cells (*s*) and neurons (*N*) are marked with letters; *asterisks* (*) indicate nuclei of satellite cells located within a putative polykaryon. *Arrowheads* point to cell boundaries detected by NCAM staining (*green*). Scale bars = 10 μm. **E:** e-g. EM analysis of acutely infected DRG. *Arrowheads* point to the cell membrane surrounding satellite cells (*s*) or the neuron cell body (*N*) or a polykaryon. *Black boxes* indicate the area shown at higher magnification. Note that despite the normal morphology of the mitochondria, the ER, and the nuclear envelope in the polykaryon, no cell membranes between the nuclei (*N*) of the polykaryon are detected. (**A-D**: Adapted by permission from Springer: Zerboni L, Reichelt M, Arvin A. Varicella-Zoster virus neurotropism in SCID mouse–human dorsal root ganglia xenografts. In: Abendroth A, Arvin A, Moffat J, eds. *Varicella-zoster virus. Current topics in microbiology and immunology*, Vol 342. Berlin, Heidelberg: Springer; 2010:255-276. Copyright © 2010 Springer-Verlag Berlin Heidelberg. **E:** Adapted from Reichelt M, Zerboni L, Arvin AM. Mechanisms of varicella-zoster virus neuropathogenesis in human dorsal root ganglia. *J Virol* 2008;82(8):3971–3983.)

spread from satellite glial cells, but RT97+ neurons are nonpermissive for replication.[483] By 1 month, infectious virus is no longer released from cells, virion assembly ceases, and VZV genome copy numbers are reduced. *ORF63* and less consistently *ORF62* continue to be transcribed but gB expression is silenced. This transition from lytic to persistent infection indicates that VZV latency can be established in human neurons in the absence of adaptive immunity, since SCID mice do not generate antigen-specific T cell or humoral immunity. VZV neurotropism was also shown by intraventricular inoculation of SCID mice.[22]

Like VZV, SVV establishes latent infection in ganglionic neurons at multiple levels of the neuraxis, but not in lung or liver.[199,322] SVV DNA, viral gene transcripts, and CD4+ and CD8+ T cells are detected in ganglia 3 days before the rash, supporting viremia as a route of access to sites of latency during acute infection; notably, VZV gene transcription declined within only 7 days after inoculation, accompanied by dramatic innate immune responses within the ganglia.[10] VZV neurotropism has also been investigated in rodent and guinea pig models.[64,70] Inoculation of cotton rats by injections adjacent to the spine and sensory ganglia with VZV mutants showed that *ORFs 1, 2, 10, 13, 14, 17, 21, 32, 47, 57, 61, 66,* and *67* were dispensable for VZV DNA persistence in ganglion tissues, whereas *ORF 4, 63,* and *66* mutants were impaired. VZV persists in the enteric neurons in the guinea pig model, as does SVV in nonhuman primates.[124,255,322]

Reactivation

The factors that trigger VZV reactivation from latency in infected neurons *in vivo* are unknown. In an *in vitro* model, inhibition of nerve growth factor induces reactivation of VZV and HSV from latently infected human neurons.[361] Three possible outcomes of reactivation are abortive infection restricted to the ganglia; transport of virus particles to skin but with lesion formation blocked by innate and adaptive immunity; and cutaneous lesion formation, manifested as zoster (see **Clinical Features**)[166] (Fig. 13.10 and e-Fig. 13.4).

The pathology of VZV reactivation in ganglia is characterized by inflammation and hemorrhagic necrosis with associated neuritis, localized leptomeningitis, unilateral segmental myelitis, and degeneration of related motor and sensory roots.[158] Demyelination is seen in areas with mononuclear cell infiltration and microglial proliferation. Intranuclear inclusions, viral DNA and proteins (Fig. 13.12), and viral particles are found in acutely infected ganglia.[63,112,129] Infectious VZV has been isolated from human ganglia only of patients with active zoster.[336] Immune cell subsets have been identified in ganglia during active VZV reactivation, with a predominance of CD4+ and CD8+ T cells[392] while ganglia obtained 1 to 5 months after zoster had an immune infiltrate composed of noncytolytic granzyme B-negative T cells and macrophages.[139] VZV-infected cells have been detected in subependymal microvessels in fatal zoster cases. VZV reactivation may be followed by vasculopathy affecting large and small vessels with resultant cortical and subcortical infarction and mixed necrotic and demyelinative lesions, particularly in deep white matter and periventricular ependyma.

The lytic phase of VZV infection of DRG xenografts in SCID mice can be considered a model of events that occur during VZV reactivation[354] (Fig. 13.12). Both neurons and satellite cells are productively infected.[486,488] Importantly, VZV induces cell–cell fusion between neurons and satellite cells and spread from satellite cells to adjacent uninfected satellite cells. Infection of these cells surrounding neuronal cell bodies facilitates access of the virus to other neuronal cell bodies. Similar cell–cell fusion has been observed in ganglia obtained at autopsy from patients with zoster.[112] During VZV reactivation, amplification by spread to other neuronal cell bodies within the ganglia presumably allows delivery of virus particles from many neurons along axons to the skin in the affected dermatome. VZV damage to both satellite cells and neurons in the ganglia helps to account for the neurologic consequences that are rare during HSV reactivation.

SVV also reactivates in a dermatomal distribution either spontaneously or after drug- or radiation-induced immunosuppression, or CD4+ T-cell depletion.[258,415] SVV glycoproteins are detected in zoster skin lesions, lungs, and multiple ganglia of most immunosuppressed monkeys, but not in control animals. Reactivation is associated with SVV infection of macrophages, dendritic cells, and T cells of lymph nodes, indicating dissemination.[414]

Postherpetic neuralgia (PHN) is a chronic pain syndrome that is common after VZV reactivation (see **Clinical Features**), and has been suggested to reflect an altered excitability of ganglionic or spinal cord neurons. PHN has been associated with diffuse and focal infiltration of ganglia by chronic inflammatory cells[450] (e-Fig. 13.4), and CD4+ T cells, CD8+ T cells, and CD20+ B cells have been reported to persist in ganglia years after zoster (Fig. 13.11).[406] VZV DNA has been detected in PBMCs of patients with PHN.[421]

Reinfection

Reinfection with VZV appears to be rare based on clinical criteria, although genotyping evidence of recombination demonstrates that it can occur.[42] Second episodes of varicella have been documented,[127] but confirmation of true reinfection with VZV as opposed to incorrect diagnosis of a previous vesicular rash is difficult. In a cohort of adults who developed varicella despite a reported previous episode, none had VZV antibodies in sera obtained before the acute illness, suggesting that the earlier exanthem was not caused by VZV.[433] Most immunocompromised patients who have had prior VZV infection and who develop signs suggestive of a second episode of varicella likely have generalized, atypical reactivation without dermatomal involvement although reinfection may occur. Immunologic evidence of reinfection based on increases in antibody and cellular immunity to VZV when immune subjects have close contact with an infected person is indirect since enhancement of adaptive immunity can occur without any viral replication, as observed when immune individuals receive inactivated varicella vaccine. Subclinical reinfection can occur despite vaccine-induced immunity since vaccinated individuals can develop zoster due to wild-type VZV.[123]

IMMUNE RESPONSE

Immune Control of Primary VZV Infection

Both the innate and adaptive arms of the immune response are required to resolve primary VZV infection. In addition to local antiviral responses mediated by epidermal cells (Fig. 13.10), NK cells are crucial as evident from case studies reporting severe, often fatal, varicella in patients with NK cell deficiency and dysfunction.[113] In immunocompetent hosts, NK cells are likely to be key responders, as suggested by increased frequencies of NK cells during active infection.[411] NK cells from non-immune individuals lyse VZV-infected fibroblasts and also produce granulysin, which has antiviral activity.[156] In addition, NK cells are rapidly recruited to sites of VZV antigen challenge in previously exposed hosts.[306]

IFN-α is detected in serum at the onset of varicella and may limit early viral replication, as suggested by its clinical efficacy in modifying the severity of varicella in immunocompromised children and by the association of more severe varicella in adults with reduced serum IFN-α.[14,434] The importance of IFNs is also underscored by acute, severe varicella in patients who have primary immunodeficiencies affecting IFN signaling pathways.[309]

The innate response to primary VZV infection also appears to involve invariant natural killer T cells (iNKT) and antigen presentation to these unusual T cells by CD1, a nonclassical MHC class I molecule, as suggested by disseminated infection after administration of varicella vaccine virus in a child who had deficient iNKT cells and CD1 expression but no other evidence of a primary immunodeficiency disorder.[25]

The initial stages of primary VZV infection before and in the first few days of rash evoke little or no adaptive immunity, as measured by antibody production or assessment of T cells that recognize VZV antigens. Nevertheless, although the virus can evade induction of and recognition by CD4+ and CD8+ T cells transiently, replication becomes contained when VZV-specific immunity is induced[12] (Fig. 13.13). Antibodies can be detected in low concentrations in some individuals at the onset of the varicella rash and are usually present within 3 days. Antibodies to VZV proteins neutralize VZV replication, either directly or with complement, and also function in ADCC.[157,195,377] IgG, IgM, and IgA antibodies are directed against many viral proteins[13] and the breadth of the VZV B-cell repertoire has been shown in identical twins.[442] However, the humoral immune response appears to have little role in controlling primary VZV infection, since children with agammaglobulinemia have uncomplicated varicella. Among healthy children, the early detection of high levels of circulating VZV-specific IgG or IgM antibodies does not predict disease severity. Moreover, children with T-cell immunodeficiencies may develop fulminant varicella, despite VZV antibody responses.[13]

The critical role of VZV-specific cell-mediated immunity in primary VZV infection is supported by correlations between the induction of virus-specific T cells and disease outcome.[12] Cellular immunity appears to be important for terminating viremia and limiting virus replication at localized cutaneous

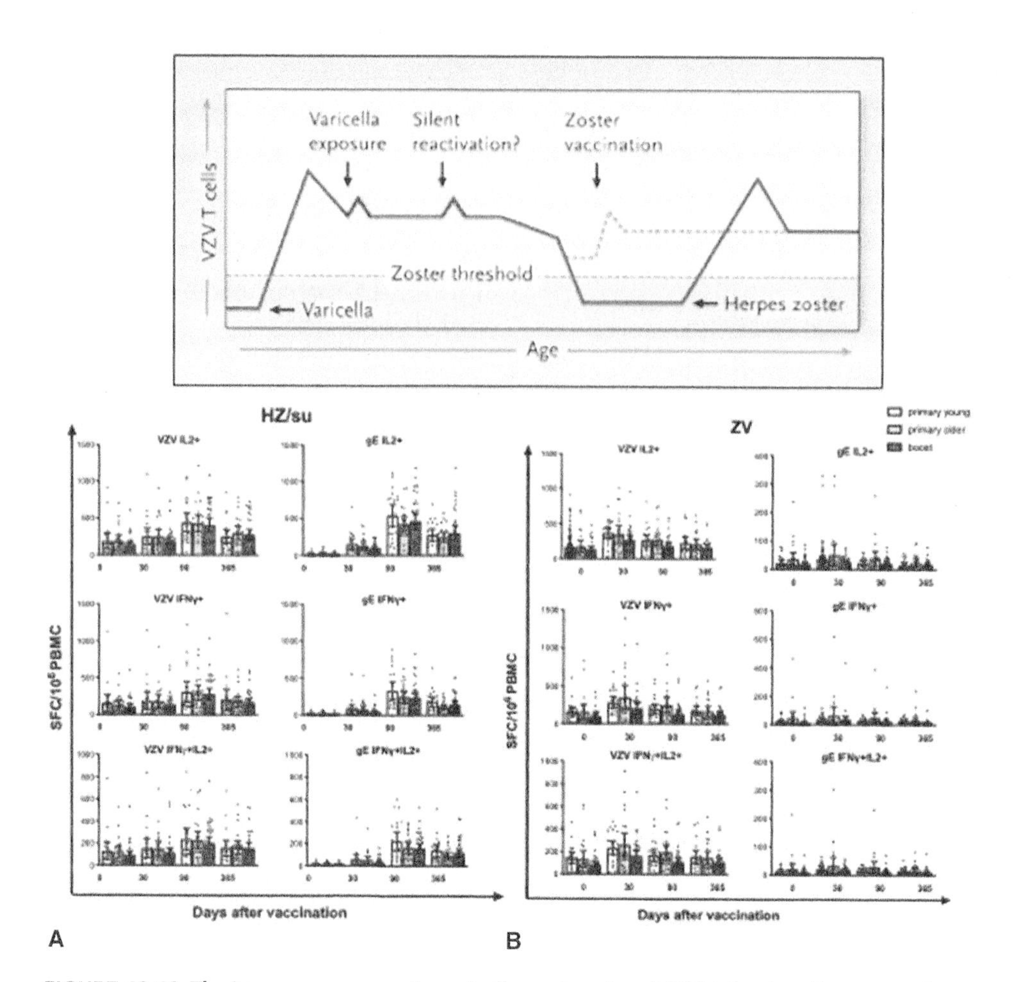

FIGURE 13.13 **The immune response to varicella–zoster virus (VZV) infection. Upper panel:** Schematic of VZV T-cell immunity. Varicella is the primary infection caused by VZV, and its resolution is associated with the induction of VZV-specific memory T cells (*blue line*); varicella vaccine also induces memory T cells. Memory immunity to VZV may be boosted periodically by exposure to varicella or silent reactivation from latency (*red peaks*). VZV-specific memory T cells decline with age. The decline below a threshold (*dashed green line*) correlates with an increased risk of zoster. The occurrence of zoster, in turn, is associated with an increase in VZV-specific T cells. Administration of zoster vaccine to older persons may prevent VZV-specific T cells from dropping below the threshold for zoster occurrence (*dashed blue line*). (From Arvin A. Aging, immunity, and the varicella-zoster virus. *N Engl J Med* 2005;352(22):2266–2267. Copyright © 2005 Massachusetts Medical Society. Reprinted with permission from Massachusetts Medical Society.) **Lower panel:** T-cell responses to recombinant subunit glycoprotein E zoster vaccine (*A*) and live attenuated zoster vaccine (*B*) by age and treatment group. Data were derived from 158 participants. Bars represent geometric mean spot-forming cells per 10^6 peripheral blood mononuclear cells and 95% confidence interval at the time points indicated at the bottom of each graph. Analytes and stimulants are indicated in the title of each graph. Abbreviations: HZ/su, recombinant subunit glycoprotein E zoster vaccine; gE, glycoprotein E; IFN-γ, interferon gamma; IL-2, interleukin 2; PBMCs, peripheral blood mononuclear cells; SFC, spot-forming cell; VZV, varicella–zoster virus; ZV, live attenuated zoster vaccine. (From Weinberg A, Kroehl ME, Johnson MJ, et al. Comparative immune responses to licensed herpes zoster vaccines. *J Infect Dis* 2018;218(suppl_2):S81–S87. Reproduced by permission of Oxford University Press.)

sites. Healthy children who had T cells that recognized VZV antigens within 24 to 72 hours experienced milder varicella.[13] T-cell proliferation in response to VZV antigen is accompanied by the production of many cytokines, including IL-2 and IFN-γ, which amplify the initial antiviral response.[179] Robust cellular immunity is elicited even when the varicella rash consists of fewer than 10 lesions. Conversely, lymphopenia and failure to develop VZV-specific T-cell proliferation in immunocompromised children correlate with persistent viremia and risk of visceral dissemination.[13] Children with immunosuppression due to underlying diseases or interventions or those with primary cellular immunodeficiency diseases experienced progressive and often fatal varicella before the availability of antiviral drugs. A similar pattern of acquisition of cell-mediated immunity and resolution of viremia and rash is observed in SVV infection.

Overall, this pattern of virus–host interaction initially favors the virus because cutaneous viral replication allows VZV transmission to other susceptible individuals, while the host is favored thereafter through the protection from illness on subsequent exposures afforded by memory B and T cells that recognize VZV antigens.

Memory Immunity

Memory immunity to VZV is required to prevent symptomatic reinfection with exogenous virus and to prevent or minimize the severity of symptomatic VZV reactivations. The extent to which memory immunity contributes to the preservation of viral latency in neurons is not known. IgG antibodies that bind to viral glycoproteins and many other VZV polypeptides and VZV-specific IgA antibodies are maintained, likely functioning as the first line of defense against reinfection.

Cell-mediated immunity to VZV proteins including gB, gC, gE, gH, gI, and the immediate early proteins IE62 and IE63, persists for years in the immunocompetent host.[12,16,365] Healthy VZV-immune adults have circulating T cells that recognize an average of 7 of 10 IE62 peptides and 6 of 10 gE peptides. Such individuals also have T cells that exhibit class I and class II MHC-restricted lysis of target cells expressing VZV antigens.[99,384] CTLs that recognize IE62 protein or gE are present at equivalent precursor frequencies in both the CD4+ and CD8+ memory T-cell populations.[16] VZV gC, gI, ORF4 protein, and ORF10 protein are also CTL targets.[12,15] VZV-specific memory T cells circulate at low frequencies of about 5 per 100,000 PBMCs in immune adults, and memory CD4+ and CD8+ CTLs specific for individual VZV proteins circulate at frequencies of about 1 per 150,000 PBMCs. Intracellular cytokine detection assays showed that the mean percentage of VZV-specific CD4+ T cells based on IFN-γ or TNF-α production was about 0.12%.[19] Immune subjects also have persistent delayed-type hypersensitivity (DTH) responses to VZV skin test antigens.

Mechanisms by which memory immunity to VZV is maintained may include exposure to VZV through close contact with an infected person, since enhanced VZV T-cell proliferation, DTH, and VZV IgG antibodies often follow such contacts, as well as endogenous reexposure to VZV antigens by subclinical reactivations (Fig. 13.13). Repeated antigenic stimulation may also result if subclinical VZV reactivations lead to viral transfer to skin or mucosal sites of replication without progressing to zoster. This possibility is supported by the recovery of cell-mediated immunity to VZV in bone marrow transplant recipients who had no clinical episodes of zoster but had subclinical reactivations detectable by PCR.[467] It is not known whether conditions necessary for CD4+ and CD8+ T-cell recognition of neurons harboring VZV are present during latency; if so, VZV immunity may be maintained by intermittent local expression of viral proteins during abortive reactivations. However, viral peptides can only be detected by T cells when present in MHC complexes, and class I MHC requires IFN-γ exposure for up-regulation on neurons. Attempts to analyze local T-cell responses during latency have been hampered by the lack of a marker for cells harboring VZV genomes.[259,491]

Long-lived memory NK cells have been suggested to play a role in antiherpesvirus immunity. Cytotoxic NK cells with a tissue resident phenotype were recruited to skin sites of VZV test antigen challenge in previously exposed hosts. This NK cell-mediated recall response, decades after initial virus exposure, indicates NK cells may contribute to a long-lived memory response to VZV.[306]

Immunity and Reactivation

T cells are present in ganglia obtained postmortem from latently infected individuals, but the extent to which VZV-specific T cells provide surveillance for early stages of reactivation in ganglionic neurons is unknown. Diminished T-cell responses to VZV antigens in older and immunocompromised individuals correlate with enhanced susceptibility to zoster.[12,243] The restoration of VZV T-cell immunity and the reduced risk of zoster in immunocompromised and elderly individuals given live attenuated and gE subunit VZV vaccines have confirmed this hypothesis[87,323] (Fig. 13.13). Age-related immunosenescence is also associated with a decrease in DTH responses to VZV antigens. The decrease in VZV-specific immunity in skin of older individuals is unlikely to be due to a defect in CD4+ T resident memory (Trm) cells, as VZV-specific CD4+ T cells were shown to be functionally competent and not altered by aging. Rather, it has been proposed that other modulatory factors in the skin such as increased PD1 receptor signaling or skin resident regulatory T cells may inhibit immune responses in the skin of older aged individuals.[430] A study of peripheral blood from zoster patients revealed that the numbers of CD3+ and CD8+ T cells decreased during aging and PHN. NK cell numbers were also reduced in older aged zoster patients compared to the middle age patient group, which may reflect NK cells being important following VZV reactivation in older age zoster patients.[454]

Zoster in young children after intrauterine or early postnatal varicella and the short interval between primary and recurrent VZV infections in HIV-infected children probably reflects suboptimal induction of VZV cell-mediated immunity.[20,96] Severe and prolonged suppression of VZV-specific cellular immunity also creates the highest risk for zoster, viremia, and dissemination. Depletion of CD4+ T cells alone was sufficient to permit the reactivation of latent SVV.[415] By contrast, susceptibility to VZV reactivation is not associated with decreasing titers of VZV IgG antibodies, even in immunocompromised patients.[453]

Upon VZV reactivation, VZV T-cell responses increase promptly, peaking at a responder cell frequency of about 10 per 100,000 PBMC at 6 weeks. The resolution of rash is also accompanied by local production of IFN-α in lesions. When reactivation was mimicked using a VZV skin test, VZV-specific central memory CD4+ T cells accumulated and proliferated at the site, as did regulatory T cells.[431] While information is limited, autopsy studies indicate that an extensive inflammatory response, including CD4+ T cells, CD8+ T cells, and NK cells, persists in ganglia for several months after zoster with or without PHN.[139] Up-regulation of CXCL10 occurs in ganglia during reactivation, and lymphocytes that express the CXCR3 receptor for CXCL10 are prominent among infiltrating cells (Fig. 13.11).[391] A persistent inflammatory response including CD4+ T cells, CD8+ T cells, and B cells was observed in ganglia of a patient with PHN.[406] Enhanced VZV T-cell immunity persists for at least 3 years after zoster and may explain why second episodes of zoster are rare except in immunocompromised patients.

EPIDEMIOLOGY

Incidence and Prevalence

VZV is a ubiquitous human pathogen with a worldwide geographic distribution. The annual incidence of varicella in the United States was equivalent to the annual birth rate (~4 million) before varicella vaccine was introduced in 1995, and the prevalence of anti-VZV IgG antibodies indicated that up to 99% of adults had been infected.[211] Universal varicella vaccine in the United States has dramatically reduced the annual epidemics.[266] By 20 to 29 years of age, only about 5% of individuals remain susceptible in geographic areas with temperate climates, in the absence of vaccination programs. In tropical regions, only about half of individuals younger than 24 years of age have had varicella. The varicella attack rate is very high among susceptible adults who emigrate from tropical areas to temperate zones.

Given the high incidence of varicella, most adults are at risk for VZV reactivation and one-third will develop zoster. In the United States, approximately 1 million cases of zoster are diagnosed annually, two-thirds of which occur in individuals older than 50 years and 9 in 10 are immunocompetent.[481] Hope-Simpson[166] observed that the incidence rose to 7.8 cases per 1,000 people older than 60 years of age, compared with 2.5 per 1,000 people 20 to 50 years of age. The risk is as high as 50% among those who reach 85 years of age. Since the risk of zoster increases with age, and the population over age 65 is expected to be 72 million in 2030, zoster and its attendant serious neurologic complications will continue to be a significant health burden.

Zoster incidence rates are equivalent between men and women but are lower in black than in white Americans. Zoster is particularly frequent among patients with leukemia, Hodgkin's and non-Hodgkin's lymphoma, small cell carcinoma of the lung, and after bone marrow transplantation (>25%) and renal transplantation (15%). HIV infection increases the risk for zoster by 15- to 25-fold regardless of age.[133] Although cancer is correlated with a higher risk of zoster, zoster in healthy individuals is not associated with an increased risk for malignancy. Patients with systemic lupus erythematosus are more susceptible. Zoster is rare in childhood, but infection *in utero*, varicella during the first year of life, and varicella in adults are associated with higher risks.[20,334]

Epidemic Patterns

While varicella cases appear to initiate most annual epidemics, episodes of zoster provide a source of reintroduction and transmission to susceptible individuals, who then develop varicella. Genotyping demonstrates the cocirculation of several VZV strains during a single varicella outbreak, indicating multiple sources of the virus.[92] Before varicella vaccination was introduced, most susceptible children became infected during annual epidemics due to efficient VZV transmission by the respiratory route and contact with high titers of infectious virus in skin lesions. The attack rate for previously uninfected household or day care center contacts exposed to varicella was about 90%, compared to 12% to 33% for more casual exposures such as school classrooms. VZV appears to be transmitted less efficiently in tropical climates although high population density may offset this pattern. Zoster is not seasonal because it originates from the reactivation of endogenous latent virus. Some reports have suggested that exposures to varicella can precipitate episodes of zoster, but there is no known mechanism by which reexposure would trigger reactivation. While zoster vaccines are available, uptake has been limited, leaving many older adults at risk for zoster.

Morbidity and Mortality

The high prevalence of VZV infection means that almost all individuals experience some VZV-related morbidity, absent vaccination. The risk for severe morbidity or mortality during primary or recurrent VZV infection depends on host factors rather than virulence characteristics of the infecting virus strain.

Varicella complications resulted in hospitalization rates of 11,000 per year in the United States (2.2 to 4.3/1,000 cases) before varicella vaccine was introduced.[265] Serious complications are least common among children 1 to 9 years of age and are 6 to 15 times higher among adults. Case fatality rates are 10 and 24 times higher in infants (6.7/100,000 cases) and adults (17.1/100,000 cases), respectively, than in children 1 to 4 years of age (0.7/100,000).[303] Serious complications are usually secondary bacterial infections, varicella pneumonia in adults, or neurologic syndromes.[115,144] CNS morbidity is higher among patients younger than 5 years and older than 20 years of age.[183] Among adults requiring intensive care, half required mechanical ventilation for an average duration of 14 days and mortality was 24% despite acyclovir therapy.[275] Before effective antiviral drugs were available, 32% to 50% of children with malignancy developed disseminated infection; varicella pneumonia occurred in 20% of cases, and the mortality rate was 7% to 17%.[114]

Varicella has been reported to occur in 0.7 to 2 per 1,000 pregnancies, with a predicted maternal mortality rate of 0.5 per 1,000 cases[108] and a risk of congenital varicella syndrome. Rarely, the pregnancy may terminate by spontaneous abortion, fetal demise, or premature delivery. The incidence of congenital varicella syndrome was 0.4% when maternal varicella occurred from 0 to 12 weeks of gestation, compared with 2% for infection from 13 to 20 weeks of gestation.[108] The virus appears to be transmitted to the fetus during the second and third trimester of maternal varicella with about the same frequency as in the first trimester, but a study found no infants with congenital varicella syndrome or other morbidity at birth if the mother had varicella between 25 and 36 weeks of gestation.[108] Infants are at risk for neonatal varicella when maternal varicella occurs at the end of gestation, with an attack rate of about 20% unless antibody prophylaxis is given, and a 30% mortality rate without antiviral therapy. Zoster is not unusual in pregnancy but it does not cause significant maternal or fetal morbidity.[108]

One in ten individuals with zoster experiences at least one zoster-related nonpain complication, while one in four experience zoster-related pain that persists 30 days or more.[481] The frequency of PHN is higher in older patients, increasing from 3% to 4% in those between 30 and 49 years of age to 21%, 29%, and 34% in patients 60 to 69, 70 to 79, and more than 80 years of age, respectively.[12,466] Data from the United States indicate a risk of PHN of 1.38 cases per 1,000 person-years in healthy adults older than 60 years.[323] The incidence of zoster-associated CNS disease, most of which are cases of VZV vasculopathy, ranges from 0.2% to 0.5%, with risk factors including older age and cranial nerve involvement during the acute zoster episode. Cerebral angiitis following zoster has a case-fatality rate as high as 20%. Immunosuppressive therapy for malignancy increases the morbidity and mortality associated with zoster, although the risk for fatal infection is less than 1%.

CLINICAL FEATURES

Varicella

Varicella follows an incubation period that ranges from 10 to 21 days. Prodromal symptoms of fever, malaise, headache, and abdominal pain often precede the appearance of the rash by 24 to 48 hours. Fever, irritability, lethargy, and anorexia are prominent during the 24 to 72 hours after the first cutaneous lesions are noted; respiratory symptoms and vomiting are unusual. Body temperature usually rises to less than 101.5°F but can be as high as 106°F. The varicella exanthem typically begins on the scalp, face, or trunk. The cutaneous lesions consist of erythematous macules that evolve within several hours to form a clear, fluid-filled vesicle surrounded by an irregular erythema margin, the classic "dew drop on a rose petal" (Fig. 13.1). Lesions in the maculopapular or vesicular stages are usually pruritic. After 24 to 48 hours, the vesicular fluid becomes turbid and crusting begins. Later crops of lesions form on the trunk and extremities and can resolve without progressing to form vesicles. Lesions of the mucous membranes of the oropharynx, conjunctivae, and vagina are common. In the final phase, the crusted lesions are sloughed as new epithelial cells are generated at the lesion site. Varicella vesicles are common on eyelids and conjunctivae, but eye disease is unusual.

New varicella lesions emerge for 3 to 6 days, with the total number of lesions ranging from less than 10 to 2,000; most children have fewer than 300 lesions. True subclinical varicella is rare.[357] Children who develop varicella after household exposure to an index case are more likely to have more severe varicella, presumably due to a higher inoculum.[102,357] Skin damage such as eczema or sunburn exacerbates the severity of the exanthem. Hypopigmentation of the skin at sites of varicella lesions often persists for weeks, but extensive scarring is unusual. Low polymorphonuclear leukocyte and lymphocyte counts during the first 72 hours of rash are followed by lymphocytosis[45]; slight elevations of liver function tests are common.

Staphylococcus aureus and *Streptococcus pyogenes* (group A β-hemolytic streptococcus) cause secondary bacterial infection of skin lesions, cellulitis, bacterial lymphadenitis, or subcutaneous abscesses[45,88,115,328] (e-Fig. 13.5). Varicella gangrenosa, a form of necrotizing fasciitis, is a life-threatening infection usually caused by *S. pyogenes*.[494] Bacteremia, usually caused by *S. aureus* or *S. pyogenes*, can lead to acute bacterial sepsis or focal infection such as pneumonia, arthritis, or osteomyelitis.

Varicella pneumonia in otherwise healthy adults presents with fever, cough, tachypnea, and dyspnea beginning about 3 days (range 1 to 6 days) after the onset of rash and may be associated with cyanosis, pleuritic chest pain, or hemoptysis (e-Fig. 13.6). Varicella pneumonia is often transient, resolving completely within 24 to 72 hours, but interstitial pneumonitis with severe hypoxemia progresses rapidly to cause respiratory failure in severe cases.[275] Varicella pneumonia is associated with active infection of the epithelial cells of the pulmonary alveoli. Infection induces mononuclear cell infiltration of the alveolar septa and edema of alveolar septal cells, along with the accumulation of exudate, formation of hyaline membranes, and cellular desquamation into the alveolar spaces, which inhibit oxygen transfer. Desquamated cells in the alveoli and bronchiolar epithelial cells contain eosinophilic intranuclear inclusions and virions. Fatal varicella pneumonia is more common in smokers and is characterized by focal necrosis.

Varicella hepatitis, a rare complication, is associated with extensive replication in the liver, lysis of hepatocytes, and inflammation. Aspirin is contraindicated in children with varicella because it predisposes to liver damage (Reye syndrome).

Varicella encephalitis or cerebellar ataxia usually occurs within 2 to 8 days.[183,253,378,432] Patients with encephalitis typically have sudden onset of seizures and altered sensorium, whereas those with cerebellar disease show irritability, nystagmus, and gait and speech disturbances. Some patients have fever, headache, and meningismus only, without altered consciousness or seizures. The cerebrospinal fluid (CSF) usually shows a mild lymphocytic pleocytosis (<100 cells/mm^3) and a slight-to-moderate protein level (<200 mg) with normal glucose. Encephalitic symptoms usually resolve rapidly (within 24 to 72 hours); ataxia can persist for days to weeks. A few cases of optic neuritis, transverse myelitis, and Guillain-Barré syndrome have been associated with varicella.[183]

Varicella encephalitis is observed most often in immunocompromised patients who have persistent viremia, suggesting a role for direct viral invasion of CNS tissue in some cases. The histopathology of brain tissue from rare cases of fatal varicella encephalitis demonstrates vasculitis of large and small vessels, demyelination, axonal damage, perivascular infiltration with mononuclear cells, microglial proliferation, and neuronal degeneration; however, histologic abnormalities are often minimal. Recovery is associated with astrocytosis surrounding affected areas.[50] In other cases, varicella-related neurologic syndromes resolve rapidly and completely, which may indicate a predominantly inflammatory or immune-mediated pathogenesis. The observation that cerebellar ataxia and encephalitis can occur during the pre-eruptive phase of varicella may indicate early transfer of VZV to neural tissues, triggering local inflammatory responses.[432] CNS disease may also result from ischemic arteriopathies; one-third of these cases in children are associated with varicella.[40]

Acute thrombocytopenia is a complication of varicella that causes petechiae and purpuric skin lesions, hemorrhage into the varicella vesicles, epistaxis, hematuria, and gastrointestinal bleeding. Hemorrhagic complications are usually transient. Purpura fulminans, caused by arterial thrombosis and hemorrhagic gangrene, is a rare but life-threatening complication. Thrombocytopenia may occur from 1 to 2 weeks or longer after varicella, as a result of direct infection of bone marrow megakaryocytes or immune-mediated processes. Platelet survival may also be reduced as a result of endothelial cell damage caused by vasculitis or transient hypersplenism, or as part of the syndrome of intravascular coagulopathy. As a postinfectious complication, thrombocytopenia may be associated with increased production but shortened platelet survival due to antiplatelet antibodies.

Varicella nephritis causes hematuria, proteinuria, diffuse edema, and decreased renal function, with or without hypertension. A few cases of nephrotic syndrome and hemolytic-uremic syndrome have been reported in children with varicella. Varicella arthritis is rare; it resolves spontaneously within 3 to

5 days with no residual joint disease. Other unusual complications of varicella include myocarditis, pericarditis, pancreatitis, and orchitis. Adrenal infection, characterized by focal necrosis, is common in fatal disseminated varicella. Renal pathology can occur, with hypercellularity of the glomeruli, epithelial proliferation, focal necrosis, and interstitial inflammation.

Varicella in High-Risk Populations

Varicella vesicles in immunocompromised children are usually larger and more numerous, and new lesion formation often continues for at least 7 days, with an average time to lesion crusting of 14 days. In one series, all of the deaths from varicella in children with leukemia occurred within 3 days after the diagnosis of varicella pneumonia.[114] Varicella hepatitis and thrombocytopenia lead to coagulopathy; hemorrhage into lesions is a sign of severe varicella, as is severe abdominal or back pain. Encephalitis is rarely the immediate cause of death. Disseminated VZV infection in children with cancer has also produced myocarditis, nephritis, pancreatitis, necrotizing splenitis, esophagitis, and enterocolitis. Neutropenia enhances susceptibility to secondary bacterial infections. Children who acquire varicella after organ transplantation are also at risk for progressive VZV infection. Children on long-term, low-dose steroid therapy for asthma are not usually at risk for serious varicella, but fatal varicella has been described in patients receiving higher doses of prednisone during the incubation period.

Untreated varicella can be fatal in children with SCID or T-cell disorders, including adenosine deaminase or nucleoside phosphorylase deficiency and cartilage hair hypoplasia and NK cell deficiencies.[113] Varicella can also be severe in children with Wiskott-Aldrich syndrome, ataxia telangiectasia, and other primary immunodeficiencies. Children with HIV infection may have unusual hyperkeratotic lesions and new lesion formation for weeks or months.[96,143]

Placental infection with chronic villitis has been described after maternal varicella in pregnancy. VZV can be transmitted to the fetus and, in rare instances, causes congenital varicella syndrome (e-Fig. 13.7). Infants with congenital varicella syndrome have unusual cutaneous defects, with cicatricial skin scars, atrophy of an extremity, microcephaly, seizures, mental retardation, intrauterine growth retardation, and other sequelae, including chorioretinitis, microophthalmia, and cataracts.[108] Varicella embryopathy exemplifies the consequences of VZV infection of spinal ganglion cells and damage to the developing autonomic nervous system. Severe microcephaly with cortical atrophy and calcification follows intrauterine encephalitis and necrosis of brain parenchyma.

Infants acquire varicella in the newborn period due to maternal varicella. Those whose lesions are present at birth or within the first 5 days of life are not at risk for dissemination, probably because of transplacental transfer of maternal IgG antibodies to VZV. Those who are born within 4 days before, or 2 days after, the onset of maternal varicella may develop progressive varicella with hepatitis, pneumonia, and coagulopathy.

Zoster

Zoster is characterized by pain and a vesicular eruption on an erythematous base in one or several dermatomes (Fig. 13.1 and e-Fig.13.4). Rash and pain usually develop within a few days of each other, although pain may precede the rash by 7 days or longer. The initial cutaneous lesions often appear in groups at one or several sites anteriorly and posteriorly within each affected dermatome; discrete vesicles resembling varicella lesions may merge to form larger, fluid-filled lesions as the exanthem evolves. Skin lesions resolve within 1 to 2 weeks, while complete cessation of pain usually takes 4 to 6 weeks. A few disseminated cutaneous lesions occasionally accompany the localized dermatomal infection even in the normal host, and VZV DNA may persist in peripheral blood up to 6 months after resolution of zoster.[344] Many patients with uncomplicated zoster have a CSF pleocytosis and elevated protein. VZV can be isolated from CSF and detected by PCR.[63,146] VZV reactivation in the immunocompromised host often causes a more extensive dermatomal rash and cell-associated viremia, which allows VZV dissemination to lungs, liver, CNS, and other organs. Dissemination can occur without rash, suggesting that T cells can become infected while trafficking through the infected ganglia. Patients with HIV infection may have chronic hyperkeratotic skin lesions (e-Fig. 13.8). Antibody-based therapies for immune-mediated diseases such as multiple sclerosis may increase risks of VZV infection.[469] Second episodes of zoster may occur, as documented in five zoster vaccine study participants from whom the same VZV strain was recovered at intervals of 12 to 28 months between reactivations.[150]

Because VZV becomes latent in any ganglion, zoster can develop in any dermatome. The trunk from T3 to L2, which is innervated by twelve pairs of ganglia, is the most frequently involved (e-Table 13.1), followed by the face and the extremities. The face, which is the second most common site, is supplied by afferent fibers only from the two trigeminal ganglia; these are the most frequently latently infected ganglia,[299] as is the case for HSV-1. In the classic study by Hope-Simpson,[166] about half of the cases involve the thoracic dermatomes, particularly T5 to T12. Lumbosacral dermatome disease was observed in 16% of these patients, predominantly in the L1 to L2 distribution. HSV reactivations occur in this region but are patchy rather than dermatomal (e-Fig. 13.4).

Zoster affects the head in approximately 19% of cases, with 97% in the trigeminal distribution.[166] In patients with trigeminal zoster, the ophthalmic division of the fifth nerve is most frequently affected (e-Fig. 13.9). The seventh cranial nerve ganglion is the next most commonly affected. Weakness of facial muscles is usually associated with lesions in the ear (Ramsay Hunt syndrome; geniculate zoster). Commonly associated with geniculate zoster are eighth-nerve deficit, fifth-nerve zoster or zoster of the occiput and neck,[223] ophthalmoplegia, and multiple lower cranial nerve palsies. Importantly, multiple forms of VZV reactivation in a trigeminal and facial distribution as well as polyneuritis cranialis may occur in the absence of rash.

PHN, the most common neurologic complication of zoster, is often defined clinically as pain that persists for at least 3 months after resolution of zoster rash.[447] Age is the most important factor in predicting the development of PHN. Genetic factors may play a role.[273] Pain is usually constant, severe, stabbing or burning, and frequently associated with allodynia (increased sensitivity to light touch). The incidence of PHN appears to be slightly higher in women[167] and after zoster involving the trigeminal ganglia. VZV reactivation can also produce chronic radicular pain without rash (zoster sine herpete) as well as other zoster-related neurologic and ocular disorders in the absence of rash.

Zoster paresis (weakness) is manifest by arm weakness, which may extend to the brachial plexus, or diaphragmatic paralysis after cervical distribution zoster, by leg weakness after lumbar or sacral distribution zoster, and by urinary retention after sacral distribution zoster. Magnetic resonance imaging (MRI) reveals involvement not only of the posterior horn and posterior roots but also of the anterior roots and anterior horn at the spinal level corresponding to the clinical deficit. The prognosis of zoster paresis varies, with near-complete recovery in the majority of cases.

VZV reactivation may also present as meningitis or meningoencephalitis. Encephalitis was associated with VZV infection and extensive fusion of astrocytes and astrocyte gliosis in the recovery phase. Many reported cases of VZV encephalitis may actually be VZV vasculopathy. Reports of VZV meningitis, meningoradiculitis, and cerebellitis (gait ataxia and tremor predominated), all in the absence of rash and confirmed by the detection of VZV DNA or anti-VZV antibody in CSF, reveal that VZV is not an uncommon cause of aseptic meningitis. CNS infections in adults have been associated with genetic disorders of DNA sensing due to mutations in the RNA polymerase III gene.[55]

VZV produces several ocular disorders, including both acute retinal necrosis (ARN) and progressive outer retinal necrosis (PORN)[192] (e-Fig. 13.10). ARN patients have periorbital pain and floaters with hazy vision and loss of peripheral vision. PORN presents with sudden painless loss of vision, floaters, and constricted visual fields with resultant retinal detachment. Diffuse retinal hemorrhages and whitening with macular involvement bilaterally are characteristic findings (e-Fig. 13.10). Although PORN can also be caused by HSV and cytomegalovirus, most cases in AIDS and other immunocompromised patients are due to VZV. PORN may be preceded by retrobulbar optic neuritis and aseptic meningitis, central retinal artery occlusion, or ophthalmic-distribution zoster and may occur together with multifocal vasculopathy or myelitis. Optic neuritis after zoster may be bilateral. Reports of visual loss in association with pain on eye movement and clinical findings of papillitis and central scotomata or optic atrophy weeks after VZV infection suggest an immunologic pathogenesis in some cases. The third nerve is affected more frequently than the sixth as a cause of zoster ophthalmoplegia. Combinations of third, fourth, and sixth nerve palsies are not unusual. Like optic neuritis, ophthalmoplegia may appear weeks to months after cutaneous signs.

VZV infection of cerebral arteries (VZV vasculopathy) is a serious complication of VZV reactivation, which causes both ischemic and hemorrhagic stroke.[297] In adults with zoster, the risk of stroke was increased by 30% within the following year[193] and 4.5-fold when zoster was in the ophthalmic distribution of the trigeminal nerve. VZV vasculopathy can present as headache, mental status changes, and focal neurologic deficits. Lesions at gray-white matter junctions are seen on brain imaging (e-Fig. 13.10). In more than two-thirds of patients, angiography reveals focal arterial stenosis and occlusion, aneurysm, or hemorrhage. Angiography showed involvement of both large and small arteries in 50% of 23 cases, small arteries in 37%, and large arteries alone in only 13%. Deep white matter lesions often predominate and are ischemic or demyelinating (e-Fig. 13.10). Vascular pathology ranges from neointimal proliferation to necrosis with and without inflammation. Infected cerebral arteries contain multinucleated giant cells, Cowdry A inclusion bodies, herpesvirus particles detected by electron microscopy, as well as VZV DNA and viral proteins. Reactivated VZV may also travel along ganglionic afferent fibers to the adventitia of cerebral arteries. Elements of VZV vasculopathy that may contribute to stroke include a thickened arterial intima composed of myofibroblasts and cells of medial smooth muscle origin, a disrupted internal elastic lamina, and decreased numbers of smooth muscle cells.[297] Most recently, VZV has been associated with vasculopathy involving extracranial arteries, including some cases of giant cell arteritis (GCA) of the temporal arteries based on VZV antigen detection and VZV DNA by PCR in biopsy tissues.[130,300] When VZV is detected, GCA is attributed to axonal transport of the virus to infect the adventitia, associated with the formation of multinucleated giant cells, transmural inflammation, and medial smooth muscle damage. Nevertheless, VZV protein expression has not been detected in other biopsy studies,[386,425] indicating that GCA has other etiologies.

VZV myelopathy, also called postinfectious myelitis, usually presents days to weeks after zoster as a self-limiting, monophasic spastic paraparesis, with or without sensory features and loss of sphincter function. The CSF usually contains a mild mononuclear pleocytosis, with a normal or slightly elevated protein. Rarely, VZV myelitis recurs. VZV myelopathy may also be an insidious, progressive, and sometimes fatal myelitis, usually in immunocompromised individuals, especially those with AIDS. MRI reveals longitudinal serpiginous enhancing lesions (e-Fig. 13.10). Pathologic and virologic analyses of the spinal cord from fatal cases have shown VZV invasion of the parenchyma and spread to adjacent nerve roots. Importantly, VZV myelitis may develop without rash. VZV-induced vasculopathy can also produce spinal cord infarction.

Zoster sine herpete is chronic radicular pain without rash, which has been virologically confirmed by detection of VZV DNA in CSF,[128] by detection of VZV DNA in blood mononuclear cells (MNCs) and anti-VZV IgG antibody in CSF, or by reduced serum/CSF ratios of anti-VZV IgG indicative of intrathecal synthesis.[35] Persistent radicular pain without rash was caused by a chronic active VZV ganglionitis of the trigeminal ganglion (e-Fig. 13.10). PORN severe unremitting eye pain, third cranial nerve palsies, retinal periphlebitis, uveitis, iridocyclitis, and disciform keratitis can occur without a zoster rash.

DIAGNOSIS

Differential Diagnosis

Varicella must be differentiated from vesicular rashes caused by enteroviruses or *S. aureus*, scabies, drug reactions, contact dermatitis, or, rarely, rickettsial pox or disseminated HSV infection. The clinical diagnosis of zoster can be difficult when acute pain and paresthesias precede the cutaneous eruption; the pain can be sufficiently severe to mimic myocardial infarction, cholecystitis, appendicitis, and other conditions. Localized contact dermatitis is the most common alternative etiology. A recurrent vesicular rash in lumbosacral dermatomes is usually HSV infection.

Laboratory Diagnosis

Laboratory techniques are most useful to guide decisions about antiviral treatment for VZV infection, especially for high-risk patients and for the differential diagnosis of neurologic disorders. The most sensitive method to identify VZV in any tissue is detection of viral DNA by PCR, although PCR may have false-positive results[241]; VZV proteins can be identified by immunohistochemical analysis of cells from cutaneous lesions prior to crusting. Infectious virus can be isolated from lesion specimens in tissue culture but cultures are often negative, especially if the specimen is not processed rapidly or the lesions are later stage. Assays for VZV IgG antibodies are most useful for determining the immune status of individuals whose clinical history of varicella is equivocal. The fluorescent-antibody membrane antigen assay (FAMA) is the most sensitive and specific method and the only method documented to predict susceptibility but is only available in research labs. Most commercial enzyme immunoassay methods have high specificity, generating few false-positive results, but 10% to 15% of immune individuals may be misidentified as susceptible. These commercial assays often do not detect antibody in recipients of the varicella vaccine, even though they have a protective immune response. Commercial VZV IgM antibody assays often lack specificity and should not be used as the only evidence of VZV-related disease.

If VZV is considered a potential cause of a neurologic disorder without rash, CSF and blood MNCs should be tested for VZV DNA by PCR and CSF for anti-VZV antibody.[131] VZV DNA is most likely to be found in patients with acute meningoencephalitis and cerebellitis and in some patients with VZV vasculopathy and myelitis. VZV vasculopathy is difficult to diagnose because many patients do not have a preceding zoster rash or CSF pleocytosis; VZV DNA PCR analysis of CSF is only 30% sensitive. Intrathecal synthesis of anti-VZV IgG antibodies is considered superior to CSF PCR for diagnosis of VZV vasculopathy, recurrent VZV myelopathy, and zoster sine herpete.

TREATMENT

While human leukocyte interferon and vidarabine were the first antiviral treatments with clinical benefit,[14,271] acyclovir and related nucleoside analog prodrugs are more effective and safer for treating both varicella and zoster.[24,33,104,123,222,250,271,418,465] Valacyclovir is a valine ester derivative of acyclovir that is de-esterified by hepatic enzymes to yield acyclovir. Famciclovir is a diacetyl derivative of penciclovir, a guanosine analog, which is enzymatically converted to penciclovir by intestinal and hepatic enzymes. These prodrugs are better absorbed from the gastrointestinal tract, allowing higher serum levels of drug after oral administration.

Molecular proof of the pivotal role of the VZV TK in the action of acyclovir and penciclovir has come from both the cloning and stable expression of the gene in TK-deficient cells and from sequencing of the VZV gene in acyclovir-resistant viral mutants.[373] Missense mutations in the TK ATP– or nucleoside-binding sites, and mutations clustered between these two sites confer acyclovir resistance. Mutations leading to expression of truncated VZV TK protein also result in drug-resistant viruses. Rarely, acyclovir resistance can be conferred by mutations in the VZV DNA polymerase. VZV strains that are resistant to both acyclovir and penciclovir retain sensitivity to the pyrophosphate analog, foscarnet. Cidofovir, an acyclic nucleoside phosphonate, is also active against acyclovir-resistant VZV strains and is an alternative to foscarnet.

Sorivudine (1-β-D-arabinofuranosyl-E-[2-bromo-vinyl] uracil) is an oral drug with potent *in vitro* activity against VZV and is effective *in vivo* in healthy adults with varicella and HIV-infected patients with zoster, but it is not licensed in the United States because of toxicity resulting from interaction with 5-fluorouracil.[36,134] However, the marginal benefit of this drug over acyclovir in HIV-infected patients with zoster suggests that early administration is more important than potency of the antiviral drug. Whereas all of the licensed antiviral drugs that inhibit VZV replication act on the viral DNA polymerase, other as yet unapproved compounds have different targets. A thiourea compound inhibits VZV by interfering with VZV ORF54 portal protein and encapsidation of viral DNA.[426] Roscovitine, an inhibitor of CDKs, also inhibits VZV replication in cultured cells.[410] Brincidofovir, the prodrug of cidofovir, has activity against acyclovir-resistant VZV.[295] New agents that target host cell proteins and restrict VZV replication *in vitro* and in human tissue xenografts have also been identified.[359]

Varicella

Early acyclovir therapy prevents progressive varicella and visceral dissemination by ensuring that cell-associated viremia is terminated, even if the host response is impaired. In addition, early therapy minimizes cutaneous disease and may therefore reduce the risk of secondary bacterial infections. Immunocompromised patients who have pneumonia, hepatitis, thrombocytopenia, or encephalitis, and adults with varicella pneumonia including pregnant women, require immediate treatment with intravenous acyclovir. Oral acyclovir ameliorates varicella in healthy children, adolescents, and adults when administered within 24 hours after the appearance of the initial cutaneous lesions.[8,102] Acyclovir therapy does not prevent the host from mounting an effective immune response to VZV, consistent with the concept that limited viral replication provides sufficient antigenic stimulation to induce VZV memory immunity.

Zoster

Acyclovir and the related drugs are beneficial therapies for zoster in healthy and immunocompromised patients. Among healthy individuals, treatment initiated within 72 hours reduces the period of continued new lesions in the involved dermatome and the time to complete healing. Antiviral treatment is especially important in immunocompromised patients because of their risk of disseminated disease and for adults with ophthalmic zoster because of their risk for developing acute uveitis and chronic keratitis. Acute neuropathic pain is reduced by early treatment with acyclovir, valacyclovir, or famciclovir; these drugs do not affect PHN. The benefits of antiviral therapy for acute rather than chronic pain suggest that different mechanisms may contribute to these two components of zoster-related pain.

Acyclovir is usually given intravenously to immunocompromised patients who are at high risk for disseminated zoster; less severely immunocompromised patients are given oral valacyclovir or famciclovir. Treatment reduces the duration of new lesion formation, acute pain, and time to complete healing; some benefit is observed even when therapy is delayed for more than 72 hours in persons still developing new lesions.[24,465] Relapse of zoster occurs in some immunocompromised patients despite antiviral treatment[177] although most respond to a second course of acyclovir, indicating that relapse usually reflects an inadequate host response rather than antiviral resistance.[177]

While not life-threatening, PHN is disabling and difficult to treat. Neuroleptic drugs and various analgesics are used to alleviate pain, but no universally accepted treatment exists. Drugs include gabapentin; pregabalin; tricyclic antidepressants such as amitriptyline, nortriptyline, maprotiline, and desipramine; and levorphanol, topical lidocaine, and rarely opiates.[184]

Patients with VZV vasculopathy can be treated with intravenous acyclovir and prednisone. Steroids are also used to treat patients with myelopathy, although some improve spontaneously. PORN is treated with intravenous acyclovir and steroids followed by oral acyclovir, or with intravitreal injections of foscarnet and oral acyclovir. Retinopathy may persist or recur despite acyclovir treatment.

PREVENTION

In most circumstances, preventing VZV transmission to susceptible individuals is difficult because patients with varicella may be contagious for 24 to 48 hours before the onset of their rash. Infection control practices, including caring for infected patients in isolation rooms with filtered air systems, are essential in hospitals that treat patients for whom varicella might be life-threatening.[145,372]

Passive Antibody Prophylaxis

VZV-specific antibodies interfere with the initial phases of VZV replication *in vivo*, as shown by the reduced varicella attack rate in individuals given VZV immunoglobulin prophylaxis shortly after exposure.[357] Passive antibodies may limit replication at initial sites of inoculation or may block or diminish cell-associated viremia or the early phase of VZV infection of epidermal cells. Anti-gH antibodies have neutralizing activity and may be important for this effect, as suggested by the restricted skin infection in SCID mice given anti-gH antibody at the time of VZV inoculation.[429]

VZV antibody prophylaxis is recommended for individuals with risk factors for serious varicella and exposure to a person with acute varicella or zoster.[8,56] Varicella zoster immunoglobulin (VariZIG)[56,101,274] or high-dose intravenous immunoglobulin should be given within 96 hours after exposure[8] although some benefit may occur with later administration.[242] Prophylaxis does not eliminate the possibility of varicella, especially with household exposure,[274] which may require antiviral therapy if the patient is at high risk. Passive antibody administration does not reduce the risk for VZV reactivation or alter the severity of varicella or zoster when given after the onset of illness.[394]

Antiviral Prophylaxis

Acyclovir given during the incubation period following exposure of susceptible individuals to VZV can prevent disease but the benefit of using acyclovir for prophylaxis has not been compared directly with acyclovir treatment of individuals in whom the varicella rash has just erupted. Daily oral acyclovir for 12 to 24 months can diminish the risk of zoster in bone marrow transplant recipients, but zoster may occur when prophylaxis is discontinued and drug-resistant VZV mutants may emerge. The alternative is prompt initiation of acyclovir for VZV reactivation.

VACCINES AND VACCINE IMMUNITY

Varicella

The live attenuated varicella vaccine is the first human herpesvirus vaccine licensed for clinical use and is recommended for routine vaccination of infants and susceptible older children and adults in the United States.[8,408,422] The vaccine virus was derived from a clinical isolate of VZV, the Oka strain, which was propagated in guinea pig embryo fibroblasts and then in WI38 human fibroblasts. In contrast to the outcome in susceptible children inoculated with infectious VZV from vesicular fluid,[37] tissue culture propagation appears to attenuate the virus so that vaccine containing as much as 17,000 plaque-forming units (pfu) per dose of infectious virus induces immunity to VZV but rarely produces clinical symptoms.[455] Attenuation is achieved even though varicella vaccine stocks contain mixtures of VZV genomes with varying mutations.[93,376] Comparing the parent Oka and vaccine Oka viruses in the SCID mouse model indicated that passage in fibroblasts reduces the ability of the virus to replicate efficiently in human skin, although T-cell tropism and neurotropism are not affected.[281,486] Less than 5% of children develop skin lesions after vaccination with Oka-derived vaccines; however, the vaccine Oka strain of VZV can be transmitted from these individuals.[236,264] (e-Fig. 13.11). Whether the virus remains attenuated after transmission is not known because of the low frequency of secondary cases.

In prelicensure trials, the live attenuated (Oka-Merck strain) vaccine was administered to more than 7,000 children and more than 1,600 healthy, susceptible adults.[232,463] In clinical trials, a single dose of vaccine containing 1,000 to 3,000 pfu of attenuated Oka virus induced seroconversion rates of more than 90% in children 12 years of age and younger and afforded complete protection against disease in about 85% of exposures. On exposure to varicella, some previously vaccinated children experience breakthrough infection, but the resulting disease usually remains mild, with fewer than 50 cutaneous lesions and no fever. Modified disease severity is consistent with priming of the host response by immunization.

The varicella vaccine also induces VZV-specific cellular immunity,[296,452,487] which is likely to be essential for its long-term protective efficacy.[99,384] Varicella immunization elicits T cells that proliferate and produce lymphokines in response to stimulation with the IE62 protein and the viral glycoproteins[19,31] and induces cytotoxic T cells that can lyse cells expressing VZV proteins.[179,384] The VZV-specific T-cell response is detectable within 10 to 14 days in most individuals,[19] whereas IgG antibodies to VZV were detected in only 40% of children tested at 2 weeks. This early T-cell response may account for the efficacy of vaccination when given immediately after exposure.[18] Varicella vaccine is also immunogenic when administered concurrently with measles–mumps–rubella (MMR) vaccines or as a quadrivalent MMR-V vaccine.[221]

Achieving high VZV IgG seroconversion rates in susceptible adolescents and adults requires two doses of the vaccine administered at an interval of at least 4 weeks,[126,296] consistent with the diminished host response to primary VZV infection and more severe varicella in adults. However, cellular immunity to VZV in adults given two doses of vaccine was significantly lower compared with children who received a single dose of vaccine, and VZV-specific T-cell proliferation correlated with lower IFN-γ responses.[179,296] Adults are also more likely than children to have transient local rash, and waning VZV antibody titers. Nevertheless, immunizing susceptible adults is important to protect against their risk of developing severe varicella.[123]

The persistence of VZV memory immunity after immunization has been difficult to assess because the continued circulation of wild-type VZV may boost vaccine-acquired immunity through exogenous exposure. However, VZV IgG and T-cell responses have been documented in 94% to 100% of varicella vaccine recipients for 7 to 10 years after vaccination, and protection has been sustained in most vaccinees.[126,232,303,423] In postlicensure surveillance done before vaccine coverage rates were high, no change in the frequency of breakthrough varicella or severity of symptoms with time after vaccination was found; however, those with low or undetectable VZV IgG titers 6 weeks after immunization were four times more likely to experience varicella.

Although the incidence of varicella is dramatically lower in all age groups in the United States, the widespread use of the varicella vaccine has meant that as many as half of the cases of varicella in well-vaccinated populations are in immunized children. Because the wild-type virus is transmissible from cases of breakthrough varicella, community outbreaks can be sustained. Prelicensure studies showed that a two-dose regimen induces higher humoral and cellular immune responses in children evaluated just after vaccination and after 1 year.[296,449] The observations of the enhanced host response to two doses, along with the surveillance data on breakthrough infections, have led to the use of a two-dose regimen in children as well as in adolescents and adults.[8] Varicella immunization using a two-dose regimen of MMR-V also enhances the primary immune response to the varicella component.

The Oka-Merck varicella vaccine has been given to children with acute leukemia in remission, reducing the attack rate after household exposure to 13%.[126] Seroconversion in these patients is associated with a high degree of protection after two doses of vaccine. Cell-mediated immunity is elicited less reliably in leukemic children given varicella vaccine, consistent with the often diminished T-cell proliferation to VZV antigens after natural varicella in immunocompromised children. Because it contains infectious virus, varicella vaccine must be given to these children with careful attention to the status of their underlying disease and immunosuppressive therapy regimens. Vaccine-related rashes occurred at about 1 month after immunization in approximately 50% of children with leukemia in remission. Rashes occurred at the site of inoculation but also as widely scattered vesicles, indicating that the vaccine virus remains capable of causing cell-associated viremia. This experience is consistent with retention of vaccine Oka tropism for T cells in the SCID mouse model. In healthy children, the limited replication of the vaccine virus at the site of subcutaneous inoculation likely allows time for induction of adaptive VZV-specific immunity before viremia can occur, whereas vaccine virus may escape from infected epithelial cells into T cells, causing viremia and varicella-like symptoms in some immunocompromised children. When children with leukemia developed rash, the vaccine virus was transmitted to their healthy, susceptible siblings, but the contacts had mild illness or asymptomatic seroconversion. The vaccine virus was not transmitted unless the immunocompromised child had rash indicating that no significant replication of the vaccine virus occurred at respiratory sites.[416] Detection by PCR of VZV in oropharyngeal secretions from children given varicella vaccine has been reported, but infectious virus has not been recovered. Immunizing susceptible, healthy household contacts of high-risk children may also reduce the risk of household exposure.[98]

Reactivation of the vaccine strain of VZV has been described in healthy vaccine recipients; however, analysis of the incidence of zoster in leukemic children who had vaccine-induced immunity and in those with past natural infection showed that the vaccine virus reactivated significantly less often than wild-type VZV.[151] Whether this observation indicates that the vaccine virus is less likely to establish latency or has less potential to cause symptomatic reactivation is not known. VZV-specific T-cell responses were higher in leukemic children who had been vaccinated but did not experience recurrent VZV compared with children who developed zoster. Vaccinated individuals can also develop zoster through subclinical infection with wild-type VZV despite vaccine-induced immunity.[149] Information about the prevalence of vaccine or wild-type VZV in neurons after immunization is limited, but VZV was detected by PCR in ganglia from children who died from trauma or nonimmunocompromising conditions.[123] As annual varicella epidemics diminish due to universal childhood vaccination programs, opportunities for superinfection with wild-type VZV will be minimal. If exogenous exposures are important for maintaining memory immunity in individuals with naturally acquired infection, then zoster could become more common in highly vaccinated populations, but accumulating evidence argues against this possible outcome.[152,153,191,470]

Zoster

The development of the varicella vaccine raised the possibility that vaccination might also be effective for reducing the risk of zoster associated with waning immunity in the elderly.[323] A high-potency preparation of the live attenuated VZV vaccine containing about 14-fold more attenuated Oka virus than the varicella vaccine reduced the burden of zoster illness in healthy adults aged 60 years and older,[323] when both incidence and severity of disease were considered together, by 61.1% ($p < 0.001$) over a median follow-up period of 3 years. The incidence of PHN was reduced by 66.5% ($p < 0.001$) and zoster incidence decreased by 51.3% ($p < 0.001$).

Administration of the live attenuated zoster vaccine induced memory B-cell responses composed of IgG and IgA antibody-secreting cells. A majority of antibodies produced were VZV–gE specific. However, the most potent neutralizing antibodies produced were gH specific, complement independent, and restricted cell–cell spread *in vitro* and may be important in controlling viral spread following VZV reactivation.[429] By contrast, most of the gE-specific antibodies did not neutralize, required complement, and could not restrict cell–cell spread.[405] VZV-specific responder cell frequencies increased from 1 per 68,000 to 1 per 40,000 in healthy adults over 55 years of age given the live attenuated vaccine, which was equivalent to the VZV responder cell numbers in naturally immune individuals aged 35 to 40 years.[243] VZV DNA was detected in saliva but transmission has not been reported. Evidence that baseline immunity to VZV and the number of regulatory T cells prior to vaccination can predict the effect of age on zoster vaccine immunogenicity suggests their importance in modulating responses.[458] Notably, CD4+ T-cell responses to VZV showed enhanced breadth after vaccination[234] and diversification of the VZV-specific T-cell receptor repertoire.[341]

Older individuals given the live attenuated zoster vaccine had diminished CD4+ and CD8+ T-cell responses[456,460]; a second dose boosted the responses.[459] A decline in the immunogenicity of the vaccine was observed in recipients every decade over the age of 50 years. Furthermore, older adults had higher proportions of VZV-specific T cells exhibiting markers of senescence and exhaustion, which may result in reduced effector responses to VZV challenge. Another study of older individuals revealed reduced generation of long-lived memory T-cell responses, which was likely due to reduced T-cell survival after the peak response to zoster vaccination.[342]

To avoid risks associated with infectious virus, a heat-inactivated preparation of varicella vaccine was given to patients receiving autologous bone marrow transplantation; recovery of VZV T-cell immunity was accelerated and zoster was less common in vaccinated transplant recipients as compared with unvaccinated controls.[155,350] The efficacy of peritransplantation vaccination of these patients with inactivated VZV vaccine was later demonstrated in placebo-controlled studies, indicating that their immunocompromised status does not block vaccine-induced immunity effective against zoster.[294,468]

Most recently, a zoster vaccine consisting of recombinant glycoprotein E with the ASO1 adjuvant had an even greater impact on clinical illness due to VZV reactivation than the live attenuated zoster vaccine, showed equivalent efficacy across all older age groups, and is now preferred for zoster prevention[57,87,235,325] (e-Fig. 13.10). Compared to the live attenuated vaccine, the recombinant gE vaccine induced a marked increase in gE-specific CD4+ T-cell frequencies and showed no age-related differences in numbers of responder T cells or cytokine production.[342] T-cell responses were higher to either vaccine in recipients when baseline responses were higher and VZV-specific IFN-γ and IL-2/IFN-γ dual positive CD4+ T-cell frequencies were equivalent, but the gE recombinant vaccine elicited higher IL-2 CD4+ T-cell frequencies as well as higher gE-specific T-cell responses.[457] These differences in immunogenicity may account for its enhanced efficacy regardless of age and the longer duration of protection compared to the live attenuated vaccine. This gE subunit vaccine is also safe for administration, immunogenic, and protective against zoster in immunocompromised patients.[88]

PERSPECTIVE

Advanced sequencing to understand the molecular evolution of the VZV genome, the capacity to map functional domains of viral proteins using structure-based discovery and targeted mutagenesis of the VZV genome, single-cell proteomics to probe VZV–host cell interactions, and use of state-of-the-art methods to document innate and adaptive immune responses in VZV-infected tissues have generated many new insights over the past decade. New approaches to probing the mechanisms by which VZV achieves tropism for human lymphocytes and myeloid lineage cells, skin epithelial and dermal cells, and neuronal cell subtypes will not only advance the understanding of the interplay of VZV with host cells but will also guide studies of other alpha herpesviruses in the human cell context. Notably, our knowledge of the complexities of VZV latency and reactivation as well as the molecular mechanisms underpinning postherpetic neuralgia remains limited. These and other questions about VZV pathogenesis will require multiparameter systems biology tools, since the processes involve many overlapping modifications of the host cell, rather than representing a single "mechanism." While exceptional progress has been made with the licensure of antiviral therapies and vaccines to prevent VZV infections, more cost-effective interventions are needed to reduce the global burden of VZV disease.

ACKNOWLEDGMENTS

The authors and editors wish to acknowledge the invaluable contributions of the late Don Gilden to the field of VZV research and clinical care and to this chapter in the previous edition of Fields Virology.

REFERENCES

1. Abendroth A, Lin I, Slobedman B, et al. Varicella-zoster virus retains major histocompatibility complex class I proteins in the Golgi compartment of infected cells. *J Virol* 2001;75:4878–4888.
2. Abendroth A, Morrow G, Cunningham AL, et al. Varicella-zoster virus infection of human dendritic cells and transmission to T cells: implications for virus dissemination in the host. *J Virol* 2001;75:6183–6192.
3. Abendroth A, Slobedman B, Lee E, et al. Modulation of major histocompatibility class II protein expression by varicella-zoster virus. *J Virol* 2000;74:1900–1907.
4. Alconada A, Bauer U, Baudoux L, et al. Intracellular transport of the glycoproteins gE and gI of the varicella-zoster virus. *J Biol Chem* 1998;273:13430–13436.
5. Ali MA, Li Q, Fischer ER, et al. The insulin degrading enzyme binding domain of varicella-zoster virus (VZV) glycoprotein E is important for cell-to-cell spread and VZV infectivity, while a glycoprotein I binding domain is essential for infection. Virology 2009;386(2):270–279.
6. Ambagala AP, Bosma T, Ali MA, et al. Varicella-zoster virus immediate-early 63 protein interacts with human antisilencing function 1 protein and alters its ability to bind histones h3.1 and h3.3. *J Virol* 2009;83:200–209.
7. Ambagala AP, Cohen JI. Varicella-Zoster virus IE63, a major viral latency protein, is required to inhibit the alpha interferon-induced antiviral response. *J Virol* 2007;81(15):7844–7851.
8. American Academy of Pediatrics. Varicella-zoster virus. In: Kimberlin DW, Brady MT, Jackson MA, et al., eds. *Red Book®*. 2018.
9. Annunziato PW, Lungu O, Panagiotidis C, et al. Varicella-zoster virus proteins in skin lesions: implications for a novel role of ORF29p in chickenpox. *J Virol* 2000;74:2005–2010.
10. Arnold N, Girke T, Sureshchandra S, et al. Acute simian varicella virus infection causes robust and sustained changes in gene expression in the sensory ganglia. *J Virol* 2016;90:10823–10843.
11. Arnold N, Girke T, Sureshchandra S, et al. Genomic and functional analysis of the host response to acute simian varicella infection in the lung. *Sci Rep* 2016;6:34164.
12. Arvin A. Aging, immunity, and the varicella-zoster virus. *N Engl J Med* 2005;352:2266–2267.
13. Arvin AM, Koropchak CM, Williams BRG, et al. The early immune response in healthy and immunocompromised subjects with primary varicella-zoster virus infection. *J Infect Dis* 1986;154:422–429.
14. Arvin AM, Kushner JH, Feldman S, et al. Human leukocyte interferon for treatment of varicella in children with cancer. *N Engl J Med* 1982;306:761–767.
15. Arvin AM, Sharp M, Moir M, et al. Memory cytotoxic T-cell responses to viral tegument and regulatory proteins encoded by open reading frames 4, 10, 29, and 62 of varicella-zoster virus. *Viral Immunol* 2002;15:507–516.
16. Arvin AM, Sharp M, Smith S, et al. Equivalent recognition of a varicella-zoster virus immediate early protein (IE62) and glycoprotein I by cytotoxic T lymphocytes of either $CD4^+$ or $CD8^+$ phenotype. *J Immunol* 1991;146:257–264.
17. Asano Y, Itakura N, Hiroishi Y, et al. Viral replication and immunologic responses in children naturally infected with varicella-zoster and in varicella vaccine recipients. *J Infect Dis* 1985;152:863–868.
18. Asano Y, Nakayama H, Yazaki T, et al. Protection against varicella in family contacts by immediate inoculation with live varicella vaccine. *Pediatrics* 1977;59:3–7.
19. Asanuma H, Sharp M, Maecker HT, et al. Frequencies of memory T cells specific for varicella-zoster virus, herpes simplex virus and cytomegalovirus determined by intracellular detection of cytokine expression. *J Infect Dis* 2000;181:859–866.

20. Baba K, Yabuuchi H, Takahashi M, et al. Increased incidence of herpes zoster in normal children infected with varicella-zoster virus during infancy: community-based follow-up study. *J Pediatr* 1986;108:373–376.
21. Baiker, A, Bagowski C, Ito H, et al. The immediate-early 63 protein of varicella-zoster virus: analysis of functional domains required for replication in vitro and T cell and skin tropism in the SCIDhu model in vivo. *J Virol* 2004;78:1181–1194.
22. Baiker A, Fabel K, Cozzio A, et al. Varicella-zoster virus infection of human neural cells in vivo. *Proc Natl Acad Sci U S A* 2004;101:10792–10797.
23. Baird NL, Bowlin JL, Hotz TJ, et al. Interferon gamma prolongs survival of varicella-zoster virus-infected human neurons in vitro. *J Virol* 2015;89:7425–7427.
24. Balfour HH, Bean B, Laskin O, et al. Acyclovir halts progression of herpes zoster in immunocompromised patients. *N Engl J Med* 1983;308:1448–1453.
25. Banovic T, Yanilla M, Simmons R, et al. Disseminated varicella infection caused by varicella vaccine strain in a child with low invariant natural killer T cells and diminished CD1d expression. *J Infect Dis* 2011;204(12):1893–1901.
26. Baudoux L, Defechereux P, Rentier B, et al. Gene activation by varicella-zoster virus IE4 protein requires its dimerization and involves both the arginine-rich sequence, the central part and the carboxy-terminal cysteine-rich region. *J Biol Chem* 2000;275:32822–32831.
27. Baudoux L, Defechereux P, Schoonbroodt S, et al. Mutational analysis of varicella-zoster virus major immediate-early protein IE62. *Nucleic Acids Res* 1995;23:1341–1349.
28. Berarducci B, Rajamani J, Reichelt M, et al. Deletion of the first cysteine-rich region of the varicella-zoster virus glycoprotein E ectodomain abolishes the gE and gI interaction and differentially affects cell-cell spread and viral entry. *J Virol* 2009;83(1):228–240.
29. Berarducci B, Rajamani J, Zerboni L, et al. Functions of the unique N-terminal region of glycoprotein E in the pathogenesis of varicella-zoster virus infection. *Proc Natl Acad Sci U S A* 2010;107(1):282–287.
30. Berarducci B, Sommer M, Zerboni L, et al. Cellular and viral factors regulate the varicella-zoster virus gE promoter during viral replication. *J Virol* 2007;81:10258–10267.
31. Besser J, Ikoma M, Fabel K, et al. Differential requirement for cell fusion and virion formation in the pathogenesis of varicella-zoster virus infection of skin and T cells. *J Virol* 2004;78:13293–13305.
32. Besser J, Sommer M, Zerboni L, et al. Differentiation of varicella-zoster virus ORF47 protein kinase and IE62 protein binding domains and their contributions to replication in human skin xenografts in the SCID-hu mouse. *J Virol* 2003;77:5964–5974.
33. Beutner KR, Friedman DJ, Forszpaniak C, et al. Valacyclovir compared with acyclovir for improved therapy for herpes zoster in immunocompetent adults. *Antimicrob Agents Chemother* 1995;39:1546–1553.
34. Bird LE, Ren J, Wright A, et al. Crystal structure of the varicella-zoster virus thymidine kinase. *J Biol Chem* 2003;278:24680–24687.
35. Blumenthal DT, Shacham-Shmueli E, Bokstein F, et al. Zoster sine herpete: virological verification by detection of anti-VZV IgG antibody in CSF. *Neurology* 2011;76:484–485.
36. Bodsworth NJ, Boag F, Burge D, et al. Evaluation of sorivudine (BV-araU) versus acyclovir in the treatment of acute localized herpes zoster in human immunodeficiency virus-infected adults. The Multinational Sorivudine Study Group. *J Infect Dis* 1997;176:103–111.
37. von Bokay J. Über den ætiologisched zusammenhang der varizellen met gewissen fällen von herpes zoster. *Wein Klin Wochenschr* 1909;22:1323.
38. Bontems S, diValentin E, Baudoux L, et al. Phosphorylation of varicella-zoster virus IE63 protein by casein kinase influences its cellular localization and gene regulation activity. *J Biol Chem* 2002;277:21050–21060.
39. Boucaud D, Yoshitake H, Hay J, et al. The varicella-zoster virus (VZV) open-reading frame 29 protein acts as a modulator of a late VZV gene promoter. *J Infect Dis* 1998;178(Suppl 1):S34–S38.
40. Braun KP, Bulder MM, Chabrier S, et al. The course and outcome of unilateral intracranial arteriopathy in 79 children with ischaemic stroke. *Brain* 2009;132:544–557.
41. Breuer J. VZV molecular epidemiology. *Curr Top Microbiol Immunol* 2010;342:15–42.
42. Breuer J. Molecular genetic insights into varicella zoster virus (VZV), the vOka vaccine strain, and the pathogenesis of latency and reactivation. *J Infect Dis* 2018;218:S75–S80.
43. Buckingham EM, Carpenter JE, Jackson W, et al. Autophagic flux without a block differentiates varicella-zoster virus infection from herpes simplex virus infection. *Proc Natl Acad Sci U S A* 2015;112:256–261.
44. Buckingham EM, Jarosinski KW, Jackson W, et al. Exocytosis of varicella-zoster virus virions involves a convergence of endosomal and autophagy pathways. *J Virol* 2016;90:8673–8685.
45. Bullowa JGM, Wishik SM. Complications of varicella. I. Their occurrence among 2534 patients. *Am J Dis Child* 1935;49:923–926.
46. Cai M, Wang S, Xing J, et al. Characterization of the nuclear import and export signals, and subcellular transport mechanism of varicella-zoster virus ORF9. *J Gen Virol* 2011;92(Pt 3):621–626.
47. Campbell TM, McSharry BP, Steain M, et al. Varicella zoster virus productively infects human natural killer cells and manipulates phenotype. *PLoS Pathog* 2018;4(4):e1006999. doi:10.1371/journal.ppat.1006999.
48. Campbell TM, McSharry BP, Steain M, et al. Abendroth functional paralysis of human natural killer cells by alphaherpesviruses. *PLoS Pathog* 2019;15:e1007784.
49. Campbell TM, McSharry BP, Steain M, et al. Varicella-Zoster virus and herpes simplex virus 1 differentially modulate NKG2D ligand expression during productive infection. *J Virol* 2015;89:7932–7943.
50. Carpenter JE, Clayton AC, Halling KC, et al. Defensive perimeter in the central nervous system: predominance of astrocytes and astrogliosis during recovery from varicella-zoster virus encephalitis. *J Virol* 2015;90:379–391.
51. Carpenter JE, Henderson EP, Grose C. Enumeration of an extremely high particle-to-PFU ratio for Varicella-zoster virus. *J Virol* 2009;83:6917–6921.
52. Carpenter JE, Hutchinson JA, Jackson W, et al. Egress of light particles among filopodia on the surface of Varicella-Zoster virus-infected cells. *J Virol* 2008;82:2821–2835.
53. Carpenter JE, Jackson W, Benetti L, et al. Autophagosome formation during varicella-zoster virus infection following endoplasmic reticulum stress and the unfolded protein response. *J Virol* 2011;85:9414–9424.
54. Carpenter JE, Jackson W, de Souza GA, et al. Insulin-degrading enzyme binds to the nonglycosylated precursor of varicella-zoster virus gE protein found in the endoplasmic reticulum. *J Virol* 2010;84:847–855.
55. Carter-Timofte ME, Hansen AF, Christiansen M, et al. Mutations in RNA Polymerase III genes and defective DNA sensing in adults with varicella-zoster virus CNS infection. *Genes Immun* 2019;20:214–223.
56. Centers for Disease Control and Prevention. A new product (VariZIG) for postexposure prophylaxis of varicella available under an investigational new drug application expanded access protocol. *MMWR Morb Mortal Wkly Rep* 2006;55:209–210.
57. Centers for Disease Control and Prevention. Prevention of herpes zoster: recommendations of the Advisory Committee on Immunization Practices (ACIP) Recommendations for use of Herpes Zoster Vaccines. *MMWR Recomm Rep* 2018;67:103–108.
58. Chaudhuri V, Sommer M, Rajamani J, et al. Functions of Varicella-zoster virus ORF23 capsid protein in viral replication and the pathogenesis of skin infection. *J Virol* 2008;82:10231–10246.
59. Che X, Oliver SL, Reichelt M, et al. ORF11 protein interacts with the ORF9 essential tegument protein in varicella-zoster virus infection. *J Virol* 2013;87:5106–5117.
60. Che X, Oliver SL, Sommer MH, et al. Identification and functional characterization of the Varicella zoster virus ORF11 gene product. *Virology* 2011;412(1):156–166.
61. Che X, Reichelt M, Sommer MH, et al. Functions of the ORF9-to-ORF12 gene cluster in varicella-zoster virus replication and in the pathogenesis of skin infection. *J Virol* 2008;82(12):5825–5834.
62. Che X, Zerboni L, Sommer MH, et al. Varicella-zoster virus open reading frame 10 is a virulence determinant in skin cells but not in T cells in vivo. *J Virol* 2006;80:3238–3248.
63. Cheatham WJ, Dolan TF Jr, Dower JC, et al. Varicella: report on two fatal cases with necropsy, virus isolation, and serologic studies. *Am J Pathol* 1956;32:1015–1035.
64. Chen JJ, Gershon AA, Li ZS, et al. Latent and lytic infection of isolated guinea pig enteric ganglia by varicella zoster virus. *J Med Virol* 2003;70(Suppl 1):S71–S78.
65. Chen D, Olivo PD. Expression of the varicella-zoster virus origin-binding protein and analysis of its site-specific DNA-binding properties. *J Virol* 1994;68:3841–3849.
66. Chen D, Stabell EC, Olivo PD. Varicella-zoster virus gene 51 complements a herpes simplex virus type 1 UL9 null mutant. *J Virol* 1995;69:4515–4518.
67. Chen JJ, Zhu Z, Gershon AA, et al. Mannose 6-phosphate receptor dependence of varicella zoster virus infection in vitro and in the epidermis during varicella and zoster. *Cell* 2004;119:915–926.
68. Christensen J, Steain M, Slobedman B, et al. Varicella-zoster virus glycoprotein I is essential for spread in dorsal root ganglia and facilitates axonal localization of structural virion components in neuronal cultures. *J Virol* 2013;87:13719–13728.
69. Clarke P, Beer T, Cohrs R, et al. Configuration of latent varicella-zoster virus DNA. *J Virol* 1995;69:8151–8154.
70. Cohen JI. Rodent models of varicella-zoster virus neurotropism. *Curr Top Microbiol Immunol* 2010;342:277–289.
71. Cohen JI, Cox E, Pesnicak L, et al. The varicella-zoster virus ORF63 latency-associated protein is critical for establishment of latency. *J Virol* 2004;78:11833–11840.
72. Cohen JI, Heffel D, Seidel K. The transcriptional activation domain of varicella-zoster virus open reading frame 62 protein is not conserved with its herpes simplex virus homolog. *J Virol* 1993;67:4246–4251.
73. Cohen JI, Krogmann T, Bontems S, et al. Regions of the varicella-zoster virus open reading frame 63 latency-associated protein important for replication in vitro are also critical for efficient establishment of latency. *J Virol* 2005;79:5069–5077.
74. Cohen JI, Krogmann T, Ross JP, et al. Varicella-zoster virus ORF4 latency-associated protein is important for establishment of latency. *J Virol* 2005;79:6969–6975.
75. Cohen JI, Nguyen H. Varicella-zoster glycoprotein I is essential for growth of virus in Vero cells. *J Virol* 1997;71:6913–6920.
76. Cohen JI, Nguyen H. Varicella-zoster ORF61 deletion mutants replicate in cell culture, but a mutant with stop codons in ORF61 reverts to wild-type virus. *Virology* 1998;246:306–316.
77. Cohen JI, Sato H, Srinivas S, et al. Varicella-zoster virus (VZV) ORF65 virion protein is dispensable for replication in cell culture and is phosphorylated by casein kinase II, but not by the VZV protein kinases. *Virology* 2001;280:62–71.
78. Cohen JI, Seidel KE. Generation of varicella-zoster virus (VZV) and viral mutants from cosmid DNAs: VZV thymidylate synthetase is not essential for replication in vitro. *Proc Natl Acad Sci U S A* 1993;90:7376–7380.
79. Cohen JI, Seidel KE. Varicella-zoster virus (VZV) open reading frame 10 protein, the homolog of the essential herpes simplex virus protein VP16, is dispensable for VZV replication in vitro. *J Virol* 1994;68:7850–7858.
80. Cohen JI, Seidel KE. Varicella-zoster virus open reading frame 1 encodes a membrane protein that is dispensable for growth of VZV in vitro. *Virology* 1995;206:835–842.
81. Cohrs RJ, Gilden DH, Gomi Y, et al. Comparison of virus transcription during lytic infection of the Oka parental and vaccine strains of Varicella-Zoster virus. *J Virol* 2006;80:2076–2082.
82. Cohrs RJ, Gilden DH, Kinchington PR, et al. Varicella-zoster virus gene 66 transcription and translation in latently infected human ganglia. *J Virol* 2003;77:6660–6665.
83. Cohrs RJ, Lee KS, Beach A, et al. Targeted genome sequencing reveals varicella-zoster virus open reading frame 12 deletion. *J Virol* 2017;91:e01141.
84. Cohrs RJ, Randall J, Smith J, et al. Analysis of individual human trigeminal ganglia for latent herpes simplex virus type 1 and varicella-zoster virus nucleic acids using real-time PCR. *J Virol* 2000;74:11464–11471.
85. Como CN, Pearce CM, Cohrs RJ, et al. Interleukin-6 and type 1 interferons inhibit varicella zoster virus replication in human neurons. *Virology* 2018;522:13–18.
86. Cox E, Reddy S, Iofin I, et al. Varicella-zoster virus ORF57, unlike its pseudorabies virus UL3.5 homolog, is dispensable for viral replication in cell culture. *Virology* 1998;250:205–209.
87. Cunningham AL, Lal H, Kovac M, et al. Efficacy of the herpes zoster subunit vaccine in adults 70 years of age or older. *N Engl J Med* 2016;375:1019–1032.

88. Dagnew AF, Ilhan O, Lee WS, et al. Immunogenicity and safety of the adjuvanted recombinant zoster vaccine in adults with haematological malignancies: a phase 3, randomised, clinical trial and post-hoc efficacy analysis. *Lancet Infect Dis* 2019;19:988–1000.
89. Davison AJ, McGeoch DJ. Evolutionary comparisons of the S segments in the genomes of herpes simplex virus type 1 and varicella-zoster virus. *J Gen Virol* 1986;67:597–611.
90. Davison AJ, Scott J. The complete DNA sequence of varicella-zoster virus. *J Gen Virol* 1986;67:1759–1816.
91. Defechereux P, Debrus S, Baudoux L, et al. Varicella-zoster virus open reading frame 4 encodes an immediate-early protein with posttranscriptional regulatory properties. *J Virol* 1997;71:7073–7079.
92. Depledge DP, Gray ER, Kundu S, et al. Evolution of cocirculating varicella-zoster virus genotypes during a chickenpox outbreak in Guinea-Bissau. *J Virol* 2014;88:13936–13946.
93. Depledge DP, Kundu S, Jensen NJ, et al. Deep sequencing of viral genomes provides insight into the evolution and pathogenesis of varicella zoster virus and its vaccine in humans. *Mol Biol Evol* 2014;31:397–409.
94. Depledge DP, Ouwendijk WJD, Sadaoka T, et al. A spliced latency-associated VZV transcript maps antisense to the viral transactivator gene 61. *Nat Commun* 2018;9:1167.
95. Depledge DP, Yamanishi K, Gomi Y, et al. Deep sequencing of distinct preparations of the live attenuated varicella-zoster virus vaccine reveals a conserved core of attenuating single-nucleotide polymorphisms. *J Virol* 2016;90:8698–8704.
96. Derryck A, LaRussa P, Steinberg S, et al. Varicella and zoster in children with human immunodeficiency virus infection. *Pediatr Infect Dis J* 1998;17:931–933.
97. Desloges N, Rahaus M, Wolff MH. Role of the protein kinase PKR in the inhibition of varicella-zoster virus replication by beta interferon and gamma interferon. *J Gen Virol* 2005;86:1–6.
98. Diaz PS, Au D, Smith S, et al. Lack of transmission of the live attenuated varicella vaccine virus to immunocompromised children after immunization of their siblings. *Pediatrics* 1991;87:166–170.
99. Diaz PS, Smith S, Hunter E, et al. T lymphocyte cytotoxicity with natural varicella-zoster virus infection and after immunization with live attenuated varicella vaccine. *J Immunol* 1989;142:636–641.
100. Disney GH, McKee TA, Preston CM, et al. The product of varicella-zoster virus gene 62 autoregulates its own promoter. *J Gen Virol* 1990;71:2999–3003.
101. Duchon JM, Levin MJ, Gershon AA. Safety and varicella outcomes in in utero-exposed newborns and preterm infants treated with varicella zoster immune globulin (VARIZIG): a subgroup analysis of an expanded-access program. *J Pediatric Infect Dis Soc* 2020;9:449–453.
102. Dunkle LM, Arvin AM, Whitley RJ, et al. A controlled trial of acyclovir for chickenpox in normal children. *N Engl J Med* 1991;325:1539–1544.
103. Duus KM, Grose C. Multiple regulatory effects of varicella-zoster virus (VZV) gL on trafficking patterns and fusogenic properties of VZV gH. *J Virol* 1996;70:8961–8971.
104. Dworkin RH, Boon RJ, Griffin DR, et al. Postherpetic neuralgia: impact of famciclovir, age, rash severity and acute pain in herpes zoster patients. *J Infect Dis* 1998;178(Suppl 1):S76–S80.
105. Ecker JR, Hyman RW. Varicella-zoster virus DNA exists as two isomers. *Proc Natl Acad Sci U S A* 1982;79:156–160.
106. Eisfeld AJ, Turse SE, Jackson SA, et al. Phosphorylation of the varicella-zoster virus (VZV) major transcriptional regulatory protein IE62 by the VZV open reading frame 66 protein kinase. *J Virol* 2006;80:1710–1723.
107. Eisfeld AJ, Yee MB, Erazo A, et al. Downregulation of class I major histocompatibility complex surface expression by varicella-zoster virus involves open reading frame 66 protein kinase-dependent and -independent mechanisms. *J Virol* 2007;81(17):9034–9049.
108. Enders G, Miller E, Cradock-Watson J, et al. Consequences of varicella and herpes zoster in pregnancy: a prospective study of 1739 cases. *Lancet* 1994;343:1547–1550.
109. Erazo A, Kinchington PR. Varicella-zoster virus open reading frame 66 protein kinase and its relationship to alphaherpesvirus US3 kinases. *Curr Top Microbiol Immunol* 2010;342:79–98.
110. Erazo A, Yee MB, Banfield BW, et al. The alphaherpesvirus US3/ORF66 protein kinases direct phosphorylation of the nuclear matrix protein matrin 3. *J Virol* 2011;85:568–581.
111. Erazo A, Yee MB, Osterrieder N, et al. Varicella-zoster virus open reading frame 66 protein kinase is required for efficient viral growth in primary human corneal stromal fibroblast cells. *J Virol* 2008;82:7653–7665.
112. Esiri MM, Tomlinson AH. Herpes zoster: demonstration of virus in trigeminal nerve and ganglion by immunofluorescence and electron microscopy. *J Neurol Sci* 1972;15:35–48.
113. Etzioni A, Eidenschenk C, Katz R, et al. Fatal varicella associated with selective natural killer cell deficiency. *J Pediatr* 2005;146:423–425.
114. Feldman S, Lott L. Varicella in children with cancer: impact of antiviral therapy and prophylaxis. *Pediatrics* 1987;80:465–572.
115. Fleisher G, Henry W, McSorley M, et al. Life-threatening complications of varicella. *Am J Dis Child* 1981;135:896–899.
116. Fossum E, Friedel CC, Rajagopala SV, et al. Evolutionarily conserved herpesviral protein interaction networks. *PLoS Pathog* 2009;5(9):e1000570.
117. François S, Sen N, Mitton B, et al. Varicella-zoster virus activates CREB, and inhibition of the pCREB-p300/CBP interaction inhibits viral replication in vitro and skin pathogenesis in vivo. *J Virol* 2016;90:8686–8697.
118. Garcia-Valcarcel M, Fowler WJ, Harper DR, et al. Cloning, expression, and immunogenicity of the assembly protein of varicella-zoster virus and detection of the products of open reading frame 33. *J Med Virol* 1997;53:332–339.
119. Garland J. Varicella following exposure to herpes zoster. *N Engl J Med* 1943;228:336–337.
120. Gary L, Gilden DH, Cohrs RJ. Epigenetic regulation of varicella-zoster virus open reading frame 62 and 63 in latently infected trigeminal ganglia. *J Virol* 2006;80:4921–4926.
121. Gerada C, Steain M, Campbell TM, et al. Granzyme B cleaves multiple herpes simplex virus 1 and varicella-zoster virus (VZV) gene products, and VZV ORF4 inhibits natural killer cell cytotoxicity. *J Virol* 2019;93:e01140.
122. Gerada C, Steain M, McSharry BP, et al. Varicella-zoster virus ORF63 protects human neuronal and keratinocyte cell lines from apoptosis and changes its localization upon apoptosis induction. *J Virol* 2018;92:e00338.
123. Gershon AA, Breuer J, Cohen JI, et al. Varicella zoster virus infection. *Nat Rev Dis Primers* 2015;1:15016.
124. Gershon M, Gershon A. Varicella-zoster virus and the enteric nervous system. *J Infect Dis* 2018;218:S113–S119.
125. Gershon AA, Sherman DL, Zhu Z, et al. Intracellular transport of newly synthesized varicella-zoster virus: final envelopment in the trans-Golgi network. *J Virol* 1994;68:6372–6390.
126. Gershon AA, Steinberg SP. Live attenuated varicella vaccine: protection in healthy adults compared with leukemic children. NIAID Varicella Vaccine Collaborative Study Group. *J Infect Dis* 1990;161:661–666.
127. Gershon AA, Steinberg SP, Gelb L. Clinical reinfection with varicella-zoster virus. *J Infect Dis* 1984;149:137–142.
128. Gilden D, Cohrs RJ, Mahalingam R, et al. Neurological disease produced by varicella zoster virus reactivation without rash. *Curr Top Microbiol Immunol* 2010;342:243–253.
129. Gilden DH, Vafai A, Shtram Y, et al. Varicella-zoster virus DNA in human sensory ganglia. *Nature* 1983;306:478–480.
130. Gilden D, White T, Boyer PJ, et al. Varicella zoster virus infection in granulomatous arteritis of the aorta. *J Infect Dis* 2016;213:1866–1871.
131. Gilden DH, Wright RR, Schneck SA, et al. Zoster sine herpete, a clinical variant. *Ann Neurol* 1994;35:530–533.
132. Girsch JH, Walters K, Jackson W, et al. Progeny varicella-zoster virus capsids exit the nucleus but never undergo secondary envelopment during autophagic flux inhibition by bafilomycin A1. *J Virol* 2019;93:e00505.
133. Glesby M, Moore RD, Chaisson RE. Clinical spectrum of herpes zoster in adults with HIV. *Clin Infect Dis* 1995;21:370–375.
134. Gnann JW Jr, Crumpacker CS, Lalezari JP, et al. Sorivudine versus acyclovir for treatment of dermatomal herpes zoster in human immunodeficiency virus-infected patients: results from a randomized, controlled clinical trial. Collaborative Antiviral Study Group/AIDS Clinical Trials Group, Herpes Zoster Study Group. *Antimicrob Agents Chemother* 1998;42:1139–1145.
135. Golani-Zaidie L, Borodianskiy-Shteinberg T, Bisht P, et al. Bioinformatically-predicted varicella zoster virus small non-coding RNAs are expressed in lytically-infected epithelial cells and neurons. *Virus Res* 2019;274:197773.
136. González-Motos V, Jürgens C, Ritter B, et al. Varicella zoster virus glycoprotein C increases chemokine-mediated leukocyte migration. *PLoS Pathog* 2017;13:e1006346.
137. Goodwin TJ, McCarthy M, Osterrieder N, et al. Three-dimensional normal human neural progenitor tissue-like assemblies: a model of persistent varicella-zoster virus infection. *PLoS Pathog* 2013;9:e1003512.
138. Gowrishankar K, Slobedman B, Cunningham AL, et al. Productive varicella-zoster virus infection of cultured intact human ganglia. *J Virol* 2007;81(12):6752–6756. doi:10.1128/JVI.02793-06.
139. Gowrishankar K, Steain M, Cunningham AL, et al. Characterization of the host immune response in human Ganglia after herpes zoster. *J Virol* 2010;84(17):8861–8870.
140. Gray WL. Simian varicella virus: molecular virology. *Curr Top Microbiol Immunol* 2010;342:291–308.
141. Grose C, Carpenter JE, Jackson W, et al. Overview of varicella-zoster virus glycoproteins gC, gH and gL. *Curr Top Microbiol Immunol* 2010;342:113–128.
142. Grose C, Yu X, Cohrs RJ, et al. Aberrant virion assembly and limited glycoprotein C production in varicella-zoster virus-infected neurons. *J Virol* 2013;87:9643–9648.
143. Grossman MC, Grossman ME. Chronic hyperkeratotic herpes zoster and human immunodeficiency virus infection. *J Am Acad Dermatol* 1993;28:306–308.
144. Guess HA, Broughton DD, Melton II LJ, et al. Population-based studies of varicella complications. *Pediatrics* 1987;78:723–727.
145. Gustafson TL, Lavely GB, Brawner ER Jr, et al. An outbreak of airborne nosocomial varicella. *Pediatrics* 1982;70:550–556.
146. Haanpaa M, Dastidar P, Weinberg A, et al. CSF and MRF findings in patients with acute herpes zoster. *Neurology* 1998;51:1405–1411.
147. Habran L, Bontems S, Di Valentin E. Varicella-zoster virus IE63 protein phosphorylation by roscovitine-sensitive cyclin-dependent kinases modulates its cellular localization and activity. *J Biol Chem* 2005;280:29135–29143.
148. Hall SL, Govero JL, Heineman TC. Intracellular transport and stability of varicella-zoster virus glycoprotein K. *Virology* 2007;358:283–290.
149. Hammerschlag MR, Gershon AA, Steinberg SP, et al. Herpes zoster in an adult recipient of live attenuated varicella vaccine. *J Infect Dis* 1989;160:535–537.
150. Harbecke R, Jensen NJ, Depledge DP, et al. Recurrent herpes zoster in the shingles prevention study: are second episodes caused by the same varicella-zoster virus strain? *Vaccine* 2020;38:150–157.
151. Hardy I, Gershon AA, Steinberg SP, et al. Varicella Vaccine Collaborative Study Group. The incidence of zoster after immunization with live attenuated varicella vaccine. A study in children with leukemia. *N Engl J Med* 1991;325:1545–1550.
152. Harpaz R, Leung JW. The epidemiology of herpes zoster in the United States during the era of varicella and herpes zoster vaccines: changing patterns among children. *Clin Infect Dis* 2019;69:345–347.
153. Harpaz R, Leung JW. The epidemiology of herpes zoster in the United States during the era of varicella and herpes zoster vaccines: changing patterns among older adults. *Clin Infect Dis* 2019;69:341–344.
154. Harper DR, Sanders EA, Ashcroft MA. Varicella-zoster virus assembly protein p32/p36 is present in DNA-containing as well as immature capsids. *J Med Virol* 1995;46:144–147.
155. Hata A, Asanuma H, Rinki M, et al. Use of an inactivated varicella vaccine in recipients of hematopoietic-cell transplants. *N Engl J Med* 2002;347:26–34.
156. Hata A, Zerboni L, Sommer M, et al. Granulysin blocks replication of varicella-zoster virus and triggers apoptosis of infected cells. *Viral Immunol* 2001;14:125–133.
157. Haumont M, Jurdan M, Kangro H, et al. Neutralizing antibody responses induced by varicella-zoster virus gE and gB glycoproteins following infection, reactivation or immunization. *J Med Virol* 1997;53:63–68.

158. Head H, Campbell AW. The pathology of herpes zoster and its bearing on sensory localisation. *Brain* 1900;23:353–361.
159. Heineman TC, Cohen JI. Deletion of the varicella-zoster virus large subunit of ribonucleotide reductase impairs the growth of virus in vitro. *J Virol* 1994;68:3317–3323.
160. Heineman TC, Cohen JI. The varicella-zoster virus (VZV) open reading frame 47 (ORF47) protein kinase is dispensable for viral replication and is not required for phosphorylation of ORF63 protein, the VZV homolog of herpes simplex virus ICP22. *J Virol* 1995;69:7367–7370.
161. Heineman TC, Hall SL. VZV gB endocytosis and Golgi localization are mediated by YXXf motifs in its cytoplasmic domain. *Virology* 2001;285:42–49.
162. Heineman TC, Hall SL. Role of the varicella-zoster virus gB cytoplasmic domain in gB transport and viral egress. *J Virol* 2002;76:591–599.
163. Heineman TC, Seidel K, Cohen JI. The varicella-zoster virus ORF66 protein induces kinase activity and is dispensable for viral replication. *J Virol* 1996;70:7312–7317.
164. Hood C, Cunningham AL, Slobedman B, et al. Varicella-zoster virus ORF63 inhibits apoptosis of primary human neurons. *J Virol* 2006;80:1025–1031.
165. Hoover S, Cohrs RJ, Rangel Z, et al. Downregulation of varicella-zoster virus (VZV) immediate-early ORF62 transcription by VZV ORF63 correlates with virus replication in vitro and with latency. *J Virol* 2006;80:3459–3468.
166. Hope-Simpson RE. The nature of herpes zoster: a long-term study and a new hypothesis. *Proc R Soc Med* 1965;58:9–20.
167. Hope-Simpson RE. Postherpetic neuralgia. *J R Coll Gen Pract* 1975;25:571–575.
168. Hu H, Cohen JI. Varicella-zoster virus open reading frame 47 (ORF47) protein is critical for virus replication in dendritic cells and for spread to other cells. *Virology* 2005;337:304–311.
169. Huch JH, Cunningham AL, Arvin AM, et al. Impact of varicella-zoster virus on dendritic cell subsets in human skin during natural infection. *J Virol* 2010;84:4060–4072.
170. Hukkanen RR, Gillen M, Grant R, et al. Simian varicella virus in pigtailed macaques (*Macaca nemestrina*): clinical, pathologic, and virologic features. *Comp Med* 2009;59:482–487.
171. Hyman RW, Ecker JR, Tenser RB. Varicella-zoster virus RNA in human trigeminal ganglia. *Lancet* 1983;83:814–816.
172. Inchauspé G, Nagpal S, Ostrove JM. Mapping of two varicella-zoster virus-encoded genes that activate the expression of viral early and late genes. *Virology* 1989;173:700–709.
173. Inoue H, Motani-Saitoh H, Sakurada K, et al. Detection of varicella-zoster virus DNA in 414 human trigeminal ganglia from cadavers by the polymerase chain reaction: a comparison of the detection rate of varicella-zoster virus and herpes simplex virus type 1. *J Med Virol* 2010;82(2):345–349.
174. Ito H, Sommer MH, Zerboni L, et al. Promoter sequences of varicella-zoster virus glycoprotein I targeted by cellular transactivating factors Sp1 and USF determine virulence in skin and T cells in SCIDhu mice in vivo. *J Virol* 2003;77:489–498.
175. Ito H, Sommer MH, Zerboni L, et al. Role of the varicella-zoster virus gene product encoded by open reading frame 35 in viral replication in vitro and in differentiated human skin and T cells in vivo. *J Virol* 2005;79:4819–4827.
176. Jackers P, Defechereux P, Baudoux L, et al. Characterization of regulatory functions of varicella-zoster virus gene 63-encoded protein. *J Virol* 1992;66:3899–3903.
177. Jacobson MA, Berger TG, Fikrig S, et al. Acyclovir-resistant varicella zoster virus infection after chronic oral acyclovir therapy in patients with the acquired immunodeficiency syndrome (AIDS). *Ann Intern Med* 1990;112:187–191.
178. Jacquet A, Haumont M, Chellun D, et al. The varicella-zoster virus glycoprotein B (gB) plays a role in virus binding to cell heparan sulfate proteoglycans. *Virus Res* 1998;53:197–207.
179. Jenkins DE, Redman RL, Lam EM, et al. Interleukin (IL)-10, IL-12, and interferon-γ production in primary and memory immune responses to varicella-zoster virus. *J Infect Dis* 1998;178:940–948.
180. Jensen NJ, Depledge DP, Ng T, et al. Analysis of sequence variation of the VZV reiteration regions. *Virology* 2020:546:38–50.
181. Jensen NJ, Rivailler P, Tseng HF, et al. Revisiting the genotyping scheme for varicella-zoster viruses based on whole-genome comparisons. *J Gen Virol* 2017;98:1434–1438.
182. Jiang HF, Wang W, Jiang X, et al. ORF7 of varicella-zoster virus is required for viral cytoplasmic envelopment in differentiated neuronal cells. *J Virol* 2017;91:e00127.
183. Johnson R, Milbourne PE. Central nervous system manifestations of chickenpox. *Can Med Assoc J* 1970;102:831–834.
184. Johnson RW, Rice AS. Clinical practice. Postherpetic neuralgia. *N Engl J Med* 2014;371(16):1526–1533.
185. Jones JO, Arvin AM. Microarray analysis of host T cell gene transcription in response to varicella-zoster virus infection of human T cells and fibroblasts in vitro and SCIDhu skin xenografts in vivo. *J Virol* 2003;77:1268–1280.
186. Jones JO, Arvin AM. Inhibition of the NF-*k*B pathway by varicella-zoster virus in vitro and in human epidermal cells in vivo. *J Virol* 2006;80:5113–5124.
187. Jones D, Blackmon A, Neff CP, et al. Varicella-zoster virus downregulates programmed death ligand 1 and major histocompatibility complex class I in human brain vascular adventitial fibroblasts, perineurial cells, and lung fibroblasts. *J Virol* 2016;90:10527–10534.
188. Jones D, Como CN, Jing L, et al. Varicella zoster virus productively infects human peripheral blood mononuclear cells to modulate expression of immunoinhibitory proteins and blocking PD-L1 enhances virus-specific CD8+ T cell effector function. *PLoS Pathog* 2019;15:e1007650.
189. Jones M, Dry IR, Frampton D, et al. RNA-seq analysis of host and viral gene expression highlights interaction between varicella zoster virus and keratinocyte differentiation. *PLoS Pathog* 2014;10:e1003896.
190. Jones JO, Sommer M, Stamatis S, et al. Mutational analysis of the varicella-zoster virus ORF62/63 intergenic region. *J Virol* 2006;80:3116–3121.
191. Jumaan AO, Yu O, Jackson LA, et al. Incidence of herpes zoster, before and after varicella-vaccination-associated decreases in the incidence of varicella, 1992–2002. *J Infect Dis* 2005;191:2002–2007.
192. Kalpoe JS, van Dehn CE, Bollemeijer JG, et al. Varicella zoster virus (VZV)-related progressive outer retinal necrosis (PORN) after allogeneic stem cell transplantation. *Bone Marrow Transplant* 2005;36:467–469.
193. Kang JH, Ho JD, Chen YH, et al. Increased risk of stroke after a herpes zoster attack: a population-based follow-up study. *Stroke* 2009;40:3443–3448.
194. Kaufer BB, Smejkal B, Osterrieder N. The varicella-zoster virus ORFS/L (ORF0) gene is required for efficient viral replication and contains an element involved in DNA cleavage. *J Virol* 2010;84(22):11661–11669.
195. Keller PM, Davison AJ, Lowe RS, et al. Identification and structure of the gene encoding gpII, a major glycoprotein of varicella-zoster virus. *Virology* 1986;152:181–191.
196. Keller PM, Davison AJ, Lowe RS, et al. Identification and sequence of the gene encoding gpIII, a major glycoprotein of varicella-zoster virus. *Virology* 1987;157:526–533.
197. Kemble GW, Annunziato P, Lunga O, et al. Open reading frame S/L of varicella-zoster virus encodes a cytoplasmic protein expressed in infected cells. *J Virol* 2000;74:11311–11321.
198. Kennedy PGE, Grinfeld E, Craigon M, et al. Transcriptional analysis of varicella-zoster virus infection using long oligonucleotide-based microarrays. *J Gen Virol* 2005;86:2673–2684.
199. Kennedy PGE, Grinfeld E, Traina-Dorge V, et al. Neuronal localization of simian varicella virus DNA in ganglia of naturally infected African green monkeys. *Virus Genes* 2004;28:273–276.
200. Kennedy PG, Grinfield E, Gow JW. Latent varicella-zoster virus is located predominantly in neurons in human trigeminal ganglia. *Proc Natl Acad Sci U S A* 1998;95:4658–4662.
201. Kennedy JJ, Steain M, Slobedman B, et al. Infection and functional modulation of human monocytes and macrophages by varicella-zoster virus. *J Virol* 2019;93:e01887.
202. Kenyon TK, Cohen JI, Grose C. Phosphorylation by the varicella-zoster virus ORF47 protein serine kinase determines whether viral gE traffics to the TGN or recycles to the cell membrane and thereby regulates viral cell-cell spread. *J Virol* 2002;76:10980–10993.
203. Kenyon TK, Grose C. VZV ORF47 serine protein kinase and its viral substrates. *Curr Top Microbiol Immunol* 2010;342:99–111.
204. Kenyon TK, Lynch J, Hay J, et al. Varicella-zoster virus ORF47 protein serine kinase: characterization of a cloned, biologically active phosphotransferase and two viral substrates, ORF62 and ORF63. *J Virol* 2001;75:8854–8858.
205. Khalil MI, Arvin AM, Jones J, et al. A sequence within the VZV OriS is a negative regulator of DNA replication and is bound by a protein complex containing the VZV ORF 29 protein. *J Virol* 2011;85:12188–12200.
206. Khalil MI, Che X, Sung P, et al. Mutational analysis of varicella-zoster virus (VZV) immediate early protein (IE62) subdomains and their importance in viral replication. *Virology* 2016;492:82–91.
207. Khalil MI, Ruyechan WT, Hay J, et al. Differential effects of Sp cellular transcription factors on viral promoter activation by varicella-zoster virus (VZV) IE62 protein. *Virology* 2015;485:47–57.
208. Khalil MI, Sommer M, Arvin A, et al. Regulation of the varicella-zoster virus ORF3 promoter by cellular and viral factors. *Virology* 2013;440:171–181.
209. Khalil MI, Sommer M, Arvin A, et al. Cellular transcription factor YY1 mediates the varicella-zoster virus (VZV) IE62 transcriptional activation. *Virology* 2014;449:244–253.
210. Khalil MI, Sommer MH, Hay J, et al. Varicella-zoster virus (VZV) origin of DNA replication oriS influences origin-dependent DNA replication and flanking gene transcription. *Virology* 2015;481:179–186.
211. Kilgore PE, Kruszon-Moran D, Seward JF, et al. Varicella in Americans from NHANES III: implications for control through routine immunization. *J Med Virol* 2003;70:S111–S1118.
212. Kim SK, Shakya AK, Kim S, et al. Functional characterization of the serine-rich tract of varicella-zoster virus IE62. *J Virol* 2015;90:959–971.
213. Kinchington PR, Bookey D, Turse SE. The transcriptional regulatory proteins encoded by varicella-zoster virus open reading frames (ORFs) 4 and 63, but not ORF61 are associated with purified virus particles. *J Virol* 1995;69:4274–4282.
214. Kinchington PR, Fite K, Seman A, et al. Virion association of IE62, the varicella-zoster virus (VZV) major transcriptional regulatory protein, requires expression of the VZV open reading frame 66 protein kinase. *J Virol* 2001;75:9106–9113.
215. Kinchington PR, Fite K, Turse SE. Nuclear accumulation of IE62, the varicella-zoster virus (VZV) major transcriptional regulatory protein, is inhibited by phosphorylation mediated by the VZV open reading frame 66 protein kinase. *J Virol* 2000;74:2265–2277.
216. Kinchington PR, Hougland JK, Arvin AM, et al. The varicella-zoster virus immediate-early protein IE62 is a major component of virus particles. *J Virol* 1992;66:359–366.
217. Kinchington PR, Inchauspé G, Subak-Sharpe JH, et al. Identification and characterization of a varicella-zoster virus DNA-binding protein by using antisera directed against a predicted synthetic oligonucleotide. *J Virol* 1988;62:802–809.
218. Kinchington PR, Ling P, Pensiero M, et al. The glycoprotein products of varicella-zoster virus gene 14 and their defective accumulation in a vaccine strain (Oka). *J Virol* 1990;64:4540–4548.
219. Kinchington PR, Reinhold WC, Casey TA, et al. Inversion and circularization of the varicella-zoster virus genome. *J Virol* 1985;56:194–200.
220. Kinchington PR, Vergnes J-P, Defechereux P, et al. Transcriptional mapping of the varicella-zoster virus regulatory genes encoding open reading frames 4 and 63. *J Virol* 1994;68:3570–3581.
221. Klein NP, Fireman B, Yih WK, et al. Vaccine Safety Datalink. Measles-mumps-rubella-varicella combination vaccine and the risk of febrile seizures. *Pediatrics* 2010;126:e1–e8.
222. Klein A, Miller KB, Sprague K, et al. A randomized, double-blind, placebo-controlled trial of valacyclovir prophylaxis to prevent zoster recurrence from months 4 to 24 after BMT. *Bone Marrow Transplant* 2011;46(2):294–299.
223. Klippel M, Aynaud R. La paralysie faciale zostérienne. *Rev Gen Clin Therapeut* 1899;13:225.
224. Kolappaswamy K, Mahalingam R, Traina-Dorge V, et al. Disseminated simian varicella virus infection in an irradiated rhesus macaque (*Macaca mulatta*). *J Virol* 2007;81:411–415.
225. Koropchak CM, Solem SM, Diaz PS, et al. Investigation of varicella-zoster virus infection of lymphocytes by in situ hybridization. *J Virol* 1989;63:2392–2395.
226. Koshizuka T, Ota M, Yamanishi K, et al. Characterization of varicella-zoster virus-encoded ORF0 gene—comparison of parental and vaccine strains. *Virology* 2010;405:280–288.
227. Koshizuka T, Sadaoka T, Yoshii H, et al. Varicella-zoster virus ORF1 gene product is a tail-anchored membrane protein localized to plasma membrane and trans-Golgi network in infected cells. *Virology* 2008;377:289–295.

228. Kost RG, Kupinsky H, Straus SE. Varicella-zoster virus gene 63: transcript mapping and regulatory activity. *Virology* 1995;209:218–224.
229. Ku CC, Padilla J, Grose C, et al. Tropism of varicella-zoster virus for human tonsillar CD4+ T lymphocytes that express activation, memory and skin homing markers. *J Virol* 2002;76:11425–11433.
230. Ku CC, Zerboni L, Ito H, et al. Varicella-zoster virus transfer to skin by T cells and modulation of viral replication by epidermal cell interferon-α. *J Exp Med* 2004;200:917–925.
231. Kurapati S, Sadaoka T, Rajbhandari L, et al. Role of the JNK pathway in varicella-zoster virus lytic infection and reactivation. *J Virol* 2017;91:e00640.
232. Kuter BJ, Weibel RE, Guess HA, et al. Oka/Merck varicella vaccine in healthy children: final report of a 2-year efficacy study and 7-year follow-up studies. *Vaccine* 1991;9:643–647.
233. Kyratsous CA, Silverstein SJ. Components of nuclear domain 10 bodies regulate varicella-zoster virus replication. *J Virol* 2009;83(9):4262–4274.
234. Laing KJ, Russell RM, Dong L, et al. Zoster vaccination increases the breadth of CD4+ T cells responsive to varicella zoster virus. *J Infect Dis* 2015;212:1022–1031.
235. Lal H, Cunningham AL, Godeaux O, et al. Efficacy of an adjuvanted herpes zoster subunit vaccine in older adults. *N Engl J Med* 2015;372:2087–2096.
236. LaRussa P, Steinberg S, Meurice F, et al. Transmission of vaccine strain varicella-zoster virus from a healthy adult with vaccine-associated rash to susceptible household contacts. *J Infect Dis* 1997;176:1072–1075.
237. Lebrun M, Lambert J, Riva L, et al. Varicella-zoster virus ORF9p binding to cellular adaptor protein complex 1 is important for viral infectivity. *J Virol* 2018;92:e00295.
238. Lebrun M, Thelen N, Thiry M, et al. Varicella-zoster virus induces the formation of dynamic nuclear capsid aggregates. *Virology* 2014;454–455:311–327.
239. Leisenfelder SA, Kinchington PR, Moffat JF. Cyclin-dependent kinase 1/cyclin B1 phosphorylates varicella-zoster virus IE62 and is incorporated into virions. *J Virol* 2008;82:12116–12125.
240. Leisenfelder SA, Moffat JF. Varicella-zoster virus infection of human foreskin fibroblast cells results in atypical cyclin expression and cyclin-dependent kinase activity. *J Virol* 2006;80:5577–5587.
241. Levin MJ. Varicella-zoster virus and virus DNA in the blood and oropharynx of people with latent or active varicella-zoster virus infections. *J Clin Virol* 2014;61:487–495.
242. Levin MJ, Duchon JM, Swamy GK, et al. Varicella zoster immune globulin (VARIZIG) administration up to 10 days after varicella exposure in pregnant women, immunocompromised participants, and infants: varicella outcomes and safety results from a large, open-label, expanded-access program. *PLoS One* 2019;14:e0217749.
243. Levin MJ, Smith JG, Kaufhold RM, et al. Decline in varicella-zoster virus (VZV)-specific cell-mediated immunity with increasing age and boosting with a high-hose VZV vaccine. *J Infect Dis* 2003;188:1336–1344.
244. Li Q, Ali MA, Cohen JI. Insulin degrading enzyme is a cellular receptor for varicella-zoster virus infection and for cell-to-cell spread of virus. *Cell* 2006;127(2):305–316.
245. Li Q, Ali MA, Wang K, et al. Insulin degrading enzyme induces a conformational change in varicella-zoster virus gE, and enhances virus infectivity and stability. *PLoS One* 2010;5:e11327.
246. Ling P, Kinchington PR, Ruyechan WT, et al. A detailed analysis of transcripts mapping to varicella-zoster virus gene 14 (glycoprotein V). *Virology* 1991;184:625–635.
247. Litwin V, Jackson W, Grose C. Receptor properties of two varicella-zoster virus glycoproteins, gpI and gpIV, homologous to herpes simplex virus gE and gI. *J Virol* 1992;66:3643–3651.
248. Liu X, Cohen JI. Varicella-zoster virus ORF12 protein activates the phosphatidylinositol 3 kinase/Akt pathway to regulate cell cycle progression. *J Virol* 2013;87:1842–1848.
249. Liu X, Cohen JI. Inhibition of Bim enhances replication of varicella-zoster virus and delays plaque formation in virus-infected cells. *J Virol* 2014;88:1381–1388.
250. Ljungman P, Lonnqvist B, Ringden O, et al. A randomized trial of oral versus intravenous acyclovir for treatment of herpes zoster in bone marrow transplant recipients. Nordic Bone Marrow Transplant Group. *Bone Marrow Transplant* 1989;4:613–615.
251. Lungu O, Panagiotidis CA, Annunziato PW, et al. Aberrant intracellular localization of varicella-zoster virus regulatory proteins during latency. *Proc Natl Acad Sci U S A* 1998;95:7080–7085.
252. Lynch JM, Kenyon TK, Grose C, et al. Physical and functional interaction between the varicella-zoster virus IE63 and IE62 proteins. *Virology* 2002;302:71–82.
253. van der Maas NA, Bondt PE, de Melker H, et al. Acute cerebellar ataxia in the Netherlands: a study on the association with vaccinations and varicella zoster infection. *Vaccine* 2009;27:1970–1973.
254. Mace EM, Hsu AP, Monaco-Shawver L, et al. Mutations in GATA2 cause human NK cell deficiency with specific loss of the CD56(bright) subset. *Blood* 2013;121:2669–2677.
255. Mahalingam R, Gershon A, Gershon M, et al. Current in vivo models of varicella-zoster virus neurotropism. *Viruses* 2019;11:E502.
256. Mahalingam R, Kennedy PGE, Gilden D. The problems of latent varicella zoster virus in human ganglia: precise cell location and viral content. *J Neurovirol* 1999;5:445–448.
257. Mahalingam R, Lasher R, Wellish M, et al. Localization of varicella-zoster virus gene 21 protein in virus-infected cells in culture. *J Virol* 1998;72:6832–6837.
258. Mahalingam R, Traina-Dorge V, Wellish M, et al. Latent simian varicella virus reactivates in monkeys treated with tacrolimus with or without exposure to irradiation. *J Neurovirol* 2010b;16:342–354.
259. Mahalingam R, Wellish M, Cohrs R, et al. Expression of protein encoded by varicella-zoster virus open reading frame 63 in latently infected human ganglionic neurons. *Proc Natl Acad Sci U S A* 1996;93:2122–2124.
260. Mahalingam R, Wellish M, Wolf Q, et al. Latent varicella-zoster virus DNA in human trigeminal and thoracic ganglia. *N Engl J Med* 1990;323:627–631.
261. Mallory S, Sommer M, Arvin AM. Mutational analysis of the role of glycoprotein I in varicella-zoster virus replication and its effects on glycoprotein E conformation and trafficking. *J Virol* 1997;71:8279–8288.
262. Maresova L, Kutinova L, Ludvikova V, et al. Characterization of interaction of gH and gL glycoproteins of varicella-zoster virus: their processing and trafficking. *J Gen Virol* 2000;81:1545–1552.
263. Maresova L, Pasieka TJ, Homan E, et al. Incorporation of three endocytosed varicella-zoster virus glycoproteins, gE, gH, and gB into the virion envelope. *J Virol* 2005;79:997–1007.
264. Marin M, Leung J, Gershon AA. Transmission of vaccine-strain varicella-zoster virus: a systematic review. *Pediatrics* 2019;144:e20191305.
265. Marin M, Meissner HC, Seward JF. Varicella prevention in the United States: a review of successes and challenges. *Pediatrics* 2008;122(3):e744–e751.
266. Marin M, Zhang JX, Seward JF. Near elimination of varicella deaths in the U.S. after implementation of the vaccination program. *Pediatrics* 2011;128:214–220.
267. Markus A, Waldman Ben-Asher H, Kinchington PR, et al. Cellular transcriptome analysis reveals differential expression of pro- and antiapoptosis genes by varicella-zoster virus-infected neurons and fibroblasts. *J Virol* 2014;88:7674–7677.
268. Markus A, Golani L, Ojha NK, et al. Varicella-Zoster virus expresses multiple small noncoding RNAs. *J Virol* 2017;91:e01710.
269. Markus A, Lebenthal-Loinger I, Yang IH, et al. An in vitro model of latency and reactivation of varicella zoster virus in human stem cell-derived neurons. *PLoS Pathog* 2015;11:e1004885.
270. Meier JL, Luo X, Sawadogo M, et al. The cellular transcription factor USF cooperates with varicella-zoster virus immediate-early protein 62 to symmetrically activate a bidirectional viral promoter. *Mol Cell Biol* 1994;10:6896–6906.
271. Merigan TC, Rand KH, Pollard RB, et al. Human leukocyte interferon for the treatment of herpes zoster in patients with cancer. *N Engl J Med* 1978;298:981–987.
272. Messaoudi I, Barron A, Wellish M, et al. Simian varicella virus infection of rhesus macaques recapitulates essential features of varicella zoster virus infection in humans. *PLoS Pathog* 2009;5(11):e1000657.
273. Meysman P, Ogunjimi B, Naulaerts S, et al. Varicella-zoster virus-derived major histocompatibility complex class I-restricted peptide affinity is a determining factor in the HLA risk profile for the development of postherpetic neuralgia. *J Virol* 2015;89:962–969.
274. Miller E, Cradock-Watson JE, Ridehalgh MK. Outcome in newborn babies given anti-varicella-zoster immunoglobulin after perinatal maternal infection with varicella-zoster virus. *Lancet* 1989;2:371–373.
275. Mirouse A, Vignon P, Piron P, et al. Severe varicella-zoster virus pneumonia: a multicenter cohort study. *Crit Care* 2017;21:137.
276. Mo C, Lee J, Sommer M, et al. The requirement of varicella-zoster virus glycoprotein E (gE) for viral replication and effects of glycoprotein I on gE in melanoma cells. *Virology* 2002;304:176–186.
277. Mo C, Schneeberger EE, Arvin AM. Glycoprotein E of varicella-zoster virus enhances cell–cell contact in polarized epithelial cells. *J Virol* 2000;74:11377–11387.
278. Mo C, Suen J, Sommer M, et al. Characterization of varicella-zoster virus glycoprotein K (open reading frame 5) and its role in virus growth. *J Virol* 1999;73:4197–4207.
279. Moffat JF, Ito H, Sommer M, et al. Glycoprotein I of varicella-zoster virus is required for viral replication in skin and T cells. *J Virol* 2002;76:8468–8471.
280. Moffat JF, Mo C, Cheng JJ, et al. Functions of C-terminal domain of varicella-zoster virus glycoprotein E in viral replication in vitro and skin and T-cell tropism in vivo. *J Virol* 2004;78:12406–12415.
281. Moffat JF, Zerboni L, Kinchington PR, et al. Attenuation of the vaccine Oka strain of varicella-zoster virus and role of glycoprotein C in alphaherpesvirus virulence demonstrated in the SCID-hu mouse. *J Virol* 1998;72:965–974.
282. Moffat JF, Zerboni L, Sommer MH, et al. The ORF47 and ORF66 putative protein kinases of varicella-zoster virus determine tropism for human T cells and skin in the SCID-hu mouse. *Proc Natl Acad Sci U S A* 1998;95:11969–11974.
283. Montalvo EA, Grose C. Neutralization epitope of varicella-zoster virus on native viral glycoprotein gp118 (VZV glycoprotein gpIII). *Virology* 1986;149:230–241.
284. Montalvo EA, Parmley RT, Grose C. Structural analysis of the varicella-zoster virus gp98-gp62 complex: posttranslational addition of N-linked and O-linked oligosaccharide moieties. *J Virol* 1985;53:761–770.
285. Mori Y, Sadaoka T. Varicella-zoster virus glycoprotein M. *Curr Top Microbiol Immunol* 2010;342:147–154.
286. Moriuchi H, Moriuchi M, Cohen JI. The varicella-zoster virus immediate-early 62 promoter contains a negative regulatory element that binds transcription factor NF-Y. *Virology* 1995;214:256–258.
287. Moriuchi H, Moriuchi M, Debrus S, et al. The acidic amino-terminal region of varicella-zoster open reading frame 4 protein is required for transactivation and can functionally replace the corresponding region of herpes simplex virus ICP27. *Virology* 1995;208:376–382.
288. Moriuchi H, Moriuchi M, Pichyangkura R, et al. Hydrophobic cluster analysis predicts an amino-terminal domain of varicella-zoster virus open reading frame 10 required for transcriptional activation. *Proc Natl Acad Sci U S A* 1995;92:9333–9337.
289. Moriuchi H, Moriuchi M, Smith HA, et al. Varicella-zoster open reading frame 61 protein is functionally homologous to herpes simplex virus type 1 ICP0. *J Virol* 1992;66:7303–7308.
290. Moriuchi H, Moriuchi M, Straus SE, et al. Varicella-zoster virus open reading frame 10 protein, the herpes simplex virus VP16 homolog, transactivates herpesvirus immediate-early gene promoters. *J Virol* 1993;67:2739–2746.
291. Moriuchi H, Moriuchi M, Straus SE, et al. Varicella-zoster virus (VZV) open reading frame 61 protein transactivates VZV gene promoters and enhances the infectivity of VZV DNA. *J Virol* 1993;67:4290–4295.
292. Morrow G, Slobedman B, Cunningham AL, et al. Varicella-zoster virus productively infects mature dendritic cells and alters their immune function. *J Virol* 2003;77:4950–4959.
293. Mueller NH, Gilden D, Cohrs RJ. Varicella-zoster virus open reading frame 48 encodes an active nuclease. *J Virol* 2013;87:11936–11938.
294. Mullane KM, Morrison VA, Camacho LH, et al. Safety and efficacy of inactivated varicella zostervirus vaccine in immunocompromised patients with malignancies: a two-arm, randomised, double-blind, phase 3 trial. *Lancet Infect Dis* 2019;19:1001–1012.
295. Mullane KM, Nuss C, Ridgeway K, et al. Brincidofovir treatment of acyclovir-resistant disseminated varicella zoster virus infection in an immunocompromised host. *Transpl Infect Dis* 2016;18:785–790.

296. Nader S, Bergen R, Sharp M, et al. Age-related differences in cell-mediated immunity to varicella-zoster virus among children and adults immunized with live attenuated varicella vaccine. *J Infect Dis* 1995;171:13–17.
297. Nagel MA, Bubak AN. Varicella zoster virus vasculopathy. *J Infect Dis* 2018;218:S107–S112.
298. Nagel MA, Choe A, Cohrs RJ, et al. Persistence of varicella zoster virus DNA in saliva after herpes zoster. *J Infect Dis* 2011;204:820–824.
299. Nagel MA, Choe A, Traktinskiy I, et al. Varicella-zoster virus transcriptome in latently infected human ganglia. *J Virol* 2011;85(5):2276–2287.
300. Nagel MA, White T, Khmeleva N, et al. Analysis of varicella-zoster virus in temporal arteries biopsy positive and negative for giant cell arteritis. *JAMA Neurol* 2015;72:1281–1287.
301. Narayanan A, Nogueira ML, Ruyechan WT, et al. Combinatorial transcription of herpes simplex virus and varicella zoster virus immediate early genes is strictly determined by the cellular coactivator HCF-1. *J Biol Chem* 2005;280:1369–1375.
302. Ng TI, Keenan L, Kinchington PR, et al. Phosphorylation of varicella-zoster virus open reading frame (ORF) 62 regulatory product by viral ORF47-associated protein kinase. *J Virol* 1994;68:1350–1359.
303. Nguyen HQ, Jumaan AO, Seward JF. Decline in mortality due to varicella after implementation of varicella vaccination in the United States. *N Engl J Med* 2005;352:450–458.
304. Niizuma T, Zerboni L, Sommer M, et al. Construction of varicella-zoster virus recombinants from parental Oka cosmids and demonstration that ORF65 protein is dispensable for infection of human skin and T cells in the SCID-hu mouse model. *J Virol* 2003;77:6062–6065.
305. Nikkels AF, Debrus S, Sadzot-Delvaux C, et al. Localization of varicella-zoster virus nucleic acids and proteins in human skin. *Neurology* 1995;45(Suppl):S47–S49.
306. Nikzad R, Angelo LS, Aviles-Padilla K, et al. Human natural killer cells mediate adaptive immunity to viral antigens. *Sci Immunol* 2019;4:eaat8116.
307. Norberg P, Depledge DP, Kundu S, et al. Recombination of globally circulating varicella zoster virus. *J Virol* 2015;89:7133–7146.
308. Nour AM, Reichelt M, Ku CC, et al. Varicella-zoster virus infection triggers formation of an interleukin-1β (il-1β)-processing inflammasome complex. *J Biol Chem* 2011;286(20):17921–17933.
309. Ogunjimi B, Zhang SY, Sørensen KB, et al. Inborn errors in RNA polymerase III underlie severe varicella zoster virus infections. *J Clin Invest* 2017;127:3543–3556.
310. Oliver SL, Brady JJ, Sommer MH, et al. An immunoreceptor tyrosine-based inhibition motif in varicella-zoster virus glycoprotein B regulates cell fusion and skin pathogenesis. *Proc Natl Acad Sci U S A* 2013;110:1911–1916.
311. Oliver SL, Sommer MH, Reichelt M, et al. Mutagenesis of varicella-zoster virus glycoprotein I (gI) identifies a cysteine residue critical for gE/gI heterodimer formation, gI structure, and virulence in skin cells. *J Virol* 2011;85(9):4095–4110.
312. Oliver SL, Sommer M, Zerboni L, et al. Mutagenesis of varicella-zoster virus glycoprotein B: putative fusion loop residues are essential for viral replication, and the furin cleavage motif contributes to pathogenesis in skin tissue in vivo. *J Virol* 2009;83:7495–7506.
313. Oliver SL, Xing Y, Chen DH, et al. The N-terminus of varicella-zoster virus glycoprotein B has a functional role in fusion. *PLoS Pathog* 2021;17(1):e1008961. doi:10.1371/journal.ppat.1008961.
314. Oliver SL, Yang E, Arvin AM. Dysregulated glycoprotein B-mediated cell-cell fusion disrupts varicella-zoster virus and host gene transcription during infection. *J Virol* 2016;91:e01613.
315. Oliver S, Yi Xing U, Chen D-H, et al. A glycoprotein B-neutralizing antibody structure at 2.8 Å uncovers a critical domain for herpesvirus fusion initiation. *Nat Commun* 2020;11:4141. doi:10.1038/s41467-020-17911-0.
316. Oliver SL, Zerboni L, Sommer M, et al. Development of recombinant varicella-zoster viruses expressing luciferase fusion proteins for live in vivo imaging in human skin and dorsal root ganglia xenografts. *J Virol Methods* 2008;154:182–193.
317. Olson JK, Grose C. Endocytosis and recycling of varicella-zoster virus Fc receptor glycoprotein gE: internalization mediated by a YXXL motif in the cytoplasmic tail. *J Virol* 1997;71:4042–4054.
318. Olson JK, Grose C. Complex formation facilitates endocytosis of the varicella-zoster virus gE:gI receptor. *J Virol* 1998;72:1542–1551.
319. Ote I, Lebrun M, Vandevenne P, et al. Varicella-zoster virus IE4 protein interacts with SR proteins and exports mRNAs through the TAP/NXF1 pathway. *PLoS One* 2009;4(11):e7882.
320. Ote I Piette J Sadzot-Delvaux C. The varicella-zoster virus IE4 protein: a conserved member of the herpesviral mRNA export factors family and a potential alternative target in antiherpetic therapies. *Biochem Pharmacol* 2010;80:1973–1980.
321. Ouwendijk WJ, Choe A, Nagel MA, et al. Restricted varicella-zoster virus transcription in human trigeminal ganglia obtained soon after death. *J Virol* 2012;86:10203–10206.
322. Ouwendijk WJ, Verjans GM. Pathogenesis of varicelloviruses in primates. *J Pathol* 2015;235:298–311.
323. Oxman MN, Levin MJ, Johnson GR, et al. Shingles prevention study group. A vaccine to prevent herpes zoster and postherpetic neuralgia in older adults. *N Engl J Med* 2005;352:2271–2284.
324. Ozaki T, Ichikawa T, Matsui Y, et al. Lymphocyte-associated viremia in varicella. *J Med Virol* 1986;19:249–253.
325. Parrino J, McNeil SA, Lawrence SJ, et al. Safety and immunogenicity of inactivated varicella-zoster virus vaccine in adults with hematologic malignancies receiving treatment with anti-CD20 monoclonal antibodies. *Vaccine* 2017;35:1764–1769.
326. Pasieka TJ, Maresova L, Grose C. A functional YNK1 motif in the short cytoplasmic tail of varicella-zoster virus glycoprotein gH mediates clathrin-dependent and antibody-independent endocytosis. *J Virol* 2003;77:4191–4204.
327. Pasieka TJ, Maresova L, Shiraki K, et al. Regulation of varicella-zoster virus-induced cell-to-cell fusion by the endocytosis-competent glycoproteins gH and gE. *J Virol* 2004;78:2884–2896.
328. Patel RA, Binns HJ, Shulman ST. Reduction in pediatric hospitalizations for varicella-related invasive group A streptococcal infections in the varicella vaccine era. *J Pediatr* 2004;144:68–74.
329. Peng H, He H, Hay J, et al. Interaction between the varicella-zoster virus IE62 major transactivator and cellular transcription factor SP1. *J Biol Chem* 2003;278:38068–38075.
330. Perera LP. The TATA motif specifies the differential activation of minimal promoters by varicella-zoster virus immediate-early regulatory protein IE62. *J Biol Chem* 2000;275:487–496.
331. Perera LP, Kaushal S, Kinchington PR, et al. Varicella-zoster open reading frame 4 encodes a transcriptional activator that is functionally different from that of herpes simplex virus homolog ICP27. *J Virol* 1994;68:2468–2477.
332. Perera LP, Mosca JD, Ruyechan WT, et al. Regulation of varicella-zoster virus gene expression in human T lymphocytes. *J Virol* 1992;66:5298–5304.
333. Perera LP, Mosca JD, Sadeghi-Zadeh M, et al. The varicella-zoster virus immediate early protein, IE62, can positively regulate its cognate promoter. *Virology* 1992;191:346–354.
334. Petursson G, Helgason S, Gudmundsson S, et al. Herpes zoster in children and adolescents. *Pediatr Infect Dis J* 1998;17:905–908.
335. Pevenstein SR, Williams RK, McChesney D, et al. Quantitation of latent varicella-zoster virus and herpes simplex virus genomes in human trigeminal ganglia. *J Virol* 1999;73:10514–10518.
336. Plotkin SA, Stein S, Snyder M, et al. Attempts to recover varicella virus from ganglia. *Ann Neurol* 1977;2:249.
337. Pontremoli C, Forni D, Clerici M, et al. Possible European origin of circulating varicella-zoster virus strains. *J Infect Dis* 2020;221:1286–1294.
338. Prazsák I, Moldován N, Balázs Z, et al. Long-read sequencing uncovers a complex transcriptome topology in varicella zoster virus. *BMC Genomics* 2018;19:873.
339. Preston VG, Kennard J, Rixon FJ, et al. Efficient herpes simplex virus type 1 (HSV-1) capsid formation directed by the varicella-zoster virus scaffolding protein requires the carboxy-terminal sequences from the HSV-1 homologue. *J Gen Virol* 1997;78:1633–1646.
340. Pugazhenthi S, Nair S, Velmurugan K, et al. Varicella zoster virus infection of differentiated human neural stem cells. *J Virol* 2011;85:6678–6686.
341. Qi Q, Cavanagh MM, Le Saux S, et al. Diversification of the antigen-specific T cell receptor repertoire after varicella zoster vaccination. *Sci Transl Med* 2016;8:332ra46.
342. Qi Q, Cavanagh MM, Le Saux S, et al. Defective T memory cell differentiation after varicella zoster vaccination in older individuals. *PLoS Pathog* 2016; 12:e1005892.
343. Qiu X, Janson CA, Culp JS, et al. Crystal structure of the varicella-zoster virus protease. *Proc Natl Acad Sci U S A* 1997;94:2874–2879.
344. Quinlivan ML, Ayres KL, Kelly PJ, et al. Persistence of varicella-zoster virus viraemia in patients with herpes zoster. *J Clin Virol* 2011;50(2):130–135.
345. Quinlivan ML, Gershon AA, Al Bassam MM, et al. Natural selection for rash-forming genotypes of the varicella-zoster vaccine virus detected within immunized human hosts. *Proc Natl Acad Sci U S A* 2007;104:208–212.
346. Quinlivan MA, Gershon AA, Nichols RA, et al. Vaccine Oka varicella-zoster virus genotypes are monomorphic in single vesicles and polymorphic in respiratory tract secretions. *J Infect Dis* 2006;193:927–930.
347. Rahaus M, Desloges N, Wolff MH. Varicella-zoster virus requires a functional PI3K/Akt/GSK-3alpha/beta signaling cascade for efficient replication. *Cell Signal* 2007;19:312–320.
348. Rahaus M, Desloges N, Yang M, et al. Transcription factor USF, expressed during the entire phase of varicella-zoster virus infection, interacts physically with the major viral transactivator IE62 and plays a significant role in virus replication. *J Gen Virol* 2003;2957–2967.
349. Reddy SM, Cox E, Iofin I, et al. Varicella-zoster virus (VZV) ORF32 encodes a phosphoprotein that is posttranslationally modified by the VZV ORF47 protein kinase. *J Virol* 1998;72:8083–8088.
350. Redman RL, Nader S, Zerboni L, et al. Early reconstitution of immunity and decreased severity of herpes zoster in bone marrow transplant recipients immunized with inactivated varicella vaccine. *J Infect Dis* 1997;176:578–585.
351. Reichelt M, Brady J, Arvin AM. The replication cycle of varicella-zoster virus: analysis of the kinetics of viral protein expression, genome synthesis, and virion assembly at the single-cell level. *J Virol* 2009;83:3904–3918.
352. Reichelt M, Joubert L, Perrino J, et al. Three-dimensional reconstruction of VZV infected cell nuclei and PML nuclear cages by serial section array scanning electron microscopy and electron tomography. *PLoS Pathog* 2012;8:e100274.
353. Reichelt M, Wang L, Sommer M, et al. Entrapment of viral capsids in nuclear PML cages is an intrinsic antiviral host defense against varicella-zoster virus. *PLoS Pathog* 2011;7:e1001266.
354. Reichelt M, Zerboni L, Arvin AM. Mechanisms of varicella-zoster virus neuropathogenesis in human dorsal root ganglia. *J Virol* 2008;82:3971–3983.
355. Riva L, Thiry M, Bontems S, et al. ORF9p phosphorylation by ORF47p is crucial for the formation and egress of varicella-zoster virus viral particles. *J Virol* 2013;87:2868–2881.
356. Riva L, Thiry M, Lebrun M, et al. Deletion of the ORF9p acidic cluster impairs the nuclear egress of varicella-zoster virus capsids. *J Virol* 2015;89:2436–2441.
357. Ross AH. Modification of chickenpox in family contacts by administration of gamma globulin. *N Engl J Med* 1962;267:369–376.
358. Ross J, Williams M, Cohen JI. Disruption of the varicella-zoster virus dUTPase and the adjacent ORF9A gene results in impaired growth and reduced syncytia formation in vitro. *Virology* 1997;234:186–195.
359. Rowe J, Greenblatt RJ, Liu D, et al. Compounds that target host cell proteins prevent varicella-zoster virus replication in culture, ex vivo, and in SCID-Hu mice. *Antiviral Res* 2010;86:276–285.
360. Ruyechan WT. Roles of cellular transcription factors in VZV replication. *Curr Top Microbiol Immunol* 2010;342:43–65.
361. Sadaoka T, Depledge DP, Rajbhandari L, et al. In vitro system using human neurons demonstrates that varicella-zoster vaccine virus is impaired for reactivation, but not latency. *Proc Natl Acad Sci U S A* 2016;113:e2403.
362. Sadaoka T, Schwartz CL, Rajbhandari L, et al. Human embryonic stem cell-derived neurons are highly permissive for varicella-zoster virus lytic infection. *J Virol* 2017;92:e01108.
363. Sadaoka T, Serada S, Kato J, et al. Varicella-zoster virus ORF49 functions in the efficient production of progeny virus through its interaction with essential tegument protein ORF44. *J Virol* 2014;88:188–201.

364. Sadaoka T Yanagi T, Yamanishi K, et al. Characterization of the varicella-zoster virus ORF50 gene, which encodes glycoprotein M. *J Virol* 2010;84:3488–3502.
365. Sadzot-Delvaux C, Kinchington P, Rentier B, et al. Recognition of the latency-associated immediate early protein IE63 of varicella-zoster virus by human memory T lymphocytes. *J Immunol* 1997;159:2802–2806.
366. Santos RA, Hatfield CC, Cole NL, et al. Varicella-zoster virus gE escape mutant VZV-MSP exhibits an accelerated cell-to-cell spread phenotype in both infected cell cultures and SCID-hu mice. *Virology* 2000;275:306–317.
367. Santos RA, Padilla JA, Hatfield C, et al. Antigenic variation of varicella zoster virus Fc receptor gE: loss of a major B cell epitope in the ectodomain. *Virology* 1998;249:21–31.
368. Sato H, Callanan LD, Pesnicak L, et al. Varicella-zoster virus (VZV) ORF17 protein induces RNA cleavage and is critical for replication of VZV at 37°C, but not 33°C. *J Virol* 2002;76:11012–11023.
369. Sato B, Ito H, Hinchliffe S, et al. Mutational analysis of open reading frames 62 and 71, encoding the varicella-zoster virus immediate-early transactivating protein, IE62, and effects on replication in vitro and in skin xenografts in the SCID-hu mouse in vivo. *J Virol* 2003;77:5607–5620.
370. Sato H, Pesnicak L, Cohen JI. Varicella-zoster virus ORF2 encodes a membrane phosphoprotein that is dispensable for viral replication and for establishment of latency. *J Virol* 2002;76:3575–3578.
371. Sato B, Sommer MH, Ito H, et al. The requirement of varicella-zoster virus immediate early 4 protein for viral replication. *J Virol* 2003;77:12369–12372.
372. Sawyer MH, Chamberlin CJ, Wu YN, et al. Detection of varicella-zoster virus DNA in air samples from hospital rooms. *J Infect Dis* 1994;169:91–94.
373. Sawyer MH, Inchauspé G, Biron KK, et al. Molecular analysis of the pyrimidine deoxyribonucleoside kinase gene of wild-type and acyclovir-resistant strains of varicella-zoster virus. *J Gen Virol* 1988;69:2585–2593.
374. Schaap A, Fortin J-F, Sommer M, et al. T-cell tropism and the role of ORF66 protein in pathogenesis of varicella-zoster virus infection. *J Virol* 2005;79:12921–12933.
375. Schaap-Nutt A, Sommer M, Che X, et al. ORF66 protein kinase function is required for T-cell tropism of varicella-zoster virus in vivo. *J Virol* 2006;80(23):11806–11816.
376. Schmid DS. Varicella-zoster virus vaccine: molecular genetics. *Curr Top Microbiol Immunol* 2010;342:323–340.
377. Schmidt NJ, Lennette EH. Neutralizing antibody responses to varicella-zoster virus. *Infect Immun* 1975;12:606–613.
378. Science M, MacGregor D, Richardson SE, et al. Central nervous system complications of varicella-zoster virus. *J Pediatr* 2014;165:779–785.
379. Sen N, Che X, Rajamani J, et al. STAT3 activation and survivin induction by varicella zoster virus promotes viral replication and skin pathogenesis. *Proc Natl Acad Sci U S A* 2012;109:600–605.
380. Sen N, Mukherjee G, Sen A, et al. Single-cell mass cytometry analysis of human tonsil T cell remodeling by varicella zoster virus. *Cell Rep* 2014;8:633–645.
381. Sen N, Sommer M, Che X, et al. Varicella-zoster virus immediate-early protein 62 blocks interferon regulatory factor 3 (IRF3) phosphorylation at key serine residues: a novel mechanism of IRF3 inhibition among herpesviruses. *J Virol* 2010;84:9240–9253.
382. Sen N, Sung P, Panda A, et al. Distinctive roles for type I and type II interferons and interferon regulatory factors in the host cell defense against varicella-zoster virus. *J Virol* 2018;92:e01151.
383. Shakya AK, O'Callaghan DJ, Kim SK. Interferon gamma inhibits varicella-zoster virus replication in a cell line-dependent manner. *J Virol* 2019;93:e00257.
384. Sharp M, Terada K, Wilson A, et al. Kinetics and viral protein specificity of the cytotoxic T lymphocyte response in healthy adults immunized with live attenuated varicella vaccine. *J Infect Dis* 1992;165:852–858.
385. Sloan E, Henriquez R, Kinchington PR, et al. Varicella-zoster virus inhibition of the NF-κB pathway during infection of human dendritic cells: role for open reading frame 61 as a modulator of NF-κB activity. *J Virol* 2012;86:1193–1202.
386. Solomon IH, Docken WP, Padera RF Jr. Investigating the association of giant cell arteritis with varicella zoster virus in temporal artery biopsies or ascending aortic resections. *J Rheumatol* 2019;46:1614–1618.
387. Sommer MH, Zagha E, Serrano OK. Mutational analysis of the repeated open reading frames, ORFs 63 and 70 and ORF 64 and 69, of varicella-zoster virus. *J Virol* 2001;75:8224–8239.
388. Spector T, Stonehueerner JG, Biron KK, et al. Ribonucleotide reductase induced by varicella-zoster virus: characterization, and potentiation of acyclovir by its inhibition. *Biochem Pharmacol* 1987;36:4341–4346.
389. Spengler ML, Ruyechan WT, Hay J. Physical interaction between two varicella-zoster virus gene regulatory proteins, IE4 and IE62. *Virology* 2000;272:375–381.
390. Stallings CL, Silverstein S. Dissection of a novel nuclear localization signal in open reading frame 29 of varicella-zoster virus. *J Virol* 2005;79:13070–13081.
391. Steain M, Gowrishankar K, Rodriguez M, et al. Upregulation of CXCL10 in human dorsal root ganglia during experimental and natural varicella-zoster virus infection. *J Virol* 2011;85:626–631.
392. Steain M, Sutherland JP, Rodriguez M, et al. Analysis of T cell responses during active varicella-zoster virus reactivation in human ganglia. *J Virol* 2014;88:2704–2716.
393. Steiner G. Zür inokulation der varicellen. *Wien Med Wochenschr* 1875;25:306.
394. Stevens DA, Merigan TC. Zoster immune globulin prophylaxis of disseminated zoster in compromised hosts. *Arch Intern Med* 1980;140:52–54.
395. Stevenson D, Colman KL, Davison AJ. Characterization of the putative protein kinases specified by varicella-zoster virus genes 47 and 66. *J Gen Virol* 1994;75:317–326.
396. Stevenson D, Colman KL, Davison AJ. Delineation of a sequence required for nuclear localization of the protein encoded by varicella-zoster virus gene 61. *J Gen Virol* 1994;75:3229–3233.
397. Stevenson D, Xue M, Hay J, et al. Phosphorylation and nuclear localization of the varicella-zoster virus gene 63 protein. *J Virol* 1996;70:658–662.
398. Storlie J, Carpenter JE, Jackson W, et al. Discordant varicella-zoster virus glycoprotein C expression and localization between cultured cells and human skin vesicles. *Virology* 2008;382(2):171–181.
399. Stow ND, Weir HM, Stow EC. Analysis of the binding sites for the varicella-zoster virus gene 51 product within the viral origin of DNA replication. *Virology* 1990;177:570–577.
400. Straus SE, Aulakh HS, Ruyechan WT, et al. Structure of varicella-zoster virus DNA. *J Virol* 1981;40:516–525.
401. Straus SE, Owens J, Ruyechan WT, et al. Molecular cloning and physical mapping of varicella-zoster virus DNA. *Proc Natl Acad Sci U S A* 1982;79:993–997.
402. Straus SE, Reinhold W, Smith HA, et al. Endonuclease analysis of viral DNA from varicella and subsequent zoster infection in the same patient. *N Engl J Med* 1984;311:1362–1364.
403. Suenaga T, Matsumoto M, Arisawa F, et al. Sialic acids on varicella-zoster virus glycoprotein B are required for cell-cell fusion. *J Biol Chem* 2015;290:19833–19843.
404. Suenaga T, Satoh T, Somboonthum P, et al. Myelin-associated glycoprotein mediates membrane fusion and entry of neurotropic herpesviruses. *Proc Natl Acad Sci U S A* 2010;107(2):866–871.
405. Sullivan NL, Reuter-Monslow MA, Sei J, et al. Breadth and functionality of Varicella-zoster virus glycoprotein-specific antibodies identified after Zostavax vaccination in humans. *J Virol* 2018;92:e00269.
406. Sutherland JP, Steain M, Buckland ME, et al. Persistence of a T cell infiltrate in human ganglia years after herpes zoster and during post-herpetic neuralgia. *Front Microbiol* 2019;10:2117.
407. Szpara M, Tafuri Y, Parsons L, et al. A wide extent of inter-strain diversity in virulent and vaccine strains of alpha-herpesviruses. *PLoS Pathog* 2011;7(10):e1002282.
408. Takahashi M, Asano Y, Kamiya H, et al. Development of varicella vaccine. *J Infect Dis* 2008;197(Suppl 2):S41–S44.
409. Takahashi MN, Jackson W, Laird DT, et al. Varicella-zoster virus infection induces autophagy in both cultured cells and human skin vesicles. *J Virol* 2009;83:5466–5476.
410. Taylor S, Kinchington PR, Brooks A, et al. Roscovitine, a cyclin-dependent kinase inhibitor, prevents replication of varicella-zoster virus. *J Virol* 2004;78:2853–2862.
411. Terada K, Kawano S, Yagi Y, et al. Alteration of T cells and natural killer cells during chickenpox in infancy. *J Clin Immunol* 1996;16:55–59.
412. Thompson R, Honess RW, Taylor L, et al. Varicella-zoster virus specifies a thymidylate synthetase. *J Gen Virol* 1987;68:1449–1455.
413. Tischer BK, Kaufer BB, Sommer M, et al. A self-excisable infectious bacterial artificial chromosome clone of varicella-zoster virus allows analysis of the essential tegument protein encoded by ORF9. *J Virol* 2007;81:13200–13208.
414. Traina-Dorge V, Doyle-Meyers LA, Sanford R, et al. Simian varicella virus is present in macrophages, dendritic cells, and T cells in lymph nodes of rhesus macaques after experimental reactivation. *J Virol* 2015;89:9817–9824.
415. Traina-Dorge V, Palmer BE, Coleman C, et al. Reactivation of simian varicella virus in rhesus macaques after CD4 T cell depletion. *J Virol* 2020;93:e01375.
416. Tsolia M, Gershon AA, Steinberg SP, et al. Live attenuated varicella vaccine: evidence that the virus is attenuated and the importance of skin lesions in transmission of varicella-zoster virus. NIAID Varicella Vaccine Collaborative Study Group. *J Pediatr* 1990;116:184–189.
417. Tyler JK, Everett RD. The DNA binding domains of the varicella-zoster gene 62 and herpes simplex virus type 1 ICP4 transactivator proteins heterodimerize and bind to DNA. *Nucleic Acids Res* 1994;22:711–721.
418. Tyring S, Barbarash RA, Nahlik JE, et al. Famciclovir for the treatment of acute herpes zoster: Effects on acute disease and postherpetic neuralgia: a randomized, double-blind, placebo-controlled trial. Collaborative Famciclovir Herpes Zoster Study Group. *Ann Intern Med* 1995;123:89–96.
419. Tyzzer EE. The histology of skin lesions in varicella. *J Med Res* 1906;14:361–392.
420. Umbach JL, Nagel MA, Cohrs RJ, et al. Analysis of human alphaherpesvirus microRNA expression in latently infected human trigeminal ganglia. *J Virol* 2009;83(20):10677–10683.
421. Vafai A, Wellish M, Gilden DH. Expression of varicella-zoster virus in blood mononuclear cells of patients with postherpetic neuralgia. *Proc Natl Acad Sci U S A* 1988;85:2767–2770.
422. Varicella and herpes zoster vaccines: WHO position paper, June 2014—Recommendations. *Vaccine* 2016;34:198–199.
423. Vazquez M, LaRussa PS, Gershon AA, et al. Effectiveness over time of varicella vaccine. *JAMA* 2004;291:851–855.
424. van Velzen M, Ouwendijk WJ, Selke S, et al. Longitudinal study on oral shedding of herpes simplex virus 1 and varicella-zoster virus in individuals infected with HIV. *J Med Virol* 2013;85:1669–1677.
425. Verdijk RM, Ouwendijk WJD, Kuijpers RWAM, et al. No evidence of varicella-zoster virus infection in temporal artery biopsies of anterior ischemic optic neuropathy patients with and without giant cell arteritis. *J Infect Dis* 2021;223(1):109-112. doi: 10.1093/infdis/jiaa566.
426. Visalli MA, House BL, Selariu A, et al. The varicella-zoster virus portal protein is essential for cleavage and packaging of viral DNA. *J Virol* 2014;88:7973–7986.
427. Visalli RJ, Knepper J, Goshorn B, et al. Characterization of the varicella-zoster virus ORF25 gene product: pORF25 interacts with multiple DNA encapsidation proteins. *Virus Res* 2009;144:58–64.
428. Vleck SE, Oliver SL, Brady J, et al. Structure-function analysis of varicella-zoster virus glycoprotein H identifies domain-specific roles for fusion and skin tropism. *Proc Natl Acad Sci U S A* 2011;108:18412–18417.
429. Vleck SE, Oliver SL, Reichelt M, et al. Anti-glycoprotein H antibody impairs the pathogenicity of varicella-zoster virus in skin xenografts in the SCID mouse model. *J Virol* 2010;84:141–152.
430. Vukmanovic-Stejic M, Sandhu D, Seidel JA, et al. The characterization of varicella zoster virus-specific T cells in skin and blood during aging. *J Invest Dermatol* 2015;135:1752–1762.
431. Vukmanovic-Stejic M, Sandhu D, Sobande TO, et al. Varicella zoster-specific CD4+Foxp3+ T cells accumulate after cutaneous antigen challenge in humans. *J Immunol* 2013;190:977–986.
432. Wagner HJ, Seidel A, Grande-Nagel I, et al. Pre-eruptive varicella encephalitis: case report and review of the literature. *Eur J Pediatr* 1998;157:814–815.
433. Wallace MR, Chamberlin CC, Zerboni L, et al. Lack of evidence for recurrent varicella in immunocompetent adults. *JAMA* 1997;278:1520–1522.
434. Wallace MR, Woelfl I, Bowler WA, et al. Tumor necrosis factor, interleukin-2 and interferon-γ in adult varicella. *J Med Virol* 1994;43:69–71.

435. Walters MS, Erazo A, Kinchington PR, et al. Histone deacetylases 1 and 2 are phosphorylated at novel sites during varicella-zoster virus infection. *J Virol* 2009;83:11502–11513.
436. Walters MS, Kinchington PR, Banfield BW, et al. Hyperphosphorylation of histone deacetylase 2 by alphaherpesvirus US3 kinases. *J Virol* 2010;84:9666–9676.
437. Walters MS, Kyratsous CA, Silverstein SJ. The RING finger domain of varicella-zoster virus ORF61p has E3 ubiquitin ligase activity that is essential for efficient autoubiquitination and dispersion of Sp100-containing nuclear bodies. *J Virol* 2010;84:6861–6865.
438. Walters MS, Kyratsous CA, Wan S, et al. Nuclear import of the varicella-zoster virus latency-associated protein ORF63 in primary neurons requires expression of the lytic protein ORF61 and occurs in a proteasome-dependent manner. *J Virol* 2008;82:8673–8686.
439. Wang ZH, Gershon MD, Lungu O, et al. Essential role played by the C-terminal domain of glycoprotein I in envelopment of varicella-zoster virus in the trans-Golgi network: interactions of glycoproteins with tegument. *J Virol* 2001;75:323–340.
440. Wang JP, Kurt-Jones EA, Shin OS, et al. Varicella-zoster virus activates inflammatory cytokines in human monocytes and macrophages via Toll-like receptor 2. *J Virol* 2005;79:12658–12666.
441. Wang K, Lau TY, Morales M, et al. Laser-capture microdissection: refining estimates of the quantity and distribution of latent herpes simplex virus 1 and varicella-zoster virus DNA in human trigeminal ganglia at the single cell level. *J Virol* 2005;79:14079–14087.
442. Wang C, Liu Y, Cavanagh MM, et al. B-cell repertoire responses to varicella-zoster vaccination in human identical twins. *Proc Natl Acad Sci U S A* 2015;112:500–505.
443. Wang L, Oliver SL, Sommer M, et al. Disruption of PML nuclear bodies is mediated by ORF61 SUMO-interacting motifs and required for varicella-zoster virus pathogenesis in skin. *PLoS Pathog* 2011;7:e1002157.
444. Wang L, Rajamani J, Sommer M, et al. Identification of a hydrophobic domain in varicella-zoster virus ORF61 necessary for ORF61 self-interaction, viral replication, and skin pathogenesis. *J Virol* 2013;87:4075–4079.
445. Wang L, Rajamani, J, Sommer M, et al. Identification of a hydrophobic domain in VZV ORF61 necessary for ORF61 self-interaction, Viral replication and Skin pathogenesis. *J Virol* 2013;87:4075–4079.
446. Wang L, Sommer M, Rajamani J, et al. Regulation of the ORF61 promoter and ORF61 functions in varicella-zoster virus replication and pathogenesis. *J Virol* 2009;83:7560–7572.
447. Wang W, Wang X, Yang L, et al. Modulation of host CD59 expression by varicella-zoster virus in human xenografts in vivo. *Virology* 2016;491:96–105.
448. Wang W, Yang L, Huang X, et al. Outer nuclear membrane fusion of adjacent nuclei in varicella-zoster virus-induced syncytia. *Virology* 2017;512:34–38.
449. Watson B, Boardman C, Laufer D, et al. Humoral and cell-mediated immune responses in healthy children after one or two doses of varicella vaccine. *Clin Infect Dis* 1995;20:316–319.
450. Watson CPN, Deck JH, Morshead C, et al. Postherpetic neuralgia: further post-mortem studies of cases with and without pain. *Pain* 1991;44:105–117.
451. Watson PN, Evans RJ. Postherpetic neuralgia: a review. *Arch Neurol* 1986;43:836–840.
452. Watson B, Gupta R, Randall T, et al. Persistence of cell-mediated and humoral immune responses in healthy children immunized with live attenuated varicella vaccine. *J Infect Dis* 1994;169:197–199.
453. Webster A, Grint P, Brenner MK, et al. Titration of IgG antibodies against varicella zoster virus before bone marrow transplantation is not predictive of future zoster. *J Med Virol* 1989;27:117–119.
454. Wei L, Zhao J, Wu W, et al. Decreased absolute numbers of CD3+ T cells and CD8+ T cells during aging in herpes zoster patients. *Sci Rep* 2017;7(1):15039
455. Weibel RE, Neff BJ, Kuter BJ, et al. Live attenuated varicella virus vaccine: efficacy trial in healthy children. *N Engl J Med* 1984;310:1409–1415.
456. Weinberg A, Canniff J, Rouphael N, et al. Varicella-zoster virus-specific cellular immune responses to the live attenuated zoster vaccine in young and older adults. *J Immunol* 2017;199:604–612.
457. Weinberg A, Kroehl ME, Johnson MJ, et al. Comparative immune responses to licensed herpes zoster vaccines. *J Infect Dis* 2018;218:S81–S87.
458. Weinberg A, Pang L, Johnson MJ, et al. The effect of age on the immunogenicity of the live attenuated zoster vaccine is predicted by baseline regulatory T cells and varicella-zoster virus-specific T cell immunity. *J Virol* 2019;93:e00305.
459. Weinberg A, Popmihajlov Z, Schmader KE, et al. Persistence of varicella-Zoster virus cell-mediated immunity after the administration of a second dose of live herpes zoster vaccine. *J Infect Dis* 2019;219:335–338.
460. Weinberg A, Zhang JH, Oxman MN, et al. Varicella-zoster virus-specific immune responses to herpes zoster in elderly participants in a trial of a clinically effective zoster vaccine. *J Infect Dis* 2009;200:1068–1077.
461. Weller TH, Stoddard MB. Intranuclear inclusion bodies in cultures of human tissue inoculated with varicella vesicle fluid. *J Immunol* 1952;68:311–319.
462. Weller TH, Witton HM, Bell EJ. The etiologic agents of varicella and herpes zoster: Isolation, propagation, and cultural characteristics in vitro. *J Exp Med* 1958;108:843–868.
463. White CJ, Kuter BJ, Hildebrand CS, et al. Varicella vaccine (VARIVAX) in healthy children and adolescents: results from clinical trials, 1987 to 1989. *Pediatrics* 1991;87:604–610.
464. White K, Peng H, Hay J, et al. Role of the IE62 consensus binding site in transactivation by the varicella-zoster virus IE62 protein. *J Virol* 2010;84:3767–3779.
465. Whitley RJ, Gnann JW Jr, Hinthorn D, et al. Disseminated herpes zoster in the immunocompromised host: a comparative trial of acyclovir and vidarabine. The NIAID collaborative antiviral study group. *J Infect Dis* 1992;165:450–455.
466. Whitley RJ, Shukla S, Crooks RJ. The identification of risk factors associated with persistent pain following herpes zoster. *J Infect Dis* 1998;178(Suppl 1):S71–S75.
467. Wilson A, Sharp M, Koropchak CM, et al. Subclinical varicella-zoster virus viremia, herpes zoster and recovery of T-cell responses to varicella-zoster viral antigens after allogeneic and autologous bone marrow transplantation. *J Infect Dis* 1992;165:119–126.
468. Winston DJ, Mullane KM, Cornely OA, et al. Inactivated varicella zoster vaccine in autologous haemopoietic stem-cell transplant recipients: an international, multicentre, randomised, double-blind, placebo-controlled trial. *Lancet* 2018;391:2116–2127.
469. Winthrop KL, Melmed GY, Vermeire S, et al. Herpes zoster infection in patients with ulcerative colitis receiving tofacitinib. *Inflamm Bowel Dis* 2018;24:2258–2265.
470. Wolfson LJ, Daniels VJ, Altland A, et al. The impact of varicella vaccination on the incidence of varicella and herpes zoster in the United States: updated evidence from observational databases, 1991–2016. *Clin Infect Dis* 2020;70:995–1002.
471. Xia D, Srinivas S, Sato H, et al. Varicella-zoster virus open reading frame 21, which is expressed during latency, is essential for virus replication but dispensable for establishment of latency. *J Virol* 2003;77:1211–1218.
472. Xing Y, Oliver SL, Nguyen T, et al. A site of varicella-zoster virus vulnerability identified by structural studies of neutralizing antibodies bound to the glycoprotein complex gHgL. *Proc Natl Acad Sci U S A* 2011;112:6056–6061.
473. Yamagishi Y, Sadaoka T, Yoshii H, et al. Varicella-zoster virus glycoprotein M homolog is glycosylated, is expressed on the viral envelope, and functions in virus cell-to-cell spread. *J Virol* 2008;82:795–804.
474. Yamamoto T, Ali MA, Liu X, et al. Activation of H2AX and ATM in varicella-zoster virus (VZV)-infected cells is associated with expression of specific VZV genes. *Virology* 2014;452–453:52–58.
475. Yang E, Arvin AM, Oliver SL. The cytoplasmic domain of varicella-zoster virus glycoprotein H regulates syncytia formation and skin pathogenesis. *PLoS Pathog* 2014;10:e1004173.
476. Yang E, Arvin AM, Oliver SL. The glycoprotein B cytoplasmic domain lysine cluster is critical for varicella-zoster virus cell-cell fusion regulation and infection. *J Virol* 2016;91:e01707.
477. Yang E, Arvin AM, Oliver SL. Role for the αV integrin subunit in varicella-zoster virus-mediated fusion and infection. *J Virol* 2016;90:7567–7578.
478. Yang M, Hay J, Ruyechan WT. The DNA element controlling expression of the varicella-zoster virus open reading frames 28 and 29 genes consists of two divergent unidirectional promoters which have a common USF site. *J Virol* 2004;78:10939–10952.
479. Yang M, Hay J, Ruyechan WT. Varicella-zoster virus IE62 protein utilizes the human mediator complex in promoter activation. *J Virol* 2008;82:12154–12163.
480. Yao Z, Jackson W, Grose C. Identification of the phosphorylation sequence in the cytoplasmic tail of the varicella-zoster virus Fc receptor glycoprotein gpI. *J Virol* 1993;67:4464–4473.
481. Yawn BP, Saddier P, Wollan PC, et al. A population-based study of the incidence and complication rates of herpes zoster before zoster vaccine introduction. *Mayo Clin Proc* 2007;82:1341–1349.
482. Yoshii H, Sadaoka K, Matsuura M, et al. Varicella-zoster virus ORF 58 gene is dispensable for viral replication in cell culture. *Virol J* 2008;5:54.
483. Zerboni L, Arvin A. Neuronal subtype and satellite cell tropism are determinants of varicella-zoster virus virulence in human dorsal root ganglia xenografts in vivo. *PLoS Pathog* 2015;11:e1004989.
484. Zerboni L, Berarducci B, Rajamani J, et al. Varicella-zoster virus glycoprotein E is a critical determinant of virulence in the SCID mouse-human model of neuropathogenesis. *J Virol* 2011;85:98–111.
485. Zerboni L, Hinchliffe S, Sommer MH, et al. Analysis of varicella zoster virus attenuation by evaluation of chimeric parent Oka/vaccine Oka recombinant viruses in skin xenografts in the SCIDhu mouse model. *Virology* 2005;332:337–346.
486. Zerboni L, Ku C-C, Jones CD, et al. Varicella-zoster virus infection of human dorsal root ganglia in vivo. *Proc Natl Acad Sci U S A* 2005;102:6490–6495.
487. Zerboni L, Nader S, Aoki K, et al. Analysis of the persistence of humoral and cellular immunity in children and adults immunized with varicella vaccine. *J Infect Dis* 1998;177:1701–1704.
488. Zerboni L, Reichelt M, Arvin A. Varicella-zoster virus neurotropism in SCID mouse-human dorsal root ganglia xenografts. *Curr Top Microbiol Immunol* 2010;342:255–276.
489. Zerboni L, Sen N, Oliver SL, et al. Molecular mechanisms of varicella zoster virus pathogenesis. *Nat Rev Microbiol* 2014;12:197–210.
490. Zerboni L, Sobel RA, Lai M, et al. Apparent expression of varicella-zoster virus proteins in latency resulting from reactivity of murine and rabbit antibodies with human blood group A determinants in sensory neurons. *J Virol* 2012;86:578–583.
491. Zerboni L, Sobel RA, Ramachandran V, et al. Expression of varicella-zoster virus immediate-early regulatory protein IE63 in neurons of latently infected human sensory ganglia. *J Virol* 2010;84:3421–3430.
492. Zerboni L, Sung P, Lee G, et al. Age-associated differences in infection of human skin in the SCID mouse model of varicella-zoster virus pathogenesis. *J Virol* 2018;9:e00002.
493. Zerboni L, Sung P, Sommer M, et al. The C-terminus of varicella-zoster virus glycoprotein M contains trafficking motifs that mediate skin virulence in the SCID-human model of VZV pathogenesis. *Virology* 2018;523:110–120.
494. Zerr DM, Alexander ER, Duchin JS, et al. A case–control study of necrotizing fasciitis during primary varicella. *Pediatrics* 1999;103:783–790.
495. Zhang Z, Rowe J, Wang W, et al. Genetic analysis of varicella-zoster virus ORF0 to ORF4 by use of a novel luciferase bacterial artificial chromosome system. *J Virol* 2007;81:9024–9033.
496. Zhang Z, Selariu A, Warden C, et al. Genome-wide mutagenesis reveals that ORF7 is a novel VZV skin-tropic factor. *PLoS Pathog* 2010;6:e1000971.
497. Zhou M, Stefan Oliver S, Kamarshi V, et al. Calcineurin phosphatase activity regulates varicella-zoster virus induced cell-cell fusion. *PLoS Pathog* 2020;16(11):e1009022.
498. Zhu Z, Gershon MD, Ambron RT, et al. Infection of cells by varicella-zoster virus: entry by mannose 6-phosphate and heparin. *Proc Natl Acad Sci U S A* 1995;92:3546–3550.
499. Zhu Z, Hao Y, Gershon MD, et al. Targeting of glycoprotein I (gE) of varicella-zoster virus to the trans-Golgi network by an AYRV sequence and an acidic amino acid-rich patch in the cytosolic domain of the molecule. *J Virol* 1996;70:6563–6575.
500. Zhu H, Zheng C, Xing J, et al. Varicella zoster virus immediate early protein ORF61 abrogated IRF3-mediated innate immune response through degradation of activated IRF3. *J Virol* 2011;85:11079–11089.
501. Zuranski T, Nawar H, Czechowski D, et al. Cell-type-dependent activation of the cellular EF-1α promoter by the varicella-zoster virus IE63 protein. *Virology* 2005;338:35–42.

CHAPTER

14 Human Herpesviruses 6A, 6B, and 7

Yasuko Mori • Danielle M. Zerr • Louis Flamand • Philip E. Pellett

HISTORY

A novel herpesvirus was discovered in 1986 in patients with lymphoproliferative disorders.[212] Initially named human B-lymphotropic virus, it was later found mainly to infect and replicate in lymphocytes of the T-cell lineage, and renamed human herpesvirus 6 (HHV-6). Subsequently, based on their sequences and biological properties, HHV-6 strains were classified into two distinct groups, which are now known as human herpesvirus 6A (HHV-6A; species *Human betaherpesvirus 6A*) and human herpesvirus 6B (HHV-6B; species *Human betaherpesvirus 6B*). HHV-6B is the major causative agent of exanthema subitum (ES; also known as roseola)[282]; HHV-6A has been associated with spontaneous abortion and Hashimoto thyroiditis, but the etiologic proof is not yet definitive.

Human herpesvirus 7 (HHV-7; species *Human betaherpesvirus 7*) was isolated in 1990 from a healthy individual whose T cells were stimulated with antibodies against CD3 and then incubated with interleukin-2 (IL-2).[70] The virus is a second causative agent of ES[240] and has been associated with febrile convulsions in young children.[272] HHV-6B and HHV-7 are ubiquitous, with more than 80% of adults having antibodies to both viruses.[3,4,21,26,45,135,271]

INFECTIOUS AGENT

Classification

HHV-6A, HHV-6B, and HHV-7 share many properties with other herpesviruses, including virion structure, genomic architecture and genetic features, high prevalence in their natural host, and the ability to establish latent infections in the host. Their lytic replication cycles (Fig. 14.1) are generally similar to that for other herpesviruses. They belong to the *Roseolovirus* genus of the betaherpesvirus subfamily, and are characterized by replication in T lymphocytes (although they can also infect other cell types), high prevalence, and association with febrile rash illness. As betaherpesviruses, roseoloviruses are related to cytomegaloviruses (CMV), including having genetically colinear genomes, encoding several subfamily-specific genes, and having protracted replication cycles. Other roseoloviruses have been identified in chimpanzees,[138] mandrills,[137] pigs,[48] and mice,[48,196] and as an endogenous virus in a Philippine tarsier.[14]

The human roseoloviruses are closely related, yet molecularly and biologically distinct viruses that differ with respect to their genome sequences, cell tropisms, interactions with cells and signaling pathways of the immune system, and epidemiology.[1,4,21,26,52,110,135]

Propagation and *In Vitro* Cell Tropism

HHV-6A and HHV-6B infect a variety of cultured human cells, such as T cells (preferentially mature CD4+), natural killer (NK) cells, γ/δ T lymphocytes, primary fetal astrocytes and dendritic cells, olfactory ensheathing cells (HHV-6A but not HHV-6B), and peripheral blood mononuclear cells (PBMC). Cell lines derived from megakaryocytes and glioblastomas, as well as neural, epithelial, and fibroblastic cells can also support limited HHV-6 replication.[26,45] Fresh isolates can be adapted to grow in continuous T-cell lines, such as HSB-2 and J-JHAN for HHV-6A, and Molt-3 and MT-4 for HHV-6B, but the genetic changes required for adaptation have not been characterized.

HHV-6A has a greater capacity than HHV-6B for replication in cultured cells of neuronal origin.[46] In primary astrocytes, HHV-6A establishes a productive lytic infection, whereas HHV-6B produces little cytopathic effect and only small amounts of viral nucleic acids, proteins, or infectious progeny, and establishes a long-term, low-level persistent infection.[53]

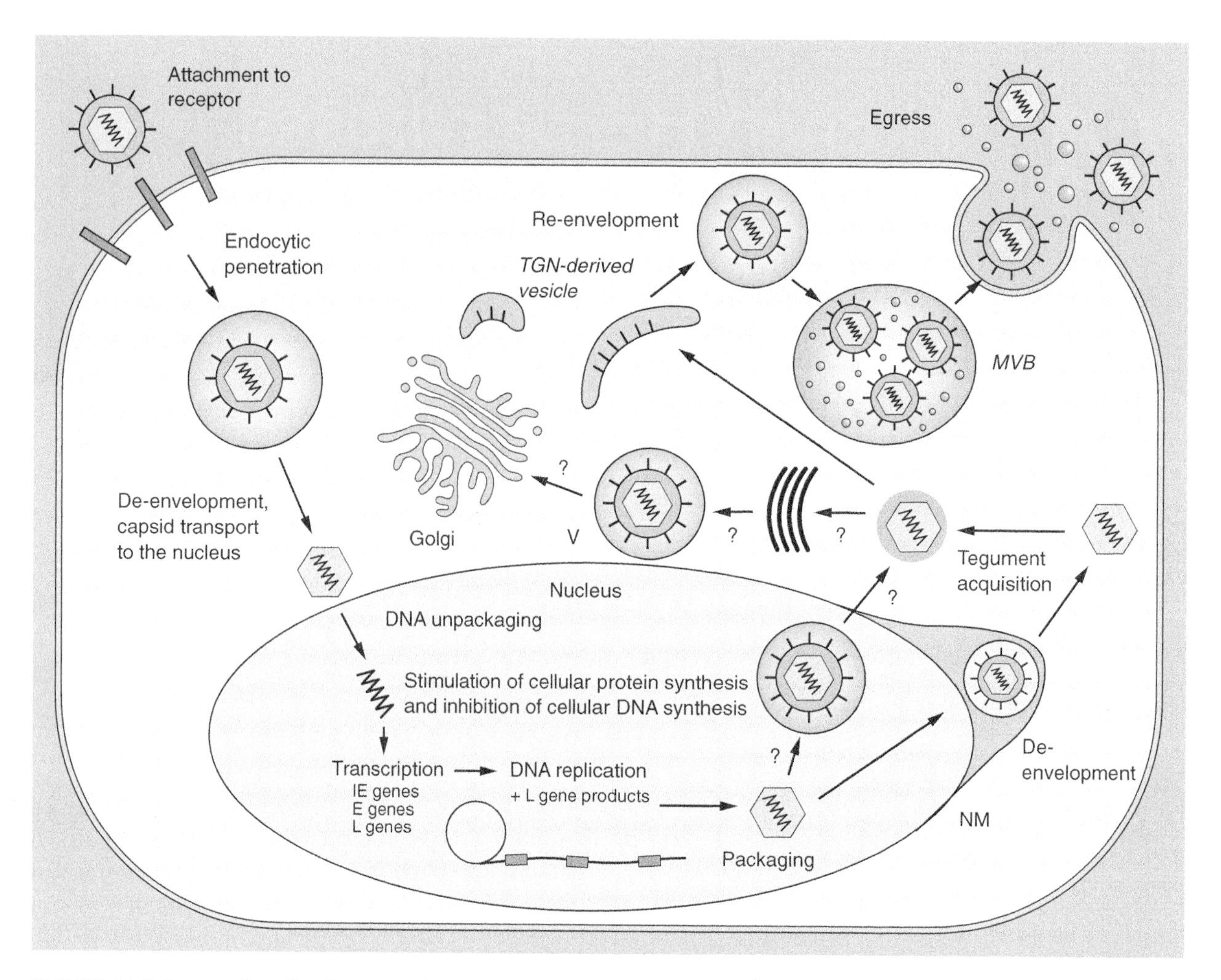

FIGURE 14.1 **Stages of replication.** A single receptor is shown, although it is likely that the virus employs multiple receptors to enable entry into a wide range of cell types. AL, annulate lamellae; G, Golgi complex; HS, heparan sulfate; Nu, nucleus; NM, nuclear membrane; R, receptor (CD46 for HHV-6A and HHV-6B, CD4 for HHV-7); V, vacuole, MVB (multivesicular body).

After the course of 30 days in an oligodendrocyte cell line, HHV-6A transitioned from a lytic state to a quiescent infection that may represent latency (reactivation was not demonstrated), whereas HHV-6B infection was nonproductive and did not persist.[5] In some cultured cells, the HHV-6 genome integrates into a host cell telomere (chromosomally integrated, or ciHHV-6), establishing a quiescent form of persistence that may represent a form of latency.[10]

In contrast, HHV-7 has a narrow *in vitro* cell tropism, thus far being restricted to primary phytohemagglutinin (PHA)-stimulated CD4+ T cells obtained from umbilical cords or PBMC, and an immature continuous T-lymphoblastoid cell line, SupT-1.[21] HHV-6A, HHV-6B, and HHV-7 induce similar cytopathic effects, characterized by ballooning refractile cells (Fig. 14.2).

Virion Structure

Roseoloviruses share the standard features of herpesvirus virions: an icosahedral capsid 90 to 110 nm in diameter that contains the 145-kb (HHV-7) and up to 170-kb (HHV-6B) double-stranded DNA (dsDNA) genome, a tegument that surrounds the capsid, and a lipid bilayer envelope studded with virus-specified membrane proteins and glycoproteins; enveloped extracellular virions are 160 to 200 nm in diameter[19,20,126,287] (Fig. 14.3).

HHV-6B capsids have atomic-level structural properties shared with evolutionary relatives that range from tailed bacteriophage (caudoviruses) to herpesviruses.[298] The HHV-6B pU11 tegument protein is a homolog of human cytomegalovirus (HCMV) pp150/pUL32, which forms a capsid-associated tegument complex (CATC) that appears to strengthen HCMV capsids to enable stable accommodation of the 236 kb HCMV genome, which is nearly 50% longer than the HHV-6B genome. Dimers of pU11 also form CATCs, but their reduced number and the nature of their interaction with the capsid suggest less need for the level of reinforcement provided by the HCMV CATC. By thin-section electron microscopy (EM), HHV-6 teguments are smooth and fill the space between the capsid and envelope, whereas HHV-7 teguments have an electron lucent space between the tegument and envelope. Immunoelectron microscopy revealed that HHV-7 pU14 is present at the outer periphery of the tegument.[232]

Mature HHV-6B virions consist of at least 29 polypeptides, including 6 in the envelope fraction and cellular p53.[26,239] As described below in the Entry section, envelope glycoproteins

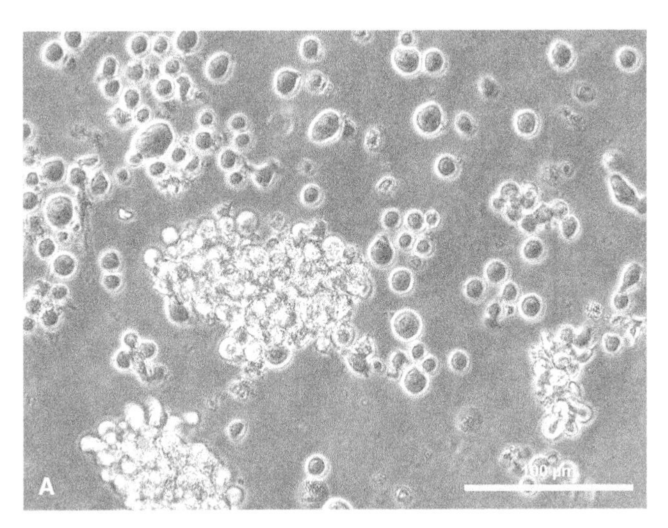

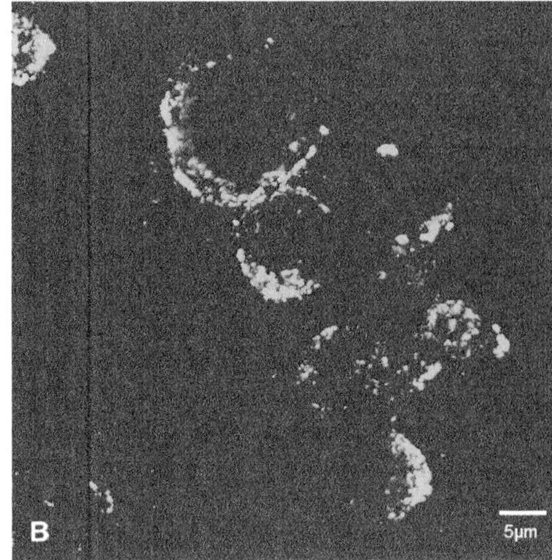

FIGURE 14.2 **Cytopathic effects induced in cord blood mononuclear cells (CBMCs) by HHV-6B. A:** Balloon-like cells are seen in CBMCs at 1 day post infection. **B:** CMBCs at 3 days post infection were stained by IFA using monoclonal antibody for HHV-6B gB. Similar cytopathic effects and staining are seen for HHV-6A, HHV-6B, and HHV-7.

include gB, and the gH/gL/gQ1, gH/gL/gQ1/gQ2, and gQ1/gQ2 complexes.

Genome Structure and Organization

Genomic Architecture

As packaged in nucleocapsids, roseolovirus genomes are composed of a central unique segment (U) bracketed by a pair of direct repeat structures, DR_L and DR_R (Fig. 14.4; e-Fig. 14.1; Table 14.1).[52,135,145,161] Some forms of HHV-6 intracellular replicative intermediates do not have duplicated DR segments; the unit form of these concatemeric or circular genomes consists of one copy of the U segment and a single DR.[23] From left to right, HHV-6 DRs consist of 25 to 29 base pairs (bp) of unique sequence, a conserved pac1 (cleavage and packaging) element, an array of heterogeneous telomere-related repeats based on the sequence TA(A/G)(C/G)(C/T)C that span about 300 bp

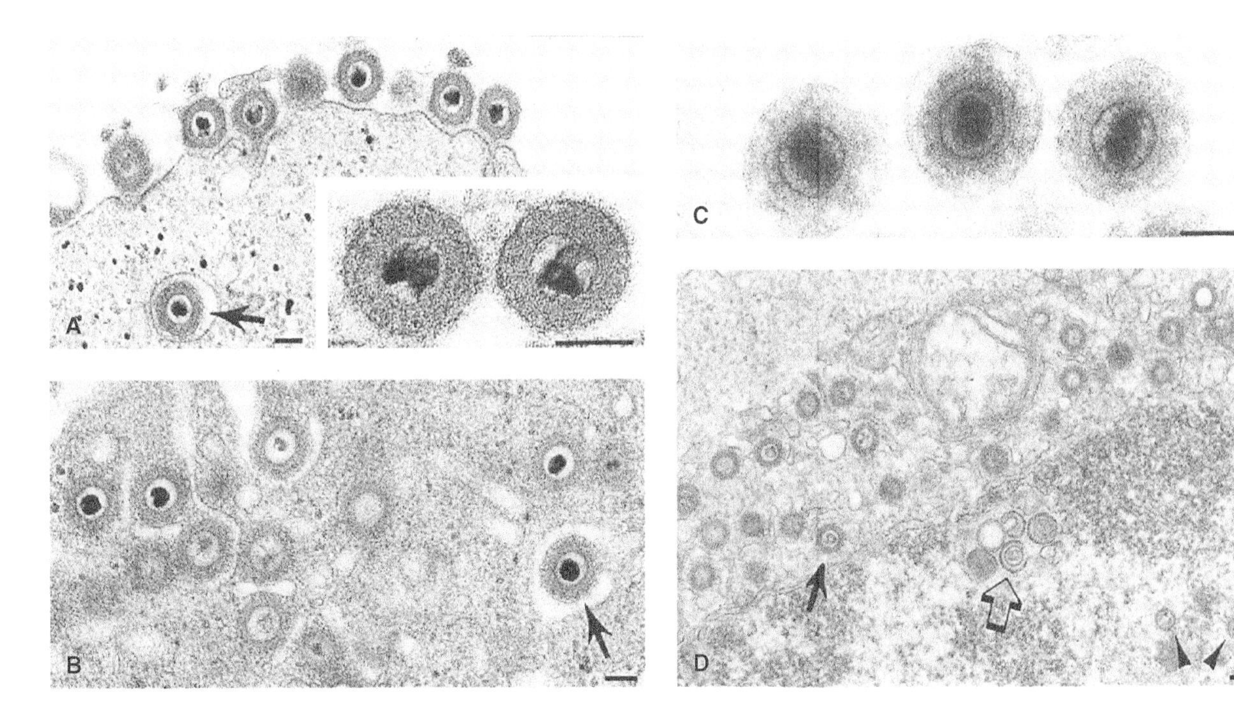

FIGURE 14.3 **Ultrastructural characteristics of HHV-6B(Z29) and HHV-7(SB) grown in human umbilical cord blood lymphocytes. A:** HHV-6B virus particles accumulated along the plasma membrane and within a vesicle (*arrow*) of an infected cell. Inset: Detail of HHV-6B virions. **B:** Tegument-coated nucleocapsids of HHV-6 within the cytoplasm and apparently budding into the cisternae of the Golgi apparatus (*arrow*). **C:** Extracellular HHV-7 virions. **D:** HHV-7 nucleocapsids within the nucleus (*arrowheads*), accumulated within the perinuclear space (*open arrow*), and surrounded by tegument within the cytoplasm (*arrow*). Bars, 100 nm. (Courtesy of C. S. Goldsmith, C. Lopez, P.E.P., and J. B. Black, Centers for Disease Control and Prevention.)

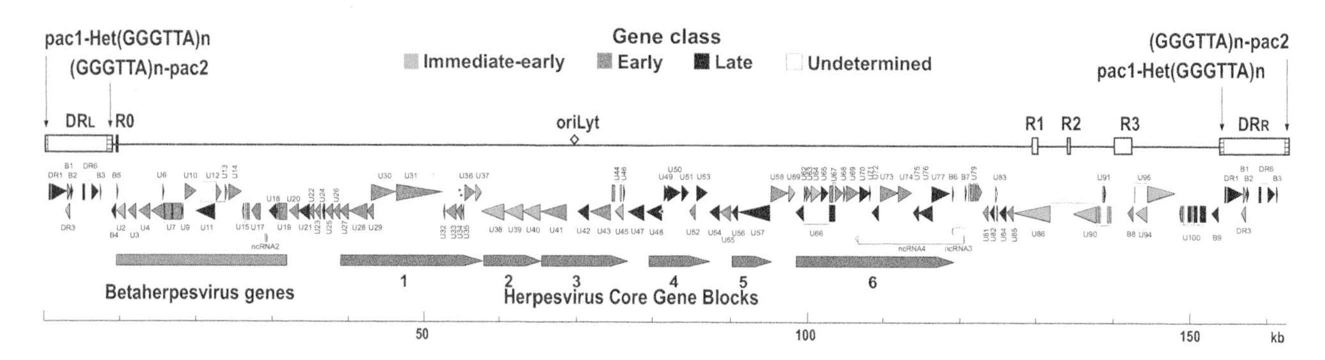

FIGURE 14.4 HHV-6B genomic and genetic architecture. The diagram is based on information from.[37,52,60,80,85,88,110,164,182] The positions and arrangements of the major internal repeat elements, the origin of replication (*oriLyt*), and the structure of the direct repeat (*DR*) termini are shown for frame (ORF) sizes, orientation, and location are indicated. ORF found in HHV-6B and not in HHV-6A are designated with "B" prefixes. Small upstream ORFs are indicated with small triangles at the N-termini of the associated large ORFs. Only a subset of known mRNA splicing events is represented. The orientation and order of the six conserved herpesvirus core gene blocks are indicated, as is the block of genes (U2 to U19) found only in betaherpesviruses.

in laboratory-passaged strains and up to 3 kb in low passage viruses, about 7 kb of unique sequence that encodes a handful of genes, an array of telomeric repeat sequences similar to sequences present at the telomeres of vertebrate chromosomes (R-TRS, [TAACCC]n), a conserved pac2 element, and 16 to 18 bp of unique sequence (Fig. 14.4, e-Fig. 14.1, and e-Fig. 14.2). The HHV-7 R-TRS is more heterogeneous than for HHV-6 (e-Fig. 14.2).[210] Despite the differences, HHV-7

TABLE 14.1 Properties of roseolovirus genomes

	HHV-6A	HHV-6B	HHV-7
%(G+C)			
DR	58	59	53
U	41	41	34
Overall	43	43	36
Length (kb)			
DR	8	8.1–13	5.8–10
U	143	145	133
Total	159	161–170	145–153
Repeat arrays (copy number and length)			
DR			
L-TRS[a]	42 × 6*h* bp	50 × 6*h* bp	20–663 × 6*h* bp
R-TRS	59 × 6 bp	78 × 6 bp	106–148 × 6*h* bp
R0	NP	13 × 14 bp	NP
R1	51 × 12 bp	54 × 12 bp	NP
R2A (HHV-7 R1)	2 × 17–18 bp	5 × 17–18 bp	2 × 84 bp plus 2 partial 64 bp[b]
R2B	1,233 bp[c]	8 × 12 bp	NP
R3 (HHV-7 R2)	28 × ~105	24–26 × ~104 bp	15–16 × 105 bp

[a]Left-terminal resolution site (L-TRS) and right-terminal resolution site (R-TRS) designate the TRS arrays near the left and right ends of direct repeat (DR), respectively.
[b]In human herpesvirus (HHV)-7(RK), the arrangement is 3 × 84 bp plus 68 bp partial repeat.
[c]HHV-6A R2 is composed of TpG dinucleotide repeats spanning 1,233 bp.
h, heterogeneous versions of repeat element; NP, not present.
Modified from Dominguez G, Dambaugh TR, Stamey FR, et al. Human herpesvirus 6B genome sequence: coding content and comparison with human herpesvirus 6A. *J Virol* 1999;73:8040–8052, with additional information from Isegawa Y, Mukai T, Nakano K, et al. Comparison of the complete DNA sequences of human herpesvirus 6 variants A and B. *J Virol* 1999;73:8053–8063; Megaw AG, Rapaport D, Avidor B, et al. The DNA sequence of the RK strain of human herpesvirus 7. *Virology* 1998;244(1):119–132; and Nicholas J. Determination and analysis of the complete nucleotide sequence of human herpesvirus 7. *J Virol* 1996;70:5975–5989.

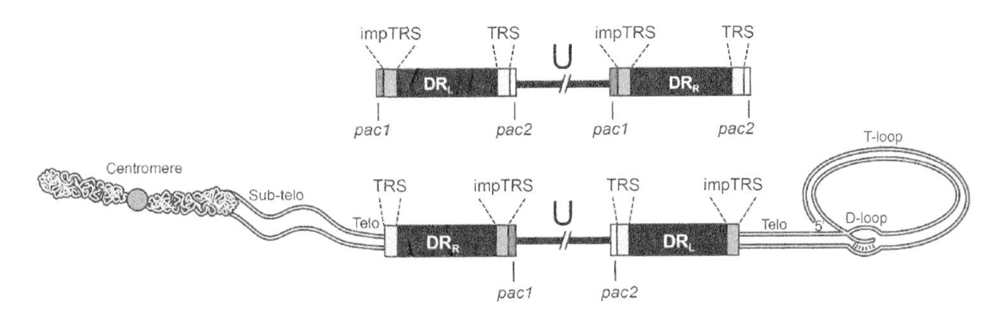

FIGURE 14.5 **Structure of HHV-6 genomes when integrated at chromosomal telomeres.**

cleavage and packaging signals are recognized and processed during HHV-6 infections, and vice versa.[149] Other repeat arrays (R0 to R3) are located in the U segment of each of the viruses[52,80,110,164,182] (Table 14.1 and Fig. 14.4 and e-Fig. 14.1). Compared with other herpesviruses, some of which have G+C contents exceeding 60%, roseoloviruses have relatively low G+C contents (Table 14.1).

The mammalian telomere-like sequences have no role in nuclear retention of viral DNA, efficiency of DNA replication, or packaging-associated DNA cleavage.[27,47] Like the similar sequences required for integration of Marek disease virus genomes into telomeres of its host cells,[119] these sequences are involved in site-specific integration of HHV-6 genomes into telomeres of host chromosomes during establishment of ciHHV-6. In ciHHV-6,[10] the virus genome is typically linked to the host chromosome with the TRS array at the DR_R end of the genome joined to the chromosomal TRS (with loss of the viral *pac2* sequence) (Fig. 14.5). A TRS is added to the imperfect telomeric repeat present at the distal end of the virus genome (with loss of *pac1*).

About 1% of humans inherit ciHHV-6 via their parental germ line,[44,118,198,257] which results in every nucleated cell harboring at least one complete HHV-6A or HHV-6B genome. In most individuals with inherited ciHHV-6 (iciHHV-6), a single chromosome is targeted, but some individuals have iciHHV-6 on chromosomes acquired from both of their parents. Persistent lineages of iciHHV-6A or iciHHV-6B have sporadically emerged in human populations over a period of thousands of years.[13,146,197,251,297] iciHHV-6A and iciHHV-6B genomes have the potential to reactivate to lytic replication with pathogenic potential.[56,277]

Although HHV-7 also has telomeric sequences, its chromosomal integration is much less common; it has not been observed to integrate into the host germ line.[203]

Genetic Structure and Genetic Relationships

Recent application of modern genome sequencing methods, coupled with deep RNA sequencing and proteomics analyses, has had multiple impacts, including more accurate genome sequences, increasing availability of genome sequences from many strains from numerous international sources, and information that demonstrates wide variation in forms and degrees of gene expression. These include pervasive RNA splicing, including over long ranges, as well as the presence of long RNAs that do not have long open reading frames comparable to the canonical protein-coding regions, but in fact abundantly express short proteins.[60,85,88] Some mRNAs that express canonical proteins contain upstream short open reading frames whose translation can modulate translation of the longer downstream ORF.[60] Maximal utility of this new information will be dependent on development of updated annotations that connect to informative sequence feature displays and to canonical literature and gene names.[85]

Protein-coding open reading frames (ORF) are present on both strands of the genome, with little overlap among adjacent ORF (Fig. 14.4 and e-Fig. 14.1). The HHV-7 genome is more compactly arranged than for HHV-6A or HHV-6B, with a similar genetic complement being encoded in a U segment that is 12 kb shorter than for HHV-6A or HHV-6B (Table 14.1). In addition to the repeat arrays, two genomic regions have no long open reading frames with obvious protein coding capacity: the region between U41 and U42 that harbors the origin of lytic DNA replication (oriLyt), and the region between U77 and U79. RNA sequencing and coupled proteomics analyses recently revealed the presence of abundant long RNAs transcribed from these regions, including mRNAs that express small proteins.[60]

Many of the genes encoded in the central portion of roseolovirus genomes are conserved among the alpha-, beta-, and gammaherpesvirus[52,80,135,164,182] (Table 14.2; Fig. 14.4; e-Fig. 14.1; and Chapter 8). A betaherpesvirus-specific gene cluster is located to the left of the core genes. Clusters of genes unique to roseoloviruses flank the core genes.

Over the conserved domains, roseoloviruses are genetically colinear with CMV, but CMV encode many genes without roseolovirus counterparts. Between HHV-6 and HHV-7, amino acid sequence identities range from 22% to 75%, most being approximately 50%. HHV-6A and HHV-6B have 90% overall nucleotide sequence identity; the 66-kb segment that spans U32 to U77 is highly conserved (95% identity), whereas the 27-kb segment spanning U86 to U100 is only 72% identical.[52]

Intraspecies sequence variation is very low. Across a 120-kb segment spanning HHV-6B genes U2 to R2, pairwise identities were greater than 99.9% across a set that included 61 clinical specimens from Japan, Uganda, and the United States, plus 64 iciHHV-6B specimens from Seattle[88]; comparable results have been seen for HHV-6A. Other than repeat copy number differences, HHV-7 strains JI and RK differ by only 179 bp (0.1%) over their genomes.

Roseoloviruses differ somewhat from each other in their genetic complement, with several small differences in coding capacity and splicing patterns between HHV-6A and HHV-6B.[60,88] DR3, U6, U22, U83, and U94 are encoded by

TABLE 14.2 HHV-6A, HHV-6B, and HHV-7 genes of known or implied functions and their HCMV homologs

HHV-6 ORF	HHV-7 ORF	HCMV ORF	Gene Block	Kinetic Class	Properties or Implied Functions
DR1	DR1			L	HCMV US22 gene family
DR3				IE	
DR6	DR6			L	HCMV US22 gene family, transactivator
U2	U2	UL23	Beta	IE	HCMV US22 gene family
U3	U3	UL24	Beta	E	HCMV US22 gene family, transactivator
U3	U4		Beta	E	
U6			Beta	L	
U7	U7	UL27/UL28	Beta	E	HCMV US22 gene family
U9	U9		Beta	E	
U10	U10		Beta	E	
U11	U11	UL32	Beta	L	Antigenic tegument protein; HHV-6A p100, HHV-6B 101K, HHV-7 89K
U12	U12	UL33	Beta	E	G-protein–coupled receptor
U13	U13		Beta	E	
U14	U14	UL25	Beta	E	Antigenic tegument protein; HHV-7 pp85, HCMV UL25/UL35 gene family
U15	U15		Beta	E	HCMV UL25/UL35 gene family
U17	U17	UL36	Beta	E	HCMV US22 gene family, IE-B
U18	U18	UL37EX3	Beta	L	IE-B
U19	U19	UL38	Beta	E	IE-B
U20	U20			E	Glycoprotein
U21	U21			L	Glycoprotein
U22				E	Glycoprotein
U23	U24			E	Glycoprotein
U24	U24			L	
U25	U25	UL43		E	HCMV US22 gene family
U26	U26	UL43		E	
U27	U27	UL44	1	E	Polymerase processivity factor (PA)
U28	U28	UL45	1	E	Ribonucleotide reductase large subunit (RR)
U29	U29	UL46	1	E	Capsid assembly and DNA maturation
U30	U30	UL47	1	E	Tegument protein
U31	U31	UL48	1	E	Large tegument protein (Teg)
U32	U32			L	Capsid protein
U33	U33	UL49	1	E	Virion protein
U34	U34	UL50	1	E	Membrane-associated phosphoprotein
U35	U35	UL51		E	DNA packaging
U36	U36	UL52	1	E	DNA packaging
U37	U37	UL53	1	IE	Putative phosphoprotein
U38	U38	UL54	2	IE	DNA polymerase (Pol)
U39	U39	UL55	2	IE	Glycoprotein B (gB)
U40	U40	UL56	2	I	Transport/capsid assembly (TP)
U41	U41	UL57	2	E	Major DNA-binding protein (MDBP)
U42	U42	UL69	3	L	Transactivator
U43	U43	UL70	3	E	Helicase/primase complex (HP)
U44	U44		3	E	

TABLE 14.2 HHV-6A, HHV-6B, and HHV-7 genes of known or implied functions and their HCMV homologs *(Continued)*

HHV-6 ORF	HHV-7 ORF	HCMV ORF	Gene Block	Kinetic Class	Properties or Implied Functions
U45	U45		3	IE	
U46	U46	UL73	3	L	Membrane protein
U47	U47	UL74		L	Glycoprotein O (gO)
U48	U48	UL75	4	L	Glycoprotein H (gH)
U49	U49	UL76	4	L	Putative fusion protein
U50	U50	UL77	4	L	DNA packaging
U51	U51	UL78	4	E	G-protein–coupled receptor
U52	U52		4	E	
U53	U53	UL80	4	L	Proteinase
U54	U54	UL82/UL83		L	Virion transactivator/tegument
U55	U55			E	
U56	U56	UL85	5	L	Capsid protein
U57	U57	UL86	5	L	Major capsid protein (MCP)
U58	U58			E	
U59	U59			IE	
U62	U62		6	IE	
U63	U63		6	E	
U64	U64	UL93	6	I	DNA packaging; tegument protein
U65	U65	UL94	6	L	Tegument protein
U66	U66	UL89	6	L	Putative terminase
U67	U67		6	E	
U68	U68		6	E	
U69	U69	UL97	6	E	Phosphotransferase; ganciclovir kinase
U70	U70	UL98	6	L	Alkaline exonuclease (Exo)
U71	U71		6	L	Myristylated virion protein
U72	U72	UL100	6	L	Glycoprotein M (gM)
U73	U73		6	E	Origin-binding protein (OBP)
U74	U74	UL102	6	E	Helicase/primase complex (HP)
U75	U75	UL102	6	L	
U76	U76	UL104	6	L	DNA packaging, virion protein
U77	U77	UL105	6	L	Helicase/primase complex (HP)
U79	U79	UL112/UL113		E	DNA replication
U81	U81	UL114		E	Uracil-DNA glycosylase
U82	U82	UL115		L	Glycoprotein L (gL)
U83				L	Intercrine cytokine
U84	U84			L	
U85	U85			IE	OX-2 homology, glycoprotein
U86	U86	UL122		IE	IE-A, transactivator
U90	U90			IE	IE-A (IE1), transactivator
U91	U91			L	
U94				IE	Parvovirus *rep* homolog (Rep)
U95	U95			IE	HCMV US22 gene family
U100	U100			L	Spliced envelope glycoprotein (HHV-6 gQ1-gQ2, HHV-7 gp65)

Based on information in.[37,52,60,80,85,88,110,164,182] Kinetic class assignments are based on.[85]
HHV, human herpesvirus; HCMV, human cytomegalovirus; ORF, open reading frame; IE, immediate early; E, early; L, late.

HHV-6A and HHV-6B, but not HHV-7. HHV-7 encodes a duplicated gene (U55A and U55B) that is encoded as a single copy by HHV-6A and HHV-6B. Relative to HCMV, genes unique to roseoloviruses include U20, U21, U23, U24, U24A, U26, and U100.

Although no amino acid sequence similarity has been identified, the general layout and splicing patterns of two HCMV immediate-early (IE) regions are conserved in the roseoloviruses. Thus, the roseolovirus IE-B domain that spans U17 to U19 corresponds to the HCMV UL36 to U38 IE locus, and the IE-A domain spanning U86 to U90 corresponds to the HCMV major IE locus.[160,182]

Every betaherpesvirus encodes several members of a family of duplicated and diverged genes that are related to HCMV US22 and are referred to as the US22 gene family.[182] For HCMV, some US22 family members are transcribed as IE genes and encode transactivating functions. In the roseoloviruses, DR2, DR6/7, U2, U3, U5, U7 (U5/7 in HHV-7), U8, U17/16, U25, and U95 are all members of this gene family. At least four of the HHV-6A US22 homologs encode transcriptional transactivators (DR6, U3, U16, and U25).

Roseoloviruses have been the subject of little genetic experimentation. Replacement of the HHV-6B U3-U7 gene cluster with a selection marker demonstrated that these genes are not essential for virus replication or latency in cultured cells.[131] HHV-6A genomes have been cloned as bacterial artificial chromosomes (BACs), which have been used in studies of viral glycoproteins[244] and the function of the telomeric repeats[267,268] and to identify a role for an HHV-6A-encoded microRNA in regulation of lytic infection.[186]

Stages of Replication

Entry

Differences in receptor recognition likely contribute to the distinct cellular tropisms of HHV-6A and HHV-6B.

A cellular receptor for HHV-6A,[215] CD46, is also a member of the regulator of complement fixation family and is expressed on the surface of all nucleated human cells. The short consensus repeats 2 and 3 of the CD46 ectodomain are required for HHV-6 receptor activity.[87] HHV-6A but not HHV-6B can mediate fusion from without (FFWO; fusion that does not require viral protein synthesis) in a variety of human cells,[174] an activity that is dependent on CD46 expression. CD46 isoforms that are alternative splice variants also may impact HHV-6 infection.[95]

Human CD134 is a cellular receptor of HHV-6B,[248] but not HHV-6A. CD134 is a member of the TNF receptor superfamily, which is a type I transmembrane protein, and a costimulator for T-cell activation. Compared with the ubiquitous expression of CD46, CD134 is mainly expressed on activated primary T cells. Another cellular protein, GP96, is important for both HHV-6A and HHV-6B entry.[154,204]

HHV-7 uses CD4 as a receptor, although the virus can infect cells that do not express detectable CD4.[21]

On the virus side, two HHV-7 glycoproteins have been identified as being able to bind cell surface proteoglycans heparan and heparan sulfate: gB, and the spliced glycoprotein encoded by U100.[45] Other virion proteins are likely involved in receptor interactions or entry, such as the gH/gL complex, which, along with products of U100, is a target for complement-independent neutralization. gQ1, a spliced product of the U97, 98, 99, and 100 ORFs, is unique to roseoloviruses.[246] The gene is expressed via complex splicing, producing a number of envelope-associated polypeptides. The HHV-6 gH/gL complex associates with the 80-kDa virion envelope form of gQ1 (gQ-80K; gQ1). A different small transcript from U97 gene encodes an unrelated protein of 37 kDa (gQ-37K; gQ2) that interacts with the gH/gL/gQ1 complex in infected cells and virions.[6]

Interaction of the virion with the CD46 or CD134 receptor is via the HHV-6A or HHV-6B gH/gL/gQ1/gQ2 complex (Fig. 14.6).[6,176,214,247,249] HHV-6A gQ1/gQ2 is critical for the CD46 interaction.[114] A short amino sequence in HHV-6A gQ1 (494aa-497aa) is important for HHV-6A gH/gL/gQ1/gQ2 complex function.[156] HHV-6B gQ1/gQ2 complex is sufficient for CD134 binding[249] while all four components of HHV-6A gH/gL/gQ1/gQ2 complex are required for CD46 binding.[242]

An amino acid residue in HHV-6B gQ1 (E127) is important for CD134 binding.[247] The ectodomain of CD134 contains four cysteine-rich domains (CRD) and a stalk domain. CRD2 is needed for HHV-6B complex binding, and 2 amino acid residues (K79 and W86) within CRD2 are key for its interaction with the HHV-6B complex, and the positive charge of K79 could associate with the negative charge of E127 of HHV-6B gQ1 and contribute to the interaction.[247,249]

HHV-6A and HHV-6B U47 are positional homologs of HCMV glycoprotein O (gO) gene. Both HHV-6 gOs are components of gH/gL-associated envelope complexes, but they are not CD46 ligands and likely play different roles than gH/gL/gQ1/gQ2.[171] gQ and gO have much greater sequence divergence between HHV-6A and HHV-6B than do other glycoproteins (76.8% and 72.1% identity, respectively), suggesting that they contribute to the biological differences between these viruses.

Lipid rafts are critical for HHV-6 entry. Depletion of cholesterol from virion and cell membranes inhibits virus infection, and HHV-6A binding to cells triggers rapid redistribution of CD46 to lipid rafts.[173,243] Envelope glycoproteins are enriched in raft fractions, and raft components are incorporated into virions.[121]

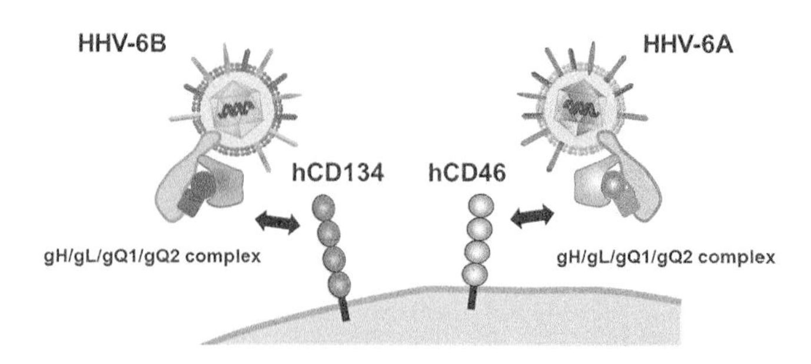

FIGURE 14.6 Virion–receptor interactions. HHV-6A and HHV-6B recognize distinct cellular receptors. The HHV-6A gH/gL/gQ1/gQ2 complex binds human CD46 and the HHV-6B complex binds human CD134.

Transcription

Herpesvirus genes generally belong to one of two main categories: latent or lytic. There are three general kinetic classes of lytic genes: immediate-early (IE; expression not dependent on *de novo* protein synthesis) genes that provide functions for regulation of gene expression, early (E; expression dependent on IE gene expression) genes that encode proteins needed for replication of the virus genome, and late (L; expression is dependent on viral DNA synthesis) genes that encode virion proteins.

Roseolovirus gene expression follows the general herpesvirus program. For HHV-6B, 8 genes are expressed as IE, 44 as Early, and 44 as Late, and 4 were biphasic[85] (Table 14.2). HHV-6A and HHV-6B U83 and U89/90 are well established as IE genes. For both loci, multiple differently regulated transcripts are expressed (e-Fig. 14.3). The U83 IE transcript is spliced and expresses a truncated version of the chemokine encoded by U83, whereas the full-length transcript is expressed as a late gene. U42 encodes a homolog of the HSV IE gene $\alpha 27$ and HCMV UL69, which is regulated as an E gene; HHV-6B U42 is not transcribed in the absence of *de novo* protein synthesis; thus, its regulation is similar to that of its HCMV counterpart. Expression of the U90 IE gene rose to more than 10 copies per cell within 8 hours, whereas a structural gene transcript (U11) took 16 hours to reach comparable levels[205]; at 72 hours after infection, U11 was expressed at several hundred copies per cell. Transcripts of the gene needed for initiation of DNA replication (U73) and the parvovirus ns1/rep homolog (U94) were expressed at much lower levels (<10 copies/cell).

Recent studies that employed deep RNA sequencing and proteomics have made it clear that, as for other herpesviruses, HHV-6A and HHV-6B transcription is very complex.[60,85,88] Important features include abundant mRNA, numerous splice isoforms that can be differentially regulated and can express diverse forms of related proteins. Some mRNAs include small ORFs that are likely to be involved in regulation of larger downstream canonical ORFs that have long been recognized. Some regions of the genomes are spanned by long RNAs that at first glance seemed to be noncoding because of the absence of long ORFs, but proteomics analyses and studies of ribosomal occupancy have made it clear that some small ORFs are indeed expressed as proteins. Much work will be required to develop frameworks for understanding the biological activities enabled by these complex forms and patterns of gene expression.

The HHV-6 R3 repeat element (R2 in HHV-7) is a potential IE enhancer. R3 is located about 300 bp upstream of the oppositely oriented U89/90 and U95 genes; it is present in more than 25 copies per genome (Table 14.1) and contains potential transcription factor-binding sites (nuclear factor kappaB [NF-κB] and AP2 in HHV-6A; PEA3 and AP2 in HHV-6B; and PEA3 in HHV-7). U95 has amino acid sequence similarity with the murine CMV (MCMV) IE2 gene and is a member of the HCMV US22 gene family. Deletion of three R3 units decreases promoter activity 15-fold, and NF-κB family members p50 and c-Rel bind to NF-κB sites in R3.[179] The HHV-6 major immediate early gene (U90-89) promoter (MIEp) is highly active in T cells; its activity is reduced in the absence of intron 1. The NF-κB-binding site in the R3 repeat is critical for this activity.[162]

Promoters of the genes encoding the HHV-6A DNA polymerase (U38) and its processivity factor (U27) were active in infected, but not in uninfected, cells; thus, they have virally responsive elements. The U38 promoter is TATA-less, and its activity is dependent on a palindromic activating transcription factor (ATF)/CREB-binding site.

Four latency-associated transcripts from the IE1/IE2 locus are oriented in the same direction as the IE1/IE2 genes and share their protein-coding regions with IE1/IE2, but have latency-specific transcription initiation sites and exons.[132] In addition, transcripts from the U94 gene (a homolog of the parvovirus ns1/rep gene) have been detected in primary PBMC that were polymerase chain reaction (PCR) positive for HHV-6 DNA, and negative for other lytic gene transcripts.[211] If a role for U94 in HHV-6 latency is identified, this would constitute a significant biologic difference from HHV-7 because HHV-7 does not encode a U94 homolog. While neither human nor murine CMV encodes a U94 homolog,[263] hints as to U94 function may come from studies of rat CMV, which encodes a U94 homolog that binds single- and dsDNA and is not essential for virus replication.[40]

MicroRNAs (miRNAs) play important roles in biological processes. HHV-6B expresses 4 miRNAs: hhv6b-miR-Ro6-1, hhv6b-miR-Ro6-2, hhv6b-miR-Ro6-3, and hhv6b-miR-Ro6-4, which are encoded at two loci within the genome (in both DRL and DRR) and are encoded in antisense orientation relative to predicted HHV-6B specific genes.[260] There is a report that the maximum levels of hhv6b-miR-Ro6-1, hhv6b-miR-Ro6-2, hhv6b-miR-Ro6-3, and hhv6b-miR-Ro6-4 in serum of patients with the drug-induced hypersensitivity syndrome/drug reaction (DIHS/ DRESS) were significantly higher than in those with maculopapular eruption (MPE) and healthy controls and the serum levels of hhv6b-miR-Ro6-2 were associated with the severity of skin lesions, indicating that the detection of their miRNAs in DIHS/ DRESS may reflect the HHV-6B reactivation.[169] HHV-6A-encoded miR-U86 is involved in regulation of viral lytic replication.[186] Numerous additional HHV-6A and HHV-6B miRNAs were recently identified whose functions have not been studied.[60]

Translation and Transport

Several HHV-6A and HHV-6B genes (e.g., U36 and U48; Fig. 14.4) were recently found to have short translated upstream ORFs near the 5′ end of mRNAs that express larger proteins from downstream ORFs.[60] Ribosomal interactions with upstream short ORFs regulate translation of downstream ORFs, and the small peptides can have independent biological activities.[61,76]

HHV-6A and HHV-6B U51 encode a G-protein–coupled receptor homolog that is expressed on the surfaces of transfected T-cell lines but in other cell lines accumulates intracellularly without being transported to the cell surface,[166] suggesting the presence of a cell-specific transport or processing function.

Virally Encoded Transcription Regulators

Roseoloviruses encode genes that regulate transcription of viral and cellular genes. These include products of HHV-6A IE-A and IE-B loci, DR6, U3, U27, and U94. Positive regulatory effects have been seen by transfection or infection in a variety of cell types on heterologous viral promoters, including the HIV-1 and human T-cell lymphoma 1 (HTLV-1) LTR,

Epstein-Barr virus (EBV) latent membrane protein 1 (LMP-1) and EBV nuclear antigen 2 (EBNA-2), HSV gD, human papillomaviruses 16 and 18, and the adenovirus E3 and E4 genes.[26,45] In addition, negative regulatory effects have been observed on cellular promoters for p53, H-ras, and CXCR4, along with mixed effects on the CD4 promoter (positive by HHV-6A and negative by HHV-7).[66] Up-regulation of the HIV-1 LTR is variously dependent on the presence of the NF-kB, AP-1, transacting response (TAR), and SP1 sites, whereas its suppression by U94 is independent of NF-kB and SP1 but dependent on the TAR element.

Functions of Immediate-Early Gene Products

Human herpesvirus 6 IE-A consists of two genetic units, IE1 and IE2, corresponding to U90-U89 and U90-U86/87, respectively.[83,195] IE2 proteins with molecular masses of 100, 85, and 55 kDa are detectable 3 days after infection, whereas IE1 proteins of greater than 170 kDa are detectable within 8 hours. IE2 is expressed via differential splicing and alternative translation initiation. IE2 proteins show a mixed cytoplasmic and nuclear localization pattern. At earlier times (8 to 48 hours after infection), it is present as intranuclear granules, whereas at later time points (72 to 120 hours after infection), IE2 coalesces into a few large immunoreactive patches. IE2 can induce the transcription of a complex promoter, such as the HIV-LTR, as well as simpler promoters, whose expression is driven by a unique set of responsive elements (*cis*-acting replication element [CRE], nuclear factor of activated T cells [NFAT], NF-κB).[86] Moreover, minimal promoters having a single TATA box or no defined eukaryotic regulatory elements can be activated by IE2, suggesting that it plays an important role in initiating the expression of several HHV-6 genes as a promiscuous transactivator.[256] HHV-6 IE2 interacts with the heterogeneous nuclear ribonucleoprotein K (hnRNP K) and the beta subunit of casein kinase 2 (CK2β).[229] IE2 localizes at cellular telomeres and viral replication compartments during infection (PMID 32320442). U95 interacts with the mitochondrial GRIM-19 protein that promotes cell death induced by IFN-β and retinoic acid.[286] Short-term HHV-6B infection of MT-4 T-lymphocytic cells induced syncytial formation, resulted in decreased mitochondrial membrane potential, and led to progressively pronounced ultrastructural changes, such as mitochondrial swelling, myelin-like figures, and a loss of cristae. The high affinity between U95 and GRIM-19 may be closely linked to the detrimental effect of HHV-6B infection on mitochondria.

The C-terminal domain of the IE2 protein is conserved among betaherpesviruses and important for the transactivation function. Structural analysis of this domain revealed a homo-dimeric form reminiscent of the DNA-binding domains of EBV EBNA1 and KSHV LANA, presenting a putative DNA-binding site that may interact with transcription factors.[184]

IE1 of HHV-6A and HHV-6B stably interact with PML bodies (also known as ND10 or nuclear promyelocytic leukemia protein [PML] oncogenic domains [POD]).[83,231] Remarkably, PML bodies remain structurally intact and associate with the IE1 protein throughout lytic HHV-6 infection, unlike other herpesviruses, which trigger PML-body dispersal. IE1 is covalently modified by conjugation to the small ubiquitin-like proteins, SUMO-1-3.[82,83,231] Recent work indicates that PML plays an important in IE1 SUMOylation.[41]

HHV-6A U16 is encoded in the IE-B region of the genome. The protein-coding region of one transcript is generated by in-frame splicing of ORF U17 and U16, and another includes ORFs U16 and U15. A third differentially spliced complementary DNA (cDNA) (U16+) was identified by 5′ rapid amplification of cDNA ends. These transcripts arise from at least two transcription initiation sites; the U17/U16 spliced transcript is expressed under IE conditions, and a multiply spliced gene product encoded by U16 is expressed as a late gene. The U17/U16 and the U16+ gene products can transactivate the HIV LTR.[68]

Replication of Genome

Nucleotide metabolism

Roseoloviruses encode several enzymes that have roles in nucleotide metabolism and provide the precursors needed for nucleic acid synthesis: ribonucleotide reductase (pU28), a phosphotransferase (pU69), alkaline exonuclease (pU70), and uracil-DNA glycosylase (pU81), but do not encode a thymidylate synthase or thymidine kinase. Roseolovirus ribonucleotide reductases consist of a single subunit homologous to the large subunit of two-subunit enzymes.

Initiation and elongation

Roseolovirus lytic DNA replication is initiated at an oriLyt that is similar to alphaherpesvirus oriLyts and markedly different from the oriLyts of CMV and gammaherpesviruses.[107,133,148,210] The oriLyts are located between the 5′ end of U41 and the 3′ end of U42. The minimal oriLyt segment is about 300 bp long, and a fully functional oriLyt is about 800 bp long. Multiple tandem iterations of the origin sequence enable more efficient replication of plasmids in transient replication assays, and confer a replication advantage on virus genomes.[50] A critical element near the center of oriLyt consists of two palindromically arranged sequences, OBP-1 and OBP-2, that are recognized by the origin-binding protein (OBP) encoded in roseoloviruses by U73 (a homolog of HSV-1 UL9). The core OBP sites flank an AT-rich sequence of about 30 bp (e-Fig. 14.4). Several positions within the OBP binding sites are conserved among the viruses that encode OBP homologs, whereas others differ in a manner that provides viral specificity. Replication efficiency is also affected by the sequence and composition of the AT-rich spacer. HHV-6A and HHV-6B are able to support replication of each other's oriLyt. Plasmids containing the HHV-6 oriLyt, however, were replicated in HHV-7-infected cells, but not vice versa, suggesting that oriLyt sequences and binding specificities differ between the viruses. It is thus surprising that the HHV-6 OBP binds strongly to the HHV-7 OBP binding sites, but the HHV-7 OBP binds strongly to only one of the HHV-6 OBP sites.[134]

In addition to OBP, roseoloviruses encode homologs of the six other virally encoded proteins needed for replication of plasmids containing an HSV oriLyt. They include the major DNA-binding protein (pU41), the DNA polymerase (pU38) and its processivity factor (pU27), and three gene products that constitute the helicase–primase complex (pU43, pU74, and pU77). In an *in vitro* DNA synthesis system that employed the single-stranded M13 genome as a template, the HHV-6A DNA polymerase alone synthesized molecules shorter than 100 nucleotides.[144] Addition of the polymerase processivity factor homolog encoded by U27 (p41), led to synthesis of molecules greater than 7,200 nucleotides in length, similar to the processivity increase produced by its homologs in other herpesviruses. The N-terminal portion of the processivity factor was required for this activity.

Genome packaging and cleavage

About 5% of genomes contained in nucleocapsids are circularized, creating a juxtaposition of direct repeat right (DRR) and direct repeat left (DRL) that results in assembly of a complete cleavage and packaging signal. The structure of such circular genomes is as follows: DRR-(TRS)n-pac2-N16–18-junction-N25–29-pac1-het(TRS)n-DRL.[47,52,79,210,223,252] Some heterogeneity is seen in the sequences of concatemeric junctions, with 1 to 8 bp of additional, possibly untemplated, DNA being inserted into some molecules.[52,223] Circularized molecules provide the template for rolling-circle replication, which leads to production of concatemers of nascent DNA suitable for packaging into capsids.[210] In the model of Frenkel and Roffman,[69] concatemers are cleaved between properly juxtaposed pac1 and pac2 sequences after a headful threshold has been reached during packaging, leading to unit-length packaged genomes. Relatively few multimeric concatemers are generated during replication, and compared with HSV, HHV-6 replication intermediates are not highly branched, suggesting less frequent homologous recombination among replicating molecules, or effects due to the presence of three oriLyts in every HSV genomes, versus one for roseoloviruses.[228]

Identification of the oriLyt and cleavage and packaging signals allowed development of amplicon systems based on HHV-6 and HHV-7[24,47] that feature T-cell replication, oriLyt, and cleavage-packaging signals and can be used for expression of foreign genes. They have potential use as gene therapy vectors.

Virion Assembly and Release

Roseolovirus virion maturation and egress appear to involve a process of successive envelopment, de-envelopment, and re-envelopment steps during nuclear egress and acquisition of the final envelope (Fig. 14.1). DNA replication and capsid assembly take place in the nucleus; nascent capsids that contain DNA appear about 3 days after infection.[20,22] A feature that is likely to be a result of the envelopment–development process is the presence of abundant nonenveloped, tegumented nucleocapsids in the cytoplasm. In some studies, particles with neither tegument nor envelope were observed in the cytoplasm[20,258]; teguments appeared to be acquired cytoplasmically in pools of electron-dense material. Membrane-bound nuclear structures that appear to be cytoplasmic invaginations (tegusomes) have been proposed as sites of tegument acquisition,[209] but given the relatively low frequency with which they are observed, this is not the major pathway. Because viral glycoproteins gB, gH-gL, and gQ1 are absent from the plasma membrane, envelopment or egress by budding directly from the plasma membrane are not likely. These glycoproteins are concentrated in cytoplasmic structures known as *annulate lamellae*,[258] which may correspond to the endosome- and TGN-related intracellular membranes where final envelopment of virions occurs.[173] HHV-6 virions collect in multivesicular bodies (MVB) that contain numerous mature virions and small exosomal vesicles.[173] MVB membranes can fuse with the plasma membrane, resulting in the release of mature virions and exosomal particles. In addition to exocytosis, mature virions can be released by cell lysis.[258]

Functions of Other Virally Encoded Gene Products

The U3-U7 gene cluster is not essential for virus replication or latency in cultured cells.[131]

U11 encodes the roseolovirus homologs of HCMV tegument protein, pp150: p100 (HHV-6A), 101K (HHV-6B), and phosphoprotein p86 (HHV-7).[181,201,232] HHV-6A U11 is incorporated into teguments in association with the product of the U14 gene (pU14); U11 is essential for virus propagation.[158]

pU14 localizes in the nucleus at early phase of infection and then relocates to the cytoplasm where it functions as a tegument protein. In the early phase, pU14 induces cell cycle arrest in G2/M phase by associating with EDD in the nucleus.[172] The substitution or deletion of 3 amino acids (L424, E425, and V426) of U14 abolishes its binding with another tegument protein, U11,[158] and results in a defect in viral maturation.[175,269] The importance of these amino acids for U14 function is suggested by its structure, in which a β hairpin contributes to the dimer interaction and likely contributes to interactions with other proteins.[269]

HHV-6B U19 can inhibit p53-dependent signaling following gamma irradiation[127] and also bind to the p53-regulating protein HDM2.[128]

The HHV-6A U21-24 gene cluster is dispensable for virus replication.[115] HHV-6A U23 is a membrane protein expressed at late phase of infection locating at the trans-Golgi network (TGN),[98] although its function is still unknown.

The gB (encoded by U39) is a conserved herpesvirus glycoprotein that is found on virions of most herpesviruses, including roseoloviruses. It has roles in attachment and penetration and is a target for complement-independent neutralization. The primary HHV-6A gB translation product of about 112 kDa is proteolytically cleaved to form disulfide-bond–linked subunits of 64 kDa and 58 kDa; for HHV-6B and HHV-7, the corresponding products were approximately 102, 59, and 50 kDa, and 112, 63, and 51 kDa, respectively. As with the gB of other herpesviruses, the extracellular domain of HHV-7 gB binds to cell surface heparan sulfate proteoglycans, indicating a role in adsorption of the virion to cells.[224] The deletion of gB cytoplasmic tail (CTD) impairs the intracellular transport of gB protein to the TGN, showing that CTD is critical for gB transportation.[157] Domain II of gB is expected to be exposed to the solvent in the trimeric form. A neutralizing monoclonal antibody targets a linear epitope on the domain II, indicating its functional importance.[266]

HHV-6 U42 is a homolog of HCMV UL69. Like pUL69, pU42 homodimerizes and shuttles from between the nucleus and cytoplasm, but pU42 does not interact with the cellular DExD/H-box helicases UAP56 and URH49, and thus does not export mRNA.[300]

As for other herpesviruses, the conserved virion glycoproteins gH and gL (encoded by ORFs U48 and U82, respectively), heterodimerize and together have roles in membrane fusion associated with both virus entry and cell-to-cell spread.[246] As mentioned, the HHV-6 gH/gL complex forms independent envelope complexes with either gQ1/gQ2 or gO.[30,171] HHV-6A gQ1 and gQ2 are essential for HHV-6A replication[242,244] while HHV-6A gO is not essential.[245]

The proteinase required for capsid maturation, DNA packaging, and virus assembly is encoded by U53. The HHV-6 proteinase, like its homologs in other herpesviruses, is translated as a precursor molecule that is autolytically processed at two sites (the release and maturation sites) to produce the mature proteinase and assembly proteins. As in the other herpesviruses, the processing sites consist of an Ala-Ser sequence. In contrast to the other herpesviruses, roseoloviruses lack an internal autocatalytic cleavage site (Ala-Ala instead of Ala-Ser), which results in their proteinase being a single-chain enzyme.[254]

HHV-6 U69 gene product (pU69) is the presumed functional homologue of HCMV UL97-encoded kinase (pUL97), which converts ganciclovir to its monophosphate metabolite in HCMV-infected cells.[45] The efficiency of ganciclovir phosphorylation in HHV-6-infected cells, and by vaccinia virus–expressed pU69, however, is relatively poor.

Viral DNA replication was reduced 50-fold, and cytopathic effects were also inhibited in T cells stably expressing short interfering RNA (siRNA) specific for the HHV-6 G-protein–coupled receptor (GPCR) homolog encoded by U51, suggesting that HHV-6 U51 is a positive regulator of virus replication.[299]

HHV-6 gM (encoded by U72) is a type III membrane protein with 7 membrane-spanning domains and a C-terminal cytoplasmic tail, and interacts with gN (encoded by U46) to form a complex for transport to the TGN.[120] Finally, the complex is incorporated into mature virions and essential for virus production.[120] The gM/gN complex interacts with the v-SNARE, VAMP3, which is incorporated into virions.[98]

The Rep68 protein of adeno-associated virus type 2 (AAV-2) is a site-specific adenosine triphosphate–dependent endonuclease and helicase and is involved in site-specific integration of the viral genome into the host genome (see Chapter 06—parvovirus chapter). Rep68's HHV-6A homolog, U94, can serve as a helper for AAV-2 replication, and can complement a point mutant of AAV-2 rep.[253] As summarized by Caselli et al.[30] (a) HHV-6 U94 transcripts have been detected in PBMC during latency; (b) activities associated with U94 include suppression of H-ras and bovine papillomavirus 1 (BPV-1) transformation and transcription from the H-ras and HIV-1 LTR promoters, the ability to bind to ssDNA and to human TATA-binding protein, the ability to inhibit the replication of HHV-6 and other betaherpesviruses (HHV-7 and HCMV), but not HSV, and (c) HHV-7 does not encode a U94 homolog, although rat CMV does. The activities of U94 in the regulation of HHV-6 replication have implications for co-reactivations and latency of human betaherpesviruses. U94 is also able to hydrolyze ATP to ADP and has a 3′ to 5′ exonuclease activity on dsDNA, and compromises the integrity of synthetic telomeric D-loop through exonuclease attack at the 3′end of the invading strand, suggesting a possible role in genome integration.[259] In addition, expression of U94 in cultured endothelial cells inhibits the formation of capillary-like structures, reduces cell migration, and blocks angiogenesis.[29] U94 is dispensable for HHV-6A chromosomal integration.[267]

U41 and U70, which enhance dsDNA break repair, were also dispensable.[275]

HHV-6B direct repeat 6 (DR6) expresses a nuclear protein that interacts with the U27-encoded viral DNA polymerase processivity factor, p41, and can induce p53-independent cell cycle arrest in G2/M.[216] HHV-6A lineages that spontaneously lost the genomic segment spanning DR1 through the first exon of DR6 appear to have a growth advantage in at least some cell lines.[25]

Fate of Host Cell

Roseolovirus infection has profound effects on host cells, including margination of chromatin, shutoff of host cell DNA synthesis, generalized stimulation of host cell protein synthesis, and development of the classic cytopathic effect of ballooning, refractile, multinucleated giant cells, as has been reviewed elsewhere.[26,45] For at least HHV-7, the multinucleated cells develop not by fusion of cells into syncytia but by polyploidization that is linked to dysregulation of cdc2 and cyclin B. This leads to an accumulation of cells in the G2 to M phase of the cell cycle, with nuclei continuing to reproduce in the absence of cell division.[219] Cytokines can be induced, including interferon-alpha (IFN-α), interleukin-1β, interleukin-15, CC chemokines, tumor necrosis factor alpha (TNF-α), and the G-protein-coupled peptide receptor, EB1. In addition, HHV-6A and HHV-6B can inhibit the proliferative responses of PBMC to antigens and mitogens.[64,102]

HHV-6 infection induces cell surface expression of CD4, which then renders NK cells susceptible to HIV-1 infection. HHV-6A, but neither HHV-6B nor HHV-7, down-regulates cell surface expression of CD3; HHV-7 sharply down-regulates CD4.[21,26,91]

HHV-6B infection induces a p53-independent G2 cell cycle arrest in human cord blood mononuclear cells that is mediated by the pDR6 viral protein.[217] HHV-6B infections of T-cell lines led to G1/S and G2/M arrests concomitant with an increased level and enhanced DNA-binding activity of p53. HHV-6B induces phosphorylation of p53 at Ser15 and Ser20 by casein kinase 1,[155] suggesting that viral suppression of T-cell proliferation links to p53 phosphorylation and accumulation. Interactions of HHV-6B pU19 with the p53-regulating protein HDM2 result in decreased p53 ubiquitination and increased levels of p53 in HHV-6-infected cells.[128] p53 mainly localizes in the cytoplasm of HHV-6-infected cells, but it translocates into the nucleus of mock-infected cells. Infected cells are resistant to UV-induced apoptosis, suggesting that HHV-6 has a mechanism for retaining p53 within the cytoplasm, providing protection from apoptosis. Since HHV-6 gene expression is enhanced in the absence of active p53,[193] p53 induction may be a cellular response to the invading pathogen. p53 interacts also with the HHV-6B U14 tegument protein, and is incorporated into viral particles.[239]

In ways that have parallels to manipulation of cellular metabolism by other herpesviruses, HHV-6A replication is enhanced by its ability to modulate infected cell metabolism in ways that result in enhanced glycolysis that is linked to increased glucose uptake, glucose consumption, and lactate production[278]; this activity is linked to viral activation of AKT-mTORC signaling.

Some parallels have emerged in studies of apoptosis induction during infections with HHV-6 and HHV-7. In fresh umbilical cord blood lymphocytes, infected cells are apoptotic,[20,106] whereas in cell lines, infected cells die by necrotic lysis and apoptosis is triggered in apparently uninfected or nonproductively infected cells.[108,221] For HHV-7, the induction and release of TRAIL by infected cells is likely responsible for apoptosis induction in uninfected bystander cells.[222] During *in vivo* primary HHV-6B infections, apoptosis was detected in 15% to 20% of circulating PBMC.[284] HHV-7 replication was enhanced in cells expressing high levels of the apoptosis suppressor, Bcl-2.[220]

HHV-6 attachment and/or entry in the absence of de novo protein synthesis can induce expression of the human endogenous retrovirus K18-encoded superantigen.[36]

In HHV-6-infected immature monocyte-derived dendritic cells, viral early and late antigens are expressed, and nucleocapsids containing a DNA core are observed, but few virions are detected in the cytoplasm. In co-cultures, HHV-6 can be transmitted from these cells to stimulated CD4+ T cells, suggesting that DCs may be the one of the first cell populations targeted by the virus and may transmit the virus to T cells.[238]

HHV-6 infection of monocytes/macrophages results in the establishment of latency with expression of latency-associated transcripts overlapping the IE locus encoding the U86-U90 genes. Latent HHV-6 can be reactivated by stimulating cells with phorbol esters.[131] Whether latently infected cells carry episomes or integrated viral genomes remains to be determined.

PATHOGENESIS AND PATHOLOGY

Detailed referencing of historical literature in this area is available in several comprehensive reviews.[4,26,65,271]

Transmission

HHV-6B and HHV-7 are ubiquitous viruses infecting most individuals during the first 2 to 3 years of life. Horizontal infection accounts for the majority of transmission events, likely via saliva and respiratory secretions (Fig. 14.7). Studies have demonstrated that family saliva-sharing behaviors are associated with earlier acquisition of HHV-6B and older siblings are associated with earlier acquisition of both HHV-6B and HHV-7.[139,208,296]

Given the young age of primary HHV-6B infection, most organ transplant recipients have acquired the virus prior to transplantation; however, the transplanted organ may be a source of HHV-6B primary infection in very young patients (Fig. 14.7).[291]

While most HHV-6B infections occur via horizontal routes, approximately 1% of the population acquires HHV-6A or B as inherited chromosomally integrated virus via the germ line.[118,198] In such individuals, an intact HHV-6A/B genome is integrated at the telomere of a chromosome, with copies of that chromosome being present in every cell in the body. While HHV-6A/B DNA has been detected in fetuses and in blood of neonates, indicating that intrauterine transmission is possible, most cases of congenital transmission of HHV-6A/B can be attributed either to genetic transmission of iciHHV-6A/B from either or both parents or to transplacental transmission of virus from mothers with iciHHV-6A/B.[93]

Primary Infection

Site of Primary Replication

Human herpesvirus 6B and HHV-7 possibly initiate infection through respiratory pathways, including lymphocyte-rich tonsils and olfactory ensheathing cells present in the nasal cavity. The high prevalence of the virus in the olfactory bulb suggests that a route of CNS entry might be via olfactory ensheathing glial cells present in the nasal cavity.[97]

Cell and Tissue Tropism

The *in vivo* host tissue range of HHV-6A/B includes lymphoid and endothelial cells, as well as cells present in the liver, central nervous system tissues, and salivary glands.[26,45]

In vivo, HHV-7 infects CD4+ T lymphocytes (believed to be the site of latent infection), and salivary gland epithelial cells (a site of productive infection and viral shedding).[21] In addition, cells expressing an HHV-7 structural antigen were detectable in lungs, skin, and mammary glands, and at reduced frequencies in liver, kidney, and tonsils; this antigen was not detected in large intestine, spleen, or brain.[124] In a recent tissue level study of the human virome, HHV-7 was detected in 37% of 203 specimens.[136]

Persistence

Human herpesvirus 6 DNA and antigens can be detected in saliva, nasal secretions, brain, lung, bone marrow progenitors, and PBMC. HHV-6 DNA was detected mainly in the monocyte fraction of PBMC from patients convalescing from

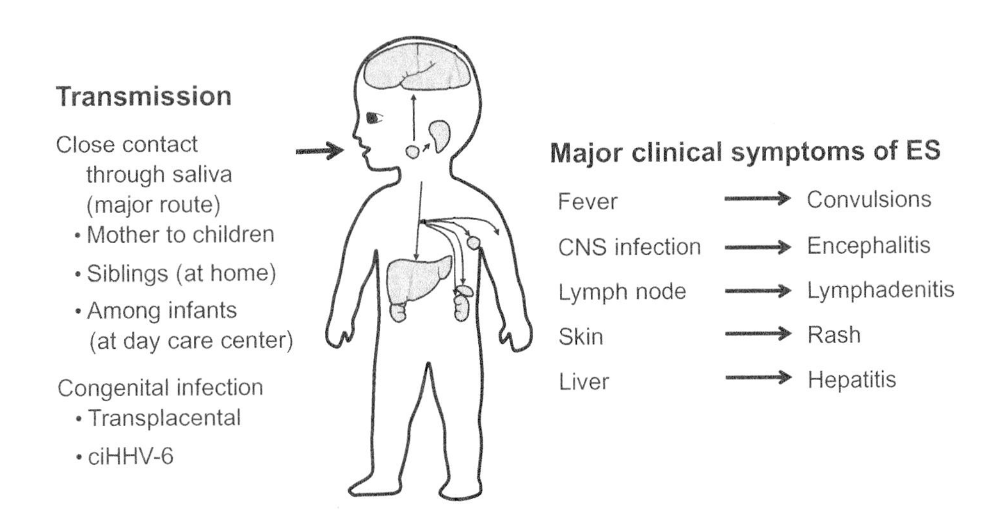

FIGURE 14.7 Pathogenesis of HHV-6B primary infection.

ES and from healthy adults, and appears to establish latency in monocytes or macrophages and CD34-positive progenitor cells.[7,130,149] As described above, latency-associated transcripts have been detected from the IE region and U94. In a prospective study, 89% of children from 1 to 12 years of age were PCR positive for HHV-6 at least one time point, with 1.2% of specimens being positive for reverse transcription PCR (RT-PCR), indicating active infection[33]; this activity was not associated with illness.

The HHV-6 variants differ with respect to their absolute and relative frequencies of detection in PBMC and cerebrospinal fluid (CSF). Of over 1,000 HHV-6 PCR-positive PBMC specimens, 2.5% were positive for HHV-6A and 99% for HHV-6B (some were positive for both). Of 84 HHV-6 PCR-positive CSF specimens, 17% were positive for HHV-6A and 86% for HHV-6B (some dual positives). Thus, HHV-6B was detected much more frequently in CSF than was HHV-6A, but the ratio of 6A to 6B was higher in CSF than in PBMCs indicating a greater relative neurotropism for HHV-6A.[92]

Germ line or iciHHV-6 enables a form of persistence in which the virus genome is present in every cell in the body. Under most circumstances, the virus appears to be quiescent, but spontaneous viral gene expression from the integrated virus does occur; U90 and U100 transcripts have been detected in tissues of several iciHHV-6-positive individuals.[197] Reactivation of iciHHV-6A with subsequent pathogenic outcomes was convincingly demonstrated in a boy with X-SCID.[56] Transplacental vertical transmission can also occur following reactivation of maternal iciHHV-6,[84] and fetal iciHHV-6 inheritance can lead to viral gene expression in the placenta and increased risk of preeclampsia.[72] It has been hypothesized that the default latency pathway for HHV-6 in individuals without germ line ciHHV-6 involves chromosomal integration in peripheral cells,[9] but this has not been demonstrated.

Human herpesvirus 7 DNA is frequently detectable in whole blood[74] and the virus establishes latent infections in CD4+ cells[70] and persistent lytic infections in salivary glands.[279] As described earlier, HHV-7 lytic antigens are present in a variety of tissues, suggesting that persistent infection occurs in many tissues *in vivo*.[124] None of three HHV-7 lytic cycle transcripts studied were detected in HHV-7 DNA-positive PBMC,[165] evidence that the virus is truly latent in these cells.

Immune Response

Immune responses to HHV-6 and HHV-7 and their immunomodulatory activities have been reviewed in detail.[45,150,270,271]

Antigens

Responses are generated to many of the virally encoded proteins. The immunodominant HHV-6 antigen in immunoblots is a virion tegument protein, pU11 (101K or p100). Responses to HHV-7 are directed predominantly to pp85 and pp89 (encoded by U14 and U11),[232] as well as to a 52 kDa species.[178] Consistent with their sequence similarities, sufficient antigenic cross-reactivity exists between HHV-6A and HHV-6B to preclude the use of conventional serologic assays for the study of variant-specific immune responses. These levels of cross-reactivity are reflected in the frequencies of cross-reactive mAb and T-cell clones.[11,21,285]

Primary Infection

Serologic studies on the association between ES and HHV-6 infection have mainly come from Japan. In patients with ES, IgM antibodies were detected on day 5 and persisted for 3 weeks but were not detectable in most sera 1 month after the onset of disease (e-Fig.14.5). The viremia during primary infection subsides coincident with the appearance of neutralizing antibodies. IgG antibodies are first detected about 7 days after onset of illness, increase for 3 weeks, and persist thereafter. HHV-6 antibody titers are boosted during infection with HHV-7 (e-Fig. 14.5). Plasma IFN-α levels are elevated during the acute febrile phase of ES compared with convalescence.[237] NK cell activity is also elevated in the exanthem phase of ES, probably induced by IL-15.[67,237] These early responses likely play pivotal roles in control of the infection.

Cellular immunity appears to be important for control of primary HHV-6 infection. Low-level *ex vivo* T-cell immune responses against HHV-6 can be detected in most healthy adults indicating a low frequency of HHV-6-specific memory T cells. However, such effector cells can be rapidly expanded *in vitro* and be of potential therapeutic benefit.[75,177] Both $CD8^+$ class I–restricted and $CD4^+$ class II–restricted T cells recognizing HHV-6A/B peptides have been identified. With a few exceptions, such as the U90 IE1 gene product, most peptides presented to T cells are derived from virion structural proteins including the U11, U14, U31, and U54 tegument proteins; the gB and gH virion envelope glycoproteins; and the U56 and U57 capsid proteins.[16,17,75,96,159] HHV-6-specific $CD4^+$ and $CD8^+$ T cells are generally polyfunctional, secreting IFN-γ and TNF-α and are cytotoxic.[16,75,105,159] Some T-cell clones with activity against HHV-6 also responded to HHV-7 and HCMV, indicating the presence of shared T-cell epitopes.[285]

In *in vitro* studies, IFN-α activity was detected in PBMC from healthy seropositive adults as early as 12 hours after exposure to HHV-6; they plateaued at days 2 to 5, and gradually decreased thereafter; the response of cord blood mononuclear cells was lower.[125] HHV-6 also induces IL-1β and TNF-α, but not IL-6 in PBMC.[63] Thus, HHV-6 can exert a strong immunomodulatory effect by stimulating cytokine production in cells of myeloid lineage. IFN-γ regulates the production of IL-10 and IL-12 at a transcriptional level mainly through inhibiting endogenous IL-10 production in HHV-6-infected monocyte–macrophage cells.[143]

Reports on the immune response during HHV-7 primary infection are scarce because HHV-7 primary infection is seldom apparent. During a documented infection, 16 days after onset, HHV-7 antibody titer rose from less than 1:10 to 1:320 by an immunofluorescence antibody (IFA) test, whereas the HHV-6 titer remained less than 1:10.[240] In a patient with two independent ES episodes within 2 months, HHV-6 and HHV-7 were sequentially isolated; seroconversion to HHV-7 during the second episode was observed 4 days after disease onset. HHV-7 infection induces IL-15 production, which then results in an enhancement of NK cell activity that may play a major role in control of the infection.[15]

Immune Modulation

Human herpesvirus 6 infects a variety of immune cells, as described previously, and has numerous immune modulatory effects *in vivo* and *in vitro*.

Infection of PBMC or T-cell–enriched cultures by HHV-6A suppressed IL-2 synthesis after mitogen stimulation, and levels of IL-2 transcripts were diminished in experiments with enriched T-cell cultures.[64] By binding calcineurin, the HHV-6B U54 tegument protein prevents the dephosphorylation and nuclear translocation of NFAT1/2, transcription factors essential for *IL-2* gene expression.[104]

Suppression of bone marrow function may be one of the most serious effects of HHV-6 infection in bone marrow transplant recipients. *In vitro*, HHV-6 infection of normal bone marrow mononuclear cells reduced the outgrowth of granulocyte–macrophage colony-forming units (GM-CFU), granulocyte–erythrocyte–macrophage–megakaryocyte colony-forming units (GEMM-CFU), erythroid burst-forming units, and marrow stromal cells by 40% to 74%.[28] Although HHV-6A was generally a more potent inhibitor than HHV-6B, it did not exhibit as significant a suppressive effect on the formation of GM colonies. In hemopoietic progenitor cells derived from human umbilical cord blood lymphocytes, HHV-6A suppressed erythroid colonies, HHV-6B suppressed erythroid and GM colonies, and HHV-7 had no effect on either lineage.[113] These results could be the consequence of the virus either encoding or inducing a soluble mediator or mediators that interfere with the responses of bone marrow to growth factors and block differentiation of macrophages from marrow precursors.[28]

Human herpesvirus 6A and HHV-6B, but not HHV-7, modestly (twofold) induced several T-cell adhesion markers, including CD2, CD4, CD11a, CD44, CD49d, and HLA antigen-DR. HHV-6B infection had little effect on CD4+ cytotoxic lymphocytes, but HHV-6A and HHV-7 decreased their activity; the inhibition by HHV-7 was overcome by lectin stimulation.[71] Thus, the three viruses differ in their effects on T cells.

Human lymphocyte antigen (HLA) class I expression on dendritic cells (DC) was down-regulated after infection with HHV-6A but not HHV-6B, whereas no significant change was seen in the expression of CD1a, CD83, and MHC class II; IE or E gene expression was required for this.[101] Preexposure to HHV-6 markedly impaired IFNγ- and lipopolysaccharide-induced DC maturation. HHV-6, but not HHV-7, dramatically suppressed the secretion of IL-12 p70 by DC, whereas the production of other cytokines that influence DC maturation (i.e., IL-10 and TNF-α) was not affected.[230] Children who acquired HHV-6 after 18 months of age were more likely to express IgE to common allergens, suggesting that early life exposure to HHV-6 might reduce allergic responses, possibly due to the virus down-regulating Th2 responses.[185] While HHV-6 infection led to reduced IL-5 expression in DC, systemic IL-5 levels are elevated during convalescence from primary infection.[292]

Human herpesvirus 6 infection of monocyte-derived immature DC induced CD80, CD83, CD86, and HLA antigen class I and class II molecules, but decreased their capacity to present alloantigens and exogenous virus antigens to T lymphocytes.[117] Levels of DC-specific intracellular adhesion molecule-grabbing nonintegrin (SIGN) messenger RNA (mRNA) and intracellular protein decreased following HHV-6 infection.[183]

The cytokine encoded by HHV-6A U83 is an agonist for multiple chemokine receptors, including CCR1, CCR4, CCR5, CCR6, and CCR8, which are present on immune effector and antigen presenting cells.[34,51] In contrast, HHV-6B U83 is monospecific and functionally activates the CCR2 receptor and serves as a chemoattractant for mononuclear cells.[153,301] HHV-6B U83 also competes with CCL2, the natural ligand of CCR2.

HHV-6 and HHV-7 U12 and U51 encode GPCR homologs. HHV-6 pU12 is a functional β-chemokine receptor, with selectivity that differs somewhat from its cellular homologs in its higher relative affinity for RANTES relative to macrophage inhibitory proteins 1α and 1β or monocyte chemoattractant protein 1.[111] When stably expressed in cell lines, HHV-6 pU51 specifically binds the CC chemokine RANTES and competes for binding with other β-chemokines, such as eotaxin and monocyte chemoattractant proteins 1, 3, and 4. In epithelial cells already secreting RANTES, U51 expression induces specific transcriptional down-regulation of RANTES.[168] pU51 constitutively activates phospholipase C. It also binds several chemokines and promotes chemotaxis and internalization of chemokines, suggesting roles in virus dissemination or host transmission by chemotaxis of infected cells to sites of chemokine secretion specific for pU51.[35,62] Suppression of pU51 expression by siRNA reduces the replication of HHV-6, demonstrating that pU51 is important for virus growth.[299]

HHV-7 U12 and U51 also encode functional calcium-mobilizing receptors for β-chemokines, which include thymus and activation-regulated chemokine, macrophage-derived chemokine, EBI1-ligand chemokine, and secondary lymphoid-tissue chemokine.[180,236] Furthermore, EBI1-ligand chemokine and secondary lymphoid-tissue chemokine induce migration in Jurkat cells stably expressing U12, but thymus and activation-regulated chemokine, macrophage-derived chemokine, do not.[236]

Human herpesvirus 6A had little direct effect on cytokine production in primary adult astrocytes, but profoundly affected the response of these cells to a mixture of proinflammatory cytokines (TNF-α, IL-1β, and IFN-γ), inducing anti-inflammatory molecules (IL10 and IL-11), chemotactic and growth factors, and regulators of type 1 IFN production.[163]

Through inhibition of IRF3 dimerization, HHV-6A and HHV-6B IE1 prevent IFN-β gene expression,[116] but HHV-6B IE1 expression, and not HHV-6A IE1, impairs IFN-α/β antiviral activity. By interacting with STAT2, HHV-6B IE1 sequesters it in the nucleus, preventing ISG3 from binding to IFN-responsive promoters resulting in improper IFN-stimulated gene (ISG) expression.

HHV-6 and HHV-7 U21 proteins bind to HLA class I molecules and divert them to endolysosomal compartments, thereby removing them from the cell surface, leading to reduced or delayed cytotoxic T-lymphocyte recognition of infected cells.[77,103]

HHV-6 and HHV-7 U24 proteins cause internalization of the T-cell receptor/CD3 complex at the cell surface, resulting in improper T-cell activation by antigen-presenting cells.[234] A PxxY motif present in HHV-6A and HHV-7 U24 is responsible for this effect. Recent results also indicate that the PxxY motif of U24 binds with strong affinity to the WW3* domain of human Nedd4.[213] U24 also down-regulates the transferrin receptor, suggesting that this viral protein acts by blocking early endosome recycling.[235]

Epidemiology

Little is known about the epidemiology and natural history of HHV-6A. In contrast, HHV-6B is ubiquitous, infecting most children in the first 2 years of life. Very young infants appear to be protected against HHV-6B infection by maternal antibody as HHV-6B seroprevalence decreases from 0 to 5 months of age, as maternal antibody wanes. Beginning at about 6 months, seroprevalence increases rapidly, with almost all children acquiring infection by 2 years of age.[191,296]

Human herpesvirus 7 infection generally occurs somewhat later than does that for HHV-6B.[280] Similar to HHV-6B, seroprevalence declines over the first 5 to 6 months, as maternal antibody wanes, and then increases through about 4 years of age. It reaches its highest level from the teens until the end of the third decade, decreasing thereafter.[241,290]

Clinical Features

Primary Infection

Clinical features of primary infection due to HHV-6A have not been described, and its epidemiology and associated clinical syndromes remain undefined.

A population-based study of young infants followed prospectively over the first 2 years of life demonstrated that HHV-6B primary infection is typically symptomatic, causing an illness characterized by fussiness (70% of affected children), fever (58%), rhinorrhea (66%), rash (31%), roseola (fever followed by a rash with defervescence, 24%), and diarrhea (26%).[296] In this study, fever, fussiness, diarrhea, rash, roseola, and visits to a physician were all more common during primary HHV-6B infections than during control periods of illness. None of the 81 children with well-defined primary infection had a seizure. In contrast, studies performed in emergency department settings have found that HHV-6B primary infection accounts for a large proportion of first-time febrile seizures (one-third in those <2 years) presenting to emergency care.[94] Among children with febrile seizures, HHV-6B primary infection has been association with more complex seizures, such as clustering seizures, prolonged seizures, partial seizures, and postictal paralysis.[233] Primary infection has also been associated with febrile status epilepticus in 22% of cases.[58]

Encephalitis/meningoencephalitis/encephalopathy can occur during primary HHV-6B infection. Of 89 cases identified in a Japanese national survey, half of the patients had neurological sequelae and 2 died.[293] In comparison to stem cell recipients, HHV-6 encephalitis during primary infection is characterized by low viral DNA levels in the CSF and differences in cytokine responses.[123]

Liver dysfunction is also associated with HHV-6 infection; although usually mild, chronic hepatitis, fatal hepatitis, and liver failure of unknown etiology that can necessitate liver transplantation have been also reported.[283] Primary HHV-6 infection has also been associated with cases of idiopathic thrombocytopenic purpura.

Primary infection with HHV-7 causes illnesses similar to those caused by HHV-6B, including roseola, high fever, and febrile seizures.[31,240,272] HHV-7 has also been associated with febrile status epilepticus in 5% of cases.[58]

Disease in Immune Compromised Patients

Because herpesviruses persist in their hosts after primary infection and can be reactivated, they are important pathogens in immune compromised hosts. Since HHV-6B and HHV-7 are acquired early in life, most instances of detection of the virus after transplantation are due to reactivation of latent virus.

Hematopoietic cell transplants

HHV-6B reactivates in approximately 40% of allogeneic hematopoietic cell transplant (HCT) recipients, most commonly within the first 4 weeks after transplantation.[188,294] HHV-6B reactivation has been associated with a number of clinical outcomes and HHV-6B is recognized as the most common cause of encephalitis in the HCT recipient.[218]

HHV-6B encephalitis occurs in approximately 1% of allogeneic HCT transplant recipients overall and 10% of cord blood transplant recipients.[99] The timeline for onset of symptoms of encephalitis is similar to the timeline for reactivation. In most studies, HHV-6B encephalitis is defined by acute encephalopathy, HHV-6B detection in the CSF, and lack of a more likely explanation. A more specific entity, posttransplant acute limbic encephalitis (PALE), accounts for a subset of HHV-6B encephalitis, and is characterized by anterograde amnesia; the syndrome of inappropriate antidiuretic hormone secretion; mild CSF pleocytosis; temporal EEG abnormalities, often reflecting clinical or subclinical seizures; and MRI findings within the hippocampus region of the brain.[226,265]

Short of overt encephalitis, HHV-6B reactivation has also been associated with delirium and neurocognitive decline in the HCT population,[295] suggesting that the neurological impact of HHV-6B may be broader than that seen with encephalitis alone. The index of suspicion for encephalitis should be high for HCT recipients with acute encephalopathy. These patients should be tested for HHV-6B using quantitative PCR of blood or plasma and CSF.[273] Empiric therapy with foscarnet or ganciclovir is recommended for treatment of HHV-6B encephalitis,[273] and should be strongly considered while awaiting results of laboratory results.

HHV-6B has been associated with a number of other outcomes following HCT including rash, bone marrow suppression, hepatitis, lower respiratory tract disease, CMV reactivation, and acute GVHD.[3,4,26,45,202,273] Whether a causal association exists between HHV-6B and these outcomes remains to be determined; however, evidence supporting a causal association between HHV-6B and lower respiratory tract disease is accumulating. For example, studies have demonstrated detection of HHV-6B in the bronchoalveolar lavage fluid of 25% to 30% of HCT recipients with lower respiratory tract disease or idiopathic pneumonia syndrome.[100,227] In one study of 553 HCT recipients who underwent a BAL for evaluation of LRTD, HHV-6B detection in BAL fluid was associated with overall mortality and death from respiratory failure.[100] In the same study, receipt of HHV-6B-active antivirals was associated with lower levels of HHV-6B in the BAL fluid and lower mortality compared to patients without detectable HHV-6B in their BAL.

The frequency of HHV-7 reactivation following HCT is less clear as rates of viral detection in the blood have been highly variable across different studies and most studies have not found specific diseases to be associated with HHV-7 reactivation.

Solid organ transplant recipients

While HHV-6B reactivation after SOT occurs at a similar frequency and on a similar timeline as HCT, disease associations are much less frequently found. HHV-6B is not a common cause of encephalitis in SOT recipients in contrast to HCT recipients, though a wide range of clinical signs, symptoms, and entities have been associated with HHV-6B in SOT recipients including fever, cytopenias, hepatitis, gastroduodenitis, colitis, pneumonitis, and graft dysfunction and rejection.[200]

HHV-7 reactivation appears to occur at a similar rate as HHV-6B following SOT.[59] In addition, like HHV-6B, the majority of reactivation events are not associated with overt disease, though reactivation has been associated with nonspecific febrile illnesses and cytopenias.[200]

To what extent HHV-6B and HHV-7 cause poor clinical outcomes after SOT is unclear. A trial of 129 liver transplant recipients who were randomized to be monitored for HHV-6B and HHV-7 DNAemia for 12 weeks after transplantation with real-time therapeutic interventions ("monitoring/intervention" group) did not show a difference in the composite outcome of opportunistic infection, graft rejection, and severe hepatitis C virus recurrence compared to the usual care control group.[59] Therapeutic interventions for detection of DNAemia included reduction in immunosuppression and preemptive antiviral therapy, at the discretion of the patient's clinicians. In the "monitoring/intervention" group, HHV-6B and HHV-7 viremia occurred in 23 of 64 patients (35.9%) and 21 of 64 patients (32.8%) patients, respectively. No cases of symptomatic HHV-6B and HHV-7 disease were identified. Despite the fact that some level of therapeutic intervention was performed in almost 60% of viremic episodes, there were no differences in cumulative incidence of the primary outcome between the "monitoring/intervention" group and the control group at 1 year (58.7% vs. 52.3%; odds ratio, 0.77; 95% confidence interval, 0.38 to 1.55) and 5 years after transplantation (79.0% vs. 70.3%; odds ratio, 0.63; 95% confidence interval, 0.28 to 1.42).

Acquired immunodeficiency syndrome

The possible role of HHV-6A and HHV-6B as cofactors in HIV infection has been considered because both viruses can infect CD4+ cells, and transactivate the HIV LTR.[26] In addition, they can induce CD4 gene transcription and expression in CD4-negative cells, which renders them susceptible to HIV infection. Furthermore, coinfections of macaques with HHV-6A and simian immunodeficiency virus (SIV) resulted in a plasma viremia that was associated with clinical manifestations that progressed to AIDS more rapidly than in monkeys infected only with SIV, providing *in vivo* evidence that HHV-6A may promote AIDS progression.[151]

It has been hypothesized that the most important issue with respect to HHV-6A- or HHV-6B-related disease in HIV-positive individuals may not be a direct effect on specific target organs, but by their contributing to immune deficiency.[152] Studies of HHV-6 serology or detection in the context of HIV-infected individuals versus controls have had variable outcomes making it very difficult to infer what role(s) HHV-6A of HHV-6B might play.[4,26]

Possible Disease Associations

Neoplasia

Human herpesvirus 6 DNA has been detected in non-Hodgkin lymphoma, Hodgkin disease, S100-positive, T-cell chronic lymphoproliferative disease, oral salivary gland carcinoma tissues, pediatric and adult glial tumors, and other neoplasias.[26,38,43,55] Although there has been no conclusive demonstration that either HHV-6A or HHV-6B causes any malignancy, the frequency of detecting HHV-6 in certain tumors suggests a possible cofactorial role in multistep carcinogenesis.

Chronic fatigue syndrome

Conflicting reports have appeared of a connection between chronic fatigue syndrome (CFS) and HHV-6 infection.[187] We do not consider the evidence to support an etiologic association.

Multiple sclerosis

Numerous studies have found that HHV-6B and HHV-6A are commensal viruses of the human brain. Studies have variably associated serum anti-HHV-6 IgG and/or IgM, and serum DNA detection with MS.[250] However, compelling results from several studies are difficult to dismiss. For example, a longitudinal study demonstrated a higher positivity of HHV6 DNA at time of relapse when compared to remission,[18] and increasing HHV6 DNA in CSF has been associated with elevated numbers of contrast-enhancing lesions on MRI.[264] In addition, a higher prevalence of anti-HHV6 CSF IgG detection has been demonstrated in patients with MS compared to patients with other neurological diseases (34% vs. 12%, $p = 0.05$).[49] A recent study of a cohort of 8,742 persons with MS and 7,215 matched controls employed serologic assays based on the HHV-6A and HHV-6B IE1 proteins, an EBV serologic assay, and analysis of HLA haplotypes.[57] For all MS subtypes and severities of disease, a positive relationship was seen in individuals with EBV and HHV-6A IE1 serological responses and the DRB1(*)13:01-DQA1(*)01:03-DQB1(*)06:03 haplotype.

Both indirect effects of HHV-6 via molecular mimicry between the virus and host myelin components as well as direct impact of the virus on the myelin-producing cells of the CNS have been hypothesized to explain the pathogenesis of MS.[250] Further research, including additional longitudinal cohort studies, ideally measuring both serological and viral levels in both CSF and peripheral circulation, and ultimately treatment trials, are needed to determine whether a true association exists.[129]

Other neurologic disorders

HHV-6 (mostly B) DNA has been detected more frequently and at higher levels in resected brain tissues from patients with mesial temporal lobe epilepsy compared to controls, suggesting that HHV-6B may have a role in pathogenesis of the condition, though results have not been consistent across all studies.[122,129,141,276]

Progressive multifocal leukoencephalopathy (PML) is a primary demyelinating disease of the CNS, occurring almost exclusively in individuals with impaired cell-mediated immunity. The JC polyoma virus has been accepted as the etiologic agent of PML, but the question of whether herpesviruses might be associated with PML has been raised. One study found HHV-6 detection in conjunction with JC virus infection associated with the demyelinative lesions of PML.[170] However, another study did not find HHV-6 in the setting of PML but did find evidence of other herpesviruses.[179]

Myocarditis

Several case reports of HHV-6-associated myocarditis and dilated cardiomyopathy in children and adults have been published; however, whether the association is causal remains to be determined as the virus can be detected in the heart tissue of healthy controls.[42,206]

Drug hypersensitivity

Drug-induced hypersensitivity syndrome (DIHS) is characterized by a severe, potentially fatal, multiorgan reaction that usually appears after prolonged exposure to certain drugs.[4,255] Clinical signs include a maculopapular rash progressing to exfoliate erythroderma, fever, and lymphadenopathy. Reactivation of herpesviruses, including HHV-6B, HHV-7, HCMV, and EBV have been detected during severe drug-induced hypersensitivity syndrome and the related illnesses, but it is uncertain whether the virus reactivation is triggered by the disease and/or contributes to the disease.

Pityriasis rosea

Pityriasis rosea has variably been associated with HHV-6 and/or HHV-7 infection or reactivation. It has also been suggested that pityriasis rosea early in pregnancy and HHV-6 viral load during pregnancy are associated with pregnancy complications.[54]

Animal Models

Animal models for HHV-6 and HHV-7 are scarce. Various groups have successfully experimentally infected various monkey species with HHV-6A/B.[142,151,281]

An *in vivo* model for immune suppression by HHV-6 was developed in severe combined immunodeficient (SCID-hu) Thy/Liv mice.[78] HHV-6A and HHV-6B efficiently infected the human thymic tissue implanted in these mice, leading to graft destruction. Virus replication was associated with severe, progressive thymocyte depletion involving all major cellular subsets. Intrathymic T progenitor cells were more severely depleted than the other subpopulations, and a preferred tropism of HHV-6 for these cells was demonstrated. Thus, thymocyte depletion by HHV-6 may be caused by infection and destruction of their immature precursors.

Mice expressing human CD46 were developed as a model to study HHV-6A infection and pathogenesis. Although intracranial injection of HHV-6A leads to long-term viral DNA persistence, the virus does not appear to replicate efficiently.[207]

Genome analysis indicates that the mouse thymic virus is a roseolovirus. Although this virus lacks the telomeric repeats found in the DRs of HHV-6 and HHV-7, this virus could prove useful to study the pathogenesis of roseolovirus in mice.[196]

In a marmoset model, intranasal inoculation with HHV-6A or HHV-6 accelerated development of experimental autoimmune encephalomyelitis (EAE), and elevated levels of viral antigens were detected in brain lesions.[140]

Diagnosis

Diagnosis of HHV-6 and HHV-7 infections has been reviewed comprehensively elsewhere.[3,4,26,90,271,273]

Differential Diagnosis

Because the symptoms of primary HHV-6B and HHV-7 are nonspecific and the infections are generally mild and self-limiting, specific laboratory diagnosis to identify primary infection is seldom warranted. HHV-6B can be detected in the CSF of healthy children at the time of primary infection, but it is a very rare cause of encephalitis in the United States. Clinicians are often faced with the question of interpreting positive results for HHV-6B since it is now included on multiplex PCR panels for meningitis and encephalitis. Other etiologies of encephalitis, particularly those that are treatable, should be aggressively pursued.

HHV-6B is the most common cause of encephalitis in HCT recipients[218]; however, other causes of encephalitis in the immunocompromised host should be considered and testing informed by the clinical setting, season, and epidemiological exposures. For example, viral pathogens, including HSV, VZV, EBV, and CMV, should be considered in all HCT recipients, while Enterovirus and arboviruses should be considered as seasonally and regionally appropriate. Bacterial and fungal (e.g., *Aspergillus* and other molds) pathogens may disseminate from the lung or other organ systems and cause central nervous system disease. Thus, evaluation of lung and sinus imaging as well as blood cultures may be indicated, depending on the clinical setting. Finally, while they are rare causes of encephalitis, tuberculosis and parasites such as toxoplasmosis should be considered in patients from endemic regions or with pretransplant evidence of infection.

Laboratory Diagnosis

Virus detection by culture

While virus culture is seldom employed for clinical diagnosis, it remains important for research purposes. HHV-6B is easily recovered from PBMC of patients with ES during the acute phase. Lymphocyte activation with either PHA or antibody to CD3 and maintenance in IL-2 is required.[282] A profound cytopathic effect develops within 7 to 10 days (Fig. 14.2). The refractile giant cells usually contain one or two nuclei; after CPE develops, the cells degenerate. Mononuclear cell–associated viremia caused by HHV-6 was detected in 66% of blood samples from children with ES between days 0 and 7 of the disease. The rate of virus isolation from mononuclear cells was 100% on days 0 to 2 (just before appearance of skin rash), 82% on day 3, 20% on day 4, 7% on days 5 to 7, and 0% on day 8 and thereafter. Cell-free virus was also detected in blood samples during the same period.[12] HHV-7 is sometimes isolated from peripheral blood of patients with ES, and can be readily isolated from saliva by using methods as described above for HHV-6. Isolation of HHV-6 from saliva is uncommon, although its DNA is often detectable there.

Detection of viral genome, transcripts, and proteins

HHV-6A, HHV-6B, and HHV-7 DNA are commonly detected by quantitative polymerase chain reaction assays (qPCR). Numerous primer sets have been described, including commercially available rapid quantitative and multiplex assays that enable identification and discrimination of HHV-6A, HHV-6B, and HHV-7 (fewer options).[3,4,90]

A multicenter external quality assessment among 51 laboratories that employ PCR for HHV-6 found that most labs use in-house quantitative assays, there was good qualitative agreement on specimens containing at least 200 copies/mL, but quantitative reporting was much more variable.[194] Widespread adoption of the WHO quantitative PCR standard for HHV-6B will hopefully contribute to improvement in the quality of quantitative PCR data.[81]

Latent and replicating virus can be discriminated by assays that combine reverse transcription and PCR (RT-PCR).[289] Such assays target spliced mRNAs, enabling easy discrimination between mRNA (short amplimer because of intron removal) and residual DNA contamination (long amplimer). Because HHV-6 DNA is usually cell associated,[2] it can be more useful to describe qPCR results in terms of a ratio between virus and cell genomes, rather than in terms of virus genome copies per volume of fluid (e.g., virus genomes per mL of blood) that can contain variable concentrations of cells.[73]

HHV-6 DNA is easily detectable by PCR in peripheral blood of patients with ES during the acute phase. Although detection of cell-free virus in serum or plasma by PCR offers the possibility of diagnosing active HHV-6 infections, PCR-based assays of plasma were not reliable for discriminating primary HHV-6 from iciHHV-6.[32] qPCR was less sensitive than culture for detecting primary infection, while RT-PCR was approximately as specific as culture for detection of primary infection.

A monoclonal antibody-based quantitative antigenemia assay enables enumeration of HHV-6B-infected cells and has been used to monitor HHV-6 activity in liver transplant recipients.[147]

iciHHV-6 presents several challenges to PCR-based methods for HHV-6 diagnosis.[39,89,90,198,274] Because at least one copy of the virus genome is present in every cell, high copy numbers will be detected in most clinical specimens, even if the virus is not actively replicating or otherwise contributing to the illness. Sufficient viral DNA can leak from lysed cells to cause false positives in bodily fluids that are normally relatively acellular. Cell lysis during serum clotting and during the period between blood collection and plasma separation can also lead to false positives in these acellular fluids. iciHHV-6 should be suspected when uncommonly high levels of HHV-6 DNA are found.[89] Persistent loads greater than 5.5 $\log_{10}$ copies/mL are consistent with iciHHV-6.[198] Droplet digital PCR enables precise determination of the ratio between virus and host genomes[225,262]; integer ratios (e.g., one or two virus genomes per haploid cell genome) are reliable indicators of iciHHV-6.

Serology

Serologic assays have little clinical utility but are valuable for studies of virus prevalence and immunological reactivity in population-based studies. Numerous HHV-6 and HHV-7 serologic assays have been described,[4,26,199] including IFA, anticomplement IFA, ELISA, neutralization (NT), radioimmunoprecipitation, and immunoblot. For detection of IgM, separation of serum IgM from IgG and IgA significantly increases the specificity, but IgM testing is not useful for clinical diagnosis.[192] The products of U11 (86 kDa) and U14 (85 kDa) were identified as sensitive and specific markers for HHV-7 serology.[232] Antibody avidity assays enable identification of recent primary infections.[272] Serologic responses to HHV-6A and HHV-6B cannot be reliably discriminated by the assays described earlier.

Prevention and Control

Given that HHV-6B and HHV-7 appear to be transmitted most commonly via saliva, in the hospital setting, standard precautions will prevent spread of HHV-6B and HHV-7. For further guidance, the European Conference on Infections in Leukaemia provides evidence-based guidelines for management of roseolovirus infections in patients with hematological malignancies and after HSCT[273] and the American Society of Transplantation provides guidance in the solid organ transplantation setting.[200]

Antivirals

Ganciclovir, phosphonoformate (foscarnet), and cidofovir (including brincidofovir) are potent inhibitors of roseolovirus replication *in vitro*, and are used clinically to treat these viruses. Acyclovir (ACV) and other thymidine kinase–dependent drugs are only marginally effective.[26,45] The inhibitory effects of IFN-α and IFN-β on HHV-6 replication were also demonstrated *in vitro*, as described earlier. Ganciclovir is activated by the phosphotransferase encoded by gene U69, which can confer ganciclovir susceptibility on recombinant baculoviruses.[8] Methods have been described for rapid identification of U69 mutations in instances of clinical resistance to ganciclovir.[109] Other compounds with *in vitro* activity against HHV-6 include CMV423, a protein tyrosine kinase inhibitor,[45] and artesunate.[167] The sensitivity of HHV-7 to the guanine analogs was different from HHV-6, suggesting a difference in selectivity of specific viral enzymes.[288]

Foscarnet and/or ganciclovir are generally considered the first-line choices for treatment of HHV-6B encephalitis.[273] Strong consideration should be given to beginning empiric therapy with an HHV-6B-active antiviral (as described below) while awaiting results from laboratory testing of CSF and blood/plasma. A retrospective study using data from the Transplant Registry Unified Management Program in Japan suggested improved outcomes when full-dose ganciclovir (5 mg/kg every 12 hours) or foscarnet (90 mg/kg every 12 hours) were used to treat HHV-6B encephalitis compared to lower doses of the same antivirals.[189] This study showed no difference in encephalitis-related outcomes in those receiving foscarnet versus ganciclovir, but there was a suggestion of improved all-cause survival in those patients receiving foscarnet. These data must be interpreted with caution given the retrospective nature of the study and the possibilities of potential confounders.

Studies of ganciclovir and foscarnet in immunocompromised hosts have demonstrated an impact on HHV-6B viral kinetics, but prospective studies of prophylactic and preemptive therapy with foscarnet have not demonstrated an impact on occurrence of encephalitis.[112,190] Thus, these strategies are generally not recommended.

Adoptively transferred HHV-6B-specific T cells can be manufactured, and results from a descriptive study of 3 patients who received infusions of such cells suggest that two of the patients may have derived some benefit.[261] Without controls, however, the true effect of this strategy remains undefined.

Further research is needed to identify effective antivirals and strategies for preventing and controlling HHV-6B infection.

PERSPECTIVE

The high prevalences of the roseoloviruses, coupled with their ability to establish lifelong infections and their relatively low associated morbidity and mortality, suggest that these highly evolved viruses have much left to teach us about host–pathogen interactions. Recent advances in diagnostics, availability of tools for genetic manipulation of the viruses, deeper understanding of virus gene expression, and advances in structural biology portend ongoing advances in our understanding of these interesting and important viruses.

REFERENCES

1. Ablashi D, Agut H, Berneman Z, et al. Human herpesvirus-6 strain groups: a nomenclature. *Arch Virol* 1993;129:363–366.
2. Achour A, Boutolleau D, Slim A, et al. Human herpesvirus-6 (HHV-6) DNA in plasma reflects the presence of infected blood cells rather than circulating viral particles. *J Clin Virol* 2007;38(4):280–285.
3. Agut H, Bonnafous P, Gautheret-Dejean A. Laboratory and clinical aspects of human herpesvirus 6 infections. *Clin Microbiol Rev* 2015;28(2):313–335.
4. Agut H, Bonnafous P, Gautheret-Dejean A. Human herpesviruses 6A, 6B, and 7. *Microbiol Spectr* 2016;4(3).

5. Ahlqvist J, Fotheringham J, Akhyani N, et al. Differential tropism of human herpesvirus 6 (HHV-6) variants and induction of latency by HHV-6A in oligodendrocytes. *J Neurovirol* 2005;11:384–394.
6. Akkapaiboon P, Mori Y, Sadaoka T, et al. Intracellular processing of human herpesvirus 6 glycoproteins Q1 and Q2 into tetrameric complexes expressed on the viral envelope. *J Virol* 2004;78(15):7969–7983.
7. Andre-Garnier E, Milpied N, Boutolleau D, et al. Reactivation of human herpesvirus 6 during ex vivo expansion of circulating CD34+ haematopoietic stem cells. *J Gen Virol* 2004;85(Pt 11):3333–3336.
8. Ansari A, Emery VC. The U69 gene of human herpesvirus 6 encodes a protein kinase which can confer ganciclovir sensitivity to baculoviruses. *J Virol* 1999;73(4):3284–3291.
9. Arbuckle JH, Medveczky PG. The molecular biology of human herpesvirus-6 latency and telomere integration. *Microbes Infect* 2011;13(8–9):731–741.
10. Arbuckle JH, Medveczky MM, Luka J, et al. The latent human herpesvirus-6A genome specifically integrates in telomeres of human chromosomes in vivo and in vitro. *Proc Natl Acad Sci U S A* 2010;107(12):5563–5568.
11. Arsenault S, Gravel A, Gosselin J, et al. Generation and characterization of a monoclonal antibody specific for human herpesvirus 6 variant A immediate-early 2 protein. *J Clin Virol* 2003;28(3):284–290.
12. Asano Y, Yoshikawa T, Suga S, et al. Viremia and neutralizing antibody response in infants with exanthem subitum. *J Pediatr* 1989;114(4):535–539.
13. Aswad A, Aimola G, Wight D, et al. Evolutionary history of endogenous Human Herpesvirus 6 reflects human migration out of Africa. *Mol Biol Evol* 2020;38:96–107.
14. Aswad A, Katzourakis A. The first endogenous herpesvirus, identified in the tarsier genome, and novel sequences from primate rhadinoviruses and lymphocryptoviruses. *PLoS Genet* 2014;10(6):e1004332.
15. Atedzoe BN, Ahmad A, Menezes J. Enhancement of natural killer cell cytotoxicity by the human herpesvirus-7 via IL-15 induction. *J Immunol* 1997;159(10):4966–4972.
16. Becerra-Artiles A, Cruz J, Leszyk JD, et al. Naturally processed HLA-DR3-restricted HHV-6B peptides are recognized broadly with polyfunctional and cytotoxic CD4 T-cell responses. *Eur J Immunol* 2019;49(8):1167–1185.
17. Becerra-Artiles A, Dominguez-Amorocho O, Stern LJ, et al. A simple proteomics-based approach to identification of immunodominant antigens from a complex pathogen: application to the CD4 T cell response against human herpesvirus 6B. *PLoS One* 2015;10(11):e0142871.
18. Berti R, Brennan MB, Soldan SS, et al. Increased detection of serum HHV-6 DNA sequences during multiple sclerosis (MS) exacerbations and correlation with parameters of MS disease progression. *J Neurovirol* 2002;8(3):250–256.
19. Biberfeld P, Kramarsky B, Salahuddin SZ, et al. Ultrastructural characterization of a new human B-lymphotropic DNA virus (HBLV) isolated from patients with lymphoproliferative disease. *J Natl Cancer Inst* 1987;79(5):933–941.
20. Black JB, Burns DA, Goldsmith CS, et al. Biologic properties of human herpesvirus 7 strain SB. *Virus Res* 1997;52:25–41.
21. Black JB, Pellett PE. Human herpesvirus 7. *Rev Med Virol* 1999;9:245–262.
22. Black JB, Sanderlin KC, Goldsmith CS, et al. Growth properties of human herpesvirus-6 strain Z29. *J Virol Methods* 1989;26:133–145.
23. Borenstein R, Frenkel N. Cloning human herpes virus 6A genome into bacterial artificial chromosomes and study of DNA replication intermediates. *Proc Natl Acad Sci U S A* 2009;106(45):19138–19143.
24. Borenstein R, Singer O, Moseri A, et al. Use of amplicon-6 vectors derived from human herpesvirus 6 for efficient expression of membrane-associated and -secreted proteins in T cells. *J Virol* 2004;78(9):4730–4743.
25. Borenstein R, Zeigerman H, Frenkel N. The DR1 and DR6 first exons of human herpesvirus 6A are not required for virus replication in culture and are deleted in virus stocks that replicate well in T-cell lines. *J Virol* 2010;84(6):2648–2656.
26. Braun DK, Dominguez G, Pellett PE. Human herpesvirus 6. *Clin Microbiol Rev* 1997;10:521–567.
27. Bulboaca GH, Deng H, Dewhurst S, et al. Telomeric sequences from human herpesvirus 6 do not mediate nuclear retention of episomal DNA in human cells. *Arch Virol* 1998;143(3):563–570.
28. Carrigan DR, Knox KK. Bone marrow suppression by human herpesvirus-6: comparison of the A and B variants of the virus [letter]. *Blood* 1995;86(2):835–836.
29. Caruso A, Caselli E, Fiorentini S, et al. U94 of human herpesvirus 6 inhibits in vitro angiogenesis and lymphangiogenesis. *Proc Natl Acad Sci U S A* 2009;106(48):20446–20451.
30. Caselli E, Bracci A, Galvan M, et al. Human herpesvirus 6 (HHV-6) U94/REP protein inhibits betaherpesvirus replication. *Virology* 2006;346(2):402–414.
31. Caserta MT, Hall CB, Schnabel K, et al. Primary human herpesvirus 7 infection: a comparison of human herpesvirus 7 and human herpesvirus 6 infections in children. *J Pediatr* 1998;133(3):386–389.
32. Caserta MT, Hall CB, Schnabel K, et al. Diagnostic assays for active infection with human herpesvirus 6 (HHV-6). *J Clin Virol* 2010;48(1):55–57.
33. Caserta MT, McDermott MP, Dewhurst S, et al. Human herpesvirus 6 (HHV6) DNA persistence and reactivation in healthy children. *J Pediatr* 2004;145(4):478–484.
34. Catusse J, Parry CM, Dewin DR, et al. Inhibition of HIV-1 infection by viral chemokine U83A via high-affinity CCR5 interactions that block human chemokine-induced leukocyte chemotaxis and receptor internalization. *Blood* 2007;109(9):3633–3639.
35. Catusse J, Spinks J, Mattick C, et al. Immunomodulation by herpesvirus U51A chemokine receptor via CCL5 and FOG-2 down-regulation plus XCR1 and CCR7 mimicry in human leukocytes. *Eur J Immunol* 2008;38(3):763–777.
36. Charvet B, Reynaud JM, Gourru-Lesimple G, et al. Induction of proinflammatory multiple sclerosis-associated retrovirus envelope protein by human herpesvirus-6A and CD46 receptor engagement. *Front Immunol* 2018;9:2803.
37. Chee MS, Bankier AT, Beck S, et al. Analysis of the protein-coding content of the sequence of human cytomegalovirus strain AD169. *Curr Top Microbiol Immunol* 1990;154:125–169.
38. Chi J, Gu B, Zhang C, et al. Human herpesvirus 6 latent infection in patients with glioma. *J Infect Dis* 2012;206:1394–1398.
39. Clark DA, Tsao EH, Leong HN, et al. Human herpesvirus 6 genome integration: a possible cause of misdiagnosis of active viral infection? *J Infect Dis* 2006;194:1021–1023.
40. van Cleef KW, Scaf WM, Maes K, et al. The rat cytomegalovirus homologue of parvoviral rep genes, r127, encodes a nuclear protein with single- and double-stranded DNA-binding activity that is dispensable for virus replication. *J Gen Virol* 2004;85(Pt 7):2001–2013.
41. Collin V, Gravel A, Kaufer BB, et al. The Promyelocytic Leukemia Protein facilitates human herpesvirus 6B chromosomal integration, immediate-early 1 protein multiSUMOylation and its localization at telomeres. *PLoS Pathog* 2020;16(7):e1008683.
42. Comar M, D'Agaro P, Campello C, et al. Human herpes virus 6 in archival cardiac tissues from children with idiopathic dilated cardiomyopathy or congenital heart disease. *J Clin Pathol* 2009;62(1):80–83.
43. Crawford JR, Santi MR, Cornelison R, et al. Detection of human herpesvirus-6 in adult central nervous system tumors: predominance of early and late viral antigens in glial tumors. *J Neurooncol* 2009;95(1):49–60.
44. Daibata M, Taguchi T, Sawada T, et al. Chromosomal transmission of human herpesvirus 6 DNA in acute lymphoblastic leukaemia. *Lancet* 1998;352(9127):543–544.
45. De Bolle L, Naesens L, De Clercq E. Update on human herpesvirus 6 biology, clinical features, and therapy. *Clin Microbiol Rev* 2005;18(1):217–245.
46. De Bolle L, Van Loon J, De Clercq E, et al. Quantitative analysis of human herpesvirus 6 cell tropism. *J Med Virol* 2005;75(1):76–85.
47. Deng H, Dewhurst S. Functional identification and analysis of cis-acting sequences which mediate genome cleavage and packaging in human herpesvirus 6. *J Virol* 1998;72(1):320–329.
48. Denner J, Bigley TM, Phan TL, et al. Comparative analysis of roseoloviruses in humans, pigs, mice, and other species. *Viruses* 2019;11(12).
49. Derfuss T, Hohlfeld R, Meinl E. Intrathecal antibody (IgG) production against human herpesvirus type 6 occurs in about 20% of multiple sclerosis patients and might be linked to a polyspecific B-cell response. *J Neurol* 2005;252(8):968–971.
50. Dewhurst S, Krenitsky DM, Dykes C. Human herpesvirus 6B origin: sequence diversity, requirement for two binding sites for origin-binding protein, and enhanced replication from origin multimers. *J Virol* 1994;68(10):6799–6803.
51. Dewin DR, Catusse J, Gompels UA. Identification and characterization of U83A viral chemokine, a broad and potent beta-chemokine agonist for human CCRs with unique selectivity and inhibition by spliced isoform. *J Immunol* 2006;176(1):544–556.
52. Dominguez G, Dambaugh TR, Stamey FR, et al. Human herpesvirus 6B genome sequence: coding content and comparison with human herpesvirus 6A. *J Virol* 1999;73:8040–8052.
53. Donati D, Martinelli E, Cassiani-Ingoni R, et al. Variant-specific tropism of human herpesvirus 6 in human astrocytes. *J Virol* 2005;79(15):9439–9448.
54. Drago F, Ciccarese G, Herzum A, et al. Pityriasis rosea during pregnancy: major and minor alarming signs. *Dermatology* 2018;234(1–2):31–36.
55. Eliassen E, Lum E, Pritchett J, et al. Human herpesvirus 6 and malignancy: a review. *Front Oncol* 2018;8:512.
56. Endo A, Watanabe K, Ohye T, et al. Molecular and virological evidence of viral activation from chromosomally integrated human herpesvirus 6A in a patient with X-linked severe combined immunodeficiency. *Clin Infect Dis* 2014;59(4):545–548.
57. Engdahl E, Gustafsson R, Huang J, et al. Increased serological response against human herpesvirus 6A Is associated with risk for multiple sclerosis. *Front Immunol* 2019;10:2715.
58. Epstein LG, Shinnar S, Hesdorffer DC, et al. Human herpesvirus 6 and 7 in febrile status epilepticus: the FEBSTAT study. *Epilepsia* 2012;53(9):1481–1488.
59. Fernandez-Ruiz M, Kumar D, Husain S, et al. Utility of a monitoring strategy for human herpesviruses 6 and 7 viremia after liver transplantation: a randomized clinical trial. *Transplantation* 2015;99(1):106–113.
60. Finkel Y, Schmiedel D, Tai-Schmiedel J, et al. Comprehensive annotations of human herpesvirus 6A and 6B genomes reveal novel and conserved genomic features. *Elife* 2020;9:e50960.
61. Finkel Y, Stern-Ginossar N, Schwartz M. Viral short ORFs and their possible functions. *Proteomics* 2018;18(10):e1700255.
62. Fitzsimons CP, Gompels UA, Verzijl D, et al. Chemokine-directed trafficking of receptor stimulus to different g proteins: selective inducible and constitutive signaling by human herpesvirus 6-encoded chemokine receptor U51. *Mol Pharmacol* 2006;69(3):888–898.
63. Flamand L, Gosselin J, D'Addario M, et al. Human herpesvirus 6 induces interleukin-1 beta and tumor necrosis factor alpha, but not interleukin-6, in peripheral blood mononuclear cell cultures. *J Virol* 1991;65(9):5105–5110.
64. Flamand L, Gosselin J, Stefanescu I, et al. Immunosuppressive effect of human herpesvirus 6 on T-cell functions: suppression of interleukin-2 synthesis and cell proliferation [published erratum appears in Blood 86:418,1995]. *Blood* 1995;85(5):1263–1271.
65. Flamand L, Komaroff AL, Arbuckle JH, et al. Review, part 1: human herpesvirus-6-basic biology, diagnostic testing, and antiviral efficacy. *J Med Virol* 2010;82(9):1560–1568.
66. Flamand L, Romerio F, Reitz MS, et al. CD4 promoter transactivation by human herpesvirus 6. *J Virol* 1998;72(11):8797–8805.
67. Flamand L, Stefanescu I, Menezes J. Human herpesvirus-6 enhances natural killer cell cytotoxicity via IL-15. *J Clin Investig* 1996;97:1373–1381.
68. Flebbe-Rehwaldt LM, Wood C, Chandran B. Characterization of transcripts expressed from human herpesvirus 6A strain GS immediate-early region B U16-U17 open reading frames. *J Virol* 2000;74(23):11040–11054.
69. Frenkel N, Roffman E. Human herpesvirus 7. In: Fields BN, ed. *Fields Virology*. 3rd ed. Philadelphia, PA: Lippencott-Raven; 1996:2609–2622.
70. Frenkel N, Schirmer EC, Wyatt LS, et al. Isolation of a new herpesvirus from CD4+ T cells. *Proc Natl Acad Sci U S A* 1990;87:748–752.
71. Furukawa M, Yasukawa M, Yakushijin Y, et al. Distinct effects of human herpesvirus 6 and human herpesvirus 7 on surface molecule expression and function of CD4+ T cells. *J Immunol* 1994;152:5768–5775.
72. Gaccioli F, Lager S, de Goffau MC, et al. Fetal inheritance of chromosomally integrated human herpesvirus 6 predisposes the mother to pre-eclampsia. *Nat Microbiol* 2020;5(7):901–908.
73. Gautheret-Dejean A, Henquell C, Mousnier F, et al. Different expression of human herpesvirus-6 (HHV-6) load in whole blood may have a significant impact on the diagnosis of active infection. *J Clin Virol* 2009;46(1):33–36.

74. Geraudie B, Charrier M, Bonnafous P, et al. Quantitation of human herpesvirus-6A, -6B and -7 DNAs in whole blood, mononuclear and polymorphonuclear cell fractions from healthy blood donors. *J Clin Virol* 2012;53(2):151–155.
75. Gerdemann U, Keukens L, Keirnan JM, et al. Immunotherapeutic strategies to prevent and treat human herpesvirus 6 reactivation after allogeneic stem cell transplantation. *Blood* 2013;121(1):207–218.
76. Glaunsinger BA. Modulation of the translational landscape during herpesvirus infection. *Annu Rev Virol* 2015;2(1):311–333.
77. Glosson NL, Hudson AW. Human herpesvirus-6A and -6B encode viral immunoevasins that downregulate class I MHC molecules. *Virology* 2007;365(1):125–135.
78. Gobbi A, Stoddart CA, Malnati MS, et al. Human herpesvirus 6 (HHV-6) causes severe thymocyte depletion in SCID-hu Thy/Liv mice. *J Exp Med* 1999;189(12):1953–1960.
79. Gompels UA, Macaulay HA. Characterization of human telomeric repeat sequences from human herpesvirus 6 and relationship to replication. *J Gen Virol* 1995;76:451–458.
80. Gompels UA, Nicholas J, Lawrence G, et al. The DNA sequence of human herpesvirus-6: structure, coding content, and genome evolution. *Virology* 1995;209:29–51.
81. Govind S, Hockley J, Morris C, Group tCS. *Collaborative Study to Establish the 1st WHO International Standard for Human Herpes Virus 6B (HHV-6B) DNA for Nucleic Acid Amplification Technique (NAT)-Based Assays*. Hertfordshire, United Kingdom: World Health Organization; 2017.
82. Gravel A, Dion V, Cloutier N, et al. Characterization of human herpesvirus 6 variant B immediate-early 1 protein modifications by small ubiquitin-related modifiers. *J Gen Virol* 2004;85(Pt 5):1319–1328.
83. Gravel A, Gosselin J, Flamand L. Human herpesvirus 6 immediate-early 1 protein is a sumoylated nuclear phosphoprotein colocalizing with promyelocytic leukemia protein-associated nuclear bodies. *J Biol Chem* 2002;277(22):19679–19687.
84. Gravel A, Hall CB, Flamand L. Sequence analysis of transplacentally acquired human herpesvirus 6 DNA is consistent with transmission of a chromosomally integrated reactivated virus. *J Infect Dis* 2013;207(10):1585–1589.
85. Gravel A, Sanders W, Fournier E, et al. Mapping HHV-6B transcriptome. *J Virol* 202124:JVI.01335-20.
86. Gravel A, Tomoiu A, Cloutier N, et al. Characterization of the immediate-early 2 protein of human herpesvirus 6, a promiscuous transcriptional activator. *Virology* 2003;308(2):340–353.
87. Greenstone HL, Santoro F, Lusso P, et al. Human herpesvirus 6 and measles virus employ distinct CD46 domains for receptor function. *J Biol Chem* 2002;277(42):39112–39118.
88. Greninger AL, Knudsen GM, Roychoudhury P, et al. Comparative genomic, transcriptomic, and proteomic reannotation of human herpesvirus 6. *BMC Genomics* 2018;19(1):204.
89. Greninger AL, Naccache SN, Pannaraj P, et al. The Brief Case: inherited chromosomally integrated human herpesvirus 6 (HHV-6) in the age of multiplex HHV-6 testing. *J Clin Microbiol* 2019;57(10).
90. Greninger AL, Sedlak RH, Jerome KR. Human herpesviruses 6A, 6B, and 7. In: Carrol KC, Pfaller MA, Landry ML, et al., eds. *Manual of Clinical Microbiology*. Vol. 2. 12th ed. ASM Press: Washington DC; 2019:1814–1825.
91. Grivel JC, Santoro F, Chen S, et al. Pathogenic effects of human herpesvirus 6 in human lymphoid tissue ex vivo. *J Virol* 2003;77(15):8280–8289.
92. Hall CB, Caserta MT, Schnabel KC, et al. Persistence of human herpesvirus 6 according to site and variant: possible greater neurotropism of variant A. *Clin Infect Dis* 1998;26(1):132–137.
93. Hall CB, Caserta MT, Schnabel KC, et al. Transplacental congenital human herpesvirus 6 infection caused by maternal chromosomally integrated virus. *J Infect Dis* 2010;201(4):505–507.
94. Hall CB, Long CE, Schnabel KC, et al. Human herpesvirus-6 infection in children. A prospective study of complications and reactivation. *N Engl J Med* 1994;331(7):432–438.
95. Hansen AS, Bundgaard BB, Biltoft M, et al. Divergent tropism of HHV-6AGS and HHV-6BPL1 in T cells expressing different CD46 isoform patterns. *Virology* 2017;502:160–170.
96. Hanson DJ, Tsvetkova O, Rerolle GF, et al. Genome-wide approach to the CD4 T-cell response to human herpesvirus 6B. *J Virol* 2019;93(14).
97. Harberts E, Yao K, Wohler JE, et al. Human herpesvirus-6 entry into the central nervous system through the olfactory pathway. *Proc Natl Acad Sci U S A* 2011;108:13734–13739.
98. Hayashi M, Yoshida K, Tang H, et al. Characterization of the human herpesvirus 6A U23 gene. *Virology* 2014;450–451:98–105.
99. Hill JA, Koo S, Guzman Suarez BB, et al. Cord-blood hematopoietic stem cell transplant confers an increased risk for human herpesvirus-6-associated acute limbic encephalitis: a cohort analysis. *Biol Blood Marrow Transplant* 2012;18(11):1638–1648.
100. Hill JA, Vande Vusse LK, Xie H, et al. Human herpesvirus 6B and lower respiratory tract disease after hematopoietic cell transplantation. *J Clin Oncol* 2019;37(29):2670–2681.
101. Hirata Y, Kondo K, Yamanishi K. Human herpesvirus 6 downregulates major histocompatibility complex class I in dendritic cells. *J Med Virol* 2001;65(3):576–583.
102. Horvat RT, Parmely MJ, Chandran B. Human herpesvirus 6 inhibits the proliferative responses of human peripheral blood mononuclear cells. *J Infect Dis* 1993;167(6):1274–1280.
103. Hudson AW, Blom D, Howley PM, et al. The ER-lumenal domain of the HHV-7 immunoevasin U21 directs class I MHC molecules to lysosomes. *Traffic* 2003;4(12):824–837.
104. Iampietro M, Morissette G, Gravel A, et al. Inhibition of interleukin-2 gene expression by human herpesvirus 6B U54 tegument protein. *J Virol* 2014;88(21):12452–12463.
105. Iampietro M, Morissette G, Gravel A, et al. Human herpesvirus 6B immediate-early I protein contains functional HLA-A*02, HLA-A*03, and HLA-B*07 class I restricted CD8(+) T-cell epitopes. *Eur J Immunol* 2014;44(12):3573–3584.
106. Ichimi R, Jin-no T, Ito M. Induction of apoptosis in cord blood lymphocytes by HHV-6. *J Med Virol* 1999;58(1):63–68.
107. Inoue N, Pellett PE. Human herpesvirus 6B origin-binding protein: DNA-binding domain and consensus binding sequence. *J Virol* 1995;69:4619–4627.
108. Inoue Y, Yasukawa M, Fujita S. Induction of T-cell apoptosis by human herpesvirus 6. *J Virol* 1997;71:3751–3759.
109. Isegawa Y, Matsumoto C, Nishinaka K, et al. PCR with quenching probes enables the rapid detection and identification of ganciclovir-resistance-causing U69 gene mutations in human herpesvirus 6. *Mol Cell Probes* 2010;24:167–177.
110. Isegawa Y, Mukai T, Nakano K, et al. Comparison of the complete DNA sequences of human herpesvirus 6 variants A and B. *J Virol* 1999;73:8053–8063.
111. Isegawa Y, Ping Z, Nakano K, et al. Human herpesvirus 6 open reading frame U12 encodes a functional beta-chemokine receptor. *J Virol* 1998;72(7):6104–6112.
112. Ishiyama K, Katagiri T, Hoshino T, et al. Preemptive therapy of human herpesvirus-6 encephalitis with foscarnet sodium for high-risk patients after hematopoietic SCT. *Bone Marrow Transplant* 2011;46(6):863–869.
113. Isomura H, Yamada M, Yoshida M, et al. Suppressive effects of human herpesvirus 6 on in vitro colony formation of hematopoietic progenitor cells. *J Med Virol* 1997;52(4):406–412.
114. Jasirwan C, Furusawa Y, Tang H, et al. Human herpesvirus-6A gQ1 and gQ2 are critical for human CD46 usage. *Microbiol Immunol* 2014;58(1):22–30.
115. Jasirwan C, Tang H, Kawabata A, et al. The human herpesvirus 6 U21-U24 gene cluster is dispensable for virus growth. *Microbiol Immunol* 2015;59(1):48–53.
116. Jaworska J, Gravel A, Flamand L. Divergent susceptibilities of human herpesvirus 6 variants to type I interferons. *Proc Natl Acad Sci U S A* 2010;107(18):8369–8374.
117. Kakimoto M, Hasegawa A, Fujita S, et al. Phenotypic and functional alterations of dendritic cells induced by human herpesvirus 6 infection. *J Virol* 2002;76(20):10338–10345.
118. Kaufer BB, Flamand L. Chromosomally integrated HHV-6: impact on virus, cell and organismal biology. *Curr Opin Virol* 2014;9:111–118.
119. Kaufer BB, Jarosinski KW, Osterrieder N. Herpesvirus telomeric repeats facilitate genomic integration into host telomeres and mobilization of viral DNA during reactivation. *J Exp Med* 2011;208(3):605–615.
120. Kawabata A, Jasirwan C, Yamanishi K, et al. Human herpesvirus 6 glycoprotein M is essential for virus growth and requires glycoprotein N for its maturation. *Virology* 2012;429(1):21–28.
121. Kawabata A, Tang H, Huang H, et al. Human herpesvirus 6 envelope components enriched in lipid rafts: evidence for virion-associated lipid rafts. *Virol J* 2009;6:127.
122. Kawamura Y, Nakayama A, Kato T, et al. Pathogenic role of human herpesvirus 6B infection in mesial temporal lobe epilepsy. *J Infect Dis* 2015;212(7):1014–1021.
123. Kawamura Y, Sugata K, Ihira M, et al. Different characteristics of human herpesvirus 6 encephalitis between primary infection and viral reactivation. *J Clin Virol* 2011;51(1):12–19.
124. Kempf W, Adams V, Mirandola P, et al. Persistence of human herpesvirus 7 in normal tissues detected by expression of a structural antigen. *J Infect Dis* 1998;178(3):841–845.
125. Kikuta H, Nakane A, Lu H, et al. Interferon induction by human herpesvirus 6 in human mononuclear cells. *J Infect Dis* 1990;162(1):35–38.
126. Klussmann JP, Krueger E, Sloots T, et al. Ultrastructural study of human herpesvirus-7 replication in tissue culture. *Virchows Archiv [B]* 1997;430:417–426.
127. Kofod-Olsen E, Moller JM, Schleimann MH, et al. Inhibition of p53-dependent, but not p53-independent, cell death by U19 protein from human herpesvirus 6B. *PLoS One* 2013;8(3):e59223.
128. Kofod-Olsen E, Pettersson S, Wallace M, et al. Human herpesvirus-6B protein U19 contains a p53 BOX I homology motif for HDM2 binding and p53 stabilization. *Virology* 2014;448:33–42.
129. Komaroff AL, Pellett PE, Jacobson S. Human herpesviruses 6A and 6B in brain diseases: association versus causation. *Clin Microbiol Rev* 2020;34(1).
130. Kondo K, Kondo T, Okuno T, et al. Latent human herpesvirus 6 infection of human monocytes/macrophages. *J Gen Virol* 1991;72:1401–1408.
131. Kondo K, Nozaki H, Shimada K, et al. Detection of a gene cluster that is dispensable for human herpesvirus 6 replication and latency. *J Virol* 2003;77(19):10719–10724.
132. Kondo K, Shimada K, Sashihara J, et al. Identification of human herpesvirus 6 latency-associated transcripts. *J Virol* 2002;76(8):4145–4151.
133. Krug LT, Inoue N, Pellett PE. Sequence requirements for interaction of human herpesvirus 7 origin binding protein with the origin of lytic replication. *J Virol* 2001;75(8):3925–3936.
134. Krug LT, Inoue N, Pellett PE. Differences in DNA binding specificity among Roseolovirus origin binding proteins. *Virology* 2001;288(1):145–153.
135. Krug LT, Pellett PE. Roseolovirus molecular biology: recent advances. *Curr Opin Virol* 2014;9:170–177.
136. Kumata R, Ito J, Takahashi K, et al. A tissue level atlas of the healthy human virome. *BMC Biol* 2020;18(1):55.
137. Lacoste V, Mauclere P, Dubreuil G, et al. Simian homologues of human gamma-2 and betaherpesviruses in mandrill and drill monkeys. *J Virol* 2000;74(24):11993–11999.
138. Lacoste V, Verschoor EJ, Nerrienet E, et al. A novel homologue of human herpesvirus 6 in chimpanzees. *J Gen Virol* 2005;86(Pt 8):2135–2140.
139. Lanphear BP, Hall CB, Black J, et al. Risk factors for the early acquisition of human herpesvirus 6 and human herpesvirus 7 infections in children. *Pediatr Infect Dis J* 1998;17(9):792–795.
140. Leibovitch EC, Caruso B, Ha SK, et al. Herpesvirus trigger accelerates neuroinflammation in a nonhuman primate model of multiple sclerosis. *Proc Natl Acad Sci U S A* 2018;115(44):11292–11297.
141. Leibovitch EC, Jacobson S. Human herpesvirus 6 as a viral trigger in mesial temporal lobe epilepsy. *J Infect Dis* 2015;212(7):1011–1013.
142. Leibovitch E, Wohler JE, Cummings Macri SM, et al. Novel marmoset (Callithrix jacchus) model of human herpesvirus 6A and 6B infections: immunologic, virologic and radiologic characterization. *PLoS Pathog* 2013;9(1):e1003138.
143. Li C, Goodrich JM, Yang X. Interferon-gamma (IFN-gamma) regulates production of IL-10 and IL-12 in human herpesvirus-6 (HHV-6)-infected monocyte/macrophage lineage. *Clin Exp Immunol* 1997;109(3):421–425.
144. Lin K, Ricciardi RP. The 41-kDa protein of human herpesvirus 6 specifically binds to viral DNA polymerase and greatly increases DNA synthesis. *Virology* 1998;250(1):210–219.

145. Lindquester GJ, Pellett PE. Properties of the human herpesvirus 6 strain Z29 genome: G + C content, length, and presence of variable-length directly repeated terminal sequence elements. *Virology* 1991;182:102–110.
146. Liu X, Kosugi S, Koide R, et al. Endogenization and excision of human herpesvirus 6 in human genomes. *PLoS Genet* 2020;16(8):e1008915.
147. Loginov R, Karlsson T, Hockerstedt K, et al. Quantitative HHV-6B antigenemia test for the monitoring of transplant patients. *Eur J Clin Microbiol Infect Dis* 2010;29(7):881–886.
148. van Loon N, Dykes C, Deng H, et al. Identification and analysis of a lytic-phase origin of DNA replication in human herpesvirus 7. *J Virol* 1997;71:3279–3284.
149. Luppi M, Barozzi P, Morris C, et al. Human herpesvirus 6 latently infects early bone marrow progenitors in vivo. *J Virol* 1999;73(1):754–759.
150. Lusso P. HHV-6 and the immune system: mechanisms of immunomodulation and viral escape. *J Clin Virol* 2006;37 Suppl 1:S4-S10.
151. Lusso P, Crowley RW, Malnati MS, et al. Human herpesvirus 6A accelerates AIDS progression in macaques. *Proc Natl Acad Sci U S A* 2007;104(12):5067–5072.
152. Lusso P, Gallo RC. Human herpesvirus 6 in AIDS. *Lancet* 1994;343:555–556.
153. Luttichau HR, Clark-Lewis I, Jensen PO, et al. A highly selective CCR2 chemokine agonist encoded by human herpesvirus 6. *J Biol Chem* 2003;278(13):10928–10933.
154. Ma J, Jia J, Jiang X, et al. gp96 Is critical for both human herpesvirus 6A (HHV-6A) and HHV-6B infections. *J Virol* 2020;94(13).
155. MacLaine NJ, Oster B, Bundgaard B, et al. A central role for CK1 in catalyzing phosphorylation of the p53 transactivation domain at serine 20 after HHV-6B viral infection. *J Biol Chem* 2008;283(42):28563–28573.
156. Maeki T, Hayashi M, Kawabata A, et al. Identification of the human herpesvirus 6A gQ1 domain essential for its functional conformation. *J Virol* 2013;87(12):7054–7063.
157. Mahmoud NF, Jasirwan C, Kanemoto S, et al. Cytoplasmic tail domain of glycoprotein B is essential for HHV-6 infection. *Virology* 2016;490:1–5.
158. Mahmoud NF, Kawabata A, Tang H, et al. Human herpesvirus 6 U11 protein is critical for virus infection. *Virology* 2016;489:151–157.
159. Martin LK, Hollaus A, Stahuber A, et al. Cross-sectional analysis of CD8 T cell immunity to human herpesvirus 6B. *PLoS Pathog* 2018;14(4):e1006991.
160. Martin MED, Nicholas J, Thomson BJ, et al. Identification of a transactivating function mapping to the putative immediate-early locus of human herpesvirus 6. *J Virol* 1991;65:5381–5390.
161. Martin MED, Thomson BJ, Honess RW, et al. The genome of human herpesvirus 6: maps of unit-length and concatemeric genomes for nine restriction endonucleases. *J Gen Virol* 1991;72:157–168.
162. Matsuura M, Takemoto M, Yamanishi K, et al. Human herpesvirus 6 major immediate early promoter has strong activity in T cells and is useful for heterologous gene expression. *Virol J* 2011;8:9.
163. Meeuwsen S, Persoon-Deen C, Bsibsi M, et al. Modulation of the cytokine network in human adult astrocytes by human herpesvirus-6A. *J Neuroimmunol* 2005;164(1–2):37–47.
164. Megaw AG, Rapaport D, Avidor B, et al. The DNA sequence of the RK strain of human herpesvirus 7. *Virology* 1998;244(1):119–132.
165. Menegazzi P, Galvan M, Rotola A, et al. Temporal mapping of transcripts in human herpesvirus-7. *J Gen Virol* 1999;80:2705–2712.
166. Menotti L, Mirandola P, Locati M, et al. Trafficking to the plasma membrane of the seven-transmembrane protein encoded by human herpesvirus 6 U51 gene involves a cell-specific function present in T lymphocytes. *J Virol* 1999;73(1):325–333.
167. Milbradt J, Auerochs S, Korn K, et al. Sensitivity of human herpesvirus 6 and other human herpesviruses to the broad-spectrum antiinfective drug artesunate. *J Clin Virol* 2009;46(1):24–28.
168. Milne RS, Mattick C, Nicholson L, et al. RANTES binding and down-regulation by a novel human herpesvirus-6 beta chemokine receptor. *J Immunol* 2000;164(5):2396–2404.
169. Miyashita K, Miyagawa F, Nakamura Y, et al. Up-regulation of human herpesvirus 6B-derived microRNAs in the serum of patients with Drug-induced Hypersensitivity Syndrome/Drug Reaction with Eosinophilia and Systemic Symptoms. *Acta Derm Venereol* 2018;98(6):612–613.
170. Mock DJ, Powers JM, Goodman AD, et al. Association of human herpesvirus 6 with the demyelinative lesions of progressive multifocal leukoencephalopathy. *J Neurovirol* 1999;5(4):363–373.
171. Mori Y, Akkapaiboon P, Yonemoto S, et al. Discovery of a second form of tripartite complex containing gH-gL of human herpesvirus 6 and observations on CD46. *J Virol* 2004;78(9):4609–4616.
172. Mori J, Kawabata A, Tang H, et al. Human herpesvirus-6 U14 induces cell-cycle arrest in G2/M phase by associating with a cellular protein, EDD. *PLoS One* 2015;10(9): e0137420.
173. Mori Y, Koike M, Moriishi E, et al. Human herpesvirus-6 induces MVB formation, and virus egress occurs by an exosomal release pathway. *Traffic* 2008;9(10):1728–1742.
174. Mori Y, Seya T, Huang HL, et al. Human herpesvirus 6 variant A but not variant B induces fusion from without in a variety of human cells through a human herpesvirus 6 entry receptor, CD46. *J Virol* 2002;76(13):6750–6761.
175. Mori J, Tang H, Kawabata A, et al. Human herpesvirus 6A U14 is important for virus maturation. *J Virol* 2016;90(3):1677–1681.
176. Mori Y, Yang X, Akkapaiboon P, et al. Human herpesvirus 6 variant A glycoprotein H-glycoprotein L-glycoprotein Q complex associates with human CD46. *J Virol* 2003;77(8):4992–4999.
177. Naik S, Nicholas SK, Martinez CA, et al. Adoptive immunotherapy for primary immunodeficiency disorders with virus-specific T lymphocytes. *J Allergy Clin Immunol* 2016;137(5):1498–1505.e1491.
178. Nakagawa N, Mukai T, Sakamoto J, et al. Antigenic analysis of human herpesvirus 7 (HHV-7) and HHV-6 using immune sera and monoclonal antibodies against HHV-7. *J Gen Virol* 1997;78:1131–1137.
179. Nakamichi K, Inoue N, Shimokawa T, et al. Detection of human herpesviruses in the cerebrospinal fluid from patients diagnosed with or suspected of having progressive multifocal leukoencephalopathy. *BMC Neurol* 2013;13:200.
180. Nakano K, Tadagaki K, Isegawa Y, et al. Human herpesvirus 7 open reading frame U12 encodes a functional beta-chemokine receptor. *J Virol* 2003;77(14):8108–8115.
181. Neipel F, Ellinger K, Fleckenstein B. Gene for the major antigenic structural protein (p100) of human herpesvirus 6. *J Virol* 1992;66:3918–3924.
182. Nicholas J. Determination and analysis of the complete nucleotide sequence of human herpesvirus 7. *J Virol* 1996;70:5975–5989.
183. Niiya H, Azuma T, Jin L, et al. Transcriptional downregulation of DC-SIGN in human herpesvirus 6-infected dendritic cells. *J Gen Virol* 2004;85(Pt 9):2639–2642.
184. Nishimura M, Wang J, Wakata A, et al. Crystal structure of the DNA-binding domain of human herpesvirus 6A immediate early protein 2. *J Virol* 2017;91(21).
185. Nordstrom I, Rudin A, Adlerberth I, et al. Infection of infants with human herpesvirus type 6 may be associated with reduced allergic sensitization and T-helper type 2 development. *Clin Exp Allergy* 2010;40(6):882–890.
186. Nukui M, Mori Y, Murphy EA. A human herpesvirus 6A-encoded microRNA: role in viral lytic replication. *J Virol* 2015;89(5):2615–2627.
187. Oakes B, Hoagland-Henefield M, Komaroff AL, et al. Human endogenous retrovirus-K18 superantigen expression and human herpesvirus-6 and human herpesvirus-7 viral loads in chronic fatigue patients. *Clin Infect Dis* 2013;56(10):1394–1400.
188. Ogata M, Kikuchi H, Satou T, et al. Human herpesvirus 6 DNA in plasma after allogeneic stem cell transplantation: incidence and clinical significance. *J Infect Dis* 2006;193(1):68–79.
189. Ogata M, Oshima K, Ikebe T, et al. Clinical characteristics and outcome of human herpesvirus-6 encephalitis after allogeneic hematopoietic stem cell transplantation. *Bone Marrow Transplant* 2017;52(11):1563–1570.
190. Ogata M, Takano K, Moriuchi Y, et al. Effects of prophylactic foscarnet on human herpesvirus-6 reactivation and encephalitis in cord blood transplant recipients: a prospective multicenter trial with an historical control group. *Biol Blood Marrow Transplant* 2018;24(6):1264–1273.
191. Okuno T, Takahashi K, Balachandra K, et al. Seroepidemiology of human herpesvirus 6 infection in normal children and adults. *J Clin Microbiol* 1989;27:651–653.
192. de Oliveira Vianna RA, Siqueira MM, Camacho LA, et al. The accuracy of anti-human herpesvirus 6 IgM detection in children with recent primary infection. *J Virol Methods* 2008;153(2):273–275.
193. Oster B, Kofod-Olsen E, Bundgaard B, et al. Restriction of human herpesvirus 6B replication by p53. *J Gen Virol* 2008;89(Pt 5):1106–1113.
194. de Pagter PJ, Schuurman R, de Vos NM, et al. Multicenter external quality assessment of molecular methods for detection of human herpesvirus 6. *J Clin Microbiol* 2010;48(7):2536–2540.
195. Papanikolaou E, Kouvatsis V, Dimitriadis G, et al. Identification and characterization of the gene products of open reading frame U86/87 of human herpesvirus 6. *Virus Res* 2002;89(1):89–101.
196. Patel SJ, Zhao G, Penna VR, et al. A murine herpesvirus closely related to ubiquitous human herpesviruses causes T-cell depletion. *J Virol* 2017;91(9).
197. Peddu V, Dubuc I, Gravel A, et al. Inherited chromosomally integrated human herpesvirus 6 demonstrates tissue-specific RNA expression in vivo that correlates with an increased antibody immune response. *J Virol* 2019;94:e01418.
198. Pellett PE, Ablashi DV, Ambros PF, et al. Chromosomally integrated human herpesvirus 6: questions and answers. *Rev Med Virol* 2011;22:144–155.
199. Pellett PE, Dollard SC. Human herpesviruses 6, 7, and 8. In: Specter S, Hodinka RL, Young SA, et al., eds. *Clinical Virology Manual.* 4th ed. Washington, DC: ASM Press; 2009:494–522.
200. Pellett Madan R, Hand J; AST Infectious Diseases Community of Practice. Human herpesvirus 6, 7, and 8 in solid organ transplantation: guidelines from the American Society of Transplantation Infectious Diseases Community of Practice. *Clin Transplant* 2019;33(9):e13518.
201. Pellett PE, Sanchez-Martinez D, Dominguez G, et al. A strongly immunoreactive virion protein of human herpesvirus 6 variant B strain Z29: identification and characterization of the gene and mapping of a variant-specific monoclonal antibody reactive epitope. *Virology* 1993;195(2):521–531.
202. Phan TL, Carlin K, Ljungman P, et al. Human herpesvirus-6B reactivation is a risk factor for grades II to IV acute graft-versus-host disease after hematopoietic stem cell transplantation: a systematic review and meta-analysis. *Biol Blood Marrow Transplant* 2018;24(11):2324–2336.
203. Prusty BK, Gulve N, Rasa S, et al. Possible chromosomal and germline integration of human herpesvirus 7. *J Gen Virol* 2017;98(2):266–274.
204. Prusty BK, Siegl C, Gulve N, et al. GP96 interacts with HHV-6 during viral entry and directs it for cellular degradation. *PLoS One* 2014;9(12):e113962.
205. Rapp JC, Krug LT, Inoue N, et al. U94, the human herpesvirus 6 homolog of the parvovirus nonstructural gene, is highly conserved among isolates and is expressed at low mRNA levels as a spliced transcript. *Virology* 2000;268:504–516.
206. Reddy S, Eliassen E, Krueger GR, et al. Human herpesvirus 6-induced inflammatory cardiomyopathy in immunocompetent children. *Ann Pediatr Cardiol* 2017;10(3):259–268.
207. Reynaud JM, Jegou JF, Welsch JC, et al. Human herpesvirus 6A infection in CD46 transgenic mice: viral persistence in the brain and increased production of proinflammatory chemokines via Toll-like receptor 9. *J Virol* 2014;88(10):5421–5436.
208. Rhoads MP, Magaret AS, Zerr DM. Family saliva sharing behaviors and age of human herpesvirus-6B infection. *J Infect* 2007;54(6):623–626.
209. Roffman E, Albert JP, Goff JP, et al. Putative site for the acquisition of human herpesvirus 6 virion tegument. *J Virol* 1990;64(12):6308–6313.
210. Romi H, Singer O, Rapaport D, et al. Tamplicon-7, a novel T-lymphotropic vector derived from human herpesvirus 7. *J Virol* 1999;73(8):7001–7007.
211. Rotola A, Ravaioli T, Gonelli A, et al. U94 of human herpesvirus 6 is expressed in latently infected peripheral blood mononuclear cells and blocks viral gene expression in transformed lymphocytes in culture. *Proc Natl Acad Sci U S A* 1998;95(23):13911–13916.
212. Salahuddin SZ, Ablashi DV, Markham PD, et al. Isolation of a new virus, HBLV, in patients with lymphoproliferative disorders. *Science* 1986;234:596–601.

213. Sang Y, Zhang R, Scott WR, et al. U24 from Roseolovirus interacts strongly with Nedd4 WW Domains. *Sci Rep* 2017;7:39776.
214. Santoro F, Greenstone HL, Insinga A, et al. Interaction of glycoprotein H of human herpesvirus 6 with the cellular receptor CD46. *J Biol Chem* 2003;278(28):25964–25969.
215. Santoro F, Kennedy PE, Locatelli G, et al. CD46 is a cellular receptor from human herpesvirus 6. *Cell* 1999;99:817–827.
216. Schleimann MH, Hoberg S, Solhoj Hansen A, et al. The DR6 protein from human herpesvirus-6B induces p53-independent cell cycle arrest in G2/M. *Virology* 2014;452–453:254–263.
217. Schleimann MH, Moller JM, Kofod-Olsen E, et al. Direct Repeat 6 from human herpesvirus-6B encodes a nuclear protein that forms a complex with the viral DNA processivity factor p41. *PLoS One* 2009;4(10):e7457.
218. Schmidt-Hieber M, Schwender J, Heinz WJ, et al. Viral encephalitis after allogeneic stem cell transplantation: a rare complication with distinct characteristics of different causative agents. *Haematologica* 2011;96(1):142–149.
219. Secchiero P, Bertolaso L, Casareto L, et al. Human herpesvirus 7 infection induces profound cell cycle perturbations coupled to disregulation of cdc2 and cyclin B and polyploidization of CD4(+) T cells. *Blood* 1998;92(5):1685–1696.
220. Secchiero P, Bertolaso L, Gibellini D, et al. Enforced expression of human bcl-2 in CD4+ T cells enhances human herpesvirus 7 replication and induction of cytopathic effects. *Eur J Immunol* 1998;28(5):1587–1596.
221. Secchiero P, Flamand L, Gibellini D, et al. Human herpesvirus 7 induces CD4+ T-cell death by two distinct mechanisms: necrotic lysis in productively infected cells and apoptosis in uninfected or nonproductively infected cells. *Blood* 1997;90:4502–4512.
222. Secchiero P, Mirandola P, Zella D, et al. Human herpesvirus 7 induces the functional up-regulation of tumor necrosis factor-related apoptosis-inducing ligand (TRAIL) coupled to TRAIL-R1 down-modulation in CD4(+) T cells. *Blood* 2001;98(8):2474–2481.
223. Secchiero P, Nicholas J, Deng H, et al. Identification of human telomeric repeat motifs at the genome termini of human herpesvirus 7: structural analysis and heterogeneity. *J Virol* 1995;69:8041–8045.
224. Secchiero P, Sun D, De Vico A, et al. Role of the extracellular domain of human herpesvirus 7 glycoprotein B in virus binding to cell surface heparan sulfate proteoglycans. *J Virol* 1997;71:4571–4580.
225. Sedlak RH, Cook L, Huang ML, et al. Identification of chromosomally integrated human herpesvirus 6 by droplet digital PCR. *Clin Chem* 2014;60(5):765–772.
226. Seeley WW, Marty FM, Holmes TM, et al. Post-transplant acute limbic encephalitis: clinical features and relationship to HHV6. *Neurology* 2007;69(2):156–165.
227. Seo S, Renaud C, Kuypers JM, et al. Idiopathic pneumonia syndrome after hematopoietic cell transplantation: evidence of occult infectious etiologies. *Blood* 2015;125(24):3789–3797.
228. Severini A, Sevenhuysen C, Garbutt M, et al. Structure of replicating intermediates of human herpesvirus type 6. *Virology* 2003;314(1):443–450.
229. Shimada K, Kondo K, Yamanishi K. Human herpesvirus 6 immediate-early 2 protein interacts with heterogeneous ribonucleoprotein K and casein kinase 2. *Microbiol Immunol* 2004;48(3):205–210.
230. Smith AP, Paolucci C, Di Lullo G, et al. Viral replication-independent blockade of dendritic cell maturation and interleukin-12 production by human herpesvirus 6. *J Virol* 2005;79(5):2807–2813.
231. Stanton R, Fox JD, Caswell R, et al. Analysis of the human herpesvirus-6 immediate-early 1 protein. *J Gen Virol* 2002;83(Pt 11):2811–2820.
232. Stefan A, De Lillo M, Frascaroli G, et al. Development of recombinant diagnostic reagents based on pp85(U14) and p86(U11) proteins to detect the human immune response to human herpesvirus 7 infection. *J Clin Microbiol* 1999;37:3980–3985.
233. Suga S, Suzuki K, Ihira M, et al. Clinical characteristics of febrile convulsions during primary HHV-6 infection [see comments]. *Arch Dis Child* 2000;82(1):62–66.
234. Sullivan BM, Coscoy L. Downregulation of the T-cell receptor complex and impairment of T-cell activation by human herpesvirus 6 u24 protein. *J Virol* 2008;82(2):602–608.
235. Sullivan BM, Coscoy L. The U24 protein from human herpesvirus 6 and 7 affects endocytic recycling. *J Virol* 2010;84(3):1265–1275.
236. Tadagaki K, Nakano K, Yamanishi K. Human herpesvirus 7 open reading frames U12 and U51 encode functional beta-chemokine receptors. *J Virol* 2005;79(11):7068–7076.
237. Takahashi K, Segal E, Kondo T, et al. Interferon and natural killer cell activity in patients with exanthem subitum. *Pediatr Infect Dis J* 1992;11(5):369–373.
238. Takemoto M, Imasawa T, Yamanishi K, et al. Role of dendritic cells infected with human herpesvirus 6 in virus transmission to CD4(+) T cells. *Virology* 2009;385(2):294–302.
239. Takemoto M, Koike M, Mori Y, et al. Human herpesvirus 6 open reading frame U14 protein and cellular p53 interact with each other and are contained in the virion. *J Virol* 2005;79(20):13037–13046.
240. Tanaka K, Kondo T, Torigoe S, et al. Human herpesvirus 7: another causal agent for roseola (exanthem subitum). *J Pediatr* 1994;125:1–5.
241. Tanaka-Taya K, Kondo T, Mukai T, et al. Seroepidemiological study of human herpesvirus-6 and -7 in children of different ages and detection of these two viruses in throat swabs by polymerase chain reaction. *J Med Virol* 1996;48:88–94.
242. Tang H, Hayashi M, Maeki T, et al. Human herpesvirus 6 glycoprotein complex formation is required for folding and trafficking of the gH/gL/gQ1/gQ2 complex and its cellular receptor binding. *J Virol* 2011;85(21):11121–11130.
243. Tang H, Kawabata A, Takemoto M, et al. Human herpesvirus-6 infection induces the reorganization of membrane microdomains in target cells, which are required for virus entry. *Virology* 2008;378(2):265–271.
244. Tang H, Kawabata A, Yoshida M, et al. Human herpesvirus 6 encoded glycoprotein Q1 gene is essential for virus growth. *Virology* 2010;407(2):360–367.
245. Tang H, Mahmoud NF, Mori Y. Maturation of human herpesvirus 6A glycoprotein O requires coexpression of glycoprotein H and glycoprotein L. *J Virol* 2015;89(9): 5159–5163.
246. Tang H, Mori Y. Human herpesvirus-6 entry into host cells. *Future Microbiol* 2010;5(7):1015–1023.
247. Tang H, Mori Y. Determinants of human CD134 essential for entry of human herpesvirus 6B. *J Virol* 2015;89(19):10125–10129.
248. Tang H, Serada S, Kawabata A, et al. CD134 is a cellular receptor specific for human herpesvirus-6B entry. *Proc Natl Acad Sci U S A* 2013;110(22):9096–9099.
249. Tang H, Wang J, Mahmoud NF, et al. Detailed study of the interaction between human herpesvirus 6B glycoprotein complex and its cellular receptor, human CD134. *J Virol* 2014;88(18):10875–10882.
250. Tao C, Simpson S, Taylor BV, et al. Association between human herpesvirus & human endogenous retrovirus and MS onset & progression. *J Neurol Sci* 2017;372:239–249.
251. Telford M, Navarro A, Santpere G. Whole genome diversity of inherited chromosomally integrated HHV-6 derived from healthy individuals of diverse geographic origin. *Sci Rep* 2018;8(1):3472.
252. Thomson BJ, Dewhurst SD, Gray D. Structure and heterogeneity of the a sequences of human herpesvirus 6 strain variants U1102 and Z29 and identification of human telomeric repeat sequences at the genomic termini. *J Virol* 1994;68:3007–3014.
253. Thomson BJ, Weindler FW, Gray D, et al. Human herpesvirus 6 (HHV-6) is a helper virus for adeno-associated virus type 2 (AAV-2) and the AAV-2 rep gene homologue in HHV-6 can mediate AAV-2 DNA replication and regulate gene expression. *Virology* 1994;204:304–311.
254. Tigue NJ, Kay J. Autoprocessing and peptide substrates for human herpesvirus 6 proteinase. *J Biol Chem* 1998;273(41):26441–26446.
255. Tohyama M, Hashimoto K. New aspects of drug-induced hypersensitivity syndrome. *J Dermatol* 2011;38(3):222–228.
256. Tomoiu A, Gravel A, Flamand L. Mapping of human herpesvirus 6 immediate-early 2 protein transactivation domains. *Virology* 2006;354(1):91–102.
257. Torelli G, Barozzi P, Marasca R, et al. Targeted integration of human herpesvirus 6 in the p arm of chromosome 17 of human peripheral blood mononuclear cells in vivo. *J Med Virol* 1995;46:178–188.
258. Torrisi MR, Gentile M, Cardinali G, et al. Intracellular transport and maturation pathway of human herpesvirus 6. *Virology* 1999;257(2):460–471.
259. Trempe F, Gravel A, Dubuc I, et al. Characterization of human herpesvirus 6A/B U94 as ATPase, helicase, exonuclease and DNA-binding proteins. *Nucleic Acids Res* 2015;43(12):6084–6098.
260. Tuddenham L, Jung JS, Chane-Woon-Ming B, et al. Small RNA deep sequencing identifies microRNAs and other small noncoding RNAs from human herpesvirus 6B. *J Virol* 2012;86(3):1638–1649.
261. Tzannou I, Papadopoulou A, Naik S, et al. Off-the-shelf virus-specific T cells to treat BK virus, human herpesvirus 6, cytomegalovirus, Epstein-Barr virus, and adenovirus infections after allogeneic hematopoietic stem-cell transplantation. *J Clin Oncol* 2017;35(31):3547–3557.
262. Vellucci A, Leibovitch EC, Jacobson S. Using droplet digital PCR to detect coinfection of human herpesviruses 6A and 6B (HHV-6A and HHV-6B) in clinical samples. *Methods Mol Biol* 2018;1768:99–109.
263. Vink C, Beuken E, Bruggeman CA. Complete DNA sequence of the rat cytomegalovirus genome. *J Virol* 2000;74:7656–7665.
264. Virtanen JO, Wohler J, Fenton K, et al. Oligoclonal bands in multiple sclerosis reactive against two herpesviruses and association with magnetic resonance imaging findings. *Mult Scler* 2014;20(1):27–34.
265. Wainwright MS, Martin PL, Morse RP, et al. Human herpesvirus 6 limbic encephalitis after stem cell transplantation. *Ann Neurol* 2001;50(5):612–619.
266. Wakata A, Kanemoto S, Tang H, et al. The neutralizing linear epitope of human herpesvirus 6A glycoprotein B does not affect virus infectivity. *J Virol* 2018;92(5).
267. Wallaschek N, Gravel A, Flamand L, et al. The putative U94 integrase is dispensable for human herpesvirus 6 (HHV-6) chromosomal integration. *J Gen Virol* 2016;97(8):1899–1903.
268. Wallaschek N, Sanyal A, Pirzer F, et al. The telomeric repeats of human herpesvirus 6A (HHV-6A) are required for efficient virus integration. *PLoS Pathog* 2016;12(5):e1005666.
269. Wang B, Nishimura M, Tang H, et al. Crystal structure of human herpesvirus 6B tegument protein U14. *PLoS Pathog* 2016;12(5):e1005594.
270. Wang FZ, Pellett PE. Human herpesviruses 6A, 6B, and 7: immunobiology and host response (freely available as PMID 21348133). In: Arvin A, Campadelli-Fiume G, Mocarski ES, et al., eds. *Human Herpesviruses: Biology, Therapy, and Immunoprophylaxis.* Cambridge: Cambridge University Press; 2006:850–874.
271. Ward KN. The natural history and laboratory diagnosis of human herpesviruses-6 and -7 infections in the immunocompetent. *J Clin Virol* 2005;32(3):183–193.
272. Ward KN, Andrews NJ, Verity CM, et al. Human herpesviruses-6 and -7 each cause significant neurological morbidity in Britain and Ireland. *Arch Dis Child* 2005;90(6):619–623.
273. Ward KN, Hill JA, Hubacek P, et al. Guidelines from the 2017 European Conference on Infections in Leukaemia for management of HHV-6 infection in patients with hematologic malignancies and after hematopoietic stem cell transplantation. *Haematologica* 2019;104(11):2155–2163.
274. Ward KN, Leong HN, Thiruchelvam AD, et al. Human herpesvirus 6 DNA levels in cerebrospinal fluid due to primary infection differ from those due to chromosomal viral integration and have implications for diagnosis of encephalitis. *J Clin Microbiol* 2007;45(4):1298–1304.
275. Wight DJ, Wallaschek N, Sanyal A, et al. Viral proteins U41 and U70 of human herpesvirus 6A are dispensable for telomere integration. *Viruses* 2018;10(11).
276. Wipfler P, Dunn N, Beiki O, et al. The viral hypothesis of mesial temporal lobe epilepsy - Is human herpes virus-6 the missing link? A systematic review and meta-analysis. *Seizure* 2018;54:33–40.
277. Wood ML, Royle NJ. Chromosomally integrated human herpesvirus 6: models of viral genome release from the telomere and impacts on human health. *Viruses* 2017;9(7).
278. Wu Z, Jia J, Xu X, et al. Human herpesvirus 6A promotes glycolysis in infected T cells by activation of mTOR signaling. *PLoS Pathog* 2020;16(6):e1008568.
279. Wyatt LS, Frenkel N. Human herpesvirus 7 is a constitutive inhabitant of adult human saliva. *J Virol* 1992;66(5):3206–3209.

280. Wyatt LS, Rodriguez WJ, Balachandran N, et al. Human herpesvirus 7: antigenic properties and prevalence in children and adults. *J Virol* 1991;65:6260–6265.
281. Yalcin S, Mukai T, Kondo K, et al. Experimental infection of cynomolgus and African green monkeys with human herpesvirus 6. *J Gen Virol* 1992;73:1673–1677.
282. Yamanishi K, Okuno T, Shiraki K, et al. Identification of human herpesvirus-6 as a causal agent for exanthem subitum. *Lancet* 1988;1:1065–1067.
283. Yang CH, Sahoo MK, Fitzpatrick M, et al. Evaluating for human herpesvirus 6 in the liver explants of children with liver failure of unknown etiology. *J Infect Dis* 2019;220(3):361–369.
284. Yasukawa M, Inoue Y, Ohminami H, et al. Apoptosis of CD4+ T lymphocytes in human herpesvirus-6 infection. *J Gen Virol* 1998;79:143–147.
285. Yasukawa M, Yakushijin Y, Furukawa M, et al. Specificity analysis of human CD4+ T-cell clones directed against human herpesvirus 6 (HHV-6), HHV-7, and human cytomegalovirus. *J Virol* 1993;67(10):6259–6264.
286. Yeo WM, Isegawa Y, Chow VT. The U95 protein of human herpesvirus 6B interacts with human GRIM-19: silencing of U95 expression reduces viral load and abrogates loss of mitochondrial membrane potential. *J Virol* 2008;82(2):1011–1020.
287. Yoshida M, Uno F, Bai ZL, et al. Electron microscopic study of a herpes-type virus isolated from an infant with exanthem subitum. *Microbiol Immunol* 1989;33(2):147–154.
288. Yoshida M, Yamada M, Chatterjee S, et al. A method for detection of HHV-6 antigens and its use for evaluating antiviral drugs. *J Virol Methods* 1996;58(1–2):137–143.
289. Yoshikawa T, Akimoto S, Nishimura N, et al. Evaluation of active human herpesvirus 6 infection by reverse transcription-PCR. *J Med Virol* 2003;70(2):267–272.
290. Yoshikawa T, Asano Y, Kobayashi I, et al. Seroepidemiology of human herpesvirus 7 in healthy children and adults in Japan. *J Med Virol* 1993;41:319–323.
291. Yoshikawa T, Ihira M, Furukawa H, et al. Four cases of human herpesvirus 6 variant B infection after pediatric liver transplantation. *Transplantation* 1998;65(9):1266–1269.
292. Yoshikawa T, Kato Y, Ihira M, et al. Kinetics of cytokine and chemokine responses in patients with primary human herpesvirus 6 infection. *J Clin Virol* 2011;50(1):65–68.
293. Yoshikawa T, Ohashi M, Miyake F, et al. Exanthem subitum-associated encephalitis: nationwide survey in Japan. *Pediatr Neurol* 2009;41(5):353–358.
294. Zerr DM, Boeckh M, Delaney C, et al. HHV-6 reactivation and associated sequelae after hematopoietic cell transplantation. *Biol Blood Marrow Transplant* 2012;18(11):1700–1708.
295. Zerr DM, Fann JR, Breiger D, et al. HHV-6 reactivation and its effect on delirium and cognitive functioning in hematopoietic cell transplantation recipients. *Blood* 2011;117(19):5243–5249.
296. Zerr DM, Meier AS, Selke SS, et al. A population-based study of primary human herpesvirus 6 infection. *N Engl J Med* 2005;352(8):768–776.
297. Zhang E, Bell AJ, Wilkie GS, et al. Inherited chromosomally integrated human herpesvirus 6 genomes are ancient, intact, and potentially able to reactivate from telomeres. *J Virol* 2017;91(22).
298. Zhang Y, Liu W, Li Z, et al. Atomic structure of the human herpesvirus 6B capsid and capsid-associated tegument complexes. *Nat Commun* 2019;10(1):5346.
299. Zhen Z, Bradel-Tretheway B, Sumagin S, et al. The human herpesvirus 6 G protein-coupled receptor homolog U51 positively regulates virus replication and enhances cell-cell fusion in vitro. *J Virol* 2005;79(18):11914–11924.
300. Zielke B, Thomas M, Giede-Jeppe A, et al. Characterization of the betaherpesviral pUL69 protein family reveals binding of the cellular mRNA export factor UAP56 as a prerequisite for stimulation of nuclear mRNA export and for efficient viral replication. *J Virol* 2011;85(4):1804–1819.
301. Zou P, Isegawa Y, Nakano K, et al. Human herpesvirus 6 open reading frame U83 encodes a functional chemokine. *J Virol* 1999;73(7):5926–5933.

CHAPTER

15 Kaposi's Sarcoma Herpesvirus

Blossom Damania • Ethel Cesarman

Kaposi's sarcoma herpesvirus (KSHV) is the eighth human herpesvirus, originally named Kaposi's sarcoma-associated herpesvirus, and also known as human herpesvirus 8 (HHV8). KSHV is the most recently identified herpesvirus among the human herpesviruses. Chang, Moore, Cesarman, and colleagues first identified the virus from AIDS-associated Kaposi's sarcoma (KS) tissues.[106] KSHV has been classified as a member of the lymphotropic gammaherpesvirus subfamily. In this chapter, we review epidemiological evidence linking the virus to multiple human cancers, and the clinical description of these viral cancers. We also discuss the latent and lytic life cycles of KSHV and the contribution of viral genes and proteins to disease pathogenesis.

KSHV: DISCOVERY AND CLASSIFICATION

KS was first described by a Hungarian dermatologist named Moritz Kaposi in the late 19th century as "*Idiopathisches multiples Pigmentsarkom der Haut.*"[298] Classically considered an indolent disease of older men, the disease was later found to be more common in the Mediterranean region as well as parts of Africa.[17] In several regions of Africa, KS afflicts children as well as adults. Prior to the emergence of HIV infection in the human population KS was considered a rare neoplasm in the United States and Western Europe. However, with the advent of pandemic HIV in the early 1980s, KS emerged as the most common AIDS-defining cancer. The linkage between KS and HIV infection first prompted speculation that HIV was the etiological agent of KS, but this was disregarded in light of many epidemiological studies. First, classical KS occurred before the

AIDS epidemic and was originally seen in HIV-negative individuals. Second, even among HIV-positive subjects, certain groups are distinctly different in their risk for KS development. KS was more widespread among patients who acquired HIV via sexual routes (e.g., men who have sex with men or MSM), compared to individuals who acquired HIV parenterally (e.g., children and hemophiliacs[41]). These data suggested that KS might be acquired by a sexually transmitted pathogen other than HIV, which initiated a hunt for the etiological agent in question. In 1994, Yuan Chang, Patrick Moore, and their colleagues[106] identified KSHV genomic DNA in KS lesions using representational difference analysis.

It is now generally accepted that there are four main classes of KS, only one of which is strongly linked to HIV infection:

1. Classic KS
2. Endemic or African KS
3. Iatrogenic KS associated with immunosuppressive therapies in transplant patients.
4. Epidemic or AIDS-related KS

Although KSHV was first identified in an endothelial-driven tumor, it was later found to be associated with lymphoproliferative disorders, which were greatly increased in AIDS patients. The KSHV genome is consistently present in two B cell lymphoproliferative diseases.[95,567] One such disease is *primary effusion lymphoma* (PEL), which is an expansion of B cells predominantly in serosal cavities such as the pericardium, pleura, and peritoneum, although infiltration of solid organs does occur. B cells in PEL are clonal in origin, as discovered by analysis of immunoglobulin rearrangements. Every PEL cell harbors KSHV DNA in the form of a circular episome. These are in multiple copies. Some PELs also harbor Epstein-Barr virus (EBV), but KSHV is the defining pathogen for a diagnosis of PEL.

PEL cell lines can be established in culture relatively easily[96] and form tumors in immunodeficient mice.[85,572] PEL cell lines were the first system where KSHV replication could be induced *in vitro*,[512] and have yielded latent and lytic antigens for serologic test development.

Another B-cell disorder associated with KSHV infection is multicentric Castleman disease (MCD). MCD is a polyclonal[170] lymphoproliferative disorder that can develop in both HIV-negative and HIV-positive individuals. MCD is an aggressive disorder that has a higher incidence in AIDS patients, where it is always associated with KSHV infection.[567] It is a systemic disease characterized by fever, loss of weight, sweats, splenomegaly, and lymphadenopathy. The KSHV viral genome is present in the B cells of the mantle zones surrounding the germinal centers. In a given germinal center, upto 30% of the mantle zone B cells appear to be infected with virus.[173,483] All the KSHV-positive cells in MCD bear lambda light chains together with IgM heavy chains.[170] In HIV-negative individuals, less than 50% of all MCD cases are linked to KSHV infection.[567]

The KSHV genomic sequence confirmed the classification of the virus as a member of the lymphotropic (or γ-) herpesviruses (Fig. 15.1). Lymphotropic herpesviruses can be further divided into two groups: the γ1 or *lymphocryptoviruses* (which includes EBV and its simian relatives) and the γ2 or *rhadinoviruses*. KSHV falls squarely into the latter category, which also includes the prototype primate virus, Herpesvirus saimiri (HVS). With the identification of additional primate rhadinoviruses, it is now evident that rhadinoviruses are represented by two different lineages, based on their biological properties and genomic organization—one lineage is represented by KSHV and a primate virus named retroperitoneal fibromatosis herpesvirus (RFHV), and a second group is represented by HVS and rhesus monkey rhadinovirus (RRV) (reviewed in Ref.[53]).

VIRION STRUCTURE

Structurally similar to virions of other herpesviruses, KSHV virions exhibit an electron-dense nucleocapsid surrounded by a lipid bilayer envelope as visualized by electron microscopy (EM). In between the capsid and envelope is a morphologically amorphous but highly organized proteinaceous layer called the tegument. The envelope is studded with viral glycoproteins—for example, glycoprotein gB is thought to engage cell surface receptors and participate directly in viral entry. The virion contains six other glycoproteins including ORF22 (gH), ORF39 (gM), ORF47 (gL), ORF53 (gN), ORF68, and K8.1.[695] Little is known regarding the architecture of the tegument. However, multiple proteins have been identified that localize to this region.[38,695] KSHV tegument proteins share the common feature in that they are delivered to the target cell along with the genome upon primary infection, and may thus contribute to early events in the replication cycle even before the synthesis of immediate-early proteins. This is also the case for the 11 viral mRNAs that are incorporated in the tegument layer.[37] These virion mRNAs are derived from viral transcripts expressed in the prior lytic cycle and are incorporated into the tegument during the process of budding and envelopment. It is likely that one or more mRNAs are selectively incorporated into the virus particle.[37,38] How such targeted recruitment might occur is unknown.

The KSHV capsid, like its HSV and HCMV counterparts, is icosahedral. A significant amount of work has been done to characterize the KSHV capsid structure in terms of its three-dimensional architecture and polypeptide composition.[462] Cryo-EM reconstruction has revealed that the icosahedral capsid is symmetric (T= 16) with 20 triangular faces. There are three types of capsid structures as identified by electron microscopy: an empty capsid shell (A-capsid), a capsid containing scaffolding protein (B-capsid), and a capsid encapsidating the viral genome (C-capsid) (Fig. 15.2).[158,462]

The capsomers are composed of hexamers and pentamers of the major capsid protein (MCP encoded by ORF25). Each capsid contains 150 hexons and 12 pentons, which are interconnected by 320 triplexes that are heterotrimer structures composed of ORF62 (1 copy) and ORF26 (2 copies). The capsomeric hexons form the capsid edges and faces, whereas the pentons are located at each capsid vertex (Fig. 15.2). The KSHV smallest capsid protein (SCP) is required for capsid assembly. It forms a crown on each hexon and cross-links adjacent MCP subunits. SCP binds MCP through hydrophobic interactions and SCP has a kinked helix that connects to neighboring MCPs[145] (Fig. 15.2). A 4.2 angstrom structure of the KSHV capsid by cryo-electron microscopy shows that the

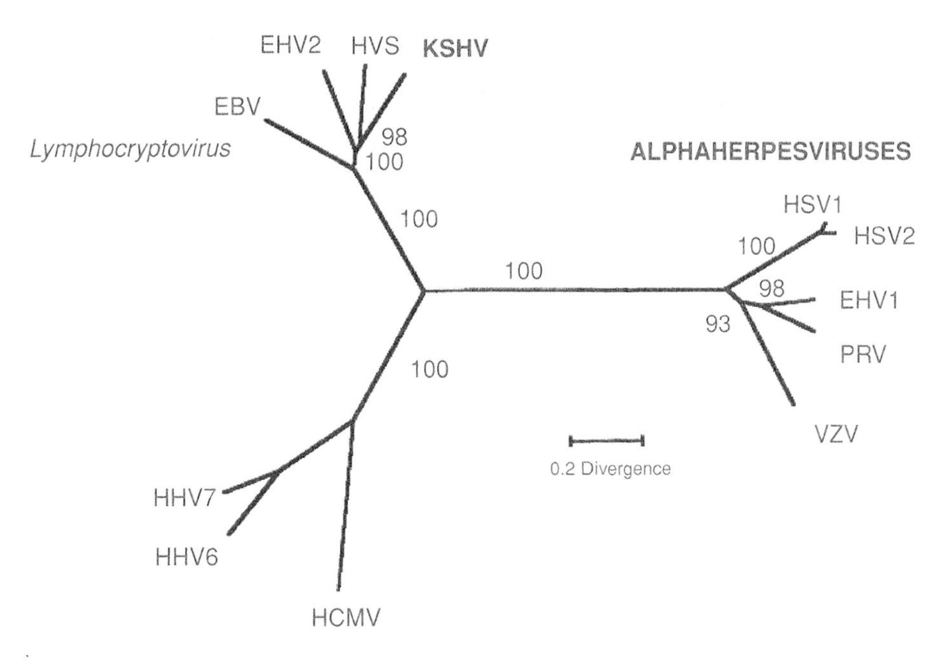

FIGURE 15.1 A radial phylogenetic tree was constructed based on comparisons of the herpesviral DNA polymerase proteins from twelve primate herpesviruses showing the relationships between members of the alpha-, beta- and gammaherpesvirus subfamilies. The human alpha herpesviruses include herpes simplex virus (HSV)1 and HSV2 and varicella–zoster virus (VZV); human beta-herpesviruses include cytomegalovirus (CMV), HHV6, and HHV7; and human gamma-herpesviruses include Kaposi's sarcoma herpesvirus (KSHV) and Epstein-Barr virus (EBV). KSHV is the first human rhadinovirus, the prototype member of which is HVS (Herpesvirus saimiri). Other viruses shown are equine herpesvirus (EHV) 1 and EHV2 and pseudorabies virus (PRV). A bar showing 0.2 divergence is depicted. (Reprinted from Moore PS, Gao SJ, Dominguez G, et al. Primary characterization of a herpesvirus agent associated with Kaposi's sarcomae. *J Virol* 1996;70(1):549–558.)

capsid contains 46 unique conformers of the MCP, the SCP and the triplex proteins Tri1 and Tri2[146] (Fig. 15.2). A hydrophobic residue containing groove present in MCP interacts with the SCP, which can cross-link with adjacent MCPs in the same hexon resulting in capsid stabilization.[146] Two Tri2 molecules and one Tri1 molecule form a triplex. The triplex binds to the capsid floor via Tri1.[146]

For the most part, the KSHV capsid resembles the features of the well-studied HSV-1 capsid, with the exception that the KSHV hexons lack the presence of a VP26 subunit, which is seen bound to the HSV-1 hexon subunits, and the KSHV triplexes appear smaller and less elongated than those of HSV-1. The viral linear genomic DNA is located inside the capsid.

THE KSHV GENOME: STRUCTURE AND ORGANIZATION

The KSHV genome is a double-stranded linear DNA that is 165 to 170 kb long.[523] The genome is composed of a central unique region of 145 kb encoding the viral open reading frames (ORFs).[523] The central region is flanked by highly GC-rich direct terminal repeats (TRs) (Fig. 15.3). Each TR unit is 85% GC rich and is 801 bp long. Commonly, viral isolates contain 20 to 25 kb of TR DNA per genome; however, the exact number of TRs present at each terminus differs.

Comparison of the KSHV genome sequence with other herpesviruses reveals blocks of highly conserved genes that are common to all herpesviruses (Fig. 15.3). These are typically genes that encode for proteins involved in viral replication or proteins that encode for structural components of the virions. In addition, there is a group of genes that show homology to the gammaherpesvirus ($\gamma 1$ and $\gamma 2$) lineage, and those that are only common to the $\gamma 2$ lineage. Finally, there are also a group of genes that are only encoded by KSHV and its simian relatives but not present in other herpesviruses from nonprimate species, for example, KSHV viral interleukin 6 (vIL-6), viral interferon regulatory factors (vIRFs), etc. (Fig. 15.3).

The KSHV ORFs are numbered in consecutive order from left (ORF 1) to right (ORF 75). KSHV contains numerous ORFs that are not conserved in other herpesviruses, and these are interspersed amongst the conserved herpesvirus genes.

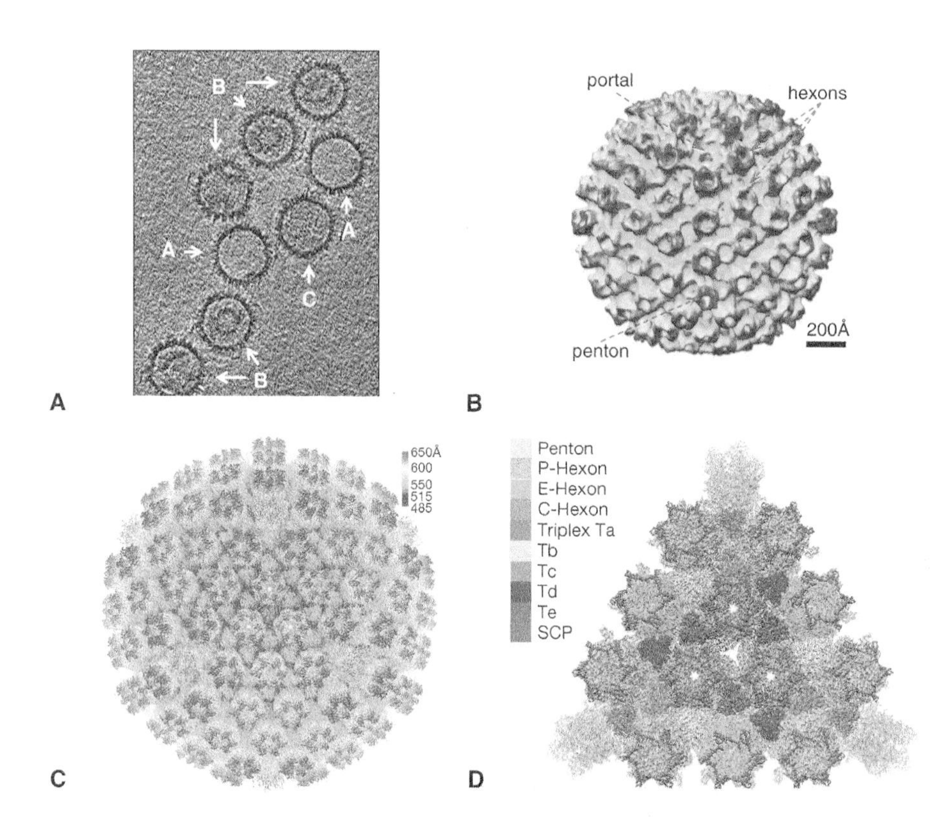

FIGURE 15.2 **KSHV A-, B-, and C-capsid. A:** Central slice of a tomogram showing the KSHV A-, B-, and C-capsid. **B:** Radially colored surface representation of an averaged KSHV capsid showing the characteristic herpesvirus capsomers, including an "umbilical" portal, 11 pentons and 150 hexons. **C:** Cryo-EM reconstruction and atomic modeling of KSHV capsid. Radially colored cryo-EM density map of KSHV capsid. **D:** Zoomed in view of one facet of the icosahedral capsid. The penton, hexon, small capsid protein (SCP), and Triplex (named Tri a/b/c/d/e) are shown. (**A and B:** Reprinted from Deng B, O'Connor CM, Kedes DH, et al. Cryo-electron tomography of Kaposi's sarcoma-associated herpesvirus capsids reveals dynamic scaffolding structures essential to capsid assembly and maturation. *J Struct Biol* 2008;161(3):419–427. Copyright © 2007 Elsevier, with permission. **C and D:** Reprinted by permission from Dai X, Gong D, Lim H, et al. Structure and mutagenesis reveal essential capsid protein interactions for KSHV replication. *Nature* 2018;553(7689):521–525. Copyright © 2018 Springer Nature.)

The KSHV unique ORFs are given "K" designations, ORFs K1-K15, numbered from left to right (Fig. 15.3). Some of the K open-reading frames encode for more than one protein due to alternative splicing and/or alternative translational initiation sites. Many of the K ORFs encode signaling molecules and proteins that are homologs of cellular genes, for example, vIL-6, vIRFs, etc. The KSHV genome also encodes for many small noncoding RNAs, including a set of micro RNAs[78,489,527] and a noncoding lytic 1.1 kb nuclear RNA named PAN that is polyadenylated.[134,578] Moreover, the KSHV genome also encodes for circular RNAs.[587,598,606]

Genetic Analysis of KSHV

Construction of mutant viruses using homologous recombination has revolutionized the study of replication and pathogenesis of herpesviruses. Two methods have been used to generate recombinant KSHV viruses. In earlier work, PEL cells were transfected with a targeting vector encoding the viral gene of interest, disrupted by a GFP cassette and selectable marker. Stable GFP-positive cells were selected, followed by viral reactivation with 12-*O*-tetradecanoylphorbol-13-acetate (TPA) and supernatants were then tested for GFP transduction capacity.[618] Others have used BACmid technology to construct a KSHV BACmid.[69,692] Recombinant viruses deleted for several open reading frames and miRNAs have been described in the literature. In addition, replication-competent, KSHV viruses with markers (GFP and RFP) to track latent (GFP) and lytic (RFP) infection have been constructed[69,616] and are highly beneficial for studies of viral infectivity. Table 15.1 lists the KSHV viral genes, proteins, and their corresponding EBV homologs.

THE VIRAL LIFE CYCLE

Viral Binding and Entry

KSHV is able to infect multiple cell types *in vitro* and *in vivo*. KSHV binds to and enters a variety of human cell lines and primary cells in culture, including transformed B cells, primary

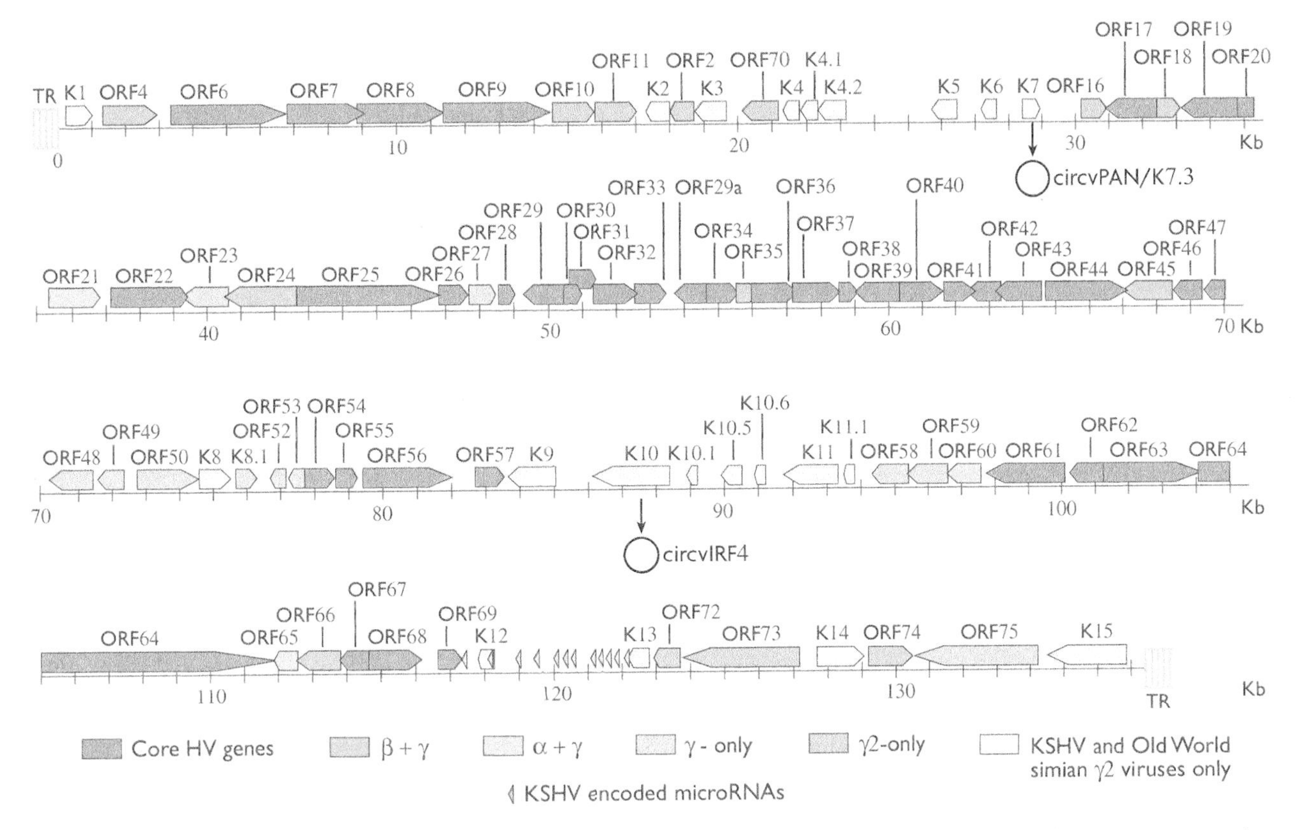

FIGURE 15.3 The KSHV (HHV8) genome map. Blocks of conserved genes between KSHV and related α, β, γ herpesviruses are indicated by the same color. *Arrows* indicate open reading frames (ORFs), with direction of *arrow* indicating direction of translation.

B cells, 293 human embryonic kidney cells, THP-1 monocytic cells, myeloid and plasmacytoid dendritic cells, primary monocytes, human foreskin fibroblasts, HeLa epithelial cells, mast cells, and endothelial cells. KSHV can also infect monkey cells such as Vero and CV-1, hamster cells such as BHK-21 and CHO cells, and mouse cells *in vitro*.

KSHV encodes for multiple envelope glycoproteins, including gB, gH, and gL. Attachment of the virion to the cell is thought to be mediated by several host receptor proteins as described below and highlighted in Figure 15.4.

Heparan Sulfate

Several glycoproteins encoded by KSHV have been shown to bind heparan sulfate present on the surface of the cell. These include KSHV gB, gH, ORF4, and gpK8.1A.[7,49,458] The fact that the virus encodes four proteins that bind to heparan sulfate highlights the importance of this protein for attachment. Binding to heparan sulfate may contribute to efficiency of infection, since soluble heparan competes and hinders binding and impairs (but does not eliminate) infectivity. Thus, similar to HSV, the role of heparan sulfate binding helps to concentrate virus particles on the cell surface, thereby increasing their effective local concentration for interactions with cell surface receptors.

Integrins

Chandran and colleagues were the first to identify an integrin binding motif—the RGD (Arg-Gly-Asp) motif, contained in the KSHV gB glycoprotein and showed that it contributes to KSHV binding and entry.[7,8] A twofold reduction in KSHV infection of endothelial and fibroblast cells was observed upon treatment with RGD peptides or antibodies against RGD-gB peptide.[8] Conversely, blocking of integrins using anti-integrin α3 or β1 antibodies, also prevented KSHV entry.[8] Moreover, integrin-independent entry has also been described for KSHV.[591]

DC-SIGN

Dendritic cell-specific intercellular adhesion molecule 3 (ICAM-3)-grabbing nonintegrin (DC-SIGN; CD209) is expressed on activated B cells, dendritic cells (DCs), and macrophages. KSHV is thought to bind DC-SIGN since KSHV infection can be blocked by an anti-DC-SIGN monoclonal antibody and soluble DC-SIGN.[507] However, similar to the situation with the integrins mentioned above, these agents did not completely prevent KSHV binding to the cell suggesting that additional binding partners may exist, for example, heparan sulfate (Fig. 15.4). The incomplete inhibition of viral entry by the integrin-blocking antibodies supports the notion that although integrins play an important role in viral entry, other host proteins may also be involved in KSHV entry.

xCT

xCT is a 12-transmembrane glutamate/cysteine exchange transporter protein that has also been proposed to be a KSHV entry receptor.[295] xCT is part of the cell surface CD98 (4F2 antigen) complex containing a common glycosylated heavy

TABLE 15.1 KSHV genes and their homologs in EBV

KSHV Gene	Other KSHV Name	EBV Gene	Function
K1			Signaling protein
ORF4	KCP		Complement binding protein
ORF6		BALF2	ssDNA binding protein
ORF7		BALF3	DNA packaging terminase
ORF8	gB	BALF4	Glycoprotein B
ORF9		BALF5	DNA polymerase
ORF10	RIF		
ORF11		Raji LF2	
K2	vIL-6		IL-6 homolog
ORF02			DHFR
K3			Membrane-associated RING-CH (MARCH) ubiquitin lig
ORF70			Thymidylate synthase
K4	vMIP-II/vCCL2		Chemokine
K5			Membrane-associated RING-CH (MARCH) ubiquitin lig
K6	vMIP-I/vCCL1		Chemokine
K7			
ORF16	vBcl-2	BHRF1	Bcl-2 homolog
ORF17		BVRF2	Protease
ORF17.5	SCAF		Scaffold protein
ORF18		BVLF1	
ORF19		BVRF1	Virion protein
ORF20		BXRF1	
ORF21	vTK	BXLF1	Thymidine kinase
ORF22	gH	BXLF2	Glycoprotein H
ORF23		BTRF1	
ORF24		BcRF1	Transcription factor
ORF25	MCP	BcLF1	Major capsid protein
ORF26	Triplex 2	BDLF1	Capsid protein
ORF27		BDLF2	
ORF28		BDLF3	
ORF29b		BDRF1	Packaging protein
ORF30		BDLF3.5	
ORF31		BDLF4	
ORF32		BGLF1	Virion protein
ORF33		BGLF2	Virion protein
ORF29a		BGRF1	Packaging protein
ORF34		BGLF3	
ORF35		BGLF3.5	
ORF36	vPK	BGLF4	Viral protein kinase
ORF37	SOX	BGLF5	Exonuclease/Host shutoff
ORF38		BBLF1	
ORF39	gM	BBRF3	Glycoprotein M

TABLE 15.1 KSHV genes and their homologs in EBV (*Continued*)

KSHV Gene	Other KSHV Name	EBV Gene	Function
ORF40		BBLF2	Primase-associated factor
ORF41		BBLF3	Primase-associated factor
ORF42		BBRF2	
ORF43		BBRF1	Capsid protein
ORF44		BBLF4	Helicase
ORF45		BKRF4	Immune evasion
ORF46		BKRF3	Uracil DNA glycosylase
ORF47	gL	BKRF2	Glycoprotein L
ORF48		BRRF2	
ORF49		BRRF1	
ORF50	RTA	BRLF1	Lytic transactivator
K8	K-bZIP		
ORF52	KicGAS	BLRF2	Tegument protein/immune evasion
ORF53		BLRF1	Glycoprotein N
ORF54		BLLF3	dUTPase
ORF55		BSRF1	
ORF56		BSLF1	Primase/DNA replication protein
ORF57	MTA	BSLF2/BMLF	Posttranscriptional regulator of gene expression
K9	vIRFI		Immune evasion
K10	vIRF4		Immune evasion
K10.5/10.6	vIRF3/LANA2		Immune evasion
K11/K11.1	vIRF2		Immune evasion
ORF58		BMRF2	
ORF59		BMRF1	Polymerase-associated processivity factor
ORF60		BaRF1	Ribonucleotide reductase, small
ORF61		BORF2	Ribonucleotide reductase, large
ORF62	Triplex I	BORF1	Capsid protein
ORF63		BOLF1	Tegument protein/immune evasion
ORF64		BPLF1	Deubiquitinase
ORF65	SCP	BFRF3	Small capsid protein
ORF66		BFRF2	
ORF67		BFRF1	Tegument protein
ORF68	gN	BFLF1	Glycoprotein N
ORF69		BFLF2	
K12	Kaposin		
K13	vFLIP		viral FLICE inhibitory protein
ORF72	vCyclin		Cyclin D homolog
ORF73	LANA		Latency-associated nuclear antigen
K14	vOX-2		CD200/OX-2 homolog
ORF74	vGPCR		viral G-protein coupled receptor
ORF75		BNRF1	Tegument protein/FGARAT
K15			Signaling protein

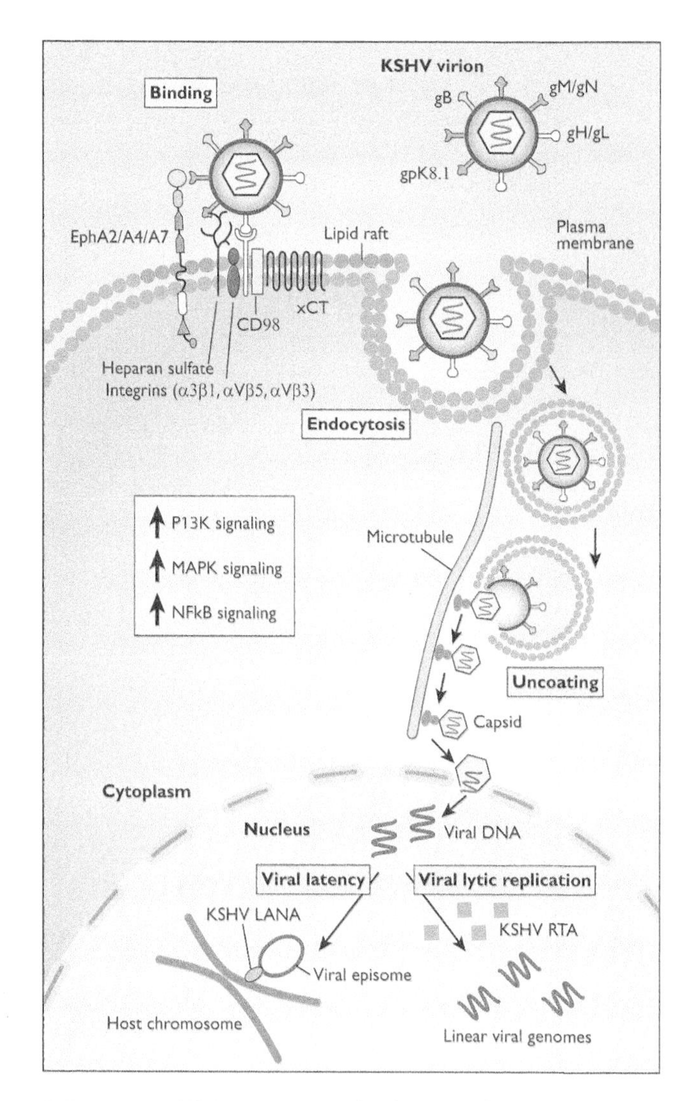

FIGURE 15.4 KSHV entry. Virion binding, attachment, and entry into the host cell. The different stages of KSHV entry are highlighted. Once the viral genome enters the nucleus, the decision to enter the latent or lytic phase of the life cycle is made.

chain and a group of 45-kDa light chains; the xCT molecule is one of the light chains. Expression of recombinant xCT protein in cells that are not permissive for infection restores permissivity to KSHV infection. Additionally, antibodies against xCT block infection.[295] Generally, xCT exists as a heterodimer with CD98, and this complex can associate with cell surface integrins, for example, α3β1. Collectively, these studies demonstrate the interactions of KSHV with closely linked cellular receptor proteins, for example, heparan sulfate, integrins, and xCT, in different cell types[609] (Fig. 15.4). Additionally, there are likely to be many different entry pathways *in vivo*. Of note, the KSHV-encoded microRNAs were reported to up-regulate xCT expression in macrophages and endothelial cells, through miR-K12-11 suppression of the transcriptional repressor, BACH-1.[498,557] The up-regulation of xCT by the KSHV miRNAs increased cell permissiveness for KSHV infection and protected infected cells from death induced by reactive nitrogen species.[498]

Ephrin Receptors

The ephrin receptor tyrosine kinase A2 (EphA2) has also been shown to be a cellular receptor for KSHV in endothelial and epithelial cells.[241] Furthermore, EphA2 was shown to interact with KSHV gH-gL.[240,241] EphrinA2 can modulate clathrin-mediated KSHV endocytosis involving integrin-associated signaling and c-Cbl polyubiquitination.[175] EphA2 was further reported to synergize with CIB1 to facilitate macropinocytic entry of KSHV in dermal endothelial cells.[30] Recently, Ephrin Receptor A4 (EphA4) was also shown to function as a KSHV entry receptor.[122]

Mechanisms of Viral Entry

Endocytosis is the predominant mode of KSHV entry *in vitro* for both adherent and nonadherent target cells. KSHV utilizes clathrin-mediated endocytosis and a low pH environment for its infectious entry into human foreskin fibroblasts (HFF) cells.[9] Studies also suggested endocytosis as the mode of KSHV entry in activated primary human B cells.[507]

Binding of the virus to the cell not only promotes viral entry but also triggers host cell signaling cascades, which may modulate the cellular microenvironment to enhance virus infection. For example, binding of the cell surface integrins by KSHV triggers phosphorylation and activation of focal adhesion kinase (FAK). This activates several signaling molecules including PI3K, Src, Rho GTPases (RhoA, Rac, and Cdc42), and Diaphanous 2 (Dia2). Downstream effector molecules of these signaling moieties are also consequently activated and include Akt, Ezrin, protein kinase C (PKC), MEK, ERK1/2 (extracellular signal-regulated kinase), NFκB, and p38MAPK.[329] Signal transduction does not need active viral replication, since UV-inactivated virions also elicit signaling, and signaling is inhibited by soluble α3β1 integrin peptides. FAK-PI3K activation induced by KSHV binding also activates Rho GTPase and induces cytoskeletal rearrangements.[545,546]

Following virion binding, cellular kinases are activated leading to the recruitment of signaling molecules to the plasma membrane. These signaling proteins then rapidly translocate to clathrin, caveolae, and other vesicles. Src-mediated phosphorylation of clathrin induces the translocation of clathrin to the plasma membrane where it interacts with AP2, Eps15, and dynamin.[425] Src-initiated phosphorylation also triggers the assembly of the plasma membrane–associated Ras activation complex leading to the downstream activation of Rho and Rab GTPases by Ras and PI3K. The Rho and Rab GTPases play critical roles in the formation and movement of endocytic vesicles. These various KSHV-induced signaling events are summarized below.

1. KSHV binding to integrin triggers FAK activation, which appears to be critical for viral entry.[322,545]
2. The activation of FAK and Pyk2 leads to the activation of the Src kinase family, which subsequently activates PI3K and Rho GTPases. Inhibitors of PI3K reduced viral entry suggesting that PI3K's activation of Rac, Rho, Cdc42, and Rab5 GTPases is critical for viral entry since they induce actin reorganization and provide the mechanical force required for endosome formation and trafficking. Induction of the downstream modulator, Akt kinase, early during the

entry process may be beneficial for triggering a pro-survival environment in the infected cell.[322,502,545]

3. PI3K and Rho GTPase activation leads to cytoskeletal rearrangements and the formation of structures such as lamellipodia (Rac), stress fibers (RhoA), and filopodia (Cdc42). This allows for microtubule acetylation and the thickening of microtubule bundles. This process is also essential for delivery of the viral capsids to the nuclear membrane via the microtubules.[459,608]
4. KSHV also activates the ERK1/2 signaling pathway and the NFκB pathway. These pathways are thought to be important for viral gene expression.[458,481,546,666]

The viral capsids traverse down the microtubules towards the nuclear membrane. Consistent with this description, microtubule-depolymerizing agents block infection.[459] It is thought that the capsid then injects the viral genomic DNA into the nucleus through the pore complex. Once the viral DNA enters the nucleus, the virus has a choice to enter either the lytic phase of its life cycle or the latent phase (Fig. 15.4). During latency, the genome is circularized and subsequently is organized into chromatin through the assembly of cellular histones, thereby making it a suitable template for host RNA polymerase II transcription. During lytic replication, the virus is in a linear state amenable for viral DNA replication.

The Innate Immune Response Following Viral Entry

Toll-like receptors (TLRs) are the first line of defense against invading pathogens. They recognize pathogen-associated molecular patterns (PAMPs) present on invading pathogens and trigger signaling cascades, which lead to the activation of type I IFN, NF-κB and many other pro-inflammatory cytokines. Some TLRs are expressed on the cell surface, for example, TLR2 and TLR4, while others are expressed in the endosome, for example, TLR 3,7,8, and 9.[6] TLRs 3, 7, and 8 are activated by RNA. TLR3 recognizes dsRNA, while TLR7 and TLR8 recognize ssRNA. It is important to note that different cell types have distinct TLR expression profiles; hence, TLR recognition of an invading pathogen is dependent on the cell type being infected.

During infection of primary human monocytes, KSHV activates TLR3 resulting in the up-regulation of TLR3 expression (both mRNA and protein are increased) and its downstream mediators, including IFN-β1 and the chemokine CXCL10 (also called IP-10).[644] As mentioned above, KSHV is known to be endocytosed in monocytes, and during this process it is possible that the viral RNA transcripts present in the tegument of the virus trigger TLR3 activation. In human plasmacytoid dendritic cells (pDCs), which are the chief IFN producing cells in the body, KSHV infection triggers the activation of TLR9, a TLR whose agonist is CpG DNA.[645] Thus, in pDCs, TLR9 is likely recognizing KSHV viral DNA. Unlike monocytes, human pDCs do not express TLR3 and only express TLR7 and TLR9. Finally, TLR4 appears to be important for recognition of KSHV in endothelial cells, since the virus can down-regulate TLR4 expression on endothelial cells.[332] Both vIRF1 and vGPCR are involved in TLR4 down-regulation.[332]

TLRs also play a role in a very different context, for example, during reactivation from latency. Stimulation of TLR7/8 in KSHV latently infected PEL cells, either by synthesized agonist (poly-Uridine) or by infection with a biologically relevant pathogen, vesicular stomatitis virus (a known activator of TLR7 and -8), led to viral reactivation and progeny virion production.[220] This represents a new role for TLR stimulation in the context of KSHV infection (which differs from the role TLRs play during primary infection) and suggests a possible physiological stimulus that can lead to viral reactivation *in vivo*.[220]

Additional sensors that detect KSHV during infection include the nucleotide-binding domain, leucine-rich repeat protein (NLR) receptors, RIG-I-like receptors (RLRs), interferon gamma–inducible protein 16 (IFI16), and cGAS-STING sensors. During primary infection, KSHV can be detected by the NLR family members, NLRP1 and NLRP3,[221] as well as IFI16.[310] The RLR family members, RIG-I and MDA5, can activate interferon signaling in response to KSHV infection.[646,688,690] In contrast, NLRX1 and adenosine deaminase acting on RNA 1 (ADAR1) was shown to be proviral and required for KSHV reactivation from latency.[396,689] Finally, another pathway important for KSHV sensing is the cGAS-STING DNA signaling pathway.[395,466,661,686]

OVERVIEW OF THE LYTIC AND LATENT PHASES OF THE KSHV LIFE CYCLE

Following successful primary infection, KSHV can establish either a lytic or a latent state in the infected cell. Subsequent to initial viral infection, the host cell microenvironment is thought to govern the decision of which life cycle phase the virus enters. The default program appears to be latency. The kinetics of lytic versus latent gene expression during primary infection was examined in KSHV-infected endothelial cells and fibroblasts.[321] ORF50/RTA levels were detected 2 hours postinfection but declined thereafter. Conversely, low levels of the latency-associated nuclear antigen (LANA) were seen at first but expression increased substantially 48 to 72 hours postinfection. The latent genes were expressed continually while lytic viral gene expression declined.[321] Thus, concurrent expression of lytic and latent genes occurs immediately following viral infection, but only latent gene expression persists. It is thought that the minimal or marginal expression of lytic genes, many of which play key roles in immune evasion, cell proliferation, and prevention of apoptosis, could be necessary for the establishment and maintenance of latent infection *in vivo*.[226,321]

Latency is the default pathway in most, if not all, experimental situations, and no virions are produced during this stage. During latency, viral gene expression is limited to only a subset of viral genes. The latent viral genome in the nucleus is replicated as an episome by host cellular DNA polymerase, and the replicated genomes are evenly distributed to the daughter cells. Although latently infected cells do not make virus, they maintain the viral genome and thus retain the potential for virus replication and virion production. Upon different exogenous stimuli, latently infected cells can undergo reactivation, a process that switches the virus from latency back into lytic replication mode. Physiological stimuli that reactivate KSHV are not well defined, but in tissue culture several molecules can reactivate the virus including phorbol esters, histone deacetylase inhibitors, TLR agonists, bacterial coinfection, natural products from endemic regions, calcium ionophores and IFN-γ.[51,220,441,512,649,681] Additionally, cell differentiation has also been shown to induce KSHV lytic replication.[290]

During lytic infection, the entire viral genome is expressed in a temporally regulated transcriptional cascade. Similar to other herpesviruses, the first genes that are expressed are known as the immediate-early (IE) genes. IE genes encode for transcriptional factors and regulatory proteins. The key lytic switch regulator is encoded by ORF50. ORF50 encodes for a protein called RTA (replication and *t*ranscription *a*ctivator). Expression of RTA is sufficient to initiate the lytic replication cycle. The second temporal class of mRNAs encode for the delayed-early (DE) genes. The function of DE genes is to ready the cell for viral DNA replication and viral protein production. The DE genes encode for proteins (enzymes, cofactors) that are involved in viral DNA replication, proteins that affect nucleotide precursor pools and host transcription, as well as proteins involved in immune evasion. Once DE expression is under way, lytic cycle DNA replication commences in the nucleus and the viral genomic DNA is replicated to produce many copies of the viral DNA per cell. Subsequent to the onset of replication, the late (L) genes are synthesized. Late genes are those that encode for viral structural proteins. These proteins are made after viral DNA replication since they are required in vast quantities. Late proteins are made after viral replication as they often need to be transcribed from genomic templates that have accumulated to a high enough copy number following viral genome replication.

After all three classes of IE, DE, and L genes are transcribed, virus assembly takes place in the nucleus. Newly replicated viral genomes are incorporated into newly synthesized viral capsids, which subsequently acquire their teguments by a poorly defined process. The capsids subsequently bud through host membranes in a series of steps in order to acquire a host-derived membranous envelope containing KSHV glycoproteins. Finally, viral progeny are released from the host cell. A more detailed view of KSHV latency and lytic life cycles is described below.

The transition to latency is not seamless. Following the first 12 hours postinfection, virus infected cells display both lytic and latent gene expression.[321] The lytic transcript profile is nontemporal in that different classes of IE, DE, and L genes are expressed simultaneously.[321] It is possible that at least some of these lytic transcripts are delivered to the cell via the incoming virion tegument, which contains eleven viral lytic mRNAs that are assimilated into the virion during assembly.[37] Alternatively, some of these transcripts could represent genuine transcription using the host cell machinery. Some studies[38,337] but not all[695] have detected small amounts of the lytic switch protein, ORF50/RTA, in virions, which may contribute to this process. However, why the presence of ORF50 does not trigger the full lytic cascade is unknown and may depend on the host cell environment and the lack of sufficient amounts of cellular proteins required for lytic replication. Virion-encapsidated viral genomes do not appear to harbor bound histones unlike the viral episomes found in latently infected cells.[573] Several lytic transcripts represent inhibitors of apoptosis and viral mediators of immune evasion.[321] Twenty-four hours postinfection, lytic gene expression declines, resulting in only latent gene transcription in the infected cell.

Approximately 24 to 48 hours postinfection, the classical latency program is established in nearly all the infected cells, except for a small percentage (1% to 5%) of cells that enter the lytic cycle. The frequency with which lytic infection ensues following *de novo* infection is related to the multiplicity of infection (MOI) and the cell type. For example, a high MOI in primary endothelial cells favors early progression into the lytic cycle. However, even under such circumstances, lytic replication tends to subside a few days postinfection, and the latency program dominates.

Our knowledge of the KSHV latent program comes from the study of PEL cell lines. These cells were originally isolated from PEL patients and subsequently propagated in cell culture.[95,512] PELs stably maintain latent KSHV genomes and they express latent viral proteins in most of the cells. Although it is likely that latent gene expression in these cultured PEL cell lines is not representative of true latency *in vivo per se*, for the most part mRNA transcripts identified in PEL are detected in other contexts, for example, cell lines infected with KSHV *in vitro* as well as primary KS tumors.[162]

KSHV gene expression is complicated by the fact that a clear demarcation of latent versus lytic genes cannot always be made. For example, some genes are said to be expressed during latency, for example, LANA, while other genes are expressed only during lytic replication, for example, RTA/ORF50. However, although RTA is only expressed during the lytic cycle, LANA expression is observed during latency and lytic replication suggesting a gray area in which some latent genes continue to be expressed at low levels during lytic replication, while other latent genes are expressed during latency and then highly up-regulated during lytic replication.

It is widely accepted that LANA; vFLIP; vCyclin; kaposins A, B, and C; and v-IRF3 (aka LANA-2) are latent genes in PEL cells,[163,516] as are the 12 pre-microRNAs (pre-miRNAs).[78,527] However there has been considerable debate about whether additional genes might also be expressed in latently infected cells, and several groups have shown that additional genes are expressed under some latent conditions. There is a class of genes that is expressed at low levels during latency but is highly up-regulated during lytic infection, for example, vIL-6, K1[59,60,81,104,483,534,570,633] and K15.[2] Originally these genes were classified as purely lytic genes, but more sensitive techniques indicate that these genes are also expressed at low levels under conditions in which there is no lytic gene expression.[2,59,60,104,633] For K1, one compounding factor is that the protein is highly variable and so antibodies against K1 from one strain may not readily recognize K1 from another strain making protein expression analysis more difficult.[59,118,633] It is also worth mentioning that in EBV, genes at the same genomic positions as K1 and K15 have been shown to be expressed during EBV types II and III latency, and encode transforming abilities raising the possibility of different latency patterns occurring during the KSHV viral life cycle.

In PEL, KSHV reactivation from latency is not one hundred percent. During reactivation, low levels of latent gene expression can be detected in the background of lytic gene expression[181,285,534] due to the fact that it is usually not possible to reactivate all of the latent cells. Thus, there is always a background of latency. Finally, some viral gene products, for example, vIRF3/LANA-2 are expressed in latent PELs but are not detected in latent KS spindle cells[516] while vIRF1 has been detected in latently infected KS cells but not in latently infected PELs.[162] In EBV, three latent transcriptional programs have been described. Hence, the fact that KSHV also has a complex gene expression pattern should not be surprising.

In the following section, we first review the general patterns of latent and/or lytic transcription and then review the functions of these viral proteins.

The Latent Phase

Latent Transcripts

In PEL cells, the major latency transcript arises from a single genomic region, located between the K12 and ORF74 open-reading frames. At least two latent promoters are active, each of which initiate synthesis of a group of transcripts (Fig. 15.5). The first transcripts discovered originated from the LANA promoter, located just upstream of the LANA gene (ORF73).[163,535] This promoter appears to be constitutively active. In transgenic mice, the LANA promoter drove LacZ expression mostly in B cells, though a few epithelial cells also demonstrated LANA expression.[182,287] LANA promoter activity can be enhanced by

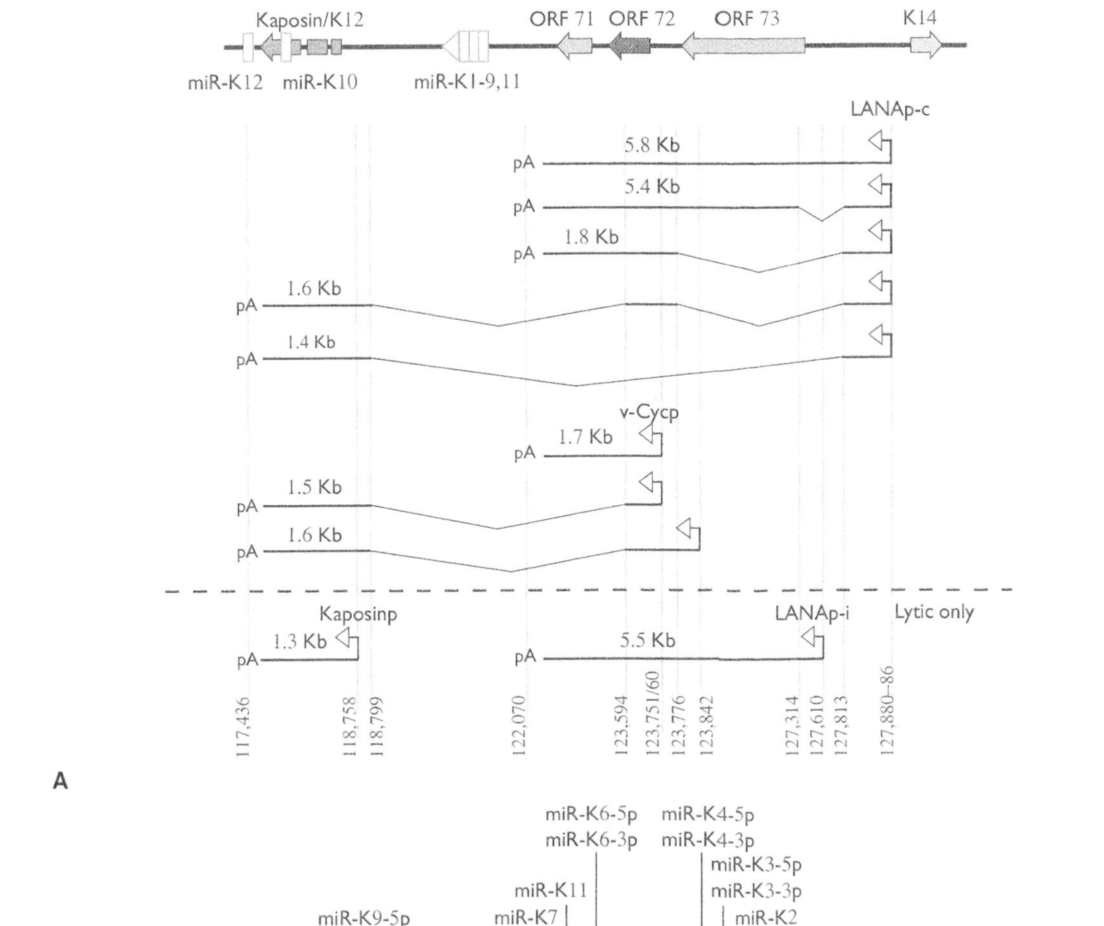

FIGURE 15.5 Map of known transcripts emanating from the main latency region of KSHV. A: *Top line* shows map of the major genomic ORFs (*arrows*), as well as the positions of most of the known microRNAs. Two major latency promoters exist: one 5′ to ORF73, the other just 5′ to ORF72; each of these can generate the indicated spliced mRNA isoforms. Additionally, a lytic cycle promoter drives transcription of a 1.3 kb kaposin (K12) transcript. All mRNAs are polyadenylated at the indicated positions. LANAp-c refers to the LANA promoter, which is expressed constitutively, and LANAp-i refers to the LANA promoter used during reactivation. (Modified by permission from Springer: Yuan Y, Renne R. Organization and Expression of the Kaposi's sarcoma-associated herpesvirus genome. In: Damania B, Pipas JM, eds. *DNA Tumor Viruses*. New York: Springer; 2009:469–493. Copyright © 2009 Springer Science + Business Media, LLC.)

exogenous expression of LANA, suggesting autoregulation of this transcript *in vivo*.[288] Additionally, there exists a second promoter element (just upstream of the latent LANA promoter) that up-regulates LANA transcription in the presence of increased RTA expression.[337,415,571] There also exists a third latency promoter embedded within the LANA-vFLIP transcription unit which drives the vCyclin and vFLIP transcript, as well as the kaposin transcript.[363,487] All these promoters also drive transcription of the viral miRNAs which are located in an intron obtained by read-through of the vFLIP-distal polyA-element and subsequent splicing.[77,527]

This is a complex region of the viral genome since it has a nested arrangement of divergent promoters of latency genes (LANA, vCyclin, vFLIP, viral miRNAs) and lytic genes (vGPCR and K14). Thus, this region has a complex structure and intricate regulation so that lytic transcripts are suppressed during latent gene expression. CTCF, a cellular protein that functions at chromatin boundaries, and cohesins, proteins that mediate sister chromatin cohesion, also bind to a specific site within the KSHV major latency control region.[574] KSHV genes regulated by the CTCF–cohesin complex are under cell cycle control, and mutation of the CTCF binding sites abolished cell cycle–regulated transcription.[121,296,366] The cohesins interact with CTCF in mid-S phase and repress CTCF-regulated genes in a cell cycle–dependent manner. Deletion of the CTCF–cohesin binding site in the KSHV genome caused an inhibition of cell growth as well as viral genome instability. Thus, CTCF and cohesins play a critical role in regulating viral gene expression during latency as well as during reactivation.[296,366,574]

The LANA promoter primarily drives transcription of three genes, ORF 73 (LANA), ORF72 (vCyclin) and ORF 71 (vFLIP), which utilizes both alternative splicing and internal translational initiation.[163] Figure 15.5 depicts the spliced mRNAs generated from this locus; all of these spliced transcripts are polyadenylated at a common site downstream of ORF 71. The ORFs 73-72-71 tricistronic mRNA exists as an unspliced transcript, and another transcript with a small splice in its 5′ untranslated region (UTR). An even more highly expressed transcript is a spliced bicistronic transcript composed of ORFs 72-71. This mRNA encodes both vCyclin (ORF72) and vFLIP (ORF71). vCyclin is translated by conventional cap-dependent initiation, while vFLIP (ORF71 or K13) translation is thought to occur through the use of an internal ribosome entry site (IRES) element located within the open-reading frame of ORF72.[224]

The second set of major latent transcripts in this region encodes for proteins from the kaposin locus (Fig. 15.5). All mRNA transcripts originating from this locus are polyadenylated at a common site downstream of ORF K12. These transcripts include both ORF K12 and the upstream direct repeat sequences named DR1 and DR2. When these mRNAs are translated they generate kaposins A, B, and C proteins.[524] Several latent promoters regulate the initiation of transcripts from this region. LANAp is an RTA/ORF50-inducible LANA promoter.[571] One transcript maps upstream of ORF 72 and is spliced to a region just upstream of the direct repeats in latent PEL.[77,363,487] Extensive transcript mapping has identified multiple spliced latent transcripts (all capable of expressing kaposins). Some of these transcripts originate from the LANA promoter through alternative splicing that removes the ORFs 71 to 73 (Fig. 15.5).[77,487] The spliced kaposin transcripts also encode for many of the viral microRNAs (miRNAs).[77,78,227,489,527] The vast majority of these miRNAs map to the region upstream of the kaposin DRs, which is essentially the intron of the latent kaposin pre-mRNAs while some miRNAs map to the mature kaposin transcript (Fig. 15.5). The miRNAs are derived by Drosha-mediated processing.

Interestingly, KSHV RNA transcripts contain N6-methyladenosine (m6A) and N6,2′-*O*-dimethyladenosine (m6Am) modifications. This is true for both the latent and lytic phases. YTH N6-Methyladenosine RNA Binding Protein 2 (YTHD2) binds to viral transcripts and stabilizes them. Depletion of YTHD2 augments lytic replication by preventing the degradation of KSHV RNA.[257,590]

KSHV Latent Proteins

Latency-Associated Nuclear Antigen

LANA, the product of ORF73,[305,306,503] is a large and multifunctional protein that is present in the nucleus of latently infected cells. LANA exhibits characteristic punctate foci in the nucleus when examined by immunofluorescence and immunohistochemistry assays. LANA is highly immunogenic and antibodies against LANA were the first utilized serologic markers of KSHV infection. LANA-specific CD8 T-cell responses have also been observed. LANA has been detected in PEL and KS tumor cells *in vivo*, in B cells in MCD, and in every latent cell type infected *in vitro*. It was recently demonstrated that EBV infection increase KSHV LANA expression and genome maintenance.[48] LANA has three major domains: an N-terminal domain involved in chromatin attachment and corepressor recruitment, a central region composed of highly acidic amino acid repeats, and a C-terminal basic region involved in DNA binding and oligomerization. LANA interacts with many viral and cellular proteins to exert its function.

The most well-characterized function of LANA is its involvement in the establishment and maintenance of the nuclear latent viral genome[27,139] (Fig. 15.6). The episomal viral genomes established in the nucleus during latency are replicated by the host DNA polymerase during cell proliferation in order to be passed on to the daughter cells. LANA plays many roles in this latent replicative process. It directly binds DNA sequences within the TRs, which contains the latent origin of replication,[26,140,203,218,254] and induces a bend. An x-ray crystal structure of the LANA C-terminal DNA binding domain (DBD) revealed that it can form a decameric ring with an exterior DNA binding surface.[168]

The LANA-TR interaction initiates semiconservative replication by recruitment of the host DNA replication machinery to the viral episome.[225,268] This also includes the recruitment of replication factor C (RFC) and the DNA polymerase clamp (proliferating cell nuclear antigen [PCNA]) loader[581] as well as Bub1.[582] Each 801-bp-long TR contains a high- and a low-affinity LANA binding site (LBS1 and LBS2, respectively). LBS1 and 2 are separated by 22 nucleotides. There is a GC-rich replication element (RE), which is LANA binding site (LBS3), that lies upstream of the LBS 1 and 2. Deletion of this element hinders origin activity[267,613] suggesting that the RE is the site for binding of cellular proteins involved in latent replication. In sum, LANA and the TR sequences recruit the host

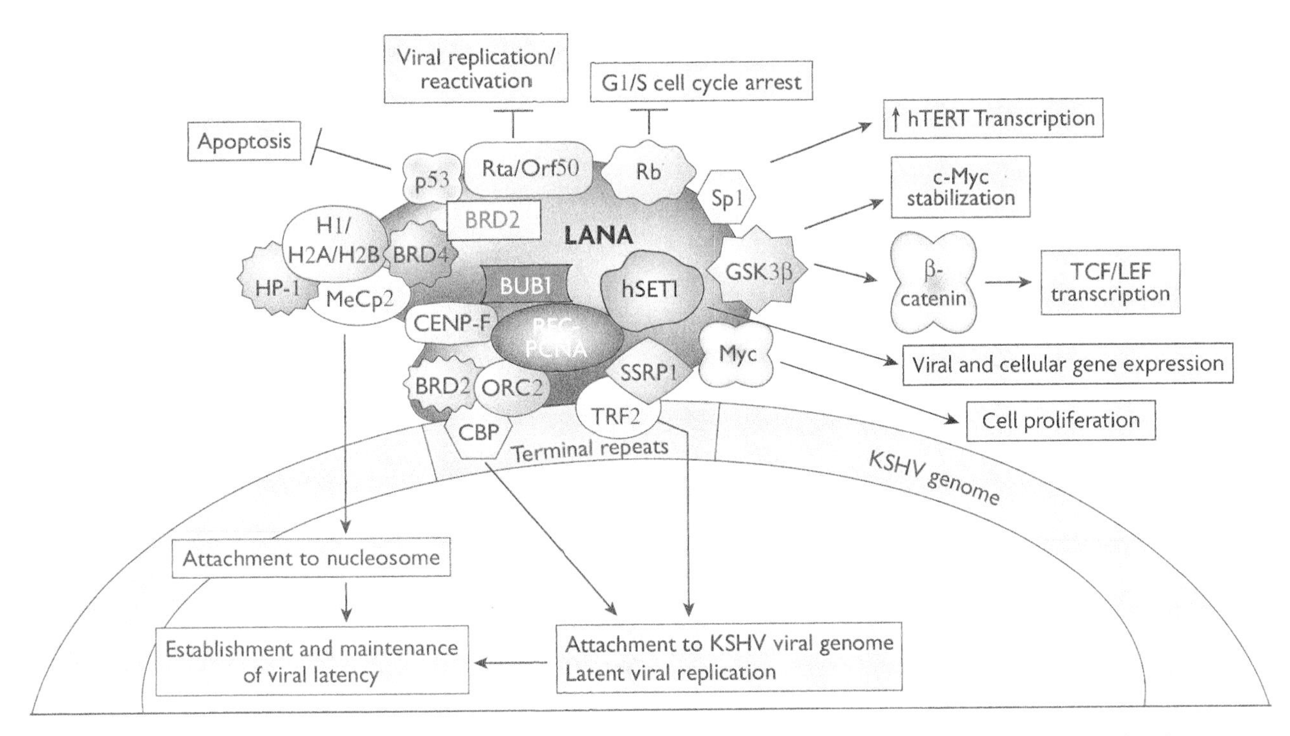

FIGURE 15.6 LANA interaction partners. Functional consequences of the interaction of LANA with other cellular and viral proteins.

cell origin recognition complex (ORC) and minichromosome maintenance (MCM) proteins.[573,612] LANA's C-terminal DBD binds the TRs at two sites which helps to recruit ORC and MCM.[203,268,573,612] Although the C terminal domain of LANA is sufficient for latent replication, the N-terminal chromosomal binding domain enhances latent replication, a fact that reveals that both replication and maintenance are interlinked.[31,268] LANA also binds to multiple viral and cellular promoters and associates with the H3K4methyltransferase hSET1 complex[270] and recruits the polycomb repressive complex (PRC) to the viral genome to suppress lytic gene expression following de novo infection[600] (Fig. 15.6).

The TRs undergo reorganization in late G_1/S phase when replication licensing and initiation occur.[573] The structure-specific recognition protein 1 (SSRP1) and telomeric repeat binding factor 2 (TRF2) bind to LANA and the TR region[269] to facilitate viral episomal replication during latency.[269] The LANA-TR interactions are similar to the EBV EBNA 1-oriP complex, although LANA does not show significant sequence homology to EBNA1, and the EBV oriP sequence is very different from the LANA binding elements of the TR. Yet, the LANA C-terminal DBD shows some similarity to EBNA-1 in terms of predicted secondary and tertiary structural motifs.[225] Viral genomes are replicated once per cell cycle in synchrony with replication of the cellular genome.[613]

Semiconservative replication is not sufficient to explain the establishment of stable KSHV latency. A mechanism must exist in proliferating cells to ensure the proper segregation of replicated KSHV genomes to the daughter cells. Here too, LANA plays a critical role. Transfected plasmids with KSHV TR elements joined to a drug-resistance selectable marker produced stable colonies at a higher frequency when LANA was present than in its absence.[27,139] Such colonies display stably maintained circular genomes over subsequent generations as is seen in PEL cultures. In interphase cells, viral genomes appear to be localized to LANA-containing dots or puncta. In mitotic cells, LANA and the viral episome colocalize to mitotic chromosomes. Thus, LANA can bind to mitotic chromosomes through its N-terminal domain. These data are suggestive of a model in which the N-terminus of LANA binds to the mitotic chromosome and tethers the viral genome (bound via its C-terminus) to this structure.[32,665,679] This allows for the segregation of the tethered latent episomes to both daughter cells following mitosis. Tethering occurs through multiple protein–protein interactions, including binding to histones H2A to H2B, H1, centromeric protein F (CENP-F), budding uninhibited by benzimidazole 1 (Bub1), Brd4, and Brd2/RING3.[3,2,136,139,253,619,665,679] Genetic evidence for this mechanism comes from the observation that a KSHV recombinant virus with a disrupted LANA gene does not generate a stable latent episome following primary infection.[674]

Viral episome maintenance is complex. In cells harboring the KSHV genome that do not make use of drug-resistance marker inserted in the viral genome, LANA, while necessary for plasmid maintenance, is not always sufficient. When LANA expression plasmids and the TRs are introduced into cells, the resulting episomes are lost during the process of cell division.[226] This suggests that viral latency requires the *in vivo* environment and continued lytic replication.[226,446] In certain cell lines, it has been shown that small subpopulation of cells do exhibit stable genomes and enter permanent latency similar to the case in PEL tumor cell lines. In these cases the viral genome undergoes epigenetic changes that enable its being stably maintained in the cell.[226,233]

Curiously, the KSHV genome also contains a cis-acting DNA element within the long unique region that can initiate and support replication of plasmids lacking LANA-binding sequences or a eukaryotic replication origin. The replication machinery proteins, ORC2 and MCM3, associate with this sequence and are required for replication of this element. Thus, KSHV can initiate DNA replication of its genome in the absence of LANA or any other viral protein.[614]

Aside from its function in maintenance of the KSHV latent genome, LANA is also involved in the dysregulation of cell growth and survival. Transgenic mice expressing LANA from the latent promoter display splenic follicular hyperplasia and increased germinal center formation[182] as well as an increased response to antigen stimulation.[253,555] Some of the older animals developed B-cell lymphomas. The slow onset of lymphomagenesis suggests that LANA itself may not be sufficient for transformation and requires additional genetic changes once LANA drives the expansion of B cells, which is likely the result of LANA-mediated proliferation or LANA's ability to augment cell survival.

There have been many biochemical studies looking at LANA interactions with cellular proteins. It has been found that LANA binds p53, and LANA-expressing cells display less activation of p53-dependent reporter genes and also are more resistant to p53-dependent apoptosis induced by γ-irradiation.[187] At the same time, most PELs respond to p53-activating DNA-damaging agents.[488] LANA expression in endothelial cells extends their life span, although this does not lead to immortalization.[640] LANA can also activate survivin[388] and pro-angiogenic pathways.[639]

LANA has been shown to bind the tumor suppressor Rb,[501] and this binding functionally inactivates Rb resulting in increased E2F-dependent reporter gene activation in the presence of LANA. LANA can also interact with GSK-3β, a kinase that phosphorylates and inactivates β-catenin by targeting it for ubiquitin-mediated degradation.[191] LANA binding to GSK-3β induces the kinase to move from the cytosol to the nucleus, allowing for cytoplasmic accumulation of β-catenin. Cytosolic β-catenin can then interact with the transcription factor, LEF, which relocates it to the nucleus, where this complex up-regulates proliferative genes, for example, cyclin D and c-myc. Additionally, LANA expression in other cell types induces S-phase entry.[191] LANA has also been reported to enhance the stability of the c-Myc protein through its effects on GSK-3β nuclear localization. In LANA-expressing cells, inactivation of nuclear GSK-3β inhibited c-Myc phosphorylation at threonine 58 and contributed to c-Myc stabilization by decreasing c-Myc ubiquitination.[73,381] Furthermore, LANA induces genetic alterations through chromosomal instability by regulating Bub1 and Shugoshin-1 (Sgo1).[339]

LANA also impacts host gene expression through binding of multiple components of the transcriptional machinery. Gene expression profiling of LANA-positive B cells identified many host genes whose expression is dysregulated by LANA.[513] LANA can transcriptionally modulate genes in the Rb/E2F pathway[13,513,656] (Fig. 15.6). Although LANA can activate transcription of some cellular genes,[13,513,656] LANA primarily mediates repression of transcription. LANA inhibits expression of TR-linked reporter genes and when fused to the DBD of GAL4, LANA does inhibit transcription of GAL4-dependent reporters.[203,539] LANA also binds the co-activator CBP to repress transcription by inhibiting its histone acetyl transferase (HAT) activity. LANA interacts with RBP-Jκ (also called CSL), and is targeted to RBP-Jκ sites in the ORF50 promoter,[336] where it again mediates repression. Further, LANA can inhibit the activated intracellular domain of notch (ICN)-mediated transactivation of ORF50 thereby preventing lytic reactivation.[338]

The physiological role of LANA-mediated repression might affect cell survival and/or proliferation. It may function in the repression of lytic cycle viral genes thereby allowing for establishment and maintenance of viral latency. This likely also applies to the many other nuclear proteins that can bind to LANA, for example, the methyl CpG binding protein (MeCP2), the bromodomain-containing RING3 protein 2 (Brd2), nuclear matrix proteins, and heterochromatin protein 1.[372,493] LANA also contributes to the epigenetic profile of KSHV episomes through the hSET1 complex.[270]

Specific caspase cleavage sites in KSHV LANA appear to thwart apoptosis and prevent caspase-1-mediated inflammasome activation.[151] Finally, LANA cytoplasmic isoforms are also generated through the use of noncanonical internal translation initiation sites within the N-terminal domain that do not encode a nuclear localization sequence.[597] The LANA cytoplasmic isoforms have been shown to inhibit the DNA sensor, cGAS[686] and also regulate the members of the MRN (Mre11-Rad50-NBS1) repair complex to inhibit DNA sensing.[408]

vCyclin

As described above, the KSHV latency transcripts also encode two other proteins in addition to LANA. ORF72 encodes vCyclin, which shows homology to cellular cyclin D. The vCyclin transcript is made by splicing out the LANA gene, yielding a bicistronic ORF 72+ 71 transcript whose 5′ gene encodes vCyclin (see Fig. 15.5). Similar to its cellular homolog, vCyclin can bind and activate CDK6.[107] However, it differs from host cyclin D in that it is less active on CDK4 and although both can induce CDK6-mediated Rb phosphorylation, the viral cyclin can also activate phosphorylation of p27, histone H1, nucleophosmin (NPM), Id-2, and cdc25a.[144,361] NPM is a nuclear phosphoprotein and a histone chaperone involved in transcription and chromatin organization. Phosphorylation of NPM by the vCyclin/CDK6 complex allows NPM to interact with LANA and regulate viral latency.[533] Exogenous vCyclin expression can promote S-phase entry in 3T3 cells, and also overcome Rb-mediated cell cycle arrest triggered by CDK inhibitors[584] (Fig. 15.7). Overall, the vCyclin/CDK6 complex is less sensitive to inhibition by CDK inhibitory proteins like p27, p21, and p16. Inactivation of p27 is mediated by phosphorylation, and p27 phosphorylation by vCyclin-CDK6 targets it for degradation, further impairing p27 control of CDK6. vCyclin can also interact with CDK9 leading to increased phosphorylation of p53 at serine 33, which results in cell cycle arrest.[105] Consistent with this report, overexpression of vCyclin in multiple cell types induces apoptosis.[473] vCyclin has been demonstrated to promote KSHV-induced cellular transformation and tumorigenesis by overriding contact inhibition.[292]

However, there are some discrepancies. For example, although vCyclin overexpression destabilizes p27, PELs routinely display high levels of p27 expression and establishing stable cell lines expressing vCyclin has been difficult since such cells often undergo apoptosis, especially if they display high levels of CDK6.[473]

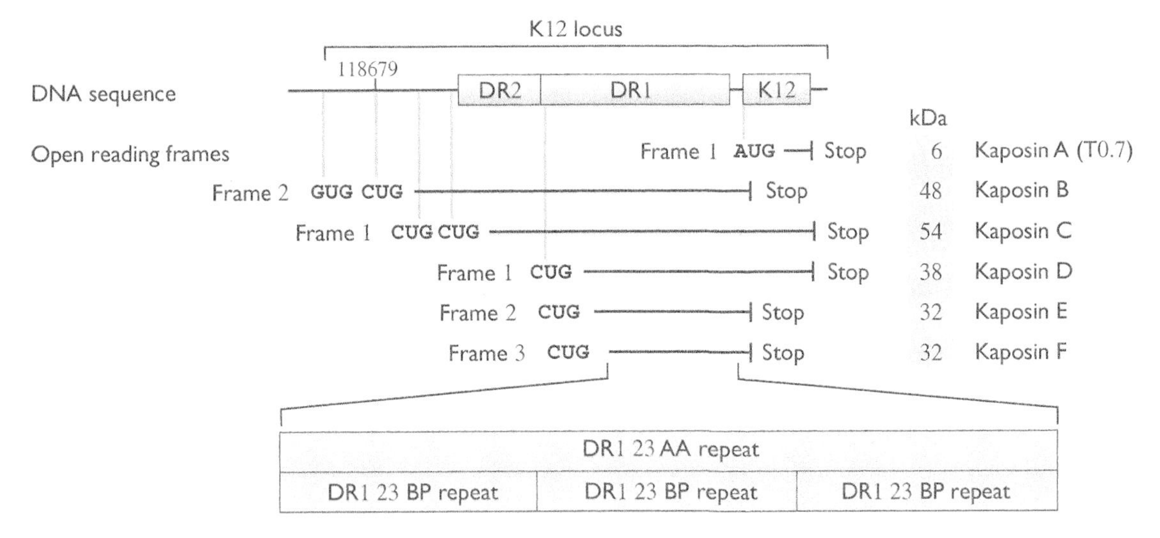

FIGURE 15.7 The coding capacity of the kaposin locus. Top line: Coding organization of kaposin mRNA. **Middle panel:** Protein products predicted from translation of each of the several CUG codons of kaposin. Kaposins A, B, and C are products of this locus. It is unclear as to whether the lower molecular weight species listed here as kaposins D,E, and F—which are regularly observed in infected cells—are in fact translated from the indicated CUG (as shown) or if they represent proteolytic end products of the larger kaposins.

vCyclin-induced apoptosis is linked to the inactivation of the antiapoptotic factor Bcl2[474] due to its phosphorylation by vCyclin/CDK6. Thus, the low levels of vCyclin protein expression during latency likely represent one way the virus avoids triggering cellular apoptosis. Alternatively, another viral protein might ablate this apoptotic effect. Along this vein, it is of interest that Verschuren et al.[615] demonstrated that loss of p53 allows for cell survival in the presence of increased levels of vCyclin. Moreover, when vCyclin was expressed in B cells in transgenic mice, lymphomas developed only in animals deleted for p53.[615] This suggests that the functional inactivation of p53 by LANA during latency (or by vIRF3; see below) might unmask the oncogenic potential of vCyclin. The antiapoptotic effects of vFLIP may also alleviate vCyclin-induced toxicity.

A different line of transgenic mice was made in which vCyclin was expressed in only the lymphatic endothelium through the use of the VEGF-R3 promoter. These mice displayed severe lymphatic dysfunction, and developed chylous ascites. The reason for this is unknown but might reflect the toxicity of vCyclin overexpression. Indeed, in human dermal microvascular endothelial cells, vCyclin induces replicative stress leading to the development of senescence and activation of the DNA damage response.[320] It has recently been shown that KSHV-infected PELs are highly dependent on cyclin D2 as well.[407]

vFLIP

KSHV vFLIP, the product of ORF 71, also referred to as K13, is the viral homolog of cellular FLIP (FLICE [protein FADD-like interleukin-1 beta-converting enzyme, now called caspase-8] inhibitory protein). KSHV vFLIP is composed of two death effector domains (DEDs) one right next to the other, which mediate homotypic protein–protein interactions with other DED-containing proteins. DEDs are present in the adaptor protein FADD, which binds the death receptor, FasR. Initiator caspases, including caspase 8 and 10 in humans, also contain two tandem DEDs, and caspase 8 is a critical player in Fas-mediated death induction. Among the cellular FLIPs, the two predominant forms are the long form ($FLIP_L$) and the short form ($FLIP_S$). vFLIP is structurally more similar to $FLIP_S$, as they both lack a caspase-like domain present in $FLIP_L$. After FasR is bound by Fas ligand present outside the cell, FasR binds FADD, which in turn recruits and activates procaspase 8, via interactions between the DED domains of FADD and the caspase, generating the death-inducing signaling complex (DISC). Caspase activation subsequently triggers the apoptotic cell death program. This process can be blocked by competitive binding by the cellular FLIP proteins.

Virally encoded FLIPs were first discovered in poxviruses and other herpesviruses, where they blunted Fas-mediated killing by preventing caspase 8 recruitment to the DISC.[592] Procaspase 8 can also be bound and inhibited. Several early studies have supported a mechanism for KSHV vFLIP.[28,39] However, the ability of vFLIP to block Fas-mediated killing has been questioned[128]; consistently observed in all studies is the observation that KSHV vFLIP up-regulates the antiapoptotic transcription factor, NFκB,[112] and that vFLIP can be found bound to NEMO (also called IKKγ) in PEL cells.[229,380,593] This complex activates IKK, leading to IkB phosphorylation and the release of active p65-p50 NFκB heterodimers. In addition, vFLIP also increases accumulation of the p52 subunit of NFκB, indicating that vFLIP can activate the alternate pathway of NFκB, which involves the proteolysis of p100 to p52.[416] These findings are concordant with the observations that (a) PEL cells exhibit high levels of NFκB activity, and inhibition of this pathway induces cell death[308]; and (b) siRNA-mediated knockdown of vFLIP promotes apoptosis in PEL.[212,228] It therefore appears that the key role of vFLIP during PEL latency is the activation of an antiapoptotic program through the up-regulation of NFkB activity. Notably, among the cellular genes that are clearly regulated by NFκB, and therefore by vFLIP, are the cellular inhibitor of apoptosis 1 and 2 proteins, as well as cellular FLIP,[228] making studies to determine whether vFLIP can inhibit FAS-mediated apoptosis complicated as the effect might be direct or indirect. vFLIP has also been demonstrated to suppress glycolysis by activating the NFκB pathway in rat mesenchymal stem cells (MSCs).[697] vFLIP itself is stabilized by Hsp90[461] and the MAVS signaling complex in peroxisomes.[127]

Several transgenic mouse models for vFLIP have been made. In one of these, where vFLIP was expressed in all B and T cells, mice showed enhanced responses to mitogenic stimuli and not surprisingly, an increased incidence of lymphoma in a small proportion of mice, but in a much higher proportion when bred with cMyc transgenic mice.[4,128] In the second report, a conditional knock-in system was used to express vFLIP in all B cells, or specifically in germinal center B cells.[28] These mice developed lymphadenopathy with increased numbers of lambda light chain–expressing plasmablasts, reminiscent of MCD, as well as tumors of B-cell origin with high frequency, albeit with an abnormal immunophenotype and histiocytic transdifferentiation. The same conditional model was used to induce vFLIP expression in endothelial cells, which led to vascular proliferation, increased circulating IL6 and IL10, and increased myeloid cells with a suppressive phenotype.[29] Expression of vFLIP in intestinal epithelial cells also led to inflammation.[521]

The proteasome inhibitor, bortezomib, blocks IkB proteolysis, impairs NFkB activation and triggers apoptosis of PEL cell lines[12,417] and in a xenograft mouse model of PEL. These data suggest that this drug might have therapeutic efficacy in PEL.

We have discussed the antiapoptotic effects of NFκB, which likely provides the selective force for maintaining KSHV vFLIP. However, NFκB is a key positive regulator of inflammatory responses. It seems paradoxical that a latency program in herpesviruses, designed for cryptic persistence, would call attention to itself by activating inflammation; but vFLIP has additional effects, which may at least partially explain this paradox. In addition to the antiapoptotic function that is thought to be mediated mainly by NFκB-regulated genes, vFLIP has been shown to protect B cells from autophagy by binding to Atg3.[352] In endothelial cells, it is required for the spindling seen after infection with KSHV.[222] It contributes to prevention of detachment-induced apoptosis (anoikis) in endothelial cells.[178] Moreover, NFκB activation may not be the only function of KSHV vFLIP. The protein also binds to RIP and TRAF2 upstream of IKK, and TRAF binding results in JNK activation.[11,229] It has also been shown that activation of NFkB hinders lytic gene expression, and inhibition of NFκB activation induces lytic reactivation. Thus, vFLIP may play an important role in maintaining stable KSHV latency.

Kaposins

The locus for kaposin was initially identified by a screen for genes that were expressed during latency in PEL cell cultures.[691] *In situ* hybridization using probes for kaposin mRNA revealed that kaposin is expressed at low levels in both uninduced BCBL-1 cells and to some degree in latent KS spindle cells.[569,577] Like several other latent loci, kaposin is also highly up-regulated during lytic replication.[524]

Kaposin mRNA encodes for three proteins due to differential translation initiation (Fig. 15.7).[524] At their 3′ end, all kaposin messages contain a small ORF (ORF K12) encoding a highly hydrophobic 60 amino acid polypeptide called *kaposin A*. Kaposin A is found in intracellular membranes and the plasma membrane.[594] Kaposin A is capable of transforming Rat-1 fibroblasts, and the resulting cell lines form tumors (fibrosarcomas) in nude mice.[445] Kaposin A binds cytohesin-1, a guanine nucleotide exchange factor (GEF) for ARF GTPases, and a regulator of cell adhesion mediated by integrins. This interaction allows for GTP binding to ARF1. Since expression of a cytohesin-1 mutant deficient in guanine nucleotide exchange reverses transformation,[314] this activity is likely to be important for transformation. Immediately upstream of the K12 ORF is a series of tandemly repeated 23-nt GC-rich elements, termed DR (*d*irect *r*epeat) 1 and DR2. This region lacks AUG codons; however, multiple proteins are generated from this region by initiation at variant CUG codons. One of these initiates upstream of the DR2 repeat cluster and terminates after the DR1 repeats and encodes a nuclear protein named kaposin B that lacks the ORF K12 polypeptide region because of a stop codon in the reading frame. Another protein, kaposin C, similarly begins 5′ to DR2 but in an alternative reading frame compared to kaposin B. Translation proceeds through the DR regions and ORF K12. This generates a transmembrane protein that contains the amino acid repeats (encoded by the DRs) fused to K12. Although the kaposins B and C DR sequences are in different frames, they share a common segment of repetitive sequence. Translation of an individual repeat induces the ribosome to enter the next repeat one nucleotide out of frame; after traversing three such repetitive sequences, the ribosome reverts back to the initial frame (Fig. 15.7). Thus, the repeat regions of kaposin B and C share two sets of common 23 amino acid repeats, flanked on both sides by sequences unique to each protein. Consequently, kaposin C is partly a membrane-bound kaposin B isoform.

Kaposin B can bind and activate MAP kinase–associated protein kinase 2 (MK2) as well as the upstream kinase, p38 MAP kinase.[420] MK2 is the major target of p38, which is a stress-inducible kinase. MK2 regulates the stability of cytoplasmic mRNAs that contain AU-rich elements (AREs) in their 3′UTRs. AREs are found in many cytokine mRNA transcripts, for example, IL-1, -3, -4, -6, TNF-alpha, GM-CSF, as well as other growth factors like VEGF, and oncogenes, for example, MYC. AU-rich mRNAs are highly unstable, but activation of the MK2/p38 kinases inhibits their turnover and thereby enhances the levels of these cytokine mRNAs. Thus, by up-regulating MK2, kaposin B prolongs the half-lives of ARE-bearing reporter transcripts and increases cytokine production[420] (Fig. 15.8). Both the DR1 and DR2 repeat regions are essential for kaposin B's function.[421] It was shown that kaposin B also enhanced stability of PROX1, a regulator of lymphatic endothelial differentiation that is up-regulated upon KSHV infection of endothelial cells. The PROX1 mRNA transcript also contains an ARE, and kaposin B enhances its stability.[678]

K10.5/vIRF3/LANA2

The KSHV genome has four genes that encode proteins of the IRF (*i*nterferon *r*egulatory *f*actor) family. IRFs are cellular transcription factors and several members, including IRF3 and IRF7, transcriptionally activate type I interferons and interferon-stimulated genes (ISGs). The viral IRF homologs (vIRFs) are encoded by ORFs K9-11 (Fig. 15.3), suggestive of the fact that they arose by duplication of one or more ancestral genes, plausibly obtained from the cellular genome. All the vIRFs are lytic proteins except for

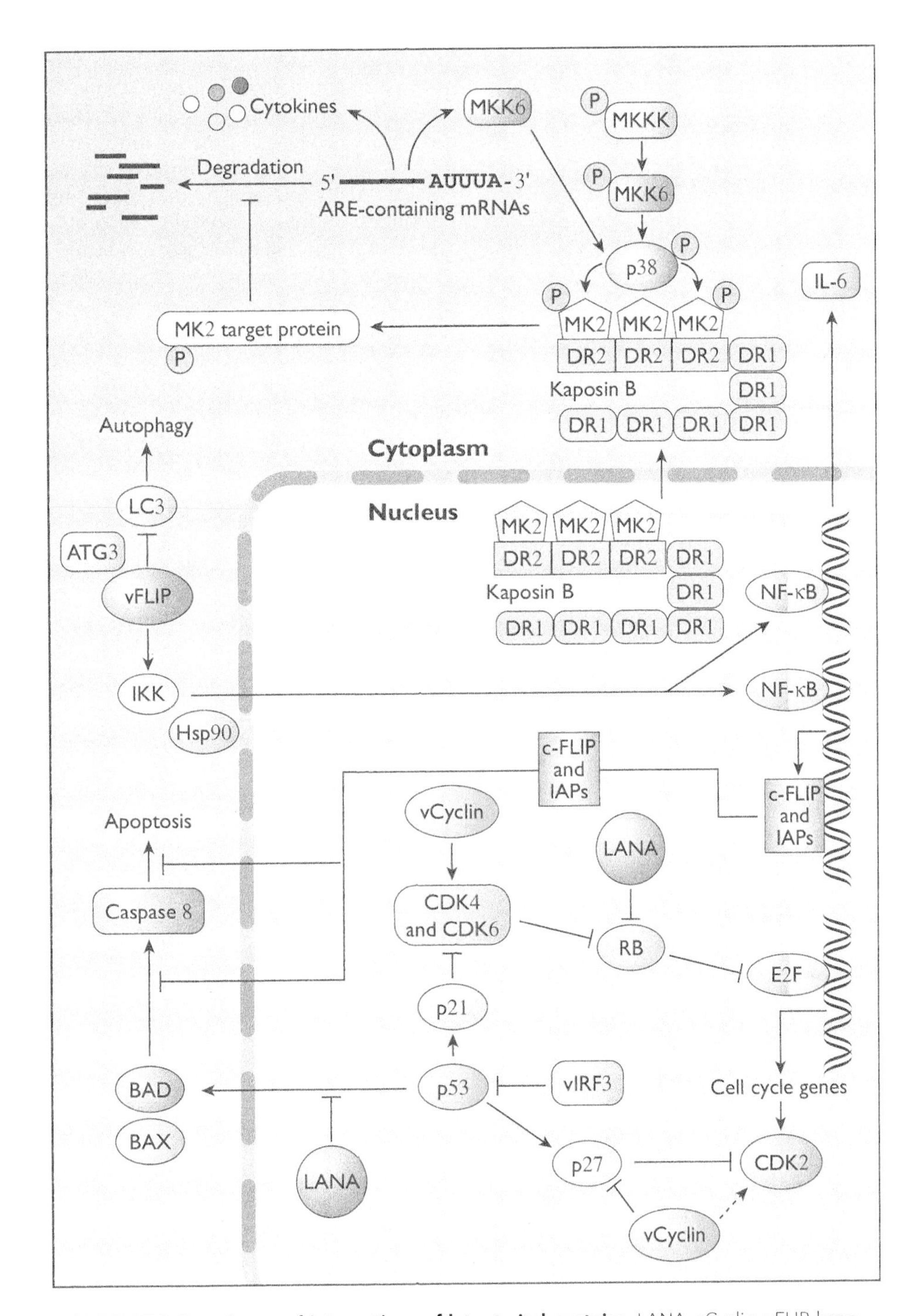

FIGURE 15.8 Functions and interactions of latent viral proteins. LANA, vCyclin, vFLIP, kaposin, and vIRF3/LANA act in concert to inhibit apoptosis and enhance cell survival and proliferative loops.

one, vIRF3 (ORF K10.5), which encodes a nuclear protein that is expressed in latent PEL but not in KS spindle cells.[162,389,516] For this reason, vIRF3 is also called latency-associated nuclear antigen 2 or LANA-2.

vIRF3 expression inhibits the IRF3/7-mediated induction of the IFN-A4 promoter in murine cells and hinders the ability of these cells to mount an IFN response to RNA virus infection.[389] KSHV vIRF3 can also bind and inactivate the function of cellular IRF7.[293] This leads to the suppression of IFN-alpha-related activities.[293]

vIRF3 also inhibits cellular IRF5 function[651] preventing its ability to induce p53-independent apoptosis and p21-mediated cell cycle arrest.[651] In concordance, vIRF3 has also been shown to bind and inactivate p53.[516] Central to its expression in PEL, a critical finding was that vIRF3 expression was required for PEL survival.[650] Knockdown of vIRF3 expression in PEL hampered cell proliferation and increased activity of caspase-3 and -7.[650] Additionally, these effects were seen even in the context of dually infected, EBV-positive, and KSHV-positive PEL lines.[650] In endothelial cells, vIRF3 appears to play a role in angiogenesis.

Hypoxia-inducible factor-1 (HIF-1), a regulator of angiogenesis, is composed of an oxygen-sensitive alpha-subunit and a constitutively expressed beta-subunit. vIRF3 can bind the HIF-1 alpha subunit to stabilize it under normoxic conditions and increase the expression of VEGF and angiogenesis in endothelial cells.[549] vIRF3 together with vIRF1 can also interact with the cellular USP7 deubiquitinase to impact the KSHV life cycle.[664] Additionally, vIRF3's interaction with HDAC5 contributes to virus-induced lymphangiogenesis.[354] vIRF3 has also been shown to interact with the host sumoylation machinery to inhibit sumoylation of tumor suppressors.[341]

Thus, vIRF3 appears to play a key role in cell survival and angiogenesis in the context of viral latency, and perhaps angiogenesis in KS lesions.

Viral microRNAs, lncRNAs, and Circular RNAs

MicroRNAs are 21 to 23 nucleotide long RNAs that regulate gene expression via base pairing to their mRNA targets. MicroRNAs (miRNAs) are generated from the cleavage of larger transcripts named pri-miRNAs, via a processing pathway involving a RNAse III-like endonuclease named Drosha located in the nucleus. These pri-miRNAs contain an imperfect inverted repeat that is cleaved by Drosha into a 65-nucleotide hairpin called a pre-miRNA, which is then transported to the cytoplasm where it is recognized by another RNAse III-like endonuclease named Dicer. Dicer cleaves off the loop of the hairpin thereby generating a partial duplex RNA molecule, which can bind to its target mRNAs. One strand of the RNA duplex is transferred to a cytoplasmic complex named RISC (RNA-induced silencing complex). In general, if base pairing of the miRNA to the target is perfect, RISC cleaves the target mRNA. However, if base pairing of the miRNA to the target is imperfect, RISC modulates translational repression of the target mRNA either through inhibiting translational initiation or elongation or through deadenylation.

Following the seminal discovery of viral microRNAs (miRNAs),[489] KSHV was found to encode eleven pre-miRNAs that arose from transcripts in the latency region (Fig. 15.5).[78,227,489,527] The miRNAs derived from these hairpins are designated as miR-K1 through miR-K11. Some of these pre-miRNAs, for example, miR-K3, 4, 6, 9, donate each of the 2 arms of the hairpin to RISC, thereby giving rise to two mature miRNAs from each pre-miRNA. Each member of the pair is referred to as "5p" or "3p" to indicate its origin from the 5′ or 3′ segment of the hairpin. Additionally, the miR-K10 miRNA undergoes RNA editing at a single site in the seed sequence generating two different miRNAs (miR-K10a and miR-K10b). Thus, although there are 12 pre-miRNA transcripts arising from the KSHV genome, these lead to the generation of 17 mature miRNAs. These miRNAs are present in KS and PEL.[470,471] There is strong sequence conservation in the genomic sequences that encode for these miRNAs and only a subset of pre-miRNAs displayed single nucleotide polymorphisms (SNPs) that could affect their biogenesis.[409]

There are many publications identifying functions for the KSHV miRNAs since their discovery. miR-K11 was found to contain an identical seed sequence to that of a cellular miRNA, miR-155.[216] Viral miR-K11 was found to suppress known targets of cellular miR-155, including the transcriptional repressor BACH1, the pro-apoptotic protein, BIRC4BP/XAF1, and the cell cycle regulator, FOS.[216] Using a transcriptional profiling approach, another group identified that the target for miR-K5 was a pro-apoptotic Bcl2-associated factor, named BCLAF1. Moreover, additional KSHV miRNAs including miRs K9, K10a and K10b were also found to target BCLAF1. Repression of BCLAF1 expression by the KSHV miRNAs was found to be important for cell survival to apoptotic stimuli[700] as was the down-regulation of tumor necrosis factor–like weak inducer of apoptosis (TWEAK) receptor, a pro-apoptotic protein that is targeted by miR-K12-10a (also known as miR-K10a).[1] miR-K1 has been shown to down-regulate p21, a protein that induces cell cycle arrest[215] and also to target IkBα.[356] Moreover, miR-K12-3 and miR-K12-7 (also called miR-K3 and miR-K7, respectively) down modulate C/EBPbeta p20 (LIP), an isoform of C/EBP that represses IL-6 and IL-10 expression. This results in up-regulation of these cytokines in cells from the myeloid lineage.[499]

One study also looked at gene expression profiling in cells stably expressing all KSHV-encoded miRNAs.[528] They found that 81 genes were changed in the presence of the viral miRNAs. One of these proteins is the anti–tumor suppressor protein, thrombospondin 1 (THBS1), whose protein levels were decreased over tenfold.[528] Reduced THBS1 expression in the presence of viral miRNAs led to decreased TGF-beta activity suggesting that the viral miRNAs contribute to tumorigenesis and angiogenesis.[528] Many of the KSHV viral miRNAs target genes regulating glycolysis, cell cycle, and apoptosis.[204]

It is known that KS is composed of poorly differentiated endothelial cells, expressing markers of both lymphatic endothelial cells (LECs) and blood vessel endothelial cells (BECs). KSHV-encoded miRNAs appear to contribute to transcriptional reprogramming by silencing the cellular transcription factor, musculoaponeurotic fibrosarcoma oncogene homolog (MAF).[243] MAF is expressed in LECs but not in BECs, where it functions as a transcriptional repressor of BEC-specific genes to maintain the differentiation status of LECs. KSHV-infected LECs show an up-regulation of BEC-specific genes through miRNA-dependent down-regulation of MAF.[243] In summary, KSHV-encoded miRNAs can influence the differentiation status of a cell in a manner similar to certain cellular miRNAs and this suggests that the viral miRNAs may contribute to the development of viral malignancies via reprogramming the differentiation pathway of the infected cell. The entire KSHV miRNA cluster impacts the cellular metabolic response by suppressing heat shock protein A9 (HSPA9), HIF and prolyl hydroxylase EGLN2.[676] KSHV miRNAs also up-regulate argininosuccinate synthase 1 (ASS1) and modulate the generation of nitric oxide (NO), which is important for the survival of KSHV infected cells.[369] KSHV viral miRNAs have also been demonstrated to target enzymes in the mevalonate pathway to repress cholesterol levels in infected cells.[542]

The viral miRNAs are also incorporated into extracellular vesicales (exosomes) that can shape the extracellular tumor environment.[424,677] The KSHV miRNAs have also been shown to suppress CASTOR1-mediated mTORC1 inhibition to promote tumorigenesis.[368]

In addition to their roles in cell survival and oncogenesis, the KSHV viral miRNAs also play a key role in regulating the lytic–latent switch. Several studies have examined the role of viral miRNAs in controlling this switch, and although all these studies find that the miRNAs enhance latency and suppress lytic replication, the mechanism by which this occurs is different in each case. For example, miR-K9* has been reported to target the 3′ UTR of the ORF50 transcript thereby enhancing latency and preventing viral reactivation.[40] Consistent with this finding, a KSHV BAC with 10 of the 12 viral miRNAs deleted displayed elevated levels of viral lytic genes, including ORF50.[387] Additionally, miR-K12-4-5p (also called miR-K4-5p) was found to target Rb-like protein 2 (Rbl2), a known repressor of DNA methyl transferase 3a and 3b (DNMT3a/b). miR-K12-4-5p reduced Rbl2 protein expression and increased DNMT1, -3a, and -3b mRNA levels to regulate genome-wide epigenetic reprogramming.[387] In further confirmation of the role of the viral miRNAs in suppressing lytic replication, deletion of 14 microRNAs from the KSHV genome also significantly enhanced viral lytic replication as a result of reduced NFκB activity.[356] The viral miRNAs were also found to decrease expression of lytic genes by targeting host transcription factors.[492]

Circular RNAs (circRNAs) encoded by KSHV were recently discovered. Multiple circRNAs were detected in cells infected individually with KSHV, as well as cells dually infected with KSHV and EBV.[587,598,606] KSHV encodes multiple circRNAs, which are located within ORFs of viral lytic genes and are induced during the lytic phase of the viral life cycle.[587,606] KSHV circRNAs were also found in KSHV-associated tumors, suggestive of the fact that these viral circRNAs may play a role in KSHV pathogenesis. Additionally, it was reported that a human circRNA, hsa_circ_0001400, is induced upon KSHV infection and can inhibit the expression of several KSHV genes.[587]

Genes Expressed at Low Levels During Latency but Highly Up-Regulated During Lytic Replication

Although K1 and vIL-6 are considered to be lytic proteins, several publications demonstrate that these proteins are expressed at low levels during latency, yet are highly up-regulated during lytic replication.[59,104,483,570,633] Using tightly latent cell lines that displayed very low levels of spontaneous lytic reactivation to perform array-based transcript profiling and limiting dilution reverse transcription PCR (RT-PCR), Chandriani et al. found that both K1 and K2/vIL-6 genes were expressed under latent conditions.[104] Additionally, the K1 promoter is active in multiple cell types in the absence of ORF50/RTA protein.[59,60,104,633] It is likely that due to their potent signaling properties, both K1 and vIL-6 need to be expressed at low levels in infected cells. Since these two genes show a distinct latent/lytic expression profile compared to other viral genes, we discuss them in a separate section below. It is likely that the K15 gene also falls in this same category[2].

K1

ORF K1 is situated at the left end of the genome and encodes for a type I transmembrane protein whose signaling function is analogous to the B cell antigen receptor complex. K1 is found in the ER and also on the plasma membrane. It contains a highly variable and glycosylated N-terminal ectodomain, a transmembrane region, and a cytoplasmic tail that sports an immunoreceptor tyrosine-based activation motif (ITAM).[346] This structure, also found in BCR and TCR signaling complexes, contains two tyrosine residues separated by characteristic spacing. Activation of the B-cell receptor by antibody binding results in phosphorylation of tyrosines by Src kinases. Phosphorylation creates binding sites for Syk kinase, which upon activation mediates downstream signaling, including PLCγ activation, calcium release, and NFATc activation, among other events. The K1 protein signals in a similar fashion, but its activity appears to be constitutive, since it signals in the absence of a ligand.[333,346] While it is possible that the K1 ectodomain binds to a ubiquitously expressed cell surface protein, constitutive activation is more likely due to self-oligomerization mediated by cysteine residues in the K1 ectodomain. K1 aggregation leads to ITAM phosphorylation, Syk kinase recruitment, and increased NFATc and AP-1 activity similar to what occurs upon BCR activation. Moreover, the activated K1 tail can interact with other signaling proteins besides Syk, including PI3-kinase (via its p85 regulatory subunit), Lyn, RAS-GAP, PLC-γ 2, vav, and Cbl.[333,350,595] PI3K activation results in phosphorylation and activation of Akt kinase.[595] Activated Akt phosphorylates the forkhead (now known as FOXO) transcription factors, sequestering them in the cytoplasm (Fig. 15.9). Since FOXOs induce apoptosis, this phosphorylation is an antiapoptotic event, and K1 expressing cells exhibit greater resistance to apoptosis induced by both Fas ligand and by the expression of FOXO proteins.[595] K1's effect on apoptosis may also be linked to its ability to bind to chaperones. K1 was shown to interact with heat shock protein 90-beta (Hsp90beta) and endoplasmic reticulum–associated Hsp40 (Erdj3/DnaJB11) by tandem affinity purification.[643] K1 expression and antiapoptotic function was highly dependent on Hsp90 and Hsp40/Erdj3 since knockdown of these proteins, as well as pharmacological inhibitors of Hsp90, dramatically reduced K1 expression.[643] Interestingly, Hsp90 inhibitors were efficacious against KS by also targeting LANA[120] and vFLIP in PEL.[461] Furthermore, in B cells, K1 expression hinders the surface transport of the BCR[348] and this may be a means by which KSHV puts the infected B cell under the control of the virus rather than the control of the BCR. In this manner, stimulation of BCR signaling does not jeopardize the viral life cycle. K1 signaling function in B cells has been shown to be regulated by its endocytosis, and these two events are intertwined.[596]

K1 is capable of transforming rodent fibroblasts and substituting for the STP oncogene in the context of HVS-mediated transformation of T cells.[347] Lymphomas and sarcomas are known to develop in K1 transgenic mice, and the lymphomas show activated Lyn kinase and are refractory to Fas-mediated apoptosis.[635] In epithelial and endothelial cells, K1 expression has been reported to induce the secretion of angiogenic factors, including vascular endothelial growth factor (VEGF) and matrix metalloproteinase-9.[630] K1 can activate the PI3K/Akt/mTOR pathway in endothelial cells and can immortalize and extend the life span of primary human umbilical vein endothelial cells (HUVECs) in culture[633] (Fig. 15.9). K1 ITAM expression was needed to activate both the VEGF/VEGFR-2 and the PI3K/Akt signaling pathways in these cells. Additionally, K1 was shown to modulate 5′ adenosine monophosphate-activated protein (AMPK) to enhance cell survival.[15] Thus, K1 appears to be important in KSHV-associated tumorigenesis and angiogenesis.

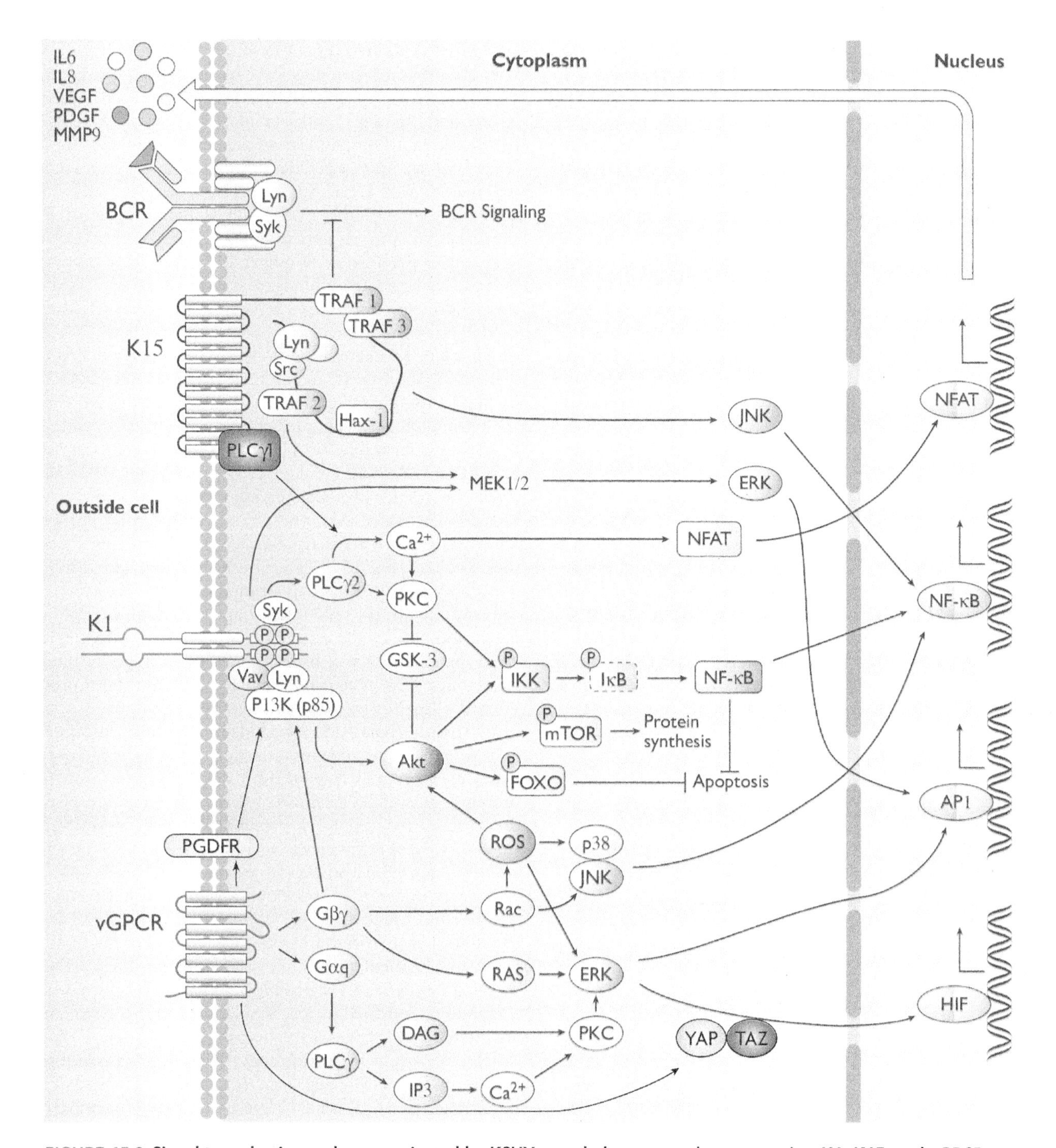

FIGURE 15.9 Signal transduction pathways activated by KSHV-encoded trans-membrane proteins, K1, K15, and vGPCR. Activation of the PI3K and MAPK pathways by viral signaling proteins leads to enhanced production of cytokines and growth factors, cell proliferation, and inhibition of cell death.

In the context of lytic replication, the ITAM of K1 has been shown to augment lytic reactivation from latency.[334] However, others have shown that the K1 ITAM is needed to suppress TPA-mediated viral reactivation in the context of PEL cells and this suppression may contribute to the establishment and/or maintenance of KSHV latency *in vivo*.[349] These differences may be explained by the experimental conditions used in each model system. A study with recombinant viruses showed that K1 deletion viruses displayed reduced lytic replication compared to WT KSHV and also yielded smaller numbers of infectious progeny. Cells infected with a K1 deleted virus showed reduced phosphorylation and activation of Akt kinase.[687]

Recently, it was demonstrated that K1 proteins from AIDS-related KS had greater transformation potential versus K1 sequences from classic KS and that this corresponded with the aggressiveness of KS seen in AIDS patients with KS versus classic KS patients.[588]

vIL-6

Cellular human IL-6 (hIL-6) signals through a heterodimeric receptor composed of a signaling subunit (gp130) and a high-affinity ligand-binding subunit (gp80/IL-6Rα). Following hIL-6 binding to this receptor complex, STATs 1 and 3 are activated. The signaling mechanism of the viral homolog, vIL-6, differs from hIL-6 in that it does not need the gp80 subunit; rather, it binds directly to gp130 to trigger signal transduction (Fig. 15.10). Although vIL-6 does not need gp80 to activate signaling, it can still interact with this subunit of the receptor complex, which appears to modulate vIL-6's activity.[266,360]

IL-6 promotes B-cell differentiation to plasma cells and also impairs B cell apoptosis in response to apoptotic-inducing signals. vIL-6 shares the antiapoptotic activities of cellular IL-6 on B cells (including PEL cells),[291] thus implicating vIL-6 in PEL and MCD pathogenesis.

Ectopic expression of vIL-6 in immortalized mouse fibroblast lines is linked to increased angiogenesis in the fibrosarcomas when these lines are transplanted into nude mice.[18] Increased angiogenesis due to VEGF induction by vIL-6 is an activity shared with cellular IL-6.[18] In PEL, vIL-6 expression was shown to be selectively activated by IFNα in the absence of full lytic replication, indicating that the virus can use vIL-6 to detect an early innate immune response. vIL-6 was also shown to blunt IFN signaling in these cells. In endothelial cells, vIL-6 expression caused an induction of Angiopoietin 2, a proangiogenic and lymphangiogenic factor[607] as well as integrin β3 (ITGB3).[517]

Several groups have shown that vIL-6 can be localized to the endoplasmic reticulum (ER)[117,118,426] where it still retains "intracrine" signaling activity by interacting with gp130 intracellularly. The ER-resident chaperone protein, calnexin, plays a role in ER localization of vIL-6.[117] Intracellular vIL-6 appears to be functional in the autocrine promotion of proliferation and survival of PEL. Additionally, secreted vIL-6 is completely N-glycosylated, and this glycosylation is required for optimal conformation of the protein and optimal signaling.[155,426]

Although a vIL-6 deletion mutant of KSHV did not affect viral latency or reactivation,[114] knockdown of vIL-6 expression in PEL led to reduced cell growth[118] suggesting that vIL-6 likely plays an important role in PEL proliferation. Taken altogether, vIL-6 can contribute to KSHV pathogenesis through an autocrine manner during latency by augmenting survival and proliferation (Fig. 15.10). During lytic replication, vIL-6 may function in a paracrine manner to promote survival of uninfected cells.

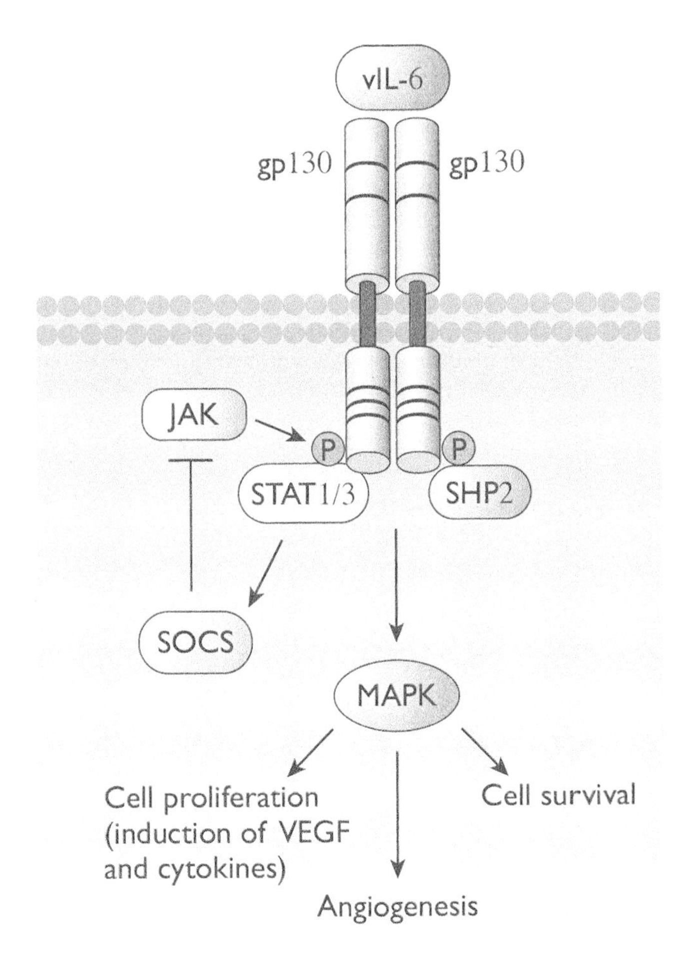

FIGURE 15.10 **KSHV vIL-6 activates IL6 receptor signaling by directly binding and activating the gp130 subunits of the IL-6 receptor complex.** This leads to increased cell survival, proliferation, and induction of pro-angiogenic factors.

The Lytic Phase

The default pathway for KSHV is latency. Hence, lytic infection, in cell culture, is most often studied by using compounds to induce reactivation from latency. In PEL cell lines, this is achieved by treatment with phorbol esters (TPA) or histone deacetylase (HDAC) inhibitors (sodium butyrate, valproic acid) which will induce lytic reactivation in approximately 30% of PEL cells as judged by lytic protein expression. Transfected RTA expression plasmids or chemically induced RTA can also be used to induce more uniform reactivation. When immunofluorescence assays (IFA) for late lytic proteins (e.g., ORF K8.1) are utilized, only half of the cells are positive, even at very late times. Thus, not every entry into lytic infection is completed successfully, and abortive lytic infection occurs some or most of the time. We currently do not comprehend why many of these reactivated PEL cells fail to enter the lytic cycle when treated with HDAC inhibitors or TPA, and why only a fraction of cells in culture undergo lytic replication. One possibility is that many cells do not support the transmission of the inducing signal, or that the signal itself is ineffective or inhibitory in cells that do not support replication. Additionally, when PEL cell lines are cultured for many weeks in tissue culture, they lose efficient inducibility by TPA and HDAC inhibitors. Similarly, passage of stable PEL cell lines with drugs such as hygromycin, neomycin etc. also hinders induction by TPA and HDAC inhibitors. Again, although it is not clear why this happens, it is important to work with cells at low passage.

In addition to PEL, other latently infected cell lines including 293, Vero, human foreskin fibroblasts (HFF), and TIME cells[335] can be induced sufficiently, while other lines (e.g., HeLa, SLK) into which a KSHV genome was transfected are only transiently inducible by chemical means.[14,36] However, inducible or forced expression of the lytic switch protein, RTA, can induce reactivation in a much wider array of lines than chemical activation.[36,448]

Epigenetic Regulation of the Latent–Lytic Switch

Several groups reported the presence of genome-wide epigenetic marks on the viral episome and their involvement in the regulation of the switch between latency and lytic replication.

These epigenetic modifications occur early following primary infection.[289] Histone modifications associated with the KSHV latent genome are involved in the regulation of latency and also control the temporal and sequential expression of genes during the viral lytic life cycle. Activating histone modifications include acetylated H3 (AcH3) and H3K4me3 while repressive histone modifications include H3K9me3 and H3K27me3. The latent viral genome contains both activating and repressive histone modifications. These marks are mutually exclusive across the latent genome.[233,599] For example, under latent conditions, the genomic region encoding the lytic gene, ORF50/RTA, contains activating H3K4me3 and repressive H3K27me3 marks that rapidly change to increasing AcH3 and H3K4me3 activating modifications and decreasing H3K27me3 modifications upon viral reactivation.[233,599] Additionally, latency-specific histone modification patterns were established following *de novo* infection, and there was rapid and widespread deposition of H3K27-me3 marks across latent genomes.[233] H3K27-me3 can be a bivalent modification that can repress transcription despite the simultaneous presence of activating marks on the genome, leaving these genes in a poised state for expression.[233] It was also observed that EZH2, the H3K27me3 histone methyltransferase, was present on the entire KSHV genome during latency, but was dissociated from the genome during ORF50-mediated reactivation. EZH2 inhibition or knockdown and expression of H3K27me3-specific histone demethylases all induced the lytic life cycle in PEL.[599] Chromatin immunoprecipitation (ChIP) assays revealed that KSHV genomes are highly methylated at CpG residues (except for the LANA promoter[116]), leading to the establishment of characteristic global DNA methylation patterns. These types of studies are still in their infancy, but thus far they revealed that the viral genome is epigenetically modified in the latent state so that transcription is generally repressed. At the same time, parts of the genome also contain activating histone modifications and the virus may therefore be poised to enter the lytic cycle once reactivation is triggered. Additionally, ORF50/RTA lytic transcription is actively repressed by LANA during latency, which is relieved upon lysine acetylation of the LANA protein.[386] BET inhibitors were shown to disrupt KSHV latency,[121] and it was also reported that Bmi regulates latency and inhibition of Bmi induces KSHV reactivation.[262]

Immediate Early (IE) Gene Expression

A single viral protein named RTA encoded by ORF50 controls reactivation from latency and the induction of lytic replication. The fact that RTA is the key lytic switch protein was derived from two types of experiments: (a) expression of ectopic RTA by itself is sufficient to induce reactivation from latency[390,579]; and (b) knocking out ORF50 function, either by dominant negative ORF50 mutants,[391] or by removal of ORF50 from the viral genome[668] prevents reactivation from latency. Thus, ORF50/RTA is the critical protein required for the induction of lytic replication. Several experiments show that (a) ORF50 is the first transcript to appear following chemical induction with TPA of PEL[390,580]; (b) the RTA/ORF50 promoter is inducible by TPA and knockdown of tousled-like kinase (TLK),[161] and (c) lytic induction is linked to demethylation of the ORF50 promoter.[116,385] ORF50 is a canonical immediate-early protein as it is transcribed in the presence of cycloheximide.[579,693] ORF50 is part of a polycistronic transcript encoding for both K8 and K8.1 genes (Fig. 15.11).

ORF50/RTA

ORF50/RTA is a viral transcription factor. Its sequence and function is highly conserved among the rhadinoviruses.[148] KSHV RTA has an amino-terminal DBD and a carboxy-terminal activation domain. A fusion of the ORF50 activation domain with a GAL4 DBD results in robust activation of GAL4 responsive promoter elements. ORF50 is phosphorylated on its C-terminal activation domain during viral replication. Moreover, phosphatase-treated ORF50 runs at a higher mobility than its predicted molecular weight, suggesting that additional, posttranslational modifications must exist.[391] ORF50 forms tetramers and higher-order multimers in solution and

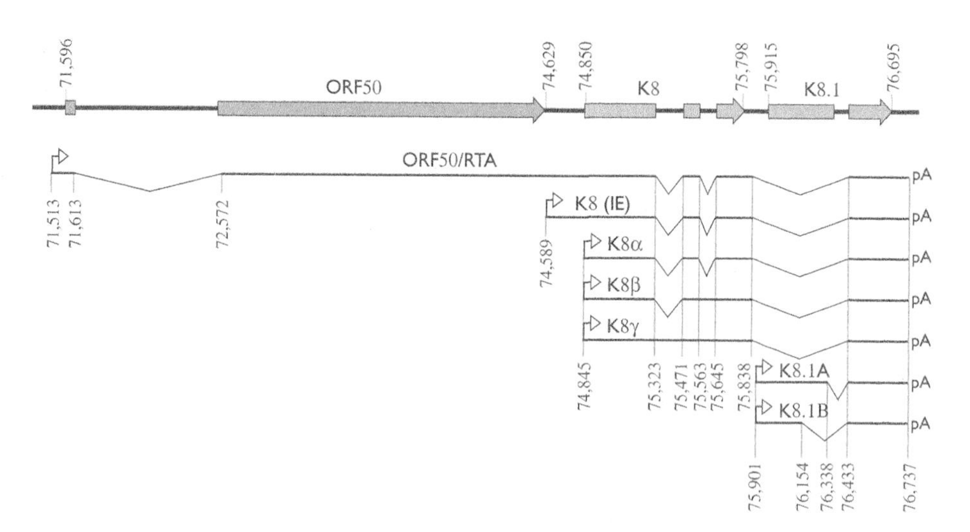

FIGURE 15.11 Map of known transcripts emanating from the main lytic region of KSHV. *Top line* shows map of the major genomic ORFs (*arrows*). ORF50, K8, and K8.1 are encoded on a polycistronic transcript. All mRNAs are polyadenylated at the indicated positions. (Modified by permission from Yuan Y, Renne R. Organization and Expression of the Kaposi's sarcoma-associated herpesvirus genome. In: Damania B, Pipas JM, eds. *DNA Tumor Viruses*. New York: Springer; 2009:469–493. Copyright © 2009 Springer Science + Business Media, LLC.)

the amino-terminal proline-rich, leucine heptapeptide repeat (LR) of ORF50 is necessary, but not sufficient, for oligomerization. Mutagenesis of this LR region revealed that ORF50 tetramers are sufficient for transactivation and viral reactivation and that ORF50 mutants that are unable to form tetramers, but can still form higher-order multimers, are either nonfunctional or reduced in function.[71]

ORF50 has been shown to bind to at least 19 sites in the KSHV viral genome.[119] These include regions of promoters, introns, and exons of KSHV genes including ORF8, K4.1, K5, PAN, ORF16, ORF29, ORF45, ORF50, K8, K10.1, ORF59, K12, LANA, K14/vGPCR, and K15, the two origins of lytic replication OriLyt-L and OriLyt-R, and the microRNA cluster.[119] ORF50 expression leads to a strong activation of delayed early (DE) promoters (8- to 300-fold depending upon the DE promoter). The highest activation by ORF50 is of the PAN (nut-1) promoter, which drives the transcription of a very abundant noncoding *p*oly*a*denylated *n*uclear transcript (PAN RNA). Several mutagenesis experiments demonstrated that the ORF50-responsive site in the PAN promoter is the sequence AAATGGGTGGCTAACCTGTCCAAAA upstream of the PAN RNA cap site. ORF50 has been shown to bind to this site *in vitro*.[108,564] A similar sequence is located just upstream of the lytic kaposin transcript.[524,565] Many other RTA-response elements (RREs) have been identified using promoter–reporter cotransfection assays in the promoters of DE viral genes (e.g., TK, ORF57/MTA, K8/RAP, K2, K9, K14, DBP), and in one late promoter (gB).[232] ORF50 can also up-regulate its own promoter. Many of the RREs share little sequence homology to the PAN/kaposin site or to each other. The RREs display low-affinity interactions with purified ORF50 protein in *in vitro* ORF50 binding assays.[565,699] Although ORF50 binds to these sites with low affinity, many of these sites are very strongly induced by ORF50 in transient transfection cell–based assays, for example, the ORF57/MTA and K14 promoters.[571]

Direct DNA binding by ORF50 is not the sole mechanism by which this protein can transcriptionally activate promoters. Two-hybrid screens of ORF50 binding cellular partners revealed that ORF50 can efficiently bind to the transcription factor, RBP-Jκ[370] (also called CBF-1 or CSL). Indeed, RBP-Jκ recognition sites are found in many promoters of ORF50-responsive genes (e.g., K8/RAP, TK, PAN, ORF57/MTA, K14, LANA, and gB).[232] In many of these promoters, RBP-Jκ sites lie adjacent to low-affinity ORF50 binding sites, suggesting that cooperative interactions may exist to enhance or stabilize the binding of ORF50 at these sites. Even reporter genes that harbor synthetic RBP-Jκ elements can be strongly activated by ORF50. This suggests that in addition to binding promoters through its sequence-specific DNA binding activity, ORF50 is also targeted to promoters through protein–protein interactions with RBP-Jκ (as well as other transcription factors) bound at the promoter. RBP-Jκ deleted fibroblasts are not supportive of ORF50-transactivation of many reporter genes, and when infected with KSHV, they show defective reactivation upon transfection of ORF50.

RBP-Jκ protein normally functions as a transcriptional repressor. ORF50 binding to RBP-Jκ converts it from a repressor to an activator via ORF50's activation domain. In uninfected cells, RBP-Jκ-directed repression is controlled by the Notch pathway. Notch is a transmembrane receptor, and activation by extracellular ligands leads to the cleavage of its juxtamembrane domain, liberating its intracellular domain (ICD). The Notch ICD moves to the nucleus, where it can bind RBP-Jκ, converting it from a repressor of transcription to an activator of transcription. This phenomenon is similar to what happens with RBP-Jκ and ORF50. Thus, KSHV has co-opted the Notch-RBP-Jκ pathway to transactivate ORF50-responsive, RBP-Jκ binding site containing promoters.

Interestingly, ORF50 binds to RBP-Jκ at two sites, and one of these is identical to the site bound by Notch ICD and EBNA2. The human Notch ICD that constitutively activates RBP-Jκ was expressed in PEL and gene expression profiling showed that this domain robustly induced expression of a number of lytic viral genes but could not evoke the full repertoire of lytic viral gene expression normally induced by ORF50 expression.[109] These results indicate that the control of viral gene expression by cellular Notch signal transduction only partially overlaps with ORF50[109] suggesting that RTA does more than merely mimic notch and that some RBP-Jκ elements in the viral genome have completely diverged from Notch signaling. This result is not surprising given that ORF50 has additional mechanisms of promoter targeting besides RBP-Jκ sites (see below). However, these results suggest that certain lytic genes can be activated in an ORF50-independent manner and under conditions when ORF50 is not expressed.

ORF50 can also interact with the transcription factor C/EBPα in the K8/RAP, ORF57/MTA and PAN promoters and with Oct-1 in the ORF50 promoter.[628] These interactions are important for ORF50 recruitment to these sites. Additionally, the binding of ORF50 to both Oct-1 and the K8 promoter leads to transactivation and viral reactivation and the ORF50/Oct-1 interaction is necessary for optimal KSHV reactivation.[91] ORF50 can also interact with STAT-3, inducing it to move to the nucleus to activate STAT-responsive genes.[237] ORF50 also binds proteins involved in histone acetylation (CBP and histone deacetylase 1)[236] and the chromatin remodeling complex, SWI/SNF and the TRAP/Mediator complex, that enables interaction of RNA pol II with many transcription factors.[238] Interactions with the histone modeling proteins occur via the C-terminal activation domain of ORF50. Mutational studies show that blocking these interactions prevents both transcriptional activation and lytic induction, confirming their importance for ORF50 function.

The spliced isoform of plasma cell transcription factor X box binding protein 1 (XBP-1s) can regulate the latency to lytic switch for KSHV.[654,682] XBP-1s is normally absent in PEL, but the induction of endoplasmic reticulum stress or hypoxia leads to production of XBP-1s and induction of the lytic cycle.[147,682] XBP-1s binds to ORF50 and activates the ORF50 promoter in a synergistic manner.[654] This interaction links lytic reactivation to plasma cell differentiation, which may be a mechanism whereby virus is produced in sites where immunoglobulin production is occurring, which include lymphoid tissues in the oral mucosa allowing virus to be shed into saliva.[654]

While most research has focused on ORF50 transactivation, several reports show that ORF50 can also bind transcriptional repressors. As mentioned above, ORF50 binds HDAC1 resulting in repression of ORF50-mediated transactivation.[236] ORF50 also binds to and is inhibited by poly(ADP-ribose) polymerase 1 (PARP-1) and Ste20-like kinase hKFC.[239] It has also been shown that ORF50 can bind a cellular zinc-finger protein named K-RBP (for KSHV RTA binding protein). K-RBP is a transcriptional repressor that was shown to repress ORF50-mediated transactivation in an HDAC-independent manner. K-RBP could also suppress ORF50-mediated lytic reactivation. In a subsequent study, it was found that ORF50 could induce ubiquitin-mediated degradation of K-RBP and ORF50 mutants that were defective in mediating K-RBP degradation were not as transcriptionally active as wild-type ORF50.[670] Interestingly, the HSV-1 ICP0 transactivator and the HCMV pp71 transactivator also induce degradation of transcriptional repressors suggesting that this may be a common mechanism by which many herpesviral lytic transactivators function.[670] Additionally, transducin-like enhancer of split 2 (TLE2) is another repressor that interacts with ORF50 and inhibits its transactivation activity and ability to induce the lytic life cycle.[252] TLE2 appears to interact with the Pro-rich domain of ORF50, which is the same site that interacts with RBP-Jκ.[252]

Finally, ORF50 has also been shown to target IRF7 through ubiquitin-mediated degradation. The degradation is mediated through ORF50's recruitment of a E3 ubiquitin ligase, RAUL, which normally imparts K48-linked ubiquitins on IRF3 and IRF7.[680] It has also been shown to down-regulate MHC II[583] and promote the degradation of TRIF thereby blocking TLR3 signaling.[429] Through down-regulation of myeloid differentiation primary response 88 (MyD88), RTA is also able to block TLR4 signaling.[377] A summary of ORF50's interactions and functions is shown in Figure 15.12.

Other Immediate-Early Genes

Detailing the kinetics of viral gene expression in the presence of cycloheximide led to the identification of several other IE genes.[693] Additional IE mRNAs encode for the products of ORF45 and K4.2, as well as a 4.5-kb RNA with partial complementarity to ORF 29. (Note: some reports refer to ORF45 and K8 as DE genes). Moreover, several transcripts antisense to ORF50 have been identified; however, their biological function is not known.[390,693] The K8 gene has two promoters, one of which is activated in the IE phase and a second promoter that is activated as a DE promoter through an ORF50-responsive RBP-Jκ site in the promoter.[631] Interestingly, the gene for KSHV ORF57/MTA, the homolog of HSV ICP27, is transcribed in the DE phase. The IE ORF45 protein functions to evade host innate immunity and is discussed separately (see below).

K8/RAP

ORFK8 is a DE protein that is member of the bZIP family of proteins, including EBV Zta and cellular transcription factors, c-jun and c-fos. K8 is also called RAP (*r*eplication-*a*ssociated *p*rotein) or K-bZIP. ORF K8 and EBV Zta share some sequence similarity[223] although unlike EBV Zta, K8 does not induce viral reactivation of KSHV or enhance ORF50-mediated reactivation from latency.

Unlike ORF50, K8 does not appear to affect promoter activity to a great extent. However, together with other proteins, K8 contributes to KSHV lytic replication and gene expression. For example, it binds to cellular bZIP proteins such

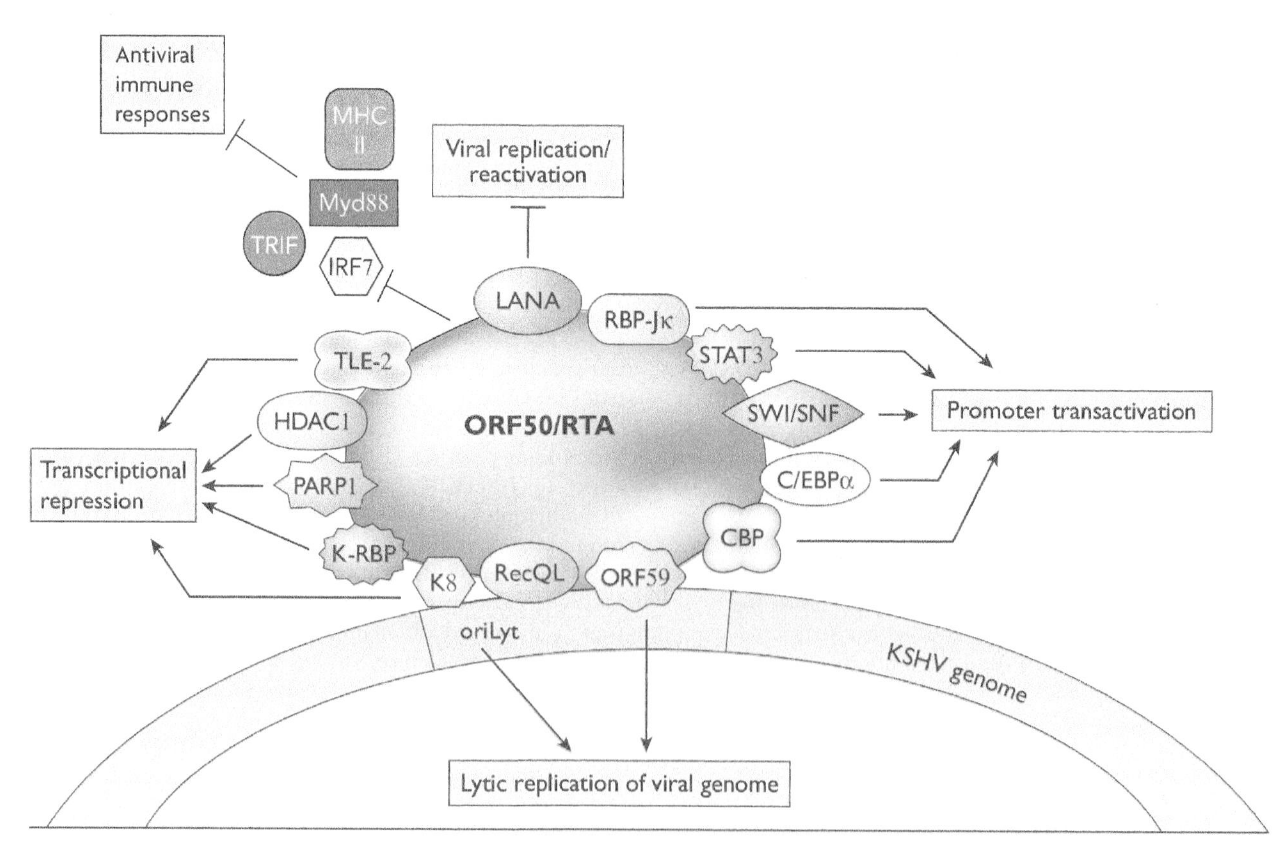

FIGURE 15.12 ORF50/RTA domains and interaction partners. Functional consequences of the interaction of ORF50 with other cellular and viral proteins.

as C/EBP-α, a transactivator that is involved in the induction of differentiation and cell cycle arrest.[658] K8 binding to C/EBP-α prolongs the half-life of C/EBP-α, thereby augmenting its function. The K8 promoter itself contains C/EBP-α binding sites and there is a positive feedback loop for both K8 and C/EBP-α during viral replication. Further, since ORF50 also binds C/EBP-α, ORF50-driven transactivation of K8 is increased by K8. Stabilization of C/EBP-α also helps ORF50 activate other viral lytic promoters with C/EBP-α binding sites such as the ORF50 and ORF57 promoters.[628] Although K8 augments C/EBP-α function, K8's effect on most other transcription factors appears to be of a repressive nature. For example, K8 hinders CBP[274] transactivation, and direct binding of K8 to ORF50 hinders its transactivation function on some promoters like those of ORF57 and ORF50, although PAN promoter activity is not affected.[280,371] RTA/ORF50 and K8 together have been reported to bind to cellular and viral genomes to modulate gene expression.[302] It is also involved in the regulation of viral DNA replication.[383]

K8 induces a prominent G1 arrest. Many herpesviruses exhibit cell cycle arrest during lytic replication, including KSHV. This is thought to occur in order to prevent cellular DNA synthesis from ensuing thereby reducing the competition for energy and nucleotide pools. K8 induces cell cycle arrest by enhancing C/EBP-α accumulation through inhibition of E2F expression and increased expression of the CDK inhibitor, p21.[658] Moreover, K8 can directly bind CDK2 complexed to cyclins A and E, and this interaction leads to impaired kinase activity.

Finally, K8 also plays important roles in viral lytic replication as it is thought to bind the lytic replication origins of KSHV. These roles will be discussed below in the lytic replication section.

Delayed-Early (DE) Gene Expression

KSHV proteins belonging to the DE class are genes whose transcription is sensitive to the effects of cycloheximide since their expression depends on the transactivation of their promoters by IE proteins. However, their expression is independent of viral DNA synthesis inhibitors. Many DE proteins, for example, DNA polymerase, thymidine kinase, ribonucleotide reductase, etc. have enzymatic functions or serve as accessory proteins (ssDNA binding protein, polymerase processivity factor, etc.). The DE proteins prepare the infected cell for viral DNA replication. Other DE proteins are involved in immune evasion (K3/MIR1, K5/MIR2, and K14), host shutoff (ORF37/SOX), nuclear–cytoplasmic transport of viral RNAs (ORF57), or modulation of signal transduction (vGPCR, K1, K15). At least two noncoding RNAs have been identified as DE transcripts—the polyadenylated nuclear (PAN) RNAs. Please note that the term delayed early (DE) is borrowed from the alpha herpesvirus literature and may not be as strictly applicable to the various environments that trigger KSHV reactivation. In most cases, the time delay is minimal.

ORF57/MTA

ORF57 also known as MTA (*m*RNA *t*ranscript *a*ccumulation) is a posttranscriptional regulator and a homolog of HSV ICP27 and EBV ORF57/MTA proteins. ORF57 moves between the nucleus and cytoplasm and enables the cytosolic accumulation of unspliced mRNAs.[312] A crystal structure of the C-terminus of ORF57 has been reported[684] and its stability has been shown to be regulated by phosphorylation and homodimerization.[401]

ORF57 interacts with Aly/REF, an export factor, to promote nuclear mRNA export.[402] ORF57 binds to intronless viral mRNAs and functions to recruit the hTREX complex (through interactions with the export adapter protein, Aly), but not the EJC, and assemble a viral ribonucleoprotein particle termed vRNP.[61,538] Aly subsequently binds the DEAD-box protein UAP56, which recruits the remaining hTREX components to the complex.[61] It has also been shown that ORF57 associates with PYM, a protein that recruits the 48S preinitiation complex to newly exported mRNAs through binding EJC. This ORF57-PYM interaction allows this complex to associate with intronless KSHV transcripts to initiate translation of viral mRNAs.[62] ORF57 also inhibits the ARS2-mediated RNA decay pathway.[522]

Unlike HSV ICP27, ORF57 does not hinder the expression of intron-containing transcripts[312] since unlike HSV, many lytic cycle KSHV genes are efficiently spliced (e.g., K8, K14, K15, ORF50, ORF57, the vIRFs, ORF29 etc.). During lytic replication, ORF57 partially colocalizes with the cellular splicing machinery in nuclear speckles and assembles into spliceosomal complexes in association with viral pre-mRNAs and essential splicing components. ORF57 binds Sm protein and interacts with snRNAs. Thus, ORF57 appears to function as a novel factor in the spliceosome-mediated splicing of viral RNA transcripts.[400]

ORF57 can bind ORF50 and augment ORF50's transactivation function on several viral promoters.[312,480] ORF57 can also promote the accumulation of nuclear PAN RNA[134,312] in an export-independent manner. ORF57 binds PAN RNA directly at an ORF57-responsive element (ORE) thereby protecting it from the cellular RNA decay pathway.[525] Another mechanism by which ORF57 has been shown to stabilize mRNAs is through inhibition of microRNA modulation of viral transcripts.[297] The vIL-6 transcript contains an MRE (ORF57/MTA-responsive element) analogous to the ORE reported previously.[525] Binding of ORF57 to the MREs in vIL-6 stabilized its message and enhanced its translation.[297] One of the MRE sites was also a binding site for miR-1293 and hence, ORF57 competes with miR-1293 for binding to vIL-6 thereby preventing its RISC-mediated degradation. ORF57 also interacts with a miR-608 binding site in the cellular human IL-6 transcript and prevents miR-608 repression of this message as well.[297] Finally, ORF57 interacts directly with the cellular protein RNA Binding Motif Protein 15 (RBM15), thereby stabilizing the ORF59 RNA transcript in the cytoplasm.[401] A genome-wide analysis of viral RNA targets of ORF57 performed by a UV cross-linking and immunoprecipitation (CLIP) assay revealed eleven viral transcripts that were targeted by ORF57 including vIL-6.[297] ORF57 has also been shown to block PKR activation and inhibit stress granule formation.[543]

Additionally, two groups have shown that the disruption of ORF57 in a KSHV BACmid resulted in the lack of expression of several lytic genes including ORF57, ORF59, K8alpha, K8.1, and PAN RNA during the viral lytic cycle and yielded no virion production.[399] It has been reported that ORF57 is cleaved by caspase-7 during reactivation. The cleaved ORF57 was hampered in aiding the expression of viral lytic genes suggesting that caspase-7 displays antiviral activity against KSHV lytic proteins.[401] ORF57 is also involved in lytic replication through the inhibition of P-bodies.[544]

Lytic Viral Replication

The delayed early phase is followed by lytic cycle DNA replication. Similar to the case with other herpesviruses, multisubunit complexes containing the core replication machinery are directed to a cis-acting replication origin called oriLyt, by an ori-specific DNA binding protein. Replication complexes are nuclear substructures where viral replication occurs and are in proximity to host ND10 domains. Replication utilizes a rolling circle mechanism, whereby linear genomes are processed and packaged into nascent capsids.

KSHV encodes 6 catalytic and accessory proteins similar to other herpesviruses, including the viral DNA polymerase (POL, encoded by ORF 9), helicase (HEL, ORF 44), polymerase processivity factor (PPF, ORF 59), primase (PRI, ORF 56), primase associated factor (PAF, ORF 40/41), and single-strand binding protein (SSB, ORF 6). When coexpressed in cells, these proteins form stable multi-subunit nuclear structures.[657] The KSHV genome contains two oriLyt regions: the left-hand origin (oriLyt L) is situated between ORFs K4.2 and K5, while the right-hand element (oriLyt R) lies between ORFs K12 and 71.[21,375] These elements promote semiconservative replication, which is suppressed by viral DNA polymerase inhibitors (e.g., phosphonoacetic acid). These two ~1.7 kb regions share striking sequence homology with one another; the right-hand element seems to be an imperfect inverted repeat of the left-hand element. Each lytic origin is composed of two subdomains: (a) a 1.1-kb region with multiple AT-rich palindrome sequences, TATA boxes, and transcription factor binding sites and (b) an adjacent region (~600 bp) composed of multiple GC-rich tandem repeats. Genetic studies have identified four critical elements required for oriLyt-L function. These include (a) a high-affinity ORF50 binding site and nearby TATA box, (b) four pairs of C/EBPα sites, (c) an 18 bp AT-rich palindrome, and (d) a 32 bp sequence of unknown function.[21,632] The RRE and TATA box are components of a promoter that drives expression of a 1.4-kb transcript. Similar features are also present in oriLyt R where the RRE and TATA element drive expression of kaposin mRNA.[524] These similarities are schematized in Figure 15.13, in which oriLytL and oriLyt R have been superimposed to highlight their commonalities. Among these motifs, the K8, C/EBP, and RREs function as key cis-acting elements.[634]

The oriLyt regions can bind K8 indirectly through the C/EBPα sites.[375] The 18 bp AT-rich palindrome is thought to be the place where initial strand unwinding occurs during the start of DNA replication. ORF50 activates the RRE-containing ori-Lyt promoter by binding to it and initiating transcription across the GC-rich tandem repeats.[634] The prereplication complex, of which ORF50 is a component, is recruited to ori-Lyt through the ORF50-RRE and the K8-C/EBP interactions with the ori-Lyt.[634]

Consistent with its function as a repressor of viral genes, a K8 deleted KSHV BAC displayed an enhanced growth phenotype in terms of virion production and the expression of lytic genes in the context of ORF50/RTA induction.[301] However, reactivation by chemical induction (TPA and sodium butyrate) yielded no virion production and an aberrant lytic profile compared to wild-type KSHV BAC.[301] Curiously, immunofluorescence staining revealed that in the absence of K8 there was a disruption of LANA subcellular localization suggesting that K8 can influence LANA localization.[301] However, another group showed that a different K8 deleted KSHV BAC displayed no difference in overall viral gene expression during lytic reactivation with TPA in epithelial cells, fibroblasts, and endothelial cells.[637] However, the K8 mutant virus–infected cells displayed lower copy numbers of latent KSHV genomes compared to wild-type KSHV–infected cells. These data suggest two possibilities—(a) K8 may be involved in abortive viral replication (leading to viral genome replication but not virion production) or (b) K8 may be involved in the maintenance of latent viral genomes[637] through modulation of LANA function as discussed above.[301,637] The former is likely to be the case since it was shown that LANA represses origin-dependent lytic DNA replication in a dose-dependent manner and that this suppression was overcome by increasing amounts of K8.[519] Additionally,

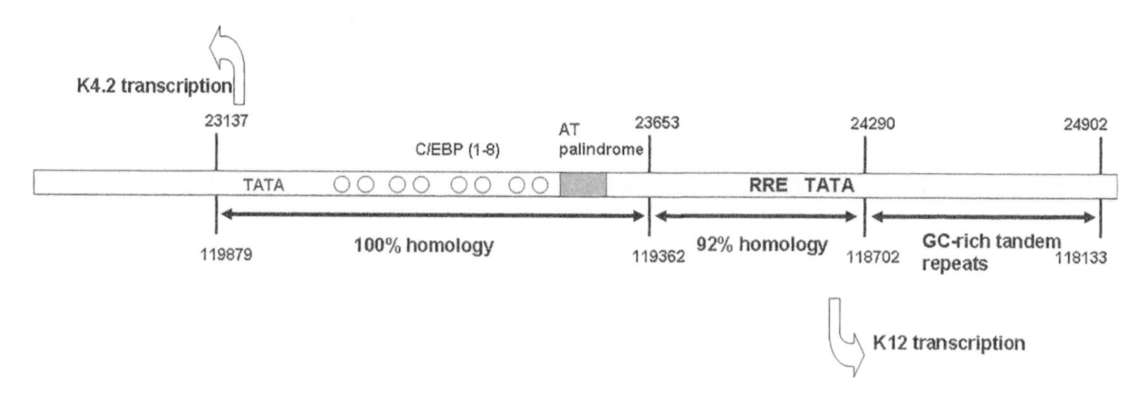

FIGURE 15.13 The structure of KSHV lytic replication origins. OriLyt-R and OriLyt-L are superimposed to reveal their commonalities. The *central bar* depicts important common sequence features. *Arrows* above the bar depict the transcripts from this region in OriLyt-L; *arrows* below the *bar* denote RNAs transcribed in oriLyt-R. Numbers refer to nucleotide sequence of each region. Degree of conservation of each domain between the two origins is indicated by percent homology. (Modified from Wang Y, Li H, Chan MY, et al. Kaposi's sarcoma-associated herpesvirus ori-Lyt-dependent DNA replication: cis-acting requirements for replication and ori-Lyt-associated RNA transcription. *J Virol* 2004;78(16):8615–8629. Copyright © 2004 American Society for Microbiology. Amended with permission from American Society for Microbiology.)

LANA alone was shown to interact with oriLyt by chromatin immunoprecipitation (ChIP) implying that the inhibition of lytic replication by LANA was mediated by direct binding.[519] This suggests a model where LANA interacts with K8 to negatively modulate the switch from latency to lytic replication. Conversely, K8 positively modulates lytic replication by relieving the LANA-mediated suppression of lytic replication.

Late Gene Expression

As with other herpesviruses, late gene transcription starts subsequent to the onset of DNA replication. The transcription of many (but not all) late genes is hindered by viral DNA synthesis inhibitors, for example, phosphonoacetic acid, ganciclovir, foscarnet, and cidofovir. Most late genes encode for structural proteins, for example, capsid and envelope proteins.[181,285,534] Late templates must either be actively replicating or have undergone a chromatin structure change that is dependent on viral replication to be activated. The KSHV ORF24 encodes for a protein that binds RNA polymerase II and recruits this polymerase to the late promoters of viral genes thereby mimicking the host TATA-box-binding protein (TBP). It was reported that ORF24 was necessary for late gene expression.[152]

FUNCTIONS OF LYTIC VIRAL PROTEINS

Modulation of Antigen Presentation by K3/MIR1 and K5/MIR2

The observation that diseases associated with KSHV infection are substantially more severe in hosts with T-cell impairment (e.g., AIDS) indicates that T cells are critical for the control of viral infection. Immune surveillance and clearance by cytotoxic T (CTL) cells is likely an important selective pressure in driving KSHV evolution with the host; therefore, it is no surprise that KSHV possesses an arsenal of proteins that evade the host's immune system.

The infected cell usually presents antigenic peptides from the virus in complex with class I major histocompatibility complex (MHC I) to CTLs. Two proteins (ORFs K3 and K5) prevent MHC-I display.[137] K3 and K5 encode for proteins called MIR1 and MIR2, respectively, for *m*odulators of *i*mmune *r*ecognition. K5/MIR2 down-regulates only HLA-A and HLA-B, while K3/MIR 1 down-regulates all four HLA allotypes (HLA-A, -B, -C, and -E)[279,575] (Fig. 15.14).

K3 and K5 are transmembrane proteins that resemble each other suggesting that they may have arisen from duplication of an ancestral gene. Each protein contains an amino-terminal variant RING finger with cysteine and histidine residues that vaguely resemble those found in PHD domain proteins. The zinc finger structure is on the cytosolic face of the membrane.[529] The KSHV MIR proteins show functional similarity to the cellular MARCH protein family, which was discovered after K3 and K5. MARCH proteins are transmembrane ubiquitin ligases that ubiquitinate and target cellular glycoproteins for lysosomal destruction[34] (Fig. 15.14). K3 and K5 appear to act during different stages of the viral life cycle. While K5 acts during viral entry into the lytic phase, K3-mediated down-regulation of MHC-I occurred during later stages of lytic replication.[70]

The MIR proteins reside in the ER membrane and augment the endocytosis of MHC-I chains that reach the cell surface[137,279] through MIR-mediated ubiquitination.[529] Ubiquitination directs these chains to the endosomes and subsequently the multivesicular body (MVB), a sorting organelle from which the MHC-I chains can be targeted for lysosomal degradation.[384,427,529] Interestingly, K3 induces lysine-63-linked polyubiquitination (instead of K48-linked polyubiquitination) of MHC class I chains, which leads to endocytosis and endolysosomal degradation.[172] This lysine-63-linked polyubiquitination required the activities of UbcH5b/c and Ubc13-conjugating enzymes.[172]

The MIR RING finger recruits E2 ubiquitin conjugases. K3 and K5 target recognition maps to the transmembrane regions of both effector and target molecules[529] Subsequently, transfer of the ubiquitin chain to lysines in the cytoplasmic tail can occur. Strikingly, K3/MIR 1 can also ubiquitinate cytosolic cysteine residues.[76]

The MIRs can also down-regulate CD1d, an MHC-related protein that presents lipids and glycolipids to classical and nonclassical natural killer (NK) T cells, which respond with the release of interferon.[376] This observation suggests that CD1d-restricted T cells likely play a role in host immunity against KSHV, but the lipid presentation and antiviral immunity is not well understood. K5/MIR2 (but not K3) also down-regulates ICAM-1 and the costimulatory molecule B7-2 (CD86).[138,278] These two proteins, which are expressed on antigen presenting cells, can bind and activate CD4-positive T cells. K5-mediated down-regulation of these proteins reduces helper T-cell costimulation[138] and impairs susceptibility to NK-cell cytotoxicity.[278] K3 and K5 also down-regulate the interferon gamma receptor 1 (IFN-gammaR1),[364] thereby preventing it from binding IFNγ released from activated T and NK cells. KSHV K5 reduces cell surface expression of the NKG2D ligands, MHC class I–related chain A (MICA), MICB, and activation-induced C-type lectin (AICL), which is a ligand for NKp80.

Although K3 and K5 appear to be functionally homologous in most cases, there are instances when K5 appears to encode additional functions not performed by K3. For instance, unlike K3, which induces ubiquitin-dependent endocytosis and degradation, K5 can induce the down-regulation of its targets through multiple pathways, including endocytosis-dependent and -independent as well as ubiquitination-dependent and -independent pathways.[428] K5 induces the degradation of nonclassical MHC class I-related (MHC-I) HFE via a polyubiquitination-mediated ESCRT1/TSG101-dependent pathway.[515] A proteomic screen performed with K5 revealed that it also targets bone marrow stromal antigen 2 (BST-2, CD316) also known as tetherin, activated leukocyte cell adhesion molecule (ALCAM, CD166), and Syntaxin-4.[35]

Independent of its role in immune modulation, K5 has also been implicated in vascular permeability during lytic infection by targeting the junctional endothelial protein, VE-cadherin, for ubiquitin-mediated degradation, thereby preventing endothelial cell adhesion.[457] Alpha-, beta- and gamma-catenins were also targeted for proteosomal destruction.[406]

Interferon Evasion by Viral Interferon Regulatory Factors

Several KSHV lytic proteins are involved in preventing the activation and function of type I interferons that are produced in response to infection. As described above, interferons are induced by PAMPs, which are recognized by innate immune sensors such as TLRs and RIG-I like receptors (RLRs), for

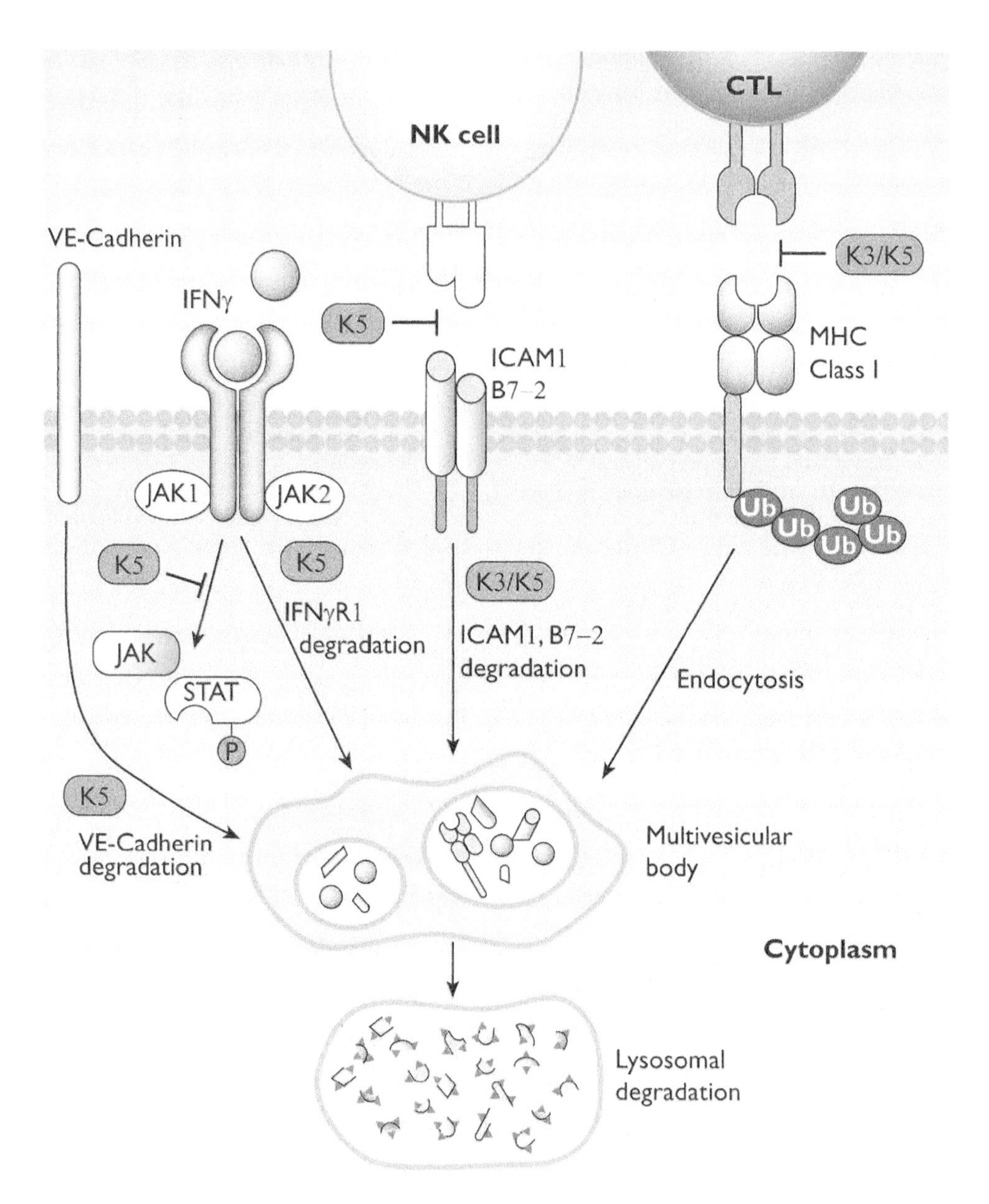

FIGURE 15.14 **Ubiquitination and degradation of cell receptors by K3/MIR1 and K5/MIR2.** The MIRs are able to induce the ubiquitination and degradation of a number of these receptors including MHC class I, ICAM-1, B7-2, and IFNγR1.

example, RIG-I and MDA-5. Activation of TLRs and RLRs leads to the activation of cellular IRFs, for example, IRF3 and IRF7 depending on which TLR is stimulated, type I interferon (IFNα and IFNβ), and inflammatory cytokines. IFN-α/β released from the cell can bind to IFNα and IFNβ receptors present on surrounding cells. This signal is transduced to the nucleus thereby stimulating the transcription of multiple IFN-sensitive genes (ISGs), which include known antiviral effectors (e.g., OAS, Mx and PKR) as well as the IRFs themselves.

IFN-α/β binding to IFN receptor leads to the phosphorylation and activation of STAT1 and STAT2. The activated STATs then bind to IRF9 (p48), and relocate to the nucleus to induce transcription from ISG promoters. Both the IFN-α/β and the ISG promoters contain IRF binding sites for many cellular IRFs.

The KSHV genome encodes four different homologs of cellular IRFs from a single locus, which is suggestive of the fact that they arose from an ancestral gene through gene duplication, followed by divergence. vIRF1, -2, -3, and -4 were named based on their order of discovery and not by their homology to a particular cellular IRF. vIRF3 is a latent gene as discussed above.

The remaining vIRFs (vIRF1, -2, and -4) are mostly expressed during the lytic cycle. Although vIRF1 is a lytic gene, it was found to be transcribed in latently infected KS cells as well.[115,162] vIRF1, -2, and -3 do not share the DBD of the cellular IRFs and hence do not bind to IRF binding sites in ISG and type I IFN promoters, although vIRF2 was shown to bind DNA.[271] In contrast to cellular IRFs, these three vIRFs hinder the function of cellular IRFs thereby suppressing IFN production (Fig. 15.15). The three vIRFs also differ in their inhibition of interferon activation mediated by TLR3.[283]

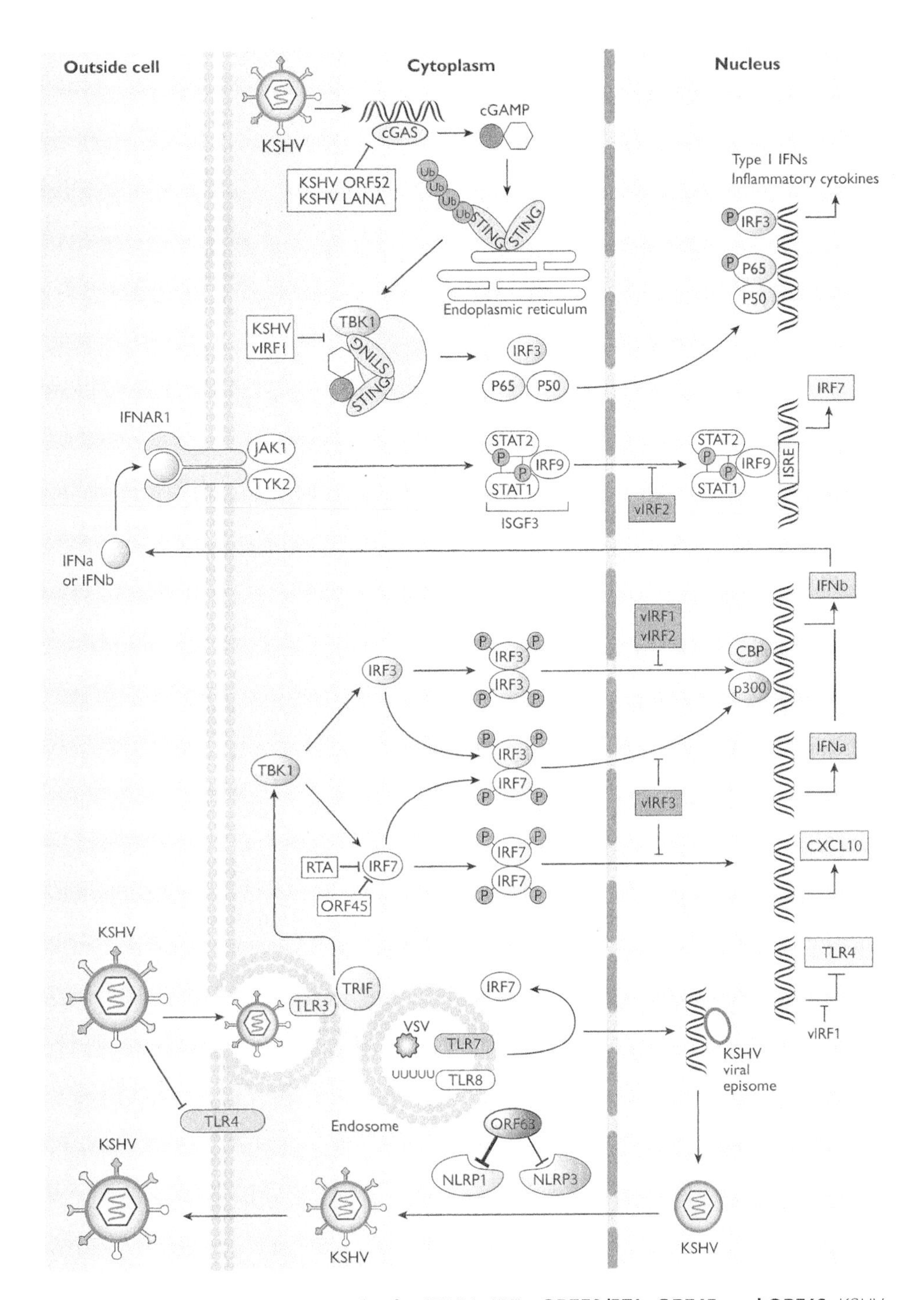

FIGURE 15.15 **Innate immune evasion by KSHV vIRFs, ORF50/RTA, ORF45, and ORF63.** KSHV entry triggers activation of TLR3 in monocytes and TLR4 in endothelial cells. Furthermore, binding of latently infected cells by TLR7/8 agonists leads to reactivation of KSHV from latency. The vIRFs block interferon activation by host cells. ORF50/RTA targets IRF7 for degradation while ORF45 inhibits IRF7 function. ORF63 inhibits activation of NLRP1 and NLRP3 innate immune sensors.

vIRF1 (encoded by ORF K9) is the most well studied vIRF and can inhibit IFN production in response to Sendai virus infection.[202] vIRF1 dimerizes with cellular IRF1 and IRF3, which prevents the cellular IRFs from transactivating the IFN promoters although DNA binding does not appear to be affected. Inhibition of IRF function is thought to occur through vIRF1's ability to bind and sequester coactivator CBP/p300 from cellular IRFs and inhibition of its HAT activity.[362,374] vIRF1 also binds HERC5, the major ubiquitin ligase for ISG15 resulting in decreased ISG15 conjugation of proteins.[284] vIRF1 is also able to block STING-mediated TBK1 activation[395] and block mitochondrial antiviral signaling protein (MAVS) mediated apoptosis and type I interferon gene expression.[273] vIRF1's ability to prevent apoptosis and evade immune responses is likely to greatly contribute to KSHV pathogenesis.

Studies have also demonstrated the ability of vIRF2 to impair IFN-dependent transcription. In the context of type I IFN, vIRF2 inhibited ISG56 activation,[192] cellular IRF1- and IRF3-mediated transcriptional activation, IFNβ promoter activity in response to double-stranded RNA and IRF3 transfection,[19] and ISRE transactivation mediated by the IFNγ family members IL28A or IL29.[192] vIRF2 was unable to inhibit IRF7-mediated transactivation of ISG promoters, as well as IFNγ promoter (pGAS) activity in response to IFNγ treatment.[192] However, it was recently reported that vIRF2-dependent regulation of the KSHV life cycle might involve up-regulated expression of interferon-induced genes, for example, IFIT proteins 1, 2, and 3, which antagonize the expression of early KSHV lytic proteins.[317]

Similar to vIRF1 and vIRF2, vIRF3 has been shown to inhibit transactivation of the IFN-α4 and IFN-α6 promoter upon Sendai virus infection as well as in the presence of exogenous IRF3 and IRF7.[389] KSHV vIRF1 and vIRF3 mediate some of their functions through interacting with the USP7 deubiquitinase.[664] vIRF3-expressing B cells show resistance to recognition by KSHV-specific CD4 T cells.[707]

KSHV vIRF4 has been shown to bind to IRF7 and inhibit IFN alpha production[275] and to target cellular IRF4 as well as interact with Myc and RTA to augment KSHV lytic replication.[353,662] vIRF4's ability to target IRF4 also results in enhancement of BCL6 expression.[683]

In addition to their ability to inhibit interferon, the vIRFs have also been shown to prevent apoptosis. vIRF1 was shown to relocalize the pro-apoptotic protein, Bim, a negative regulator of KSHV replication, to the nucleus.[125] This nuclear sequestration of Bim prevents apoptosis during viral replication, thereby leading to increased viral production during the lytic phase.[125] Furthermore, vIRF1 expression in mouse fibroblasts can induce cellular transformation, which is probably due to the fact that vIRF1 can also bind p53 and inhibit apoptosis.[202,452] vIRF1 co-precipitates with p53 and inhibits p53-driven transcription and targets, for example, p21 and Bax.[452] Expression of vIRF1 can also lead to a decrease in total p53 levels, due to vIRF1 directed ubiquitination and degradation of p53.[548] This activity required the p53 E3 ligase, MDM2. Inhibition of p53-mediated apoptosis may be a mechanism through which KSHV is able to establish latency. In addition to vIRF1, vIRF3 and vIRF4 also interfere with p53 signaling. Like vIRF1, vIRF3 was shown to interact with p53 *in vitro* and reduce p53 reporter activity.[516] vIRF3 also decreased apoptosis and activation of caspase 8 mediated by p53[516] and inhibited apoptosis in response to Fas and TRAIL.[652] Finally, vIRF4 interferes with the p53 pathway by interacting with MDM2 to increase MDM2 protein levels[351] through the inhibition of MDM2 autoubiquitination and prevention of MDM2 proteosomal degradation.[351] Interestingly, both vIRF1 and vIRF4 induce MDM2-mediated p53 degradation but through different mechanisms. For a more detailed review of the function of the four vIRFs please see review article.[282] Finally, vIRF2 was shown to activate the phosphatidylinositol 3-kinase(PI3K)/Akt pathway, inhibiting FOXO3A-mediated caspase-3 cleavage and apoptosis.[311] Furthermore, KSHV vIRF3 was detected in over 40% of various KS lesions and was demonstrated to function as a pro-lymphangiogenic factor by blocking the phosphorylation-dependent cytosolic translocation of HDAC5.[354]

Two other KSHV proteins, which are not homologs of cellular IRFs, can also block IRF action. ORF50 was shown to induce IRF7 degradation as described earlier. Additionally, the IE protein ORF45, can interact with IRF7 and prevent its phosphorylation and nuclear translocation[694] (Fig. 15.15). ORF45 interacts with an inhibitory domain in IRF7,[536] which keeps IRF7 in a closed inhibitory state. Since ORF45 is a tegument protein, in theory it should be able to hinder type I interferon activation pretty soon after viral infection. A KSHV recombinant virus deleted for ORF45 exhibited lower viral replicative capacity compared to wild-type virus.[696] ORF45 has also been shown to interact with p90 ribosomal S6 kinases (RSKs), RSK1 and RSK2, and strongly stimulates their kinase activities leading to ERK activation.[328]

Overall, KSHV encodes a battery of viral proteins dedicated to the ablation of IRF activation, and their function is testimony to the significant role innate immunity plays in the viral life cycle (Fig. 15.15).

Modulation of Inflammatory Pathways

In addition to the viral IRF proteins, KSHV also encodes for virally encoded CC chemokines: vCCL1 (formerly known as v-MIP-I, the product of ORF K6), vCCL-2 (vMIP-II, from ORF K4), and vCCL-3 (v-MIP-III, from ORF K4.1). Although chemokines are generally positive mediators of immune and inflammatory responses, the receptor preferences for the KSHV-encoded chemokines are consistent with their function as inhibitors of inflammation in response to viral infection. The CD4 T-cell subset of Th1 cells shape antiviral cytotoxic immune responses by promoting IL2, TNFα, and IFNγ induction, which can activate macrophages and promote the development of CD8+ CTL responses. Th2 cells on the other hand promote induction of IL4, IL5, IL6, IL10, and IL13, in order to elicit B-cell differentiation and humoral immunity (as well as allergic-type responses). Th2 cells also polarize immunity away from cytotoxic responses regulated by Th1 cells. The chief chemokine receptor on Th1 cells is CCR5, while Th2 cells express CCR3, CCR4, and CCR8 receptors. KSHV vCCL-1 signals through CCR8; vCCL-2 signals through CCR8 and CCR3; and vCCL-3 signals through CCR4.[467,576] In summary, the KSHV chemokines activate chemokine receptors that are distributed on Th2 cells. Moreover, vCCL-2 can interact with other chemokine receptors including CCR1, CCR2, CCR5, CXCR1, CXCR2, and CXCR4. However, binding of vCCL-2 to these receptors does not activate signaling but rather inhibits signal transduction by these receptor proteins in the presence of their chemokine ligands. For example, binding of RANTES and MIP-1α to activate CCR5 is inhibited by low amounts of vCCL-2. Thus, vCCL-2 appears to promote Th2 responses and also inhibit Th1 responses (Fig. 15.16). Consistent with this observation, KS lesions contain more Th2 T cells (CCR3+) than Th1 T cells (CCR5+).[642] Moreover, treatment of LCMV-infected mice with vCCL-2 inhibits CD8 T-cell migration into the lesion and impairs local inflammation.

Apart from their anti-inflammatory properties, the viral chemokines can also promote angiogenic responses and induce VEGF from PEL.[379] Additionally, the vCCLs can promote cell survival in an autocrine and paracrine manner—the vCCLs inhibit the expression of the pro-apoptotic protein, Bim, during KSHV lytic replication.[124]

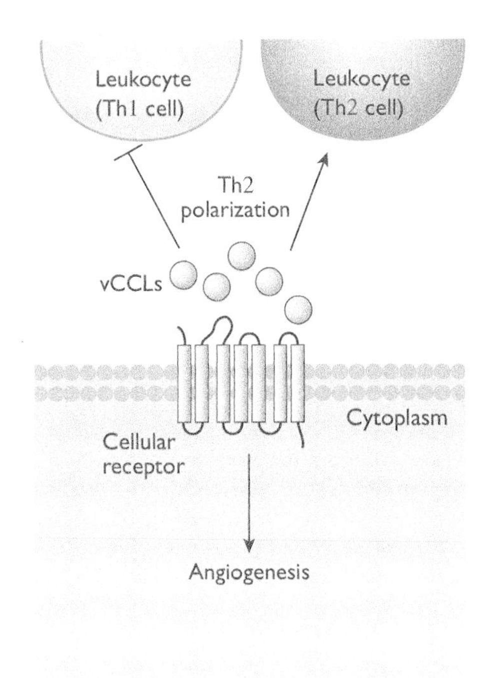

FIGURE 15.16 The KSHV encoded viral chemokines (vCCLs) block Th1 responses and augment Th2 responses. These viral chemokines have also been shown to activate angiogenic pathways.

KSHV K14 encodes a glycoprotein of the Ig superfamily that resembles cellular CD200 (also known as OX2). CD200 is expressed on many cell types (B, T, and endothelial cells) and its receptor (CD200R) is located on cells of the myeloid lineage (basophils, neutrophils and monocyte–macrophages). Cellular CD200 is a negative regulator of inflammation and myeloid cells, and CD200 knockout mice have an increase in monocytes and macrophages, macrophage and microglial activation, and increased susceptibility to experimentally induced autoimmune disease.[260] Soluble recombinant KSHV K14/vOX2 protein binds to CD200R.[186] There is some discrepancy in the literature regarding the inflammatory nature of K14. One study observed proinflammatory signaling by K14,[129] but other studies found K14/vOX2 suppresses markers of myeloid activation including suppression of TNF-α production by activated macrophages, decreased MCP-1 and IL8 production by a monocytic cell line, reduced oxidative burst in primary neutrophils triggered with a phagocytic stimulus, and a blunted release of histamine from basophils activated by Fc-ε receptor cross-linking.[186,514] Both cellular CD200 and vOX2 were reported to have a T cell–attenuating role resulting in the negative regulation of antigen-specific T-cell responses.[432]

KSHV encodes a viral protein, ORF63, with homology to the nucleotide-binding and oligomerization, leucine-rich repeat (NLR) family of proteins.[221] NLRs mediate antiviral immune responses to many different invading viruses. Some NLRs form a large molecular structure called an inflammasome upon activation. The inflammasome contains oligomerized NLRs, apoptotic-associated speck-like protein (ASC), and procaspase-1. Activation of this complex results in the autocatalytic processing of procaspase-1 to caspase-1. Activated caspase-1 subsequently cleaves the precursors of proinflammatory cytokines, pro-IL-1β and pro-IL-18, to their biologically active forms, IL-1β and IL-18, respectively. ORF63 is a tegument protein and hence is present in the incoming virion. ORF63 could bind and inhibit the association of the NLR family member, NLRP1, with procaspase-1 and prevent the processing of pro-caspase-1 and subsequent processing of pro-IL-1β and pro-IL18 (Fig. 15.15).[221] ORF63 inhibition of NLRP1 was found to be important during reactivation from latency and primary infection.[221]

Moreover, the KSHV ORF64 protein encodes a viral deubiquitinase,[213] that has been shown to inhibit the innate immune sensor, RIG-I.[277]

Signaling Proteins

K15

The coding regions adjacent to the KSHV TRs encode two signaling proteins: K1 and K15. K1 (described above) is located at the left end of the genome while at the right end of the genome lies ORF K15, which encodes for another transmembrane signaling protein. Expression of K15 is highly increased during lytic growth, and its expression during latency has been controversial. It was initially named latency-associated membrane protein (LAMP)[211] and is expressed at low levels during latency.[2,547] K15 mRNAs originate from alternatively spliced transcripts that include 8 or less exons, encoding up to 12 TM domains and a cytosolic tail.[126,211] All spliced variants encode the carboxy-terminal tail linked to varying numbers of transmembrane domains. The full-length proteins contain 8 exons (12 TM). All the K15 protein variants are found on intracellular membranes and the plasma membrane. A subset of K15 in the plasma membrane is associated with lipid rafts.[65] The K15 cytoplasmic region can be tyrosine-phosphorylated and appears to inhibit B-cell receptor (BCR) signal transduction.[126] The cytosolic tail contains a SH2 binding motif (YEEVL), and the Y is phosphorylated *in vivo* by the Src family of kinases. The cytoplasmic domain contains an SH3-binding region, and another motif (YASIL) represents an endocytosis signal and a potential site of tyrosine phosphorylation.

The cytoplasmic tail also contains a TRAF binding site (ATQPTDD). K15 binds TRAFs 1, 2, and 3 and constitutively activates NFκB, JNK, and ERK, MAPK signaling pathways, leading to up-regulation of the transcription factor, AP-1.[65,211] Activation of NFκB involves the recruitment of NFκB—inducing kinase (NIK) to K15.[250] In this manner, K15 is capable of inducing the expression of an array of cytokines and chemokines, including IL-8, IL-6, CCL20, CCL2, CXCL3, and IL-1α/β, Dscr1, and Cox-2[66] (Fig. 15.9).

Activation of MAPK signaling might be important for mediating lytic replication since MAPK activation is necessary for full lytic induction and reactivation from latency.[132,481,546,667] K15 also interacts with the protein HAX-1, an antiapoptotic factor, suggesting another mechanism (besides NFκB induction) by which K15 contributes to enhanced cell survival.[547] K15 can interact with Lyn and Hck kinases.[491] Thus, K15 appears to contribute to KSHV pathogenesis through the up-regulation of multiple inflammatory cytokines and the activation of multiple signaling pathways (Fig. 15.9). K15 also recruits PLCγ1, and thereby activates Calcineurin/NFAT1-dependent RCAN1 expression to induce angiogenesis.[25,217] Finally, KSHV K15 has been shown to be expressed in KS tumor biopsies and to be required for viral lytic replication.[2]

vGPCR

In addition to K1 and K15 discussed above, KSHV encodes a third transmembrane signaling molecule encoded by ORF74, a viral G-protein coupled receptor (vGPCR). It is a member of the family of seven transmembrane G-protein coupled chemokine receptors. Expression of this protein is dependent on ORF50 and is restricted to the lytic cycle. The protein displays constitutive signaling activity in the absence of ligand, although its activity can be stimulated further by chemokines, for example, GRO-α, and down-regulated by chemokines, for example, CXCL10/IP10.[20,207] The resulting signaling activates the PI3K/Akt/mTOR and p38 pathways,[435,559,563] as well as upregulates NFκB activity, angiogenesis, and cell proliferation[24,244] (Fig. 15.9). Indeed, vGPCR-deleted recombinant viruses are impaired for viral replication and vGPCR's function in lytic replication is dependent on its ability to signal through G-α(q) and activate MAPK signaling.[532]

Due to this potent signaling activity, vGPCR activates expression of many host genes. Among these are Rac1[437] and VEGF,[24,562] a critical mediator of vascular permeability and angiogenesis. vGPCR can also activate PDGF receptor.[94] KSHV vGPCR can promote tumorigenesis by activating the oncogenes, YAP/TAZ through inhibition of the tumor suppressive Hippo pathway.[382] Further, expression of vGPCR in mice in several different cell lineages generates focal angioproliferative lesions that have some features in common with KS.[234,436,669] What is a notable commonality among two of the models where expression was evaluated at the cellular level is that vGPCR was expressed only in a small proportion of the cells in the lesions, which has led to the belief that in KS lesions, expression by a few lytic cells can induce pathology through paracrine mechanisms. Because vGPCR can be linked to both proliferation and angiogenesis, it may be a key element in KS pathogenesis.[23,562] Additionally, siRNA suppression of vGPCR in the context of the whole viral genome also inhibited angiogenesis and tumorigenicity.[446] Interestingly, transgenic mice that express the constitutively active form of the small GTPase Rac1 develop KS-like lesions.[394] Transcription profiling showed many consistencies between KS tumors and the Rac1 tumors. The tumorigenesis seen in the Rac1 model was dependent on activation of Akt signaling, ROS-induced proliferation, and HIF-1 alpha. Furthermore, inhibitors of ROS reduced tumorigenesis in this model.[394] The contribution of lytic genes to oncogenesis is further discussed in the section on KSHV pathogenesis.

ORF36/vPK

ORF36 encodes for a viral protein kinase (vPK) that is a serine–threonine kinase.[247] vPK expression is induced by hypoxic environments due to the fact its promoter contains hypoxia-inducible elements[247] and vPK expression has been observed in 59% of KS biopsies.[264]

vPK is present in both the nucleus and cytoplasm,[330] and it can modulate signal transduction pathways. vPK can bind and phosphorylate the histone acetyltransferase TIP60,[365] which is a protein involved in the DNA damage response. Both mitogen-activated kinases 4 (MKK4) and 7 (MKK7) are phosphorylated by vPK resulting in c-Jun N-terminal kinase (JNK) phosphorylation and consequently phosphorylation of c-Jun transcription factor.[242]

vPK can also phosphorylate cyclin-dependent kinase substrates, retinoblastoma, and lamin A/C.[330] In addition, vPK shows some homology to cellular ribosomal protein S6 kinase (S6KB1) and can phosphorylate ribosomal S6 protein.[46] Moreover, vPK transgenic mice show an eightfold increase in the incidence of B-cell non-Hodgkin lymphoma (NHL) compared to age-matched wild-type mice.[16]

Host Shutoff

Many previous attempts to examine the effects of lytic replication on host gene expression in KSHV were hindered by the low frequency of lytic replication in chemically induced PEL lines. However, systems now exist where lytic reactivation is seen in the majority of cultured cells.[448,616] This is typically performed by infecting cultured cells with KSHV at high MOI after which cells are allowed to establish latency; these cells are subsequently superinfected at a high MOI using baculoviral or adenoviral vectors expressing ORF50. This induces the lytic cycle in the vast majority of cells in culture. Under these conditions, the majority of lytically infected cells display some degree of inhibition of host gene expression 10 to 12 hours postinfection. The principal block appears to be at the level of host mRNA accumulation.[210] This phenomenon can be attributed to a single protein encoded by ORF37.

KSHV ORF37 encodes for a DE protein named SOX (*s*hut-*o*ff e*x*onuclease). Homologs of SOX exist in other herpesviruses as well. In HSV, the SOX homolog is not involved in host shutoff (which instead is mediated by ICP27 and VHS). The KSHV SOX protein retains DNA exonuclease activity similar to its HSV counterpart, but this function can be genetically separated from its function in host RNA shutoff.[210] There is a coordinated destruction of cellular mRNAs by SOX and the mammalian exonuclease Xrn1.[142] Cleavage sites of SOX are specific and are defined by a degenerate sequence motif containing a small number of conserved residues rather than a strong consensus sequence.[193] Importantly, a small subset of host mRNAs escape SOX-mediated turnover. The cellular IL-6 message is one of these transcripts. Mapping studies have shown that the 3′ untranslated region of IL-6 mRNA contains elements that allow it to escape from SOX-induced degradation and that these elements are protected by the binding of a ribonucleoprotein complex.[444] The length of polyadenylated tails is emerging as a distinct marker of mRNA fate and differences from the canonical length lead to either degradation or nuclear retention. KSHV SOX stimulates RNA turnover through polyadenylation-linked mRNA turnover.[345] Inhibition of poly(A) tail formation blocks ORF37/SOX activity and transcripts in SOX-expressing cells exhibit extended poly(A) polymerase II generated poly(A) tails. The poly(A) binding proteins (PABPs) were also shown to be essential for SOX function.[345] Exactly how selectivity for host mRNAs is achieved by SOX, while viral transcripts are spared, remains to be elucidated.

KSHV PATHOGENESIS

In this section we review the cellular and molecular mechanisms that underlie KSHV's relationship with its associated cancers.

Molecular Pathogenesis of KS

Histologically, KS tumors are highly complex and unlike most classical cancers that arise as a clonal outgrowth of a single cell type.[509] This makes KS different from traditional forms of cancer, where the malignant cell is of a clear, distinct type. In KS, the chief proliferating cell is called the "*spindle cell*," which is named after its spindle-like shape. As mentioned above, the spindle cells are of endothelial lineage, since they express many markers of endothelial origin, including factor XIII, CD31, CD34, CD36, En-4, and PAL-E.[17,97,256,509] However, some spindle cells lack the presence of factor VIII, which is a marker of differentiated vascular endothelium. Spindle cells also display heterogeneity in marker expression.[509] For example, some spindle cells in KS biopsies stain for factor VIII, while other cells stain for smooth muscle α-actin.

Gene expression profiling studies of infected endothelial cells[89,243,261,629] found that latent viral infection reprograms expression of endothelial markers, inducing the vascular endothelium to express lymphatic markers such as PROX1, while the lymphatic endothelium displays a more vascular-like profile. On the basis of microRNA profiling it has been shown that there exist multiple distinct stages of endothelial cell reprogramming by KSHV, most significantly associated with the down-regulation of mir-221.[470] In view of the stage-wise reprogramming, which endothelial cell type represents the actual progenitor of the KS spindle cell is still unclear; it is still possible that multiple types of endothelial cells could give rise to the KS spindle cell following viral infection. The resultant KS spindle cell may be shaped as much by the viral infection as by the microenvironment. Gene expression profiling of KS tumor biopsies have shown multiple subtypes of KS lesions—those that express just the latency transcripts and those that express both latency and lytic transcripts.[264]

KSHV-infected endothelial cells have also been found to up-regulate several signal transduction pathways including the PI3K/Akt/mTOR pathway and JAK2/STAT3 pathway.[442,627] STAT3 activation was mediated by gp130 receptor, a common receptor of the IL-6 cytokine family. Both Akt and STAT3 were necessary for KSHV-induced lymphatic reprogramming of endothelial cells.[442]

In addition to spindle cells, KS lesions also contain infiltrating T cells, B cells, monocytes, and aberrant, slit-like neovascular spaces. The neovascular spaces are lined with both infected and uninfected endothelial cells.[173] They don't contain pericyte or smooth muscle cells and are very susceptible to leakage and rupture. Because of these features, KS lesions often exhibit hemorrhage, with erythrophagocytosis by inflammatory cells in the interstitial spaces. The KSHV-infected endothelial cells display increased vascular permeability—lytic infection is associated with VE-cadherin degradation[177,406,497] attributed to the actions of K5 and vGPCR, while latent infection is associated with increased Rac1 activation and ROS generation leading to disruption of endothelial junctions due to the phosphorylation of VE-cadherin.[231] Thus, the histologic appearance of KS probably results from at least four different processes—proliferation, inflammation, reprogramming, and angiogenesis. These processes are intertwined but distinguishable. These distinctions are important because KSHV contributes through different genetic mechanisms to each of these disease components.

KS can occur in a variety of sites. It is frequently localized to the skin, and in the sporadic classical form, it may be restricted to the lower extremities. In the skin, the dermis is involved, with sparing of the overlying epidermis.[483] While progression is not quite linear, and patients may present with lesions in all stages, in general terms, cutaneous KS is thought to begin as a *patch* lesion, with histologically demonstrable spindle cells that are not necessarily the predominant cell type; inflammatory cells and neovascular elements are also abundant at this stage. The lesion may progress through a plaque-like stage to the *nodular* stage, with the proportion of spindle cells becoming progressively larger as the lesion progresses. By the nodular stage, spindle cells fill up most of the lesion. The spindle cell progressively dominates during the course of KS and is therefore considered to be the key tumor cell.

In immunocompetent adults, classical KS is frequently indolent. However, in immunocompromised hosts, KS is highly aggressive, with widespread involvement of lymphoreticular structures and multiple organs such as the GI tract, the lung, and skin. Pulmonary KS has a grave prognosis since it is often accompanied by death from respiratory failure. Analysis of KS spindle cell clonality has revealed that KS lesions are either oligo- or polyclonal.[294] Although clonality is observed in some KS lesions,[500] the lesion is generally thought to be oligo- or polyclonal throughout much of its development, including progression to macroscopically visible KS. One striking feature is how frequently the individual lesions in a KS patient appear to have arisen independently. This is different than that observed in most classical cancers and underscores the uniqueness of KS. This scenario is reminiscent of that seen with EBV-driven post-transplantation lymphoproliferative disorders, where lesions can be polyclonal, showing a possible progression to monoclonality, and when there are multiple lesions, they may be of different clonal origin a single patient.[99,316] Cellular pre-miRNA profiling of KSHV-infected endothelial cells and KS tumors revealed that as cells infected with KSHV transition from immortalization to fully tumorigenic, there was a loss of mir-221 expression and a gain of mir-15 expression.[470] Additionally, expression of mir-140 and the KSHV viral miRNAs increased proportionally with the degree of transformation.[470] Additionally, down-regulation of multiple tumor suppressor miRNAs was observed in KS and PEL.[471] Since the tumor suppressor proteins themselves are, for the most part, not mutated in these tumors, regulation of their expression in KS and PEL highlighted a novel, alternative mechanism of transformation.[471]

KS spindle cells exhibit only a few of the hallmarks of transformation. KS cells are very dependent upon growth factors and cytokines when cultured *in vitro*. KS also do not display genetic instability, although this may reflect the nature of viral cancers, which tend to show less genetic instability (e.g., p53 mutations) in general. KS spindle cells are diploid and do not display microsatellite instability, although certain advanced AIDS-KS tumors can display these characteristics. The KS spindle cells are dependent on cytokines and growth factors (perhaps from infiltrating inflammatory cells) in their microenvironment for their proliferation, but they themselves can generate angiogenic and proinflammatory factors to recruit additional blood vessels to the site of the infected lesion. Thus, KS is highly dependent on its microenvironment for growth and survival.

The Role of Hypoxia in KS Biology

One descriptive observation involving KS was that it often (but not always) develops in the lower extremities, such as the feet, where tissue may be less oxygenated. A seminal finding revealed that low oxygen conditions, that is, hypoxia, lead to the reactivation of KSHV replication from latently infected PEL.[149] Hypoxia augmented vIL-6 secretion as did several compounds that increase the levels of HIF-1. Hypoxia also increased expression of the viral kinase, KSHV ORF36, and the thymidine kinase encoded by ORF21.[150] HIF-1 is a master regulator of angiogenesis and is activated posttranscriptionally by hypoxia, leading to increased protein stability of HIF-1alpha and/or HIF-2alpha, which are two subunits that constitute HIF-1. Consistent with this hypothesis, the KSHV genome contains several hypoxia response elements (HREs).[246] The ORF50/RTA and the ORF34 promoters contain HREs, which under hypoxic conditions are activated by HIF-1 alpha and/or HIF-2 alpha.[246] As mentioned above, XBP-1s can reactivate KSHV from latency and it has been reported that hypoxia also induces active XBP-1s.[147]

Additionally, in the context of primary KSHV infection, there is an increase in HIF activity under normoxic conditions.[90] Both HIF-1alpha and HIF-2alpha proteins are elevated in KSHV-infected cells.[90] KSHV also appears to utilize a portion of the hypoxic cellular response—for example, during KSHV infection there is a significant portion of hypoxia-induced changes in cellular gene expression.[621]

Impact of KSHV Infection on Metabolic Pathways

KSHV infection of endothelial cells has been shown to increase aerobic glycolysis (leading to lactate secretion) and decrease oxidative phosphorylation in the cell. This effect is common to tumors and is known as the "Warburg effect." Inhibitors of glycolysis appear to enhance cell death of KSHV-infected cells.[156] Additionally, KSHV also induces lipogenesis for survival of latent infection in endothelial cells.[157] Latent KSHV infection was shown to result in increased levels of intracellular glutamine and enhanced glutamine uptake through the glutamine transporter, SLC1A5.[530] Thus, multiple pathways including glycolysis, glutaminolysis, and fatty acid synthesis (FAS) are up-regulated by KSHV infection of endothelial cells and inhibitors of these pathways block the production of infectious virus from lytically infected cells, each at a different stage of viral replication.[531] Interestingly, in KSHV-induced cellular transformation of rat primary MSCs, glycolysis is suppressed and KSHV appears to accelerate glutamine metabolism.[698] These differences might be due to a difference in cell types.

In B cell–derived PEL, both aerobic glycolysis and FAS are significantly up-regulated compared to primary B cells, and PEL were more sensitive to the FAS inhibitor, C75.[45]

Molecular Pathogenesis of PEL and MCD

Gene expression profiling demonstrated that PEL display a distinct profile from all other NHL that is neither related to germinal center (GC) nor to memory B cells.[313] The mRNA profile of PEL was defined as plasmablastic because it showed features of both immunoblasts (similar to EBV-transformed lymphoblastoid cells) and plasma cells (similar to multiple myeloma cells).[313] Another group reported that the stage of B-cell development represented by PEL closely resembles that of malignant plasma cells.[286] The unfolded protein response is partially activated in PEL (XBP-1) and genes overexpressed in PEL include those involved in inflammation, cell adhesion, and invasion.[286] KSHV-infected PEL have also been found to up-regulate the PI3K/Akt/mTOR signaling pathway,[44,554,602] as well as higher levels of B-Raf and angiogenic VEGF-A as compared to other lymphoma subtypes. MEK inhibition reduced VEGF-A expression in PEL.[10] In PEL, Interleukin 1 receptor-associated kinase 1 (IRAK1) appears to be essential for KSHV PEL.[671] NFkB is also active in PEL cells, but knock-out of single genes in this pathway do no result in PEL cell death.[407] In contrast, PEL cells are dependent on IRF4, MDM2, cyclin D2, cellular FLIP, and MCL1. Genome-wide comparative genome hybridization (CGH) found consistent deletions in fragile sites that encode the FHIT and WWOX tumor suppressor genes.[520] In terms of viral gene expression, most of the PEL cells express latent genes, for example, LANA, vCyclin, vFLIP, vIRF3 etc.[181,453] However, between 1% and 5% of PEL cells spontaneously reactivate in culture and display lytic gene expression.

MCD is associated with both latent and lytic infection. In MCD, latent (LANA) and lytic (ORF59, K8, and K10) viral proteins are expressed.[483] One protein that is constitutively expressed in a significant proportion of KSHV-infected cells in MCD is vIL-6, which as described above is expressed during latency and is highly up-regulated during lytic infection. It is thought that expression of lytic proteins contributes extensively to the pathobiology of MCD.

KSHV Gene Expression in KS and PEL

KSHV viral DNA is present in all KS tumors, regardless of type of KS or disease stage. As mentioned above, KSHV specifically targets the spindle cell compartment within the tumor.[173,569] However, when passaged *in vitro*, the spindle cells generally lose the viral genome. It has been reported that monocytes in the lesion can also be infected by KSHV[52,477] as well as some epithelial cells.[185,483,569] *In situ* hybridization for latent mRNA transcripts suggest that most KS spindle cells are latently infected; however, a small subpopulation (<1% to 2%) express markers of lytic infection in some lesions.[163,173,299,569,577] With the exception of vIRF3, all latent genes expressed in PEL are also found as latent genes in KS.[516]

Similar to EBV, it is thought that the latency program drives tumorigenesis. Early (patch) lesions of KS have only a small proportion of spindle-like cells that are LANA positive (<10%), while in more progressed lesions a variable, but higher, proportion of spindle cells are latently infected.[173,569] The *in vitro* properties of the latent proteins (e.g., the inhibition of p53 and Rb by LANA, the induction of NFκB by vFLIP, the stimulation of CDK6 by vCyclin, and the up-regulation of β-catenin by LANA) are commensurate with transformation, growth advantage, and survival. However, it is important to note that many of these functions were identified in experiments involving overexpression of individual viral proteins. When most transformed cell lines are infected with KSHV, the resulting latent infection does not greatly impact their biology.[36,335] However, when KSHV infects primary (or immortalized) human endothelial cells, the virus replicates for the first few days (usually with significant CPE) and spreads through the monolayer. Over the next 7 to 10 days postinfection, lytic replication subsides and most of the cells are latently infected. The resulting LANA-positive cells exhibit a change in morphology, that is, elongation to a spindle morphology similar to that seen in KS tumors *in vivo*. In most cases, primary human cells are not immortalized by KSHV. However, efficient cellular transformation of primary rat mesenchymal precursor cells has been observed.[439] Similarly, most KSHV-positive primary endothelial cells cannot form tumors in nude mice or grow in soft agar. However, Renne and colleagues did isolate a KSHV-infected immortalized endothelial line (TIVE) in which KSHV-infected cells were tumorigenic and grew out many weeks following infection.[14] These KSHV-infected TIVE cells do give rise to tumors in nude mice.[14] However, this cell line appears to represent the exception to the rule, rather than the norm.

The above results may simply reflect the paucity of culture conditions to successfully propagate KSHV-infected endothelial cells. Indeed, a similar situation is observed in EBV where epithelial cells like nasopharyngeal carcinoma (NPC) cells lose the EBV genome during passage in tissue culture.[165] This is despite the fact that EBV-infected B lymphoma cells do not lose the virus during similar passage as is the analogous situation with KSHV-infected B lymphoma cells. Thus, in contrast to B lymphoproliferative cells, it is generally not possible to establish cell lines from either NPC or KS that retain the EBV and KSHV episomes respectively, during passage in tissue culture. However, *in vivo*, every KS and NPC tumor cell retains the viral genome.

Early studies showed that KSHV infection of primary B cells *in vitro* is inefficient and, in contrast to EBV, does not lead to immortalization. Infection efficiency was enhanced when primary B cells were activated and expressed DC-SIGN.[507] When KSHV DNA was transfected into BJAB B cells, the virus was maintained as an episome and could establish latency with a low level (1% to 5%) of underlying spontaneous lytic replication.[113] The latent viral gene profile was similar to that observed in PEL and the virus could be reactivated to produce infectious progeny virions.[113] *In vivo*, it appears that KSHV can infect B cells and *in vitro* infection of primary tonsillar B cells has shown that activated T cells help to promote and stabilize latency[447] and that these infected B cells predominantly express lambda light chain.[249] Analysis of specific B-cell lineages from human tonsils infected with KSHV revealed that infection of immunoglobulin κ (Igκ) naïve B cells induces expression of Igλ, with eventual loss of Igκ.[601]

Recently, a number of papers have examined the coinfection of EBV and KSHV in B cells. It was reported that persistent KSHV infection increases EBV-associated lymphomagenesis in humanized mice through enhancement of EBV lytic gene expression.[423] Another report showed that EBV enhances genome maintenance of KSHV in B cells[48] and supports optimal coinfection of B cells with KSHV.[183]

The Unprecedented Role for Viral Lytic Proteins in KSHV Oncogenesis

The latency program has traditionally been associated with tumorigenesis (as is the case with EBV). Hence, it was surprising that independent evidence from clinical studies suggested that both lytic replication and latency play an important role in KS development. In the case of patients with advanced AIDS, the administration of ganciclovir (GCV)—a drug that blocks lytic, but not latent KSHV infection—prevented the onset of new KS tumors.[412] This is a striking result because these patients were infected with HIV and KSHV for many years; the fact that the administration of GCV blocks tumor appearance suggests that viral reactivation may be necessary to support KS development. Further, patients with KS typically display circulating KSHV DNA in the peripheral blood.[79] Two other antiviral drugs, however, failed to affect already established KS lesions.[326,378] One could speculate that dependence of KSHV lytic genes exists during the initial stages of lesion formation. Subsequently fully tumorigenic spindle cell clones may emerge, in which host cell mutations lead to independence of KSHV lytic proteins.

How might lytic replication contribute to KS tumor development?

The lytic and latent phases of the viral life cycle go hand in hand. Without lytic proteins, the virus cannot replicate, survive in the human population, or exert paracrine effects on neighboring uninfected cells in the tumor microenvironment. Without latent proteins, the virus cannot persist in the infected host and establish latency for the lifetime of the infected host. Thus, these two phases of the viral life cycle are interdependent on one another, and the cumulative pathogenesis seen with KSHV infection is a contribution of both lytic and latent genes. Albeit there is no firm answer to the question of how lytic genes contribute to KS tumor development, several (nonexclusive) possibilities can be considered:

1. Latent KSHV infection is not clearly immortalizing *in vitro* using current culture conditions, which distinguishes it from EBV. If spindle cells do not proliferate indefinitely, then for a tumor mass to grow, KSHV-positive cells that die must be replaced by newly infected cells. The source of such cells could be generated from *de novo* infection of endothelial cells with virus produced from lytically replicating cells.
2. When recently infected cells bearing latent KSHV genomes undergo sustained proliferation *in vitro*, they lose their viral genome.[226] This is supported by the consistent observation that when infected KS spindle cells are explanted from clinical specimens and placed in culture under conditions that favor their proliferation and expansion, they rapidly lose their viral episomes but retain their transformed nature.[184] Thus, lytic replication may be continuously needed for KS development to infect and restore latent infection to spindle cells that have lost their viral genomes. Some experimental evidence indicates that selective pressures exist *in vivo* to retain the KSHV genome, and these are different from those of explanted KSHV-infected cells in culture.[14,446]
3. The third way that lytic KSHV replication may contribute to KS pathogenesis is through activation of three processes required for KS development: proliferation, inflammation, and angiogenesis. Since fully lytically infected cells die, they are not able to contribute to the proliferative component of the disease. However, in the context of abortive lytic replication, the lytically infected cells can produce paracrine factors that support the inflammatory and angiogenic nature of the lesion. As described before, KSHV encodes multiple secreted signaling proteins expressed during the lytic cycle—examples include the three viral CC chemokines and vGPCR.

The viral chemokines exhibit chemotactic properties for both Th2 cells[576] and endothelial cells.[245] Polarization of local T cells away from Th1 responses might inhibit antitumor cytotoxic responses, while the effect of viral chemokines on endothelial chemotaxis suggests that KS lesions are likely to recruit more endothelial cells for latent or lytic infection. Indeed, the application of the viral chemokines to chick chorioallantoic membranes stimulates angiogenesis.[576] Moreover, vGPCR is a potent signaling protein as discussed above and is capable of activating pro-survival, pro-angiogenic, and pro-proliferative cellular pathways.

4. Finally, it is also possible that some lytic proteins are expressed outside of the traditional lytic cycle—if not during the canonical latent phase, then in response to an extracellular signal or microenvironment cue, which allows the lytic gene to be expressed in the absence of other lytic genes. An example of this is that hypoxic conditions have been shown to turn on expression of viral genes like ORF36.[247]

Conversely, one conundrum is the ability of a subset of latent proteins to up-regulate inflammatory cytokines. Several latent proteins are linked to the induction of inflammatory responses including vFLIP, K15, and kaposin B, as described above. Cytokines play important roles in KS and MCD pathogenesis, and it is likely that these viral proteins induce cytokine production in KS and MCD. Although understandable from a pathogenesis standpoint, from an evolutionary point of view it appears contradictory that KSHV would embed such proinflammatory biology in the heart of its latency program. In contrast, many viruses encode proteins that prevent inflammatory responses or evade those they cannot ablate. This conundrum remains unresolved. It is possible that cytokines are important to maintain latency in naturally infected cells *in vivo*, or for sustaining the viability of latent cells. Alternatively, an inflammatory microenvironment may help to recruit KSHV-permissive cells to sites of viral infection, thereby facilitating viral spread from cells undergoing lytic reactivation. The fact that some of the latent viral proteins also possess antiapoptotic activity suggests that these viral proteins acting in concert may negate the negative effects of proinflammatory cytokines, while the positive effects of these cytokines, for example, recruitment of target cells, are retained. In addition, there is increasing experimental evidence suggesting that expression of lytic genes (at least vGPCR) in small subsets of cells can augment the proliferation or tumorigenicity of cells expressing latent genes (such as vFLIP and vCyclin).[436,438]

The identity of the origin of the KSHV-infected tumor cells remains unresolved. One report suggested that bone marrow precursors serve as a reservoir for KSHV.[484] Primary MSCs in human bone marrow were shown to be susceptible to KSHV in tissue culture.[484] A recent report provides evidence that KS might actually originate from MSCs through KSHV-induced mesenchymal-to-endothelial transition.[367]

Human CD34+ hematopoietic progenitor cells (HPCs) were also subjected to KSHV infection and differentiated *in vitro*.[659] Infection of CD34+ HPCs with a recombinant GFP-containing KSHV followed by reconstitution with KSHV-infected CD34+ HPCs showed that the virus could be detected in human CD14+ and CD19+ cells recovered from NOD/SCID mouse bone marrow and spleen following infection.[659] These results suggest that KSHV can establish persistence in CD34+ HPCs and this may serve as a KSHV reservoir to allow the virus to be disseminated to B cells and monocytes after differentiation.[659]

EXPERIMENTAL SYSTEMS FOR STUDYING KSHV

Animal Models

KSHV does not establish persistent infection in mice; hence humanized mouse models have been used. Early studies showed that C.B-17 SCID mice implanted with human fetal thymus and liver grafts (SCID-hu Thy/Liv mice) were susceptible to KSHV infection, with an early phase of lytic replication and subsequent sustained latency.[164] Viral gene expression in CD19+ B lymphocytes was observed, and infection was inhibited by ganciclovir. However, no disease was evident in the infected animals.[164] Another humanized model of NOD/SCID mice with functional human hematopoietic tissue grafts (NOD/SCID-hu mice) was also injected with KSHV. A portion of these animals generated human KSHV-specific antibodies. Antiviral treatment of the NOD/SCID-hu mice with ganciclovir led to prolonged but reversible suppression of KSHV DNA and RNA levels, suggesting that KSHV can establish latent infection *in vivo*.[485] Human CD34+ cells have been infected *in vitro* and followed in immunodeficient mice, also without any disease.[659] A humanized BLT (bone marrow, liver, and thymus) mouse (hu-BLT) model generated from NOD/SCID/IL2rγ mice showed that KSHV can establish infection in human B cells and macrophages.[638]

Viruses related to KSHV from other species, for example, murine herpesvirus 68 (MHV68), rhesus monkey rhadinovirus (RRV), and HVS, are used as experimental models of KSHV pathogenesis (reviewed in Ref.[166]). However, *in vivo*, KSHV infection is restricted to the human population and no natural infection of any other species has been identified. KSHV is not successfully transmitted to small animal experimental hosts. Implantation of PEL cells into immunodeficient mice leads to tumor engraftment, but not to spread of virus or infection in murine tissues. As described above, SCID/hu mice transplanted with human lymphoid tissues display infected human B cells within the implant, but there is no spread to the surrounding mouse tissue, and no disease state developed in these animals.[164]

KSHV can be successfully transmitted to New World primates, specifically common marmosets (*Callithrix jacchus*).[110] Infected common marmosets displayed antibody reactivity to KSHV, and LANA protein and KSHV genomic DNA could be detected in PBMCs from these animals indicating that KSHV could establish persistent infection in these animals.[110] One KSHV-infected animal developed a KS-like skin lesion consisting of spindle cells and infiltrating leukocytes.[110]

Xenograft models have been very useful for the study of pathogenesis, and to test a variety of potential therapies. Xenograft models of PEL have been reported by several laboratories,[166] and PEL cell lines expressing firefly luciferase have allowed *in vivo* tracking of tumor growth (BC3-NFκB-luc). Xenograft models of KS have also been reported, but these have used cell lines, such as SLK, KS Y-1, and KS-IMM, obtained from KS patients but lacking KSHV. Other cell implantation models include injection of human endothelial cells that have been infected with KSHV *in vitro*,[14] and mouse bone marrow cells that have been transduced with a KSHV BAC.[446] These models have provided interesting biological insights and are particularly important because they assess the effect in the context of the entire virus. A related system, which has been used to evaluate the interaction of cells expressing a lytic gene (vGPCR) and cells expressing latent genes (vFLIP and vCYC), is the implantation in mice of endothelial cells transduced to express viral genes.[436] These important studies have confirmed that KSHV can produce vascular tumors, that vGPCR is a critical viral gene for this process, and that there is a selective pressure *in vivo* for viral maintenance.

Cell Culture Models of Infection

In order to determine parameters of KSHV tropism and transmission, many different cell culture systems have been developed as experimental models to examine these events. The first successful cultivation of cells containing KSHV utilized PEL from AIDS patients with advanced disease.[96,511] These cells grew as ascites tumors in the KS patients and were readily established in cell culture. A panel of these lines has now been established, from both EBV-positive and EBV-negative cases of PEL. These cell lines have complex, hyper-diploid karyotypes with multiple structural abnormalities, a few of which are recurrent (trisomy 7, trisomy 12, and aberrations in the proximal long arm of chromosome 1 (1q)).[520,653] However, in general, they do not contain structural alterations in common genes involved in lymphomagenesis (such as MYC, p52, RAS).[451] PEL cells predominantly harbor latent KSHV episomes[511] with only a handful of latent viral genes being expressed, and virus is not produced. However, in most experimental systems, 1% to 5% of PEL cells display lytic replication with the viral genome being expressed in a temporally regulated fashion, resulting in viral DNA replication and yielding infectious virions as described above. The viral titers are quite low, but can be greatly increased by the addition of chemical inducers (e.g., phorbol esters) or the histone deacetylase inhibitors (e.g., sodium butyrate and valproic acid).[430,512] Chemical inducers reactivate 15% to 30% of latent PEL, which begin to exhibit lytic gene expression. Virions isolated from PEL have been utilized for structural studies of the virus particle and for studies of infection studies *in vitro* and animal infectivity studies *in vivo*. These cell lines have also been utilized for serologic assays.

While cell lines established from patients with advanced KS do exist (SLK, KS Y-1, and KS-IMM), these lack the KSHV genome, and are therefore not useful for virological studies. Thus, immortalized endothelial cell lines have been generated that contain the KSHV genome. While these in general do not result in stable viral infection, a few cell lines have been generated that do appear to maintain the virus and grow indefinitely. The first such system used dermal microvascular endothelial cells immortalized with HPV E6 and E7, prior to infection with KSHV.[443] Another important cell culture system was generated by infecting telomerized endothelial cells (TIVE), to generate long-term cultures (TIVE-LTC).[14] A different cell line—latently-infected SLK cells that are tightly latent—has been shown to be efficiently induced by doxycycline. These cells seem to produce increased quantities of infectious KSHV virions.[448]

Most KSHV-infected cells *in vitro* result in viral latency and not lytic replication. These include common cell lines, for example, HeLa and HEK293.[36,618] Human cell lines of fibroblastic, endothelial and epithelial lineages, monocytes, and rodent cell lines (3T3 and BHK) can all support latent infection *in vitro*.[36,265a,335,443] Thus, the entry machinery for KSHV is likely distributed across different cell types and infection in culture is highly amenable and often does not parallel the pattern of infection seen *in vivo*. Established cell lines (e.g., HEK293, TIME, Vero, HFF) that are readily infected can also be induced to reactivate by the same chemical stimuli mentioned above for PEL (e.g., TPA or sodium butyrate). A workhorse cell line in the field is the inducible iSLK.219 cell, which allows for doxycycline-induced KSHV reactivation from latency.[448] A B-cell version of this was also developed.[300]

Oral Infection Model

KSHV has been shown to infect epithelial cells, including those from the oral cavity.[176,290,540,617] Indeed, KSHV has been detected in the saliva of KSHV seropositive individuals[50,318,486] and is also known to be transmitted orally to children from KSHV-positive breast-feeding mothers.[64,154,419] Tissue culture–based infection of oral keratinocyte raft cultures with a recombinant KSHV virus resulted in latent infection in the basal layer, but when these keratinocytes differentiated, lytic replication was induced and virions were produced at the epithelial surface.[290] Interestingly, early keratinocyte differentiation did not result in lytic replication in cells attached to a substratum and only occurred in the suprabasal cell layer.[540] Consistent with this model of adherence-dependent latency, keratinocytes that were differentiated in a suspension activated lytic KSHV.[540] It appears that the engagement of integrins on the KSHV-infected cell surface plays a key role in maintaining latency and preventing reactivation. *In vivo*, it is likely that virus present in oral epithelial cells is subsequently transmitted to tonsillar B cells (such as those mentioned above) where the virus can establish lifelong latency.

KSHV can infect both T and B cells from primary tonsillar explant cultures.[249,447,449] T cells, however, do not support lytic replication (they display abortive replication), while B cells spontaneously produce substantial amounts of infectious virus. When mixed cultures of B cells and activated T cells were exposed to KSHV, virus production was not seen unless the T cells were removed from the cultures or the culture was spiked with immune suppressants. Thus it appears that oropharyngeal activated T cells recognize ligands on KSHV-infected B cells suppressing lytic replication and thereby promoting latency.[249,447,449] Furthermore, when human tonsillar cells were infected with KSHV and analyzed using multispectral imaging flow cytometry (MIFC), LANA expression was mostly seen in cells that expressed the lambda light chain of the B-cell receptor.[249] The KSHV-infected B cells displayed increased expression of Ki67 and IgM and IL-6 receptor. They proliferated and also displayed blast morphology. All these characteristics are similar to those seen with MCD, which are IgM lambda-expressing plasmablasts.[249] The preference for lambda light chains is not due to preferential infection of B cells expressing this type of Ig, because KSHV can infect both kappa and lambda light chain–expressing tonsillar B cells. However, kappa-expressing cells begin coexpressing lambda light chains soon after infection (being double positive), and eventually many become only lambda light chain positive.[601] This is accompanied by regulation of Rag proteins, which account for induction of V(D) J recombination and receptor revision. Thus, it is likely that oral transmission of KSHV leads to latent infection of a subset of tonsillar B cells that become IgM lambda positive and can expand and resemble plasmablasts.

Taken altogether, these observations suggest several possibilities through which KSHV could establish infection in endothelial cells and B cells *in vivo*. A putative model is shown in Figure 15.17.

1. It is possible that the virus first infects the oral epithelium from which it is shed into the saliva and can then subsequently infect either endothelial cells or B cells in the oral submucosa.[176,447,540]
2. It is equally possible that the virus can directly infect B cells (and plausibly endothelial cells) in the oral submucosa through a break in the mucosal epithelium as described previously for KSHV infection of tonsillar B cells.[447]
3. Since KSHV-infected monocytes and macrophages have been detected *in vivo*,[52,477,556] it is also conceivable that KSHV can directly infect these cells in the oral submucosa or indirectly through the oral keratinocytes as described above.
4. Although KSHV has not been detected in dendritic cells *in vivo*, it can infect these cells *in vitro*,[255,506] which raises the possibility that these cells might also be directly or indirectly infected by KSHV in the oral submucosa. Alternatively. KSHV-infected monocytes may be able to differentiate into dendritic cells.

It is important to note that the above described model is based on different tissue culture studies and correlative measures of viral loads in various compartments *in vivo*. However, it provides some insight into how KSHV can establish latency in B cells and endothelial cells *in vivo*.

EPIDEMIOLOGY

Age

KSHV infection can occur at any age, beginning in early childhood. KS was reported to afflict children in endemic regions indicating that viral transmission can occur during childhood.[558] Studies evaluating the age in which viral transmission occurs have been possible in sub-equatorial Africa, where prevalence of KSHV is highest. Transmission is unlikely to occur during delivery, since a study in an endemic area found no evidence of KSHV in cord blood.[84] However, seroconversion can

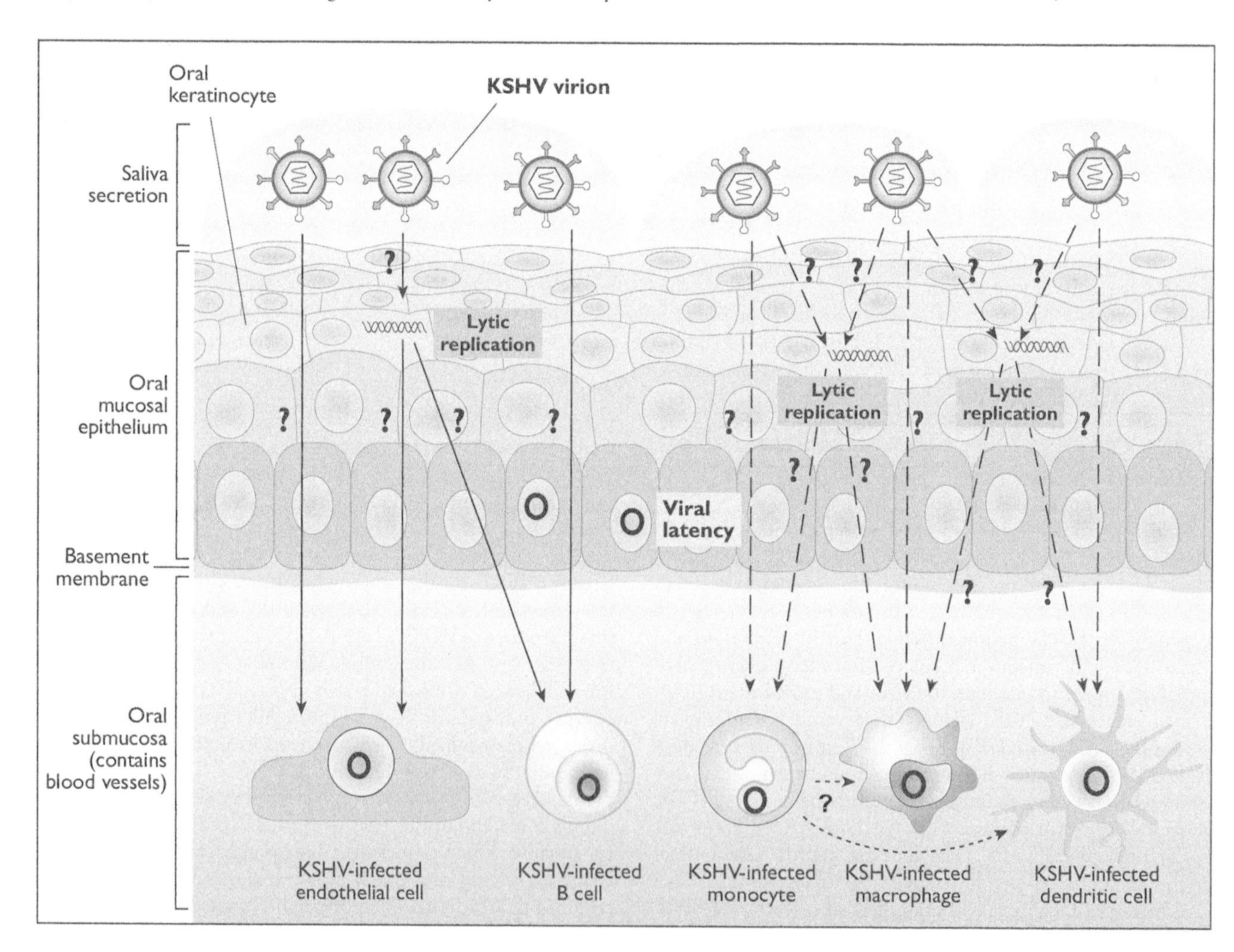

FIGURE 15.17 **Hypothetical model of KSHV infection in the oral cavity.** This model is based on various tissue culture studies and correlative measures of viral loads in different compartments *in vivo*. A number of scenarios are depicted to indicate how KSHV establishes latency in B cells and endothelial cells following primary infection.

begin soon thereafter; studies have largely shown that infection occurs at an early age, arguing for nonsexual transmission. The presence of antibodies to KSHV increases gradually with age (reviewed in Ref.[97]), with as many as 15% of children under 2 years of age having been exposed to KSHV in endemic areas (Fig. 15.18). One study in rural Uganda showed that 90% of children are seropositive for KSHV by the age of 15.[464] Closely following puberty, seroprevalence of KSHV continues to rise through early to mid-adulthood, which is a pattern suggestive of inefficient heterosexual transmission[22,179] with close to half of the population being seropositive by the age of 50.[74] There is a strong familial association, with a higher likelihood of a child being positive if the mother or a sibling is positive for the virus. A large study (>2,500 participants) was conducted to address whether possible sociodemographic, behavioral, and biological factors were associated with transmission in rural Uganda. This study confirmed that in highly endemic regions, infection is mostly acquired from intrafamilial contacts in childhood, and that it continues into adulthood most likely through nonsexual routes.[75] The finding of childhood transmission routes has more recently been confirmed by assessing seroconversion in Zambia. Increased risk of seroconversion was found as a consequence of sharing of utensils between a child with a primary caregiver, having more KSHV-infected household members and five or more children in the household.[143]

Routes of Transmission

KSHV has been found in maternal saliva and in breast milk in endemic areas, arguing for an oral/salivary route of transmission in African children.[64,154,403,419] The presence of KSHV in saliva is not correlated with KSHV viremia, but it increases with age and is more common in males, as found in a study from Uganda.[455]

Analysis of a cohort of Italian patients with classic KS and their first-degree relatives showed that infection in these was significantly higher than in healthy controls, and these included spouses, siblings, and offspring. These relatives were found to contain viral DNA in their saliva, indicating that close contact contributes to the spread of KSHV, and that this spread can occur via nonsexual routes, although sexual transmission in the spouses could not be excluded.[405]

In contrast to endemic areas (Africa and the Mediterranean Basin), in Western Europe and the United States, which are zones of low prevalence (seropositivity 1% to 7%), infection

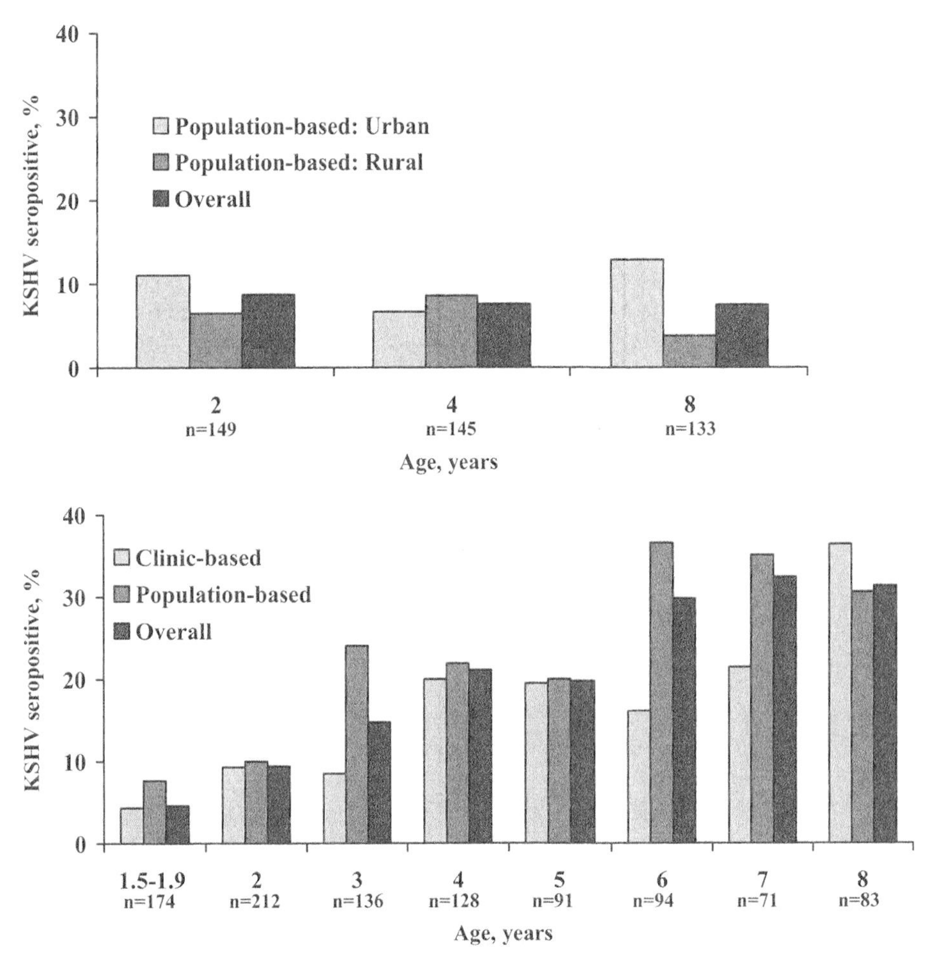

FIGURE 15.18 **KSHV seroprevalence among children in South Africa (top) and Uganda (bottom), by age.** *n* values underneath bars refer to the overall number of children in each age group. (From Butler LM, Dorsey G, Hladik W, et al. Kaposi sarcoma-associated herpesvirus (KSHV) seroprevalence in population-based samples of African children: evidence for at least 2 patterns of KSHV transmission. *J Infect Dis* 2009;200(3):430–438. Reproduced by permission of Infectious Diseases Society of America.)

is generally acquired sexually: prepubertal children are uninfected, while infection rates rise in adulthood, coinciding with sexual activity. Sexual transmission occurs efficiently among men who have sex with men (MSM) where seroprevalence can range from 25% to 60%[111,201,303,553,560]; in this group, there is a clear linkage to infection and the number of sexual partners.[411] Seroprevalence rates tend to be lower among women than men,[304] though rates of infection among female attendees of STD clinics and commercial sex workers are elevated,[82,303] suggesting that heterosexual transmission to females occurs. The finding that virus is consistently detected in saliva,[486,617] and only sometimes in genital secretions,[486] favors an important role for salivary virus-mediated sexual transmission.

The possibility of blood-borne transmission through blood transfusion has been witnessed, and there is evidence that it may occur, albeit rarely.[258] One prospective observational cohort study of transfusion recipients was conducted in Uganda, where the seroprevalence among blood donors was very high, leukocyte reduction was not used, and blood storage time was usually short. In this study, an estimated 12 of the 425 patients who received KSHV-seropositive blood were infected by transfusion. Other studies have confirmed that in some settings transfusion may lead to acquisition of KSHV, and a few case reports have documented transfusion-associated KS.[3,478,636] In contrast, a study in the United States that evaluated a historical cohort of participants in the Transfusion-Transmitted Viruses Study showed that there was no statistically significant difference in KSHV seroconversion in the transfusion and nontransfusion groups.[83] The question of whether organ transplants should be screened has also been raised. While the incidence of KS is highly increased in organ transplant recipients, this is mostly due to reactivation as a consequence of the immunosuppressive therapy. However, molecular studies have documented that the KSHV originated from the donor in some instances.[167,190,392,620] A study found that among 454 organ recipients (281 renal, 116 liver, and 57 heart) close to 30% of recipients seroconverted among those where the donor was seropositive for KSHV. Only liver transplant recipients developed KSHV viremia (close to 4% of recipients). In this study, two liver and one kidney transplant recipients developed KS.[344]Thus, some investigators have advocated for screening for organ transplantation, and for blood transfusion in endemic areas, but there are no formal guidelines.

Morbidity and Mortality

The major disease caused by KSHV is KS, and the incidence of this disease globally varies. In the early AIDS epidemic, KS incidence skyrocketed, and was reported to be 20,000 times more frequent in HIV-infected patients with AIDS than in the general population. The use of combination antiretroviral therapy (cART) starting in the mid 1990s dramatically decreased the incidence of AIDS-related KS.[518] The overall incidence of KS in Western countries decreased from around 15 per 1,000 person-years to 5 per 1,000 person years between 1992 and 1999.[281] The current rates of KS were reported recently in a large study with over 200,000 patients that included 42 cohorts from 57 countries. Incidence rates per 100,000 person-years were 237 in North America, 244 in Latin America, 180 in Europe, 52 in Asia Pacific, and 280 in South Africa.[5] KS risk was approximately 2 times higher in heterosexual men than in women and 6 times higher in MSM than in women.[5] Globally, it appears that while incidence of AIDS-related KS has dramatically decreased, the rates have mostly reached a plateau, without reaching pre-HIV levels,[325,418,672] and there is anecdotal evidence and case reports that KS is presenting in people living with HIV who are treated with combined antiretroviral therapy (cART) and with controlled HIV loads and CD4 counts.[309,611] There is also evidence that risk groups of individuals presenting with classic KS may be changing, as documented by a retrospective cohort study of classic KS in Paris between 2006 and 2015 that reported that less than 40% of patients were of Mediterranean origin and 28% were MSM.[159]

In sub-Saharan Africa, the incidence of KS increased close to 20-fold when the AIDS epidemic began. The effect of cART on the incidence of AIDS-related KS in sub-Saharan Africa is difficult to quantitate since not much data are available.[98,541] However, we know that most of the global burden of KS is currently happening in Sub-Saharan Africa. According to Cancer Today,[276] the annual incidence of KS is currently estimated to be 41,799, with 32,446 of these deaths occurring in Africa, while the annual mortality is estimated to be of 19,902 cases, where 17,659 are in Africa.

Origin and Spread of Epidemics

KS has been grouped into four major epidemiological forms[195]: Classic KS affecting elderly men of Mediterranean or eastern European Jewish ancestry; endemic KS, existing in parts of Central and Eastern Africa, described long before the HIV pandemic and often affecting children with disseminated lymphadenopathy[43,472,558]; iatrogenic KS, developing in immunosuppressed individuals such as after an organ transplant or for autoimmune disorders[551]; and epidemic or AIDS-KS, a major AIDS-defining malignancy. In the western world, AIDS-KS predominantly affects HIV-infected gay men. However, in Africa, since the spread of HIV, epidemic KS has become more common in both genders, with a lowering of the male to female ratio.[623] The incidence of childhood KS has risen more than 40-fold in the era of AIDS in endemic regions.[702]

Lymphadenopathies linked to KSHV infection, namely PEL and MCD, are much more common in HIV-infected individuals. While MCD is increasingly recognized in Africa,[214] KSHV-associated lymphomas appear to be extraordinarily rare in regions that are endemic for KSHV, even in individuals with HIV infection.[180]

Prevalence and Seroepidemiology

Strong epidemiological studies suggest that KSHV infection is absolutely required for the development of Kaposi's sarcoma. Studies that utilized the measurement of antiviral antibodies demonstrated that these antibodies are made during primary infection, but since primary infection gives way to latent infection in the host, seropositivity is a marker for not only past exposure but also the presence of ongoing viral latent infection.

Like the disease incidence, the prevalence varies globally. As individuals with KS have higher anti-KSHV antibody titers than do individuals without KS, the overall seroprevalence may be underestimated. However, despite this caveat and some regional exceptions, there is a strong concordance between KSHV seroprevalence rates and incidence of KS. Different tests have been used to determine seroprevalence, and these are variably reliable, with some assays overestimating, and others underestimating, the true prevalence. Thus, some studies are difficult to interpret. Since KSHV encodes multiple latent and

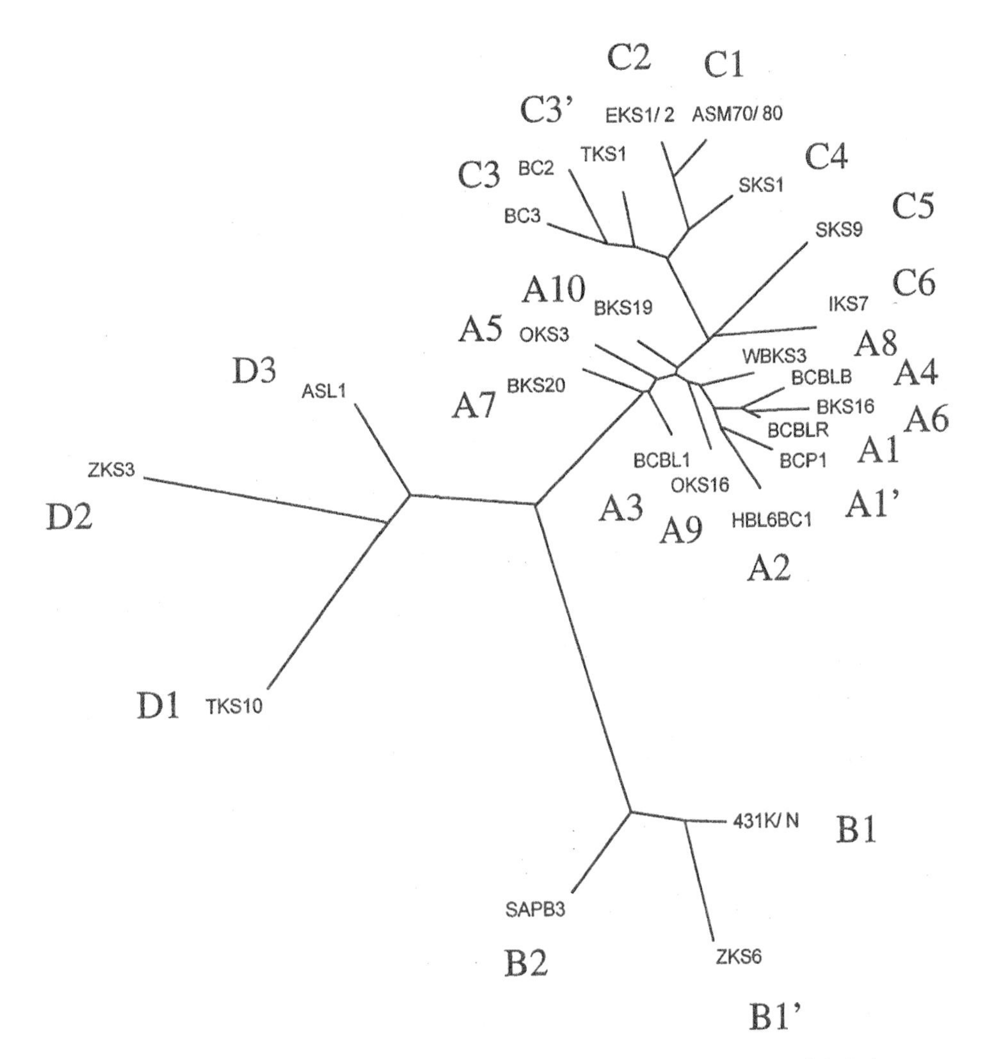

FIGURE 15.19 Clades of KSHV based on ORF K1 sequence differences. A and C clades cluster together and are typically found in Europe and the United States. B clade isolates are from sub-Saharan Africa, and D clades are from Australia and the Pacific islands. The subgroups within each individual clade are denoted by numbers following the clade letter, for example, C1 to C6. Many of the isolates shown here are from commonly used PEL cell lines, including BCBL-1, BC-1, BC-3, and BCP-1. (Reprinted from Zong J, Ciufo DM, Viscidi R, et al. Genotypic analysis at multiple loci across Kaposi's sarcoma herpesvirus (KSHV) DNA molecules: clustering patterns, novel variants and chimerism. *J Clin Virol* 2002;23(3):119–148. Copyright © 2002 Elsevier, with permission.)

lytic antigenic proteins,[103] assays have variably targeted these antigens. The earlier studies used immunofluorescence using latently infected PEL cells, or PEL cells treated with TPA to induce lytic replication.[201,303,358,553] Newer generation methods rely on enzyme-linked immunosorbent assays (ELISAs) using recombinant proteins or peptides, most frequently LANA (ORF73), which is the major latently expressed antigen, or the lytic antigens K8.1 and ORF65. Usually testing for both LANA and at least one lytic antigen is encouraged, because infected subjects may have detectable antibodies to one or the other,[47,431] and develop seroreactivity to these antigens at different times.

In an assessment of which proteins encoded by KSHV induce an antibody response, 72 KSHV ORFs were used to make recombinant proteins and tested in people with KSHV-associated diseases. In addition to LANA and K8.1, ORF38, ORF61, ORF59, and K5 were found to elicit significant responses.[331] Given that many studies from different areas used variable methodology to assess the seroprevalence, one analysis using a single method was conducted to determine the presence of antibodies among a cohort of over 6,000 people in sub-Saharan Africa testing for antibodies to LANA and K8.1. This study showed age, higher rates of coinfection occurring in rural areas, geographical variation (highest seroprevalence in West Nile, Uganda, of 70%, and lowest in Nigeria, of 23%), and gender (higher in men than in women) impacted seroprevalence.[490] This study also nicely confirmed that variations in KSHV seropositivity parallel the cumulative incidence of KS. Regional variation was also shown in a study evaluating seroprevalence in China, where higher rates were found in the Uygur, Mongolian, and Kazar ethnic groups, in which most of the cases of KS occur, as compared to the Han people.[636]

Nearly all KS patients are seropositive for KSHV with current testing techniques. Prospective studies suggest that KSHV infection predates AIDS-KS development and is a strong predictor of KS risk. Fifty percent of men infected with both HIV and KSHV, who received no effective treatment for either agent, develop KS within 10 years.[411] The association of KSHV infection with KS is also evident from the fact that KSHV viral genomic DNA and viral antigens are present in all cases of HIV-positive or HIV-negative KS.[272,440] These data indicate that KSHV is the etiological agent of KS and that KSHV is the *sine qua non* of KS—patients that do not have KSHV infection will not develop KS. Treatment of AIDS patients at high risk for KS with ganciclovir reduces KS incidence and further bolsters this conclusion.[412]

When comparing three time periods in a rural Uganda cohort (1990–1991, 1999–2000, and 2007–2008) for prevalence, titer, and temporal trends, a modest reduction was found in prevalence in the most recent period, which was more pronounced in children.[464] If this trend holds true, there may be hope for eventual decrease in this population, where the vast majority are infected with this virus. This report also found higher seroprevalence rates in males than females. Notably, boys tend to shed more KSHV in saliva than girls as determined by a study in Uganda.[463]

Geographical Distribution and Genetic Diversity

KSHV infection is found at variable rates all worldwide, with rates lowest in Western Europe and America and highest in Africa.[97,153,410,537,648] In Europe, however, KSHV is more prevalent in the Mediterranean region, for example, Italy and Spain.[197,647] KSHV isolates from different regions in the world show differences that help explain KSHV evolution and its relationship with its human host. As described in Figure 15.3, large blocks of KSHV sequence are highly conserved and do not exhibit much variation from different isolates. However, some genomic regions in the virus display remarkable sequence variability, which makes them useful as markers for strain diversity and markers to track epidemiological spread. These include regions surrounding the internal sequence repeats and the coding regions directly adjacent to the left- and right-hand TRs namely ORFs K1 and K15, respectively. The biochemical functions of these transmembrane proteins have been discussed earlier, and here we discuss their sequence variability in the context of KSHV evolution.

ORF K1 is a transmembrane protein whose N-terminal cysteine-rich ectodomain is highly variable; amino acid differences in K1 between geographically disparate isolates range from 30% to 60% of the total residues in the K1 ectodomain[704,705] (Fig. 15.19). Importantly, the cysteine residues, N-linked glycosylation sites, and signaling motifs in the cytoplasmic tail are not changed, which reflects the important nature of these amino acids for K1 function. A vast degree of sequence variation occurs in the hypervariable regions of K1, named V1 and V2, in which amino acids surge to 60%. It is assumed that host immune pressure drives this variability, but another hypothesis is that this diversity might have been driven by the need to recognize highly polymorphic cell surface proteins.[706] K1 sequence variation allows for the separation of KSHV isolates into four major subtypes (A, B, C, and D) (Fig. 15.19). These subgroup identifications are also supported by sequence variations in other genomic loci.[705,706] However, it is important to note that the viral strains are stable in a given individual since different samplings recovered from a single patient taken at various time points often yield identical sequences. The A and C subgroups are viral isolates from KSHV-infected subjects in Europe, the United States, the Middle East, and Asia, while subgroup B strains are viral isolates from sub-Saharan Africa; type D strains are found primarily in Australia, South Asia, and the Pacific islands. These data indicate that KSHV is an ancient human infectious agent that entered the human population at or around the time that modern humans arose in Africa in the early Pleistocene Age.[251] The diversification of the main branches (A/C, B, and D) is thought to occur from isolation and founder effects associated with proposed migrations of humans out of Africa—the first (ca 100,000 years ago) disseminating subtype B through sub-Saharan Africa, the second (ca 60,000 years ago) spread subtype D to South Asia, and onto Australia and the Pacific islands, and the third (ca. 35,000 years ago) carried subgroups A and C to Europe and northern Asia, and onto the Americas.[706] Alternative interpretations of these findings exist as well, but seem less likely.[422] The clustering of subtypes with ethnic and geographic population also implies that the virus is primarily transmitted in a familial pattern (e.g., vertically from parent to child and horizontally among siblings), with wider horizontal transmission being less efficient. Of course, in the context of the AIDS epidemic, viral spread occurred by a predominantly sexual route.

There is additional sequence diversity at the right-most end of the viral coding region—in the K15 coding sequence. Here, the A and C subgroups (and only rare B isolates) display two allelic variants, termed P (for prototype) and M (for minority). The K15 alleles show large sequence differences that sometimes can extend into the adjacent ORF 75 gene (and sometimes up to 20 kb from the right-hand TRs).[496,706] A functional ORF K15 gene is preserved in both P and M alleles. The P and M K15 isolates only share 33% amino acid identity. This extensive sequence divergence is consistent with the notion that the allelic variants were generated from recombination events with an unknown progenitor herpesviral genome during the course of evolution. The fact that both M and P alleles exist among KSHV subgroups A and C suggests that this recombination event likely occurred after the first two waves of emigration from Africa, but occurred soon after this, which allowed for dissemination of these alleles to both the Middle East and northern Europe.[705] Additional alleles (N and Q) at the right-hand end of the genome have been identified.[706]

The impact of the different strains in pathogenesis has been analyzed in different defined geographical areas, mostly based on K1 sequencing. One study in Brazil showed a significant predominance of A genotypes in KS lesions from HIV-positive patients, whereas C genotypes were found mostly in the HIV-negative setting.[504] In China, subtype A was significantly more frequent in mucosal KS lesions than subtype C.[685] One study in Italy showed that patients with rapid progression of KS and higher blood viral loads contained type A KSHV, while C type was mainly present in slow progressing patients.[404]

Cofactors

Although KSHV infection is necessary for KS to develop, it is not sufficient and cofactors have been identified. Globally, the presence of antibodies to KSHV is much more common than KS, indicating that on average only about one in 10,000 infected people gets the disease. The most important cofactor is clearly HIV infection. It is not yet completely clear if immunodeficiency itself is the main determinant of KS, or whether

HIV has a more direct role. Individuals with iatrogenic immunosuppression, particularly renal transplant patients, also have an increased risk for KS, but not as great as that seen with HIV infection. This may reflect differences in KSHV infection rates, rather than HIV-specific causes, or differences in immune dysfunction, but a direct role for HIV as a cofactor has not been excluded. KS is clearly more common in males than females, which is more dramatic in classic KS. The reasons for this gender disparity are not known.

Potential contributions from host genetic factors have been reported, including genetic polymorphisms of inflammatory and immune-response genes. Classic KS risk is associated with diplotypes of interleukin 8 receptor β (IL8RB), IL13[68] and certain human leukocyte antigen (HLA) haplotypes.[141,169] Transplant KS risk is associated with an IL6 promoter polymorphism,[205] and genotypes of FcgammaRIIIA may influence the development of KS in HIV-infected men.[355] Thus far, these association studies have only shown a relatively small overall increased risk and have not included very large patient cohorts.

Environmental exposures have also been evaluated and found to have an effect on KSHV seroprevalence, or incidence of KS. These include regional variations associated with certain volcanic soils, arthropod bites, and living in rural areas.[490,504,685,701] In Sub-Equatorial Africa, malaria in particular has been shown to increase KSHV seropositivity[454,456] and shedding in saliva.[455] Helminth infection, in particular *S. mansoni* and hookworms, have also been found to be associated with higher KSHV seropositivity.[456,625]

These data suggest that common host genetic variants, in addition to coinfections, environmental factors, gender, timing, and possibly routes of infection, all contribute to the oncogenic outcome of KSHV infection.

CLINICAL DISEASE

Kaposi's Sarcoma

Clinical Features

Moritz Kaposi first described five patients with a hemorrhagic sarcoma of the skin and mucous membranes, but also involving internal organs as appreciated during postmortem examination.[298] While he described an aggressive tumor, this form was eventually recognized to be a rare, frequently indolent disease confined to the skin, and mostly occurring in older men of Mediterranean and Eastern European origin and referred to as sporadic or classic KS. An endemic form of KS was recognized and described by the early sixties, occurring in sub-Saharan Africa.[398] While African KS was histologically indistinguishable from the sporadic form, it tended to be more aggressive, and a lymphadenopathic form was documented to occur in children.[558] Subsequently, patients receiving immunosuppressive agents, such as solid organ transplant recipients, were also found to develop KS, which has been designated iatrogenic KS.[248] With the advent of AIDS, KS was found to occur with greatly increased frequency, therefore called epidemic KS. In the context of HIV infection, KS was reported to occur mostly in men who have sex with men (MSM), and have a much more aggressive clinical behavior, with frequent dissemination to internal organs.[188] Increasingly, an additional epidemiologic form of KS has been recognized, which is in HIV-negative MSM.[160,189,340,508]

Kaposi's sarcoma can have a variable clinical presentation, ranging from limited to fulminant disease, where in general it tends to be more indolent in sporadic KS and more aggressive in Africans and in individuals with AIDS.[97] The main clinical features in the different epidemiological forms are listed in Table 15. 2. Cutaneous lesions are most common in the lower extremities, face and genitalia, but can appear anywhere[123] (Fig. 15.20). In the context of HIV infection, the appearance of cutaneous KS lesions in visible areas may be indicative of AIDS and carry a heavy psychosocial burden because of existing stigma. Cutaneous KS lesions are typically multifocal and have the appearance of papules, patches, plaques, or nodules, and there can be fungating lesions and tumors. Among these, the patch lesions are considered early-stage lesions and other forms are considered more advanced. However, while these definitions are useful as dermatologic descriptors, in practice these distinctions frequently do not reflect disease progression; several forms can appear simultaneously. There can be patch-type lesions constituting large areas, or nodules with limited disease. Lymphedema may be extensive and debilitating. KS can also involve noncutaneous sites. Particularly common is involvement of the oral cavity, which can be the initial site of presentation. KS can also affect practically all internal organs, most frequently the gastrointestinal tract, lungs, and lymph nodes. In children, lymph node involvement signifies a poor prognosis subset, while in adults, focal lymph node involvement is quite common and does not signify the same poor prognosis as other visceral disease.[450]

A clinical classification scheme was proposed for AIDS-related KS by the AIDS Clinical Trials Group (ACTG) Oncology Committee.[323,324] This staging system incorporates extent of tumor, where T0 (good risk) is when KS is confined to skin and/or lymph nodes and/or minimal oral disease (i.e., nonnodular KS confined to the palate), and T1 (poor risk) is when there is any of the following: tumor-associated edema or ulceration, extensive oral KS, gastrointestinal KS, or KS in other nonnodal viscera. Other criteria in this classification are severity of immunodeficiency (I0 and I1 with a cutoff of <200 CD4 cells per cubic millimeter) and presence of systemic symptoms. This classification was validated prospectively in the pre-cART era[324]; this study found that the combination of poor immune response and tumor stage most accurately predicted survival. Subsequently, a prospective evaluation of the ACTG staging system conducted in the cART era showed that the combination of poor tumor stage and systemic illness identified patients with unfavorable prognosis[460] (Table 15.3. For classic KS, the classification focuses on tumor only and is based on a case series of 300 patients (Table 15.4). There are no staging systems specifically for iatrogenic or endemic KS.[63]

Early lesions can be mistaken clinically for purpura, hematomas, hemangiomas, and dermatofibromas, so a biopsy and histological confirmation is necessary, especially when lesions that are not entirely typical of KS occur. It is important to rule out mimics, such as bacillary angiomatosis and angiosarcoma when KS is associated with systemic symptoms. Other diseases that can be confused with KS clinically include lymphangioma, hemangioendothelioma, hemangiopericytoma, and pyogenic granuloma.

TABLE 15.2 Comparison of the epidemiological forms of Kaposi's sarcoma

Form of Kaposi's Sarcoma (KS)	Clinical Presentation	Risk Factors	Progression
Acquired immune deficiency syndrome (AIDS) related (also known as epidemic)	Multiple cutaneous lesions on the limbs, trunk, and face. Mucosal lesions are common (identified in 20% of cases) and visceral involvement is seen in 15% of cases. Patients can also present with tumor-associated edema.	The risk of KS rises with declining CD4 cell counts and falls with the use of combination antiretroviral therapy (cART).	May follow an indolent course but visceral involvement is not uncommon and may be aggressive. It may regress with effective cART.
Iatrogenic	Often presents as cutaneous KS lesions but both mucosal and, rarely, visceral disease can occur.	Occurs following solid organ allograft; the risk of occurrence correlates with the level of immunosuppression. Hence, the risk of occurrence is higher in multi-organ transplants and with greater human leukocyte antigen (HLA) mismatching.	Usually localized but may involve organs. It may regress with the reduction of immunosuppression or with modification of the immunosuppressive regimen.
Endemic	Children often present with multiple lymph nodes with lymphedema and a very aggressive natural history of the disease, including visceral dissemination. Adults present with lower limb lesions that resemble classic KS..	Occurs most commonly in sub-Saharan Africa in HIV-seronegative individuals	In children, progression is often aggressive with widespread lymphadenopathy and visceral involvement. In adults, progression is indolent or locally invasive but occasionally has visceral involvement.
Classic (also known as sporadic KS)	Typically confined to lower limbs with few lesions. Visceral and mucosal disease is rare and usually occurs in the gastrointestinal tract.	Occurs in middle-aged and elderly individuals and is more common in men than in women. Ethnic groups from regions of high Kaposi's sarcoma herpesvirus prevalence (Middle East, Eastern Europe, Mediterranean) are at increased risk.	Usually indolent; rarely aggressive and disseminated
HIV-negative MSM (men who have sex with men)	May occur at any skin sites, usually with few lesions. Visceral and mucosal disease is rare.	HIV-negative MSM who are young or middle aged and are not immunocompromised.	Usually indolent, although disseminated disease has been described

From Cesarman E, Damania B, Krown SE, et al. Kaposi sarcoma. *Nat Rev Dis Primers* 2019;5(1):9.

Laboratory Diagnosis

Diagnostic confirmation of KS is done through histopathology, as there are currently no blood tests for this disease, mostly because viremia is highly variable, and seropositivity does not necessarily indicate a diagnosis of KS. The histologic features of KS are essentially very heterogeneous and indistinguishable.[97] In skin, it affects the dermis, and similar to the clinical appearance of cutaneous KS, there is a range in the cellularity and microscopic appearance of the lesions. Lesions are characterized by the presence of jagged, thin-walled, and poorly formed dilated vascular spaces with large endothelial cells that may protrude into the lumen (Fig. 15.21). Between these vascular spaces is a spindle cell proliferation that can range from sparse to significant, sometimes forming sheets and extending irregularly in various directions. These spindle cells are considered to be the KS tumor cells. The elongated nuclei vary in size, and some are atypical, thus resembling a fibrosarcoma. However, the presence of narrow irregular, angulated slits containing erythrocytes among the spindle-shaped cells is a distinguishing feature of KS. These can be intertwined with normal vascular channels as well as lymphatic channels, some of which may show considerable cystic dilatation. There is a variable but consistently present inflammatory mononuclear cell infiltrate, composed of lymphocytes, plasma cells, and macrophages. Red blood cells and hemosiderin pigment are frequently present, often extravasated between the spindle cells. Small granules of intracytoplasmic or extracellular hyalin material may be identified. Granules of hemosiderin can also be seen within the spindle-shaped cells as a result of phagocytosis.[72,131] Confirmation of a diagnosis of KS is most commonly done by immunohistochemistry in formalin-fixed paraffin-embedded tissues using commercially available monoclonal antibodies to the KSHV latent nuclear antigen, LANA (ORF73). Since this protein is essential for viral episome maintenance, it is expressed by all the KSHV-infected cells. Using immunohistochemistry for LANA, KSHV is detected in a variable proportion of the spindle cells and endothelial cells lining the vascular spaces (Fig. 15.21). KSHV can also be detected by PCR in KS biopsies. Given that most cases of KS occur in Sub-Equatorial Africa, where there is a scarcity of pathology resources, new methods for easier and more affordable molecular testing of KSHV for the diagnosis of KS in poor-resource settings have been developed and are currently being evaluated.[561]

Clinical Course

The clinical course of disease can be highly variable. In general, initial presentation is usually a mild to moderate disease without symptomatic visceral symptoms, lymphatic obstruction or

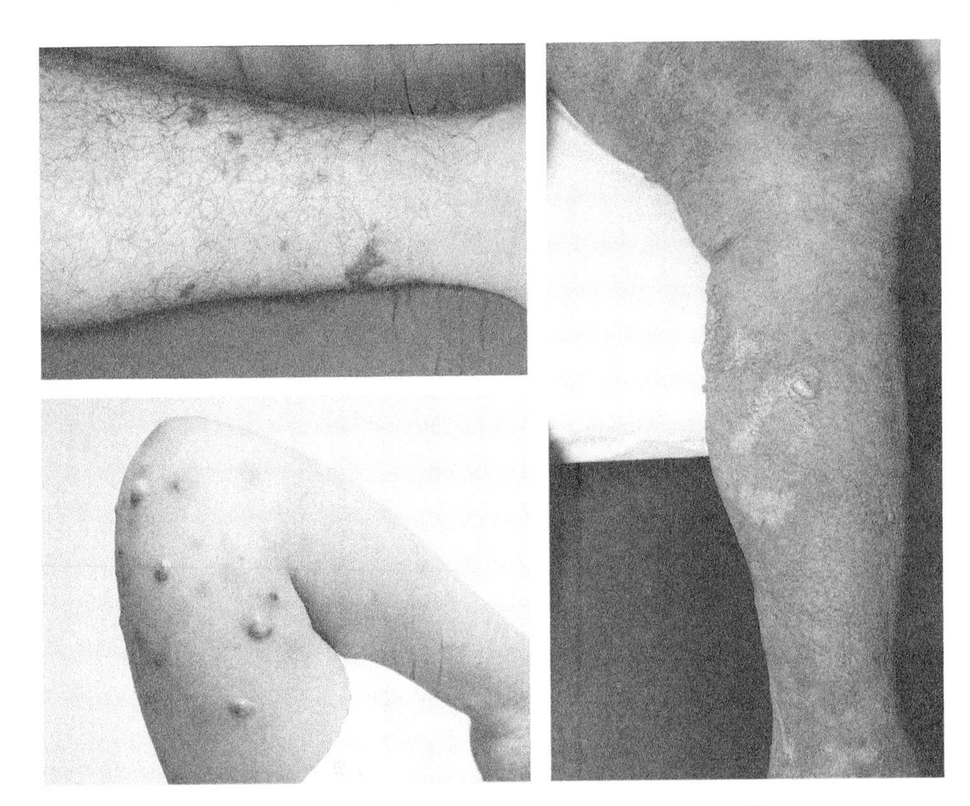

FIGURE 15.20 Cutaneous lesions of Kaposi's sarcoma. Upper left: Leg of HIV-negative patient with patch lesions. **Lower left:** Multiple nodules in arm of individual with AIDS. **Right:** HIV-infected individual with extensive involvement of lower extremities by KS. (Courtesy of Dr. Susan Krown.)

function-altering edema, difficulty swallowing or chewing, or any other functionally disabling manifestation, and has good clinical outcomes. It can be stable, have marked exacerbations, or even regress, especially in posttransplant patients in whom immunosuppressive therapy can be adjusted and HIV-infected individuals who begin antiretroviral therapy. The latter is likely due to the improvement of the immunological response to KSHV and possibly due to decreased circulating HIV-associated pro-angiogenic and inflammatory cytokines.[196]

Interestingly, in some patients, KS may progress dramatically, and even be fatal, upon treatment with antiretrovirals, due to an immune reconstitution inflammatory syndrome (IRIS).[133] Currently, diagnostic criteria for KS-IRIS include evidence of progressive KS within 12 weeks of initiating cART in parallel with the suppression of HIV-RNA levels by ≥0.5 to 1 log10 and/or an increase in CD4 T-cell counts by at least 50 cells/μL compared to pre-cART levels. Early systemic chemotherapy

TABLE 15.3 The modified AIDS Clinical Trials Group staging of AIDS-related KS

TIS Staging of KS	Good Risk (T0)	Poor Risk (T1)
(T) Tumor	Confined to skin and/or lymph nodes, or minimal oral disease	Tumor-associated edema or ulceration, extensive oral Kaposi's sarcoma (KS), gastrointestinal KS or KS in other nonnodal viscera
(I) Immune status	CD4 cell count >150/mm^3	CD4 cell count <150/mm^3
(S) Systemic illness	Karnofsky performance status >70	Karnofsky performance status <70 or other HIV-related illness

From Cesarman E, Damania B, Krown SE, et al. Kaposi sarcoma. *Nat Rev Dis Primers* 2019;5(1):9.

TABLE 15.4 Staging of classic Kaposi's sarcoma

Stage	Description	Features
Stage 1	Maculonodular	Small macules and nodules primarily confined to the lower extremities
Stage 2	Infiltrative	Plaques mainly involving lower extremities, sometimes associated with a few nodules
Stage 3	Florid	Multiple angiomatous plaques and nodules involving the lower extremities that are often ulcerated
Stage 4	Disseminated	Multiple angiomatous nodules and plaques extending beyond the lower extremities

From Cesarman E, Damania B, Krown SE, et al. Kaposi sarcoma. *Nat Rev Dis Primers* 2019;5(1):9.

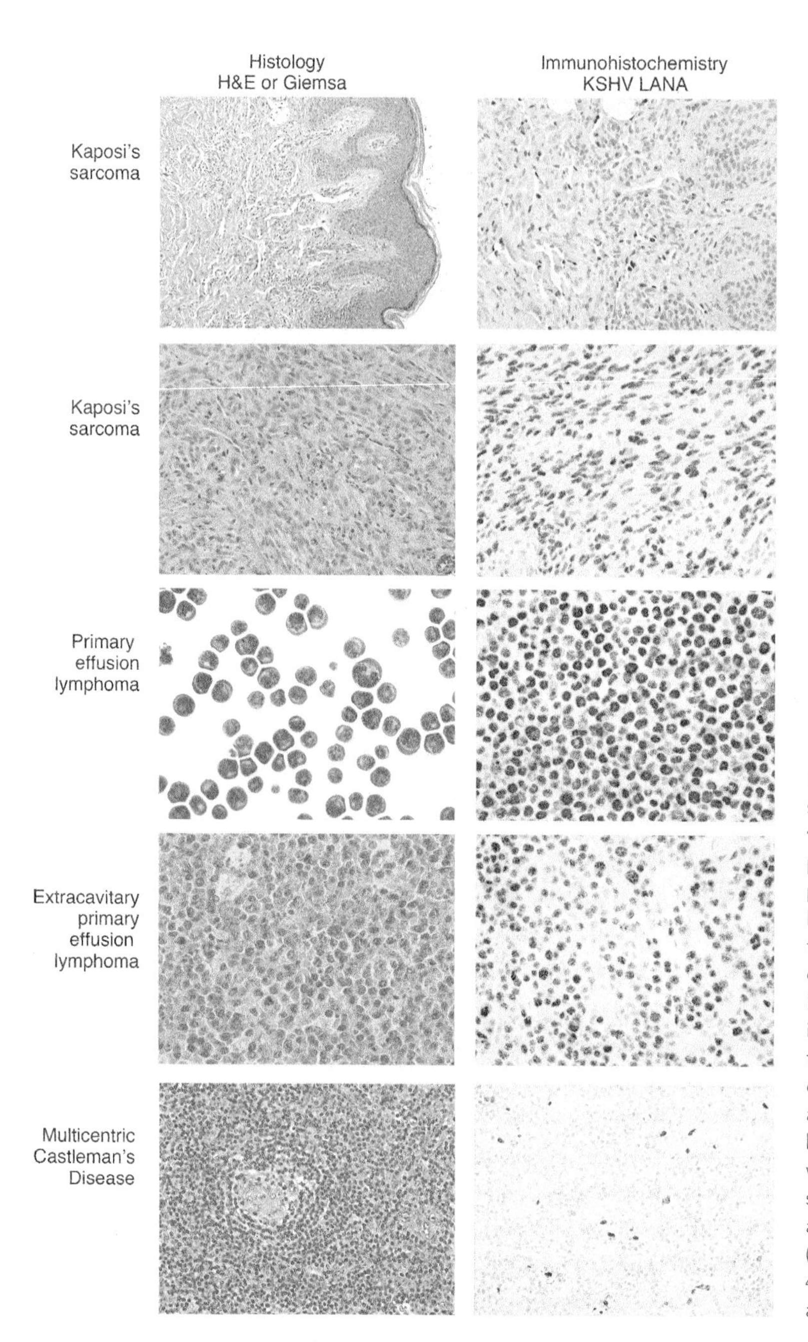

FIGURE 15.21 **Histologic features of Kaposi's sarcoma, primary effusion lymphoma and multicentric Castleman disease.** Skin biopsies of two different patients with KS are shown, illustrating the spindle cell proliferation and presence of irregular vascular spaces. **Left columns** are hematoxilin and eosin (H&E) staining of formalin fixed, paraffin-embedded tissues and the **right column** shows immunohistochemical (IHC) staining for LANA, demonstrating broad variability in the number of infected cells. The **third row** shows a cytospin preparation stained with Giemsa of a primary effusion lymphoma on the left, and IHC for LANA in the right, performed on a PEL cell block. The **fourth row** shows H&E staining of a biopsy from a patient with a non-Hodgkin lymphoma that was positive for KSHV LANA (right), therefore subclassified as extracavitary PEL. The lower row exemplifies a case of MCD, with scattered LANA-positive cells. (Original magnification, left column rows 1–2: 20x and 40x, rows 3–4: 60x, row 5: 20x; right column rows 1–2 and 5: 40x and rows 3–4 60x.)

can be effective in suppressing IRIS-associated flares,[265,357] but it has also been demonstrated that patients with IRIS not receiving chemotherapy can have good clinical outcomes if they survive the initial period of KS-IRIS.[622] KS-IRIS incidence and mortality were reported to be higher in Sub-Saharan Africa than in the United Kingdom, and this difference was attributed to more advanced KS and lower chemotherapy availability.[359] But it is also likely that careful management of systemic disease and coinfections in patients with IRIS improves the clinical outcome of these patients.

Treatment

cART has reduced the incidence of AIDS-KS in developed countries and can induce AIDS-KS regression in some individuals. Up to 80% of patients with T0 stage KS who were not previously treated with cART will require no other treatment for KS besides continued cART over 10 years.[58] HIV protease inhibitors have been shown to display direct antitumor activity,[434] but non–protease-inhibitor-containing antiretroviral combinations also induce KS regression.[56] However, KS remains a clinical problem,[465] and patients can present with HIV-KS in spite of having good HIV control and high CD4 counts.

Clinical staging is important for the decision on how to treat AIDS-KS.[97] cART should be given to patients with T0 early stage disease (if not already receiving this treatment for HIV), to which KS will often respond (i.e., lesions will shrink by 50% or more in size and/or number) within 6 to 12 months. T1 advanced-stage or progressive AIDS-related KS is best treated with liposomal anthracyclines, such as Doxil, in combination with cART. Another useful chemotherapeutic agent is paclitaxel. This is particularly important for cases with anthracycline-resistant disease and in health care settings where liposomal anthracyclines are not available, or the cost is prohibitive. One head-to-head comparison of pegylated liposomal doxorubicin and paclitaxel in the treatment of advanced AIDS-related KS showed no significant differences in response rate,[130] but paclitaxel has more toxicities. While clinical trials are still at an early stage and are small and limited, assessment of pathogenesis-directed therapies is ongoing. One notable example is the use of the mTOR inhibitor, rapamycin, given that KSHV activates this pathway. Complete regression of cutaneous KS was reported in patients with transplant-associated KS when the immunosuppressive therapy was switched to rapamycin.[80,568] Good response rates have been confirmed by other investigators in the majority of patients with transplant KS (cutaneous and visceral) when rapamycin was used as the immunosuppressive regimen.[235,343,703] Rapamycin has also shown some clinical responses in AIDS-KS,[327] but data regarding treatment with rapamycin in patients with KS in other risk groups are very limited.[230] It is difficult to know with certainty if the effects are due to changes in immune response to KSHV as a result of changing the immunosuppressive therapy, or to direct effects on the KSHV-infected lesional cells, or both. Recently, it was demonstrated that the use of MLN0128, another mTOR inhibitor, circumvents rapamycin and chemoresistant PEL.[87]

Additional pathogenesis-related treatments have shown promise in small clinical trials: imatinib, which inhibits tyrosine kinase–mediated transmembrane receptor signaling to prevent KS cell proliferation and angiogenesis[319]; bevacizumab, a monoclonal antibody inhibiting VEGF, which is an angiogenic growth factor that is highly expressed in KS lesions[605]; interleukin-12, a cytokine that enhances immune responses, mediates antiangiogenic effects, and down-regulates vGPCR activity[673]; immunomodulatory imide drugs (IMiDs), including thalidomide, lenalidomide, and pomalidomide, all of which possess anti-inflammatory, antiangiogenic and immunomodulatory properties[495]; and proteasome inhibitors, such as bortezomib,[510] which may promote the KSHV lytic cycle and/or inhibit NFκB signaling.

Primary Effusion Lymphoma

Soon after the discovery of KSHV in KS, viral sequences were also identified in a unique type of lymphoma,[95] referred to as PEL. Given the initial descriptive name of body cavity–based lymphoma (BCBL), many of the PEL cell lines are designated BC or BCBL. The first reported cases of malignant lymphoma occurring as body cavity effusions were described as AIDS-associated lymphohematopoietic neoplasms containing EBV and displaying an indeterminate immunophenotype.[315] In this first report of three cases, two were lymphomatous effusions, and a B-cell lineage was demonstrated by using DNA-based clonality assays. Subsequent studies recognized that these lymphomatous effusions occurred relatively frequently in HIV-infected individuals.[219,626] However, they were thought of as unusual AIDS-related lymphomas, and it only became clear that they represent a quite distinct clinicopathological entity with the recognition of the presence of KSHV within them.[451] As described above, the presence of KSHV in this subset of lymphomas allowed the development of cell lines that have been used as a tool for its propagation, for serologic assays and for viral purification. PELs contain many KSHV genomes, ranging from 40 to 80 copies per cell, a feature that has facilitated analysis of this virus.

PELs possess quite distinctive clinicopathologic features. Most importantly, they commonly present as lymphomatous effusions in body cavities, which are usually the pleural, peritoneal, or pericardial cavities, but can also occur in unusual sites, such as an artificial cavity related to the capsule of a breast implant or cerebrospinal fluid.[433,526] Although they are more common in HIV-positive males, HIV-negative men and women can also develop a PEL.[451,526] Because some KSHV-negative lymphomas, such as BL, can involve body cavities as lymphomatous effusions, and KSHV-positive lymphomas can present as solid-tissue masses, diagnostic criteria for PEL have been proposed.[451,505] These criteria include immunoblastic–anaplastic large-cell morphology (Fig. 15.21), null-cell phenotype (including the lack of B cell–associated antigen and immunoglobulin expression in most cases), and B-cell genotype. The expression of CD138/Syndecan-1[194] and hypermutation of the immunoglobulin genes[414] indicated that PELs are at a preterminal stage of B-cell differentiation. This assumption was confirmed by gene expression profiling of PEL,[286,313,479] as these studies found that PEL resembled plasma cells and had a profile between multiple myeloma and EBV-associated immunoblastic lymphoma.

Lymphomas containing KSHV can also arise with the first presentation as a solid tissue mass, nodal or extranodal, similar to other AIDS-related non-Hodgkin lymphomas. While some of these patients subsequently develop a lymphomatous effusion, others apparently do not. These cases may be diagnosed as diffuse large cell, immunoblastic, or anaplastic large cell lymphomas, in which the presence of KSHV in practically all the tumor cells has been demonstrated (Fig. 15.21).[101] Most of these are immunoblastic in appearance, have a high mitotic rate and variable amounts of apoptotic debris. Since these lymphomas have some of the defining features of PEL, including a similar morphology, they lack expression of B-cell antigens and immunoglobulin, and they are frequently coinfected with EBV, they have been classified as a variant of PEL, called either extracavitary PEL or solid PEL.

The almost invariable presence of KSHV in PELs suggests that it is necessary for the development of this disease. But like in the case of KS, infection by KSHV is necessary but clearly not sufficient, as PELs are very rare tumors, even in populations with high KSHV seroprevalence. The true incidence of PEL is not known, but based on retrospective analyses of specimens seen in a pathology department, it is estimated to constitute approximately 4% of AIDS-related lymphomas and 0.4% of all AIDS unrelated diffuse large cell NHLs. Therefore, it is evident that KSHV infection represents only one of several events involved in the development of PEL. Another cofactor appears to be EBV, because many PELs contain both viral genomes. Analysis of the pattern of EBV gene expression in PELs revealed that only EBNA1 was expressed, corresponding to Latency I,[263,586] and expression of at least one EBV microRNA (BART2) has been shown.[469,663] In spite of the limited EBV gene expression in PEL, it has been shown that EBV plays a role in dually infected PEL since dominant-negative variants of EBNA-1 inhibit colony formation of PEL cells.[397]

The cellular genome of PEL has not been well characterized, likely due to the rarity of these disease. These tumors have complex cytogenetics but lack structural alterations in common lymphoma-associated oncogenes (MYC, BCL2, RAS, TP53, etc.), with the possible exception of mutations in the regulatory region of BCL-6 (the relevance of which is unclear because PELs do not express BCL6).[86,451] Two fragile site tumor suppressor genes FHIT and WWOX were found deleted in the majority of PEL cell lines.[520] Recurrent cytogenetic alterations are present, namely trisomy 7, trisomy 12, and aberrations in the proximal long arm of chromosome 1 (1q).[653] Mutational signatures revealed by DNA sequencing have shown an APOBEC signature in PEL, consistent with a cellular defense against viral infection.[624] These observations suggest that KSHV is the critical element for the development of PEL, which is supported by the essential role of several latent viral genes in this disease.

Survival with conventional chemotherapy was initially reported to be very poor, with a median survival of approximately 6 months.[451,552] Nevertheless, there are case reports of good outcomes with antiviral therapy, bortezomib, or rituximab[54,208,259,373,476,550] or pleurodesis with bleomycin.[675] A recent retrospective analysis of 20 patients seen at the NIH provides the best current appraisal of the viral, immunological, and clinical features of PEL.[393] These patients were diagnosed between 2000 and 2013 and treated with EPOCH. The main observations include more hypoalbuminemia, thrombocytopenia, and elevated IL-10 levels than patients with AIDS-related diffuse large B-cell lymphoma (DLBCL). The median overall survival was 22 months, with a plateau in survival after 2 years and a three-year cancer-specific survival of 47%. EBV+ cases had better survival and patients with elevated IL-6 had inferior survival. The outcomes in this study are better than in previous reports, but still quite poor. Clinical trials using pomalidomide or lenalidomide and EPOCH-R are ongoing and may lead to improved survival.

Multicentric Castleman Disease

Castleman disease is an atypical lymphoproliferative disorder that encompasses various clinicopathologic entities. There have been both pathological and clinical classifications, which overlap partially. Two distinct histopathologic subtypes were described prior to the identification of KSHV: the more common hyaline vascular type and the plasma cell type.[307] Clinically, Castleman disease can be localized, or the patient may have multiple enlarged lymph nodes, therefore called "multicentric" Castleman disease (MCD). Approximately 90% of patients with MCD have the plasma cell type morphology. Systemic constitutional symptoms in MCD include fevers, malaise, wasting, hypoalbuminemia, cytopenias, and hyponatremia.[641] There is a strong risk for these patients to develop malignancies, most commonly KS and NHL, and soon after the discovery of KSHV, association of this virus with MCD was described.[567] Approximately half of MCD cases from immunocompetent individuals have detectable KSHV, while in individuals with HIV, almost all patients with MCD have KSHV in involved lymph nodes. Currently MCD is divided into idiopathic and KSHV-associated categories, which are considered to be different disease entities with overlapping histologic features.

The presence of both KS and MCD in a single lymph node is not uncommon in HIV-positive patients. Notably, MCD, also called multicentric angiofollicular hyperplasia in early publications, is characterized histologically by a vascular proliferation, which is reminiscent of KS. One study showed that KSHV-positive endothelial cells can also be found in MCD lymph nodes, in both HIV-positive and HIV-negative patients.[67] The KSHV-infected B cells can be numerous, coalesce, and form microlymphomas or frank lymphomas. KSHV-infected plasmablasts are B cells that are monotypic but polyclonal, almost invariably expressing IgM-lambda.[170] These infected cells are different from PEL cells in terms of B-cell differentiation, in that they lack somatic hypermutation of the Ig genes and they express cytoplasmic Ig but lack expression of CD138 and variably express CD27.[102,170] Therefore, it appears that even if both PEL and MCD originate from KSHV-infected pre–terminally differentiated B cells, infected cells in MCD arise from extrafollicular B cells that did not undergo a germinal center reaction, whereas PELs may originate from cells that have traversed the germinal center. An explanation for the Ig lambda restriction is that KSHV induces up-regulation of Rag proteins leading to Ig recombination in a process called B-cell receptor revision.[601] Since kappa light chains rearrange first, receptor revision leads to subsequent recombination leading to V(D)J recombination and expression of lambda light chains.

Lymphomas arising in KSHV-associated MCD have been described mainly as occurring in HIV-positive patients,[174] and were originally called plasmablastic lymphomas and subsequently lymphoma arising in KSHV-associated MCD.[585] More recently, this has been replaced by "HHV8-positive diffuse large B-cell lymphoma, not otherwise specified" in the current WHO classification.[585] These lymphomas are usually associated with MCD, but not always. They are usually EBV negative, do not contain mutations in the immunoglobulin genes, and are thought to arise from naïve IgM lambda-expressing B cells rather than terminally differentiated B cells. A different rare entity has also been reported, called germinotropic lymphoproliferative disorder, in which germinal center B cells are coinfected with EBV and KSHV.[171] It appears that KSHV-associated lymphoid proliferations encompass a set of entities ranging from MCD, to microlymphomas, to monoclonal B-cell expansion with a range of clinical and pathological features, which may be overlapping among these different entities.[610]

Systemic symptoms in MCD are believed to be a result of production of excess cytokines, and in particular interleukin-6 (IL-6), and probably both the cellular and viral versions of this cytokine contribute to pathogenesis. vIL-6 has been demonstrated to be expressed in MCD in scattered plasmablasts surrounding the lymphoid follicles.[81,482,570] Lytic antigens are also expressed more frequently in KSHV-infected cells in MCD than in other disorders associated with this virus, indicating that lytic viral replication may be a feature of MCD.[299] It is possible that MCD falls in the spectrum of KSHV-associated lymphadenopathies, as KSHV-infected cells can be found in lymph node biopsies in patients with HIV-associated lymphadenopathy that lack all the defining pathologic characteristics of MCD.[100]

Median survival of HIV-associated MCD in the pre-cART era was approximately of 14 months.[475] A variety of approaches have been used for the treatment of patients with MCD, including cytotoxic chemotherapy, with variable success.[55] Evidence of lytic viral expression has led to testing of ganciclovir or other antiviral therapy, with mixed results.[92,135] The best responses have been obtained with the advent of two different antibody therapies. A humanized anti–human interleukin-6 (IL-6) receptor monoclonal antibody (tocilizumab) has been reported to result in clinical responses in two studies of patients in Japan, but the patients did not have AIDS, and only two patients were positive for KSHV.[468,566] Larger studies have used the humanized monoclonal anti-CD20 antibody, rituximab, which has resulted in successful treatment with responses in approximately 70% of patients.[42,57,135,206] The mechanism of action is not very clear, since KSHV-infected cells in MCD frequently lack expression of CD20.[102] The use of rituximab monotherapy for good performance status patients without organ involvement and rituximab with chemotherapy for more aggressive disease has been recommended[55] although rituximab was reported to exacerbate or unmask KS.[57] A report demonstrated that targeting lytic proteins, ORF21 and ORF36 with valganciclovir and zidovudine, respectively, showed very promising results.[604]

KSHV Inflammatory Cytokine Syndrome

An inflammatory syndrome with symptoms very similar to those of MCD has been described in patients with HIV and KS, but in the absence of generalized lymphadenopathy and without a pathologic diagnosis of MCD.[603] This entity was called KSHV inflammatory cytokine syndrome (KICS). These patients frequently have elevated levels of IL-6 and IL-10,[88,589] and may have other KSHV-associated tumors, such as KS or PEL. Outcome is poor, with a median survival of 13 months.[494] It is unclear how best to treat this disease.

PREVENTION AND CONTROL

Prevention of KSHV infection is challenging, especially in endemic areas where the prevalence rate is high, and transmission occurs mainly through saliva within families. Immunization would be ideal, but to this date, no candidate vaccines have been developed. As with EBV, it is difficult to use live, attenuated viruses because of the establishment of persistent infection and the potential danger of malignancy development.[660] So far, the clearly successful approach in individuals with HIV has been the use of antiretroviral therapy, which has led to a marked decrease in the incidence of KS. This decrease in the incidence of KS is believed to be due to improvement in immune function, but a direct role on KS or KSHV has also been proposed.[198] Several reports have shown regression of AIDS KS following treatment with protease inhibitor–based therapy, suggesting that this approach may be better for patients with AIDS and a high risk of KS than the use of nucleoside or nonnucleoside reverse transcriptase inhibitors.[342,413,655] However, one relatively small prospective study found that both regimens with and without protease inhibitors can decrease KSHV viremia and result in clinical improvement of KS, which occurred more commonly in patients that had undetectable or very low HIV loads.[209] Since a direct effect of HIV infection in KS pathogenesis has been proposed (e.g., due to paracrine angiogenic effects of Tat), it could be argued that control of HIV infection itself may be partly responsible for the beneficial effects of antiretroviral therapy.[33] Nevertheless, there is evidence that protease inhibitors have a direct role on KSHV. In particular, nelfinavir has been found to inhibit KSHV replication using a recombinant virus assay at concentrations that are achieved in plasma with standard oral dosing.[199] Nelfinavir has also been found to reduce viral shedding, potentially limiting transmission.[200]

Prevention of KS may also be possible in high-risk individuals using inhibitors of lytic replication, such as valganciclovir, which has been found to reduce KSHV shedding.[93] One study where ganciclovir was used for the treatment of CMV retinitis in patients with HIV showed that the incidence of KS was markedly reduced by 75%.[412] While oral valganciclovir did not show beneficial effects on HIV-negative patients with established KS, it appears that compounds that inhibit KSHV lytic replication may have a role in preventing the spread of KSHV and the development of KS. However, ganciclovir-associated toxicities make this approach impractical as a preventive strategy.

A preventive approach would be ideal to reduce the global burden of KS, and studies are under way to tackle this issue. An eventual HIV vaccine could greatly diminish the global incidence of KS, and development of a KSHV vaccine can potentially eliminate it altogether. In contrast to most malignancies, the geographic location of the majority of KS patients in low-resource countries makes these studies challenging. Nevertheless, our increased understanding of the pathobiology of KS and our increased armamentarium of targeted agents and immunomodulators makes preventing and curing KSHV-associated diseases an achievable goal.

ACKNOWLEDGMENTS

We thank S. Krown for medical images. We thank K. Christensen for scientific illustrations. We thank members of the Damania laboratory for proofreading. We had a strict limit on the number of references and profusely apologize for not including all possible literature citations. Please refer to the previous KSHV chapter edition from 2013 for some earlier citations we could not cite in this chapter.

REFERENCES

1. Abend JR, Uldrick T, Ziegelbauer JM. Regulation of tumor necrosis factor-like weak inducer of apoptosis receptor protein (TWEAKR) expression by Kaposi's sarcoma-associated herpesvirus microRNA prevents TWEAK-induced apoptosis and inflammatory cytokine expression. *J Virol* 2010;84(23):12139–12151.
2. Abere B, Mamo TM, Hartmann S, et al. The Kaposi's sarcoma-associated herpesvirus (KSHV) non-structural membrane protein K15 is required for viral lytic replication and may represent a therapeutic target. *PLoS Pathog* 2017;13(9):e1006639.
3. Aboulafia D, Mathisen G, Mitsuyasu R. Aggressive Kaposi's sarcoma and campylobacter bacteremia in a female with transfusion associated AIDS. *Am J Med Sci* 1991;301(4):256–258.
4. Ahmad A, Groshong JS, Matta H, et al. Kaposi sarcoma-associated herpesvirus-encoded viral FLICE inhibitory protein (vFLIP) K13 cooperates with Myc to promote lymphoma in mice. *Cancer Biol Ther* 2010;10(10):1033–1040.
5. AIDS-defining Cancer Project Working Group for IeDEA and COHERE in EuroCoord. Comparison of Kaposi sarcoma risk in human immunodeficiency virus-positive adults across 5 continents: a multiregional multicohort study. *Clin Infect Dis* 2017;65(8):1316–1326.
6. Akira S, Takeda K. Toll-like receptor signalling. *Nat Rev Immunol* 2004;4(7):499–511.
7. Akula SM, Wang FZ, Vieira J, et al. Human herpesvirus 8 interaction with target cells involves heparan sulfate. *Virology* 2001;282(2):245–255.
8. Akula SM, Pramod NP, Wang FZ, et al. Integrin alpha3beta1 (CD 49c/29) is a cellular receptor for Kaposi's sarcoma-associated herpesvirus (KSHV/HHV-8) entry into the target cells. *Cell* 2002;108(3):407–419.
9. Akula SM, Naranatt PP, Walia NS, et al. Kaposi's sarcoma-associated herpesvirus (human herpesvirus 8) infection of human fibroblast cells occurs through endocytosis. *J Virol* 2003;77(14):7978–7990.
10. Akula SM, Ford PW, Whitman AG, et al. B-Raf-dependent expression of vascular endothelial growth factor-A in Kaposi sarcoma-associated herpesvirus-infected human B cells. *Blood* 2005;105(11):4516–4522.
11. An J, Sun Y, Sun R, et al. Kaposi's sarcoma-associated herpesvirus encoded vFLIP induces cellular IL-6 expression: the role of the NF-kappaB and JNK/AP1 pathways. *Oncogene* 2003;22(22):3371–3385.

12. An J, Sun Y, Fisher M, et al. Antitumor effects of bortezomib (PS-341) on primary effusion lymphomas. *Leukemia* 2004;18(10):1699–1704.
13. An FQ, Compitello N, Horwitz E, et al. The latency-associated nuclear antigen of Kaposi's sarcoma-associated herpesvirus modulates cellular gene expression and protects lymphoid cells from p16 INK4A-induced cell cycle arrest. *J Biol Chem* 2005;280(5):3862–3874.
14. An FQ, Folarin HM, Compitello N, et al. Long-term-infected telomerase-immortalized endothelial cells: a model for Kaposi's sarcoma-associated herpesvirus latency in vitro and in vivo. *J Virol* 2006;80(10):4833–4846.
15. Anders PM, Zhang Z, Bhende PM, et al. The KSHV K1 Protein Modulates AMPK Function to Enhance Cell Survival. *PLoS Pathog* 2016;12(11):e1005985.
16. Anders PM, Montgomery ND, Montgomery SA, et al. Human herpesvirus-encoded kinase induces B cell lymphomas in vivo. *J Clin Invest* 2018;128(6):2519–2534.
17. Antman K, Chang Y. Kaposi's sarcoma. *N Engl J Med* 2000;342(14):1027–1038.
18. Aoki Y, Jaffe ES, Chang Y, et al. Angiogenesis and hematopoiesis induced by Kaposi's sarcoma-associated herpesvirus-encoded interleukin-6. *Blood* 1999;93(12):4034–4043.
19. Areste C, Mutocheluh M, Blackbourn DJ. Identification of caspase-mediated decay of interferon regulatory factor-3, exploited by a Kaposi sarcoma-associated herpesvirus immunoregulatory protein. *J Biol Chem* 2009;284(35):23272–23285.
20. Arvanitakis L, Geras-Raaka E, Varma A, et al. Human herpesvirus KSHV encodes a constitutively active G-protein-coupled receptor linked to cell proliferation. *Nature* 1997;385(6614):347–350.
21. AuCoin DP, Colletti KS, Cei SA, et al. Amplification of the Kaposi's sarcoma-associated herpesvirus/human herpesvirus 8 lytic origin of DNA replication is dependent upon a cis-acting AT-rich region and an ORF50 response element and the trans-acting factors ORF50 (K-Rta) and K8 (K-bZIP). *Virology* 2004;318(2):542–555.
22. Baeten JM, Chohan BH, Lavreys L, et al. Correlates of human herpesvirus 8 seropositivity among heterosexual men in Kenya. *AIDS* 2002;16(15):2073–2078.
23. Bais C, Santomasso B, Coso O, et al. G-protein-coupled receptor of Kaposi's sarcoma-associated herpesvirus is a viral oncogene and angiogenesis activator. *Nature* 1998;391(6662):86–89.
24. Bais C, Van Geelen A, Eroles P, et al. Kaposi's sarcoma associated herpesvirus G protein-coupled receptor immortalizes human endothelial cells by activation of the VEGF receptor-2/ KDR. *Cancer Cell* 2003;3(2):131–143.
25. Bala K, Bosco R, Gramolelli S, et al. Kaposi's sarcoma herpesvirus K15 protein contributes to virus-induced angiogenesis by recruiting PLCgamma1 and activating NFAT1-dependent RCAN1 expression. *PLoS Pathog* 2012;8(9):e1002927.
26. Ballestas ME, Kaye KM. Kaposi's sarcoma-associated herpesvirus latency-associated nuclear antigen 1 mediates episome persistence through cis-acting terminal repeat (TR) sequence and specifically binds TR DNA. *J Virol* 2001;75(7):3250–3258.
27. Ballestas ME, Chatis PA, Kaye KM. Efficient persistence of extrachromosomal KSHV DNA mediated by latency-associated nuclear antigen. *Science* 1999;284(5414):641–644.
28. Ballon G, Chen K, Perez R, et al. Kaposi sarcoma herpesvirus (KSHV) vFLIP oncoprotein induces B cell transdifferentiation and tumorigenesis in mice. *J Clin Invest* 2011;121(3):1141–1153.
29. Ballon G, Akar G, Cesarman E. Systemic expression of Kaposi sarcoma herpesvirus (KSHV) Vflip in endothelial cells leads to a profound proinflammatory phenotype and myeloid lineage remodeling in vivo. *PLoS Pathog* 2015;11(1):e1004581.
30. Bandyopadhyay C, Valiya-Veettil M, Dutta D, et al. CIB1 synergizes with EphrinA2 to regulate Kaposi's sarcoma-associated herpesvirus macropinocytic entry in human microvascular dermal endothelial cells. *PLoS Pathog* 2014;10(2):e1003941.
31. Barbera AJ, Ballestas ME, Kaye KM. The Kaposi's sarcoma-associated herpesvirus latency-associated nuclear antigen 1 N terminus is essential for chromosome association, DNA replication, and episome persistence. *J Virol* 2004;78(1):294–301.
32. Barbera AJ, Chodaparambil JV, Kelley-Clarke B, et al. The nucleosomal surface as a docking station for Kaposi's sarcoma herpesvirus LANA. *Science* 2006;311(5762):856–861.
33. Barillari G, Ensoli B. Angiogenic effects of extracellular human immunodeficiency virus type 1 Tat protein and its role in the pathogenesis of AIDS-associated Kaposi's sarcoma. *Clin Microbiol Rev* 2002;15(2):310–326.
34. Bartee E, Mansouri M, Hovey Nerenberg BT, et al. Downregulation of major histocompatibility complex class I by human ubiquitin ligases related to viral immune evasion proteins. *J Virol* 2004;78(3):1109–1120.
35. Bartee E, McCormack A, Fruh K. Quantitative membrane proteomics reveals new cellular targets of viral immune modulators. *PLoS Pathog* 2006;2(10):e107.
36. Bechtel JT, Liang Y, Hvidding J, et al. Host range of Kaposi's sarcoma-associated herpesvirus in cultured cells. *J Virol* 2003;77(11):6474–6481.
37. Bechtel J, Grundhoff A, Ganem D. RNAs in the virion of Kaposi's sarcoma-associated herpesvirus. *J Virol* 2005;79(16):10138–10146.
38. Bechtel JT, Winant RC, Ganem D. Host and viral proteins in the virion of Kaposi's sarcoma-associated herpesvirus. *J Virol* 2005;79(8):4952–4964.
39. Belanger C, Gravel A, Tomoiu A, et al. Human herpesvirus 8 viral FLICE-inhibitory protein inhibits Fas-mediated apoptosis through binding and prevention of procaspase-8 maturation. *J Hum Virol* 2001;4(2):62–73.
40. Bellare P, Ganem D. Regulation of KSHV lytic switch protein expression by a virus-encoded microRNA: an evolutionary adaptation that fine-tunes lytic reactivation. *Cell Host Microbe* 2009;6(6):570–575.
41. Beral V, Peterman TA, Berkelman RL, et al. Kaposi's sarcoma among persons with AIDS: a sexually transmitted infection? *Lancet* 1990;335(8682):123–128.
42. Bestawros A, Michel R, Seguin C, et al. Multicentric Castleman's disease treated with combination chemotherapy and rituximab in four HIV-positive men: a case series. *Am J Hematol* 2008;83(6):508–511.
43. Bhagwat GP, Naik KG, Sachdeva R, et al. Disseminated lymphadenopathic Kaposi's sarcoma in Zambian children. *Med J Zambia* 1980;14(4):61–63.
44. Bhatt AP, Bhende PM, Sin SH, et al. Dual inhibition of PI3K and mTOR inhibits autocrine and paracrine proliferative loops in PI3K/Akt/mTOR-addicted lymphomas. *Blood* 2010;115(22):4455–4463.
45. Bhatt AP, Jacobs SR, Freemerman AJ, et al. Dysregulation of fatty acid synthesis and glycolysis in non-Hodgkin lymphoma. *Proc Natl Acad Sci U S A* 2012;109(29):11818–11823.
46. Bhatt AP, Wong JP, Weinberg MS, et al. A viral kinase mimics S6 kinase to enhance cell proliferation. *Proc Natl Acad Sci U S A* 2016;113(28):7876–7881.
47. Biggar RJ, Engels EA, Whitby D, et al. Antibody reactivity to latent and lytic antigens to human herpesvirus-8 in longitudinally followed homosexual men. *J Infect Dis* 2003;187(1):12–18.
48. Bigi R, Landis JT, An H, et al. Epstein-Barr virus enhances genome maintenance of Kaposi sarcoma-associated herpesvirus. *Proc Natl Acad Sci U S A* 2018;115(48):E11379–E11387.
49. Birkmann A, Mahr K, Ensser A, et al. Cell surface heparan sulfate is a receptor for human herpesvirus 8 and interacts with envelope glycoprotein K8.1. *J Virol* 2001;75(23):11583–11593.
50. Blackbourn DJ, Lennette ET, Ambroziak J, et al. Human herpesvirus 8 detection in nasal secretions and saliva. *J Infect Dis* 1998;177(1):213–216.
51. Blackbourn DJ, Fujimura S, Kutzkey T, et al. Induction of human herpesvirus-8 gene expression by recombinant interferon gamma. *AIDS* 2000;14(1):98–99.
52. Blasig C, Zietz C, Haar B, et al. Monocytes in Kaposi's sarcoma lesions are productively infected by human herpesvirus 8. *J Virol* 1997;71(10):7963–7968.
53. Blossom D., et al., eds. EBV and KSHV-related herpesviruses in non-human primates. In: *Human Herpesviruses: Biology, Therapy, and Immunoprophylaxis.* Cambridge: Cambridge University Press; 2007:Chapter 61.
54. Boulanger E, Agbalika F, Maarek O, et al. A clinical, molecular and cytogenetic study of 12 cases of human herpesvirus 8 associated primary effusion lymphoma in HIV-infected patients. *Hematol J* 2001;2(3):172–179.
55. Bower M. How I treat HIV-associated multicentric Castleman disease. *Blood* 2010;116(22):4415–4421.
56. Bower M, Palmieri C, Dhillon T. AIDS-related malignancies: changing epidemiology and the impact of highly active antiretroviral therapy. *Curr Opin Infect Dis* 2006;19(1):14–19.
57. Bower M, Newsom-Davis T, Naresh K, et al. Clinical features and outcome in HIV-associated multicentric Castleman's disease. *J Clin Oncol* 2011;29(18):2481–2486.
58. Bower M, Dalla Pria A, Coyle C, et al. Prospective stage-stratified approach to AIDS-related Kaposi's sarcoma. *J Clin Oncol* 2014;32(5):409–414.
59. Bowser BS, DeWire SM, Damania B. Transcriptional regulation of the K1 gene product of Kaposi's sarcoma-associated herpesvirus. *J Virol* 2002;76(24):12574–12583.
60. Bowser BS, Morris S, Song MJ, et al. Characterization of Kaposi's sarcoma-associated herpesvirus (KSHV) K1 promoter activation by Rta. *Virology* 2006;348(2):309–327.
61. Boyne JR, Colgan KJ, Whitehouse A. Recruitment of the complete hTREX complex is required for Kaposi's sarcoma-associated herpesvirus intronless mRNA nuclear export and virus replication. *PLoS Pathog* 2008;4(10):e1000194.
62. Boyne JR, Jackson BR, Taylor A, et al. Kaposi's sarcoma-associated herpesvirus ORF57 protein interacts with PYM to enhance translation of viral intronless mRNAs. *EMBO J* 2010;29(11):1851–1864.
63. Brambilla L, Boneschi V, Taglioni M, et al. Staging of classic Kaposi's sarcoma: a useful tool for therapeutic choices. *Eur J Dermatol* 2003;13(1):83–86.
64. Brayfield BP, Kankasa C, West JT, et al. Distribution of Kaposi sarcoma-associated herpesvirus/human herpesvirus 8 in maternal saliva and breast milk in Zambia: implications for transmission. *J Infect Dis* 2004;189(12):2260–2270.
65. Brinkmann MM, Glenn M, Rainbow L, et al. Activation of mitogen-activated protein kinase and NF-kappaB pathways by a Kaposi's sarcoma-associated herpesvirus K15 membrane protein. *J Virol* 2003;77(17):9346–9358.
66. Brinkmann MM, Pietrek M, Dittrich-Breiholz O, et al. Modulation of host gene expression by the K15 protein of Kaposi's sarcoma-associated herpesvirus. *J Virol* 2007;81(1):42–58.
67. Brousset P, Cesarman E, Meggetto F, et al. Colocalization of the viral interleukin-6 with latent nuclear antigen-1 of human herpesvirus-8 in endothelial spindle cells of Kaposi's sarcoma and lymphoid cells of multicentric Castleman's disease. *Hum Pathol* 2001;32(1):95–100.
68. Brown EE, Fallin D, Ruczinski I, et al. Associations of classic Kaposi sarcoma with common variants in genes that modulate host immunity. *Cancer Epidemiol Biomarkers Prev* 2006;15(5):926–934.
69. Brulois KF, Chang H, Lee AS, et al. Construction and manipulation of a new Kaposi's sarcoma-associated herpesvirus bacterial artificial chromosome clone. *J Virol* 2012;86(18):9708–9720.
70. Brulois K, Toth Z, Wong LY, et al. Kaposi's sarcoma-associated herpesvirus K3 and K5 ubiquitin E3 ligases have stage-specific immune evasion roles during lytic replication. *J Virol* 2014;88(16):9335–9349.
71. Bu W, Carroll KD, Palmeri D, et al. Kaposi's sarcoma-associated herpesvirus/human herpesvirus 8 ORF50/Rta lytic switch protein functions as a tetramer. *J Virol* 2007;81(11):5788–5806.
72. Bubman D, Cesarman E. Pathogenesis of Kaposi's sarcoma. *Hematol Oncol Clin North Am* 2003;17(3):717–745.
73. Bubman D, Guasparri I, Cesarman E. Deregulation of c-Myc in primary effusion lymphoma by Kaposi's sarcoma herpesvirus latency-associated nuclear antigen. *Oncogene* 2007;26(34):4979–4986.
74. Butler LM, Were WA, Balinandi S, et al. Human herpesvirus 8 infection in children and adults in a population-based study in rural Uganda. *J Infect Dis* 2010;203(5):625–634.
75. Butler LM, Were WA, Balinandi S, et al. Human herpesvirus 8 infection in children and adults in a population-based study in rural Uganda. *J Infect Dis* 2011;203(5):625–634.
76. Cadwell K, Coscoy L. Ubiquitination on nonlysine residues by a viral E3 ubiquitin ligase. *Science* 2005;309(5731):127–130.
77. Cai X, Cullen BR. Transcriptional origin of Kaposi's sarcoma-associated herpesvirus microRNAs. *J Virol* 2006;80(5):2234–2242.
78. Cai X, Lu S, Zhang Z, et al. Kaposi's sarcoma-associated herpesvirus expresses an array of viral microRNAs in latently infected cells. *Proc Natl Acad Sci U S A* 2005;102(15):5570–5575.
79. Campbell TB, Borok M, White IE, et al. Relationship of Kaposi sarcoma (KS)-associated herpesvirus viremia and KS disease in Zimbabwe. *Clin Infect Dis* 2003;36(9):1144–1151.
80. Campistol JM, Gutierrez-Dalmau A, Torregrosa JV. Conversion to sirolimus: a successful treatment for posttransplantation Kaposi's sarcoma. *Transplantation* 2004;77(5):760–762.

81. Cannon JS, Nicholas J, Orenstein JM, et al. Heterogeneity of viral IL-6 expression in HHV-8-associated diseases. *J Infect Dis* 1999;180(3):824–828.
82. Cannon MJ, Dollard SC, Smith DK, et al. Blood-borne and sexual transmission of human herpesvirus 8 in women with or at risk for human immunodeficiency virus infection. *N Engl J Med* 2001;344(9):637–643.
83. Cannon MJ, Operskalski EA, Mosley JW, et al. Lack of evidence for human herpesvirus-8 transmission via blood transfusion in a historical US cohort. *J Infect Dis* 2009;199(11):1592–1598.
84. Capan-Melser M, Mombo-Ngoma G, Akerey-Diop D, et al. Epidemiology of human herpes virus 8 in pregnant women and their newborns—a cross-sectional delivery survey in Central Gabon. *Int J Infect Dis* 2015;39:16–19.
85. Carbone A, Cilia AM, Gloghini A, et al. Establishment of HHV-8-positive and HHV-8-negative lymphoma cell lines from primary lymphomatous effusions. *Int J Cancer* 1997;73(4):562–569.
86. Carbone A, Cilia AM, Gloghini A, et al. Establishment and characterization of EBV-positive and EBV-negative primary effusion lymphoma cell lines harbouring human herpesvirus type-8. *Br J Haematol* 1998;102(4):1081–1089.
87. Caro-Vegas C, Bailey A, Bigi R, et al. Targeting mTOR with MLN0128 overcomes rapamycin and chemoresistant primary effusion lymphoma. *MBio* 2019;10(1).
88. Caro-Vegas C, Sellers S, Host KM, et al. Runaway Kaposi sarcoma-associated herpesvirus replication correlates with systemic IL-10 levels. *Virology* 2020;539:18–25.
89. Carroll PA, Brazeau E, Lagunoff M. Kaposi's sarcoma-associated herpesvirus infection of blood endothelial cells induces lymphatic differentiation. *Virology* 2004;328(1):7–18.
90. Carroll PA, Kenerson HL, Yeung RS, et al. Latent Kaposi's sarcoma-associated herpesvirus infection of endothelial cells activates hypoxia-induced factors. *J Virol* 2006;80(21):10802–10812.
91. Carroll KD, Khadim F, Spadavecchia S, et al. Direct interactions of Kaposi's sarcoma-associated herpesvirus/human herpesvirus 8 ORF50/Rta protein with the cellular protein octamer-1 and DNA are critical for specifying transactivation of a delayed-early promoter and stimulating viral reactivation. *J Virol* 2007;81(16):8451–8467.
92. Casper C, Nichols WG, Huang ML, et al. Remission of HHV-8 and HIV-associated multicentric Castleman disease with ganciclovir treatment. *Blood* 2004;103(5):1632–1634.
93. Casper C, Krantz EM, Corey L, et al. Valganciclovir for suppression of human herpesvirus-8 replication: a randomized, double-blind, placebo-controlled, crossover trial. *J Infect Dis* 2008;198(1):23–30.
94. Cavallin LE, Ma Q, Naipauer J, et al. KSHV-induced ligand mediated activation of PDGF receptor-alpha drives Kaposi's sarcomagenesis. *PLoS Pathog* 2018;14(7):e1007175.
95. Cesarman E, Chang Y, Moore PS, et al. Kaposi's sarcoma-associated herpesvirus-like DNA sequences in AIDS-related body-cavity-based lymphomas. *N Engl J Med* 1995;332(18):1186–1191.
96. Cesarman E, Moore PS, Rao PH, et al. In vitro establishment and characterization of two acquired immunodeficiency syndrome-related lymphoma cell lines (BC-1 and BC-2) containing Kaposi's sarcoma-associated herpesvirus-like (KSHV) DNA sequences. *Blood* 1995;86(7):2708–2714.
97. Cesarman E, Damania B, Krown SE, et al. Kaposi sarcoma. *Nat Rev Dis Primers* 2019;5(1):9.
98. Chaabna K, Bray F, Wabinga HR, et al. Kaposi sarcoma trends in Uganda and Zimbabwe: a sustained decline in incidence? *Int J Cancer* 2013;133(5):1197–1203.
99. Chadburn A, Cesarman E, Liu YF, et al. Molecular genetic analysis demonstrates that multiple posttransplantation lymphoproliferative disorders occurring in one anatomic site in a single patient represent distinct primary lymphoid neoplasms. *Cancer* 1995;75(11):2747–2756.
100. Chadburn A, Nador R, Cesarman E, et al. Kaposi's sarcoma-associated herpesvirus (KSHV) infection in progressive HIV-related lymphadenopathy (HIV-LAP). *J Acquir Immune Defic Syndr Hum Retrovirol* 1998;17(4):A19.
101. Chadburn A, Hyjek E, Mathew S, et al. KSHV-positive solid lymphomas represent an extra-cavitary variant of primary effusion lymphoma. *Am J Surg Pathol* 2004;28(11):1401–1416.
102. Chadburn A, Hyjek EM, Tam W, et al. Immunophenotypic analysis of the Kaposi sarcoma herpesvirus (KSHV; HHV-8)-infected B cells in HIV+ multicentric Castleman disease (MCD). *Histopathology* 2008;53(5):513–524.
103. Chandran B, Smith MS, Koelle DM, et al. Reactivities of human sera with human herpesvirus-8-infected BCBL-1 cells and identification of HHV-8-specific proteins and glycoproteins and the encoding cDNAs. *Virology* 1998;243(1):208–217.
104. Chandriani S, Ganem D. Array-based transcript profiling and limiting-dilution reverse transcription-PCR analysis identify additional latent genes in Kaposi's sarcoma-associated herpesvirus. *J Virol* 2010;84(11):5565–5573.
105. Chang PC, Li M. Kaposi's sarcoma-associated herpesvirus K-cyclin interacts with Cdk9 and stimulates Cdk9-mediated phosphorylation of p53 tumor suppressor. *J Virol* 2008;82(1):278–290.
106. Chang Y, Cesarman E, Pessin MS, et al. Identification of herpesvirus-like DNA sequences in AIDS-associated Kaposi's sarcoma. *Science* 1994;266(5192):1865–1869.
107. Chang Y, Moore PS, Talbot SJ, et al. Cyclin encoded by KS herpesvirus. *Nature* 1996;382(6590):410.
108. Chang PJ, Shedd D, Gradoville L, et al. Open reading frame 50 protein of Kaposi's sarcoma-associated herpesvirus directly activates the viral PAN and K12 genes by binding to related response elements. *J Virol* 2002;76(7):3168–3178.
109. Chang H, Dittmer DP, Shin YC, et al. Role of Notch signal transduction in Kaposi's sarcoma-associated herpesvirus gene expression. *J Virol* 2005;79(22):14371–14382.
110. Chang H, Wachtman LM, Pearson CB, et al. Non-human primate model of Kaposi's sarcoma-associated herpesvirus infection. *PLoS Pathog* 2009;5(10):e1000606.
111. Chatlynne LG, Ablashi DV. Seroepidemiology of Kaposi's sarcoma-associated herpesvirus (KSHV). *Semin Cancer Biol* 1999;9(3):175–185.
112. Chaudhary PM, Jasmin A, Eby MT, et al. Modulation of the NF-kappa B pathway by virally encoded death effector domains-containing proteins. *Oncogene* 1999;18(42):5738–5746.
113. Chen L, Lagunoff M. Establishment and maintenance of Kaposi's sarcoma-associated herpesvirus latency in B cells. *J Virol* 2005;79(22):14383–14391.
114. Chen L, Lagunoff M. The KSHV viral interleukin-6 is not essential for latency or lytic replication in BJAB cells. *Virology* 2007;359(2):425–435.
115. Chen J, Ueda K, Sakakibara S, et al. Transcriptional regulation of the Kaposi's sarcoma-associated herpesvirus viral interferon regulatory factor gene. *J Virol* 2000;74(18):8623–8634.
116. Chen J, Ueda K, Sakakibara S, et al. Activation of latent Kaposi's sarcoma-associated herpesvirus by demethylation of the promoter of the lytic transactivator. *Proc Natl Acad Sci U S A* 2001;98(7):4119–4124.
117. Chen D, Choi YB, Sandford G, et al. Determinants of secretion and intracellular localization of human herpesvirus 8 interleukin-6. *J Virol* 2009;83(13):6874–6882.
118. Chen D, Sandford G, Nicholas J. Intracellular signaling mechanisms and activities of human herpesvirus 8 interleukin-6. *J Virol* 2009;83(2):722–733.
119. Chen J, Ye F, Xie J, et al. Genome-wide identification of binding sites for Kaposi's sarcoma-associated herpesvirus lytic switch protein, RTA. *Virology* 2009;386(2):290–302.
120. Chen W, Sin SH, Wen KW, et al. Hsp90 inhibitors are efficacious against Kaposi Sarcoma by enhancing the degradation of the essential viral gene LANA, of the viral co-receptor EphA2 as well as other client proteins. *PLoS Pathog* 2012;8(11):e1003048.
121. Chen HS, De Leo A, Wang Z, et al. BET-inhibitors disrupt Rad21-dependent conformational control of KSHV latency. *PLoS Pathog* 2017;13(1):e1006100.
122. Chen J, Zhang X, Schaller S, et al. Ephrin receptor A4 is a new Kaposi's sarcoma-associated herpesvirus virus entry receptor. *MBio* 2019;10(1).
123. Cheung MC, Pantanowitz L, Dezube BJ. AIDS-related malignancies: emerging challenges in the era of highly active antiretroviral therapy. *Oncologist* 2005;10(6):412–426.
124. Choi YB, Nicholas J. Autocrine and paracrine promotion of cell survival and virus replication by human herpesvirus 8 chemokines. *J Virol* 2008;82(13):6501–6513.
125. Choi YB, Nicholas J. Bim nuclear translocation and inactivation by viral interferon regulatory factor. *PLoS Pathog* 2010;6(8):e1001031.
126. Choi JK, Lee BS, Shim SN, et al. Identification of the novel K15 gene at the rightmost end of the Kaposi's sarcoma-associated herpesvirus genome. *J Virol* 2000;74(1):436–446.
127. Choi YB, Choi Y, Harhaj EW. Peroxisomes support human herpesvirus 8 latency by stabilizing the viral oncogenic protein vFLIP via the MAVS-TRAF complex. *PLoS Pathog* 2018;14(5):e1007058.
128. Chugh P, Matta H, Schamus S, et al. Constitutive NF-kappaB activation, normal Fas-induced apoptosis, and increased incidence of lymphoma in human herpes virus 8 K13 transgenic mice. *Proc Natl Acad Sci U S A* 2005;102(36):12885–12890.
129. Chung YH, Means RE, Choi JK, et al. Kaposi's sarcoma-associated herpesvirus OX2 glycoprotein activates myeloid-lineage cells to induce inflammatory cytokine production. *J Virol* 2002;76(10):4688–4698.
130. Cianfrocca M, Lee S, Von Roenn J, et al. Randomized trial of paclitaxel versus pegylated liposomal doxorubicin for advanced human immunodeficiency virus-associated Kaposi sarcoma: evidence of symptom palliation from chemotherapy. *Cancer* 2010;116(16):3969–3977.
131. Cockerell CJ. Histopathological features of Kaposi's sarcoma in HIV infected individuals. *Cancer Surv* 1991;10:73–89.
132. Cohen A, Brodie C, Sarid R. An essential role of ERK signalling in TPA-induced reactivation of Kaposi's sarcoma-associated herpesvirus. *J Gen Virol* 2006;87(Pt 4):795–802.
133. Connick E, Kane MA, White IE, et al. Immune reconstitution inflammatory syndrome associated with Kaposi sarcoma during potent antiretroviral therapy. *Clin Infect Dis* 2004;39(12):1852–1855.
134. Conrad NK, Steitz JA. A Kaposi's sarcoma virus RNA element that increases the nuclear abundance of intronless transcripts. *EMBO J* 2005;24(10):1831–1841.
135. Corbellino M, Bestetti G, Scalamogna C, et al. Long-term remission of Kaposi sarcoma-associated herpesvirus-related multicentric Castleman disease with anti-CD20 monoclonal antibody therapy. *Blood* 2001;98(12):3473–3475.
136. Correia B, Cerqueira SA, Beauchemin C, et al. Crystal structure of the gamma-2 herpesvirus LANA DNA binding domain identifies charged surface residues which impact viral latency. *PLoS Pathog* 2013;9(10):e1003673.
137. Coscoy L, Ganem D. Kaposi's sarcoma-associated herpesvirus encodes two proteins that block cell surface display of MHC class I chains by enhancing their endocytosis. *Proc Natl Acad Sci U S A* 2000;97(14):8051–8056.
138. Coscoy L, Ganem D. A viral protein that selectively downregulates ICAM-1 and B7-2 and modulates T cell costimulation. *J Clin Invest* 2001;107(12):1599–1606.
139. Cotter MA, II, Robertson ES. The latency-associated nuclear antigen tethers the Kaposi's sarcoma-associated herpesvirus genome to host chromosomes in body cavity-based lymphoma cells. *Virology* 1999;264(2):254–264.
140. Cotter MA, II, Subramanian C, Robertson ES. The Kaposi's sarcoma-associated herpesvirus latency-associated nuclear antigen binds to specific sequences at the left end of the viral genome through its carboxy-terminus. *Virology* 2001;291(2):241–259.
141. Cottoni F, Masala MV, Santarelli R, et al. Susceptibility to human herpesvirus-8 infection in a healthy population from Sardinia is not directly correlated with the expression of HLA-DR alleles. *Br J Dermatol* 2004;151(1):247–249.
142. Covarrubias S, Gaglia MM, Kumar GR, et al. Coordinated destruction of cellular messages in translation complexes by the gammaherpesvirus host shutoff factor and the mammalian exonuclease Xrn1. *PLoS Pathog* 2011;7(10):e1002339.
143. Crabtree KL, Wojcicki JM, Minhas V, et al. Association of household food- and drink-sharing practices with human herpesvirus 8 seroconversion in a Cohort of Zambian children. *J Infect Dis* 2017;216(7):842–849.
144. Cuomo ME, Knebel A, Morrice N, et al. p53-Driven apoptosis limits centrosome amplification and genomic instability downstream of NPM1 phosphorylation. *Nat Cell Biol* 2008;10(6):723–730.
145. Dai X, Gong D, Xiao Y, et al. CryoEM and mutagenesis reveal that the smallest capsid protein cements and stabilizes Kaposi's sarcoma-associated herpesvirus capsid. *Proc Natl Acad Sci U S A* 2015;112(7):E649–E656.
146. Dai X, Gong D, Lim H, et al. Structure and mutagenesis reveal essential capsid protein interactions for KSHV replication. *Nature* 2018;553(7689):521–525.
147. Dalton-Griffin L, Wilson SJ, Kellam P. X-box binding protein 1 contributes to induction of the Kaposi's sarcoma-associated herpesvirus lytic cycle under hypoxic conditions. *J Virol* 2009;83(14):7202–7209.
148. Damania B, Jeong JH, Bowser BS, et al. Comparison of the Rta/Orf50 transactivator proteins of gamma-2-herpesviruses. *J Virol* 2004;78(10):5491–5499.

149. Davis DA, Rinderknecht AS, Zoeteweij JP, et al. Hypoxia induces lytic replication of Kaposi sarcoma-associated herpesvirus. *Blood* 2001;97(10):3244–3250.
150. Davis DA, Singer KE, Reynolds IP, et al. Hypoxia enhances the phosphorylation and cytotoxicity of ganciclovir and zidovudine in Kaposi's sarcoma-associated herpesvirus infected cells. *Cancer Res* 2007;67(14):7003–7010.
151. Davis DA, Naiman NE, Wang V, et al. Identification of caspase cleavage sites in KSHV latency-associated nuclear antigen and their effects on caspase-related host defense responses. *PLoS Pathog* 2015;11(7):e1005064.
152. Davis ZH, Verschueren E, Jang GM, et al. Global mapping of herpesvirus-host protein complexes reveals a transcription strategy for late genes. *Mol Cell* 2015;57(2):349–360.
153. de Sanjose S, Marshall V, Sola J, et al. Prevalence of Kaposi's sarcoma-associated herpesvirus infection in sex workers and women from the general population in Spain. *Int J Cancer* 2002;98(1):155–158.
154. Dedicoat M, Newton R, Alkharsah KR, et al. Mother-to-child transmission of human herpesvirus-8 in South Africa. *J Infect Dis* 2004;190(6):1068–1075.
155. Dela Cruz CS, Viswanathan SR, El-Guindy AS, et al. Complex N-linked glycans on Asn-89 of Kaposi sarcoma herpes virus-encoded interleukin-6 mediate optimal function by affecting cytokine protein conformation. *J Biol Chem* 2009;284(43):29269–29282.
156. Delgado T, Carroll PA, Punjabi AS, et al. Induction of the Warburg effect by Kaposi's sarcoma herpesvirus is required for the maintenance of latently infected endothelial cells. *Proc Natl Acad Sci U S A* 2010;107(23):10696–10701.
157. Delgado T, Sanchez EL, Camarda R, et al. Global metabolic profiling of infection by an oncogenic virus: KSHV induces and requires lipogenesis for survival of latent infection. *PLoS Pathog* 2012;8(8):e1002866.
158. Deng B, O'Connor CM, Kedes DH, et al. Cryo-electron tomography of Kaposi's sarcoma-associated herpesvirus capsids reveals dynamic scaffolding structures essential to capsid assembly and maturation. *J Struct Biol* 2008;161(3):419–427.
159. Denis D, Seta V, Regnier-Rosencher E, et al. A fifth subtype of Kaposi's sarcoma, classic Kaposi's sarcoma in men who have sex with men: a cohort study in Paris. *J Eur Acad Dermatol Venereol* 2018;32(8):1377–1384.
160. Denis D, Seta V, Regnier-Rosencher E, et al. A fifth subtype of Kaposi's sarcoma, classic Kaposi's sarcoma in men who have sex with men: a cohort study in Paris. *J Eur Acad Dermatol Venereol* 2018;32(8):1377–1384.
161. Dillon PJ, Gregory SM, Tamburro K, et al. Tousled-like kinases modulate reactivation of gammaherpesviruses from latency. *Cell Host Microbe* 2013;13(2):204–214.
162. Dittmer DP. Transcription profile of Kaposi's sarcoma-associated herpesvirus in primary Kaposi's sarcoma lesions as determined by real-time PCR arrays. *Cancer Res* 2003;63(9):2010–2015.
163. Dittmer D, Lagunoff M, Renne R, et al. A cluster of latently expressed genes in Kaposi's sarcoma-associated herpesvirus. *J Virol* 1998;72(10):8309–8315.
164. Dittmer D, Stoddart C, Renne R, et al. Experimental transmission of Kaposi's sarcoma-associated herpesvirus (KSHV/HHV-8) to SCID-hu Thy/Liv mice. *J Exp Med* 1999;190(12):1857–1868.
165. Dittmer DP, Hilscher CJ, Gulley ML, et al. Multiple pathways for Epstein-Barr virus episome loss from nasopharyngeal carcinoma. *Int J Cancer* 2008;123(9):2105–2112.
166. Dittmer DP, Damania B, Sin SH. Animal models of tumorigenic herpesviruses—an update. *Curr Opin Virol* 2015;14:145–150.
167. Dollard SC, Douglas D, Basavaraju SV, et al. Donor-derived Kaposi's sarcoma in a liver-kidney transplant recipient. *Am J Transplant* 2018;18(2):510–513.
168. Domsic JF, Chen HS, Lu F, et al. Molecular basis for oligomeric-DNA binding and episome maintenance by KSHV LANA. *PLoS Pathog* 2013;9(10):e1003672.
169. Dorak MT, Yee LJ, Tang J, et al. HLA-B, -DRB1/3/4/5, and -DQB1 gene polymorphisms in human immunodeficiency virus-related Kaposi's sarcoma. *J Med Virol* 2005;76(3):302–310.
170. Du MQ, Liu H, Diss TC, et al. Kaposi sarcoma-associated herpesvirus infects monotypic (IgM lambda) but polyclonal naive B cells in Castleman disease and associated lymphoproliferative disorders. *Blood* 2001;97(7):2130–2136.
171. Du MQ, Diss TC, Liu H, et al. KSHV- and EBV-associated germinotropic lymphoproliferative disorder. *Blood* 2002;100(9):3415–3418.
172. Duncan LM, Piper S, Dodd RB, et al. Lysine-63-linked ubiquitination is required for endolysosomal degradation of class I molecules. *EMBO J* 2006;25(8):1635–1645.
173. Dupin N, Fisher C, Kellam P, et al. Distribution of human herpesvirus-8 latently infected cells in Kaposi's sarcoma, multicentric Castleman's disease, and primary effusion lymphoma. *Proc Natl Acad Sci U S A* 1999;96(8):4546–4551.
174. Dupin N, Diss TL, Kellam P, et al. HHV-8 is associated with a plasmablastic variant of Castleman disease that is linked to HHV-8-positive plasmablastic lymphoma. *Blood* 2000;95(4):1406–1412.
175. Dutta D, Chakraborty S, Bandyopadhyay C, et al. EphrinA2 regulates clathrin mediated KSHV endocytosis in fibroblast cells by coordinating integrin-associated signaling and c-Cbl directed polyubiquitination. *PLoS Pathog* 2013;9(7):e1003510.
176. Duus KM, Lentchitsky V, Wagenaar T, et al. Wild-type Kaposi's sarcoma-associated herpesvirus isolated from the oropharynx of immune-competent individuals has tropism for cultured oral epithelial cells. *J Virol* 2004;78(8):4074–4084.
177. Dwyer J, Le Guelte A, Galan Moya EM, et al. Remodeling of VE-cadherin junctions by the human herpes virus 8 G-protein coupled receptor. *Oncogene* 2010;30(2):190–200.
178. Efklidou S, Bailey R, Field N, et al. vFLIP from KSHV inhibits anoikis of primary endothelial cells. *J Cell Sci* 2008;121(Pt 4):450–457.
179. Eltom MA, Mbulaiteye SM, Dada AJ, et al. Transmission of human herpesvirus 8 by sexual activity among adults in Lagos, Nigeria Aids 2002;16(18):2473–2478.
180. Engels EA, Mbulaiteye SM, Othieno E, et al. Kaposi sarcoma-associated herpesvirus in non-Hodgkin lymphoma and reactive lymphadenopathy in Uganda. *Hum Pathol* 2007;38(2):308–314.
181. Fakhari FD, Dittmer DP. Charting latency transcripts in Kaposi's sarcoma-associated herpesvirus by whole-genome real-time quantitative PCR. *J Virol* 2002;76(12): 6213–6223.
182. Fakhari FD, Jeong JH, Kanan Y, et al. The latency-associated nuclear antigen of Kaposi sarcoma-associated herpesvirus induces B cell hyperplasia and lymphoma. *J Clin Invest* 2006;116(3):735–742.
183. Faure A, Hayes M, Sugden B. How Kaposi's sarcoma-associated herpesvirus stably transforms peripheral B cells towards lymphomagenesis. *Proc Natl Acad Sci U S A* 2019;116(33):16519–16528.
184. Flamand L, Zeman RA, Bryant JL, et al. Absence of human herpesvirus 8 DNA sequences in neoplastic Kaposi's sarcoma cell lines. *J Acquir Immune Defic Syndr Hum Retrovirol* 1996;13(2):194–197.
185. Foreman KE, Bacon PE, Hsi ED, et al. In situ polymerase chain reaction-based localization studies support role of human herpesvirus-8 as the cause of two AIDS-related neoplasms: Kaposi's sarcoma and body cavity lymphoma. *J Clin Invest* 1997;99(12):2971–2978.
186. Foster-Cuevas M, Wright GJ, Puklavec MJ, et al. Human herpesvirus 8 K14 protein mimics CD200 in down-regulating macrophage activation through CD200 receptor. *J Virol* 2004;78(14):7667–7676.
187. Friborg J, Jr., Kong W, Hottiger MO, et al. p53 inhibition by the LANA protein of KSHV protects against cell death. *Nature* 1999;402(6764):889–894.
188. Friedman-Kien AE. Disseminated Kaposi's sarcoma syndrome in young homosexual men. *J Am Acad Dermatol* 1981;5(4):468–471.
189. Friedman-Kien AE, Saltzman BR, Cao YZ, et al. Kaposi's sarcoma in HIV-negative homosexual men. *Lancet* 1990;335(8682):168–169.
190. Fu W, Merola J, Malinis M, et al. Successful treatment of primary donor-derived human herpesvirus-8 infection and hepatic Kaposi Sarcoma in an adult liver transplant recipient. *Transpl Infect Dis* 2018;20(5):e12966.
191. Fujimuro M, Wu FY, ApRhys C, et al. A novel viral mechanism for dysregulation of beta-catenin in Kaposi's sarcoma-associated herpesvirus latency. *Nat Med* 2003;9(3):300–306.
192. Fuld S, Cunningham C, Klucher K, et al. Inhibition of interferon signaling by the Kaposi's sarcoma-associated herpesvirus full-length viral interferon regulatory factor 2 protein. *J Virol* 2006;80(6):3092–3097.
193. Gaglia MM, Rycroft CH, Glaunsinger BA. Transcriptome-wide cleavage site mapping on cellular mRNAs reveals features underlying sequence-specific cleavage by the viral ribonuclease SOX. *PLoS Pathog* 2015;11(12):e1005305.
194. Gaidano G, Gloghini A, Gattei V, et al. Association of Kaposi's sarcoma-associated herpesvirus-positive primary effusion lymphoma with expression of the CD138/syndecan-1 antigen. *Blood* 1997;90(12):4894–4900.
195. Gallo RC. The enigmas of Kaposi's sarcoma. *Science* 1998;282(5395):1837–1839.
196. Gallo RC. Some aspects of the pathogenesis of HIV-1-associated Kaposi's sarcoma. *J Natl Cancer Inst Monogr* 1998(23):55–57.
197. Gambus G, Bourboulia D, Esteve A, et al. Prevalence and distribution of HHV-8 in different subpopulations, with and without HIV infection, in Spain. *AIDS* 2001;15(9):1167–1174.
198. Gantt S, Casper C. Human herpesvirus 8-associated neoplasms: the roles of viral replication and antiviral treatment. *Curr Opin Infect Dis* 2011;24(4):295–301.
199. Gantt S, Carlsson J, Ikoma M, et al. The HIV protease inhibitor nelfinavir inhibits Kaposi sarcoma-associated herpesvirus replication in vitro. *Antimicrob Agents Chemother* 2011;55(6):2696–2703.
200. Gantt S, Cattamanchi A, Krantz E, et al. Reduced human herpesvirus-8 oropharyngeal shedding associated with protease inhibitor-based antiretroviral therapy. *J Clin Virol* 2014;60(2):127–132.
201. Gao SJ, Kingsley L, Li M, et al. KSHV antibodies among Americans, Italians and Ugandans with and without Kaposi's sarcoma. *Nat Med* 1996;2(8):925–928.
202. Gao SJ, Boshoff C, Jayachandra S, et al. KSHV ORF K9 (vIRF) is an oncogene which inhibits the interferon signaling pathway. *Oncogene* 1997;15(16):1979–1985.
203. Garber AC, Hu J, Renne R. Latency-associated nuclear antigen (LANA) cooperatively binds to two sites within the terminal repeat, and both sites contribute to the ability of LANA to suppress transcription and to facilitate DNA replication. *J Biol Chem* 2002;277(30):27401–27411.
204. Gay LA, Sethuraman S, Thomas M, et al. Modified cross-linking, ligation, and sequencing of hybrids (qCLASH) identifies Kaposi's sarcoma-associated herpesvirus MicroRNA targets in endothelial cells. *J Virol* 2018;92(8):e02138-17.
205. Gazouli M, Zavos G, Papaconstantinou I, et al. The interleukin-6–174 promoter polymorphism is associated with a risk of development of Kaposi's sarcoma in renal transplant recipients. *Anticancer Res* 2004;24(2C):1311–1314.
206. Gerard L, Berezne A, Galicier L, et al. Prospective study of rituximab in chemotherapy-dependent human immunodeficiency virus associated multicentric Castleman's disease: ANRS 117 CastlemaB Trial. *J Clin Oncol* 2007;25(22):3350–3356.
207. Gershengorn MC, Geras-Raaka E, Varma A, et al. Chemokines activate Kaposi's sarcoma-associated herpesvirus G protein-coupled receptor in mammalian cells in culture. *J Clin Invest* 1998;102(8):1469–1472.
208. Ghosh SK, Wood C, Boise LH, et al. Potentiation of TRAIL-induced apoptosis in primary effusion lymphoma through azidothymidine-mediated inhibition of NF-kappa B. *Blood* 2003;101(6):2321–2327.
209. Gill J, Bourboulia D, Wilkinson J, et al. Prospective study of the effects of antiretroviral therapy on Kaposi sarcoma—associated herpesvirus infection in patients with and without Kaposi sarcoma. *J Acquir Immune Defic Syndr* 2002;31(4):384–390.
210. Glaunsinger B, Chavez L, Ganem D. The exonuclease and host shutoff functions of the SOX protein of Kaposi's sarcoma-associated herpesvirus are genetically separable. *J Virol* 2005;79(12):7396–7401.
211. Glenn M, Rainbow L, Aurade F, et al. Identification of a spliced gene from Kaposi's sarcoma-associated herpesvirus encoding a protein with similarities to latent membrane proteins 1 and 2A of Epstein-Barr virus. *J Virol* 1999;73(8):6953–6963.
212. Godfrey A, Anderson J, Papanastasiou A, et al. Inhibiting primary effusion lymphoma by lentiviral vectors encoding short hairpin RNA. *Blood* 2005;105(6):2510–2518.
213. Gonzalez CM, Wang L, Damania B. Kaposi's sarcoma-associated herpesvirus encodes a viral deubiquitinase. *J Virol* 2009;83(19):10224–10233.
214. Gopal S, Fedoriw Y, Montgomery ND, et al. Multicentric Castleman's disease in Malawi. *Lancet* 2014;384(9948):1158.

215. Gottwein E, Cullen BR. A human herpesvirus microRNA inhibits p21 expression and attenuates p21-mediated cell cycle arrest. *J Virol* 2010;84(10):5229–5237.
216. Gottwein E, Mukherjee N, Sachse C, et al. A viral microRNA functions as an orthologue of cellular miR-155. *Nature* 2007;450(7172):1096–1099.
217. Gramolelli S, Weidner-Glunde M, Abere B, et al. Inhibiting the recruitment of PLCgamma1 to Kaposi's sarcoma herpesvirus K15 protein reduces the invasiveness and angiogenesis of infected endothelial cells. *PLoS Pathog* 2015;11(8):e1005105.
218. Grant MJ, Loftus MS, Stoja AP, et al. Superresolution microscopy reveals structural mechanisms driving the nanoarchitecture of a viral chromatin tether. *Proc Natl Acad Sci U S A* 2018;115(19):4992–4997.
219. Green I, Espiritu E, Ladanyi M, et al. Primary lymphomatous effusions in AIDS: a morphological, immunophenotypic, and molecular study. *Mod Pathol* 1995;8(1):39–45.
220. Gregory SM, West JA, Dillon PJ, et al. Toll-like receptor signaling controls reactivation of KSHV from latency. *Proc Natl Acad Sci U S A* 2009;106(28):11725–11730.
221. Gregory SM, Davis BK, West JA, et al. Discovery of a viral NLR homolog that inhibits the inflammasome. *Science* 2011;331(6015):330–334.
222. Grossmann C, Podgrabinska S, Skobe M, et al. Activation of NF-kappaB by the latent vFLIP gene of Kaposi's sarcoma-associated herpesvirus is required for the spindle shape of virus-infected endothelial cells and contributes to their proinflammatory phenotype. *J Virol* 2006;80(14):7179–7185.
223. Gruffat H, Portes-Sentis S, Sergeant A, et al. Kaposi's sarcoma-associated herpesvirus (human herpesvirus-8) encodes a homologue of the Epstein-Barr virus bZip protein EB1. *J Gen Virol* 1999;80 (Pt 3):557–561.
224. Grundhoff A, Ganem D. Mechanisms governing expression of the v-FLIP gene of Kaposi's sarcoma-associated herpesvirus. *J Virol* 2001;75(4):1857–1863.
225. Grundhoff A, Ganem D. The latency-associated nuclear antigen of Kaposi's sarcoma-associated herpesvirus permits replication of terminal repeat-containing plasmids. *J Virol* 2003;77(4):2779–2783.
226. Grundhoff A, Ganem D. Inefficient establishment of KSHV latency suggests an additional role for continued lytic replication in Kaposi sarcoma pathogenesis. *J Clin Invest* 2004;113(1):124–136.
227. Grundhoff A, Sullivan CS, Ganem D. A combined computational and microarray-based approach identifies novel microRNAs encoded by human gamma-herpesviruses. *RNA* 2006;12(5):733–750.
228. Guasparri I, Keller SA, Cesarman E. KSHV vFLIP is essential for the survival of infected lymphoma cells. *J Exp Med* 2004;199(7):993–1003.
229. Guasparri I, Wu H, Cesarman E. The KSHV oncoprotein vFLIP contains a TRAF-interacting motif and requires TRAF2 and TRAF3 for signalling. *EMBO Rep* 2006;7(1):114–119.
230. Guenova E, Metzler G, Hoetzenecker W, et al. Classic Mediterranean Kaposi's sarcoma regression with sirolimus treatment. *Arch Dermatol* 2008;144(5):692–693.
231. Guilluy C, Zhang Z, Bhende PM, et al. Latent KSHV infection increases the vascular permeability of human endothelial cells. *Blood* 2011;118(19):5344–5354.
232. Guito J, Lukac DM. KSHV reactivation and novel implications of protein isomerization on lytic switch control. *Viruses* 2015;7(1):72–109.
233. Gunther T, Grundhoff A. The epigenetic landscape of latent Kaposi sarcoma-associated herpesvirus genomes. *PLoS Pathog* 2010;6(6):e1000935.
234. Guo HG, Sadowska M, Reid W, et al. Kaposi's sarcoma-like tumors in a human herpesvirus 8 ORF74 transgenic mouse. *J Virol* 2003;77(4):2631–2639.
235. Gutierrez-Dalmau A, Sanchez-Fructuoso A, Sanz-Guajardo A, et al. Efficacy of conversion to sirolimus in posttransplantation Kaposi's sarcoma. *Transplant Proc* 2005;37(9): 3836–3838.
236. Gwack Y, Byun H, Hwang S, et al. CREB-binding protein and histone deacetylase regulate the transcriptional activity of Kaposi's sarcoma-associated herpesvirus open reading frame 50. *J Virol* 2001;75(4):1909–1917.
237. Gwack Y, Hwang S, Lim C, et al. Kaposi's Sarcoma-associated herpesvirus open reading frame 50 stimulates the transcriptional activity of STAT3. *J Biol Chem* 2002;277(8):6438–6442.
238. Gwack Y, Baek HJ, Nakamura H, et al. Principal role of TRAP/mediator and SWI/SNF complexes in Kaposi's sarcoma-associated herpesvirus RTA-mediated lytic reactivation. *Mol Cell Biol* 2003;23(6):2055–2067.
239. Gwack Y, Nakamura H, Lee SH, et al. Poly(ADP-ribose) polymerase 1 and Ste20-like kinase hKFC act as transcriptional repressors for gamma-2 herpesvirus lytic replication. *Mol Cell Biol* 2003;23(22):8282–8294.
240. Hahn AS, Desrosiers RC. Binding of the Kaposi's sarcoma-associated herpesvirus to the ephrin binding surface of the EphA2 receptor and its inhibition by a small molecule. *J Virol* 2014;88(16):8724–8734.
241. Hahn AS, Kaufmann JK, Wies E, et al. The ephrin receptor tyrosine kinase A2 is a cellular receptor for Kaposi's sarcoma-associated herpesvirus. *Nat Med* 2012;18(6): 961–966.
242. Hamza MS, Reyes RA, Izumiya Y, et al. ORF36 protein kinase of Kaposi's sarcoma herpesvirus activates the c-Jun N-terminal kinase signaling pathway. *J Biol Chem* 2004;279(37):38325–38330.
243. Hansen A, Henderson S, Lagos D, et al. KSHV-encoded miRNAs target MAF to induce endothelial cell reprogramming. *Genes Dev* 2010;24(2):195–205.
244. Hanson J. Standardization of proximal femur BMD measurements. International Committee for Standards in Bone Measurement. *Osteoporos Int* 1997;7(5):500–501.
245. Haque NS, Fallon JT, Taubman MB, et al. The chemokine receptor CCR8 mediates human endothelial cell chemotaxis induced by I-309 and Kaposi sarcoma herpesvirus-encoded vMIP-I and by lipoprotein(a)-stimulated endothelial cell conditioned medium. *Blood* 2001;97(1):39–45.
246. Haque M, Davis DA, Wang V, et al. Kaposi's sarcoma-associated herpesvirus (human herpesvirus 8) contains hypoxia response elements: relevance to lytic induction by hypoxia. *J Virol* 2003;77(12):6761–6768.
247. Haque M, Wang V, Davis DA, et al. Genetic organization and hypoxic activation of the Kaposi's sarcoma-associated herpesvirus ORF34–37 gene cluster. *J Virol* 2006;80(14): 7037–7051.
248. Harwood AR, Osoba D, Hofstader SL, et al. Kaposi's sarcoma in recipients of renal transplants. *Am J Med* 1979;67(5):759–765.
249. Hassman LM, Ellison TJ, Kedes DH. KSHV infects a subset of human tonsillar B cells, driving proliferation and plasmablast differentiation. *J Clin Invest* 2011;121(2):752–768.
250. Havemeier A, Gramolelli S, Pietrek M, et al. Activation of NF-kappaB by the Kaposi's sarcoma-associated herpesvirus K15 protein involves recruitment of the NF-kappaB-inducing kinase, IkappaB kinases, and phosphorylation of p65. *J Virol* 2014;88(22):13161–13172.
251. Hayward GS. KSHV strains: the origins and global spread of the virus. *Semin Cancer Biol* 1999;9(3):187–199.
252. He Z, Liu Y, Liang D, et al. Cellular corepressor TLE2 inhibits replication-and-transcription- activator-mediated transactivation and lytic reactivation of Kaposi's sarcoma-associated herpesvirus. *J Virol* 2010;84(4):2047–2062.
253. Hellert J, Weidner-Glunde M, Krausze J, et al. A structural basis for BRD2/4-mediated host chromatin interaction and oligomer assembly of Kaposi sarcoma-associated herpesvirus and murine gammaherpesvirus LANA proteins. *PLoS Pathog* 2013;9(10):e1003640.
254. Hellert J, Weidner-Glunde M, Krausze J, et al. The 3D structure of Kaposi sarcoma herpesvirus LANA C-terminal domain bound to DNA. *Proc Natl Acad Sci U S A* 2015;112(21): 6694–6699.
255. Hensler HR, Rappocciolo G, Rinaldo CR, et al. Cytokine production by human herpesvirus 8-infected dendritic cells. *J Gen Virol* 2009;90(Pt 1):79–83.
256. Herndier B, Ganem D. The biology of Kaposi's sarcoma. *Cancer Treat Res* 2001;104: 89–126.
257. Hesser CR, Karijolich J, Dominissini D, et al. N6-methyladenosine modification and the YTHDF2 reader protein play cell type specific roles in lytic viral gene expression during Kaposi's sarcoma-associated herpesvirus infection. *PLoS Pathog* 2018;14(4):e1006995.
258. Hladik W, Dollard SC, Mermin J, et al. Transmission of human herpesvirus 8 by blood transfusion. *N Engl J Med* 2006;355(13):1331–1338.
259. Hocqueloux L, Agbalika F, Oksenhendler E, et al. Long-term remission of an AIDS-related primary effusion lymphoma with antiviral therapy. *AIDS* 2001;15(2):280–282.
260. Hoek RM, Ruuls SR, Murphy CA, et al. Down-regulation of the macrophage lineage through interaction with OX2 (CD200). *Science* 2000;290(5497):1768–1771.
261. Hong YK, Foreman K, Shin JW, et al. Lymphatic reprogramming of blood vascular endothelium by Kaposi sarcoma-associated herpesvirus. *Nat Genet* 2004;36(7):683–685.
262. Hopcraft SE, Pattenden SG, James LI, et al. Chromatin remodeling controls Kaposi's sarcoma-associated herpesvirus reactivation from latency. *PLoS Pathog* 2018;14(9):e1007267.
263. Horenstein MG, Nador RG, Chadburn A, et al. Epstein-Barr virus latent gene expression in primary effusion lymphomas containing Kaposi's sarcoma-associated herpesvirus/human herpesvirus-8. *Blood* 1997;90(3):1186–1191.
264. Hosseinipour MC, Sweet KM, Xiong J, et al. Viral profiling identifies multiple subtypes of Kaposi's sarcoma. *MBio* 2014;5(5):e0163314.
265. Hosseinipour MC, Kang M, Krown SE, et al. As-needed vs immediate etoposide chemotherapy in combination with antiretroviral therapy for mild-to-moderate AIDS-associated Kaposi sarcoma in resource-limited settings: A5264/AMC-067 randomized clinical trial. *Clin Infect Dis* 2018;67(2):251–260.
265a. Host KM, et al. Kaposi's Sarcoma-Associated Herpesvirus Increases PD-L1 and Proinflammatory Cytokine Expression in Human Monocytes. *MBio* 2017;8(5):e00917-17.
266. Hu F, Nicholas J. Signal transduction by human herpesvirus 8 viral interleukin-6 (vIL-6) is modulated by the nonsignaling gp80 subunit of the IL-6 receptor complex and is distinct from signaling induced by human IL-6. *J Virol* 2006;80(21):10874–10878.
267. Hu J, Renne R. Characterization of the minimal replicator of Kaposi's sarcoma-associated herpesvirus latent origin. *J Virol* 2005;79(4):2637–2642.
268. Hu J, Garber AC, Renne R. The latency-associated nuclear antigen of Kaposi's sarcoma-associated herpesvirus supports latent DNA replication in dividing cells. *J Virol* 2002;76(22):11677–11687.
269. Hu J, Liu E, Renne R. Involvement of SSRP1 in latent replication of Kaposi's sarcoma-associated herpesvirus. *J Virol* 2009;83(21):11051–11063.
270. Hu J, Yang Y, Turner PC, et al. LANA binds to multiple active viral and cellular promoters and associates with the H3K4methyltransferase hSET1 complex. *PLoS Pathog* 2014;10(7):e1004240.
271. Hu H, Dong J, Liang D, et al. Genome-wide mapping of the binding sites and structural analysis of Kaposi's sarcoma-associated herpesvirus viral interferon regulatory factor 2 reveal that it is a DNA-binding transcription factor. *J Virol* 2016;90(3):1158–1168.
272. Huang YQ, Li JJ, Kaplan MH, et al. Human herpesvirus-like nucleic acid in various forms of Kaposi's sarcoma. *Lancet* 1995;345(8952):759–761.
273. Hwang KY, Choi YB. Modulation of mitochondrial antiviral signaling by human herpesvirus 8 interferon regulatory factor 1. *J Virol* 2016;90(1):506–520.
274. Hwang S, Gwack Y, Byun H, et al. The Kaposi's sarcoma-associated herpesvirus K8 protein interacts with CREB-binding protein (CBP) and represses CBP-mediated transcription. *J Virol* 2001;75(19):9509–9516.
275. Hwang SW, Kim D, Jung JU, et al. KSHV-encoded viral interferon regulatory factor 4 (vIRF4) interacts with IRF7 and inhibits interferon alpha production. *Biochem Biophys Res Commun* 2017;486(3):700–705.
276. IARC. *Cancer Today*. https://gco.iarc.fr/today/home.
277. Inn KS, Lee SH, Rathbun JY, et al. Inhibition of RIG-I-mediated signaling by Kaposi's sarcoma-associated herpesvirus-encoded deubiquitinase ORF64. *J Virol* 2011;85(20): 10899–10904.
278. Ishido S, Choi JK, Lee BS, et al. Inhibition of natural killer cell-mediated cytotoxicity by Kaposi's sarcoma-associated herpesvirus K5 protein. *Immunity* 2000;13(3):365–374.
279. Ishido S, Wang C, Lee BS, et al. Downregulation of major histocompatibility complex class I molecules by Kaposi's sarcoma-associated herpesvirus K3 and K5 proteins. *J Virol* 2000;74(11):5300–5309.
280. Izumiya Y, Ellison TJ, Yeh ET, et al. Kaposi's sarcoma-associated herpesvirus K-bZIP represses gene transcription via SUMO modification. *J Virol* 2005;79(15):9912–9925.
281. International Collaboration on HIV, Cancer. Highly active antiretroviral therapy and incidence of cancer in human immunodeficiency virus-infected adults. *J Natl Cancer Inst* 2000;92(22):1823–1830.

282. Jacobs S, Damania B. The viral interferon regulatory factors of KSHV: immunosuppressors or oncogenes? *Front Immunol* 2011;2:19.
283. Jacobs SR, Gregory SM, West JA, et al. The viral interferon regulatory factors of kaposi's sarcoma-associated herpesvirus differ in their inhibition of interferon activation mediated by toll-like receptor 3. *J Virol* 2013;87(2):798–806.
284. Jacobs SR, Stopford CM, West JA, et al. Kaposi's sarcoma-associated herpesvirus viral interferon regulatory factor 1 interacts with a member of the interferon-stimulated gene 15 pathway. *J Virol* 2015;89(22):11572–11583.
285. Jenner RG, Alba MM, Boshoff C, et al. Kaposi's sarcoma-associated herpesvirus latent and lytic gene expression as revealed by DNA arrays. *J Virol* 2001;75(2):891–902.
286. Jenner RG, Maillard K, Cattini N, et al. Kaposi's sarcoma-associated herpesvirus-infected primary effusion lymphoma has a plasma cell gene expression profile. *Proc Natl Acad Sci U S A* 2003;100(18):10399–10404.
287. Jeong JH, Hines-Boykin R, Ash JD, et al. Tissue specificity of the Kaposi's sarcoma-associated herpesvirus latent nuclear antigen (LANA/orf73) promoter in transgenic mice. *J Virol* 2002;76(21):11024–11032.
288. Jeong JH, Orvis J, Kim JW, et al. Regulation and autoregulation of the promoter for the latency-associated nuclear antigen of Kaposi's sarcoma-associated herpesvirus. *J Biol Chem* 2004;279(16):16822–16831.
289. Jha HC, Lu J, Verma SC, et al. Kaposi's sarcoma-associated herpesvirus genome programming during the early stages of primary infection of peripheral blood mononuclear cells. *MBio* 2014;5(6).
290. Johnson AS, Maronian N, Vieira J. Activation of Kaposi's sarcoma-associated herpesvirus lytic gene expression during epithelial differentiation. *J Virol* 2005;79(21):13769–13777.
291. Jones KD, Aoki Y, Chang Y, et al. Involvement of interleukin-10 (IL-10) and viral IL-6 in the spontaneous growth of Kaposi's sarcoma herpesvirus-associated infected primary effusion lymphoma cells. *Blood* 1999;94(8):2871–2879.
292. Jones T, Ramos da Silva S, Bedolla R, et al. Viral cyclin promotes KSHV-induced cellular transformation and tumorigenesis by overriding contact inhibition. *Cell Cycle* 2014;13(5):845–858.
293. Joo CH, Shin YC, Gack M, et al. Inhibition of interferon regulatory factor 7 (IRF7)-mediated interferon signal transduction by the Kaposi's sarcoma-associated herpesvirus viral IRF homolog vIRF3. *J Virol* 2007;81(15):8282–8292.
294. Judde JG, Lacoste V, Briere J, et al. Monoclonality or oligoclonality of human herpesvirus 8 terminal repeat sequences in Kaposi's sarcoma and other diseases. *J Natl Cancer Inst* 2000;92(9):729–736.
295. Kaleeba JA, Berger EA. Kaposi's sarcoma-associated herpesvirus fusion-entry receptor: cystine transporter xCT. *Science* 2006;311(5769):1921–1924.
296. Kang H, Lieberman PM. Cell cycle control of Kaposi's sarcoma-associated herpesvirus latency transcription by CTCF-cohesin interactions. *J Virol* 2009;83(12):6199–6210.
297. Kang JG, Pripuzova N, Majerciak V, et al. Kaposi's sarcoma-associated herpesvirus ORF57 promotes escape of viral and human interleukin-6 from microRNA-mediated suppression. *J Virol* 2011;85(6):2620–2630.
298. Kaposi M. Idiopathisches multiples Pigmentsarkom der Haut. *Arch Dermatol Syph* 1872;4:265–273.
299. Katano H, Sato Y, Kurata T, et al. Expression and localization of human herpesvirus 8-encoded proteins in primary effusion lymphoma, Kaposi's sarcoma, and multicentric Castleman's disease. *Virology* 2000;269(2):335–344.
300. Kati S, Hage E, Mynarek M, et al. Generation of high-titre virus stocks using BrK.219, a B-cell line infected stably with recombinant Kaposi's sarcoma-associated herpesvirus. *J Virol Methods* 2015;217:79–86.
301. Kato-Noah T, Xu Y, Rossetto CC, et al. Overexpression of the kaposi's sarcoma-associated herpesvirus transactivator K-Rta can complement a K-bZIP deletion BACmid and yields an enhanced growth phenotype. *J Virol* 2007;81(24):13519–13532.
302. Kaul R, Purushothaman P, Uppal T, et al. KSHV lytic proteins K-RTA and K8 bind to cellular and viral chromatin to modulate gene expression. *PLoS One* 2019;14(4):e0215394.
303. Kedes DH, Operskalski E, Busch M, et al. The seroepidemiology of human herpesvirus 8 (Kaposi's sarcoma-associated herpesvirus): distribution of infection in KS risk groups and evidence for sexual transmission. *Nat Med* 1996;2(8):918–924.
304. Kedes DH, Ganem D, Ameli N, et al. The prevalence of serum antibody to human herpesvirus 8 (Kaposi sarcoma-associated herpesvirus) among HIV-seropositive and high-risk HIV-seronegative women. *JAMA* 1997;277(6):478–481.
305. Kedes DH, Lagunoff M, Renne R, et al. Identification of the gene encoding the major latency-associated nuclear antigen of the Kaposi's sarcoma-associated herpesvirus. *J Clin Invest* 1997;100(10):2606–2610.
306. Kellam P, Boshoff C, Whitby D, et al. Identification of a major latent nuclear antigen, LNA-1, in the human herpesvirus 8 genome. *J Hum Virol* 1997;1(1):19–29.
307. Keller AR, Hochholzer L, Castleman B. Hyaline-vascular and plasma-cell types of giant lymph node hyperplasia of the mediastinum and other locations. *Cancer* 1972;29(3):670–683.
308. Keller SA, Schattner EJ, Cesarman E. Inhibition of NF-kappaB induces apoptosis of KSHV-infected primary effusion lymphoma cells. *Blood* 2000;96(7):2537–2542.
309. Kerkemeyer KLS, Mar A, Lai FYX. Kaposi's Sarcoma occurring in HIV infection controlled on HAART. *Am J Med* 2019.
310. Kerur N, Veettil MV, Sharma-Walia N, et al. IFI16 acts as a nuclear pathogen sensor to induce the inflammasome in response to Kaposi Sarcoma-associated herpesvirus infection. *Cell Host Microbe* 2011;9(5):363–375.
311. Kim Y, Cha S, Seo T. Activation of the phosphatidylinositol 3-kinase/Akt pathway by viral interferon regulatory factor 2 of Kaposi's sarcoma-associated herpesvirus. *Biochem Biophys Res Commun* 2016;470(3):650–656.
312. Kirshner JR, Lukac DM, Chang J, et al. Kaposi's sarcoma-associated herpesvirus open reading frame 57 encodes a posttranscriptional regulator with multiple distinct activities. *J Virol* 2000;74(8):3586–3597.
313. Klein U, Gloghini A, Gaidano G, et al. Gene expression profile analysis of AIDS-related primary effusion lymphoma (PEL) suggests a plasmablastic derivation and identifies PEL-specific transcripts. *Blood* 2003;101(10):4115–4121.
314. Kliche S, Nagel W, Kremmer E, et al. Signaling by human herpesvirus 8 kaposin A through direct membrane recruitment of cytohesin-1. *Mol Cell* 2001;7(4):833–843.
315. Knowles DM, Inghirami G, Ubriaco A, et al. Molecular genetic analysis of three AIDS-associated neoplasms of uncertain lineage demonstrates their B-cell derivation and the possible pathogenetic role of the Epstein-Barr virus. *Blood* 1989;73(3):792–799.
316. Knowles DM, Cesarman E, Chadburn A, et al. Correlative morphologic and molecular genetic analysis demonstrates three distinct categories of posttransplantation lymphoproliferative disorders. *Blood* 1995;85(2):552–565.
317. Koch S, Damas M, Freise A, et al. Kaposi's sarcoma-associated herpesvirus vIRF2 protein utilizes an IFN-dependent pathway to regulate viral early gene expression. *PLoS Pathog* 2019;15(5):e1007743.
318. Koelle DM, Huang ML, Chandran B, et al. Frequent detection of Kaposi's sarcoma-associated herpesvirus (human herpesvirus 8) DNA in saliva of human immunodeficiency virus-infected men: clinical and immunologic correlates. *J Infect Dis* 1997;176(1):94–102.
319. Koon HB, Krown SE, Lee JY, et al. Phase II trial of imatinib in AIDS-associated Kaposi's sarcoma: AIDS Malignancy Consortium Protocol 042. *J Clin Oncol* 2014;32(5):402–408.
320. Koopal S, Furuhjelm JH, Jarviluoma A, et al. Viral oncogene-induced DNA damage response is activated in Kaposi sarcoma tumorigenesis. *PLoS Pathog* 2007;3(9):1348–1360.
321. Krishnan HH, Naranatt PP, Smith MS, et al. Concurrent expression of latent and a limited number of lytic genes with immune modulation and antiapoptotic function by Kaposi's sarcoma-associated herpesvirus early during infection of primary endothelial and fibroblast cells and subsequent decline of lytic gene expression. *J Virol* 2004;78(7):3601–3620.
322. Krishnan HH, Sharma-Walia N, Streblow DN, et al. Focal adhesion kinase is critical for entry of Kaposi's sarcoma-associated herpesvirus into target cells. *J Virol* 2006;80(3):1167–1180.
323. Krown SE, Metroka C, Wernz JC. Kaposi's sarcoma in the acquired immune deficiency syndrome: a proposal for uniform evaluation, response, and staging criteria. AIDS Clinical Trials Group Oncology Committee. *J Clin Oncol* 1989;7(9):1201–1207.
324. Krown SE, Testa MA, Huang J. AIDS-related Kaposi's sarcoma: prospective validation of the AIDS Clinical Trials Group staging classification. AIDS Clinical Trials Group Oncology Committee. *J Clin Oncol* 1997;15(9):3085–3092.
325. Krown SE, Lee JY, Dittmer DP. More on HIV-associated Kaposi's sarcoma. *N Engl J Med* 2008;358(5):535–536; author reply 536.
326. Krown SE, Dittmer DP, Cesarman E. Pilot study of oral valganciclovir therapy in patients with classic kaposi sarcoma. *J Infect Dis* 2011;203(8):1082–1086.
327. Krown SE, Roy D, Lee JY, et al. Rapamycin with antiretroviral therapy in AIDS-associated Kaposi sarcoma: an AIDS Malignancy Consortium study. *J Acquir Immune Defic Syndr* 2012;59(5):447–454.
328. Kuang E, Wu F, Zhu F. Mechanism of sustained activation of ribosomal S6 kinase (RSK) and ERK by kaposi sarcoma-associated herpesvirus ORF45: multiprotein complexes retain active phosphorylated ERK AND RSK and protect them from dephosphorylation. *J Biol Chem* 2009;284(20):13958–13968.
329. Kumar B, Chandran B. KSHV entry and trafficking in target cells-hijacking of cell signal pathways, actin and membrane dynamics. *Viruses* 2016;8(11).
330. Kuny CV, Chinchilla K, Culbertson MR, et al. Cyclin-dependent kinase-like function is shared by the beta- and gamma- subset of the conserved herpesvirus protein kinases. *PLoS Pathog* 2010;6(9):e1001092.
331. Labo N, Miley W, Marshall V, et al. Heterogeneity and breadth of host antibody response to KSHV infection demonstrated by systematic analysis of the KSHV proteome. *PLoS Pathog* 2014;10(3):e1004046.
332. Lagos D, Vart RJ, Gratrix F, et al. Toll-like receptor 4 mediates innate immunity to Kaposi sarcoma herpesvirus. *Cell Host Microbe* 2008;4(5):470–483.
333. Lagunoff M, Majeti R, Weiss A, et al. Deregulated signal transduction by the K1 gene product of Kaposi's sarcoma-associated herpesvirus. *Proc Natl Acad Sci U S A* 1999;96(10):5704–5709.
334. Lagunoff M, Lukac DM, Ganem D. Immunoreceptor tyrosine-based activation motif-dependent signaling by Kaposi's sarcoma-associated herpesvirus K1 protein: effects on lytic viral replication. *J Virol* 2001;75(13):5891–5898.
335. Lagunoff M, Bechtel J, Venetsanakos E, et al. De novo infection and serial transmission of Kaposi's sarcoma-associated herpesvirus in cultured endothelial cells. *J Virol* 2002;76(5):2440–2448.
336. Lan K, Kuppers DA, Robertson ES. Kaposi's sarcoma-associated herpesvirus reactivation is regulated by interaction of latency-associated nuclear antigen with recombination signal sequence-binding protein Jkappa, the major downstream effector of the Notch signaling pathway. *J Virol* 2005;79(6):3468–3478.
337. Lan K, Kuppers DA, Verma SC, et al. Induction of Kaposi's sarcoma-associated herpesvirus latency-associated nuclear antigen by the lytic transactivator RTA: a novel mechanism for establishment of latency. *J Virol* 2005;79(12):7453–7465.
338. Lan K, Murakami M, Choudhuri T, et al. Intracellular-activated Notch1 can reactivate Kaposi's sarcoma-associated herpesvirus from latency. *Virology* 2006;351(2):393–403.
339. Lang F, Sun Z, Pei Y, et al. Shugoshin 1 is dislocated by KSHV-encoded LANA inducing aneuploidy. *PLoS Pathog* 2018;14(9):e1007253.
340. Lanternier F, Lebbe C, Schartz N, et al. Kaposi's sarcoma in HIV-negative men having sex with men. *AIDS* 2008;22(10):1163–1168.
341. Laura MV, de la Cruz-Herrera CF, Ferreiros A, et al. KSHV latent protein LANA2 inhibits sumo2 modification of p53. *Cell Cycle* 2015;14(2):277–282.
342. Lebbe C, Blum L, Pellet C, et al. Clinical and biological impact of antiretroviral therapy with protease inhibitors on HIV-related Kaposi's sarcoma. *AIDS* 1998;12(7):F45–F49.
343. Lebbe C, Euvrard S, Barrou B, et al. Sirolimus conversion for patients with posttransplant Kaposi's sarcoma. *Am J Transplant* 2006;6(9):2164–2168.
344. Lebbe C, Porcher R, Marcelin AG, et al. Human herpesvirus 8 (HHV8) transmission and related morbidity in organ recipients. *Am J Transplant* 2013;13(1):207–213.
345. Lee YJ, Glaunsinger BA. Aberrant herpesvirus-induced polyadenylation correlates with cellular messenger RNA destruction. *PLoS Biol* 2009;7(5):e1000107.

346. Lee H, Guo J, Li M, et al. Identification of an immunoreceptor tyrosine-based activation motif of K1 transforming protein of Kaposi's sarcoma-associated herpesvirus. *Mol Cell Biol* 1998;18(9):5219–5228.
347. Lee H, Veazey R, Williams K, et al. Deregulation of cell growth by the K1 gene of Kaposi's sarcoma-associated herpesvirus. *Nat Med* 1998;4(4):435–440.
348. Lee BS, Alvarez X, Ishido S, et al. Inhibition of intracellular transport of B cell antigen receptor complexes by Kaposi's sarcoma-associated herpesvirus K1. *J Exp Med* 2000;192(1):11–21.
349. Lee BS, Paulose-Murphy M, Chung YH, et al. Suppression of tetradecanoyl phorbol acetate-induced lytic reactivation of Kaposi's sarcoma-associated herpesvirus by K1 signal transduction. *J Virol* 2002;76(23):12185–12199.
350. Lee BS, Lee SH, Feng P, et al. Characterization of the Kaposi's sarcoma-associated herpesvirus K1 signalosome. *J Virol* 2005;79(19):12173–12184.
351. Lee HR, Toth Z, Shin YC, et al. Kaposi's sarcoma-associated herpesvirus viral interferon regulatory factor 4 targets MDM2 to deregulate the p53 tumor suppressor pathway. *J Virol* 2009;83(13):6739–6747.
352. Lee JS, Li Q, Lee JY, et al. FLIP-mediated autophagy regulation in cell death control. *Nat Cell Biol* 2009;11(11):1355–1362.
353. Lee HR, Doganay S, Chung B, et al. Kaposi's sarcoma-associated herpesvirus viral interferon regulatory factor 4 (vIRF4) targets expression of cellular IRF4 and the Myc gene to facilitate lytic replication. *J Virol* 2014;88(4):2183–2194.
354. Lee HR, Li F, Choi UY, et al. Deregulation of HDAC5 by viral interferon regulatory factor 3 plays an essential role in Kaposi's sarcoma-associated herpesvirus-induced lymphangiogenesis. *MBio* 2018;9(1).
355. Lehrnbecher TL, Foster CB, Zhu S, et al. Variant genotypes of FcgammaRIIIA influence the development of Kaposi's sarcoma in HIV-infected men. *Blood* 2000;95(7):2386–2390.
356. Lei X, Bai Z, Ye F, et al. Regulation of NF-kappaB inhibitor IkappaBalpha and viral replication by a KSHV microRNA. *Nat Cell Biol* 2010;12(2):193–199.
357. Leidner RS, Aboulafia DM. Recrudescent Kaposi's sarcoma after initiation of HAART: a manifestation of immune reconstitution syndrome. *AIDS Patient Care STDS* 2005;19(10):635–644.
358. Lennette ET, Blackbourn DJ, Levy JA. Antibodies to human herpesvirus type 8 in the general population and in Kaposi's sarcoma patients. *Lancet* 1996;348(9031):858–861.
359. Letang E, Lewis JJ, Bower M, et al. Immune reconstitution inflammatory syndrome associated with Kaposi sarcoma: higher incidence and mortality in Africa than in the UK. *AIDS* 2013;27(10):1603–1613.
360. Li H, Nicholas J. Identification of amino acid residues of gp130 signal transducer and gp80 alpha receptor subunit that are involved in ligand binding and signaling by human herpesvirus 8-encoded interleukin-6. *J Virol* 2002;76(11):5627–5636.
361. Li M, Lee H, Yoon DW, et al. Kaposi's sarcoma-associated herpesvirus encodes a functional cyclin. *J Virol* 1997;71(3):1984–1991.
362. Li M, Damania B, Alvarez X, et al. Inhibition of p300 histone acetyltransferase by viral interferon regulatory factor. *Mol Cell Biol* 2000;20(21):8254–8263.
363. Li H, Komatsu T, Dezube BJ, et al. The Kaposi's sarcoma-associated herpesvirus K12 transcript from a primary effusion lymphoma contains complex repeat elements, is spliced, and initiates from a novel promoter. *J Virol* 2002;76(23):11880–11888.
364. Li Q, Means R, Lang S, et al. Downregulation of gamma interferon receptor 1 by Kaposi's sarcoma-associated herpesvirus K3 and K5. *J Virol* 2007;81(5):2117–2127.
365. Li R, Zhu J, Xie Z, et al. Conserved herpesvirus kinases target the DNA damage response pathway and TIP60 histone acetyltransferase to promote virus replication. *Cell Host Microbe* 2011;10(4):390–400.
366. Li DJ, Verma D, Mosbruger T, et al. CTCF and Rad21 act as host cell restriction factors for Kaposi's sarcoma-associated herpesvirus (KSHV) lytic replication by modulating viral gene transcription. *PLoS Pathog* 2014;10(1):e1003880.
367. Li Y, Zhong C, Liu D, et al. Evidence for Kaposi sarcoma originating from mesenchymal stem cell through KSHV-induced mesenchymal-to-endothelial transition. *Cancer Res* 2018;78(1):230–245.
368. Li T, Ju E, Gao SJ. Kaposi sarcoma-associated herpesvirus miRNAs suppress CASTOR1-mediated mTORC1 inhibition to promote tumorigenesis. *J Clin Invest* 2019;129(8):3310–3323.
369. Li T, Zhu Y, Cheng F, et al. Oncogenic Kaposi's sarcoma-associated herpesvirus upregulates argininosuccinate synthase 1, a rate-limiting enzyme of the citrulline-nitric oxide cycle, to activate the STAT3 pathway and promote growth transformation. *J Virol* 2019;93(4).
370. Liang Y, Chang J, Lynch SJ, et al. The lytic switch protein of KSHV activates gene expression via functional interaction with RBP-Jkappa (CSL), the target of the Notch signaling pathway. *Genes Dev* 2002;16(15):1977–1989.
371. Liao W, Tang Y, Lin SF, et al. K-bZIP of Kaposi's sarcoma-associated herpesvirus/human herpesvirus 8 (KSHV/HHV-8) binds KSHV/HHV-8 Rta and represses Rta-mediated transactivation. *J Virol* 2003;77(6):3809–3815.
372. Lim C, Lee D, Seo T, et al. Latency-associated nuclear antigen of Kaposi's sarcoma-associated herpesvirus functionally interacts with heterochromatin protein 1. *J Biol Chem* 2003;278(9):7397–7405.
373. Lim ST, Rubin N, Said J, et al. Primary effusion lymphoma: successful treatment with highly active antiretroviral therapy and rituximab. *Ann Hematol* 2005;84(8):551–552.
374. Lin R, Genin P, Mamane Y, et al. HHV-8 encoded vIRF-1 represses the interferon antiviral response by blocking IRF-3 recruitment of the CBP/p300 coactivators. *Oncogene* 2001;20(7):800–811.
375. Lin CL, Li H, Wang Y, et al. Kaposi's sarcoma-associated herpesvirus lytic origin (ori-Lyt)-dependent DNA replication: identification of the ori-Lyt and association of K8 bZip protein with the origin. *J Virol* 2003;77(10):5578–5588.
376. Lindow M, Nansen A, Bartholdy C, et al. The virus-encoded chemokine vMIP-II inhibits virus-induced Tc1-driven inflammation. *J Virol* 2003;77(13):7393–7400.
377. Lingel A, Ehlers E, Wang Q, et al. Kaposi's sarcoma-associated herpesvirus reduces cellular myeloid differentiation primary-response gene 88 (MyD88) expression via modulation of its RNA. *J Virol* 2016;90(1):180–188.
378. Little RF, Merced-Galindez F, Staskus K, et al. A pilot study of cidofovir in patients with kaposi sarcoma. *J Infect Dis* 2003;187(1):149–153.
379. Liu C, Okruzhnov Y, Li H, et al. Human herpesvirus 8 (HHV-8)-encoded cytokines induce expression of and autocrine signaling by vascular endothelial growth factor (VEGF) in HHV-8-infected primary-effusion lymphoma cell lines and mediate VEGF-independent antiapoptotic effects. *J Virol* 2001;75(22):10933–10940.
380. Liu L, Eby MT, Rathore N, et al. The human herpes virus 8-encoded viral FLICE inhibitory protein physically associates with and persistently activates the Ikappa B kinase complex. *J Biol Chem* 2002;277(16):13745–13751.
381. Liu J, Martin HJ, Liao G, et al. The Kaposi's sarcoma-associated herpesvirus LANA protein stabilizes and activates c-Myc. *J Virol* 2007;81(19):10451–10459.
382. Liu G, Yu FX, Kim YC, et al. Kaposi sarcoma-associated herpesvirus promotes tumorigenesis by modulating the Hippo pathway. *Oncogene* 2015;34(27):3536–3546.
383. Liu D, Wang Y, Yuan Y. Kaposi's sarcoma-associated herpesvirus K8 is an RNA binding protein that regulates viral DNA replication in coordination with a noncoding RNA. *J Virol* 2018;92(7).
384. Lorenzo ME, Jung JU, Ploegh HL. Kaposi's sarcoma-associated herpesvirus K3 utilizes the ubiquitin-proteasome system in routing class major histocompatibility complexes to late endocytic compartments. *J Virol* 2002;76(11):5522–5531.
385. Lu F, Zhou J, Wiedmer A, et al. Chromatin remodeling of the Kaposi's sarcoma-associated herpesvirus ORF50 promoter correlates with reactivation from latency. *J Virol* 2003;77(21):11425–11435.
386. Lu F, Day L, Gao SJ, et al. Acetylation of the latency-associated nuclear antigen regulates repression of Kaposi's sarcoma-associated herpesvirus lytic transcription. *J Virol* 2006;80(11):5273–5282.
387. Lu F, Stedman W, Yousef M, et al. Epigenetic regulation of Kaposi's sarcoma-associated herpesvirus latency by virus-encoded microRNAs that target Rta and the cellular Rbl2-DNMT pathway. *J Virol* 2010;84(6):2697–2706.
388. Lu J, Jha HC, Verma SC, et al. Kaposi's sarcoma-associated herpesvirus-encoded LANA contributes to viral latent replication by activating phosphorylation of survivin. *J Virol* 2014;88(8):4204–4217.
389. Lubyova B, Pitha PM. Characterization of a novel human herpesvirus 8-encoded protein, vIRF-3, that shows homology to viral and cellular interferon regulatory factors. *J Virol* 2000;74(17):8194–8201.
390. Lukac DM, Renne R, Kirshner JR, et al. Reactivation of Kaposi's sarcoma-associated herpesvirus infection from latency by expression of the ORF 50 transactivator, a homolog of the EBV R protein. *Virology* 1998;252(2):304–312.
391. Lukac DM, Kirshner JR, Ganem D. Transcriptional activation by the product of open reading frame 50 of Kaposi's sarcoma-associated herpesvirus is required for lytic viral reactivation in B cells. *J Virol* 1999;73(11):9348–9361.
392. Luppi M, Barozzi P, Guaraldi G, et al. Human herpesvirus 8-associated diseases in solid-organ transplantation: importance of viral transmission from the donor. *Clin Infect Dis* 2003;37(4):606–607; author reply 607.
393. Lurain K, Polizzotto MN, Aleman K, et al. Viral, immunologic, and clinical features of primary effusion lymphoma. *Blood* 2019;133(16):1753–1761.
394. Ma Q, Cavallin LE, Yan B, et al. Antitumorigenesis of antioxidants in a transgenic Rac1 model of Kaposi's sarcoma. *Proc Natl Acad Sci U S A* 2009;106(21):8683–8688.
395. Ma Z, Jacobs SR, West JA, et al. Modulation of the cGAS-STING DNA sensing pathway by gammaherpesviruses. *Proc Natl Acad Sci U S A* 2015;112(31):E4306–E4315.
396. Ma Z, Hopcraft SE, Yang F, et al. NLRX1 negatively modulates type I IFN to facilitate KSHV reactivation from latency. *PLoS Pathog* 2017;13(5):e1006350.
397. Mack AA, Sugden B. EBV is necessary for proliferation of dually infected primary effusion lymphoma cells. *Cancer Res* 2008;68(17):6963–6968.
398. Maclean CM. Kaposi's sarcoma in Nigeria. *Br J Cancer* 1963;17:195–205.
399. Majerciak V, Pripuzova N, McCoy JP, et al. Targeted disruption of Kaposi's sarcoma-associated herpesvirus ORF57 in the viral genome is detrimental for the expression of ORF59, K8alpha, and K8.1 and the production of infectious virus. *J Virol* 2007;81(3):1062–1071.
400. Majerciak V, Yamanegi K, Allemand E, et al. Kaposi's sarcoma-associated herpesvirus ORF57 functions as a viral splicing factor and promotes expression of intron-containing viral lytic genes in spliceosome-mediated RNA splicing. *J Virol* 2008;82(6):2792–2801.
401. Majerciak V, Kruhlak M, Dagur PK, et al. Caspase-7 cleavage of Kaposi sarcoma-associated herpesvirus ORF57 confers a cellular function against viral lytic gene expression. *J Biol Chem* 2010;285(15):11297–11307.
402. Malik P, Blackbourn DJ, Clements JB. The evolutionarily conserved Kaposi's sarcoma-associated herpesvirus ORF57 protein interacts with REF protein and acts as an RNA export factor. *J Biol Chem* 2004;279(31):33001–33011.
403. Malope BI, Pfeiffer RM, Mbisa G, et al. Transmission of Kaposi sarcoma-associated herpesvirus between mothers and children in a South African population. *J Acquir Immune Defic Syndr* 2007;44(3):351–355.
404. Mancuso R, Biffi R, Valli M, et al. HHV8 a subtype is associated with rapidly evolving classic Kaposi's sarcoma. *J Med Virol* 2008;80(12):2153–2160.
405. Mancuso R, Brambilla L, Agostini S, et al. Intrafamiliar transmission of Kaposi's sarcoma-associated herpesvirus and seronegative infection in family members of classic Kaposi's sarcoma patients. *J Gen Virol* 2011;92(Pt 4):744–751.
406. Mansouri M, Rose PP, Moses AV, et al. Remodeling of endothelial adherens junctions by Kaposi's sarcoma-associated herpesvirus. *J Virol* 2008;82(19):9615–9628.
407. Manzano M, Patil A, Waldrop A, et al. Gene essentiality landscape and druggable oncogenic dependencies in herpesviral primary effusion lymphoma. *Nat Commun* 2018;9(1):3263.
408. Mariggio G, Koch S, Zhang G, et al. Kaposi Sarcoma Herpesvirus (KSHV) Latency-Associated Nuclear Antigen (LANA) recruits components of the MRN (Mre11-Rad50-NBS1) repair complex to modulate an innate immune signaling pathway and viral latency. *PLoS Pathog* 2017;13(4):e1006335.
409. Marshall V, Parks T, Bagni R, et al. Conservation of virally encoded microRNAs in Kaposi sarcoma—associated herpesvirus in primary effusion lymphoma cell lines and in patients with Kaposi sarcoma or multicentric Castleman disease. *J Infect Dis* 2007;195(5):645–659.

410. Martin JN. Diagnosis and epidemiology of human herpesvirus 8 infection. *Semin Hematol* 2003;40(2):133–142.
411. Martin JN, Ganem DE, Osmond DH, et al. Sexual transmission and the natural history of human herpesvirus 8 infection. *N Engl J Med* 1998;338(14):948–954.
412. Martin DF, Kuppermann BD, Wolitz RA, et al. Oral ganciclovir for patients with cytomegalovirus retinitis treated with a ganciclovir implant. Roche Ganciclovir Study Group. *N Engl J Med* 1999;340(14):1063–1070.
413. Martinelli C, Zazzi M, Ambu S, et al. Complete regression of AIDS-related Kaposi's sarcoma-associated human herpesvirus-8 during therapy with indinavir. *AIDS* 1998;12(13):1717–1719.
414. Matolcsy A, Nador RG, Cesarman E, et al. Immunoglobulin VH gene mutational analysis suggests that primary effusion lymphomas derive from different stages of B cell maturation. *Am J Pathol* 1998;153(5):1609–1614.
415. Matsumura S, Fujita Y, Gomez E, et al. Activation of the Kaposi's sarcoma-associated herpesvirus major latency locus by the lytic switch protein RTA (ORF50). *J Virol* 2005;79(13):8493–8505.
416. Matta H, Chaudhary PM. Activation of alternative NF-kappa B pathway by human herpes virus 8-encoded Fas-associated death domain-like IL-1 beta-converting enzyme inhibitory protein (vFLIP). *Proc Natl Acad Sci U S A* 2004;101(25):9399–9404.
417. Matta H, Chaudhary PM. The proteasome inhibitor bortezomib (PS-341) inhibits growth and induces apoptosis in primary effusion lymphoma cells. *Cancer Biol Ther* 2005;4(1):77–82.
418. Maurer T, Ponte M, Leslie K. HIV-associated Kaposi's sarcoma with a high CD4 count and a low viral load. *N Engl J Med* 2007;357(13):1352–1353.
419. Mbulaiteye S, Marshall V, Bagni RK, et al. Molecular evidence for mother-to-child transmission of Kaposi sarcoma-associated herpesvirus in Uganda and K1 gene evolution within the host. *J Infect Dis* 2006;193(9):1250–1257.
420. McCormick C, Ganem D. The kaposin B protein of KSHV activates the p38/MK2 pathway and stabilizes cytokine mRNAs. *Science* 2005;307(5710):739–741.
421. McCormick C, Ganem D. Phosphorylation and function of the kaposin B direct repeats of Kaposi's sarcoma-associated herpesvirus. *J Virol* 2006;80(12):6165–6170.
422. McGeoch DJ, Davison AJ. The descent of human herpesvirus 8. *Semin Cancer Biol* 1999;9(3):201–209.
423. McHugh D, Caduff N, Barros MHM, et al. Persistent KSHV infection increases EBV-associated tumor formation in vivo via enhanced EBV lytic gene expression. *Cell Host Microbe* 2017;22(1):61–73 e67.
424. McNamara RP, Chugh PE, Bailey A, et al. Extracellular vesicles from Kaposi Sarcoma-associated herpesvirus lymphoma induce long-term endothelial cell reprogramming. *PLoS Pathog* 2019;15(2):e1007536.
425. McPherson PS, Kay BK, Hussain NK. Signaling on the endocytic pathway. *Traffic* 2001;2(6):375–384.
426. Meads MB, Medveczky PG. Kaposi's sarcoma-associated herpesvirus-encoded viral interleukin-6 is secreted and modified differently than human interleukin-6: evidence for a unique autocrine signaling mechanism. *J Biol Chem* 2004;279(50):51793–51803.
427. Means RE, Ishido S, Alvarez X, et al. Multiple endocytic trafficking pathways of MHC class I molecules induced by a Herpesvirus protein. *EMBO J* 2002;21(7):1638–1649.
428. Means RE, Lang SM, Jung JU. The Kaposi's sarcoma-associated herpesvirus K5 E3 ubiquitin ligase modulates targets by multiple molecular mechanisms. *J Virol* 2007;81(12):6573–6583.
429. Meyer F, Ehlers E, Steadman A, et al. TLR-TRIF pathway enhances the expression of KSHV replication and transcription activator. *J Biol Chem* 2013;288(28):20435–20442.
430. Miller G, Heston L, Grogan E, et al. Selective switch between latency and lytic replication of Kaposi's sarcoma herpesvirus and Epstein-Barr virus in dually infected body cavity lymphoma cells. *J Virol* 1997;71(1):314–324.
431. Minhas V, Crabtree KL, Chao A, et al. Early childhood infection by human herpesvirus 8 in Zambia and the role of human immunodeficiency virus type 1 coinfection in a highly endemic area. *Am J Epidemiol* 2008;168(3):311–320.
432. Misstear K, Chanas SA, Rezaee SA, et al. Suppression of antigen-specific T cell responses by the Kaposi's sarcoma-associated herpesvirus viral OX2 protein and its cellular orthologue, CD200. *J Virol* 2012;86(11):6246–6257.
433. Moatamed NA, Song SX, Apple SK, et al. Primary effusion lymphoma involving the cerebrospinal fluid. *Diagn Cytopathol* 2011;40(7):635–638.
434. Monini P, Sgadari C, Toschi E, et al. Antitumour effects of antiretroviral therapy. *Nat Rev Cancer* 2004;4(11):861–875.
435. Montaner S, Sodhi A, Pece S, et al. The Kaposi's sarcoma-associated herpesvirus G protein-coupled receptor promotes endothelial cell survival through the activation of Akt/protein kinase B. *Cancer Res* 2001;61(6):2641–2648.
436. Montaner S, Sodhi A, Molinolo A, et al. Endothelial infection with KSHV genes in vivo reveals that vGPCR initiates Kaposi's sarcomagenesis and can promote the tumorigenic potential of viral latent genes. *Cancer Cell* 2003;3(1):23–36.
437. Montaner S, Sodhi A, Servitja JM, et al. The small GTPase Rac1 links the Kaposi sarcoma-associated herpesvirus vGPCR to cytokine secretion and paracrine neoplasia. *Blood* 2004;104(9):2903–2911.
438. Montaner S, Sodhi A, Ramsdell AK, et al. The Kaposi's sarcoma-associated herpesvirus G protein-coupled receptor as a therapeutic target for the treatment of Kaposi's sarcoma. *Cancer Res* 2006;66(1):168–174.
439. Moody R, Zhu Y, Huang Y, et al. KSHV microRNAs mediate cellular transformation and tumorigenesis by redundantly targeting cell growth and survival pathways. *PLoS Pathog* 2013;9(12):e1003857.
440. Moore PS, Chang Y. Detection of herpesvirus-like DNA sequences in Kaposi's sarcoma in patients with and without HIV infection. *N Engl J Med* 1995;332(18):1181–1185.
441. Morris TL, Arnold RR, Webster-Cyriaque J. Signaling cascades triggered by bacterial metabolic end products during reactivation of Kaposi's sarcoma-associated herpesvirus. *J Virol* 2007;81(11):6032–6042.
442. Morris VA, Punjabi AS, Lagunoff M. Activation of Akt through gp130 receptor signaling is required for Kaposi's sarcoma-associated herpesvirus-induced lymphatic reprogramming of endothelial cells. *J Virol* 2008;82(17):8771–8779.
443. Moses AV, Fish KN, Ruhl R, et al. Long-term infection and transformation of dermal microvascular endothelial cells by human herpesvirus 8. *J Virol* 1999;73(8):6892–6902.
444. Muller M, Hutin S, Marigold O, et al. A ribonucleoprotein complex protects the interleukin-6 mRNA from degradation by distinct herpesviral endonucleases. *PLoS Pathog* 2015;11(5):e1004899.
445. Muralidhar S, Pumfery AM, Hassani M, et al. Identification of kaposin (open reading frame K12) as a human herpesvirus 8 (Kaposi's sarcoma-associated herpesvirus) transforming gene. *J Virol* 1998;72(6):4980–4988.
446. Mutlu AD, Cavallin LE, Vincent L, et al. In vivo-restricted and reversible malignancy induced by human herpesvirus-8 KSHV: a cell and animal model of virally induced Kaposi's sarcoma. *Cancer Cell* 2007;11(3):245–258.
447. Myoung J, Ganem D. Active lytic infection of human primary tonsillar B cells by KSHV and its noncytolytic control by activated CD4+ T cells. *J Clin Invest* 2011;121(3):1130–1140.
448. Myoung J, Ganem D. Generation of a doxycycline-inducible KSHV producer cell line of endothelial origin: maintenance of tight latency with efficient reactivation upon induction. *J Virol Methods* 2011;174(1–2):12–21.
449. Myoung J, Ganem D. Infection of primary human tonsillar lymphoid cells by KSHV reveals frequent but abortive infection of T cells. *Virology* 2011;413(1):1–11.
450. Myskowski PL, Niedzwiecki D, Shurgot BA, et al. AIDS-associated Kaposi's sarcoma: variables associated with survival. *J Am Acad Dermatol* 1988;18(6):1299–1306.
451. Nador RG, Cesarman E, Chadburn A, et al. Primary effusion lymphoma: a distinct clinicopathologic entity associated with the Kaposi's sarcoma-associated herpes virus. *Blood* 1996;88(2):645–656.
452. Nakamura H, Li M, Zarycki J, et al. Inhibition of p53 tumor suppressor by viral interferon regulatory factor. *J Virol* 2001;75(16):7572–7582.
453. Nakamura H, Lu M, Gwack Y, et al. Global changes in Kaposi's sarcoma-associated virus gene expression patterns following expression of a tetracycline-inducible Rta transactivator. *J Virol* 2003;77(7):4205–4220.
454. Nalwoga A, Cose S, Nash S, et al. Relationship between anemia, malaria coinfection, and Kaposi sarcoma-associated herpesvirus seropositivity in a population-based study in rural Uganda. *J Infect Dis* 2018;218(7):1061–1065.
455. Nalwoga A, Nakibuule M, Marshall V, et al. Risk factors for Kaposi's sarcoma associated herpesvirus (KSHV) DNA in blood and in saliva in rural Uganda. *Clin Infect Dis* 2020;71(4):1055–1062.
456. Nalwoga A, Webb EL, Chihota B, et al. Kaposi's sarcoma-associated herpesvirus seropositivity is associated with parasite infections in Ugandan fishing communities on Lake Victoria islands. *PLoS Negl Trop Dis* 2019;13(10):e0007776.
457. Nanes BA, Grimsley-Myers CM, Cadwell CM, et al. p120-catenin regulates VE-cadherin endocytosis and degradation induced by the Kaposi sarcoma-associated ubiquitin ligase K5. *Mol Biol Cell* 2017;28(1):30–40.
458. Naranatt PP, Akula SM, Zien CA, et al. Kaposi's sarcoma-associated herpesvirus induces the phosphatidylinositol 3-kinase-PKC-zeta-MEK-ERK signaling pathway in target cells early during infection: implications for infectivity. *J Virol* 2003;77(2):1524–1539.
459. Naranatt PP, Krishnan HH, Smith MS, et al. Kaposi's sarcoma-associated herpesvirus modulates microtubule dynamics via RhoA-GTP-diaphanous 2 signaling and utilizes the dynein motors to deliver its DNA to the nucleus. *J Virol* 2005;79(2):1191–1206.
460. Nasti G, Talamini R, Antinori A, et al. AIDS-related Kaposi's Sarcoma: evaluation of potential new prognostic factors and assessment of the AIDS Clinical Trial Group Staging System in the Haart Era—the Italian Cooperative Group on AIDS and Tumors and the Italian Cohort of Patients Naive From Antiretrovirals. *J Clin Oncol* 2003;21(15):2876–2882.
461. Nayar U, Lu P, Goldstein RL, et al. Targeting the Hsp90-associated viral oncoproteome in gammaherpesvirus-associated malignancies. *Blood* 2013;122(16):2837–2847.
462. Nealon K, Newcomb WW, Pray TR, et al. Lytic replication of Kaposi's sarcoma-associated herpesvirus results in the formation of multiple capsid species: isolation and molecular characterization of A, B, and C capsids from a gammaherpesvirus. *J Virol* 2001;75(6):2866–2878.
463. Newton R, Labo N, Wakeham K, et al. Determinants of gammaherpesvirus shedding in saliva among Ugandan children and their mothers. *J Infect Dis* 2018;218(6):892–900.
464. Newton R, Labo N, Wakeham K, et al. Kaposi sarcoma-associated herpesvirus in a rural Ugandan Cohort, 1992–2008. *J Infect Dis* 2018;217(2):263–269.
465. Nguyen HQ, Magaret AS, Kitahata MM, et al. Persistent Kaposi sarcoma in the era of highly active antiretroviral therapy: characterizing the predictors of clinical response. *AIDS* 2008;22(8):937–945.
466. Ni G, Ma Z, Wong JP, et al. PPP6C negatively regulates STING-dependent innate immune responses. *MBio* 2020;11(4).
467. Nicholas J. Human gammaherpesvirus cytokines and chemokine receptors. *J Interferon Cytokine Res* 2005;25(7):373–383.
468. Nishimoto N, Kanakura Y, Aozasa K, et al. Humanized anti-interleukin-6 receptor antibody treatment of multicentric Castleman disease. *Blood* 2005;106(8):2627–2632.
469. O'Hara AJ, Vahrson W, Dittmer DP. Gene alteration and precursor and mature microRNA transcription changes contribute to the miRNA signature of primary effusion lymphoma. *Blood* 2008;111(4):2347–2353.
470. O'Hara AJ, Chugh P, Wang L, et al. Pre-micro RNA signatures delineate stages of endothelial cell transformation in Kaposi sarcoma. *PLoS Pathog* 2009;5(4):e1000389.
471. O'Hara AJ, Wang L, Dezube BJ, et al. Tumor suppressor microRNAs are underrepresented in primary effusion lymphoma and Kaposi sarcoma. *Blood* 2009;113(23):5938–5941.
472. Oettle AG. Geographical and racial differences in the frequency of Kaposi's sarcoma as evidence of environmental or genetic causes. *Acta Unio Int Contra Cancrum* 1962;18:330–363.
473. Ojala PM, Tiainen M, Salven P, et al. Kaposi's sarcoma-associated herpesvirus-encoded v-cyclin triggers apoptosis in cells with high levels of cyclin-dependent kinase 6. *Cancer Res* 1999;59(19):4984–4989.
474. Ojala PM, Yamamoto K, Castanos-Velez E, et al. The apoptotic v-cyclin-CDK6 complex phosphorylates and inactivates Bcl-2. *Nat Cell Biol* 2000;2(11):819–825.
475. Oksenhendler E, Duarte M, Soulier J, et al. Multicentric Castleman's disease in HIV infection: a clinical and pathological study of 20 patients. *AIDS* 1996;10(1):61–67.

476. Oksenhendler E, Clauvel JP, Jouveshomme S, et al. Complete remission of a primary effusion lymphoma with antiretroviral therapy. *Am J Hematol* 1998;57(3):266.
477. Orenstein JM, Alkan S, Blauvelt A, et al. Visualization of human herpesvirus type 8 in Kaposi's sarcoma by light and transmission electron microscopy. *AIDS* 1997;11(5):F35–F45.
478. Padilla S, Rivera-Perlman Z, Solomon L. Kaposi's sarcoma in transfusion-associated acquired immunodeficiency syndrome. A case report and review of the literature. *Arch Pathol Lab Med* 1990;114(1):40–42.
479. Palarcik J. Clavicular fractures (group of patients treated in the Traumatological Research Institute in 1986–1989). *Czech Med* 1991;14(3):184–190.
480. Palmeri D, Spadavecchia S, Carroll KD, et al. Promoter- and cell-specific transcriptional transactivation by the Kaposi's sarcoma-associated herpesvirus ORF57/Mta protein. *J Virol* 2007;81(24):13299–13314.
481. Pan H, Xie J, Ye F, et al. Modulation of Kaposi's sarcoma-associated herpesvirus infection and replication by MEK/ERK, JNK, and p38 multiple mitogen-activated protein kinase pathways during primary infection. *J Virol* 2006;80(11):5371–5382.
482. Parravicini C, Corbellino M, Paulli M, et al. Expression of a virus-derived cytokine, KSHV vIL-6, in HIV-seronegative Castleman's disease. *Am J Pathol* 1997;151(6):1517–1522.
483. Parravicini C, Chandran B, Corbellino M, et al. Differential viral protein expression in Kaposi's sarcoma-associated herpesvirus-infected diseases: Kaposi's sarcoma, primary effusion lymphoma, and multicentric Castleman's disease. *Am J Pathol* 2000;156(3):743–749.
484. Parsons CH, Szomju B, Kedes DH. Susceptibility of human fetal mesenchymal stem cells to Kaposi sarcoma-associated herpesvirus. *Blood* 2004;104(9):2736–2738.
485. Parsons CH, Adang LA, Overdevest J, et al. KSHV targets multiple leukocyte lineages during long-term productive infection in NOD/SCID mice. *J Clin Invest* 2006;116(7):1963–1973.
486. Pauk J, Huang ML, Brodie SJ, et al. Mucosal shedding of human herpesvirus 8 in men. *N Engl J Med* 2000;343(19):1369–1377.
487. Pearce M, Matsumura S, Wilson AC. Transcripts encoding K12, v-FLIP, v-cyclin, and the microRNA cluster of Kaposi's sarcoma-associated herpesvirus originate from a common promoter. *J Virol* 2005;79(22):14457–14464.
488. Petre CE, Sin SH, Dittmer DP. Functional p53 signaling in Kaposi's sarcoma-associated herpesvirus lymphomas: implications for therapy. *J Virol* 2007;81(4):1912–1922.
489. Pfeffer S, Sewer A, Lagos-Quintana M, et al. Identification of microRNAs of the herpesvirus family. *Nat Methods* 2005;2(4):269–276.
490. Pfeiffer RM, Wheeler WA, Mbisa G, et al. Geographic heterogeneity of prevalence of the human herpesvirus 8 in sub-Saharan Africa: clues about etiology. *Ann Epidemiol* 2010;20(12):958–963.
491. Pietrek M, Brinkmann MM, Glowacka I, et al. Role of the Kaposi's sarcoma-associated herpesvirus K15 SH3 binding site in inflammatory signaling and B-cell activation. *J Virol* 2010;84(16):8231–8240.
492. Plaisance-Bonstaff K, Choi HS, Beals T, et al. KSHV miRNAs decrease expression of lytic genes in latently infected PEL and endothelial cells by targeting host transcription factors. *Viruses* 2014;6(10):4005–4023.
493. Platt GM, Simpson GR, Mittnacht S, et al. Latent nuclear antigen of Kaposi's sarcoma-associated herpesvirus interacts with RING3, a homolog of the Drosophila female sterile homeotic (fsh) gene. *J Virol* 1999;73(12):9789–9795.
494. Polizzotto MN, Uldrick TS, Wyvill KM, et al. Clinical features and outcomes of patients with symptomatic Kaposi Sarcoma herpesvirus (KSHV)-associated inflammation: prospective characterization of KSHV inflammatory cytokine syndrome (KICS). *Clin Infect Dis* 2016;62(6):730–738.
495. Polizzotto MN, Uldrick TS, Wyvill KM, et al. Pomalidomide for symptomatic Kaposi's sarcoma in people with and without HIV infection: a phase I/II study. *J Clin Oncol* 2016;34(34):4125–4131.
496. Poole LJ, Zong JC, Ciufo DM, et al. Comparison of genetic variability at multiple loci across the genomes of the major subtypes of Kaposi's sarcoma-associated herpesvirus reveals evidence for recombination and for two distinct types of open reading frame K15 alleles at the right-hand end. *J Virol* 1999;73(8):6646–6660.
497. Qian LW, Greene W, Ye F, et al. Kaposi's sarcoma-associated herpesvirus disrupts adherens junctions and increases endothelial permeability by inducing degradation of VE-cadherin. *J Virol* 2008;82(23):11902–11912.
498. Qin Z, Freitas E, Sullivan R, et al. Upregulation of xCT by KSHV-encoded microRNAs facilitates KSHV dissemination and persistence in an environment of oxidative stress. *PLoS Pathog* 2010;6(1):e1000742.
499. Qin Z, Kearney P, Plaisance K, et al. Pivotal advance: Kaposi's sarcoma-associated herpesvirus (KSHV)-encoded microRNA specifically induce IL-6 and IL-10 secretion by macrophages and monocytes. *J Leukoc Biol* 2010;87(1):25–34.
500. Rabkin CS, Janz S, Lash A, et al. Monoclonal origin of multicentric Kaposi's sarcoma lesions. *N Engl J Med* 1997;336(14):988–993.
501. Radkov SA, Kellam P, Boshoff C. The latent nuclear antigen of Kaposi sarcoma-associated herpesvirus targets the retinoblastoma-E2F pathway and with the oncogene Hras transforms primary rat cells. *Nat Med* 2000;6(10):1121–1127.
502. Raghu H, Sharma-Walia N, Veettil MV, et al. Lipid rafts of primary endothelial cells are essential for Kaposi's sarcoma-associated herpesvirus/human herpesvirus 8-induced phosphatidylinositol 3-kinase and RhoA-GTPases critical for microtubule dynamics and nuclear delivery of viral DNA but dispensable for binding and entry. *J Virol* 2007;81(15):7941–7959.
503. Rainbow L, Platt GM, Simpson GR, et al. The 222- to 234-kilodalton latent nuclear protein (LNA) of Kaposi's sarcoma-associated herpesvirus (human herpesvirus 8) is encoded by orf73 and is a component of the latency-associated nuclear antigen. *J Virol* 1997;71(8):5915–5921.
504. Ramos da Silva S, Ferraz da Silva AP, Bacchi MM, et al. KSHV genotypes A and C are more frequent in Kaposi sarcoma lesions from Brazilian patients with and without HIV infection, respectively. *Cancer Lett* 2011;301(1):85–94.
505. Raphaël M, Said J, Borisch B, et al. Lymphomas associated with HIV infection. In: Swerdlow SH, Campo E, Harris NL, et al., eds. *WHO Classification of Tumours of Haematopoietic and Lymphoid Tissues*. Lyon, France: IARC Press; 2008:340–342.
506. Rappocciolo G, Jenkins FJ, Hensler HR, et al. DC-SIGN is a receptor for human herpesvirus 8 on dendritic cells and macrophages. *J Immunol* 2006;176(3):1741–1749.
507. Rappocciolo G, Hensler HR, Jais M, et al. Human herpesvirus 8 infects and replicates in primary cultures of activated B lymphocytes through DC-SIGN. *J Virol* 2008;82(10):4793–4806.
508. Rashidghamat E, Bunker CB, Bower M, et al. Kaposi sarcoma in HIV-negative men who have sex with men. *Br J Dermatol* 2014;171(5):1267–1268.
509. Regezi JA, MacPhail LA, Daniels TE, et al. Human immunodeficiency virus-associated oral Kaposi's sarcoma. A heterogeneous cell population dominated by spindle-shaped endothelial cells. *Am J Pathol* 1993;143(1):240–249.
510. Reid EG, Suazo A, Lensing SY, et al. Pilot trial AMC-063: safety and efficacy of bortezomib in AIDS-associated Kaposi sarcoma. *Clin Cancer Res* 2020;26(3):558–565.
511. Renne R, Lagunoff M, Zhong W, et al. The size and conformation of Kaposi's sarcoma-associated herpesvirus (human herpesvirus 8) DNA in infected cells and virions. *J Virol* 1996;70(11):8151–8154.
512. Renne R, Zhong W, Herndier B, et al. Lytic growth of Kaposi's sarcoma-associated herpesvirus (human herpesvirus 8) in culture. *Nat Med* 1996;2(3):342–346.
513. Renne R, Barry C, Dittmer D, et al. Modulation of cellular and viral gene expression by the latency-associated nuclear antigen of Kaposi's sarcoma-associated herpesvirus. *J Virol* 2001;75(1):458–468.
514. Rezaee SA, Gracie JA, McInnes IB, et al. Inhibition of neutrophil function by the Kaposi's sarcoma-associated herpesvirus vOX2 protein. *AIDS* 2005;19(16):1907–1910.
515. Rhodes DA, Boyle LH, Boname JM, et al. Ubiquitination of lysine-331 by Kaposi's sarcoma-associated herpesvirus protein K5 targets HFE for lysosomal degradation. *Proc Natl Acad Sci U S A* 2010;107(37):16240–16245.
516. Rivas C, Thlick AE, Parravicini C, et al. Kaposi's sarcoma-associated herpesvirus LANA2 is a B-cell-specific latent viral protein that inhibits p53. *J Virol* 2001;75(1):429–438.
517. Rivera-Soto R, Dissinger NJ, Damania B. Kaposi's sarcoma-associated herpesvirus viral interleukin-6 signaling upregulates integrin beta3 levels and is dependent on STAT3. *J Virol* 2020;94(5).
518. Roshan R, Labo N, Trivett M, et al. T-cell responses to KSHV infection: a systematic approach. *Oncotarget* 2017;8(65):109402–109416.
519. Rossetto C, Yamboliev I, Pari GS. Kaposi's sarcoma-associated herpesvirus/human herpesvirus 8 K-bZIP modulates latency-associated nuclear protein-mediated suppression of lytic origin-dependent DNA synthesis. *J Virol* 2009;83(17):8492–8501.
520. Roy D, Sin SH, Damania B, et al. Tumor suppressor genes FHIT and WWOX are deleted in primary effusion lymphoma (PEL) cell lines. *Blood* 2011;118(7):e32–e39.
521. Ruder B, Murtadak V, Sturzl M, et al. Chronic intestinal inflammation in mice expressing viral Flip in epithelial cells. *Mucosal Immunol* 2018;11(6):1621–1629.
522. Ruiz JC, Hunter OV, Conrad NK. Kaposi's sarcoma-associated herpesvirus ORF57 protein protects viral transcripts from specific nuclear RNA decay pathways by preventing hMTR4 recruitment. *PLoS Pathog* 2019;15(2):e1007596.
523. Russo JJ, Bohenzky RA, Chien MC, et al. Nucleotide sequence of the Kaposi sarcoma-associated herpesvirus (HHV8). *Proc Natl Acad Sci U S A* 1996;93(25):14862–14867.
524. Sadler R, Wu L, Forghani B, et al. A complex translational program generates multiple novel proteins from the latently expressed kaposin (K12) locus of Kaposi's sarcoma-associated herpesvirus. *J Virol* 1999;73(7):5722–5730.
525. Sahin BB, Patel D, Conrad NK. Kaposi's sarcoma-associated herpesvirus ORF57 protein binds and protects a nuclear noncoding RNA from cellular RNA decay pathways. *PLoS Pathog* 2010;6(3):e1000799.
526. Said JW, Tasaka T, Takeuchi S, et al. Primary effusion lymphoma in women: report of two cases of Kaposi's sarcoma herpes virus-associated effusion-based lymphoma in human immunodeficiency virus-negative women. *Blood* 1996;88(8):3124–3128.
527. Samols MA, Hu J, Skalsky RL, et al. Cloning and identification of a microRNA cluster within the latency-associated region of Kaposi's sarcoma-associated herpesvirus. *J Virol* 2005;79(14):9301–9305.
528. Samols MA, Skalsky RL, Maldonado AM, et al. Identification of cellular genes targeted by KSHV-encoded microRNAs. *PLoS Pathog* 2007;3(5):e65.
529. Sanchez DJ, Coscoy L, Ganem D. Functional organization of MIR2, a novel viral regulator of selective endocytosis. *J Biol Chem* 2002;277(8):6124–6130.
530. Sanchez EL, Carroll PA, Thalhofer AB, et al. Latent KSHV Infected Endothelial Cells Are Glutamine Addicted and Require Glutaminolysis for Survival. *PLoS Pathog* 2015;11(7):e1005052.
531. Sanchez EL, Pulliam TH, Dimaio TA, et al. Glycolysis, glutaminolysis, and fatty acid synthesis are required for distinct stages of Kaposi's sarcoma-associated herpesvirus lytic replication. *J Virol* 2017;91(10).
532. Sandford G, Choi YB, Nicholas J. Role of ORF74-encoded viral G protein-coupled receptor in human herpesvirus 8 lytic replication. *J Virol* 2009;83(24):13009–13014.
533. Sarek G, Jarviluoma A, Moore HM, et al. Nucleophosmin phosphorylation by v-cyclin-CDK6 controls KSHV latency. *PLoS Pathog* 2010;6(3):e1000818.
534. Sarid R, Flore O, Bohenzky RA, et al. Transcription mapping of the Kaposi's sarcoma-associated herpesvirus (human herpesvirus 8) genome in a body cavity-based lymphoma cell line (BC-1). *J Virol* 1998;72(2):1005–1012.
535. Sarid R, Wiezorek JS, Moore PS, et al. Characterization and cell cycle regulation of the major Kaposi's sarcoma-associated herpesvirus (human herpesvirus 8) latent genes and their promoter. *J Virol* 1999;73(2):1438–1446.
536. Sathish N, Zhu FX, Golub EE, et al. Mechanisms of autoinhibition of IRF-7 and a probable model for inactivation of IRF-7 by Kaposi's sarcoma-associated herpesvirus protein ORF45. *J Biol Chem* 2011;286(1):746–756.
537. Schulz TF. Epidemiology of Kaposi's sarcoma-associated herpesvirus/human herpesvirus 8. *Adv Cancer Res* 1999;76:121–160.
538. Schumann S, Jackson BR, Yule I, et al. Targeting the ATP-dependent formation of herpesvirus ribonucleoprotein particle assembly as an antiviral approach. *Nat Microbiol* 2016;2:16201.
539. Schwam DR, Luciano RL, Mahajan SS, et al. Carboxy terminus of human herpesvirus 8 latency-associated nuclear antigen mediates dimerization, transcriptional repression, and targeting to nuclear bodies. *J Virol* 2000;74(18):8532–8540.

540. Seifi A, Weaver EM, Whipple ME, et al. The lytic activation of KSHV during keratinocyte differentiation is dependent upon a suprabasal position, the loss of integrin engagement, and calcium, but not the interaction of cadherins. *Virology* 2011;410(1):17–29.
541. Semeere AS, Busakhala N, Martin JN. Impact of antiretroviral therapy on the incidence of Kaposi's sarcoma in resource-rich and resource-limited settings. *Curr Opin Oncol* 2012;24(5):522–530.
542. Serquina AKP, Kambach DM, Sarker Oet al. Viral MicroRNAs repress the cholesterol pathway, and 25-hydroxycholesterol inhibits infection. *MBio* 2017;8(4).
543. Sharma NR, Majerciak V, Kruhlak MJ, et al. KSHV inhibits stress granule formation by viral ORF57 blocking PKR activation. *PLoS Pathog* 2017;13(10):e1006677.
544. Sharma NR, Majerciak V, Kruhlak MJ, et al. KSHV RNA-binding protein ORF57 inhibits P-body formation to promote viral multiplication by interaction with Ago2 and GW182. *Nucleic Acids Res* 2019;47(17):9368–9385.
545. Sharma-Walia N, Naranatt PP, Krishnan HH, et al. Kaposi's sarcoma-associated herpesvirus/human herpesvirus 8 envelope glycoprotein gB induces the integrin-dependent focal adhesion kinase-Src-phosphatidylinositol 3-kinase-rho GTPase signal pathways and cytoskeletal rearrangements. *J Virol* 2004;78(8):4207–4223.
546. Sharma-Walia N, Krishnan HH, Naranatt PP, et al. ERK1/2 and MEK1/2 induced by Kaposi's sarcoma-associated herpesvirus (human herpesvirus 8) early during infection of target cells are essential for expression of viral genes and for establishment of infection. *J Virol* 2005;79(16):10308–10329.
547. Sharp TV, Wang HW, Koumi A, et al. K15 protein of Kaposi's sarcoma-associated herpesvirus is latently expressed and binds to HAX-1, a protein with antiapoptotic function. *J Virol* 2002;76(2):802–816.
548. Shin YC, Nakamura H, Liang X, et al. Inhibition of the ATM/p53 signal transduction pathway by Kaposi's sarcoma-associated herpesvirus interferon regulatory factor 1. *J Virol* 2006;80(5):2257–2266.
549. Shin YC, Joo CH, Gack MU, et al. Kaposi's sarcoma-associated herpesvirus viral IFN regulatory factor 3 stabilizes hypoxia-inducible factor-1 alpha to induce vascular endothelial growth factor expression. *Cancer Res* 2008;68(6):1751–1759.
550. Siddiqi T, Joyce RM. A case of HIV-negative primary effusion lymphoma treated with bortezomib, pegylated liposomal doxorubicin, and rituximab. *Clin Lymphoma Myeloma* 2008;8(5):300–304.
551. Siegel JH, Janis R, Alper JC, et al. Disseminated visceral Kaposi's sarcoma. Appearance after human renal homograft operation. *JAMA* 1969;207(8):1493–1496.
552. Simonelli C, Spina M, Cinelli R, et al. Clinical features and outcome of primary effusion lymphoma in HIV-infected patients: a single-institution study. *J Clin Oncol* 2003;21(21):3948–3954.
553. Simpson GR, Schulz TF, Whitby D, et al. Prevalence of Kaposi's sarcoma associated herpesvirus infection measured by antibodies to recombinant capsid protein and latent immunofluorescence antigen. *Lancet* 1996;348(9035):1133–1138.
554. Sin SH, Roy D, Wang L, et al. Rapamycin is efficacious against primary effusion lymphoma (PEL) cell lines in vivo by inhibiting autocrine signaling. *Blood* 2007;109(5):2165–2173.
555. Sin SH, Fakhari FD, Dittmer DP. The viral latency-associated nuclear antigen augments the B-cell response to antigen in vivo. *J Virol* 2010;84(20):10653–10660.
556. Sirianni MC, Vincenzi L, Fiorelli V, et al. gamma-Interferon production in peripheral blood mononuclear cells and tumor infiltrating lymphocytes from Kaposi's sarcoma patients: correlation with the presence of human herpesvirus-8 in peripheral blood mononuclear cells and lesional macrophages. *Blood* 1998;91(3):968–976.
557. Skalsky RL, Samols MA, Plaisance KB, et al. Kaposi's sarcoma-associated herpesvirus encodes an ortholog of miR-155. *J Virol* 2007;81(23):12836–12845.
558. Slavin G, Cameron HM, Forbes C, et al. Kaposi's sarcoma in East African children: a report of 51 cases. *J Pathol* 1970;100(3):187–199.
559. Smit MJ, Verzijl D, Casarosa P, et al. Kaposi's sarcoma-associated herpesvirus-encoded G protein-coupled receptor ORF74 constitutively activates p44/p42 MAPK and Akt via G(i) and phospholipase C-dependent signaling pathways. *J Virol* 2002;76(4):1744–1752.
560. Smith NA, Sabin CA, Gopal R, et al. Serologic evidence of human herpesvirus 8 transmission by homosexual but not heterosexual sex. *J Infect Dis* 1999;180(3):600–606.
561. Snodgrass R, Gardner A, Semeere A, et al. A portable device for nucleic acid quantification powered by sunlight, a flame or electricity. *Nat Biomed Eng* 2018;2(9):657–665.
562. Sodhi A, Montaner S, Patel V, et al. The Kaposi's sarcoma-associated herpes virus G protein-coupled receptor up-regulates vascular endothelial growth factor expression and secretion through mitogen-activated protein kinase and p38 pathways acting on hypoxia-inducible factor 1alpha. *Cancer Res* 2000;60(17):4873–4880.
563. Sodhi A, Chaisuparat R, Hu J, et al. The TSC2/mTOR pathway drives endothelial cell transformation induced by the Kaposi's sarcoma-associated herpesvirus G protein-coupled receptor. *Cancer Cell* 2006;10(2):133–143.
564. Song MJ, Brown HJ, Wu TT, et al. Transcription activation of polyadenylated nuclear rna by rta in human herpesvirus 8/Kaposi's sarcoma-associated herpesvirus. *J Virol* 2001;75(7):3129–3140.
565. Song MJ, Deng H, Sun R. Comparative study of regulation of RTA-responsive genes in Kaposi's sarcoma-associated herpesvirus/human herpesvirus 8. *J Virol* 2003;77(17):9451–9462.
566. Song SN, Tomosugi N, Kawabata H, et al. Down-regulation of hepcidin resulting from long-term treatment with an anti-IL-6 receptor antibody (tocilizumab) improves anemia of inflammation in multicentric Castleman disease. *Blood* 2010;116(18):3627–3634.
567. Soulier J, Grollet L, Oksenhendler E, et al. Kaposi's sarcoma-associated herpesvirus-like DNA sequences in multicentric Castleman's disease. *Blood* 1995;86(4):1276–1280.
568. Stallone G, Schena A, Infante B, et al. Sirolimus for Kaposi's sarcoma in renal-transplant recipients. *N Engl J Med* 2005;352(13):1317–1323.
569. Staskus KA, Zhong W, Gebhard K, et al. Kaposi's sarcoma-associated herpesvirus gene expression in endothelial (spindle) tumor cells. *J Virol* 1997;71(1):715–719.
570. Staskus KA, Sun R, Miller G, et al. Cellular tropism and viral interleukin-6 expression distinguish human herpesvirus 8 involvement in Kaposi's sarcoma, primary effusion lymphoma, and multicentric Castleman's disease. *J Virol* 1999;73(5):4181–4187.
571. Staudt MR, Dittmer DP. Promoter switching allows simultaneous transcription of LANA and K14/vGPCR of Kaposi's sarcoma-associated herpesvirus. *Virology* 2006;350(1):192–205.
572. Staudt MR, Kanan Y, Jeong JH, et al. The tumor microenvironment controls primary effusion lymphoma growth in vivo. *Cancer Res* 2004;64(14):4790–4799.
573. Stedman W, Deng Z, Lu F, et al. ORC, MCM, and histone hyperacetylation at the Kaposi's sarcoma-associated herpesvirus latent replication origin. *J Virol* 2004;78(22):12566–12575.
574. Stedman W, Kang H, Lin S, et al. Cohesins localize with CTCF at the KSHV latency control region and at cellular c-myc and H19/Igf2 insulators. *EMBO J* 2008;27(4):654–666.
575. Stevenson PG, Efstathiou S, Doherty PC, et al. Inhibition of MHC class I-restricted antigen presentation by gamma 2-herpesviruses. *Proc Natl Acad Sci U S A* 2000;97(15):8455–8460.
576. Stine JT, Wood C, Hill M, et al. KSHV-encoded CC chemokine vMIP-III is a CCR4 agonist, stimulates angiogenesis, and selectively chemoattracts TH2 cells. *Blood* 2000;95(4):1151–1157.
577. Sturzl M, Blasig C, Schreier A, et al. Expression of HHV-8 latency-associated T0.7 RNA in spindle cells and endothelial cells of AIDS-associated, classical and African Kaposi's sarcoma. *Int J Cancer* 1997;72(1):68–71.
578. Sun R, Lin SF, Gradoville L, et al. Polyadenylylated nuclear RNA encoded by Kaposi sarcoma-associated herpesvirus. *Proc Natl Acad Sci U S A* 1996;93(21):11883–11888.
579. Sun R, Lin SF, Gradoville L, et al. A viral gene that activates lytic cycle expression of Kaposi's sarcoma-associated herpesvirus. *Proc Natl Acad Sci U S A* 1998;95(18):10866–10871.
580. Sun R, Lin SF, Staskus K, et al. Kinetics of Kaposi's sarcoma-associated herpesvirus gene expression. *J Virol* 1999;73(3):2232–2242.
581. Sun Z, Xiao B, Jha HC, et al. Kaposi's sarcoma-associated herpesvirus-encoded LANA can induce chromosomal instability through targeted degradation of the mitotic checkpoint kinase Bub1. *J Virol* 2014;88(13):7367–7378.
582. Sun Z, Jha HC, Robertson ES. Bub1 in complex with LANA recruits PCNA to regulate Kaposi's sarcoma-associated herpesvirus latent replication and DNA translesion synthesis. *J Virol* 2015;89(20):10206–10218.
583. Sun Z, Jha HC, Pei YG, et al. Major histocompatibility complex class II HLA-DRalpha is downregulated by Kaposi's sarcoma-associated herpesvirus-encoded lytic transactivator RTA and MARCH8. *J Virol* 2016;90(18):8047–8058.
584. Swanton C, Mann DJ, Fleckenstein B, et al. Herpes viral cyclin/Cdk6 complexes evade inhibition by CDK inhibitor proteins. *Nature* 1997;390(6656):184–187.
585. Swerdlow SH, Campo E, Harris NL, et al. *WHO Classification of Tumours of Haematopoietic and Lymphoid Tissues*. Lyon, France: IARC; 2017.
586. Szekely L, Chen F, Teramoto N, et al. Restricted expression of Epstein-Barr virus (EBV)-encoded, growth transformation-associated antigens in an EBV- and human herpesvirus type 8-carrying body cavity lymphoma line. *J Gen Virol* 1998;79(Pt 6):1445–1452.
587. Tagawa T, Gao S, Koparde VN, et al. Discovery of Kaposi's sarcoma herpesvirus-encoded circular RNAs and a human antiviral circular RNA. *Proc Natl Acad Sci U S A* 2018;115(50):12805–12810.
588. Tamanaha-Nakasone A, Uehara K, Tanabe Y, et al. K1 gene transformation activities in AIDS-related and classic type Kaposi's sarcoma: correlation with clinical presentation. *Sci Rep* 2019;9(1):6416.
589. Tamburro KM, Yang D, Poisson J, et al. Vironome of Kaposi sarcoma associated herpesvirus-inflammatory cytokine syndrome in an AIDS patient reveals co-infection of human herpesvirus 8 and human herpesvirus 6A. *Virology* 2012;433(1):220–225.
590. Tan B, Liu H, Zhang S, et al. Viral and cellular N(6)-methyladenosine and N(6),2'-O-dimethyladenosine epitranscriptomes in the KSHV life cycle. *Nat Microbiol* 2018;3(1):108–120.
591. TerBush AA, Hafkamp F, Lee HJ, et al. A Kaposi's sarcoma-associated herpesvirus infection mechanism is independent of integrins alpha3beta1, alphaVbeta3, and alphaVbeta5. *J Virol* 2018;92(17).
592. Thome M, Schneider P, Hofmann K, et al. Viral FLICE-inhibitory proteins (FLIPs) prevent apoptosis induced by death receptors. *Nature* 1997;386(6624):517–521.
593. Tolani B, Matta H, Gopalakrishnan R, et al. NEMO is essential for Kaposi's sarcoma-associated herpesvirus-encoded vFLIP K13-induced gene expression and protection against death receptor-induced cell death, and its N-terminal 251 residues are sufficient for this process. *J Virol* 2014;88(11):6345–6354.
594. Tomkowicz B, Singh SP, Cartas M, et al. Human herpesvirus-8 encoded Kaposin: subcellular localization using immunofluorescence and biochemical approaches. *DNA Cell Biol* 2002;21(3):151–162.
595. Tomlinson CC, Damania B. The K1 protein of Kaposi's sarcoma-associated herpesvirus activates the Akt signaling pathway. *J Virol* 2004;78(4):1918–1927.
596. Tomlinson CC, Damania B. Critical role for endocytosis in the regulation of signaling by the Kaposi's sarcoma-associated herpesvirus K1 protein. *J Virol* 2008;82(13):6514–6523.
597. Toptan T, Fonseca L, Kwun HJ, et al. Complex alternative cytoplasmic protein isoforms of the Kaposi's sarcoma-associated herpesvirus latency-associated nuclear antigen 1 generated through noncanonical translation initiation. *J Virol* 2013;87(5):2744–2755.
598. Toptan T, Abere B, Nalesnik MA, et al. Circular DNA tumor viruses make circular RNAs. *Proc Natl Acad Sci U S A* 2018;115(37):E8737–E8745.
599. Toth Z, Maglinte DT, Lee SH, et al. Epigenetic analysis of KSHV latent and lytic genomes. *PLoS Pathog* 2010;6(7):e1001013.
600. Toth Z, Papp B, Brulois K, et al. LANA-mediated recruitment of host polycomb repressive complexes onto the KSHV genome during de novo infection. *PLoS Pathog* 2016;12(9):e1005878.
601. Totonchy J, Osborn JM, Chadburn A, et al. KSHV induces immunoglobulin rearrangements in mature B lymphocytes. *PLoS Pathog* 2018;14(4):e1006967.
602. Uddin S, Hussain AR, Al-Hussein KA, et al. Inhibition of phosphatidylinositol 3'-kinase/AKT signaling promotes apoptosis of primary effusion lymphoma cells. *Clin Cancer Res* 2005;11(8):3102–3108.
603. Uldrick TS, Wang V, O'Mahony D, et al. An interleukin-6-related systemic inflammatory syndrome in patients co-infected with Kaposi sarcoma-associated herpesvirus and HIV but without Multicentric Castleman disease. *Clin Infect Dis* 2010;51(3):350–358.

604. Uldrick TS, Polizzotto MN, Aleman K, et al. High-dose zidovudine plus valganciclovir for Kaposi sarcoma herpesvirus-associated multicentric Castleman disease: a pilot study of virus-activated cytotoxic therapy. *Blood* 2011;117(26):6977–6986.
605. Uldrick TS, Wyvill KM, Kumar P, et al. Phase II study of bevacizumab in patients with HIV-associated Kaposi's sarcoma receiving antiretroviral therapy. *J Clin Oncol* 2012;30(13):1476–1483.
606. Ungerleider NA, Jain V, Wang Y, et al. Comparative analysis of gammaherpesvirus circular RNA repertoires: conserved and unique viral circular RNAs. *J Virol* 2019;93(6).
607. Vart RJ, Nikitenko LL, Lagos D, et al. Kaposi's sarcoma-associated herpesvirus-encoded interleukin-6 and G-protein-coupled receptor regulate angiopoietin-2 expression in lymphatic endothelial cells. *Cancer Res* 2007;67(9):4042–4051.
608. Veettil MV, Sharma-Walia N, Sadagopan S, et al. RhoA-GTPase facilitates entry of Kaposi's sarcoma-associated herpesvirus into adherent target cells in a Src-dependent manner. *J Virol* 2006;80(23):11432–11446.
609. Veettil MV, Sadagopan S, Sharma-Walia N, et al. Kaposi's sarcoma-associated herpesvirus forms a multimolecular complex of integrins (alphaVbeta5, alphaVbeta3, and alpha3beta1) and CD98-xCT during infection of human dermal microvascular endothelial cells, and CD98-xCT is essential for the postentry stage of infection. *J Virol* 2008;82(24):12126–12144.
610. Vega F, Miranda RN, Medeiros LJ. KSHV/HHV8-positive large B-cell lymphomas and associated diseases: a heterogeneous group of lymphoproliferative processes with significant clinicopathological overlap. *Mod Pathol* 2020;33(1):18–28.
611. Verdecia J, Warda F, Rechcigl K, et al. Kaposi sarcoma with musculoskeletal manifestations in a well-controlled HIV patient. *IDCases* 2019;17:e00571.
612. Verma SC, Choudhuri T, Kaul R, et al. Latency-associated nuclear antigen (LANA) of Kaposi's sarcoma-associated herpesvirus interacts with origin recognition complexes at the LANA binding sequence within the terminal repeats. *J Virol* 2006;80(5):2243–2256.
613. Verma SC, Choudhuri T, Robertson ES. The minimal replicator element of the Kaposi's sarcoma-associated herpesvirus terminal repeat supports replication in a semiconservative and cell-cycle-dependent manner. *J Virol* 2007;81(7):3402–3413.
614. Verma SC, Lan K, Choudhuri T, et al. An autonomous replicating element within the KSHV genome. *Cell Host Microbe* 2007;2(2):106–118.
615. Verschuren EW, Hodgson JG, Gray JW, et al. The role of p53 in suppression of KSHV cyclin-induced lymphomagenesis. *Cancer Res* 2004;64(2):581–589.
616. Vieira J, O'Hearn PM. Use of the red fluorescent protein as a marker of Kaposi's sarcoma-associated herpesvirus lytic gene expression. *Virology* 2004;325(2):225–240.
617. Vieira J, Huang ML, Koelle DM, et al. Transmissible Kaposi's sarcoma-associated herpesvirus (human herpesvirus 8) in saliva of men with a history of Kaposi's sarcoma. *J Virol* 1997;71(9):7083–7087.
618. Vieira J, O'Hearn P, Kimball L, et al. Activation of Kaposi's sarcoma-associated herpesvirus (human herpesvirus 8) lytic replication by human cytomegalovirus. *J Virol* 2001;75(3):1378–1386.
619. Viejo-Borbolla A, Ottinger M, Bruning E, et al. Brd2/RING3 interacts with a chromatin-binding domain in the Kaposi's Sarcoma-associated herpesvirus latency-associated nuclear antigen 1 (LANA-1) that is required for multiple functions of LANA-1. *J Virol* 2005;79(21):13618–13629.
620. Vijgen S, Wyss C, Meylan P, et al. Fatal outcome of multiple clinical presentations of human herpesvirus 8-related disease after solid organ transplantation. *Transplantation* 2016;100(1):134–140.
621. Viollet C, Davis DA, Tekeste SS, et al. RNA sequencing reveals that Kaposi sarcoma-associated herpesvirus infection mimics hypoxia gene expression signature. *PLoS Pathog* 2017;13(1):e1006143.
622. Volkow P, Cesarman-Maus G, Garciadiego-Fossas P, et al. Clinical characteristics, predictors of immune reconstitution inflammatory syndrome and long-term prognosis in patients with Kaposi sarcoma. *AIDS Res Ther* 2017;14(1):30.
623. Wabinga HR, Parkin DM, Wabwire-Mangen F, et al. Cancer in Kampala, Uganda, in 1989–91: changes in incidence in the era of AIDS. *Int J Cancer* 1993;54(1):26–36.
624. Wagener R, Alexandrov LB, Montesinos-Rongen M, et al. Analysis of mutational signatures in exomes from B-cell lymphoma cell lines suggest APOBEC3 family members to be involved in the pathogenesis of primary effusion lymphoma. *Leukemia* 2015;29(7):1612–1615.
625. Wakeham K, Webb EL, Sebina I, et al. Parasite infection is associated with Kaposi's sarcoma associated herpesvirus (KSHV) in Ugandan women. *Infect Agent Cancer* 2011;6(1):15.
626. Walts AE, Shintaku IP, Said JW. Diagnosis of malignant lymphoma in effusions from patients with AIDS by gene rearrangement. *Am J Clin Pathol* 1990;94(2):170–175.
627. Wang L, Damania B. Kaposi's sarcoma-associated herpesvirus confers a survival advantage to endothelial cells. *Cancer Res* 2008;68(12):4640–4648.
628. Wang SE, Wu FY, Fujimuro M, et al. Role of CCAAT/enhancer-binding protein alpha (C/EBPalpha) in activation of the Kaposi's sarcoma-associated herpesvirus (KSHV) lytic-cycle replication-associated protein (RAP) promoter in cooperation with the KSHV replication and transcription activator (RTA) and RAP. *J Virol* 2003;77(1):600–623.
629. Wang HW, Trotter MW, Lagos D, et al. Kaposi sarcoma herpesvirus-induced cellular reprogramming contributes to the lymphatic endothelial gene expression in Kaposi sarcoma. *Nat Genet* 2004;36(7):687–693.
630. Wang L, Wakisaka N, Tomlinson CC, et al. The Kaposi's sarcoma-associated herpesvirus (KSHV/HHV-8) K1 protein induces expression of angiogenic and invasion factors. *Cancer Res* 2004;64(8):2774–2781.
631. Wang Y, Chong OT, Yuan Y. Differential regulation of K8 gene expression in immediate-early and delayed-early stages of Kaposi's sarcoma-associated herpesvirus. *Virology* 2004;325(1):149–163.
632. Wang Y, Li H, Chan MY, et al. Kaposi's sarcoma-associated herpesvirus ori-Lyt-dependent DNA replication: cis-acting requirements for replication and ori-Lyt-associated RNA transcription. *J Virol* 2004;78(16):8615–8629.
633. Wang L, Dittmer DP, Tomlinson CC, et al. Immortalization of primary endothelial cells by the K1 protein of Kaposi's sarcoma-associated herpesvirus. *Cancer Res* 2006;66(7):3658–3666.
634. Wang Y, Tang Q, Maul GG, et al. Kaposi's sarcoma-associated herpesvirus ori-Lyt-dependent DNA replication: dual role of replication and transcription activator. *J Virol* 2006;80(24):12171–12186.
635. Wang S, Wang S, Maeng H, et al. K1 protein of human herpesvirus 8 suppresses lymphoma cell Fas-mediated apoptosis. *Blood* 2007;109(5):2174–2182.
636. Wang X, He B, Zhang Z, et al. Human herpesvirus-8 in northwestern China: epidemiology and characterization among blood donors. *Virol J* 2010;7:62.
637. Wang Y, Sathish N, Hollow C, et al. Functional characterization of Kaposi's sarcoma-associated herpesvirus open reading frame K8 by bacterial artificial chromosome-based mutagenesis. *J Virol* 2011;85(5):1943–1957.
638. Wang LX, Kang G, Kumar P, et al. Humanized-BLT mouse model of Kaposi's sarcoma-associated herpesvirus infection. *Proc Natl Acad Sci U S A* 2014;111(8):3146–3151.
639. Wang X, He Z, Xia T, et al. Latency-associated nuclear antigen of Kaposi sarcoma-associated herpesvirus promotes angiogenesis through targeting notch signaling effector Hey1. *Cancer Res* 2014;74(7):2026–2037.
640. Watanabe T, Sugaya M, Atkins AM, et al. Kaposi's sarcoma-associated herpesvirus latency-associated nuclear antigen prolongs the life span of primary human umbilical vein endothelial cells. *J Virol* 2003;77(11):6188–6196.
641. Waterston A, Bower M. Fifty years of multicentric Castleman's disease. *Acta Oncol* 2004;43(8):698–704.
642. Weber KS, Grone HJ, Rocken M, et al. Selective recruitment of Th2-type cells and evasion from a cytotoxic immune response mediated by viral macrophage inhibitory protein-II. *Eur J Immunol* 2001;31(8):2458–2466.
643. Wen KW, Damania B. Hsp90 and Hsp40/Erdj3 are required for the expression and anti-apoptotic function of KSHV K1. *Oncogene* 2010;29(24):3532–3544.
644. West J, Damania B. Upregulation of the TLR3 pathway by Kaposi's sarcoma-associated herpesvirus during primary infection. *J Virol* 2008;82(11):5440–5449.
645. West JA, Gregory SM, Sivaraman V, et al. Activation of plasmacytoid dendritic cells by Kaposi's sarcoma-associated herpesvirus. *J Virol* 2011;85(2):895–904.
646. West JA, Wicks M, Gregory SM, et al. An important role for mitochondrial antiviral signaling protein in the Kaposi's sarcoma-associated herpesvirus life cycle. *J Virol* 2014;88(10):5778–5787.
647. Whitby D, Luppi M, Barozzi P, et al. Human herpesvirus 8 seroprevalence in blood donors and lymphoma patients from different regions of Italy. *J Natl Cancer Inst* 1998;90(5):395–397.
648. Whitby D, Marshall VA, Bagni RK, et al. Genotypic characterization of Kaposi's sarcoma-associated herpesvirus in asymptomatic infected subjects from isolated populations. *J Gen Virol* 2004;85(Pt 1):155–163.
649. Whitby D, Marshall VA, Bagni RK, et al. Reactivation of Kaposi's sarcoma-associated herpesvirus by natural products from Kaposi's sarcoma endemic regions. *Int J Cancer* 2007;120(2):321–328.
650. Wies E, Mori Y, Hahn A, et al. The viral interferon-regulatory factor-3 is required for the survival of KSHV-infected primary effusion lymphoma cells. *Blood* 2008;111(1):320–327.
651. Wies E, Hahn AS, Schmidt K, et al. The Kaposi's sarcoma-associated herpesvirus-encoded vIRF-3 inhibits cellular IRF-5. *J Biol Chem* 2009;284(13):8525–8538.
652. Williamson SJ, Nicol SM, Sturzl M, et al. Azidothymidine sensitizes primary effusion lymphoma cells to Kaposi sarcoma-associated herpesvirus-specific CD4+ T cell control and inhibits vIRF3 function. *PLoS Pathog* 2016;12(11):e1006042.
653. Wilson KS, McKenna RW, Kroft SH, et al. Primary effusion lymphomas exhibit complex and recurrent cytogenetic abnormalities. *Br J Haematol* 2002;116(1):113–121.
654. Wilson SJ, Tsao EH, Webb BL, et al. X box binding protein XBP-1s transactivates the Kaposi's sarcoma-associated herpesvirus (KSHV) ORF50 promoter, linking plasma cell differentiation to KSHV reactivation from latency. *J Virol* 2007;81(24):13578–13586.
655. Wit FW, Sol CJ, Renwick N, et al. Regression of AIDS-related Kaposi's sarcoma associated with clearance of human herpesvirus-8 from peripheral blood mononuclear cells following initiation of antiretroviral therapy. *AIDS* 1998;12(2):218–219.
656. Wong LY, Matchett GA, Wilson AC. Transcriptional activation by the Kaposi's sarcoma-associated herpesvirus latency-associated nuclear antigen is facilitated by an N-terminal chromatin-binding motif. *J Virol* 2004;78(18):10074–10085.
657. Wu FY, Ahn JH, Alcendor DJ, et al. Origin-independent assembly of Kaposi's sarcoma-associated herpesvirus DNA replication compartments in transient cotransfection assays and association with the ORF-K8 protein and cellular PML. *J Virol* 2001;75(3):1487–1506.
658. Wu FY, Wang SE, Tang QQ, et al. Cell cycle arrest by Kaposi's sarcoma-associated herpesvirus replication-associated protein is mediated at both the transcriptional and posttranslational levels by binding to CCAAT/enhancer-binding protein alpha and p21(CIP-1). *J Virol* 2003;77(16):8893–8914.
659. Wu W, Vieira J, Fiore N, et al. KSHV/HHV-8 infection of human hematopoietic progenitor (CD34+) cells: persistence of infection during hematopoiesis in vitro and in vivo. *Blood* 2006;108(1):141–151.
660. Wu TT, Blackman MA, Sun R. Prospects of a novel vaccination strategy for human gamma-herpesviruses. *Immunol Res* 2010;48(1–3):122–146.
661. Wu JJ, Li W, Shao Y, et al. Inhibition of cGAS DNA sensing by a herpesvirus virion protein. *Cell Host Microbe* 2015;18(3):333–344.
662. Xi X, Persson LM, O'Brien MW, et al. Cooperation between viral interferon regulatory factor 4 and RTA to activate a subset of Kaposi's sarcoma-associated herpesvirus lytic promoters. *J Virol* 2012;86(2):1021–1033.
663. Xia T, O'Hara A, Araujo I, et al. EBV microRNAs in primary lymphomas and targeting of CXCL-11 by ebv-mir-BHRF1–3. *Cancer Res* 2008;68(5):1436–1442.
664. Xiang Q, Ju H, Li Q, et al. Human herpesvirus 8 interferon regulatory factors 1 and 3 mediate replication and latency activities via interactions with USP7 deubiquitinase. *J Virol* 2018;92(7).
665. Xiao B, Verma SC, Cai Q, et al. Bub1 and CENP-F can contribute to Kaposi's sarcoma-associated herpesvirus genome persistence by targeting LANA to kinetochores. *J Virol* 2010;84(19):9718–9732.

666. Xie J, Pan H, Yoo S, et al. Kaposi's sarcoma-associated herpesvirus induction of AP-1 and interleukin 6 during primary infection mediated by multiple mitogen-activated protein kinase pathways. *J Virol* 2005;79(24):15027–15037.
667. Xie J, Ajibade AO, Ye F, et al. Reactivation of Kaposi's sarcoma-associated herpesvirus from latency requires MEK/ERK, JNK and p38 multiple mitogen-activated protein kinase pathways. *Virology* 2008;371(1):139–154.
668. Xu Y, AuCoin DP, Huete AR, et al. A Kaposi's sarcoma-associated herpesvirus/human herpesvirus 8 ORF50 deletion mutant is defective for reactivation of latent virus and DNA replication. *J Virol* 2005;79(6):3479–3487.
669. Yang TY, Chen SC, Leach MW, et al. Transgenic expression of the chemokine receptor encoded by human herpesvirus 8 induces an angioproliferative disease resembling Kaposi's sarcoma. *J Exp Med* 2000;191(3):445–454.
670. Yang Z, Yan Z, Wood C. Kaposi's sarcoma-associated herpesvirus transactivator RTA promotes degradation of the repressors to regulate viral lytic replication. *J Virol* 2008;82(7):3590–3603.
671. Yang D, Chen W, Xiong J, et al. Interleukin 1 receptor-associated kinase 1 (IRAK1) mutation is a common, essential driver for Kaposi sarcoma herpesvirus lymphoma. *Proc Natl Acad Sci U S A* 2014;111(44):E4762–E4768.
672. Yarchoan R, Uldrick TS. HIV-associated cancers and related diseases. *N Engl J Med* 2018;378(22):2145.
673. Yarchoan R, Pluda JM, Wyvill KM, et al. PART IV. Cytokine and hormone immunotherapy treatment of AIDS-related Kaposi's sarcoma with interleukin-12: rationale and preliminary evidence of clinical activity. *Crit Rev Immunol* 2007;27:401–414.
674. Ye FC, Zhou FC, Yoo SM, et al. Disruption of Kaposi's sarcoma-associated herpesvirus latent nuclear antigen leads to abortive episome persistence. *J Virol* 2004;78(20):11121–11129.
675. Yiakoumis X, Pangalis GA, Kyrtsonis MC, et al. Primary effusion lymphoma in two HIV-negative patients successfully treated with pleurodesis as first-line therapy. *Anticancer Res* 2011;30(1):271–276.
676. Yogev O, Lagos D, Enver T, et al. Kaposi's sarcoma herpesvirus microRNAs induce metabolic transformation of infected cells. *PLoS Pathog* 2014;10(9):e1004400.
677. Yogev O, Henderson S, Hayes MJ, et al. Herpesviruses shape tumour microenvironment through exosomal transfer of viral microRNAs. *PLoS Pathog* 2017;13(8):e1006524.
678. Yoo J, Kang J, Lee HN, et al. Kaposin-B enhances the PROX1 mRNA stability during lymphatic reprogramming of vascular endothelial cells by Kaposi's sarcoma herpes virus. *PLoS Pathog* 2010;6(8):e1001046.
679. You J, Srinivasan V, Denis GV, et al. Kaposi's sarcoma-associated herpesvirus latency-associated nuclear antigen interacts with bromodomain protein Brd4 on host mitotic chromosomes. *J Virol* 2006;80(18):8909–8919.
680. Yu Y, Hayward GS. The ubiquitin E3 ligase RAUL negatively regulates type i interferon through ubiquitination of the transcription factors IRF7 and IRF3. *Immunity* 2010;33(6):863–877.
681. Yu Y, Black JB, Goldsmith CS, et al. Induction of human herpesvirus-8 DNA replication and transcription by butyrate and TPA in BCBL-1 cells. *J Gen Virol* 1999;80 (Pt 1):83–90.
682. Yu F, Feng J, Harada JN, et al. B cell terminal differentiation factor XBP-1 induces reactivation of Kaposi's sarcoma-associated herpesvirus. *FEBS Lett* 2007;581(18):3485–3488.
683. Yu HR, Kim YJ, Lee HR. KSHV vIRF4 enhances BCL6 transcription via downregulation of IRF4 expression. *Biochem Biophys Res Commun* 2018;496(4):1128–1133.
684. Yuan F, Gao ZQ, Majerciak V, et al. The crystal structure of KSHV ORF57 reveals dimeric active sites important for protein stability and function. *PLoS Pathog* 2018;14(8):e1007232.
685. Zhang D, Pu X, Wu W, et al. Genotypic analysis on the ORF-K1 gene of human herpesvirus 8 from patients with Kaposi's sarcoma in Xinjiang, China. *J Genet Genomics* 2008;35(11):657–663.
686. Zhang G, Chan B, Samarina N, et al. Cytoplasmic isoforms of Kaposi sarcoma herpesvirus LANA recruit and antagonize the innate immune DNA sensor cGAS. *Proc Natl Acad Sci U S A* 2016;113(8):E1034–E1043.
687. Zhang Z, Chen W, Sanders MK, et al. The K1 protein of Kaposi's sarcoma-associated herpesvirus augments viral lytic replication. *J Virol* 2016;90(17):7657–7666.
688. Zhang Y, Dittmer DP, Mieczkowski PA, et al. RIG-I detects Kaposi's sarcoma-associated herpesvirus transcripts in a RNA polymerase III-independent manner. *MBio* 2018;9(4).
689. Zhang H, Ni G, Damania B. ADAR1 facilitates KSHV lytic reactivation by modulating the RLR-dependent signaling pathway. *Cell Rep* 2020;31(4):107564.
690. Zhao Y, Ye X, Dunker W, et al. RIG-I like receptor sensing of host RNAs facilitates the cell-intrinsic immune response to KSHV infection. *Nat Commun* 2018;9(1):4841.
691. Zhong W, Wang H, Herndier B, et al. Restricted expression of Kaposi sarcoma-associated herpesvirus (human herpesvirus 8) genes in Kaposi sarcoma. *Proc Natl Acad Sci U S A* 1996;93(13):6641–6646.
692. Zhou FC, Zhang YJ, Deng JH, et al. Efficient infection by a recombinant Kaposi's sarcoma-associated herpesvirus cloned in a bacterial artificial chromosome: application for genetic analysis. *J Virol* 2002;76(12):6185–6196.
693. Zhu FX, Cusano T, Yuan Y. Identification of the immediate-early transcripts of Kaposi's sarcoma-associated herpesvirus. *J Virol* 1999;73(7):5556–5567.
694. Zhu FX, King SM, Smith EJ, et al. A Kaposi's sarcoma-associated herpesviral protein inhibits virus-mediated induction of type I interferon by blocking IRF-7 phosphorylation and nuclear accumulation. *Proc Natl Acad Sci U S A* 2002;99(8):5573–5578.
695. Zhu FX, Chong JM, Wu L, et al. Virion proteins of Kaposi's sarcoma-associated herpesvirus. *J Virol* 2005;79(2):800–811.
696. Zhu FX, Sathish N, Yuan Y. Antagonism of host antiviral responses by Kaposi's sarcoma-associated herpesvirus tegument protein ORF45. *PLoS One* 2010;5(5):e10573.
697. Zhu Y, Ramos da Silva S, He M, et al. An oncogenic virus promotes cell survival and cellular transformation by suppressing glycolysis. *PLoS Pathog* 2016;12(5):e1005648.
698. Zhu Y, Li T, Ramos da Silva S, et al. A critical role of glutamine and asparagine gamma-nitrogen in nucleotide biosynthesis in cancer cells hijacked by an oncogenic virus. *MBio* 2017;8(4).
699. Ziegelbauer J, Grundhoff A, Ganem D. Exploring the DNA binding interactions of the Kaposi's sarcoma-associated herpesvirus lytic switch protein by selective amplification of bound sequences in vitro. *J Virol* 2006;80(6):2958–2967.
700. Ziegelbauer JM, Sullivan CS, Ganem D. Tandem array-based expression screens identify host mRNA targets of virus-encoded microRNAs. *Nat Genet* 2009;41(1):130–134.
701. Ziegler JL. Endemic Kaposi's sarcoma in Africa and local volcanic soils. *Lancet* 1993;342(8883):1348–1351.
702. Ziegler JL, Katongole-Mbidde E. Kaposi's sarcoma in childhood: an analysis of 100 cases from Uganda and relationship to HIV infection. *Int J Cancer* 1996;65(2):200–203.
703. Zmonarski SC, Boratynska M, Rabczynski J, et al. Regression of Kaposi's sarcoma in renal graft recipients after conversion to sirolimus treatment. *Transplant Proc* 2005;37(2):964–966.
704. Zong JC, Metroka C, Reitz MS, et al. Strain variability among Kaposi sarcoma-associated herpesvirus (human herpesvirus 8) genomes: evidence that a large cohort of United States AIDS patients may have been infected by a single common isolate. *J Virol* 1997;71(3):2505–2511.
705. Zong JC, Ciufo DM, Alcendor DJ, et al. High-level variability in the ORF-K1 membrane protein gene at the left end of the Kaposi's sarcoma-associated herpesvirus genome defines four major virus subtypes and multiple variants or clades in different human populations. *J Virol* 1999;73(5):4156–4170.
706. Zong J, Ciufo DM, Viscidi R, et al. Genotypic analysis at multiple loci across Kaposi's sarcoma herpesvirus (KSHV) DNA molecules: clustering patterns, novel variants and chimerism. *J Clin Virol* 2002;23(3):119–148.
707. Zuo J, Hislop AD, Leung CS, et al. Kaposi's sarcoma-associated herpesvirus-encoded viral IRF3 modulates major histocompatibility complex class II (MHC-II) antigen presentation through MHC-II transactivator-dependent and -independent mechanisms: implications for oncogenesis. *J Virol* 2013;87(10):5340–5350.

CHAPTER

16 *Poxviridae*: The Viruses and Their Replication

Bernard Moss • Geoffrey L. Smith

INTRODUCTION

The *Poxviridae* comprise a fascinating family of complex DNA viruses that replicate entirely in the cytoplasm of vertebrate or invertebrate cells. Two members of the family, variola virus (VARV), and molluscum contagiosum virus (MOCV) are obligate human pathogens, and others such as monkeypox virus (MPXV) are transmitted from animal hosts to humans and cause severe disease. VARV was the cause of smallpox, a once common and highly lethal disease that altered human history. Smallpox was eradicated in 1977 through a dedicated effort spearheaded by the World Health Organization, nearly two centuries after the introduction of highly effective prophylactic inoculations with cowpox virus (CPXV) and vaccinia virus (VACV). In addition to public health value, vaccination contributed to present concepts of infectious disease and immunity. From a historical perspective, VACV was the first animal virus seen microscopically, grown in tissue culture, accurately titered, physically purified, and chemically analyzed. Moreover, the general view of virus particles as packets of nucleic acid was revised following the discovery of RNA synthetic activity in purified poxvirus (POXV) virions. This finding sparked investigations that led to the discovery of transcriptase and reverse transcriptase activities in RNA viruses and to the elucidation of structural features of viral and eukaryotic mRNA, including the 5′ cap and 3′ poly(A) tail. Recombinant DNA technology eliminated obstacles to working with large viruses, and considerable progress has been made in elucidating the virus replication cycle. Discoveries of virus-encoded proteins that affect cell growth and modulate immune defense mechanisms continue to provide new insights into virus/host relationships. In addition, the development of POXVs as live recombinant expression vectors provides a powerful tool for immunologists and biochemists as well as an alternative approach to the development of vaccines and therapeutics against a variety of infectious agents and cancer.

CLASSIFICATION

Distinguishing properties of the family *Poxviridae* include a cytoplasmic site of replication and a large complex enveloped virion, which contains enzymes that synthesize mRNA and a genome composed of a linear double-stranded DNA molecule of 128 to 380 kilobase pairs (kbp) with a hairpin loop at each end. POXVs are divided into the subfamilies *Chordopoxvirinae* and *Entomopoxvirinae*, based on vertebrate and insect host range (Table 16.1). DNA sequencing and bioinformatic analysis confirm the genetic relationship between the POXV subfamilies and further suggest that POXVs are distantly related to *Asfarviridae*, *Ascoviridae*, *Iridoviridae*, and *Phycodnaviridae* and the giant viruses *Mimiviridae*, *Marseilleviridae*, *Pandoraviridae*, and *Pithoviridae*.[366] These nucleocytoplasmic large DNA viruses (NCLDV) are believed to form a monophyletic group

TABLE 16.1 Family *Poxviridae*

Subfamily	Genus	Species[a]	DNA Genome
Chordopoxvirinae	*Avipoxvirus*	*Canarypox, Fowlpox*[b] *(FWPV), Juncopox, Mynahpox, Pigeonpox, Psittacinepox, Quailpox, Sparrowpox, Starlingpox, Turkeypox*	270 kbp, G + C ~35%
	Capripoxvirus	*Goatpox, Lumpy skin disease, Sheeppox*[b]	150 kbp, G + C 25%
	Centapoxvirus	*Yokapox*[b]	176 kbp, G + C 26%
	Cervidopoxvirus	*Mule deerpox*[b]	170 kbp, G + C 27%
	Crocodylipoxvirus	*Nile crocodilepox*[b]	190 kbp, G + C 62%
	Leporipoxvirus	*Hare fibroma, Myxoma,*[b] *Rabbit fibroma, Squirrel fibroma*	160 kbp, G + C 40%
	Macropoxvirus	*Eastern kangaroopox,*[b] *Western kangaroopox*	173 kbp, G + C 58%
	Molluscipoxvirus	*Molluscum contagiosum*[b]	190 kbp, G + C ~60%
	Mustelpoxvirus	*Sea otterpox*[b]	128 kbp, G + C 31%
	Orthopoxvirus	*Camelpox (CMLV), Cowpox (CPXV), Ectromelia (ECTV), Monkeypox (MPXV), Raccoonpox, Skunkpox, Taterapox (TATV), Vaccinia*[b] *(VACV), Variola (VARV), Volepox*	190 kbp, G + C 36%
	Oryzopoxvirus	*Cotia*[b]	185 kbp, G + C 24%
	Parapoxvirus	*Bovine papular stomatitis, Orf,*[b] *Parapoxvirus of red deer, Pseudocowpox*	140 kbp, G + C 64%
	Pteropoxvirus	*Pteropox*[b]	134 kbp, G + C 34%
	Salmonpoxvirus	*Salmon gillpox*[b]	242 kbp, GC 38%
	Sciuripoxvirus	*Squirrelpox*[b]	148 kbp G + C 67%
	Suipoxvirus	*Swinepox*[b]	146 kbp, G + C 28%
	Vespertilionpoxvirus	*Eptesipox*[b]	177 kbp, G + C 24%
	Yatapoxvirus	*Tanapox, Yaba monkey tumor*[b]	135 kbp, G + C 30%
Entomopoxvirinae	*Alphaentomopoxvirus*	*Anomala cuprea, Aphodius tasmaniae, Demodema boranensis, Dermolepida albohirtum, Figulus subleavis, Geotrupes sylvaticus, Melolontha melolontha*[b]	246 kbp, G + C 20%
	Betaentomopoxvirus	*Acrobasis zelleri, Adoxophyes honmai, Amsacta moorei,*[b] *Arphia conspersa, Choristoneura biennis, C. conflicta, C. diversuma, C. fumiferana, C. rosacea, Chorizagrotis auxiliars, Heliothis armiger, Locusta migratoria, Mythimna separata, Oedaleus senegalensis, Operophtera brumata, Schistocerca gregaria*	228–307 kbp, G + C 20%
	Deltaentomopoxvirus	*Melanoplus sanguinipes*	236 kbp, G + C 18%
	Gammaentomopoxvirus	*Aedes aegypti, Camptochironomus tentans, Chironomus attenuatus, C. luridus,*[b] *C. plumosus, Goeldichironomus haloprasimus*	~250–380 kbp

[a]Four-letter abbreviations of species used in text appear in parentheses.
[b]Prototypal member.

based mainly on the presence of about 40 genes that can be traced back to their last common ancestor.

The subfamily *Chordopoxvirinae* consists of 18 genera (Table 16.1). Members of the same genus are genetically and antigenically related and have a similar morphology and host range. Salmon gill poxvirus is the deepest representative of the *Chordopoxvirinae*.[263] The orthopoxviruses (OPXVs) have been studied most intensively. The species names frequently refer to the host from which the virus was first isolated rather than the reservoir species, for example, rodents are reservoirs for CPXV and MPXV. VACV, the prototype OPXV, has been propagated as the smallpox vaccine and its natural host remains unknown, although vaccine-derived strains are currently circulating in cattle in Brazil and occasionally infect humans.[179] DNA sequencing reveals that genes common to camelpox virus (CMLV), CPXV, ectromelia virus (ECTV), MPXV, taterapox (TATV), VACV, and VARV share greater than 90% nucleotide identity, whereas OPXVs indigenous to the USA (e.g., raccoonpox, skunkpox, and volepox virus) exhibit greater genetic divergence. CPXV contains all genes present in other OPXVs, suggesting that it resembles the ancestral member of this genus, whereas other species have genes that are deleted or disrupted. Recent analyses suggest that more than one species of OPXV have been grouped under the CPXV species.[239] The entomopoxviruses are divided into four genera based in part on the insect host of isolation (Table 16.1).

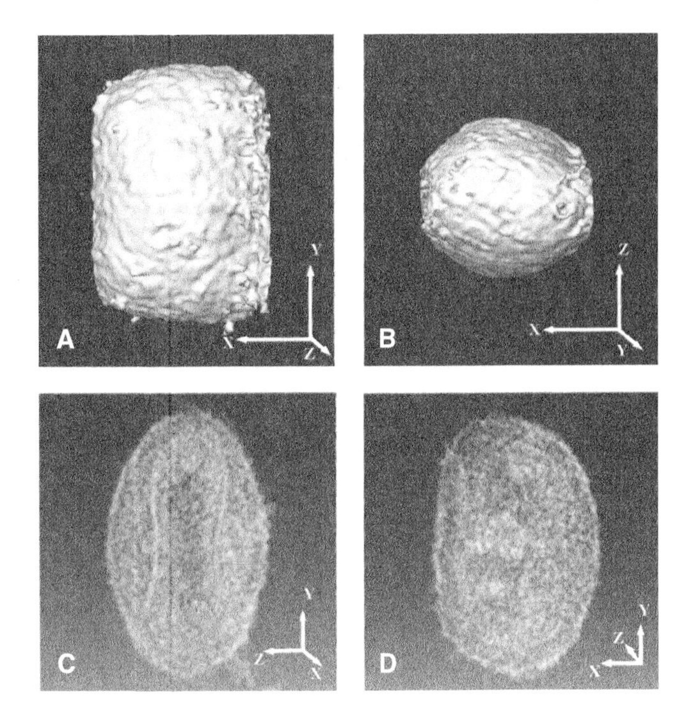

FIGURE 16.1 Reconstructions of VACV MV. A and B: Volumetric representations highlighting the outer shape and size of the virions in two orthogonal views along perpendicular axes. **C and D:** Translucent representations showing the complex internal structure of the core. In one orientation **(C)**, the dumbbell shape of the core is seen. (Reprinted with permission from Cyrklaff M, Risco C, Fernández JJ, et al. Cryo-electron tomography of vaccinia virus. *Proc Natl Acad Sci U S A* 2005;102(8):2772–2777. Copyright © 2005 National Academy of Sciences, U.S.A. Ref.[158])

VIRION STRUCTURE

Morphology

The basic infectious form of a POXV is the mature virion (MV), which has a barrel shape and is composed of an outer membrane, a dumbbell-shaped core, and lateral bodies within the concavities.[168] For VACV, dimensions of approximately 360 × 270 × 250 nm were derived by cryoelectron tomography[158] (Fig. 16.1). The thickness (5 to 6 nm) and density of the outer layer is consistent with one lipid membrane bilayer, the outside of which appears corrugated because of irregular protrusions extending 3 to 5 nm. The core wall seems to be composed of two layers with an overall thickness of 18 to 19 nm. The inner layer appears continuous, except for a small number of channels. The outer layer has a palisade structure made of T-shaped spikes (8 nm in length and 5 nm wide) that are anchored in a putative inner membrane. Freeze fracture and deep etch electron microscopy confirm both the outer structure of the virion as consisting of a single membrane bilayer with surface corrugations and the palisade structure of the core wall but evidence for an inner membrane was not found.[292] The ultrastructure of the core appears to consist of two phases: the denser layer just under the core wall has a fiber-like morphology suggesting nucleoprotein. Cylindrical elements that may take an S-shape representing nucleoprotein have been visualized within POXV cores.[333,548]

Chemical Composition

The mass of a VACV MV is 9.5 fg.[279] The principal components of the MV are protein, lipid, and DNA, accounting for 90%, 5%, and 3.2%, respectively, of the dry weight.[817] In contrast, about one-third of fowlpox virus (FWPV) virions is lipid.[417] The lipid components of VACV MVs are predominantly cholesterol and phospholipids,[145] whereas FWPV virions also contain squalene and cholesterol esters.[417] Carbohydrate is present in the VACV extracellular virion (EV) as a constituent of glycoproteins. Spermine and spermidine[384] and trace amounts of RNA[594] have been found in VACV MVs.

Genome

POXVs have linear double-stranded DNA genomes that vary from 140 kbp in parapoxviruses to over 300 kbp in some avipoxviruses. The ends of the genome consist of identical but oppositely oriented sequences referred to as inverted terminal repetitions (ITRs). The ITRs include an A+T-rich, incompletely base-paired, hairpin loop that connects the two DNA strands[53]; a highly conserved region of less than 100 bp that contains sequences required for the resolution of replicating concatemeric forms of DNA[190,458]; sets of short, tandemly repeated sequences; and up to several open reading frames (ORFs). The ends of the VACV genome are depicted in Figure 16.2. The ITRs are variable in length due to deletions, repetitions, and transpositions.

Complete genome sequences have been reported for at least one member of each chordopoxvirus and three entomopoxvirus genera. Nearly 100 genes are conserved in all chordopoxviruses and about half of these can be recognized in entomopoxviruses.[742] Based on the above, several generalizations can be made: genes are largely nonoverlapping, tend to occur in blocks pointing toward the nearer end of the genome, are usually located in the central region if highly conserved and concerned with essential

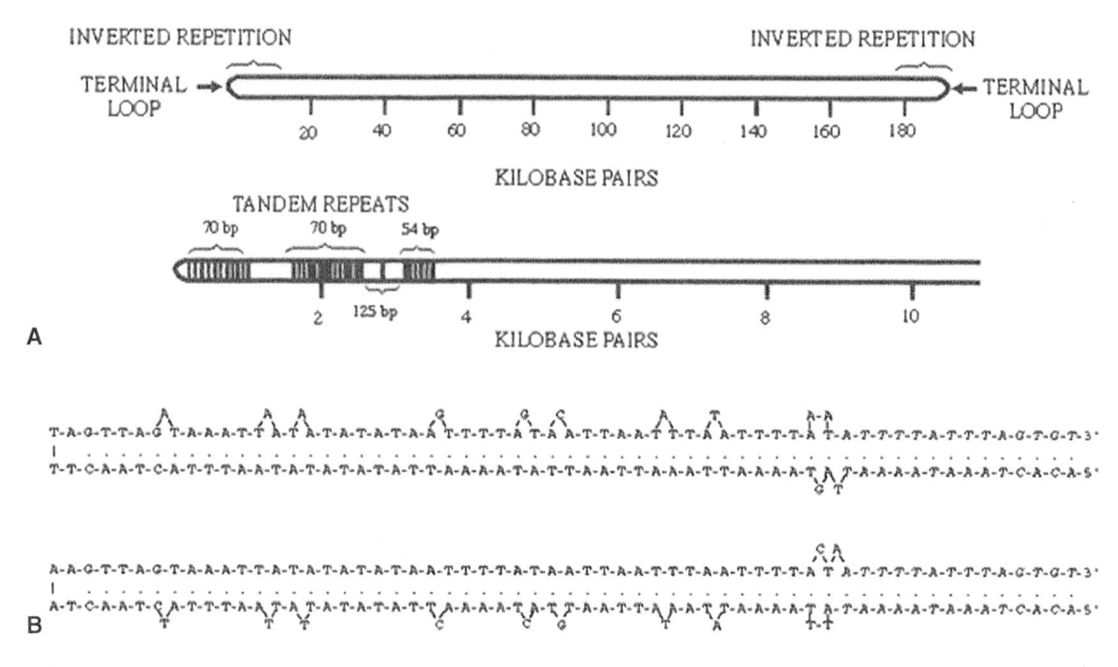

FIGURE 16.2 **Structural features of VACV genome. A:** Representation of the entire linear double-stranded DNA genome and an expansion of the 10,000-bp inverted terminal repetition. (A republished with permission of John Wiley & Sons from Moss B, Winters E, Jones EV. Replication of vaccinia virus. In: Cozzarelli N, ed. *Mechanisms of DNA Replication and Recombination*. New York: A.R. Liss; 1983:449–461; permission conveyed through Copyright Clearance Center, Inc. Ref.[485]) **B:** Nucleotide sequences of the inverted and complementary forms of the terminal loops. (Reprinted from Baroudy BM, Venkatesan S, Moss B. Incompletely base-paired flip-flop terminal loops link the two DNA strands of the vaccinia virus genome into one uninterrupted polynucleotide chain. *Cell* 1982;28(2):315–324. Copyright © 1982 Elsevier. With permission. Ref.[53])

replication functions, and are usually located in the end regions if variable and concerned with host interactions. An ORF map of the VACV genome is shown in Figure 16.3. The arrangement of the central genes is remarkably similar in all chordopoxviruses. A convention for naming VACV ORFs, originating prior to sequencing the entire genome and used for the complete sequence of the Copenhagen (CPN) strain of VACV, consists of using the HindIII restriction endonuclease DNA fragment letter, followed by the ORF number (from left to right except for HindIII C) within the fragment, and L or R, depending on the direction of transcription. Protein names correspond to ORF names, except that L or R is dropped. In addition, ORFs have been numbered successively from one end of the genome to the other in most subsequent complete POXV genome sequences; nevertheless, the old letter designations have been retained as common names for homologs to provide continuity in the literature. The ORF number of the Western Reserve (WR) strain of VACV, which has been used for the majority of biochemical and genetic studies, is included in tables.

Polypeptide Components

Consistent with their size and complex structure, POXV virions contain a multitude of polypeptides.[150] Approximately 80 virus-encoded polypeptides have been identified by mass spectrometry[507,580] and approximately 30 have been localized near the exterior of purified MVs by surface-specific labeling, sensitivity to proteases, extraction with nonionic detergents, or reactivity with virus-neutralizing antibodies. Several methods have been used to investigate membrane protein interactions including chemical cross-linking.[462] The surface proteins can be divided structurally into those with transmembrane domains and those without and functionally into those required for attachment, entry, disulfide bond formation, morphogenesis, and virulence (Table 16.2). None of the MV membrane proteins have signal peptides or are glycosylated, suggesting novel trafficking mechanisms.

Virus cores isolated by sedimentation following treatment of MVs with a nonionic detergent and reducing agent contain approximately 50 polypeptides. Of these, approximately 30 are enzymes of which at least half directly participate in early mRNA biosynthesis (Table 16.3); the nonenzymatic proteins may be primarily involved in morphogenesis and structure (Table 16.4). F17, L4, A3, and A10 are particularly abundant. L4 and the transcription system have been localized to the nucleocapsid; A3, A4, and A10 to the core wall; and F17, G4, and H1 to the lateral bodies.[490,619] Cross-linking reveals numerous interactions between core proteins.[462]

Evidence for a distinct extracellular form of VACV first came from vaccine-related studies. Antibodies to inactivated MVs did not protect rodents against an OPXV infection as well as antibodies to live virus or inactivated EVs.[90] Subsequent studies showed that the EV has an additional outer membrane, which is a target of protective antibodies, and consequently a lower buoyant density.[590] The additional membrane contains several unique glycosylated proteins (A33, A34, A56, B5, K2) and one nonglycosylated (F13) (Table 16.5). Of the six EV membrane proteins, only A34 and F13 are conserved in all chordopoxviruses. Although EVs are usually considered to be MVs with an additional membrane, that is not precisely true. There is evidence that MVs contain at least two surface proteins A26 and A25 that are absent from EVs.[736]

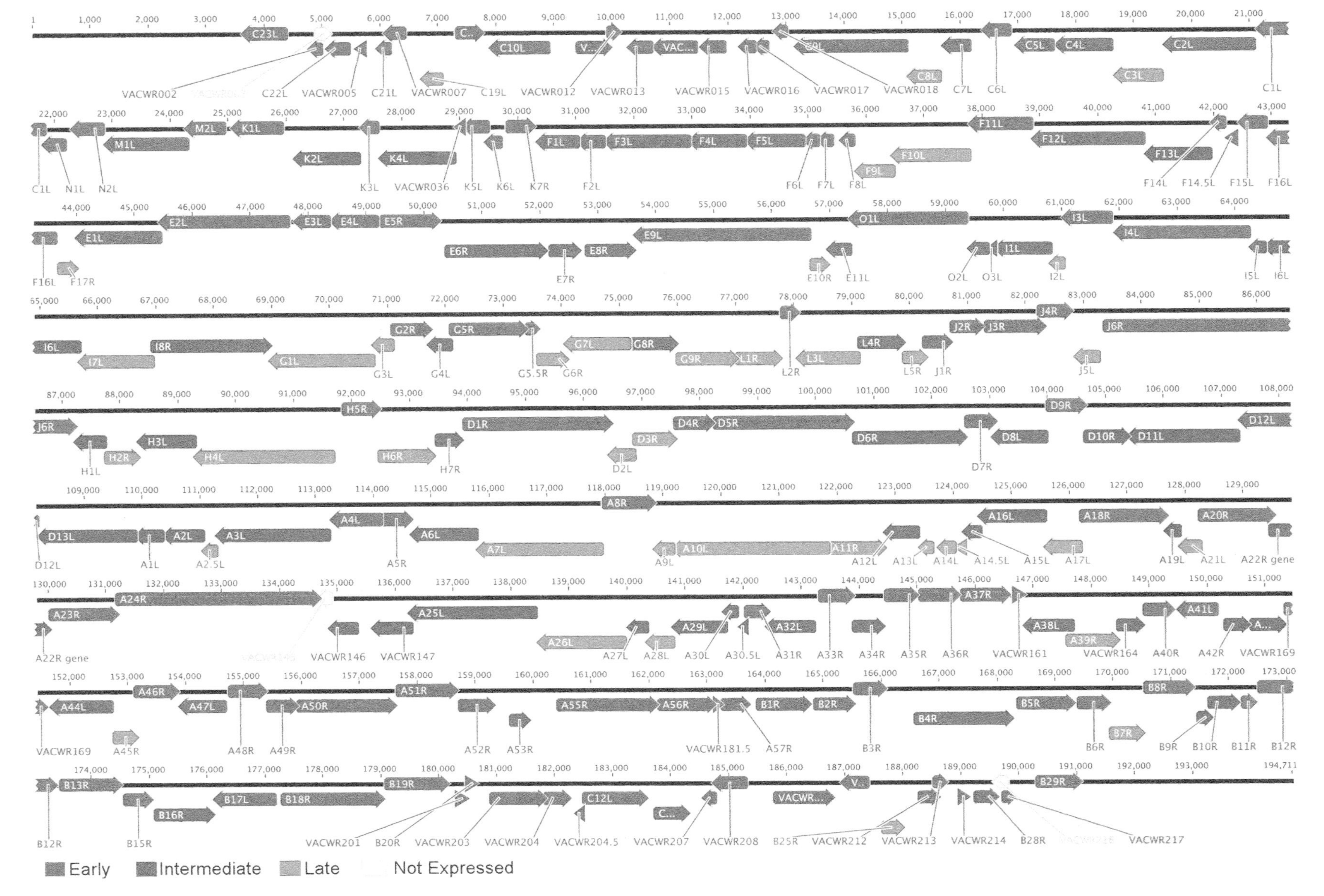

FIGURE 16.3 Transcriptional map of the VACV genome. VACV WR ORFs are shown as *colored arrows* indicating the direction of transcription. When applicable, the common (Copenhagen) HindIII fragment letter/number name was used to identify ORFs; otherwise, the VACV WR number was provided. The numbers from 1 to 194,711 indicate the nucleotide positions on the VACV genome. Each ORF has been assigned the stage at which its earliest expression can be detected; additional promoter elements that potentially contribute to later stages of gene expression are not indicated. (Adapted from Yang Z, Reynolds SE, Martens CA, et al. Expression profiling of the intermediate and late stages of poxvirus replication. *J Virol* 2011;85(19):9899–9908. Ref.[810])

TABLE 16.2 VACV MV membrane-associated proteins

ORF[a] COP	WR	kDA	T[b]	C[c]	TM[d]	Properties	References
Cell attachment							
A26L	149	58	L		—	Binds laminin, assoc A27, fusion suppressor	(130,140)
A27L	150	13	I		—	Binds heparan, assoc A17, N[e]	(132,761)
D8L	113	35	I		N	Binds chondroitin, N	(307)
H3L	101	38	I	P	C	Binds heparan, N	(395)
Cell entry							
A16L	136	43	I	P	C	EFC[f]; paralog G9, J5, S-S[g]	(517)
A21L	140	14	L	P	N	EFC, S-S	(723)
A28L	151	16	L	P	N	EFC, N, S-S	(640)
F9L	048	24	L	P	C	EFC, S-S	(98,203)
G3L	079	13	L	P	N	EFC	(731)
G9R	087	39	L	P	C	EFC; paralog A16, J5, S-S	(516)
H2R	100	22	L	P	N	EFC, S-S	(638)
J5L	097	15	L	P	C	EFC; paralog A16, G9, S-S	(639)
L1R	088	27	L	P	C	EFC, N, S-S	(75,699)
L5R	092	15	L	P	C	EFC, S-S	(722)
O3L	069.5	4	I	C	N	EFC	(612)
REDOX							
A2.5L	121	9	L	C	—	S-S to E10, G4	(633)
E10R	066	11	L	P	—	ERV/ALR family, S-S to A2.5	(642)
G4L	081	14	I	P	—	Thioredoxin family, S-S to A2.5	(40,700,778)
Morphogenesis							
A9L	128	12	L	P	N	Post-IV[h]	(812)
A13L	132	8	L	C	N	Post-IV, N	(738)
A14L	133	10	L	C	N, C	Pre-IV, assoc A17	(737)
A17L	137	23	L	C	N, C	Pre-IV, assoc A14, N	(737)
D13L	118	62	I	P	—	Pre-IV, lattice scaffold, assoc A17	(76,709)
I2L	071	8	L	C	C	Post-IV	(321,509)
Virulence							
A14.5L	134	6	L	C	N, C	Virulence	(74)
F14.5L	53.5	6	I		N	Cell adhesion, virulence	(331)
I5L	074	9	I	C	N, C	Virulence	(683)

[a]Copenhagen (COP) or WR ORF designation.
[b]Time of synthesis: Intermediate (I) or Late (L).
[c]Conservation in all POXV (P) or chordopoxviruses (C).
[d]Transmembrane domain (TM).
[e]Target of neutralizing antibody (N).
[f]Entry–fusion complex (EFC).
[g]Intramolecular disulfide.
[h]Pre-IV and Post-IV refer to requirement before or after formation of immature virion, respectively.

CELL ENTRY

General Considerations

Studies of POXV entry are usually carried out with VACV, which can enter most tissue culture cells suggesting either the absence of a specific receptor or receptors that are ubiquitous. A special feature of POXVs is the existence of two infectious forms: MVs (also called intracellular mature virion, IMV), which have a single outer membrane containing the proteins necessary for fusion, and EVs, which have an additional membrane that is disrupted prior to entry. Although the MV is the more abundant form, the EV is specialized for spread from

TABLE 16.3 VACV core-associated enzymes and transcription factors

Enzyme/Factor	COP[a]	WR[b]	kDa	T[c]	C[d]	Comments	References
Transcription and mRNA modification							
RNA polymerase						Multisubunit	(52)
RPO 147	J6R	098	147	E	P	RPB1 homolog	(103)
RPO 132	A24R	144	132	E	P	RPB2 homolog	(24)
RPO 35	A29L	152	35	E	P	No cell homolog	(26)
RPO 30	E4L	060	30	E	C	SII elongation factor homolog	(5)
RPO 22	J4R	096	22	E	C	RPB5 homolog	(103)
RPO 19	A5R	124	19	E	P	RPB6 homolog	(9)
RPO 18	D7R	112	18	E	P	RPB7 homolog	(7)
RPO 7	G5.5R	083	7	E	C	RPB10 homolog	(25)
RAP94	H4L	102	94	L	P	RNA pol associated, early transcription	(8)
Early transcription factor (VETF)						Promoter binding, DNA-depend ATPase	(105)
Large subunit	A7L	126	82	L	P	Interacts with promoter core	(127,258)
Small subunit	D6R	111	74	I	P	Helicase motif	(101,258)
Capping enzyme						RNA triphosphatase, guanylyltransferase, guanine-7-methyltransferase	(430)
Large subunit	D1R	106	82	E	P	Catalytic activities	(473)
Small subunit	D12L	117	33	E	P	Stimulates methyltransferase	(510)
Cap 2′-methyltransferase	J3R	039	39	E	P	Ribose methyltransferase; poly(A) polymerase subunit	(621)
Poly(A) polymerase						Adds As to 3′ ends of mRNAs	(483)
Large subunit	E1L	057	55	E	P	Catalytic activity	(256)
Small subunit	J3R	039	39	E	P	Stimulatory activity; methyltransferase	(256)
Nucleoside triphosphate phosphohydrolase I (NPH I)	D11	116	72	I	P	DNA-dependent ATPase	(526)
Nucleoside triphosphate phosphohydrolase II (NPH II)	I8R	077	77	I	P	DNA/RNA-dependent NTPase, helicase	(526)
DNA topoisomerase	H6R	104	37	L	P	Sequence-specific nicking, early transcription	(659)
DNA helicase	A18R	138	57	E	P	DNA-dependent ATPase	(660)
Other roles							
Holliday junction resolvase	A22R	142	22	I	P	RuvC homolog; resolves concatemer junctions	(248)
FEN1-like nuclease	G5R	082	50	E	P	DNA recombination	(636)
DNA packaging ATPase	A32L	155	31	I	P	Related to phage enzyme	(126)
Protein kinase 1	B1R	183	34	E	—	Serine/threonine	(397)
Protein kinase 2	F10L	049	52	L	P	Serine/threonine	(396)
Protein phosphatase	H1L	099	34	I		Tyr/Ser	(277)
Protease 1	I7L	076	49	L	P	Putative cysteine protease	(113)
Protease 2	G1L	078	68	L	P	Putative metalloprotease	(32)
Glutaredoxin	O2L	069	12	I	—	Cofactor ribonucleotide reductase	(10)
DNA nicking–joining	K4L	035	49	I	—	Nonessential, role unknown	(215)
Superoxide dismutase	A45R	171	14	L	—	Nonessential, inactive catalytic site, role unknown	(21)

[a]Copenhagen (COP) ORF name.
[b]Western Reserve (WR) ORF number.
[c]Time of synthesis: early, intermediate, or late.
[d]Conservation in all POXV (P) or chordopoxviruses (C).

TABLE 16.4 VACV core-associated nonenzymatic proteins

ORF[a]		kDa	T[b]	C[c]	Properties	References
COP	WR					
A3L	122	73	I	P	4b precursor, I7-dependent cleavage, morphogenesis	(481,598,750)
A4L	123	31	E	C	F10-dependent phosphorylation, morphogenesis	(155,587,783)
A10L	129	102	L	P	4a precursor, I7-dependent cleavage, morphogenesis	(481,751,789)
A12L	131	20	I	C	I7-dependent cleavage, morphogenesis	(806)
A15L	135	11	I	C	Component of 7-protein complex, morphogenesis	(707)
A30L	153	9	I	C	Component of 7-protein complex, morphogenesis	(455,711)
D2L	107	17	L	C	Component of 7-protein complex, morphogenesis	(707)
D3R	108	28	L	C	Component of 7-protein complex, morphogenesis	(707)
E8R	064	32	I	C	ts mutant virion decreased transcription	(346)
E11L	067	15	I		ts mutant noninfectious virions	(766)
F17R	065	11	E	C	Phosphoprotein, morphogenesis	(541,789,826)
G7L	085	42	L	C	Component of 7-protein complex, morphogenesis	(455,708)
H5R	103	22	E	C	Interacts with A20, transcription, morphogenesis	(64,78,194,369,440)
I6L	075	43	I	C	Telomere binding, DNA packaging	(193,275)
J1R	093	18	I	C	Component of 7-protein complex, morphogenesis	(139,141)
L3L	090	41	L	P	ts virions defective in core transcription	(581)
L4R	091	28	I	P	Single-strand DNA/RNA binding, core transcription, I7-depend cleavage	(31,60,780)

[a]Copenhagen (COP) or WR ORF designation.
[b]Time of synthesis: early, intermediate or late.
[c]Conservation in all POXV (P) or chordopoxviruses (C).

TABLE 16.5 VACV WV and EV membrane proteins

COP[a]	WR[b]	kDa	T[c]	C[d]	TM[e]	Properties	References
A33R	156	21	E*		N, T2	EV, glycosylated, phosphorylated, associated with A36, actin tail formation	(595,793)
A34R	157	20	I	Ch	N, T2	EV, N-gly, lectin-like, associated with A36 and B5, actin tail formation, EV release	(82,600,791)
A36R	159	25	E*		N, T1	WV only, phosphorylated, associated with A33, A34, cellular Nck and kinesin, actin tail formation and movement on microtubules	(614,748,794)
A56R	181	35	E*		C, T1	EV, hemagglutinin, glycosylated, associated with K2, EFC proteins and C3, prevents syncytia and superinfection	(631,649,732,759)
B5R	187	35	E*		C, T1	EV, glycosylated, associated with A34, A36, F13, WV formation	(290,770)
E2L	058	86	L	Ch	—	WV only, movement on microtubules	(124,207,208)
F12L	051	73	E*	Ch	—	WV only, movement on microtubules	(747,820)
F13L	052	42	I	Ch	—	EV, palmitylated, phospholipase domain, associated with B5, WV formation	(80,620)
K2L	033	42	I		—	EV, signal peptide, associates with A56, prevents syncytia formation and superinfection	(732,758,759)

[a]Copenhagen (COP) ORF name.
[b]Western reserve (WR) ORF number.
[c]Time of synthesis: E*, early plus intermediate or late.
[d]Conserved in all chordopoxviruses (Ch).
[e]Transmembrane domain: N-terminal (N), C-terminal (C), Type 1 (T1), Type 2 (T2).

cell-to-cell and within an infected host. VACV encodes at least four attachment proteins and eleven that comprise the entry fusion complex (EFC) (Table 16.2). Additional descriptions and references may be found in recent reviews.[476,618]

MV Entry

Enveloped viruses typically enter cells by fusion with the plasma or endocytic membrane. VACV MVs use both entry mechanisms (Fig. 16.4A and B), perhaps contributing to their ability to enter most cells. OPXVs that have not undergone extensive *in vitro* passaging preferentially employ the endosomal pathway.[68] Endosomal acidification promotes entry of the virus core into the cytoplasm following actin-dependent macropinocytosis or fluid-phase uptake of the large virus particles,[313,453,725] although there is some disagreement regarding later steps in the endosomal trafficking pathway.[306,588] Preferential use of the endosomal pathway depends in part on the A26 protein, which binds components of the EFC and acts as a suppressor of neutral pH fusion.[131] Low pH activation of MVs[724] can be explained by conformational changes of A26.[130]

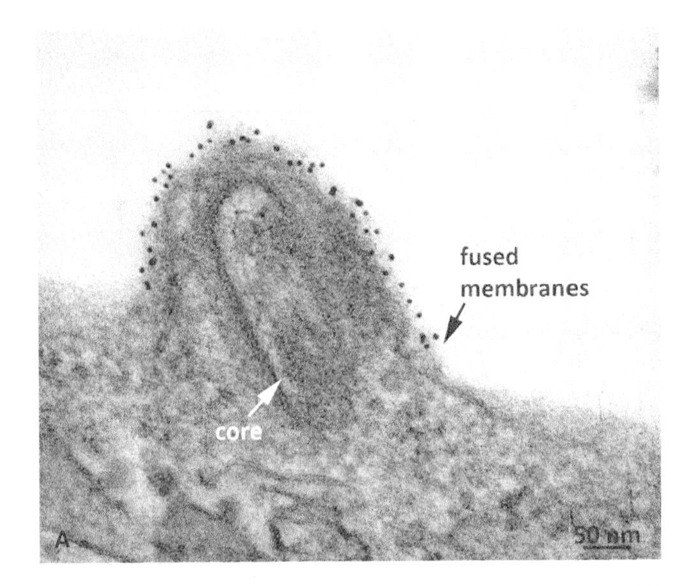

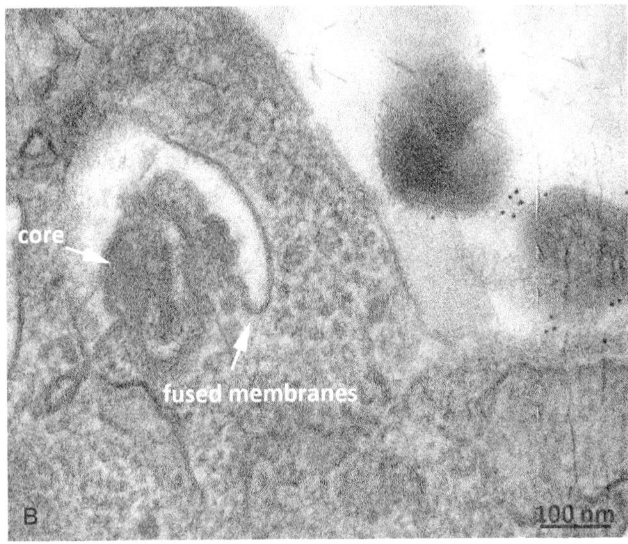

FIGURE 16.4 **VACV MVs fusing with plasma and endosomal membranes.** VACV MVs were deposited on the cell surface by spinoculation and incubated at 37°C for 30 minutes. Unpermeabilized cells were incubated with antibody to the D8 membrane protein and labeled with Protein A conjugated to gold spheres. The gold particles are present on the viral membrane that has fused with the plasma membrane **(A)** but not on the viral membrane that has fused with the endosomal membrane **(B)**. (Images provided by A. Weisberg.)

The four VACV attachment proteins are D8, which binds chondroitin sulfate[307]; A27 and H3, which bind heparan sulfate[143,395]; and A26, which binds laminin.[140] The attachment proteins provide some redundancy as individually they are not essential. Only D8 and H3 have transmembrane domains. A26 and A27 interact with each other, and the A17 transmembrane protein anchors the latter.[302,761] The crystal structure of a truncated trimeric form of A27[132] and the tetrameric ectodomain of D8 with a crevice predicted to be the chondroitin-binding site[435] have been solved.

The eleven protein components of the entry–fusion complex (EFC) listed in Table 16.2 are dedicated to entry and conserved in all POXVs.[478,639] The EFC proteins, A16, G9, and J5, are related in sequence as are L1 and F9 suggesting they derive from common genes early in POXV evolution. The EFC proteins vary in size from 4 to 43 kDa, are nonglycosylated, and resemble neither type 1 nor type 2 fusion proteins of other viruses. Except for G3 and O3, the EFC proteins contain conserved intramolecular disulfide bonds that are formed by a cytoplasmic redox system, which is also encoded by all POXVs and will be described below. The EFC proteins are not required for attachment of virions to cells, although the purified L1 ectodomain can bind to the cell surface and reduce MV entry.[237] Entry of VACV is a two-step process comprising lipid mixing (hemifusion) followed by pore formation. Most of the EFC proteins are needed for the first step and all for the second.[382] The anatomy of the complex has not yet been determined, although some interacting partners have been identified and the related atomic structures of L1[699] and F9[203] have been determined (Table 16.2). L1 contains a hydrophobic cavity capable of shielding a myristate moiety suggesting a myristate switch model.[238] The VACV A17 and A27 proteins have also been implicated in membrane fusion,[362] possibly by localizing the entry proteins at the tips of the virion.[268]

Interaction of the MV with the cell surface triggers a signaling cascade that results in membrane rearrangements and the formation of actin-containing protrusions that envelope the virus and are important for fusion of viral and cellular membranes.[382,453] The lipid composition of the cell membrane is important as depletion of cholesterol inhibits virus penetration.[144] Specific fusion activation receptors have not been confidently determined, although the epidermal growth factor receptor[427] and chemokine receptors[379] have been suggested. Infectivity can be increased by incubating MVs with phosphatidylserine,[324] and an apoptotic mimicry model with a role for a specific phosphatidylserine receptor has been suggested based on reconstitution of delipidated virus.[453] However, phospholipids not known to signal apoptotic uptake can also reconstitute infectivity, indicating that the putative receptor has broad specificity or that the phospholipids have a different role in enhancement of infectivity.[380]

Superinfection exclusion mechanisms prevent fusion of MVs with infected cells that have the A56-K2 heterodimer on the plasma membrane at late times after infection; the mechanism involves interaction of A56-K2 with the A16 and G9 subunits of the EFC.[758] Another mode of superinfection exclusion prevents membrane fusion and entry at earlier times after infection.[381]

EV Entry and Virus Spread

Efficient cell-to-cell spread of VACV is mediated largely by EVs (sometimes called cell-associated EVs or CEVs) that adhere to the cell surface at the ends of long, mobile, finger-like projections that are formed by actin polymerization as illustrated in Figure 16.5.[81,694] Spread to uninfected cells may be enhanced by a repulsion mechanism that hinders superinfection of cells that express the A33 and A36 proteins on the plasma membrane and generate new actin protrusions.[206] Deletion of the A33R, A34R, or A36R ORF (Table 16.5) prevents actin tail formation and reduces the efficiency of virus spread.[600,604,791] However, mutations of the A33, A34, or A36 proteins, which cause enhanced release of free EVs, can overcome a deficiency in actin tail formation restoring spread.[81,351]

For technical reasons, most entry studies of EVs have been carried out with free particles, even though the outer membrane is fragile and not always intact. EVs may enter by endocytosis[322,617] or by fusion at the plasma membrane beneath a disrupted EV membrane.[387] Disruption at the plasma membrane is dependent on polyanionic molecules or low pH and requires the membrane glycoproteins A34 and B5.[387,589]

Cell–Cell Fusion

Two types of cell–cell fusion have been described: fusion from within and fusion from without. The former occurs late in infection, is dependent on progeny virions on the cell surface, and is triggered by lowering the pH or mutations in the A56 hemagglutinin or K2 glycoprotein.[631,733] Fusion from without is induced by infecting cells at a high multiplicity and then lowering the pH, which causes changes in the A26 protein also discussed above. Both types of cell–cell fusion require the EFC and mimic the entry pathway.[758] Unmutated A56-K2 prevents fusion by interacting with the A16-G9 components of the EFC.

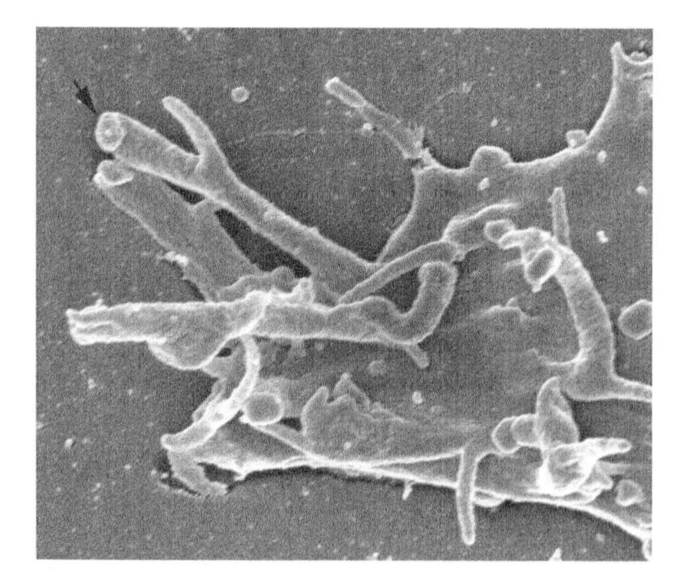

FIGURE 16.5 Scanning electron microscopy of cell infected with VACV. BS-C-1 cells were infected with VACV for 20 hours and then fixed and coated with palladium gold. The *arrow* points to an EV at the tip of a virus-induced actin-containing microvillus. (Image kindly provided by A. Weisberg.)

GENE EXPRESSION

Programmed Expression of POXV Genes

Studies primarily with VACV have led to an understanding of the POXV gene expression program (Fig. 16.6), which occurs exclusively in the cytoplasm: (a) A complete early transcription system is present within the core of virus particles, providing for the synthesis of viral early mRNAs soon after infection; (b) the early mRNAs encode enzymes and factors needed for synthesis of viral DNA and for transcription of the intermediate class of genes; (c) the intermediate gene transcripts encode enzymes and factors for late gene expression; (d) the products of the late genes include the early transcription factors, which are packaged with the viral RNA polymerase (vRNAP) and other enzymes in progeny virions. Most reports refer to postreplicative gene products as late without distinguishing between intermediate and late classes, although progress in resolving them has been made[810] as shown in the transcription map (Fig. 16.3).

Regulation of Early-Stage Transcription

Infectious POXV particles contain a transcription system that synthesizes mRNAs that are capped, methylated, and polyadenylated.[344,773] A large number of virus-encoded enzymes and factors that are directly involved in the synthesis or modification of mRNA have been isolated. These include a multisubunit DNA-dependent vRNAP, vRNAP-associated protein of 94-kDa (RAP94), early transcription factor (VETF), capping and methylating enzymes, poly(A) polymerase, nucleotide phosphohydrolase I (NPH I), and topoisomerase (Table 16.3). Additional virion-associated enzymes may participate in transcription within the virus core or remain after carrying out roles in virion assembly, protein processing, or DNA packaging.

Following entry into the cytoplasm, virus cores are transported on microtubules to a juxtanuclear region[125,422] and mRNA synthesis is detected within 20 minutes[44] (Fig. 16.7). RNA/DNA hybridization studies revealed that about half of the VACV genome is transcribed prior to DNA replication,[86,525] and genome tiling and deep RNA sequencing have corroborated this.[38,808] The 118 early ORFs that have been identified tend to cluster near the two ends of the genome (Fig. 16.3). Early genes can be divided into two groups based on kinetic cluster analysis of transcripts and temporal proteomic analysis,[38,679] but both groups are transcribed in the presence of protein synthesis inhibitors and are classified as immediate early.[808] The cessation of early gene expression coincides with disruption of the virus core, a process known as uncoating that will be discussed later. If uncoating is prevented by protein synthesis inhibitors, early mRNA synthesis is increased and prolonged,[44,795] suggesting that under normal conditions, core disassembly leads to inactivation of the early transcription apparatus.

The rapid decline of steady-state early mRNA levels (Fig. 16.7) is due to an enhanced rate of mRNA degradation in addition to cessation of transcription. Removal of the cap by the D9 and D10 decapping enzymes[530-533] is followed by activity of the cellular 5′exonuclease Xrn1.[110,411] Rapid mRNA turnover may be advantageous in eliminating cellular mRNA and decreasing viral early mRNA to enhance translation of

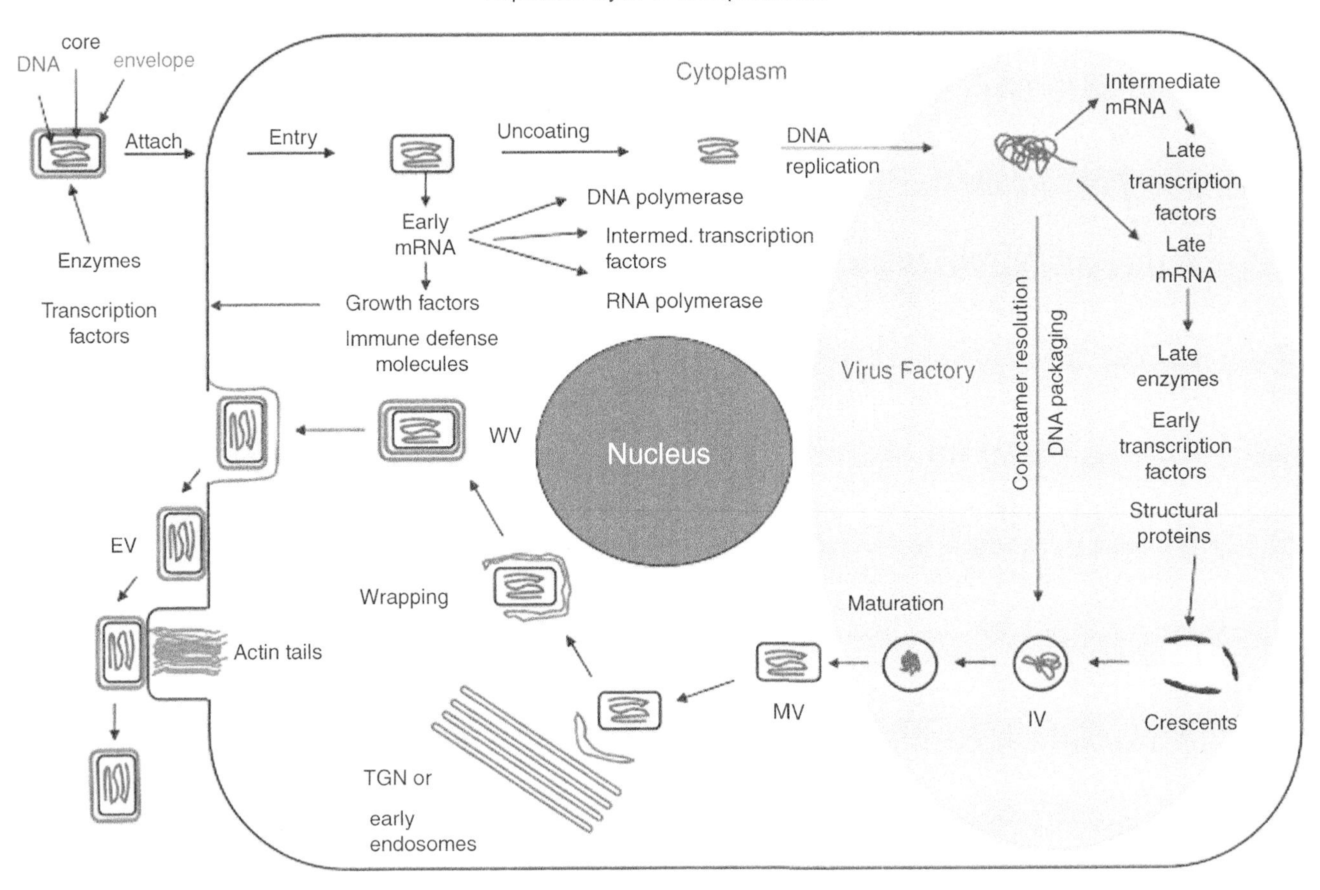

FIGURE 16.6 Replication cycle of VACV. Virions, containing a double-stranded DNA genome, enzymes, and transcription factors, attach to cells and fuse with the cell membrane, releasing cores into the cytoplasm. The cores synthesize early mRNAs that are translated into a variety of proteins, including growth factors, immune defense molecules, enzymes, and factors for DNA replication and intermediate transcription. Uncoating occurs and the DNA is replicated to form concatemeric molecules. Intermediate genes in the progeny DNA are transcribed, and the mRNAs are translated to form late transcription factors. Late genes are transcribed and the mRNAs are translated to form virion structural proteins, enzymes, and early transcription factors. Assembly begins with the formation of discrete membrane structures. Concatemeric DNA intermediates are resolved into unit genomes and packaged in immature virions. Maturation proceeds to the formation of infectious intracellular mature virions (MVs). The virions are wrapped by modified trans-Golgi and endosomal cisternae, and the wrapped virions (WVs) are transported to the periphery of the cell via microtubules. Fusion of the wrapped virions with the plasma membrane results in release of extracellular enveloped virions (EVs).

intermediate and late transcripts. Another important role of the decapping enzymes is to prevent the accumulation of double-stranded RNA (dsRNA).[411]

Early-Stage Promoters and Termination Signals

Transcription of early genes is determined by an A/T-rich sequence upstream of the RNA start site. Saturation mutagenesis of a VACV early promoter defined a critical core region, from −13 to −25 relative to the RNA start site.[173] The consensus core sequence derived from an analysis of the region upstream of all annotated early start sites[807] is consistent with the mutagenesis studies (Fig. 16.8). Transcription initiation occurs with a purine, predominantly 12 to 17 nucleotides downstream of the core region. Many more transcription starts than annotated ORFs have been revealed by deep sequencing, but their significance is not yet understood. Promoter motifs are conserved between POXV genera, explaining genetic reactivation, which consists of rescue of a heat-inactivated POXV by coinfection with a second UV-inactivated POXV of a different genus.[233,283] An explanation is that heat-killed POXVs provide intact templates and the UV-inactivated POXVs provide the transcription apparatus and early gene products.

The transcription of VACV early genes usually stops 20 to 50 bp downstream of the sequence TTTTTNT (T5NT)[815] and the transcripts are then polyadenylated. Mechanistically, termination is mediated by U5NU in RNA.[658] The T5NT sequences are present near the ends of most but not all viral early genes. When absent, the mRNA tail may extend through the next gene downstream. *In vivo* studies suggested that the efficiency of termination following a single T5NT is about 80%,[213] although in some cases, it may be less due to RNA secondary structure.[415] T5NT sequences have been noted near the ends of putative early genes of other POXV genera suggesting a similar role in termination. A VACV genome-wide analysis of the 3′ ends of early mRNAs revealed that about two-thirds have a T5NT sequence implying an additional termination mechanism for the remainder.[807] A pyrimidine-rich sequence in the coding strand up to position −25 relative to the polyadenylation site was found regardless of the presence of T5NT, suggesting that it may also facilitate termination.

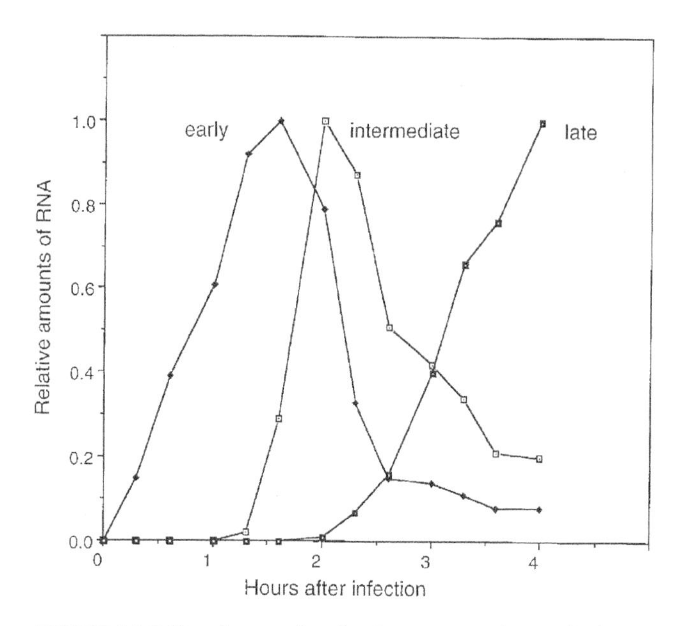

FIGURE 16.7 **Steady-state levels of representative early, intermediate, and late-stage mRNAs in VACV-infected cells.** Total RNA was isolated from infected HeLa cells at various times after infection and hybridized to antisense RNA probes specific for the 5′-ends of mRNAs encoded by the C11R (early), G8R (intermediate), or F17R (late) ORFs.[44] After ribonuclease digestion, the protected probe fragments were analyzed by polyacrylamide gel electrophoresis and the radioactivity quantified. The numbers were normalized to the peak value in each case.

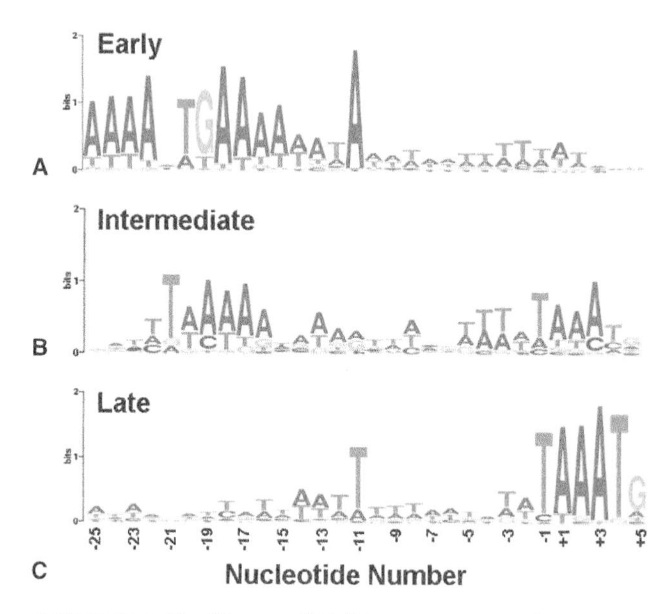

FIGURE 16.8 **Motif logos of VACV promoters.** Motifs represent early genes **(A)**, intermediate genes **(B)**, and late genes **(C)**. +1 represents the RNA start site. (Adapted from Yang Z, Bruno DP, Martens CA, et al. Genome-wide analysis of the 5′ and 3′ ends of vaccinia virus early mRNAs delineates regulatory sequences of annotated and anomalous transcripts. *J Virol* 2011;85(12):5897–5909; Yang Z, Reynolds SE, Martens CA, et al. Expression profiling of the intermediate and late stages of poxvirus replication. *J Virol* 2011;85(19):9899–9908. Refs.[807,810])

Enzymes and Factors for Early-Stage Transcription

The vRNAP has eight subunits ranging from 7- to 147-kDa[52] with 20% or less amino acid identities to host RNA polymerase II subunits.[271,359] RPO30 is an exception with approximately 23% identity to eukaryotic transcription elongation factor SII (TFIIS), which has 3′ exonuclease activity that relieves stalled polymerase. The VACV elongation complex also has a 3′ RNase activity that permits resumption of transcription by stalled polymerase likely mediated by RPO30.[281] The structure of the VACV vRNAP was recently solved by cryo-electron microscopy (EM)[271] and ribbon diagrams of the elongating core enzyme showing the positions of the template DNA and RNA are seen in Figure 16.9A.

The core vRNAP is insufficient to transcribe VACV genome templates, and additional factors present in a larger enzyme complex are needed.[104] The structure of the holoenzyme determined by cryo-EM (Fig. 16.9B) reveals 7 polypeptides in addition to the 8 subunits of vRNAP.[271] The RAP94 polypeptide encoded by the H4L gene serves as a bridge between vRNAP and transcription and processing factors.[271,824] Biochemical studies demonstrated that RAP94 is specifically required for transcription of early promoter templates[6,196] and partially resembles RNA polymerase II transcription factor TFIIB.[271] Synthesis of RAP94 occurs late, at the time of virion assembly, consistent with its role in early transcription. In contrast, the genes encoding the core vRNAP subunits are expressed both pre- and post-DNA replication because they are also needed for intermediate and late transcription.

VETF, a heterodimer of 82- and 70-kDa subunits, is a specific early transcription factor.[105,258] Like RAP94, VETF is synthesized only late during infection. The protein binds to the core region of early promoters and to DNA downstream of the RNA start site, thereby altering the conformation of the DNA.[102,127,814] A DNA-dependent ATPase activity associated with the small subunit of VETF has a role post-promoter binding.[282,392] VETF associates with vRNAP through direct interaction with RAP94[271,809] (Fig. 16.9B).

Early viral transcripts made *in vivo* or *in vitro* are capped[85,773] and polyadenylated[344] like eukaryotic mRNAs. RNAs synthesized by virus cores contain a cap I structure that consists of a terminal 7-methylguanosine connected via a triphosphate bridge to a 2′-*O*-methylribonucleoside. The N^7-methylguanosine component of the cap is required for mRNA stability and translation of VACV mRNA,[495] whereas ribose methylation prevents inhibition of translation by the interferon (IFN)-inducible IFIT proteins.[166] The VACV capping enzyme was the first such enzyme to be purified and characterized.[429,430,753] The steps in cap formation are (a) removal of the terminal phosphate of the triphosphate end of the nascent RNA to form a pp(5′)N-terminus, (b) transfer of a GMP residue from GTP to form G(5′)ppp(5′)N-, (c) transfer of a methyl group from *S*-adenosylmethionine to produce m^7G(5′)ppp(5′)N-, and (d) transfer of a second methyl group to form m^7G(5′)ppp(5′)Nm. The first three reactions are catalyzed by the virus-encoded 127-kDa capping enzyme heterodimer.[428] The capping enzyme large subunit forms a covalent lysyl-GMP intermediate.[657] The RNA triphosphatase, guanylyltransferase, and N^7-methyltransferase activities all reside in the large subunit; the small subunit binds to the methyltransferase domain and stimulates the activity of the latter allosterically.[375] Both subunits are expressed early in infection.[473,510] The capping enzyme is associated with the

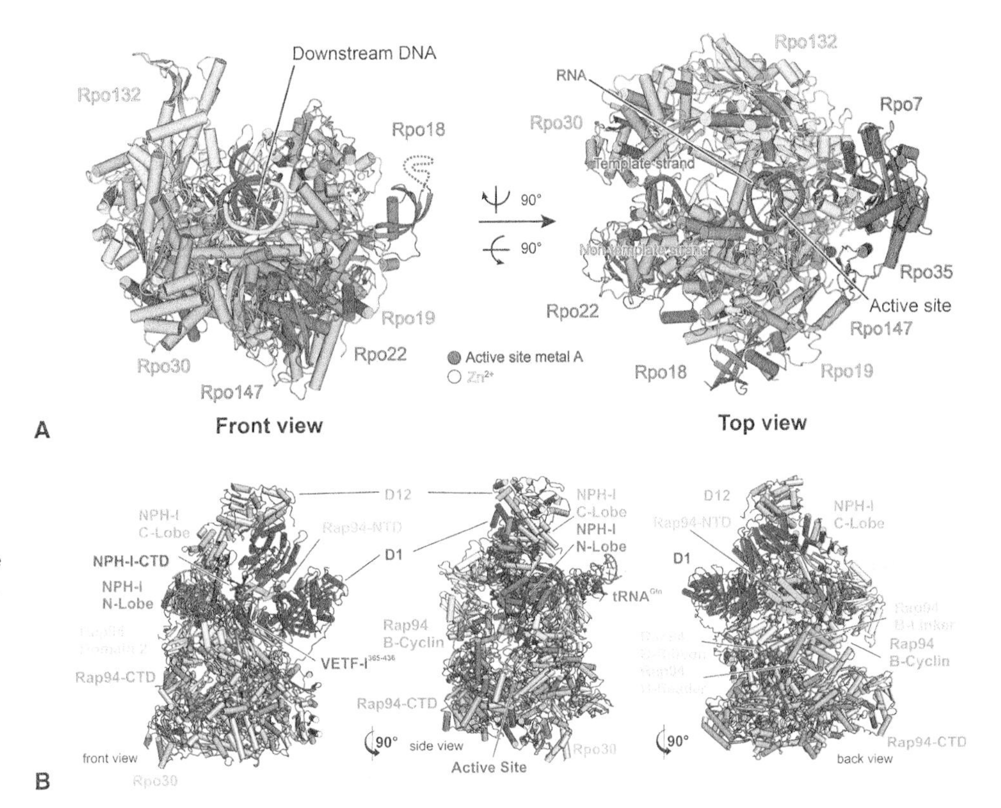

FIGURE 16.9 vRNAP. A: vRNAP core structure showing arrangement of subunits. (Reprinted from Hillen HS, Bartuli J, Grimm C, et al. Structural Basis of Poxvirus Transcription: Transcribing and Capping Vaccinia Complexes. *Cell* 2019;179(7):1525–1536.e12. Copyright © 2019 Elsevier. With permission. Ref.[293]) **B:** Overview of the complete vRNAP model. vRNAP core in gray; associated proteins in colors. (Reprinted from Grimm C, Hillen HS, Bedenk K, et al. Structural Basis of Poxvirus Transcription: Vaccinia RNA Polymerase Complexes. *Cell* 2019;179(7):1537–1550.e19. Copyright © 2019 Elsevier. With permission. Ref.[271])

VACV vRNAP through interaction with RAP94 (Fig. 16.9B) and capping occurs during transcription when the nascent RNA chains are approximately 30 nucleotides long.[280]

Ribose methylation of the penultimate nucleoside is mediated by a separate viral nucleoside 2′-MTase.[51] This MTase is a 39-kDa protein that exists as a monomeric species and also as the VP39 subunit of poly(A) polymerase.[621] High-resolution X-ray crystal structures of the MTase complexed to its methyl donor and mRNA cap have been obtained.[299] Viral mRNAs synthesized *in vivo* have additional base and ribose methylations that are catalyzed by cellular enzymes.[85]

The enzyme that catalyzes poly(A) tail formation is a heterodimer of virus-encoded 55- and 39-kDa subunits called VP55 and VP39, respectively.[256,489] VP55 binds to uridylate sequences near the end of the RNA chain and catalyzes the processive addition of approximately 30 adenylate residues before changing to slow and nonprocessive addition.[260,813] VP39 binds poly(A) and stimulates VP55 to add additional adenylates.[259] The processivity and MTase activities of VP39 are independent since mutated forms that lack MTase retain adenylyltransferase stimulatory activity.[622,648] Genetic and biochemical studies indicate an additional role of VP39 as an RNA elongation factor for intermediate and late RNA synthesis.[386,798] The finding that the capping enzyme/termination factor and the ribose MTase/poly(A) polymerase processivity factor function at the 5′ and 3′ ends of the mRNA is intriguing. The association of such apparently disparate functions in the same enzymes may provide a specific advantage or represent an economical use of proteins.

Both capping enzyme and NPH I are needed to release nascent mRNA containing a U5NU sequence from the transcription complex in an ATP-dependent reaction.[142,296] The physical interaction of NPH I with RAP94 (Fig. 16.9B) explains the specificity of this termination system for early transcripts.[271,550] NPH I also serves as a polymerase elongation factor to facilitate read-through of intrinsic pause sites.[195]

The minimal components for synthesis of correctly initiated, terminated, capped, and polyadenylated mRNAs were defined by *in vitro* reconstitution assays. However, several additional proteins are needed within the virus core. These include the DNA topoisomerase,[162] NPH II,[274] the H1 serine/tyrosine phosphatase,[406] the L4 DNA-RNA binding protein,[780] and the L3[581] and E8[346] proteins. E11, a previously described core protein known to be required for infectivity,[766] interacts with RAP94 and associates with the vRNAP complex.[271] The *in vitro* activity of the topoisomerase, which relaxes supercoiled DNA, has been studied extensively.[576]

Regulation of Intermediate-Stage Transcription

Amino acid labeling and transcription studies indicate the existence of an intermediate class of genes that are expressed after DNA replication but before expression of stringent late genes[44,757] (Fig. 16.7). The number of VACV genes belonging to the intermediate class is estimated to be about 53.[810] Three of the intermediate genes (A1L, A2L, and G8R) encode late-stage transcription factors,[352] and others include DNA binding/packaging and core-associated proteins.

Because the intermediate transcription factors are early proteins, the DNA replication requirement for intermediate gene expression may result from inaccessibility of the genome within the infecting particles. This hypothesis is consistent with transfection experiments showing that transfected genomic DNA or recombinant plasmids can serve as a template for intermediate and late transcription in the absence of DNA replication.[352]

Intermediate-Stage Promoters

Mutagenesis of intermediate promoters indicates two important regions: a 14-bp core element separated by 10 or 11 bp from a 4-bp TAAA initiator element.[45,360] The intermediate promoter core element like that of early promoters is A/T rich.

A consensus (Fig. 16.8) has been derived from an analysis of the sequences preceding 53 intermediate ORFs.[810] Intermediate-stage RNAs are initiated within the AAA triplet, but additional A residues are incorporated by vRNAP slippage.

Enzymes and Factors for Intermediate-Stage Transcription

Intermediate promoter templates can be transcribed by extracts prepared from cells infected with VACV in the presence of an inhibitor of DNA replication indicating that all necessary proteins are synthesized early in infection.[757] Further studies indicate a role for both viral and cellular proteins. The viral proteins include the vRNAP lacking RAP94; free RPO30 called VITF-1[597]; capping enzyme, which acts by a mechanism that does not involve cap formation[285,756]; and a heterodimer composed of polypeptides encoded by the A8R and A23R genes referred to as VITF-3[607] (Table 16.6). Neither VITF-1 nor VITF-3 has been shown to have ATPase activity or exhibit sequence-specific DNA binding. An additional requirement is for *in vitro* transcription can be fulfilled by two cellular proteins, Ras-GTPase–activating protein SH3 domain-binding protein (G3BP) and cytoplasmic activation/proliferation-associated protein (p137), which form a complex.[349] However, as yet, there are no *in vivo* studies confirming their specific role in transcription. On the other hand, *in vivo* experiments employing RNAi and dominant negative inhibitors suggest that the cellular TATA-binding protein has a positive role in VACV intermediate and late gene expression and that YY1 has a negative role by binding to promoter and initiator elements, respectively.[360,361] However, *in vitro* experiments confirming a direct action have not been reported. In addition, neither was found by mass spectrometry of proteins cross-linked to viral DNA.[634] A reliance on cellular proteins is surprising since POXVs transcription occurs in the cytoplasm, and they encode their own vRNAP and other transcription factors.

TABLE 16.6 Viral stage-specific transcription factors

Stage	Factor	ORF[a] COP	ORF[a] WR	kDa	T[b]	C[c]	References
Early	VETF	A7L	126	82	L	P	(258)
		D6R	111	74	L	P	(258)
	RAP94	H4L	102	94	L	P	(8)
Inter	VITF-1	E4L	060	30	E	C	(597)
	VITF-3	A8R	127	34	E	C	(607)
		A23R	143	45	E	P	(607)
	Cap enzyme	D1R	106	97	E	P	(756)
		D12L	117	33	E	P	(756)
Late	VLTF-1	G8R	086	30	I	C	(352)
	VLTF-2	A1L	119	17	I	P	(352)
	VLTF-3	A2L	120	26	I	P	(352)
	VLTF-4	H5R	103	22	E	C	(369)

[a]Copenhagen (COP) or Western Reserve (WR) ORF designation.
[b]Time of synthesis: early (E), intermediate (I), or late (L).
[c]Conservation in all POXV (P) or chordopoxviruses (C).

Further studies provided evidence for virus-encoded positive and negative regulators of intermediate and/or late transcription elongation. The VACV A18 DNA helicase acts as a negative transcription elongation and a transcript release factor.[376,802] A18R mutations increase read-through of neighboring genes and increase levels of dsRNA. The G2 protein acts as a positive elongation factor as inactivating mutations result in intermediate and late mRNAs that are truncated.[77] Moreover, mutation of G2R can compensate for A18R mutations.[151] Physical interactions between G2, A18, and H5 (a late transcription factor) were demonstrated by a variety of methods.[78,440] J3, which is the cap 2′-O-MTase and the VP39 subunit of the poly(A) polymerase, also is an mRNA elongation factor.[386,798]

Regulation of Late-Stage Transcription

Transcription of late genes quickly follows that of intermediate genes and persists till the end of the virus life cycle (Fig. 16.7). Short half-lives of late mRNAs[513,628] emphasize the need for continued high-level transcription. A recent study distinguished intermediate and late genes and identified 38 that belong to the latter class, which encode proteins involved in morphogenesis, the virion membrane, and early transcription.[810] In addition, many intermediate genes also exhibit varying amounts of late expression. Although distributed throughout the genome, late-stage genes cluster in the central region (Fig. 16.3).

Late-Stage Promoters and RNA Processing Signal

Late-stage promoters consist of a core sequence of about 20 bp with some consecutive T residues, separated by a region of approximately 6 bp from a highly conserved TAAAT element within which transcription initiates.[174] A synthetic promoter with exclusively T-residues forming the core sequence was stronger than natural late promoters tested and any mutations of TAAAT severely decreased transcription. A consensus promoter (Fig. 16.8) derived from the sequence upstream of 38 late genes is consistent with the mutational analysis.[810] A G or A usually follows the late promoter TAAAT sequence: in the former case, the TAAATG transcription initiation sequence and the ATG translation initiation codon overlap. The seeming absence of an untranslated RNA leader and in some cases a poor Kozak consensus translation initiation sequence were puzzling until it was found that late mRNAs have a 5′ capped, heterogeneous-length, poly(A) leader sequence formed by RNA polymerase slippage.[535,626] Poly(A) leaders are also present on intermediate mRNAs and mRNAs of a few early genes that have a TAAAT initiation site,[807] suggesting that slippage on an AAA sequence is an intrinsic property of the vRNAP. The 5′ poly(A) may provide a translational benefit.[199]

Most postreplicative transcripts are long, heterogeneous and lack defined 3′-ends.[152,421] Terminal heterogeneity, combined with transcription from both DNA strands, causes overlapping of transcripts explaining their ability to self-anneal or anneal with early transcripts to form dsRNA.[87,147,752] The early termination signal is not recognized even though T5NT is frequently present within the coding region of postreplicative genes. A few exceptions to the general 3′ heterogeneity of late mRNAs occur.[33] The CPXV late mRNA encoding the A-type inclusion protein has a defined 3′-end. The DNA sequence at this position encodes an RNA cis-acting signal for RNA 3′-end formation that can function independently of either the nature of the promoter or the RNA polymerase responsible for generating the primary RNA.[304] Cleavage also generates the 3′ end of F17R transcripts[160] and endoribonuclease activity directly or indirectly associated with the product of the H5R gene can cleave this RNA,[161] which is then polyadenylated. Therefore, POXVs employ at least two mechanisms of RNA 3′-end formation. The first, operative at early times in viral replication, terminates transcription downstream of an RNA signal, whereas the second, operative at late times, involves RNA site-specific cleavage.

Enzymes and Factors for Late-Stage Transcription

The vRNAP catalyzes late mRNA synthesis in conjunction with specific factors. Late transcription factors (Table 16.4) were identified by the systematic transfection of cloned viral DNA fragments: ORFs A1L, A2L, and G8R were necessary and sufficient for transactivation of a transfected late promoter reporter gene in VACV-infected cells that were blocked in DNA replication.[352] An intermediate promoter regulates each of these late transcription factor genes, which is consistent with a cascade model of regulation. *In vitro* studies confirmed that the products of the G8R, A1L, and A2L genes are VACV late transcription factors,[316,534,796] and they have been named VLTF-1, VLTF-2, and VLTF-3, respectively. Temperature-sensitive and null mutations of A1L or G8R block late gene expression.[123,827] Yeast two-hybrid studies indicate interactions between G8 and itself and with A1.[440] *In vitro* studies indicated that the product of the early H5R gene, named VLTF-4, stimulated late transcription several-fold,[369] and interactions between H5 and other late transcription factors has been described.[192] H5 also appears to have a role in transcript elongation.[78] *In vitro* transcription assays suggest a role for a host factor originally called VLTF-X and shown to consist of the heterogeneous nuclear ribonucleoproteins A2/B1 and RBM3.[797]

Proteins cross-linked to newly replicated VACV DNA were identified by mass spectrometry.[634] In addition to DNA replication proteins, to be discussed below, the following proteins involved in intermediate and late RNA synthesis and processing were found supporting their roles *in vivo*: the four largest vRNAP subunits (RPO147, RPO132, RPO35, and RPO30), two intermediate transcription factors (A23 and A8), two capping enzyme subunits (D1 and D12), the 2′-O MTase (J3), the elongation factor (G2), the late transcription factors (G8, A1, and A2), and H5.

Regulation of Translation

Although POXV gene expression is mainly regulated at the transcriptional and mRNA degradation levels, perturbations of signaling pathways also has translational effects[447] and will be discussed further in the section on viral defense molecules. While early and postreplicative mRNAs like those of eukaryotes have cap I or II 5′ ends,[85] the 5′ poly(A) leader may reduce the requirements for certain translation initiation factors.[199,650] The VACV B1 kinase phosphorylates residues in the small ribosomal subunit protein RACK1 to facilitate translation of mRNAs with poly(A) leaders.[334] Postreplicative mRNAs are translated in or adjacent to virus factories,[347,816] although local translation has been shown to occur at the sites of A-type inclusions.[348] Viral protein synthesis depends on an adequate source of amino acids. A recent study shows that in the absence of glutamine, asparagine becomes limiting.[523]

DNA REPLICATION

General Features

POXV DNA replication takes place in the cytoplasm and occurs even when cells have been enucleated.[544,560] Uncoating, which depends on *de novo* protein synthesis, is required to release the DNA from the virus core to serve as a template.[337] The D5 helicase/primase is required for this process,[357] and two viral ankyrin-repeat proteins may also have roles.[402,410] Proteasome inhibitors prevent uncoating as well as DNA replication by mechanisms that are not yet understood.[454,611]

Discrete cytoplasmic foci of replication, termed factories, are discerned by light and electron microscopic autoradiography.[118,284] During the first few hours of infection, the factories are delimited by ER membranes.[719] DNA replication begins 1 to 2 hours after VACV infection, and by 3 to 4 hours, the nucleoside analog EdU is incorporated almost exclusively into cytoplasmic DNA factories (Fig. 16.10). Each factory can be initiated by a single virion, although factories merge together with time.[347,398] About 10,000 genomes are synthesized per cell of which half are ultimately packaged into virions.[338]

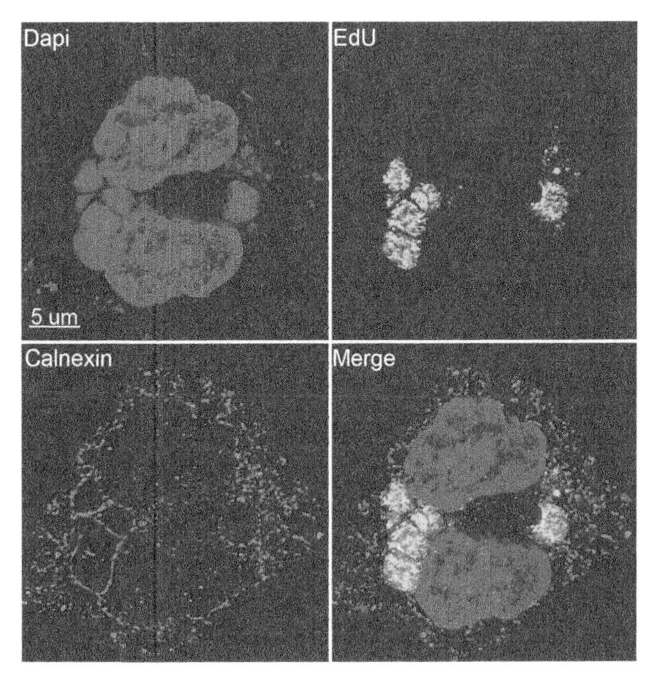

FIGURE 16.10 Localization of nascent viral DNA. A549 cells were incubated for 10 minutes with EdU at 3.5 hours after VACV infection and then fixed, permeabilized, and reacted with Alexa Fluor 488 azide to reveal newly synthesized DNA. The cells were then incubated with rabbit polyclonal antibody to calnexin (Santa Cruz) followed by secondary antibody conjugated to Alexa Fluor 594 and DAPI to visualize ER and total DNA, respectively. (Reprinted from Senkevich TG, Katsafanas GC, Weisberg A, et al. Identification of vaccinia virus replisome and transcriptome proteins by isolation of proteins on nascent DNA coupled with mass spectrometry. *J Virol* 2017;91(19):e01015–17. Ref.[634])

Efforts to locate a specific POXV origin of replication using a plasmid assay in transfected cells were unsuccessful; surprisingly, any circular DNA replicates in cells infected with Shope fibroma virus (SFV)[191] or VACV.[460] Further studies demonstrated that origin-independent plasmid replication occurs in virus factory areas and requires each protein needed for genome replication confirming the specificity of this activity.[182] Using a transfection assay in which the template is a linear DNA molecule containing VACV hairpin ends, a specific enhancing effect of the terminal 200 bp of the viral genome was found.[211] Deep sequencing of short single-stranded DNA fragments enriched for RNA-primed nascent strands from VACV-infected cells identified a bidirectional origin within the hairpin loop at one end of the VACV genome and within the concatemeric junction of replication intermediates, although the possibility of additional origins was not excluded.[645]

DNA Replication Models

The unique terminal structure of the POXV genome,[53] evidence that nicking and initiation occurs near the ends of the molecule,[552] the presence of telomeric junction fragments,[54,492] and high molecular weight DNA[189,459] suggested the model depicted in Figure 16.11: a nick at one or both ends of the genome provides a free 3′-end for priming replication. The replicated DNA strand then folds back on itself, and the replication complex copies the remainder of the genome. Concatemer junctions form after replication through the hairpin; very large branched concatemers can arise by initiating new rounds of replication before resolution occurs. After the onset of late-stage transcription, unit-length genomes are resolved and the incompletely base-paired terminal loops, with inverted and complementary sequences, are regenerated. Despite the attractiveness of this model, neither the site of nicking nor an essential nicking enzyme needed to initiate DNA replication has been identified.[215]

A more conventional model posits RNA priming and semidiscontinuous DNA synthesis at replication forks. Early reports of VACV DNA covalently linked to RNA and the chasing of short DNA into larger molecules suggested lagging strand synthesis.[222,553] Initially, this model was not favored because the viral DNA ligase was found to be nonessential,[148,354] and there was no evidence for a primase. The subsequent discovery of a viral primase and the finding that a cellular DNA ligase substitutes for the absent viral enzyme revived interest in this model.[180,527] Evidence for a bidirectional origin of genome replication near the end of the genome supports leading and lagging strand synthesis at replication forks[645] as illustrated in Figure 16.12. The two models are not mutually exclusive as it is possible that POXVs use multiple mechanisms to achieve replication of their large genomes.

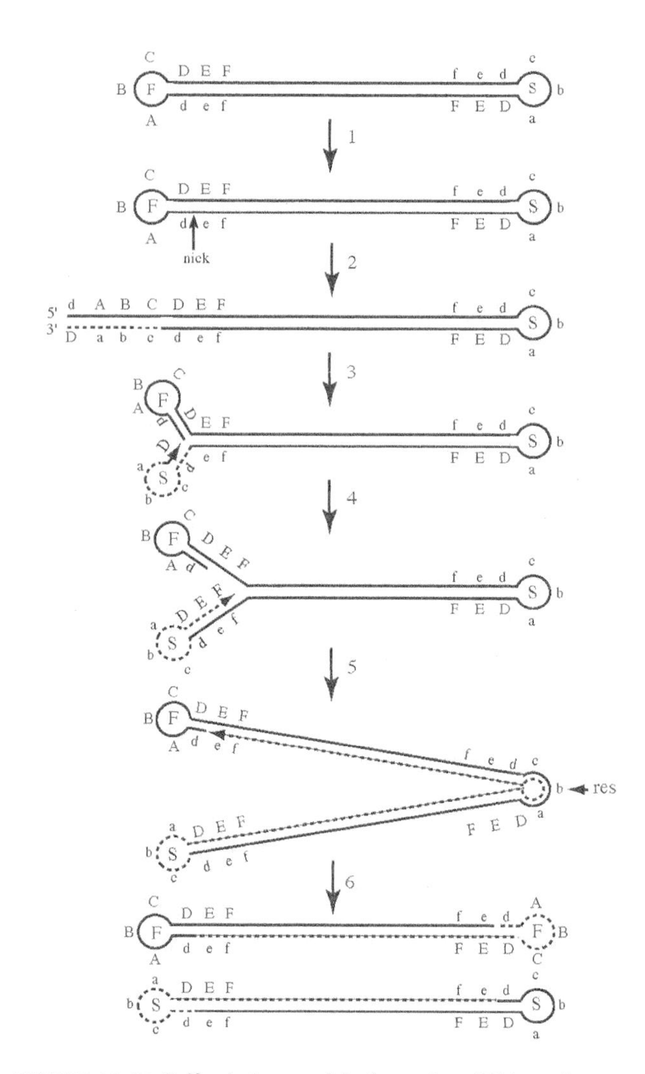

FIGURE 16.11 Self-priming model of poxvirus DNA replication. F and S within the hairpin loops refer to the fast and slow electrophoretic mobilities of DNA fragments containing inverted and complementary hairpin sequences as shown in Figure 16.2. *Dashed lines* indicate newly synthesized DNA with *arrowheads* at the 3′ OH ends. Complementary sequences are depicted by upper and lower case letters. The resolution site (res) within the concatemer junction is indicated. (Adapted with permission of John Wiley & Sons from Moss B, Winters E, Jones EV. Replication of vaccinia virus. In: Cozzarelli N, ed. *Mechanisms of DNA Replication and Recombination*. New York: A.R. Liss; 1983:449–461; permission conveyed through Copyright Clearance Center, Inc. Ref.[485])

Enzymes Involved in DNA Precursor Metabolism

Some POXVs encode several enzymes involved in the synthesis of deoxyribonucleotides to enhance DNA replication in resting cells with suboptimal precursor pools, whereas others lack some or all of these. Inactivation of these enzymes has been used for construction of oncolytic poxviruses that selectively kill proliferating cancer cells.[439] In OPXVs, these enzymes include a TK,[43] thymidylate kinase,[674] ribonucleotide reductase,[665,715] and dUTPase.[100] VACV and some OPXVs also contain a gene encoding an inactive guanylate kinase.[264,673] Leporipoxviruses are missing genes encoding the large subunit of ribonucleotide reductase and thymidylate kinase,[119,782] and MOCV is missing genes for all of the enzymes involved in DNA precursor metabolism perhaps contributing to its limited host range.[635] FWPV encodes a protein related to human deoxycytidine kinase that is not present in the other POXVs.[364] Entomopoxvirus Melanoplus sanguinipes lacks all of the previously described POXV genes involved in nucleotide metabolism but has a thymidylate synthetase homolog.[2] However, a TK gene is present in other entomopoxviruses.[276,419]

POXV TKs are 20 to 25 kDa and related in sequence to corresponding eukaryotic enzymes (35% to 70% amino acid identity). The structure of VACV TK is similar to human TK,

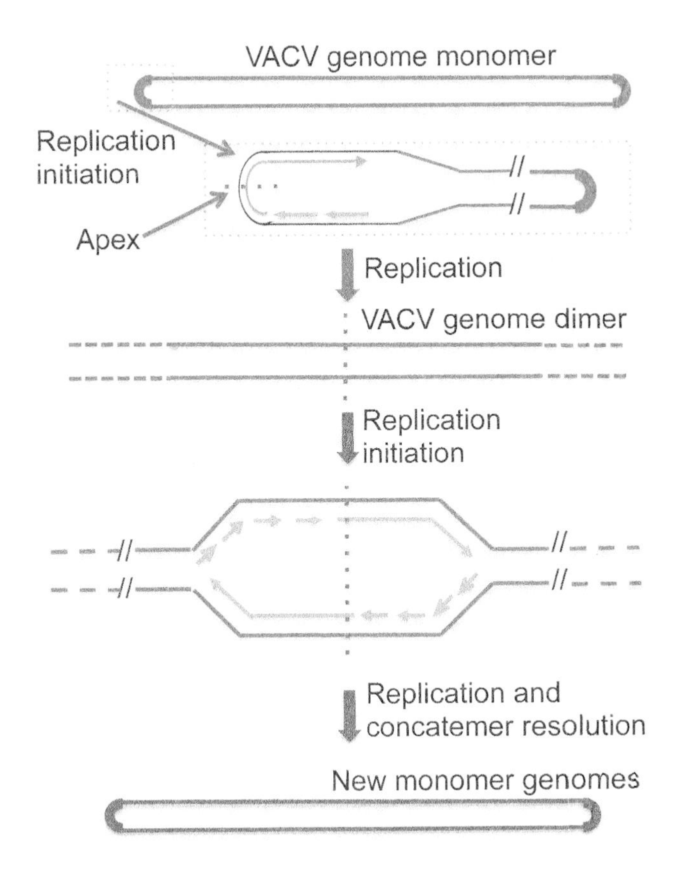

FIGURE 16.12 Model depicting replication origins at the terminal hairpin and concatemer junction. The VACV genome monomer with hairpin ends that is packaged in virus particles is shown at the top. DNA synthesis initiating within one hairpin is shown below. Replication results in the formation of a dimer by conversion of the incompletely base-paired hairpins into completely base-paired concatemer junctions. In this model, the concatemer junction serves as a bidirectional origin. Finally, the concatemers are resolved into unit genomes by the Holliday junction resolvase. Leading strands are shown as *blue arrows* and lagging strand fragments as *short green arrows*. The apex of the concatemer junction is indicted by *red dashes*. (Reprinted with permission from Senkevich TG, Bruno D, Martens C, et al. Mapping vaccinia virus DNA replication origins at nucleotide level by deep sequencing. *Proc Natl Acad Sci U S A* 2015;112(35):10908–10913. Ref.[645])

but there are differences in the association with dTTP that might be exploited for antivirals.[216] The enzyme exists as a tetramer, has ATP and Mg^{2+}-binding domains, and is susceptible to feedback inhibition by dTDP or dTTP.[79] The TK gene is regulated by an early promoter, as befits its role in increasing precursors for DNA replication.[774] Although the TK gene is not required for virus growth in tissue culture cells, deletion mutants are severely attenuated *in vivo*.[109]

Thymidylate kinase catalyzes the next step in TMP metabolism. The VACV gene encodes a 23-kDa protein that can complement *Saccharomyces cerevisiae* mutants deficient in the homologous enzyme.[317] The protein is expressed early in infection and is not required for virus replication in tissue culture. VACV thymidylate kinase has a 42% identity with its human homolog but differs in substantial ways and has broader substrate specificity.[39,117]

Ribonucleotide reductase, an enzyme that converts ribonucleoside diphosphates to deoxyribonucleoside diphosphates, is synthesized soon after VACV infection.[667] The small catalytic subunit and the large regulatory subunit resemble their eukaryotic counterparts structurally (70% to 80% identity) and functionally.[305,666] Catalytic activity is inhibited by hydroxyurea preventing DNA replication, and drug-resistant mutants generate direct tandem repeats of the gene encoding the catalytic subunit.[669] Mutation of the large subunit prevents induced ribonucleotide reductase activity in tissue culture cells without affecting replication.[138] However, the mutant virus was mildly attenuated in a mouse model. In contrast to OPXVs, many chordopoxviruses only encode the large subunit, which complexes with the cellular small subunit to form active ribonucleotide reductase.[243]

Hydrolysis of dUTP by the VACV dUTPase provides dUMP, an intermediate in the biosynthesis of TTP, and might also minimize dUTP incorporation into DNA.[100] The protein is synthesized early in infection[668] and is nonessential for virus replication in dividing cells.[546] The dUTPase is important in quiescent cells, particularly in the absence of the viral uracil DNA glycosylase.[181] The structure of VACV dUTPase is similar to the human homolog.[603]

Viral Proteins Involved in DNA Replication

Genetic and biochemical studies led to the identification of viral proteins that carry out genome replication.[159,377] The VACV DNA polymerase holoenzyme consists of the 116 kDa catalytic subunit E9 with a heterodimer of A20 and D4, which promotes processive DNA replication.[128,214,328,693] The core enzyme belongs to the B family of replicative polymerases, has 3′ proofreading exonuclease activity, and is the target of several inhibitors two of which (cidofovir and brincidofovir) are promising therapeutics for smallpox. Important features of these proteins were derived from high-resolution structures of E9 in complex with the N-terminal domain of D4 and of D4 in complex with the N-terminal domain of A20.[712]

In addition to serving as a processivity factor, D4 is a functional uracil DNA glycosylase[95,697] with structural features common to Family I enzymes.[623] These enzymes function in DNA repair by removing uracil residues that have been introduced into DNA, either through misincorporation of dUTP or through the deamination of cytosine. Mutagenesis studies demonstrated that the requirement for DNA replication is independent of its glycosylase activity.[183] Nevertheless, VACV mutants with enzymatically inactive UDG are attenuated in mice indicating that the repair function is beneficial, consistent with the preservation of the catalytic site in all POXV orthologs.

The VACV 49-kDa A20 protein has no nonpoxvirus homologs, and a role in DNA replication was first suggested by a yeast two-hybrid analysis, which demonstrated an interaction with the DNA replication proteins D4 and D5 and also H5.[328,440] The association of A20 and D4 with DNA polymerase imparts processivity.[159]

D5, a 90-kDa protein, has both nucleic acid-independent nucleoside triphosphatase[225] and primase activities[180,330] that are essential for DNA replication.[93,180] Helicase activity is predicted but not yet demonstrated. As previously noted, the triphosphatase domain of D5 also contributes to release of DNA from the core.[357]

VACV I3 is a 34-kDa phosphoprotein that forms octameric complexes on single-stranded DNA[729] and is essential for VACV genome replication.[269]

VACV encodes a functional ATP-dependent DNA ligase that is not essential for replication in tissue culture, although it imparts resistance to DNA-damaging agents and is important for virulence.[148,353] The ability of VACV to replicate in the absence of the viral DNA ligase depends on the recruitment of cellular DNA ligase I, which is responsible for joining Okazaki fragments.[527] However, replication of ligase-deficient VACV is greatly reduced and delayed in resting primary cells, correlating with initial low levels of ligase I and subsequent viral induction and localization of ligase I in virus factories.[527] By encoding its own ligase VACV can "jump-start" DNA synthesis in resting cells and enhance replication.

B1 is a 35-kDa serine/threonine protein kinase that is expressed early in infection, packaged in virions and fosters viral DNA replication by phosphorylating the cellular protein called barrier to autointegration factor (BAF).[518] B1 is a homolog of cellular protein kinases, which can substitute for the viral enzyme. An early protein encoded by the H5R gene is a substrate for the B1 kinase,[64] and interactions between these proteins was demonstrated by the yeast two-hybrid system.[440] H5 is a multifunctional protein with a role in DNA replication[94] as well as transcription, mRNA processing, and morphogenesis.

Each of the viral proteins involved in DNA replication plus the FEN-1–like nuclease G5, the telomere-binding protein I1, and components of the intermediate and late transcription systems were identified by mass spectrometry of proteins cross-linked to newly replicated viral DNA.[634] In that study, the cellular protein Top2B was found in equal abundance with and dependent on the VACV DNA ligase. Top2A and PCNA were identified at lower abundance than the viral proteins.

Photolyases, which protect DNA from ultraviolet radiation by excision of cyclobutane pyrimidine dimers, are encoded by avipoxviruses and leporipoxviruses as well as entomopoxviruses.[70,501,690]

While it is generally believed that VACV DNA synthesis is mediated exclusively by viral proteins, there is evidence that cytoplasmic activation of the ATR/ATM arms of the DNA damage response promote genome replication.[558]

Concatemer Resolution

The replication of the POXV genome involves the formation of concatemers and their resolution into unit–length molecules.[54,492] The concatemer junction consists of a precise duplex copy of the hairpin loop present at the ends of mature DNA genomes.[457] The conversion of circular plasmids containing concatemer junctions into linear molecules with hairpin termini when transfected into POXV-infected cells allowed determination of the structural and sequence requirements for resolution of concatemer junctions.[443,458] The minimal requirement for resolution is two copies of the sequence T_6-N_{7-9}-T/C-A_3-T/A present in an inverted repeat orientation on either side of an extended double-stranded copy of the hairpin loop.

In supercoiled plasmids, the concatemer junction can form a cruciform structure resembling a four-way Holliday junction (HJ) recombination intermediate.[200,457] This suggested that the putative concatemer resolving enzyme would be a HJ resolvase. Bioinformatic analyses led to the discovery of motifs and structural elements that are critical for activity of *Escherichia coli* RuvC HJ resolvase in ORFs that are conserved in all POXV genomes.[248] Moreover, the RuvC homolog encoded by the VACV A22R ORF specifically cleaves HJs.[248] Like RuvC, A22 is a dimer in solution and when bound to HJ structures but exhibits less cleavage sequence specificity.[157,250] A VACV-inducible A22 null mutant was defective in processing concatemers into unit–length genomes with hairpin ends under nonpermissive conditions, indicating that the enzyme is required for resolution, although additional proteins may also be involved in determining site specificity.[249]

Type I DNA topoisomerases form a covalent link with DNA and relieve supercoils during replication, transcription, recombination, and other activities. POXVs encode a type 1 topoisomerase that has served as a model for this class of enzymes.[647,659,805] The topoisomerase is unusual in that it exhibits some sequence specificity.[656] *In vitro*, the topoisomerase can carry out a variety of reactions including strand transfer, transesterification, recombination, and cleavage and ligation of a variety of DNA structures including a HJ.[520,632] A VACV topoisomerase deletion mutant has impaired early transcription, but DNA replication and concatemer resolution still occur.[162] The topoisomerase is regulated by a late promoter, which is consistent with a role in transcription or DNA processing.

Homologous Recombination

Recombination can occur during coinfection[231] and has occurred naturally between SFV, which produces benign fibromas in rabbits, and myxoma virus (MYXV), the agent of myxomatosis, to form malignant rabbit fibroma virus,[83] and between individual capripoxviruses.[257] Recombination between the terminal sequences of POXV DNA may explain variations in the number of tandem repeats as well as translocations and mirror image deletions.[442,493] Most extraordinarily, field and vaccine strains of FWPV carry a near full length and apparently infectious integrated avian retrovirus genome.[291] The existence of families of related proteins in poxviruses suggests the occurrence of gene duplications in the past. Moreover, experimental evolution studies reveal the occurrence of transient gene duplications that enhance expression, referred to as an accordion model.[217,669] Viral genomes rapidly eliminate direct repeats with the formation of intra- and intermolecular recombination products.[48]

Recombination can also occur between viral genomic DNA and transfected subgenomic DNA fragments, and this has been exploited to map and construct mutations and to insert genes for expression.[480] Single- and double-crossover products resulting from recombination between transfected plasmids and viral genomes[689] and inter- and intramolecular plasmid or bacteriophage DNA recombinants[224,529] have been detected in POXV-infected cells.

Recombination does not require postreplicative gene products.[456,781] There is evidence that the DNA polymerase participates directly in recombination and that the 3′ exonuclease and DNA joining activities are involved.[242] The protein encoded by the G5R gene, which is conserved in all POXVs and expressed early in infection, belongs to the FEN1 family of exo/endo nucleases.[165,329] Deletion of VACV G5R reduces the yield of infectious virus by two orders of magnitude.[636] Although the amount of viral DNA produced in the absence of G5 is similar to that made by wild-type virus, the mean size is approximately one-fourth of the genome length. Experiments with transfected plasmids show that G5 is required for double-strand break repair by homologous recombination, suggesting a similar role during VACV genome replication.[636]

The chordopoxviruses, except for avipoxviruses, encode homologs of serine recombinases.[1] However, only the crocodile

POXV contains all amino acids that comprise the catalytic active site, and deletion of the VACV F16 homolog had no effect on replication in cultured cells.[637]

VIRION ASSEMBLY

Overview

The initial stages of virion assembly occur in virus factories. Assembly can be divided into the following stages: (a) formation of membrane crescents and spherical immature virions (IVs) containing the core protein precursors, genome, and an outer spicule layer; (b) loss of the spicules, organization of the core, and conversion to a brick-shaped mature virions (MVs); (c) enclosure of some MVs by two additional membranes to form wrapped virions (WVs) also called intracellular enveloped virions (IEVs); and (d) movement of WVs to the periphery and exocytosis to form EVs.[150] A thin section transmission electron microscopic image of a cell infected with VACV and enlarged pictures of virions at successive stages of assembly and egress are shown in Figures 16.13 and 16.14, respectively. Deep etch electron microscopy revealed that the outer spicule layer is a honeycomb lattice composed of the D13 protein viewed on edge (Fig. 16.15).[292,709]

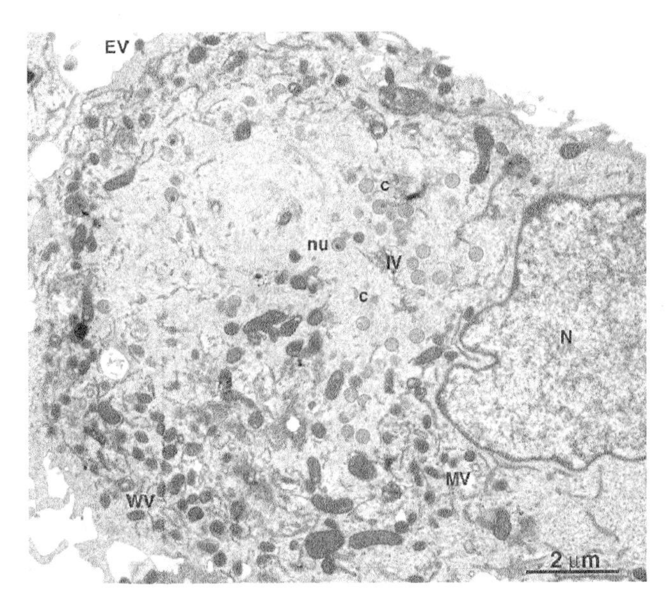

FIGURE 16.13 Transmission electron microscopy of cell infected with VACV. N, cell nucleus; c, viral crescent; IV, immature virion; nu, DNA nucleoid within IV; MV, mature virion; WV, wrapped virion; EV, extracellular enveloped virion. (Image kindly provided by A. Weisberg.)

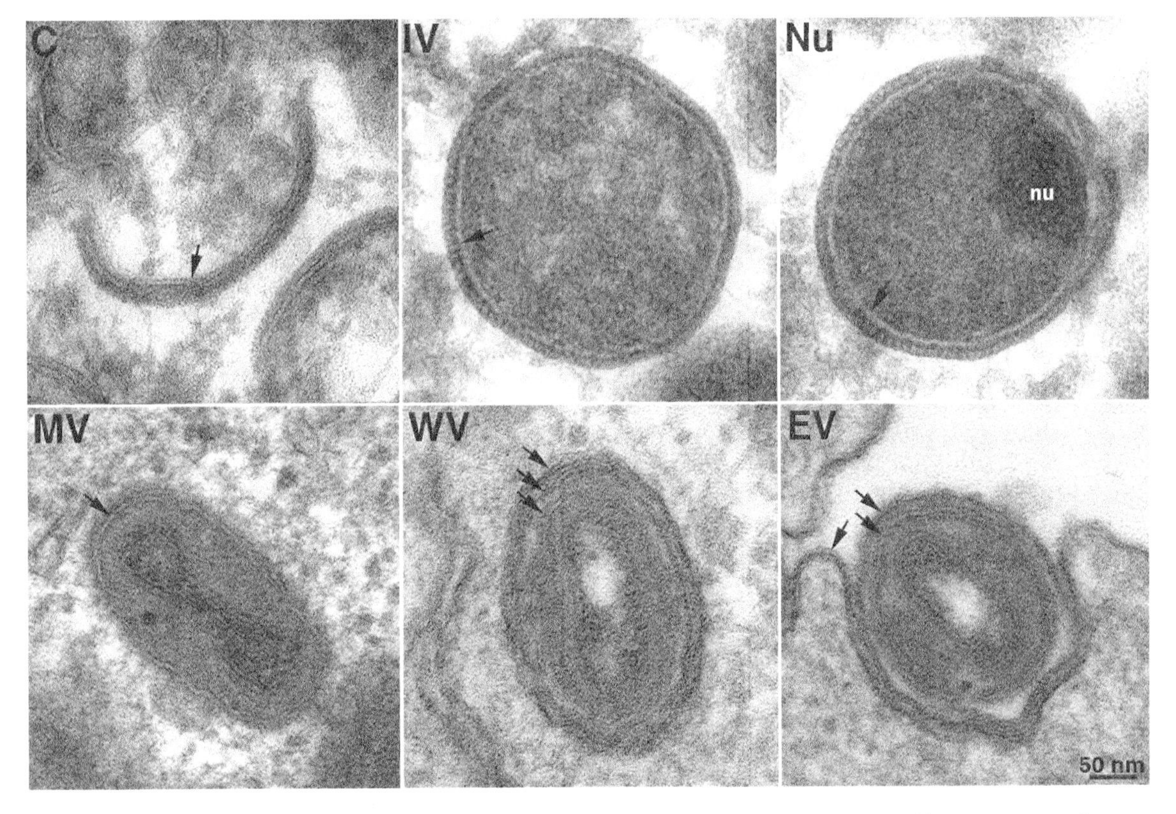

FIGURE 16.14 Stages of VACV morphogenesis. Infected cells were cryosectioned and viewed by transmission electron microscopy. In the panels showing crescent stage (C), immature virion (IV), immature virion with nucleoid (Nu), and mature virion (MV), the *arrow* points to the single outer membrane. Note the presence of the thick "spicule layer" comprising the D13 lattice on the outside of the crescent and IVs. In the panel showing the wrapped virion (WV), the *inner arrow* points to the MV membrane and the two *outer arrows* to the double wrapping membrane. In the panel showing the extracellular enveloped virion (EV), one *arrow* points to the outer wrapping membrane that has fused with the plasma membrane; the other *arrows* point to the MV membrane and remaining EV wrapper. (Images kindly provided by A. Weisberg.)

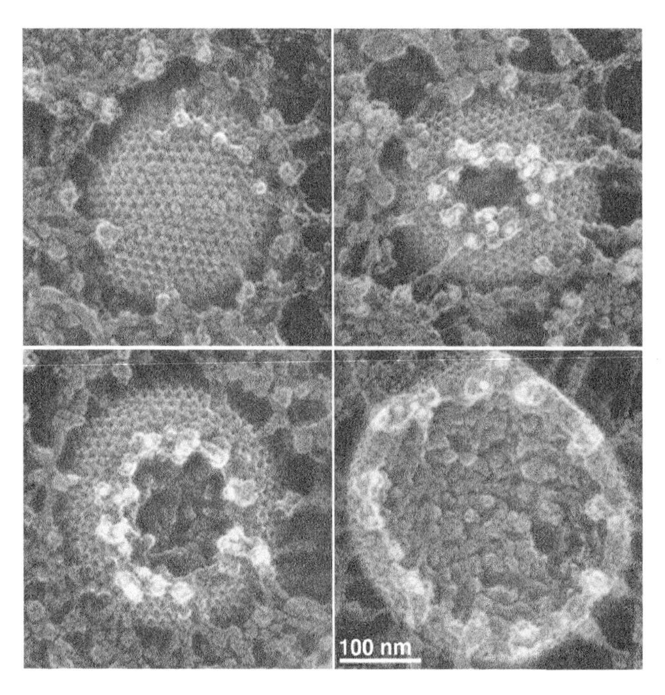

FIGURE 16.15 **Deep etch electron microscopy of immunogold-labeled IVs.** Thawed cryosections of IVs were labeled with antibody to the D13 scaffold protein and Protein A conjugated to gold spheres and then were processed for deep etch electron microscopy. IVs that were uncut or cut at various depths off their equator are shown. The gold particles look white as a result of contrast reversal. (Republished with permission of Rockefeller University Press from Szajner P, Weisberg AS, Lebowitz J, et al. External scaffold of spherical immature poxvirus particles is made of protein trimers, forming a honeycomb lattice. *J Cell Biol* 2005;170(6):971–981; permission conveyed through Copyright Clearance Center, Inc. Ref.[709])

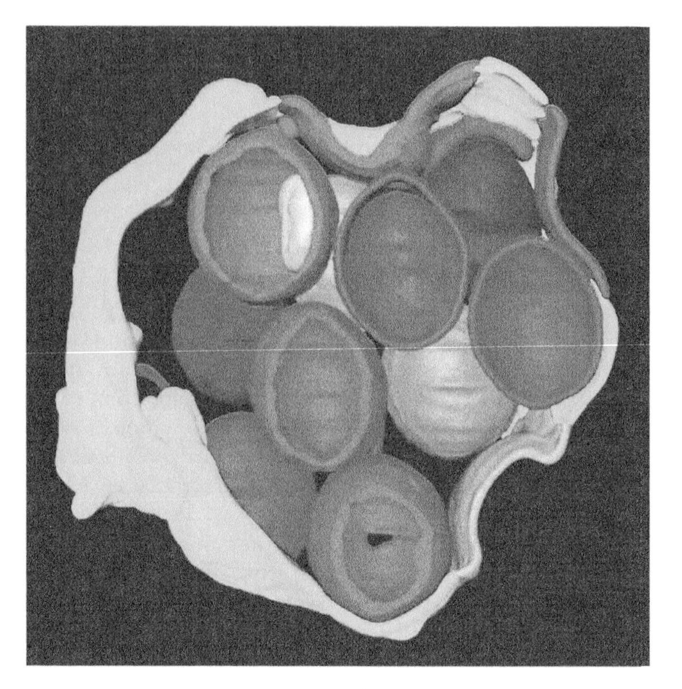

FIGURE 16.16 **Three-dimensional rendering of a cluster of crescent and IV-like structures associated with ER.** Cells were infected with an A30.5R deletion mutant and sections prepared for transmission electron microscopy and tomography. Curved viral membranes are colored *violet* and smooth ER is *green*. Crescent-like membranes are continuous with ER, and IV-like forms are in lumen. (Reprinted with permission from Weisberg AS, Maruri-Avidal L, Bisht H, et al. Enigmatic origin of the poxvirus membrane from the endoplasmic reticulum shown by 3D imaging of vaccinia virus assembly mutants. *Proc Natl Acad Sci U S A* 2017;114(51):E11001–E11009. Ref.[775])

Formation of Crescent and IV Membranes

Microscopic images showing crescents composed of a single bilayer open to the cytoplasm and with no apparent connection to cellular organelles led to the idea that the viral membrane forms *de novo*.[167,292] Such an open architecture, however, is contrary to the idea that stable membranes have sealed ends and arise from preexisting membranes; the latter perception led to a series of now discounted reports proposing that the IV has a double membrane. An alternative explanation for the failure to see connections between cellular and viral membranes is that they are transient. Supporting this explanation are experiments showing that normal-looking IVs are absent and connections between ER and viral membranes persist when expression of any one of five VACV proteins (A6, A11, A30.5, H7, and L2) are repressed.[433,775] Under these conditions, crescent-like membranes containing viral proteins are connected to the ER membrane and appear to bud into expanded ER lumens where spherical IV-like structures accumulate (Fig. 16.16). The five conserved proteins are referred to as viral membrane assembly proteins (VMAPs). L2, A30.5, and A11 have C-terminal hydrophobic domains, whereas A6 and H7 do not. The structure of A6, however, suggests that the C-terminal domain forms a cage that could enclose glycerophospholipids.[537] During a normal infection, L2, A30.5, and A11 localize at the edges of viral crescents, which might coat and protect the single viral membrane, as well as on the adjacent ER.[431,432] A model for viral membrane formation is that following insertion of viral proteins A17 and A14 into the ER, the VMAPs create or stabilize ER scissions possibly in collaboration with cellular proteins leading to the formation of the single membranes of the crescents and IVs.[477] A17 and A14 are major interacting components of the IV membrane[737] and small vesicles accumulate and crescent formation is reduced or abrogated if synthesis of either is repressed.[592,593,727,792]

Additional biochemical and microscopic studies support an ER origin of the viral membrane. Blockade of the COPII ER exit pathway by dominant negative inhibitors of the Sar1 GTPase[318] and the drug brefeldin A[735] have no effect on formation of IVs or MVs ruling out a post-ER membrane origin. However, none of the viral proteins incorporated into purified MVs have a signature of ER translocation, such as signal peptide cleavage or glycosylation. However, a heterologous signal peptide fused to the N-terminal region of a VACV membrane protein was cleaved and the truncated protein localized in IVs and MVs providing evidence for a functional pathway between the ER and viral membranes.[319]

Several proteins in addition to A17, A14, and the VMAPs that are required for the formation of crescents and IVs have been identified. The formation of masses of electron dense "viroplasm" resembling the interior of IVs with few or no crescent membranes represents a characteristic phenotype of cells infected with conditional lethal F10 kinase,[726,765] H5,[194] and G5[163] mutants. H5 and G5 have other roles, so their action in crescent formation may be indirect. F10 phosphorylates the A14 and A17 IV membrane proteins,[73,197] and the kinase activity is required for its function in morphogenesis.[562,710]

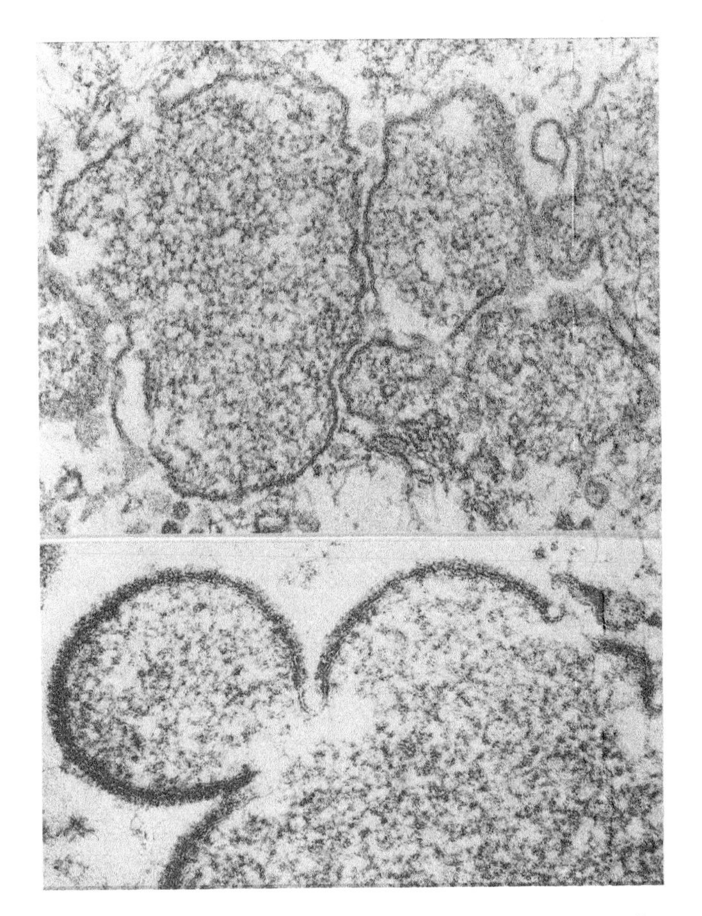

FIGURE 16.17 Electron micrographs of thin sections of cell infected with VACV in the presence of rifampicin. Upper panel: HeLa cells were fixed and sectioned at 8 hours after infection in the presence of rifampicin. **Lower panel:** Cells were fixed and sectioned at 10 minutes after removal of rifampicin. Note the thin uncoated single membrane bilayer loop connecting the more rigid crescent-like membranes that have acquired the D13 honey-comb lattice layer. (Reprinted from Grimley PM, Rosenblum EN, Mims SJ, et al. Interruption by rifampin of an early stage in vaccinia virus morphogenesis: accumulation of membranes which are precursors of virus envelopes. *J Virol* 1970;6(4):519–533. Ref.[270])

In the presence of the antibiotic rifampicin, irregular viral membranes that lack the honeycomb lattice accumulate (Fig. 16.17).[482,497] Within minutes after removal of the drug, the single membrane bilayer becomes coated with the protein forming the honeycomb and assumes a crescent shape (Fig. 16.17) even in the presence of RNA or protein synthesis inhibitors, suggesting that rifampicin directly interferes with assembly.[270] The gene responsible for resistance of mutant viruses to rifampicin was mapped to the D13L ORF, which encodes a 65-kDa protein,[46,134,713] and a recent structural study shows a direct interaction of D13 and rifampicin.[252] When expression of D13 is repressed, morphogenesis of the viral envelope is blocked at the same stage as occurs with rifampicin.[825] The D13 protein forms trimers that assemble to form the honeycomb lattice, which gives the IVs a spherical shape (Fig. 16.15).[709] The structure of D13 is similar to the capsids of other viruses and phage suggesting a common origin.[41,320] D13 interacts with the N-terminal region of A17 to form the scaffold.[76] The A17 protein resembles cellular reticulon proteins and also contributes to the curvature of the IV membrane.[220]

Association of the Genome, Core Proteins, and Transcription Complex With IVs

Electron micrographs show DNA nucleoids that appear to be entering IVs before complete membrane closure.[472] When morphogenesis is interrupted at a pre-IV stage, the viral DNA concatemers are processed normally, but mature DNA accumulates in large crystalloid structures.[270] Although concatemer resolution occurs in the absence of viral morphogenesis, DNA processing is required for morphogenesis.[249] A DNA packaging role for the A32 protein was predicted because of sequence similarity to the products of gene I of filamentous single-strand DNA bacteriophages and to the IVa2 gene of adenovirus, both of which are ATPases involved in DNA packaging.[365] This hypothesis was confirmed by the finding that repression of A32 synthesis blocked VACV genome packaging.[126] DNA packaging also fails to occur under nonpermissive conditions in cells infected with a *ts* mutant that mapped to the I6 telomere-binding protein of VACV.[193,275] Mutation of a second telomere-binding protein encoded by the I1 ORF, however, causes a defect at a later stage of morphogenesis.[275,358] Conditional lethal mutants of the A13 protein, which is a component of the virion membrane, also display a defect in genome packaging and DNA crystalloids associated with membrane accumulate.[738] How the membrane protein, telomere-binding protein and ATPase enable genome incorporation is unknown.

The dense viroplasm that is engulfed during the extension of the crescent into the IV contains unprocessed core proteins. Insight into the association of the core proteins with the crescent membrane has been obtained through use of conditional lethal VACV mutants. Eight core proteins A15, A30, D2, D3, F10, G7, J1, and F17 are each required for the association of crescent membranes with the granular viroplasm.[707,779] Similar phenotypes occur when expression of the A10 and E6 core proteins are repressed.[92,289,582,826] However, the mechanism enabling the association of core proteins with the membrane remains to be determined.

Packaging of the transcription apparatus is dependent on RAP94, the RNA polymerase-associated protein required for transcription of early genes.[824] When expression of RAP94 is repressed, morphologically normal but noninfectious virus particles form. These particles contain the genome and structural proteins as well as the early transcription factor VETF but lack the vRNAP, poly(A) polymerase, capping enzyme, topoisomerase, NPH I, and NPH II. Such a specific effect could be explained by the presence of a multienzyme complex that associates with promoter-bound VETF through RAP94. Physical association of RAP94 with NPH I[466] and VETF[809] have been demonstrated. Moreover, the cryo EM structure of the vRNAP holoenzyme[271] shows that VETF, capping enzyme, and NPH I interact directly with RAP94.[271] Repression of synthesis of VETF, however, leads to a more severe defect with accumulation of immature virus particles.[311,312] Association of VETF with promoter sequences in the genome would facilitate packaging of the transcription complex, which would be poised to initiate transcription of early genes.

Removal of the D13 Scaffold and Proteolytic Processing of Virion Proteins

Transition of spherical IVs to more compact and barrel-shaped MVs involves loss of the D13 scaffold (Fig. 16.15). Disassembly of the D13 scaffold correlates with processing of A17 by the I7 protease; when I7 expression is repressed, D13 is retained on aberrant virus particles.[76] Disassembly of the scaffold and transition to MVs fails to occur when expression of A9 is repressed[812] and with a ts A6 mutant at the nonpermissive temperature.[449] There is also some accumulation of IVs and delayed formation of MVs when the H3L ORF is deleted.[164,395]

In addition to processing of A17, at least five core proteins (A3, A10, A12, G7, and L4) undergo proteolytic cleavages. Processing of A17 depends on formation of the IV membrane,[583] whereas cleavage of core proteins occurs at a later step in morphogenesis.[350,481] In each case, cleavage occurs at the consensus sequence AG↓X.[750] The I7 protease is responsible for cleavage of the above proteins based on the phenotype of ts mutants[342,464] and conserved cysteine protease active site mutants.[31,113] The product of the G1L ORF contains a motif HXXEH that is found in some metalloproteases and conserved in all chordopoxviruses. Conditional lethal G1 mutants are blocked in morphogenesis, but processing of the known membrane and core proteins is not affected.[32,288] Nevertheless, mutagenesis of the putative active site abrogates the ability of G1 to complement a null mutant and G1 itself appears to be proteolytically processed.[390]

Intramolecular Disulfide Bond Pathway

The cytoplasmic domains of some MV membrane proteins contain intramolecular disulfide bonds. Because disulfide bonds usually form in the ER, this raised the possibility that POXVs encode novel oxidoreductases. Indeed, A2.5, E10, and G4 form a unique cytoplasmic disulfide bond pathway.[633,641,642,778] The atomic structure of G4 has been solved; the protein crystallized as a dimer that buried the Cys-X-X-Cys active site, which could protect the reactive disulfides from reduction in the cytoplasm.[40,700] Repression of any one of the three redox proteins results in a block in virion maturation. Nine of the eleven EFC proteins have intramolecular disulfides formed by the cytoplasmic redox system (Table 16.2). Both the entry proteins and the redox system are conserved in all POXVs suggesting their codevelopment. Some core proteins also contain intramolecular bonds, which form by a different mechanism within the developing virion and are reduced following infection.[412]

Occlusion of MVs

The MVs of some chordopoxviruses (e.g., CPXV, ECTV, raccoonpox virus, and FWPV) become occluded in dense protein matrices[247] within the cytoplasm, which are referred to as A-type inclusions (ATIs) to differentiate them from virus factories, which are sometimes called B-type inclusions.[345] Presumably, ATIs that are released following degeneration of infected cells protect the enclosed MVs from the environment. There is, however, suggestions that loss of the ATI protein enhances the dissemination of virus within a host,[343] which may account for the absence of ATI by VARV and MPXV. The major ATI protein of CPXV is a 160-kDa myristoylated species that may represent up to 4% of the total cell protein at late times after infection.[241,536] Early EM images revealed polyribosomes decorating ATIs.[323] Follow-up studies demonstrated local translation of ATI mRNAs around the inclusions, which could prevent premature ATI aggregation and inclusion of MVs within factories.[348]

CPXV A26 mutants form inclusions without virions implicating a role for the latter protein.[444,736] A26 has a bridging role between the ATI protein and A27, which is tethered to MVs through interaction with A17.[303] Although VACV does not form ATIs, a homologous truncated protein is encoded by some strains.[27,175] Interestingly, neither the A26 nor A25 is present in EVs.[736]

Entomopoxvirus virions are also occluded.[71] Following ingestion by a larval host, infectious particles may be released in the alkaline pH of the gut. The sequences of homologous occlusion proteins, called spheroidin or spherulin, have been deduced from the ORFs of several entomopoxviruses.[2,608] These proteins are cysteine-rich, have a mass of approximately 100 kDa, and lack homology to fusolin, an abundant 50-kDa spindle body protein of entomopoxviruses,[169] the A-type inclusion protein of chordopoxviruses, or the polyhedrin protein of baculoviruses.

FORMATION OF EV

Overview

The EV is an extracellular form of POXV that consists essentially of a MV with an additional membrane that is important for virus dissemination.[90,539] For OPXVs, the extra membrane is frequently formed by an intracellular MV wrapping process followed by exocytosis,[540] whereas FPXV exits the cell predominantly by budding.[89]

Wrapping

Some MVs are wrapped by an additional double membrane (Fig. 16.14) that is important for intracellular movement and EV formation. Both the trans-Golgi and endosomal cisternae have been implicated in the formation of the wrapping membrane.[294,616,720] The discovery of retrograde transport of the F13 protein from endosomes to the trans-Golgi apparatus implicates both membrane compartments.[286,664] Eight viral proteins have been associated with either the wrapping or EV membrane (Table 16.5). Of these, A36 and F12 are associated exclusively with the outermost WV membrane that fuses with the plasma membrane and therefore are not retained in the EV. With the exception of E2, F12, F13, and K2, the proteins have a transmembrane anchor. A56, A33, A34, B5, and K2 are glycosylated and exposed on the outer EV surface, whereas F13 is palmitoylated, has a putative phospholipase motif that is essential for its role in wrapping, and is on the inner surface.[273,596,620] F13 is the target of TPOXX (Tecovirimat, ST-246), a therapeutic against smallpox licensed by the US Federal Drug Administration in 2018.[272] F12 associates with E2,[207] and A36[336] and K2 associates with A56.[732] Complex interactions between the A33, A34, and B5 proteins determine the composition of the EV membrane.[469] A33 has unique C-type lectin domains that could interact with other viral or cell proteins.[372,701]

Deletion of any of the genes encoding WV or EV membrane proteins, except A56 and K2, results in a small plaque phenotype indicating decreased virus spread. A56 and K2 are also located on the plasma membrane and deletion mutants have a syncytial phenotype that can be explained by the abrogation of A56/K2 binding to the A16/G9 components of the EFC.[759] Studies with mutant VACVs indicate that several proteins are required for efficient wrapping and that severe effects are caused by repression or inactivation of the A27 MV protein,[591,769] the F13 protein,[80] and the B5 glycoprotein.[219,790]

Intracellular Movement and Exocytosis

The movement of MVs to the wrapping sites depends on microtubules, but the viral attachment protein is not known. Whether A27 is required for movement as well as wrapping *per se* is disputed.[605,769] Movement of WVs to the periphery of the cell occurs on microtubules.[253,300,586,772] A36 exposed on the surface of the WV interacts with the cargo-binding domain of the light chain of kinesin (KLC), a microtubule motor protein.[332,771] Movement is enhanced by interactions of the F12/E2 complex, which binds predominantly to KLC isoform 2,[124] whereas A36 binds KLC isoform 1.[246]

When the WVs arrive near the periphery of the cell, their migration through the dense cortical actin is facilitated by the action of F11 in preventing RhoA signaling.[36,154] The outer of the two wrapping membranes fuses with the plasma membrane to liberate the EV with one more membrane than a MV (Fig. 16.14). The externalization of VACV resembles vesicle exocytosis, but the detailed mechanism has not been determined. A role of the ESCRT machinery has been suggested.[301]

Only a minority of the externalized virus is found in the medium, whereas most adhere to the cell surface. The ratio of adherent to released virions varies in different VACV strains,[538] and the high amount of released EVs for the IHD-J strain is due to a single amino acid substitution in the putative lectin-binding domain of A34.[82] Mutations in A33, B5, and A36 also enhance release,[351,677] and the host Abl-family tyrosine kinases and host phosphoinositide 5-phosphatase SHIP2 are involved.[446,577] On cell monolayers, adherent EVs can mediate efficient cell-to-cell spread due to actin tails discussed below, whereas the released EVs provide long-range dissemination.[81]

Actin Tail Formation

Efficient cell-to-cell spread of EVs depends on their location at the tip of motile, actin-containing microvilli, which have been visualized by fluorescence and electron microscopy[156,295,694] (Fig. 16.6). The proteins encoded by the A33R, A34R, and A36R ORFs are required for the formation of the actin-containing microvilli, and their absence results in a small plaque phenotype.[595,604,791,794] Nucleation of the actin tails depends on tyrosine phosphorylation of the A36 protein of OPXVs and functional homologs of other POXVs by Src or Abl family kinases.[389] The phosphorylated A36 protein interacts with the adaptor protein Nck, which results in the recruitment of the Ena/VASP family member N-WASP to the site of actin assembly.

VIRUS–HOST INTERACTIONS

Tropism and Host Range

Individual POXVs frequently have a narrow host range capable of maintaining their survival in the wild, although they may occasionally infect and cause disease in other species. Indeed, the eradication of smallpox would not have succeeded if there were a wild animal reservoir. Occasionally, infection of an unnatural host, for example, the European rabbit by MYXV,[232] results in a high mortality. Tropism and virulence are frequently based on the genus- and species-specific properties of defense genes rather than the essential ones conserved in all or most POXVs. This is reflected in the broader species specificity for cultured cells than whole animals. Where restriction occurs, it is usually at a post-entry step.[441] An interesting example of tropism is the ability to infect primary mouse fibroblasts and mice by MYXV only if the IFN response is abrogated.[763] Under certain nonpermissive conditions of OPXV infection, viral macromolecular synthesis may be inhibited. Examples are the abortive VACV infection of drosophila cells restricted at the stage of viral DNA replication[69] and Chinese hamster ovary cells restricted at the stage of intermediate protein synthesis, which can be overcome by the CPXV gene encoding a 77-kDa protein.[308,568,686] CPXV CP77 is related to a family of VACV host range proteins that have ankyrin repeats and include C7 and K1[545] and which have overlapping functions.[393,569,819] In addition, VACV K1L deletion mutants are blocked at the stage of early protein synthesis in rabbit RK13 cells and VACV double K1L and C7L mutants exhibit a similar defect in human cells. A human genome-wide RNAi screen and coprecipitation studies identified human sterile alpha domain-containing 9 (SAMD9) and the paralog SAMD9L as IFN-induced host restriction factors that are antagonized by the C7 family of proteins.[404,452,661,663] Members of this family of host range genes are present in other POXV genera including sheeppox virus, Yaba-like disease virus (YLDV), MYXV, and swinepox virus (SWPV).[405,448,450] VACV strain modified virus Ankara (MVA), which was extensively passaged in chicken embryo fibroblasts, is unable to replicate in most mammalian cells due to gene loss or mutation,[34] which prevents late stages of morphogenesis.[703] The virus proteins lost from MVA that counteract the putative host restriction factors have been identified as C12 and C16.[407,543] C12, also known as serine protease inhibitor 1, is a host range gene for rabbitpox virus and other VACV strains.[470,651] A human genome-wide RNAi screen identified three host proteins (IRF2, FAM111A, and RFC3) as restriction factors for rabbitpox C12 deletion mutants.[522]

Effects on the Cytoskeleton

Infection of tissue culture cells with VACV and other OPXVs results in profound morphological changes consisting of rounding, cell–cell dissociation, and migration. These cytopathic effects involve alterations in microtubules, actin, and intermediate filaments.[235,461,551,615] VACV induces cell motility[606] that requires F11 protein-mediated inhibition of RhoA signaling.[471,743]

Effects on Host Macromolecular Synthesis

A rapid and profound reduction in cell protein synthesis follows VACV infection.[223,484] Several factors may contribute to the switch from host to viral protein synthesis, and the relative contribution of each factor may depend on the virus multiplicity, cell type, and time of analysis. Inhibition of host protein synthesis frequently remains incomplete until after DNA replication, suggesting a major role of a viral intermediate or late protein. The primary factor in the shut off of host protein synthesis is a profound reduction in cellular mRNA. After several hours, most of the mRNA present in the cytoplasm of infected cells is viral[86,808] due to accelerated degradation of host mRNAs[65,585,628] coupled with active virus transcription and inhibition of host RNA synthesis and transport.[542,561,786] The accelerated degradation of host and viral mRNAs is initiated by the expression of the viral decapping enzymes D9 and D10[531–533,655,684,685] and completed by host cell exonuclease activity.

VACV also hijacks cellular translation initiation factors to expression sites within cytoplasmic factories, which may contribute to suppression of cell protein synthesis.[347] The abundance of the cellular translational repressor 4E binding protein decreases during VACV infection enhancing translation of viral mRNAs.[760] VACV protein WR 169 is a protein synthesis inhibitor excluded from virus factories that may also contribute to host shut-off.[695] At high virus multiplicities, inhibition of host protein synthesis can occur in the absence of viral gene expression, implicating a virion protein.[438,475,547] Other studies suggested that small poly (A)-containing RNA molecules are involved.[116] VACV also inhibits nuclear DNA replication.[340,634] This effect may be indirect, although a role for VACV-encoded deoxyribonucleases was suggested.[198]

The VACV protein WR C16 (CPN C10) binds to prolyl hydroxylase domain-containing protein 2 (PHD2) to stabilize HIF-1α and induce a hypoxic response under normoxia[437] that results in reprogramming of central energy metabolism.[436]

Interactions With the Ubiquitin-Proteasome System

Ubiquitylation is a posttranslational modification that regulates cellular processes by several mechanisms including protein degradation. The exploitation of the ubiquitin–proteasome system by POXVs has been reviewed.[58] Studies with inhibitors suggested that OPXVs require the ubiquitin proteasome system for uncoating cores and DNA replication.[611,714] In addition, VACV exploits the proteasome to degrade cellular factors that restrict virus replication; out of 265 cell proteins reduced greater than twofold during infection, 70% were degraded in a proteasome-dependent manner.[679] A few POXVs encode ubiquitin-like genes, but many more encode modulators of the ubiquitin–proteasome system, including E3 ubiquitin ligases,[314,424,505] and ankyrin/F-box-like proteins.[335,680,681,687,776] Some of the ankyrin/F-box–like proteins interact with the SKP1 component of the SCF ubiquitin ligase complex to commandeer the cell proteasome machinery. Although many of these modulators of ubiquitin are required for virulence, the functions of most remain unknown. One exception is VACV C9; the ankyrin repeat domain binds IFITs and the F-box interacts with SCF ubiquitin ligase complex, which together mediate the degradation of the IFITs.[410] POXVs also encode BTB-kelch proteins that are predicted Cullin 3 E3 adapters.[47,61,240,363,785] The VACV BTB-kelch protein A55 binds Cullin 3 directly and with high affinity.[245,521] VACV C6 binds to histone deacetylase (HDAC)4 and mediates its proteasome-dependent degradation by a mechanism not yet defined.[414,679]

Stimulatory Effects on Cell Pathways

To enhance their replication, POXVs may stimulate certain host pathways, for example, MAPK and P13K/Akt.[29,678,764] FWPV,[135] SFV,[654] Yaba virus,[511] and MOCV[559] induce hyperplasia and tumors. VACV protein B14 is a MAPK activator.[721] In the case of OPXVs and leporipoxviruses, the hyperplastic effect is due to secretion of a homolog of epidermal growth factor, which binds to ErbB receptors and enhances virulence.[108,133,399,519,696,734] A gene encoding a mitogenic polypeptide with homology to mammalian vascular endothelial growth factor is present in the ORFV genome and may account for the extensive vascularization of lesions and virulence.[613,788] VACV protein A49 activates the wnt signaling pathway by binding β-TrCP and thereby stabilizing β-catenin.[178]

VIRAL DEFENSE MOLECULES

Overview

The first line of host defense against viruses consists of nonspecific, innate mechanisms involving IFNs, chemokines, cytokines, signaling pathways, complement activation, and natural killer cells. Subsequently, antigen-specific cytotoxic T lymphocytes (CTLs) and antibodies become important. However, POXVs encode multiple proteins that help evade innate and adaptive immune responses. These may be grouped according to their site of action, inside or outside the infected cell, structural similarity, or which host defense pathway they antagonize. Secreted proteins may be related to cellular soluble binding proteins (BPs) for specific cytokines or IFNs, or cellular receptors that have lost their transmembrane anchor sequences and have been termed viroceptors.[740] Numerous intracellular proteins interfere with signaling or effector pathways. In contrast to the highly conserved mechanisms of entry, gene expression, and genome replication that are employed by all POXVs, there is considerable diversity in POXV defense genes, which are adapted to specific hosts. Many of these genes were acquired from their hosts and retain recognizable motifs despite extensive modification, whereas others may represent acquisition of new functions by proteins.

Extracellular Defense Proteins

Secreted defense molecules have been reported for many poxviruses, and 12 have been described for VACV (Table 16.7). Some may also bind to both infected or uninfected cells via interactions with other viral proteins or cell surface glycosaminoglycans. Secreted proteins may not only protect the infected cell from immune attack but also diminish the inflammatory response more widely to aid virus spread and transmission.

Complement Regulatory Proteins

VACV and other OPXVs encode a secreted complement control protein (VCP), consisting largely of tandem, inexact copies of a 60-amino acid short consensus repeat found in cellular complement regulatory proteins, that inhibits the classical and alternative pathways of complement activation by binding and inactivating C4B and C3B and accelerating the decay of C3 convertases.[4,367,368,445,602] Although VCP is secreted, some of it is retained on the surface of infected cells by binding to heparin-like molecules[244] and to the VACV A56 protein.[187] Both the VACV and ECTV complement control proteins contribute to virulence.[262,326] Interestingly, the VARV ortholog of VCP is more potent than the VACV version in inhibiting human complement[400,599] and strain variation in the MPXV ortholog may contribute to differences in virulence.[394,401] Although the VACV B5 EV membrane protein also has short consensus repeats, there is no evidence that it has complement inhibitory activity. Host proteins incorporated into the EV membrane may also inhibit complement activation.[749]

TABLE 16.7 VACV secreted proteins

Cop[a]	WR[b]	kDa	Time[c]	Properties	References
A39R	163/4[d]	50-55	L	Related to semaphorin SEMA7A, virulence factor, restricts NK cell response	(149,251,403)
A41L	166	30	E	Chemokine-binding protein, virulence factor	(42,506)
A53R[d]	186[d]	20	L	TNF-binding protein, CrmC VACV strain Lister, USSR, and Evans	(12,572)
—	—	18	L	TNF-binding protein, CrmE, VACV strain USSR, secreted and on cell surface, virulence factor	(572,609)
B8R	190	42	E	IFN-γ–binding protein, virulence factor	(16,488,512,691,706)
B16R[d]	197	50–60	L	IL-1β–binding protein, virulence factor, regulates body temperature	(14,15,688)
B19R	200	60–65	E	Type I IFN-binding protein, secreted and on cell surface by binding GAGs, virulence factor	(19,146,468,705)
C3L	025	35	E	Complement control protein (VCP), virulence factor, binds C3b and C4b, inhibits complement activation, secreted and on cell surface, binds to A56	(187,261,327,367,368)
K2L	033	48–50	E	Serine protease inhibitor, fusion inhibitor, binds A56 on cell and EV surface	(106,768)
C11R	009/210	19	E	Vaccinia growth factor (VGF), virulence factor	(84,99,108,696)
—	013	13	E	IL-18–binding protein, virulence factor	(88,676,704)
C23L	001/218	35	E/L	Chemokine-binding protein, binds CC chemokines, virulence factor	(17,122,265,575,630,670)
M2L	031	33	E	Binds B7.1 (CD80) and B7.2 (CD86) T-cell costimulatory proteins to block T-cell activation	(679,767)

[a]Copenhagen (COP) ORF name.
[b]Western Reserve (WR) ORF number.
[c]Time of synthesis: E, early; L, late.
[d]Gene fragmented and nonfunctional.

IFN-Binding Proteins

Type I IFN BPs encoded by VACV and other OPXVs are present in the supernatants and on the surface of cells and are important for virulence.[146,188,705] Glycosaminoglycans help retain the IFN BPs to the surface of infected and uninfected cells so enabling virus spread to cells not rendered resistant to virus infection by IFN signaling.[19,468] The VACV type I IFN BP (Copenhagen B19, WR B18/200) and orthologs are Ig family proteins with limited sequence similarity to regions of the IL-1 receptor family[672] but not to the ligand-binding subunits of IFN receptors. Nevertheless, these proteins neutralize human IFN-α, -β, and -ω and have broad species specificity.[705] MYXV encodes a protein important for virulence that is related in sequence to VACV B18 but is smaller, membrane bound and apparently cannot bind IFN.[55] Antibodies that bind the ECTV-type I IFN BP greatly attenuate infection *in vivo* showing the importance of these soluble virus proteins for disease progression.[804]

Proteins that bind to type II IFNs are secreted by POXVs of several different genera. The IFN-γ BPs of MYXV and OPXVs are related in sequence to the extracellular domain of the IFN-γ receptor.[16,488,741] Deletion of the MYXV and VACV IFN-γ BP attenuate disease in rabbits.[487,691,706] Because of the low affinity of the VACV IFN-γ BP for mouse IFN-γ compared to human IFN-γ, this cytokine would have a more profound inhibitory effect on VACV in mice compared to humans, which may be important for interpreting disease models.[728] The type I IFN inhibitor encoded by Yaba monkey tumor virus also inhibits type III IFN.[315]

IL-18 BPs

IL-18 induces IFN-γ and acts in synergy with IL-12 to induce NK cell activation, T-cell activation, and Th1 response polarization. MOCV, OPXVs, Yaba monkey tumor virus, and some other POXVs encode secreted proteins with amino acid similarity to the mammalian IL-18 BP and which bind and inactivate IL-18.[88,451,502,676,704,799,800] Despite limited sequence identity, similar amino acids of the human and viral residues interact with IL-18.[371] The MOCV IL-18 BP is secreted as a full-length form that binds cell surface glycosaminoglycans through the C-terminal tail and a furin-cleaved form with only the IL-18 binding domain.[801] ECTV and VACV IL-18 BP deletion mutants exhibit decreased virulence compared with wild-type virus.[88,574,704]

Soluble Tumor Necrosis Factor BPs

Tumor necrosis factors (TNFs) bind to their cognate receptors and induce pro-inflammatory responses or death of virus-infected cells. Leporipoxviruses,[624] OPXVs,[12,309,413,572,609] and yatapoxviruses[107] encode up to four soluble TNF receptors with varying binding specificities, time of expression during infection, and presence on the cell surface.[554-556] The VACV CrmE protein shares structural features with mammalian type 2 TNF receptors,[266] whereas the tanapox and Yaba-like virus TNF BPs have sequence similarity with MHC class 1 molecules.[107,564,811] CPXV and ECTV also encode a soluble homolog of CD30, another member of the TNF receptor family, which inhibits interaction of CD30 with its ligand.[524,610] Some OPXV TNF BPs also bind chemokines via a distinct C-terminal domain (see below).

Soluble IL-1β Receptor Homologs

IL-1β mediates a broad-spectrum response to virus infection by binding to a high-affinity cell receptor leading to activation of NF-κB. OPXVs encode homologs of the IL-1 receptor that bind IL-1β.[13,15,688] Depending on the virus dose and route of inoculation, deletion of the gene can reduce or enhance virulence. Expression of the IL-1β BP by VACV prevented induction of a febrile response.[13] In some VACV strains and all sequenced VARVs, the corresponding gene is rendered nonfunctional by frameshift mutations.[221]

Chemokine Inhibitors

A principal role of chemokines (CKs) is to coordinate the activation and migration of leukocytes to sites of virus infection by establishing concentration gradients on endothelial cells. CKs bind to endothelial cells via a glycosaminoglycan (GAG)-binding domain and to CK receptors on leukocytes via a CK receptor–binding domain. POXVs encode soluble CK BPs, transmembrane CK receptors, and CK mimics. The soluble CK BPs lack sequence similarity to CK receptors and interfere with the CK response in two ways. One group, typified by CC type CK BPs from CPXV, VACV, and MYXV (vCKBP/vCCI and M-T1), bind to CKs via the CK receptor binding domain and so prevent CKs binding to CK receptors on leukocytes.[18,265,670] The second group, exemplified by VACV protein A41[42,506] and MYXV M-T7,[378] bind to CKs via the GAG-binding domain. This prevents the establishment of CK concentration gradients to diminish leukocyte recruitment to sites of infection. Another group of CK BPs (CrmB and CrmD) were identified first as TNF BPs, but also bind CKs by a C-terminal domain.[20] Orthologs of either or both are expressed by CPXV, ECTV, and VARV. Blocking both TNF and CK binding to cognate receptors simultaneously has synergistic anti-inflammatory benefit, and antibody against ECTV CrmD alone can protect against mousepox.[20] Secreted CK BPs are encoded by OPXVs, leporipoxviruses, and parapoxviruses.[17,112,122,265,385,575,629,630,670] The structures of several POXV CK BPs have been solved and the binding sites determined.[37,42,821]

Several POXVs encode homologs of the CK receptor CCR8. The Yaba-like disease virus protein is inserted into the plasma membrane, binds human CCL1, and activates signal-regulated kinases.[499] A recombinant VACV expressing the Yaba-like disease virus CCR8 homolog is attenuated in mice.[498]

CK homologs are encoded by MOCV and FWPV. The MOCV-encoded homolog is predicted to be a CK antagonist based on the absence of the conserved N-terminal region[635] and binding specifically to the CCR8 CK receptor and competitively inhibiting binding of I-309, the natural ligand.[416] Other reports, based mainly on chemotaxis assays, suggested a broader activity.[170,186,370]

Other Cytokine-Binding Proteins and Homologs

Some parapoxviruses encode a secreted protein that binds granulocyte–macrophage colony-stimulating factor and IL-2.[184,185] ORFV encodes an IL-10 homolog with a high degree of identity to ovine IL-10.[236,325] The ORFV IL-10 suppresses macrophage activation and exerts an immunosuppressive effect.[787] Some chordopoxviruses secrete a semaphorin homolog with proinflammatory properties that interacts with plexin C1.[3,149,251,403]

Secreted Inhibitors of NK and T-Cell Activation

NK cells and CTLs have important roles in combating OPXV infections.[228,528] CPXV and MPXV encode a secreted class I MHC-like protein that acts as a competitive antagonist of the NKG2D activating receptor and inhibits NKG2D-dependent killing by NK cells.[120] Another secreted CPXV protein called M2, which is conserved in VARV, MPXV, and some VACVs, binds the T-cell costimulatory ligands B7.1 (CD80) and B7.2 (CD86) to compete with binding of CD28 and CTLA4 and thereby diminish T-cell activation.[767] CPXV lacking M2 induced stronger antiviral $CD4^+$ and $CD8^+$ T-cell responses. The B22 protein homologs of VARV and MPXV render human T cells unresponsive to stimulation of the T-cell receptor by MHC-dependent antigen presentation, and MPXV and ECTV deletion mutants are attenuated in monkeys and mice, respectively.[22,584]

Intracellular Defense Proteins

Poxviruses encode many intracellular proteins that target innate immunity. These vary between poxvirus genera and antagonize diverse signaling pathways or antiviral factors. Often these proteins are encoded in the terminal regions of the genome, are expressed early during infection, and are nonessential for virus replication in cell culture. These proteins may affect virus virulence *in vivo* and modulate the development of virus-specific immunological memory.[11] It is not uncommon for a single virus to encode multiple proteins that target a single pathway. These diverse proteins are grouped here according to the pathways they target.

Inhibitors of Cell Pattern Recognition Receptor and Cytokine Stimulated Signaling Pathways

Pattern recognition receptors (PRRs) detect pathogen-associated molecular patterns (PAMPs) and thereafter activate innate immune signaling pathways leading to the expression of cytokines, CKs, and IFNs. Viral PAMPS include cytoplasmic DNA, single-stranded RNA with triphosphate ends, dsRNA, and viral proteins. POXVs interfere with these innate immune defenses at multiple levels including blocking interaction of the PRR and PAMP, inhibiting the signaling pathways, targeting the up-regulated cytokines, CKs and IFNs, and blocking the signaling pathways these host factors activate or the function of antiviral proteins they induce.

Inhibitors of RNA and DNA Sensing

To diminish recognition of viral RNA by PRRs, POXVs either synthesize viral mRNAs that are indistinguishable from host mRNAs by encoding capping, methylating, and polyadenylating enzymes, or minimize the level or availability of dsRNA produced by convergent overlapping transcription (predominantly late during infection). dsRNA is sequestered by the dsRNA-binding protein E3[129] and reduced by the decapping enzymes D9 and D10 that remove the 5′-caps from dsRNAs leading to their degradation and, consequently, diminishing the PKR- and RNase L-mediated antiviral responses.[408,411]

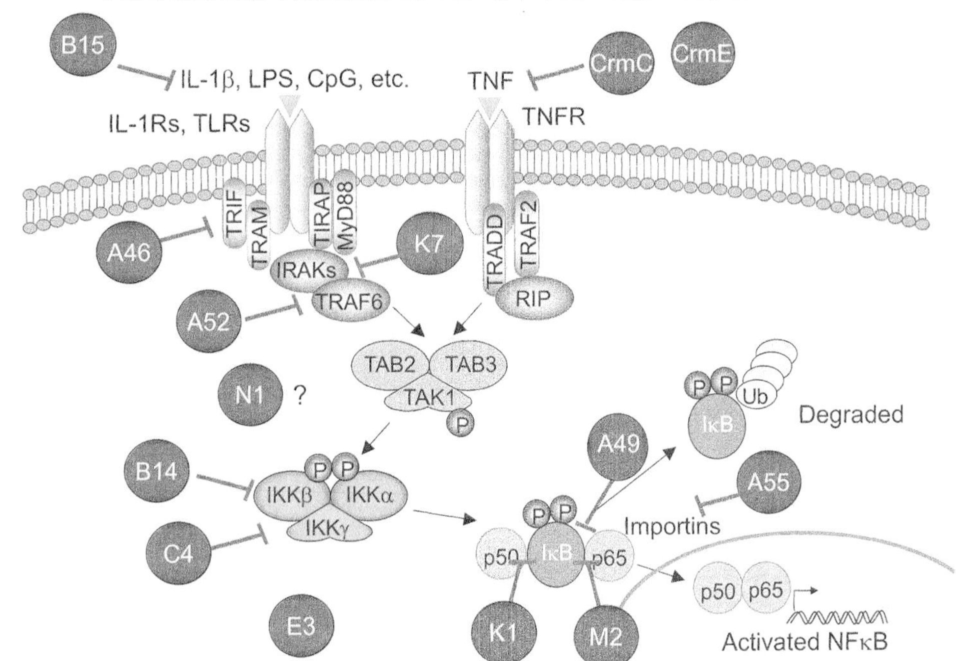

FIGURE 16.18 VACV inhibitors of NF-κB. Schematic showing simplified pathway of NF-κB activation following engagement of IL-1, TNF, or TLR ligands with their cognate receptors. Individual VACV proteins that inhibit activation of the pathway at specific places are indicated with *red circles*. Note B15 is from VACV strain WR. CrmC and CrmE are from VACV strains Lister, USSR, and Evans. Protein E3 binds dsRNA. The site of action of N1 is uncertain.

POXVs synthesize DNA in the cytoplasm that may be detected by DNA sensors such as cGAS, DNA-PK, IFI16, DAI, AIM2, RNA polymerase III, DDX36, DDX41, and Mre11. In response, POXVs have evolved countermeasures. DNA-PK is targeted by VACV proteins WR C16 (CPN C10)[549] and C4[627] that bind the Ku heterodimer to diminish DNA binding by this PRR. Evidence for additional downstream inhibitors[255] was followed by the discovery of poxins (VACV protein B2) in a wide range of poxviruses. These are 2′-3′-cGAMP nucleases that destroy this second messenger produced by cGAS after its engagement with dsDNA, and so prevent STING-TBK1-IRF3 activation.[212] RNA polymerase III-mediated sensing is counteracted by the dsRNA-binding protein E3.[426,744] Many other POXV inhibitors target the IFN regulatory factors (IRFs), NF-κB, and AP-1 pathways that are activated by these and other PRRs such as toll-like receptors (TLRs), RIG-like receptors (RLRs), and NOD-like receptors (NLRs).

Inhibitors of NF-κB Signal Transduction

The NF-κB complex comprises a family of dimeric transcription factors that have a central role in responding to viral infections and mediating an inflammatory response. NF-κB exists in an inactive complex with IκBα in the cytoplasm until the latter is phosphorylated by Iκ kinase (IKK) complex, polyubiquitylated, and then degraded by the proteasome. POXVs can trigger NF-κB activation but use a variety of mechanisms to suppress this. Modified VACV Ankara (MVA), a highly attenuated strain of VACV used as a safe smallpox vaccine and as a vector for other vaccines, has suffered multiple deletions and lost the ability to prevent NF-κB activation due to dsRNA triggering of PKR in some cells.[418,515,652] Restoration of the N1L or M2L genes prevents induction of NF-κB by the PKR or ERK2 pathway, respectively.[254,297,418,784] The importance of NF-κB for innate immune signaling is underscored by the many inhibitors that POXVs express to inhibit its activation. This is illustrated well by VACV, which encodes greater than 10 inhibitors of this pathway (A46, A49, A52, A55, B14, C4, E3, K1, K7, M2, and N1) that act at different stages (Fig. 16.18) (for review[671]) and additional inhibitors remain to be identified.[702] Protein A46 binds to the TLR/IL-1R (TIR) domain of TLRs and the signaling adaptors TRAM, TRIF, MAL, and Myd88 to block signaling.[91,692] Proteins A52[91,287] and K7[625] act downstream of NF-κB and each binds TRAF6 and IRAK2 to inhibit TLR/IL-1R-induced signaling. A46, A52, and K7 inhibit TLR/IL-1R-induced NF-κB signaling but not TNF-induced signaling, whereas other VACV inhibitors act at or downstream of the convergence of these pathways and so have broader inhibitory activity. Protein B14 binds to IKKβ, to block IKKβ phosphorylation and so prevent phosphorylation of IκBα.[66,137] ORFV protein 024 also prevents phosphorylation of IKKβ and IKKα but does not bind the IKK proteins.[201] Protein N1 also inhibits NF-κB activation although the report that it binds to the IKK complex[204] is disputed.[137,153] Mutation of the N1 dimerization interface abrogates NF-κB inhibition,[177] but its mechanism of action remains unknown. Protein C4 also inhibits the pathway at or close to the IKK complex.[218] Protein A49 mimics IκBα and, via a motif conserved between these proteins, binds to the E3 ligase β-TrCP.[425] This prevents ubiquitylation and proteasomal degradation of IκBα and so IκBα remains bound to NF-κB subunits in the cytoplasm. A49 is an inducible inhibitor of NF-κB that requires activation by phosphorylation.[504] The kinase IKKβ activates both NF-κB signaling and A49 to inhibit NF-κB signaling.[504] Protein K1, a host range protein with ANK repeats, also prevents the degradation of IκBα.[652] The translocation of p65 into the nucleus is inhibited by VACV protein A55, which binds to the importin KPNA2.[521] Proteins M2[254] and E3[496] inhibit activation of NF-κB via the ERK2 and PKR pathways, respectively. NF-κB inhibitors A46,[229,230] A49,[503] A52 and B14,[267] K7,[341] and N1[35,153] are structurally related and have a Bcl-2 fold. A surprising feature of VACV NF-κB inhibitors is that, where tested, each one contributes to virulence despite the presence of other inhibitors[59,61,67,136,218,287,425,692] suggesting multiple functions.

Other OPXVs contain orthologs of several of these VACV inhibitors and some additional inhibitors. For instance, VARV protein G1 and its orthologs (CPXV 006, ECTV 002, and MPXV 003) have ANK repeats and bind to the NF-κB p105 subunit and to SCP1 to inhibit pathway activation.[465,467] ECTV ANK proteins 002, 005, 154, and 165 also interact with SCP1, stabilize IκBα, and prevent p65 nuclear translocation.[111,745,746] Another group of ANK proteins have a C-terminal BC domain (ECTV 010, CPXV 016 and 019, raccoonpox virus 011, and skunkpox virus 202) and bind to cullin 2 and inhibit NF-κB activation or other signaling pathways.[514] NF-κB inhibitors in other POXV genera include ORFV protein 121 that binds to and inhibits the phosphorylation and nuclear translocation of NF-κB,[202] MC160, that inhibits TNFα-induced NF-κB activation by association with Hsp90 to increase IKKα degradation and by interaction with procaspase-8,[508] and MYXV protein MO13 that binds NF-κB.[566]

Inhibitors of IRF-3 Activation

The IRF-3 pathway is also targeted by several POXV proteins, and several of these are also inhibitors of NF-κB. VACV dsRNA-binding protein E3 prevents PKR-dependent activation of IRF-3 and mitogen-activated protein kinases.[822,823] VACV protein A46 binds to TRIF and TRAM and thereby prevents activation of IRF-3 and IFN-β expression.[692] Four additional VACV Bcl-2 proteins, N1, K7, C6, and N2, each inhibit IRF-3 activation at or downstream of the kinases TANK-binding kinase 1 (TBK1) and IKKε that function at the convergence of several pathways leading to IRF-3 activation. N1 associates with TBK1,[204] and K7 binds directly to the DEAD-box helicase DDX3 that promotes activation of the IRF-3 pathway at the level of TBK-1 and IKKe.[625] C6 binds to the TBK-1 adaptors TANK, SINTBAD, and NAP1 to restrict IRF-3 activation,[739] and N2 acts after IRF-3 nuclear translocation to inhibit *ifnb* gene transcription within the nucleus.[234] The concerted inhibition of both IRF-3 and NF-κB activation by many POXVs restricts the production of pro-inflammatory cytokines, CKs, and IFNs. Additional POXV inhibitors target IFN-induced signaling and the function of IFN-stimulated gene (ISG) products with antiviral activity.

Inhibitors of IFN Pathways

Secreted proteins that bind type I, II, or III IFNs and block IFNs binding to their cellular receptors have been described above. A notable feature of these extracellular viral proteins is their ability to block the action of IFNs whether these are produced by the infected cell or uninfected cells recruited to the site of infection. POXVs also encode proteins that prevent IFN signaling and the function of IFN stimulated gene (ISG) products. The VACV dual specificity H1 phosphatase inhibits phosphorylation of the STAT1 and STAT2 transcription factors and block type I and II IFN-mediated immune responses.[406,423,500] MYXV inhibits type I IFN by blocking the activity of Janus kinase Tyke2, upstream of STATs.[762] VACV protein C6 associates with STAT2 and inhibits type I IFN signaling after STAT1-STAT2 phosphorylation, dimerization, nuclear translocation, and binding of the IFN-stimulated gene factor 3 (ISGF3) complex to promoters bearing the IFN-stimulated response element (ISRE).[698] Further analysis showed that C6 binds and induces the proteasomal degradation of histone deacetylase (HDAC)4, and that HDAC4 is needed for type I IFN signaling. Following IFN stimulation, HDAC4 is recruited to the ISRE-bearing promoters and is needed for the recruitment of STAT2.[414]

Inhibition of IFN-Stimulated Gene Products

IFNs induce the expression of hundreds of ISGs and several of these are antagonized by POXVs. The first examples were PKR and 2′5′-oligoadenylate synthetase (OAS). These host proteins are up-regulated by IFN but require dsRNA for their activation. Once activated by dsRNA present during infection, PKR phosphorylates eukaryotic translation initiation factor 2 alpha (eIF2α) to block protein synthesis. OAS synthesizes 2′-5′-linked oligoadenylates that activate RNase L, which then cleaves rRNA, tRNA, and mRNA and thereby also prevents protein synthesis. The action of both proteins is antagonized by VACV protein E3[129] and also by related dsRNA-binding proteins from other POXV genera, such as MYXV protein M029.[563,565] E3L deletion mutants show host range restriction and enhanced apoptosis, RNA degradation, and IFN sensitivity.[62,356] The C-terminal domain of E3 contains the dsRNA-binding domain and the N-terminal segment contains a Z-DNA–binding domain important for virulence.[374] The antiviral action of PKR is also antagonized by a truncated viral version of eIF2α (e.g., VACV K3 and MYXV M156), which inhibits eIF-2α phosphorylation by PKR.[171,172,567] Deletion of K3L increases the IFN sensitivity of VACV.[63,383] Thus, E3 and K3 proteins have overlapping roles in blocking IFN action.

The VACV C7-like family of host range genes encoded by several POXV genera mediate resistance to the IFN-induced antiviral factor SAMD9.[405,450,661,662,819] VACV protein C9 induces resistance to IFN treatment by binding to components of the SCF (CUL1, SKP1, and F-box) and signalosome/deneddylation complexes and to IFITs and inducing their proteasomal degradation.[409,410] VACV induces greater than twofold down-regulation of 265 cellular proteins during infection, and the majority including many ISGs are degraded by proteasome-mediated proteolysis.[679] VACV strategies to interfere with IFN is the subject of a recent review.[675]

Apoptosis Inhibitors

POXVs encode a variety of proteins that inhibit apoptosis by different mechanisms to prevent activation of the extrinsic pathway, for example, TNF, Fas ligand, or intrinsic pathway mediated by mitochondria. CrmA, a viral member of the serine protease inhibitor (serpin) superfamily initially described as an inhibitor of IL-1β converting enzyme caspase 1,[570] blocks apoptosis activated through Fas and TNF receptors[205,355,463,716] and potently inhibit caspase-8, the apical caspase in these pathways.[828] CrmA deletion mutants replicate normally in most cell lines without inducing apoptosis but do induce apoptosis in a pig kidney cell line.[420,571] The effect on virulence caused by deletion of CrmA or related SPI-2 has varied in different animal models.[355,718]

MOCV encodes two FLIP proteins with death effector domains (DEDs).[635] DEDs are also present in cellular FADD and procaspase-8 and mediate their interaction following the binding of TNF or FasL to their receptors. One of the MOCV DED proteins, MC159, has been shown to bind FADD and

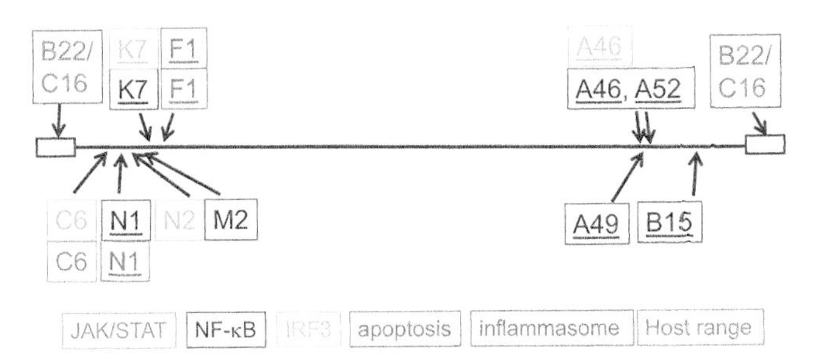

FIGURE 16.19 The VACV Bcl-2 family. The VACV genome is depicted as a *black line* with the inverted terminal repeats as *black boxes*. The positions of VACV CPN genes encoding Bcl-2–like proteins are shown with *arrows* and the function(s) of the encoded proteins indicated by *color*. Note several proteins have multiple functions. Proteins *underlined* have had their structure solved by x-ray crystallography or nuclear magnetic resonance. Note B15 CPN is B14 in strain WR. C16/B22 are diploid due to being in the ITR.

protect transfected cells against death effector filament formation and apoptosis induced by Fas and other members of the TNF receptor superfamily.[72,310,391,494,717,730]

Some POXVs encode Bcl-2-like proteins (e.g., VACV F1, MYXV M11, ORFV 125, FPV 039, deerpox virus 022) that prevent cytochrome c release from mitochondria by preventing Bak and Bax activation.[28,49,50,121,210,226,373,557,777] Those encoded by VACV are shown in Figure 16.19. F1 is also a caspase 9 inhibitor indicating that it is a multifunctional apoptosis inhibitor.[818] VACV protein N1 is another Bcl-2 antiapoptotic protein[153,177] although a relatively weak inhibitor compared to some other VACV proteins.[754] M1, a VACV ankyrin repeat protein, encodes an inhibitor of apoptosis that associates with the apoptosome.[601]

Several POXV proteins prevent apoptosis by additional mechanisms. GAAP (Golgi Anti-Apoptotic Protein) is encoded by CMLV, some strains of VACV, and eukaryotes and can inhibit apoptosis mediated by extrinsic and intrinsic pathways.[278] The ECTV p28 protein contains a RING finger motif that is required for virulence in mice,[643] acts upstream of caspase 3 to block UV-induced apoptosis,[96] and has been shown to be an E3 ubiquitin ligase.[314] Over expression of the SFV ring finger protein N1 can also block apoptosis induced by UV light.[97] MOCV encodes a selenocysteine-containing protein, MC66, that is homologous to cellular glutathione peroxidase and which can protect cells against the cytotoxic effects of hydrogen peroxide, which could be produced by inflammatory cells and UV irradiation.[653] A putative glutathione peroxidase is also encoded by FWPV.[3] The MYXV M-T4 localizes to the ER of infected cells and is required for virulence and to prevent induction of apoptosis in a rabbit CD4+T cell line or primary rabbit lymphocytes.[57,298] The MYXV M-T5 protein has a single ankyrin motif, is related to OPXV host range genes, and is required to prevent apoptosis in a rabbit CD4+ T-cell line.[486] VACV E3L deletion mutants induced apoptosis in HeLa cells through failure to inhibit PKR and RNase L as discussed above.[356,388]

Inhibitors of Antigen Presentation

CPXV encodes two proteins that down-regulate MHC class I presentation by distinct mechanisms. CPXV203 retains fully assembled MHC class I by exploiting the KDEL-mediated ER retention pathway, whereas CPXV12 binds to the peptide-loading complex and inhibits peptide loading on MHC class I molecules.[114,115] The VACV A35 protein inhibits MHC class II antigen presentation by an unknown mechanism.[578,579]

Additional POXV Defense Proteins

The VACV β-hydroxysteroid dehydrogenase contributes to virulence by inhibiting an effective inflammatory response.[573] The mechanism of action of many other POXV proteins that are not required for replication in cell culture but reduce virulence in animal models remain to be determined.[56,209,227,644,682,683]

ADAPTIVE IMMUNE RESPONSE TO POXVIRUSES

Adaptive humoral and cell-mediated immune responses are important in clearing poxvirus infections, and knowledge in this area helps to understand the efficacy of vaccines and the design of new ones. Not surprisingly given their large size and complexity, there are numerous antigens, and consequently protective antibodies are directed toward both the MV and EV forms. As in other areas, most information has been obtained for OPXVs, and this has been the subject of several reviews.[11,479,491,646,803]

ANTIVIRALS

In view of the large number of viral proteins involved in cytoplasmic replication, there are many potential targets for antivirals, and some have been investigated over the years.[176] Two potent antivirals have reached the stage of clinical testing. Cidofovir is an acyclic nucleoside analog that is incorporated into the growing DNA strand and inhibits the 5′-to-3′ chain extension and 3′-to-5′ exonuclease activities of VACV DNA polymerase.[30] Cidofovir (Vistide) has been approved to treat cytomegalovirus retinitis in AIDS patients. An orally available derivative of cidofovir, Brincidofovir, is being tested for both cytomegalovirus and poxvirus applications. The other antiviral is ST-246, which inhibits the wrapping of MVs and formation of EVs by targeting the F13 protein[339] and has been approved under the name TPOXX (Tecovirimat) as a treatment for smallpox and monkeypox.[272]

EXPRESSION VECTORS

Several attributes of POXVs have led to their extensive use as expression vectors.[474] These include relative ease of formation and isolation of recombinant viruses, capacity for large amounts of DNA, relatively high cytoplasmic expression, and wide host range. Expression has been achieved either by using POXV promoters or by employing bacteriophage RNA polymerases and cognate promoters. Recombinant viruses have been used for the synthesis of proteins *in vivo* or *in vitro* and as vaccine candidates to prevent infectious disease and treat cancer.[434] In particular, there has been a recent emphasis on the attenuated MVA primarily for safety reasons[755] and the combination of MVA with DNA priming.[23]

ACKNOWLEDGMENTS

Thanks to Andrea Weisberg of the Laboratory of Viral Diseases for electron microscopic images. The contribution of B.M. was supported by the Division of Intramural Research, National Institute of Allergy and Infectious Diseases, National Institutes of Health. The G.L.S. laboratory has been supported by grants from the UK Medical Research Council and the Wellcome Trust.

REFERENCES

1. Afonso CL, Tulman ER, Delhon G, et al. Genome of crocodilepox virus. *J Virol* 2006;80(10):4978–4991.
2. Afonso CL, Tulman ER, Lu Z, et al. The genome of Melanoplus sanguinipes entomopoxvirus. *J Virol* 1999;73(1):533–552.
3. Afonso CL, Tulman ER, Lu Z, et al. The genome of fowlpox virus. *J Virol* 2000;74(8):3815–3831.
4. Ahmad M, Raut S, Pyaram K, et al. Domain swapping reveals complement control protein modules critical for imparting cofactor and decay-accelerating activities in vaccinia virus complement control protein. *J Immunol* 2010;185(10):6128–6137.
5. Ahn B-Y, Gershon PD, Jones EV, et al. Identification of *rpo30*, a vaccinia virus RNA polymerase gene with structural similarity to a eukaryotic transcription factor. *Mol Cell Biol* 1990;10:5433–5441.
6. Ahn B-Y, Gershon PD, Moss B. RNA-polymerase associated protein RAP94 confers promoter specificity for initiating transcription of vaccinia virus early stage genes. *J Biol Chem* 1994;269:7552–7557.
7. Ahn B-Y, Jones EV, Moss B. Identification of the vaccinia virus gene encoding an 18-kilodalton subunit of RNA polymerase and demonstration of a 5′ poly(A) leader on its early transcript. *J Virol* 1990;64:3019–3024.
8. Ahn B-Y, Moss B. RNA polymerase-associated transcription specificity factor encoded by vaccinia virus. *Proc Natl Acad Sci U S A* 1992;89:3536–3540.
9. Ahn B-Y, Rosel J, Cole NB, et al. Identification and expression of *rpo19*, a vaccinia virus gene encoding a 19-kiloDalton DNA-dependent RNA polymerase subunit. *J Virol* 1992;66:971–982.
10. Ahn B-Y, Moss B. Glutaredoxin homolog encoded by vaccinia virus is a virion-associated enzyme with thioltransferase and dehydroascorbate reductase activities. *Proc Natl Acad Sci U S A* 1992;89(15):7060–7064.
11. Albarnaz JD, Torres AA, Smith GL. Modulating vaccinia virus immunomodulators to improve immunological memory. *Viruses* 2018;10(3):101.
12. Alcami A, Khanna A, Paul NL, et al. Vaccinia virus strains Lister, USSR and Evans express soluble and cell-surface tumour necrosis factor receptors. *J Gen Virol* 1999;80:949–959.
13. Alcami A, Smith GL. A mechanism for inhibition of fever by a virus. *Proc Natl Acad Sci U S A* 1996;93:11029–11034.
14. Alcami A, Smith GL. Soluble interferon-gamma receptors encoded by poxviruses. *Comp Immunol Microbiol Infect Dis* 1996;19(4):305–317.
15. Alcami A, Smith GL. A soluble receptor for interleukin-1b encoded by vaccinia virus—a novel mechanism of virus modulation of the host response to infection. *Cell* 1992;71(1):153–167.
16. Alcami A, Smith GL. Vaccinia, cowpox, and camelpox viruses encode soluble gamma interferon receptors with novel broad species specificity. *J Virol* 1995;69:4633–4639.
17. Alcami A, Symons JA, Collins PD, et al. Blockade of chemokine activity by a soluble chemokine binding protein from vaccinia virus. *J Immunol* 1998;160(2):624–633.
18. Alcami A, Symons JA, Khanna A, et al. Poxviruses: capturing cytokines and chemokines. *Semin Virol* 1998;8(5):419–427.
19. Alcami A, Symons JA, Smith GL. The vaccinia virus soluble alpha/beta interferon (IFN) receptor binds to the cell surface and protects cells from the antiviral effects of IFN. *J Virol* 2000;74(23):11230–11239.
20. Alejo A, Ruiz-Arguello MB, Ho Y, et al. A chemokine-binding domain in the tumor necrosis factor receptor from variola (smallpox) virus. *Proc Natl Acad Sci U S A* 2006;103(15):5995–6000.
21. Almazan F, Tscharke DC, Smith GL. The vaccinia virus superoxide dismutase-like protein (A45R) is a virion component that is nonessential for virus replication. *J Virol* 2001;75(15):7018–7029.
22. Alzhanova D, Hammarlund E, Reed J, et al. T cell inactivation by poxviral B22 family proteins increases viral virulence. *PLoS Pathog* 2014;10(5):e1004123.
23. Amara RR, Villinger F, Altman JD, et al. Control of a mucosal challenge and prevention of AIDS by a multiprotein DNA/MVA vaccine. *Science* 2001;292(5514):69–74.
24. Amegadzie B, Holmes M, Cole NB, et al. Identification, sequence, and expression of the gene encoding the second-largest subunit of the vaccinia virus DNA polymerase. *Virology* 1991;180:88–98.
25. Amegadzie BY, Ahn BY, Moss B. Characterization of a 7-kilodalton subunit of vaccinia virus DNA-dependent RNA polymerase with structural similarities to the smallest subunit of eukaryotic RNA polymerase-II. *J Virol* 1992;66(5):3003–3010.
26. Amegadzie BY, Cole N, Ahn BY, et al. Identification, sequence and expression of the gene encoding a Mr 35,000 subunit of the vaccinia virus DNA-dependent RNA polymerase. *J Biol Chem* 1991;266:13712–13718.
27. Amegadzie BY, Sisler JR, Moss B. Frame-shift mutations within the vaccinia virus A-type inclusion protein gene. *Virology* 1992;186:777–782.
28. Anasir MI, Caria S, Skinner MA, et al. Structural basis of apoptosis inhibition by the fowlpox virus protein FPV039. *J Biol Chem* 2017;292(22):9010–9021.
29. Andrade AA, Silva PNG, Pereira A, et al. The vaccinia virus-stimulated mitogen-activated protein kinase (MAPK) pathway is required for virus multiplication. *Biochem J* 2004;381:437–446.
30. Andrei G, Snoeck R. Cidofovir activity against poxvirus infections. *Viruses* 2010;2(12):2803–2830.
31. Ansarah-Sobrinho C, Moss B. Role of the I7 protein in proteolytic processing of vaccinia virus membrane and core components. *J Virol* 2004;78:6335–6343.
32. Ansarah-Sobrinho C, Moss B. Vaccinia virus G1 protein, a predicted metalloprotease, is essential for morphogenesis of infectious virions but not for cleavage of major core proteins. *J Virol* 2004;78:6855–6863.
33. Antczak JB, Patel DD, Ray CA, et al. Site-specific RNA cleavage generates the 3′ end of a poxvirus late mRNA. *Proc Natl Acad Sci U S A* 1992;89:12033–12037.
34. Antoine G, Scheiflinger F, Dorner F, et al. The complete genomic sequence of the modified vaccinia Ankara strain: comparison with other orthopoxviruses. *Virology* 1998;244(2):365–396.
35. Aoyagi M, Zhai DY, Jin CF, et al. Vaccinia virus N1L protein resembles a B cell lymphoma-2 (Bcl-2) family protein. *Protein Sci* 2007;16(1):118–124.
36. Arakawa Y, Cordeiro JV, Schleich S, et al. The release of vaccinia virus from infected cells requires RhoA-mDia modulation of cortical actin. *Cell Host Microbe* 2007;1(3):227–240.
37. Arnold PL, Fremont DH. Structural determinants of chemokine binding by an ectromelia virus-encoded decoy receptor. *J Virol* 2006;80(15):7439–7449.
38. Assarsson E, Greenbaum JA, Sundstrom M, et al. Kinetic analysis of a complete poxvirus transcriptome reveals an immediate-early class of genes. *Proc Natl Acad Sci U S A* 2008;105(6):2140–2145.
39. Auvynet C, Topalis D, Caillat C, et al. Phosphorylation of dGMP analogs by vaccinia virus TMP kinase and human GMP kinase. *Biochem Biophys Res Commun* 2009;388(1):6–11.
40. Bacik JP, Hazes B. Crystal structures of a poxviral glutaredoxin in the oxidized and reduced states show redox-correlated structural changes. *J Mol Biol* 2007;365(5):1545–1558.
41. Bahar MW, Graham SC, Stuart DI, et al. Insights into the evolution of a complex virus from the crystal structure of vaccinia virus D13. *Structure* 2011;19(7):1011–1020.
42. Bahar MW, Kenyon JC, Putz MM, et al. Structure and function of A41, a vaccinia virus chemokine binding protein. *PLoS Pathog* 2008;4(1):e5.
43. Bajszar G, Wittek R, Weir JP, et al. Vaccinia virus thymidine kinase and neighboring genes: mRNAs and polypeptides of wild type virus and putative nonsense mutants. *J Virol* 1983;45:62–72.
44. Baldick CJ Jr, Moss B. Characterization and temporal regulation of mRNAs encoded by vaccinia virus intermediate stage genes. *J Virol* 1993;67:3515–3527.
45. Baldick CJ, Keck JG, Moss B. Mutational analysis of the core, spacer and initiator regions of vaccinia virus intermediate class promoters. *J Virol* 1992;66:4710–4719.
46. Baldick CJ, Moss B. Resistance of vaccinia virus to rifampicin conferred by a single nucleotide substitution near the predicted NH_2 terminus of a gene encoding an M_r 62,000 polypeptide. *Virology* 1987;156:138–145.
47. Balinsky CA, Delhon G, Afonso CL, et al. Sheeppox virus kelch-like gene SPPV-019 affects virus virulence. *J Virol* 2007;81(20):11392–11401.
48. Ball LA. High frequency recombination in vaccinia virus DNA. *J Virol* 1987;61:1788–1795.
49. Banadyga L, Lam SC, Okamoto T, et al. Deerpox virus encodes an inhibitor of apoptosis that regulates Bak and Bax. *J Virol* 2011;85(5):1922–1934.
50. Banadyga L, Veugelers K, Campbell S, et al. The fowlpox virus BCL-2 homologue, FPV039, interacts with activated bax and a discrete subset of BH3-only proteins to inhibit apoptosis. *J Virol* 2009;83(14):7085–7098.
51. Barbosa E, Moss B. mRNA(nucleoside-2′-)-methyltransferase from vaccinia virus. Characteristics and substrate specificity. *J Biol Chem* 1978;253:7698–7702.
52. Baroudy BM, Moss B. Purification and characterization of a DNA-dependent RNA polymerase from vaccinia virions. *J Biol Chem* 1980;255:4372–4380.
53. Baroudy BM, Venkatesan S, Moss B. Incompletely base-paired flip-flop terminal loops link the two DNA strands of the vaccinia virus genome into one uninterrupted polynucleotide chain. *Cell* 1982;28:315–324.
54. Baroudy BM, Venkatesan S, Moss B. Structure and replication of vaccinia virus telomeres. *Cold Spring Harb Symp Quant Biol* 1983;47:723–729.
55. Barrett JW, Sypula J, Wang F, et al. M135R is a novel cell surface virulence factor of myxoma virus. *J Virol* 2007;81(1):106–114.
56. Barrett JW, Werden SJ, Wang FA, et al. Myxoma virus M130R is a novel virulence factor required for lethal myxomatosis in rabbits. *Virus Res* 2009;144(1–2):258–265.
57. Barry M, Hnatiuk S, Mossman K, et al. The myxoma virus M-T4 gene encodes a novel RDEL-containing protein that is retained within the endoplasmic reticulum and is important for the productive infection of lymphocytes. *Virology* 1997;239:360–377.
58. Barry M, van Buuren N, Burles K, et al. Poxvirus exploitation of the ubiquitin-proteasome system. *Viruses* 2010;2(10):2356–2380.
59. Bartlett N, Symons JA, Tscharke DC, et al. The vaccinia virus N1L protein is an intracellular homodimer that promotes virulence. *J Gen Virol* 2002;83:1965–1976.
60. Bayliss CD, Smith GL. Vaccinia virion protein VP8, the 25 kDa product of the L4R gene, binds single-stranded DNA and RNA with similar affinity. *Nucleic Acids Res* 1997;25(20):3984–3990.
61. Beard PM, Froggatt GC, Smith GL. Vaccinia virus keltch protein A55 is a 64 kDa intracellular factor that affects virus-induced cytopathic effect and the outcome of infection in a murine intradermal model. *J Gen Virol* 2006;87:1521–1529.
62. Beattie E, Paoletti E, Tartaglia J. Distinct patterns of IFN sensitivity observed in cells infected with vaccinia K3L⁻ and E3L⁻ mutant viruses. *Virology* 1995;210:254–263.
63. Beattie E, Tartaglia J, Paoletti E. Vaccinia virus encoded eIF-2a homolog abrogates the antiviral effect of interferon. *Virology* 1991;183:419–422.

64. Beaud G, Beaud R, Leader DP. Vaccinia virus gene H5R encodes a protein that is phosphorylated by the multisubstrate vaccinia virus B1R protein kinase. *J Virol* 1995;69:1819–1826.
65. Becker Y, Joklik WK. Messenger RNA in cells infected with vaccinia virus. *Proc Natl Acad Sci U S A* 1964;51:577–584.
66. Benfield CTO, Mansur DS, McCoy LE, et al. Mapping the I kappa B kinase beta (IKK beta)-binding interface of the B14 protein, a vaccinia virus inhibitor of IKK beta-mediated activation of nuclear factor kappa B. *J Biol Chem* 2011;286(23):20727–20735.
67. Benfield CTO, Ren HW, Lucas SJ, et al. Vaccinia virus protein K7 is a virulence factor that alters immune response to infection. *J Gen Virol* 2013;94:1647–1657.
68. Bengali Z, Satheshkumar PS, Moss B. Orthopoxvirus species and strain differences in cell entry. *Virology* 2012;433(2):506–512.
69. Bengali Z, Satheshkumar PS, Yang Z, et al. Drosophila S2 cells are non-permissive for vaccinia virus DNA replication following entry via low pH-dependent endocytosis and early transcription. *PLoS One* 2011;6(2):e17248.
70. Bennett CJ, Webb M, Willer DO, et al. Genetic and phylogenetic characterization of the type II cyclobutane pyrimidine dimer photolyases encoded by Leporipoxviruses. *Virology* 2003;315(1):10–19.
71. Bergoin M, Devauchelle G, Vago C. Electron microscopy study of the pox-like virus of Melolontha melolontha L (Coleptera, Scarabeidae) virus morphogenesis. *Arch Gesamte Virusforsch* 1969;28:285–302.
72. Bertin J, Armstrong RC, Ottilie S, et al. DED-containing herpesvirus and poxvirus proteins inhibit both Fas- and TNFR1-induced apoptosis. *Proc Natl Acad Sci U S A* 1997;94:1172–1176.
73. Betakova T, Wolffe EJ, Moss B. Regulation of vaccinia virus morphogenesis: phosphorylation of the A14L and A17L membrane proteins and C-terminal truncation of the A17L protein are dependent on the F10L protein kinase. *J Virol* 1999;73:3534–3543.
74. Betakova T, Wolffe EJ, Moss B. Vaccinia virus A14.5L gene encodes a hydrophobic 53-amino acid virion membrane protein that enhances virulence in mice and is conserved amongst vertebrate poxviruses. *J Virol* 2000;74:4085–4092.
75. Bisht H, Weisberg AS, Moss B. Vaccinia virus L1 protein is required for cell entry and membrane fusion. *J Virol* 2008;82:8687–8694.
76. Bisht H, Weisberg AS, Szajner P, et al. Assembly and disassembly of the capsid-like external scaffold of immature virions during vaccinia virus morphogenesis. *J Virol* 2009;83: 9140–9150.
77. Black EP, Condit RC. Phenotypic characterization of mutants in vaccinia virus gene G2R, a putative transcription elongation factor. *J Virol* 1996;70:47–54.
78. Black EP, Moussatche N, Condit RC. Characterization of the interactions among vaccinia virus transcription factors G2R, A18R, and H5R. *Virology* 1998;245(2):313–322.
79. Black ME, Hruby DE. A single amino acid substitution abolishes feedback inhibition of vaccinia virus thymidine kinase. *J Biol Chem* 1992;267(14):9743–9748.
80. Blasco R, Moss B. Extracellular vaccinia virus formation and cell-to-cell virus transmission are prevented by deletion of the gene encoding the 37,000 Dalton outer envelope protein. *J Virol* 1991;65:5910–5920.
81. Blasco R, Moss B. Role of cell-associated enveloped vaccinia virus in cell-to-cell spread. *J Virol* 1992;66(7):4170–4179.
82. Blasco R, Sisler JR, Moss B. Dissociation of progeny vaccinia virus from the cell membrane is regulated by a viral envelope glycoprotein: effect of a point mutation in the lectin homology domain of the A34R gene. *J Virol* 1993;67:3319–3325.
83. Block W, Upton C, McFadden G. Tumorigenic poxviruses: genomic organization of malignant rabbit virus, a recombinant between Shope fibroma virus and myxoma virus. *Virology* 1985;140:113–124.
84. Blomquist MC, Hunt LT, Barker WC. Vaccinia virus 19-kilodalton protein: relationship to several mammalian proteins, including two growth factors. *Proc Natl Acad Sci U S A* 1984;81:7363–7367.
85. Boone RF, Moss B. Methylated 5′ terminal sequences of vaccinia virus mRNA species made in vivo at early and late times after infection. *Virology* 1977;79:67–80.
86. Boone RF, Moss B. Sequence complexity and relative abundance of vaccinia virus mRNA's synthesized in vivo and in vitro. *J Virol* 1978;26:554–569.
87. Boone RF, Parr RP, Moss B. Intermolecular duplexes formed from polyadenylated vaccinia virus RNA. *J Virol* 1979;30:365–374.
88. Born TL, Morrison LA, Esteban DJ, et al. A poxvirus protein that binds to and inactivates IL-18, and inhibits NK cell response. *J Immunol* 2000;164(6):3246–3254.
89. Boulanger D, Smith T, Skinner MA. Morphogenesis and release of fowlpox virus. *J Gen Virol* 2000;81(Pt 3):675–687.
90. Boulter EA, Appleyard G. Differences between extracellular and intracellular forms of poxvirus and their implications. *Prog Med Virol* 1973;16:86–108.
91. Bowie A, Kiss-Toth E, Symons JA, et al. A46R and A52R from vaccinia virus are antagonists of host IL-1 and toll-like receptor signaling. *Proc Natl Acad Sci U S A* 2000;97:10162–10167.
92. Boyd O, Turner PC, Moyer RW, et al. The E6 protein from vaccinia virus is required for the formation of immature virions. *Virology* 2010;399(2):201–211.
93. Boyle KA, Arps L, Traktman P. Biochemical and genetic analysis of the vaccinia virus D5 protein: multimerization-dependent ATPase activity is required to support viral DNA replication. *J Virol* 2007;81(2):844–859.
94. Boyle KA, Greseth MD, Traktman P. Genetic confirmation that the H5 protein is required for vaccinia virus DNA replication. *J Virol* 2015;89(12):6312–6327.
95. Boyle KA, Stanitsa ES, Greseth MD, et al. Evaluation of the role of the vaccinia virus uracil DNA glycosylase and A20 proteins as intrinsic components of the DNA polymerase holoenzyme. *J Biol Chem* 2011;286(28):24702–24713.
96. Brick DJ, Burke RD, Minkley AA, et al. Ectromelia virus virulence factor p28 acts upstream of caspase-3 in response to UV light-induced apoptosis. *J Gen Virol* 2000;81(Pt 4):1087–1097.
97. Brick DJ, Burke RD, Schiff L, et al. Shope fibroma virus RING finger protein N1R binds DNA and inhibits apoptosis. *Virology* 1998;249(1):42–51.
98. Brown E, Senkevich TG, Moss B. Vaccinia virus F9 virion membrane protein is required for entry but not virus assembly, in contrast to the related l1 protein. *J Virol* 2006;80(19):9455–9464.
99. Brown JP, Twardzik DR, Marquardt H, et al. Vaccinia virus encodes a polypeptide homologous to epidermal growth factor and transforming growth factor. *Nature* 1985;313:491–492.
100. Broyles SS. Vaccinia virus encodes a functional dUTPase. *Virology* 1993;195:863–865.
101. Broyles SS, Fesler BS. Vaccinia virus gene encoding a component of the viral early transcription factor. *J Virol* 1990;64:1523–1529.
102. Broyles SS, Li J. The small subunit of the vaccinia virus early transcription factor contacts the transcription promoter DNA. *J Virol* 1993;67:5677–5680.
103. Broyles SS, Moss B. Homology between RNA polymerases of poxviruses, prokaryotes, and eukaryotes: nucleotide sequence and transcriptional analysis of vaccinia virus genes encoding 147-kDa and 22-kDa subunits. *Proc Natl Acad Sci U S A* 1986;83:3141–3145.
104. Broyles SS, Moss B. Sedimentation of an RNA polymerase complex from vaccinia virus that specifically initiates and terminates transcription. *Mol Cell Biol* 1987;7(1):7–14.
105. Broyles SS, Yuen L, Shuman S, et al. Purification of a factor required for transcription of vaccinia virus early genes. *J Biol Chem* 1988; 263:10754–10760.
106. Brum LM, Turner PC, Devick H, et al. Plasma membrane localization and fusion inhibitory activity of the cowpox virus serpin SPI-3 require a functional signal sequence and the virus encoded hemagglutinin. *Virology* 2003;306(2):289 302.
107. Brunetti CR, Paulose-Murphy M, Singh R, et al. A secreted high-affinity inhibitor of human TNF from Tanapox virus. *Proc Natl Acad Sci U S A* 2003;100(8):4831–4836.
108. Buller RML, Chakrabarti S, Moss B, et al. Cell proliferative response to vaccinia virus is mediated by VGF. *Virology* 1988;164:182–192.
109. Buller RML, Smith GL, Cremer K, et al. Decreased virulence of recombinant vaccinia virus expression vectors is associated with a thymidine kinase-negative phenotype. *Nature* 1985;317:813–815.
110. Burgess HM, Mohr I. Cellular 5′-3′ mRNA exonuclease Xrn1 controls double-stranded RNA accumulation and anti-viral responses. *Cell Host Microbe* 2015;17(3):332–344.
111. Burles K, Irwin CR, Burton RL, et al. Initial characterization of vaccinia virus B4 suggests a role in virus spread. *Virology* 2014;456:108–120.
112. Burns JM, Dairaghi DJ, Deitz M, et al. Comprehensive mapping of poxvirus vCCI chemokine-binding protein—expanded range of ligand interactions and unusual dissociation kinetics. *J Biol Chem* 2002;277(4):2785–2789.
113. Byrd CM, Bolken TC, Hruby DE. Molecular dissection of the vaccinia virus I7L core protein proteinase. *J Virol* 2003;77(20):11279–11283.
114. Byun M, Verweij MC, Pickup DJ, et al. Two mechanistically distinct immune evasion proteins of cowpox virus combine to avoid antiviral CD8 T cells. *Cell Host Microbe* 2009;6(5): 422–432.
115. Byun M, Wang X, Pak M, et al. Cowpox virus exploits the endoplasmic reticulum retention pathway to inhibit MHC class I transport to the cell surface. *Cell Host Microbe* 2007;2(5):306–315.
116. Cacoullos N, Bablanian R. Role of polyadenylated RNA sequences (POLADS) in vaccinia virus infection: correlation between accumulation of POLADS and extent of shut-off in infected cells. *Cell Mol Biol Res* 1993;39(7):657–664.
117. Caillat C, Topalis D, Agrofoglio LA, et al. Crystal structure of poxvirus thymidylate kinase: an unexpected dimerization has implications for antiviral therapy. *Proc Natl Acad Sci U S A* 2008;105(44):16900–16905.
118. Cairns J. The initiation of vaccinia infection. *Virology* 1960;11:603–623.
119. Cameron C, Hota-Mitchell S, Chen L, et al. The complete DNA sequence of myxoma virus. *Virology* 1999;264(2):298–318.
120. Campbell JA, Trossman DS, Yokoyama WM, et al. Zoonotic orthopoxviruses encode a high-affinity antagonist of NKG2D. *J Exp Med* 2007;204(6):1311–1317.
121. Campbell S, Hazes B, Kvansakul M, et al. Vaccinia virus F1L interacts with Bak using highly divergent Bcl-2 homology domains and replaces the function of Mcl-1. *J Biol Chem* 2010;285(7):4695–4708.
122. Carf A, Smith CA, Smolak PJ, et al. Structure of a soluble secreted chemokine inhibitor vCCI (p35) from cowpox virus. *Proc Natl Acad Sci U S A* 1999;96(22):12379–12383.
123. Carpenter MS, DeLange AM. Identification of a temperature-sensitive mutant of vaccinia virus defective in late but not intermediate gene expression. *Virology* 1992;188:233–244.
124. Carpentier DCJ, Gao WND, Ewles H, et al. Vaccinia virus protein complex F12/E2 interacts with kinesin light chain isoform 2 to engage the kinesin-1 motor complex. *PLoS Pathog* 2015;11(3):e1004723.
125. Carter GC, Rodger G, Murphy BJ, et al. Vaccinia virus cores are transported on microtubules. *J Gen Virol* 2003;84(Pt 9):2443–2458.
126. Cassetti MC, Merchlinsky M, Wolffe EJ, et al. DNA packaging mutant: repression of the vaccinia virus A32 gene results in noninfectious, DNA-deficient, spherical, enveloped particles. *J Virol* 1998;72:5769–5780.
127. Cassetti MC, Moss B. Interaction of the 82-kDa subunit of the vaccinia virus early transcription factor heterodimer with the promoter core sequence directs downstream DNA binding of the 70-kDa subunit. *Proc Natl Acad Sci U S A* 1996;93:7540–7545.
128. Challberg MD, Englund PT. Purification and properties of the deoxyribonucleic acid polymerase induced by vaccinia virus. *J Biol Chem* 1979;254:7812–7819.
129. Chang HW, Watson JC, Jacobs BL. The E3L gene of vaccinia virus encodes an inhibitor of the interferon-induced, double-stranded RNA-dependent protein kinase. *Proc Natl Acad Sci U S A* 1992;89(11):4825–4829.
130. Chang HW, Yang CH, Luo YC, et al. Vaccinia viral A26 protein is a fusion suppressor of mature virus and triggers membrane fusion through conformational change at low pH. *PLoS Pathog* 2019;15(6):e1007826.
131. Chang SJ, Shih AC, Tang YL, et al. Vaccinia mature virus fusion regulator A26 protein binds to A16 and G9 proteins of the viral entry fusion complex and dissociates from mature virions at low pH. *J Virol* 2012;86(7):3809–3818.
132. Chang TH, Chang SJ, Hsieh FL, et al. Crystal structure of vaccinia viral A27 protein reveals a structure critical for its function and complex formation with protein. *PLoS Pathog* 2013;9(8):e1003563.
133. Chang W, Macaulay C, Hu S-L, et al. Tumorigenic poxviruses: characterization of the expression of an epidermal growth factor related gene in Shope fibroma virus. *Virology* 1990;179:926–930.
134. Charity JC, Katz E, Moss B. Amino acid substitutions at multiple sites within the vaccinia virus D13 scaffold protein confer resistance to rifampicin. *Virology* 2007;359(1):227–232.

135. Cheevers WP, O'Callaghan DJ, Randall CC. Biosynthesis of host and viral deoxyribonucleic acid during hyperplastic fowlpox-infection *in vivo*. *J Virol* 1968;2:421–429.
136. Chen RAJ, Jacobs N, Smith GL. Vaccinia virus strain Western Reserve protein B14 is an intracellular virulence factor. *J Gen Virol* 2006;87:1451–1458.
137. Chen RAJ, Ryzhakov G, Cooray S, et al. Inhibition of I kappa B kinase by vaccinia virus virulence factor B14. *PLoS Pathog* 2008;4(2):E22.
138. Child SJ, Palumbo G, Buller RM, et al. Insertional inactivation of the large subunit of ribonucleotide reductase encoded by vaccinia virus is associated with reduced virulence in vivo. *Virology* 1990;174:625–629.
139. Chiu WL, Chang W. Vaccinia virus J1R protein: a viral membrane protein that is essential for virion morphogenesis. *J Virol* 2002;76(19):9575–9587.
140. Chiu WL, Lin CL, Yang MH, et al. Vaccinia virus 4c (A26L) protein on intracellular mature virus binds to the extracellular cellular matrix laminin. *J Virol* 2007;81(5):2149–2157.
141. Chiu WL, Szajner P, Moss B, et al. Effects of a temperature sensitivity mutation in the J1R protein component of a complex required for vaccinia virus assembly. *J Virol* 2005;79(13):8046–8056.
142. Christen LA, Piacente S, Mohamed MR, et al. Vaccinia virus early gene transcription termination factors VTF and Rap94 interact with the U9 termination motif in the nascent RNA in a transcription ternary complex. *Virology* 2008;376(1):225–235.
143. Chung C-S, Hsiao J-C, Chang Y-S, et al. A27L protein mediates vaccinia virus interaction with cell surface heparin sulfate. *J Virol* 1998;72:1577–1585.
144. Chung CS, Huang CY, Chang W. Vaccinia virus penetration requires cholesterol and results in specific viral envelope proteins associated with lipid rafts. *J Virol* 2005;79(3):1623–1634.
145. Cluett EB, Machamer CE. The envelope of vaccinia virus reveals an unusual phospholipid in Golgi complex membranes. *J Cell Sci* 1996;109 (Pt 8):2121–2131.
146. Colamonici OR, Domanski P, Sweitzer SM, et al. Vaccinia virus B18R gene encodes a type I interferon-binding protein that blocks interferon alpha transmembrane signaling. *J Biol Chem* 1995;270(27):15974–15978.
147. Colby C, Jurale C, Kates JR. Mechanism of synthesis of vaccinia virus double-stranded ribonucleic acid in vivo and in vitro. *J Virol* 1971;7:71–76.
148. Colinas RJ, Goebel SJ, Davis SW, et al. A DNA ligase gene in the Copenhagen strain of vaccinia virus is nonessential for viral replication and recombination. *Virology* 1990;179: 267–275.
149. Comeau MR, Johnson R, DuBose RF, et al. A poxvirus-encoded semaphorin induces cytokine production from monocytes and binds to a novel cellular semaphorin receptor, VESPR. *Immunity* 1998;8(4):473–482.
150. Condit RC, Moussatche N, Traktman P. In a nutshell: structure and assembly of the vaccinia virion. *Adv Virus Res* 2006;66:31–124.
151. Condit RC, Xiang Y, Lewis JI. Mutation of vaccinia virus gene G2R causes suppression of gene A18R ts mutants: implication for control of transcription. *Virology* 1996;220:10–19.
152. Cooper JA, Wittek R, Moss B. Extension of the transcriptional and translational map of the left end of the vaccinia virus genome to 21 kilobase pairs. *J Virol* 1981;39:733–745.
153. Cooray S, Bahar MW, Abrescia NGA, et al. Functional and structural studies of the vaccinia virus virulence factor N1 reveal a Bcl-2-like anti-apoptotic protein. *J Gen Virol* 2007;88:1656–1666.
154. Cordeiro JV, Guerra S, Arakawa Y, et al. F11-mediated inhibition of RhoA signalling enhances the spread of vaccinia virus in vitro and in vivo in an intranasal mouse model of infection. *PLoS One* 2009;4(12):e8506.
155. Cudmore S, Blasco R, Vincentelli R, et al. A vaccinia virus core protein, p39, is membrane associated. *J Virol* 1996;70:6909–6921.
156. Cudmore S, Cossart P, Griffiths G, et al. Actin-based motility of vaccinia virus. *Nature* 1995;378:636–638.
157. Culyba MJ, Minkah N, Hwang Y, et al. DNA branch nuclease activity of vaccinia A22 resolvase. *J Biol Chem* 2007;282(48):34644–34652.
158. Cyrklaff M, Risco C, Fernandez JJ, et al. Cryo-electron tomography of vaccinia virus. *Proc Natl Acad Sci U S A* 2005;102(8):2772–2777.
159. Czarnecki MW, Traktman P. The vaccinia virus DNA polymerase and its processivity factor. *Virus Res* 2017;234:193–206.
160. D'Costa SM, Antczak JB, Pickup DJ, et al. Post-transcription cleavage generates the 3′ end of F17R transcripts in vaccinia virus. *Virology* 2004;319(1):1–11.
161. D'Costa SM, Bainbridge TW, Condit RC. Purification and properties of the vaccinia virus mRNA processing factor. *J Biol Chem* 2008;283(9):5267–5275.
162. Da Fonseca F, Moss B. Poxvirus DNA topoisomerase knockout mutant exhibits decreased infectivity associated with reduced early transcription. *Proc Natl Acad Sci U S A* 2003;100(20):11291–11296.
163. Da Fonseca FG, Weisberg AS, Caeiro MF, et al. Vaccinia virus mutants with alanine substitutions in the conserved G5R gene fail to initiate morphogenesis at the nonpermissive temperature. *J Virol* 2004;78(19):10238–10248.
164. da Fonseca FG, Wolffe EJ, Weisberg A, et al. Effects of deletion or stringent repression of the H3L envelope gene on vaccinia virus replication. *J Virol* 2000;74(16): 7518–7528.
165. Da Silva M, Shen L, Tcherepanov V, et al. Predicted function of the vaccinia virus G5R protein. *Bioinformatics* 2006;22(23):2846–2850.
166. Daffis S, Szretter KJ, Schriewer J, et al. 2′-O methylation of the viral mRNA cap evades host restriction by IFIT family members. *Nature* 2010;468(7322):452–456.
167. Dales S, Mosbach EH. Vaccinia as a model for membrane biogenesis. *Virology* 1968;35:564–583.
168. Dales S, Siminovitch L. The development of vaccinia virus in Earle's L strain cells as examined by electron microscopy. *J Biophys Biochem Cytol* 1961;10:475–503.
169. Dall D, Sriskantha A, Verra A, et al. A gene encoding a highly expressed spindle body protein of Heliothis armigera entomopoxvirus. *J Gen Virol* 1993;74:1811–1818.
170. Damon I, Murphy PM, Moss B. Broad spectrum chemokine antagonist activity of a human poxvirus chemokine homolog. *Proc Natl Acad Sci U S A* 1998;95:6403–6407.
171. Dar AC, Sicheri F. X-ray crystal structure and functional analysis of vaccinia virus K3L reveals molecular determinants for PKR subversion and substrate recognition. *Mol Cell* 2002;10(2):295–305.
172. Davies MV, Elroy-Stein O, Jagus R, et al. The vaccinia virus K3L gene product potentiates translation by inhibiting double-stranded-RNA-activated protein kinase and phosphorylation of the alpha subunit of eukaryotic initiation factor 2. *J Virol* 1992;66:1943–1950.
173. Davison AJ, Moss B. The structure of vaccinia virus early promoters. *J Mol Biol* 1989;210:749–769.
174. Davison AJ, Moss B. The structure of vaccinia virus late promoters. *J Mol Biol* 1989;210:771–784.
175. De Carlos A, Paez E. Isolation and characterization of mutants of vaccinia virus with a modified 94-kDa inclusion protein. *Virology* 1991;185:768–778.
176. De Clercq E. Historical perspectives in the development of antiviral agents against poxviruses. *Viruses* 2010;2(6):1322–1339.
177. Maluquer de Motes C, Cooray S, Ren HW, et al. Inhibition of apoptosis and NF-kappa B activation by vaccinia protein N1 occur via distinct binding surfaces and make different contributions to virulence. *PLoS Pathog* 2011;7(12):e1002430.
178. Maluquer de Motes C, Smith GL. Vaccinia virus protein A49 activates Wnt signalling by targeting the E3 ligase beta-TrCP. *J Gen Virol* 2017;98(12):3086–3092.
179. de Oliveira JS, Figueiredo PD, Costa GB, et al. Vaccinia virus natural infections in Brazil: the good, the bad, and the ugly. *Viruses* 2017;9(11):340.
180. De Silva FS, Lewis W, Berglund P, et al. Poxvirus DNA primase. *Proc Natl Acad Sci U S A* 2007;104(47):18724–18729.
181. De Silva FS, Moss B. Effects of vaccinia virus uracil DNA glycosylase catalytic site and deoxyuridine triphosphatase deletion mutations individually and together on replication in active and quiescent cells and pathogenesis in mice. *Virol J* 2008;5:145.
182. De Silva FS, Moss B. Origin-independent plasmid replication occurs in vaccinia virus cytoplasmic factories and requires all five known poxvirus replication factors. *Virol J* 2005;2(1):23.
183. De Silva FS, Moss B. Vaccinia virus uracil DNA glycosylase has an essential role in DNA synthesis that is independent of its glycosylase activity: catalytic site mutations reduce virulence but not virus replication in cultured cells. *J Virol* 2003;77:159–166.
184. Deane D, McInnes CJ, Percival A, et al. Orf virus encodes a novel secreted protein inhibitor of granulocyte- macrophage colony-stimulating factor and interleukin-2. *J Virol* 2000;74(3):1313–1320.
185. Deane D, Ueda N, Wise LM, et al. Conservation and variation of the parapoxvirus GM-CSF-inhibitory factor (GIF) proteins. *J Gen Virol* 2009;90(Pt 4):970–977.
186. DeBruyne LA, Li K, Bishop DK, et al. Gene transfer of virally encoded chemokine antagonists vMIP-II and MC148 prolongs cardiac allograft survival and inhibits donor-specific immunity. *Gene Ther* 2000;7(7):575–582.
187. DeHaven BC, Girgis NM, Xiao YH, et al. Poxvirus complement control proteins are expressed on the cell surface through an intermolecular disulfide bridge with the viral A56 protein. *J Virol* 2010;84(81):11245–11254.
188. Del Mar Fernandez de Marco M, Alejo A, Hudson P, et al. The highly virulent variola and monkeypox viruses express secreted inhibitors of type I interferon. *FASEB J* 2010;24:1479–1488.
189. DeLange AM. Identification of temperature-sensitive mutants of vaccinia virus that are defective in conversion of concatemeric replicative intermediates to the mature linear DNA genome. *J Virol* 1989;63:2437–2444.
190. DeLange AM, McFadden G. Efficient resolution of replicated poxvirus telomeres to native hairpin structures requires two inverted symmetrical copies of a core target DNA sequence. *J Virol* 1987;61:1957–1963.
191. DeLange AM, McFadden G. Sequence-nonspecific replication of transfected plasmid DNA in poxvirus-infected cells. *Proc Natl Acad Sci U S A* 1986;83:614–618.
192. Dellis S, Strickland KC, McCrary WJ, et al. Protein interactions among the vaccinia virus late transcription factors. *Virology* 2004;329(2):328–336.
193. DeMasi J, Du S, Lennon D, et al. Vaccinia virus telomeres: interaction with the viral I1, I6, and K4 proteins. *J Virol* 2001;75(21):10090–10105.
194. DeMasi J, Traktman P. Clustered charge-to-alanine mutagenesis of the vaccinia virus H5 gene: isolation of a dominant, temperature-sensitive mutant with a profound defect in morphogenesis. *J Virol* 2000;74(5):2393–2405.
195. Deng L, Shuman S. Vaccinia NPH-I, a DExH-box ATPase, is the energy coupling factor for mRNA transcription termination. *Genes Dev* 1998;12(4):538–546.
196. Deng S, Shuman S. A role for the H4 subunit of vaccinia RNA polymerase in transcription initiation at a viral early promoter. *J Biol Chem* 1994;269:14323–14329.
197. Derrien M, Punjabi A, Khanna R, et al. Tyrosine phosphorylation of A17 during vaccinia virus infection: involvement of the H1 phosphatase and the F10 kinase. *J Virol* 1999;73(9):7287–7296.
198. des Gouttes Olgiati D, Pogo BG, Dales S. Biogenesis of vaccinia: specific inhibition of rapidly labeled host DNA in vaccinia inoculated cells. *Virology* 1976;71(1):325–335.
199. Dhungel P, Cao S, Yang Z. The 5′-poly(A) leader of poxvirus mRNA confers a translational advantage that can be achieved in cells with impaired cap-dependent translation. *PLoS Pathog* 2017;13(8):e1006602.
200. Dickie P, Morgan AR, McFadden G. Cruciform extrusion in plasmids bearing the replicative intermediate configuration of a poxvirus telomere. *J Mol Biol* 1987;196(3):541–558.
201. Diel DG, Delhon G, Luo S, et al. A novel inhibitor of the NF-kappa B signaling pathway encoded by the parapoxvirus Orf virus. *J Virol* 2010;84(8):3962–3973.
202. Diel DG, Luo S, Delhon G, et al. Orf virus ORFV121 encodes a novel inhibitor of NF-kappa B that contributes to virus virulence. *J Virol* 2011;85(5):2037–2049.
203. Diesterbeck US, Gittis AG, Garboczi DN, et al. The 2.1 angstrom structure of protein F9 and its comparison to L1, two components of the conserved poxvirus entry-fusion complex. *Sci Rep* 2018;8:16807.
204. DiPerna G, Stack J, Bowie AG, et al. Poxvirus protein N1L targets the I-kappaB kinase complex, inhibits signaling to NF-kappaB by the tumor necrosis factor superfamily of receptors, and inhibits NF-kappaB and IRF3 signaling by toll-like receptors. *J Biol Chem* 2004;279(35):36570–36578.
205. Dobbelstein M, Shenk T. Protection against apoptosis by the vaccinia virus SPI-2 (B13R) gene product. *J Virol* 1996;70:6479–6485.
206. Doceul V, Hollinshead M, van der Linden L, et al. Repulsion of superinfecting virions: a mechanism for rapid virus spread. *Science* 2010;327(5967):873–876.

207. Dodding MP, Newsome TP, Collinson LM, et al. An E2-F12 complex is required for IEV morphogenesis during vaccinia infection. *Cell Microbiol* 2009;11(5):808–824.
208. Domi A, Weisberg AS, Moss B. Vaccinia virus E2L null mutants exhibit a major reduction in extracellular virion formation and virus spread. *J Virol* 2008;82(9):4215–4226.
209. Dorfleutner A, Talbott SJ, Bryan NB, et al. A Shope Fibroma virus PYRIN-only protein modulates the host immune response. *Virus Genes* 2007;35(3):685–694.
210. Douglas AE, Corbett KD, Berger JM, et al. Structure of M11L: a myxoma virus structural homolog of the apoptosis inhibitor, Bcl-2. *Protein Sci* 2007;16(4):695–703.
211. Du S, Traktman P. Vaccinia virus DNA replication: two hundred base pairs of telomeric sequence confer optimal replication efficiency on minichromosome templates. *Proc Natl Acad Sci U S A* 1996;93:9693–9698.
212. Eaglesham JB, Pan YD, Kupper TS, et al. Viral and metazoan poxins are cGAMP-specific nucleases that restrict cGAS-STING signalling. *Nature* 2019;566(7743):259–263.
213. Earl PL, Hügin AW, Moss B. Removal of cryptic poxvirus transcription termination signals from the human immunodeficiency virus type 1 envelope gene enhances expression and immunogenicity of a recombinant vaccinia virus. *J Virol* 1990;64:2448–2451.
214. Earl PL, Jones EV, Moss B. Homology between DNA polymerases of poxviruses, herpesviruses, and adenoviruses: nucleotide sequence of the vaccinia virus DNA polymerase gene. *Proc Natl Acad Sci U S A* 1986;83:3659–3663.
215. Eckert D, Williams O, Meseda CA, et al. Vaccinia virus nicking-joining enzyme is encoded by K4L (VACWR035). *J Virol* 2005;79(24):15084–15090.
216. El Omari K, Solaroli N, Karlsson A, et al. Structure of vaccinia virus thymidine kinase in complex with dTTP: insights for drug design. *BMC Struct Biol* 2006;6:9.
217. Elde NC, Child SJ, Eickbush MT, et al. Poxviruses deploy genomic accordions to adapt rapidly against host antiviral defenses. *Cell* 2012;150(4):831–841.
218. Ember SW, Ren H, Ferguson BJ, et al. Vaccinia virus protein C4 inhibits NF-kappaB activation and promotes virus virulence. *J Gen Virol* 2012;93(Pt 10):2098–2108.
219. Engelstad M, Smith GL. The vaccinia virus 42-kDa envelope protein is required for the envelopment and egress of extracellular virus and for virus virulence. *Virology* 1993;194:627–637.
220. Erlandson KJ, Bisht H, Weisberg AS, et al. Poxviruses encode a reticulon-like protein that promotes membrane curvature. *Cell Rep* 2016;14(9):2084–2091.
221. Esposito JJ, Sammons SA, Frace AM, et al. Genome sequence diversity and clues to the evolution of variola (smallpox) virus. *Science* 2006;313(5788):807–812.
222. Esteban M, Flores L, Holowczak JA. Model for vaccinia virus DNA replication. *Virology* 1977;83:467–473.
223. Esteban M, Metz DH. Early virus protein synthesis in vaccinia virus-infected cells. *J Gen Virol* 1973;19:201–216.
224. Evans DH, Stuart D, McFadden G. High levels of genetic recombination among cotransfected plasmid DNAs in poxvirus-infected mammalian cells. *J Virol* 1988;62:367–375.
225. Evans E, Klemperer N, Ghosh R, et al. The vaccinia virus D5 protein, which is required for DNA replication, is a nucleic acid-independent nucleotide triphosphatase. *J Virol* 1995;69:5353–5361.
226. Everett H, Barry M, Lee SF, et al. M11L: a novel mitochondria-localized protein of myxoma virus that blocks apoptosis of infected leukocytes. *J Exp Med* 2000;191(9):1487–1498.
227. Fahy AS, Clark RH, Glyde EF, et al. Vaccinia virus protein C16 acts intracellularly to modulate the host response and promote virulence. *J Gen Virol* 2008;89:2377–2387.
228. Fang M, Lanier LL, Sigal LJ. A role for NKG2D in NK cell-mediated resistance to poxvirus disease. *PLoS Pathog* 2008;4(2):e30.
229. Fedosyuk S, Bezerra GA, Radakovics K, et al. Vaccinia virus immunomodulator A46: a lipid and protein-binding scaffold for sequestering host TIR-domain proteins. *PLoS Pathog* 2016;12(12):e1006079.
230. Fedosyuk S, Grishkovskaya I, Ribeiro ED, et al. Characterization and structure of the vaccinia virus NF-kappa B antagonist A46. *J Biol Chem* 2014;289(6):3749–3762.
231. Fenner F, Comben BM. Genetic studies with mammalian poxviruses. I. Demonstration of recombination between two strains of poxviruses. *Virology* 1958;5:530–548.
232. Fenner F, Ross J. *Myxomatosis* Oxford: Oxford University Press; 1994.
233. Fenner F, Woodroofe GM. The reactivation of poxviruses. II. The range of reactivating viruses. *Virology* 1960;11:185–201.
234. Ferguson BJ, Benfield CTO, Ren HW, et al. Vaccinia virus protein N2 is a nuclear IRF3 inhibitor that virulence. *J Gen Virol* 2013;94:2070–2081.
235. Ferreira LR, Moussatche N, Moura Neto V. Rearrangement of intermediate filament network of BHK-21 cells infected with vaccinia virus. *Arch Virol* 1994;138(3–4):273–285.
236. Fleming SB, Anderson IE, Thomson J, et al. Infection with recombinant orf viruses demonstrates that the viral interleukin-10 is a virulence factor. *J Gen Virol* 2007;88:1922–1927.
237. Foo CH, Lou H, Whitbeck JC, et al. Vaccinia virus L1 binds to cell surfaces and blocks virus entry independently of glycosaminoglycans. *Virology* 2009;385(2):368–382.
238. Foo CH, Whitbeck JC, Ponce-de-Leon M, et al. The myristate moiety and amino-terminus of the vaccinia virus L1 constitute a bipartite functional region needed for entry. *J Virol* 2012;86:5437–5451.
239. Franke A, Pfaff F, Jenckel M, et al. Classification of cowpox viruses into several distinct clades and identification of a novel lineage. *Viruses* 2017;9(6):142.
240. Froggatt GC, Smith GL, Beard PM. Vaccinia virus gene F3L encodes an intracellular protein that affects the innate immune response. *J Gen Virol* 2007;88(Pt 7):1917–1921.
241. Funahashi S, Sato T, Shida H. Cloning and characterization of the gene encoding the major protein of the A-type inclusion body of cowpox virus. *J Gen Virol* 1988;69:35–47.
242. Gammon DB, Evans DH. The 3′-to-5′ exonuclease activity of vaccinia virus DNA polymerase is essential and plays a role in promoting virus genetic recombination. *J Virol* 2009;83(9):4236–4250.
243. Gammon DB, Gowrishankar B, Duraffour S, et al. Vaccinia virus-encoded ribonucleotide reductase subunits are differentially required for replication and pathogenesis. *PLoS Pathog* 2010;6(7):e1000984.
244. Ganesh VK, Smith SA, Kotwal GJ, et al. Structure of vaccinia complement protein in complex with heparin and potential implications for complement regulation. *Proc Natl Acad Sci U S A* 2004;101(24):8924–8929.
245. Gao C, Pallett MA, Croll TI, et al. Molecular basis of cullin-3 (Cul3) ubiquitin ligase subversion by vaccinia virus protein A55. *J Biol Chem* 2019;294(16):6416–6429.
246. Gao WND, Carpentier DCJ, Ewles HA, et al. Vaccinia virus proteins A36 and F12/E2 show strong preferences for different kinesin light chain isoforms. *Traffic* 2017;18(8):505–518.
247. Gao Y, Cui Y, Fox T, et al. Structures and operating principles of the replisome. *Science* 2019;363(6429):eaav7003.
248. Garcia AD, Aravind L, Koonin EV, et al. Bacterial-type DNA Holliday junction resolvases in eukaryotic viruses. *Proc Natl Acad Sci U S A* 2000;97(16):8926–8931.
249. Garcia AD, Moss B. Repression of vaccinia virus Holliday junction resolvase inhibits processing of viral DNA into unit-length genomes. *J Virol* 2001;75(14):6460–6471.
250. Garcia AD, Otero J, Lebowitz J, et al. Quaternary structure and cleavage specificity of a poxvirus Holliday junction resolvase. *J Biol Chem* 2006;281(17):11618–11626.
251. Gardner JD, Tscharke DC, Reading PC, et al. Vaccinia virus semaphorin A39R is a 50–55 kDa secreted glycoprotein that affects the outcome of infection in a murine intradermal model. *J Gen Virol* 2001;82(Pt 9):2083–2093.
252. Garriga D, Headey S, Accurso C, et al. Structural basis for the inhibition of poxvirus assembly by the antibiotic rifampicin. *Proc Natl Acad Sci U S A* 2018;115(33):8424–8429.
253. Geada MM, Galindo I, Lorenzo MM, et al. Movements of vaccinia virus intracellular enveloped virions with GFP tagged to the F13L envelope protein. *J Gen Virol* 2001;82(Pt 11):2747–2760.
254. Gedey R, Jin XL, Hinthong O, et al. Poxviral regulation of the host NF-kappa B response: the vaccinia virus M2L protein inhibits induction of NF-kappa B activation via an ERK2 pathway in virus-infected human embryonic kidney cells. *J Virol* 2006;80(17):8676–8685.
255. Georgana I, Sumner RP, Towers GJ, et al. Virulent poxviruses inhibit DNA sensing by preventing STING activation. *J Virol* 2018;92(10):e02145-17.
256. Gershon PD, Ahn BY, Garfield M, et al. Poly(A) polymerase and a dissociable polyadenylation stimulatory factor encoded by vaccinia virus. *Cell* 1991;66(6):1269–1278.
257. Gershon PD, Kitching RP, Hammond JM, et al. Poxvirus genetic recombination during natural virus transmission. *J Gen Virol* 1989;70:485–489.
258. Gershon PD, Moss B. Early transcription factor subunits are encoded by vaccinia virus late genes. *Proc Natl Acad Sci U S A* 1990;87:4401–4405.
259. Gershon PD, Moss B. Stimulation of poly(A) tail elongation by the VP39 subunit of the vaccinia virus-encoded poly(A) polymerase. *J Biol Chem* 1993;268(3):2203–2210.
260. Gershon PD, Moss B. Uridylate-containing RNA sequences determine specificity for binding and polyadenylation by the catalytic subunit of vaccinia virus poly(A) polymerase. *EMBO J* 1993;12(12):4705–4714.
261. Girgis NM, Dehaven BC, Fan X, et al. Cell surface expression of the vaccinia virus complement control protein is mediated by interaction with the viral A56 protein and protects infected cells from complement attack. *J Virol* 2008;82(9):4205–4214.
262. Girgis NM, DeHaven BC, Xiao YH, et al. The vaccinia virus complement control protein modulates adaptive immune responses during infection. *J Virol* 2011;85(6):2547–2556.
263. Gjessing MC, Yutin N, Tengs T, et al. Salmon gill poxvirus, the deepest representative of the chordopoxvirinae. *J Virol* 2015;89(18):9348–9367.
264. Goebel SJ, Johnson GP, Perkus ME, et al. The complete DNA sequence of vaccinia virus. *Virology* 1990;179:247–266; 517–563.
265. Graham KA, Lalani AS, Macen JL, et al. The T1/35kDa family of poxvirus-secreted proteins bind chemokines and modulate leukocyte influx into virus-infected tissues. *Virology* 1997;229:12–24.
266. Graham SC, Bahar MW, Abrescia NGA, et al. Structure of CrmE, a virus-encoded tumour necrosis factor receptor. *J Mol Biol* 2007;372(3):660–671.
267. Graham SC, Bahar MW, Cooray S, et al. Vaccinia virus proteins A52 and B14 share a Bcl-2-like fold but have evolved to inhibit NF-kappa B rather than apoptosis. *PLoS Pathog* 2008;4(8):e1000128.
268. Gray RDM, Albrecht D, Beerli C, et al. Nanoscale polarization of the entry fusion complex of vaccinia virus drives efficient fusion. *Nat Microbiol* 2019;4(10):1636–1644.
269. Greseth MD, Czarnecki MW, Bluma MS, et al. Isolation and characterization of v delta I3 confirm that vaccinia virus SSB plays an essential role in viral replication. *J Virol* 2018;92(2).
270. Grimley PM, Rosenblum EN, Mims SJ, et al. Interruption by rifampin of an early stage in vaccinia virus morphogenesis: accumulation of membranes which are precursors of virus envelopes. *J Virol* 1970;6:519–533.
271. Grimm C, Hillen HS, Bedenk K, et al. Structural basis of poxvirus transcription: vaccinia RNA polymerase complexes. *Cell* 2019;179(7):1537–1550.e19.
272. Grosenbach DW, Honeychurch K, Rose EA, et al. Oral tecovirimat for the treatment of smallpox. *N Engl J Med* 2018;379(1):44–53.
273. Grosenbach DW, Ulaeto DO, Hruby DE. Palmitylation of the vaccinia virus 37-kDa major envelope antigen. Identification of a conserved acceptor motif and biological relevance. *J Biol Chem* 1997;272(3):1956–1964.
274. Gross CH, Shuman S. Vaccinia virions lacking the RNA helicase nucleoside triphosphate hydrolase II are defective in early transcription. *J Virol* 1996;70:8549–8570.
275. Grubisha O, Traktman P. Genetic analysis of the vaccinia virus I6 telomere-binding protein uncovers a key role in genome encapsidation. *J Virol* 2003;77(20):10929–10942.
276. Gruidl ME, Hall RL, Moyer RW. Mapping and molecular characterization of a functional thymidine kinase from Amsacta moorei entomopoxvirus. *Virology* 1992;186:507–516.
277. Guan K, Broyles SS, Dixon JE. A Tyr/Ser protein phosphatase encoded by vaccinia virus. *Nature* 1991;350:359–362.
278. Gubser C, Bergamaschi D, Hollinshead M, et al. A new inhibitor of apoptosis from vaccinia virus and eukaryotes. *PLoS Pathog* 2007;3(2):246–259.
279. Gupta A, Akin D, Bashir R. Single virus particle mass detection using microresonators with nanoscale thickness. *Appl Phys Lett* 2004;84(11):1976–1978.
280. Hagler J, Shuman S. A freeze-frame view of eukaryotic transcription during elongation and capping of nascent mRNA. *Science* 1992;255:983–986.
281. Hagler J, Shuman S. Nascent RNA cleavage by purified ternary complexes of vaccinia RNA polymerase. *J Biol Chem* 1993;268(3):2166–2173.
282. Hagler J, Shuman S. Ternary complex formation by vaccinia virus RNA polymerase at an early viral promoter: analysis by native gel electrophoresis. *J Virol* 1992;66:2982–2989.

283. Hanafusa H, Hanafusa T, Kamahora J. Transformation phenomena in the pox group viruses. II. Transformation between several members of the pox group. *Biken's J* 1959;2:85–91.
284. Harford C, Hamlin A, Riders E. Electron microscopic autoradiography of DNA synthesis in cell infected with vaccinia virus. *Exp Cell Res* 1966;42:50–57.
285. Harris N, Rosales R, Moss B. Transcription initiation factor activity of vaccinia virus capping enzyme is independent of mRNA guanylylation. *Proc Natl Acad Sci U S A* 1993;90:2860–2864.
286. Harrison K, Haga IR, Jowers TP, et al. Vaccinia virus uses retromer-independent cellular retrograde transport pathways to facilitate the wrapping of intracellular mature virions during virus morphogenesis. *J Virol* 2016;90(22):10120–10132.
287. Harte MT, Haga IR, Maloney G, et al. The poxvirus protein A52R targets toll-like receptor signaling complexes to suppress host defense. *J Exp Med* 2003;197(3):343–351.
288. Hedengren-Olcott M, Byrd CM, Watson J, et al. The vaccinia virus G1L putative metalloproteinase is essential for viral replication in vivo. *J Virol* 2004;78(18):9947–9953.
289. Heljasvaara R, Rodriguez D, Risco C, et al. The major core protein P4a (A10L gene) of vaccinia virus is essential for correct assembly of viral DNA into the nucleoprotein complex to form immature viral particles. *J Virol* 2001;75(13):5778–5795.
290. Herrera E, del Mar Lorenzo M, Blasco R, et al. Functional analysis of vaccinia virus B5R protein: essential role in virus envelopment is independent of a large portion of the extracellular domain. *J Virol* 1998;72(1):294–302.
291. Hertig C, Coupar BEH, Boyle DB. Field and vaccine strains of fowlpox virus carry integrated sequences from the avian retrovirus: reticuloendotheliosis virus. *Virology* 1997;235:367–376.
292. Heuser J. Deep-etch EM reveals that the early poxvirus envelope is a single membrane bilayer stabilized by a geodetic "honeycomb" surface coat. *J Cell Biol* 2005;169:269–283.
293. Hillen HS, Bartuli J, Grimm C, et al. Structural basis of poxvirus transcription: transcribing and capping vaccinia complexes. *Cell* 2019;179(7):1525–1536.e12.
294. Hiller G, Weber K. Golgi-derived membranes that contain an acylated viral polypeptide are used for vaccinia virus envelopment. *J Virol* 1985;55:651–659.
295. Hiller G, Weber K, Schneider L, et al. Interaction of assembled progeny pox viruses with the cellular cytoskeleton. *Virology* 1979;98:142–153.
296. Hindman R, Gollnick P. Nucleoside triphosphate phosphohydrolase I (NPH I) functions as a 5′ to 3′ translocase in transcription termination of vaccinia early genes. *J Biol Chem* 2016;291(28):14826–14838.
297. Hinthong O, Jin XL, Shisler JL. Characterization of wild-type and mutant vaccinia virus M2L proteins' abilities to localize to the endoplasmic reticulum and to inhibit NF-kappa B activation during infection. *Virology* 2008;373(2):248–262.
298. Hnatiuk S, Barry M, Zeng W, et al. Role of the C-terminal RDEL motif of the myxoma virus MT-4 protein in terms of apoptosis regulation and viral pathogenesis. *Virology* 1999;263:290–306.
299. Hodel AE, Gershon PD, Shi X, et al. The 1.8 Å structure of vaccinia protein VP39: a bifunctional enzyme that participates in the modification of both mRNA ends. *Cell* 1996;85:247–256.
300. Hollinshead M, Rodger G, Van Eijl H, et al. Vaccinia virus utilizes microtubules for movement to the cell surface. *J Cell Biol* 2001;154(2):389–402.
301. Honeychurch KM, Yang G, Jordan R, et al. The vaccinia virus F13L YPPL motif is required for efficient release of extracellular enveloped virus. *J Virol* 2007;81(13):7310–7315.
302. Howard AR, Senkevich TG, Moss B. Vaccinia virus A26 and A27 proteins form a stable complex tethered to mature virions by association with the A17 transmembrane protein. *J Virol* 2008;82(24):12384–12391.
303. Howard AR, Weisberg AS, Moss B. Congregation of orthopoxvirus virions in cytoplasmic A-type inclusions is mediated by interactions of a bridging protein (A26p) with a matrix protein (ATIp) and a virion membrane-associated protein (A27p). *J Virol* 2010;84(15):7592–7602.
304. Howard ST, Ray CA, Patel DD, et al. A 43-nucleotide RNA cis-acting element governs the site- specific formation of the 3′ end of a poxvirus late mRNA. *Virology* 1999;255(1):190–204.
305. Howell ML, Sanders-Loehr J, Loehr TM, et al. Cloning of the vaccinia virus ribonucleotide reductase small subunit gene. Characterization of the gene product expressed in *Escherichia coli*. *J Biol Chem* 1992;267:1705–1711.
306. Hsiao JC, Chu LW, Lo YT, et al. Intracellular transport of vaccinia virus in HeLa cells requires WASH-VPEF/FAM21-retromer complexes and recycling molecules Rab11 and Rab22. *J Virol* 2015;89(16):8365–8382.
307. Hsiao JC, Chung CS, Chang W. Vaccinia virus envelope D8L protein binds to cell surface chondroitin sulfate and mediates the adsorption of intracellular mature virions to cells. *J Virol* 1999;73(10):8750–8761.
308. Hsiao JC, Chung CS, Drillien R, et al. The cowpox virus host range gene, CP77, affects phosphorylation of eIF2 alpha and vaccinia viral translation in apoptotic HeLa cells. *Virology* 2004;329(1):199–212.
309. Hu F-Q, Smith CA, Pickup DJ. Cowpox virus contains two copies of an early gene encoding a soluble secreted form of the type II TNF receptor. *Virology* 1994;204:343–356.
310. Hu S, Vincenz C, Buller M, et al. A novel family of viral death effector domain-containing molecules that inhibit both CD-95 and tumor necrosis factor receptor-1-induced apoptosis. *J Biol Chem* 1997;272:9621–9624.
311. Hu X, Carroll LJ, Wolffe EJ, et al. *De novo* synthesis of the early transcription factor 70-kDa subunit is required for morphogenesis of vaccinia virions. *J Virol* 1996;70:7669–7677.
312. Hu X, Wolffe EJ, Weisberg AS, et al. Repression of the A8L gene, encoding the early transcription factor 82-kilodalton subunit, inhibits morphogenesis of vaccinia virions. *J Virol* 1998;72:104–112.
313. Huang CY, Lu TY, Bair CH, et al. A novel cellular protein, VPEF, facilitates vaccinia virus penetration into HeLa cells through fluid phase endocytosis. *J Virol* 2008;82(16):7988–7999.
314. Huang JN, Huang Q, Zhou XL, et al. The poxvirus p28 virulence factor is an E3 ubiquitin ligase. *J Biol Chem* 2004;279(52):54110–54116.
315. Huang JY, Smirnov SV, Lewis-Antes A, et al. Inhibition of type I and type III interferons by a secreted glycoprotein from Yaba-like disease virus. *Proc Natl Acad Sci U S A* 2007;104(23):9822–9827.
316. Hubbs AE, Wright CF. The A2L intermediate gene product is required for in vitro transcription from a vaccinia virus late promoter. *J Virol* 1996;70:327–331.
317. Hughes SJ, Johnston LH, Decarlos A, et al. Vaccinia virus encodes an active thymidylate kinase that complements a cdc8 mutant of *Saccharomyces cerevisiae*. *J Biol Chem* 1991;266(30):20103–20109.
318. Husain M, Moss B. Evidence against an essential role of COPII-mediated cargo transport to the endoplasmic reticulum-Golgi intermediate compartment in the formation of the primary membrane of vaccinia virus. *J Virol* 2003;77:11754–11766.
319. Husain M, Weisberg AS, Moss B. Existence of an operative pathway from the endoplasmic reticulum to the immature poxvirus membrane. *Proc Natl Acad Sci U S A* 2006;103(51):19506–19511.
320. Hyun JK, Accurso C, Hijnen M, et al. Membrane remodeling by the double-barrel scaffolding protein of poxvirus. *PLoS Pathog* 2011;7(9):e1002239.
321. Hyun SI, Weisberg A, Moss B. Deletion of the vaccinia virus I2 protein interrupts virion morphogenesis leading to retention of the scaffold protein and mislocalization of membrane-associated entry proteins. *J Virol* 2017;91(15):e00558-17.
322. Ichihashi Y. Extracellular enveloped vaccinia virus escapes neutralization. *Virology* 1996;217:478–485.
323. Ichihashi Y, Dales S. Biogenesis of poxviruses: relationship between a translation complex and formation of A-type inclusions. *Virology* 1973;51(2):297–319.
324. Ichihashi Y, Oie M. The activation of vaccinia virus infectivity by the transfer of phosphatidylserine from the plasma membrane. *Virology* 1983;130:306–317.
325. Imlach W, McCaughan CA, Mercer AA, et al. Orf virus-encoded interleukin-10 stimulates the proliferation of murine mast cells and inhibits cytokine synthesis in murine peritoneal macrophages. *J Gen Virol* 2002;83(Pt 5):1049–1058.
326. Isaacs SN, Kotwal GJ, Moss B. Vaccinia virus complement-control protein prevents antibody-dependent complement-enhanced neutralization of infectivity and contributes to virulence. *Proc Natl Acad Sci U S A* 1992;89:628–632.
327. Isaacs SN, Wolffe EJ, Payne LG, et al. Characterization of a vaccinia virus-encoded 42-kilodalton class I membrane glycoprotein component of the extracellular virus envelope. *J Virol* 1992;66:7217–7224.
328. Ishii K, Moss B. Mapping interaction sites of the A20R protein component of the vaccinia virus DNA replication complex. *Virology* 2002;303:232–239.
329. Iyer LA, Balaji S, Koonin EV, et al. Evolutionary genomics of nucleo-cytoplasmic large DNA viruses. *Virus Res* 2006;117(1):156–184.
330. Iyer LM, Koonin EV, Leipe DD, et al. Origin and evolution of the archaeo-eukaryotic primase superfamily and related palm-domain proteins: structural insights and new members. *Nucleic Acids Res* 2005;33(12):3875–3896.
331. Izmailyan R, Chang W. Vaccinia virus WR53.5/F14.5 protein is a new component of intracellular mature virus and is important for calcium-independent cell adhesion and vaccinia virus virulence in mice. *J Virol* 2008;82(20):10079–10087.
332. Jeshtadi A, Burgos P, Stubbs CD, et al. Interaction of poxvirus intracellular mature virion proteins with the TPR domain of kinesin light chain in live infected cells revealed by two-photon-induced fluorescence resonance energy transfer fluorescence lifetime imaging microscopy. *J Virol* 2010;84(24):12886–12894.
333. Jesus DM, Moussatche N, Condit RC. An improved high pressure freezing and freeze substitution method to preserve the labile vaccinia virus nucleocapsid. *J Struct Biol* 2016;195(1):41–48.
334. Jha S, Rollins MG, Fuchs G, et al. Trans-kingdom mimicry underlies ribosome customization by a poxvirus kinase. *Nature* 2017;546(7660):651–655.
335. Johnston JB, Wang G, Barrett JW, et al. Myxoma virus M-T5 protects infected cells from the stress of cell cycle arrest through its interaction with host cell cullin-1. *J Virol* 2005;79(16):10750–10763.
336. Johnston SC, Ward BM. Vaccinia virus protein F12 associates with intracellular enveloped virions through an interaction with A36. *J Virol* 2009;83(4):1708–1717.
337. Joklik WK. The intracellular uncoating of poxvirus DNA. II. The molecular basis of the uncoating process. *J Mol Biol* 1964;8:277–288.
338. Joklik WK, Becker Y. The replication and coating of vaccinia DNA. *J Mol Biol* 1964;10:452–474.
339. Jordan R, Leeds JM, Tyavanagimatt S, et al. Development of ST-246 for treatment of poxvirus infections. *Viruses* 2010;2(11):2409–2435.
340. Jungwirth C, Launer J. Effects of poxvirus infection on host cell deoxyribonucleic acid synthesis. *Virology* 1968;2:401–408.
341. Kalverda AP, Thompson GS, Vogel A, et al. Poxvirus K7 protein adopts a Bcl-2 fold: biochemical mapping of Its interactions with human DEAD box RNA helicase DDX3. *J Mol Biol* 2009;385(3):843–853.
342. Kane EM, Shuman S. Vaccinia virus morphogenesis is blocked by a temperature sensitive mutation in the I7 gene that encodes a virion component. *J Virol* 1993;67:2689–2698.
343. Kastenmayer RJ, Maruri-Avidal L, Americo JL, et al. Elimination of A-type inclusion formation enhances cowpox virus replication in mice: implications for orthopoxvirus evolution. *Virology* 2014;452:59–66.
344. Kates J, Beeson J. Ribonucleic acid synthesis in vaccinia virus. II. Synthesis of polyriboadenylic acid. *J Mol Biol* 1970;50:19–23.
345. Kato S, Takahashi M, Kameyama S, et al. A study on the morphological and cyto-immunological relationship between the inclusions of variola, cowpox, rabbitpox, vaccinia (variola origin) and vaccinia IHD, and a consideration of the term "Guarnieri body". *Biken's J* 1959;2:353–363.
346. Kato SE, Condit RC, Moussatche N. The vaccinia virus E8R gene product is required for formation of transcriptionally active virions. *Virology* 2007;367(2):398–412.
347. Katsafanas GC, Moss B. Colocalization of transcription and translation within cytoplasmic poxvirus factories coordinates viral expression and subjugates host functions. *Cell Host Microbe* 2007;2(4):221–228.

348. Katsafanas GC, Moss B. Specific anchoring and local translation of poxviral ATI mRNA at cytoplasmic inclusion bodies. *J Virol* 2020;94(4):e01671-19.
349. Katsafanas GC, Moss B. Vaccinia virus intermediate stage transcription is complemented by Ras-GTPase-activating protein SH3 domain-binding protein (G3BP) and cytoplasmic activation/proliferation-associated protein (p137) individually or as a heterodimer. *J Biol Chem* 2004;279(50):52210–55217.
350. Katz E, Moss B. Vaccinia virus structural polypeptide derived from a high-molecular-weight precursor: formation and integration into virus particles. *J Virol* 1970;6(6):717–726.
351. Katz E, Ward BM, Weisberg AS, et al. Mutations in the vaccinia virus A33R and B5R envelope proteins that enhance release of extracellular virions and eliminate formation of actin-containing microvilli without preventing tyrosine phosphorylation of the A36R protein. *J Virol* 2003;77(22):12266–12275.
352. Keck JG, Baldick CJ, Moss B. Role of DNA replication in vaccinia virus gene expression: a naked template is required for transcription of three late transactivator genes. *Cell* 1990;61:801–809.
353. Kerr SM, Johnston LH, Odell M, et al. Vaccinia DNA ligase complements Saccharomyces cerevisiae Cdc9, localizes in cytoplasmic factories and affects virulence and virus sensitivity to DNA damaging agents. *EMBO J* 1991;10(13):4343–4350.
354. Kerr SM, Smith GL. Vaccinia virus DNA ligase is nonessential for virus replication: recovery of plasmids from virus-infected cells. *Virology* 1991;180:625–632.
355. Kettle S, Alcami A, Khanna A, et al. Vaccinia virus serpin B13R (SPI-2) inhibits interleukin-1-b converting enzyme and protects virus-infected cells from TNF- and Fas-mediated apoptosis, but does not prevent IL-1b-induced fever. *J Gen Virol* 1997;78:677–685.
356. Kibler KV, Shors T, Perkins KB, et al. Double-stranded RNA is a trigger for apoptosis in vaccinia virus-infected cells. *J Virol* 1997;71:1992–2003.
357. Kilcher S, Schmidt FI, Schneider C, et al. siRNA screen of early poxvirus genes identifies the AAA+ ATPase D5 as the virus genome-uncoating factor. *Cell Host Microbe* 2014;15(1):103–112.
358. Klemperer N, Ward J, Evans E, et al. The vaccinia virus I1 protein is essential for the assembly of mature virions. *J Virol* 1997;71:9285–9294.
359. Knutson BA, Broyles SS. Expansion of poxvirus RNA polymerase subunits sharing homology with corresponding subunits of RNA polymerase II. *Virus Genes* 2008;36(2):307–311.
360. Knutson BA, Liu X, Oh J, et al. Vaccinia virus intermediate and late promoter elements are targeted by the TATA-binding protein. *J Virol* 2006;80(14):6784–6793.
361. Knutson BA, Oh J, Broyles SS. Downregulation of vaccinia virus intermediate and late promoters by host transcription factor YY1. *J Gen Virol* 2009;90:1592–1599.
362. Kochan G, Escors D, Gonzalez JM, et al. Membrane cell fusion activity of the vaccinia virus A17-A27 protein complex. *Cell Microbiol* 2008;10:1149–1164.
363. Kochneva G, Kolosova I, Maksyutova T, et al. Effects of deletions of kelch-like genes on cowpox virus biological properties. *Arch Virol* 2005;150(9):1857–1870.
364. Koonin EV, Senkevich TG. Fowlpox virus encodes a protein related to human deoxycytidine kinase: further evidence for independent acquisition of genes for enzymes of nucleotide metabolism by different viruses. *Virus Genes* 1993;7(3):289–295.
365. Koonin EV, Senkevich TG, Chernos VI. Gene A32 protein product of vaccinia virus may be an ATPase involved in viral DNA packaging as indicated by sequence comparisons with other putative viral ATPases. *Virus Genes* 1993;7:89–94.
366. Koonin EV, Yutin N. Evolution of the large nucleocytoplasmic DNA viruses of eukaryotes and convergent origins of viral gigantism. *Adv Virus Res* 2019;103:167–202.
367. Kotwal GJ, Isaacs SN, Mckenzie R, et al. Inhibition of the complement cascade by the major secretory protein of vaccinia virus. *Science* 1990;250(4982):827–830.
368. Kotwal GJ, Moss B. Vaccinia virus encodes a secretory polypeptide structurally related to complement control proteins. *Nature* 1988;335:176–178.
369. Kovacs GR, Moss B. The vaccinia virus H5R gene encodes late gene transcription factor 4: purification, cloning and overexpression. *J Virol* 1996;70:6796–6802.
370. Krathwohl MD, Hromas R, Brown DR, et al. Functional characterization of the C-C chemokine-like molecules encoded by molluscum contagiosum virus types 1 and 2. *Proc Natl Acad Sci U S A* 1997;94:9875–9880.
371. Krumm B, Meng XZ, Li YC, et al. Structural basis for antagonism of human interleukin 18 by poxvirus interleukin 18-binding protein. *Proc Natl Acad Sci U S A* 2008;105(52):20711–20715.
372. Krupovic M, Cvirkaite-Krupovic V, Bamford DH. Protein A33 responsible for antibody-resistant spread of vaccinia virus is homologous to C-type lectin-like proteins. *Virus Res* 2010;151(1):97–101.
373. Kvansakul M, Yang H, Fairlie WD, et al. Vaccinia virus anti-apoptotic F1L is a novel Bcl-2-like domain-swapped dimer that binds a highly selective subset of BH3-containing death ligands. *Cell Death Differ* 2008;15(10):1564–1571.
374. Kwon JA, Rich A. Biological function of the vaccinia virus Z-DNA-binding protein E3L: gene transactivation and antiapoptotic activity in HeLa cells. *Proc Natl Acad Sci U S A* 2005;102(36):12759–12764.
375. Kyrieleis OJP, Chang J, de la Pena M, et al. Crystal structure of vaccinia virus mRNA capping enzyme provides insights into the mechanism and evolution of the capping apparatus. *Structure* 2014;22(3):452–465.
376. Lackner CA, Condit RC. Vaccinia virus gene A18R DNA helicase is a transcript release factor. *J Biol Chem* 2000;275(2):1485–1494.
377. Lackner CA, D'Costa SM, Buck C, et al. Complementation analysis of the Dales collection of vaccinia virus temperature-sensitive mutants. *Virology* 2003;305(2):240–259.
378. Lalani AS, Graham K, Mossman K, et al. The purified myxoma virus gamma interferon receptor homolog M-T7 interacts with the heparin-binding domains of chemokines. *J Virol* 1997;71:4356–4363.
379. Lalani AS, Masters J, Zeng W, et al. Use of chemokine receptors by poxviruses. *Science* 1999;286(5446):1968–1971.
380. Laliberte JP, Moss B. Appraising the apoptotic mimicry model and the role of phospholipids for poxvirus entry. *Proc Natl Acad Sci U S A* 2009;106(41):17517–17521.
381. Laliberte JP, Moss B. A novel mode of poxvirus superinfection exclusion that prevents fusion of the lipid bilayers of viral and cellular membranes. *J Virol* 2014;88(17): 9751–9768.
382. Laliberte JP, Weisberg AS, Moss B. The membrane fusion step of vaccinia virus entry is cooperatively mediated by multiple viral proteins and host cell components. *PLoS Pathog* 2011;7(12):e1002446.
383. Langland JO, Jacobs BL. The role of the PKR-inhibitory genes, E3L and K3L, in determining vaccinia virus host range. *Virology* 2002;299(1):133–141.
384. Lanzer W, Holowczak JA. Polyamines in vaccinia virions and polypeptides released from viral cores by acid extraction. *J Virol* 1975;16(5):1254–1264.
385. Lateef Z, Baird MA, Wise LM, et al. The chemokine-binding protein encoded by the poxvirus orf virus inhibits recruitment of dendritic cells to sites of skin inflammation and migration to peripheral lymph nodes. *Cell Microbiol* 2010;12(5):665–676.
386. Latner DR, Xiang Y, Lewis JI, et al. The vaccinia virus bifunctional gene J3 (nucleoside-2′-O-)- methyltransferase and poly(A) polymerase stimulatory factor is implicated as a positive transcription elongation factor by two genetic approaches. *Virology* 2000;269(2):345–355.
387. Law M, Carter GC, Roberts KL, et al. Ligand-induced and non-fusogenic dissolution of a viral membrane. *Proc Natl Acad Sci U S A* 2006;103:5989–5994.
388. Lee SB, Esteban M. The interferon-induced double-stranded RNA-activated protein kinase induces apoptosis. *Virology* 1994;199:491–496.
389. Leite F, Way M. The role of signalling and the cytoskeleton during vaccinia virus egress. *Virus Res* 2015;209:87–99.
390. Leite FGG, Bergthaler A, Skern T. Vaccinia virus G1 protein: absence of autocatalytic self-processing. *Arch Virol* 2017;162(9):2803–2808.
391. Li FY, Jeffrey PD, Yu JW, et al. Crystal structure of a viral FLIP—insights into FLIP-mediated inhibition of death receptor signaling. *J Biol Chem* 2006;281(5):2960–2968.
392. Li J, Broyles SS. The DNA-dependent ATPase activity of vaccinia virus early gene transcription factor is essential for its transcription activation function. *J Biol Chem* 1993;268(27): 20016–20021.
393. Li YC, Meng XZ, Xiang Y, et al. Structure function studies of vaccinia virus host range protein K1 reveal a novel functional surface for ankyrin repeat proteins. *J Virol* 2010;84(7):3331–3338.
394. Likos AM, Sammons SA, Olson VA, et al. A tale of two clades: monkeypox viruses. *J Gen Virol* 2005;86:2661–2672.
395. Lin CL, Chung CS, Heine HG, et al. Vaccinia virus envelope H3L protein binds to cell surface heparan sulfate and is important for intracellular mature virion morphogenesis and virus infection in vitro and in vivo. *J Virol* 2000;74(7):3353–3365.
396. Lin S, Broyles SS. Vaccinia protein kinase 2: a second essential serine/threonine protein kinase encoded by vaccinia virus. *Proc Natl Acad Sci U S A* 1994;91:7653–7657.
397. Lin S, Chen W, Broyles SS. The vaccinia virus B1R gene product is a serine/threonine protein kinase. *J Virol* 1992;66:2717–2723.
398. Lin YCJ, Evans DH. Vaccinia virus particles mix inefficiently, and in a way that would restrict viral recombination, in coinfected cells. *J Virol* 2010;84(5):2432–2443.
399. Lin YZ, Ke XH, Tam JP. Synthesis and structure-activity study of myxoma virus growth factor. *Biochemistry* 1991;30(13):3310–3314.
400. Liszewski MK, Bertram P, Leung MK, et al. Smallpox inhibitor of complement enzymes (SPICE): regulation of complement activation on cells and mechanism of its cellular attachment. *J Immunol* 2008;181(6):4199–4207.
401. Liszewski MK, Leung MK, Hauhart R, et al. Structure and regulatory profile of the monkeypox inhibitor of complement: comparison to homologs in vaccinia and variola and evidence for dimer formation. *J Immunol* 2006;176(6):3725–3734.
402. Liu B, Panda D, Mendez-Rios JD, et al. Identification of poxvirus genome uncoating and DNA replication factors with mutually redundant roles. *J Virol* 2018;92(7):e02152-17.
403. Liu H, Juo ZS, Shim AH, et al. Structural basis of semaphorin-plexin recognition and viral mimicry from Sema7A and A39R complexes with PlexinC1. *Cell* 2010;142(5):749–761.
404. Liu J, McFadden G. SAMD9 is an innate antiviral host factor with stress response properties that can be antagonized by poxviruses. *J Virol* 2015;89(3):1925–1931.
405. Liu J, Wennier S, Zhang LL, et al. M062 is a host range factor essential for myxoma virus pathogenesis and functions as an antagonist of host SAMD9 in human cells. *J Virol* 2011;85(7):3270–3282.
406. Liu K, Lemon B, Traktman P. The dual-specificity phosphatase encoded by vaccinia virus, VH1, is essential for viral transcription in vivo and in vitro. *J Virol* 1995;69:7823–7834.
407. Liu R, Mendez-Rios JD, Peng C, et al. SPI-1 is a missing host-range factor required for replication of the attenuated modified vaccinia Ankara (MVA) vaccine vector in human cells. *PLoS Pathog* 2019;15(5):e1007710.
408. Liu R, Moss B. Opposing roles of double-stranded RNA effector pathways and viral defense proteins revealed with CRISPR/Cas9 knock-out cell lines and vaccinia virus mutants. *J Virol* 2016;90(17):7864–7879.
409. Liu R, Moss B. Vaccinia virus C9 ankyrin repeat/F-Box protein is a newly identified antagonist of the type I interferon-induced antiviral state. *J Virol* 2018;92(9):e00053-18.
410. Liu R, Olano LR, Mirzakhanyan Y, et al. Vaccinia virus ankyrin-repeat/F-Box protein targets interferon-induced IFITs for proteasomal degradation. *Cell Rep* 2019;29(4):816–828.e8.
411. Liu SW, Katsafanas GC, Liu R, et al. Poxvirus decapping enzymes enhance virulence by preventing the accumulation of dsRNA and the induction of innate antiviral responses. *Cell Host Microbe* 2015;17(3):320–331.
412. Locker JK, Griffiths G. An unconventional role for cytoplasmic disulfide bonds in vaccinia virus proteins. *J Cell Biol* 1999;144(2):267–279.
413. Loparev VN, Parsons JM, Knight JC, et al. A third distinct tumor necrosis factor receptor of orthopoxviruses. *Proc Natl Acad Sci U S A* 1998;95(7):3786–3791.
414. Lu Y, Stuart JH, Talbot-Cooper C, et al. Histone deacetylase 4 promotes type I interferon signaling, restricts DNA viruses, and is degraded via vaccinia virus protein C6. *Proc Natl Acad Sci U S A* 2019;116(24):11997–12006.
415. Luo Y, Shuman S. Antitermination of vaccinia virus early transcription: possible role of RNA secondary structure. *Virology* 1991;185:432–436.
416. Luttichau HR, Stine J, Boesen TP, et al. A highly selective CC chemokine receptor (CCR)8 antagonist encoded by the poxvirus molluscum contagiosum. *J Exp Med* 2000;191(1):171–179.
417. Lyles DS, Randall CC, Gafford LG, et al. Cellular fatty acids during fowlpox virus infection of three different host systems. *Virology* 1976;70:227–229.

418. Lynch HE, Ray CA, Oie KL, et al. Modified vaccinia virus Ankara can activate NF-kappaB transcription factors through a double-stranded RNA-activated protein kinase (PKR)-dependent pathway during the early phase of virus replication. *Virology* 2009;391(2):177–186.
419. Lytvyn V, Fortin Y, Banville M, et al. Comparison of the thymidine kinase genes from 3 entomopoxviruses. *J Gen Virol* 1992;73(Pt 12):3235–3240.
420. Macen J, Takahashi A, Moon KB, et al. Activation of caspases in pig kidney cells infected with wild-type and crmA/SPI-2 mutants of cowpox and rabbitpox viruses. *J Virol* 1998;72:3524–3533.
421. Mahr A, Roberts BE. Arrangement of late RNAs transcribed from a 7.1 kilobase *Eco R1* vaccinia virus DNA fragment. *J Virol* 1984;49:510–520.
422. Mallardo M, Schleich S, Krijnse-Locker J. Microtubule-dependent organization of vaccinia virus core-derived early mRNAs into distinct cytoplasmic structures. *Mol Biol Cell* 2001;12(12):3875–3891.
423. Mann BA, Huang JH, Li P, et al. Vaccinia virus blocks Stat1-dependent and Stat1-independent gene expression induced by type I and type II interferons. *J Interferon Cytokine Res* 2008;28(6):367–380.
424. Mansouri M, Bartee E, Gouveia K, et al. The PHD/LAP-domain protein M153R of myxomavirus is a ubiquitin ligase that induces the rapid internalization and lysosomal destruction of CD4. *J Virol* 2003;77(2):1427–1440.
425. Mansur DS, Maluquer de Motes C, Unterholzner L, et al. Poxvirus targeting of E3 ligase beta-TrCP by molecular mechanism to inhibit NF-kappa B activation and promote immune and virulence. *PLoS Pathog* 2013;9(2):e1003183.
426. Marq JB, Hausmann S, Luban J, et al. The double-stranded RNA binding domain of the vaccinia virus E3L protein inhibits both RNA- and DNA-induced activation of interferon beta. *J Biol Chem* 2009;284(38):25471–25478.
427. Marsh YV, Eppstein DA. Vaccinia virus and the EGF receptor: a portal of entry for infectivity? *J Cell Biochem* 1987;34:239–245.
428. Martin SA, Moss B. Modification of RNA by mRNA guanylyltransferase and mRNA (guanine-7-)methyl-transferase from vaccinia virions. *J Biol Chem* 1975;250:9330–9335.
429. Martin SA, Moss B. mRNA guanylyltransferase and mRNA (guanine-7)methyltransferase from vaccinia virions. Donor and acceptor substrate activities. *J Biol Chem* 1976;251:7313–7321.
430. Martin SA, Paoletti E, Moss B. Purification of mRNA guanylyltransferase and mRNA (guanine 7-)methyltransferase from vaccinia virus. *J Biol Chem* 1975;250:9322–9329.
431. Maruri-Avidal L, Weisberg AS, Bisht H, et al. Analysis of viral membranes formed in cells infected by a vaccinia virus L2-deletion mutant suggests their origin from the endoplasmic reticulum. *J Virol* 2013;87(3):1861–1871.
432. Maruri-Avidal L, Weisberg AS, Moss B. Association of the vaccinia virus A11 protein with the endoplasmic reticulum and crescent precursors of immature virions. *J Virol* 2013;87:10195–11206.
433. Maruri-Avidal L, Weisberg AS, Moss B. Direct formation of vaccinia virus membranes from the endoplasmic reticulum in the absence of the newly characterized L2-interacting protein A30.5. *J Virol* 2013;87:12313–12326.
434. Mastrangelo MJ, Eisenlohr LC, Gomella L, et al. Poxvirus vectors: orphaned and underappreciated. *J Clin Invest* 2000;105(8):1031–1034.
435. Matho MH, Maybeno M, Benhnia MRE, et al. Structural and biochemical characterization of the vaccinia virus envelope protein D8 and its recognition by the antibody LA5. *J Virol* 2012;86(15):8050–8058.
436. Mazzon M, Castro C, Roberts LD, et al. A role for vaccinia virus protein C16 in reprogramming cellular energy metabolism. *J Gen Virol* 2015;96:395–407.
437. Mazzon M, Peters NE, Loenarz C, et al. A mechanism for induction of a hypoxic response by vaccinia. *Proc Natl Acad Sci U S A* 2013;110(30):12444–12449.
438. Mbuy GN, Morris RE, Bubel HC. Inhibition of cellular protein synthesis by vaccinia virus surface tubules. *Virology* 1982;116(1):137–147.
439. McCart JA, Ward JM, Lee J, et al. Systemic cancer therapy with a tumor selective vaccinia virus mutant lacking thymidine kinase and vaccinia growth factor. *Cancer Res* 2001;61:8751–8757.
440. McCraith S, Holtzman T, Moss B, et al. Genome-wide analysis of vaccinia virus protein-protein interactions. *Proc Natl Acad Sci U S A* 2000;97:4879–4884.
441. McFadden G. Poxvirus tropism. *Nat Rev Microbiol* 2005;3(3):201–213.
442. McFadden G, Dales S. Biogenesis of poxviruses: mirror image deletions in vaccinia virus DNA. *Cell* 1979;18:101–108.
443. McFadden G, Stuart D, Upton C, et al. Replication and resolution of poxvirus telomeres. *Cancer Cells* 1988;6:77–85.
444. McKelvey TA, Andrews SC, Miller SE, et al. Identification of the orthopoxvirus p4c gene, which encodes a structural protein that directs intracellular mature virus particles into A-type inclusions. *J Virol* 2002;76(22):11216–11225.
445. McKenzie R, Kotwal GJ, Moss B, et al. Regulation of complement activity by vaccinia virus complement-control protein. *J Infect Dis* 1992;166(6):1245–1250.
446. McNulty S, Powell K, Erneux C, et al. The host phosphoinositide 5-phosphatase SHIP2 regulates dissemination of vaccinia virus. *J Virol* 2011;85(14):7402–7410.
447. Meade N, DiGiuseppe S, Walsh D. Translational control during poxvirus infection. *Wiley Interdiscip Rev RNA* 2019;10(2):e1515.
448. Meng XZ, Chao J, Xiang Y. Identification from diverse mammalian poxviruses of host-range regulatory genes functioning equivalently to vaccinia virus C7L. *Virology* 2008;372(2):372–383.
449. Meng XZ, Embry A, Sochia D, et al. Vaccinia virus A6L encodes a virion core protein required for formation of mature virion. *J Virol* 2007;81(3):1433–1443.
450. Meng XZ, Krumm B, Li YC, et al. Structural basis for antagonizing a host restriction factor by C7 family of poxvirus host-range proteins. *Proc Natl Acad Sci U S A* 2015;112(48):14858–14863.
451. Meng XZ, Leman M, Xiang Y. Variola virus IL-18 binding protein interacts with three human IL-18 residues that are part of a binding site for human IL-18 receptor alpha subunit. *Virology* 2007;358(1):211–220.
452. Meng XZ, Zhang FS, Yan B, et al. A paralogous pair of mammalian host restriction factors form a critical host barrier against poxvirus infection. *PLoS Pathog* 2018;14(2):e1006884.
453. Mercer J, Helenius A. Vaccinia virus uses macropinocytosis and apoptotic mimicry to enter host cells. *Science* 2008;320(5875):531–535.
454. Mercer J, Snijder B, Sacher R, et al. RNAi screening reveals proteasome- and cullin3-dependent stages in vaccinia virus infection. *Cell Rep* 2012;2(4):1036–1047.
455. Mercer J, Traktman P. Genetic and cell biological characterization of the vaccinia virus A30 and G7 phosphoproteins. *J Virol* 2005;79(11):7146–7161.
456. Merchlinsky M. Intramolecular homologous recombination in cells infected with temperature-sensitive mutants of vaccinia virus. *J Virol* 1989;63:2030–2035.
457. Merchlinsky M, Garon C, Moss B. Molecular cloning and sequence of the concatemer junction from vaccinia virus replicative DNA: viral nuclease cleavage sites in cruciform structures. *J Mol Biol* 1988;199:399–413.
458. Merchlinsky M, Moss B. Nucleotide sequence required for resolution of the concatemer junction of vaccinia virus DNA. *J Virol* 1989;63:4354–4361.
459. Merchlinsky M, Moss B. Resolution of vaccinia virus DNA concatemer junctions requires late gene expression. *J Virol* 1989;63:1595–1603.
460. Merchlinsky M, Moss B. Sequence-independent replication and sequence-specific resolution of plasmids containing the vaccinia virus concatemer junction: requirements for early and late trans-acting factors. In: Kelly T, Stillman B, eds. *Cancer Cells 6/Eukaryotic DNA Replication*. Cold Spring Harbor, NY: Cold Spring Harbor Laboratory; 1988:87–93.
461. Meyer RK, Burger MM, Tschannen R, et al. Actin filament bundles in vaccinia virus infected fibroblasts. *Arch Virol* 1981;67(1):11–18.
462. Mirzakhanyan Y, Gershon P. The Vaccinia virion: filling the gap between atomic and ultrastructure. *PLoS Pathog* 2019;15(1):e1007508.
463. Miura M, Friedlander RM, Yuan J. Tumor necrosis factor-induced apoptosis is mediated by a CrmA-sensitive cell death pathway. *Proc Natl Acad Sci U S A* 1995;92(18):8318–8322.
464. Moerdyk MJ, Byrd CM, Hruby DE. Analysis of vaccinia virus temperature-sensitive I7L mutants reveals two potential functional domains. *Virol J* 2006;3:64.
465. Mohamed MR, McFadden G. NF kappa B inhibitors strategies from poxviruses. *Cell Cycle* 2009;8(19):3125–3132.
466. Mohamed MR, Niles EG. Interaction between nucleoside triphosphate phosphohydrolase I and the H4L subunit of the viral RNA polymerase is required for vaccinia virus early gene transcript release. *J Biol Chem* 2000;275(33):25798–25804.
467. Mohamed MR, Rahman MM, Lanchbury JS, et al. Proteomic screening of variola virus reveals a unique NF-kappa B inhibitor that is highly conserved among pathogenic orthopoxviruses. *Proc Natl Acad Sci U S A* 2009;106(22):9045–9050.
468. Montanuy I, Alejo A, Alcami A. Glycosaminoglycans mediate retention of the poxvirus type I interferon binding protein at the cell surface to locally block interferon antiviral responses. *FASEB J* 2011;25(6):1960–1971.
469. Monticelli SR, Earley AK, Tate J, et al. The ectodomain of the vaccinia virus glycoprotein A34 is required for cell binding by extracellular virions and contains a large region capable of interaction with glycoprotein B5. *J Virol* 2019;93(4):e01343-18.
470. Moon KB, Turner PC, Moyer RW. SPI-1-Dependent host range of rabbitpox virus and complex formation with cathepsin G is associated with serpin motifs. *J Virol* 1999;73(11):8999–9010.
471. Morales I, Carbajal MA, Bohn S, et al. The vaccinia virus F11L gene product facilitates cell detachment and promotes migration. *Traffic* 2008;9(8):1283–1298.
472. Morgan C. The insertion of DNA into vaccinia virus. *Science* 1976;193:591—592.
473. Morgan JR, Cohen LK, Roberts BE. Identification of the DNA sequences encoding the large subunit of the mRNA capping enzyme of vaccinia virus. *J Virol* 1984;52:206–214.
474. Moss B. Genetically engineered poxviruses for recombinant gene expression, vaccination, and safety. *Proc Natl Acad Sci U S A* 1996;93:11341–11348.
475. Moss B. Inhibition of HeLa cell protein synthesis by the vaccinia virion. *J Virol* 1968;2(10):1028–1037.
476. Moss B. Membrane fusion during poxvirus entry. *Semin Cell Dev Biol* 2016;60:89–96.
477. Moss B. Origin of the poxviral membrane: a 50-year-old riddle. *PLoS Pathog* 2018;14(6):e1007002.
478. Moss B. Poxvirus cell entry: how many proteins does it take? *Viruses* 2012;4(5):688–707.
479. Moss B. Smallpox vaccines: targets of protective immunity. *Immunol Rev* 2011;239(1):8–26.
480. Moss B. Vaccinia virus: a tool for research and vaccine development. *Science* 1991;252:1662–1667.
481. Moss B, Rosenblum EN. Protein cleavage and poxvirus morphogenesis: tryptic peptide analysis of core precursors accumulated by blocking assembly with rifampicin. *J Mol Biol* 1973;81:267–269.
482. Moss B, Rosenblum EN, Katz E, et al. Rifampicin: a specific inhibitor of vaccinia virus assembly. *Nature* 1969;224:1280–1284.
483. Moss B, Rosenblum EN, Paoletti E. Polyadenylate polymerase from vaccinia virions. *Nat New Biol* 1973;245:59–63.
484. Moss B, Salzman NP. Sequential protein synthesis following vaccinia virus infection. *J Virol* 1968;2:1016–1027.
485. Moss B, Winters E, Jones EV. Replication of vaccinia virus. In: Cozzarelli N, ed. *Mechanics of DNA Replication and Recombination*. New York: A. Liss; 1983:449–461.
486. Mossman K, Lee SF, Barry M, et al. Disruption of M-T5, a novel myxoma virus gene member of the poxvirus host range superfamily, results in dramatic attenuation of myxomatosis in infected European rabbits. *J Virol* 1996;70:4394–4410.
487. Mossman K, Nation P, Macen J, et al. Myxoma virus M-T7, a secreted homolog of the interferon-g receptor, is a critical virulence factor for the development of myxomatosis in European rabbits. *Virology* 1996;215:17–30.
488. Mossman K, Upton C, Buller RM, et al. Species specificity of ectromelia virus and vaccinia virus interferon-gamma binding proteins. *Virology* 1995;208(2):762–769.
489. Moure CM, Bowman BR, Gershon PD, et al. Crystal structures of the vaccinia virus polyadenylate polymerase heterodimer: insights into ATP selectivity and processivity. *Mol Cell* 2006;22(3):339–349.

490. Moussatche N, Condit RC. Fine structure of the vaccinia virion determined by controlled degradation and immunolocalization. *Virology* 2015;475:204–218.
491. Moutaftsi M, Tscharke DC, Vaughan K, et al. Uncovering the interplay between CD8, CD4 and antibody responses to complex pathogens. *Future Microbiol* 2010;5(2):221–239.
492. Moyer RW, Graves RL. The mechanism of cytoplasmic orthopoxvirus DNA replication. *Cell* 1981;27:391–401.
493. Moyer RW, Graves RL, Rothe CT. The white pock (μ) mutants of rabbit poxvirus. III. The terminal DNA sequence duplication and transposition in rabbit poxvirus. *Cell* 1980;22:545–553.
494. Murao LE, Shisler JL. The MCV MC159 protein inhibits late, but not early, events of TNF-alpha-induced NF-kappa B activation. *Virology* 2005;340(2):255–264.
495. Muthukrishnan S, Moss B, Cooper JA, et al. Influence of 5′ terminal cap structure on the initiation of translation of vaccinia virus mRNA. *J Biol Chem* 1978;253:1710–1715.
496. Myskiw C, Arsenio J, van Bruggen R, et al. Vaccinia virus E3 suppresses expression of diverse cytokines through inhibition of the PKR, NF-kappa B, and IRF3 pathways. *J Virol* 2009;83(13):6757–6768.
497. Nagayama A, Pogo BGT, Dales S. Biogenesis of vaccinia: separation of early stages from maturation by means of rifampicin. *Virology* 1970;40:1039–1051.
498. Najarro P, Gubser C, Hollinshead M, et al. Yaba-like disease virus chemokine receptor 7L, a CCR8 orthologue. *J Gen Virol* 2006;87:809–816.
499. Najarro P, Lee HJ, Fox J, et al. Yaba-like disease virus protein 7L is a cell-surface receptor for chemokine CCL1. *J Gen Virol* 2003;84:3325–3336.
500. Najarro P, Traktman P, Lewis JA. Vaccinia virus blocks gamma interferon signal transduction: viral VH1 phosphatase reverses Stat1 activation. *J Virol* 2001;75(7):3185–3196.
501. Nalcacioglu R, Dizman YA, Vlak JM, et al. Amsacta moorei entomopoxvirus encodes a functional DNA photolyase (AMV025). *J Invertebr Pathol* 2010;105(3):363–365.
502. Nazarian SH, Rahman MM, Werden SJ, et al. Yaba monkey tumor virus encodes a functional inhibitor of interleukin-18. *J Virol* 2008;82(1):522–528.
503. Neidel S, Maluquer de Motes C, Mansur DS, et al. Vaccinia virus protein A49 is an unexpected member of the B-cell lymphoma (Bcl)-2 protein family. *J Biol Chem* 2015;290(10):5991–6002.
504. Neidel S, Ren HW, Torres AA, et al. NF-kappa B activation is a turn on for vaccinia virus phosphoprotein A49 to turn off NF-kappa B activation. *Proc Natl Acad Sci U S A* 2019;116(12):5699–5704.
505. Nerenberg BTH, Taylor J, Bartee E, et al. The poxviral RING protein p28 is a ubiquitin ligase that targets ubiquitin to viral replication factories. *J Virol* 2005;79(1):597–601.
506. Ng A, Tscharke DC, Reading PC, et al. The vaccinia virus A41L protein is a soluble 30 kDa glycoprotein that affects virus virulence. *J Gen Virol* 2001;82(Pt 9):2095–2105.
507. Ngo T, Mirzakhanyan Y, Moussatche N, et al. Protein primary structure of the vaccinia virion at increased resolution. *J Virol* 2016;90(21):9905–9919.
508. Nichols DB, Shisler JL. Poxvirus MC160 protein utilizes multiple mechanisms to inhibit NF-kappa B activation mediated via components of the tumor necrosis factor receptor 1 signal transduction pathway. *J Virol* 2009;83(7):3162–3174.
509. Nichols RJ, Stanitsa E, Unger B, et al. The vaccinia I2L gene encodes a membrane protein with an essential role in virion entry. *J Virol* 2008;82(20):10247–10261.
510. Niles EG, Lee-Chen G-J, Shuman S, et al. Vaccinia virus gene D12L encodes the small subunit of the viral mRNA capping enzyme. *Virology* 1989;172:513–522.
511. Niven JSF, Armstrong JA, Andrewes CH, et al. Subcutaneous "growths" in monkeys produced by a poxvirus. *J Pathol Bacteriol* 1961;81:1–10.
512. Nuara AA, Walter LJ, Logsdon NJ, et al. Structure and mechanism of IFN-gamma antagonism by an orthopoxvirus IFN-gamma-binding protein. *Proc Natl Acad Sci U S A* 2008;105(6):1861–1866.
513. Oda K, Joklik WK. Hybridization and sedimentation studies on "early" and "late" vaccinia messenger RNA. *J Mol Biol* 1967;27:395–419.
514. Odon V, Georgana I, Holley J, et al. Novel class of viral ankyrin proteins targeting the host E3 ubiquitin ligase cullin-2. *J Virol* 2018;92(23):e01374-18.
515. Oie KL, Pickup DJ. Cowpox virus and other members of the orthopoxvirus genus interfere with the regulation of nf-kappa b activation. *Virology* 2001:288(1):175–187.
516. Ojeda S, Domi A, Moss B. Vaccinia virus G9 protein is an essential component of the poxvirus entry-fusion complex. *J Virol* 2006;80(19):9822–9830.
517. Ojeda S, Senkevich TG, Moss B. Entry of vaccinia virus and cell-cell fusion require a highly conserved cysteine-rich membrane protein encoded by the A16L gene. *J Virol* 2006;80:51–61.
518. Olson AT, Rico AB, Wang ZG, et al. Deletion of the vaccinia virus B1 kinase reveals essential functions of this enzyme complemented partly by the homologous cellular kinase VRK2. *J Virol* 2017;91(15):e00635-17.
519. Opgenorth A, Strayer D, Upton C, et al. Deletion of the growth factor gene related to EGF and TGF-alpha reduces virulence of malignant rabbit fibroma virus. *Virology* 1992;186(1):175–191.
520. Palaniyar N, Gerasimopoulos E, Evans DH. Shops fibroma virus DNA topoisomerase catalyses Holliday junction resolution and hairpin formation in vitro. *J Mol Biol* 1999;287(1):9–20.
521. Pallett MA, Ren H, Zhang RY, et al. Vaccinia virus BBK E3 ligase adaptor A55 targets importin-dependent NF-kappaB activation and inhibits CD8(+) T-cell memory. *J Virol* 2019;93(10).
522. Panda D, Fernandez DJ, Lal M, et al. Triad of human cellular proteins, IRF2, FAM111A, and RFC3, restrict replication of orthopoxvirus SPI-1 host-range mutants. *Proc Natl Acad Sci U S A* 2017;114(14):3720–3725.
523. Pant A, Cao S, Yang Z. Asparagine is a critical limiting metabolite for vaccinia virus protein synthesis during glutamine deprivation. *J Virol* 2019;93(13).
524. Panus JF, Smith CA, Ray CA, et al. Cowpox virus encodes a fifth member of the tumor necrosis factor receptor family: a soluble, secreted CD30 homologue. *Proc Natl Acad Sci U S A* 2002;99(12):8348–8353.
525. Paoletti E, Grady LJ. Transcriptional complexity of vaccinia virus in vivo and in vitro. *J Virol* 1977;23:608–615.
526. Paoletti E, Moss B. Two nucleic acid-dependent nucleoside triphosphate phosphohydrolases from vaccinia virus. Nucleotide substrate and polynucleotide cofactor specificities. *J Biol Chem* 1974;249:3281–3286.
527. Paran N, De Silva FS, Senkevich TG, et al. Cellular DNA ligase I is recruited to cytoplasmic vaccinia virus factories and masks the role of the vaccinia ligase in viral DNA replication. *Cell Host Microbe* 2009;6(6):563–569.
528. Parker AK, Parker S, Yokoyama WM, et al. Induction of natural killer cell responses by ectromelia virus controls infection. *J Virol* 2007;81(8):4070–40799.
529. Parks RJ, Evans DH. Effect of marker distance and orientation on recombinant formation in poxvirus-infected cells. *J Virol* 1991;65:1263–1272.
530. Shors T, Keck, JG, Moss B, Down regulation of gene expression by the vaccinia virus D10 protein. *J Virol* 1999;73:791–796.
531. Parrish S, Moss B. Characterization of a second vaccinia virus mRNA-decapping enzyme conserved in poxviruses. *J Virol* 2007;81(23):12973–12978.
532. Parrish S, Moss B. Characterization of a vaccinia virus mutant with a deletion of the D10R gene encoding a putative negative regulator of gene expression. *J Virol* 2006;80(2):553–561.
533. Parrish S, Resch W, Moss B. Vaccinia virus D10 protein has mRNA decapping activity, providing a mechanism for control of host and viral gene expression. *Proc Natl Acad Sci U S A* 2007;104:2139–2144.
534. Passarelli AL, Kovacs GR, Moss B. Transcription of a vaccinia virus late promoter template: requirement for the product of the A2L intermediate-stage gene. *J Virol* 1996;70:4444–4450.
535. Patel DD, Pickup DJ. Messenger RNAs of a strongly-expressed late gene of cowpox virus contains a 5′-terminal poly(A) leader. *EMBO J* 1987;6:3787–3794.
536. Patel DD, Pickup DJ, Joklik WK. Isolation of cowpox virus A-type inclusions and characterization of their major protein component. *Virology* 1986;149:174–189.
537. Pathak PK, Peng SX, Meng XZ, et al. Structure of a lipid-bound viral membrane assembly protein reveals a modality for enclosing the lipid bilayer. *Proc Natl Acad Sci U S A* 2018;115(27):7028–7032.
538. Payne LG. Identification of the vaccinia hemagglutinin polypeptide from a cell system yielding large amounts of extracellular enveloped virus. *J Virol* 1979;31:147–155.
539. Payne LG. Significance of extracellular virus in the in vitro and in vivo dissemination of vaccinia virus. *J Gen Virol* 1980;50:89–100.
540. Payne LG, Kristenson K. Mechanism of vaccinia virus release and its specific inhibition by N_1-isonicatinoyl-N_2-3-methyl-4-chlorobenzoylhydrazine. *J Virol* 1979;32:614–622.
541. Pedersen K, Snijder EJ, Schleich S, et al. Characterization of vaccinia virus intracellular cores: implications for viral uncoating and core structure. *J Virol* 2000;74(8):3525–3536.
542. Pedley S, Cooper RJ. The inhibition of HeLa cell RNA synthesis following infection with vaccinia virus. *J Gen Virol* 1984;65:1687–1697.
543. Peng C, Moss B. Repair of a previously uncharacterized second host-range gene contributes to full replication of modified vaccinia virus Ankara (MVA) in human cells. *Proc Natl Acad Sci U S A* 2020;117(7):3759–3767.
544. Pennington TH, Follett EA. Vaccinia virus replication in enucleated BSC-1 cells: particle production and synthesis of viral DNA and proteins. *J Virol* 1974;13:488–493.
545. Perkus ME, Goebel SJ, Davis SW, et al. Vaccinia virus host range genes. *Virology* 1990;179:276–286.
546. Perkus ME, Goebel SJ, Davis SW, et al. Deletion of 55 open reading frames from the termini of vaccinia virus. *Virology* 1991;180:406–410.
547. Person-Fernandez A, Beaud G. Purification and characterization of a protein synthesis inhibitor associated with vaccinia virus. *J Biol Chem* 1986;261:8283–8289.
548. Peters D, Müller G. The fine structure of the DNA containing core of vaccinia virus. *Virology* 1963;21:266–269.
549. Peters NE, Ferguson BJ, Mazzon M, et al. A mechanism for the inhibition of DNA-PK-mediated DNA sensing by a virus. *PLoS Pathog* 2013;9(10):e1003649.
550. Piacente SC, Christen LA, Mohamed MR, et al. Effect of selected mutations in the C-terminal region of the vaccinia virus nucleoside triphosphate phosphohydrolase I on binding to the H4L subunit of the viral RNA polymerase and early gene transcription termination in vitro. *Virology* 2003;310(1):109–117.
551. Ploubidou A, Moreau V, Ashman K, et al. Vaccinia virus infection disrupts microtubule organization and centrosome function. *EMBO J* 2000;19(15):3932–3944.
552. Pogo BGT, O'Shea M, Freimuth P. Initiation and termination of vaccinia virus DNA replication. *Virology* 1981;108:241–248.
553. Pogo BGT, O'Shea MT. The mode of replication of vaccinia virus DNA. *Virology* 1978;84:1–8.
554. Pontejo SM, Alejo A, Alcami A. Comparative biochemical and functional analysis of viral and human secreted tumor necrosis factor (TNF) decoy receptors. *J Biol Chem* 2015;290(26):15973–15984.
555. Pontejo SM, Alejo A, Alcami A. Poxvirus-encoded TNF decoy receptors inhibit the biological activity of transmembrane TNF. *J Gen Virol* 2015;96(10):3118–3123.
556. Pontejo SM, Sanchez C, Ruiz-Arguello B, et al. Insights into ligand binding by a viral tumor necrosis factor (TNF) decoy receptor yield a selective soluble human type 2 TNF receptor. *J Biol Chem* 2019;294(13):5214–5227.
557. Postigo A, Cross JR, Downward J, et al. Interaction of F1L with the BH3 domain of Bak is responsible for inhibiting vaccinia-induced apoptosis. *Cell Death Differ* 2006;13(10):1651–1662.
558. Postigo A, Ramsden AE, Howell M, et al. Cytoplasmic ATR activation promotes vaccinia virus genome replication. *Cell Rep* 2017;19(5):1022–1032.
559. Postlethwaite R. Molluscum contagiosum. A review. *Arch Environ Health* 1970;21:432–452.
560. Prescott DM, Kates J, Kirkpatrick JB. Replication of vaccinia virus DNA in enucleated L-cells. *J Mol Biol* 1971;59:505–508.
561. Puckett C, Moss B. Selective transcription of vaccinia virus genes in template dependent soluble extracts of infected cells. *Cell* 1983;35:441–448.
562. Punjabi A, Traktman P. Cell biological and functional characterization of the vaccinia virus F10 kinase: implications for the mechanism of virion morphogenesis. *J Virol* 2005;79(4):2171–2190.

563. Rahman MM, Bagdassarian E, Ali MAM, et al. Identification of host DEAD-box RNA helicases that regulate cellular tropism of oncolytic Myxoma virus in human cancer cells. *Sci Rep* 2017;7:15710.
564. Rahman MM, Jeng D, Singh R, et al. Interaction of human TNF and beta 2-microglobulin with Tanapox virus-encoded TNF inhibitor, TPV-2L. *Virology* 2009;386(2):462–468.
565. Rahman MM, Liu J, Chan WM, et al. Myxoma virus protein M029 is a dual function immunomodulator inhibits PKR and also conscripts RHA/DHX9 to promote expanded tropism and viral replication. *PLoS Pathog* 2013;9(7):e1003465.
566. Rahman MM, Mohamed MR, Kim M, et al. Co-regulation of NF-kappa B and inflammasome-mediated inflammatory responses by myxoma virus pyrin domain-containing protein M013. *PLoS Pathog* 2009;5(10):e1000635.
567. Ramelot TA, Cort JR, Yee AA, et al. Myxoma virus immunomodulatory protein M156R is a structural mimic of eukaryotic translation initiation factor eIF2 alpha. *J Mol Biol* 2002;322(5):943–954.
568. Ramsey-Ewing A, Moss B. Restriction of vaccinia virus replication in CHO cells occurs at the stage of viral intermediate protein synthesis. *Virology* 1995;206(2):984–993.
569. Ramsey-Ewing AL, Moss B. Complementation of a vaccinia virus host range K1L gene deletion by the non-homologous CP77 gene. *Virology* 1996;222:75–86.
570. Ray CA, Black RA, Kronheim SR, et al. Viral inhibition of inflammation—cowpox virus encodes an inhibitor of the interleukin-1b converting enzyme. *Cell* 1992;69(4): 597–604.
571. Ray CA, Pickup DJ. The mode of death of pig kidney cells infected with cowpox virus is governed by the expression of the CrmA gene. *Virology* 1996;217(1):384–391.
572. Reading PC, Khanna A, Smith GL. Vaccinia virus CrmE encodes a soluble and cell surface tumor necrosis factor receptor that contributes to virus virulence. *Virology* 2002;292(2):285–298.
573. Reading PC, Moore JB, Smith GL. Steroid hormone synthesis by vaccinia virus suppresses the inflammatory response to infection. *J Exp Med* 2003;197(10):1269–1278.
574. Reading PC, Smith GL. Vaccinia virus interleukin-18-binding protein promotes virulence by reducing gamma interferon production and natural killer and T-cell activity. *J Virol* 2003;77(18):9960–9968.
575. Reading PC, Symons JA, Smith GL. A soluble chemokine-binding protein from vaccinia virus reduces virus virulence and the inflammatory response to infection. *J Immunol* 2003;170(3):1435–1442.
576. Reed B, Yakovleva L, Shuman S, et al. Characterization of DNA binding by the isolated N-terminal domain of vaccinia virus DNA topoisomerase IB. *Biochemistry* 2017;56(26):3307–3317.
577. Reeves PM, Bommarius B, Lebeis S, et al. Disabling poxvirus pathogenesis by inhibition of Abl-family tyrosine kinases. *Nat Med* 2005;11(7):731–739.
578. Rehm KE, Connor RF, Jones GJB, et al. Vaccinia virus decreases major histocompatibility complex (MHC) class II antigen presentation, T-cell priming, and peptide association with MHC class II. *Immunology* 2009;128(3):381–392.
579. Rehm KE, Connor RF, Jones GJB, et al. Vaccinia virus A35R inhibits MHC class II antigen presentation. *Virology* 2010;397(1):176–186.
580. Resch W, Hixson KK, Moore RJ, et al. Protein composition of the vaccinia virus mature virion. *Virology* 2007;358(1):233–247.
581. Resch W, Moss B. The conserved poxvirus L3 virion protein is required for transcription of vaccinia virus early genes. *J Virol* 2005;79(23):14719–14729.
582. Resch W, Weisberg AS, Moss B. Expression of the highly conserved vaccinia virus E6 protein is required for virion morphogenesis. *Virology* 2009;386:478–485.
583. Resch W, Weisberg AS, Moss B. Vaccinia virus nonstructural protein encoded by the A11R gene is required for formation of the virion membrane. *J Virol* 2005;79(11):6598–6609.
584. Reynolds SE, Earl PL, Minai M, et al. A homolog of the variola virus B22 membrane protein contributes to ectromelia virus pathogenicity in the mouse footpad model. *Virology* 2017;501:107–114.
585. Rice AP, Roberts BE. Vaccinia virus induces cellular mRNA degradation. *J Virol* 1983;47:529–539.
586. Rietdorf J, Ploubidou A, Reckmann I, et al. Kinesin dependent movement on microtubules precedes actin based motility of vaccinia virus. *Nat Cell Biol* 2001;3:992–1000.
587. Risco C, Rodriguez JR, Demkowicz W, et al. The vaccinia virus 39-kDa protein forms a stable complex with the p4a/4a major core protein early in morphogenesis. *Virology* 1999;265:375–386.
588. Rizopoulos Z, Balistreri G, Kilcher S, et al. Vaccinia virus Infection requires maturation of macropinosomes. *Traffic* 2015;16(8):814–831.
589. Roberts KL, Breiman A, Carter GC, et al. Acidic residues in the membrane-proximal stalk region of vaccinia virus protein B5 are required for glycosaminoglycan-mediated disruption of the extracellular enveloped virus outer membrane. *J Gen Virol* 2009;90:1582–1591.
590. Roberts KL, Smith GL. Vaccinia virus morphogenesis and dissemination. *Trends Microbiol* 2008;16(10):472–479.
591. Rodriguez JF, Smith GL. IPTG-dependent vaccinia virus: Identification of a virus gene enabling virion envelopment by a Golgi membrane and egress. *Nucleic Acids Res* 1990;18:5347–5351.
592. Rodriguez JR, Risco C, Carrascosa JL, et al. Characterization of early stages in vaccinia virus membrane biogenesis: implications of the 21-kilodalton protein and a newly identified 15-kilodalton envelope protein. *J Virol* 1997;71(3):1821–1833.
593. Rodriguez JR, Risco C, Carrascosa JL, et al. Vaccinia virus 15-kilodalton (A14L) protein is essential for assembly and attachment of viral crescents to virosomes. *J Virol* 1998;72:1287–1296.
594. Roening G, Holowczak JA. Evidence for the presence of RNA in the purified virions of vaccinia virus. *J Virol* 1974;14:704–708.
595. Roper R, Wolffe EJ, Weisberg A, et al. The envelope protein encoded by the A33R gene is required for formation of actin-containing microvilli and efficient cell-to-cell spread of vaccinia virus. *J Virol* 1998;72:4192–4204.
596. Roper RL, Moss B. Envelope formation is blocked by mutation of a sequence related to the HKD phospholipid metabolism motif in the vaccinia virus F13L protein. *J Virol* 1999;73(2):1108–1117.
597. Rosales R, Harris N, Ahn B-Y, et al. Purification and identification of a vaccinia virus-encoded intermediate stage promoter-specific transcription factor that has homology to eukaryotic transcription factor SII (TFIIS) and an additional role as a viral RNA polymerase subunit. *J Biol Chem* 1994;269:14260–14267.
598. Rosel J, Moss B. Transcriptional and translational mapping and nucleotide sequence analysis of a vaccinia virus gene encoding the precursor of the major core polypeptide 4b. *J Virol* 1985;56:830–838.
599. Rosengard AM, Liu Y, Nie Z, et al. Variola virus immune evasion design: expression of a highly efficient inhibitor of human complement. *Proc Natl Acad Sci U S A* 2002;99(13):8808–8813.
600. Rottger S, Frischknecht F, Reckmann I, et al. Interactions between vaccinia virus IEV membrane proteins and their roles in IEV assembly and actin tail formation. *J Virol* 1999;73(4):2863–2875.
601. Ryerson MR, Richards MM, Kvansakul M, et al. Vaccinia virus encodes a novel inhibitor of apoptosis that associates with the apoptosome. *J Virol* 2017;91(23):e01385-17.
602. Sahu A, Isaacs SN, Soulika AM, et al. Interaction of vaccinia virus complement control protein with human complement proteins: factor I-mediated degradation of C3b to iC3b1 inactivates the alternative complement pathway. *J Immunol* 1998;160(11): 5596–5604.
603. Samal A, Schormann N, Cook WJ, et al. Structures of vaccinia virus dUTPase and its nucleotide complexes. *Acta Crystallogr D Biol Crystallogr* 2007;63:571–580.
604. Sanderson CM, Frischknecht F, Way M, et al. Roles of vaccinia virus EEV-specific proteins in intracellular actin tail formation and low pH-induced cell-cell fusion. *J Gen Virol* 1998;79(Pt 6):1415–1425.
605. Sanderson CM, Hollinshead M, Smith GL. The vaccinia virus A27L protein is needed for the microtubule- dependent transport of intracellular mature virus particles. *J Gen Virol* 2000;81:47–58.
606. Sanderson CM, Way M, Smith GL. Virus-induced cell motility. *J Virol* 1998;72:1235–1243.
607. Sanz P, Moss B. Identification of a transcription factor, encoded by two vaccinia virus early genes, that regulates the intermediate stage of viral gene expression. *Proc Natl Acad Sci U S A* 1999;96(6):2692–2697.
608. Sanz P, Veyrunes J-C, Cousserans F, et al. Cloning and sequencing of the Spherulin gene, the occlusion body major polypeptide of the Melolontha melolontha entomopoxvirus (MmEPV). *Virology* 1994;202:449–457.
609. Saraiva M, Alcami A. CrmE, a novel soluble tumor necrosis factor receptor encoded by poxviruses. *J Virol* 2001;75(1):226–233.
610. Saraiva M, Smith P, Fallon PG, et al. Inhibition of type 1 cytokine-mediated inflammation by a soluble CD30 homologue encoded by ectromelia (mousepox) virus. *J Exp Med* 2002;196(6):829–839.
611. Satheshkumar PS, Anton LC, Sanz P, et al. Inhibition of the ubiquitin-proteasome system prevents vaccinia virus DNA replication and expression of intermediate and late genes. *J Virol* 2009;83(6):2469–2479.
612. Satheshkumar PS, Moss B. Characterization of a newly identified 35 amino acid component of the vaccinia virus entry/fusion complex conserved in all chordopoxviruses. *J Virol* 2009;83:12822–12832.
613. Savory LJ, Stacker SA, Fleming SB, et al. Viral vascular endothelial growth factor plays a critical role in orf virus infection. *J Virol* 2000;74(22):10699–10706.
614. Scaplehorn N, Holmstrom A, Moreau V, et al. Grb2 and Nck act cooperatively to promote actin-based motility of vaccinia virus. *Curr Biol* 2002;12(9):740–745.
615. Schepis A, Schramm B, de Haan Cornelis AM, et al. Vaccinia virus-induced microtubule-dependent cellular rearrangements. *Traffic* 2006;7(3):308–323.
616. Schmelz M, Sodeik B, Ericsson M, et al. Assembly of vaccinia virus: the second wrapping cisterna is derived from the trans Golgi network. *J Virol* 1994;68:130–147.
617. Schmidt FI, Bleck CK, Helenius A, et al. Vaccinia extracellular virions enter cells by macropinocytosis and acid-activated membrane rupture. *EMBO J* 2011;30:3647–3661.
618. Schmidt FI, Bleck CK, Mercer J. Poxvirus host cell entry. *Curr Opin Virol* 2012;2(1): 20–27.
619. Schmidt FI, Bleck CKE, Reh L, et al. Vaccinia virus entry is followed by core activation and proteasome-mediated release of the immunomodulatory effector lateral bodies. *Cell Rep* 2013;4(3):464–476.
620. Schmutz C, Rindisbacher L, Galmiche MC, et al. Biochemical analysis of the major vaccinia virus envelope antigen. *Virology* 1995;213:19–27.
621. Schnierle BS, Gershon PD, Moss B. Cap-specific mRNA (nucleoside-$O^{2'}$-)-methyltransferase and poly(A) polymerase stimulatory activities of vaccinia virus are mediated by a single protein. *Proc Natl Acad Sci U S A* 1992;89:2897–2901.
622. Schnierle BS, Gershon PD, Moss B. Mutational analysis of a multifunctional protein, with mRNA 5′ cap-specific (nucleoside-2′-O-)-methyltransferase and 3′ adenylyltransferase stimulatory activities, encoded by vaccinia virus. *J Biol Chem* 1994;269:20700–20706.
623. Schormann N, Zhukovskaya N, Bedwell G, et al. Poxvirus uracil-DNA glycosylase-An unusual member of the family I uracil-DNA glycosylases. *Protein Sci* 2016;25(12):2113–2131.
624. Schreiber M, Rajarathnam K, McFadden G. Myxoma virus T2 protein, a tumor necrosis factor (TNF) receptor homolog, is secreted as a monomer and dimer that each bind rabbit TNFalpha, but the dimer is a more potent TNF inhibitor. *J Biol Chem* 1996;271(23):13333–13341.
625. Schroder M, Baran M, Bowie AG. Viral targeting of DEAD box protein 3 reveals its role in TBK1/IKKepsilon-mediated IRF activation. *EMBO J* 2008;27(15):2147–2157.
626. Schwer B, Visca P, Vos JC, et al. Discontinuous transcription or RNA processing of vaccinia virus late messengers results in a 5′ poly(A) leader. *Cell* 1987;50:163–169.
627. Scutts SR, Ember SW, Ren HW, et al. DNA-PK is targeted by multiple vaccinia virus proteins to inhibit DNA sensing. *Cell Rep* 2018;25(7):1953–1965.e5.
628. Sebring ED, Salzman NP. Metabolic properties of early and late vaccinia messenger ribonucleic acid. *J Virol* 1967;1:550–575.
629. Seet BT, McCaughan CA, Handel TM, et al. Analysis of an orf virus chemokine-binding protein: shifting ligand specificities among a family of poxvirus viroceptors. *Proc Natl Acad Sci U S A* 2003;100(25):15137–15142.

630. Seet BT, Singh R, Paavola C, et al. Molecular determinants for CC-chemokine recognition by a poxvirus CC-chemokine inhibitor. *Proc Natl Acad Sci U S A* 2001;98(16):9008–9013.
631. Seki M, Oie M, Ichihashi Y, et al. Hemadsorption and fusion inhibition activities of hemagglutinin analyzed by vaccinia virus mutants. *Virology* 1990;175:372–384.
632. Sekiguchi J, Seeman NC, Shuman S. Resolution of Holliday junctions by eukaryotic DNA topoisomerase I. *Proc Natl Acad Sci U S A* 1996;93:785–789.
633. Senkevich T, White C, Weisberg A, et al. Expression of the vaccinia virus A2.5L redox protein is required for virion morphogenesis. *Virology* 2002;300(2):296–303.
634. Senkevich TG, Katsafanas G, Weisberg A, et al. Identification of vaccinia virus replisome and transcriptome proteins by iPOND coupled with mass spectrometry. *J Virol* 2017;91(19):e01015-17.
635. Senkevich TG, Koonin EV, Bugert JJ, et al. The genome of molluscum contagiosum virus: analysis and comparison with other poxviruses. *Virology* 1997;233:19–42.
636. Senkevich TG, Koonin EV, Moss B. Predicted poxvirus FEN1-like nuclease required for homologous recombination, double-strand break repair and full-size genome formation. *Proc Natl Acad Sci U S A* 2009;106(42):17921–17926.
637. Senkevich TG, Koonin EV, Moss B. Vaccinia virus F16 protein, a predicted catalytically inactive member of the prokaryotic serine recombinase superfamily, is targeted to nucleoli. *Virology* 2011;417:334–342.
638. Senkevich TG, Moss B. Vaccinia virus H2 protein is an essential component of a complex involved in virus entry and cell-cell fusion. *J Virol* 2005;79:4744–4754.
639. Senkevich TG, Ojeda S, Townsley A, et al. Poxvirus multiprotein entry-fusion complex. *Proc Natl Acad Sci U S A* 2005;102(51):18572–18577.
640. Senkevich TG, Ward BM, Moss B. Vaccinia virus entry into cells is dependent on a virion surface protein encoded by the A28L gene. *J Virol* 2004;78(5):2357–2366.
641. Senkevich TG, White CL, Koonin EV, et al. Complete pathway for protein disulfide bond formation encoded by poxviruses. *Proc Natl Acad Sci U S A* 2002;99:6667–6672.
642. Senkevich TG, White CL, Koonin EV, et al. A viral member of the ERV1/ALR protein family participates in a cytoplasmic pathway of disulfide bond formation. *Proc Natl Acad Sci U S A* 2000;97:12068–12073.
643. Senkevich TG, Wolffe EJ, Buller ML. Ectromelia virus RING finger protein is localized in virus factories and is required for virus replication in macrophages. *J Virol* 1995;69:4103–4111.
644. Senkevich TG, Wyatt LS, Weisberg AS, et al. A conserved poxvirus NlpC/P60 superfamily protein contributes to vaccinia virus virulence in mice but not to replication in cell culture. *Virology* 2008;374(2):506–514.
645. Senkevicha TG, Bruno D, Martens C, et al. Mapping vaccinia virus DNA replication origins at nucleotide level by deep sequencing. *Proc Natl Acad Sci U S A* 2015;112(35):10908–10913.
646. Sette A, Grey H, Oseroff C, et al. Definition of epitopes and antigens recognized by vaccinia specific immune responses: their conservation in variola virus sequences, and use as a model system to study complex pathogens. *Vaccine* 2009;27:G21–G26.
647. Shaffer R, Traktman P. Vaccinia virus encapsidates a novel topoisomerase with the properties of a eucaryotic type I enzyme. *J Biol Chem* 1987;262:9309–9315.
648. Shi X, Yao P, Jose T, et al. Methyltransferase-specific domains within VP39, a bifunctional protein which participates in the modification of both mRNA ends. *RNA* 1996;2:88–101.
649. Shida H. Nucleotide sequence of the vaccinia virus hemagglutinin gene. *Virology* 1986;150:451–462.
650. Shirokikh NE, Spirin AS. Poly(A) leader of eukaryotic mRNA bypasses the dependence of translation on initiation factors. *Proc Natl Acad Sci U S A* 2008;105(31):10738–10743.
651. Shisler JL, Isaacs SN, Moss B. Vaccinia virus serpin-1 deletion mutant exhibits a host range defect characterized by low levels of intermediate and late mRNAs. *Virology* 1999;262(2):298–311.
652. Shisler JL, Jin XL. The vaccinia virus K1L gene product inhibits host NF-kB activation by preventing IkBa degradation. *J Virol* 2004;78(7):3553–3560.
653. Shisler JL, Senkevich TG, Berry MJ, et al. Ultraviolet-induced cell death blocked by a selenoprotein from a human dermotropic poxvirus. *Science* 1998;279(5347):102–105.
654. Shope RE. A filtrable virus causing a tumor—like condition in rabbits and its relationship to virus myxomatosum. *J Exp Med* 1932;56:803–822.
655. Shors T, Keck JG, Moss B. Down regulation of gene expression by the vaccinia virus D10 protein. *J Virol* 1999;73(1):791–796.
656. Shuman S. Site-specific DNA cleavage by vaccinia virus DNA topoisomerase-I—role of nucleotide sequence and DNA secondary structure. *J Biol Chem* 1991;266(3):1796–1803.
657. Shuman S, Hurwitz J. Mechanism of mRNA capping by vaccinia virus guanylyltransferase: characterization of an enzyme-guanylate intermediate. *Proc Natl Acad Sci U S A* 1981;78:187–191.
658. Shuman S, Moss B. Bromouridine triphosphate inhibits transcription termination and mRNA release by vaccinia virions. *J Biol Chem* 1989;264:21356–21360.
659. Shuman S, Moss B. Identification of a vaccinia virus gene encoding a type I DNA topoisomerase. *Proc Natl Acad Sci U S A* 1987;84:7478–7482.
660. Simpson DA, Condit RC. Vaccinia virus gene A18R encodes an essential DNA helicase. *J Virol* 1995;69:6131–6139.
661. Sivan G, Glushakow-Smith SG, Katsafanas GC, et al. Human host range restriction of the vaccinia virus C7/K1 double deletion mutant is mediated by an atypical mode of translation inhibition. *J Virol* 2018;92(23):e01329-18.
662. Sivan G, Martin SE, Myers TG, et al. Human genome-wide RNAi screen reveals a role for nuclear pore proteins in poxvirus morphogenesis. *Proc Natl Acad Sci U S A* 2013;110(9):3519–3524.
663. Sivan G, Ormanoglu P, Buehler EC, et al. Identification of restriction factors by human genome-wide RNA interference screening of viral host range mutants exemplified by discovery of SAMD9 and WDR6 as inhibitors of the vaccinia virus K1L-C7L-mutant. *MBio* 2015;6(4):e01122.
664. Sivan G, Weisberg AS, Americo JL, et al. Retrograde transport from early endosomes to the trans-Golgi network enables membrane wrapping and egress of vaccinia virions. *J Virol* 2016;90:8891–8905.
665. Slabaugh M, Roseman N, Davis R, et al. Vaccinia virus-encoded ribonucleotide reductase: sequence conservation of the gene for the small subunit and its amplification in hydroxyurea-resistant mutants. *J Virol* 1988;62(2):519–527.
666. Slabaugh MB, Davis RE, Roseman NA, et al. Vaccinia virus ribonucleotide reductase expression and isolation of the recombinant large subunit. *J Biol Chem* 1993;268(24):17803–17810.
667. Slabaugh MB, Johnson TL, Mathews CK. Vaccinia virus induces ribonucleotide reductase in primate cells. *J Virol* 1984;52(2):507–514.
668. Slabaugh MB, Roseman NA. Retroviral protease-like gene in the vaccinia virus genome. *Proc Natl Acad Sci U S A* 1989;86(11):4152–4155.
669. Slabaugh MB, Roseman NA, Mathews CK. Amplification of the ribonucleotide reductase small subunit gene: analysis of novel joints and the mechanism of gene duplication in vaccinia virus. *Nucleic Acids Res* 1989;17(17):7073–7088.
670. Smith CA, Smith TD, Smolak PJ, et al. Poxvirus genomes encode a secreted, soluble protein that preferentially inhibits b chemokine activity yet lacks sequence homology to known chemokine receptors. *Virology* 1997;236:316–327.
671. Smith GL, Benfield CTO, Maluquer de Motes C, et al. Vaccinia virus immune evasion: mechanisms, virulence and immunogenicity. *J Gen Virol* 2013;94:2367–2392.
672. Smith GL, Chan YS. Two vaccinia virus proteins structurally related to the interleukin-1 receptor and the immunoglobulin superfamily. *J Gen Virol* 1991;72(Pt 3):511–518.
673. Smith GL, Chan YS, Howard ST. Nucleotide sequence of 42 kbp of vaccinia virus strain WR from near the right inverted terminal repeat. *J Gen Virol* 1991;72(Pt 6):1349–1376.
674. Smith GL, de Carlos A, Chan YS. Vaccinia virus encodes a thymidylate kinase gene: sequence and transcriptional mapping. *Nucleic Acids Res* 1989;17:7581–7590.
675. Smith GL, Talbot-Cooper C, Lu YX. How does vaccinia virus interfere with interferon? In: Kielian M, Mettenleiter TC, Roossinck MJ, eds. *Advances in Virus Research*, Vol 100. Academic Press, Cambridge, MA. 2018:355–378.
676. Smith VP, Bryant NA, Alcami A. Ectromelia, vaccinia and cowpox viruses encode secreted interleukin-18-binding proteins. *J Gen Virol* 2000;81(Pt 5):1223–1230.
677. Snetkov X, Weisswange I, Pfanzelter J, et al. NPF motifs in the vaccinia virus protein A36 recruit intersectin-1 to promote Cdc42:N-WASP-mediated viral release from infected cells. *Nat Microbiol* 2016;1(10):16141.
678. Soares JAP, Leite FGG, Andrade LG, et al. Activation of the PI3K/Akt pathway early during vaccinia and cowpox virus infections is required for both host survival and viral replication. *J Virol* 2009;83(13):6883–6899.
679. Soday L, Lu Y, Albarnaz JD, et al. Quantitative temporal proteomic analysis of vaccinia virus infection reveals regulation of histone deacetylases by an interferon antagonist. *Cell Rep* 2019;27(6):1920–1933.e7.
680. Sonnberg S, Fleming SB, Mercer AA. A truncated two-alpha-helix F-box present in poxvirus ankyrin-repeat proteins is sufficient for binding the SCF1 ubiquitin ligase complex. *J Gen Virol* 2009;90:1224–1228.
681. Sonnberg S, Seet BT, Pawson T, et al. Poxvirus ankyrin repeat proteins are a unique class of F-box proteins that associate with cellular SCF1 ubiquitin ligase complexes. *Proc Natl Acad Sci U S A* 2008;105(31):10955–10960.
682. Sood CL, Moss B. Vaccinia virus A43R gene encodes an orthopoxvirus-specific late non-virion type-1 membrane protein that is dispensable for replication but enhances intradermal lesion formation. *Virology* 2010;396(1):160–168.
683. Sood CL, Ward JM, Moss B. Vaccinia virus encodes a small hydrophobic virion membrane protein (I5) that enhances replication and virulence in mice. *J Virol* 2008;82:10071–10078.
684. Souliere MF, Perreault JP, Bisaillon M. Characterization of the vaccinia virus D10 decapping enzyme provides evidence for a two-metal-ion mechanism. *Biochem J* 2009;420:27–35.
685. Souliere MF, Perreault JP, Bisaillon M. Insights into the molecular determinants involved in cap recognition by the vaccinia virus D10 decapping enzyme. *Nucleic Acids Res* 2010;38(21):7599–7610.
686. Spehner D, Gillard S, Drillien R, et al. A cowpox virus gene required for multiplication in Chinese hamster ovary cells. *J Virol* 1988;62:1297–1304.
687. Sperling KM, Schwantes A, Schnierle BS, et al. The highly conserved orthopoxvirus 68k ankyrin-like protein is part of a cellular SCF ubiquitin ligase complex. *Virology* 2008;374(2):234–239.
688. Spriggs MK, Hruby DE, Maliszewski CR, et al. Vaccinia and cowpox viruses encode a novel secreted interleukin-1-binding protein. *Cell* 1992;71(1):145–152.
689. Spyropoulos DD, Roberts BE, Panicali DL, et al. Delineation of the viral products of recombination in vaccinia virus-infected cells. *J Virol* 1988;62:1046–1054.
690. Srinivasan V, Tripathy DN. The DNA repair enzyme, CPD-photolyase restores the infectivity of UV-damaged fowlpox virus isolated from infected scabs of chickens. *Vet Microbiol* 2005;108(3–4):215–223.
691. Sroller V, Ludvikova V, Maresova L, et al. Effect of IFN-gamma receptor gene deletion on vaccinia virus virulence. *Arch Virol* 2001;146(2):239–249.
692. Stack J, Haga IR, Schroder M, et al. Vaccinia virus protein Toll-like-interleukin-1 A46R targets multiple receptor adaptors and contributes to virulence. *J Exp Med* 2005;201(6):1007–1018.
693. Stanitsa ES, Arps L, Traktman P. Vaccinia virus uracil DNA glycosylase interacts with the A20 protein to form a heterodimeric processivity factor for the viral DNA polymerase. *J Biol Chem* 2006;281:3439–3451.
694. Stokes GV. High-voltage electron microscope study of the release of vaccinia virus from whole cells. *J Virol* 1976;18:636–643.
695. Strnadova P, Ren HW, Valentine R, et al. Inhibition of translation initiation by protein 169: a vaccinia virus strategy to suppress innate and adaptive immunity and alter virus virulence. *PLoS Pathog* 2015;11(9):e1005151.
696. Stroobant P, Rice AP, Gullick WJ, et al. Purification and characterization of vaccinia virus growth factor. *Cell* 1985;42:383–393.
697. Stuart DT, Upton C, Higman MA, et al. A poxvirus-encoded uracil DNA glycosylase is essential for virus viability. *J Virol* 1993;67:2503–2512.
698. Stuart JH, Sumner RP, Lu YX, et al. Vaccinia virus protein C6 inhibits type I IFN signalling in the nucleus and binds to the transactivation domain of STAT2. *PLoS Pathog* 2016;12(12):e1005955.

699. Su HP, Garman SC, Allison TJ, et al. The 1.51-A structure of the poxvirus L1 protein, a target of potent neutralizing antibodies. *Proc Natl Acad Sci U S A* 2005;102(12):4240–4245.
700. Su HP, Lin DYW, Garboczi DN. The structure of G4, the poxvirus disulfide oxidoreductase essential for virus maturation and infectivity. *J Virol* 2006;80(15):7706–7713.
701. Su HP, Singh K, Gittis AG, et al. The structure of the poxvirus A33 protein reveals a dimer of unique C-type lectin-like domains. *J Virol* 2010;84(5):2502–2510.
702. Sumner RP, Maluquer de Motes C, Veyer DL, et al. Vaccinia virus inhibits NF-kappa B-dependent gene expression downstream of p65 translocation. *J Virol* 2014;88(6):3092–3102.
703. Sutter G, Moss B. Nonreplicating vaccinia vector efficiently expresses recombinant genes. *Proc Natl Acad Sci U S A* 1992;89(22):10847–10851.
704. Symons JA, Adams E, Tscharke DC, et al. The vaccinia virus C12L protein inhibits mouse IL-18 and promotes virus virulence in the murine intranasal model. *J Gen Virol* 2002;83(Pt 11):2833–2844.
705. Symons JA, Alcami A, Smith GL. Vaccinia virus encodes a soluble type 1 interferon receptor of novel structure and broad species specificity. *Cell* 1995;81:551–560.
706. Symons JA, Tscharke DC, Price N, et al. A study of the vaccinia virus interferon-gamma receptor and its contribution to virus virulence. *J Gen Virol* 2002;83:1953–1964.
707. Szajner P, Jaffe H, Weisberg AS, et al. A complex of seven vaccinia virus proteins conserved in all chordopoxviruses is required for the association of membranes and viroplasm to form immature virions. *Virology* 2004;330(2):447–459.
708. Szajner P, Jaffe H, Weisberg AS, et al. Vaccinia virus G7L protein interacts with the A30L protein and is required for association of viral membranes with dense viroplasm to form immature virions. *J Virol* 2003;77(6):3418–3429.
709. Szajner P, Weisberg AS, Lebowitz J, et al. External scaffold of spherical immature poxvirus particles is made of protein trimers, forming a honeycomb lattice. *J Cell Biol* 2005;170(6): 971–981.
710. Szajner P, Weisberg AS, Moss B. Evidence for an essential catalytic role of the F10 protein kinase in vaccinia virus morphogenesis. *J Virol* 2004;78:257–265.
711. Szajner P, Weisberg AS, Wolffe EJ, et al. Vaccinia virus A30L protein is required for association of viral membranes with dense viroplasm to form immature virions. *J Virol* 2001;75(13):5752–5761.
712. Tarbouriech N, Ducournau C, Hutin S, et al. The vaccinia virus DNA polymerase structure provides insights into the mode of processivity factor binding. *Nat Commun* 2017;8: 1455.
713. Tartaglia J, Piccini A, Paoletti E. Vaccinia virus rifampicin-resistance locus specifies a late 63,000 Da gene product. *Virology* 1986;150:45–54.
714. Teale A, Campbell S, Van Buuren N, et al. Orthopoxviruses require a functional ubiquitin-proteasome system for productive replication. *J Virol* 2009;83:2099–2108.
715. Tengelsen LA, Slabaugh MB, Bibler JK, et al. Nucleotide sequence and molecular genetic analysis of the large subunit of ribonucleotide reductase encoded by vaccinia virus. *Virology* 1988;164:121–131.
716. Tewari M, Telford WG, Miller RA, et al. CrmA, a poxvirus-encoded serpin, inhibits cytotoxic T-lymphocyte-mediated apoptosis. *J Biol Chem* 1995;270(39):22705–22708.
717. Thome M, Schneider P, Hofmann K, et al. Viral flice-inhibitory proteins (FLIPs) prevent apoptosis induced by death receptors. *Nature* 1997;386:517–521.
718. Thompson JP, Turner PC, Ali AN, et al. The effects of serpin gene mutations on the distinctive pathobiology of cowpox and rabbitpox virus following intranasal inoculation of balb/c mice. *Virology* 1993;197:328–338.
719. Tolonen N, Doglio L, Schleich S, et al. Vaccinia virus DNA replication occurs in endoplasmic reticulum- enclosed cytoplasmic mini-nuclei. *Mol Biol Cell* 2001;12(7):2031–2046.
720. Tooze J, Hollinshead M, Reis B, et al. Progeny vaccinia and human cytomegalovirus particles utilize early endosomal cisternae for their envelopes. *Eur J Cell Biol* 1993;60(1): 163–178.
721. Torres AA, Albarnaz JD, Bonjardim CA, et al. Multiple Bcl-2 family immunomodulators from vaccinia virus regulate MAPK/AP-1 activation. *J Gen Virol* 2016;97:2346–2351.
722. Townsley A, Senkevich TG, Moss B. The product of the vaccinia virus L5R gene is a fourth membrane protein encoded by all poxviruses that is required for cell entry and cell-cell fusion. *J Virol* 2005;79:10988–10998.
723. Townsley A, Senkevich TG, Moss B. Vaccinia virus A21 virion membrane protein is required for cell entry and fusion. *J Virol* 2005;79:9458–9469.
724. Townsley AC, Moss B. Two distinct low-pH steps promote entry of vaccinia virus. *J Virol* 2007;81(16):8613–8620.
725. Townsley AC, Weisberg AS, Wagenaar TR, et al. Vaccinia virus entry into cells via a low pH-dependent-endosomal pathway. *J Virol* 2006;80:8899–8908.
726. Traktman P, Caligiuri A, Jesty SA, et al. Temperature-sensitive mutants with lesions in the vaccinia virus F10 kinase undergo arrest at the earliest stage of morphogenesis. *J Virol* 1995;69:6581–6587.
727. Traktman P, Liu K, DeMasi J, et al. Elucidating the essential role of the A14 phosphoprotein in vaccinia virus morphogenesis: construction and characterization of a tetracycline-inducible recombinant. *J Virol* 2000;74(8):3682–3695.
728. Trilling M, Le VTK, Zimmermann A, et al. Gamma interferon-induced interferon regulatory factor 1-dependent antiviral response inhibits vaccinia virus replication in mouse but not human fibroblasts. *J Virol* 2009;83(8):3684–3695.
729. Tseng M, Palaniyar N, Zhang WD, et al. DNA binding and aggregation properties of the vaccinia virus I3L gene product. *J Biol Chem* 1999;274(31):21637–21644.
730. Tsukumo SI, Yonehara S. Requirement of cooperative functions of two repeated death effector domains in caspase-8 and in MC159 for induction and inhibition of apoptosis, respectively. *Genes Cells* 1999;4(9):541–549.
731. Turner PC, Dilling BP, Prins C, et al. Vaccinia virus temperature-sensitive mutants in the A28 gene produce non-infectious virions that bind to cells but are defective in entry. *Virology* 2007;366(1):62–72.
732. Turner PC, Moyer RW. The cowpox virus fusion regulator proteins SPI-3 and hemagglutinin interact in infected and uninfected cells. *Virology* 2006;347(1):88–99.
733. Turner PC, Moyer RW. Orthopoxvirus fusion inhibitor glycoprotein SPI-3 (open reading frame K2L) contains motifs characteristic of serine protease inhibitors that are not required for control of cell fusion. *J Virol* 1995;69:5978–5987.
734. Tzahar E, Moyer JD, Waterman H, et al. Pathogenic poxviruses reveal viral strategies to exploit the ErbB signaling network. *EMBO J* 1998;17(20):5948–5963.
735. Ulaeto D, Grosenbach D, Hruby DE. Brefeldin A inhibits vaccinia virus envelopment but does not prevent normal processing and localization of the putative envelopment receptor P37. *J Gen Virol* 1995;76(Pt 1):103–111.
736. Ulaeto D, Grosenbach D, Hruby DE. The vaccinia virus 4c and A-type inclusion proteins are specific markers for the intracellular mature virus particle. *J Virol* 1996;70:3372–3375.
737. Unger B, Mercer J, Boyle KA, et al. Biogenesis of the vaccinia virus membrane: genetic and ultrastructural analysis of the contributions of the A14 and A17 proteins. *J Virol* 2013;87(2):1083–1097.
738. Unger B, Traktman P. Vaccinia virus morphogenesis: A13 phosphoprotein is required for assembly of mature virions. *J Virol* 2004;78(16):8885–8901.
739. Unterholzner L, Sumner RP, Baran M, et al. Vaccinia virus protein C6 is a virulence factor that binds TBK-1 adaptor proteins and inhibits activation of IRF3 and IRF7. *PLoS Pathog* 2011;7(9):e1002247.
740. Upton C, Macen JL, Schreiber M, et al. Myxoma virus expresses a secreted protein with homology to the tumor necrosis factor receptor gene family that contributes to viral virulence. *Virology* 1991;184:370–382.
741. Upton C, Mossman K, McFadden G. Encoding of a homolog of the IFN-g receptor by myxoma virus. *Science* 1992;258(5086):1369–1373.
742. Upton C, Slack S, Hunter AL, et al. Poxvirus orthologous clusters: toward defining the minimum essential poxvirus genome. *J Virol* 2003;77(13):7590–7600.
743. Valderrama F, Cordeiro JV, Schleich S, et al. Vaccinia virus-induced cell motility requires F11L-mediated inhibition of RhoA signaling. *Science* 2006;311(5759):377–381.
744. Valentine R, Smith GL. Inhibition of the RNA polymerase III-mediated dsDNA-sensing pathway of innate immunity by vaccinia virus protein E3. *J Gen Virol* 2010;91:2221–2229.
745. van Buuren N, Burles K, Schriewer J, et al. EVM005: an ectromelia-encoded protein with dual roles in NF-kappa B inhibition and virulence. *PLoS Pathog* 2014;10(8):e1004326.
746. van Buuren N, Couturier B, Xiong Y, et al. Ectromelia virus encodes a novel family of F-Box proteins that interact with the SCF complex. *J Virol* 2008;82(20):9917–9927.
747. van Eijl H, Hollinshead M, Rodger G, et al. The vaccinia virus F12L protein is associated with intracellular enveloped virus particles and is required for their egress to the cell surface. *J Gen Virol* 2002;83:195–207.
748. van Eijl H, Hollinshead M, Smith GL. The vaccinia virus A36R protein Is a type Ib membrane protein present on intracellular but not extracellular enveloped virus particles. *Virology* 2000;271(1):26–36.
749. Vanderplasschen A, Mathew E, Hollinshead M, et al. Extracellular enveloped vaccinia virus is resistant to complement because of incorporation of host complement control proteins into its envelope. *Proc Natl Acad Sci U S A* 1998;95(13):7544–7549.
750. Vanslyke JK, Franke CA, Hruby DE. Proteolytic maturation of vaccinia virus core proteins—identification of a conserved motif at the N termini of the 4b and 25K virion proteins. *J Gen Virol* 1991;72(Pt 2):411–416.
751. VanSlyke JK, Whitehead SS, Wilson EM, et al. The multistep proteolytic maturation pathway utilized by vaccinia virus P4a protein: a degenerate conserved cleavage motif within core proteins. *Virology* 1991;183:467–478.
752. Varich NL, Sychova IV, Kaverin NV, et al. Transcription of both DNA strands of vaccinia virus genome in vivo. *Virology* 1979;96:412–430.
753. Venkatesan S, Gershowitz A, Moss B. Modification of the 5′-end of mRNA: association of RNA triphosphatase with the RNA guanylyltransferase-RNA (guanine-7)methyltransferase complex from vaccinia virus. *J Biol Chem* 1980;255:903–908.
754. Veyer DL, Maluquer de Motes C, Sumner RP, et al. Analysis of the anti-apoptotic activity of four vaccinia virus proteins demonstrates that B13 is the most potent inhibitor in isolation and during viral infection. *J Gen Virol* 2014;95:2757–2768.
755. Volz A, Sutter G. Modified vaccinia virus Ankara: history, value in basic research, and current perspectives for vaccine development. In: Kielian M, Mettenleiter TC, Roossinck MJ, eds. *Advances in Virus Research*, Vol 97. Academic Press, Cambridge, MA. 2017:187–243.
756. Vos JC, Sasker M, Stunnenberg HG. Vaccinia virus capping enzyme is a transcription initiation factor. *EMBO J* 1991;10:2553–2558.
757. Vos JC, Stunnenberg HG. Derepression of a novel class of vaccinia virus genes upon DNA replication. *EMBO J* 1988;7:3487–3492.
758. Wagenaar TR, Moss B. Expression of the A56 and K2 proteins is sufficient to inhibit vaccinia virus entry and cell fusion. *J Virol* 2009;83(4):1546–1554.
759. Wagenaar TR, Ojeda S, Moss B. Vaccinia virus A56/K2 fusion regulatory protein interacts with the A16 and G9 subunits of the entry fusion complex. *J Virol* 2008;82(11):5153–5160.
760. Walsh D, Arias C, Perez C, et al. Eukaryotic translation initiation factor 4F architectural alterations accompany translation initiation factor redistribution in poxvirus-infected cells. *Mol Cell Biol* 2008;28(8):2648–2658.
761. Wang DR, Hsiao JC, Wong CH, et al. Vaccinia viral protein A27 is anchored to the viral membrane via a cooperative interaction with viral membrane protein A17. *J Biol Chem* 2014;289(10):6639–6655.
762. Wang F, Barrett JW, Shao Q, et al. Myxoma virus selectively disrupts type I interferon signaling in primary human fibroblasts by blocking the activation of the Janus kinase Tyk2. *Virology* 2009;387(1):136–146.
763. Wang F, Ma YY, Barrett JW, et al. Disruption of Erk-dependent type I interferon induction breaks the myxoma virus species barrier. *Nat Immunol* 2004;5(12):1266–1274.
764. Wang G, Barrett JW, Stanford M, et al. Infection of human cancer cells with myxoma virus requires Akt activation via interaction with a viral ankyrin-repeat host range factor. *Proc Natl Acad Sci U S A* 2006;103(12):4640–4645.
765. Wang S, Shuman S. Vaccinia virus morphogenesis is blocked by temperature-sensitive mutations in the F10 gene, which encodes protein kinase 2. *J Virol* 1995;69:6376–6388.
766. Wang SP, Shuman S. A temperature sensitive mutation of the vaccinia virus E11 gene encoding a 15-kDa component. *Virology* 1996;216:252–257.
767. Wang XL, Piersma SJ, Elliott JI, et al. Cowpox virus encodes a protein that binds B7.1 and B7.2 and subverts T cell costimulation. *Proc Natl Acad Sci U S A* 2019;116(42): 21113–21119.

768. Wang YX, Turner PC, Ness TL, et al. The cowpox virus SPI-3 and myxoma virus SERP1 serpins are not functionally interchangeable despite their similar proteinase inhibition profiles in vitro. *Virology* 2000;272(2):281–292.
769. Ward BM. Visualization and characterization of the intracellular movement of vaccinia virus intracellular mature virions. *J Virol* 2005;79:4755–4763.
770. Ward BM, Moss B. Golgi network targeting and plasma membrane internalization signals in vaccinia virus B5R envelope protein. *J Virol* 2000;74(8):3771–3780.
771. Ward BM, Moss B. Vaccinia virus A36R membrane protein provides a direct link between intracellular enveloped virions and the microtubule motor kinesin. *J Virol* 2004;78(5):2486–2493.
772. Ward BM, Moss B. Vaccinia virus intracellular movement is associated with microtubules and independent of actin tails. *J Virol* 2001;75:11651–11663.
773. Wei CM, Moss B. Methylated nucleotides block 5′-terminus of vaccinia virus mRNA. *Proc Natl Acad Sci U S A* 1975;72:318–322.
774. Weir JP, Moss B. Determination of the promoter region of an early vaccinia virus gene encoding thymidine kinase. *Virology* 1987;158:206–210.
775. Weisberg AS, Maruri-Avidal L, Bisht H, et al. Enigmatic origin of the poxvirus membrane from the endoplasmic reticulum shown by 3D imaging of vaccinia virus assembly mutants. *Proc Natl Acad Sci U S A* 2017;114(51):E11001–E11009.
776. Werden SJ, Lanchbury J, Shattuck D, et al. The myxoma Virus M-T5 ankyrin repeat host range protein is a novel adaptor that coordinately links the cellular signaling pathways mediated by Akt and Skp1 in virus-infected cells. *J Virol* 2009;83(23):12068–12083.
777. Westphal D, Ledgerwood EC, Tyndall JDA, et al. The orf virus inhibitor of apoptosis functions in a Bcl-2-like manner, binding and neutralizing a set of BH3-only proteins and active Bax. *Apoptosis* 2009;14(11):1317–1330.
778. White CL, Senkevich TG, Moss B. Vaccinia virus G4L glutaredoxin is an essential intermediate of a cytoplasmic disulfide bond pathway required for virion assembly. *J Virol* 2002;76(2):467–472.
779. Wickramasekera NT, Traktman P. Structure/function analysis of the vaccinia virus F18 phosphoprotein, an abundant core component required for virion maturation and infectivity. *J Virol* 2010;84(13):6846–6860.
780. Wilcock D, Smith GL. Vaccinia virions lacking core protein VP8 are deficient in early transcription. *J Virol* 1996;70:934–943.
781. Willer DO, Mann MJ, Zhang WD, et al. Vaccinia virus DNA polymerase promotes DNA pairing and strand-transfer reactions. *Virology* 1999;257(2):511–523.
782. Willer DO, McFadden G, Evans DH. The complete genome sequence of Shope (rabbit) fibroma virus. *Virology* 1999;264(2):319–343.
783. Williams O, Wolffe EJ, Weisberg AS, et al. Vaccinia virus WR gene A5L is required for morphogenesis of mature virions. *J Virol* 1999;73(6):4590–4599.
784. Willis KL, Patel S, Xiang Y, et al. The effect of the vaccinia K1 protein on the PKR-eIF2 alpha pathway in RK13 and HeLa cells. *Virology* 2009;394(1):73–81.
785. Wilton BA, Campbell S, Van Buuren N, et al. Ectromelia virus BTB/kelch proteins, EVM150 and EVM167, interact with cullin-3-based ubiquitin ligases. *Virology* 2008;374(1):82–99.
786. Wilton S, Dales S. Relationship between RNA polymerase II and efficiency of vaccinia virus replication. *J Virol* 1989;63:1540–1548.
787. Wise L, McCaughan C, Tan CK, et al. Orf virus interleukin-10 inhibits cytokine synthesis in activated human THP-1 monocytes, but only partially impairs their proliferation. *J Gen Virol* 2007;88:1677–1682.
788. Wise LM, Ueda N, Dryden NH, et al. Viral vascular endothelial growth factors vary extensively in amino acid sequence, receptor-binding specificities, and the ability to induce vascular permeability yet are uniformly active mitogens. *J Biol Chem* 2003;278(39):38004–38014.
789. Wittek R, Hanggi M, Hiller G. Mapping of a gene coding for a major late structural polypeptide on the vaccinia virus genome. *J Virol* 1984;49:371–378.
790. Wolffe EJ, Isaacs SN, Moss B. Deletion of the vaccinia virus B5R gene encoding a 42-kilodalton membrane glycoprotein inhibits extracellular virus envelope formation and dissemination. *J Virol* 1993;67:4732–4741.
791. Wolffe EJ, Katz E, Weisberg A, et al. The A34R glycoprotein gene is required for induction of specialized actin-containing microvilli and efficient cell-to-cell transmission of vaccinia virus. *J Virol* 1997;71:3904–3915.
792. Wolffe EJ, Moore DM, Peters PJ, et al. Vaccinia virus A17L open reading frame encodes an essential component of nascent viral membranes that is required to initiate morphogenesis. *J Virol* 1996;70:2797–2808.
793. Wolffe EJ, Weisberg A, Moss B. The vaccinia virus A33R protein provides a chaperone function for viral membrane localization and tyrosine phosphorylation of the A36R protein. *J Virol* 2001;75:303–310.
794. Wolffe EJ, Weisberg AS, Moss B. Role for the vaccinia virus A36R outer envelope protein in the formation of virus-tipped actin-containing microvilli and cell-to-cell virus spread. *Virology* 1998;244:20–26.
795. Woodson B. Vaccinia mRNA synthesis under conditions which prevent uncoating. *Biochem Biophys Res Commun* 1967;27:169–175.
796. Wright CF, Coroneos AM. Purification of the late transcription system of vaccinia virus: identification of a novel transcription factor. *J Virol* 1993;67:7264–7270.
797. Wright CF, Oswald BW, Dellis S. Vaccinia virus late transcription is activated in vitro by cellular heterogeneous nuclear ribonucleoproteins. *J Biol Chem* 2001;276:40680–40686.
798. Xiang Y, Latner DR, Niles EG, et al. Transcription elongation activity of the vaccinia virus J3 protein in vivo is independent of poly(A) polymerase stimulation. *Virology* 2000;269(2):356–369.
799. Xiang Y, Moss B. Correspondence of the functional epitopes of poxvirus and human interleukin-18-binding proteins. *J Virol* 2001;75(20):9947–9954.
800. Xiang Y, Moss B. IL-18 binding and inhibition of interferon gamma induction by human poxvirus-encoded proteins. *Proc Natl Acad Sci U S A* 1999;96(20):11537–11542.
801. Xiang Y, Moss B. Molluscum contagiosum virus interleukin-18 (IL-18) binding protein Is secreted as a full-length form that binds cell surface glycosaminoglycans through the C-terminal tail and a furin-cleaved form with only the IL-18 binding domain. *J Virol* 2003;77(4):2623–2630.
802. Xiang Y, Simpson DA, Spiegel J, et al. The vaccinia virus A18R DNA helicase is a postreplicative negative transcription elongation factor. *J Virol* 1998;72(9):7012–7023.
803. Xiao YH, Isaacs SN. Therapeutic vaccines and antibodies for treatment of orthopoxvirus infections. *Viruses* 2010;2(10):2381–2403.
804. Xu RH, Rubio D, Roscoe F, et al. Antibody inhibition of a viral type 1 interferon decoy receptor cures a viral disease by restoring interferon signaling in the liver. *PLoS Pathog* 2012;8(1):e1002475.
805. Yakovleva L, Chen SX, Hecht SM, et al. Chemical and traditional mutagenesis of vaccinia DNA topoisomerase provides insights to cleavage site recognition and transesterification chemistry. *J Biol Chem* 2008;283(23):16093–16103.
806. Yang SJ, Hruby DE. Vaccinia virus A12L protein and its AG/A proteolysis play an important role in viral morphogenic transition. *Virol J* 2007;4.
807. Yang Z, Bruno DP, Martens CA, et al. Genome-wide analysis of the 5′ and 3′ ends of vaccinia virus early mRNAs delineates regulatory sequences of annotated and anomalous transcripts. *J Virol* 2011;85(12):5897–5909.
808. Yang Z, Bruno DP, Martens CA, et al. Simultaneous high-resolution analysis of vaccinia virus and host cell transcriptomes by deep RNA sequencing. *Proc Natl Acad Sci U S A* 2010;107(25):11513–11518.
809. Yang Z, Moss B. Interaction of the vaccinia virus RNA polymerase-associated 94-kilodalton protein with the early transcription factor. *J Virol* 2009;83(23):12018–12026.
810. Yang Z, Reynolds SE, Martens CA, et al. Expression profiling of the intermediate and late stages of poxvirus replication. *J Virol* 2011;85:9899–9908.
811. Yang ZR, West AP, Bjorkman PJ. Crystal structure of TNF alpha complexed with a poxvirus MHC-related TNF binding protein. *Nat Struct Mol Biol* 2009;16(11):1189–1191.
812. Yeh WW, Moss B, Wolffe EJ. The vaccinia virus A9L gene encodes a membrane protein required for an early step in virion morphogenesis. *J Virol* 2000;74:9701–9711.
813. Yoshizawa JM, Li C, Gershon PD. Saltatory forward movement of a Poly(A) polymerase during Poly(A) tail addition. *J Biol Chem* 2007;282(26):19144–19151.
814. Yuen L, Davison AJ, Moss B. Early promoter-binding factor from vaccinia virions. *Proc Natl Acad Sci U S A* 1987;84:6069–6073.
815. Yuen L, Moss B. Oligonucleotide sequence signaling transcriptional termination of vaccinia virus early genes. *Proc Natl Acad Sci U S A* 1987;84:6417–6421.
816. Zaborowska I, Kellner K, Henry M, et al. Recruitment of host translation initiation factor eIF4G by the vaccinia virus ssDNA-binding protein I3. *Virology* 2012;425(1):11–22.
817. Zartouw HT. The chemical composition of vaccinia virus. *J Gen Microbiol* 1964;34:115–123.
818. Zhai DY, Yu E, Jin CF, et al. Vaccinia virus protein F1L is a caspase-9 inhibitor. *J Biol Chem* 2010;285(8):5569–5580.
819. Zhang F, Meng X, Townsend MB, et al. Identification of CP77 as the third orthopoxvirus SAMD9 and SAMD9L inhibitor with a unique specificity for a rodent SAMD9L. *J Virol* 2019;93(12):e00225-19.
820. Zhang J, Pekosz A, Lamb RA. Influenza virus assembly and lipid raft microdomains: a role for the cytoplasmic tails of the spike glycoproteins. *J Virol* 2000;74(10):4634–4644.
821. Zhang L, DeRider M, McCornack MA, et al. Solution structure of the complex between poxvirus-encoded CC chemokine inhibitor vCCI and human MIP-1 beta. *Proc Natl Acad Sci U S A* 2006;103(38):13985–13990.
822. Zhang P, Jacobs BL, Samuel CE. Loss of protein kinase PKR expression in human HeLa cells complements the vaccinia virus E3L deletion mutant phenotype by restoration of viral protein synthesis. *J Virol* 2008;82(2):840–848.
823. Zhang P, Langland JO, Jacobs BL, et al. Protein kinase PKR-dependent activation of mitogen-activated protein kinases occurs through mitochondrial adapter IPS-1 and is antagonized by vaccinia virus E3L. *J Virol* 2009;83(11):5718–5725.
824. Zhang Y, Ahn B-Y, Moss B. Targeting of a multicomponent transcription apparatus into assembling vaccinia virus particles requires RAP94, an RNA polymerase-associated protein. *J Virol* 1994;68:1360–1370.
825. Zhang Y, Moss B. Immature viral envelope formation is interrupted at the same stage by lac operator-mediated repression of the vaccinia virus D13L gene and by the drug rifampicin. *Virology* 1992;187:643–653.
826. Zhang Y, Moss B. Vaccinia virus morphogenesis is interrupted when expression of the gene encoding an 11-kilodalton phosphorylated protein is prevented by the *Escherichia coli lac* repressor. *J Virol* 1991;65:6101–6110.
827. Zhang YF, Keck JG, Moss B. Transcription of viral late genes is dependent on expression of the viral intermediate gene G8R in cells infected with an inducible conditional-lethal mutant vaccinia virus. *J Virol* 1992;66(11):6470–6479.
828. Zhou Q, Snipas S, Orth K, et al. Target protease specificity of the viral serpin CrmA. Analysis of five caspases. *J Biol Chem* 1997;272(12):7797–7800.

CHAPTER

17 Poxviruses

Panayampalli S. Satheshkumar • Inger K. Damon

INTRODUCTION

The family *Poxviridae* is extensive, with member species infecting insects (*Entomopoxvirinae*) and vertebrates (*Chordopoxvirinae*). This chapter focuses on vertebrate poxviruses (Table 17.1). Genera of poxviruses with species described to cause human illness are *Orthopoxvirus, Parapoxvirus, Yatapoxvirus,* and *Molluscipoxvirus.* The majority of human pathogenic poxvirus infections are zoonoses; only variola virus (VARV) and molluscum contagiosum (MCV) virus are sole human pathogens. The appearance and general structure of poxvirus virions is depicted in Figure 17.1.

ORTHOPOXVIRUSES

History

The orthopoxviruses are perhaps best known for their most notorious member, VARV, the causative agent of human smallpox. Smallpox was a febrile rash illness with a variable mortality rate extending to 30% to 40% in some outbreaks. The disease was understood to be a sole human pathogen; extensive experimental studies infecting closely related species failed to produce a viral infection that could be sustained in other host species. Recognition that an infectious agent that caused lesions on the skin and mucosal surfaces on cows and their caretakers could be used to prevent VARV infection was published by Jenner in 1798.[121] The viruses, cowpox- and later likely horsepox,[191] and vaccinia were used in the 19th and 20th centuries to prevent VARV infection; the use of the former virus (cowpox), the Latin for cow being vacca led to the term "vaccination." Previously, material derived from convalescent smallpox patients, usually scab material, was used either as an intranasal or percutaneous preparation (termed inoculation) to prevent smallpox in humans.[73] Ultimately, this, in part, led to our early understanding of the genus *Orthopoxvirus* (where at least cowpox virus, CPXV) was used to cross-protect against smallpox.[15] In addition, the unsuccessful use of infectious material from "spurious" lesions[159] for smallpox vaccinations, which were later recognized to be of parapoxvirus origin (termed paravaccinia or pseudocowpox), led to the recognition of this distinct group of poxviruses. Vaccinia virus (VACV), however, is the most comprehensively studied of the orthopoxviruses.

The history of smallpox and its eradication program has been chronicled in detail[73] and is available from the World Health Organization (WHO) Web site. Perhaps the earliest, most reliable accounts of smallpox are from China in the fourth century AD; contained in writings that distinguish the disease from measles, report that smallpox was endemic in the region,

TABLE 17.1 Host range and geographic distribution of genera and unclassified members of the subfamily *Chordopoxvirinae*

Genus and Species	Reservoir Host	Geographic Distribution	Other Infected Hosts
Orthopoxvirus			
Camelpox virus	Camels	Africa, Asia	Nil
Cowpox virus	Bank voles *Clethrionomys glareolus*, long-tailed field mouse *Apodemus sylvaticus*	Europe, western Asia	Cats, cattle, humans, zoo animals
Akhmeta virus	Rodents?	Europe	Cattle?
AK2015 (from Alaska)	?	Northern United States (Alaska)	?
Ectromelia virus	Rodents	Europe	Nil
Horsepox virus	?	Central Asia	Horses
Monkeypox virus	? Unknown—likely rodent	Western and central Africa	Monkeys, zoo animals, humans, prairie dogs
Raccoonpox virus	Raccoons	(Eastern) United States	Nil
Skunkpox virus	Skunks	(Western) United States	Nil
Taterapox virus	Gerbils (*Tatera kempii*)	Western Africa	Nil
Uasin Gishu virus	?	Eastern Africa	Horses
Vaccinia virus	?	?	Humans, rabbits, cows, river buffaloes (*Bubalis*)
Variola virus	Humans	Eradicated (formerly worldwide)	Nil
Volepox virus	California vole (*Microtus californicus*)	Western United States	Nil
Parapoxvirus			
Ausdyk virus	Camels	Africa, Asia	Nil
Bovine popular stomatitis virus	Cattle (beef)	Worldwide	Humans
Orf virus	Sheep, goats	Worldwide	Ruminants, humans
Pseudocowpox virus	Cattle (dairy)	Worldwide	Humans
Red deer poxvirus	Red deer	New Zealand	Nil
Seal parapoxvirus	Seals	Worldwide	Humans
Capripoxvirus			
Sheeppox virus	Sheep	Asia, Africa	Nil
Goatpox virus	Goats	Asia, Africa	Nil
Lumpy skin disease virus	? African cape buffalo	Africa	Cattle (*Bos taurus, Bos indicus*)
Suipoxvirus			
Swinepox virus	Swine	Worldwide	Nil
Leporipoxvirus			
Myxoma virus	*Sylvilagus brasiliensis* *Sylvilagus bachmani*	South America, western United States	*Oryctolagus*, other leporids
Fibroma virus	*Sylvilagus floridanus*	Eastern United States	*Oryctolagus*
Hare Fibroma virus	*Lepus capensis*	Europe	Nil
Squirrel fibroma virus	*Sciurus carolinensis*	Eastern United States	? Woodchuck
Western squirrel fibroma virus	*Sciurus griseus*	California	Nil
Yatapoxvirus			
Tanapox virus		Eastern and central Africa	Humans
Yaba poxvirus	? Primates	Western Africa	Humans
Molluscipoxvirus			
Molluscum contagiosum virus	Humans	Worldwide	Nil

(Continued)

TABLE 17.1 Host range and geographic distribution of genera and unclassified members of the subfamily *Chordopoxvirinae* (*Continued*)

Genus and Species	Reservoir Host	Geographic Distribution	Other Infected Hosts
Unclassified			
Crocodilepox	Crocodiles	Australia, South Africa	Nil
	Caimans	Florida	Nil
	Quokkas		
Cotia poxvirus	? Mice	Brazil	Nil
Squirrelpox virus	Grey squirrel	? Europe	*Sciurus vulgaris* (red squirrel)
Deerpox virus	? *Odocoileus hemionus* (North American mule deer)	North America	*Odocoileus hemionus* (North American mule deer)[121]
Mucocutaneous disease			
Avipoxvirus			
Many species	Birds	Worldwide	
NY014		Northern United States	
Murmansk virus	Root vole	Russia	
Salmon gill poxvirus	Salmon	Norway	
Eptestipox virus	*Eptesicus fuscus* (big brown bat)	United States	
Batpox virus	*Miniopterus schreibersii bassani* (Southern bent-wing bat)	Australia	
Batpox virus	*Pteropus scapulatus* (Little red flying fox)	Australia	
Batpox virus	*Eidolon helvum* (fruit bat)	Africa	
Hypsugopoxvirus	*Hypsugo savii* (insectivorous bat)	Europe	
Western grey kangaroo poxvirus, WKPV	*Macropus fuliginosus*	Australia	
Eastern grey kangaroo poxvirus, EKPV	*Macropus giganteus*	Australia	
Cetacean poxvirus	Dolphins	Europe	
Sea otter poxvirus	*Enhydra lutris kenyoni*	United States	

and report the disease was introduced from the west in 48 AD.[73] Early practices from the 10th to the 18th centuries to control disease included quarantine, intranasal insufflation with powdered smallpox scabs, and cutaneous inoculation with pulverized smallpox scabs. With the recognition that vaccination with cowpox or vaccinia would diminish iatrogenic VARV cases, improvements in disease control were seen. By 1953, smallpox had been eliminated from Europe. The development of freeze-dried vaccine preparations permitted vaccination in areas outside the cold chain. Largely through the global efforts in improvement of public health surveillance and disease control methods and the design and implementation of WHO-sponsored vaccination programs, the disease smallpox was declared eradicated in 1980 by the WHO. The last naturally occurring cases of smallpox occurred in the Indian subcontinent in 1975 and in the Horn of Africa in 1977. Remaining stocks of VARV were subsequently moved to two designated WHO Collaborating Centers for Smallpox and Other Poxvirus Infections with maximum containment laboratory facilities. The dismantling of population-based vaccination programs began in 1980. The eradication of smallpox and the discontinuation of vaccination programs likely contribute to the increase in observations of other human orthopoxvirus infections since 1980. Also, it has enhanced the concerns that if unknown stocks of VARV exist and were to be used, the effects on our current population would be profound.

Infectious Agent

By electron microscopy, the orthopoxviruses are large brick-shaped particles; as with all other poxviruses, the virus replicates and matures within the cytoplasm of the host cell. The viral steps involved in entry, fusion, morphogenesis, and release of virus are described in Chapter 16 as well as in a number of detailed reviews.[181,219] By light microscopy, cytopathic effects in monkey kidney cell lines are apparent and profound. Cell rounding and detachment from neighbor cells is followed by formation of elongated cellular lamellipodia[227]; ultimately, cells detach from the substrate. Similar to other poxvirus genomes, the nuclear material is a covalently closed double-stranded genome. Genome length ranges from 170 to 250 kilobase pairs, and its composition is 34% G+C. The central 90 kbp of the central region is highly conserved and contains virion structural genes and enzymes responsible for its DNA replication and mRNA transcription; the terminal regions are varied across species and encode genes involved in the host–pathogen

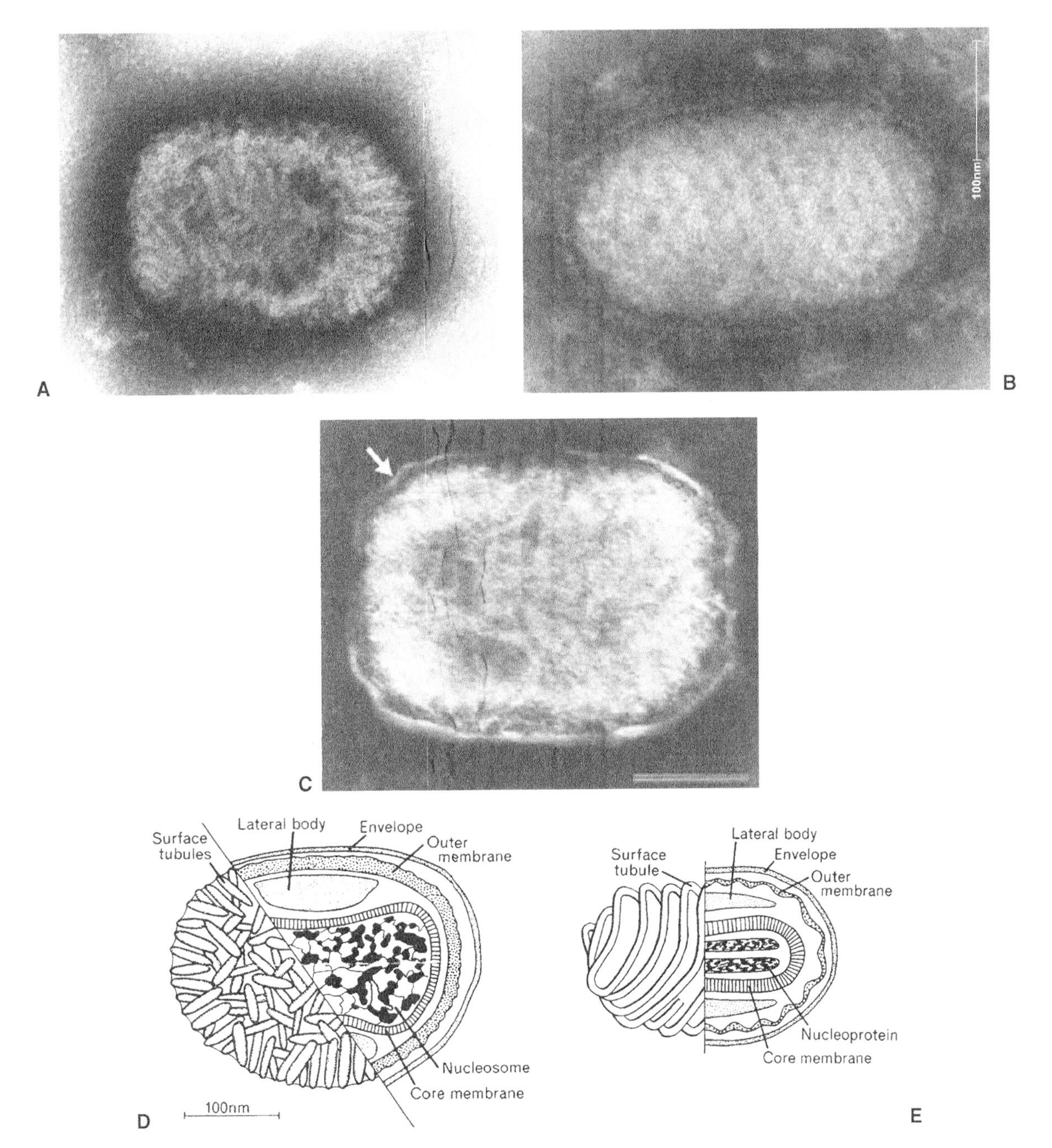

FIGURE 17.1 Negative stain electron microscopic appearance of orthopoxviruses **(A)**, parapoxviruses **(B)**, and yatapoxviruses **(C)**. Schematic diagram of structure of orthopoxvirus virion in **(D)** and of parapoxvirus virion in **(E)**. The structure of the yatapoxvirus and molluscipoxvirus virions is similar to that of the orthopoxvirus virion. As seen in **(C)**, clinical material from the yatapoxvirus tanapox often contains virion forms with enveloped virions (extracellular enveloped virions [EEVs]; see *arrow*). Knobby, brick-shaped virion forms, consistent with mature virions (MVs), are more often seen in clinical material from orthopoxvirus infections. Parapoxviruses are ovoid and smaller, with a distinctive criss-cross filament pattern derived from the wrapping of a surface tubule **(B)**. *Bars* indicate 100 nm. **D:** Drawing of a brick-shaped virion typical of an orthopoxvirus. Viral genome DNA and several proteins within the core are organized as a nucleosome. The core has a 9-nm-thick membrane with a regular subunit structure. By negative stain techniques, the virion core assumes a dumbbell shape with large lateral bodies occupying the concavities. The core and lateral bodies are enclosed within a lipoprotein structure, the outer membrane, which is 12 nm thick. The outer membrane surface appears to consist of irregularly shaped tubules that produce the knobby or mulberry-like M form seen in **(A)**. The majority of infectious virions remain cell associated; others acquire an additional envelope composed of host cellular membrane and virus-specific proteins. These associate on the cell surface to spread to neighboring cells or are released as EEVs to allow more distant spread. **E:** Schematic drawing of parapoxvirus virion showing wrapping pattern of the outer protein tubule, which appears to wrap around the virus. (**A:** Courtesy of Centers for Disease Control and Prevention. **B:** Courtesy of A. Likos. **C:** From Dhar AD, Werchniak AE, Li Y, et al. Tanapox infection in a college student. *N Engl J Med* 2004;350(4):361–366. Copyright © 2004 Massachusetts Medical Society. Reprinted with permission from Massachusetts Medical Society. **D and E:** Reprinted by permission from Springer: Fenner F, Nakano JH. *Poxviridae*: the poxviruses. In: Lenette EH, Halonen P, Murphy FA, eds. *Laboratory Diagnosis of Infectious Diseases: Principles and Practice*. Vol II. Viral, Rickettsial and Chlamydial Diseases. New York, NY: Springer-Verlag; 1988:177–210. Copyright © 1988 Springer-Verlag New York Inc.)

TABLE 17.2 Biologic properties of orthopoxviruses that can infect humans

Property	Variola	Monkeypox	Vaccinia	Cowpox
Host range	Narrow	Broad	Broad	Broad
Pocks of the chorioallantoic membrane (CAM)	Small, opaque, white	Small, opaque, hemorrhagic	Strains vary; large, opaque, white or hemorrhagic	Large, hemorrhagic
Ceiling growth temperature on CAM (°C)	37.5–38.5	39	41	40
Rabbit skin lesion	Small transient, nontransmissible	Indurated, hemorrhagic	Strains very; indurated nodule, sometimes hemorrhagic	Large, indurated hemorrhagic
Lethality for:				
Mice	Low	High	High to very high	Variable
Chick embryo	Low	Medium	Very high	High
A-type inclusion bodies	No	No	No	Yes
B-type inclusion bodies	Yes	Yes	Yes	Yes
Genome DNA size (kbp)	186	191	192	220

interaction. In addition to nucleic acid-based techniques, classification of orthopoxviral species has also been accomplished based on various biological properties (Table 17.2). These include the presence (or absence) of acidophilic-type inclusion (ATI) bodies, cytoplasmic structures containing collections of virions, and seen in cowpox, ectromelia, raccoonpox, volepox, and skunkpox infections. However, as additional sequence information becomes available, classification of viruses is becoming more complex. For instance, phylogenetic analysis of strains within species was initially supportive for at least two clades of CPXV.[92] A recent analysis, using additional CPXV genome sequences, demonstrates four distinct clades.[39,78] Current information is supportive of two clades of monkeypox virus[47,158] and two or three clades of VARV.[68,155,197] The majority of the orthopoxviruses appears to have a broad host range, although the spectrum of disease may vary, depending on what host is infected. This is exemplified by cowpox, which causes discrete localized lesions on the udders of cows but appears to cause a systemic disease in cats. The exception is VARV, which as we understand the virus, was a sole pathogen of humans and humans appeared to be the sole host. A review on the cellular host range of poxviruses is available.[171,193,197,265]

Pathogenesis and Pathology

Orthopoxvirus infections can be classified as systemic or localized (at the site of virus entry) illnesses. Generalized disease usually manifests with rash. The type of infection that results is dependent on the species of orthopoxvirus, the route of entry, and the genus/species of susceptible animal and its immune status. For this chapter, infections of humans and models to understand infections of normal host humans are largely described. In some cases, understanding of the natural pathogenesis is limited due to the lack of data on the disease pathogenesis in its natural host. The most obvious example is VARV. Although clinical descriptions of disease are well notated from early medical writings, the specifics of human pathogenesis are largely derived from inferences evaluating other (e.g., ectromelia, which causes mousepox infection in mice, rabbitpox in rabbits, and monkeypox in nonhuman primates) orthopoxvirus virus species infections of various animal models.[36,44,84,129] Other respiratory challenge animal models of orthopoxvirus disease are the intranasal vaccinia and intranasal or aerosol CPXV challenges of mice.[101,167] These appear to primarily cause upper and lower respiratory infection; virus antigen predominates in the sinuses, intranasal passages, trachea, airways, and lungs. Some evidence of viremic spread is suggested by occasional lesions in the skin or bone marrow.

Nonetheless, the use of animal models of systemic or localized disease, in combination, will be useful in determining efficacy of various therapeutic and/or prophylactic disease mitigation and prevention strategies. Intranasal or aerosol challenge models have been developed using many of the orthopoxviruses in different animal species to represent a respiratory route of infection. Different routes of exposure result in differences in disease pathogeneses, involve some different sets of viral proteins, and provide information relevant to understanding disease acquired via contact versus respiratory routes of transmission.[254] Contact transmission has been classically modeled in the footpad model of infection of mouse species with ectromelia,[69] and more recently, in the dermal ear model with vaccinia, which also provides a model for understanding the immune response to multiple puncture immunization in eliciting (vaccination) protection against smallpox. Models of specific disease manifestations in various immunocompromised hosts have also been developed in order to evaluate the effect of various host factors in both disease pathogenesis and response to, containment of, and clearance of pathogen.

Systemic Disease Pathogenesis

Entry

The cellular receptor used by poxviruses for entry into their host cells is unknown. Member viruses have a broad tropism for entry into tissue culture cells; usually it is the later steps that inhibit completion of the viral maturation process to produce infectious progeny and affect "host range".[171,200] A summary of *in vitro* research on *in vitro* (orthopoxvirus) viral entry and fusion mechanisms is available.[180,181] The portal of entry for orthopoxvirus infection is usually considered to be percutaneous (via contact) or the respiratory tract. Oral routes of exposure have also been reported if very large doses of ectromelia virus (ECTV) are administered[72] to mice; this has been proposed to be a potential route of exposure for cats to cowpox and squirrels to monkeypox.[75] However, investigations associated around a laboratory-associated outbreak in a mouse colony suggested that the natural route of transmission is through abrasions in the skin after exposure to infected animals or contaminated fomites.[263] The route of infection also affects the disease course. Inoculation of variola, when unsuccessful as a form of disease prevention and caused iatrogenic disease, demonstrated a compressed time from infection to illness with respect to that seen with respiratory acquired disease. Transmission of human smallpox is thought to occur via an upper respiratory route of infection, which is consistent with the typical time frame of disease; infection via contact with contaminated fomites has also been observed. The exposure route/portal of entry for human monkeypox infection may be either percutaneous or upper respiratory; the clinical disease course varies with route of infection.[215] To model a respiratory route of exposure, a variety of aerosol challenges with various orthopoxviruses have been used to infect various animal species; these may produce initial stages of disease that occur in lower portions of the respiratory tract than seen in natural human infection. An alternative exposure route has been intranasal challenges.[84,94,116,167,217,267] For one North American orthopoxvirus, volepox, mechanical arthropod vectors have been suggested as a route of transmission to California voles[213]; this has not been observed in other orthopoxviruses, although it is a route of transmission, and portal of entry, for fowlpox and *Capripoxvirus* and *Leporipoxvirus* species. Importantly, in rabbitpox virus challenge studies, natural respiratory/airborne transmission appeared to occur over 12 feet.[267]

Site of Primary Replication

When the skin is the portal of entry, studies with ectromelia have suggested that the virus needs to be introduced to the dermis if systemic infection is to eventually ensue.[218] Virus replicates in the Malpighian layer of the epidermis, and dermal infection consisted of fibroblasts and histiocytes; the latter were likely responsible for subsequent movement of virus to the lymphatics to initiate the course of events required for systemic illness.

When the respiratory tract has been used as portal of entry, in experimental aerosol infections, likely dependent on particle size, a combination of upper and lower respiratory tract infection has occurred. Viral replication occurred in alveolar macrophages and small bronchioles, then moving to regional pulmonary lymph nodes. Epidemiologic understanding of the natural human infections with VARV to cause smallpox suggests that the common method of transmission was via a respiratory route. Primary infection is believed to have occurred within the mucosal surfaces of the nasopharyngeal tract, then moving to the regional lymphatics by extrapolation from that seen with ectromelia and rabbitpox virus studies. A recent review of aerosolized rabbitpox virus infection in rabbits is available.[262]

Virus Spread

Our understanding of orthopoxvirus spread after initial infection and spread to regional lymphatics comes again from studies of ectromelia in mice, rabbitpox in rabbits, and monkeypox in nonhuman primates. The use of fluorescent-antibody stains of fixed tissues and titers of infectious virus in organs at various time points in disease has provided the majority of this information. With reporter viruses expressing firefly luciferase gene, live imaging and progression of viral spread is monitored with imagers limiting the need for serial sacrifice.[5,163,274] Virus moves from the regional lymphatics to the bloodstream to cause a primary viremia, then multiplies in the spleen, liver, bone marrow, and other reticuloendothelial organs. After this, a second viremic period ensues, followed by seeding of distant sites, specifically the skin, and generation of the characteristic generalized rash. Virus particles are mostly cell associated during viremic phases of disease. In ectromelia, the virus replication in the macrophages of the liver spreads to the parenchymal cells of the liver causing necrosis; similar pronounced replication and effect of virus is found in spleen and bone marrow. In certain inbred mouse species, the disease is so pronounced at this stage that mortality ensues prior to development of rash.[36]

Experimental challenge studies of monkeypox virus infection, which clinically resembles smallpox more than mousepox, have been done in several species of animals, including nonhuman primates, and have demonstrated infectivity and pathogenesis through a number of routes of infection, including aerosol, intranasal, or parenteral administrations.[44,113,185,275] Initially, after aerosol infection in cynomolgus macaques, there is regional lymph node uptake and replication of virus in lymphoid organs, followed by viremia. An eruption begins, with lesions forming macules, papules, vesicles, pustules, and crusts to scar formation from days 6 to 23 of infection. Areas of inflammation and cell necrosis have been seen in tonsils, lymph nodes, digestive tract, testes, ovaries, kidneys, liver, and lungs. Epithelial degeneration, necrosis, and intracytoplasmic bodies have been seen in skin and mucous membranes. Based on the infection and transmission of MPXV in prairie dogs observed during 2003 U.S. outbreak, several studies characterized prairie dogs as a model for MPXV/systemic orthopoxvirus disease pathogenesis.[112,114,116] MPXV infection in prairie dogs closely resembles that of human symptoms including a prodromal period and skin lesions making it an attractive model to check the effect of vaccines and antivirals.[131,244] Similarly, other potential reservoir hosts of MPXV, dormice, Gambian rats and African rope squirrels, were susceptible to MPXV infection.[70,115,234] As a mouse model, the CAST/EiJ strain was identified to be highly susceptible to MPXV infection and useful to study MPXV pathogenesis.[4] Use of high doses of variola in nonhuman primate challenges, via parenteral route of administration, produced a severe illness with hemorrhagic manifestations of disease.[120] Apoptosis and a disregulated cytokine response are believed to be responsible for what has previously been referred to as the "toxemia" of smallpox. Despite several attempts, other rodent animal models to study VARV pathogenesis, like prairie dogs and CAST-EiJ mice, did not replicate classical systemic orthopoxvirus illness signs and symptoms, although CAST-EiJ manifest adaptive humoral responses to infection.[40,80]

Pathology

Cytoplasmic inclusion bodies are a typical histopathological feature of orthopoxvirus infections. Two morphologies (Fig. 17.2) are manifest: A-type inclusion bodies, where virions are clustered within an intracytoplasmic structure (Fig. 17.2D), or B-type inclusions (Guarneri bodies), which are perinuclear and contain the viroplasm and maturing viral particles. Not all

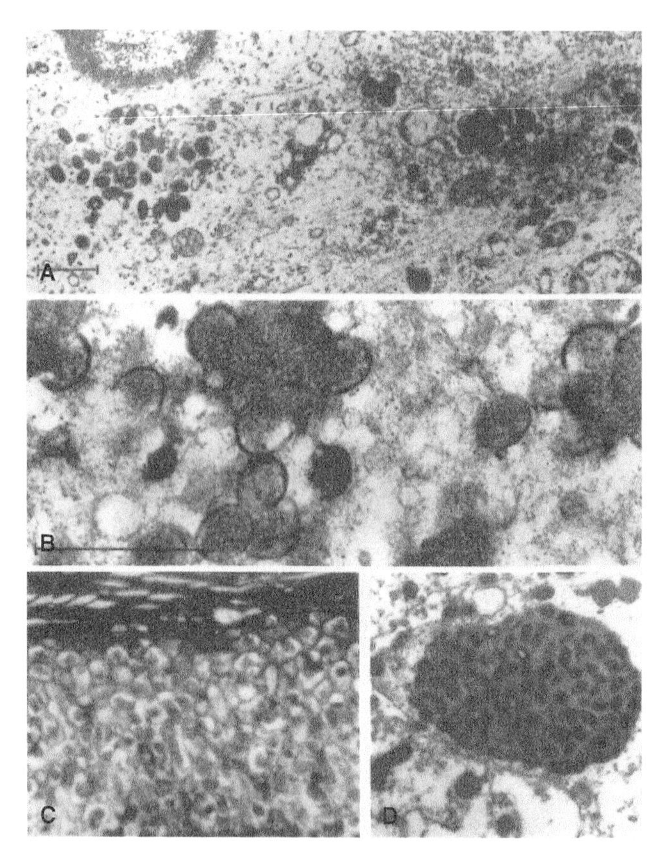

FIGURE 17.2 Cytoplasmic inclusion bodies produced by poxviruses. A and **B:** Electron micrographs of viral cytoplasmic factories that manifest by light microscopy as B-type inclusions; these structures are basophilic by hematoxylin-and-eosin staining. In **(A)**, rounded structures, the immature virions (IVs), are seen on the right, and the nonenveloped intracellular virions (IMVs) are seen on the left. In **(B)**, a higher-power magnification demonstrating the IVs and the earlier crescent-shaped progenitor forms. **C and D:** A-type inclusion bodies (ATIs) visualized by light microscopy **(C)** and electron microscopy **(D)**. **C:** Hematoxylin-and-eosin staining of mouse skin demonstrating eosinophilic intracytoplasmic structures in the skin of a mouse infected with ectromelia. **D:** Electron micrograph of mature cowpox virions within an ATI. (**A:** From Payne LG, Kristenson K. Mechanism of vaccinia virus release and its specific inhibition by N1-isonicotinoyl-N2-3-methyl-4-chlorobenzoylhydrazine. *J Virol* 1979;32(2):614–622. Copyright © 1979 American Society for Microbiology. Reproduced with permission from American Society for Microbiology. **B:** From Stern W, Pogo BG, Dales S. Biogenesis of poxviruses: analysis of the morphogenetic sequence using a conditional lethal mutant defective in envelope self-assembly. *Proc Natl Acad Sci USA* 1977;74(5):2162–2166. Reprinted with permission from Beatriz GT Pogo, MD. **C:** reprinted from Fenner F. Mousepox. In: Foster HL, Small JD, Fox JG, eds. *The Mouse in Biomedical Research*, Vol. II: Diseases. San Diego, Calif: Academic Press; 1982:209–230. Copyright © 1982 Elsevier. With permission. **D:** Photo courtesy of Y. Ichihashi.)

orthopoxviruses form A-type inclusions; a longer predicted form of the A-type protein (ATI) (130–160 kD vs. 90 kD) appears to be required. In cowpox, the A-type inclusion is termed a Downie body; in ectromelia, it is termed a Marchal body. The North American orthopoxviruses also form A-type inclusions. Notably, VARV, MPXV, VACV, and horsepox virus encode truncated ATI open reading frames and do not form inclusion bodies. In animal studies, loss of ATI or inclusion body formation was correlated to enhanced virulence/pathogenesis.[130]

In humans, it is the rash that has been extensively studied during smallpox disease pathogenesis. The viral lesion primarily develops in the epidermis, although early changes of capillary dilation, endothelial cell swelling, and perivascular cuffing with lymphocytes, macrophages, plasma cells, and eosinophils are seen in the papillary layer of the dermis prior to development of the rash lesion. Subsequently, within the epidermis, the cells of the Malpighian layer swell and vacuolate to undergo ballooning degeneration. B-type inclusions could be seen in the cytoplasm. The cytoplasm continues to enlarge, loss of nuclear material is noted, and coalescence of vacuoles via cell rupture creates reticulating degeneration of the middle and upper layers of the stratum spinosum. In the next stages, the vesicle is formed. Cells of the lower stratum spinosum and basal layer exhibit nuclear condensation and nuclei fragment. The cavity of the vesicle (later the pustule) thus develops adjacent to the dermis, permitting the "deep-seated" feel of the smallpox pustular lesions. The cavity retains some cellular remnants that create a multiloculated appearance, also adding to the firmness of the lesion. When polymorphonuclear cells move into the cavity, pustulation occurs. High titers of virus are found within the lesions.[31] In mucosal surfaces, the absence of a horny layer allowed the necrosis caused by proliferation of virus within the epithelium to create ulcers and led to liberation of large quantities of virus into the oropharynx.[228]

Evaluation of other organs in human smallpox has been done in select autopsies from cases where death was attributed to ordinary or hemorrhagic forms of smallpox.[31] Some of the observations from autopsies of ordinary smallpox case deaths have been that, unlike ectromelia, liver and spleen do not show as extensive evidence of viral replication and necrosis that is seen in ectromelia infection of susceptible mice. In general, mild pathological changes are seen in the lungs. This is in contrast to the more severe lung pathology seen in apparent cowpox infection of captive felines, which caused death and was associated with severe bronchopneumonia.[166] Similarly, pulmonary disease has been seen in respiratory rabbitpox infection of rabbits, where in addition to subpleural nodules, focal areas of consolidation were noted.[88]

The pathology of the localized lesions of cowpox in humans has been studied. The lesions are characterized by a marked inflammatory and erythematous response.[17] The bulk of the lesion is caused by hypertrophy and proliferation of the basal cell layer of the epidermis, together with massive inflammatory infiltration. Infection usually spreads into follicles, and typical A-type inclusions are usually seen.

Immune Response: Primary Infection

Early responses to virus infection are the production of interferons, nitric oxide, and elicitation of natural killer (NK) and macrophage cellular functions prior to the development of adaptive, antigen-directed B- and T-cell responses. Both complement pathways are also activated by the host in response to virus infection. Studies of ECTV infection in various mice deficient in one or more immune response pathways demonstrate the importance of IFN-γ, granzymes A and B, perforin, and CD4 and CD8 T cells in clearance of primary infection. Antibody is also essential.[45,46,198] Additional studies in other orthopoxviruses demonstrate successful clearance of a primary orthopoxvirus infection to be dependent on the adequate production of interferon-γ and Th1 cytokines[208] to promote an effective cytotoxic T-lymphocyte (CTL) effector response. Experiments where high levels of IL-4 are produced early in infection, expressed from recombinant challenge poxvirus, show delayed or inhibited ability of the host to clear the recombinant poxvirus and evade antiviral inhibition.[7,118,239] In secondary infection, as in the circumstance of infection post vaccination with a heterologous orthopoxvirus, antibody alone may be sufficient.[199] This latter finding has also been demonstrated in vaccine provided protection for monkeypox infection.[63]

Macrophages and NK cells are involved in early responses to infection and are used for clearance of orthopoxvirus infections.[71,128] The secreted interferons are needed for containment of primary orthopoxvirus infections.[163,222] The cellular secretion of tumor necrosis factor is another host response to orthopoxvirus infection. Viral infection can induce apoptosis, and the poxviruses have a number of strategies to inhibit apoptosis, which are also involved in host range, that have been reviewed[97,265] and are described in Chapter 16. One of the strategies that the orthopoxviruses have evolved is soluble secreted proteins to bind the host cytokines, complement C3b and C4b, chemokines, interferons, and their receptors. These include viral proteins that bind TNF, IL-1β, and IFN-γ via secretion of an ortholog of the mammalian protein that lacks its intermembranous and signaling portions. The orthopoxviral proteins that bind the type I interferons, as well as those that bind IL-18 (which regulates IFN-γ) and the chemokines, have apparently evolved to develop a structure distinct from the mammalian receptors for these immune response proteins; the IL-18–binding proteins have similarity to the mammalian IL-18 regulatory-binding proteins.

Studies designed to better define the pathogenesis of adverse effects of current replicative vaccinia used as smallpox vaccine in individuals with atopic dermatitis (AD) provide additional information about the early steps in viral pathogenesis and the normal and aberrant host innate immune responses, as well as factors important in containment of viral infection to produce localized disease. In AD, there is an abundant Th2 response.[21] Human skin explant models have been developed to understand eczema vaccinatum (EV), the dissemination of vaccine virus in individuals with AD.[107] In human AD skin, an abundance of Th2 cytokines IL-4 and IL-13 (with respect to normal skin) diminish the effectiveness of an innate immune response to VACV, in a STAT-6–dependent manner, allowing increased replication of virus. In normal skin, viral replication is inhibited by cathelicidins. In human keratinocytes infected by vaccinia, the cathelicidin LL-37 is down-regulated through the effects of IL-4 and IL-13.[108] Limited animal models for AD have been developed to study pathogenesis of OPXV infections. ECTV infection in an AD mouse model developed EV with large skin lesions and high viral loads, and disease could be treated with antivirals and antibodies. The use of the replication-deficient modified vaccinia Ankara (MVA) for preexposure vaccination and protection from lethal ECTV challenge has been demonstrated in this model.[2]

The orthopoxviruses have strategies to inhibit intracellular antiviral effects of the interferons.[243] All orthopoxviruses sequenced to date have a homolog of the vaccinia E3L protein, and most have a homolog of the K3L protein. The E3L gene is truncated in MPXV and Volepox, even though MPXV is still pathogenic in humans. E3L homologs bind dsRNA and have at least two functions: one is to inactivate the IFN-induced dsRNA-dependent protein kinase (PKR) and the other is to inactivate 2′5′-oligoadenylate synthetase. K3L mimics eIF-2α, which prevents eIF-2α phosphorylation and inhibits autophosphorylation (activation) of PKR. Interestingly, this gene is absent from most strains of MPXV. E3L inhibition of PKR also interferes with its proapoptotic functions[19,138,152] to affect cellular host range of VACV. VACV lacking E3L, grown in nonpermissive cells significantly expand the K3L region of genome, after continuous passages, to compensate for the lack of E3.[64] This type of genomic accordion (expansion or reduction of genomes based on the selective pressures) is documented in other cases, as well, demonstrating an effective mechanism to overcome host cell inhibition by poxviruses.[67] Of note, one set of monkeypox clinical samples, associated with the emergence of monkeypox in South Sudan, contained a sizeable genomic duplication of multiple ORFs; the significance of this is unknown.[184] A number of orthopoxvirus proteins have also been identified that interfere in various intracellular steps of the IL-1R and TLR signaling pathways, ultimately regulating the NF-κB pathway[179] and interferon regulatory factors (IRFs). Two vaccinia proteins appear to act early in the pathway and target multiple nonoverlapping TLR pathways; A52R and A46R both block NF-κB activation. A VACV with A52R deleted appears attenuated *in vivo*. A46R inhibits TRIF-dependent signaling to inhibit IRF3 activation and TRIF-dependent gene induction.[247] TRIF may have an additional role in inhibition of vaccinia replication in the macrophage.[105] The product of the vaccinia A52 ORF has the ability to block NF-κB activation via a number of pathways. Additional vaccinia proteins (K1L and N1L) block specific steps further downstream in the signaling pathway for NF-κB activation.[60,241]

The orthopoxviruses also express proteins that interfere with various steps in apoptosis.[205] The vaccinia F1L protein interferes with mitochondrial components of the apoptotic cascade[264] through interaction with Bak. The serpin, SPI-2 (vaccinia) or crmA (cowpox), inhibits caspases 1 and 8; the latter effect protects target cells against CTL lysis induced by the Fas pathway.

The host–pathogen relationship of orthopoxviruses is complex and involves many host and viral factors. Using siRNA or genetic screens using insertional inactivation, requirement of host proteins and exploitation of host cell pathways for OPXV infection were characterized.[18,164,176,210,242] These studies demonstrate a multitude of different mechanism adopted by OPXV for establishing successful infection. Host responses to pathogenic and nonpathogenic orthopoxvirus infections examined using microarray techniques[33,93] provide additional information regarding complex host–pathogen interactions. In variola parenterally infected nonhuman primates, which models aspects of the second viremia and subsequent disease course in severe forms of smallpox,[120] peripheral blood mononuclear cell transcripts showed an increase in interferon-associated gene transcripts not evident in animals that rapidly succumbed to infection.[226] There was also a significant up-regulation of Ig gene transcripts. Overall, there were minimal TNF-α and NF-κB responses.

Immune Response: Vaccination

The protective effects of smallpox vaccination and correlates of protection remain an area of active investigation.[76] Vaccinia strains provided an effective strategy for use as a live viral vaccine to prevent smallpox and to facilitate disease eradication. Smallpox disease was declared eradicated 40 years ago, at a time when the current advances in immunology were not available to dissect the mechanisms of protection. Although some studies demonstrated high levels of neutralizing antibody after vaccination or smallpox infection were protective,[229] other studies have demonstrated the level of CD8+ T-cell memory correlates with protection from subsequent viral disease.[268] A number of studies have demonstrated long-lived Ig and T-cell responses to smallpox vaccination[99,100]; individuals vaccinated in childhood demonstrate long-lived B-cell memory response, a longer duration of CD4 T-cell memory than CD8 T-cell memory,[3,51] which may be important for long-term B-cell memory.

However, previous remote childhood smallpox vaccination was not completely protective against acquisition of the related disease monkeypox when it was introduced in the United States in 2003.[127] Studies with ECTV infection in mice demonstrate the requirement of a virus-neutralizing antibody response, even in the absence of CD8+ T cells, in order to control a pathogenic virus challenge after immunization.

Release From Host

For smallpox, data on virus shedding show infectious virus in the oropharyngeal secretions, with lesser amounts in the urine and conjunctivae.[230] Levels of virus in oropharyngeal secretions were highest just after rash onset between 3 to 4 days post fever onset, the clinical manifestation of the secondary viremia; however, virus could be detected up to 2 weeks post fever onset in cases with more pronounced rash (confluent disease). Virus could be detected in urine over approximately the same time period during illness. In localized orthopoxvirus infections, such as vaccination with VACV (smallpox vaccination), virus can be found at the lesion until the scab separates.[143]

Epidemiology

Of the orthopoxviruses that infect humans, only VARV is not a zoonotic infection. Interhuman transmission of VARV occurred through the inhalation of large airborne respiratory droplets, containing infectious virus from infected persons. Transmission usually required prolonged face to face or other close contact, although airborne transmission over longer distances had been reported.[73] Transmission via fomites or contact with the infectious material from the rash also occurred. Aggregate data, collected during the smallpox eradication campaign, suggest a secondary attack rate of 58.4% in unvaccinated close or household contacts and a secondary attack rate of 3.8% in previously vaccinated close or household contacts.[73] Case fatality rates for variola major varied with the type of disease manifest, but aggregate rates of 10% to 30% in various outbreaks have been recorded. Severity of disease correlated with rash burden and was also more severe in children and pregnant women. Variola alastrim minor, a variant of VARV with a case fatality rate of less than 1%, but manifest with apparent similar epidemiologic features of human-to-human transmission.

Monkeypox has a more complex epidemiology; two genetically discrete virus clades have been described,[47,158] with apparent distinct clinical and epidemiologic parameters. Identification of human infections, in Western and Central Africa, was first made in 1970. Investigations in 1980s in the Congo Basin country Zaire, now the Democratic Republic of Congo (DRC), demonstrated that human-to-human transmission of monkeypox was less than that of smallpox. The secondary attack rate in unvaccinated contacts of monkeypox cases were calculated to be 9.3% versus 37% to 88% for smallpox.[123] Prior smallpox vaccination (3–19 years previously) appeared to be 85% protective at preventing disease acquisition in contacts and also ameliorated disease severity. Overall, although the majority of cases identified acquired disease from a presumed animal exposure(s), only 28% of cases were ascribed to person-to-person transmission. A case fatality rate of approximately 10% was observed in unvaccinated persons; the majority of fatalities and severest disease manifestations was observed in children younger than the age of 5. Serosurveys suggested that subclinical infection may have occurred in up to 28% of close contacts of monkeypox patients in some communities, which may have contributed to the rarity of sustained generations of human-to-human transmission in household and other close contact situations.

Because the majority of cases were believed to have acquired disease through animal exposures, case–control studies were attempted in the 1980s to determine the source of infection. These were not definitive because the population appeared to have multiple daily contacts with the same animals in settlements, forests, or cleared agricultural areas. Among primary cases, recent close contact via hunting, skinning, killing, cooking, or playing with carcasses was identified to *Cercopithecus, Colobus*, and *Cercocebus* primate; *Cricetomys* terrestrial rodent; and *Funisciurus* and *Heliosciurus* squirrel species. Ecologic studies, usually using convenience samples of animals collected in areas surrounding human cases in West and Central Africa, demonstrated orthopoxvirus and sometimes monkeypox-specific seroprevalence in various members of these species but were not reported for *Cricetomys* species. This work has been comprehensively reviewed.[123] Virus was only found in one euthanized, moribund squirrel species *Funisciurus anerythrus*. The prevailing hypothesis was that squirrel species were the likely reservoir of disease. Near the end of the 1980s, disease surveillance and associated studies waned after modeling studies based on the epidemiologic observations of secondary attack rates from human-to-human exposure suggested that limited number of transmission events were feasible, even with low population immunity provided by waning immunization rates in the populations of Central Africa. The virus had not, therefore, adapted to survive solely through human infection and would not manifest with the same human-to-human transmission dynamics of smallpox. This work also led to the recommendations to not continue routine smallpox vaccination in individuals considered at risk for monkeypox infection.

A re-emergence of disease was noted in 1996 in the DRC; a salient observation from a series of investigations was that more cases were derived from secondary human-to-human contact (88%) than seen in 1981 to 1986 investigations (28%). This was, in part, attributed to a larger population of humans fully susceptible to disease because of the cessation of routine smallpox vaccination in 1980 after smallpox eradication. Another observation was that disease epidemiology showed more cases in the older child/young adult population.[111] Disease mortality (1%) was observed to be lower than previously seen in 1981 to 1986. This may have been due to a smaller demographic of very young children (ages 0–4 years) being infected, may have been due to technical limitations on the investigations, or may have been due to the inclusion of chickenpox cases in the case definition. Whereas previous ecologic serosurveys of animal populations had implicated tree squirrels as having significant orthopoxvirus seroreactivity, these investigations were the first to show orthopoxvirus seroprevalence in terrestrial rodents (*Cricetomys emini*) and in one domestic pig (*Sus scrofa*) sampled. Outbreaks of monkeypox, some with apparent high interhuman transmissibility,[150] and ongoing surveillance documents an increased incidence of monkeypox in regions of the Congo Basin.[216] In addition, MPXV was detected in several West African countries in the 21st century after the absence of reported cases for several decades (Fig. 17.3).[22,214]

Monkeypox virus was introduced to the United States (U.S.) in 2003 via a consignment of wild-captured animals from the West African country of Ghana. The virus was identified as belonging to a distinct clade of monkeypox, which included previous West African monkeypox isolates and isolates derived from earlier outbreaks in primate colonies. Detailed comparison of the clinical and epidemiologic characteristics of the U.S. cases (imported from West Africa) with DRC cases from 1981 to 1986 demonstrated significant differences in human disease manifestation[158]; pronounced rash and more severe illness were seen in the Congo Basin cases. Controlling for age and vaccination status, disease severity remained more extreme in the Congo Basin than in the U.S. case patients. Monkeypox-related mortality and human-to-human transmission were only seen in the Congo Basin, but a recent outbreak of MPXV WA clade in Nigeria demonstrated human-to-human transmissions.[270] In addition, travel-related monkeypox cases spread to the United Kingdom, Israel, and Singapore from MPXV outbreak in West Africa demonstrating, again, the potential risk for introduction

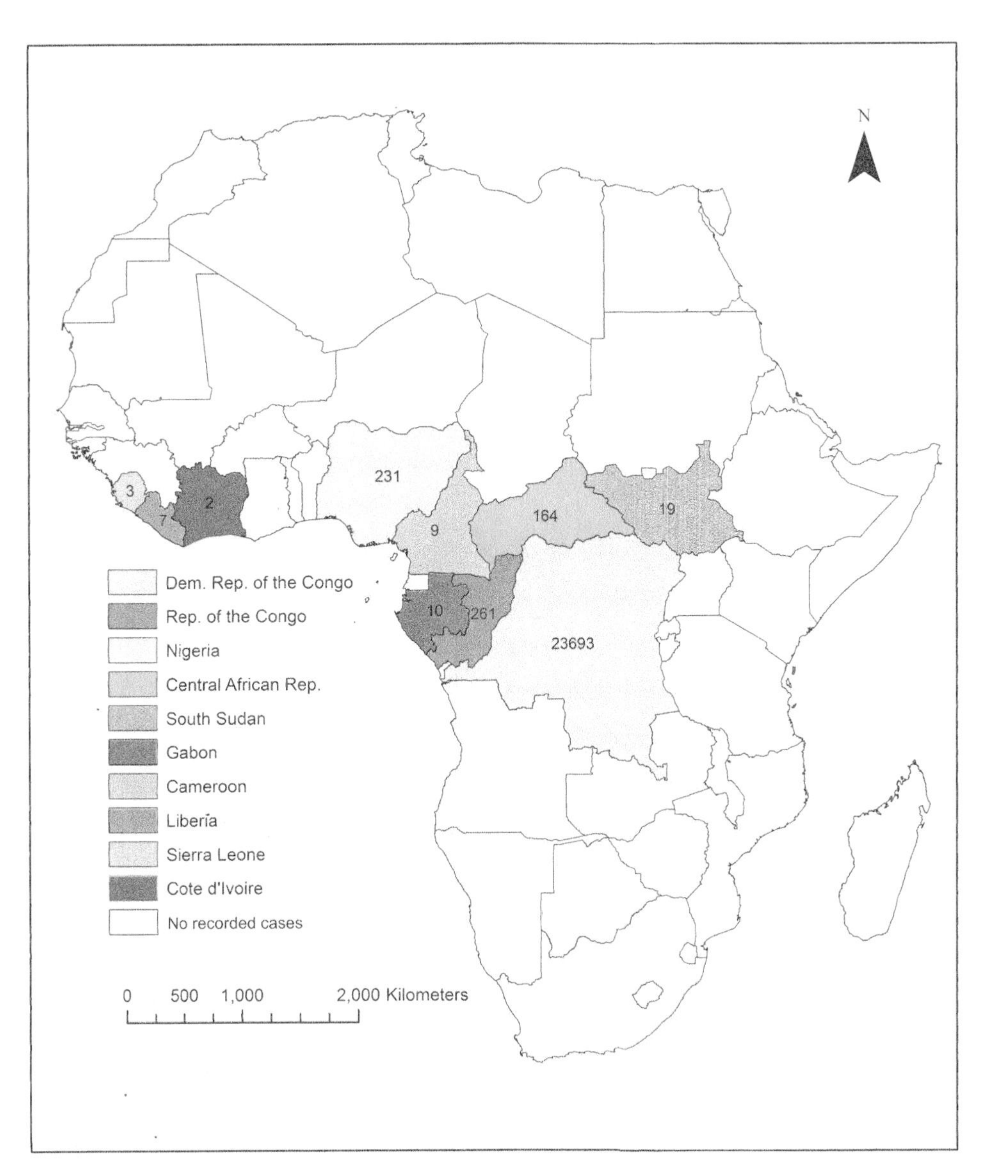

FIGURE 17.3 Human monkeypox cases reported from Africa between 1970 and 2018. (Reprinted from Beer EM, Rao VB. A systematic review of the epidemiology of human monkeypox outbreaks and implications for outbreak strategy. *PLoS Negl Trop Dis* 2019;13(10):e0007791. https://creativecommons.org/licenses/by/4.0/.)

outside the endemic area.[66,189,258] In toto, these data are suggestive of at least two populations of monkeypox viruses being maintained in Africa.

Cowpox

Cowpox is a virus found in Europe and Asia that is maintained in rodents; in Britain, these are bank voles and woodmice (Table 17.1).[23,41,43] The domestic cat is one common source of human infection,[24] and this probably explains the occurrence of cases in children; 26% of 54 cases identified between 1969 and 1993 were in children younger than 12 years.[17] Most feline and human cases occur between July and October, with only occasional cases between January and June. Human cases occur in which no source is traced, but despite detailed investigations, only three human cases in Britain since 1968 have been traced to a bovine source, and no case of bovine cowpox has been detected since 1976.

Cowpox virus has a wide host range, and an interesting finding has been the occurrence of cowpox in a variety of captive exotic species in European zoos. Susceptible animals have included cheetahs, lions, anteaters, rhinoceros, elephants, and okapi, and infection has occasionally been transmitted to animal handlers.[16,203,204] Recent outbreaks of human infections with CPXV in Europe have been traced to rat populations used in the pet trade.[38] A large number of novel CPXV infections and associated strains have been recently recognized and isolated in Germany and from Europe. Additionally, two OPXVs similar to CPXV, but phylogenetically distant, have been identified from Georgia and Italy.[78,90,261]

Vaccinia

The origin of vaccinia is unknown, and no natural host for the virus is known. However, a number of vaccinia variants have been described. Buffalopox has been described in India; human infection results from contact with infected animals. It is not known whether buffaloes are a reservoir or whether other wildlife is involved, as with cowpox. Similarly, there have been increasing reports of VACVs infecting cattle handlers in Brazil. Cantagalo virus has been classified as a vaccinia variant, but other similar nonidentical vaccinia-like viruses have also been reported in the region.[53,56,57,153,252] VACV infections were detected in Colombia among cattle handlers, and DNA sequence confirmed distinct strain but most closely grouped with VACV strains from Brazil.[257] Studies have begun to investigate the disease ecology of these viruses.[1]

Other Orthopoxviruses

A number of novel orthopoxviruses have been identified in the past years. These include NY-014,[145] the causative agent of a renal transplant patients' slowly progressive rash illness, and Alaskapox, the cause of a localized rash illness in an Alaska resident.[246] Little is understood about the exposure related to these infections, and the genomes have been characterized.[82,245]

Clinical Features

Variola: Smallpox

Naturally acquired VARV infection caused a systemic febrile rash illness; the course of clinical features is schematically diagrammed in Figure 17.4. For ordinary smallpox, the most common clinical presentation, after an asymptomatic incubation period of 10 to 14 days (range, 7–17), was fever, which quickly rose to about 103°F, sometimes with dermal petechiae. Associated constitutional symptoms included backache, headache, vomiting, and prostration. Within a day or two after incubation, a systemic rash appeared that was characteristically centrifugally distributed (i.e., lesions were present in greater numbers on the oral mucosa, face, and extremities than on the trunk). Lesions were commonly manifested on the palms and

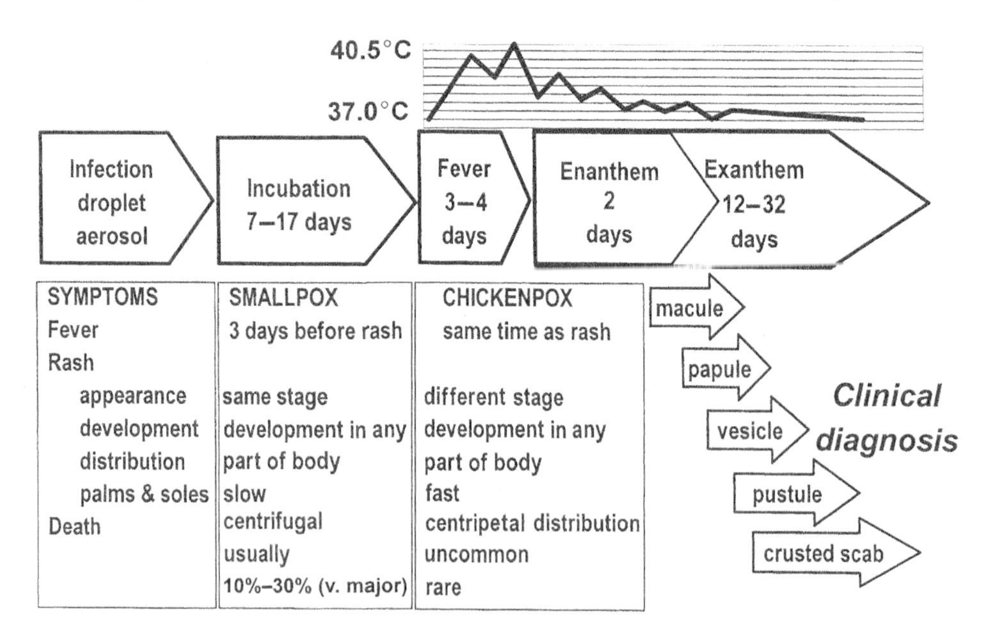

FIGURE 17.4 **The clinical development of discrete ordinary smallpox.** After respiratory droplet exposure and infection, an asymptomatic incubation period of 7 to 17 days precedes prodromal symptoms of high fever and malaise. Subsequently, rash develops 2 to 4 days after the prodrome. The fever diminishes at the onset of rash development. The characteristics of smallpox and chickenpox rash are contrasted.

soles. The rash lesions were initially macular and then advanced to the papular stage, enlarging and progressing to a vesicle by day 4 to 5 and a pustule by day 7; lesions were encrusted and scabby by day 14 and then sloughed off. Skin lesions were deep seated and in the same stage of development in any one area of the body. Images of the classic presentation of ordinary smallpox are depicted in Figure 17.5. Milder and more severe forms of the rash were also documented. Less severe manifestations (modified smallpox or variola sine eruptione) occurred in some vaccinated individuals, whereas hemorrhagic or flatpox types of smallpox are believed to have developed as a result of an impaired immune response of patients.

Variola major smallpox was differentiated into four main clinical types: (a) ordinary smallpox (~90% of cases) produced viremia, fever, prostration, and rash; mortality rates were generally proportionate with the extent of rash and ranged, using the WHO classification, from less than 10% for ordinary discrete to 50% to 75% for the rarer ordinary confluent presentation; (b) (vaccine) modified smallpox (5% of cases) produced a mild prodrome with few skin lesions in previously vaccinated people and had a mortality rate of less than 10%; (c) flat smallpox (5% of cases) produced slowly developing focal lesions with generalized infection and had an approximate fatality rate of 80%; and (d) hemorrhagic smallpox (<1% of cases) induced bleeding into the skin and the mucous membranes and was invariably fatal within a week of onset. Notably, prior vaccination did not appear to protect from mortality associated with the more severe flat or hemorrhagic forms of disease. A discrete type of the ordinary form, with typical febrile prodrome and rash, resulted from alastrim variola minor infection.[73]

The WHO established a system for classifying smallpox case types on the basis of disease presentation and rash burden. The hemorrhagic and flat types are briefly described previously. The ordinary type was subgrouped into three categories, which were based on the extent of rash on the face and the body: confluent, semiconfluent, and discrete. In ordinary confluent disease, no area of skin was visible between vesiculopustular rash lesions on the trunk or the face. In ordinary semiconfluent and discrete disease, patches of normal skin were visible between rash lesions on the trunk and face, respectively. Disease modified by vaccine presented with sparse numbers of lesions. Survival from infection conferred lifelong immunity.

Monkeypox

In humans, clinical disease is believed to result from either respiratory, percutaneous, or permucosal exposures. Classical descriptions from the active surveillance program in Zaire, now the DRC, have historically provided most of our understanding

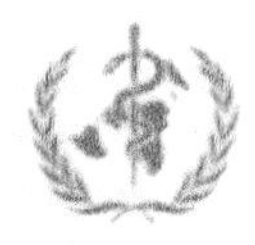
SMALLPOX
RECOGNITION CARD

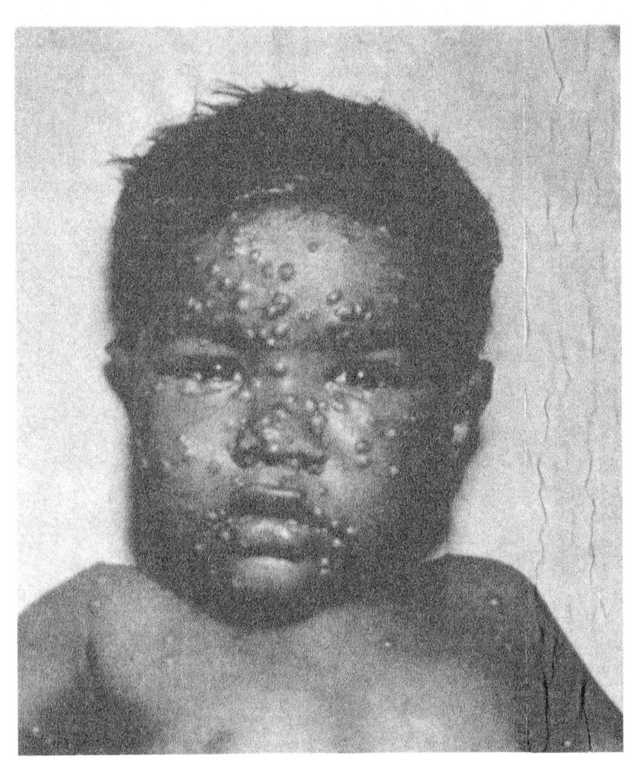
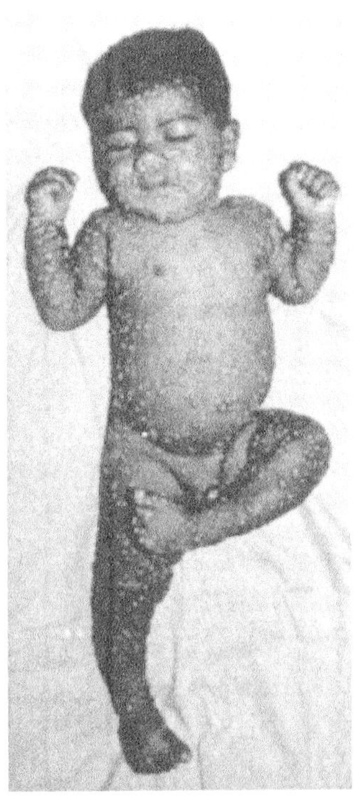
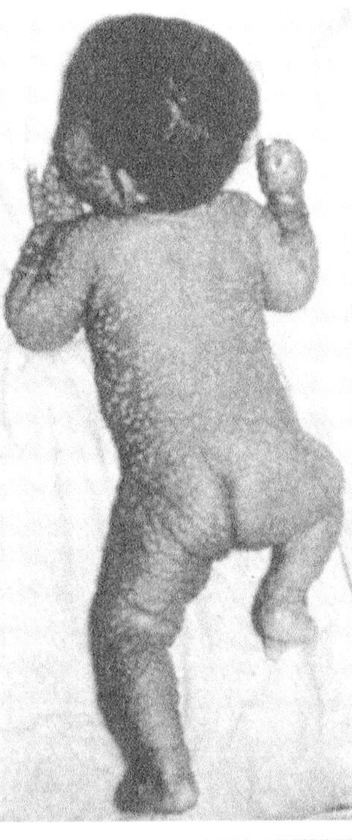
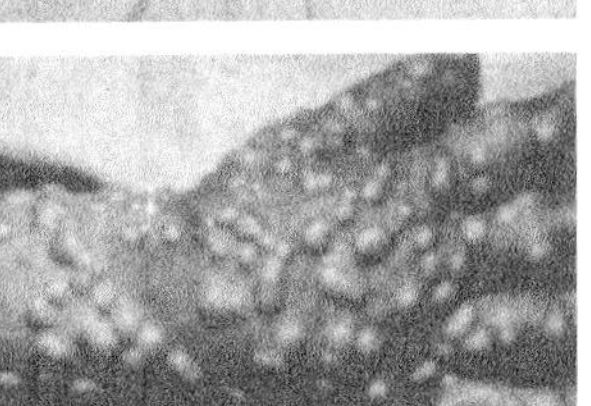
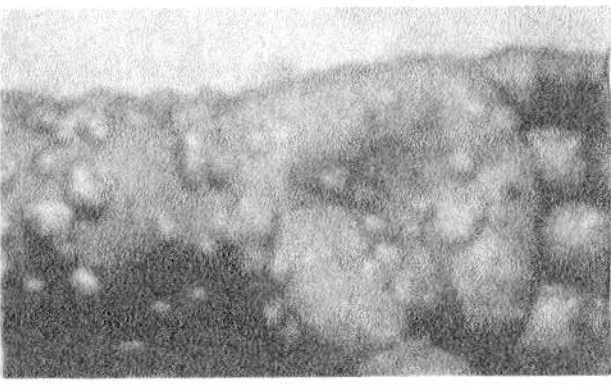

FIGURE 17.5 The rash of smallpox. The smallpox recognition card used during the Intensified Smallpox Eradication Programme of the World Health Organization, showing the nature and distribution of the rash of ordinary smallpox. (Reprinted with permission from Fenner F, Henderson DA, Arita I, et al. *Smallpox and its Eradication*. Geneva: World Health Organization; 1988.)

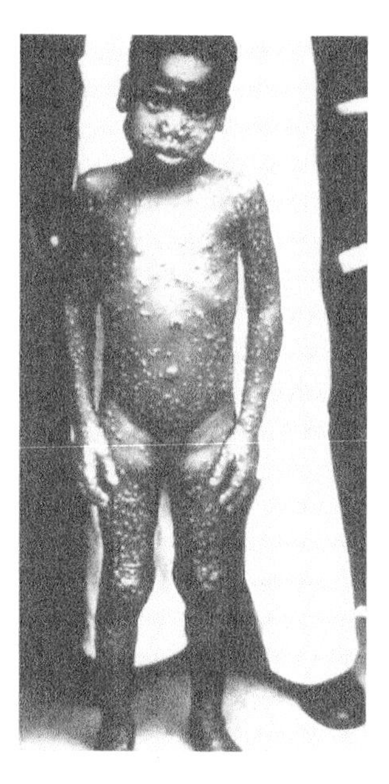
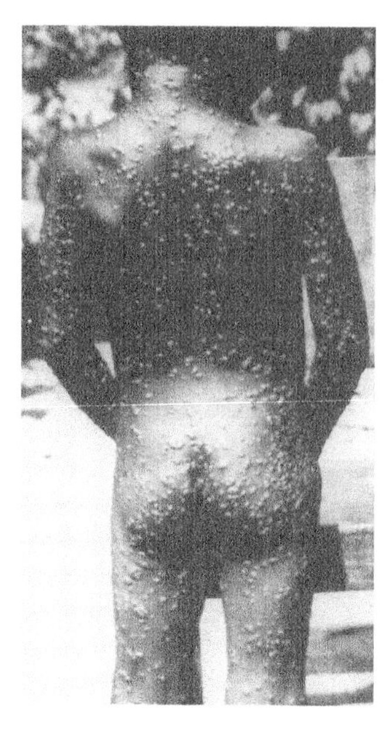

FIGURE 17.6 Human monkeypox. The day 8 appearance of monkeypox rash on a 7-year-old girl from the Democratic Republic of Congo. Prominent lymphadenopathy is apparent at the angle of the chin and in the inguinal areas. (Reprinted with permission from Breman JG, Kalisa R, Steniowski MV, et al. Human monkeypox, 1970–79. *Bull World Health Organ* 1980;58(2):165–182.)

of human monkeypox. Following an incubation period of 7 to 17 days (mean, 12 days), a prodrome of fever, headache, backache, and fatigue begins. The cutaneous eruption evolves similar to that of smallpox. Lesions evolve in the same stage in any one part of the body from macules, papules, vesicles, pustules, and then crust and scar. This is apparently more common in unvaccinated individuals[123]; in previously vaccinated individuals, pleomorphic presentation of rash lesions was observed. Following resolution of the rash, hypopigmentation is followed by hyperpigmentation of the scarred lesions. Pronounced lymphadenopathy clinically distinguishes monkeypox from smallpox. Lymphadenopathy in the facial area: cervical, postauricular, submandibular, and inguinal can be quite pronounced. Images of the typical presentation of human monkeypox in the DRC are in Figure 17.6.

Vaccinia Virus

Multiple-puncture VACV infection, using a bifurcated needle, is currently used in the smallpox vaccination regimen used for laboratory workers using replication-competent orthopoxviruses[201,224] and public health care personnel and military in the United States. Most commonly, the infection progresses through a standard course of events from vesicle to pustule (Fig. 17.7). However, of all vaccines used today, the smallpox vaccine, composed of live replicative VACV, has one of the highest rates of adverse events.[50] Major complications include progressive vaccinia, EV, generalized vaccinia, postvaccinial encephalitis, accidental infection, and carditis (Fig. 17.8). Recently, replication-deficient Modified Vaccinia Ankara vaccine (JYNNEOS) was approved by the U.S. Food and Drug Administration (FDA) as smallpox vaccine for smallpox and monkeypox preexposure vaccination; previously, the vaccine had been approved for use to prevent smallpox in Europe (Imvamune) and Canada (Imvanex).

Progressive vaccinia, previously called vaccinia necrosum or vaccinia gangrenosum, is a rare and often fatal vaccine complication in persons with severe deficiencies of cellular immunity.[32] In 1968 in the United States, there were 5 cases among 6 million primary vaccinees and 6 cases among 8.6 million revaccinated persons[146]; 4 of these 11 patients died. Progressive vaccinia is characterized by progressive, often painless growth and spread of the vaccine virus beyond the inoculation site, often leading to necrosis, sometimes with metastases to other body sites.[79] The possibility of progressive vaccinia should be considered if the vaccination site lesion continues to progress and expand without apparent healing more than 15 days after vaccination.[188] Initially, limited or no inflammation is present at the inoculation site, and histopathological examination shows an absence of inflammatory cells.[132]

EV can occur in people with a history of AD (eczema), irrespective of disease severity or activity. This complication is the clinical result of local spread or dissemination from the primary vaccination site in such persons or the result of the skin of an individual with AD contacting the unscabbed vaccination site of another person.[79,187] A localized or generalized papular, vesicular, or pustular rash anywhere on the body or localized to previous eczematous lesions is the clinical presentation of EV. Systemic illness with fever, malaise, and lymphadenopathy may occur. In the national U.S. surveillance of smallpox vaccination

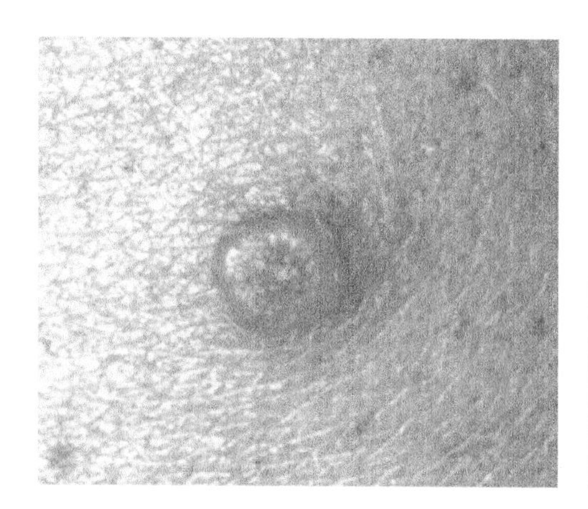
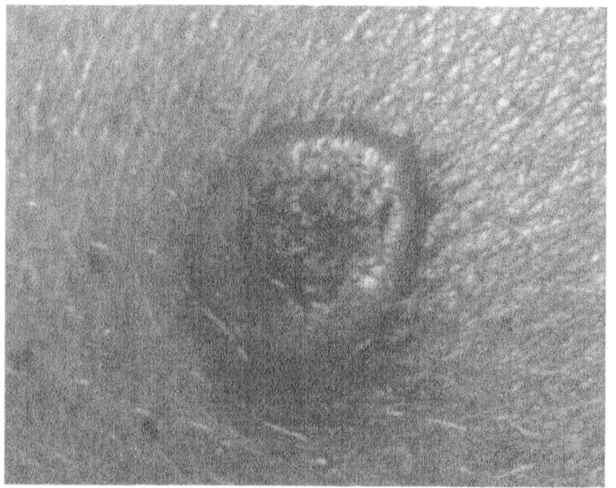

FIGURE 17.7 Primary response to vaccination: typical vesiculopustular response, maximal at 8 to 11 days. *Left:* day 7; *right:* day 11. (Courtesy of J. R. L. Forsyth.)

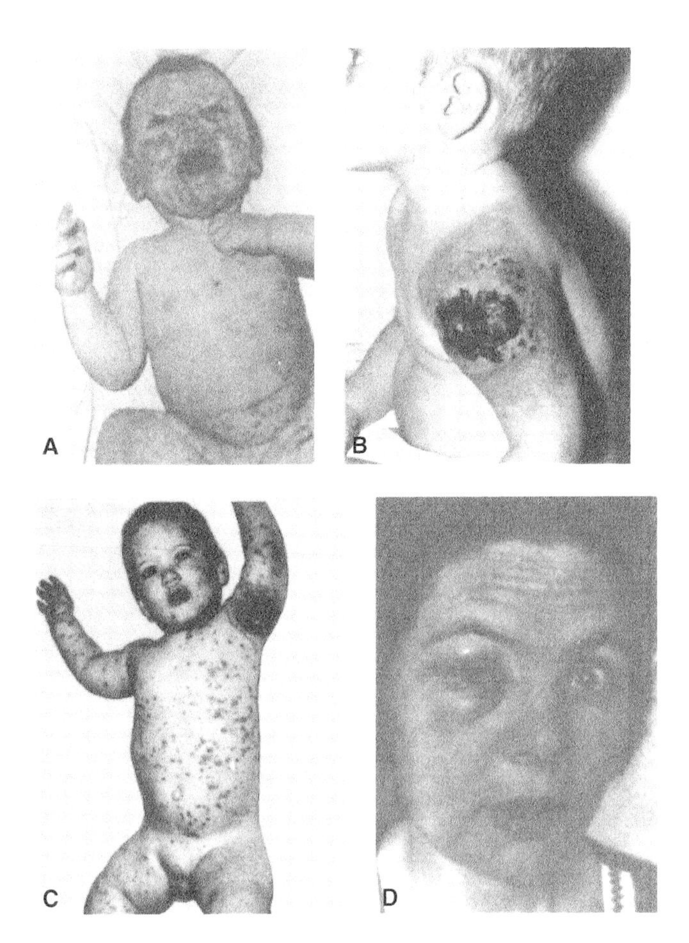

FIGURE 17.8 Severe complications of vaccination. A: Eczema vaccinatum in the unvaccinated contact of a vaccinated sibling. **B:** Progressive vaccinia, previously known as vaccinia necrosum, in a child with a congenital defect in cell-mediated immunity. **C:** Generalized vaccinia 10 days after vaccination. **D:** Ocular vaccinia. (Reprinted with permission from Fenner F, Henderson DA, Arita I, et al. *Smallpox and its Eradication*. Geneva: World Health Organization; 1988.)

that was done in 1968, there were 66 cases (no deaths) of EV among 14.5 million vaccinees (4.6 cases per million) and 60 cases (one death) among their several million contacts.[146] In one study, early vaccinia immune globulin (VIG) administration reduced mortality from 30% to 40% to 7%.[134]

Generalized vaccinia is a nonspecific term that is used to describe a vesicular rash that develops after vaccination. Excluding dissemination associated with EV and progressive vaccinia, it has been extremely rare to document virus in these lesions.[133] True generalized vaccinia is believed to represent the end product of viremic spread of virus, and no predisposing factors have been identified. Generalized vaccinia was estimated to occur in about 242 of every 1 million primary vaccinations[146]; likely many of the historic reports also included allergic and inflammatory responses to the vaccine.[259]

Postvaccination encephalomyelitis (PVEM) is a rare but serious complication that usually occurs in primary vaccinees. The frequency of its occurrence differed widely from country to country and with the strain of VACV used in the vaccine. The incidence of PVEM was lower with the NYCBOH VACV strain (the U.S. vaccine strain) than with the strain used in other countries.[73] No predisposing factors for PVEM are known, although host factors are believed to be important; the pathophysiology of PVEM is not well understood. Patients have variably displayed clinical and diagnostic features suggestive of a postimmunization demyelinating encephalomyelitis or direct viral invasion of the nervous system. This postvaccination reaction typically occurs 11 to 15 days following vaccination. Symptoms of PVEM include fever, headache, vomiting, confusion, delirium, disorientation, restlessness, drowsiness or lethargy, seizures, and coma. The cerebral spinal fluid can demonstrate elevated pressure but generally has a normal cell count and chemistry profile.[248] Infants younger than 2 years old can also develop a rare, postvaccination encephalopathy (PVE) similar to PVEM. Acute onset of PVE occurs earlier in the postvaccination period (6–10 days after vaccination), presents with the same symptoms as PVEM, and may also include hemiplegia and aphasia. Diagnosis of PVE or PVEM is one of exclusion because there are no specific diagnostic tests to confirm the diagnosis of this complication, and there are many other infectious and toxic etiologies that can result in similar clinical symptoms. Accidental infection occurs when virus from the vaccination site is transferred to another site or to another person via intimate skin contact. This usually occurs in primary vaccinees rather than revaccinees. Accidental self-inoculation, which most commonly occurs on the face, mouth, lips, or genitalia, is usually not serious and requires no specific treatment. Inoculation of the eye or eyelid is more serious and can be sight threatening if not evaluated and treated appropriately. In the 5 years between 1963 and 1968, ocular vaccinia was observed in 348 persons, 259 were vaccinees, and 66 were contacts of vaccinees. Of these, 22 had evidence of corneal involvement and 11 experienced permanent defects.[146,225]

Cardiac adverse events had not been reported before 2003 in any person vaccinated with the NYCBOH strain. Myocarditis and pericarditis were documented in 18 of 230,734 primary vaccinees immunized with the NYCBOH strain in 2002 and 2003.[98] Arrhythmias and myocardial ischemia have also been described recently, but the association with vaccination is not as clear. A review of the development of the current U.S. licensed replicative vaccine, derived from the NYCBOH strain and known as ACAM2000, and associated adverse events, has been published.[87]

VACVs in the Indian subcontinent (buffalopox), Brazil (Cantagalo virus, and related strains Aracatuba virus, Belo Horizonte virus, Passatempo virus, and others) and Colombia have been described to cause human infection in handlers of buffalo or cattle.[57] Up to 10 lesions have been described on the hands or arms of the human handlers; fever, lymphadenopathy, backache, and fatigue have also been associated symptoms. Transmission is believed to occur via unprotected contact with active lesions present on animal teats and udders. Interhuman transmission of buffalopox to family members has been reported to occur via contact.[142]

Cowpox

Cowpox also causes localized lesions in humans (Fig. 17.9D), and lesions in cows are typically found on their teats and udders (Fig. 17.9A). Most information is available from a detailed analysis of 54 human cases investigated during 1969 to 1993.[17] Lesions are generally restricted to the hands and face, and most patients (72%) have only one lesion. Multiple lesions may be

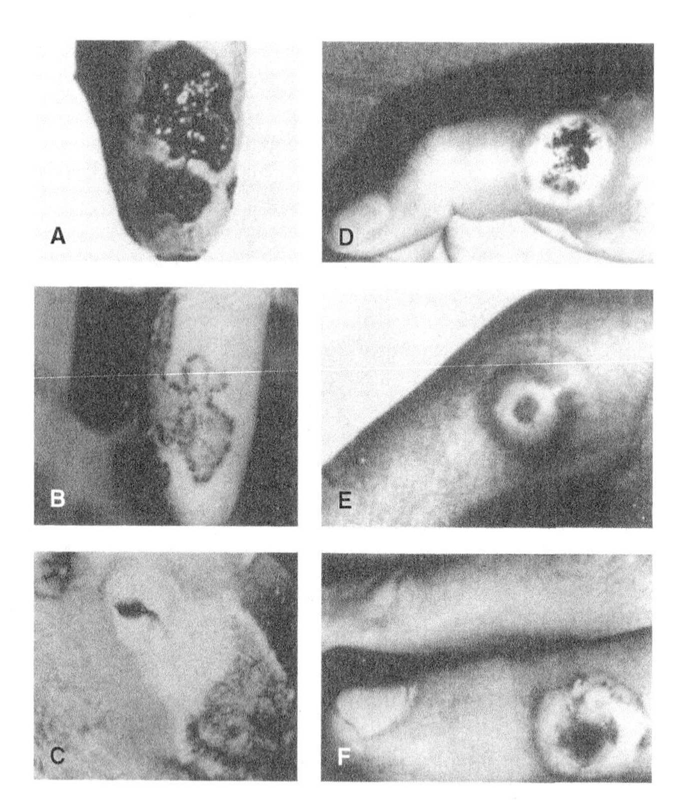

FIGURE 17.9 Cowpox, pseudocowpox, and orf virus infections of animals **(A–C)** and the lesions caused by these viruses on the digits of humans **(D–F). A:** A Cowpox ulcer on teat of cow, 7 days after onset of symptoms. **B:** Pseudocowpox (milker's nodule) virus infection of cow teat. **C:** Orf virus scabby mouth in a lamb. **D:** Cowpox. **E:** Milker's nodule. **F:** Orf. (**A and B:** Courtesy of E. P. J. Gibbs; **C:** Courtesy of A. J. Robinson; **D:** Courtesy of A. D. McNae; **E and F:** Courtesy of J. Nagington.)

caused by multiple primary inoculations, autoinoculation, and rarely by lymphatic or viremic spread. Occasionally, a very severe infection, and death, may occur usually in immunosuppressed individuals.[81]

The lesion passes through macular, papular, vesicular, and pustular stages before forming a hard black crust. The lesion is usually quite painful, and erythema and edema are common at the late vesicular and pustular stages (Fig. 17.9A). There is usually lymphadenitis, fever, and general malaise, often referred to as "flulike." These features are usually severe in children, and absence from school or work is common; 16 of 54 patients (30%) were hospitalized. Most cases take 6 to 8 weeks to recover; in some cases, it may take up to 12 weeks. Scarring is usually permanent.

Diagnosis

Differentiating Smallpox From Other Diseases and Conditions

Prior to its eradication, smallpox as a clinical entity was relatively easy to recognize, but other exanthematous illnesses were mistaken for this disease. For example, the rash of severe chickenpox, caused by varicella-zoster virus, was often misdiagnosed as that of smallpox. However, chickenpox produces a centripetally distributed rash and rarely appears on the palms and soles. In addition, in the case of chickenpox, prodromal fever and systemic manifestations are mild, if they manifest at all; the lesions are superficial in nature; and lesions in different developmental stages may present in the same area of the body. Other diseases and conditions that could be confused with vesicular-stage smallpox include monkeypox, generalized vaccinia, disseminated herpes zoster, disseminated herpes simplex virus infection, drug reactions (eruptions), erythema multiforme, enteroviral infections, scabies, insect bites, impetigo, and MCV. Diseases confused with hemorrhagic smallpox included acute leukemia, meningococcemia, and idiopathic thrombocytopenic purpura. The Centers for Disease Control and Prevention (CDC), in collaboration with numerous professional organizations, has developed an algorithm for evaluating patients for smallpox. The algorithm assists in differential diagnoses of the vesiculopustular stage of rash. The algorithm and additional laboratory testing information are available at https://www.cdc.gov/smallpox/lab-personnel/laboratory-procedures/rash-testing.html. An evaluation of the algorithm has been published.[238]

Laboratory

A variety of diagnostic strategies are available for the laboratory diagnosis of orthopoxvirus infections. Negative stain electron microscopy cannot differentiate the virions of orthopoxvirus from those of yatapox or molluscipox, but the clinical and epidemiologic information will likely aid interpretation. Some of the classic methods for distinguishing orthopoxvirus species are depicted in Table 17.2. Protein-based diagnostics can be used to detect the genus, but for the most part cannot identify individual species.[54] An IgM capture serologic assay may provide a useful tool for assessing orthopoxvirus disease incidence[126] and may provide utility in assessing infectious etiologies of encephalitic symptoms associated with orthopoxviruses.[236]

The majority of tests which are able to differentiate orthopoxvirus species, however, rely on nucleic acid testing. Identification of orthopoxvirus species can be accomplished through morphologic observations of virus pock growth on chorioallantoic membrane of embryonated eggs. A number of nucleic acid test strategies have been developed and published; the majority are polymerase chain reaction (PCR) based.[144,156,157,196,233] More recently, whole genome high-throughput DNA sequencing methods are used to obtain genome sequences to more fully characterize these viruses.

Prevention and Control

Vaccination has been the historic tool for control of interhuman transmissible orthopoxvirus infections. The successful eradication of smallpox, declared in 1980 by the WHO, was largely due to the effective use of vaccinia vaccine strains worldwide in an extensive immunization program. Classical public health tools of surveillance and isolation of cases were supported by vaccination programs. Vaccination could also be used postexposure to provide protection; greatest protection was afforded if provided within days of contact to a patient[168] and if the contact had previously been vaccinated.[103] For laboratory workers, vaccination is recommended in some countries[224] for those using any orthopoxvirus capable of causing disease in humans; in others, only for those working with the more human pathogenic orthopoxviruses. Because of the adverse events associated with the use of current VACV vaccine strains, evaluation of vaccination regimens using attenuated vaccinia strains[135,170,178] or subunit vaccines have been undertaken. In the United States, FDA approved MVA-based smallpox vaccine, a nonreplicating virus in mammalian cells with improved safety profile even in contraindicated individuals.

Recent work has also focused on the development of antiorthopoxvirus therapeutic strategies. Compounds with direct antiviral effects, as well as others that inhibit viral use of cellular functions, have been evaluated and demonstrate efficacy in various animal model systems of orthopoxvirus challenge.[29,109,136,147,207,211,212] At least two antiviral agents, with different mechanisms of antiviral action, are moving into advanced stages of research and development for orthopoxvirus treatment. A DNA polymerase inhibitor, cidofovir, and an orally bioavailable derivative brincidofovir™ of the parent compound have activity against orthopoxviruses in tissue culture, and in treatment of various orthopoxvirus-animal model challenges. ST-246 (Tecovirimat™ or TPOXX™), a novel compound which functions to inhibit later stages of viral maturation and egress, has been shown effective against orthopoxviruses in similar studies. TPOXX™ is now approved by FDA for smallpox treatment. These antivirals have been used investigationally with VIG, for the treatment of severe vaccinia infections related to vaccination.[8,9,260,273] Additionally, the efficacy of monoclonal antibodies to substitute for VIG in prophylactic treatment is currently under investigation.[182]

PARAPOXVIRUS

History

Parapoxvirus infections are widespread, worldwide in sheep, goats, and cattle. Human infections from these sources are a common occupational hazard for those in contact with infected animals or, less commonly, fomites. The current International Committee on Taxonomy of Viruses (ICTV) recognized that members of the genus *Parapoxvirus* are orf virus (ORFV), bovine papular stomatitis virus (BPSV), pseudocowpoxvirus (PCPV), and parapoxvirus of red deer in New Zealand (PVNZ). BPSV and PCPV are maintained in cattle, while ORFV is maintained in sheep and goats, but all three are zoonoses. A squirrel parapoxvirus had been described by electron microscopic morphology as a parapoxvirus, but genome sequencing suggests that it is an unclassified poxvirus.[249] Distinct parapoxvirus infections of, and viral species from, red deer in New Zealand[106,220] have been characterized. PVNZ has not been observed to infect humans. In the United States, a novel deer-associated parapoxvirus was characterized as the cause of cutaneous infections in two hunters. The viruses appear related to pseudocowpox viruses.[223] Other tentative members of the genus are camel contagious ecthyma virus or chamois contagious ecthyma virus, which causes a disease initially called Ausdyk or camel contagious ecthyma in camels; this may also be the virus responsible for cases of "camelpox" described in humans in the Middle East.[124] Another tentative member is seal parapoxvirus.[20,253] A poxvirus infection of reindeer[139] has been classified as an ORFV and demonstrated the ability of orf to cross species barriers.

Human infection with ORFV is termed orf. Most commonly, the disease is transmitted from sheep or goats. The disease in animals is alternately referred to as orf, contagious pustular dermatitis, contagious ecthyma, or scabby mouth. Disease in sheep was recognized as early as 1787; the earliest known report of human disease was made in 1879. Human infection with PCPV is commonly called milker's nodule. The disease is transmitted from dairy cattle and is referred to as paravaccinia or pseudocowpox in these animals. Notably, this disease was not formally distinguished from that caused by the orthopoxvirus cowpox until the end of the 19th century, although Jenner did recognize "spurious" forms of cowpox on cow teats, described in the late 1700s as "pustular sores" lacking "bluish or livid tint".[121] Human disease with BPSV is termed *bovine papular stomatitis* and is transmitted from beef cattle; the disease name when virus infects cattle is the same. Initial descriptions of disease in beef cattle were published in 1884; transmission of infection, causing illness in humans, was described in 1953.[195] Subsequent reports demonstrated that humans could transmit disease to cattle.[42] Human disease with seal parapoxvirus is called sealpox and is transmitted from seals. Human infection of a seal handler was first reported in 1987[104]; the virus was first detected in seals and sea lions in 1969.[269]

Infectious Agent

By negative stain electron microscopy, parapoxviruses appear ovoid with a criss-cross surface appearance (Fig. 17.1), generated by the genus' characteristic outer spiral tubule structure. The particles of ORFV are 260 nm long by 160 nm wide; pseudocowpox virions appear a bit larger 300 nm by 190 nm. The viruses obtained from clinical materials grow most readily on primary ovine or bovine cell culture systems and do not grow in embryonated eggs. A few strains have been laboratory adapted to grow on VERO cells or MRC-5 cells; this has been associated with genome changes and attenuation of the virus.

The separation of the parapoxviruses into at least four distinct groups has been based on natural host range, pathology, and nucleic acid methods, including restriction endonuclease, DNA/DNA hybridization, and, most recently, partial or full gene or genome sequence analyses.[58,177,249] As with other poxviruses, the latter studies have shown that the parapoxviruses share extensive homology between central regions of their genomes but much lower levels of relatedness within the genome termini. The high G+C content of parapoxvirus DNA is in contrast to most other poxviruses (except for molluscipoxvirus) and suggests that a significant genetic divergence from other genera of this family has occurred. DNA sequencing of the genome of two parapoxviruses, species BPSV and ORFV, has allowed a detailed comparison with the fully sequenced genomes of other *Chordopoxviruses*. These studies have provided a genetic map of ORFV and BPSV and revealed that within the central core of the genome, 88 ORF are conserved with the other sequenced *Chordopoxviruses*.[58] This conservation is not maintained in the genome termini where insertions, deletions, and translocations have occurred. Studies have demonstrated a great degree of diversity within species via comparison of three complete orf genome sequences.[177]

Pathogenesis and Pathology

Most of the work on the pathogenesis of parapoxvirus infections comes from studies of orf and paravaccinia viruses. Most animal models have used ORFV in sheep; however, there is detailed literature on the pathological appearance of human orf lesions. Infection occurs via cuts and scratches and remains localized. After entry through nonintact epithelium, virus replicates in the regenerating epidermal keratinocytes.[172] Lesions are produced by hypertrophy and proliferation of epidermal cells, often marked, and leukocyte infiltration. Histologic examination shows many small multilocular vesicles within the dermis; true macrovesicles rarely occur.[125,271] In the first 2 weeks, the epidermis shows ballooning degeneration in the keratinocytes, and the dermis shows newly formed thin-walled blood vessels with an inflammatory infiltrate. As the infection progresses, in weeks 2 to 3, the intraepidermal vesicles described previously are seen in some cases, with intraepidermal bullous lesions in others. At this point, keratotic material could be visualized on the skin surface. Viral particles were only visualized in the epidermis and were present in the greatest numbers in the first 2 weeks after infection.[125]

The immune response in natural human infection has been investigated.[271] There is a vigorous but short-lived cell-mediated response and a relatively poor and short-lived humoral response. This is consistent with the occurrence of second infections in 8% to 12% of individuals.[221,271] Studies of the immune response to orf infection in sheep have been reviewed.[95] Immunohistochemical studies of lesions demonstrate large numbers of neutrophils, lymphocytes (T and B), and dendritic cells surrounding virus-infected epidermal cells.[6] In comparison of primary versus reinfection lesions, the appearance of CD8+ T cells and B cells are later in primary infection than in reinfection; CD4+ T cells are the predominant cell present in either lesion. Virus replication is decreased in reinfection lesions with respect to that seen in primary lesions. Studies of cytokine response demonstrated γ-IFN mRNA+ cells and some TNF-α mRNA+ cells in reinfection, but not in primary infection. Cellular depletion studies[161] have suggested that CD4+ T cells, IFN-γ, and some CD8+ T-cell responses and some humeral components are necessary for host resolution of infection. Passive antibody transfer, however, does not appear to protect young animals from infection[35] nor does there appear to be a predominant neutralizing antibody response to orf infection.[52]

The parapoxvirus genomes are predicted to express several proteins involved in the host–pathogen interaction; the majority of those studied have been in the context of ORFV. ORFV expresses a homolog of the mammalian vascular endothelial growth factor (VEGF), which has been demonstrated to be a viral virulence factor. The absence of the orf protein produces an attenuated virus[232]; it is hypothesized that the viral protein stimulates keratinocyte growth likely to provide cell substrate for viral replication; in addition, it inhibits apoptosis.[232] The product of a viral gene, OVIFNR, a homolog of vaccinia E3L, prevents inhibition of host protein synthesis to permit virus utilization of the protein synthetic apparatus. The mechanism for this is protein binding to dsRNA formed during viral infection, preventing PKR kinase activation and subsequent eIF-2 phosphorylation. Other virally encoded proteins are postulated to evade or modulate the host immune response. These include proteins that inhibit GM-CSF and mimic IL-10. *In vitro* studies implicate the orf expressed IL-10 homolog in impairment of an effective immunologic memory response and is a virulence factor.[77,149] A chemokine-binding protein expressed by the virus can interfere with recruitment of dendritic cells to the site of orf infection.[148]

Epidemiology

Human infections with parapoxviruses are an occupational hazard of farm workers, abattoir workers, veterinary surgeons and students, and so on. It is most common in the lambing and calving seasons, and more commonly reported in sheep workers than in cattle workers; this probably reflects differences in animal husbandry. Of 191 cases with a known source surveyed from 1978 to 1995, 84% had an ovine source and 16% were from cattle. During the same period, 32 cases occurred in abattoir workers.[16]

Factors responsible for ongoing transmission have been attributed both to the environmental stability of ORFV in scab material (although infectivity wanes over time) and to the manifestation of chronic infections in some animals.[160] There is no known latency state for this or any other poxvirus. Transmission of virus to humans and to animals is via direct contact with lesions or with fomites.

Clinical Features

The progressive stages of human infection have been described in detail,[125,151,271] and illustrations have also been provided[45] (Fig. 17.9 B, C, E, and F). Lesions start as erythematous papules and progress to a "target" stage. This, seen 1 to 2 weeks after infection, has a red center surrounded by a white halo and an outer inflamed halo. This progresses to a nodular then papillomatous stage, which often has a "weeping" surface. In some patients, this may enlarge and persist for some weeks before resolving and may cause some concern. The lesion resolves via a crusting stage, which may last some weeks. Very large granulomatous lesions, usually in immunocompromised individuals, can occur.

Most patients have only one lesion, but multiple primary lesions may occur. Systemic reaction is relatively uncommon, and the lesion is often not particularly painful. Lymphadenopathy is present in some patients, and lymphangitis is also observed but is relatively uncommon. *Erythema multiforme* was reported in one-third of patients reported in one case series.[125] But, because many ordinary uncomplicated cases of orf go unreported, the actual incidence of *E. multiforme* is probably low.

Diagnosis

Differential

Differential diagnosis of parapoxvirus lesions can include ecthyma gangrenosum (a pseudomonas infection of immunocompromised persons), cutaneous anthrax, erysipeloid, and tularemia or tumor. Clinical diagnosis of uncomplicated cases in patients with a known animal contact should not cause difficulties but has been confused with anthrax. However, farmworkers and so on recognize the infection and tend not to seek medical attention for routine cases. Consequently, a disproportionately large number of reported cases have no known contact with infected animals. Of approximately 500 cases surveyed from 1978 to 1995, some 45% had no such contact. Clinical diagnosis of such cases, particularly if severe or prolonged, may be difficult. In particular, large weeping granulomatous or papillomatous lesions may be misdiagnosed as malignancies.

Laboratory

With negative stain electron microscopy, virions with the characteristic morphology of parapoxviruses are usually easily seen in lesion extracts, and this provides a rapid, certain diagnosis of the genus. The virus can be grown in cell culture, but this is not attempted routinely in laboratories that do not maintain primary ovine or bovine cultures.

A number of methods derived from limited or complete genomic analysis have been used for nucleic acid detection (PCR) and laboratory diagnosis of infection.[117,156,251] Species-specific and species-generic protein-based diagnostics for parapoxviruses have also been developed.[52]

Prevention and Control

Most workers at risk get infected at some stage, and reinfection is not uncommon. Individuals should take care not to spread infection by autoinoculation or to contacts, including animals. The vaccine used to control orf in sheep is fully virulent and has caused human infection. Work is underway to create live attenuated viruses that can be used as vaccines. Treatment options are limited; anecdotal reports have described the use of topical cidofovir,[169] or topical imiquimod. Other options may be topical formulations of interferon-modulating compounds such as imiquimod.

MOLLUSCUM CONTAGIOSUM

MCV virus causes a disease characterized by one or more benign, self-limited skin "tumor(s)" or papular eruption(s), occurs worldwide, and is regarded as a specific human infection.[28] There is no evidence of disease transmission between humans and other animals, although lesions resembling molluscum and containing pox virions have been detected in species other than humans (e.g., horses, chimpanzees).

Infectious Agent

Four subtypes of MCV, characterized by restriction endonuclease digests, have been described previously.[183] Disease presentation by all subtypes appears to be similar. The genomic sequence of both MCV subtypes, I and II, are determined.[237,277] The MCV genome encodes a number of novel gene products involved in its pathogenesis and evasion of the immune system, including, among others, an IL-18–binding protein and apoptosis inhibitors.[237,240] Attempts at propagating the virus in tissue culture have been unsuccessful.

Pathogenesis and Pathology

MCV does not cause systemic disease and remains localized at the site of inoculation. MCV lesions have long been known to have a distinctive pathology. Description of the characteristic molluscum bodies, or Henderson-Patterson bodies, was made in 1841 by Henderson and Patterson. A good review of the histopathological features of the infection is available[206] (Fig. 17.10A). The onset of infection occurs when virus begins replicating, extending upward, in the lower layers of the epidermis.[202] The asymptomatic incubation period is variable but can be protracted. As the infection progresses, the epidermis hypertrophies and extends down into the underlying dermal strata. Characteristic inclusions (molluscum bodies) are formed in the prickle cell layer and gradually enlarge as the cells age and migrate to the surface. These cells are replaced by hyperplasia of the basal cell layer; few to no viral structures are seen in the stratum basale. The structure of the basement membrane remains intact; the hypertrophied epidermal cells, with their cytoplasm occupied by a large acidophilic granular mass (i.e., the molluscum body), project above the skin to appear as a tumor. Little to no inflammatory infiltrate is seen until late in disease, just prior to natural resolution of the lesion.

Clinical Features

Molluscum infection occurs as a result of MCV coming in contact with nonintact skin. The characteristic lesion begins as a small papule and, when mature, is a discrete, 2- to 5-mm diameter, smooth, dome-shaped, pearly or flesh-colored nodule, which is often umbilicated (Fig. 17.10B). A cheesy, off-white or yellowish material is easily expressed from lesions. There are usually 1 to 20 lesions, but there may occasionally be hundreds. Because of multiple simultaneous infections or mechanical spread, the lesions may become confluent along the line of a scratch, and satellite lesions are sometimes seen.

In children, molluscum lesions occur mainly on the trunk and proximal extremities, and in adults, they tend to occur on the trunk, pubic area, and thighs; however, in all cases, infection can be transmitted to other parts by autoinoculation. In males infected with human immunodeficiency virus (HIV), molluscum lesions appear to occur along the beard line, and with persons with infections involving the face, there have been reports of ocular involvement. Individual lesions last for about 2 months, but the disease usually lasts 6 to 9 months. More severe and prolonged infection tends to occur in individuals with impaired cell-mediated immunity, including persons with HIV infection.[85]

Diagnosis

The clinical appearance of molluscum lesions in normal cases is generally sufficiently characteristic to permit clinical diagnosis. Brick-shaped virions can usually be seen in large numbers if the cheesy material expressed from the lesion is examined by negative-stain transmission electron microscopy. The virus

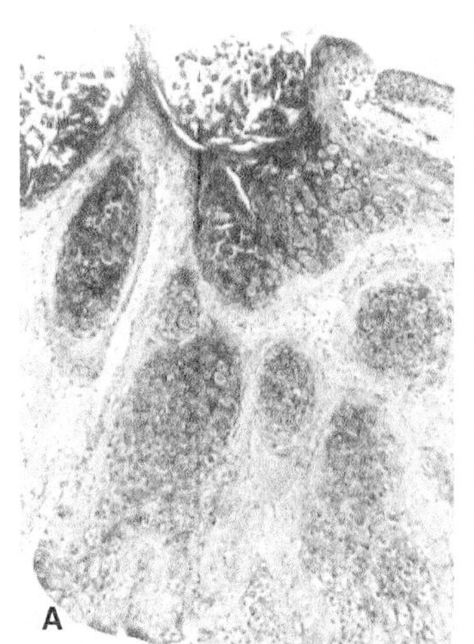

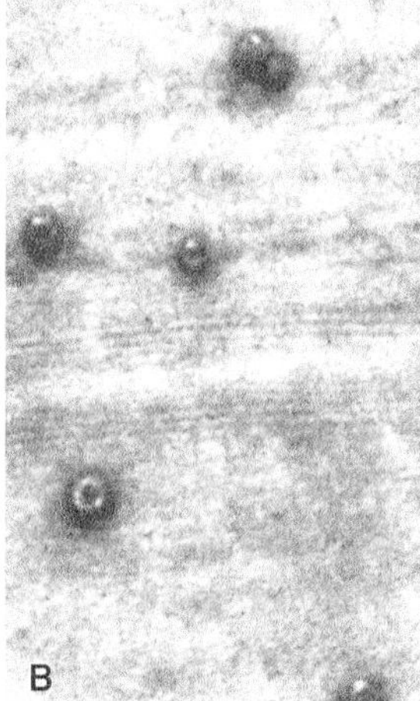

FIGURE 17.10 Molluscum contagiosum. A: Section of a skin lesion visualized by hematoxylin-and-eosin staining. **B:** Lesions of molluscum contagiosum in a human. (Courtesy of D. Lowy.)

has not been cultured in standard tissue culture systems. The characteristic histopathology of molluscum lesions and PCR are described for use in identifying MCV infections.[156,250]

Epidemiology

MCV virus occurs worldwide, affecting mostly children and immunocompromised.[194] Traditional modes of transmission are associated with mild skin trauma such as abrasions, direct contact with a lesion, and, in some cases, fomites (e.g., shared towels); however, there is increasing evidence that the disease is sexually transmitted and that genital lesions are more common than lesions elsewhere on the body.[28] The disease presents a significant concern for individuals whose children are in day care or school situations, where potential transmission to other children may exist. Secondary spread of lesions may occur by autoinoculation (excoriation of primary lesions and spread to areas of normal skin) and shaving. No known animal reservoir exists.

Prevention and Control

The covering of lesions and the use of proper hand hygiene after contact with lesions should prevent transmission in most situations.

MCV infection is benign and recovery is usually spontaneous, but treatment may be sought for cosmetic reasons, particularly for facial or multiple lesions. Various treatments have been tried, including cryotherapy, mechanical curettage, and chemical treatments, such as podophyllin/podofilox, cantharidin, iodine, and tretinoin. Irritation has been a side effect of many of the chemical treatments. Topical application of a 3% Cidofovir antiviral cream or suspension has been reported to be beneficial, as has the use of potentially immune-modulating cimetidine or topical imiquimod therapy.[49] The absence of well-controlled trials makes it difficult to assess the efficacy of various therapeutic regimens. For individuals with AIDS and molluscum, the use of highly active antiretroviral therapy, with improvement of CD4 cell counts, appears to be efficacious.

YATAPOXVIRUSES

History

Human infection with tanapox virus, a species of the genus *Yatapoxvirus*, was first recognized in the Tana River area of Kenya in 1957 and was best characterized during post smallpox eradication surveillance efforts. An account of 264 laboratory-confirmed cases from Zaire (now the DRC), with color illustrations, is available,[122] as is information on the virus itself.[141] The genome of the virus has been sequenced. Yaba-like disease of monkeys is caused by the same virus that causes tanapox in humans[62] and was responsible for outbreaks in three primate centers where animal handlers were infected. There have been a few reports of human disease outside Africa that have been published and illustrate the need to consider poxvirus etiologies of illness in travelers returning from, and emigrants from, areas where the virus is endemic.[59]

Yaba monkey tumor virus (YMTV), the other member of the genus, was recovered from rhesus monkeys in Nigeria.[190] Although no naturally occurring human infections have been reported, the virus does cause disease if injected subcutaneously or intradermally in humans or nonhuman primates.[86]

Pathogenesis and Pathology

The pathogenesis of tanapox or Yaba-like disease is incompletely understood. The clinical features, described here, are suggestive of some systemic phase of disease. The ultimate skin lesion shows epidermal thickening with marked ballooning degeneration; eosinophilic inclusions are often visible. YMTV causes localized histocytic "tumors" at the site of inoculation. After inoculation into the dermis, an accumulation of proliferating spindle-shaped cells begins about 1 week later. This continues for 4 to 6 weeks, resulting in the formation of a "tumor." The lesion can become superinfected with bacteria. Virus remains cell associated, and the lesion appears to regress as mononuclear cells move from the periphery into the lesion.[190]

The genomes of both species encode a novel TNF-binding protein, distinct from the receptor homolog expressed in orthopoxviruses. Studies of the protein expressed from tanapox demonstrate its high affinity for human, not murine or rabbit, TNF.[34,235] This and other unique immune-modulatory proteins expressed by one or both members of this genus likely affect their pathogenesis.

Epidemiology

Tanapox virus is restricted to Africa, principally to Kenya and the DRC, and is thought to have a simian reservoir.[61] Cases of direct primate-to-human transmission, via a break in skin, have been described in animal handlers, although such cases appear to be extremely rare.[96] Several factors have led to speculation that an insect or arthropod intermediary may be involved in transmission of tanapox virus to humans. Persons confirmed to have tanapox infection have denied contact with nonhuman primates but have reported arthropod and culcine mosquito bites prior to infection; in patients who developed multiple lesions, there was no evidence that the virus had been spread mechanically.[122] Furthermore, the seasonal variation of human tanapox infections follows the activity of local arthropod populations. No human-to-human transmission has been reported.

Clinical Features

Tanapox infection begins with a short febrile (38°C to 39°C) illness of 2 to 4 days that is sometimes accompanied by headache, backache, or prostration. The eruption of a lesion is often heralded by pruritis at the site of the outbreak. The lesion appears as a hyperpigmented macule, often with central elevation, and the macule then evolves to a papule, with palpable induration. Fever and systemic symptoms wane as the lesion manifests. The papule then becomes more "pock-like" but contains no fluid; umbilication or the formation of a pseudo-crust has been reported at this stage. Typically, the papule evolves into a firm, deep-seated, elevated nodule (Fig. 17.11A). At the end of the first week, the lesion is surrounded by erythema and indurated skin. Regional lymphangitis is common at this stage. During the next stage, lesions either ulcerate or become larger nodules (up to 2 cm in diameter) (Fig. 17.11B). In the African series, the maximum lesion size was usually reached within 2 weeks and then the local inflammatory response began to wane, and the lesion began to granulate. Resolution of lesions occurred within 6 weeks.[122]

Most cases (78% in one series) involve a solitary nodule; however, as many as 10 lesions on one individual have been described. Most lesions (72%) occur on the lower extremities, and the fewest occur in the face and areas normally covered by clothing. Infection appears to confer lifelong immunity.[122]

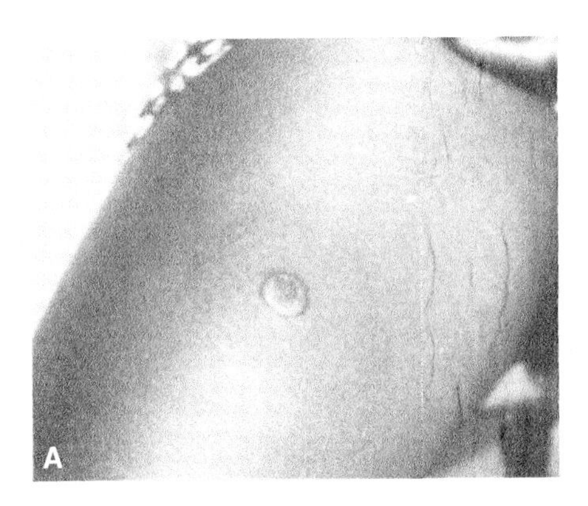

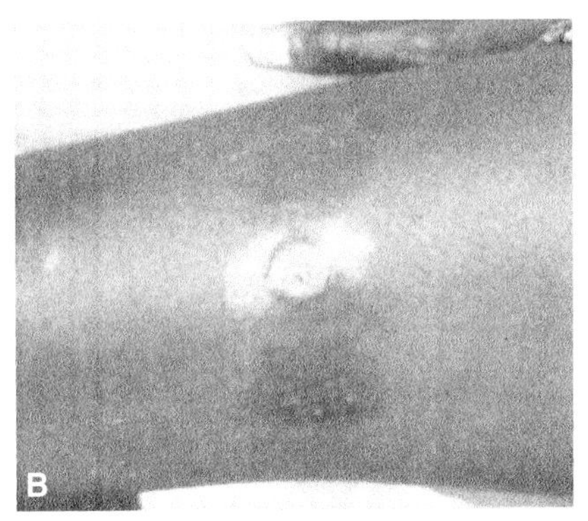

FIGURE 17.11 Lesions of tanapox in a Congolese youth. A: Day 10 of rash. **B:** Day 31 of rash. (Courtesy of Z. Jezek.)

Diagnosis

The limited geographic distribution of tanapox virus and the patient's travel history should be considered in the diagnosis of tanapox infection. Unique clinical features that allow for the differentiation of tanapox from other orthopoxvirus infections are the nodular nature of the rash lesion, the paucity of lesions, the benign disease course, and the protracted course of rash resolution. The solid nodular/ulcerated lesions are larger and develop more slowly than those of monkeypox, but they are smaller and develop more rapidly than those of tropical ulcers.

Tanapox virus can be detected by electron microscopy, and the virions usually appear enveloped, but this finding would not exclude the possibility of infection with other morphologically similar brick-shaped poxviruses; nucleic acid testing[59,276] on lesion extract could be used for that purpose. Tanapox virus grows in a number of cell lines (e.g., owl monkey kidney, Vero, MRC-5, BSC-1) but not on chorioallantoic membrane.

OTHER POXVIRUSES

This section discusses poxviruses of veterinary importance or of other interest.

Orthopoxviruses

Camelpox

Camelpox virus has a host range that is apparently restricted to *Camelus dromedarius*. The illness it causes is a systemic disease with generalized rash in dromedary camels. The disease is enzootic in camels. Geographically, the virus can be found anywhere in the native geographic distribution of the host in Asia and Africa. Case fatality rates as high as 28% in outbreaks have been noted,[124] young animals are more susceptible to severe disease manifestations, and extensive chains of transmission between camels could be documented. Another study in Somalia evaluated 295 cases of camelpox in 1,052 camels. The case fatality rate was highest in animals up to 1 year of age (13.5%), and only 2.8% in animals 4 years of age. The genome sequence shows a high degree of similarity with that of VARV[91]; despite this and the clinical similarity of camelpox disease in camels with smallpox in humans, camelpox is generally not considered to be a zoonotic disease of humans.[124] However, in human cases, (from India and South Sudan), localized lesions on the hands of camel handlers to a camelpox-like virus were reported.[26,137] Although virus was not isolated from the human lesions, genetic characterization of amplicons from one human lesion was similar to that of amplicons obtained from the camels' camelpox virus isolates. Additional surveillance is needed to understand the significance of these observations.

Camelpox disease has been experimentally studied using intradermal inoculation. By day 5, papules appear at the primary inoculation site and then form vesicles and pustules and crust by days 9 to 10. In camels, a generalized rash manifests between days 9 and 11, which is preceded by fever. The rash is most pronounced on the mouth, nose, eyes, and oral cavity. Fewer lesions are seen on the extremities. The illness can last for 2 to 5 weeks. Diagnostics historically involved evaluation of characteristic morphology on chorioallantoic membrane, in addition to electron microscopy and nucleic acid techniques. Nucleic acid PCR-based techniques are increasingly used.[26]

Prevention and control have been reported through the use of live attenuated camelpox viruses.[266] The sequences of these vaccine virus strains are not yet available, but genome restriction maps show similarity to the pathogenic strains.

Ectromelia

Ectromelia was first described in 1930.[165] The reservoir or natural hosts have been minimally characterized; virus has been reported from wild rodents.[89] Our epidemiologic understanding of this pathogen comes from studies of outbreaks of disease in captive mouse colonies; fundamental biological and genetic studies of this pathogen have provided a detailed understanding of factors involved in the host–pathogen interaction.

At least two forms of clinical "natural" disease may manifest. A rapidly fatal form that results in extensive necrosis of the liver and spleen and death occurs shortly after symptom onset; no rash is seen. Some animals do survive, however, and, if this is the case, a generalized rash can be seen (Fig. 17.12A). Characteristic organ pathology is imaged in Figure 17.12B and C. A more chronic form with ulcerating lesions of the feet tail and snout is seen in other animals. C57Bl/6 and AKR mice are highly resistant, whereas Balb/c and other inbred species are far more susceptible. Much is known about the host genetic determinants for disease presentation, and this has been reviewed.[69]

Taterapox

This virus has been isolated once in the West African country of Dahomey, now known as Benin. The virus was isolated from an apparently healthy gerbil (*Tatera kempii*) in 1968, at

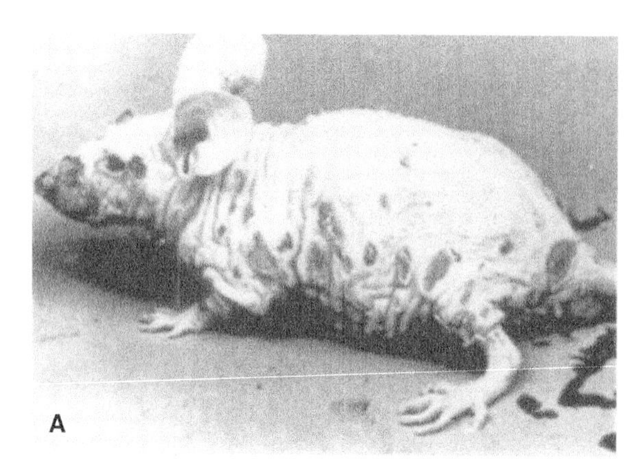

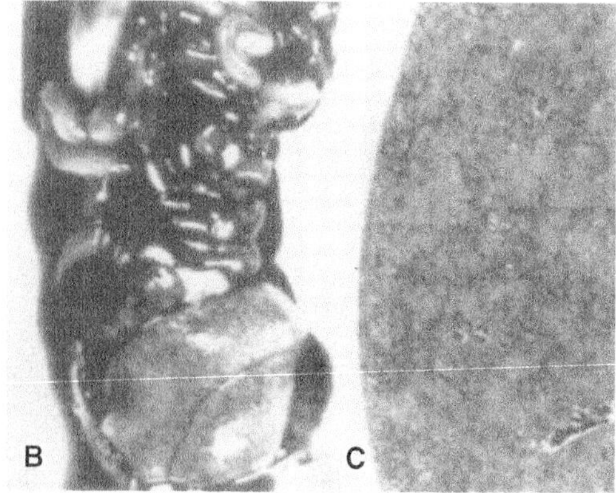

FIGURE 17.12 **Lesions of mousepox in mice. A:** The generalized rash in a susceptible hairless nonathymic mouse. **B:** Swelling and necrosis of liver and spleen and hemorrhagic intestine in a susceptible mouse that died prior to appearance of rash. **C:** Histologic appearance of necrotic liver. (**A:** Courtesy of Zentralinstiutut fur Versuchstiere, Hanover, Germany; **B and C:** Republished with permission of American Association for Laboratory Animal Science from Allen AM, Clarke GL, Ganaway JR, et al. Pathology and diagnosis of mousepox. *Lab Anim Sci* 1981;31(5 Pt 2):599–608; permission conveyed through Copyright Clearance Center, Inc.)

the time of a human smallpox outbreak. Identification as an orthopoxvirus was accomplished after liver and spleen homogenates used to inoculate suckling mouse brain–induced illness, and infectivity was blocked via administration of hyperimmune vaccinia mouse ascitic fluid. The virus had biological properties most similar to those of variola alastrim minor. The sequence of the virus is closely related to that of variola.[68] Neither 1 nonhuman primate nor 12 gerbils showed signs of viral dissemination in organs after parenteral or intracerebral inoculation.[162] This suggests that this orthopoxvirus has evolved to have a "successful" parasitic relationship and further suggests that other "nonpathogenic" orthopoxviruses exist.

North American Orthopoxviruses

Raccoonpox, skunkpox, and volepox are the North American orthopoxviruses. In general, these too have been isolated from fairly asymptomatic animals or animals with localized lesions. The viruses have been propagated in monkey kidney cell lines; A-type inclusions are evident, whereas full-genome sequence information is not yet available. Raccoonpox was identified in the upper respiratory tissues of 2 of 92 healthy-appearing raccoons trapped in Maryland. Twenty-two of these animals appeared to have orthopoxvirus seroreactivity.[140] Volepox was isolated from a skin lesion on a vole (*Microtus californicus*) in the San Francisco Bay Area of California; serosurveys of voles suggested that the virus was enzootic. Experimental infection of seronegative voles demonstrated development of a localized lesion and antiorthopoxvirus seroconversion after challenge via footpad or tail inoculation.[213]

Capripoxviruses

The capripoxviruses are somewhat larger, by electron microscopy, than other poxviruses with dimensions of 300 × 270 × 200 nm. A number of strains of each species have been sequenced; the genome is approximately 154 kbp in size. Three species of capripoxvirus have been categorized. The diseases sheeppox, goatpox, and lumpy skin are caused by the viruses of similar names (Table 17.1). Representative strains of these viruses have been sequenced.

Lumpy skin disease was first identified in 1929 in Zambia; the virus infection has largely remained restricted to the African continent[186] but has emerged in the Middle East. Illness consistent with sheeppox is recorded as early as 2 AD.[209] Reports of goatpox were first made in Norway in 1879. Sheeppox and goatpox diseases are considered to have a significant impact on domesticated animals. Geographically, they currently cause disease in Southwest Asia, on the Indian subcontinent, and in central and northern Africa. There is increasing concern for the agricultural, and economic, impact of this emerging infectious disease.[10]

Transmission of lumpy skin disease is mechanical through arthropod bites; virus has been detected in two species of biting flies, and one of these, the stable fly (*Stomoxys calcitrans*), has been shown capable of transmitting disease.[175] The reservoir host is postulated to be the African Cape buffalo. Experimentally infected young buffalo and wildebeest failed to show disease or a rise in antibody titers after infection.[272] However, LSDV seroprevalence in wild-caught buffalo has been low.[55] Within susceptible species, *Bos taurus* and *Bos indicus* mortality is usually 1% to 2%. Transmission of sheeppox and goatpox within domestic flocks is considered to be airborne[209]; additional evidence supports mechanical arthropod transmission by *S. calcitrans*. Scabs contain infectious material for months permitting fomite transmission. Sheeppox and goatpox are notifiable diseases in many countries. The spread of disease within a flock can infect up to 75% of the animals. Morbidity and mortality are highest in young animals and in lactating females, and overall mortality rates of 10% to 58% are reported.

Lumpy skin disease primarily affects species *Bos taurus* and *Bos indicus* and presents with a febrile prodrome followed, 10 days later, by cutaneous manifestations and lymphadenopathy. The skin lesions initially appear as raised nodules in the dermis and epidermis, which subsequently ulcerate and can become superinfected. In the oropharynx and mucosal surfaces, the nodules appear yellow-grey. Edema of the extremities and lymphadenitis are associated features. Recovery is slow, lasting up to 1 month.

Generally, sheeppox and goatpox are host (sheep and goat, respectively) specific, although clinical disease symptoms have been reported in both species during some outbreaks. An asymptomatic incubation period of 1 to 2 weeks is followed by febrile prodrome (up to 108°F) of mucosal swelling of the eyelids and mucosal discharge from the nose. Decreased appetite and occasionally arched back stance is noted. One to two days following prodromal symptoms, generalized appearance of approximately 1-cm lesions over the corpus develop (Fig. 17.13A and B), which progress through macular, popular, vesicular, and pustular stages; these are most obvious on areas with the least amount of hair. The lesions persist for 3 to 4 weeks and eventually scab over. Generalization of rash is more pronounced in young animals ages 4 to 5 months than it is in adult animals. Oral lesions ulcerate, and, in some animals, lesions in the lower respiratory tract are seen.

Diagnosis of capripoxvirus infections is often made on a clinical basis; differential diagnosis of lumpy skin disease includes consideration of bovine herpesvirus 2. Control strategies have largely used vaccination. Sheeppox and goatpox viruses can be grown in primary culture from ovine bovine or caprine sources. Cytoplasmic inclusion bodies are characteristic.

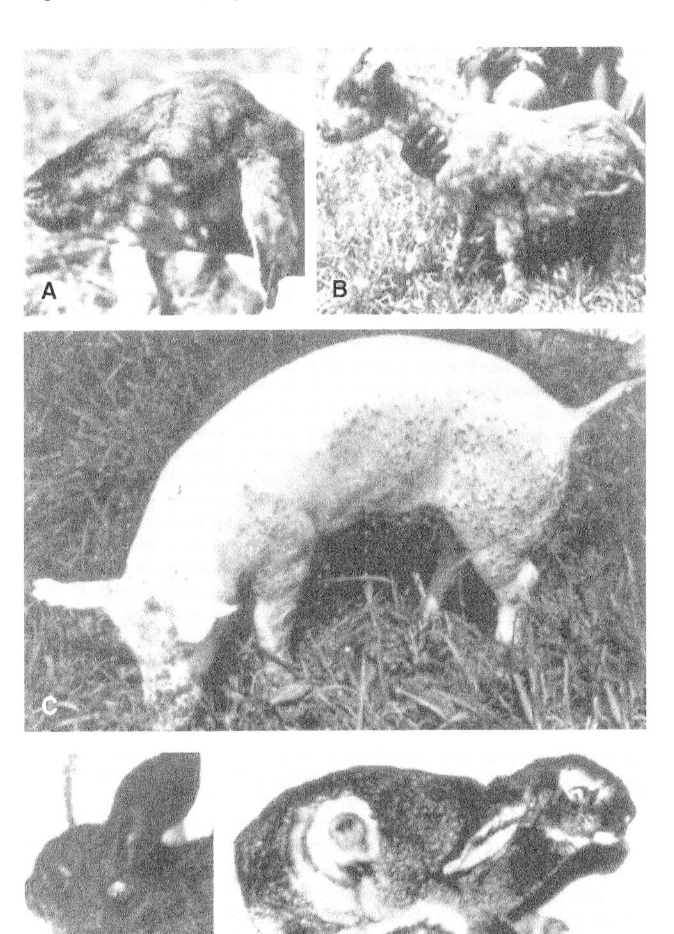

FIGURE 17.13 Infections of domestic animals with poxviruses of other genera. Capripoxvirus infection in sheep **(A)** (sheeppox) and in goats **(B)** (goatpox). **C:** Swinepox infection demonstrating generalized lesions. Myxoma virus in its native host the Californian rabbit *Sylvilagus bachmani* **(D)** and in the European rabbit *Oryctalogus cuniculi* **(E)**. **A–D**: republished with permission of John Wiley & Sons from Robinson AJ, Kerr PJ. Poxvirus Infections. In: Williams ES, Barker IK, eds. *Infectious Diseases of Wild Mammals*. 3rd ed. Ames, Iowa: Iowa State University Press; 2001:179–201; permission conveyed through Copyright Clearance Center, Inc. **A and B:** Courtesy of M. Bonniwell; **C:** Courtesy of R. Miller; **D:** Courtesy of D. C. Regnery.)

Additional laboratory diagnostics, including ELISA and PCR-based techniques, are available and have been reviewed.[209]

Prevention and control of capripoxvirus disease involve vaccination strategies. For lumpy skin diseases, strategies have included the use of sheeppox or goatpox, attenuated by tissue culture passage, or an attenuated strain of lumpy skin disease virus (strain Neethling). A review of the epidemiology and vaccination control issues is available.[110] Control of sheeppox and goatpox disease has been attempted with live attenuated and inactivated viral vaccines. However, inactivated vaccines provide only short-term protection, and the safety of live attenuated vaccines is questionable; they can cause generalized disease and death in some animals.

Suipoxvirus

An episodic viral disease of pigs with worldwide distribution, the swinepox genome, has been sequenced. The virus is currently the sole member of the *Suipoxvirus* genus and is phylogenetically most similar to species of the *Capripoxvirus* genus. Clinical disease can be heralded by low-grade fever, followed by papules, which over the course of 1 to 2 days per stage of development, progress to vesicles and pustules with umbilication (Fig. 17.13C). Crusting and scabbing of lesions ensues over the following 7 days. The duration of clinical disease can be 3 weeks. Mechanical transmission of disease between pigs occurs via the pig louse (*Haematopinus suis*). Disease control is provided by appropriate hygienic animal husbandry practices and control of the louse population.

Leporipoxvirus

The leporipoxvirus virions are brick shaped, with a size of 300 × 250 × 200 nm. Genome size is approximately 160 kbp and is 40% G+C in content. The viruses can infect multiple tissue culture cell lines. Myxoma virus is an obligate rabbit pathogen that demonstrates features that typify a general understanding of the distinction between reservoir host species and non–reservoir-susceptible species. Viral infection results in a localized "fibroma" infection in its reservoir species (Fig. 17.13D), the South American rabbit (*Sylvilagus brasiliensis*), causes a systemic, lethal disease in nonreservoir European rabbits (*Oryctolagus cuniculus*); and has coevolved with this new host. After intentional introduction of myxoma to control feral rabbit populations in Europe and Australia (the susceptible nonreservoir hosts), initial success of the program resulted in 99% mortality; however, milder virus variants emerged, and the surviving rabbits became more resistant to the effects of infection.[74]

In species susceptible to generalized disease, the illness proceeds along an aggressive course. Early clinical signs of illness are blepharoconjunctivitis and swelling of the muzzle and anogenital regions; symptoms are fever and listlessness. Within 48 hours of development of clinical signs and symptoms, animals can die; if they survive past this time point, the classic myxomas, subcutaneous swellings, develop (Fig. 17.13E). The disease is mechanically transmitted by arthropod vector bites or experimentally by intradermal injection; it can also be transmitted by droplets.

The pathogenesis in nonreservoir species follows deposition of virus into the dermis. Virus replicates in MHC-II dendritic-like cells, moves, within cells, to the draining lymph node within 24 hours to replicate in the lymph node,[27] then disseminates to the epidermis of the skin, lung, testis, and spleen. Virus from the primary lesion also moves to epidermis. A number of myxoma genes have been characterized to affect virulence and disease pathogenesis, usually via inflammatory and immune response modulation, and have been reviewed.[13,14,278] Proteins that modulate TNF, γ-IFN, and chemokines; bind CC chemokines; and inhibit apoptosis are expressed.

The fibroma viruses cause small, localized tumors—the fibroma. The host range (Table 17.1) is restricted. To date, rabbit fibroma, squirrel fibroma, and hare fibroma diseases are described, caused by rabbit fibroma (also called Shope fibroma), squirrel fibroma, and hare fibroma viruses, respectively. These have been reviewed.[14]

Control and prevention of disease is facilitated through immunization. Vaccination and protection of rabbits from myxomatosis can be provided using a related species, fibroma virus, or through the use of attenuated myxoma viruses.

Avipoxvirus

The virions of the *Avipoxvirus* genus are brick shaped, with dimensions of 330 × 280 × 200 nm. The genome size is one of the largest, about 300 kbp in size. There are a large number of avipoxviruses, mostly described by the avian species where infection has been evident to cause illness. The viruses do not cause illness or true replicative infection in mammalian hosts or mammalian cell lines but are able to present antigen to the immune system. For this reason, some have become important research vaccine vehicles. Currently, the ICTV classifies a number of avipoxvirus species: fowlpox virus, canarypox virus, juncopox virus, mynahpox virus, psittacinepox virus, quailpox virus, sparrowpox virus, starlingpox virus, turkeypox virus, and pigeonpox virus. Unclassified members are penguinpox virus, peacockpox virus, and crowpox virus.

The disease fowlpox has been best characterized. Two forms of disease manifest, and it is likely that the different manifestations are due to different routes of exposure. The first to be described manifests with largely cutaneous manifestations on the comb, wattles, and around the beak; other lesions can be evident on the limbs and cloacae. Most likely, disease results via the mechanical transmission of virus from a biting arthropod to the fowl. The lesions that develop are nodular and yellowish, and can coalesce and present a nidus for secondary bacterial infection. Lesions usually resolve in 3 weeks. Avian species with large combs are more susceptible to this form of disease than those with small combs. The other form of fowlpox has also been referred to as "diphtheric" disease. Transmission is likely via respiratory droplets between members of a flock in close proximity. The infectious lesions present in the mucosal surfaces of the airway and can coalesce to create a pseudomembrane and cause death by asphyxiation. Mortality is usually low in healthy flocks, but in flocks under stress, such as those that are egg laying, mortality can range to 50%.[30]

Novel Unclassified Poxviruses

In recent years, several novel poxviruses and new viral strains have been identified and genome sequenced. Bats are known to be a reservoir for multitude of different virus families, poxviruses are no exception, isolated from different geographic locations (Africa, Australia, Europe, and North America).[11,37,65,102,154,174,192] The viral genomes varies from 133 to 176 kb, are phylogenetically divergent, and exhibit diverse and unique clinical symptoms (progressive tenosynovitis and osteoarthritis). These bat poxviruses are tentatively classified into new genus, pteropoxvirus.[255] While poxvirus infections from marsupials were identified previously, only recently viruses were isolated and sequenced from kangaroos from different regions of Australia.[25,173,231] The genome of these viruses are around 170 kb and encode the majority of the conserved genes encoded by chordopoxviruses and are grouped under a putative new genus termed thylacopoxvirus (*thylakos*—sac or pouch). New poxvirus strains from cetaceans were identified recently, expanding the number of phylogenetically distinct strains that could tentatively be classified into genus cetacean poxvirus.[12,48] First reports of poxviruses from mustelid sp. (sea otters) were published a few years back followed with complete genome sequence of sea otterpox virus.[119,256] The genome of sea otterpox virus is the smallest known poxviral genome (127, 879 bp; 62 bp shorter than the previously determined seal parapoxvirus).[119] Salmon gill poxvirus isolated from Atlantic salmon now represent one of the most divergent and distinctive chordopoxviruses sequenced. The 241 kb genome codes for more than half the genes not previously observed in other poxviruses and lacks several of the conserved genes including the proteins required for membrane formation and morphogenesis.[83] These unclassified chordopoxviruses demonstrates greater genetic variability observed in poxviruses and the need to characterize further to understand different mechanisms adapted by poxviruses to exploit various hosts. While majority of these viruses are isolated from clinical cases, next-generation methods like pathogen discovery using metagenomics could lead to more discoveries in future.[11]

REFERENCES

1. Abrahao JS, Guedes MI, Trindade GS, et al. One more piece in the VACV ecological puzzle: could peridomestic rodents be the link between wildlife and bovine vaccinia outbreaks in Brazil? *PLoS One* 2009;4:e7428.
2. Achdout H, Lustig S, Israely T, et al. Induction, treatment and prevention of eczema vaccinatum in atopic dermatitis mouse models. *Vaccine* 2017;35:4245–4254.
3. Amara RR, Nigam P, Sharma S, et al. Long-lived poxvirus immunity, robust CD4 help, and better persistence of CD4 than CD8 T cells. *J Virol* 2004;78:3811–3816.
4. Americo JL, Moss B, Earl PL. Identification of wild-derived inbred mouse strains highly susceptible to monkeypox virus infection for use as small animal models. *J Virol* 2010;84:8172–8180.
5. Americo JL, Sood CL, Cotter CA, et al. Susceptibility of the wild-derived inbred CAST/Ei mouse to infection by orthopoxviruses analyzed by live bioluminescence imaging. *Virology* 2014;449:120–132.
6. Anderson IE, Reid HW, Nettleton PF, et al. Detection of cellular cytokine mRNA expression during orf virus infection in sheep: differential interferon-gamma mRNA expression by cells in primary versus reinfection skin lesions. *Vet Immunol Immunopathol* 2001;83:161–176.
7. Andrew ME, Coupar BE. Biological effects of recombinant vaccinia virus-expressed interleukin 4. *Cytokine* 1992;4:281–286.
8. Anonymous. Human vaccinia infection after contact with a raccoon rabies vaccine bait - Pennsylvania, 2009. *MMWR Morb Mortal Wkly Rep* 2009;58:1204–1207.
9. Anonymous. Progressive vaccinia in a military smallpox vaccinee - United States, 2009. *MMWR Morb Mortal Wkly Rep* 2009;58:532–536.
10. Babiuk S, Bowden TR, Boyle DB, et al. Capripoxviruses: an emerging worldwide threat to sheep, goats and cattle. *Transbound Emerg Dis* 2008;55:263–272.
11. Baker KS, Leggett RM, Bexfield NH, et al. Metagenomic study of the viruses of African straw-coloured fruit bats: detection of a chiropteran poxvirus and isolation of a novel adenovirus. *Virology* 2013;441:95–106.
12. Barnett J, Dastjerdi A, Davison N, et al. Identification of novel cetacean poxviruses in cetaceans stranded in South West England. *PLoS One* 2015;10:e0124315.
13. Barrett JW, Cao JX, Hota-Mitchell S, et al. Immunomodulatory proteins of myxoma virus. *Semin Immunol* 2001;13:73–84.
14. Barrett JW, McFadden G, eds. *Genus Leporipoxvirus*. Basel, Switzerland: Birkhauser; 2007.
15. Baxby D. The origins of vaccinia virus. *J Infect Dis* 1977;136:453–455.
16. Baxby D, Bennett M. Poxvirus zoonoses. *J Med Microbiol* 1997;46:17–20, 28–33.
17. Baxby D, Bennett M, Getty B. Human cowpox 1969–1993: a review based on 54 cases. *Br J Dermatol* 1994;131:598-6-7.
18. Beard PM, Griffiths SJ, Gonzalez O, et al. A loss of function analysis of host factors influencing Vaccinia virus replication by RNA interference. *PLoS One* 2014;9:e98431.

19. Beattie E, Kauffman EB, Martinez H, et al. Host-range restriction of vaccinia virus E3L-specific deletion mutants. *Virus Genes* 1996;12:89–94.
20. Becher P, Konig M, Muller G, et al. Characterization of sealpox virus, a separate member of the parapoxviruses. *Arch Virol* 2002;147:1133–1140.
21. Becker Y. Vaccinia virus pathogenicity in atopic dermatitis is caused by allergen-induced immune response that prevents the antiviral cellular and humoral immunity. *Virus Genes* 2003;27:269–282.
22. Beer EM, Rao VB. A systematic review of the epidemiology of human monkeypox outbreaks and implications for outbreak strategy. *PLoS Negl Trop Dis* 2019;13:e0007791.
23. Bennett M, Crouch AJ, Begon M, et al. Cowpox in British voles and mice. *J Comp Pathol* 1997;116:35–44.
24. Bennett M, Gaskell CJ, Gaskell RM, et al. Poxvirus infection in the domestic cat: some clinical and epidemiological observations. *Vet Rec* 1986;118:387–390.
25. Bennett M, Tu SL, Upton C, et al. Complete genomic characterisation of two novel poxviruses (WKPV and EKPV) from western and eastern grey kangaroos. *Virus Res* 2017;242:106–121.
26. Bera BC, Shanmugasundaram K, Barua S, et al. Zoonotic cases of camelpox infection in India. *Vet Microbiol* 2011;152:29–38.
27. Best SM, Kerr PJ. Coevolution of host and virus: the pathogenesis of virulent and attenuated strains of myxoma virus in resistant and susceptible European rabbits. *Virology* 2000;267:36–48.
28. Birthistle K, Carrington D. Molluscum contagiosum virus. *J Infect* 1997;34:21–28.
29. Bolken TC, Hruby DE. Tecovirimat for smallpox infections. *Drugs Today (Barc)* 2010;46:109–117.
30. Boyle D, ed. *Genus Avipoxvirus*. Basel, Switzerland: Birkhauser; 2007.
31. Bras G. The morbid anatomy of smallpox. *Doc Med Geogr Trop* 1952;4(4):303–351.
32. Bray M, Wright ME. Progressive vaccinia. *Clin Infect Dis* 2003;36:766–774.
33. Brum LM, Lopez MC, Varela JC, et al. Microarray analysis of A549 cells infected with rabbitpox virus (RPV): a comparison of wild-type RPV and RPV deleted for the host range gene, SPI-1. *Virology* 2003;315:322–334.
34. Brunetti CR, Paulose-Murphy M, Singh R, et al. A secreted high-affinity inhibitor of human TNF from Tanapox virus. *Proc Natl Acad Sci U S A* 2003;100:4831–4836.
35. Buddle BM, Pulford HD. Effect of passively-acquired antibodies and vaccination on the immune response to contagious ecthyma virus. *Vet Microbiol* 1984;9:515–522.
36. Buller RM, Palumbo GJ. Poxvirus pathogenesis. *Microbiol Rev* 1991;55:80–122.
37. Calisher CH, Childs JE, Field HE, et al. Bats: important reservoir hosts of emerging viruses. *Clin Microbiol Rev* 2006;19:531–545.
38. Campe H, Zimmermann P, Glos K, et al. Cowpox virus transmission from pet rats to humans, Germany. *Emerg Infect Dis* 2009;15:777–780.
39. Carroll D, Emerson G, Li Y, et al. Chasing Jenner's vaccine: revisiting cowpox virus classification. *PLOS One*. 2011;6(8):e23086.
40. Carroll DS, Olson VA, Smith SK, et al. Orthopoxvirus variola infection of Cynomys ludovicianus (North American black tailed prairie dog). *Virology* 2013;443:358–362.
41. Carslake D, Bennett M, Hazel S, et al. Inference of cowpox virus transmission rates between wild rodent host classes using space-time interaction. *Proc Biol Sci* 2006;273:775–782.
42. Carson CA, Kerr KM, Grumbles LC. Bovine papular stomatitis: experimental transmission from man. *Am J Vet Res* 1968;29:1783–1790.
43. Chantrey J, Meyer H, Baxby D, et al. Cowpox: reservoir hosts and geographic range. *Epidemiol Infect* 1999;122:455–460.
44. Chapman JL, Nichols DK, Martinez MJ, et al. Animal models of orthopoxvirus infection. *Vet Pathol* 2010;47:852–870.
45. Chaudhri G, Panchanathan V, Bluethmann H, et al. Obligatory requirement for antibody in recovery from a primary poxvirus infection. *J Virol* 2006;80:6339–6344.
46. Chaudhri G, Panchanathan V, Buller RM, et al. Polarized type 1 cytokine response and cell-mediated immunity determine genetic resistance to mousepox. *Proc Natl Acad Sci U S A* 2004;101:9057–9062.
47. Chen N, Li G, Liszewski MK, et al. Virulence differences between monkeypox virus isolates from West Africa and the Congo basin. *Virology* 2005;340:46–63.
48. Cocumelli C, Fichi G, Marsili L, et al. Cetacean poxvirus in two striped dolphins (Stenella coeruleoalba) stranded on the Tyrrhenian Coast of Italy: histopathological, ultrastructural, biomolecular, and ecotoxicological findings. *Front Vet Sci* 2018;5:219.
49. Coloe J, Burkhart CN, Morrell DS. Molluscum contagiosum: what's new and true? *Pediatr Ann* 2009;38:321–325.
50. Cono J, Casey CG, Bell DM. Smallpox vaccination and adverse reactions. Guidance for clinicians. *MMWR Recomm Rep* 2003;52:1–28.
51. Crotty S, Felgner P, Davies H, et al. Cutting edge: long-term B cell memory in humans after smallpox vaccination. *J Immunol* 2003;171:4969–4973.
52. Czerny CP, Waldmann R, Scheubeck T. Identification of three distinct antigenic sites in parapoxviruses. *Arch Virol* 1997;142:807–821.
53. da Fonseca FG, Trindade GS, Silva RL, et al. Characterization of a vaccinia-like virus isolated in a Brazilian forest. *J Gen Virol* 2002;83:223–228.
54. Damon I. Poxviruses that infect humans. In: Murray PJ, Baron EJ, Jorgensen G, Landry M, Pfaller, eds. *Manual of Clinical Microbiology*. Washington, DC: ASM Press; 2011.
55. Davies FG. Lumpy skin disease, an African capripox virus disease of cattle. *Br Vet J* 1991;147:489–503.
56. de Souza Trindade G, da Fonseca FG, Marques JT, et al. Aracatuba virus: a vaccinialike virus associated with infection in humans and cattle. *Emerg Infect Dis* 2003;9:155–160.
57. de Souza Trindade G, Drumond BP, Guedes MI, et al. Zoonotic vaccinia virus infection in Brazil: clinical description and implications for health professionals. *J Clin Microbiol* 2007;45:1370–1372.
58. Delhon G, Tulman ER, Afonso CL, et al. Genomes of the parapoxviruses ORF virus and bovine papular stomatitis virus. *J Virol* 2004;78:168–177.
59. Dhar AD, Werchniak AE, Li Y, et al. Tanapox infection in a college student. *N Engl J Med* 2004;350:361–366.
60. DiPerna G, Stack J, Bowie AG, et al. Poxvirus protein N1L targets the I-kappaB kinase complex, inhibits signaling to NF-kappaB by the tumor necrosis factor superfamily of receptors, and inhibits NF-kappaB and IRF3 signaling by toll-like receptors. *J Biol Chem* 2004;279:36570–36578.
61. Downie AW. The epidemiology of tanapox and yaba virus infections. *J Med Microbiol* 1972;5:Pxiv.
62. Downie AW, Espana C. Comparison of Tanapox virus and Yaba-like viruses causing epidemic disease in monkeys. *J Hyg (Lond)* 1972;70:23–32.
63. Edghill-Smith Y, Golding H, Manischewitz J, et al. Smallpox vaccine-induced antibodies are necessary and sufficient for protection against monkeypox virus. *Nat Med* 2005;11:740–747.
64. Elde NC, Child SJ, Eickbush MT, et al. Poxviruses deploy genomic accordions to adapt rapidly against host antiviral defenses. *Cell* 2012;150:831–841.
65. Emerson GL, Nordhausen R, Garner MM, et al. Novel poxvirus in big brown bats, northwestern United States. *Emerg Infect Dis* 2013;19:1002–1004.
66. Erez N, Achdout H, Milrot E, et al. Diagnosis of imported monkeypox, Israel, 2018. *Emerg Infect Dis* 2019;25:980–983.
67. Erlandson KJ, Cotter CA, Charity JC, et al. Duplication of the A17L locus of vaccinia virus provides an alternate route to rifampin resistance. *J Virol* 2014;88:11576–11585.
68. Esposito JJ, Sammons SA, Frace AM, et al. Genome sequence diversity and clues to the evolution of variola (smallpox) virus. *Science* 2006;313:807–812.
69. Esteban DJ, Buller RM. Ectromelia virus: the causative agent of mousepox. *J Gen Virol* 2005;86:2645–2659.
70. Falendysz EA, Lopera JG, Doty JB, et al. Characterization of Monkeypox virus infection in African rope squirrels (Funisciurus sp.). *PLoS Negl Trop Dis* 2017;11:e0005809.
71. Fang M, Lanier LL, Sigal LJ. A role for NKG2D in NK cell-mediated resistance to poxvirus disease. *PLoS Pathog* 2008;4:e30.
72. Fenner F. Studies in infectious ectromelia virus. II. Natural transmission: the portal of entry of the virus. *Aust J Exp Biol Med Sci* 1947;25:275–282.
73. Fenner F, Henderson DA, Arita I, et al. *Smallpox and its Eradication*. Geneva: World Health Organization; 1988.
74. Fenner F, Ratcliffe FN. *Myxomatosis*. London: Cambridge University Press; 1965.
75. Fenner F, Wittek R, Dumbell K. *The Pathogenesis, Pathology, and Immunology of Orthopoxvirus Infections: The Orthopoxviruses*. New York: Academic Press; 1989.
76. Fischer MA, Norbury CC. Initiation of primary anti-vaccinia virus immunity in vivo. *Immunol Res* 2007;37:113–133.
77. Fleming SB, Anderson IE, Thomson J, et al. Infection with recombinant orf viruses demonstrates that the viral interleukin-10 is a virulence factor. *J Gen Virol* 2007;88:1922–1927.
78. Franke A, Pfaff F, Jenckel M, et al. Classification of cowpox viruses into several distinct clades and identification of a novel lineage. *Viruses* 2017;9(6):142.
79. Fulginiti VA, Papier A, Lane JM, et al. Smallpox vaccination: a review, part II. Adverse events. *Clin Infect Dis* 2003;37:251–271.
80. Gallardo-Romero NF, Hutson CL, Carroll D, et al. Use of live Variola virus to determine whether CAST/EiJ mice are a suitable surrogate animal model for human smallpox. *Virus Res* 2019;275:197772. doi:10.1016/j.virusres.2019.197772.
81. Gazzani P, Gach JE, Colmenero I, et al. Fatal disseminated cowpox virus infection in an adolescent renal transplant recipient. *Pediatr Nephrol* 2017;32:533–536.
82. Gigante CM, Gao J, Tang S, et al. Genome of Alaskapox virus, a novel orthopoxvirus isolated from Alaska. *Viruses* 2019;11(8):708.
83. Gjessing MC, Yutin N, Tengs T, et al. Salmon gill poxvirus, the deepest representative of the chordopoxvirinae. *J Virol* 2015;89:9348–9367.
84. Goff AJ, Chapman J, Foster C, et al. A novel respiratory model of infection with monkeypox virus in cynomolgus macaques. *J Virol* 2011;85:4898–4909.
85. Gottlieb SL, Myskowski PL. Molluscum contagiosum. *Int J Dermatol* 1994;33:453–461.
86. Grace JT Jr, Mirand EA. Yaba virus infection in humans. *Exp Med Surg* 1965;23:213–216.
87. Greenberg RN, Kennedy JS. ACAM2000: a newly licensed cell culture-based live vaccinia smallpox vaccine. *Expert Opin Investig Drugs* 2008;17:555–564.
88. Greene HSN. Rabbitpox. II. Pathology of the epidemic disease. *J Exp Med* 1934;60(4):441–455.
89. Groppel KH. The occurrence of ectromelia (mousepox)in wild mice. *Arch Exp Vet* 1962;16:243–278.
90. Gruber CEM, Giombini E, Selleri M, et al. Whole genome characterization of orthopoxvirus (OPV) abatino, a zoonotic virus representing a putative novel clade of old world orthopoxviruses. *Viruses* 2018;10(10):546.
91. Gubser C, Smith GL. The sequence of camelpox virus shows it is most closely related to variola virus, the cause of smallpox. *J Gen Virol* 2002;83:855–872.
92. Gubser C, Hue S, Kellam P, et al. Poxvirus genomes: a phylogenetic analysis. *J Gen Virol* 2004;85:105–117.
93. Guerra S, Lopez-Fernandez LA, Conde R, et al. Microarray analysis reveals characteristic changes of host cell gene expression in response to attenuated modified vaccinia virus Ankara infection of human HeLa cells. *J Virol* 2004;78:5820–5834.
94. Hahon N. Smallpox and related poxvirus infections in the simian host. *Bacteriol Rev* 1961;25:459–476.
95. Haig DM, McInnes CJ. Immunity and counter-immunity during infection with the parapoxvirus orf virus. *Virus Res* 2002;88:3–16.
96. Hall AS, McNulty WP Jr. A contagious pox disease in monkeys. *J Am Vet Med Assoc* 1967;151:833–838.
97. Haller SL, Peng C, McFadden G, et al. Poxviruses and the evolution of host range and virulence. *Infect Genet Evol* 2014;21:15–40.
98. Halsell JS, Riddle JR, Atwood JE, et al. Myopericarditis following smallpox vaccination among vaccinia-naive US military personnel. *JAMA* 2003;289:3283–3289.
99. Hammarlund E, Lewis MW, Hanifin JM, et al. Antiviral immunity following smallpox virus infection: a case–control study. *J Virol* 2010;84:12754–12760.
100. Hammarlund E, Lewis MW, Hansen SG, et al. Duration of antiviral immunity after smallpox vaccination. *Nat Med* 2003;9:1131–1137.
101. Hayasaka D, Ennis FA, Terajima M. Pathogeneses of respiratory infections with virulent and attenuated vaccinia viruses. *Virol J* 2007;4:22.
102. Hayman DT. Bats as viral reservoirs. *Annu Rev Virol* 2016;3:77–99.

103. Heiner GG, Fatima N, McCrumb FR Jr. A study of intrafamilial transmission of smallpox. *Am J Epidemiol* 1971;94:316–326.
104. Hicks BD, Worthy GA. Sealpox in captive grey seals (Halichoerus grypus) and their handlers. *J Wildl Dis* 1987;23:1–6.
105. Hoebe K, Du X, Georgel P, et al. Identification of Lps2 as a key transducer of MyD88-independent TIR signalling. *Nature* 2003;424:743–748.
106. Horner GW, Robinson AJ, Hunter R, et al. Parapoxvirus infections in New Zealand farmed red deer (Cervus elaphus). *N Z Vet J* 1987;35:41–45.
107. Howell MD, Gallo RL, Boguniewicz M, et al. Cytokine milieu of atopic dermatitis skin subverts the innate immune response to vaccinia virus. *Immunity* 2006;24:341–348.
108. Howell MD, Jones JF, Kisich KO, et al. Selective killing of vaccinia virus by LL-37: implications for eczema vaccinatum. *J Immunol* 2004;172:1763–1767.
109. Huggins J, Goff A, Hensley L, et al. Nonhuman primates are protected from smallpox virus or monkeypox virus challenges by the antiviral drug ST-246. *Antimicrob Agents Chemother* 2009;53:2620–2625.
110. Hunter P, Wallace D. Lumpy skin disease in southern Africa: a review of the disease and aspects of control. *J S Afr Vet Assoc* 2001;72:68–71.
111. Hutin YJ, Williams RJ, Malfait P, et al. Outbreak of human monkeypox, Democratic Republic of Congo, 1996 to 1997. *Emerg Infect Dis* 2001;7:434–438.
112. Hutson CL, Carroll DS, Self J, et al. Dosage comparison of Congo Basin and West African strains of monkeypox virus using a prairie dog animal model of systemic orthopoxvirus disease. *Virology* 2010;402:72–82.
113. Hutson CL, Damon IK. Monkeypox virus infections in small animal models for evaluation of anti-poxvirus agents. *Viruses* 2010;2:2763–2776.
114. Hutson CL, Gallardo-Romero N, Carroll DS, et al. Transmissibility of the monkeypox virus clades via respiratory transmission: investigation using the prairie dog-monkeypox virus challenge system. *PLoS One* 2013;8:e55488.
115. Hutson CL, Nakazawa YJ, Self J, et al. Laboratory investigations of African pouched rats (Cricetomys gambianus) as a potential reservoir host species for Monkeypox virus. *PLoS Negl Trop Dis* 2015;9:e0004013.
116. Hutson CL, Olson VA, Carroll DS, et al. A prairie dog animal model of systemic orthopoxvirus disease using West African and Congo Basin strains of monkeypox virus. *J Gen Virol* 2009;90:323–333.
117. Inoshima Y, Morooka A, Sentsui H. Detection and diagnosis of parapoxvirus by the polymerase chain reaction. *J Virol Methods* 2000;84:201–208.
118. Jackson RJ, Ramsay AJ, Christensen CD, et al. Expression of mouse interleukin-4 by a recombinant ectromelia virus suppresses cytolytic lymphocyte responses and overcomes genetic resistance to mousepox. *J Virol* 2001;75:1205–1210.
119. Jacob JM, Subramaniam K, Tu SL, et al. Complete genome sequence of a novel sea otterpox virus. *Virus Genes* 2018;54:756–767.
120. Jahrling PB, Hensley LE, Martinez MJ, et al. Exploring the potential of variola virus infection of cynomolgus macaques as a model for human smallpox. *Proc Natl Acad Sci U S A* 2004;101:15196–15200.
121. Jenner E. *An Enquiry into the Causes and Effects of Variolae Vaccinae, a Disease Discovered in Some of the Western Counties of England, Particularly Gloucerstershire, and Known by the Name of Cowpox.* London: Sampson Low; 1798.
122. Jezek Z, Arita I, Szczeniowski M, et al. Human tanapox in Zaire: clinical and epidemiological observations on cases confirmed by laboratory studies. *Bull World Health Organ* 1985;63:1027–1035.
123. Jezek Z, Fenner F. *Human Monkeypox*, vol 1. New York: Karger; 1988.
124. Jezek Z, Kriz B, Rothbauer V. Camelpox and its risk to the human population. *J Hyg Epidemiol Microbiol Immunol* 1983;27:29–42.
125. Johannessen JV, Krogh HK, Solberg I, et al. Human orf. *J Cutan Pathol* 1975;2:265–283.
126. Karem KL, Reynolds M, Braden Z, et al. Characterization of acute-phase humoral immunity to monkeypox: use of immunoglobulin M enzyme-linked immunosorbent assay for detection of monkeypox infection during the 2003 North American outbreak. *Clin Diagn Lab Immunol* 2005;12:867–872.
127. Karem KL, Reynolds M, Hughes C, et al. Monkeypox-induced immunity and failure of childhood smallpox vaccination to provide complete protection. *Clin Vaccine Immunol* 2007;14:1318–1327.
128. Karupiah G, Buller RM, Van Rooijen N, et al. Different roles for CD4+ and CD8+ T lymphocytes and macrophage subsets in the control of a generalized virus infection. *J Virol* 1996;70:8301–8309.
129. Karupiah G, Panchanathan V, Sakala IG, et al. Genetic resistance to smallpox: lessons from mousepox. *Novartis Found Symp* 2007;281:129–136; discussion 136–40, 208–9.
130. Kastenmayer RJ, Maruri-Avidal L, Americo JL, et al. Elimination of A-type inclusion formation enhances cowpox virus replication in mice: implications for orthopoxvirus evolution. *Virology* 2014;452–453:59–66.
131. Keckler MS, Carroll DS, Gallardo-Romero NF, et al. Establishment of the black-tailed prairie dog (Cynomys ludovicianus) as a novel animal model for comparing smallpox vaccines administered preexposure in both high- and low-dose monkeypox virus challenges. *J Virol* 2011;85:7683–7698.
132. Keidan SE, McCarthy K, Haworth JC. Fatal generalized vaccinia with failure of antibody production and absence of serum gamma globulin. *Arch Dis Child* 1953;28:110–116.
133. Kelly CD, Egan C, Davis SW, et al. Laboratory confirmation of generalized vaccinia following smallpox vaccination. *J Clin Microbiol* 2004;42:1373–1375.
134. Kempe CH. Studies smallpox and complications of smallpox vaccination. *Pediatrics* 1960;26:176–189.
135. Kennedy RB, Ovsyannikova IG, Jacobson RM, et al. The immunology of smallpox vaccines. *Curr Opin Immunol* 2009;21:314–320.
136. Kern ER. In vitro activity of potential anti-poxvirus agents. *Antiviral Res* 2003;57:35–40.
137. Khalafalla AI, Abdelazim F. Human and dromedary camel infection with camelpox cirus in Eastern Sudan. *Vector Borne Zoonotic Dis* 2017;17:281–284.
138. Kibler KV, Shors T, Perkins KB, et al. Double-stranded RNA is a trigger for apoptosis in vaccinia virus-infected cells. *J Virol* 1997;71:1992–2003.
139. Klein J, Tryland M. Characterisation of parapoxviruses isolated from Norwegian semi-domesticated reindeer (Rangifer tarandus tarandus). *Virol J* 2005;2:79.
140. Knight JC, Goldsmith CS, Tamin A, et al. Further analyses of the orthopoxviruses volepox virus and raccoon poxvirus. *Virology* 1992;190:423–433.
141. Knight JC, Novembre FJ, Brown DR, et al. Studies on Tanapox virus. *Virology* 1989;172:116–124.
142. Kolhapure RM, Deolankar RP, Tupe CD, et al. Investigation of buffalopox outbreaks in Maharashtra State during 1992–1996. *Indian J Med Res* 1997;106:441–446.
143. Koplan JP, Marton KI. Smallpox vaccination revisited. Some observations on the biology of vaccinia. *Am J Trop Med Hyg* 1975;24:656–663.
144. Kurth A, Nitsche A. Detection of human-pathogenic poxviruses. *Methods Mol Biol* 2011;665:257–278.
145. Lakis NS, Li Y, Abraham JL, et al. Novel poxvirus infection in an immune suppressed patient. *Clin Infect Dis* 2015;61:1543–1548.
146. Lane JM, Ruben FL, Neff JM, et al. Complications of smallpox vaccination, 1968. *N Engl J Med* 1969;281:1201–1208.
147. Lanier R, Trost L, Tippin T, et al. Development of CMX001 for the treatment of poxvirus infections. *Viruses* 2010;2:2740–2762.
148. Lateef Z, Baird MA, Wise LM, et al. The chemokine-binding protein encoded by the poxvirus orf virus inhibits recruitment of dendritic cells to sites of skin inflammation and migration to peripheral lymph nodes. *Cell Microbiol* 2010;12:665–676.
149. Lateef Z, Fleming S, Halliday G, et al. Orf virus-encoded interleukin-10 inhibits maturation, antigen presentation and migration of murine dendritic cells. *J Gen Virol* 2003;84:1101–1109.
150. Learned LA, Reynolds MG, Wassa DW, et al. Extended interhuman transmission of monkeypox in a hospital community in the Republic of the Congo, 2003. *Am J Trop Med Hyg* 2005;73:428–434.
151. Leavell UW Jr, McNamara MJ, Muelling R, et al. Orf. Report of 19 human cases with clinical and pathological observations. *JAMA* 1968;204:657–664.
152. Lee SB, Esteban M. The interferon-induced double-stranded RNA-activated protein kinase induces apoptosis. *Virology* 1994;199:491–496.
153. Leite JA, Drumond BP, Trindade GS, et al. Passatempo virus, a vaccinia virus strain, Brazil. *Emerg Infect Dis* 2005;11:1935–1938.
154. Lelli D, Lavazza A, Prosperi A, et al. Hypsugopoxvirus: a novel poxvirus isolated from hypsugo savii in Italy. *Viruses* 2019;11(6):568.
155. Li Y, Carroll DS, Gardner SN, et al. On the origin of smallpox: correlating variola phylogenics with historical smallpox records. *Proc Natl Acad Sci U S A* 2007;104:15787–15792.
156. Li Y, Meyer H, Zhao H, et al. GC content-based pan-pox universal PCR assays for poxvirus detection. *J Clin Microbiol* 2010;48:268–276.
157. Li Y, Olson VA, Laue T, et al. Detection of monkeypox virus with real-time PCR assays. *J Clin Virol* 2006;36:194–203.
158. Likos AM, Sammons SA, Olson VA, et al. A tale of two clades: monkeypox viruses. *J Gen Virol* 2005;86:2661–2672.
159. Lipschutz B, ed. *Handbuch der Haut und Geschlechtskrankenheiten.* Berlin, Germany: Springer; 1932.
160. Livingston CW, Hardy WT. Longevity of contagious ecthyma virus. *J Am Vet Med Assoc* 1960;137:651.
161. Lloyd JB, Gill HS, Haig DM, et al. In vivo T-cell subset depletion suggests that CD4+ T-cells and a humoral immune response are important for the elimination of orf virus from the skin of sheep. *Vet Immunol Immunopathol* 2000;74:249–262.
162. Lourie B, Nakano JH, Kemp GE, et al. Isolation of poxvirus from an African Rodent. *J Infect Dis* 1975;132:677–681.
163. Luker KE, Hutchens M, Schultz T, et al. Bioluminescence imaging of vaccinia virus: effects of interferon on viral replication and spread. *Virology* 2005;341:284–300.
164. Luteijn RD, van Diemen F, Blomen VA, et al. A genome-wide haploid genetic screen identifies heparan sulfate-associated genes and the macropinocytosis modulator TMED10 as factors supporting vaccinia virus infection. *J Virol* 2019;93(13):e02160-18.
165. Marchal J. Infectious ectromelia. *J Pathol Bacteriol* 1930;33:713–728.
166. Marennikova SS, Maltseva NN, Korneeva VI, et al. Outbreak of pox disease among carnivora (felidae) and edentata. *J Infect Dis* 1977;135:358–366.
167. Martinez MJ, Bray MP, Huggins JW. A mouse model of aerosol-transmitted orthopoxviral disease: morphology of experimental aerosol-transmitted orthopoxviral disease in a cowpox virus-BALB/c mouse system. *Arch Pathol Lab Med* 2000;124:362–377.
168. Massoudi MS, Barker L, Schwartz B. Effectiveness of postexposure vaccination for the prevention of smallpox: results of a delphi analysis. *J Infect Dis* 2003;188:973–976.
169. McCabe D, Weston B, Storch G. Treatment of orf poxvirus lesion with cidofovir cream. *Pediatr Infect Dis J* 2003;22:1027–1028.
170. McCurdy LH, Larkin BD, Martin JE, et al. Modified vaccinia Ankara: potential as an alternative smallpox vaccine. *Clin Infect Dis* 2004;38:1749–1753.
171. McFadden G. Poxvirus tropism. *Nat Rev Microbiol* 2005;3:201–213.
172. McKeever DJ, Jenkinson DM, Hutchison G, et al. 1988. Studies of the pathogenesis of orf virus infection in sheep. *J Comp Pathol* 99:317–328.
173. McKenzie RA, Fay FR, Prior HC. Poxvirus infection of the skin of an eastern grey kangaroo. *Aust Vet J* 1979;55:188–190.
174. McLelland DJ, Reardon T, Bourne S, et al. Outbreak of skin nodules associated with Riouxgolvania beveridgei (Nematoda: Muspiceida) in the southern bentwing bat (Miniopterus schreibersii bassanii), South Australia. *J Wildl Dis* 2013;49:1009–1013.
175. Mellor PS, Kitching RP, Wilkinson PJ. Mechanical transmission of capripox virus and African swine fever virus by Stomoxys calcitrans. *Res Vet Sci* 1987;43:109–112.
176. Mercer J, Snijder B, Sacher R, et al. RNAi screening reveals proteasome- and Cullin3-dependent stages in vaccinia virus infection. *Cell Rep* 2012;2:1036–1047.
177. Mercer AA, Ueda N, Friederichs SM, et al. Comparative analysis of genome sequences of three isolates of Orf virus reveals unexpected sequence variation. *Virus Res* 2006;116:146–158.
178. Meseda CA, Mayer AE, Kumar A, et al. Comparative evaluation of the immune responses and protection engendered by LC16m8 and Dryvax smallpox vaccines in a mouse model. *Clin Vaccine Immunol* 2009;16:1261–1271.
179. Mohamed MR, McFadden G. NFkB inhibitors: strategies from poxviruses. *Cell Cycle* 2009;8:3125–3132.

180. Moss B. Membrane fusion during poxvirus entry. *Semin Cell Dev Biol* 2016;60:89–96.
181. Moss B. Poxvirus entry and membrane fusion. *Virology* 2006;344:48–54.
182. Mucker EM, Wollen-Roberts SE, Kimmel A, et al. Intranasal monkeypox marmoset model: prophylactic antibody treatment provides benefit against severe monkeypox virus disease. *PLoS Negl Trop Dis* 2018;12:e0006581.
183. Nakamura J, Muraki Y, Yamada M, et al. Analysis of molluscum contagiosum virus genomes isolated in Japan. *J Med Virol* 1995;46:339–348.
184. Nakazawa Y, Emerson GL, Carroll DS, et al. Phylogenetic and ecologic perspectives of a monkeypox outbreak, southern Sudan, 2005. *Emerg Infect Dis* 2013;19:237–245.
185. Nalca A, Livingston VA, Garza NL, et al. Experimental infection of cynomolgus macaques (Macaca fascicularis) with aerosolized monkeypox virus. *PLoS One* 2010;5(9):e12880.
186. Nawathe DR, Gibbs EP, Asagba MO, et al. Lumpyskin disease in Nigeria. *Trop Anim Health Prod* 1978;10:49–54.
187. Nell P, Kohl KS, Graham PL, et al. Eczema vaccinatum as an adverse event following exposure to vaccinia virus: case definition & guidelines of data collection, analysis, and presentation of immunization safety data. *Vaccine* 2007;25:5725–5734.
188. Nell P, Kohl KS, Graham PL, et al. Progressive vaccinia as an adverse event following exposure to vaccinia virus: case definition and guidelines of data collection, analysis, and presentation of immunization safety data. *Vaccine* 2007;25:5735–5744.
189. Ng OT, Lee V, Marimuthu K, et al. A case of imported monkeypox in Singapore. *Lancet Infect Dis* 2019;19:1166.
190. Niven JS, Armstrong JA, Andrewes CH, et al. Subcutaneous "growths" in monkeys produced by a poxvirus. *J Pathol Bacteriol* 1961;81:1–14.
191. Noyce RS, Lederman S, Evans DH. Construction of an infectious horsepox virus vaccine from chemically synthesized DNA fragments. *PLoS One* 2018;13:e0188453.
192. O'Dea MA, Tu SL, Pang S, et al. Genomic characterization of a novel poxvirus from a flying fox: evidence for a new genus? *J Gen Virol* 2016;97:2363–2375.
193. Oliveira GP, Rodrigues RAL, Lima MT, et al. Poxvirus host range genes and virus-host spectrum: a critical review. *Viruses* 2017;9(11):331.
194. Olsen JR, Gallacher J, Piguet V, et al. Epidemiology of molluscum contagiosum in children: a systematic review. *Fam Pract* 2014;31:130–136.
195. Olson C Jr, Palionis T. The transmission of proliferative stomatitis of cattle. *J Am Vet Med Assoc* 1953;123:419–426.
196. Olson VA, Laue T, Laker MT, et al. Real-time PCR system for detection of orthopoxviruses and simultaneous identification of smallpox virus. *J Clin Microbiol* 2004;42:1940–1946.
197. Pajer P, Dresler J, Kabickova H, et al. Characterization of two historic smallpox specimens from a Czech museum. *Viruses* 2017;9(8):200.
198. Panchanathan V, Chaudhri G, Karupiah G. Interferon function is not required for recovery from a secondary poxvirus infection. *Proc Natl Acad Sci U S A* 2005;102:12921–12926.
199. Panchanathan V, Chaudhri G, Karupiah G. Antiviral protection following immunization correlates with humoral but not cell-mediated immunity. *Immunol Cell Biol* 2010;88:461–467.
200. Perkus ME, Goebel SJ, Davis SW, et al. Vaccinia virus host range genes. *Virology* 1990;179:276–286.
201. Petersen BW, Harms TJ, Reynolds MG, et al. Use of vaccinia virus smallpox vaccine in laboratory and health care personnel at risk for occupational exposure to orthopoxviruses - recommendations of the Advisory Committee on Immunization Practices (ACIP), 2015. *MMWR Morb Mortal Wkly Rep* 2016;65:257–262.
202. Pierard-Franchimont C, Legrain A, Pierard GE. Growth and regression of molluscum contagiosum. *J Am Acad Dermatol* 1983;9:669–672.
203. Pilaski J, Rosen-Wolff A. Poxvirus infection in zoo-kept mammals. In: Darai G, ed. *Virus Diseases in Captive and Laboratory Animals*. Boston, MA: Martenjus-Nijhoff; 1988:84–100.
204. Pilaski J, Rosen A, Darai G. Comparative analysis of the genomes of orthopoxviruses isolated from elephant, rhinoceros, and okapi by restriction enzymes. Brief report. *Arch Virol* 1986;88:135–142.
205. Pogo BG, Melana SM, Blaho J. Poxvirus infection and apoptosis. *Int Rev Immunol* 2004;23:61–74.
206. Postlethwaite R. Molluscum contagiosum. *Arch Environ Health* 1970;21:432–452.
207. Quenelle DC, Prichard MN, Keith KA, et al. Synergistic efficacy of the combination of ST-246 with CMX001 against orthopoxviruses. *Antimicrob Agents Chemother* 2007;51:4118–4124.
208. Ramshaw IA, Ramsay AJ, Karupiah G, et al. Cytokines and immunity to viral infections. *Immunol Rev* 1997;159:119–135.
209. Rao TV, Bandyopadhyay SK. A comprehensive review of goat pox and sheep pox and their diagnosis. *Anim Health Res Rev* 2000;1:127–136.
210. Realegeno S, Puschnik AS, Kumar A, et al. Monkeypox virus host factor screen using haploid cells identifies essential role of GARP complex in extracellular virus formation. *J Virol* 2017:91.
211. Reeves PM, Bommarius B, Lebeis S, et al. Disabling poxvirus pathogenesis by inhibition of Abl-family tyrosine kinases. *Nat Med* 2005;11:731–739.
212. Reeves PM, Smith SK, Olson VA, et al. Variola and monkeypox viruses utilize conserved mechanisms of virion motility and release that depend on abl and SRC family tyrosine kinases. *J Virol* 2011;85:21–31.
213. Regnery DC. Isolation and partial characterization of an orthopoxvirus from a California vole (Microtus californicus). Brief report. *Arch Virol* 1987;94:159–162.
214. Reynolds MG, Doty JB, McCollum AM, et al. Monkeypox re-emergence in Africa: a call to expand the concept and practice of One Health. *Expert Rev Anti Infect Ther* 2019;17:129–139.
215. Reynolds MG, Yorita KL, Kuehnert MJ, et al. Clinical manifestations of human monkeypox influenced by route of infection. *J Infect Dis* 2006;194:773–780.
216. Rimoin AW, Mulembakani PM, Johnston SC, et al. Major increase in human monkeypox incidence 30 years after smallpox vaccination campaigns cease in the Democratic Republic of Congo. *Proc Natl Acad Sci U S A* 2010;107:16262–16267.
217. Roberts JA. Histopathogenesis of mousepox. I. Respiratory infection. *Br J Exp Pathol* 1962;43:451–461.
218. Roberts JA. Histopathogenesis of mousepox. II. Cutaneous infection. *Br J Exp Pathol* 1962;43:462–468.
219. Roberts KL, Smith GL. Vaccinia virus morphogenesis and dissemination. *Trends Microbiol* 2008;16:472–479.
220. Robinson AJ, Mercer AA. Parapoxvirus of red deer: evidence for its inclusion as a new member in the genus parapoxvirus. *Virology* 1995;208:812–815.
221. Robinson AJ, Petersen GV. Orf virus infection of workers in the meat industry. *N Z Med J* 1983;96:81–85.
222. Rodriguez JR, Rodriguez D, Esteban M. Interferon treatment inhibits early events in vaccinia virus gene expression in infected mice. *Virology* 1991;185:929–933.
223. Roess AA, Galan A, Kitces E, et al. Novel deer-associated parapoxvirus infection in deer hunters. *N Engl J Med* 2010;363:2621–2627.
224. Rotz L, Dotson DA, Damon I, et al. Vaccinia (smallpox) vaccine: recommendations of the Advisory Committee on Immunization Practices (ACIP), 2001. *MMWR Recomm Rep* 2001;50:1–25.
225. Ruben FL, Lane JM. Ocular vaccinia. An epidemiologic analysis of 348 cases. *Arch Ophthalmol* 1970;84:45–48.
226. Rubins KH, Hensley LE, Jahrling PB, et al. The host response to smallpox: analysis of the gene expression program in peripheral blood cells in a nonhuman primate model. *Proc Natl Acad Sci U S A* 2004;101:15190–15195.
227. Sanderson CM, Smith GL. Vaccinia virus induces Ca2+–independent cell-matrix adhesion during the motile phase of infection. *J Virol* 1998;72:9924–9933.
228. Sarkar JK, Mitra AC, Mukherjee MK, et al. Virus excretion in smallpox. 1. Excretion in the throat, urine, and conjunctiva of patients. *Bull World Health Organ* 1973;48:517–522.
229. Sarkar JK, Mitra AC, Chakravarty MS. Relationship of clinical severity, antibody level, and previous vaccination state in smallpox. *Trans R Soc Trop Med Hyg* 1972;66:789–792.
230. Sarkar JK, Mitra AC, Mukherjee MK, et al. Isolation of virus from the urine, conjunctiva and throat of smallpox cases. *Bull Calcutta Sch Trop Med* 1972;20:37–39.
231. Sarker S, Roberts HK, Tidd N, et al. Molecular and microscopic characterization of a novel Eastern grey kangaroopox virus genome directly from a clinical sample. *Sci Rep* 2017;7:16472.
232. Savory LJ, Stacker SA, Fleming SB, et al. Viral vascular endothelial growth factor plays a critical role in orf virus infection. *J Virol* 2000;74:10699–10706.
233. Schroeder K, Nitsche A. Multicolour, multiplex real-time PCR assay for the detection of human-pathogenic poxviruses. *Mol Cell Probes* 2010;24:110–113.
234. Schultz DA, Sagartz JE, Huso DL, et al. Experimental infection of an African dormouse (Graphiurus kelleni) with monkeypox virus. *Virology* 2009;383:86–92.
235. Seet BT, Johnston JB, Brunetti CR, et al. Poxviruses and immune evasion. *Annu Rev Immunol* 2003;21:377–423.
236. Sejvar JJ, Chowdary Y, Schomogyi M, et al. Human monkeypox infection: a family cluster in the midwestern United States. *J Infect Dis* 2004;190:1833–1840.
237. Senkevich TG, Bugert JJ, Sisler JR, et al. Genome sequence of a human tumorigenic poxvirus: prediction of specific host response-evasion genes. *Science* 1996;273:813–816.
238. Seward JF, Galil K, Damon I, et al. Development and experience with an algorithm to evaluate suspected smallpox cases in the United States, 2002–2004. *Clin Infect Dis* 2004;39:1477–1483.
239. Sharma DP, Ramsay AJ, Maguire DJ, et al. Interleukin-4 mediates down regulation of antiviral cytokine expression and cytotoxic T-lymphocyte responses and exacerbates vaccinia virus infection in vivo. *J Virol* 1996;70:7103–7107.
240. Shisler JL. Immune evasion strategies of molluscum contagiosum virus. *Adv Virus Res* 2015;92:201–252.
241. Shisler JL, Jin XL. The vaccinia virus K1L gene product inhibits host NF-kappaB activation by preventing IkappaBalpha degradation. *J Virol* 2004;78:3553–3560.
242. Sivan G, Martin SE, Myers TG, et al. Human genome-wide RNAi screen reveals a role for nuclear pore proteins in poxvirus morphogenesis. *Proc Natl Acad Sci U S A* 2013;110:3519–3524.
243. Smith GL, Talbot-Cooper C, Lu Y. How Does Vaccinia Virus Interfere With Interferon? *Adv Virus Res* 2018;100:355–378.
244. Smith SK, Self J, Weiss S, et al. Effective antiviral treatment of systemic orthopoxvirus disease: ST-246 treatment of prairie dogs infected with monkeypox virus. *J Virol* 2011;85:9176–9187.
245. Smithson C, Meyer H, Gigante CM, et al. Two novel poxviruses with unusual genome rearrangements: NY_014 and Murmansk. *Virus Genes* 2017;53:883–897.
246. Springer YP, Hsu CH, Werle ZR, et al. Novel orthopoxvirus infection in an Alaska resident. *Clin Infect Dis* 2017;64:1737–1741.
247. Stack J, Haga IR, Schroder M, et al. Vaccinia virus protein A46R targets multiple Toll-like-interleukin-1 receptor adaptors and contributes to virulence. *J Exp Med* 2005;201:1007–1018.
248. Tenembaum S, Chitnis T, Ness J, et al. Acute disseminated encephalomyelitis. *Neurology* 2007;68:S23-S36.
249. Thomas K, Tompkins DM, Sainsbury AW, et al. A novel poxvirus lethal to red squirrels (Sciurus vulgaris). *J Gen Virol* 2003;84:3337–3341.
250. Thompson CH. Identification and typing of molluscum contagiosum virus in clinical specimens by polymerase chain reaction. *J Med Virol* 1997;53:205–211.
251. Torfason EG, Gunadottir S. Polymerase chain reaction for laboratory diagnosis of orf virus infections. *J Clin Virol* 2002;24:79–84.
252. Trindade GS, da Fonseca FG, Marques JT, et al. Belo Horizonte virus: a vaccinia-like virus lacking the A-type inclusion body gene isolated from infected mice. *J Gen Virol* 2004;85:2015–2021.
253. Tryland M, Klein J, Nordoy ES, et al. Isolation and partial characterization of a parapoxvirus isolated from a skin lesion of a Weddell seal. *Virus Res* 2005;108:83–87.
254. Tscharke DC, Reading PC, Smith GL. Dermal infection with vaccinia virus reveals roles for virus proteins not seen using other inoculation routes. *J Gen Virol* 2002;83:1977–1986.
255. Tu SL, Nakazawa Y, Gao J, et al. Characterization of Eptesipoxvirus, a novel poxvirus from a microchiropteran bat. *Virus Genes* 2017;53:856–867.

256. Tuomi PA, Murray MJ, Garner MM, et al. Novel poxvirus infection in northern and southern sea otters (Enhydra lutris kenyoni and Enhydra lutris neiris), Alaska and California, USA. *J Wildl Dis* 2014;50:607–615.
257. Usme-Ciro JA, Paredes A, Walteros DM, et al. Detection and molecular characterization of zoonotic poxviruses circulating in the Amazon region of Colombia, 2014. *Emerg Infect Dis* 2017;23:649–653.
258. Vaughan A, Aarons E, Astbury J, et al. Two cases of monkeypox imported to the United Kingdom, September 2018. *Euro Surveill* 2018;23(38):1800509.
259. Vellozzi C, Lane JM, Averhoff F, et al. Generalized vaccinia, progressive vaccinia, and eczema vaccinatum are rare following smallpox (vaccinia) vaccination: United States surveillance, 2003. *Clin Infect Dis* 2005;41:689–697.
260. Vora S, Damon I, Fulginiti V, et al. Severe eczema vaccinatum in a household contact of a smallpox vaccinee. *Clin Infect Dis* 2008;46:1555–1561.
261. Vora NM, Li Y, Geleishvili M, et al. Human infection with a zoonotic orthopoxvirus in the country of Georgia. *N Engl J Med* 2015;372:1223–1230.
262. Voss TG, Roy CJ. Use of the aerosol rabbitpox virus model for evaluation of anti-poxvirus agents. *Viruses* 2010;2:2096–2107.
263. Wallace GD, Werner RM, Golway PL, et al. Epizootiology of an outbreak of mousepox at the National Institutes of Health. *Lab Anim Sci* 1981;31:609–615.
264. Wasilenko ST, Banadyga L, Bond D, et al. The vaccinia virus F1L protein interacts with the proapoptotic protein Bak and inhibits Bak activation. *J Virol* 2005;79:14031–14043.
265. Werden SJ, Rahman MM, McFadden G. Poxvirus host range genes. *Adv Virus Res* 2008;71:135–171.
266. Wernery U, Zachariah R. Experimental camelpox infection in vaccinated and unvaccinated dromedaries. *Zentralbl Veterinarmed B* 1999;46:131–135.
267. Westwood JC, Boulter EA, Bowen ET, et al. Experimental respiratory infection with poxviruses. I. Clinical virological and epidemiological studies. *Br J Exp Pathol* 1966;47:453–465.
268. Wherry EJ, Ahmed R. Memory CD8 T-cell differentiation during viral infection. *J Virol* 2004;78:5535–5545.
269. Wilson TM, Cheville NF, Karstad L. Seal pox. Case history. *Wildl Dis* 1969;5:412–418.
270. Yinka-Ogunleye A, Aruna O, Dalhat M, et al.; Team CDCMO. Outbreak of human monkeypox in Nigeria in 2017–18: a clinical and epidemiological report. *Lancet Infect Dis* 2019;19:872–879.
271. Yirrell DL, Vestey JP, Norval M. Immune responses of patients to orf virus infection. *Br J Dermatol* 1994;130:438–443.
272. Young E, Basson PA, Weiss KE. Experimental infection of game animals with lumpy skin disease virus (prototype strain Neethling). *Onderstepoort J Vet Res* 1970;37:79–87.
273. Yu J RS. Efficacy of three key antiviral drugs used to treat orthopoxvirus infections: a systematic review. *Global Biosecurity* 2019;1:29–73.
274. Zaitseva M, Kapnick SM, Scott J, et al. Application of bioluminescence imaging to the prediction of lethality in vaccinia virus-infected mice. *J Virol* 2009;83:10437–10447.
275. Zaucha GM, Jahrling PB, Geisbert TW, et al. The pathology of experimental aerosolized monkeypox virus infection in cynomolgus monkeys (Macaca fascicularis). *Lab Invest* 2001;81:1581–1600.
276. Zimmermann P, Thordsen I, Frangoulidis D, et al. Real-time PCR assay for the detection of tanapox virus and yaba-like disease virus. *J Virol Methods* 2005;130:149–153.
277. Zorec TM, Kutnjak D, Hosnjak L, et al. New insights into the evolutionary and genomic landscape of molluscum contagiosum virus (MCV) based on nine MCV1 and six MCV2 complete genome sequences. *Viruses* 2018;10(11):586.
278. Zuniga MC. A pox on thee! Manipulation of the host immune system by myxoma virus and implications for viral-host co-adaptation. *Virus Res* 2002;88:17–33.

CHAPTER

18 Hepadnaviridae

Christoph Seeger • Fabien Zoulim • William S. Mason

HISTORY

Highly transmissible liver disease has been known for several thousand years. A major cause is hepatitis A virus (HAV), a picornavirus that infects the liver and is shed in feces. Evidence for a distinct form of hepatitis, transmitted from blood and body fluids, began appearing in the 19th and early 20th centuries. This 2nd form was finally accepted following outbreaks of hepatitis after vaccination for measles, mumps, and yellow fever in the 1930s and 1940s. These vaccines all contained convalescent serum or plasma, or human serum added as a "stabilizer," which inadvertently contained an infectious agent. Plasma, blood transfusions, and repeated use of nonsterile needles were also identified as causes of hepatitis outbreaks, and the disease was shown to have a viral etiology (reviewed in Refs.[18,195,590]). Originally identified as hepatitis B or serum hepatitis, in distinction to the disease caused by hepatitis A virus, this newly recognized disease was later discovered to be two separate diseases. Once tests were available for hepatitis B virus (HBV), a unique DNA virus discovered during the 1960s, it became clear that there was a second form of serum hepatitis, thereafter called nonA nonB hepatitis. A virus with structural similarities to flaviviruses was identified in the late 1980s as the major cause of nonA nonB hepatitis, and named hepatitis C virus (HCV).[40,90]

The discovery of HBV came during attempts to track genetic differences in human populations. Blumberg and colleagues were using sera from multiply transfused individuals as sources of antibody to human serum proteins. The idea was that these sera would contain antibodies that bound to proteins differing in sequence from those of the transfusion recipients. During the course of these studies, a new antigen, named "Australia antigen," was identified in serum from an Australian Aborigine.[31] Because this antigen was found to be common in leukemia patients and in Down syndrome patients, who have a high risk of leukemia, it was hypothesized that the antigen predicted leukemia risk. However, a Down syndrome patient initially negative for Australia antigen was observed to seroconvert and seroconversion was correlated with a mild case of hepatitis. At about the same time, a member of Blumberg's laboratory experienced a mild case of hepatitis following contact with contaminated material, again with the appearance of Australia antigen in the blood.[32,33]

The Australia antigen was quickly associated with serum hepatitis in a wider group, including a significant fraction of posttransfusion hepatitis cases. At the time, posttransfusion hepatitis occurred in at least 10% to 30% of multiply transfused individuals. Screening blood banks for contaminated blood (Australia antigen-positive) resulted in an approximately twofold decline in the incidence of posttransfusion hepatitis. The remaining cases were mostly due to HCV. For the discovery of HBV, Blumberg received the Nobel Prize in Medicine.[34]

The ability to carry out retrospective studies with assays for Australia antigen confirmed a long held suspicion that HBV was responsible for a chronic hepatitis leading to cirrhosis and liver cancer in many parts of the world. The Australia antigen, purified from the serum of infected individuals, also proved to be an effective vaccine, with greater than 90% efficacy in inducing an antibody response in adults. However, universal vaccination still remains a goal rather than accomplished fact.[241] The WHO estimates that there are approximately 257 million people worldwide who are chronically infected with HBV, of whom approximately 1 million are estimated to die annually of chronic liver disease or hepatocellular carcinoma (https://www.who.int/news-room/fact-sheets/detail/hepatitis-b).

EM studies revealed that Australia antigen is carried by subviral spherical particles, with a diameter of approximately 22 nm, and to a lesser extent, by approximately 22 nm rod-like particles (Fig. 18.1). Sera contain a much smaller amount of spherical virus with a diameter of approximately 42 nm, termed the Dane particle.[108] Australia antigen is a component not just of the 22 nm particles but also of the virus envelope.[190] Treatment with nonionic detergent releases a spherical capsid with a diameter of approximately 32 nm from the virus. Robinson and colleagues showed that the capsids contain a circular viral DNA of about 3,000 bp, as well as an endogenous DNA polymerase activity that synthesizes virus DNA when virions are treated with nonionic detergent and incubated in the presence of dNTPs.[235,426,427] Summers showed that the circular DNA is only partially double stranded, one strand being incomplete, and that the circular conformation is maintained by a short cohesive overlap between the 5′ ends of the two DNA strands. This incomplete strand is extended, and the single strand gap is at least partially filled-in by the endogenous DNA polymerase activity.[480]

In the next few years, the endogenous DNA polymerase activity facilitated the discovery of several HBV-like viruses (Fig. 18.2) including woodchuck hepatitis virus (WHV) in eastern woodchucks (*Marmota monax*),[481] duck hepatitis B virus (DHBV) in domestic ducks in China[533,583] and the United States,[335] and ground squirrel hepatitis virus (GSHV) in Beechey ground squirrels (*Spermophilus beecheyi*).[331] Shortly thereafter, hepatitis B–like viruses related to these original isolates were identified in Richarson's (*Spermophilus richardsonii*)[346] and arctic ground squirrels (Spermophylus parryi kennicotti),[501] ducks and geese,[74,173] cranes,[404] storks,[408] and herons.[468] More recently, HBV-like viruses have been discovered in additional mammalian and avian hosts, as well as in fish and frogs.[121,182] DNA sequence elements distantly related to HBV have also been found integrated in the genomes of a variety of species including birds, snakes, turtles, and crocodiles but so far not in mammals.[158,479]

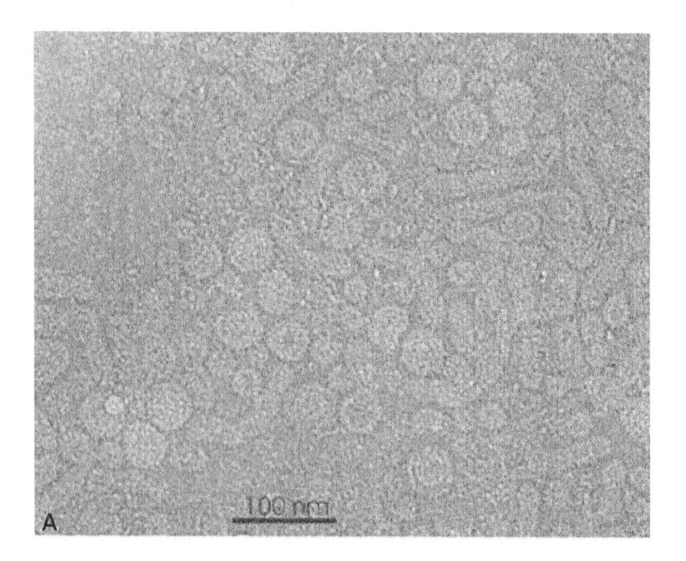

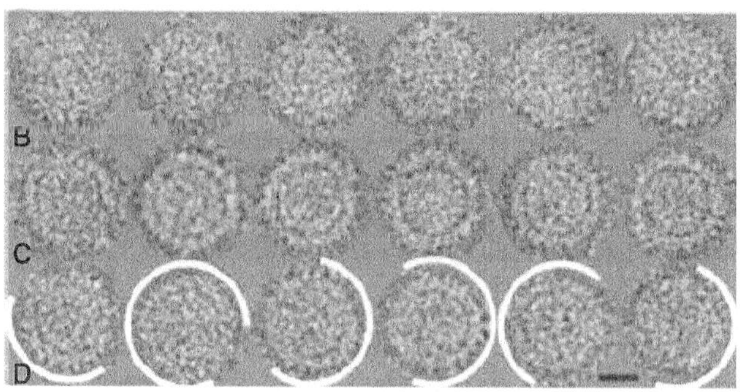

FIGURE 18.1 **CryoEM of viral particles from a chronically infected patient. A:** 42-nm Dane particles, and 22-nm filamentous and spherical subviral particles are seen. **B and C:** Particles with compact and gapped morphology, respectively. **D:** Particles with mixed morphology. Gapped areas are delineated in *white*. (From Seitz S, Urban S, Antoni C, et al. Cryo-electron microscopy of hepatitis B virions reveals variability in envelope capsid interactions. *EMBO J* 2007;26(18):4160–4167. Copyright © 2007 European Molecular Biology Organization. Reprinted by permission of John Wiley & Sons, Inc.)

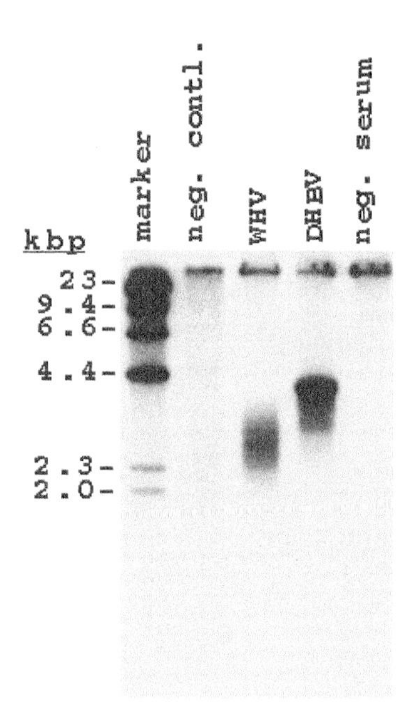

FIGURE 18.2 **Detection of hepatitis B–like viruses using an endogenous DNA polymerase assay.** Serum samples from a woodchuck and duck were centrifuged to pellet virus. The pellet was suspended in a DNA polymerase reaction cocktail containing radiolabeled nucleotides and incubated at 37°C. SDS-pronase was then added, and after digestion at 37°C to free DNA from protein, the products were subjected to gel electrophoresis in 1.5% agarose. Radiolabeled DNA was detected by autoradiography. The marker is bacteriophage lambda DNA digested with the restriction endonuclease Hind III. WHV DNA migrates faster than DHBV DNA because the incomplete strand of WHV was only partially filled in by the endogenous DNA polymerase reaction.

CLASSIFICATION OF VIRUSES WITHIN THE HEPADNAVIRUS FAMILY

The hepatitis B–like viruses are assigned to the family *Hepadnaviridae* (hepatitis DNA virus), for which (human) HBV is the prototype. This family currently contains five genera, the orthohepadnaviruses, infecting mammals, the avihepadnaviruses, infecting birds, and more recently identified, the metahepadnaviruses and parahepadnaviruses, infecting fish, and the herpetohepadnaviruses, infecting reptiles and amphibians[121,182,325] (Fig. 18.3). Designation of the *Hepadnaviridae* as a new family of viruses is based on the extremely small size of the viral genomes (3 to 3.3 kbp), the novel arrangement of open

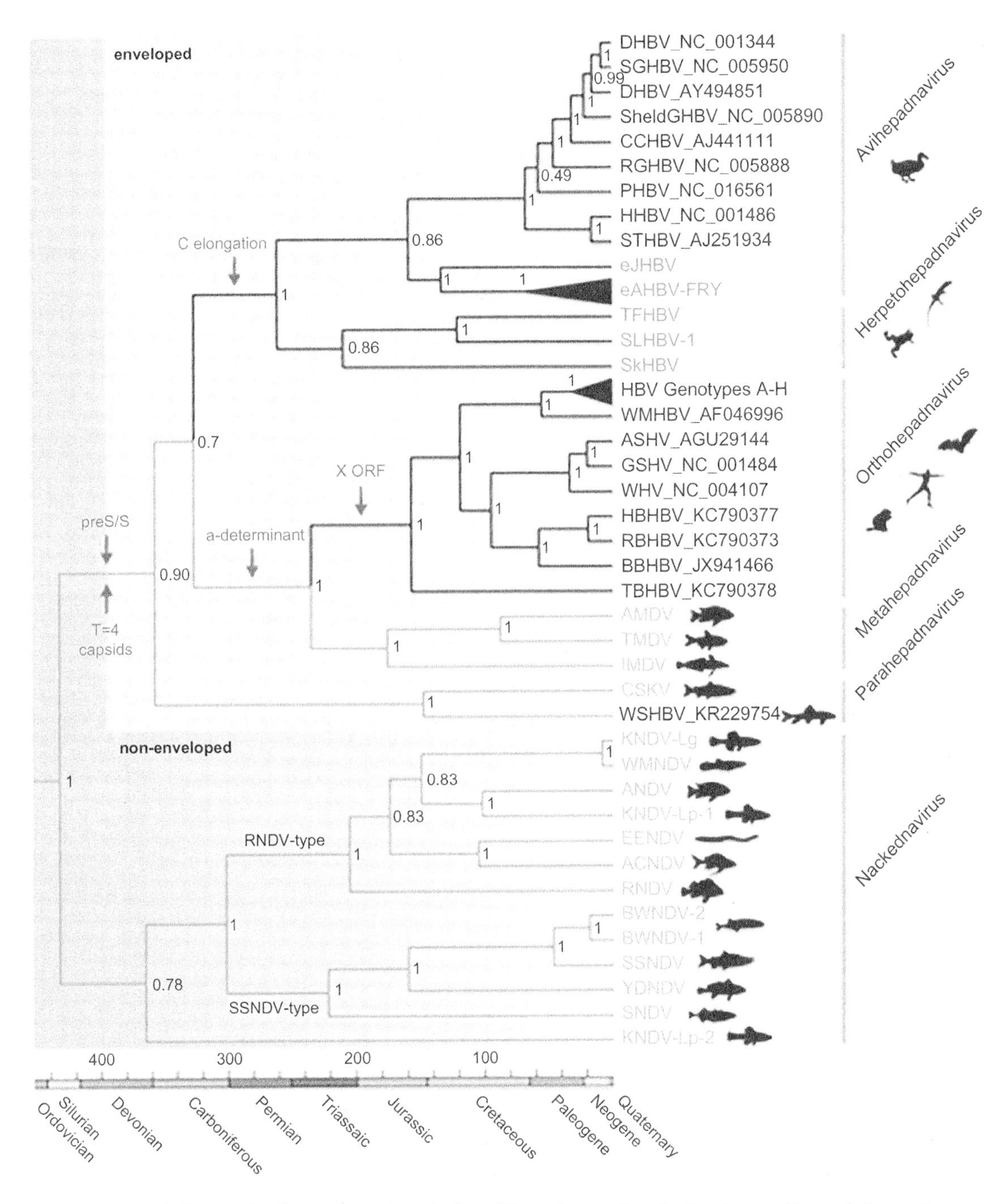

FIGURE 18.3 **Phylogenetic alignment and evolution of hepadna- and nackednaviruses.** The evolutionary time scale is shown in millions of years for the appearance of nackednaviruses (no envelope gene), parahepdnaviruses and metahepadnaviruses (fish), herpetohepadnaviruses (amphibians, reptiles), avihepadnaviruses (birds), and orthohepadnaviruses (mammals). The phylogenetic tree was based on protein sequence alignments of conserved regions in the terminal protein (TP), reverse transcriptase (RT), and RnaseH (RH) domains of the polymerase (P) gene. (eprinted from Lauber C, Seitz S, Mattei S, et al. Deciphering the origin and evolution of hepatitis B viruses by means of a family of non-enveloped fish viruses. *Cell Host Microbe* 2017;22(3):387–399.e6. https://creativecommons.org/licenses/by/4.0/.)

reading frames, and the unique replication strategy, differing almost completely from other viruses replicating by reverse transcription. Assignment to five genera was based on the strong DNA sequence similarities within genera but not between genera. The recently discovered fish nackednaviruses,[274] unlike all other HBV-like viruses, do not encode viral envelope proteins and may belong to a distinct virus family.

A maximum sequence divergence of about 40% is found among the orthohepadnaviruses,[151,449] compared to about 20% among avihepadnaviruses.[173] Assignment to separate species within the avihepadnavirus has been based historically upon differences in viral sequence as well as in host range. Three species have been assigned in the avihepadnavirus group, DHBV, heron hepatitis B virus (HHBV), and parrot hepatitis B virus.[400,438] Among the orthohepadnaviruses, virus isolates very closely related to HBV are found in all apes, including chimpanzees, gorillas, orangutans, and gibbons. At present, these primate isolates are considered subtypes of HBV rather than distinct species. Primate viruses related to HBV have also been isolated, in the New World, from the woolly[270,272] and capuchin monkeys.[112] Other HBV-related viruses recently found in antelope, bats, cats, and shrews may, along with the woodchuck, ground squirrel, woolly monkey, and capuchin monkey viruses, bring the orthohepadnavirus species assignments up to 11[4,161,267,368,417] (Fig. 18.3).

Because of their potential clinical importance, numerous studies have been performed to gain information on the number and geographic distribution of HBV genotypes infecting humans. Ten HBV genotypes, A to J, have been identified, with isolates belonging to different genotypes showing pairwise differences greater than 8% and less than 17%. Distinct genotypes have also been found in great apes. Different genotypes in humans tend to have distinct geographic distributions and possibly distinct clinical manifestations.[306] These are discussed later in this chapter.

VIRION STRUCTURE

HBV is a spherical virus with an outer diameter of approximately 42 nm (Fig. 18.1). The inner shell of the virus has a diameter of approximately 32 nm and is made up of 120 dimers of the core protein. The dimers form the icosahedral capsid with a triangulation number T = 4. A small fraction of capsids consists of only 90 dimers with a triangulation number T = 3.[100,124,552] It is not known whether virions with the smaller capsids are infectious or represent dead-end products caused by an aberrant assembly process. The capsid is covered with a lipoprotein membrane made up of three forms of the viral envelope protein, large (L), middle (M), and small (S) (Fig. 18.4), acquired together with host lipids during budding into multivesicular bodies (MVB) (Fig. 18.5). The L, M, and S proteins are present in the virus envelope at a ratio of about 1:1:4.[190] A model based on the analyses of virions and capsids by electron cryomicroscopy predicts that virions with

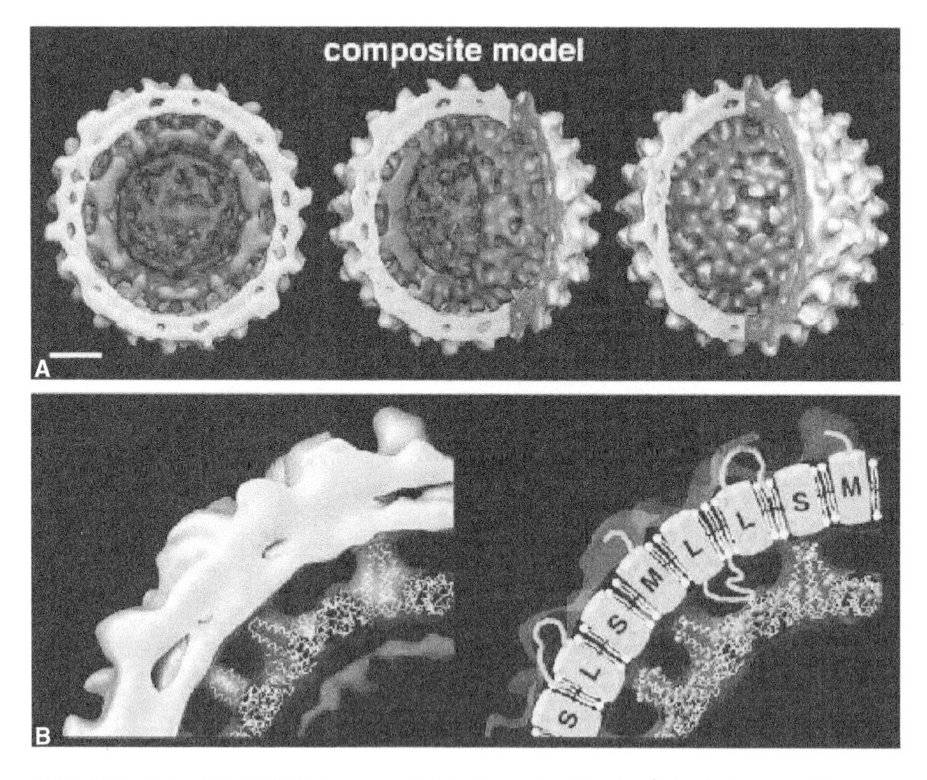

FIGURE 18.4 Model of HBV virions. **A:** HBV virion with a T = 4 icosahedral capsid (*blue*) with 120 spikes and an outer envelope with protein projections. **B:** X-ray crystal structure of a capsid docked into the cryo-EM density map of the virion capsid **(left)**. *S, M,* and *L* refer to the three envelope proteins described in the text. Amino acids around the base of the spikes in core proteins that are important for envelopment of core particles are shown in green.[277,385] (Reprinted from Dryden KA, Wieland SF, Whitten-Bauer C, et al. Native hepatitis B virions and capsids visualized by electron cryomicroscopy. *Mol Cell* 2006;22(6):843–850. Copyright © 2006 Elsevier. With permission.)

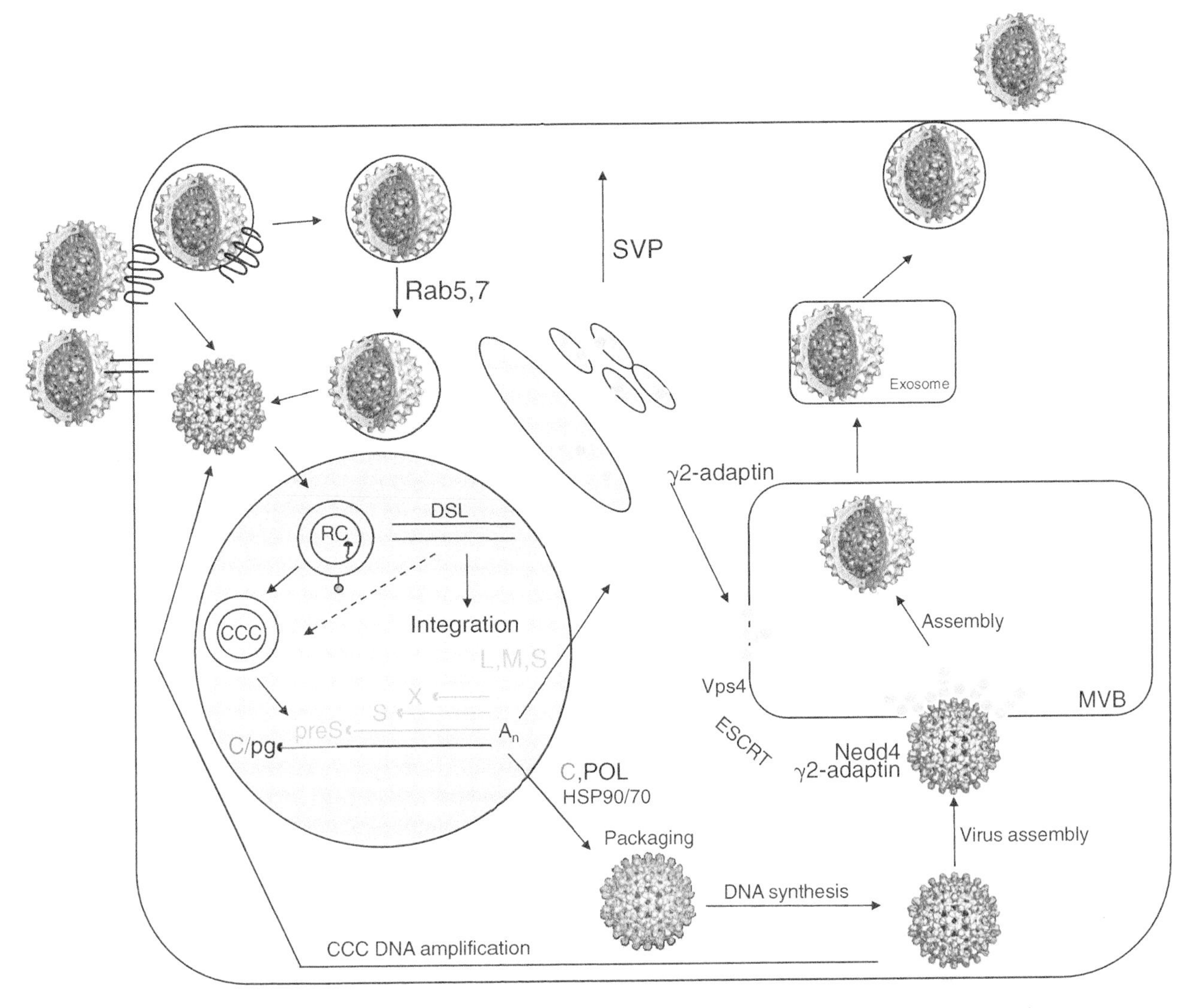

FIGURE 18.5 Hepadnavirus life cycle. Envelope proteins are shown in yellow, DNA-containing capsids in *blue* and RNA-containing capsids in *red*. Early in infection, when envelope protein concentrations are low, capsids enter the cccDNA amplification pathway. Envelope proteins enter the ER and assemble into subviral particles (*SVP*) or transfer to *MVBs* where virion assembly is believed to occur. Mature virions might exit cells through exosomes (for details and references see the text).

T = 4 capsids carry 120 dimers formed by core proteins.[124,453] Virions from patient sera exhibit morphological variation: they appear either as compact or as gapped particles, which differ in the distance between the capsid and membrane[453] (Fig. 18.1). Capsids contain a single copy of the partially double-stranded DNA genome, which is covalently linked to the viral reverse transcriptase (RT) at the 5′ end of the complete strand (Fig. 18.6). The RT provides the endogenous DNA polymerase activity, discussed earlier[235,480] (Fig. 18.2). There is also evidence for the presence of cellular proteins including one or more serine kinases within the virus.[5] The virus has a buoyant density of 1.24 to 1.26 g/cm^3 in CsCl and an $s_{20,w}$ of 280S. The titers of HBV can vary significantly among patients ranging up to 10^{10} per mL in blood.

As noted, HBV infections also lead to the production of noninfectious subviral particles (SVP) (Fig. 18.1). The 22 nm spheres, which represent the most abundant particles released into the blood from infected hepatocytes, have been claimed to reach titers of more than 10^{12} per mL.[370,586] Cryo-EM studies of the isometric subviral particles isolated from serum revealed that the spheres have an octahedral symmetry, different from the icosahedral structure of Dane particles.[159] The spheres are composed of 48 dimer subunits that assemble into two classes of particles that differ in size, presumably caused by the heterogeneity of the subunits. Spheres contain M and S proteins at a ratio of about 1:2 and only trace amounts of L.[191] The 22 nm rod-like particles found in the blood (tubes, filamentous particles) contain approximately equal amounts of M and L. Their surface exhibits spike-like features composed of homo and heterodimers of L, M, and S proteins which, like virus, are in the ratio 1:1:4.[457] However, in contrast to octahedral isometric 22 nm spheres, rod-like particles isolated from patient sera do not have an ordered structure.[457]

Subviral particles contain 40% lipid and sugar by mass and have a buoyant density of 1.18 g/cm^3 in CsCl. Their exact role in the HBV life cycle is not known. One possibility is that, by adsorbing virus-neutralizing antibodies, they facilitate virus spread and maintenance in the host.

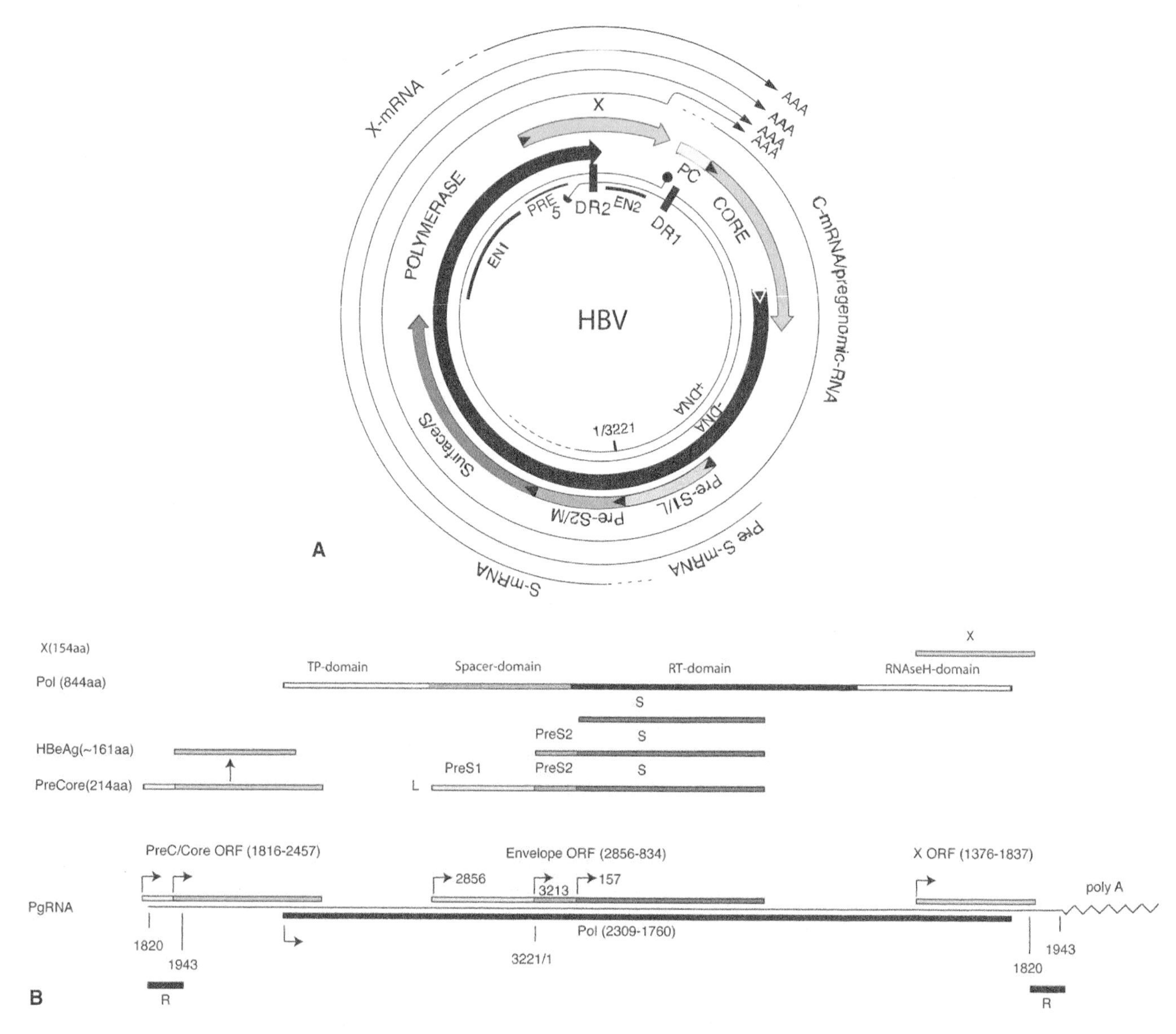

FIGURE 18.6 Genome structure and organization. The relaxed circular DNA genome of HBV with a complete minus strand and incomplete plus strand is shown in **panel A** (inner circle), along with the known mRNAs, all of which end at a common polyadenylation signal located in the core open reading frame. All open reading frames have a clockwise direction. The single-stranded gap in the plus strand is filled in by the viral RT, which is covalently attached to the 5′ end of minus strand DNA. The proteins produced from each open reading frame are illustrated in **panel B**, using pgRNA, a terminally redundant mRNA that is reverse transcribed to produce viral DNA, as a map reference. Map coordinates are from the sequence reported by Valenzuela et al.[520] (accession number X02763), with numbering from a unique EcoR1 restriction endonuclease site. R, large terminal redundancy; PgRNA, pregenomic RNA; DR, direct repeat; EN, enhancer, PRE, post transcriptional regulatory element.

GENOME STRUCTURE AND ORGANIZATION

The structure of the HBV genome and the organization of open reading frames on viral DNA is shown in Figure 18.6. All of the ORFs are in the same direction (clockwise in this illustration), defining minus and plus strands of viral DNA. Within virions, minus strand DNA is complete and spans the entire genome, in contrast to plus strands, which extend to about two-thirds of the genome length and have variable 3′ ends.[321,480] In this regard, avihepadnaviruses differ from orthohepadnaviruses because they normally extend plus strands almost all the way to the location of the modified 5′ end.[304] The protein primer of minus strand synthesis and the RNA primer of plus strand synthesis remain attached throughout virus maturation. Minus strands are covalently linked to the viral RT, which is also their protein primer, through a phospho-tyrosine bond. Plus strands contain a short RNA oligomer primer derived from the 5′ end of pregenome (pg) RNA, the template for minus strand DNA synthesis. Minus strands exhibit a small 8 to 9 nucleotide-long terminal redundancy, termed r, which is required for the formation of relaxed circular (rc) DNA during plus strand DNA synthesis.[304,451,546] A small fraction (5% to 20%) of virus contains double-stranded linear (dsl) DNA in lieu of rcDNA, a consequence of *in situ* priming of plus strand DNA synthesis[473] (see below). Virions with DSL DNA are infectious but can lose important sequences from their ends during initiation of infection and appear, therefore, to play only a minor role in hepadnavirus replication.[562,563] However, they can integrate into chromosomes by illegitimate recombination. Integrated HBV DNA may play a role in hepatocarcinogenesis,[517] as discussed later in this chapter.

The genetic organization of HBV is complex. The genome contains four promoters, two enhancer elements, and a single polyadenylation signal to regulate transcription of viral RNAs. In addition, there are four open reading frames and several *cis* acting signals that are required for viral DNA replication (Fig. 18.6). All viral transcripts are encoded by the minus strand and are capped and polyadenylated. Transcription regulatory regions are present within open reading frames and are active following the transport of the viral genome into the cell nucleus, where it is converted into a covalently closed circular DNA form, called cccDNA.

The major transcripts that are detected by Northern blot analyses of HBV infected livers are 3.5 kb, 2.4 kb, and 2.1 kb in length and termed pre-C/C, pre-S, and S mRNAs, respectively.[69] In addition, a minor transcript, X mRNA, about 0.7 kb, has occasionally been detected by Northern blot analysis in infected tissues and more consistently, in cells transfected with subgenomic HBV DNA. Avihepadnaviruses express three major transcripts analogous in length to the three major mRNAs of mammalian hepadnaviruses.[54] All hepadnavirus transcripts share a common 3′ end created by a polyadenylation signal located in the core gene. Fine mapping of the 3.5 kb preC/C mRNAs revealed three different 5′ ends bracketing the initiation codon of the pre-C gene, indicating that translation of the overlapping pre-C and core genes occurs from separate transcripts (Fig. 18.6).[69] The two longer RNAs, beginning upstream of the pre-C initiation codon, are referred to as pre-core (pre-C) mRNAs and the shorter, beginning downstream, is pregenome RNA. PgRNA is the template for the translation of the core and RT proteins and, as the name indicates, is also the template for viral DNA synthesis via reverse transcription.[359] In contrast, the function of the pre-C mRNAs appears to be limited to the translation of the pre-C gene. As with the large, terminally redundant mRNAs, S mRNAs also have heterogeneous 5′ ends flanking the initiation codon of preS2 and, hence permitting the translation of either the M or S protein.[68] The pre-S transcript has a unique 5′ end and supports the translation of L. In addition to the four promoters, two enhancers, EN1 and EN2, regulate transcription of the viral RNAs (Fig. 18.6). The X transcript can generally not be detected by Northern blot from infected tissue due to its low abundance and small size.

The core protein is a cytoplasmic, basic phosphoprotein with a molecular weight (MW) of 21 kd that assembles into subviral capsids. Historically, core antigenicity was recognized, and diagnostic assays to monitor ongoing or resolved infections were developed. The pre-C protein is best known by its serological name: e-antigen or HBeAg. Although the pre-C gene includes the entire core protein open reading frame and upstream coding sequences, the polypeptide is shorter than the core protein due to posttranslational processing and has a MW of only 15 kd. The mature pre-C protein exhibits distinct antigenic properties from the core protein. Pre-C is not required for viral replication but might exert a role in the regulation of the immune response against HBV, particularly against the core protein.[82,508] HBeAg is also an important diagnostic tool that can be used to determine the status of ongoing HBV infections.

The pol gene encodes the viral RT, which is the sole enzyme encoded by hepadnaviruses. It consists of three functional domains and a hinge region, known as the "spacer," and has a MW of about 90 kd. The N-terminus encodes the terminal protein (TP) domain, which acts as the primer for minus strand DNA synthesis. The C-terminal region encodes DNA polymerase and RNAseH domains.

The Pre-S/S genes overlap the hinge region and RT domains of the pol gene, albeit in a different reading frame. They encode three integral transmembrane envelope glycoproteins with distinct N-terminal domains. The shortest, the S protein, contains the major antigenic determinants of Australia antigen, which led to the discovery of HBV and provided the reagent for the development of diagnostic tools for the detection of HBV infections and of vaccines against HBV infections.[34] A fraction of S protein is modified by asparagine (N)-linked oligosaccharides, increasing the apparent MW of the protein from 24 to 27 kd.[330] The 31 kd M protein represents a larger form of HBsAg with a 55 amino acid N-terminal, glycosylated extension, referred to as PreS2, translated from an in-frame initiation codon. It represents about 10% to 15% of total envelope proteins in infected cells. A specific function for this protein is not yet known, as it is not essential for virion assembly.[49] Recent studies suggest that the 55 amino acids that distinguish M from S may serve primarily a spacer function between S and the PreS1 domain of L.[365]

The 42 kd L protein is a myristoylated polypeptide translated from the first initiation codon of the PresS/S open reading frame.[396] The extra amino acids at the N-terminus, relative to M, define the PreS1 domain. Although it represents only 1% to 2% of total surface proteins in infected cells, L is enriched in virions and rod-like 22 nm subviral particles, where it represents approximately 17% of the envelope proteins.[190] In contrast, spherical subviral particles are primarily composed of M and S proteins. Consistent with its distribution, L protein provides the primary ligand for the viral receptor. In contrast to the mammalian hepadnaviruses, avihepadnaviruses encode only two, nonglycosylated envelope proteins, corresponding to L and S of HBV. DHBV subviral particles are pleomorphic, roughly spherical, with diameters ranging from 35 to 60 nm,[335] as compared to the approximately 40 nm HBV virion.

The smallest viral gene, found in mammalian hepadnaviruses, encodes HBx (also called X) with a MW of 17 kd. The X gene overlaps, in a different reading frame, the C-terminal portion of the polymerase and two transcriptional control elements, EN2 and core promoter. Except for the spacer region in the polymerase, X is the least conserved hepadnavirus protein. It has a short half-life in the range of a few hours in primary human hepatocyte cultures (PHH) and accumulates primarily in the nucleus.[256] X expression is required for efficient HBV replication *in vivo*.[80,577,588] This is because HBx induces degradation of the cellular Smc5/6 complex, which otherwise directly or indirectly inhibits transcription from cccDNA.[114]

STAGES OF REPLICATION

Attachment to Hepatocytes

Critical viral and cellular factors for target cell binding and initiation of infection comprise a ca. 60 aa-long segment in S and the myristoylated N-terminal PreS1 domain of L on virions, which are required for attachment of HBV to the low affinity receptor heparan sulfate proteoglycan (HSPG) and the high-affinity receptor, sodium taurocholate cotransporting polypeptide (NTCP). Hepatocyte specificity is provided by NTCP, which is encoded by the solute carrier family 10 member 1 (SLC10A1) gene[488,556] and is expressed almost exclusively by hepatocytes. Moreover, for DHBV (but not HBV), infection may depend upon a conserved peptide translocation motif (TLM), which is located near the N-terminus of preS1.[476]

The most compelling evidence for a role of the myristoylated PreS1 domain in L in attachment to hepatocytes stems from genetic experiments with chimeric envelope proteins between closely related hepadnaviruses that exhibit different host-range specificity, such as DHBV and its close relative, HHBV, or HBV and woolly monkey hepatitis B virus (WMHBV).[91,214] These studies revealed that the specificity of these viruses for their cognate hepatocytes segregates with the N-terminal half of the PreS1 domain. Consistent with these observations, infectivity of DHBV and HBV can be neutralized by anti-PreS1 antibodies, and infection of hepatocytes can be blocked by peptides homologous to portions of the PreS1 region of the L protein.[398,519] For HBV, the most potent preS1-derived peptide spans aa 2 to 47 and carries myristic acid at the N-terminus akin to the natural L protein.[398] Using this lipopeptide as bait, Yan and coworkers identified the liver bile acid transporter NTCP as the *bona fide* high-affinity HBV receptor.[298,556] NTCP is an integral membrane glycoprotein expressed on basolateral membranes of hepatocytes where it is required for sodium-dependent uptake of bile salts. Ectopic expression of NTCP in the HepG2 cell line, for instance, confers susceptibility to HBV infections.

A study with hepatitis delta virus (HDV, Chapter 19), a viroid-like satellite of HBV that requires HBV envelop proteins to infect hepatocytes, provided initial evidence that a second determinant required for infectivity maps to the external hydrophilic loop of the S domain in L.[218,488] Subsequently, HSPG was invoked as a low-affinity receptor for HBV that "captures" virus particles to facilitate their binding to NTCP.[284,436,448] Some controversy exists concerning the site responsible for binding to HPSG. Based on genetic data, it coincides with the "a determinant," which is found in the S domain of all HBV genotypes and contains immunodominant virus-neutralization epitopes.[226,488] However, it has also been claimed that trypsin-mediated cleavage of PreS1 from the virus surface can abolish binding of virions to heparin, suggesting that PreS1 plays a role in binding to HPSG[448] (Fig. 18.6).

Identification of NTCP as the HBV receptor provided opportunities to investigate the basis of the remarkable species specificity of hepadnaviruses, limiting HBV and HDV infections to human, great apes, and the tree shrew (*Tupaia belangeri*) hepatocytes.[366] For receptor studies, HDV has been particularly useful because its species selectivity appears to be solely dependent on the binding of PreS1 in L to NTCP. In contrast, HBV infections are also restricted at subsequent steps in viral entry. Genetic analyses identified two domains in NTCP (aa 84 to 87 and 157 to 165) that are critical for PreS1 lipoprotein binding and HBV/HDV infectivity.[556,557] Replacement of aa 84 to 87 in mouse NTCP with the human residues confers susceptibility to HDV infection in mice.[189] Cloning and expression of the woodchuck NTCP ortholog in HepG2 cells revealed an additional amino acid residue (aa 263) that is critical for infection and species specificity, explaining why chimpanzees could not be infected with WHV.[149] It should be noted that it is not yet known whether NTCP is a receptor for WHV or GSHV in their natural hosts. Finally, genetic analyses of NTCP indicated that its roles in bile acid transport and HBV/HDV infection can be genetically separated.[149]

Whether duck NTCP plays a role in infection by DHBV is unknown. Carboxypeptidase D (CPD) was proposed to act as a species specific, but not liver-specific receptor that binds DHBV particles and recombinant L protein.[258] The DHBV-CPD interaction requires the PreS1-specific domain of the envelope protein and is inhibited by PreS1-specific neutralizing antibodies.[509] Many of the characteristics of CPD are consistent with its proposed role as a viral receptor. However, experimental expression of CPD in cell lines that can support DHBV replication from transfected DNA has not, so far, made these cells susceptible to DHBV infection.

Based on current knowledge about the viral and cellular determinants required for HBV infection, a model for entry and uncoating can be envisaged (Fig. 18.5). HBV reaches hepatocytes through the space of Disse and attaches with preS1 or the "a determinant" in L to the low-affinity receptor HSPG. Subsequently, the lipomyristolated 45 amino acids at the N-terminus of PreS1 in L attach to the hepatocyte-specific receptor NTCP. In turn, NTCP binds to EGFR, which then triggers entry into hepatocytes by receptor-mediated endocytosis. This model further predicts that uncoating occurs through fusion of the HBV envelope with endosomal membranes, releasing nucleocapsids into the cytoplasm for transport to the nucleus.

Entry, Intracellular Trafficking, and Uncoating

Infection by DHBV and by HBV appears to be pH independent because it can occur in the presence of lysosomotropic agents or after pretreatment of virus at low pH.[180,422] A screen with bioactive ligands identified EGFR as an additional factor for HBV internalization into primary human hepatocytes (PHH) cultures and HepG2 cells expressing NTCP[215] (Fig. 18.6). Studies with HepaRG cells, which under certain conditions become susceptible to HBV infection, have invoked roles for caveolin-1 and in particular Rab-5 and Rab-7, known to play a role in routing cargo from the cytoplasmic membrane to early and late endosomes.[323] How HBV evades lysosomal degradation still remains unresolved. After fusion of HBV with endosomal membranes, capsids are transported to the cell nucleus.[232] Experiments with capsids produced in either hepatoma cells or *Escherichia coli* provided evidence for a model where core particles migrate along microtubules to the nuclear periphery. From there, capsids enter the nuclear basket in an Importin α/β-dependent process and bind to nucleoporin 153.[412,445] The model predicts that capsids disintegrate within the nuclear pore complex and release rcDNA into the nucleus,[411] where it is converted into cccDNA, the template for transcription of the viral RNAs[412,445] (Fig. 18.7).

Several questions remain concerning HBV attachment and entry into hepatocytes: for example, how do significant amounts of HBV ever reach the liver considering that HSPG are ubiquitously expressed? This point is particularly intriguing because less than 10 HBV particles can initiate an infection in chimpanzees.[11] Another unresolved issue concerns the identity of cofactors that play a role in HBV entry and delivery of rcDNA to the nucleus. Expression of human NTCP in mouse, rat, or dog hepatocytes does not confer susceptibility to HBV infections, indicating that additional factors are required for early steps of the HBV replication cycle.[287] A defect in transport of capsids to the cell nucleus or release of viral DNA into the nucleus possibly makes these cells refractory to productive HBV infections. This view is in agreement with observations made with transgenic mice that efficiently produce HBV DNA-containing capsids in the cytoplasm but do not accumulate cccDNA in the nucleus.[168] Interestingly, cultured AML12 cells derived from hepatocytes of a transgenic mouse overexpressing human transforming growth factor alpha (TGFα) support efficient cccDNA synthesis from cytoplasmic nucleocapsids produced from an integrated HBV expression vector.[102] The ability of these cells to produce cccDNA was attributed to the presence of unstable capsids, implying that uncoating of nucleocapsids is controlled by host factors. This view is supported by results demonstrating that expression of human NTCP in AML12 cells confers some permissiveness to HBV infection.[286] However, cccDNA formation following infection is several orders of magnitude lower compared to HepG2-NTCP cells indicating that additional restrictions occur on the ultimate formation of cccDNA. Hence, it is possible that binding of human NTCP to another protein required for endocytosis, for example, EGFR,[215] produces some level of species specificity. Remarkably, expression of human NTCP in macaque and pig hepatocytes confers permissiveness to HBV infections, indicating that subtle differences in the makeup of the intracellular environment can have a profound effect on capsid migration, disassembly, and delivery of viral DNA into the cell nucleus.[287] Purified orthohepadnavirus DNAs are infectious in their respective hosts, including HBV in the chimpanzee, implying that delivery of rcDNA into the nucleus is sufficient for initiation of productive infections.[450,545]

Transcription

Orthohepadnaviruses contain four promoters that control the transcription of the 3.5-kb preC and pgRNAs and the subgenomic 2.4 kb, 2.1 kb, and 0.7 kb RNAs; PreS1, S, and X, respectively (Fig. 18.8). All promoters, except for preS1, lack a TATA box and hence produce transcripts with heterogeneous 5′ ends, which in the case of the S and preC/C promoters encode distinct proteins: M and S, and pre-C and core/pol,

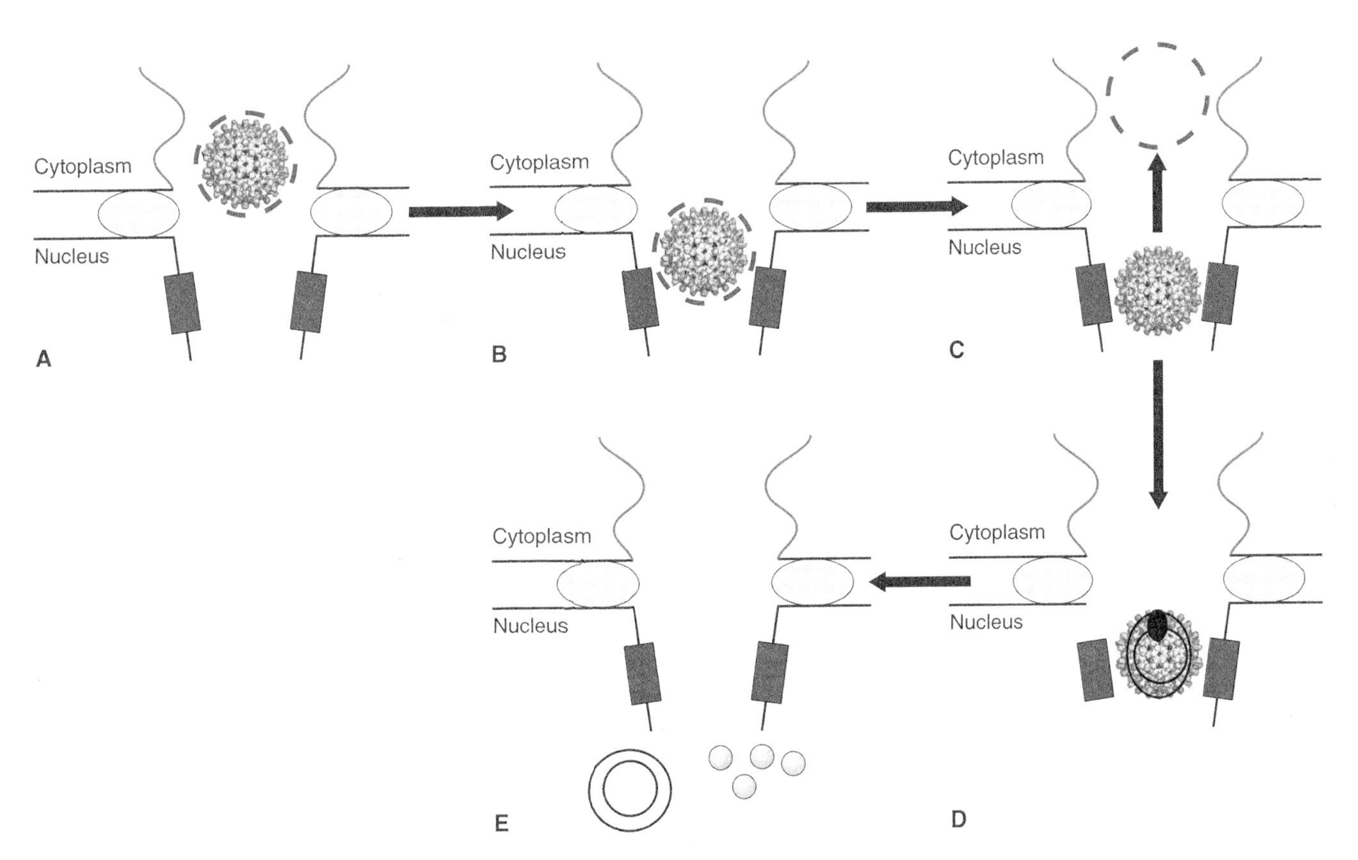

FIGURE 18.7 Transport of capsids through the nuclear core complex. A: Capsids in complex with the nuclear transport receptors Importin α and β (*purple dashed circle*) attach to the nuclear pore (*grey oval*). **B:** The complex passes the nuclear pore and becomes arrested by interaction between importin β and Nup153 (*red box*). **C:** RanGTP dissociates the nuclear transport receptors from the capsid which then interact with the nuclear transport receptors Nup153. **D:** Capsids disintegrate by a still elusive mechanism. **E:** rcDNA and capsid subunits diffuse into the nucleus. RcDNA is converted to cccDNA. (Adapted from Schmitz A, Schwarz A, Foss M, et al. Nucleoporin 153 arrests the nuclear import of hepatitis B virus capsids in the nuclear basket. *PLoS Pathog* 2010;6(1):e1000741. https://creativecommons.org/licenses/by/3.0/.)

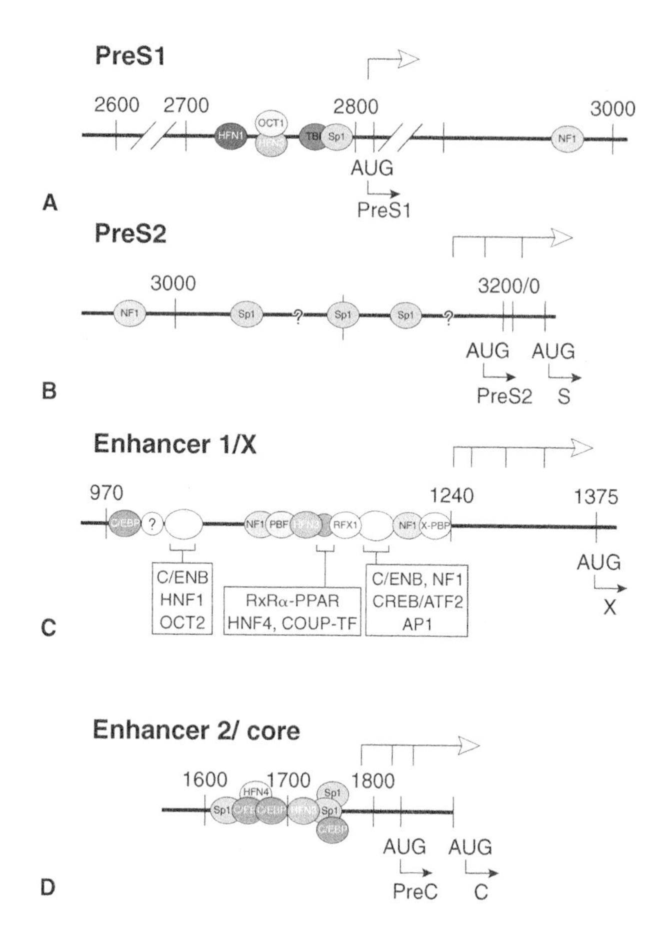

FIGURE 18.8 **Transcription factor–binding sites.** The figure shows the binding sites for transcription factors on the preS1 and preS2 promoters **(A and B)**, enhancer 1 and the X promoter **(C)**, and enhancer 2 and the pre-core/core promoter **(D)**. Transcription start sites are indicated with arrows (for details and references, see the text).

respectively. The possibility that the PreC/C promoter actually consists of two distinct promoter elements has been suggested by genetic experiments and by analyses of naturally occurring mutants that fail to express HBeAg.[462]

While the transcripts encoding preC/pgRNA, PreS1, and S were identified and characterized with RNA isolated from infected liver tissue of human patients and ground squirrels infected with HBV and GSHV, respectively,[69,133] X transcripts could first only be detected in tissue culture cells transfected with subgenomic HBV DNA constructs.[458,581] More recent global mapping of capped 5′ ends of HBV RNAs isolated from livers of HBV-infected patients provided convincing evidence for the presence of capped HBx transcripts and unexpectedly for shorter transcripts potentially encoding a shorter HBx protein initiating at a conserved AUG codon in the body of the X open reading frame.[9]

A single polyadenylation signal located in the core gene regulates the formation of the 3′ ends of all HBV transcripts. In the case of Pre-C/C RNAs, RNA polymerase II bypasses the poly A signal once, leading to the formation of terminally redundant transcripts (Fig. 18.6). Sequences located close to the 5′ end of the transcript play a role in the suppression of premature polyadenylation during the first passage by RNA polymerase II.[433]

The two enhancers, EN1, located upstream of the X region, and EN2, overlapping the pre-C/C promoter, regulate the transcription of the four promoters. Consistent with the hepatotropic nature of hepadnaviruses, all transcriptional regulatory elements of HBV, except for the S promoter, contain binding sites for liver-enriched transcription factors (Fig. 18.8; for a more comprehensive description, see Ref.[462]) For instance, the PreS1 promoter contains binding sites for the liver-enriched factors HNF1 and HNF3.

EN1, a complex enhancer less than 300 nucleotides in length, harbors binding sites for liver-enriched factors HNF1, HNF3, and C/EBP (Fig. 18.8). In addition, the pre-C/C promoter and both enhancers contain binding sites for nuclear receptors (NRs) including HNF4-α, retinoid X receptor alpha (RXR-α), peroxisome proliferators-activated receptor alpha (PPARα), the chicken ovalbumin upstream promoter transcription factors (COUP-TF) 1 and 2, and others. It should be noted that a clear separation between the binding sites on the pre-C/C promoter and EN2 is not possible because of the overlap between the two elements. Ectopic expression of RXR-α and PPARA-α in NIH3T3 cells can induce the expression of pgRNA and the accumulation of HBV replication intermediates that otherwise are not produced in these cells, underscoring the significance of NRs in the control of viral gene expression.[205,492,570] Curiously, substantial differences in the organization of the transcriptional control elements seem to exist among mammalian hepadnaviruses. For example, WHV does not appear to bear an element corresponding to HBV enhancer EN1.[118]

Under physiological conditions, cccDNA is associated with histones and other proteins to form a mini-chromosome.[35,36,360] Nucleosomal spacing on cccDNA is 180 and 150 nucleotides for HBV and DHBV, respectively, compared to 200 in liver chromatin. *In vitro* reconstitution experiments provided evidence for a role of the HBV core protein in altering the cccDNA chromatin structure.[36]

Genome-wide analysis of posttranslational modifications (PTM) of histones on cccDNA from HBV-infected PHH, HepG2/NTCP cells, and HBV-infected liver tissue demonstrated enrichment of PTMs normally associated with cellular transcriptional activation, including H3K4me3, H3K27ac, H3K36me3, and H3K122ac at positions overlapping the four viral promoters.[513] Transcriptionally inactive cccDNA produced by HBx deficient virus exhibits biochemical properties common to heterochromatin which, for cccDNA, can be reversed upon ectopic expression of HBx.[423] IFN-α-induced repression of cccDNA transcription is accompanied by a reduction of activating PTMs and not, as expected, by an increase in deposition of repressive PTMs.[513] It is conceivable that prolonged treatment with IFN-α leads to the replacement of active PTMs perhaps following recruitment of histone deacetylase 1 to cccDNA.[25]

The major mammalian and avian hepadnavirus transcripts are unspliced. In HBV and WHV, transport of unspliced viral RNA from the nucleus to the cytoplasm is regulated by a posttranscriptional *cis* regulatory element (PRE) overlapping EN1 and a portion of the X gene.[122,206] A screen to identify small molecule inhibitors of HBV surface antigen expression identified a compound, RG7834, that prevents accumulation of pgRNA and surface RNAs.[349] The compound inactivates the noncanonical poly(A) polymerases TENT4A and TENT4B (also known as PAPD5 and PAPD7).[350] Genetic studies revealed that these proteins bind to a stem-loop structure termed SLα in PRE and that this binding promotes RNA polyadenylation and, in turn, accumulation of pgRNA and surface mRNAs.[582] A second host-factor, ZCCHC14, is another component of an apparently larger complex binding to PRE to stabilize pgRNA and surface mRNAs by an yet unknown mechanism.[211]

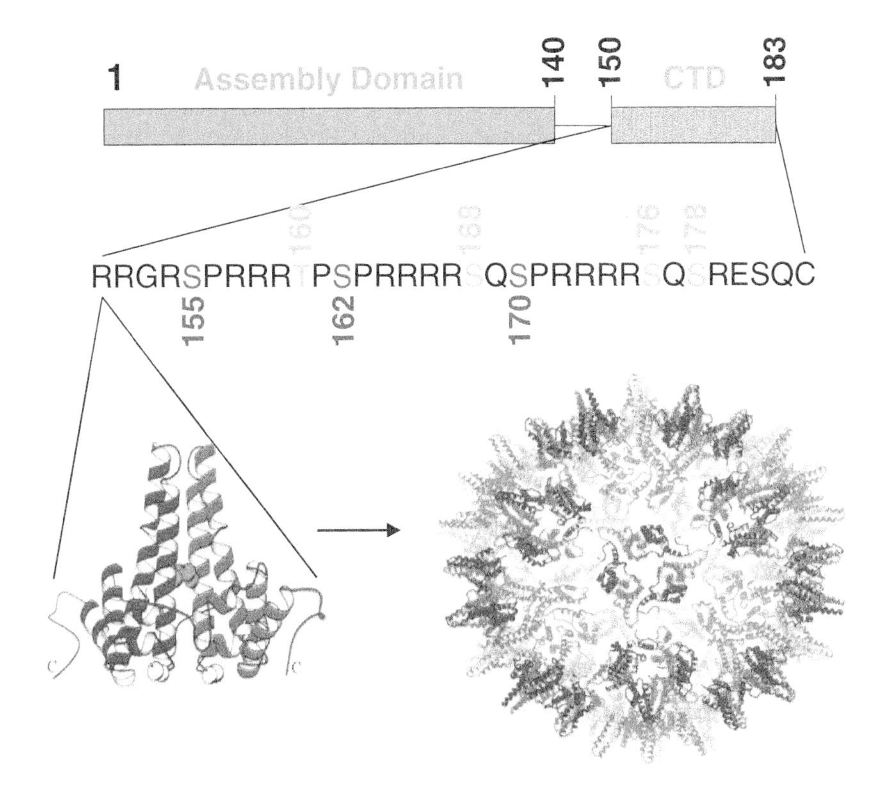

FIGURE 18.9 Structures of the HBV capsid. The assembly and C-terminal domains (*CTD*) of the HBV core protein are separated by a linker region. Major and minor phosphorylation sites in the CTD are marked in *red* and *orange*, respectively. The atomic structure of dimer subunits shows Cys-61 (*green*) forming the disulfide bridge between the monomers and amino acid sequences of arginine-rich C-terminal domains. Assembly of the dimers produces icosahedral capsids. (Adapted from Wynne SA, Crowther RA, Leslie AG. The crystal structure of the human hepatitis B virus capsid. *Mol Cell* 1999;3(6):771–780. Copyright © 1999 Elsevier. With permission. Ref.[552])

A functional PRE element has not been identified in avian hepadnaviruses. Instead, they contain positive and negative effectors of transcription (pet, net) that regulate the synthesis of pgRNA.[207] Pet spans a 60 nucleotide-long sequence near the 5′ end of pgRNA, whereas net is located downstream of the polyadenylation signal. Pet prevents net-induced termination of transcription of nascent pregenomes during the first passage of the RNA polymerase through the polyadenylation site. Like PRE, pet acts in an orientation-specific fashion, but its mode of action remains elusive. Evidence for the presence of a spliced transcript has been obtained with DHBV.[376] It contains a short sequence from the 5′ end of pgRNA fused to PreS mRNA and appears to be required for replication in primary hepatocytes and ducks. However, the exact role of this transcript for viral replication is still unclear.

Viral Proteins

Translation of HBV proteins is controlled by initiation codons located closest to the 5′ end of the relevant mRNA. An exception is the polymerase protein. It is translated from an internal AUG codon on pgRNA (Fig. 18.6). Although many other viruses (i.e., picornaviruses, hepaciviruses) control internal initiation of translation with internal ribosome entry sites (IRES), hepadnaviruses do not have an IRES. Moreover, pol is not translated by a mechanism depending on a plus one frameshift from the core to the polymerase gene, as it has been described for certain retroviruses, because stop codons or frame shift mutations placed upstream of the initiation site have no effect on translation.[72,441] Some experimental data are consistent with a model predicting leaky scanning where a small fraction of ribosomes recruited at the 5′ end of pgRNA bypass the core AUG codon and scan the transcript until they reach the initiation AUG of the pol ORF.[144,305] Other reports favored a ribosomal shunting mechanism for DHBV pol translation; however, the sequence motifs comprising the "donor" and "acceptor" sites have not yet been identified.[64]

Core

The core protein of HBV is a 183 to 185 aa-long polypeptide of MW 21 kd with an assembly domain (aa 1 to 140) followed by a linker region and an arginine-rich C-terminal domain (CTD) (aa 150 to 183) (Fig. 18.9). Avihepadnaviruses encode core proteins that are approximately 80 aa longer than HBV core, with similar properties except for an approximately 45 aa-long insertion in the central domain of the polypeptide that forms the "spike" characteristic of viral capsids, and additional amino acids in the arginine-rich carboxy terminus.[43] Cryoelectron microscopy and X-ray crystallography helped reveal the structure of capsids produced in *E. coli*.[38,97,552] The folding of the core polypeptide chain is primarily α-helical and, unlike other viral capsid proteins, lacks β-sheets (Fig. 18.9). Two juxtaposed alpha helices (α3, α4) connected by a loop represent the central domain of the monomeric structure. Dimerization leads to the formation of a 4-helix bundle that assumes the shape of an inverted T, where the stem constitutes the dimer interface and forms the spikes on the surface of capsids. The tips of the arms form the contact points, primarily located in α5, for the polymerization of the dimers into capsids. During an infection, the majority of capsids are assembled from 120 dimer subunits into a T = 4 structure with a diameter of approximately 34 nm. Capsid formation is thought to be a slow process where capsid dimers might first assemble into trimeric structures followed by addition of dimers to complete the capsid shell.[585] Capsids used for the structural studies were composed of core proteins lacking about 30 aa from the C-terminus including serine phosphorylation sites and, as a consequence, exhibited an increased fraction of particles consisting of 90 dimers with T = 3 and a diameter of approximately 30 nm. A structural analysis of the peptide that links the shell-forming core domain with the C-terminal region was consistent with a model predicting that the C-terminal "protamine" domain provides a mobile platform for viral DNA synthesis inside capsids.[538]

The 34 amino acid long carboxy-terminal domain (CTD) contains seven conserved serine and threonine phosphorylation sites and several arginine-rich motifs harboring nuclear localization signals[130,227,233,266,293,299] (Fig. 18.9). One or several cellular enzymes must mediate the phosphorylation because none of the viral proteins exhibit kinase activity. In cellular extracts, the SR protein–specific kinases 1 and 2 (SRPK1, SRPK2) associate with cores and phosphorylate the serine residues in the three SPRRR motifs.[111] Several other kinases, including cyclin dependent kinase 2 (CDK2), protein kinase C, and a 46 kd serine kinase, can phosphorylate cores *in vitro*.[157] The potential role of CDK2 in serine phosphorylation of the CTD was further substantiated through identification of the kinase in cytoplasmic core particles and by results indicating that CDK2 inhibitors could block the capsid-associated serine protein kinase activity.[316] Hence, CDK2 might be at least one of the enzymes responsible for the kinase activity in Dane particles first described approximately 40 years ago.[5]

Experiments with DHBV revealed that DNA replication is accompanied by the gradual dephosphorylation in the core protein, which might contribute to a reorganization of the C-terminus.[19,392] The nature of the phosphatase(s) is not yet known. As suggested for DHBV, all steps of HBV DNA synthesis may be regulated by serine and threonine phosphorylation in the core protein, implying that this mechanism is shared by all members of the *Hepadnaviridae*.[266,292] Genetic studies demonstrated that the arginine clusters in the SPRRR motifs play a role in packaging of pregenomic (pg) RNA, and in DNA replication and perhaps in the recruitment of SRPK1 and SRPK2 ([292]and below). Although the exact role of the charged arginine residues in DNA replication is not known, they might play a role in regulating the spatial organization of pg RNA and minus strand DNA to facilitate viral DNA synthesis.[277] Finally, the rigidity of capsids appears to change as a consequence of DNA synthesis because mature DNA containing particles exhibit increased protease and DNase sensitivities.[101] Such maturation-dependent destabilization of HBV capsids might be required for capsid uncoating. It can be augmented by mutations in both the NTD and linker regions of HBc and result in enhanced cccDNA amplification.[103]

The complexity of the capsid assembly process provides excellent targets for the development of novel antiviral drugs in addition to the already available nucleoside analogues (NUCs) targeting the polymerase. Heteroaryldihydropyrimidines (HAP)[117] and phenylpropanamides (PP)[245] are two classes of chemical compounds with demonstrated antiviral activity in tissue culture cells, in experimental animals, and in ongoing clinical trials.[136,261,572] PP compounds accelerate capsid assembly resulting in the formation of empty capsids lacking pg RNA, while HAP compounds lead to misassembly of capsids. Interestingly, both classes of compounds bind to the core protein dimer–dimer interface.[239,247] More recently, it was found that a third class of compounds, sulfamoylbenzamide (SBA), also target capsids, exhibiting an activity akin to HAP compounds.[59,327] A remarkable property of capsid inhibitors that sets them apart from nucleoside analogues is that they can also interfere with the process of capsid disassembly and, as a consequence, the conversion of rcDNA to cccDNA.[27,59]

As mentioned earlier in this chapter, a second product derived from the core region is precore or HBeAg protein. It is translated from pre-C mRNA with 5′ ends located a few nucleotides upstream of the first AUG in the pre-C/core open reading frame (Fig. 18.6). A signal sequence directs the translation of HBeAg to membranes of the endoplasmic reticulum (ER). As a consequence, the protein enters the secretory pathway, where it undergoes a second cleavage event that removes about 34 aa from its C-terminus, before it is secreted from infected cells as a 15 kd protein.[154,383,472] Expression of precore is not required for the establishment of productive infections in experimentally infected woodchucks and ducks.[71,79] However, a role in progression to chronic infection in humans is likely, as *de novo* infection generally selects for reemergence of wtHBV, with mutants defective in HBeAg production only becoming prevalent late in infection.[45] This supports the notion that HBeAg transiently suppresses the immune response to the virus, thereby increasing the frequency of chronic infections, which might explain the conservation of this gene. It is assumed that this function is no longer required to maintain chronicity, once established.[82,508]

Envelope

The three envelope proteins, L, M, and S, encoded by the mammalian hepadnaviruses have two principal functions: (a) they provide the protein components of the virus envelope and (b) they assemble into aggregates that are secreted as subviral particles. L and M differ from S in their N-terminal regions (Figs. 18.6 and 18.10). As a consequence of the common S region, the three proteins share several features: they contain two topogenic signals I and II that determine their orientation in lipid bilayers, a hydrophobic C-terminal region that is most likely embedded in ER membranes and a common N-glycosylation site (Asn-146) in S. Like a conventional signal sequence, signal I is located at the N-terminus of S, but is not proteolytically processed. Signal II is a hydrophobic domain acting as a stop-transfer sequence and a signal sequence. As a result, the two hydrophobic domains form a hairpin structure with a cytosolic loop.[128,129] The presence of a third hydrophobic domain invokes the theoretical possibility of two additional transmembrane passages. In addition to the common glycosylation site located downstream from signal II, the M protein harbors a second N-glycosylation site (Asn-4) near its N-terminus.[190] This site is also present in L, but not used, because of the cytoplasmic location of the preS2 domain of L. Some HBV genotypes contain o-glycans (Thr-37) in the preS2 domain of both L and M proteins.[444] L and M proteins contain modified N-termini. L carries a myristate group at Gly-2,[396] whereas M is N-terminally acetylated.[443] The role of M in HBV replication is not yet understood, because this protein is not required for the production of Dane particles and for infection of primary hepatocyte cultures with HBV or HDV.[137,365,487] In avihepadnaviruses, L-proteins are also myristoylated, but not glycosylated.[407] Instead they become phosphorylated in the preS1 domain.[165]

A major feature of L is that it exists in two conformations that differ in the localization of the N-terminal domain (Fig. 18.10). In the first, called i-PreS, the N-terminus, including signal I, is located in the cytosol,[50,381,403] where it is required for binding to capsids and for the assembly of virions. In the second, called e-PreS, the N-terminus is exposed on the surface of viral particles where it plays a role in the infection of hepatocytes.[403] The conformational change from internal to external is facilitated by interactions of L with the molecular chaperones Hsc70/Hsp40 and BiP.[264] However, the details of the mechanism regulating this step are not yet understood. Major determinants for infectivity of HBV are located in the N-terminal domain of L containing the binding site for NTCP and possibly HPSG.[30,278,556] However, as discussed earlier, the binding site for HPSG remains controversial.[276,436,488]

Following integration into membranes, envelope proteins form intermediates that include homo- and hetero-dimers stabilized by covalent disulfide bridges between different cysteine residues in the S domain and subsequently assemble into either subviral or Dane particles[210] (Fig. 18.5). S and M proteins contain the necessary signals for the export process because they can be secreted independently. In contrast, when synthesized in the absence of the other two envelope proteins, L is retained in intracellular membranes, suggesting that it carries a retention signal that prevents, in the absence of S and M, the export process controlled by its S domain.[84,395]

In addition to their roles as envelope proteins, L and M can activate, *in trans*, the transcription from selected promoters in transfected cells.[67,240] This function was initially described for naturally occurring mutants of these proteins with C terminal truncations. Because truncated forms of L and M were initially identified in tissues from chronically infected patients, it has been speculated that they contribute to the development of hepatocellular carcinoma (HCC). Later work showed that the complete L protein could also transactivate selected promoters.[142,192,193] This may be indirectly related to the fact that accumulation of L protein in the ER can lead to ER stress and, in consequence, increase expression of M and S.[209,554] This presumably facilitates L secretion and relieves ER stress. Mutations in the M domain have also been claimed to cause defects in host DNA repair.[198] Thus, the HBV envelope proteins may ultimately reflect adaptations to facilitate survival of infected hepatocytes but might, in the long term, lead to oncogenic transformation of rare infected hepatocytes.[263]

Reverse Transcriptase

Hepadnaviral polymerases have an approximate MW of 90 kd and consist of three functional domains: the terminal protein (TP) required for the priming of minus strand DNA synthesis, and the reverse transcriptase (RT) and RNAseH for DNA synthesis and degradation of pgRNA. A spacer (hinge) separates the TP from the other two domains (Fig. 18.11). The spacer region appears to have no other function than to provide a flexible connection between the TP and RT domains.[14,73] As will be discussed later in this chapter, the reverse transcriptase is the target for all currently FDA approved antiviral therapies with the exception of IFN-α.

Hepadnaviral polymerases are strictly template specific, which is a direct consequence of the mechanism for the activation of the enzyme. It requires binding of the polypeptide to a packaging signal, termed epsilon, located at the 5′ end of pgRNA (a second copy of epsilon is located near the 3′ end but does not play a role in replication, Fig. 18.12B). As is discussed later in this chapter, binding of the polymerase to epsilon leads to the priming of reverse transcription from a tyrosine residue (Y65) in the TP domain.[269,528,539] This results in the formation of a covalent link between the polymerase and the nascent viral minus strand. *In vitro* enzymatically active polymerase was first produced with the DHBV enzyme translated in rabbit reticulocyte lysates and led to the discovery that the interaction between the polymerase

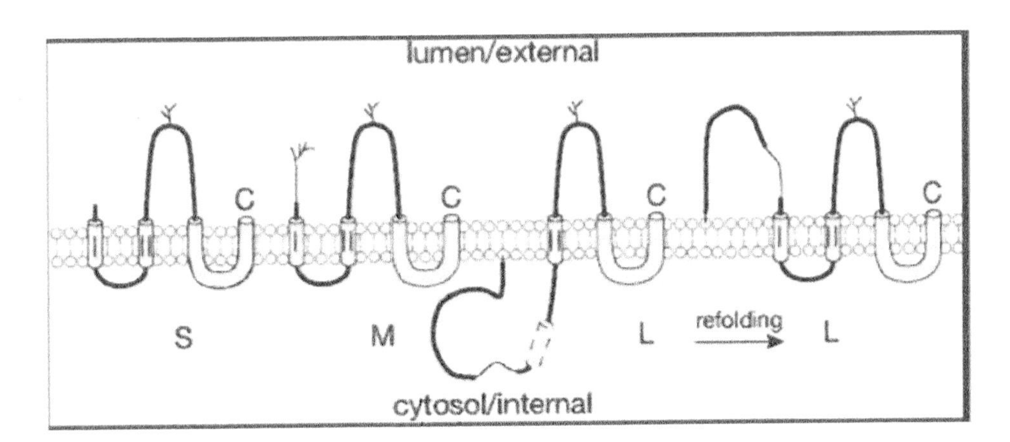

FIGURE 18.10 Proposed membrane topology of HBV envelope proteins. The orientation of the transmembrane domains (TM) is identical in S and M and the refolded L proteins. The external hydrophilic domain of S between amino acids 99 and 168 is illustrated at the left, along with the "a" determinant and the glycosylation site (branched structure) at asparagine 146. All proteins share a hydrophobic C-terminal domain that is embedded in membranes. M bears a second glycosylation site at its N-terminal extension (thin line). In contrast to the refolded product of L (e-preS), in the primary product of L (i-PreS), TM I is located in the cytosol where the N terminus is attached to membranes by the modification with myristic acid (for details see text). (Adapted from Bruss V. Envelopment of the hepatitis B virus nucleocapsid. *Virus Res* 2004;106(2):199–209. Copyright © 2004 Elsevier. With permission. Ref.[51])

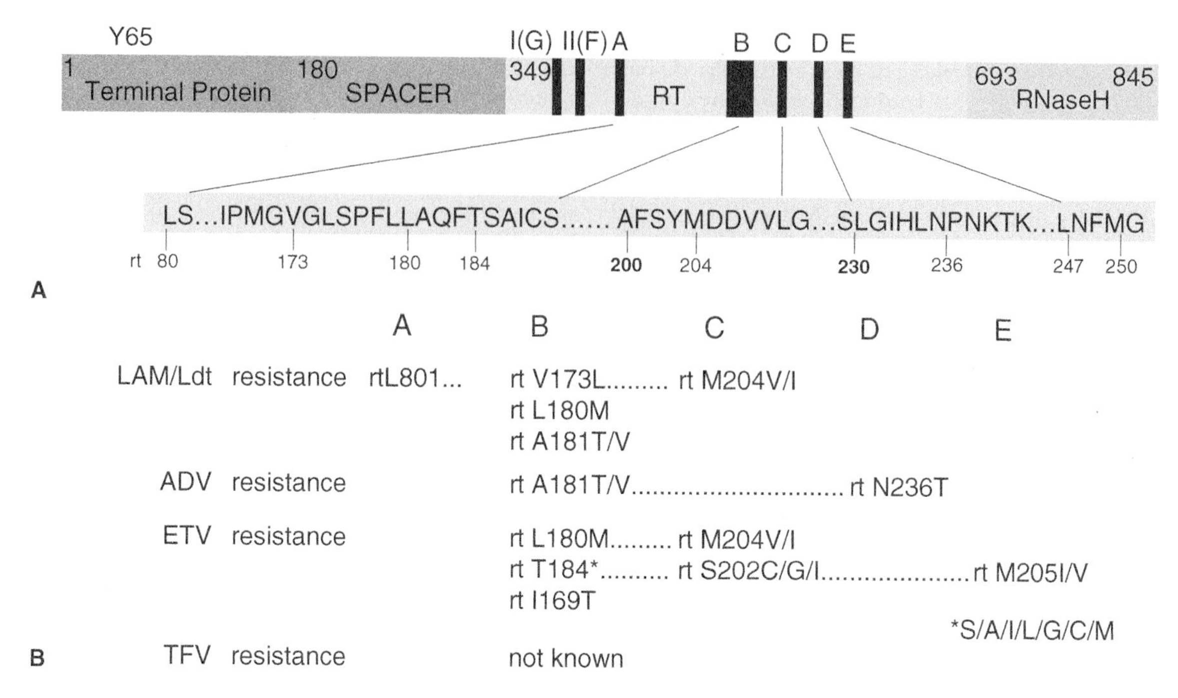

FIGURE 18.11 Physical organization of the HBV polymerase and resistance to nucleoside analogs. A: Domains of the pol protein. The polymerase contains three main functional domains, the terminal protein domain (TP), the reverse transcriptase domain (RT), and the RNaseH domain (A). Functional domains within the RT have been assigned based on structural modeling using the crystal structure of the HIV RT as a guide.[110] By this analogy, domains A, C, and D would appear to be involved in deoxynucleotide binding and polymerization. The B domain is thought to participate in template binding and the E domain in binding of the primer strand. **B:** Resistance mutations. The figure shows the location of amino acid mutations that confer resistance to lamivudine (LAM) and telbivudine (LdT), adefovir (ADV), and entecavir (ETC). (Adapted from Zoulim F, Locarnini S. Hepatitis B virus resistance to nucleos(t)ide analogues. *Gastroenterology* 2009;137(5):1593–1608. Copyright © 2009 AGA Institute. With permission.)

and epsilon RNA is dependent on chaperones including heat shock proteins 90 (Hsp90), Hsp70, and p23.[201,202,470] Consistent with these observations, both DHBV and HBV replication are sensitive to geldanamycin and its derivatives, which bind to the N-terminal ATP-binding domain of Hsp90.[202,204] Similarly, novobiocin, which binds to the C-terminus of Hsp90, inhibits HBV replication.[204] Moreover, Hsp90, p23 and three additional chaperones, Hsp70, Hsp40, and Hop can activate DHBV and HBV polymerases to bind to epsilon RNA *in vitro* and, in the case of the DHBV polymerase, restore the protein-priming activity.[203,204] With HBV, the protein-priming activity has been demonstrated in insect cells[268] and following isolation from cells as a ribonucleoprotein (RNP) complex.[225] With DHBV, enzymatically active polymerase can also be expressed in yeast.[494]

The function of the chaperones is not completely understood, because structural information about the polymerases of hepadnaviruses is lacking. It is possible that they stabilize an energetically unfavorable conformation of the polymerase and, in this way, facilitate the binding of polymerase with epsilon RNA[63,469] (Fig. 18.12A). Consistent with such a model is the observation that DHBV polymerases with deletions of the RNAseH domain can exhibit protein-priming activities in the absence of cellular factors.[534] Thus, these domains might hold the polymerase in a "closed" conformation that, in the absence of chaperones, prevents the interaction with the packaging signal.

It is likely that a single polymerase polypeptide catalyzes one complete round of DNA replication because assembly of the polymerase into capsids depends on its interaction with epsilon sequences on pgRNA, which would indicate that polymerase and RNA templates are present at equimolar amounts in subviral particles.[16,578] Consistent with such a model, experiments meant to quantify polymerase levels in HBV capsids revealed a molar ratio of approximately 0.7 polymerase molecules per virion DNA.[16]

HBx

WHV X is required for efficient infection and replication of WHV in woodchucks and by inference X is required in all hosts permissive for infection by orthohepadnaviruses.[80,415,577,588] Moreover, the requirement for HBx in establishing viremia has been reproduced with the immune-deficient chimeric mouse model demonstrating that X is required for the HBV life cycle even in the absence of a functional immune system.[515] Expression of this polypeptide has been assessed in the livers and primary hepatocyte cultures from WHV-infected woodchucks where it can accumulate to 40,000 to 80,000 molecules per cell in the cytoplasm.[106] In PHHs, HBx accumulates primarily in the cell nucleus and has a short half live of approximately 3 hours.[256] For a long time, the exact role of X for the HBV life cycle has been difficult to elucidate because the protein interacts with many cellular factors including the proteasome and its activity varies depending on the cell lines used for a study (reviewed in[462]). However, the discovery that HBx was required for transcription of cccDNA in PHH and HepaRG cells demonstrated the significance of HBx in the life cycle of HBV and provided an explanation for its essential role in infectivity *in vivo* noted earlier.[314]

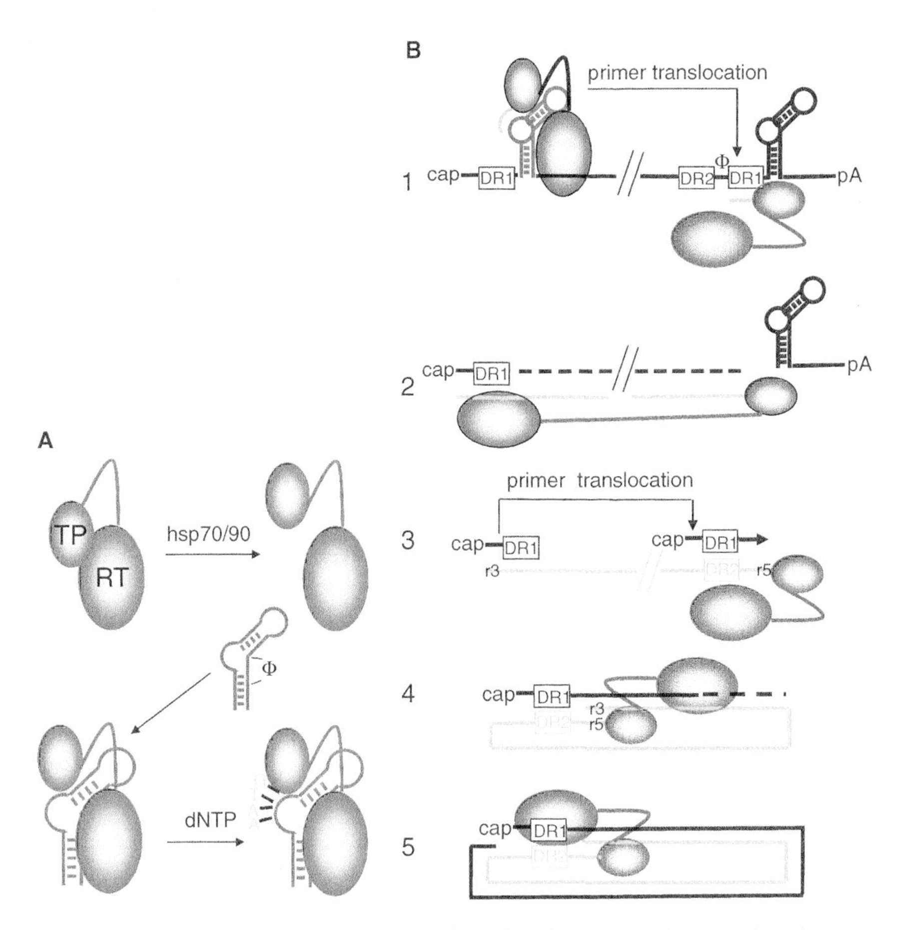

FIGURE 18.12 Genome replication. A: Binding of epsilon RNA to the TP and RT domains of the polymerase facilitated by chaperones (hsp70/90) and initiation of reverse transcription at the bulge of epsilon RNA as described in the text. Phi (F) depicts the RNA sequence on epsilon proposed to be required for circularization of pgRNA (see part B). **B:** The figure depicts five important steps in viral DNA synthesis: (*1*) Transfer of the DNA primer from epsilon to DR1 near the 3′ end of pgRNA; (*2*) Elongation of minus strand DNA and digestion of pgRNA by RNaseH of the polymerase; (*3*) Transfer of the capped RNA primer from DR1 to DR2 and synthesis of plus strand DNA to the 5′ end of minus strand DNA; (*4*) Template switch of the nascent plus strand with the help of the small terminal redundancies, r5 and r3, resulting in circularization of the genome; (*5*) Completion of plus strand DNA as described in the text. The figure was not drawn to scale. For steps *1* to *3*, pgRNA and minus strand DNA are depicted in a linear confirmation.

Several groups reported that expression of X proteins from both HBV and WHV inhibits nucleotide excision repair (NER) through binding to DNA damage–binding protein 1 (DDB1).[23,221,281,460] Subsequent studies provided evidence for an HBx-DDB1 complex binding to cullin4A-RING (CUL4A) ubiquitin ligase. This association is mediated by DDB1 acting as an adaptor protein.[399] Structural data have revealed an α-helical motif at position 88 to 100 in HBx that binds to the BPA-BPC domains of DDB1,[296] and validated the HBx-CUL4A interaction,[297] suggesting that HBx might act as a bridge linking the CUL4A-DDB1 complex to a substrate that is then ubiquitinated by the CUL4A-RING ubiquitin ligase (Fig. 18.13). Consistent with such a model, the structural maintenance of chromosomes 5/6 (Smc5/6) complex normally required for DNA repair and chromosome stability was identified as a substrate for the CUL4A-DDB1-HBx complex.[114,353] Besides Smc5 and Smc6, the complex contains the four kleisins Nse1-4. Consistent with a direct role of the complex in silencing HBV cccDNA, depletion of Smc5 or Smc6 rescued transcription of HBx-deficient virus.[114,353] So far, structural data about the binding of HBx to any of the Smc5/6 complex components remains elusive.

Smc5/6 restriction of HBV transcription requires colocalization of the complex with nuclear PML bodies (nuclear domain 10 (ND10)) where the Smc5/6 complex is believed to bind directly or indirectly to cccDNA.[114,373] Genetic analysis of HBx function identified a region spanning aa 45 to 140 essential for Smc5/6 ubiquination and degradation. This domain comprises a conserved CCCH motif defined by a cluster of three cysteine residues at positions 61, 69, and 137 and a histidine at position 139 proposed to form a zinc-binding motif.[415]

It is still difficult to assess whether Smc5/6 ubiquination and degradation is the only function of HBx for the HBV life cycle or whether any of the many other reported activities are

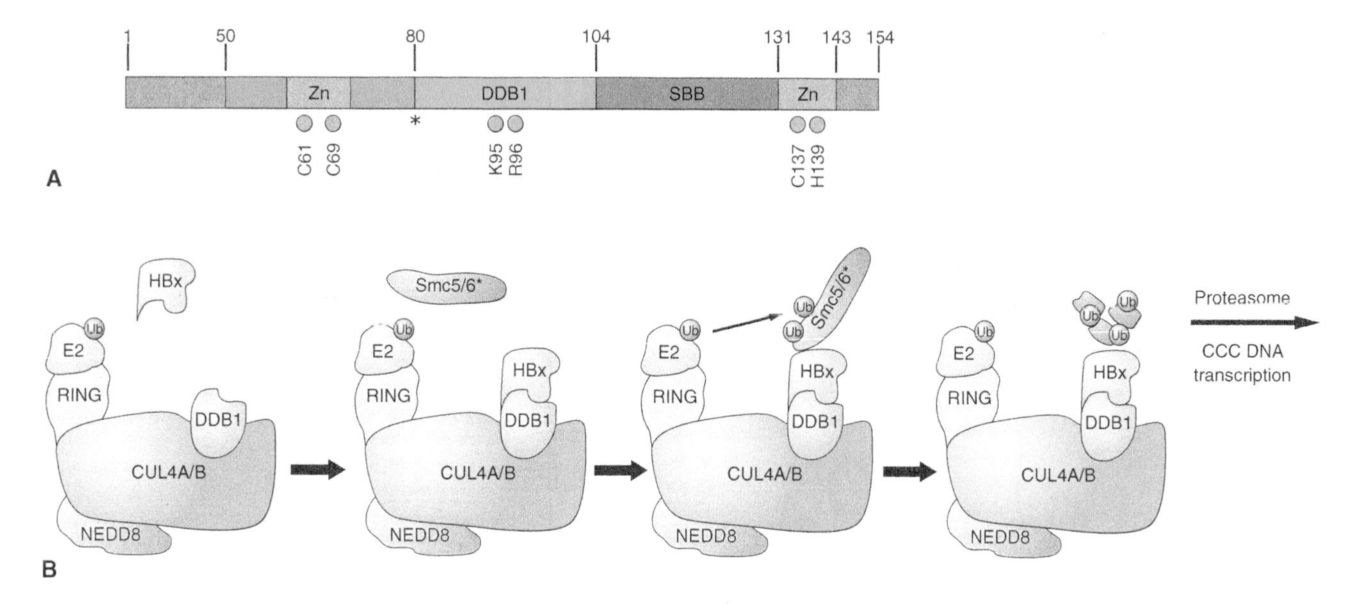

FIGURE 18.13 Formation of the HBx-Smc5/6 complex. A: Schematic representation of HBx based on ref.[415] depicting the two domains forming the Zn-binding motif (Zn), the DDB1-binding motif,[297] and a hypothetical smc–binding box (SBB). The N- and C-terminal domains spanning aa 1 to 50 and 143 to 154, respectively, are not required for HBx function. **B:** The model for HBx function stipulates that HBx binds to the CUL4A-DDB1 complex with the DDB1 domain and recruits the smc5/6 complex, which is subsequently ubiquinated and degraded by the proteasome.[114,297] *Asterisk* denotes conserved methionine (aa 79) that could lead to the expression of a truncated HBx protein.[9] Panels A and B are not to scale.

relevant for HBV infections. For example, what is the role of the relatively weak transactivator activity for promoters with NF-κB, AP-1, AP-2, c/EBP, ATF/CREB, or NFAT binding sites that has been observed in tissue culture cells[463,466]? Because Smc5/6 is required for DNA repair and genome stability, it is conceivable that at least some of the effects attributed to HBx in the past were derived indirectly as a consequence of HBx-mediated inactivation of the Smc5/6 complex, triggering stress responses and even cell death in established cell limes. An important unresolved issue is whether a small form of HBx expressed from one of the conserved internal AUGs is expressed and whether it has an activity in transcriptional regulation in infected hepatocytes as observed earlier in transfected tissue culture cells (Fig. 18.13).[260]

Replication of Genomic Nucleic Acid

Formation of cccDNA

The first step in the hepadnavirus replication cycle is the conversion of genomic rcDNA into cccDNA (Fig. 18.5). Although knowledge concerning the mechanisms responsible for this step is still incomplete, a comparison of the two DNA forms can be used to establish a model for cccDNA formation. It predicts that the polymerase and one of the terminally redundant segments on the minus strand, termed r, are removed prior to the ligation of the two minus strand ends. Similarly, a capped RNA oligomer present at the 5′ end of plus strand DNA must be removed and the incomplete plus strands extended before the ends can be joined. Cellular DNA polymerases most likely elongate the 3′ end of plus strands because RT inhibitors do not block cccDNA formation from rcDNA.[147,348] Reverse genetic experiments with DHBV suggested that an endonuclease removes the 5′ end of minus strand DNA leading to the formation of a protein-free rcDNA, which can be detected in HNF1α null HBV transgenic mice and in tissue culture cells.[153,174,416,465] Identification of rcDNA species harboring covalently closed minus strand DNA suggests that plus strand DNA repair occurs after ligation of the ends of minus strand DNA.[318] So far, investigations aimed at identifying cellular DNA repair enzymes responsible for the conversion of rc- to cccDNA revealed possible roles for the Y-DNA polymerase kappa (polK), DNA ligases I and III, and the Flap endonuclease 1.[246,313,409] More recently, DNA polymerase alpha (pol α) has been shown to be required for cccDNA synthesis when rcDNA in cytoplasmic core particles enter a retrograde pathway leading to cccDNA amplification, as described below.[493] Curiously, pol α does not appear to play a role in the production of cccDNA from rcDNA following *de novo* infection, indicating that distinct pathways might lead to cccDNA formation depending on the origin of the rcDNA-containing core particle. Tyrosyl-DNA-phosphatase 2 (Tdp2) can cleave the tyrosine-DNA linking the RT to the 5′ end of minus strand DNA *in vitro* and based on RNAi experiments was invoked to act as a host factor involved in HBV cccDNA formation.[252] However, HepG2-NTCP cells deficient in Tdp2 expression are permissive for HBV replication.[104] Whether the conversion of rc- to cccDNA in hepatocytes *in vivo* relies on the same enzymes as identified in hepatoma cells is not yet known.

Packaging of pgRNA

pgRNA has dual functions in viral replication. It acts both as the mRNA for the translation of the core and polymerase polypeptides and as the template for genome replication. The transition from the first to the second function is triggered by the binding of the polymerase to the packaging signal, epsilon, at the 5′ end of the mRNA (Fig. 18.14A). In turn, this reaction creates a signal for the assembly of this ribonucleoprotein complex (RNP) into capsids. Polymerases preferentially bind to their own mRNA, possibly while translation is still ongoing, which increases the chance for packaging and replication of biologically intact pgRNA.[17,194] The interaction between the polymerase and epsilon RNA requires cellular chaperones as described earlier. While structurally intact polymerase is required for RNA packaging, DNA polymerization activity *per se* is not required for this process, indicating that the RNP can induce assembly without a requirement for DNA synthesis.[15,73,194] A more recent study revealed that N6-methyladenosine modification within the packaging signal epsilon on pg RNA might increase reverse transcription of pgRNAs.[213] Packaging of pg RNA is inhibited by IFN-α by mechanisms that are not yet known.[542]

Based on secondary structure predictions, epsilon contains two inverted repeats that can fold into an RNA hairpin with a basal and an apical stem that are separated by a bulge (Fig. 18.12). The upper stem is capped by a loop.[228] RNA footprint analysis of free and bound epsilon RNA suggested that binding of the polymerase could induce a single-stranded conformation in the upper stem.[22] Again, it should be noted that due to a terminal redundancy (R), epsilon RNA is present at both ends of pgRNA. However, genetic experiments showed that only the 5′ copy provides a binding site for the polymerase and is required for packaging. Consistent with these results, evidence has been obtained that the nearby cap structure on pgRNA may play a role in RNA packaging. These results also evoked the possibility that the polymerase might interact with translation factors to induce a transition from translation to replication.[220] In support of this idea, evidence has been obtained that translation of pre-C RNA, with passage of 80S ribosomes through epsilon, prevents its packaging[359]; the AUG for core is downstream of epsilon.

In contrast to the mammalian hepadnaviruses, packaging in the avian viruses requires, in addition to epsilon, a second pregenome sequence, termed region II, located about 900 nucleotides downstream of epsilon and spanning approximately 300 nucleotides.[60,382] The role of this downstream sequence in RNA packaging is not yet understood.

In addition to the chaperones required for RNA packaging described previously, the human cytidine deaminase APOBEC3G can be incorporated into viral particles through binding to the viral reverse transcriptase at least when APOBEC3G is expressed at high levels.[362,363] Ectopic expression of several members of the APOBEC family of proteins inhibits HBV replication.[431] Notably, unlike the inhibition by APOBEC of retrovirus and retroposon replication,[430] inhibition of HBV is not dependent upon the catalytic activity of the deaminase. Instead it appears that the protein inhibits virus replication during an early step of minus strand DNA synthesis, perhaps by binding to viral RNA or the polymerase.[362]

Minus Strand DNA Synthesis

The first step in minus strand DNA synthesis is the priming reaction that leads to the formation of a covalent link between a tyrosine residue in the TP domain of the polymerase and dGMP (Fig. 18.12A).[271,528,539,587] The template for this protein-priming reaction is a C residue located in the bulge of epsilon. Although *in vitro* priming can occur immediately following the

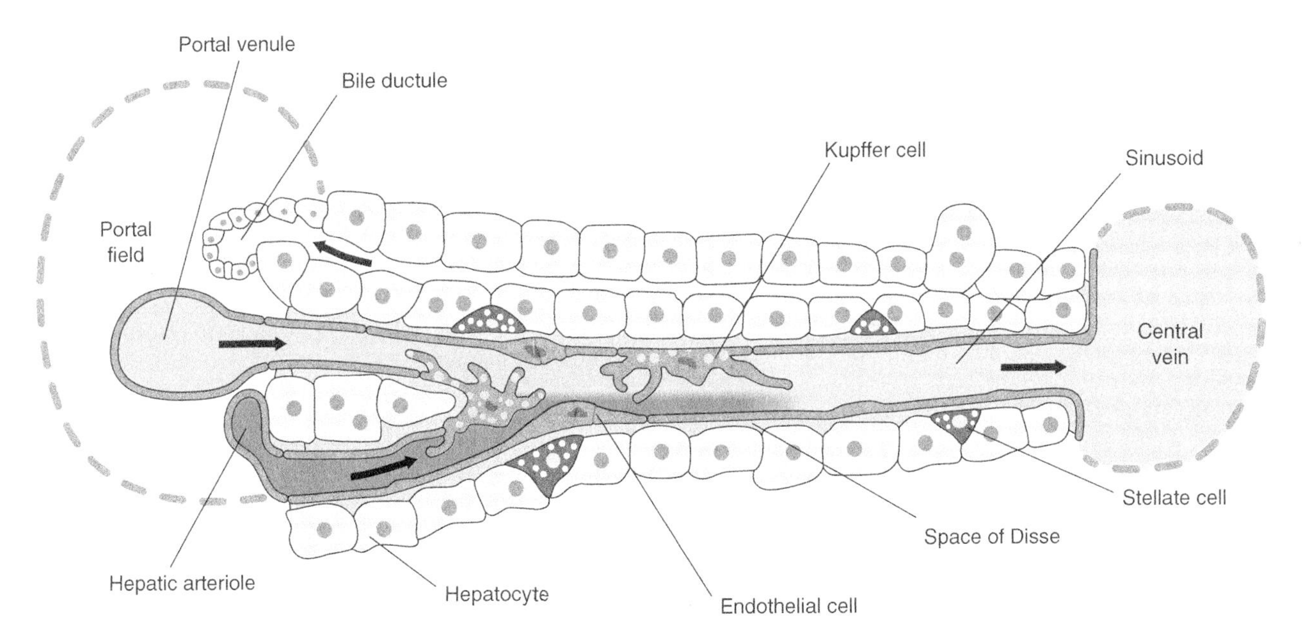

FIGURE 18.14 Structure of the liver lobule. Two dimensional representation of a small portion of a liver lobule with various cell types present (hepatic stellate cells, localized between sinusoidal endothelial cells and hepatocytes, within the space of Disse, are not shown). Blood enters the lobule from the hepatic artery and portal vein and flows through the sinusoids bounded by plates of hepatocytes, exiting at the central vein. Hepatocytes produce bile, which is released into bile canaliculi, small channels formed where the apical surfaces of hepatocytes make contact, flows to the Canals of Hering and then to bile ductules. From there, it flows to larger ducts and exits the liver. The origin of hepatic progenitor cells, which normally only appear during certain conditions of acute and chronic liver injury, is also illustrated. The exact location of progenitor cells in the healthy liver is uncertain, with different lines of evidence pointing to either bile duct epithelium or cells in the Canals of Hering. In the actual lobule, many plates of hepatocytes connect the portal triad to the central vein, though only two are shown here. (Adapted from Frevert U, Engelmann S, Zougbédé S, et al. Intravital observation of Plasmodium berghei sporozoite infection of the liver. *PLoS Biol* 2005;3(6):e192. https://creativecommons.org/licenses/by/2.0/.)

binding of the RT to epsilon in the absence of core protein, the exact sequence of events in infected cells is not known. Thus, priming could occur prior to, during, or after the assembly of capsids. To complete the priming reaction, the polymerase copies the next two or three nucleotides from the bulge of epsilon. As a consequence of this mechanism, the polymerase remains covalently linked to the 5′ end of minus strand DNA during all subsequent steps of viral DNA synthesis, virus assembly, and release.[156,347]

To continue DNA synthesis, the 3 to 4 nt DNA oligomer is transferred to the 3′ end of pgRNA, where it anneals with a complementary sequence motif located in a 10 to 12 nucleotide-long region known as DR1 (Fig. 18.12B, step 1).[529] However, the 3- to 4-nucleotide acceptor site by itself is too short to specify the transfer to DR1. Additional sequences on pgRNA are necessary to control the translocation of the DNA primer to DR1. The selection of the natural site is most likely facilitated by the structural arrangement of pgRNA in the capsid. The acceptor site and epsilon RNA presumably must be held in close physical proximity to facilitate the transfer of the 3- to 4-nt oligomer across the pregenome. Indeed, a short cis-acting element, termed phi, located upstream of the acceptor site at DR1 is required for accurate minus strand DNA synthesis from DR1 in HBV, but not DHBV.[1,328] Phi can basepair with the 5′ region of epsilon RNA, thereby stabilizing the predicted structural conformation of pgRNA required for the transfer of the short minus strand. Following the translocation reaction, minus strand DNA synthesis continues all the way to the 5′ end of the RNA template (step 2). During this reaction, pgRNA is degraded by the RNaseH activity present near the C-terminus of the polymerase.[451] Due to the location of DR1 within the terminal redundancy on the pregenome, the completed minus strand DNA bears the short terminal redundancy, r. As described below, r plays a role in the circularization of the viral genome.[304,451,546]

Plus Strand DNA Synthesis

Plus strand DNA is primed by an 18-nucleotide-long, capped RNA oligomer derived from the 5′ end of pgRNA. The oligomer contains a complete copy of DR1 and represents a product of the RNAseH activity of the polymerase (Fig. 18.12B, step 3).[303,311] As a consequence of this priming mechanism, plus strand DNA synthesis can only begin after minus strand DNA synthesis is complete. To prime plus strand DNA synthesis, the RNA oligomer must first translocate to and anneal with DR2, located near the 5′ end of the minus strand DNA and identical in sequence to DR1.[303,451,546] As expected, mutations that disrupt the homology between DR1 and DR2 block the formation of rcDNA and instead favor an *in situ* DNA priming reaction from the non–translocated primer, leading to the formation of double stranded linear (dsl) DNA.[95,473,561] DSL DNA is produced even under natural conditions, albeit with a low frequency of about 5% to 20% of rcDNA (Fig. 18.5).

The mechanism responsible for the transfer of the RNA primer to DR2 is not completely understood. The most likely scenario is that the regions encompassing DR1 and DR2 on minus strand DNA are juxtaposed to facilitate the transfer of the primer from DR1 to DR2. Studies with DHBV and HBV revealed the presence of three sequence motifs on the minus strands, which have the potential to form short duplexes that might stabilize a secondary structure required for plus-strand primer translocation.[177,291,309] Mutations that would be expected to disrupt the formation of these duplexes inhibited rcDNA, but not dsl DNA synthesis. In addition, capsid proteins might impose certain structural constraints on minus strands and thereby play a role in primer transfer.

Following the priming reaction at DR2, plus strand DNA synthesis ensues until it reaches the 5′ end of minus strand DNA. At this point, a template switch (i.e., circularization) is required for the continuation of DNA synthesis (Fig. 18.12B, step 4). The template switch is facilitated by the aforementioned terminally redundant sequences, r, in minus strand DNA. The structural requirements for this reaction must be complicated, because the polymerase attached to the 5′ end of the minus strand accommodates both ends of the minus strand DNA in close proximity. In spite of the expected steric constraints, the polymerase can copy the entire r5 region, including the dGMP residue that is covalently linked to the RT and then induce the necessary template switch to r3.[310] As with priming at DR2, this event also depends on the formation of small duplexes on distant sites in minus strand DNA, indicating that the two critical steps in plus strand DNA synthesis might be controlled by the same mechanism.[187,351]

In mammalian hepadnaviruses plus strand DNA synthesis is incomplete and reaches approximately half the genome length prior to virion formation.[426,480] The cause and significance of the premature termination of plus strand synthesis remains obscure. Perhaps the arrest in DNA synthesis is caused by steric factors imposed by the capsid and by the polymerase itself. For instance, DHBV capsids assembled with core proteins with truncated C-termini are defective in plus-strand elongation,[568] demonstrating that capsid structure can influence elongation of plus strand DNA. In addition, the coating of capsids with envelope proteins probably leads to the depletion of the dNTP pool prior to the completion of DNA synthesis. This latter possibility is supported by the fact that plus strand DNA can be extended in an *in vitro* reaction in the presence of precursor dNTPs and nonionic detergents that disrupt the viral envelope[235,480] (Fig. 18.2). In contrast to orthohepadnaviruses, plus strand DNA synthesis in wild-type avihepadnaviruses is virtually complete,[304] except that the polymerase does not displace the RNA primer from DR2, so DR2 has to be copied prior to cccDNA formation.

Amplification and Stability of cccDNA

The fate of newly made DNA-containing capsids in the cytoplasm of infected cells is twofold: The particles either enter a retrograde pathway for delivery to the cell nucleus and release of rcDNA or assemble with envelope proteins into virions and enter the secretory pathway (Fig. 18.5). The first pathway amplifies the copy number of cccDNA.[518,551] Using DHBV, cccDNA amplification in cultures of nondividing hepatocytes was shown to occur early in an infection when the cytoplasmic concentration of viral envelope proteins is still low.[483,484] The final, average cccDNA copy number per nucleus, *in vivo*, has an estimated range between 1 and 20 copies per hepatocyte[224,230,344] but exhibits large variation among individual hepatocytes.[576] Transport of newly made capsids from the cytoplasm to the nucleus does not require envelope proteins because cccDNA amplification still occurs when hepatocytes are infected with viral mutants that are unable to synthesize these proteins.[483,484] Instead, signals generated on capsids during their maturation might play a role in the retrograde transport. In fact, in the complete absence of envelope proteins, the retrograde transport leads to nonphysiological overamplification of cccDNA than can be toxic to hepatocytes.[289,290] It remains unclear if envelope proteins regulate HBV cccDNA amplification.

Critical issues with important implications for antiviral therapies with inhibitors of viral DNA replication are whether cccDNA has a half-life in resting hepatocytes and hence, whether ongoing cccDNA synthesis is required to maintain a steady-state within a nondividing cell and whether cccDNA can survive mitosis of hepatocytes. In cultured primary woodchuck and human hepatocytes, differentiated HepaRG cells and DMSO-treated nondividing HepG2-NTCP cells cccDNA appears to be very stable with long half-lives comparable to that of infected hepatocytes.[107,249,315,348] The view that cccDNA stability is high is also supported by studies of competition in infected liver between strains of DHBV with different replication rates and during Antiviral Therapy in infected woodchucks. Competition between the DHBV strains essentially stops in the fully infected adult liver, where cell turnover is low, suggesting that cccDNA has a low turnover rate in infected cells.[575] A kinetic analysis of WHV cccDNA in experimentally infected woodchucks treated with the RT inhibitor L-FMAU ([1-(2-fluoro-5-methyl-beta-L-arabinofuranosyl) uracil] suggested a half-live for cccDNA of 33 to 50 days, which corresponded to the expected loss of hepatocytes during that period.[584] Similarly, long half-lives of cccDNA ranging from 38 to 68 days were reported from experiments with ducks infected with DHBV and treated with a combination of the RT inhibitors lamivudine and dideoxyguanosine.[2,319]

A caveat with interpretation of results obtained with animals treated with RT inhibitors lies in the uncertainty about the completeness of inhibition of viral replication in infected livers.[418] Sporadic reduction in therapeutically effective concentrations in a fraction of hepatocytes could permit low-level viral replication and as a consequence replenishment of the cccDNA load. Thus, whether cccDNA is lost or partitioned to daughter cells during cell division is still not resolved. HBV does not appear to encode a protein that could tether cccDNA to chromosomes as it has been reported for human papilloma and other DNA viruses.[26,123] Hence, it would be expected that cccDNA were lost during division of hepatocytes, which probably occurs during recovery from infections as discussed later in this chapter. A recent study with HBV-infected hepatocytes that were serially transplanted into human hepatocyte chimeric uPA mice indicated that cccDNA is diluted and lost during hepatocyte proliferation.[6] However, even in the presence of the entry inhibitor Myrcludex-B or the RT inhibitor lamivudine, cccDNA persists in a small fraction of hepatocytes. Also, an earlier report revealed significant cccDNA loss during proliferation of tupaia hepatocytes infected with WMHBV in uPa chimeric mice in the absence of an antiviral.[320] On the other hand, a study with HBV-infected patients undergoing antiviral therapies with nucleoside analogs that inhibit viral DNA synthesis suggested that cccDNA may be stable in the chronically infected liver and survive through mitosis.[540] Experiments with tissue culture cells generally favor a model where cccDNA can survive mitosis and partition to daughter cells.[176,295] cccDNA also appeared to survive mitosis in primary woodchuck hepatocyte cultures derived from a chronically infected woodchuck that were treated with the nucleoside analogue adefovir dipivoxil and EGF, to block viral DNA synthesis and induce cell proliferation.[107] Again, a caveat exists with studies involving antiviral therapies due to the possibility of break-through DNA synthesis and replenishment of the cccDNA pool obscuring the detection of a more significant cccDNA loss.

Virus Assembly and Release

Assembly of Dane particles occurs in at least two distinct steps: The formation of capsids that contain pgRNA and reverse transcriptase and the formation of enveloped virus particles that contain the viral DNA genome. During the completion of viral DNA synthesis, capsids gain the ability to interact with envelope proteins[210,390] (Fig. 18.5). Interestingly, empty capsids, but not RNA or minus strand containing capsids, interact efficiently with envelope proteins.[370] This interaction must occur independently of the phosphorylation state of capsids, because secreted empty particles are hyperphosphorylated, whereas rcDNA containing particles are hypophosphorylated.[371] As explained earlier, genetic evidence pointed to a mechanism where DNA synthesis is accompanied with successive dephosphorylation of capsids.[392] A more recent study revealed that RNA containing capsids are hypophosphorylated suggesting that partial dephosphorylation of the carboxy terminal domain might occur concomitantly with RNA packaging rather than DNA synthesis.[317,580]

DNA containing core particles assemble with envelope proteins at membranes of the late endosomal multivesicular bodies (MVPs) resulting in the formation and release of infectious virus (Dane) particles.[265,535] The N-terminal domain of L plays an important role in this step, because M and S proteins alone cannot support translocation of capsids across membranes.[288] Based on biochemical and structural studies, PreS1 binds to gamma2-adaptin (γ2).[186,229] In turn, γ2 might bind through its ubiquitin recognition motif to ubiquinated Nedd4, an alleged binding partner of capsids.[432] Such a preassembly complex appears to provide a substrate for the endosomal sorting complex required for the transport (ESCRT) complex at the MVB[535,265] Moreover, Vps4 ATPase and AIP1/ALIX, known MVB-associated proteins, are required for HBV budding.[242,265,535] Following budding into MVBs, virions must enter the exosome pathway to exit the cell.

Besides DNA-containing particles, hepatocytes also secrete empty enveloped virion-like particles. Empty particles were first recognized in plasma of HBV infected patients as a population of Dane particles with lower density in CsCl and devoid of the nucleic acid and endogenous polymerase activity associated with the population with virions of higher density.[155,236,434] Notably, empty virions were more abundant than DNA-containing virions suggesting that they might represent defective interfering particles. The significance of these early observations was obscured by the prevailing notion that viral DNA synthesis provided signals necessary for the interaction between capsids and envelope proteins and hence for the formation and secretion of Dane particles.[482] However, experiments with viral DNA synthesis inhibitors and mutants defective in polymerase activity validated the original observations.[370] A revised model for Dane particle formation stipulates that capsids containing RNA or minus strand DNA exhibit a blocking signal preventing their interaction with envelope proteins.[370] Hence, the elusive signal proposed to trigger envelopment of core particles might be represented by a negative signal on

RNA and minus strand containing capsids, a hypothesis awaiting further investigation. A more recent study indicated that secretion of rcDNA-containing virions and genome-free particles employ both common and distinct interaction determinants on capsid and envelope proteins.[372] Also, it is not known if empty particles have a role in HBV biology. It should be noted that none of these restrictions is absolute; for example, a small fraction of secreted virus particles contain pgRNA or minus strand DNA.[326]

In contrast to virions, formation and secretion of 22 nm SVPs occurs through the ER-Golgi compartment independently of the MVB.[389] Consistent with this view, dominant-negative mutants of Vps4 and AIP1 do not prevent SVP release from cells.[265,535] EM studies indicated that disulfide-linked S dimers accumulate as filaments in the perinuclear space of the ER from where they must be transferred by unknown mechanisms to the ER-Golgi intermediate compartment (ERGIC).[389] Subsequently, filaments reorganize into spheres that enter the constitutive secretory pathway. It is also possible that SVPs use different exit strategies depending on the ratio of L:M:S.

PATHOGENESIS AND PATHOLOGY

Infection of the Liver

The main cellular target of HBV is the hepatocyte, the parenchymal cell of the liver, and the only liver cell that expresses NTCP, an HBV receptor. In humans, hepatocytes are the only cell type convincingly shown to replicate the virus. Structurally, the liver is composed of microscopic lobules into which blood enters from the hepatic artery and portal vein, which are situated in a region known as the portal triad, and exits via the hepatic vein (Fig. 18.14). Hepatocytes comprise 60% to 70% of liver cell mass. Other cells include bile ductular epithelial cells, sinusoidal endothelial cells, hepatic stellate cells (Ito cells), and Kupffer cells, the resident liver macrophages. Nonparenchymal cells of the liver do not appear to have a direct role in infection of hepatocytes, although an indirect role in virus transport to hepatocytes has been suggested based on experiments with DHBV.[42]

Hepatocytes are long-lived and self-renewing, with a half-life exceeding 6 months under normal conditions, and in adults a correspondingly low proliferation rate.[166,257,322,454,525,547] As a consequence, following *de novo* infection of adults, HBV primarily infects hepatocytes arrested in G0, though cycling hepatocytes are presumably infected in neonates. Infection occurs at the basolateral membrane consistent with the site of expression of NTCP, which is required for uptake of conjugated bile acids.[7]

Though hepatocytes are considered a self-renewing population in the normal liver, under conditions of severe injury, or where hepatocyte proliferation is blocked, for instance by a toxic chemical, facultative progenitor cells, considered to be located in the Canal of Hering, were considered to give rise to oval cells that proliferated and ultimately differentiated into hepatocytes.[507] Possible progenitor cells were also found in the bone marrow,[361] though their quantitative contribution to hepatocyte replacement and their relationship to progenitor cells attributed to the Canals of Hering were unclear. It has also been suggested that self-renewal in the normal liver is due to division of hepatocytes surrounding the central vein.[527] However, the prevailing concept is that most or all mature hepatocytes participate in renewal in the healthy liver. In addition, data suggest that mature hepatocytes may dedifferentiate under conditions of stress, proliferate, and then redifferentiate to mature hepatocytes, again questioning the role of stem cells in hepatocyte maintenance.[167] In this scenario, the mature hepatocyte population in adults is a closed population that can evolve to compensate for hepatotoxic conditions. Consistent with this notion, clonal outgrowth of hepatocyte lineages has been observed in genetic diseases impacting hepatocytes[334] and during the progression of chronic hepatitis B.[338,516]

Hepatocyte replacement in response to killing of infected hepatocytes by antiviral cytotoxic T cells (CTL) during transient (acute self-limiting) hepadnavirus infections also appears to be primarily through division of other hepatocytes.[224,230,485] Possible replacement from undifferentiated progenitors has been suggested to occur during late stages of chronic infections, by which time the liver may be highly damaged,[150,197,429] but mature hepatocyte proliferation also occurs, and current information would suggest that the undifferentiated cells represent dedifferentiated hepatocytes.[167] The fate of HBV during hepatocyte proliferation is difficult to assess because proliferation occurs under varying local conditions produced by the level of liver inflammation and cytokine production, factors that are believed to affect the stability of cytoplasmic capsids, nuclear cccDNA, and viral RNAs, as well as RNA packaging. Even less is known about whether a fraction of proliferating hepatocytes becomes refractory to reinfection. In any case, immune clearance of virus from most of the hepatocyte population does not appear to depend on coproduction of virus-neutralizing antibodies.

Cell and Tissue Tropism

Early immunohistochemical studies of human tissues other than the liver suggested that exocrine and endocrine cells of the pancreas can be infected, though this was not shown to reflect productive infection. However, evidence for HBV DNA replication intermediates in the spleen was also described for humans and chimpanzees. Evidence for infection, gene transcription, and viral replication in peripheral blood mononuclear cells (PBMCs) has also been reported. Data in support of infection in bone marrow, as evidenced by the presence of HBsAg and 3 kbp rcDNA, but not DNA replication intermediates, has also been presented. The idea that any of these observations reflect actual infection of blood cells has, however, been challenged by a study that failed to detect cccDNA in these cells, suggesting instead that viral DNA and antigen signals, and by inference, virus replication reported in these studies arose from observations of passively adsorbed virus.[250] At present, the question of whether PBMCs, or any other site outside the liver of HBV carriers, are productively infected, or just accumulate HBV that was produced in the liver remains elusive.

The issue of extrahepatic replication has also been addressed in woodchucks infected with WHV. The most convincing evidence of extrahepatic infection was obtained from a study with PBLs. Although PBLs did not replicate WHV *in vivo*, they produced typical viral DNA replication intermediates and released virus when stimulated with lipopolysaccharide *in vitro* and thus appear to be latently infected *in vivo*.[253,254]

The best evidence for active *in vivo* replication in cells other than hepatocytes comes from studies of ducks infected with DHBV, where replication intermediates were found in subsets of cells in the spleen, kidney, and pancreas, as well as bile duct epithelial cells of the liver,[148,183,196,223,279,367,490] and of the yolk sac during embryonic development.[491] Viral DNA also accumulates in the spleen, due to passive accumulation of virus by follicular dendritic cells[223]; evidence for DNA replication intermediates[490] and cccDNA[173] in the spleen has also been reported, though DNA replication intermediates were not observed in the latter study.

Immune Response

A remarkable aspect of the hepadnavirus life cycle is that virus infection and spread can occur in the absence of a measurable innate immune response, which only becomes evident after the appearance of the adaptive immune response, which may appear after several weeks of infection. Transcriptome analysis of liver tissue obtained from three HBV-infected chimpanzees demonstrated that genes known to be expressed upon activation of pattern recognition receptors or interferons remained at basal levels.[544] Subsequent studies using single-cell analyses of HBV-infected HepG2-NTCP, HepaRG cells and PHH confirmed the observations made in the chimpanzee model and also demonstrated that the observed lack of an innate immune response was not due to an inhibitory viral activity.[85,356,373] These observations are not entirely surprising because HBV does not produce known ligands for intracellular pattern recognition sensors such as uncapped RNA, or DNA exposed to the cytoplasm.

Indeed, a number of studies suggest that the liver can regulate or at least protect itself against the host immune response.[421] First, in some species including rats, pigs, and mice, liver transplantation between allogeneic animals induces tolerance to grafts of other tissues from the same donor that would normally be rejected, suggesting that the liver has immunoregulatory properties, possibly attributable to hepatic dendritic cells.[504,505] Second, a number of different cell types in the liver appear to have the ability to present antigen in a suboptimal context, in some cases leading to immune tolerance or a weak immune response.[99,248,506] Third, the adaptive immune response to a number of human viruses that are thought to infect, predominately hepatocytes, including HAV, HBV, HCV, and hepatitis E virus (HEV), only becomes robust enough to induce high levels of cell death and virus clearance 4 to 8 weeks after infection. During this time, the entire hepatocyte population may become infected by HBV.[543] A similar pattern has been seen following DHBV infection of ducks and WHV infection of woodchucks.[224,230] These observations suggest that scanning of hepatocytes by the immune system is low and has been attributed to low expression of major histocompatibility class I (MHC I) genes and limited access of circulating lymphocytes to hepatocytes, despite the occurrence of fenestrations in the liver endothelial cells.[171] The possibility that liver cells other than hepatocytes may induce at least partial tolerance to viral antigens could also contribute to the prolonged course of transient and chronic infections.

HBV infection, replication, and virus shedding are not cytopathic to hepatocytes. This may be another reason the immune response to infected cells is slow to evolve, often not appearing until weeks after essentially every hepatocyte is infected,[248,503,541] which may take weeks to months depending upon the infecting viral dose. The result of this massive infection is that a strong immune reaction, with killing of large numbers of hepatocytes, is typically seen during the clearance phase of such an infection.[485] About 95% of immunocompetent adults are able to mount such a response, resolving the infection within a few weeks once clearance begins. Unfortunately, about 5% of adults and most children under the age of 1 year are unable to resolve the infection (Fig. 18.15, see Fig. 18.17). Instead, chronic hepatitis B with ongoing liver injury may occur, mediated by a T-cell immune response targeting hepatocytes that express viral antigens.[28,88,152] Chronic infections, with persistence of readily detectable levels of serum virus and surface antigen particles, are generally lifelong. Antiviral T cells are rare in these patients compared to patients that have previously recovered from a transient HBV infection.[420] In addition, in chronically infected patients, a certain degree of T-cell function defect is reported which may contribute to viral persistence. It is suggested to result from T-cell exhaustion by high antigen concentrations that promote HBV-specific T-cell dysfunction by affecting phenotype and function of peripheral and intrahepatic T cells.[109,141]

Nonetheless, virus titers in the blood often decline during the course of a chronic infection, from as high as 10^{10} per mL to as little as a few hundred per mL. One explanation is that antiviral cytokines produced during chronic hepatitis suppress virus replication,[342] as also seems to occur during the clearance phase of transient infections.[230,485,503,541,543] Another possibility is that persistent killing of infected hepatocytes by antiviral CTLs selects for the clonal outgrowth of hepatocytes that have lost the ability to support high levels of virus replication.[336]

Results of placebo-controlled trials of antiviral agents suggest that approximately 5% of patients each year experience spontaneous decline of virus titer and HBe seroconversion and enter the remission/inactive hepatitis phase.[119,262,329,566] However, unlike clearance of a transient infection, the serum of a chronic HBV carrier undergoing spontaneous remission generally remains HBsAg positive, most likely because many hepatocytes contain both low amounts of cccDNA and integrated viral DNA with an intact S coding region.[550]

The mechanisms of clearance of transient infections have been investigated in detail in clinical studies as well as through the use of experimental models including HBV-infected chimpanzees, WHV-infected woodchucks, and DHBV-infected ducks. A key point in these studies is to explain how the liver recovers after infection of all hepatocytes and how hepatocytes in the recovered liver are derived mostly from previously infected hepatocytes.[337,485] From these studies, it is generally agreed that virus clearance requires the coordinated action of several components of the immune response[169,337,485,543,560]: (a) A cytolytic response by CD8-positive cells recognizing infected hepatocytes expressing viral antigens; (b) A noncytolytic response whereby the CD8-positive cells and other, non–antigen-specific cells recruited to the sites of inflammation, produce TH1 cytokines such as IFN-γ, TNF-α, and interleukin 12 (IL-12) that exhibit a direct antiviral effect, suppressing virus reproduction in the infected hepatocytes,[459] in part by blocking assembly of DNA replication complexes[176,384,388,425,446,447,544]; (c) hepatocyte proliferation to generate new cells to replace those killed by the antiviral response and repopulate the liver, with the idea that cccDNA may not efficiently survive through mitosis.

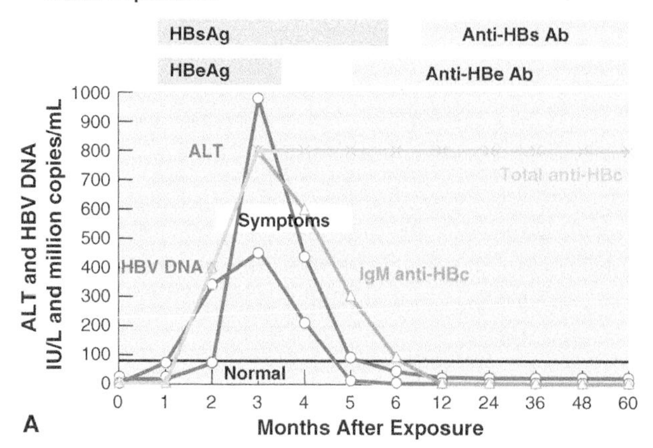

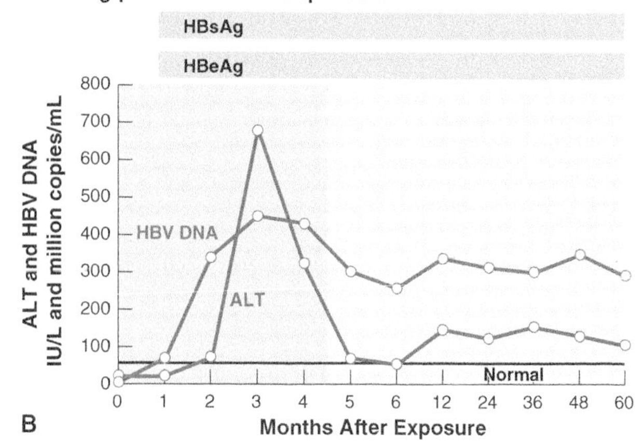

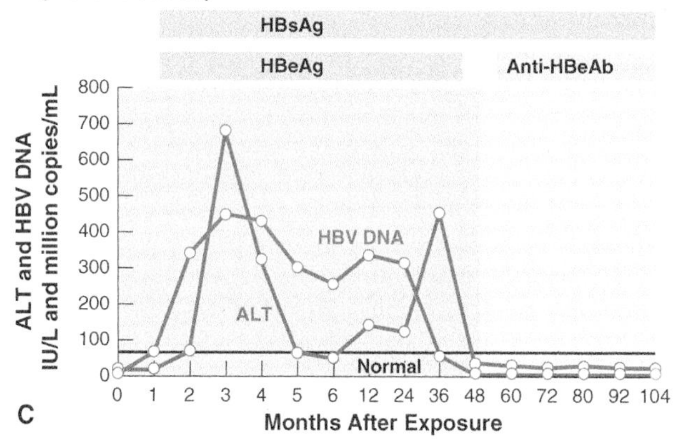

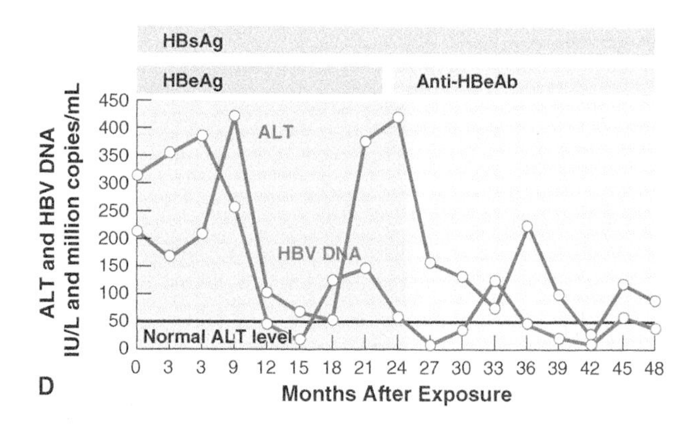

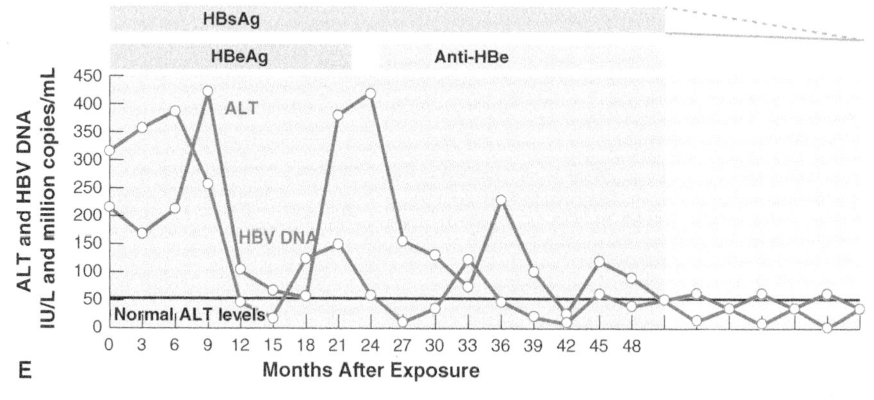

FIGURE 18.15 **Serological profiles of HBV infections. A:** Laboratory diagnosis of acute hepatitis B. Acute hepatitis is diagnosed in patients with jaundice or fatigue and high ALT levels. Evidence of transient HBV infection is obtained by the detection of HBsAg and anti-HBc IgM antibody. Viral replication is authenticated by the detection of serum HBeAg and HBV DNA. Resolution of infection is accompanied by the decline in viral load, seroconversion to anti-HBe, and normalization of ALT levels. Subsequently, HBs seroconversion is observed and represents a serological marker of the cure of the infection. **B:** Laboratory diagnosis of chronic hepatitis B associated with wild-type virus infection. Chronic HBV infection is diagnosed by the persistence of serum HBsAg and markers of viral replication (i.e., serum HBeAg and HBV DNA). Depending on the phase of disease, ALT levels may be normal (i.e., HBeAg-positive chronic *infection*) or elevated (i.e., HBeAg-positive chronic *hepatitis*). **C:** Laboratory diagnosis of transition of chronic hepatitis B to the inactive carrier state (i.e., HBeAg-negative chronic *infection*). HBe seroconversion is associated with the loss of serum HBeAg, the appearance of anti-HBeAb, the decline of serum HBV DNA levels, and the normalization of ALT levels. A flare in ALT levels sometimes precedes it, suggesting that HBe seroconversion may be associated with an immune-mediated hepatocyte lysis. HBe seroconversion is associated with an improved clinical outcome, and the patients are classified inactive carriers.

Another factor that has been considered is the innate immune response mediated by NK and NKT cells, possibly induced or triggered by ER-associated endogenous antigenic lipids that might be generated by HBV-induced secretory phospholipase.[125,140,574] However, as alluded to above, experimental HBV infection of chimpanzees does not induce a detectable innate response in the liver prior to the appearance of the adaptive response,[541] suggesting factors in the innate response critical to virus clearance are, in the context of *de novo* HBV infection, secondary to the adaptive T-cell response. The role of virus-neutralizing antibodies has also been considered. At present, anti-HBsAg antibodies are considered to prevent reinfection of the recovered liver by residual virus. Evidence that B cells play a major role during the recovery phase, when virus-infected hepatocytes are being cleared from the liver, is less compelling, as HBsAg appears to have a suppressive effect on maturation of HBsAg-specific B cells.[53,435] In addition, antibodies to the viral envelope are often not detectable before virus is cleared from the liver.[138,230,401]

An issue that is least understood is how cccDNA is cleared from the liver. Although the existence of cytokine-mediated, noncytocidal, clearance has been invoked,[169,315] the evidence for this occurring *in vivo* remains problematic because of the difficulty of quantifying hepatocyte turnover. Results of a study with HBV transgenic, HNF1alpha-deficient, mice that produce cccDNA suggested that this DNA is sensitive to noncytolytic purging by antiviral cytokines,[10] but unfortunately, the contribution of hepatocyte death to this finding was unclear. Studies of acute infection of chimpanzees have also been interpreted to argue the importance of noncytolytic clearance of HBV DNA replication intermediates and cccDNA. However, interpretation of cccDNA decline is again problematic because of the difficulty of quantifying the large amount of hepatocyte destruction during virus clearance.[170,175,337,354,485,503,543] Thus, the roles of noncytopathic clearance versus clearance by hepatocyte death versus clearance due to a failure to survive mitosis remain unresolved.

HBV Reactivation

Despite the fact that many patients will undergo spontaneous HBsAg seroconversion after acute infection or HBeAg seroconversion during the course of chronic infection and will be in a state of "immune control" of the infection, HBV infection persists in the majority of these patients whose liver still harbor low amounts of cccDNA. Thus, HBV infection is a model of viral persistence where remission is the result of a fine equilibrium between antiviral immune responses and the maintenance of viral minichromosomes at low copy numbers. Several clinical situations have shown that this equilibrium (or "immune control") may be challenged when patients undergo immune suppression or if escape variants are selected.

In patients undergoing immunosuppressive therapies (i.e., chemotherapy, biotherapies for autoimmune diseases, B-cell selective monoclonal Ab-based therapies (anti-CD19/20; e.g., Rituximab and Ofatumumab) for lymphomas or other diseases), HBV replication may reactivate from the reservoir of infected hepatocytes harboring cccDNA.[81,259] In these situations, viral reactivation may occur in inactive carriers and even in patients who previously lost HBsAg. Several studies have shown the presence of very low levels of cccDNA in the liver after HBsAg seroconversion.[341,540] For these reasons, international clinical guidelines recommend antiviral prophylaxis in patients undergoing immunosuppressive therapy as follows[127]: (a) all candidates for chemotherapy and immunosuppressive therapy should be tested for HBV markers prior to immunosuppression, (b) all HBsAg-positive patients should receive nucleos(t)ide analogue therapy as treatment or prophylaxis, (c) HBsAg-negative, anti-HBc–positive subjects should receive anti-HBV prophylaxis if they are at high risk of HBV reactivation. In patients undergoing liver transplantation with an anti-HBc positive donor, there is a potential risk for transmitting the infection to the recipient even in the absence of detectable viremia due to presence of cccDNA in the donor hepatocytes and reactivation of viral infection because of the recipient's immunosuppressive context.[89] Antiviral prophylaxis reduces the risk from 47.8% to 12% in naive recipients and from 15.2% to 3.4% in anti-HBc–positive recipients.[89] Finally, several clinical observations showed that HBs variants may escape HBsAb neutralization and result in viral reactivation, especially in case of immune suppression.[94,437]

In the case of HBV and HCV coinfections, serum HBV DNA levels are usually low possibly due to indirect mechanisms mediated by an innate immune response induced by HCV. With the advent of efficient direct-acting antivirals (DAA) that cure almost 100% of chronic HCV carriers, several cases of HBV reactivation have been observed after elimination of HCV in both HBsAg-positive and in anti-HBc–positive patients.[526,564] Thus, international clinical guidelines recommend (a) that HBsAg-positive patients undergoing DAA therapy should be considered for concomitant nucleos(t)ide analogue prophylaxis until week 12 post DAA and (b) that HBsAg-negative, anti-HBc–positive patients undergoing DAA should be monitored and tested for HBV reactivation in case of ALT elevation.

Cirrhosis and Hepatocellular Carcinoma

Chronic Infections

About 5 years after the discovery of HBV, Sherlock and colleagues looked for a link between HBV infection and HCC.[456] In a cohort of 17 chronically infected males, 5 presented

D: Laboratory diagnosis of HBeAg-negative chronic hepatitis. In some patients, pre-C mutants are selected at the time of HBe seroconversion, and the disease continues to progress with a typical fluctuation of serum HBV DNA and ALT levels. This stage of chronic hepatitis B, which was historically described in the Mediterranean basin, is usually referred to as HBeAg-negative chronic hepatitis B. **E:** After achieving spontaneous or treatment-induced remission, some patients may lose serum HBsAg; serum HBV DNA is undetectable and ALT levels are normal. HBs Ab may become positive but not always. It is expected that in the liver compartment, cccDNA persists and may be responsible for viral reactivation in case of immune depression. This phase is called "functional cure"; it is associated with a decreased risk of hepatocellular carcinoma and represents the new end point for novel therapies in clinical development.

with HCC. Definitive support for the hypothesis that HBV plays a primary role in the development of HCC came from epidemiologic studies,[340,405] and particularly from a prospective study by Beasley and colleagues, who followed more than 22,000 Taiwanese men.[21] The relative lifetime risk for HBsAg–positive males was found to be about 20 compared to uninfected individuals.[135] An even stronger correlation between chronic hepadnavirus infection and HCC was found in WHV–infected woodchucks.[481] Investigations with captive woodchucks showed that WHV induced HCC in essentially 100% of neonatally infected woodchucks within 2 to 4 years and in 20% of those that resolved the infection after neonatal inoculation.[255,495,496] In contrast, the chimpanzee did not prove to be a model for hepatocellular carcinoma, as only a few cases of HCC have been reported in HBV-infected chimpanzees and only in chimpanzees coinfected with either HDV or HCV.[402]

In humans, liver cancer usually develops after several decades of infection and is often preceded by cirrhosis of the liver (Fig. 18.16). Consistent with the distribution of chronic HBV infections around the globe, HCC is one of the two or three most common malignant neoplasms in people living in China, Taiwan and southeast Asia as well as in sub-Saharan Africa. The field has been driven by two hypotheses, one positing a direct effect of the virus in cancer development, the other predicting that HCC formation is a consequence of persistent liver injury caused by the immune response against infected hepatocytes and hence, attributing an indirect role to the virus. In reality, both may contribute to HCC.

The vast majority of tumors contain integrated HBV DNA and, since hepatocytes are the only liver cells clearly susceptible to HBV, it is assumed that most tumors arise by dedifferentiation of mature hepatocytes. While it cannot be excluded that some tumors arise from undifferentiated progenitor cells present in the liver, present findings are most consistent with the concept that the majority of tumors arise from HBV-infected hepatocytes.

Cellular Factors and HCC

Models explaining HCC development in HBV patients entirely via indirect mechanisms take into consideration a hallmark of HBV infections, death, and compensatory regeneration of hepatocytes. Hepatocytes, as noted above, appear to constitute a mostly self-renewing population. Progenitor cell proliferation may also be seen late in infection, especially in the tumor bearing and cirrhotic livers, but these progenitors may arise from dedifferentiated hepatocytes. While hepatocyte death and compensatory proliferation to maintain liver mass are inconsequential on a sporadic basis, persistent liver injury due to CTL killing observed in chronic hepatitis B can cause substantial fibrosis and cirrhosis of the liver. The progression to cirrhosis may be interrupted, and even reversed, if the infection is controlled by antiviral therapies.[300,386,424,428,567] Cirrhosis often precedes HCC, but whether this means that cirrhosis contributes to oncogenesis or that both cirrhosis and HCC are a consequence of infection and persistent hepatocyte destruction is unresolved. It is noteworthy that alcohol abuse, storage diseases, and chronic HCV infections have the same effects, and all are risk factors for HCC.[334] That is, independent of the cause, chronic liver disease is associated with an increased risk of HCC.

Whole-genome sequencing of HCC DNA obtained from HBV-infected patients identified the Wnt/beta-catenin and JAK/STAT pathways as potential oncogenic drivers in approximately half of the cases examined.[231] The same study revealed TP53 mutations in over one-third of HCCs. However, a direct link between those events and HBV infection does not yet appear to exist.

The importance of chronic liver injury in HCC has been documented in many studies with mouse models. For instance, transgenic mice expressing levels of the HBV L-protein that are toxic to hepatocytes developed HCC.[87] It was suggested that a contributing factor in emergence of HCC in this model was free radicals generated by the large number of macrophages activated in response to the high rate of apoptosis, leading to extensive DNA damage in surviving hepatocytes. The idea that oxidative

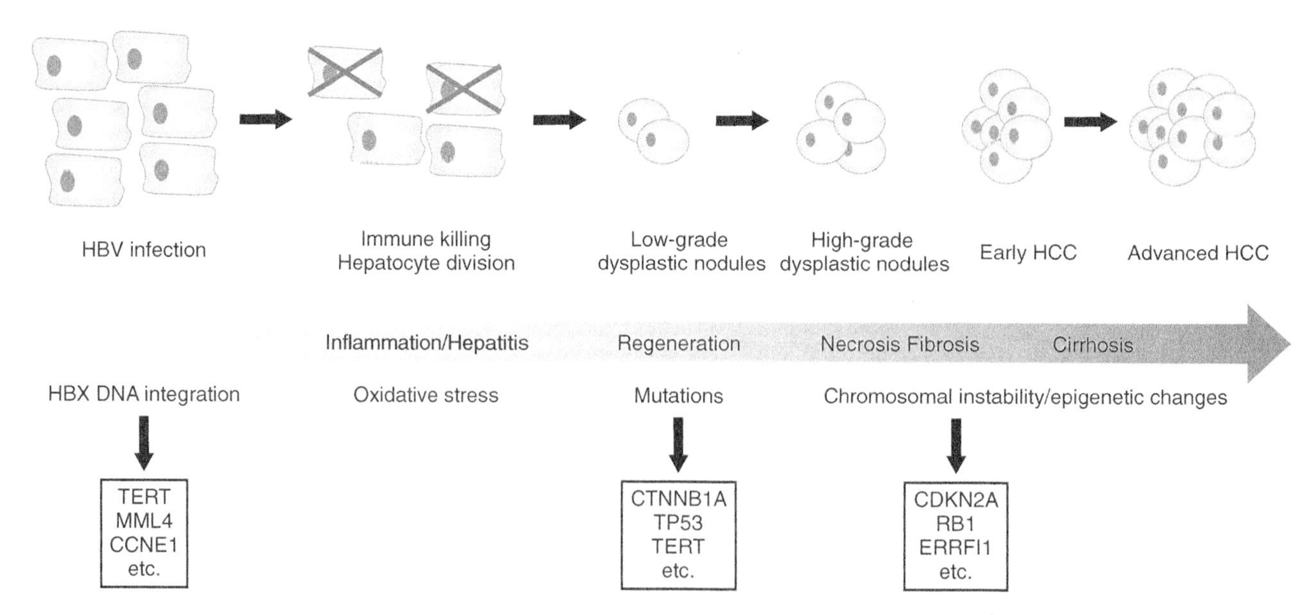

FIGURE 18.16 Model for HCC development. Schematic representation of HCC development initiated by HBV infections (see text for a detailed description and references).

DNA damage was occurring was supported by the detection of deoxyguanosine adducts on DNA isolated from the livers of these mice.[181] These data support the notion that HCC is not just due to the effects of L overexpression on the hepatocytes, leading to a high level of hepatocyte death and compensatory proliferation, but also to hepatocyte DNA damage attributable to free radical formation by activated macrophages.[334]

In a perhaps more relevant model of the events occurring during chronic HBV infections, studies were carried out with transgenic mice expressing low levels of L, which did not cause any apparent liver disease. When the immune system of these mice was ablated and replaced with bone marrow cells from syngeneic nontransgenic mice, the resulting immune response led to liver cell injury and HCC.[357] Moreover, inoculation of the mice with anti-fas ligand antibodies reduced the incidence of HCC, establishing a possible correlation between the rate of hepatocyte death, compensatory proliferation, and development of HCC.[358]

Viral Factors and HCC

Evidence for a direct role of HBV in human HCC was fueled by the observation that DNA from HCC contained integrated HBV DNA and that tumors were clonal with respect to the viral integration site.[41,70,134,455] This discovery suggested a model of insertional mutagenesis, as found by retrovirologists, in which activation of proto-oncogenes was caused by nearby provirus integration.[188,391] However, initial efforts to identify proto-oncogenes adjacent to integrated HBV DNA were not met with clear candidates, save for a few isolated cases, where integration sites were found adjacent to or within coding regions of candidate proto-oncogenes including cyclin A, erb-A, or retinoic acid receptor beta.[115,116,530] Subsequent genomic analyses using Alu-PCR–based amplification of sequences adjacent to HBV integration sites revealed several cancer-related genes including human telomerase (hTERT), which was identified as a recurrent site of HBV integration[352] (Fig. 18.16). Massive parallel sequencing of DNA derived from over 100 HCC tissue samples identified approximately 20 recurrent HBV integration targets in HCCs including hTERT, the histone H3K4 methyltransferase (MLL4), and cyclin E1 (CCNE1).[61,283,486,579] However, most of the individual recurrent sites were only found in a small percentage of tumors.

HBV integration occurs preferentially within or near the DR1 and DR2 segments of the viral genome[222,486, 579] Integration has been associated with increased expression of genes adjacent to integration sites, disruption of coding regions, and DNA copy number alterations.[222,486] Thus, HBV integration events are not limited to transcriptional deregulation but can also cause chromosomal instability.[222,579] It is also possible that HBV DNA alters the expression of some genes that are distant from the integration site, perhaps by altering the structure of chromosomes as observed with N-myc2 activation in woodchuck HCCs, which has been attributed to WHV integrations over 100 kb distal to the gene.[52,146]

Further evidence for a direct viral role in HCC development was obtained from studies with GSHV infections in woodchucks. HCC in GSHV-infected ground squirrels develops in about 50% of animals beyond 4 years of infection[105,332,333] (compared to 100% of WHV-infected woodchucks by 3 years). Delayed onset of HCC development is also observed in woodchucks infected with GSHV compared with the WHV-infected woodchucks, suggesting that the difference in pathogenesis between WHV and GSHV in their natural hosts might be a property of the viruses rather than the hosts.[452] Tumors from WHV-infected woodchucks revealed very different results from those reported with HBV in humans. The majority of these HCCs overexpress N-myc2, a functional pseudogene of N-myc1[145,410] that is not normally expressed in the liver.[145,184,216] C-myc and N-myc1 are more rarely overexpressed in woodchuck HCCs. N-myc1 or C-myc overexpression in woodchuck HCCs is typically associated with nearby integration of WHV DNA, while overexpression of N-myc2 may be due either to nearby integration[145,184] or to integration in the distal *b3n*[47,48] or *win*[146] loci.

The majority of ground squirrel HCCs overexpress C-myc.[184,511] However, C-myc overexpression in the ground squirrel does not correlate with nearby integration of GSHV DNA, though it sometimes correlates with copy number amplification of the C-myc locus. Interestingly, the pattern of DNA integration and myc activation, in HCCs that arise in woodchucks infected with GSHV, is more typical of that seen in ground squirrels infected with GSHV. This suggests that N-myc activation in WHV-infected woodchucks characterizes WHV infections rather than hepadnavirus infections of the woodchuck *per se*. Transcriptional activation of N-myc and C-Myc have not been reported to characterize human HCCs, suggesting that myc activation may play a more central role in rodent than primate HCCs.[511] This does not, however, preclude the possibility that genes regulated by myc play a central role in human HCC.[237]

Alternative models, consistent with a direct role of HBV in human HCC, posit that one or several viral gene products are oncogenic. Although the long latency period observed for HCC development indicates that HBV gene products cannot transform hepatocytes in a single hit event, the hypothesis gained momentum with the discovery that transgenic mice expressing HBx developed HCC.[243] The success of this model depended on the selection of the mouse strain, CD1, known to develop spontaneous hepatomas at an increased rate compared to other mouse strains and high expression levels of the transgene that are not observed during natural infections.[251] Thus, it appears that X promotes but does not necessarily initiate carcinogenesis. In agreement with this notion, an HBx transgene did not promote HCC in another genetic background but, interestingly, these mice were more susceptible to HCC induction by diethylnitrosamine (DEN) than nontransgenic controls,[461] which was subsequently attributed to increased proliferation of altered hepatocytes in the absence of elevated host gene mutation rates.[324] In addition, an HBx transgene accelerated development of HCC in C-myc transgenic mice.[497] One possibility is that these different *in vivo* activities attributed to HBx reflect its ability to degrade the cellular Smc5/6 complex, which plays a key role in chromosome maintenance and repair. Finally, it is important to note that in the past investigations on HBx expression in HCCs have been hampered by the lack of antibodies that can reliably detect expression of the protein.

The discovery of the transactivation function of truncated M envelope proteins also supported a viral oncogene hypothesis (i.e., Ref.[442]). Truncated M proteins are not produced by wild-type HBV but are produced by naturally occurring mutants. Overexpression of the truncated M protein with the help of the albumin promoter in transgenic mice activated the c-Raf/Erk2 signal transduction pathway and, in turn, increased hepatocyte proliferation.[193] These mice developed very small liver tumors by 1 to 2 years of age. Interestingly, Su and colleagues have suggested that L/M protein mutants are responsible for development of a class of preneoplastic lesion consisting of ground glass hepatocytes[478] as well as HCC.[565]

In summary, the details of HBV-induced liver cancer remain elusive. We can infer that the combination of alterations in hepatocyte physiology caused on one side by viral gene expression and on the other by changes in the microenvironment of hepatocytes due to inflammation results in the proliferation and eventual transformation of hepatocytes. Viral mechanisms that could contribute to hepatocyte transformation include changes in host gene expression caused by HBx, truncated M (or L), and integrated HBV DNA, and inhibition of DNA repair pathways. Cellular mechanism include hepatocyte killing by CTLs, induction of DNA damage via reactive oxygen (and nitrogen) radicals produced by macrophages, and expression of cytokines that in conjunction with viral gene expression provide a proliferative stimulus to hepatocytes.

EPIDEMIOLOGY

Global Prevalence

Disease caused by HBV has a worldwide distribution. Serum HBsAg prevalence of ≥8% defines highly endemic areas, 5% to 7% defines high intermediate, 2% to 4% low intermediate, and less than 2% defines low endemic areas. In 1995, it was estimated that more than 2 billion people globally had a history of HBV infection, though a majority had recovered. In 2015, the global prevalence of chronic HBV infection in the general population was estimated at 3.5%, or about 257 million individuals, making it the most common chronic viral infection (https://www.who.int/hepatitis/publications/global-hepatitis-report2017/en/). HBsAg seroprevalence varies considerably among the WHO Regions, with the highest in Africa (6.1%) and the Western Pacific (6.2%). HBV-induced mortality (887,220 deaths/year globally; 337,454 due to HCC; 462,690 due to cirrhosis and 87,076 due to acute hepatitis) is now twice that of malaria (429,000 deaths/year (https://www.who.int/news-room/fact-sheets/detail/malaria)) and HBV represents the seventh highest cause of mortality worldwide. HBV is responsible for greater than 50% of the hepatocellular carcinomas (HCCs) worldwide and up to 10% of liver transplants.[132,160,471] HCC caused by HBV predominated over other important causes of HCC (such as HCV) in countries where the prevalence of chronic HBV infection is high.

Most of the burden of HBV-related disease results from infections acquired in infancy, through perinatal or early childhood exposure to HBV. This is because infection acquired at an early age is much more likely to become chronic than infection acquired later in life. The risk of chronic infection remains high until after 5 years of age, when the rate stabilizes at around 5%.

Coinfection with other viruses occurs most frequently in high HBV endemic areas. About 2.7 million of the 36.7 million people infected with HIV worldwide are coinfected with HBV. Approximately 10% to 15% of patients with chronic HBV infection are coinfected with HCV. HDV infection occurs exclusively in HBV-infected individuals, and approximately 5% of HBV-infected persons are infected with HDV.

WHO estimates that only 10% of the 257 million people living with HBV have been diagnosed and as few as 1% are being adequately treated worldwide. Studies performed in highly endemic areas have shown that screening and treatment programs would be cost-effective but would require national health programs with adequate resources in order to have a significant public health impact.[285] WHO recognizes the importance of hepatocellular carcinoma and other HBV-related diseases as global public health problems and reiterates its recommendation that hepatitis B vaccines should be included in national immunization programs. WHO has defined several objectives to eliminate viral hepatitis as a public health issue by 2030 (https://www.who.int/hepatitis/strategy2016-2021/ghss-hep/en/).

Main Routes of Transmission

The main routes of HBV infection involve exposure to blood or blood-derived products, such as during childbirth from an HBV-positive mother, blood transfusion, or other potential sources of percutaneous exposure, including sexual intercourse.[282] The greatest sources of infection worldwide are from infected mothers to newborns or to or among very young children. The risk of vertical transmission from mothers varies depending on geographical regions. In Asia, the rate of perinatal transmission is as high as 90%, because many of the pregnant women who are chronically infected have high titers reaching up to 10^{10} Dane particles per mL blood.[474] In North America, Western Europe and Africa, the risk of vertical transmission from chronically infected mothers is only about 10%, which correlates with reports that infected mothers in these regions usually have a low viral load. These differences in viral loads are likely a result of different natural histories of chronic infections in different parts of the world, with neonatal infections that become chronic leading to a more persistent high-level viremia than infections later in life. That is, women infected at birth would have a higher viremia as they age and would be more likely to pass the infections to the neonate than women infected later during the first few years of life. The observed high rate of chronicity in Africa appears mostly due to horizontal spread to young children from playmates and adults involved in their care, rather than directly from infected mothers during birth.[163]

The risk of HBV transmission by blood transfusion has decreased dramatically since the early 1970s because of the exclusion of paid donors and the introduction of serological screening of volunteer blood donors for serum HBsAg and anti-HBc immunoglobulins. In the United States, the risk of HBV transmission via blood products is now one out of 63,000 transfusions, down from 15% in the 1960s.[8,162] Issues remain with the failure to identify infected blood donors because of the serological window during the incubation period following infection, the presence of some rare HBsAg variants that are not detected by the serologic assay for HBsAg, particularly when concurrent testing for anti-HBc is not performed, and the problem of so-called occult HBV infections, in which neither HBsAg nor anti-HBc is detected by serologic testing. Thus, the feasibility of nucleic acid testing (NAT) of blood donations in pools of up to 96 samples for HCV, HBV, and HIV-1 has been explored. Currently, the diagnostics industry provides commercial HCV, HIV-1, and HBV NAT tests on automated platforms. These have further decreased the risk of transmission of these viruses via blood transfusion, at least in countries where these platforms are available. However, in many endemic countries, serological assays are the only assays that are affordable for screening of blood donations.[139]

In contrast to blood transfusion, percutaneous infection of young people and adults via intravenous drug use, tattoos, acupuncture, ear piercing, razor sharing, etc., remain major modes of HBV transmission. Sexual transmission still represents 40% of the new cases of acute hepatitis B in many developed countries, while the role of intravenous drug use seems to be decreasing with time, currently representing 6% to 10% of new cases. HBV can also be transmitted by accidental needle stick in the health care setting.[8,162] Nosocomial transmission represents approximately 10% of the new cases of HBV infection, usually as the consequence of invasive treatment or diagnostic procedures. The risk of accidental transmission by the percutaneous route is estimated to be 30% from highly viremic patients. Transmission from health care worker to patients may also occur.[185] Other cases of nosocomial transmission have been reported in hemodialysis centers, and in the setting of organ transplantation, even from donors who only have anti-HBc antibodies. When found alone, anti-HBc antibodies are usually a marker of a past infection from which an individual has recovered. However, HBV infection following a liver graft, presumably by reactivation of residual virus present in the donor liver, is observed in more than 50% of cases when the donor has antibodies to HBcAg but no other serological markers of HBV infection.[113] As discussed later, this is consistent with other studies indicating that residual amounts of HBV remain for years or decades after clearance of transient infections. Finally, horizontal transmission can be observed among institutionalized persons via close bodily contact, leading to HBV infection through skin breaks and mucous membranes.[522]

HBV Genotypes

At least 10 HBV genotypes have been recognized, named A to J, along with nearly 40 subgenotypes, named with the genotype letter followed by a digit (e.g., A1, C2).[306,414] The genomes of genotypes I and J are likely genotype C recombinants. Genotype A is found in North America, Europe, South-East Africa, and India; genotypes B and C in Asia and Oceania; genotype D, the most widespread, in North America, North Africa, Europe, the Middle-East, and Oceania; genotype E in West Africa; genotype F in South America and Polynesia; genotypes G and H in Central and South America; genotype I in Vietnam and Laos; and genotype J in Japan. Genotype G is often found as a coinfection with genotype A.[477] There is evidence that HBV genome variability and genotypes can influence clinical and virological parameters, for example, viral load, course of disease, and prognosis of treatment.

Despite being close at the genome level, HBV subgenotypes have very distinct geographical distributions, as noted above, and geographical locations appear to correlate with routes of transmission and virological features. A striking example of such differences is shown by subgenotypes A1 and A2. Subgenotype A1 is found in Africa and Southern Asia, while A2 is found in Europe and North America. A1 transmission is perinatal or in early life, while A2 is mainly acquired by adults parenterally or sexually. A1 is linked to rapid progression to chronic liver disease and HCC. Thus, the differentiation between subgenotype A1 and A2 appears to be correlated with the epidemiology and outcomes of infections.

Certain mutations associated with viral genotypes may also influence disease outcomes, development of HCC, and treatment outcomes. For instance, genotype D is observed mainly in the Mediterranean basin and is associated with a higher prevalence of pre-C mutants in chronically infected individuals (i.e., HBeAg negative patients) as well as a lower response rate to IFN therapy compared to genotype A[55,164]; other clinical studies have suggested an association of genotype C with a more severe chronic liver disease and a poorer response rate to IFN therapy.[234,569] In a landmark Risk Evaluation of Viral Load Elevation and Associated Liver Disease/Cancer-HBV (REVEAL-HBV) study from Taiwan[559] performed in a large community cohort, male gender, high serum alanine aminotransferase (ALT), older age, positive HBeAg, higher HBV-DNA levels, and precore mutation were independently associated with a higher risk of HCC. In addition, genotype C was associated with an increased risk of HCC compared to genotype B, with an adjusted hazard ratio of 2.35 (95% CI = 1.68 to 3.30, $p < 0.001$).

In brief, these results and analysis of the literature show that the risk of HCC development is multifactorial and that many epidemiological, geographical, host and virological aspects may be intrinsically linked to viral genotypes and clinical outcomes.[414] Using predictive factors of HCC such as genotype C, nomograms and scoring systems have been developed to assess HCC risk in patients (i.e., Ref.[549]). However, validation of scoring systems for different parts of the world based on different cohorts of patients with different HBV (sub)genotypes, ethnicity, etc. remains an important goal.[414]

CLINICAL FEATURES

Clinical Manifestations

The natural history of chronic hepatitis B (CHB), particularly after infection of neonates or young children, can be schematically divided into five phases, which are not necessarily sequential (Fig. 18.17).[127] (a) The HBeAg-positive chronic infection phase, characterized by HBeAg positivity and high titers of serum HBV DNA, often up to 10^{9-10} IU/mL, normal levels of aminotransferases, and mild or no liver necroinflammation. During this phase, the rate of spontaneous HBeAg loss is very low. This first phase is more frequent and more prolonged in subjects infected neonatally or in the first years of life. Because of high levels of viremia, these patients are highly contagious. This phase was previously designated immune tolerant, but this designation has been revoked for many reasons including the realization that low levels of immune-mediated liver damage may be occurring. (b) HBeAg-positive chronic hepatitis, characterized by HBeAg positivity, often lower titers of serum HBV DNA (but >2,000 IU/mL), increased or fluctuating levels of aminotransferases, moderate or severe liver necroinflammation, and more rapid progression of fibrosis compared to the chronic infection phase. In this phase, the rate of spontaneous HBeAg loss is enhanced but may still occur at a late stage when fibrosis has already developed. This phase may begin after many years of the chronic infection phase. (c) HBeAg-negative chronic infection may follow seroconversion from HBeAg to

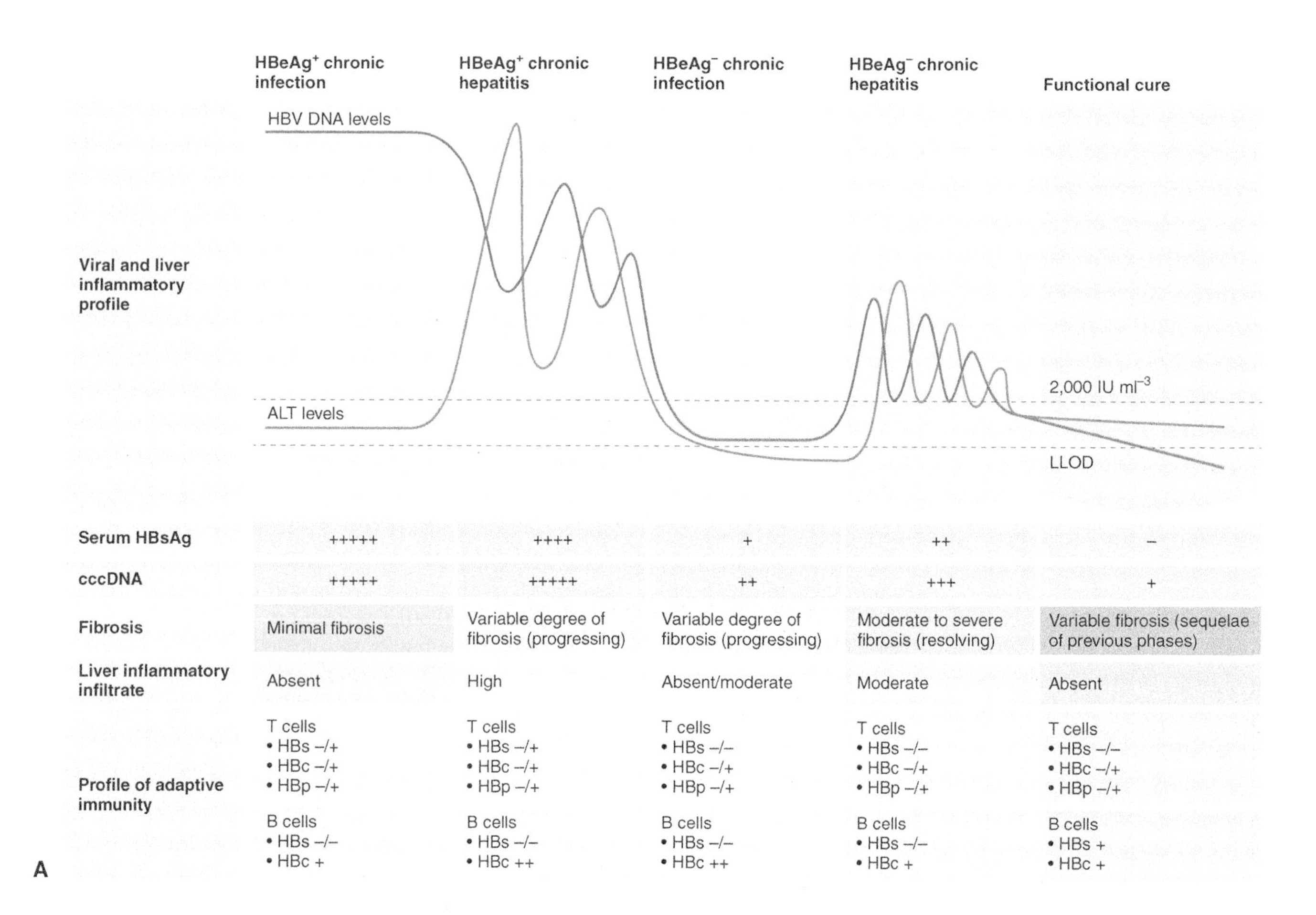

	HBeAg-positive Chronic infection	HBeAg-positive Chronic hepatitis	HBeAg-negative Chronic infection	HBeAg-negative Chronic hepatitis
HBsAg	High	High/intermediate	Low	Intermediate
HBeAg	Positive	Positive	Negative	Negative
HBV DNA	>10E7 IU/mL	10E4-10E7 IU/mL	<2,000 IU/mL°°	>2,000 IU/mL
ALT	Normal	Elevated	Normal	Elevated*
Liver disease	None/minimal	Moderate/severe	None	Moderate/severe
Old terminology	Immune tolerant	Immune reactive HBeAg positive	Inactive carrier	HBeAg negative Chronic hepatitis

*Persistently or intermittently

B °°HBV-DNA levels can be between 2,000 and 20,00 IU/mL in some patients without signs of chronic hepatitis

FIGURE 18.17 Natural history of hepatitis. A: Following acute infection, approximately 95% of adults and 5% to 10% of newborns recover, while the remainder evolve toward chronic viral infection (see ref. 136). **B.** Depending on the vigor of the immune response, chronic infection can follow several phases including the HBeAg-positive chronic infection, HBeAg-positive chronic hepatitis, HBeAg-negative chronic infection, and HBeAg-negative chronic hepatitis phases (see ref. 127). These phases may not be stable over time, and patients often evolve from one phase to the other. The major risk of chronic hepatitis is the evolution toward cirrhosis and hepatocellular carcinoma (Fig. **18.16**).

anti-HBe antibody. It is characterized by very low or undetectable serum HBV DNA (virus) levels (<2,000 IU/mL) and normal aminotransferases, but still detectable levels of serum HBsAg. As a result of immunological control of the infection, this state confers a more favorable long-term outcome with a lower risk of cirrhosis or HCC. This phase was formerly called the "inactive carrier" stage. HBsAg loss and seroconversion to anti-HBs antibody may occur spontaneously, usually after several years with persistently undetectable HBV DNA. (d) HBeAg-negative chronic hepatitis may also follow seroconversion from HBeAg to anti-HBe antibody during phase 2. It is characterized by a pattern of fluctuating levels of HBV DNA and aminotransferases and active hepatitis. It is important but sometimes difficult to distinguish true inactive HBV carriers from patients with active HBeAg-negative chronic hepatitis who, at the time of examination, are in a phase of short-term remission. (e) The HBsAg-negative phase. Low-level HBV replication may persist with detectable HBV DNA in the liver. It usually follows the HBe seroconversion phase. Generally, anti-HBc antibodies with or without anti-HBs are detectable. HBsAg loss, especially if it occurs before the age of 50, is associated with improvement of the long-term outcome with reduced risk of cirrhosis, hepatic decompensation, and HCC. This scenario is almost identical with the clearance of transient infections, since anti-HBs antibodies will help prevent virus rebound. As with clearance of transient infections, HBV DNA may still be detected in serum, though generally at very low titers (<10 IU/mL) and in the liver by the presence of low levels of cccDNA.[341,540] Also, as with transient infections, such infections may reactivate with immunosuppression. Moreover, these patients remain at elevated risk of developing HCC,[413] likely because extensive preneoplastic changes are already prevalent at the time of HBsAg loss.

Variants and HBeAg-Negative Chronic Hepatitis B

Since HBV is under selective pressure from the immune system, HBV variants typically emerge over the course of a chronic infection.[172] These variants are assumed to facilitate immune evasion and have been detected throughout the viral genome. Because both B- and T-cell epitopes may be mutated, it is unclear if emergence of these variants occurs through virus spread or selective survival of hepatocytes infected by the mutants, or both. This issue is complicated by the fact that virus-free hepatocytes emerge even when there is abundant virus in the blood stream (such cells might still have integrated HBV DNA). In the setting of the natural history of the disease, the most studied of these mutants are those that no longer express HBeAg. These variants harbor mutations in the precore region and/or in the basal core promoter (Fig. 18.8). When these mutants become predominant, infections are characterized by the presence of HBsAg and undetectable HBeAg and may be associated either with chronic infection or, with chronic hepatitis[37,179] (Fig. 18.15D). Again, like HBeAg-positive hepatitis, HBeAg-negative chronic hepatitis B is associated with a high risk of liver fibrosis, cirrhosis, and HCC.[37,164,179]

Because of RNA folding constraints placed on the epsilon region of pgRNA (Fig. 18.12), pre-C stop codon mutations that abolish preC protein synthesis and hence, HBeAg production, would also inhibit virus replication in some HBV genotypes. This restricts their occurrence to HBV genotypes in which the mutations do not negatively impact epsilon folding and, therefore, virus replication, or by the requirement of compensatory mutations. In practice, these pre-C mutations are mainly observed in patients chronically infected with HBV genotype D.[294] Patients infected with other HBV genotypes may also present with HBeAg-negative chronic hepatitis B, in these cases mainly caused by mutations in the preC/C promoter.[378] Mutations in the preC/C promoter are not HBV genotype restricted.[164,307,387]

HBeAg Seroconversion

Seroconversion to anti-HBe antibody generally occurs during resolution of acute self-limited infections.[20,355,512] Moreover, as noted above, loss of HBeAg often occurs during the course of chronic infections, sometimes but not always with the concurrent appearance of anti-HBe antibodies. Loss of HBeAg from serum, even in the absence of anti-HBe antibodies, usually reflects a decline in the amount of virus in the liver. Thus, the loss of serum HBeAg in chronically infected individuals, either with or without the concomitant appearance of anti-HBeAg, may signal a major drop in virus titers and a reduction in disease activity as patients enter a remission phase. However, in other patients, it may be associated with an ongoing disease activity because it simply reflects immune selection for virus that has lost the capacity to produce HBeAg, or suppression of virus replication by antiviral cytokines. In either case, HBeAg seroconversion is an indication that virus production has either ceased or significantly declined.

Occult HBV Infections

Occult HBV infection (OBI) is defined as the presence of replication competent HBV DNA (i.e., HBV cccDNA) in the liver and/or HBV DNA in blood of persons testing negative for hepatitis B surface antigen (HBsAg) by currently available assays. Based on the HBV-specific antibody profiles, OBI may be categorized as: (a) Seropositive-OBI—anti-HBc and/or anti-HBs positive; (b) Seronegative-OBI—anti-HBc and anti-HBs negative.[413] Among individuals with OBI, prevalence of detectable HBV DNA in serum/plasma varies depending on the population studied, the sensitivity of the assay used, and whether blood samples at one or more time-points are tested. Many studies have found that HBV DNA is only intermittently detected, and with low concentration, usually less than 1000 virions/mL.[62,467]

In persons with seropositive-OBI, HBsAg may have become negative either following the resolution of acute hepatitis B, or after decades of HBsAg-positive chronic HBV infection with or without disease. It is unknown whether patients with chronic HBV infection/disease, who become HBsAg negative following Antiviral Therapy are immunologically comparable to patients who spontaneously clear HBsAg. Persons with seronegative-OBI, estimated to comprise between 1% and 20% of all OBI patients,[57,510] might have either progressively lost hepatitis B antibodies or have been hepatitis B antibody negative since the beginning of the infection. The latter condition has been described in the woodchuck model of occult WHV infection.[343]

A subset of individuals considered OBI are actually infected with HBV S variants carrying mutations in the S gene ("S-escape" mutations), resulting in the production of modified HBsAg that is not recognized by some commercially available HBsAg assays. Circulating HBV DNA levels in these patients may be comparable to those detected in HBsAg-positive individuals. Additional HBV variants with mutations in the S-gene promoter and splice variants have also been reported to affect HBsAg production/secretion and to be responsible for some cases of OBI.[131] There are still many unresolved issues regarding (a) the development of more sensitive, standardized, and validated assays for the detection of HBV DNA in blood and in liver and more sensitive assays for HBsAg to diagnose OBI, (b) the clinical and public health implications for the risk of transmission, liver disease progression, and development of HCC, (c) the recommendations for preventing HBV reactivation in persons with OBI.[413]

DIAGNOSIS

Differential

Diagnosis of Acute Hepatitis B

Acute hepatitis, which may occur during resolution of a transient infection, or during a hepatic flare in chronic infection, is diagnosed in patients with jaundice or fatigue and high ALT levels. Evidence of HBV involvement is obtained by the detection of HBsAg and anti-HBc IgM. Coinfection with HDV should be also checked since acute coinfection may lead to a more severe course of acute hepatitis. However, other infectious agents need to be considered as causes of a *de novo* flare of liver disease activity, including HCV, HAV, and hepatitis E virus (HEV), and rare cases of acute viral hepatitis caused by herpes simplex virus, cytomegalovirus, or parvovirus infections. These other agents are also potential causes of a hepatic flare in HBV carriers experiencing an unexpected exacerbation of liver disease. If all factors suggest involvement of HBV alone, transient infection is indicated by disappearance of HBsAg in the weeks immediately following the flare of acute liver disease, followed by resolution of the infection (Fig. 18.15A). In contrast, a "spontaneous" acute flare of disease activity during a chronic HBV infection can be preceded by months of high titer viremia but little or no overt liver disease. These flares are typically due to changing HBV/immune system interactions, not to superinfections.

Diagnosis of Chronic Hepatitis B

Chronic HBV infections are usually asymptomatic for most of their course. The diagnosis of chronic hepatitis B is usually made by the detection of serum HBsAg for greater than 6 months and possibly by elevation in ALT levels (Fig. 18.15B-D).[126,312] Nausea, loss of appetite, and jaundice may occur during acute hepatic flares in chronic hepatitis B. However, a hepatic flare may be completely asymptomatic and diagnosed only by a close monitoring of HBV DNA and ALT levels in the serum. HBcAg is highly immunogenic and the appearance in the circulation of anti-HBc IgM is usually the first immunological sign of a transient HBV infection. Typical serological profiles of HBV infections are shown in Figures 18.15 and 18.17.

Laboratory

Assays

The most rigorous way of determining the presence of circulating HBV is to assay for viral DNA. The lower threshold for risk of active hepatitis and liver damage is considered to be around 10^4 viral genome equivalent per mL of serum, equivalent to approximately 2,000 IU/mL.[58,92,126,308] Figure 18.17 shows the evolution of viral load during the natural history of infection and underlines the necessity of highly sensitive and quantitative assays to monitor viral load in the different phases of the disease. In patients who have lost HBsAg from serum and may have an occult infection, virus titers are usually very low and therefore can escape detection even by PCR-based assays.[413]

The development of quantitative assays for HBsAg detection revealed that chronically infected patients as well as those at the peak of a transient infection can have HBsAg titers of greater than 10^{12} particles per mL, or greater than 500 μg of protein per mL.[370,586] Clinical assays can detect as little as 0.2 ng (or 0.05 IU/mL) of HBsAg per mL of serum, providing a highly sensitive assay for HBV infection. HBsAg levels in serum were found to correlate with HBV DNA levels during transient infections, but this correlation breaks down during the course of a chronic infection.[219,364] This may be due in part to expression of HBsAg from integrated HBV DNA, especially in patients with longer duration of infection in the HBeAg-negative phase (Fig. 18.15D). In fact, RNAseq analysis of liver tissue from HBV-infected chimpanzee showed that in contrast to HBeAg-positive animals, in HBeAg-negative chimpanzees, most viral transcripts were truncated at their 3′ end because of HBV DNA integration. This suggests that in the HBeAg-negative chronic infection phase, HBsAg is mainly expressed from integrated DNA, rather than from cccDNA.[550]

A number of secondary assays for HBV infection are available. IgG reactive to HBcAg is a marker of past or ongoing infection and is therefore found in both resolved infections and in chronically infected individuals. Anti-HBc IgM is typically found during transient infections and may be detected, at low levels, during acute exacerbation of chronic infections[178,394,586] (see Fig. 18.15). HBeAg is found in the blood of transiently infected individuals as well as in chronically infected individuals with high virus titers (that is, HBeAg-positive chronic infection and HBeAg-positive chronic hepatitis phases.[127]

Finally, sensitive real-time PCR assays for quantification of viral DNA in serum are available with a cut off as low as approximately 30 to 50 viral genome copies per mL, or approximately 10 IU/mL.[86,502] The combination of serological markers including quantification of HBsAg and HBV DNA in serum has improved the diagnosis of inactive carriers, which usually have a low viral load (HBsAg < 1,000 IU/mL and HBV DNA < 2,000 IU/mL).[46] In patients who have lost HBsAg in serum after resolution of a transient infection or during the course of chronic HBV infection (i.e., who are HBsAg (−) and anti-HBc Ab (+), either with or without anti-HBs Ab), detection of serum HBV DNA by sensitive PCR assays may reflect the persistence of infected hepatocytes after the clinical resolution of the disease[413] (Fig. 18.17).

As noted above, significant amounts of HBsAg may be produced from both integrated HBV DNA and cccDNA during chronic infection. Thus, HBsAg measurements do not provide a useful measure of the amount of transcriptionally active cccDNA in the liver.[550] In particular, assays are required to predict functional cure characterized by the loss of HBsAg and/or cccDNA and/or transcriptional inactivation of cccDNA (Fig. 18.15E).[77,499] This has prompted the development of new assays and biomarkers to better quantify transcriptionally active cccDNA and/or the number of infected hepatocytes harboring transcriptionally active cccDNA. To date, the most advanced biomarkers are hepatitis B virus core-related antigen (HBcrAg) and viral RNAs circulating in the blood stream.

HBcrAg

HBcrAg is a composite biomarker that comprises HBcAg, HBeAg, and a 22 kDa truncated core-related protein (p22cr). p22cr is an aberrantly processed PreCore protein containing the entire PreC region including the intact signal peptide but lacking the C-terminal arginine-rich domain described earlier in this chapter (Fig. 18.6).[244] The three proteins share a common sequence of 149 amino acids forming a linear epitope that can be recognized by a monoclonal antibody after denaturation. A pretreatment is required to release all core-related antigens from immune complexes or enveloped particles because the assay can detect all capsid-containing particles (HBcAg), either virions or free capsids, p22cr-related particles and secreted HBeAg. Unlike HBsAg, HBcrAg quantification should not be influenced by translation from integrated viral sequences, which generally lack the upstream core promoter, and hence could be a more accurate surrogate marker to quantify transcriptional cccDNA. In some patients, a correlation could be established between HBcrAg levels and intrahepatic amount of cccDNA, cccDNA transcriptional activity, fibrosis, and necroinflammatory activity scores.[500] However, improvement of the sensitivity of this test will be required prior to its use in evaluating novel antiviral compounds under clinical development.[500] For this and other reasons, the HBcrAg assay is not yet approved by the FDA and has not received CE-certification, although it has been available as a fully automated quantitative assay in Japan since 2014 and as a research tool on other parts of the world.

Serum Viral RNA

HBV RNAs can be detected in the serum of patients at levels ranging between 0.1% to 1% of HBV DNA levels in the absence of antiviral treatment.[56,521,531] Circulating HBV RNA was initially observed in a form of HBV DNA-RNA hybrid molecules.[345] Circulating polyadenylated HBV RNAs in sera of HBV-infected patients could be detected with rapid amplification of complementary DNA (cDNA)-ends (RACE).[250] The current (unproven) view is that serum viral RNAs mainly circulate as viral particles containing pgRNAs, and thus, they may represent a biomarker of the pool of transcriptionally active cccDNA.[77] Assays to quantify pgRNA in serum are being developed by diagnostics companies.

PREVENTION AND CONTROL

Treatment

General Considerations

Historically, clinical guidelines recommend against antiviral treatment during the HBeAg-positive chronic infection phase because patients have only minimal liver disease (inflammation and/or fibrosis) detectable by histologic examination of liver biopsies.[126,312] Also, the results of therapeutic trials with IFN-α, or with early nucleos(t)ide analogue (NUC) inhibitors of the viral DNA polymerase, showed that patients with high HBV DNA load and normal ALT levels have almost no chance of HBe seroconversion or sustained virologic response as a result of treatment[126,312]; that is, the infection rebounds when treatment is withdrawn. Whether inapparent liver injury that occurs in the HBeAg-positive chronic infection phase contributes to disease progression and, in particular HCC is not known.[241,338] Thus, new clinical guidelines have expanded treatment indications in these patients to those who have a clinically detectable higher risk of disease progression, that is, family history of HCC or cirrhosis, or if they have extrahepatic manifestations.[127,498] It is expected that treatment guidelines will continue to evolve as more data become available about HBeAg-positive chronic infection, and new antiviral drugs with better efficacy are evaluated in clinical studies.

So far, Antiviral Therapy is recommended primarily for patients with active liver disease who have a significant risk of liver disease progression in the short term, and not for patients that do not have elevated ALTs and/or histologic evidence of inflammatory liver disease.[126,312] These included (a) patients with ALTs above the upper limit of normal, virus titers greater than 2,000 IU/mL and moderate necroinflammation and fibrosis, (b) patients with virus titers greater than 20,000 IU/mL and ALTs greater than two times the upper limit for normal, irrespective of histologic assessment, and (c) patients with cirrhosis (but with NUCs, not interferon, which may cause liver failure in patients with diminished liver reserve due to the cirrhosis). Newer guidelines also include considering treatment for all patients older than 30.[127] To a certain extent, the earlier decision not to treat asymptomatic patients was due the fact that antiviral resistance developed rapidly to NUCs such as lamivudine, which has not been a major problem with the newer NUCs such as entecavir and tenofovir (Fig. 18.11). For this reason, entecavir and tenofovir are now the only NUCs that are recommended as a first-line therapy. In patients with previous exposure to lamivudine, tenofovir is recommended while entecavir is not because of cross-resistance between lamivudine and entecavir. Entecavir at higher dosage could be used in case of previous lamivudine failure but is not the preferred option in that situation.

Irrespective of the possible benefits of starting Antiviral Therapy earlier, there are major reasons for not delaying therapy once active liver disease is diagnosed: if HBV replication and elevation of ALT levels are ongoing, there is a proven risk of progression to cirrhosis and hepatocellular carcinoma (Fig. 18.16).[300,419,558,571] Antiviral Therapy, particularly with NUCs, decrease viral load, normalize ALT levels, induce a remission of the disease,[589] and reduce the progression of cirrhosis and HCC.[78,212,300] A possible reason for starting antiviral treatment earlier is that treatment according to current guidelines reduces but does not eliminate the HCC risk; whether or not earlier treatment would reduce the HCC risk further is not yet known.

With the use of the current generation of antiviral drugs within the treatment guidelines, Antiviral Therapy may lead to HBeAg-seroconversion, long-term viral suppression/control, and off-treatment control by the immune system, especially in patients in the HBeAg-positive chronic hepatitis phase (e.g., ~20% to 30% vs. a spontaneous rate of ~5%[92,566]). A decrease in virus load is usually associated with the appearance of anti-HBe antibodies. HBsAg usually remains at high levels in the serum. Liver histology usually reveals remission of liver disease activity, and arrest or reversal of fibrosis/cirrhosis progression as long as viral load remains low and ALT levels remain normal[76,120] (Fig. 18.15E).

IFN-α or NUC therapy-induced HBV DNA reduction below 2,000 IU/mL is associated with disease remission. Sustained virus suppression increases the chance of HBe seroconversion in HBeAg-positive patients and the additional possibility of HBsAg loss in both HBeAg-positive and HBeAg-negative patients.[127] The most reliable indication that therapy can be terminated is a confirmed loss of HBsAg,[98] while the development of anti-HBsAb does not seem to be required to achieve a sustained HBsAg loss, also called "functional cure" (Fig. 18.15E).

Interferon (IFN) Therapy

The principle immunological treatment for hepatitis B is IFN-α, which has been used since the 1980s. Although IFN-α has a direct antiviral effect, suppressing HBV replication, its major effect is considered immunologic, inducing, and/or abetting a hepatic flare that resolves the infection and establishes immunologic control that prevents virus rebound. This treatment only has lasting effects in patients with immunologically active liver disease, augmenting an already active host response against the virus.

In HBeAg-positive chronic hepatitis B, treatment with standard IFN-α or its pegylated form can lead to HBeAg seroconversion, loss of viral DNA, and clinical remission in approximately 20% to 30% of patients.[217,273,369,548] Clinical benefit appears to be long term in these responding patients, including a decreased risk of progression to cirrhosis and hepatocellular carcinoma. HBsAg loss may occur several years after treatment cessation. However, IFN-α treatment is not particularly well tolerated, provoking a "flu-like" syndrome in many individuals. In addition, IFN-α needs to be injected subcutaneously every week for the pegylated form for 12 months and thus causes additional discomfort to the patient. It is however the only medication which can be administered with a finite duration. Attempts to combine IFN-α and NUCs with different schedules of administration (combination, sequential administration) did not show any significant clinical advantage compared to monotherapies in most clinical trials. Such combinations are thus not recommended by current practice guidelines.[3,127,498]

In patients with end-stage cirrhosis and little liver reserve, IFN-α treatment is not recommended because it increases the risk of liver failure due to immune killing of the remaining functional hepatocytes and because of the increased risk of bacterial infections. In contrast, NUC therapy can benefit these patients, with control of viral replication, accompanied by significant improved liver functions.[301,302]

One group reported a direct effect of high doses of IFN-α or activation of the lymphotoxin β receptor, with a super-agonistic antibody, in reducing the stability of cccDNA in HepaRG cells and primary human hepatocyte cultures by a mechanism involving APOBEC3A and 3B-mediated cytidine deamination.[315,553] However, other laboratories could not validate the original observation (i.e., Refs.[356,513]). In contrast, identification of G to A transitions in viral DNA isolated from sera of chronically infected HBV patients provided strong evidence for deamination of cytosine residues in particular in the region of the genome that is single stranded, consistent with the known substrate preference of APOBEC enzymes.[489] However, the frequency of hypermutated genomes is generally low and most likely insignificant for HBV persistence in infected patients.[24] The highest frequencies have been reported from patients with advanced cirrhosis in the presence of high cytokine levels.[524] IFN-a was also shown to modify cccDNA-associated chromatin and to induce repressive epigenetic marks leading to decreased transcriptional activity both in cultured hepatocytes and liver humanized mouse models.[25]

Nucleoside Analogue (NUC) Therapy

To date, FDA-approved NUCs belong to one of three structural groups: L-nucleosides (lamivudine and telbivudine), alkyl phosphonates (adefovir dipivoxil and tenofovir disoproxil fumarate, and the prodrugs of tenofovir, tenofovir alafenamide), and D-cyclopentanes (entecavir).[3,127,498] NUC therapy represents the primary choice for treatment of chronic HBV. The effect of treatment with inhibitors of viral DNA synthesis is to stop viral DNA replication within hepatocytes and prevent release of infectious particles into the bloodstream. The half-life of circulating virus particles is relatively short, around 24 hours, and the decline in virus titers predictable.[375] The half-life of DNA replication intermediates has not been studied in great detail but is probably a few days. However, the rate of loss of cccDNA that maintains the hepatocyte infections is much slower, with a half-life in the liver of a few days to several months according to the strength of the host immune response. Therefore, NUC therapies necessitate long-term treatment.[375,514,540] cccDNA loss is believed to reflect, primarily, the death of infected hepatocytes rather than intracellular instability, at least in the context of chronic infections.[584] Hence, NUCs that inhibit HBV DNA synthesis inhibit the replacement of cccDNA as some infected hepatocytes die and others proliferate to maintain liver cell number.[584] A key question is if cccDNA survives when hepatocytes divide, or if it is lost at mitosis. This question remains unresolved, with evidence for[584] and against[6] survival *in vivo*. One possible explanation of the claim of survival during NUC therapy, as yet unresolved, is that cccDNA is lost at mitosis but is replaced by cytoplasmic DNA replication intermediates that are produced at low levels during NUC therapy, particularly during S-phase.[418] Results of mathematical modeling based on cccDNA monitoring of NUC suppressed patients suggest that new rounds of infection may occur during NUC therapy despite clinically efficient viral suppression.[39]

In liver transplant recipients with HBV recurrence in the liver graft, IFN-a is contra-indicated because of the risk of inducing liver graft rejection. Both tenofovir and entecavir have shown a clinical benefit that seems to be superior to that obtained with earlier NUCs.[93,393,439] The prevention of HBV recurrence after transplantation relies nowadays on pretransplantation Antiviral Therapy with NUCs to decrease viral load, and post-transplant hepatitis B immune globulin (HBIG) and NUC administration to prevent HBV recurrence. With such prophylactic protocols, the risk of HBV recurrence defined by HBsAg positivity after transplantation has decreased from 20% to 30% to below 5%.

The optimal NUCs are tenofovir and entecavir, to which resistance rarely if ever develops in treatment naive patients[75,464] (that is, patients that have not developed resistance to early NUCs, which can increase the risk of developing resistance to subsequent NUC therapies). Treatment with these drugs with a high barrier of resistance in patients over 30, as with early NUCs, prevents or reduces significantly the development of fibrosis and cirrhosis but does not eliminate the risk of HCC. Because of the limited systematic studies in patients less than 30, it is unclear if additional benefits would accrue if treatment was started much earlier, particularly in patients still in the HBeAg-positive chronic infection phase.[241] Overall, the rate of HBsAg loss that would allow treatment cessation is very low, that is, approximately 10% of patients in selected cohorts.[98]

Drugs in Clinical Development

With a better knowledge of the viral life cycle and the improvement of experimental study models, it has been possible to characterize viral and immune targets to develop new drugs with the aim of achieving higher rates of functional cure with finite duration treatments. A number of drugs are being evaluated in preclinical models or early phases of clinical development (Phase 1b and Phase 2 clinical trials). The main targets and drug classes are posted on https://www.hepb.org/treatment-and-management/drug-watch/.

Direct-acting antivirals include viral entry inhibitors, strategies targeting cccDNA (by either elimination or transcriptional silencing), agents targeting viral RNAs (siRNAs, antisense oligonucleotides, and locked nucleic acids), core allosteric modulators (CAM), and inhibitors of HBsAg release, namely nucleic acid polymers. Immune-based strategies under evaluation include (a) boosters of innate immunity: TLR-7, TLR-8, and RIG-I agonists, (b) check-point inhibitors: PD1 and PDL1 blockers, and (c) specific immune stimulation by therapeutic vaccines. All these strategies are being evaluated in combination with NUCs in Phase 1b and Phase 2a studies.

Currently, it is believed that a combination of strategies blocking viral replication in addition to decreasing HBsAg expression will be needed for efficient therapeutic vaccination. It is not yet known what will be the position of innate immunity boosters and checkpoint inhibitors in these strategies. Several trials are evaluating triple combinations of NUCs with capsid inhibitors and TLR7 agonists, or NUCs with capsid inhibitors and siRNA.

With respect to chronic HBV/HDV infections for which only peg-IFN is recommended by international societies, several drugs are in clinical evaluation and entering phase 3 clinical trials: (a) myrcludex-B, an entry inhibitor, that works on both HBV and HDV; it showed significant drop in serum HDV RNA and ALT improvement either in monotherapy or in combination with peg-IFN, the latter showing faster and deeper declines in HDV titers; (b) lonafarnib, a prenylation inhibitor preventing the assembly and release of HDV, which is being developed in combination with peg-IFN, with the need for ritonavir to boost its metabolism and decrease side effects; and (c) nucleic acid polymers to inhibit HBsAg release, also in combination with peg-IFN.

Vaccines

Based on the difficulties in treating chronic HBV infection, including high cost, the emergence of drug-resistant mutants, and the risk of development of HCC, the efficacy of vaccine prevention is a strong incentive for mass vaccination programs worldwide.[339] At the end of 2018, hepatitis B vaccine for infants had been introduced nationwide in 189 countries. Global coverage with 3 doses of hepatitis B vaccine is estimated at 84% and is as high as 90% in the Western Pacific. In addition, 109 countries introduced one dose of hepatitis B vaccine to newborns within the first 24 hours of life, and the global coverage is 42% (http://www.who.int/mediacentre/factsheets/fs378/en/). This will contribute to a reduction in HBV incidence but more effective neonatal vaccination will be required for HBV elimination. The UN 2030 Agenda for Sustainable Development includes "combat hepatitis" within one of its goals. In May 2016, the Global Health Sector Strategy on Viral Hepatitis set targets for 2020 and 2030: to reduce new cases of chronic HBV infection by 30% by 2020, which is equivalent to HBsAg prevalence of 1% among children aged 5 years, and to achieve 0.1% prevalence of HBV infection in children aged 5 years by 2030 (https://www.who.int/immunization/sage/Guidelines_development_recommendations.pdf?ua=1).

Similar goals have been formulated by the WHO (https://www.who.int/hepatitis/topics/hepatitis-b/en/).

Vaccines containing S alone have been produced historically by processing of HBsAg purified from plasma of HBV carriers. It is now produced from the yeast *Saccharomyces cerevisiae* expressing S from recombinant DNA. The vaccine contains the immunodominant "a" determinant of HBsAg in S. New formulations of vaccines are now available in hexavalent form to protect from multiple pathogens. A recent variant of the HBV vaccine includes a Toll-like receptor 9 agonist.[440] Vaccines are administered in the deltoid muscle and are highly immunogenic, inducing a protective anti-HBs antibody titer (>10 IU/mL) in more than 95% of children or young adults usually with a three-dose schedule.[8,275,523] About 5% of those vaccinated fail to respond with development of antibodies to the vaccine. Several factors seem responsible, including genetically determined nonresponsiveness, age over 40 years, high body mass index, and immunosuppression.[8,275,523] In immune suppressed patients, a schedule with 4 administrations is recommended (Day 0, months 1 and 2, and booster at month 12). Vaccination is associated with rare side effects, most commonly pain or soreness at the injection site. Neurological disorders such as multiple sclerosis, Guillain-Barré syndrome, and transverse myelitis have not been causally linked to the HBV vaccine.[12,96] A new recombinant hepatitis B vaccine with a CpG DNA adjuvant acting as a TLR9 agonist (Heplisav-B) has been recently approved by the FDA and EMA with a two-dose schedule increasing the rate of seroprotection.

Vaccine escape mutants have been reported in follow-up studies of individuals receiving HBsAg vaccines composed of the S protein. Vaccinated individuals typically mount a very strong antibody response to the immunodominant "a" determinant (Fig. 18.10) located in the exposed hydrophilic domain of S between amino acids 99 and 168.[129,397,475] The "a" determinant itself has been mapped from amino acids 124 to 147,[13,29,44,406,536] though some authors have extended the domain a few amino acids upstream and/or downstream. Two loops bounded by disulfide bridges are inferred by some authors to exist between cys124 and cys137, and cys139 and cys147, but other pairings have also been suggested.[83] The "a" determinant is highly conserved and is found in all genotypes of HBV.[374] Vaccine escape represents a distinct phenomenon, in which a vaccinated individual develops chronic HBV infection and is seropositive for HBsAg despite the presence of antibodies to the group-specific "a" determinant of HBsAg that were induced by the vaccine. This is possible because HBsAg present in the serum of these patients lacks the group-specific "a" determinant, generally as a result of missense mutations in the region of S that encodes amino acids 124 to 147 (Fig. 18.11).

Most studies of vaccine escape have involved at-risk children and infants who were either vaccinated or received vaccine plus HBIG, which is strongly reactive to the "a" determinant of HBsAg. For instance, in the 1980s, a follow-up study of childhood vaccination in Italy revealed vaccinees who became HBsAg positive despite the presence of a strong antibody response to HBsAg. The incidence was rare, involving about 2% of the children of HBsAg-positive mothers, or with HBsAg-positive family contacts.[65,573] More detailed analysis of virus from one patient revealed a point mutation encoding a gly145arg substitution at amino acid 145 of the S protein.[65] Analysis with monoclonal antibodies to the "a" determinant of wild-type HBV revealed a loss of binding to the mutant HBsAg.[65,537] Subsequent studies in other populations with high HBV endemicity confirmed the rare occurrence of vaccine escape mutants in children, including the glyc145arg substitution in "a," other substitutions or insertions in "a," and mutations within the external hydrophilic domain, but outside of "a".[66,143,199,208,238,280,377,379,380,555] Vaccine escape variants have also been detected in unvaccinated children and adults with circulating virus as well as anti-HBs,[199,555] possibly reflecting past or concurrent infection with wild-type and mutant virus. One concern was that these mutant viruses may become an increasing fraction of the pool of HBV carriers and an increasing risk for vaccinated individuals,[199] but recent studies and clinical field experience suggest that this scenario may not be correct.[200] However, a systematic molecular survey performed in China observed that newly selected mutations outside the major hydrophilic region but associated with changing antigenicity, such as lys21ser and lys98val, circulated among younger Chinese patients that had received neonatal HBV vaccination,[532] thus arguing for a continuous monitoring of HBV vaccine escape mutants in highly endemic areas where widescale vaccination is ongoing.

PERSPECTIVE

HBV biology is multifaceted and touches upon many areas in the basic and clinical sciences. Among them are liver biology, immunology, virology, and Antiviral Therapy. During the past three decades, we have witnessed major progress in all areas. Investigations on viral DNA replication have uncovered the mechanism for HBV persistence in the infected liver, which is based on continuous rounds of cccDNA amplification. Studies in animal models have provided insights into the course of natural infections and into the process of viral clearance. The revelations that clearance depends on a strong cytotoxic T-cell response that can eliminate infected hepatocyte and that hepatocytes may comprise a closed cell population may explain why current nucleoside-based antiviral therapies can attenuate, but not cure chronic HBV infections.

In spite of the great progress, many gaps in knowledge remain to be filled. The mechanisms for the disassembly of viral capsids, delivery of the genome into the cell nucleus, and formations of cccDNA need to be clarified in much greater detail. Although the role of X protein in maintaining transcriptionally active cccDNA is now known, we still do not know how or if X directly impacts other aspects of hepatocyte biology, including oncogenic transformation. Indeed the role of HBV in HCC emergence is still mostly a matter of speculation. While antiviral therapies can attenuate virus replication and disease progression, the development of a cure may require a much better understanding of the immune response against HBV and the ability to therapeutically augment that response to permanently suppress HBV replication. Moreover, the role of cytokines in the resolution of acute and progression of chronic infections needs to be better understood. These and other questions will have to be addressed to complete the picture of HBV biology that has come only partially into focus over the past forty years.

ACKNOWLEDGMENTS

We thank Jianming Hu for a critical reading of the manuscript.

REFERENCES

1. Abraham TM, Loeb DD. Base pairing between the 5′ half of epsilon and a cis-acting sequence, phi, makes a contribution to the synthesis of minus-strand DNA for human hepatitis B virus. *J Virol* 2006;80(9):4380–4387.
2. Addison WR, Walters KA, Wong WW, et al. Half-life of the duck hepatitis B virus covalently closed circular DNA pool in vivo following inhibition of viral replication. *J Virol* 2002;76(12):6356–6363.
3. Agarwal K, Brunetto M, Seto WK, et al. 96 weeks treatment of tenofovir alafenamide vs. tenofovir disoproxil fumarate for hepatitis B virus infection. *J Hepatol* 2018;68(4):672–681.
4. Aghazadeh M, Shi M, Barrs VR, et al. A novel hepadnavirus identified in an immunocompromised domestic cat in Australia. *Viruses* 2018;10(5):269.
5. Albin C, Robinson WS. Protein kinase activity in hepatitis B virus. *J Virol* 1980;34(1):297–302.
6. Allweiss L, Volz T, Giersch K, et al. Proliferation of primary human hepatocytes and prevention of hepatitis B virus reinfection efficiently deplete nuclear cccDNA in vivo. *Gut* 2018;67(3):542–552.
7. Alrefai WA, Gill RK. Bile acid transporters: structure, function, regulation and pathophysiological implications. *Pharm Res* 2007;24(10):1803–1823.
8. Alter MJ. Epidemiology and prevention of hepatitis B. *Semin Liver Dis* 2003;23(1):39–46.
9. Altinel K, Hashimoto K, Wei Y, et al. Single-nucleotide resolution mapping of hepatitis B virus promoters in infected human livers and hepatocellular carcinoma. *J Virol* 2016;90(23):10811–10822.
10. Anderson AL, Banks KE, Pontoglio M, et al. Alpha/beta interferon differentially modulates the clearance of cytoplasmic encapsidated replication intermediates and nuclear covalently closed circular hepatitis B virus (HBV) DNA from the livers of hepatocyte nuclear factor 1{alpha}-Null HBV transgenic mice. *J Virol* 2005;79(17):11045–11052.
11. Asabe S, Wieland SF, Chattopadhyay PK, et al. The size of the viral inoculum contributes to the outcome of hepatitis B virus infection. *J Virol* 2009;83(19):9652–9662.
12. Ascherio A, Zhang SM, Hernan MA, et al. Hepatitis B vaccination and the risk of multiple sclerosis. *N Engl J Med* 2001;344(5):327–332.
13. Ashton-Rickardt PG, Murray K. Mutations that change the immunological subtype of hepatitis B virus surface antigen and distinguish between antigenic and immunogenic determination. *J Med Virol* 1989;29(3):204–214.
14. Bartenschlager R, Schaller H. The amino-terminal domain of the hepadnaviral P-gene encodes the terminal protein (genome-linked protein) believed to prime reverse transcription. *EMBO J* 1988;7(13):4185–4192.
15. Bartenschlager R, Junker-Niepmann M, Schaller H. The P gene product of hepatitis B virus is required as a structural component for genomic RNA encapsidation. *J Virol* 1990;64(11):5324–5332.
16. Bartenschlager R, Kuhn C, Schaller H. Expression of the P-protein of the human hepatitis B virus in a vaccinia virus system and detection of the nucleocapsid-associated P-gene product by radiolabelling at newly introduced phosphorylation sites. *Nucleic Acids Res* 1992;20(2):195–202.
17. Bartenschlager R, Schaller H. Hepadnaviral assembly is initiated by polymerase binding to the encapsidation signal in the viral RNA genome. *EMBO J* 1992;11(9):3413–3420.
18. Bartholomeusz A, Tehan BG, Chalmers DK. Comparisons of the HBV and HIV polymerase, and antiviral resistance mutations. *Antiviral Therapy* 2004;9(2):149–160.
19. Basagoudanavar SH, Perlman DH, Hu J. Regulation of hepadnavirus reverse transcription by dynamic nucleocapsid phosphorylation. *J Virol* 2007;81(4):1641–1649.
20. Beasley RP, Trepo C, Stevens CE, et al. The e antigen and vertical transmission of hepatitis B surface antigen. *Am J Epidemiol* 1977;105(2):94–98.
21. Beasley RP, Lin CC, Hwang LY, et al. Hepatocellular carcinoma and hepatitis B virus. *Lancet* 1981;2:1129–1133.
22. Beck J, Nassal M. Sequence- and structure-specific determinants in the interaction between the RNA encapsidation signal and reverse transcriptase of avian hepatitis B viruses. *J Virol* 1997;71(7):4971–4980.
23. Becker SA, Lee TH, Butel JS, et al. Hepatitis B virus X protein interferes with cellular DNA repair. *J Virol* 1998;72(1):266–272.
24. Beggel B, Munk C, Daumer M, et al. Full genome ultra-deep pyrosequencing associates G-to-A hypermutation of the hepatitis B virus genome with the natural progression of hepatitis B. *J Viral Hepat* 2013;20(12):882–889.
25. Belloni L, Allweiss L, Guerrieri F, et al. IFN-alpha inhibits HBV transcription and replication in cell culture and in humanized mice by targeting the epigenetic regulation of the nuclear cccDNA minichromosome. *J Clin Invest* 2012;122(2):529–537.
26. Bentley P, Tan MJA, McBride AA, et al. The SMC5/6 complex interacts with the papillomavirus E2 protein and influences maintenance of viral episomal DNA. *J Virol* 2018;92(15):e00356-18.
27. Berke JM, Dehertogh P, Vergauwen K, et al. Capsid assembly modulators have a dual mechanism of action in primary human hepatocytes infected with hepatitis B virus. *Antimicrob Agents Chemother* 2017;61(8):e00560-17.
28. Bertoletti A, Naoumov NV. Translation of immunological knowledge into better treatments of chronic hepatitis B. *J Hepatol* 2003;39(1):115–124.
29. Bhatnagar PK, Papas E, Blum HE, et al. Immune response to synthetic peptide analogues of hepatitis B surface antigen specific for the a determinant. *Proc Natl Acad Sci U S A* 1982;79(14):4400–4404.
30. Blanchet M, Sureau C. Infectivity determinants of the hepatitis B virus pre-S domain are confined to the N-terminal 75 amino acid residues. *J Virol* 2007;81(11):5841–5849.
31. Blumberg BS, Alter HJ, Visnich S. A "new" antigen in leukemia sera. *JAMA* 1965;191:541–546.
32. Blumberg BS, Gerstley BJS, Hungerford DA, et al. A serum antigen (Australia antigen) in Down's syndrome, leukemia and hepatitis. *Ann Intern Med* 1967;66:924–931.
33. Blumberg BS, Sutnick AI, London WT. Hepatitis and leukemia: their relation to Australia antigen. *Bull N Y Acad Med* 1968;44(12):1566–1586.
34. Blumberg BS. Australia antigen and the biology of hepatitis B. *Science* 1977;197:17–25.
35. Bock CT, Schranz P, Schroder CH, et al. Hepatitis B virus genome is organized into nucleosomes in the nucleus of the infected cell. *Virus Genes* 1994;8(3):215–229.

36. Bock CT, Schwinn S, Locarnini S, et al. Structural organization of the hepatitis B virus minichromosome. *J Mol Biol* 2001;307(1):183–196.
37. Bonino F, Brunetto MR. Chronic hepatitis B e antigen (HBeAg) negative, anti-HBe positive hepatitis B: an overview. *J Hepatol* 2003;39(Suppl 1):S160–S163.
38. Bottcher B, Wynne SA, Crowther RA. Determination of the fold of the core protein of hepatitis B virus by electron cryomicroscopy [see comments]. *Nature* 1997;386(6620):88–91.
39. Boyd A, Lacombe K, Lavocat F, et al. Decay of ccc-DNA marks persistence of intrahepatic viral DNA synthesis under tenofovir in HIV-HBV co-infected patients. *J Hepatol* 2016;65(4):683–691.
40. Bradley DW, Krawczynski K, Ebert JW, et al. Parenterally transmitted non-A, non-B hepatitis: virus-specific antibody response patterns in hepatitis C virus-infected chimpanzees. *Gastroenterology* 1990;99(4):1054–1060.
41. Brechot C, Pourcel C, Louise A, et al. Presence of integrated hepatitis B virus DNA sequences in cellular DNA of human hepatocellular carcinoma. *Nature* 1980;286(5772):533–535.
42. Breiner KM, Schaller H, Knolle PA. Endothelial cell-mediated uptake of a hepatitis B virus: a new concept of liver targeting of hepatotropic microorganisms. *Hepatology* 2001;34(4 Pt 1): 803–808.
43. Bringas R. Folding and assembly of hepatitis B virus core protein: a new model proposal. *J Struct Biol* 1997;118(3):189–196.
44. Brown SE, Howard C, Zuckerman AJ, et al. Affinity of antibody responses in man to hepatitis B vaccine determined with synthetic peptides. *Lancet* 1984;2:184–187.
45. Brunetto MR, Rodriguez UA, Bonino F. Hepatitis B virus mutants. *Intervirology* 1999;42(2–3):69–80.
46. Brunetto MR, Oliveri F, Colombatto P, et al. Hepatitis B surface antigen serum levels help to distinguish active from inactive hepatitis B virus genotype D carriers. *Gastroenterology* 2010;139(2):483–490.
47. Bruni R, D'Ugo E, Giuseppetti R, et al. Activation of the N-myc2 oncogene by woodchuck hepatitis virus integration in the linked downstream b3n locus in woodchuck hepatocellular carcinoma. *Virology* 1999;257(2):483–490.
48. Bruni R, D'Ugo E, Argentini C, et al. Scaffold attachment region located in a locus targeted by hepadnavirus integration in hepatocellular carcinomas. *Cancer Detect Prev* 2003;27(3):175–181.
49. Bruss V, Ganem D. The role of envelope proteins in hepatitis B virus assembly. *Proc Natl Acad Sci U S A* 1991;88(3):1059–1063.
50. Bruss V, Lu X, Thomssen R, et al. Post-translational alterations in transmembrane topology of the hepatitis B virus large envelope protein. *EMBO J* 1994;13(10):2273–2279.
51. Bruss V. Envelopment of the hepatitis B virus nucleocapsid. *Virus Res* 2004;106(2):199–209.
52. Buendia MA, Neuveut C. Hepatocellular carcinoma. *Cold Spring Harb Perspect Med* 2015;5(2):a021444.
53. Burton AR, Pallett LJ, McCoy LE, et al. Circulating and intrahepatic antiviral B cells are defective in hepatitis B. *J Clin Invest* 2018;128(10):4588–4603.
54. Buscher M, Reiser W, Will H, et al. Transcripts and the putative RNA pregenome of duck hepatitis B virus: implications for reverse transcription. *Cell* 1985;40(3):717–724.
55. Buster EH, Hansen BE, Lau GK, et al. Factors that predict response of patients with hepatitis B e antigen-positive chronic hepatitis B to peginterferon-alfa. *Gastroenterology* 2009;137(6):2002–2009.
56. Butler EK, Gersch J, McNamara A, et al. Hepatitis B virus serum DNA and RNA levels in nucleos(t)ide analog-treated or untreated patients during chronic and acute infection. *Hepatology* 2018;68(6):2106–2117.
57. Cacciola I, Pollicino T, Squadrito G, et al. Occult hepatitis B virus infection in patients with chronic hepatitis C liver disease. *N Engl J Med* 1999;341(1):22–26.
58. Cacciola I, Pollicino T, Squadrito G, et al. Quantification of intrahepatic hepatitis B virus (HBV) DNA in patients with chronic HBV infection. *Hepatology* 2000;31(2):507–512.
59. Cai D, Mills C, Yu W, et al. Identification of disubstituted sulfonamide compounds as specific inhibitors of hepatitis B virus covalently closed circular DNA formation. *Antimicrob Agents Chemother* 2012;56(8):4277–4288.
60. Calvert J, Summers J. Two regions of an avian hepadnavirus RNA pregenome are required in cis for encapsidation. *J Virol* 1994;68(4):2084–2090.
61. Cancer Genome Atlas Research Network. Electronic address: wheeler@bcm.edu, Cancer Genome Atlas Research Network; Ally A, et al. Comprehensive and integrative genomic characterization of hepatocellular carcinoma. *Cell* 2017;169(7):1327–1341.e1323.
62. Candotti D, Assennato SM, Laperche S, et al. Multiple HBV transfusion transmissions from undetected occult infections: revising the minimal infectious dose. *Gut* 2019; 68(2):313–321.
63. Cao F, Badtke MP, Metzger LM, et al. Identification of an essential molecular contact point on the duck hepatitis B virus reverse transcriptase. *J Virol* 2005;79(16):10164–10170.
64. Cao F, Tavis JE. RNA elements directing translation of the duck hepatitis B virus polymerase via ribosomal shunting. *J Virol* 2011;85(13):6343–6352.
65. Carman WF, Zanetti AR, Karayiannis P, et al. Vaccine-induced escape mutant of hepatitis B virus. *Lancet* 1990;336(8711):325–329.
66. Carman WF, Van Deursen FJ, Mimms LT, et al. The prevalence of surface antigen variants of hepatitis B virus in Papua New Guinea, South Africa, and Sardinia. *Hepatology* 1997;26(6):1658–1666.
67. Caselmann WH, Meyer M, Kekule AS, et al. A trans-activator function is generated by integration of hepatitis B virus preS/S sequences in human hepatocellular carcinoma DNA. *Proc Natl Acad Sci U S A* 1990;87(8):2970–2974.
68. Cattaneo R, Will H, Hernandez N, et al. Signals regulating hepatitis B surface antigen transcription. *Nature* 1983;305:336–338.
69. Cattaneo R, Will H, Schaller H. Hepatitis B virus transcription in the infected liver. *EMBO J* 1984;3(9):2191–2196.
70. Chakraborty PR, Ruiz-Opazo N, Shouval D, et al. Identification of integrated hepatitis B virus DNA and expression of viral RNA in HBsAg-producing human hepatocellular carcinoma cell line. *Nature* 1980;286:531–533.
71. Chang C, Enders G, Sprengel R, et al. Expression of the precore region of an avian hepatitis B virus is not required for viral replication. *J Virol* 1987;61(10):3322–3325.
72. Chang LJ, Pryciak P, Ganem D, et al. Biosynthesis of the reverse transcriptase of hepatitis B viruses involves de novo translational initiation not ribosomal frameshifting. *Nature* 1989;337(6205):364–368.
73. Chang LJ, Hirsch RC, Ganem D, et al. Effects of insertional and point mutations on the functions of the duck hepatitis B virus polymerase. *J Virol* 1990;64(11):5553–5558.
74. Chang SF, Netter HJ, Bruns M, et al. A new avian hepadnavirus infecting snow geese (Anser caerulescens) produces a significant fraction of virions containing single-stranded DNA. *Virology* 1999;262(1):39–54.
75. Chang TT, Lai CL, Kew Yoon S, et al. Entecavir treatment for up to 5 years in patients with hepatitis B e antigen-positive chronic hepatitis B. *Hepatology* 2010;51(2):422–430.
76. Chang TT, Liaw YF, Wu SS, et al. Long-term entecavir therapy results in the reversal of fibrosis/cirrhosis and continued histological improvement in patients with chronic hepatitis B. *Hepatology* 2010;52(3):886–893.
77. Charre C, Levrero M, Zoulim F, et al. Non-invasive biomarkers for chronic hepatitis B virus infection management. *Antiviral Res* 2019;169:104553.
78. Chen CJ, Yang HI, Su J, et al. Risk of hepatocellular carcinoma across a biological gradient of serum hepatitis B virus DNA level. *JAMA* 2006;295(1):65–73.
79. Chen HS, Kew MC, Hornbuckle WE, et al. The precore gene of the woodchuck hepatitis virus genome is not essential for viral replication in the natural host. *J Virol* 1992;66(9):5682–5684.
80. Chen HS, Kaneko S, Girones R, et al. The woodchuck hepatitis virus X gene is important for establishment of virus infection in woodchucks. *J Virol* 1993;67(3):1218–1226.
81. Chen MH, Chen MH, Chou CT, et al. Low but long-lasting risk of reversal of seroconversion in patients with rheumatoid arthritis receiving immunosuppressive therapy. *Clin Gastroenterol Hepatol* 2020;18(11):2573–2581.e1.
82. Chen MT, Billaud JN, Sallberg M, et al. A function of the hepatitis B virus precore protein is to regulate the immune response to the core antigen. *Proc Natl Acad Sci U S A* 2004;101(41):14913–14918.
83. Chen YC, Delbrook K, Dealwis C, et al. Discontinuous epitopes of hepatitis B surface antigen derived from a filamentous phage peptide library. *Proc Natl Acad Sci U S A* 1996;93(5):1997–2001.
84. Cheng KC, Smith GL, Moss B. Hepatitis B virus large surface protein is not secreted but is immunogenic when selectively expressed by recombinant vaccinia virus. *J Virol* 1986;60(2):337–344.
85. Cheng X, Xia Y, Serti E, et al. Hepatitis B virus evades innate immunity of hepatocytes but activates cytokine production by macrophages. *Hepatology* 2017;66(6):1779–1793.
86. Chevaliez S, Bouvier-Alias M, Laperche S, et al. Performance of version 2.0 of the Cobas AmpliPrep/Cobas TaqMan real-time PCR assay for hepatitis B virus DNA quantification. *J Clin Microbiol* 2010;48(10):3641–3647.
87. Chisari FV, Klopchin K, Moriyama T, et al. Molecular pathogenesis of hepatocellular carcinoma in hepatitis B virus transgenic mice. *Cell* 1989;59(6):1145–1156.
88. Chisari FV, Ferrari C. Hepatitis B virus immunopathogenesis. *Annu Rev Immunol* 1995;13:29–60.
89. Cholongitas E, Papatheodoridis GV, Burroughs AK. Liver grafts from anti-hepatitis B core positive donors: a systematic review. *J Hepatol* 2010;52(2):272–279.
90. Choo QL, Kuo G, Weiner AJ, et al. Isolation of a cDNA clone derived from a blood-borne non-A, non-B viral hepatitis genome. *Science* 1989;244(4902):359–362.
91. Chouteau P, Le Seyec J, Cannie I, et al. A short N-proximal region in the large envelope protein harbors a determinant that contributes to the species specificity of human hepatitis B virus. *J Virol* 2001;75(23):11565–11572.
92. Chu CJ, Hussain M, Lok AS. Quantitative serum HBV DNA levels during different stages of chronic hepatitis B infection. *Hepatology* 2002;36(6):1408–1415.
93. Coffin CS, Terrault NA. Management of hepatitis B in liver transplant recipients. *J Viral Hepat* 2007;14(Suppl 1):37–44.
94. Colson P, Borentain P, Coso D, et al. Hepatitis B virus reactivation in HBsAg-negative patients is associated with emergence of viral strains with mutated HBsAg and reverse transcriptase. *Virology* 2015;484:354–363.
95. Condreay LD, Wu TT, Aldrich CE, et al. Replication of DHBV genomes with mutations at the sites of initiation of minus- and plus-strand DNA synthesis. *Virology* 1992;188(1):208–216.
96. Confavreux C, Suissa S, Saddier P, et al. Vaccinations and the risk of relapse in multiple sclerosis. Vaccines in Multiple Sclerosis Study Group. *N Engl J Med* 2001;344(5):319–326.
97. Conway JF, Cheng N, Zlotnick A, et al. Visualization of a 4-helix bundle in the hepatitis B virus capsid by cryo-electron microscopy.[comment]. *Nature* 1997;386(6620):91–94.
98. Cornberg M, Lok AS-F, Terrault NA, et al. Guidance for design and endpoints of clinical trials in chronic hepatitis B—report from the 2019 EASL-AASLD HBV Treatment Endpoints Conference. *Hepatology* 2020;72(3):539–557.
99. Crispe IN. The liver as a lymphoid organ. *Annu Rev Immunol* 2009;27:147–163.
100. Crowther RA, Kiselev NA, Bottcher B, et al. Three-dimensional structure of hepatitis B virus core particles determined by electron cryomicroscopy. *Cell* 1994;77:943–950.
101. Cui X, Ludgate L, Ning X, et al. Maturation-associated destabilization of hepatitis B virus nucleocapsid. *J Virol* 2013;87(21):11494–11503.
102. Cui X, Guo JT, Hu J. Hepatitis B virus covalently closed circular DNA formation in immortalized mouse hepatocytes associated with nucleocapsid destabilization. *J Virol* 2015;89(17):9021–9028.
103. Cui X, Luckenbaugh L, Bruss V, et al. Alteration of mature nucleocapsid and enhancement of covalently closed circular DNA formation by hepatitis B virus core mutants defective in complete-virion formation. *J Virol* 2015;89(19):10064–10072.
104. Cui X, McAllister R, Boregowda R, et al. Does tyrosyl DNA phosphodiesterase-2 play a role in hepatitis B virus genome repair? *PLoS One* 2015;10(6):e0128401.
105. Cullen JM, Marion PL. Non-neoplastic liver disease associated with chronic ground squirrel hepatitis virus infection. *Hepatology* 1996;23(6):1324–1329.
106. Dandri M, Schirmacher P, Rogler CE. Woodchuck hepatitis virus X protein is present in chronically infected woodchuck liver and woodchuck hepatocellular carcinomas which are permissive for viral replication. *J Virol* 1996;70(8):5246–5254.

107. Dandri M, Burda MR, Will H, et al. Increased hepatocyte turnover and inhibition of woodchuck hepatitis B virus replication by adefovir in vitro do not lead to reduction of the closed circular DNA. *Hepatology* 2000;32:139–146.
108. Dane DS, Cameron CH, Briggs M. Virus-like particles in serum of patients with Australia-antigen-associated hepatitis. *Lancet* 1970;1:695–698.
109. Das A, Hoare M, Davies N, et al. Functional skewing of the global CD8 T cell population in chronic hepatitis B virus infection. *J Exp Med* 2008;205(9):2111–2124.
110. Das K, Xiong X, Yang H, et al. Molecular modeling and biochemical characterization reveal the mechanism of hepatitis B virus polymerase resistance to lamivudine (3TC) and emtricitabine (FTC). *J Virol* 2001;75(10):4771–4779.
111. Daub H, Blencke S, Habenberger P, et al. Identification of SRPK1 and SRPK2 as the major cellular protein kinases phosphorylating hepatitis B virus core protein. *J Virol* 2002;76(16):8124–8137.
112. de Carvalho Dominguez Souza BF, Konig A, Rasche A, et al. A novel hepatitis B virus species discovered in capuchin monkeys sheds new light on the evolution of primate hepadnaviruses. *J Hepatol* 2018;68(6):1114–1122.
113. de Villa VH, Chen YS, Chen CL. Hepatitis B core antibody-positive grafts: recipient's risk. *Transplantation* 2003;75(3 Suppl):S49-S53.
114. Decorsiere A, Mueller H, van Breugel PC, et al. Hepatitis B virus X protein identifies the Smc5/6 complex as a host restriction factor. *Nature* 2016;531(7594):386–389.
115. Dejean A, Bougueleret L, Grzeschik KH, et al. Hepatitis B virus DNA integration in a sequence homologous to v-erb-A and steroid receptor genes in a hepatocellular carcinoma. *Nature* 1986;322(6074):70–72.
116. Dejean A, de The H. Hepatitis B virus as an insertional mutagene in a human hepatocellular carcinoma. *Mol Biol Med* 1990;7(3):213–222.
117. Deres K, Schroder CH, Paessens A, et al. Inhibition of hepatitis B virus replication by drug-induced depletion of nucleocapsids. *Science* 2003;299(5608):893–896.
118. Di Q, Summers J, Burch JB, et al. Major differences between WHV and HBV in the regulation of transcription. *Virology* 1997;229(1):25–35.
119. Dienstag JL, Schiff ER, Wright TL, et al. Lamivudine as initial treatment for chronic hepatitis B in the United States. *N Engl J Med* 1999;341(17):1256–1263.
120. Dienstag JL, Goldin RD, Heathcote EJ, et al. Histological outcome during long-term lamivudine therapy. *Gastroenterology* 2003;124(1):105–117.
121. Dill JA, Camus AC, Leary JH, et al. Distinct viral lineages from fish and amphibians reveal the complex evolutionary history of hepadnaviruses. *J Virol* 2016;90(17):7920–7933.
122. Donello JE, Loeb JE, Hope TJ. Woodchuck hepatitis virus contains a tripartite posttranscriptional regulatory element. *J Virol* 1998;72(6):5085–5092.
123. Dresang LR, Vereide DT, Sugden B. Identifying sites bound by Epstein-Barr virus nuclear antigen 1 (EBNA1) in the human genome: defining a position-weighted matrix to predict sites bound by EBNA1 in viral genomes. *J Virol* 2009;83(7):2930–2940.
124. Dryden KA, Wieland SF, Whitten-Bauer C, et al. Native hepatitis B virions and capsids visualized by electron cryomicroscopy. *Mol Cell* 2006;22(6):843–850.
125. Dunn C, Peppa D, Khanna P, et al. Temporal analysis of early immune responses in patients with acute hepatitis B virus infection. *Gastroenterology* 2009;137(4):1289–1300.
126. EASL. EASL Clinical practice guidelines: management of chronic hepatitis B. *J Hepatol* 2009;50(2):227–242.
127. EASL. EASL 2017 Clinical practice guidelines on the management of hepatitis B virus infection. *J Hepatol* 2017;67(2):370–398.
128. Eble BE, Lingappa VR, Ganem D. Hepatitis B surface antigen: an unusual secreted protein initially synthesized as a transmembrane polypeptide. *Mol Cell Biol* 1986;6(5):1454–1463.
129. Eble BE, MacRae DR, Lingappa VR, et al. Multiple topogenic sequences determine the transmembrane orientation of the hepatitis B surface antigen. *Mol Cell Biol* 1987;7(10):3591–3601.
130. Eckhardt SG, Milich DR, McLachlan A. Hepatitis B virus core antigen has two nuclear localization sequences in the arginine-rich carboxyl terminus. *J Virol* 1991;65(2): 575–582.
131. El Chaar M, Candotti D, Crowther RA, et al. Impact of hepatitis B virus surface protein mutations on the diagnosis of occult hepatitis B virus infection. *Hepatology* 2010;52(5):1600–1610.
132. El-Serag HB. Epidemiology of viral hepatitis and hepatocellular carcinoma. *Gastroenterology* 2012;142(6):1264–1273 e1261.
133. Enders GH, Ganem D, Varmus H. Mapping the major transcripts of ground squirrel hepatitis virus: the presumptive template for reverse transcriptase is terminally redundant. *Cell* 1985;42(1):297–308.
134. Esumi M, Aritaka T, Arii M, et al. Clonal origin of human hepatoma determined by integration of hepatitis B virus DNA. *Cancer Res* 1986;46:5767–5771.
135. Evans AA, Chen G, Ross EA, et al. Eight-year follow-up of the 90,000-person Haimen City cohort: I. Hepatocellular carcinoma mortality, risk factors, and gender differences. *Cancer Epidemiol Biomarkers Prev* 2002;11(4):369–376.
136. Fanning GC, Zoulim F, Hou J, et al. Therapeutic strategies for hepatitis B virus infection: towards a cure. *Nat Rev Drug Discov* 2019;19(4):291.
137. Fernholz D, Galle PR, Stemler M, et al. Infectious hepatitis B virus variant defective in pre-S2 protein expression in a chronic carrier. *Virology* 1993;194(1):137–148.
138. Ferrell LD, Theise ND, Scheuer PJ. Acute & chronic viral hepatitis. In: MacSween RNM, Burt AD, Portmann BC, et al., eds. *Pathology of the Liver*. 4th ed. Edinburgh: Churchill Livingstone Press; 2002:313–362.
139. Fiedler SA, Oberle D, Chudy M, et al. Effectiveness of blood donor screening by HIV, HCV, HBV-NAT assays, as well as HBsAg and anti-HBc immunoassays in Germany (2008–2015). *Vox Sang* 2019;114(5):443–450.
140. Fisicaro P, Valdatta C, Boni C, et al. Early kinetics of innate and adaptive immune responses during hepatitis B virus infection. *Gut* 2009;58(7):974–982.
141. Fisicaro P, Valdatta C, Massari M, et al. Antiviral intrahepatic T-cell responses can be restored by blocking programmed death-1 pathway in chronic hepatitis B. *Gastroenterology* 2010;138(2):682–693.
142. Foo NC, Yen TS. Activation of promoters for cellular lipogenic genes by hepatitis B virus large surface protein. *Virology* 2000;269(2):420–425.
143. Fortuin M, Karthigesu V, Allison L, et al. Breakthrough infections and identification of a viral variant in Gambian children immunized with hepatitis B vaccine. *J Infect Dis* 1994;169(6):1374–1376.
144. Fouillot N, Tlouzeau S, Rossignol JM, et al. Translation of the hepatitis B virus P gene by ribosomal scanning as an alternative to internal initiation. *J Virol* 1993;67(8):4886–4895.
145. Fourel G, Trepo C, Bougueleret L, et al. Frequent activation of N-myc genes by hepadnavirus insertion in woodchuck liver tumours. *Nature* 1990;347(6290):294–298.
146. Fourel G, Couturier J, Wei Y, et al. Evidence for long-range oncogene activation by hepadnavirus insertion. *EMBO J* 1994;13(11):2526–2534.
147. Fourel I, Saputelli J, Schaffer P, et al. The carbocyclic analog of 2'-deoxyguanosine induces a prolonged inhibition of duck hepatitis B virus DNA synthesis in primary hepatocyte cultures and in the liver. *J Virol* 1994;68(2):1059–1065.
148. Freiman JS, Jilbert AR, Dixon RJ, et al. Experimental duck hepatitis B virus infection: pathology and evolution of hepatic and extrahepatic infection. *Hepatology* 1988;8(3):507–513.
149. Fu L, Hu H, Liu Y, et al. Woodchuck sodium taurocholate cotransporting polypeptide supports low-level hepatitis B and D virus entry. *Virology* 2017;505:1–11.
150. Fu X-X, Su CY, Lee Y, et al. Insulinlike growth factor II expression and oval cell proliferation associated with hepatocarcinogenesis in woodchuck hepatitis virus carriers. *J Virol* 1988;62:3422–3430.
151. Galibert F, Chen TN, Mandart E. Nucleotide sequence of a cloned woodchuck hepatitis virus genome: comparison with the hepatitis B virus sequence. *J Virol* 1982;41(1):51–65.
152. Ganem D, Prince AM. Hepatitis B virus infection—natural history and clinical consequences. *N Engl J Med* 2004;350:1118–1129.
153. Gao W, Hu J. Formation of hepatitis B virus covalently closed circular DNA: removal of genome-linked protein. *J Virol* 2007;81(12):6164–6174.
154. Garcia PD, Ou JH, Rutter WJ, et al. Targeting of the hepatitis B virus precore protein to the endoplasmic reticulum membrane: after signal peptide cleavage translocation can be aborted and the product released into the cytoplasm. *J Cell Biol* 1988;106(4):1093–1104.
155. Gerin JL, Ford EC, Purcell RH. Biochemical characterization of Australia antigen. Evidence for defective particles of hepatitis B virus. *Am J Pathol* 1975;81(3):651–668.
156. Gerlich WH, Robinson WS. Hepatitis B virus contains protein attached to the 5' terminus of its complete DNA strand. *Cell* 1980;21(3):801–809.
157. Gerlich WH, Goldmann U, Muller R, et al. Specificity and localization of the hepatitis B virus-associated protein kinase. *J Virol* 1982;42(3):761–766.
158. Gilbert C, Feschotte C. Genomic fossils calibrate the long-term evolution of hepadnaviruses. *PLoS Biol* 2010;8(9):e1000495.
159. Gilbert RJ, Beales L, Blond D, et al. Hepatitis B small surface antigen particles are octahedral. *Proc Natl Acad Sci U S A* 2005;102:14783–14788.
160. Global Burden of Disease Liver Cancer Collaboration; Akinyemiju T, Abera S, et al. The burden of primary liver cancer and underlying etiologies from 1990 to 2015 at the global, regional, and national level: results from the Global Burden of Disease Study 2015. *JAMA Oncol* 2017;3(12):1683–1691.
161. Gogarten JF, Ulrich M, Bhuva N, et al. A novel orthohepadnavirus identified in a Dead Maxwell's Duiker (Philantomba maxwellii) in Tai National Park, Cote d'Ivoire. *Viruses* 2019;11(3):279.
162. Goldstein ST, Alter MJ, Williams IT, et al. Incidence and risk factors for acute hepatitis B in the United States, 1982–1998: implications for vaccination programs. *J Infect Dis* 2002;185(6):713–719.
163. Graber-Stiehl I. The silent epidemic killing more people than HIV, malaria or TB. *Nature* 2018;564(7734):24–26.
164. Grandjacques C, Pradat P, Stuyver L, et al. Rapid detection of genotypes and mutations in the pre-core promoter and the pre-core region of hepatitis B virus genome: correlation with viral persistence and disease severity. *J Hepatol* 2000;33(3):430–439.
165. Grgacic EVL, Anderson DA. The large surface protein of duck hepatitis B virus is phosphorylated in the pre-S domain. *J Virol* 1994;68:7344–7350.
166. Grisham JW. A morphologic study of deoxyribonucleic acid synthesis and cell proliferation in regenerating rat liver; autoradiography with thymidine-H3. *Cancer Res* 1962;22:842–849.
167. Grompe M. Liver stem cells, where art thou? *Cell Stem Cell* 2014;15(3):257–258.
168. Guidotti LG, Martinez V, Loh YT, et al. Hepatitis B virus nucleocapsid particles do not cross the hepatocyte nuclear membrane in transgenic mice. *J Virol* 1994;68(9):5469–5475.
169. Guidotti LG, Chisari FV. Cytokine-induced viral purging—role in viral pathogenesis. *Curr Opin Microbiol* 1999;2(4):388–391.
170. Guidotti LG, Rochford R, Chung J, et al. Viral clearance without destruction of infected cells during acute HBV infection. *Science* 1999;284(5415):825–829.
171. Guidotti LG, Inverso D, Sironi L, et al. Immunosurveillance of the liver by intravascular effector CD8(+) T cells. *Cell* 2015;161(3):486–500.
172. Gunther S, Fischer L, Pult I, et al. Naturally occurring variants of hepatitis B virus. *Adv Virus Res* 1999;52:25–137.
173. Guo H, Mason WS, Aldrich CE, et al. Identification and classification of avihepadnaviruses isolated from exotic anseriformes maintained in captivity. *J Virol* 2005;79:2729–2742.
174. Guo H, Jiang D, Zhou T, et al. Characterization of the intracellular deproteinized relaxed circular DNA of hepatitis B virus: an intermediate of covalently closed circular DNA formation. *J Virol* 2007;81(22):12472–12484.
175. Guo J-T, Zhou H, Liu C, et al. Apoptosis and regeneration of hepatocytes during recovery from transient hepadnavirus infection. *J Virol* 2000;74:1495–1505.
176. Guo JT, Pryce M, Wang X, et al. Conditional replication of duck hepatitis B virus in hepatoma cells. *J Virol* 2003;77:1885–1893.
177. Habig JW, Loeb DD. Small DNA hairpin negatively regulates in situ priming during duck hepatitis B virus reverse transcription. *J Virol* 2002;76(3):980–989.
178. Hadziyannis SJ, Hadziyannis AS, Dourakis S, et al. Clinical significance of quantitative anti-HBc IgM assay in acute and chronic HBV infection. *Hepatogastroenterology* 1993;40(6):588–592.
179. Hadziyannis SJ, Vassilopoulos D. Hepatitis B e antigen-negative chronic hepatitis B. *Hepatology* 2001;34(4 Pt 1):617–624.

180. Hagelstein J, Fathinejad F, Stremmel W, et al. pH-independent uptake of hepatitis B virus in primary human hepatocytes. *Virology* 1997;229(1):292–294.
181. Hagen TM, Huang S, Curnutte J, et al. Extensive oxidative DNA damage in hepatocytes of transgenic mice with chronic active hepatitis destined to develop hepatocellular carcinoma. *Proc Natl Acad Sci U S A* 1994;91(26):12808–12812.
182. Hahn CM, Iwanowicz LR, Cornman RS, et al. Characterization of a novel hepadnavirus in the white sucker (Catostomus commersonii) from the Great Lakes Region of the United States. *J Virol* 2015;89(23):11801–11811.
183. Halpern MS, England JM, Deery DT, et al. Viral nucleic acid synthesis and antigen accumulation in pancreas and kidney of Pekin ducks infected with duck hepatitis B virus. *Proc Natl Acad Sci U S A* 1983;80(15):4865–4869.
184. Hansen LJ, Tennant BC, Seeger C, et al. Differential activation of myc gene family members in hepatic carcinogenesis by closely related hepatitis B viruses. *Mol Cell Biol* 1993;13(1):659–667.
185. Harpaz R, Von SL, Averhoff FM, et al. Transmission of hepatitis B virus to multiple patients from a surgeon without evidence of inadequate infection control [see comments]. *N Engl J Med* 1996;334(9):549–554.
186. Hartmann-Stuhler C, Prange R. Hepatitis B virus large envelope protein interacts with gamma2-adaptin, a clathrin adaptor-related protein. *J Virol* 2001;75(11):5343–5351.
187. Havert MB, Ji L, Loeb DD. Analysis of duck hepatitis B virus reverse transcription indicates a common mechanism for the two template switches during plus-strand DNA synthesis. *J Virol* 2002;76(6):2763–2769.
188. Hayward WS, Neel BG, Astrin SM. Activation of a cellular onc gene by promoter insertion in ALV-induced lymphoid leukosis. *Nature* 1981;290(5806):475–480.
189. He W, Cao Z, Mao F, et al. Modification of three amino acids in sodium taurocholate cotransporting polypeptide renders mice susceptible to infection with hepatitis D virus in vivo. *J Virol* 2016;90(19):8866–8874.
190. Heermann KH, Goldmann U, Schwartz W, et al. Large surface proteins of hepatitis B virus containing the pre-s sequence. *J Virol* 1984;52(2):396–402.
191. Heermann KH, Kruse F, Seifer M, et al. Immunogenicity of the gene S and Pre-S domains in hepatitis B virions and HBsAg filaments. *Intervirology* 1987;28(1):14–25.
192. Hildt E, Saher G, Bruss V, et al. The hepatitis B virus large surface protein (LHBs) is a transcriptional activator. *Virology* 1996;225(1):235–239.
193. Hildt E, Munz B, Saher G, et al. The PreS2 activator MHBs(t) of hepatitis B virus activates c-raf-1/Erk2 signaling in transgenic mice. *EMBO J* 2002;21(4):525–535.
194. Hirsch RC, Lavine JE, Chang LJ, et al. Polymerase gene products of hepatitis B viruses are required for genomic RNA packaging as well as for reverse transcription. *Nature* 1990;344(6266):552–555.
195. Hollinger FB, Liang TJ. Hepatitis B virus. Hepadnaviridae: the viruses and their replication. In: Knipe DM, et al., eds. *Fields Virology*. Vol 2. 4th ed. Philadelphia, PA: Lippincott Williams & Wilkins; 2001:2971–3036.
196. Hosoda K, Omata M, Uchiumi K, et al. Extrahepatic replication of duck hepatitis B virus: more than expected. *Hepatology* 1990;11(1):44–48.
197. Hsia CC, Evarts RP, Nakatsukasa H, et al. Occurrence of oval-type cells in hepatitis B virus-associated human hepatocarcinogenesis. *Hepatology* 1992;16(6):1327–1333.
198. Hsieh YH, Chang YY, Su IJ, et al. Hepatitis B virus pre-S2 mutant large surface protein inhibits DNA double-strand break repair and leads to genome instability in hepatocarcinogenesis. *J Pathol* 2015;236(3):337–347.
199. Hsu HY, Chang MH, Liaw SH, et al. Changes of hepatitis B surface antigen variants in carrier children before and after universal vaccination in Taiwan. *Hepatology* 1999;30(5):1312–1317.
200. Hsu HY, Chang MH, Ni YH, et al. No increase in prevalence of hepatitis B surface antigen mutant in a population of children and adolescents who were fully covered by universal infant immunization. *J Infect Dis* 2010;201(8):1192–1200.
201. Hu J, Seeger C. Hsp90 is required for the activity of a hepatitis B virus reverse transcriptase. *Proc Natl Acad Sci U S A* 1996;93(3):1060–1064.
202. Hu J, Toft DO, Seeger C. Hepadnavirus assembly and reverse transcription require a multi-component chaperone complex which is incorporated into nucleocapsids. *EMBO J* 1997;16(1):59–68.
203. Hu J, Toft D, Anselmo D, et al. In vitro reconstitution of functional hepadnavirus reverse transcriptase with cellular chaperone proteins. *J Virol* 2002;76(1):269–279.
204. Hu J, Flores D, Toft D, et al. Requirement of heat shock protein 90 for human hepatitis B virus reverse transcriptase function. *J Virol* 2004;78(23):13122–13131.
205. Huan B, Siddiqui A. Retinoid X receptor RXR alpha binds to and trans-activates the hepatitis B virus enhancer. *Proc Natl Acad Sci U S A* 1992;89(19):9059–9063.
206. Huang J, Liang T. A novel hepatitis B virus (HBV) genetic element with rev response element-like properties that is essential for expression of HBV gene products. *Mol Cell Biol* 1993;13(12):7476–7486.
207. Huang M, Summers J. pet, a small sequence distal to the pregenome cap site, is required for expression of the duck hepatitis B virus pregenome. *J Virol* 1994;68(3):1564–1572.
208. Huang X, Lu D, Ji G, et al. Hepatitis B virus (HBV) vaccine-induced escape mutants of HBV S gene among children from Qidong area, China. *Virus Res* 2004;99(1):63–68.
209. Huang ZM, Tan T, Yoshida H, et al. Activation of hepatitis B virus S promoter by a cell type-restricted IRE1-dependent pathway induced by endoplasmic reticulum stress. *Mol Cellular Biology* 2005;25(17):7522–7533.
210. Huovila AP, Eder AM, Fuller SD. Hepatitis B surface antigen assembles in a post-ER, pre-Golgi compartment. *J Cell Biol* 1992;118(6):1305–1320.
211. Hyrina A, Jones C, Chen D, et al. A genome-wide CRISPR screen identifies ZCCHC14 as a host factor required for hepatitis B surface antigen production. *Cell Rep* 2019;29(10):2970–2978 e2976.
212. Iloeje UH, Yang HI, Su J, et al. Predicting cirrhosis risk based on the level of circulating hepatitis B viral load. *Gastroenterology* 2006;130(3):678–686.
213. Imam H, Khan M, Gokhale NS, et al. N6-methyladenosine modification of hepatitis B virus RNA differentially regulates the viral life cycle. *Proc Natl Acad Sci U S A* 2018;115(35):8829–8834.
214. Ishikawa T, Ganem D. The pre-S domain of the large viral envelope protein determines host range in avian hepatitis B viruses. *Proc Natl Acad Sci U S A* 1995;92(14):6259–6263.
215. Iwamoto M, Saso W, Sugiyama R, et al. Epidermal growth factor receptor is a host-entry cofactor triggering hepatitis B virus internalization. *Proc Natl Acad Sci U S A* 2019;116(17):8487–8492.
216. Jacob JR, Sterczer A, Toshkov IA, et al. Integration of woodchuck hepatitis and N-myc rearrangement determine size and histologic grade of hepatic tumors. *Hepatology* 2004;39(4):1008–1016.
217. Janssen HL, van Zonneveld M, Senturk H, et al. Pegylated interferon alfa-2b alone or in combination with lamivudine for HBeAg-positive chronic hepatitis B: a randomised trial. *Lancet* 2005;365(9454):123–129.
218. Jaoude GA, Sureau C. Role of the antigenic loop of the hepatitis B virus envelope proteins in infectivity of hepatitis delta virus. *J Virol* 2005;79(16):10460–10466.
219. Jaroszewicz J, Calle Serrano B, Wursthorn K, et al. Hepatitis B surface antigen (HBsAg) levels in the natural history of hepatitis B virus (HBV)-infection: a European perspective. *J Hepatol* 2010;52(4):514–522.
220. Jeong JK, Yoon GS, Ryu WS. Evidence that the 5′-end cap structure is essential for encapsidation of hepatitis B virus pregenomic RNA. *J Virol* 2000;74(12):5502–5508.
221. Jia L, Wang XW, Harris CC. Hepatitis B virus X protein inhibits nucleotide excision repair. *Int J Cancer* 1999;80(6):875–879.
222. Jiang Z, Jhunjhunwala S, Liu J, et al. The effects of hepatitis B virus integration into the genomes of hepatocellular carcinoma patients. *Genome Res* 2012;22(4):593–601.
223. Jilbert AR, Freiman JS, Gowans EJ, et al. Duck hepatitis B virus DNA in liver, spleen, and pancreas: analysis by in situ and Southern blot hybridization. *Virology* 1987;158(2):330–338.
224. Jilbert AR, Wu T-T, England JM, et al. Rapid resolution of duck hepatitis B virus infections occurs after massive hepatocellular involvement. *J Virol* 1992;66:1377–1388.
225. Jones SA, Boregowda R, Spratt TE, et al. In vitro epsilon RNA-dependent protein priming activity of human hepatitis B virus polymerase. *J Virol* 2012;86(9):5134–5150.
226. Julithe R, Abou-Jaoude G, Sureau C. Modification of the hepatitis B virus envelope protein glycosylation pattern interferes with secretion of viral particles, infectivity, and susceptibility to neutralizing antibodies. *J Virol* 2014;88(16):9049–9059.
227. Jung J, Hwang SG, Chwae YJ, et al. Phosphoacceptors threonine 162 and serines 170 and 178 within the carboxyl-terminal RRRS/T motif of the hepatitis B virus core protein make multiple contributions to hepatitis B virus replication. *J Virol* 2014;88(16):8754–8767.
228. Junker-Niepmann M, Bartenschlager R, Schaller H. A short cis-acting sequence is required for hepatitis B virus pregenome encapsidation and sufficient for packaging of foreign RNA. *EMBO J* 1990;9(10):3389–3396.
229. Jurgens MC, Voros J, Rautureau GJ, et al. The hepatitis B virus preS1 domain hijacks host trafficking proteins by motif mimicry. *Nat Chem Biol* 2013;9(9):540–547.
230. Kajino K, Jilbert AR, Saputelli J, et al. Woodchuck hepatitis virus infections: very rapid recovery after a prolonged viremia and infection of virtually every hepatocyte. *J Virol* 1994;68(9):5792–5803.
231. Kan Z, Zheng H, Liu X, et al. Whole-genome sequencing identifies recurrent mutations in hepatocellular carcinoma. *Genome Res* 2013;23(9):1422–1433.
232. Kann M, Bischof A, Gerlich WH. In vitro model for the nuclear transport of the hepadnavirus genome. *J Virol* 1997;71(2):1310–1316.
233. Kann M, Sodeik B, Vlachou A, et al. Phosphorylation-dependent binding of hepatitis B virus core particles to the nuclear pore complex. *J Cell Biol* 1999;145(1):45–55.
234. Kao JH, Wu NH, Chen PJ, et al. Hepatitis B genotypes and the response to interferon therapy. *J Hepatol* 2000;33(6):998–1002.
235. Kaplan PM, Greenman RL, Gerin JL, et al. DNA polymerase associated with human hepatitis B antigen. *J Virol* 1973;12(5):995–1005.
236. Kaplan PM, Ford EC, Purcell RH, et al. Demonstration of subpopulations of Dane particles. *J Virol* 1976;17(3):885–893.
237. Kaposi-Novak P, Libbrecht L, Woo HG, et al. Central role of c-Myc during malignant conversion in human hepatocarcinogenesis. *Cancer Res* 2009;69(7):2775–2782.
238. Karthigesu VD, Allison LM, Fortuin M, et al. A novel hepatitis B virus variant in the sera of immunized children. *J Gen Virol* 1994;75(Pt 2):443–448.
239. Katen SP, Tan Z, Chirapu SR, et al. Assembly-directed antivirals differentially bind quasi-equivalent pockets to modify hepatitis B virus capsid tertiary and quaternary structure. *Structure* 2013;21(8):1406–1416.
240. Kekule AS, Lauer U, Meyer M, et al. The preS2/S region of integrated hepatitis B virus DNA encodes a transcriptional transactivator. *Nature* 1990;343(6257):457–461.
241. Kennedy PTF, Litwin S, Dolman GE, et al. Immune tolerant chronic hepatitis B: the unrecognized risks. *Viruses* 2017;9(5):96.
242. Kian Chua P, Lin MH, Shih C. Potent inhibition of human Hepatitis B virus replication by a host factor Vps4. *Virology* 2006;354(1):1–6.
243. Kim CM, Koike K, Saito I, et al. HBx gene of hepatitis B virus induces liver cancer in transgenic mice. *Nature* 1991;351(6324):317–320.
244. Kimura T, Ohno N, Terada N, et al. Hepatitis B virus DNA-negative dane particles lack core protein but contain a 22-kDa precore protein without C-terminal arginine-rich domain. *J Biol Chem* 2005;280(23):21713–21719.
245. King RW, Ladner SK, Miller TJ, et al. Inhibition of human hepatitis B virus replication by AT-61, a phenylpropenamide derivative, alone and in combination with (−)beta-L-2′,3′-dideoxy-3′-thiacytidine [published erratum appears in Antimicrob Agents Chemother 1999 Mar;43(3):726]. *Antimicrob Agents Chemother* 1998;42(12):3179–3186.
246. Kitamura K, Que L, Shimadu M, et al. Flap endonuclease 1 is involved in cccDNA formation in the hepatitis B virus. *PLoS Pathog* 2018;14(6):e1007124.
247. Klumpp K, Lam AM, Lukacs C, et al. High-resolution crystal structure of a hepatitis B virus replication inhibitor bound to the viral core protein. *Proc Natl Acad Sci U S A* 2015;112(49):15196–15201.
248. Knolle PA, Thimme R. Hepatic immune regulation and its involvement in viral hepatitis infection. *Gastroenterology* 2014;146(5):1193–1207.
249. Ko C, Chakraborty A, Chou WM, et al. Hepatitis B virus genome recycling and de novo secondary infection events maintain stable cccDNA levels. *J Hepatol* 2018;69(6):1231–1241.

250. Kock J, Theilmann L, Galle P, et al. Hepatitis B virus nucleic acids associated with human peripheral blood mononuclear cells do not originate from replicating virus. *Hepatology* 1996;23(3):405–413.
251. Koike K, Moriya K, Iino S, et al. High-level expression of hepatitis B virus HBx gene and hepatocarcinogenesis in transgenic mice. *Hepatology* 1994;19(4):810–819.
252. Koniger C, Wingert I, Marsmann M, et al. Involvement of the host DNA-repair enzyme TDP2 in formation of the covalently closed circular DNA persistence reservoir of hepatitis B viruses. *Proc Natl Acad Sci U S A* 2014;111(40):E4244–E4253.
253. Korba BE, Cote PJ, Gerin JL. Mitogen-induced replication of woodchuck hepatitis virus in cultured peripheral blood lymphocytes. *Science* 1988;241(4870):1213–1216.
254. Korba BE, Cote PJ, Shapiro M, et al. In vitro production of infectious woodchuck hepatitis virus by lipopolysaccharide-stimulated peripheral blood lymphocytes. *J Infect Dis* 1989;160(4):572–576.
255. Korba BE, Wells FV, Baldwin B, et al. Hepatocellular carcinoma in woodchuck hepatitis virus-infected woodchucks: presence of viral DNA in tumor tissue from chronic carriers and animals serologically recovered from acute infections. *Hepatology* 1989;9(3):461–470.
256. Kornyeyev D, Ramakrishnan D, Voitenleitner C, et al. Spatiotemporal analysis of hepatitis B virus X protein in primary human hepatocytes. *J Virol* 2019;93(16):e00248-19.
257. Koukoulis G, Rayner A, Tan K-H, et al. Immunolocalization of regenerating cells after submassive liver necrosis using PCNA staining. *J Pathol* 1992;166:359–368.
258. Kuroki K, Eng F, Ishikawa T, et al. gp180, a host cell glycoprotein that binds duck hepatitis B virus particles, is encoded by a member of the carboxypeptidase gene family. *J Biol Chem* 1995;270(25):15022–15028.
259. Kusumoto S, Arcaini L, Hong X, et al. Risk of HBV reactivation in patients with B-cell lymphomas receiving obinutuzumab or rituximab immunochemotherapy. *Blood* 2019;133(2):137–146.
260. Kwee L, Lucito R, Aufiero B, et al. Alternate translation initiation on hepatitis B virus X mRNA produces multiple polypeptides that differentially transactivate class II and III promoters. *J Virol* 1992;66(7):4382–4389.
261. Lahlali T, Berke JM, Vergauwen K, et al. Novel potent capsid assembly modulators regulate multiple steps of the hepatitis B virus life cycle. *Antimicrob Agents Chemother* 2018;62(10).
262. Lai CL, Chien RN, Leung NW, et al. A one-year trial of lamivudine for chronic hepatitis B. Asia Hepatitis Lamivudine Study Group [see comments]. *N Engl J Med* 1998;339(2):61–68.
263. Lai MW, Yeh CT. The oncogenic potential of hepatitis B virus rtA181T/surface truncation mutant. *Antivir Ther* 2008;13(7):875–879.
264. Lambert C, Prange R. Chaperone action in the posttranslational topological reorientation of the hepatitis B virus large envelope protein: implications for translocational regulation. *Proc Natl Acad Sci U S A* 2003;100(9):5199–5204.
265. Lambert C, Doring T, Prange R. Hepatitis B virus maturation is sensitive to functional inhibition of ESCRT-III, Vps4, and gamma 2-adaptin. *J Virol* 2007;81(17):9050–9060.
266. Lan YT, Li J, Liao W, et al. Roles of the three major phosphorylation sites of hepatitis B virus core protein in viral replication. *Virology* 1999;259(2):342–348.
267. Lanave G, Capozza P, Diakoudi G, et al. Identification of hepadnavirus in the sera of cats. *Sci Rep* 2019;9(1):10668.
268. Lanford RE, Notvall L, Beames B. Nucleotide priming and reverse transcriptase activity of hepatitis B virus polymerase expressed in insect cells. *J Virol* 1995;69(7):4431–4439.
269. Lanford RE, Notvall L, Lee H, et al. Transcomplementation of nucleotide priming and reverse transcription between independently expressed TP and RT domains of the hepatitis B virus reverse transcriptase. *J Virol* 1997;71(4):2996–3004.
270. Lanford RE, Chavez D, Brasky KM, et al. Isolation of a hepadnavirus from the woolly monkey, a New World primate. *Proc Natl Acad Sci U S A* 1998;95(10):5757–5761.
271. Lanford RE, Kim YH, Lee H, et al. Mapping of the hepatitis B virus reverse transcriptase TP and RT domains by transcomplementation for nucleotide priming and by protein-protein interaction. *J Virol* 1999;73(3):1885–1893.
272. Lanford RE, Chavez D, Barrera A, et al. An infectious clone of woolly monkey hepatitis B virus. *J Virol* 2003;77(14):7814–7819.
273. Lau GK, Piratvisuth T, Luo KX, et al. Peginterferon Alfa-2a, lamivudine, and the combination for HBeAg-positive chronic hepatitis B. *N Engl J Med* 2005;352(26):2682–2695.
274. Lauber C, Seitz S, Mattei S, et al. Deciphering the origin and evolution of hepatitis B viruses by means of a family of non-enveloped fish viruses. *Cell Host Microbe* 2017;22(3):387–399.e386.
275. Lavanchy D. Hepatitis B virus epidemiology, disease burden, treatment, and current and emerging prevention and control measures. *J Viral Hepat* 2004;11(2):97–107.
276. Le Duff Y, Blanchet M, Sureau C. The pre-S1 and antigenic loop infectivity determinants of the hepatitis B virus envelope proteins are functionally independent. *J Virol* 2009;83(23):12443–12451.
277. Le Pogam S, Chua PK, Newman M, et al. Exposure of RNA templates and encapsidation of spliced viral RNA are influenced by the arginine-rich domain of human hepatitis B virus core antigen (HBcAg 165–173). *J Virol* 2005;79:1871–1887.
278. Le Seyec J, Chouteau P, Cannie I, et al. Infection process of the hepatitis B virus depends on the presence of defined sequence in the pre-S1 domain. *J Virol* 1999;73:2052–2057.
279. Lee JY, Culvenor JG, Angus P, et al. Duck hepatitis B virus replication in primary bile duct epithelial cells. *J Virol* 2001;75(16):7651–7661.
280. Lee PI, Chang LY, Lee CY, et al. Detection of hepatitis B surface gene mutation in carrier children with or without immunoprophylaxis at birth. *J Infect Dis* 1997;176(2):427–430.
281. Lee TH, Elledge SJ, Butel JS. Hepatitis B virus X protein interacts with a probable cellular DNA repair protein. *J Virol* 1995;69(2):1107–1114.
282. Lee WM. Hepatitis B virus infection. *N Engl J Med* 1997;337(24):1733–1745.
283. Lee WY, Bachtiar M, Choo CCS, et al. Comprehensive review of Hepatitis B Virus-associated hepatocellular carcinoma research through text mining and big data analytics. *Biol Rev Camb Philos Soc* 2019;94(2):353–367.
284. Leistner CM, Gruen-Bernhard S, Glebe D. Role of glycosaminoglycans for binding and infection of hepatitis B virus. *Cell Microbiol* 2008;10(1):122–133.
285. Lemoine M, Shimakawa Y, Njie R, et al. Acceptability and feasibility of a screen-and-treat programme for hepatitis B virus infection in The Gambia: the Prevention of Liver Fibrosis and Cancer in Africa (PROLIFICA) study. *Lancet Glob Health* 2016;4(8):e559–e567.
286. Lempp FA, Qu B, Wang YX, et al. Hepatitis B virus infection of a mouse hepatic cell line reconstituted with human sodium taurocholate cotransporting polypeptide. *J Virol* 2016;90(9):4827–4831.
287. Lempp FA, Wiedtke E, Qu B, et al. Sodium taurocholate cotransporting polypeptide is the limiting host factor of hepatitis B virus infection in macaque and pig hepatocytes. *Hepatology* 2017;66(3):703–716.
288. Lenhoff RJ, Summers J. Coordinate regulation of replication and virus assembly by the large envelope protein of an avian hepadnavirus. *J Virol* 1994;68(7):4565–4571.
289. Lenhoff RJ, Luscombe CA, Summers J. Acute liver injury following infection with a cytopathic strain of duck hepatitis B virus. *Hepatology* 1999;29(2):563–571.
290. Lentz TB, Loeb DD. Roles of the envelope proteins in the amplification of cccDNA and completion of synthesis of the plus-strand DNA in hepatitis B virus. *J Virol* 2011;85(22):11916–11927.
291. Lewellyn EB, Loeb DD. Base pairing between cis-acting sequences contributes to template switching during plus-strand DNA synthesis in human hepatitis B virus. *J Virol* 2007;81(12):6207–6215.
292. Lewellyn EB, Loeb DD. The arginine clusters of the carboxy-terminal domain of the core protein of hepatitis B virus make pleiotropic contributions to genome replication. *J Virol* 2011;85(3):1298–1309.
293. Li HC, Huang EY, Su PY, et al. Nuclear export and import of human hepatitis B virus capsid protein and particles. *PLoS Pathog* 2010;28:e1001162.
294. Li J-S, Tong S-P, Wen Y-M, et al. Hepatitis B virus genotype A rarely circulates as an HBe-minus mutant: possible contribution of a single nucleotide in the precore region. *J Virol* 1993;67:5402–5410.
295. Li M, Sohn JA, Seeger C. Distribution of hepatitis B virus nuclear DNA. *J Virol* 2017;92(1):e01391-17.
296. Li T, Chen X, Garbutt KC, et al. Structure of DDB1 in complex with a paramyxovirus V protein: viral hijack of a propeller cluster in ubiquitin ligase. *Cell* 2006;124:105–117.
297. Li T, Robert EI, van Breugel PC, et al. A promiscuous alpha-helical motif anchors viral hijackers and substrate receptors to the CUL4-DDB1 ubiquitin ligase machinery. *Nat Struct Mol Biol* 2010;17(1):105–111.
298. Li W. The hepatitis B virus receptor. *Annu Rev Cell Dev Biol* 2015;31:125–147.
299. Liao W, Ou JH. Phosphorylation and nuclear localization of the hepatitis B virus core protein: significance of serine in the three repeated SPRRR motifs. *J Virol* 1995;69(2):1025–1029.
300. Liaw YF, Sung JJ, Chow WC, et al. Lamivudine for patients with chronic hepatitis B and advanced liver disease. *N Engl J Med* 2004;351(15):1521–1531.
301. Liaw YF, Raptopoulou-Gigi M, Cheinquer H, et al. Efficacy and safety of entecavir versus adefovir in chronic hepatitis B patients with hepatic decompensation: a randomized open-label study. *Hepatology* 2011;54(1):91–100.
302. Liaw YF, Sheen IS, Lee CM, et al. Tenofovir disoproxil fumarate (TDF), emtricitabine/TDF, and entecavir in patients with decompensated chronic hepatitis B liver disease. *Hepatology* 2011;53(1):62–72.
303. Lien JM, Aldrich CE, Mason WS. Evidence that a capped oligoribonucleotide is the primer for duck hepatitis B virus plus-strand DNA synthesis. *J Virol* 1986;57(1):229–236.
304. Lien JM, Petcu DJ, Aldrich CE, et al. Initiation and termination of duck hepatitis B virus DNA synthesis during virus maturation. *J Virol* 1987;61(12):3832–3840.
305. Lin CG, Lo SJ. Evidence for involvement of a ribosomal leaky scanning mechanism in the translation of the hepatitis B virus pol gene from the viral pregenome RNA. *Virology* 1992;188(1):342–352.
306. Lin CL, Kao JH. Hepatitis B virus genotypes and variants. *Cold Spring Harb Perspect Med* 2015;5(5):a021436.
307. Lindh M, Hannoun C, Dhillon AP, et al. Core promoter mutations and genotypes in relation to viral replication and liver damage in East Asian hepatitis B virus carriers. *J Infect Dis* 1999;179(4):775–782.
308. Lindh M, Horal P, Dhillon AP, et al. Hepatitis B virus DNA levels, precore mutations, genotypes and histological activity in chronic hepatitis B. *J Viral Hepat* 2000;7(4):258–267.
309. Liu N, Tian R, Loeb DD. Base pairing among three cis-acting sequences contributes to template switching during hepadnavirus reverse transcription. *Proc Natl Acad Sci U S A* 2003;100(4):1984–1989.
310. Loeb DD, Gulya KJ, Tian R. Sequence identity of the terminal redundancies on the minus-strand DNA template is necessary but not sufficient for the template switch during hepadnavirus plus-strand DNA synthesis. *J Virol* 1997;71(1):152–160.
311. Loeb DL, Hirsch RC, Ganem D. Sequence-independent RNA cleavages generate the primers for plus strand DNA synthesis in hepatitis B viruses: implications for other reverse transcribing elements. *EMBO J* 1991;10:3533–3540.
312. Lok AS, McMahon BJ. Chronic hepatitis B: update 2009. *Hepatology* 2009;50(3):661–662.
313. Long Q, Yan R, Hu J, et al. The role of host DNA ligases in hepadnavirus covalently closed circular DNA formation. *PLoS Pathog* 2017;13(12):e1006784.
314. Lucifora J, Arzberger S, Durantel D, et al. Hepatitis B virus X protein is essential to initiate and maintain virus replication after infection. *J Hepatol* 2011;55(5):996–1003.
315. Lucifora J, Xia Y, Reisinger F, et al. Specific and nonhepatotoxic degradation of nuclear hepatitis B virus cccDNA. *Science* 2014;343(6176):1221–1228.
316. Ludgate L, Ning X, Nguyen DH, et al. Cyclin-dependent kinase 2 phosphorylates S/T-P sites in hepadnavirus core protein C-terminal domain and is incorporated into viral capsids. *J Virol* 2012;86(22):12237–12250.
317. Ludgate L, Liu K, Luckenbaugh L, et al. Cell-free hepatitis B virus capsid assembly dependent on the core protein C-terminal domain and regulated by phosphorylation. *J Virol* 2016;90(12):5830–5844.
318. Luo J, Cui X, Gao L, et al. Identification of an intermediate in hepatitis B virus covalently closed circular (CCC) DNA formation and sensitive and selective CCC DNA detection. *J Virol* 2017;91(17):e00539-17.
319. Luscombe C, Pedersen J, Uren E, et al. Long-term ganciclovir chemotherapy for congenital duck hepatitis B virus infection in vivo: effect on intrahepatic-viral DNA, RNA, and protein expression. *Hepatology* 1996;24:766–773.

320. Lutgehetmann M, Volz T, Kopke A, et al. In vivo proliferation of hepadnavirus-infected hepatocytes induces loss of covalently closed circular DNA in mice. *Hepatology* 2010;52(1):16–24.
321. Lutwick LI, Robinson WS. DNA synthesized in the hepatitis B Dane particle DNA polymerase reaction. *J Virol* 1977;21(1):96–104.
322. MacDonald RA. "Lifespan" of liver cells. *Arch Intern Med* 1960;107:335–343.
323. Macovei A, Petrareanu C, Lazar C, et al. Regulation of hepatitis B virus infection by Rab5, Rab7, and the endolysosomal compartment. *J Virol* 2013;87(11):6415–6427.
324. Madden CR, Finegold MJ, Slagle BL. Hepatitis B virus X protein acts as a tumor promoter in development of diethylnitrosamine-induced preneoplastic lesions. *J Virol* 2001;75(8):3851–3858.
325. Magnius L, Mason WS, Taylor J, et al. ICTV virus taxonomy profile: *Hepadnaviridae*. *J Gen Virol* 2020;101(6):571–572.
326. Mak LY, Seto WK, Fung J, et al. New biomarkers of chronic hepatitis B. *Gut Liver* 2019;13(6):589–595.
327. Mani N, Cole AG, Phelps JR, et al. Preclinical profile of AB-423, an inhibitor of hepatitis B virus pregenomic RNA encapsidation. *Antimicrob Agents Chemother* 2018;62(6):e00082-18.
328. Maquire ML, Loeb DD. cis-Acting sequences that contribute to synthesis of minus-strand DNA are not conserved between hepadnaviruses. *J Virol* 2010;84:12824–12831.
329. Marcellin P, Chang TT, Lim SG, et al. Adefovir dipivoxil for the treatment of hepatitis B e antigen-positive chronic hepatitis B. *N Engl J Med* 2003;348(9):808–816.
330. Marion PL, Salazar FH, Alexander JJ, et al. Polypeptides of hepatitis B virus surface antigen produced by a hepatoma cell line. *J Virol* 1979;32(3):796–802.
331. Marion PL, Oshiro LS, Regnery DC, et al. A virus in Beechey ground squirrels that is related to hepatitis B virus of humans. *Proc Natl Acad Sci U S A* 1980;77(5):2941–2945.
332. Marion PL, Van DM, Knight SS, et al. Hepatocellular carcinoma in ground squirrels persistently infected with ground squirrel hepatitis virus. *Proc Natl Acad Sci U S A* 1986;83(12):4543–4546.
333. Marion PL, Popper H, Azcarraga RR, et al. Ground squirrel hepatitis virus and hepatocellular carcinoma. In: Robinson W, Koike K, Will H, eds. *Hepadnaviruses*. New York: A.R. Liss, Inc.; 1987:337–348.
334. Marongiu F, Doratiotto S, Montisci S, et al. Liver repopulation and carcinogenesis: two sides of the same coin? *Am J Pathol* 2008;172:857–864.
335. Mason WS, Seal G, Summers J. Virus of Pekin ducks with structural and biological relatedness to human hepatitis B virus. *J Virol* 1980;36(3):829–836.
336. Mason WS, Jilbert AR, Summers J. Clonal expansion of hepatocytes during chronic woodchuck hepatitis virus infection. *Proc Natl Acad Sci U S A* 2005;102:1139–1144.
337. Mason WS, Xu C, Low HC, et al. The amount of hepatocyte turnover that occurred during resolution of transient hepadnavirus infections was lower when virus replication was inhibited with entecavir. *J Virol* 2009;83(4):1778–1789.
338. Mason WS, Gill US, Litwin S, et al. HBV DNA Integration and clonal hepatocyte expansion in chronic hepatitis B patients considered immune tolerant. *Gastroenterology* 2016;151(5):986–998.e984.
339. Mast EE, Alter MJ, Margolis HS. Strategies to prevent and control hepatitis B and C virus infections: a global perspective. *Vaccine* 1999;17(13–14):1730–1733.
340. Maupas P, Werner B, Larouze B, et al. Antibody to hepatitis-B core antigen in patients with primary hepatic carcinoma. *Lancet* 1975;2(7923):9–11.
341. Maynard M, Parvaz P, Durantel S, et al. Sustained HBs seroconversion during lamivudine and adefovir dipivoxil combination therapy for lamivudine failure. *J Hepatol* 2005;42(2):279–281.
342. Meuleman P, Libbrecht L, Wieland S, et al. Immune suppression uncovers endogenous cytopathic effects of the hepatitis B virus. *J Virol* 2006;80(6):2797–2807.
343. Michalak TI, Pardoe IU, Coffin CS, et al. Occult lifelong persistence of infectious hepadnavirus and residual liver inflammation in woodchucks convalescent from acute viral hepatitis. *Hepatology* 1999;29(3):928–938.
344. Miller RH, Robinson WS. Hepatitis B virus DNA in nuclear and cytoplasmic fractions of infected human liver. *Virology* 1984;137:390–399.
345. Miller RH, Tran CT, Robinson WS. Hepatitis B virus particles of plasma and liver contain viral DNA-RNA hybrid molecules. *Virology* 1984;139(1):53–63.
346. Minuk GY, Shaffer EA, Hoar DI, et al. Ground squirrel hepatitis virus (GSHV) infection and hepatocellular carcinoma in the Canadian Richardson ground squirrel (Spermophilus richardsonii). *Liver* 1986;6(6):350–356.
347. Molnar-Kimber KL, Summers JW, Mason WS. Mapping of the cohesive overlap of duck hepatitis B virus DNA and of the site of initiation of reverse transcription. *J Virol* 1984;51(1):181–191.
348. Moraleda G, Saputelli J, Aldrich CE, et al. Lack of effect of Antiviral Therapy in nondividing hepatocyte cultures on the closed circular DNA of woodchuck hepatitis virus. *J Virol* 1997;71(12):9392–9399.
349. Mueller H, Wildum S, Luangsay S, et al. A novel orally available small molecule that inhibits hepatitis B virus expression. *J Hepatol* 2018;68(3):412–420.
350. Mueller H, Lopez A, Tropberger P, et al. PAPD5/7 are host factors that are required for hepatitis B virus RNA stabilization. *Hepatology* 2019;69(4):1398–1411.
351. Mueller-Hill K, Loeb DD. cis-Acting sequences 5E, M, and 3E interact to contribute to primer translocation and circularization during reverse transcription of avian hepadnavirus DNA. *J Virol* 2002;76(9):4260–4266.
352. Murakami Y, Saigo K, Takashima H, et al. Large scaled analysis of hepatitis B virus (HBV) DNA integration in HBV related hepatocellular carcinomas. *Gut* 2005;54(8):1162–1168.
353. Murphy CM, Xu Y, Li F, et al. Hepatitis B virus X protein promotes degradation of SMC5/6 to enhance HBV replication. *Cell Rep* 2016;16(11):2846–2854.
354. Murray JM, Wieland SF, Purcell RH, et al. Dynamics of hepatitis B virus clearance in chimpanzees. *Proc Natl Acad Sci U S A* 2005;102(49):17780–17785.
355. Mushahwar IK, Overby LR, Frosner G, et al. Prevalence of hepatitis B e antigen and its antibody as detected by radioimmunoassays. *J Med Virol* 1978;2(2):77–87.
356. Mutz P, Metz P, Lempp FA, et al. HBV bypasses the innate immune response and does not protect HCV from antiviral activity of interferon. *Gastroenterology* 2018;154(6):1791–1804.e1722.
357. Nakamoto Y, Guidotti LG, Kuhlen CV, et al. Immune pathogenesis of hepatocellular carcinoma. *J Exp Med* 1998;188(2):341–350.
358. Nakamoto Y, Kaneko S, Fan H, et al. Prevention of hepatocellular carcinoma development associated with chronic hepatitis by anti-fas ligand antibody therapy. *J Exp Med* 2002;196(8):1105–1111.
359. Nassal M, Junker-Niepmann M, Schaller H. Translational inactivation of RNA function: discrimination against a subset of genomic transcripts during HBV nucleocapsid assembly. *Cell* 1990;63(6):1357–1363.
360. Newbold JE, Xin H, Tencza M, et al. The covalently closed duplex form of the hepadnavirus genome exists in situ as a heterogeneous population of viral minichromosomes. *J Virol* 1995;69(6):3350–3357.
361. Newsome PN, Hussain MA, Theise ND. Hepatic oval cells: helping redefine a paradigm in stem cell biology. *Curr Top Dev Biol* 2004;61:1–28.
362. Nguyen DH, Gummuluru S, Hu J. Deamination-independent inhibition of hepatitis B virus reverse transcription by APOBEC3G. *J Virol* 2007;81(9):4465–4472.
363. Nguyen DH, Hu J. Reverse transcriptase- and RNA packaging signal-dependent incorporation of APOBEC3G into hepatitis B virus nucleocapsids. *J Virol* 2008;82(14):6852–6861.
364. Nguyen T, Thompson AJ, Bowden S, et al. Hepatitis B surface antigen levels during the natural history of chronic hepatitis B: a perspective on Asia. *J Hepatol* 2010;52(4):508–513.
365. Ni Y, Sonnabend J, Seitz S, et al. The pre-s2 domain of the hepatitis B virus is dispensable for infectivity but serves a spacer function for L-protein-connected virus assembly. *J Virol* 2010;84(8):3879–3888.
366. Ni Y, Lempp FA, Mehrle S, et al. Hepatitis B and D viruses exploit sodium taurocholate co-transporting polypeptide for species-specific entry into hepatocytes. *Gastroenterology* 2014;146(4):1070–1083.
367. Nicoll AJ, Angus PW, Chou ST, et al. Demonstration of duck hepatitis B virus in bile duct epithelial cells: implications for pathogenesis and persistent infection. *Hepatology* 1997;25(2):463–469.
368. Nie FY, Tian JH, Lin XD, et al. Discovery of a highly divergent hepadnavirus in shrews from China. *Virology* 2019;531:162–170.
369. Niederau C, Heintges T, Lange S, et al. Long-term follow-up of HBeAg-positive patients treated with interferon alfa for chronic hepatitis B. *N Engl J Med* 1996;334(22):1422–1427.
370. Ning X, Nguyen D, Mentzer L, et al. Secretion of genome-free hepatitis B virus—single strand blocking model for virion morphogenesis of para-retrovirus. *PLoS Pathog* 2011;7(9):e1002255.
371. Ning X, Basagoudanavar SH, Liu K, et al. Capsid phosphorylation state and hepadnavirus virion secretion. *J Virol* 2017;91(9):e00092-17.
372. Ning X, Luckenbaugh L, Liu K, et al. Common and distinct capsid and surface protein requirements for secretion of complete and genome-free hepatitis B virions. *J Virol* 2018;92(14):e00272-18.
373. Niu C, Livingston CM, Li L, et al. The Smc5/6 complex restricts HBV when localized to ND10 without inducing an innate immune response and is counteracted by the HBV X protein shortly after infection. *PLoS One* 2017;12(1):e0169648.
374. Norder H, Courouce AM, Coursaget P, et al. Genetic diversity of hepatitis B virus strains derived worldwide: genotypes, subgenotypes, and HBsAg subtypes. *Intervirology* 2004;47(6):289–309.
375. Nowak MA, Bonhoeffer S, Hill AM, et al. Viral dynamics in hepatitis B virus infection. *Proc Natl Acad Sci U S A* 1996;93(9):4398–4402.
376. Obert S, Zachmann BB, Deindl E, et al. A splice hepadnavirus RNA that is essential for virus replication. *EMBO J* 1996;15(10):2565–2574.
377. Okamoto H, Yano K, Nozaki Y, et al. Mutations within the S gene of hepatitis B virus transmitted from mothers to babies immunized with hepatitis B immune globulin and vaccine. *Pediatr Res* 1992;32(3):264–268.
378. Okamoto H, Tsuda F, Akahane Y, et al. Hepatitis B virus with mutations in the core promoter for an e antigen-negative phenotype in carriers with antibody to e antigen. *J Virol* 1994;68(12):8102–8110.
379. Oon CJ, Lim GK, Ye Z, et al. Molecular epidemiology of hepatitis B virus vaccine variants in Singapore. *Vaccine* 1995;13(8):699–702.
380. Oon CJ, Chen WN, Koh S, et al. Identification of hepatitis B surface antigen variants with alterations outside the "a" determinant in immunized Singapore infants. *J Infect Dis* 1999;179:259–263.
381. Ostapchuk P, Hearing P, Ganem D. A dramatic shift in the transmembrane topology of a viral envelope glycoprotein accompanies hepatitis B viral morphogenesis. *EMBO J* 1994;13(5):1048–1057.
382. Ostrow KM, Loeb DD. Characterization of the cis-acting contributions to avian hepadnavirus RNA encapsidation. *J Virol* 2002;76(18):9087–9095.
383. Ou JH, Laub O, Rutter WJ. Hepatitis B virus gene function: the precore region targets the core antigen to cellular membranes and causes the secretion of the e antigen. *Proc Natl Acad Sci U S A* 1986;83(6):1578–1582.
384. Pagliaccetti NE, Chu EN, Bolen CR, et al. Lambda and alpha interferons inhibit hepatitis B virus replication through a common molecular mechanism but with different in vivo activities. *Virology* 2010;401(2):197–206.
385. Pairan A, Bruss V. Functional surfaces of the hepatitis B virus capsid. *J Virol* 2009;83(22):11616–11623.
386. Papatheodoridis GV, Petraki K, Cholongitas E, et al. Impact of interferon-alpha therapy on liver fibrosis progression in patients with HBeAg-negative chronic hepatitis B. *J Viral Hepat* 2005;12(2):199–206.
387. Parekh S, Zoulim F, Ahn SH, et al. Genome replication, virion secretion, and e antigen expression of naturally occurring hepatitis B virus core promoter mutants. *J Virol* 2003;77(12):6601–6612.
388. Pasquetto V, Wieland SF, Uprichard SL, et al. Cytokine-sensitive replication of hepatitis B virus in immortalized mouse hepatocyte cultures. *J Virol* 2002;76(11):5646–5653.
389. Patient R, Hourioux C, Sizaret PY, et al. Hepatitis B virus subviral envelope particle morphogenesis and intracellular trafficking. *J Virol* 2007;81(8):3842–3851.
390. Patzer EJ, Nakamura GR, Yaffe A. Intracellular transport and secretion of hepatitis B surface antigen in mammalian cells. *J Virol* 1984;51(2):346–353.

391. Payne GS, Bishop JM, Varmus HE. Multiple arrangements of viral DNA and an activated host oncogene in bursal lymphomas. *Nature* 1982;295:209–214.
392. Perlman DH, Berg EA, O'Connor PB, et al. Reverse transcription-associated dephosphorylation of hepadnavirus nucleocapsids. *Proc Natl Acad Sci U S A* 2005;102:9020–9025.
393. Perrillo R, Rakela J, Dienstag J, et al. Multicenter study of lamivudine therapy for hepatitis B after liver transplantation. Lamivudine Transplant Group. *Hepatology* 1999;29(5):1581–1586.
394. Perrillo RP, Chau KH, Overby LR, et al. Anti-hepatitis B core immunoglobulin M in the serologic evaluation of hepatitis B virus infection and simultaneous infection with type B, delta agent, and non-A, non-B viruses. *Gastroenterology* 1983;85(1):163–167.
395. Persing DH, Varmus HE, Ganem D. Inhibition of secretion of hepatitis B surface antigen by a related presurface polypeptide. *Science* 1986;234(4782):1388–1391.
396. Persing DH, Varmus HE, Ganem D. The preS1 protein of hepatitis B virus is acylated at its amino terminus with myristic acid. *J Virol* 1987;61(5):1672–1677.
397. Persson B, Argos P. Prediction of transmembrane segments in proteins utilising multiple sequence alignments. *J Mol Biol* 1994;237(2):182–192.
398. Petersen J, Dandri M, Mier W, et al. Prevention of hepatitis B virus infection in vivo by entry inhibitors derived from the large envelope protein. *Nat Biotechnol* 2008;26(3):335–341.
399. Petroski MD, Deshaies RJ. Function and regulation of cullin-RING ubiquitin ligases. *Nat Rev Mol Cell Biol* 2005;6(1):9–20.
400. Piasecki T, Harkins GW, Chrzastek K, et al. Avihepadnavirus diversity in parrots is comparable to that found amongst all other avian species. *Virology* 2013;438(2):98–105.
401. Ponzetto A, Cote PJ, Ford EC, et al. Core antigen and antibody in woodchucks after infection with woodchuck hepatitis virus. *J Virol* 1984;52(1):70–76.
402. Porter BF, Goens SD, Brasky KM, et al. A case report of hepatocellular carcinoma and focal nodular hyperplasia with a myelolipoma in two chimpanzees and a review of spontaneous hepatobiliary tumors in non-human primates. *J Med Primatol* 2004;33(1):38–47.
403. Prange R, Streeck RE. Novel transmembrane topology of the hepatitis B virus envelope proteins. *EMBO J* 1995;14(2):247–256.
404. Prassolov A, Hohenberg H, Kalinina T, et al. New hepatitis B virus of cranes that has an unexpected broad host range. *J Virol* 2003;77(3):1964–1976.
405. Prince AM, Szmuness W, Michon J, et al. A case/control study of the association between primary liver cancer and hepatitis B infection in Senegal. *Int J Cancer* 1975;16(3):376–383.
406. Prince AM, Ikram H, Hopp TP. Hepatitis B virus vaccine: identification of HBsAg/a and HBsAg/d but not HBsAg/y subtype antigenic determinants on a synthetic immunogenic peptide. *Proc Natl Acad Sci U S A* 1982;79:579–582.
407. Pugh JC, Sninsky JJ, Summers JW, et al. Characterization of a pre-S polypeptide on the surfaces of infectious avian hepadnavirus particles. *J Virol* 1987;61(5):1384–1390.
408. Pult I, Netter HJ, Bruns M, et al. Identification and analysis of a new hepadnavirus in white storks. *Virology* 2001;289(1):114–128.
409. Qi Y, Gao Z, Xu G, et al. DNA polymerase kappa is a key cellular factor for the formation of covalently closed circular DNA of hepatitis B virus. *PLoS Pathog* 2016;12(10):e1005893.
410. Quignon F, Renard CA, Tiollais P, et al. A functional N-myc2 retroposon in ground squirrels: implications for hepadnavirus-associated carcinogenesis. *Oncogene* 1996;12(9):2011–2017.
411. Rabe B, Vlachou A, Pante N, et al. Nuclear import of hepatitis B virus capsids and release of the viral genome. *Proc Natl Acad Sci U S A* 2003;100(17):9849–9854.
412. Rabe B, Delaleau M, Bischof A, et al. Nuclear entry of hepatitis B virus capsids involves disintegration to protein dimers followed by nuclear reassociation to capsids. *PLoS Pathog* 2009;5(8):e1000563.
413. Raimondo G, Locarnini S, Pollicino T, et al. Update of the statements on biology and clinical impact of occult hepatitis B virus infection. *J Hepatol* 2019;71(2):397–408.
414. Rajoriya N, Combet C, Zoulim F, et al. How viral genetic variants and genotypes influence disease and treatment outcome of chronic hepatitis B. Time for an individualised approach?. *J Hepatol* 2017;67(6):1281–1297.
415. Ramakrishnan D, Xing W, Beran RK, et al. Hepatitis B virus X protein function requires zinc binding. *J Virol* 2019;93(16):e00250-19.
416. Raney AK, Eggers CM, Kline EF, et al. Nuclear covalently closed circular viral genomic DNA in the liver of hepatocyte nuclear factor 1 alpha-null hepatitis B virus transgenic mice. *J Virol* 2001;75(6):2900–2911.
417. Rasche A, Lehmann F, Konig A, et al. Highly diversified shrew hepatitis B viruses corroborate ancient origins and divergent infection patterns of mammalian hepadnaviruses. *Proc Natl Acad Sci U S A* 2019;116(34):17007–17012.
418. Reaiche-Miller GY, Thorpe M, Low HC, et al. Duck hepatitis B virus covalently closed circular DNA appears to survive hepatocyte mitosis in the growing liver. *Virology* 2013;446(1–2):357–364.
419. Realdi G, Fattovich G, Hadziyannis S, et al. Survival and prognostic factors in 366 patients with compensated cirrhosis type B: a multicenter study. The Investigators of the European Concerted Action on Viral Hepatitis (EUROHEP). *J Hepatol* 1994;21(4):656–666.
420. Rehermann B, Lau D, Hoofnagle JH, et al. Cytotoxic T lymphocyte responsiveness after resolution of chronic hepatitis B virus infection. *J Clin Investig* 1996;97(7):1655–1665.
421. Rehermann B, Thimme R. Insights from antiviral therapy into immune responses to hepatitis B and C virus infection. *Gastroenterology* 2019;156(2):369–383.
422. Rigg RJ, Schaller H. Duck hepatitis B virus infection of hepatocytes is not dependent on low pH. *J Virol* 1992;66(5):2829–2836.
423. Riviere L, Gerossier L, Ducroux A, et al. HBx relieves chromatin-mediated transcriptional repression of hepatitis B viral cccDNA involving SETDB1 histone methyltransferase. *J Hepatol* 2015;63(5):1093–1102.
424. Rizzetto M, Tassopoulos NC, Goldin RD, et al. Extended lamivudine treatment in patients with HBeAg-negative chronic hepatitis B. *J Hepatol* 2005;42(2):173–179.
425. Robek MD, Boyd BS, Wieland SF, et al. Signal transduction pathways that inhibit hepatitis B virus replication. *Proc Natl Acad Sci U S A* 2004;101(6):1743–1747.
426. Robinson WS, Clayton DA, Greenman RL. DNA of a human hepatitis B virus candidate. *J Virol* 1974;14(2):384–391.
427. Robinson WS, Greenman RL. DNA polymerase in the core of the human hepatitis B virus candidate. *J Virol* 1974;13(6):1231–1236.
428. Rockey DC. Antifibrotic therapy in chronic liver disease. *Clin Gastroenterol Hepatol* 2005;3(2):95–107.
429. Rogler CE, Chisari FV. Cellular and molecular mechanisms of hepatocarcinogenesis. *Semin Liver Dis* 1992;12(3):265–278.
430. Rosler C, Kock J, Malim MH, et al. Comment on "Inhibition of hepatitis B virus replication by APOBEC3G". *Science* 2004;305(5689):1403; author reply 1403.
431. Rosler C, Kock J, Kann M, et al. APOBEC-mediated interference with hepadnavirus production. *Hepatology* 2005;42(2):301–309.
432. Rost M, Mann S, Lambert C, et al. Gamma-adaptin, a novel ubiquitin-interacting adaptor, and Nedd4 ubiquitin ligase control hepatitis B virus maturation. *J Biol Chem* 2006;281(39):29297–29308.
433. Russnak RH. Regulation of polyadenylation in hepatitis B viruses: stimulation by the upstream activating signal PS1 is orientation-dependent, distance-independent, and additive. *Nucleic Acids Res* 1991;19(23):6449–6456.
434. Sakamoto Y, Yamada G, Mizuno M, et al. Full and empty particles of hepatitis B virus in hepatocytes from patients with HBsAg-positive chronic active hepatitis. *Lab Invest* 1983;48(6):678–682.
435. Salimzadeh L, Le Bert N, Dutertre CA, et al. PD-1 blockade partially recovers dysfunctional virus-specific B cells in chronic hepatitis B infection. *J Clin Invest* 2018;128(10):4573–4587.
436. Salisse J, Sureau C. A function essential to viral entry underlies the hepatitis B virus "a" determinant. *J Virol* 2009;83(18):9321–9328.
437. Salpini R, Piermatteo L, Battisti A, et al. A hyper-glycosylation of HBV surface antigen correlates with HBsAg-negativity at immunosuppression-driven HBV reactivation in vivo and hinders HBsAg recognition in vitro. *Viruses* 2020;12(2):251.
438. Schaefer S. Hepatitis B virus taxonomy and hepatitis B virus genotypes. *World J Gastroenterol* 2007;13(1):14–21.
439. Schiff ER, Lai CL, Hadziyannis S, et al. Adefovir dipivoxil therapy for lamivudine-resistant hepatitis B in pre- and post-liver transplantation patients. *Hepatology* 2003;38(6):1419–1427.
440. Schillie S, Vellozzi C, Reingold A, et al. Prevention of hepatitis B virus infection in the United States: recommendations of the Advisory Committee on Immunization Practices. *MMWR Recomm Rep* 2018;67(1):1–31.
441. Schlicht HJ, Radziwill G, Schaller H. Synthesis and encapsidation of duck hepatitis B virus reverse transcriptase do not require formation of core-polymerase fusion proteins. *Cell* 1989;56(1):85–92.
442. Schluter V, Meyer M, Hofschneider PH, et al. Integrated hepatitis B virus X and 3' truncated preS/S sequences derived from human hepatomas encode functionally active transactivators. *Oncogene* 1994;9(11):3335–3344.
443. Schmitt S, Glebe D, Alving K, et al. Analysis of the pre-S2 N- and O-linked glycans of the M surface protein from human hepatitis B virus. *J Biol Chem* 1999;274(17):11945–11957.
444. Schmitt S, Glebe D, Tolle TK, et al. Structure of pre-S2 N- and O-linked glycans in surface proteins from different genotypes of hepatitis B virus. *J Gen Virol* 2004;85 (Pt 7):2045–2053.
445. Schmitz A, Schwarz A, Foss M, et al. Nucleoporin 153 arrests the nuclear import of hepatitis B virus capsids in the nuclear basket. *PLoS Pathog* 2010;6(1):e1000741.
446. Schultz U, Chisari FV. Recombinant duck interferon gamma inhibits duck hepatitis B virus replication in primary hepatocytes. *J Virol* 1999;73(4):3162–3168.
447. Schultz U, Summers J, Staeheli P, et al. Elimination of duck hepatitis B virus RNA-containing capsids in duck interferon-alpha-treated hepatocytes. *J Virol* 1999;73(7):5459–5465.
448. Schulze A, Gripon P, Urban S. Hepatitis B virus infection initiates with a large surface protein-dependent binding to heparan sulfate proteoglycans. *Hepatology* 2007;46(6):1759–1768.
449. Seeger C, Ganem D, Varmus HE. Nucleotide sequence of an infectious molecularly cloned genome of ground squirrel hepatitis virus. *J Virol* 1984;51(2):367–375.
450. Seeger C, Ganem D, Varmus HE. The cloned genome of ground squirrel hepatitis virus is infectious in the animal. *Proc Natl Acad Sci U S A* 1984;81(18):5849–5852.
451. Seeger C, Ganem D, Varmus HE. Biochemical and genetic evidence for the hepatitis B virus replication strategy. *Science* 1986;232(4749):477–484.
452. Seeger C, Baldwin B, Hornbuckle WE, et al. Woodchuck hepatitis virus is a more efficient oncogenic agent than ground squirrel hepatitis virus in a common host. *J Virol* 1991;65(4):1673–1679.
453. Seitz S, Urban S, Antoni C, et al. Cryo-electron microscopy of hepatitis B virions reveals variability in envelope capsid interactions. *EMBO J* 2007;26(18):4160–4167.
454. Seki S, Sakaguchi H, Kawakita N, et al. Detection of proliferating liver cells in various diseases by a monoclonal antibody against DNA polymerase-alpha: with special reference to the relationship between hepatocytes and sinusoidal cells. *Hepatology* 1991;14:781–788.
455. Shafritz DA, Shouval D, Sherman HI, et al. Integration of hepatitis B virus DNA into the genome of liver cells in chronic liver disease and hepatocellular carcinoma. Studies in percutaneous liver biopsies and post-mortem tissue specimens. *N Engl J Med* 1981;305(18):1067–1073.
456. Sherlock S, Fox RA, Niazi SP, et al. Chronic liver disease and primary liver-cell cancer with hepatitis-associated (Australia) antigen in serum. *Lancet* 1970;1(7659):1243–1247.
457. Short JM, Chen S, Roseman AM, et al. Structure of hepatitis B surface antigen from subviral tubes determined by electron cryomicroscopy. *J Mol Biol* 2009;390(1):135–141.
458. Siddiqui A, Jameel S, Mapoles J. Expression of the hepatitis B virus X gene in mammalian cells. *Proc Natl Acad Sci U S A* 1987;84(8):2513–2517.
459. Sitia G, Isogawa M, Iannacone M, et al. MMPs are required for recruitment of antigen-nonspecific mononuclear cells into the liver by CTLs. *J Clin Investig* 2004;113(8):1158–1167.
460. Sitterlin D, Bergametti F, Transy C. UVDDB p127-binding modulates activities and intracellular distribution of hepatitis B virus X protein. *Oncogene* 2000;19(38):4417–4426.
461. Slagle BL, Lee TH, Medina D, et al. Increased sensitivity to the hepatocarcinogen diethylnitrosamine in transgenic mice carrying the hepatitis B virus X gene. *Mol Carcinog* 1996;15(4):261–269.
462. Slagle BL, Bouchard MJ. Hepatitis B virus X and regulation of viral gene expression. *Cold Spring Harb Perspect Med* 2016;6(3):a021402.

463. Slagle BL, Bouchard MJ. Role of HBx in hepatitis B virus persistence and its therapeutic implications. *Curr Opin Virol* 2018;30:32–38.
464. Snow-Lampart A, Chappell B, Curtis M, et al. No resistance to tenofovir disoproxil fumarate detected after up to 144 weeks of therapy in patients monoinfected with chronic hepatitis B virus. *Hepatology* 2011;53(3):763–773.
465. Sohn JA, Litwin S, Seeger C. Mechanism for CCC DNA synthesis in hepadnaviruses. *PLoS One* 2009;4(11):e8093.
466. Spandau DF, Lee C-H. Trans-activation of viral enhancers by the hepatitis B virus X protein. *J Virol* 1988;62:427–434.
467. Spreafico M, Berzuini A, Foglieni B, et al. Poor efficacy of nucleic acid testing in identifying occult HBV infection and consequences for safety of blood supply in Italy. *J Hepatol* 2015;63(5):1068–1076.
468. Sprengel R, Kaleta EF, Will H. Isolation and characterization of a hepatitis B virus endemic in herons. *J Virol* 1988;62:932–937.
469. Stahl M, Beck J, Nassal M. Chaperones activate hepadnavirus reverse transcriptase by transiently exposing a C-proximal region in the terminal protein domain that contributes to epsilon RNA binding. *J Virol* 2007;81(24):13354–13364.
470. Stahl M, Retzlaff M, Nassal M, et al. Chaperone activation of the hepadnaviral reverse transcriptase for template RNA binding is established by the Hsp70 and stimulated by the Hsp90 system. *Nucleic Acids Res* 2007;35(18):6124–6136.
471. Stanaway JD, Flaxman AD, Naghavi M, et al. The global burden of viral hepatitis from 1990 to 2013: findings from the Global Burden of Disease Study 2013. *Lancet* 2016;388(10049):1081–1088.
472. Standring DN, Ou JH, Masiarz FR, et al. A signal peptide encoded within the precore region of hepatitis B virus directs the secretion of a heterogeneous population of e antigens in Xenopus oocytes. *Proc Natl Acad Sci U S A* 1988;85(22):8405–8409.
473. Staprans S, Loeb DD, Ganem D. Mutations affecting hepadnavirus plus-strand DNA synthesis dissociate primer cleavage from translocation and reveal the origin of linear viral DNA. *J Virol* 1991;65(3):1255–1262.
474. Stevens CE, Neurath RA, Beasley RP, et al. HBeAg and anti-HBe detection by radioimmunoassay: correlation with vertical transmission of hepatitis B virus in Taiwan. *J Med Virol* 1979;3(3):237–241.
475. Stirk HJ, Thornton JM, Howard CR. A topological model for hepatitis B surface antigen. *Intervirology* 1992;33(3):148–158.
476. Stoeckl L, Funk A, Kopitzki A, et al. Identification of a structural motif crucial for infectivity of hepatitis B viruses. *Proc Natl Acad Sci U S A* 2006;103(17):6730–6734.
477. Stuyver L, De Gendt S, Van Geyt C, et al. A new genotype of hepatitis B virus: complete genome and phylogenetic relatedness. *J Gen Virol* 2000;81(Pt 1):67–74.
478. Su IJ, Wang HC, Wu HC, et al. Ground glass hepatocytes contain pre-S mutants and represent preneoplastic lesions in chronic hepatitis B virus infection. *J Gastroenterol Hepatol* 2008;23(8 Pt 1):1169–1174.
479. Suh A, Weber CC, Kehlmaier C, et al. Early mesozoic coexistence of amniotes and hepadnaviridae. *PLoS Genet* 2014;10(12):e1004559.
480. Summers J, O'Connell A, Millman I. Genome of hepatitis B virus: restriction enzyme cleavage and structure of DNA extracted from Dane particles. *Proc Natl Acad Sci U S A* 1975;72(11):4597–4601.
481. Summers J, Smolec JM, Snyder R. A virus similar to human hepatitis B virus associated with hepatitis and hepatoma in woodchucks. *Proc Natl Acad Sci U S A* 1978;75(9):4533–4537.
482. Summers J, Mason WS. Replication of the genome of a hepatitis B-like virus by reverse transcription of an RNA intermediate. *Cell* 1982;29(2):403–415.
483. Summers J, Smith PM, Horwich AL. Hepadnavirus envelope proteins regulate covalently closed circular DNA amplification. *J Virol* 1990;64(6):2819–2824.
484. Summers J, Smith PM, Huang MJ, et al. Morphogenetic and regulatory effects of mutations in the envelope proteins of an avian hepadnavirus. *J Virol* 1991;65(3):1310–1317.
485. Summers J, Jilbert AR, Yang W, et al. Hepatocyte turnover during resolution of a transient hepadnaviral infection. *Proc Natl Acad Sci U S A* 2003;100:11652–11659.
486. Sung WK, Zheng H, Li S, et al. Genome-wide survey of recurrent HBV integration in hepatocellular carcinoma. *Nat Genet* 2012;44(7):765–769.
487. Sureau C, Guerra B, Lee H. The middle hepatitis B virus envelope protein is not necessary for infectivity of hepatitis delta virus. *J Virol* 1994;68(6):4063–4066.
488. Sureau C, Salisse J. A conformational heparan sulfate binding site essential to infectivity overlaps with the conserved hepatitis B virus a-determinant. *Hepatology* 2013;57(3):985–994.
489. Suspene R, Guetard D, Henry M, et al. Extensive editing of both hepatitis B virus DNA strands by APOBEC3 cytidine deaminases in vitro and in vivo. *Proc Natl Acad Sci U S A* 2005;102(23):8321–8326.
490. Tagawa M, Omata M, Yokosuka O, et al. Early events in duck hepatitis B virus infection. Sequential appearance of viral deoxyribonucleic acid in the liver, pancreas, kidney, and spleen. *Gastroenterology* 1985;89(6):1224–1229.
491. Tagawa M, Robinson WS, Marion PL. Duck hepatitis B virus replicates in the yolk sac of developing embryos. *J Virol* 1987;61(7):2273–2279.
492. Tang H, McLachlan A. Transcriptional regulation of hepatitis B virus by nuclear hormone receptors is a critical determinant of viral tropism. *Proc Natl Acad Sci U S A* 2001;98(4):1841–1846.
493. Tang L, Sheraz M, McGrane M, et al. DNA Polymerase alpha is essential for intracellular amplification of hepatitis B virus covalently closed circular DNA. *PLoS Pathog* 2019;15(4):e1007742.
494. Tavis JE, Ganem D. Expression of functional hepatitis B virus polymerase in yeast reveals it to be the sole viral protein required for correct initiation of reverse transcription. *Proc Natl Acad Sci U S A* 1993;90(9):4107–4111.
495. Tennant BC. Animal models of hepadnavirus-associated hepatocellular carcinoma. *Clin Liver Dis* 2001;5(1):43–68.
496. Tennant BC, Gerin JL. The woodchuck model of hepatitis B virus infection. *ILAR J* 2001;42(2):89–102.
497. Terradillos O, Billet O, Renard CA, et al. The hepatitis B virus X gene potentiates c-myc-induced liver oncogenesis in transgenic mice. *Oncogene* 1997;14(4):395–404.
498. Terrault NA, Lok ASF, McMahon BJ, et al. Update on prevention, diagnosis, and treatment of chronic hepatitis B: AASLD 2018 hepatitis B guidance. *Hepatology* 2018;67(4):1560–1599.
499. Testoni B, Levrero M, Zoulim F. Challenges to a cure for HBV infection. *Semin Liver Dis* 2017;37(3):231–242.
500. Testoni B, Lebosse F, Scholtes C, et al. Serum hepatitis B core-related antigen (HBcrAg) correlates with covalently closed circular DNA transcriptional activity in chronic hepatitis B patients. *J Hepatol* 2019;70(4):615–625.
501. Testut P, Renard CA, Terradillos O, et al. A new hepadnavirus endemic in arctic ground squirrels in Alaska. *J Virol* 1996;70(7):4210–4219.
502. Thibault V, Pichoud C, Mullen C, et al. Characterization of a new sensitive PCR assay for quantification of viral DNA isolated from patients with hepatitis B virus infections. *J Clin Microbiol* 2007;45(12):3948–3953.
503. Thimme R, Wieland S, Steiger C, et al. CD8(+) T cells mediate viral clearance and disease pathogenesis during acute hepatitis B virus infection. *J Virol* 2003;77(1):68–76.
504. Thomson AW, Drakes ML, Zahorchak AF, et al. Hepatic dendritic cells: immunobiology and role in liver transplantation. *J Leukoc Biol* 1999;66(2):322–330.
505. Thomson AW, O'Connell PJ, Steptoe RJ, et al. Immunobiology of liver dendritic cells. *Immunol Cell Biol* 2002;80(1):65–73.
506. Thomson AW, Knolle PA. Antigen-presenting cell function in the tolerogenic liver environment. *Nat Rev Immunol* 2010;10(11):753–766.
507. Thorgeirsson SS, Grisham JW. Overview of recent experimental studies on liver stem cells. *Semin Liver Dis* 2003;23(4):303–312.
508. Tian Y, Kuo CF, Akbari O, et al. Maternal-derived hepatitis B virus e antigen alters macrophage function in offspring to drive viral persistence after vertical transmission. *Immunity* 2016;44(5):1204–1214.
509. Tong S, Li J, Wands JR. Interaction between duck hepatitis B virus and a 170-kilodalton cellular protein is mediated through a neutralizing epitope of the pre-S region and occurs during viral infection. *J Virol* 1995;69(11):7106–7112.
510. Torbenson M, Thomas DL. Occult hepatitis B. *Lancet Infect Dis* 2002;2(8):479–486.
511. Transy C, Fourel G, Robinson WS, et al. Frequent amplification of c-myc in ground squirrel liver tumors associated with past or ongoing infection with a hepadnavirus. *Proc Natl Acad Sci U S A* 1992;89(9):3874–3878.
512. Trepo CG, Magnius LO, Schaefer RA, et al. Detection of e antigen and antibody: correlations with hepatitis B surface and hepatitis B core antigens, liver disease, and outcome in hepatitis B infections. *Gastroenterology* 1976;71(5):804–808.
513. Tropberger P, Mercier A, Robinson M, et al. Mapping of histone modifications in episomal HBV cccDNA uncovers an unusual chromatin organization amenable to epigenetic manipulation. *Proc Natl Acad Sci U S A* 2015;112(42):E5715–E5724.
514. Tsiang M, Rooney JF, Toole JJ, et al. Biphasic clearance kinetics of hepatitis B virus from patients during adefovir dipivoxil therapy. *Hepatology* 1999;29(6):1863–1869.
515. Tsuge M, Hiraga N, Akiyama R, et al. HBx protein is indispensable for development of viraemia in human hepatocyte chimeric mice. *J Gen Virol* 2010;91(Pt 7):1854–1864.
516. Tu T, Mason WS, Clouston AD, et al. Clonal expansion of hepatocytes with a selective advantage occurs during all stages of chronic hepatitis B virus infection. *J Viral Hepat* 2015;22(9):737–753.
517. Tu T, Budzinska MA, Vondran FWR, et al. Hepatitis B virus DNA integration occurs early in the viral life cycle in an in vitro infection model via sodium taurocholate cotransporting polypeptide-dependent uptake of enveloped virus particles. *J Virol* 2018;92(11):e02007-17.
518. Tuttleman JS, Pourcel C, Summers J. Formation of the pool of covalently closed circular viral DNA in hepadnavirus-infected cells. *Cell* 1986;47(3):451–460.
519. Urban S, Gripon P. Inhibition of duck hepatitis B virus infection by a myristoylated pre-S peptide of the large viral surface protein. *J Virol* 2002;76(4):1986–1990.
520. Valenzuela P, Quiroga M, Zalvidar J, et al. The nucleotide sequence of the hepatitis B viral genome and the identification of the major viral genes. In: Fields BN, Jaenisch R, Fox CF, eds. *Animal Virus Genetics*. New York: Academic Press; 1980:57–70.
521. van Bommel F, Bartens A, Mysickova A, et al. Serum hepatitis B virus RNA levels as an early predictor of hepatitis B envelope antigen seroconversion during treatment with polymerase inhibitors. *Hepatology* 2015;61(1):66–76.
522. Van Damme P, Cramm M, Van der Auwera JC, et al. Horizontal transmission of hepatitis B virus. *Lancet* 1995;345(8941):27–29.
523. Van Damme P. Hepatitis B: vaccination programmes in Europe—an update. *Vaccine* 2001;19(17–19):2375–2379.
524. Vartanian JP, Henry M, Marchio A, et al. Massive APOBEC3 editing of hepatitis B viral DNA in cirrhosis. *PLoS Pathog* 2010;6(5):e1000928.
525. Vemura RP, Aragona E, Gupta S. Analysis of hepatocellular proliferation: study of archival liver tissue is facilitated by an endogenous marker of DNA replication. *Hepatology* 1992;16:968–973.
526. Vionnet J, Pascual M, Testoni B, et al. Late hepatitis B reactivation following direct-acting antiviral-based treatment of recurrent hepatitis C in an anti-HBc-positive liver transplant recipient. *Hepatology* 2018;67(2):791–793.
527. Wang B, Zhao L, Fish M, et al. Self-renewing diploid Axin2(+) cells fuel homeostatic renewal of the liver. *Nature* 2015;524(7564):180–185.
528. Wang GH, Seeger C. The reverse transcriptase of hepatitis B virus acts as a protein primer for viral DNA synthesis. *Cell* 1992;71(4):663–670.
529. Wang GH, Seeger C. Novel mechanism for reverse transcription in hepatitis B viruses. *J Virol* 1993;67(11):6507–6512.
530. Wang J, Chenivesse X, Henglein B, et al. Hepatitis B virus integration in a cyclin A gene in a hepatocellular carcinoma. *Nature* 1990;343(6258):555–557.
531. Wang J, Shen T, Huang X, et al. Serum hepatitis B virus RNA is encapsidated pregenome RNA that may be associated with persistence of viral infection and rebound. *J Hepatol* 2016;65(4):700–710.
532. Wang J, Qiu J, Zhu Y, et al. Molecular evolution of hepatitis B vaccine escape variants in China, during 2000–2016. *Vaccine* 2017;35(43):5808–5813.
533. Wang N, Sun Z, Pang Q, et al. Liver cancer, liver disease background and virus-like particles in serum among ducks from high incidence area of human hepatocellular carcinoma. *Clin J Oncol* 1980;2:176–178 (In Chinese).

534. Wang X, Qian X, Guo HC, et al. Heat shock protein 90-independent activation of truncated hepadnavirus reverse transcriptase. *J Virol* 2003;77(8):4471–4480.
535. Watanabe T, Sorensen EM, Naito A, et al. Involvement of host cellular multivesicular body functions in hepatitis B virus budding. *Proc Natl Acad Sci U S A* 2007;104(24):10205–10210.
536. Waters JA, Brown SE, Steward MW, et al. Analysis of the antigenic epitopes of hepatitis B surface antigen involved in the induction of a protective antibody response. *Virus Res* 1991;22(1):1–12.
537. Waters JA, Kennedy M, Voet P, et al. Loss of the common "A" determinant of hepatitis B surface antigen by a vaccine-induced escape mutant. *J Clin Invest* 1992;90:2543–2547.
538. Watts NR, Conway JF, Cheng N, et al. The morphogenic linker peptide of HBV capsid protein forms a mobile array on the interior surface. *EMBO J* 2002;21(5):876–884.
539. Weber M, Bronsema V, Bartos H, et al. Hepadnavirus P protein utilizes a tyrosine residue in the TP domain to prime reverse transcription. *J Virol* 1994;68(5):2994–2999.
540. Werle-Lapostolle B, Bowden S, Locarnini S, et al. Persistence of cccDNA during the natural history of chronic hepatitis B and decline during adefovir dipivoxil therapy. *Gastroenterology* 2004;126(7):1750–1758.
541. Wieland S, Thimme R, Purcell RH, et al. Genomic analysis of the host response to hepatitis B virus infection. *Proc Natl Acad Sci U S A* 2004;101(17):6669–6674.
542. Wieland SF, Guidotti LG, Chisari FV. Intrahepatic induction of alpha/beta interferon eliminates viral RNA-containing capsids in hepatitis B virus transgenic mice. *J Virol* 2000;74:4165–4173.
543. Wieland SF, Spangenberg HC, Thimme R, et al. Expansion and contraction of the hepatitis B virus transcriptional template in infected chimpanzees. *Proc Natl Acad Sci U S A* 2004;101:2129–2134.
544. Wieland SF, Eustaquio A, Whitten-Bauer C, et al. Interferon prevents formation of replication-competent hepatitis B virus RNA-containing nucleocapsids. *Proc Natl Acad Sci U S A* 2005;102(28):9913–9917.
545. Will H, Cattaneo R, Koch H, et al. Cloned HBV DNA causes hepatitis in chimpanzees. *Nature* 1982;299:740–742.
546. Will H, Reiser W, Weimer T, et al. Replication strategy of human hepatitis B virus. *J Virol* 1987;61(3):904–911.
547. Wolf HK, Michalopoulos GK. Hepatocyte regeneration in acute fulminant and nonfulminant hepatitis: a study of proliferating cell nuclear antigen expression. *Hepatology* 1992;15(4):707–713.
548. Wong DKH, Cheung AM, O'Rourke K, et al. Effect of alpha-interferon treatment in patients with hepatitis B e antigen-positive chronic hepatitis B. *Ann Intern Med* 1993;119:312–323.
549. Wong VW, Chan SL, Mo F, et al. Clinical scoring system to predict hepatocellular carcinoma in chronic hepatitis B carriers. *J Clin Oncol* 2010;28(10):1660–1665.
550. Wooddell CI, Yuen MF, Chan HL, et al. RNAi-based treatment of chronically infected patients and chimpanzees reveals that integrated hepatitis B virus DNA is a source of HBsAg. *Sci Transl Med* 2017;9(409):eaan0241.
551. Wu TT, Coates L, Aldrich CE, et al. In hepatocytes infected with duck hepatitis B virus, the template for viral RNA synthesis is amplified by an intracellular pathway. *Virology* 1990;175(1):255–261.
552. Wynne SA, Crowther RA, Leslie AG. The crystal structure of the human hepatitis B virus capsid. *Mol Cell* 1999;3(6):771–780.
553. Xia Y, Stadler D, Lucifora J, et al. Interferon-gamma and tumor necrosis factor-alpha produced by T cells reduce the HBV persistence form, cccDNA, without cytolysis. *Gastroenterology* 2016;150(1):194–205.
554. Xu Z, Jensen G, Yen TS. Activation of hepatitis B virus S promoter by the viral large surface protein via induction of stress in the endoplasmic reticulum. *J Virol* 1997;71(10):7387–7392.
555. Yamamoto K, Horikita M, Tsuda F, et al. Naturally occurring escape mutants of hepatitis B virus with various mutations in the S gene in carriers seropositive for antibody to hepatitis B surface antigen. *J Virol* 1994;68(4):2671–2676.
556. Yan H, Zhong G, Xu G, et al. Sodium taurocholate cotransporting polypeptide is a functional receptor for human hepatitis B and D virus. *Elife* 2012;1:e00049.
557. Yan H, Peng B, He W, et al. Molecular determinants of hepatitis B and D virus entry restriction in mouse sodium taurocholate cotransporting polypeptide. *J Virol* 2013;87(14):7977–7991.
558. Yang HI, Lu SN, Liaw YF, et al. Hepatitis B e antigen and the risk of hepatocellular carcinoma. *N Engl J Med* 2002;347(3):168–174.
559. Yang HI, Yeh SH, Chen PJ, et al. Associations between hepatitis B virus genotype and mutants and the risk of hepatocellular carcinoma. *J Natl Cancer Inst* 2008;100(16):1134–1143.
560. Yang PL, Althage A, Chung J, et al. Immune effectors required for hepatitis B virus clearance. *Proc Natl Acad Sci U S A* 2010;107(2):798–802.
561. Yang W, Summers J. Illegitimate replication of linear hepadnavirus DNA through nonhomologous recombination. *J Virol* 1995;69(7):4029–4036.
562. Yang W, Mason WS, Summers J. Covalently closed circular viral DNA formed from two types of linear DNA in woodchuck hepatitis virus-infected liver. *J Virol* 1996;70(7):4567–4575.
563. Yang W, Summers J. Infection of ducklings with virus particles containing linear double-stranded duck hepatitis B virus DNA: illegitimate replication and reversion. *J Virol* 1998;72(11):8710–8717.
564. Yeh ML, Huang CF, Huang CI, et al. Hepatitis B-related outcomes following direct-acting Antiviral Therapy in Taiwanese patients with chronic HBV/HCV co-infection. *J Hepatol* 2020;73(1):62–71.
565. Yen TT, Yang A, Chiu WT, et al. Hepatitis B virus PreS2-mutant large surface antigen activates store-operated calcium entry and promotes chromosome instability. *Oncotarget* 2016;7(17):23346–23360.
566. Yim HJ, Lok AS. Natural history of chronic hepatitis B virus infection: what we knew in 1981 and what we know in 2005. *Hepatology* 2006;43(2 Suppl 1):S173–S181.
567. Yoshida EM, Ramji A, Chatur N, et al. Regression of cirrhosis associated with hepatitis B e (HBe) antigen-negative chronic hepatitis B infection with prolonged lamivudine therapy. *Eur J Gastroenterol Hepatol* 2004;16(3):355–358.
568. Yu M, Summers J. A domain of the hepadnavirus capsid protein is specifically required for DNA maturation and virus assembly. *J Virol* 1991;65(5):2511–2517.
569. Yu MW, Yeh SH, Chen PJ, et al. Hepatitis B virus genotype and DNA level and hepatocellular carcinoma: a prospective study in men. *J Natl Cancer Inst* 2005;97(4):265–272.
570. Yu X, Mertz JE. Distinct modes of regulation of transcription of hepatitis B virus by the nuclear receptors HNF4alpha and COUP-TF1. *J Virol* 2003;77(4):2489–2499.
571. Yuen MF, Yuan HJ, Wong DK, et al. Prognostic determinants for chronic hepatitis B in Asians: therapeutic implications. *Gut* 2005;54(11):1610–1614.
572. Yuen MF, Gane EJ, Kim DJ, et al. Antiviral activity, safety, and pharmacokinetics of capsid assembly modulator NVR 3-778 in patients with chronic HBV infection. *Gastroenterology* 2019;156(5):1392–1403.e1397.
573. Zanetti AR, Tanzi E, Manzillo G, et al. Hepatitis B variant in Europe. *Lancet* 1988;2(8620):1132–1133.
574. Zeissig S, Murata K, Sweet L, et al. Hepatitis B virus-induced lipid alterations contribute to natural killer T cell-dependent protective immunity. *Nat Med* 2012;18(7):1060–1068.
575. Zhang YY, Summers J. Low dynamic state of viral competition in a chronic avian hepadnavirus infection. *J Virol* 2000;74(11):5257–5265.
576. Zhang YY, Zhang BH, Theele D, et al. Single-cell analysis of covalently closed circular DNA copy numbers in a hepadnavirus-infected liver. *Proc Natl Acad Sci U S A* 2003;100(21):12372–12377.
577. Zhang Z, Torii N, Hu Z, et al. X-deficient woodchuck hepatitis virus mutants behave like attenuated viruses and induce protective immunity in vivo. *J Clin Investig* 2001;108(10):1523–1531.
578. Zhang Z, Tavis JE. The duck hepatitis B virus reverse transcriptase functions as a full-length monomer. *J Biol Chem* 2006;281(47):35794–35801.
579. Zhao LH, Liu X, Yan HX, et al. Genomic and oncogenic preference of HBV integration in hepatocellular carcinoma. *Nat Commun* 2016;7:12992.
580. Zhao Q, Hu Z, Cheng J, et al. Hepatitis B virus core protein dephosphorylation occurs during pregenomic RNA encapsidation. *J Virol* 2018;92(13):e02139-17.
581. Zheng YW, Riegler J, Wu J, et al. Novel short transcripts of hepatitis B virus X gene derived from intragenic promoter. *J Biol Chem* 1994;269(36):22593–22598.
582. Zhou T, Block T, Liu F, et al. HBsAg mRNA degradation induced by a dihydroquinolizinone compound depends on the HBV posttranscriptional regulatory element. *Antiviral Res* 2018;149:191–201.
583. Zhou YZ. A virus possibly associated with hepatitis and hepatoma in ducks. *Shanghai Med J* 1980;3:641–644.
584. Zhu Y, Yamamoto T, Cullen J, et al. Kinetics of hepadnavirus loss from the liver during inhibition of viral DNA synthesis. *J Virol* 2001;75:311–322.
585. Zlotnick A, Johnson JM, Wingfield PW, et al. A theoretical model successfully identifies features of hepatitis B virus capsid assembly. *Biochemistry* 1999;38(44):14644–14652.
586. Zoulim F, Mimms L, Floreani M, et al. New assays for quantitative determination of viral markers in management of chronic hepatitis B virus infection. *J Clin Microbiol* 1992;30(5):1111–1119.
587. Zoulim F, Seeger C. Reverse transcription in hepatitis B viruses is primed by a tyrosine residue of the polymerase. *J Virol* 1994;68(1):6–13.
588. Zoulim F, Seeger C. Woodchuck hepatitis virus X protein is required for viral infection in vivo. *J Virol* 1994;68:2026–2030.
589. Zoulim F. Antiviral Therapy of chronic hepatitis B. *Antiviral Res* 2006;71(2–3):206–215.
590. Zuckerman AJ, Howard CR. *Hepatitis Viruses of Man.* New York: Academic Press, Inc.; 1979.

CHAPTER 19 Hepatitis D (Delta) Virus

Camille Sureau • Paul Dény

HISTORY

The first evidence of hepatitis delta virus (HDV) in humans was reported in 1977 by Mario Rizzetto, a resolute gastroenterologist at the University of Turin, Italy, who was caring for patients suffering from chronic hepatitis related to hepatitis B virus (HBV) infection.[146] Using simple techniques of immunohistochemistry for examination of liver biopsies, Rizzetto and colleagues observed that a serum positive for antibodies directed to the HBV core antigen (HBcAg) reacted with liver specimens positive for HBV surface antigen (HBsAg), which had been previously documented as negative for HBcAg. It was initially thought to be a new HBV antigen but was subsequently proven distinct from the known HBsAg, HBcAg, or HBV e antigen (HBeAg), and given the name of delta antigen, now referred to as hepatitis delta antigen (HDAg). The new antigen was present only in liver cell nuclei of HBsAg carriers, but its staining and that of HBcAg in liver biopsy specimens were mutually exclusive. HDAg was detected neither in HBsAg-negative patients suffering from chronic hepatitis nor in patients with self-limited acute hepatitis B or asymptomatic HBV carriers. Soon thereafter, the HDAg-bearing protein was found associated with a small RNA as internal elements of a virus-like particle coated with the HBV envelope proteins.[148] The viral particle was proven transmissible in the chimpanzee model but only in the presence of HBV coinfection.[147] In 1986, the cloning and sequencing of the HDAg-associated RNA, now known as HDV RNA, unveiled the uniqueness of this entity among animal virus genomes known at the time,[181] but it also revealed structural features typical of some plant subviral agents called viroids, suggesting an evolutionary relationship.[54] The circular single-stranded HDV RNA was the smallest among known mammalian viral genomes, and its sequence presented no homology with that of the helper HBV. Overall, the characteristics of the delta agent did not fulfill the criteria for the definition of a virus, but it was nonetheless referred to as HDV.

As early as 1980, an assay was developed for serological detection of anti-HDAg antibodies,[151] which revealed a high prevalence of HDV infection among polytransfused HBsAg carriers and intravenous drug addicts.[150] HDV infection was first documented as highly endemic in the south part of Italy and then in several South American countries.[144] HDV infection was often associated with the most severe form of acute and chronic hepatitis, in particular among indigenous populations in Ecuador and Venezuela.[26,117,164] To date, chronic hepatitis D (CHD) is not only one the most severe liver diseases in humans, but one of the most difficult to treat. There is no curative therapy for HDV infection and no HDV-specific vaccine available, but HDV infection can be prevented upon HBV vaccination of individuals who are not already HBV infected.

CLASSIFICATION

According to the Baltimore classification system, the HDV RNA genome is a single-stranded RNA (ssRNA) of negative polarity. However, unlike other RNA viruses, the genome does not encode an RNA polymerase. HDV is currently assigned to the *Deltavirus* genus.[116] The origin of HDV RNA has been subject to different evolutionary theories. As an obligate satellite of HBV, it was initially speculated to have evolved—or coevolved with HBV—in humans. One hypothesis was that ribozyme originated from introns in the human cytoplasmic polyadenylation element–binding protein 3 gene, and the HDAg coding sequence from that of a cell protein ancestor.[21,158] Another hypothesis proposed that HDV RNA derived from host circular RNAs or from plant viroids, or virusoids.[175]

These speculations should now be reconsidered in light of the recent discovery of several HDV-like RNAs in species very distant to humans. A first HDV-like RNA has been identified in ducks, which shares with its human counterpart many features such as circular conformation, self-complementarity, the presence of putative ribozymes, and a coding capacity for a protein whose sequence displays 32% similarity to that of the HDAg protein.[186] Another HDV-like RNA was identified in two specimens of the *Boa constrictor* species that were affected with central nervous system disorder.[73] It was detected in two offspring and in a water python (*Liasis mackloti savuensis*) of the same snake colony, suggesting transmission. More HDV-like RNAs have since been described in the newt, toad, fish, and termite.[30] For none of the above did the corresponding transcriptomes contain HBV-like sequences. Although identifiable avian viral sequences were identified in the duck transcriptome, there is currently no proof that the HDV-like RNAs are genomes of virus satellites. Now that HDV-like agents have been discovered in species very distant to humans, it is likely that a common ancestor with HDV arose early in the history of the Metazoa, therefore long before the appearance of HDV in humans.[30,79]

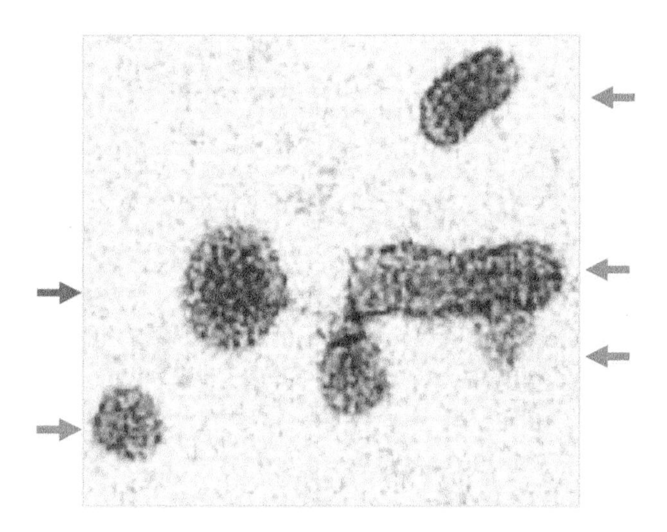

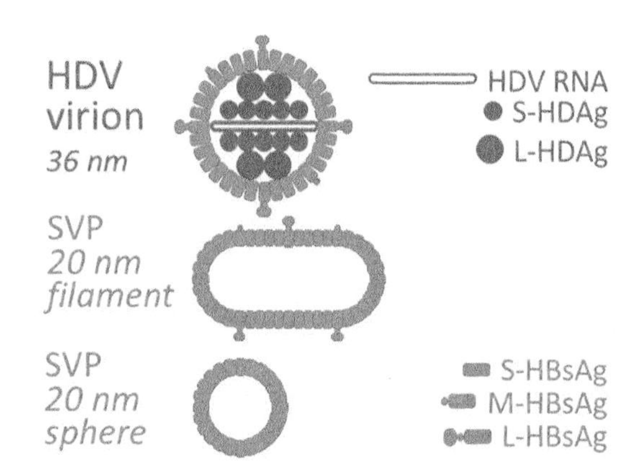

FIGURE 19.1 The HDV virion. Top panel: View of HDV virion by electron microscopy. (Modified with permission from Gudima S, He Y, Meier A, et al. Assembly of hepatitis delta virus: particle characterization, including the ability to infect primary human hepatocytes. *J Virol* 2007;81(7):3608-3617.) *Blue arrow* indicates HDV virion; *red arrows* indicate HBV subviral particles (SVPs). **Bottom panel:** Schematic representation of the HDV virion and HBV SVPs. The HDV virion consists of two types of components: (a) the viral envelope of HBV origin (in *red*), including the HBV envelope proteins S-HBsAg, M-HBsAg, and L-HBsAg and (b) the ribonucleoprotein (RNP) (in *blue*) that consists of the circular genomic HDV RNA associated to multiple copies of the HDV-encoded S- and L-HDAg proteins.

VIRION STRUCTURE

Upon electron microscopy examination of negatively stained preparations, the HDV virion appears (Fig. 19.1) as a spherical particle with an average diameter of 36 nm.[17,64,70] By ultracentrifugation in CsCl gradient, its buoyant density is at 1.24 to 1.25 g/cm^3.[148,169] The virion displays a chimeric architecture consisting of an outer coat of HBV envelope proteins, and an inner ribonucleoprotein (RNP) made of HDV-specific elements, that is, the genomic HDV RNA and multiple copies of HDAg proteins.[17,70,148] The viral envelope is identical to that of HBV subviral particles (SVPs) in including cell-derived lipids associated with HBV envelope proteins,[170] but there is no indication that lipids are organized as a bilayer. Assuming a surface density identical to that of SVPs, an HDV virion would bear approximately 100 copies of envelope proteins.[95] Electron microscopy images of the RNP revealed a spherical, core-like structure of approximately 20 nm in diameter, but no evidence of icosahedral symmetry. The three types of HBV envelope proteins that are typically produced in huge amounts by HBV-infected cells, and exported for the most part as SVPs, are present in the HDV envelope. All three bear the HBsAg and are designated small (S-HBsAg), middle (M-HBsAg), and large (L-HBsAg) proteins.[22] It was initially reported that S-, M-, and L-HBsAg were present at a ratio of 95:5:1, respectively, at the surface of HDV, as opposed to a 4:1:1 in the envelope of HBV virion.[16] Yet, considering that HDV particles can be assembled *in vitro* with S-HBsAg only,[180] it is likely that this ratio be very heterogeneous. In addition to providing HDV with an export system, the HBV envelope proteins confer an efficient protection of the RNP and stability of the virion in the extracellular space since HDV can survive after 30 hours at 60°C.[91] Obviously, there is a need for more detailed information on the 3D structure of the HDV virion, in particular with regard to the inner RNP.

GENOME STRUCTURE AND ORGANIZATION

The HDV genome is a circular, ssRNA of approximately 1,700 nucleotides in size (Fig. 19.2) and the smallest among the known mammalian viral genomes.[181] It is present in abundance

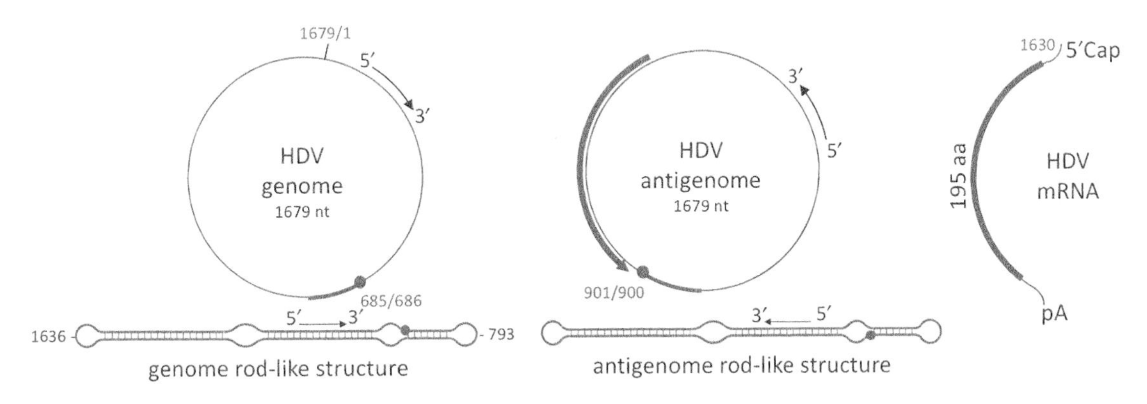

FIGURE 19.2 Representation of HDV RNA species in HDV-infected cells. Genome and antigenome are circular single-stranded RNA. Both can fold into unbranched rod-like structures. Each HDV RNA strand contains a ribozyme sequence for self-cleavage (closed *circle*) at position 685/686 in the genomic strand and 901/900 in antigenomic strand. *Arrows* on the RNA strands indicate the 5′ to 3′ direction. The mRNA, of antigenomic polarity, contains the open reading frame for HDAg protein (*thick purple line*).

in cell nuclei, along with its replication intermediate, and exact complementary, the antigenomic RNA. Both RNA strands adopt a quasi-double-stranded conformation, also referred to as rod-like structure, by self-annealing with 74% of their nucleotides; 60% of which are G or C. The unbranched rod includes interspersed double-stranded helical segments and internal loops and bulges. Genome and antigenome contain an 85-nucleotide in length ribozyme structure for self-cleavage activity. Circular conformation, self-annealing capacity, and the presence of ribozymes are characteristics of plant viroids and essential to replication.[174]

The genetic organization of the HDV genome includes several open reading frames (ORFs), but only one, present in the antigenomic strand, is known to be translated into a protein, (HDAg). HDV is thus a negative sense RNA virus. The HDAg protein is produced as two isoforms referred to as small-HDAg protein (S-HDAg) of 195 amino acids in length, and large-HDAg (L-HDAg) that differs from S-HDAg by 19 or 20 additional amino acid residues at the carboxyl terminus.

The rod-like structure of HDV RNA can be schematically divided in two distinct domains: a "ribozyme domain" with a high degree of sequence conservation between genotypes and a larger "coding domain" that includes the HDAg ORF sequence and its complementary strand in the rod-like conformation.

REPLICATION

In Vitro Experimental Models

The study of HBV and HDV has long been impeded in the absence of an efficient tissue culture system able to sustain chronic infection. This is due, in part, to the very narrow tropism of these viruses for the human liver and to the difficulties in recapitulating human hepatocyte differentiation *in vitro*. The first *in vitro* models for HBV and HDV were based on human hepatoma cell lines, such as HepG2 and Huh-7, that are fully permissive to replication and production of infectious particles but not susceptible to infection for lack of entry factors expression. Until 2002, the early steps of HBV infection could only be observed *in vitro* using primary cultures of chimpanzee or human hepatocytes.[60,168] Then, Gripon and colleagues isolated a HBV-susceptible cell line—HepaRG—that was amenable to direct infection with HBV[61] and HDV.[83] This technical breakthrough opened the way to the exploration of the viral entry mechanism and to the screening of antivirals directed to the early steps of infection. Nonetheless, for a yet unexplained reason, the HepaRG cells do not sustain chronic infection, that is, simultaneous susceptibility and permissivity. As a result, in standard laboratory practices, permissive Huh-7 or HepG2 cell lines have been used for analysis of replication and virus assembly, and HepaRG cells for the study of HBV/HDV entry.[170] Then in 2012, the landmark discovery by Yan and colleagues[195] that the human sodium taurocholate cotransporting polypeptide (hNTCP), a bile acid transporter expressed at the basolateral membrane of hepatocytes, acted as a liver-specific receptor for HBV and HDV was a long-awaited information for the HBV/HDV research field. From that point on, hNTCP-expressing cell lines could be created that were amenable to high-throughput screening approaches aimed at identifying novel host factors involved in viral entry or new antiviral drugs.[82,163,179] As a result, the entire replication cycle of HDV could be recapitulated by generating cell lines that constitutively express HBV envelope proteins, the hNTCP receptor, and antigenomic RNAs from an integrated copy of HDV cDNA.[100,128]

Mechanism of Attachment

For both HBV and HDV, hepatotropism is, for the most part, governed by the HBV envelope proteins activity at viral entry, and, as a result, the two viruses engage identical cellular entry factors at the initial step of attachment and subsequent binding to high-affinity receptor(s). This assumption has been confirmed by numerous experiments, and the HDV *in vitro* infection model has been utilized extensively to study the HBV envelope proteins function at viral entry.[14,159,171] As a matter of fact, the HDV model was critical to the identification of hNTCP as a high-affinity receptor for HBV/HDV.[195]

The first step in the HDV entry process is mediated by an interaction between the viral envelope proteins and heparan sulfate proteoglycans (HSPGs), such as Glypican-5, at the surface of human hepatocytes (Fig. 19.3).[93,161,171,178] An HSPG-binding domain is present in the surface-exposed antigenic loop (AGL) of the HBV envelope proteins, which also

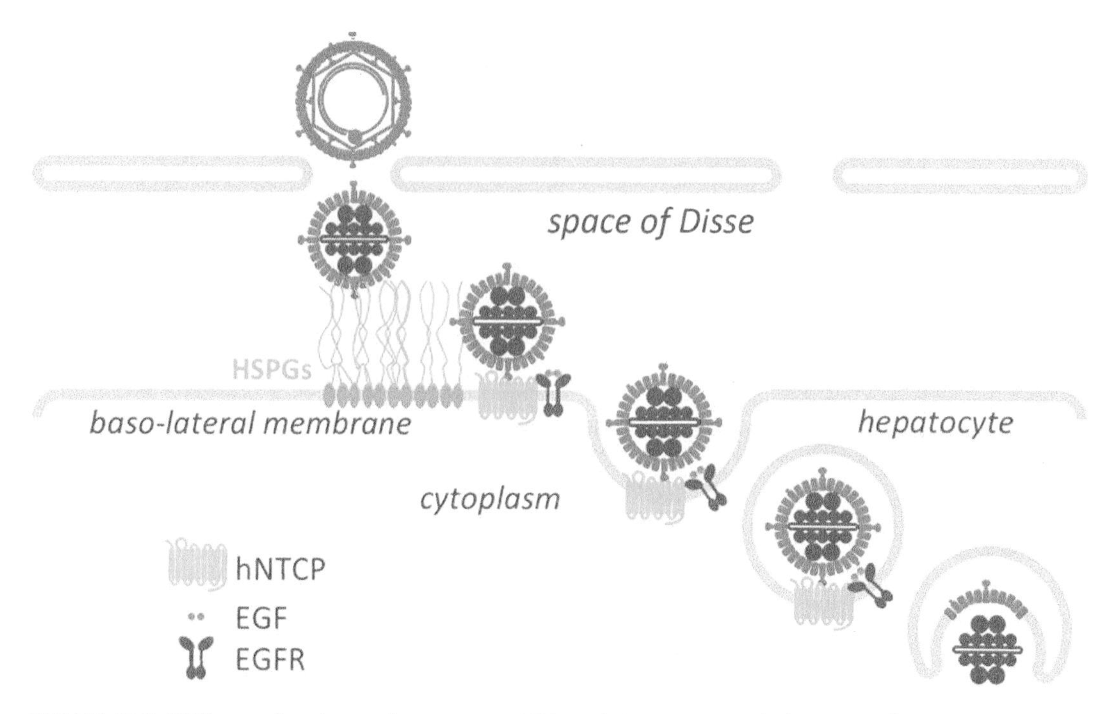

FIGURE 19.3 HDV entry into human hepatocytes. HDV and HBV virions reach the space of Disse through fenestrations of the sinusoidal endothelium. Virions first attached to heparan sulfate proteoglycans (HSPGs) at the basolateral membrane of hepatocytes then bind to hNTCP and are recruited to the NTCP–EGFR before translocation from the cell surface to the intramembrane vesicles upon stimulation with EGF.

bears the conserved immunodominant antigenic a-determinant of HBsAg.[2,159] The a-determinant elicits the most neutralizing antibodies (anti-HBs antibodies) in case of self-resolving infection, or in response to HB vaccination. It was the first identified HBV marker,[15] but its relevance to a function in the HBV life cycle had never been unveiled until the demonstration of its contribution to infectivity.[83] The HSPG-binding domain, and overlapping a-determinant, are both dependent upon a specific conformation of the AGL polypeptide stabilized by intra- and interchain disulfide bonds.[159,171] The AGL also bears an N-linked glycosylation site at N146, which is never fully functional, leading to a near-to 1:1 ratio of nonglycosylated/glycosylated isoforms for each type of envelope protein. An explanation to this peculiar pattern is that nonglycosylated N146 is essential for infectivity, while the glycosylated form is instrumental in shielding the a-determinant from neutralizing antibodies.[85]

Mechanism of Entry

After low-affinity attachment to HSPGs at the basolateral membrane of hepatocytes, the pre-S1 domain of L-HBsAg binds with high affinity to the HBV-specific receptor, hNTCP (Fig. 19.3).[127,195] The critical role of pre-S1 at viral entry was first demonstrated using the HDV model when HDV virions lacking L-HBsAg in the viral envelope were found noninfectious.[167] Adding back a small number of L-HBsAg proteins, estimated at approximately 3 to 4 per virion, was sufficient to restore infectivity.[95] The hNTCP-binding site consists of amino acids (aas) 9 to 15 in the pre-S1 domain (position in HBV genotype D ayw3), but binding requires the integrity of the N-terminal 75 amino acids sequence of pre-S1 and its acylation with myristic acid.[14,59] Interestingly enough, a synthetic myristoylated pre-S1 peptide can block HDV/HBV infection *in vitro* at subnanomolar concentrations.[59] It is actually proposed as a potent entry inhibitor under evaluation in clinical trials in HDV chronic carriers.[108]

Internalization

After its binding to hNTCP, HBV/HDV is internalized through the EGFR endocytosis pathway as a consequence of hNTCP interacting with EGFR, irrespective of the presence of the virus (Fig. 19.3).[82] Upon stimulation with EGF, the virus–hNTCP–EGFR complex is translocated, with EGFR, from the plasma membrane to endocytic vesicles, possibly using a clathrin-mediated pathway.[77] Whether a subsequent membrane fusion occurs upon acidification in intracellular vesicles for release of the RNP into the cytoplasm is presently unknown. Trafficking of the RNP into the cytoplasm is also poorly documented, but entry into the nucleus is directed by the presence of a nuclear localization signal (NLS) in the HDAg proteins.[27]

mRNA Synthesis

Postentry, the HDV genome is delivered to the nucleus and serves as a template for initiation of antigenomic RNA synthesis by cellular RNA pol II (Fig. 19.4). The nascent antigenomic RNA can proceed through two distinct pathways: (a) synthesis of an mRNA for translation into HDAg proteins or (b) synthesis of full-length antigenomic RNA that serves as replication intermediate. However, there is no switch from an early synthesis of mRNA to a late production of antigenomic RNA, the two phenomena being independent of each other and likely carried out by different machineries in different nuclear compartments.[68,107,121] Yet, whether the antigenome is synthesized by a polymerase other than pol II is a point of contention. The

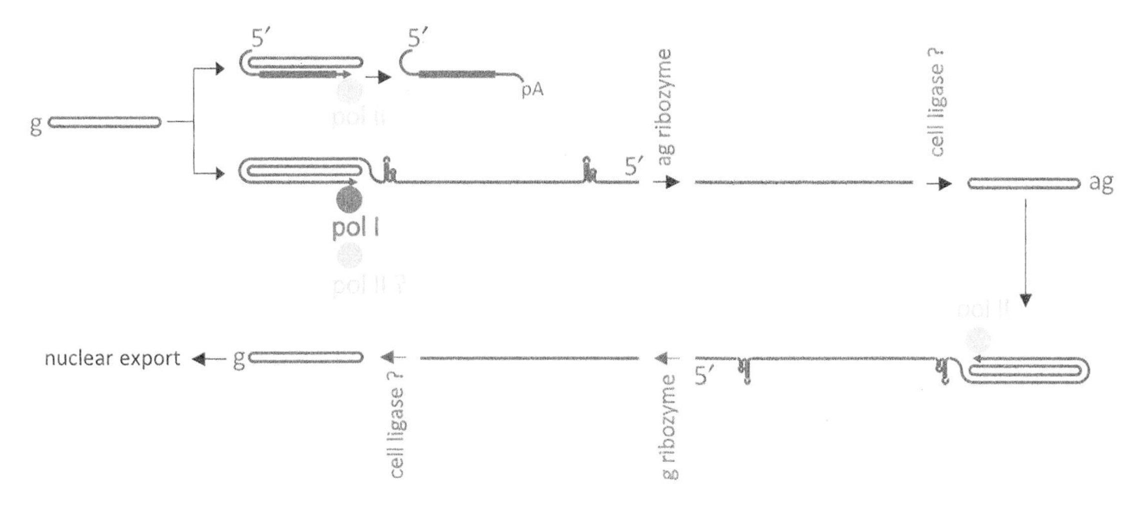

FIGURE 19.4 Rolling-circle mechanism of HDV RNA replication. Incoming genome (g) serves as template for synthesis of HDV mRNA by cellular polymerase II (pol II) and for synthesis of antigenomic RNA (ag) by pol I or pol II through a rolling-circle mechanism of replication. Neosynthesized linear antigenomic RNA is cleaved by the embedded ag ribozymes to linear unit-length molecule that is then circularized upon intramolecular ligation (cell ligase?). In turn, circular ag RNA serves as template for synthesis of genomic RNA through a second mechanism of rolling-circle amplification by pol II. HDV genomic polarity is indicated in *blue*, and antigenomic in *purple*.

HDAg mRNA is 800 nt in size and is processed in response to a polyadenylation signal AAUAAA.[65,75] Its 5′ end is capped and maps to nucleotide 1,630—or 1,631—corresponding to the left tip of the genomic rod-like structure suggesting the presence of a promoter upstream of this position.[63,121] HDAg mRNA accumulates at up to 1,000 copies per cell, a level approximately 1 and 2 log10 below that of antigenomic and genomic RNAs, respectively.[129]

Translation

Even though full-length antigenomic RNA bears the HDAg ORF, translation of HDAg proteins occurs exclusively from HDAg mRNAs.[107] In fact, two distinct mRNAs are produced during replication that differ from each other by only one nucleotide. At the early phase of replication, the mRNA codes for the 195 amino acids long S-HDAg protein, whereas at a later phase, the amber UAG codon for S-HDAg is changed to UGG for tryptophan leading to a longer ORF for L-HDAg with 19 additional codons at the 3′ end. The sequence modification occurs upon editing of UAG, not on the HDAg mRNA itself, but on the full-length antigenomic RNA.[111] It is carried out by the adenosine deaminase acting on RNA 1 (ADAR1) that converts adenosine of the UAG termination codon for S-HDAg to inosine, which is in turn recognized as guanosine by the RNA polymerase (Fig. 19.5). S-HDAg is active in promoting HDV RNA replication early in infection, whereas L-HDAg acts at a later stage to down-regulate replication and promote HDV virion assembly.[31]

The N-terminus of both S- and L-HDAg proteins is involved in the formation of dimers by establishing an intermolecular antiparallel coiled-coil interaction (Fig. 19.6).[200] Both proteins also contain an NLS[5,27,192] and two arginine-rich motifs (ARMs) with RNA-binding properties.[99] However, the major determinant for direct binding to the rod-like form of HDV RNA resides within the N-terminal 78 amino acids of HDAg proteins.[36]

The C-terminal 19 amino acids sequence unique to L-HDAg contains a CXXQ farnesylation signal that is crucial to virion assembly in allowing the farnesylated L-HDAg to interact with the HBV envelope proteins at the endoplasmic reticulum (ER) membrane.[89] In addition, the proline-rich, C-terminal sequence of L-HDAg contains a nuclear export signal (NES) and a clathrin-binding motif, both reported as instrumental in virion assembly.[98,134] Surprisingly, beside the C-terminal CXXQ farnesylation signal sequence and the presence of least four diversely scattered proline residues, the 19-amino acid C-terminus of L-HDAg is not well conserved among the different HDV genotypes.[142]

S-HDAg is subjected to several posttranslational modifications that orchestrate genome replication within the nucleus.[78,176] Methylation at Arg-13,[102] acetylation at Lys-72,[123] phosphorylation at Ser-177,[74] and sumoylation at multiple lysine residues[176] directly participate to the complex trafficking of the different forms of HDV RNA within the nucleus and between nucleus and cytoplasm.[9,78] Genomic RNA and mRNA synthesis require a S-HDAg protein that is acetylated, methylated, and phosphorylated. By contrast, antigenome synthesis does not require S-HDAg modifications.[176]

Replication of HDV RNA

HDV RNA replication takes place in the cell nucleus, and it is likely the function of the S-HDAg NLS to target the incoming RNP to the nucleus (Fig. 19.7). Since the HDAg protein is not an RNA-dependent polymerase (RdRp), the host RNA polymerase II (pol II)—a normally DNA-dependent enzyme—is first recruited for synthesis of a complementary antigenomic RNA in the nucleoplasm.[29,122] Polymerization can lead either to synthesis of the HDAg mRNA when the polyadenylation signal on the genome template is recognized by pol II, or to the production of longer-than-unit antigenomic RNA when it is ignored.[129] There is a consensus for mRNA synthesis being carried out by pol II in the nucleoplasm, but it is still uncertain whether pol II or pol I/III performs the rolling circle mechanism of antigenomic RNA synthesis, and whether the latter takes place in the nucleolus, an organelle in which pol I normally transcribes DNA into ribosomal RNA (Fig. 19.8).[177]

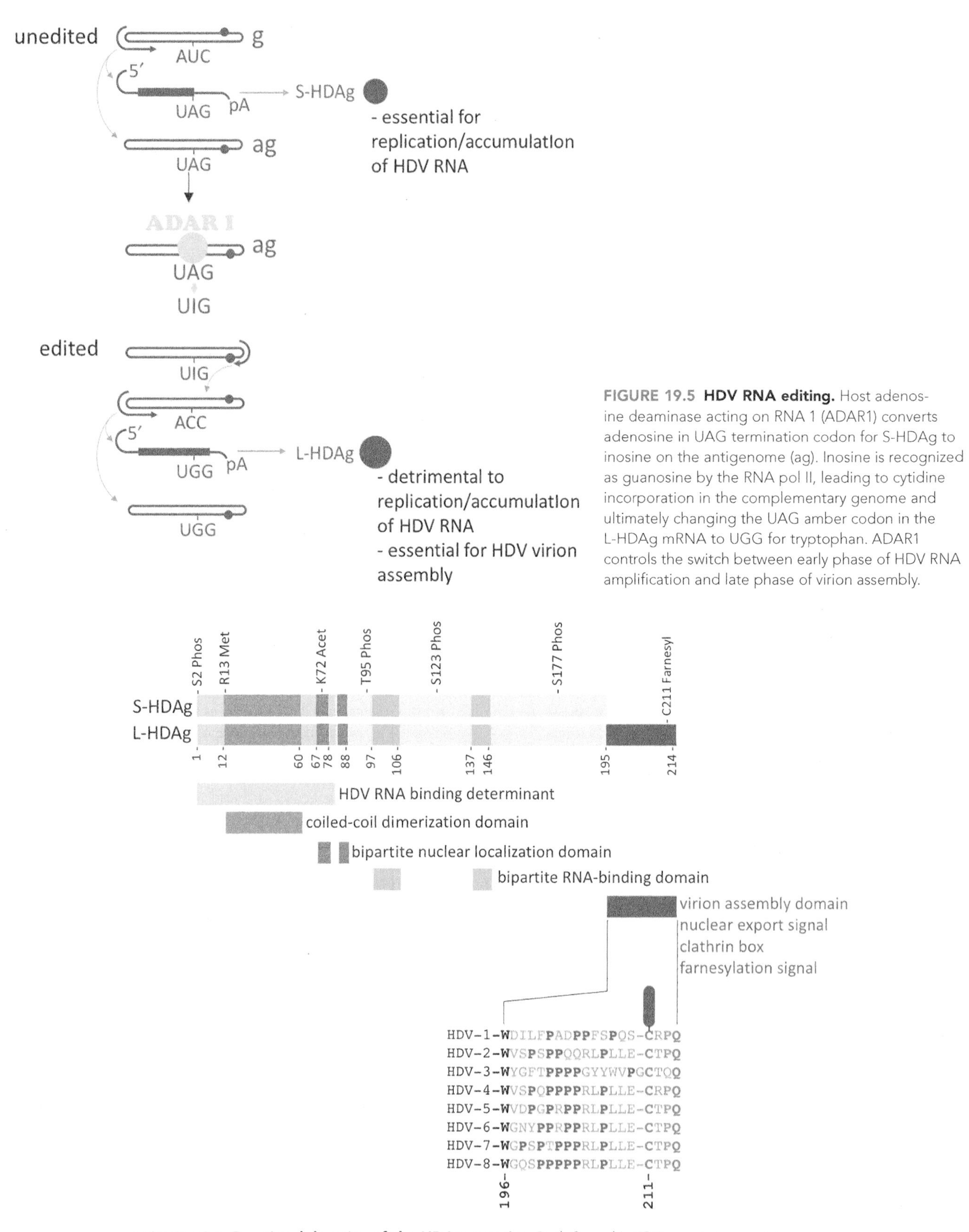

FIGURE 19.5 HDV RNA editing. Host adenosine deaminase acting on RNA 1 (ADAR1) converts adenosine in UAG termination codon for S-HDAg to inosine on the antigenome (ag). Inosine is recognized as guanosine by the RNA pol II, leading to cytidine incorporation in the complementary genome and ultimately changing the UAG amber codon in the L-HDAg mRNA to UGG for tryptophan. ADAR1 controls the switch between early phase of HDV RNA amplification and late phase of virion assembly.

FIGURE 19.6 Functional domains of the HDAg proteins. Both S- and L-HDAg proteins contain a coiled-coil dimerization domain and a nuclear localization domain (NLS). The C-terminus of L-HDAg includes a nuclear export domain (NES), a farnesylation signal, and assembly domain. The farnesyl group covalently linked to cysteine-211 is represented (*thick blue line*). The C-terminus of L-HDAg is not well conserved among HDV genotypes, except for the presence of at least four proline residues, and the CXXQ farnesylation signal. Posttranslational modifications on S-HDAg are indicated: phosphorylation (Phos); methylation (Met); and acetylation (Acet). S-HDAg is also sumoylated at multiple lysine residues.

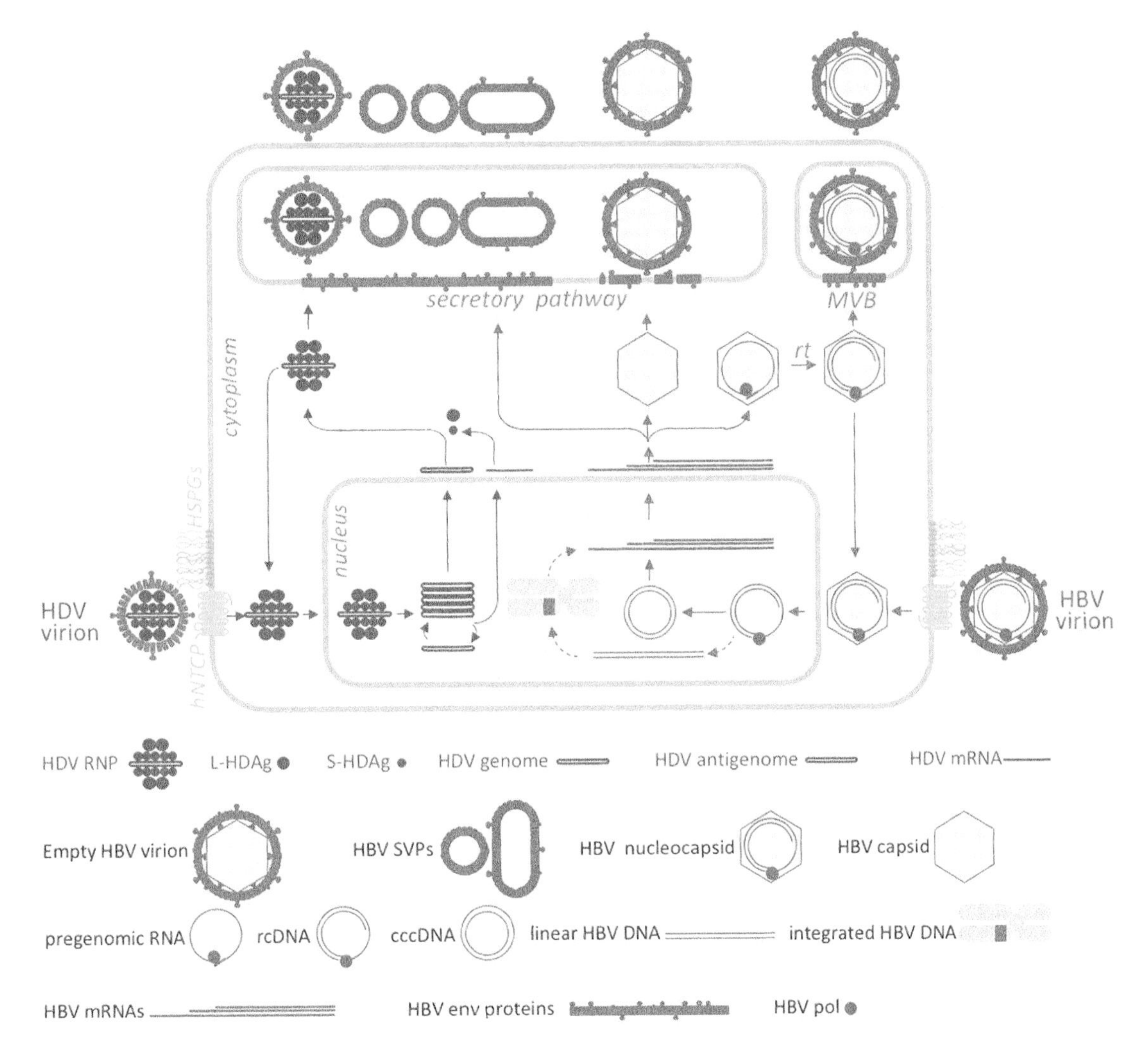

FIGURE 19.7 Schematic representation of the HDV/HBV replication cycle. Upon infection, the HDV RNP is directed to the nucleus for replication. The intrinsic HDV replication pathway is indicated in *blue* and the HBV-specific pathway in *red*. SVP, subviral particles; HSPGs, heparan sulfate proteoglycans; hNTCP, human sodium taurocholate cotransporting polypeptide; L-HDAg, large HDAg protein; S-HDAg, small HDAg protein; MVB, multivesicular body pathway; rt, reverse transcription.

The neosynthesized, and greater-than-unit length antigenomic RNA, is then rapidly processed into monomers by the embedded ribozyme. The self-cleavage product is a linear molecule that can ligate on itself to form a circular RNA. In turn, the circular antigenome serves as a template for synthesis of genomic RNA catalyzed by cellular pol II in transcription factories of the nucleoplasm, through a rolling-circle mechanism that also includes self-cleavage and circularization by intramolecular ligation.[92] Overall, the replication strategy of HDV RNA resembles that of some plant viroids but differs from the latter in including the synthesis of an mRNA.[75]

S-HDAg is central to HDV RNA replication. Beside its role as a structural protein, it displays several characteristics of a transcription factor, such as the presence of coiled-coil and helix-loop-helix domains and a propensity to posttranslational phosphorylation, acetylation, methylation, and sumoylation. S-HDAg shows limited sequence similarity to negative elongation factor A (NELF-A),[193] and in an *in vitro* transcription model, S-HDAg binding to Pol II increases the rate of RNA synthesis and fidelity by promoting elongation upon displacement of NELF.[194] S-HDAg can also interact with cellular transcription factor YY1 and its associated acetyltransferases CBP and p300 in a large nuclear complex, which has the capacity to modulate HDV RNA replication.[80] Furthermore, a recent report shows that acetylation of S-HDAg is crucial for replication in allowing the protein to interact with cellular chromatin remodeling factors. More precisely, S-HDAg acetylated at lysine 72 can bind to the bromodomain associated to zinc-finger protein-2B (BAZ2B), an integral component of chromatin remodeling imitation switch complexes (ISWI) that include BAZ2B-associated remodeling factors (BRFs). Acetylated S-HDAg would thus mimic acetylated histone H3 to recruit chromatin remodelers and pol II on the HDV genome. These findings are in agreement with pol II carrying out RNA synthesis—HDAg mRNA and eventually antigenome—from genomic template.[1,123]

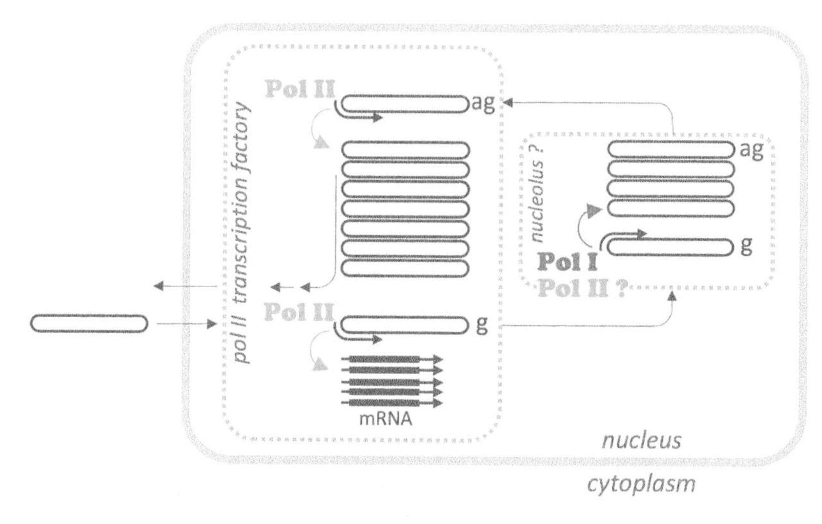

FIGURE 19.8 Intranuclear replication of HDV RNA. Genomic HDV RNA (g) and messenger RNA (mRNA) are synthesized by cellular RNA polymerase II (Pol-II) in pol II transcription factories of the nucleoplasm. Antigenomic (ag) RNA is synthesized by Pol-II—possibly Pol-I—in the nucleolus. HDV mRNAs are exported to the cytoplasm for synthesis of HDAg proteins. Genomic HDV RNA is exported through a Crm1-independent pathway.

HDV ribozymes are essential elements of the genome replication mechanism (Fig. 19.9). They are embedded in both genomic and antigenomic RNAs; they differ from each other by their nucleic acid sequences but adopt a similar secondary structure, referred to as nested double pseudoknot that is quite distinct from that of hammerhead or hairpin ribozymes of viroids or satellites of plant viruses.[47,143] The auto-cleavage reaction is a transesterification mediated by divalent metal ions, which converts a 3′-5′ phosphodiester bond to a 2′-3′ cyclic monophosphate group and a 5′ hydroxyl group. Self-cleavage activity is assisted by HDAg proteins and easily observed *in vitro*, requiring a minimal size of approximately 85 nucleotides for activity.[143] After the discovery of HDV, several cellular HDV-like ribozymes have been found to play a role in

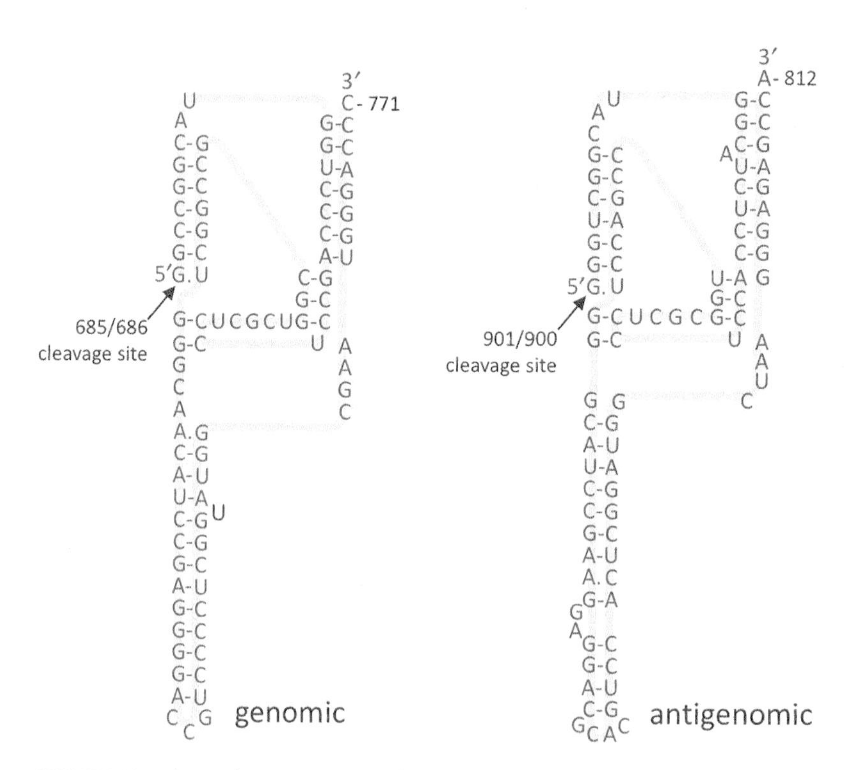

FIGURE 19.9 Secondary structures of genomic and antigenomic HDV ribozymes. Numbering of the nucleotides is indicated as positions on the genomic strand of HDV-1 (GeneBank accession number M21012.1).

a variety of biological events in different branches of life, raising the possibility of HDV RNA itself derived from the cell transcriptome.[185] The latter is notorious to contain abundant amounts of circular RNA species that can be exported from the nucleus through a circular RNA nuclear export pathway.[101]

Indirectly, ADAR1 regulates HDV RNA replication by controlling the switch between an early phase of active replication and a late phase of replication suppression and viral assembly (Fig. 19.5).[24] *In vitro*, the two known isoforms of ADAR1, that is, nuclear ADAR1-S and cytoplasmic ADAR1-L, can mediate editing. However, ADAR1-S is believed to perform most of the editing in the nucleus, whereas ADAR1-L would act only in response to IFN-alpha stimulation.[69]

Overall, the mechanism of HDV genome replication is based on a complex trafficking of both viral RNAs and proteins within the nucleus—from RNA pol II transcription factories to nucleolus—and between nucleus and cytoplasm. It can be tentatively summarized as indicated in Figure 19.8. After transport of the incoming RNP to the nucleus through the action of S-HDAg NLS, the HDV genome is either use as template for mRNA synthesis by pol II in the nucleoplasm, or directed to the nucleolus for synthesis of full-length antigenomic RNA by pol II or pol I/III.[62,115] Neosynthesized antigenomic RNA then migrates from nucleoli to RNA pol II transcription factories in the nucleoplasm for synthesis of genomic RNA. While antigenomes are retained in the nucleus, genomes are rapidly exported to the cytoplasm through a Crm1-independent pathway.[115] A disruption of nuclear paraspeckles and the delocalization of the paraspeckles protein 1 to the cytoplasm has been described to occur upon HDV replication, but it is uncertain to what degree it participates to the cytoplasmic sorting of HDV RNA.[9]

HDV genome replication appears very efficient if one considers the accumulation of up to 300,000 genomes per cell, 50,000 antigenomes, and approximately 1,000 copies of mRNA. Nonetheless, the peak of viral RNA accumulation generally occurs over a long period of time post entry—6 to 9 days—suggesting that the recruited host RNA polymerases are in fact substantially impeded when using a single-stranded HDV RNA instead of their natural double-stranded cellular DNA as template.

HDV Virion Assembly

The Assembly of HDV RNP

A possible scenario for RNP assembly is that HDAg proteins would first form dimers through antiparallel coiled coils (residues 13 to 48) prior to formation of octamers and binding to rod-like HDV RNA.[104,200] This arrangement is reminiscent of the histone octamer structure in nucleosomes. An octamer binding requires a minimum of approximately 300 nt in length of HDV RNA folded as an unbranched rod.[94,104] In *in vitro* assembled RNPs, the viral RNA is flexible enough to bend and condense with HDAg proteins. The flexibility of the rod structure is likely to result from the presence of unpaired bases.[58]

The cellular compartment in which genome-bearing RNPs are assembled prior to envelopment in the cytoplasm is not known. During replication in the nucleus, the genomic RNA—and not antigenomic—is actively exported to the cytoplasm, possibly complexed with S-HDAg, but independently of L-HDAg.[115] Yet, L-HDAg must integrate cytoplasmic RNP that are predestined to virion assembly because its farnesylated C-terminus drives the RNP to the ER membrane where the HBV envelope proteins accumulate. Then, binding of HDV RNP to envelope proteins is thought to involve a proline-rich sequence located just upstream of the farnesylation site.[89] The same C-terminus of L-HDAg contains an NES and a clathrin box, both eventually instrumental in particle morphogenesis, but it is still unclear how these elements fit into the virion assembly process.[76,89,98] Whether formation of genome-bearing RNPs takes place in the nucleus or cytoplasm and whether assembly of HDV virions require a direct binding of the C-terminal sequence of L-HDAg to HBV envelope proteins is presently unknown.

Upon electron microscopy examination, the HDV RNPs appear as spheres of approximately 20 nm in diameter with no apparent icosahedral symmetry. The molar ratio of HDAg proteins to HDV RNA in a virion-associated RNP was first measured at 70,[156] in agreement with the estimation by Lin and colleagues of approximately 32 to 40 HDAg subunits per HDV RNA,[104] but in a subsequent study, this number was revised to 220.[62]

Assembly and Release of HDV Virions

For cell egress, as for entry, HDV relies on the assistance of the HBV envelope proteins (Fig. 19.7). This is in fact the only HBV contribution to the HDV life cycle, because HDV can propagate in a liver free of HBV replication, in which production of S- and L-HBsAg proteins is directed by integrated HBV DNA sequences.[48,49]

The distinctive feature of the HBV life cycle that makes this virus the ideal partner for HDV resides in the unique properties of its envelope proteins. They are produced in amounts far exceeding the need for HBV virion assembly; they self-assemble at the ER membrane and are secreted in abundance as SVPs.[72] HBV virion assembly is a rare event in comparison with SVPs, leading to an average infectious serum containing approximately 10^{12} to 10^{13} SVPs per mL for only 10^8 to 10^9 virions (Fig. 19.7). For comparison, at the peak of an acute HDV infection, titers of HDV virions can reach 10^{11} per mL. Thus, paradoxically, HDV makes a more efficient use of HBV envelope proteins than does HBV.

The HBV envelope proteins are membrane-spanning glycoproteins that differ from each other by the size of their N-terminal ectodomain (Fig. 19.10).[72] L-HBsAg contains an N-terminal pre-S1, central pre-S2, and C-terminal S domains. M-HBsAg is shorter than L-HBsAg in lacking pre-S1, whereas S-HBsAg lacks both pre-S1 and pre-S2. Synthesis occurs at the ER membrane, and SVPs bud at a pre-Golgi intermediate compartment, before export through the secretory pathway.[137] Assembly of HBV virions requires L-HBsAg—in addition to S-HBsAg—because it bears the matrix domain for HBV nucleocapsid envelopment. But the high proportion of L-HBsAg required for assembly of HBV virion prevents its spontaneous budding in the post-ER lumen, which is achieved only with the assistance of the host endosomal sorting complex required for transport (ESCRT) in the late endosomal multivesicular bodies (MVBs).[184]

In contrast to HBV, HDV virion assembly can be achieved by the sole S-HBsAg protein, resulting in S-HBsAg-coated HDV particles that are noninfectious for lacking

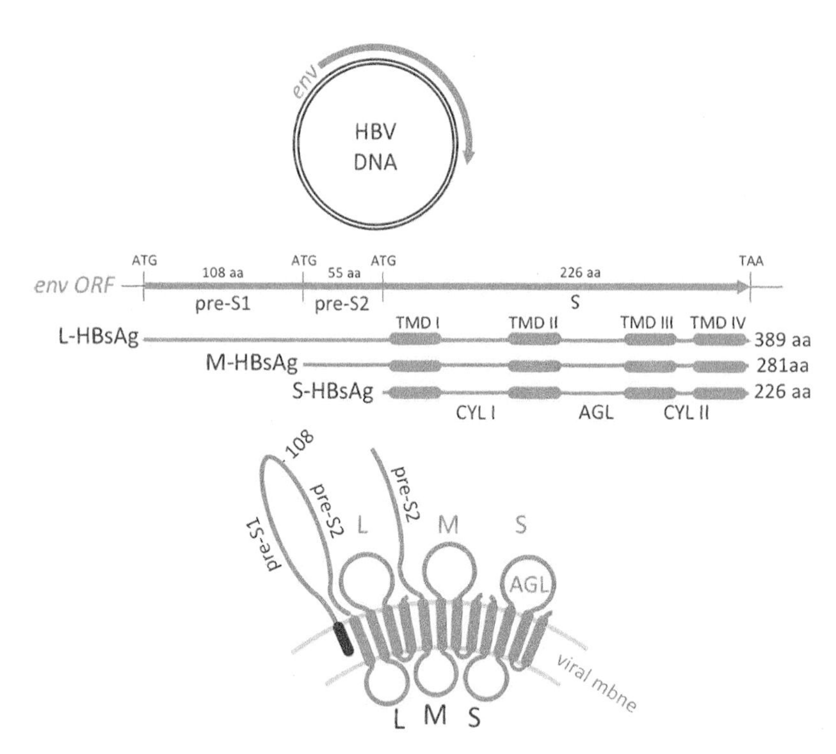

FIGURE 19.10 **The HBV envelope proteins.** The open reading frame for the HBV envelope proteins is indicated on the HBV genome (**top panel**). The L-HBsAg, M-HBsAg, and S-HBsAg proteins are translated from three in-frame initiation sites located at the amino terminus of the pre-S1, pre-S2, and S domains, respectively (**middle panel**). *Thick red lines* indicate transmembrane domains (TMDs). *Thick black line* represents myristic acid covalently linked to the L-HBsAg N-terminus. Secondary structure model (**bottom panel**) for L-, M-, and S-HBsAg at the viral membrane (mbne) is represented, including in the antigenic loop (AGL) and the pre-S1 and pre-S2 domains. CYL-I and II, cytosolic domain I and II, respectively.

L-HBsAg (Fig. 19.11).[167] The signal for binding to HDV RNP within S-HBsAg, referred to as HDV matrix domain, (Fig. 19.12) maps to the carboxyl terminus of the protein and consists of aromatic residues W196, W199, Y200, and W201 that are conserved in the envelope proteins of all *Orthohepadnaviruses*.[89] In nature, HDV infection occurs only in association with HBV, but it can be experimentally conducted in woodchucks infected with the woodchuck

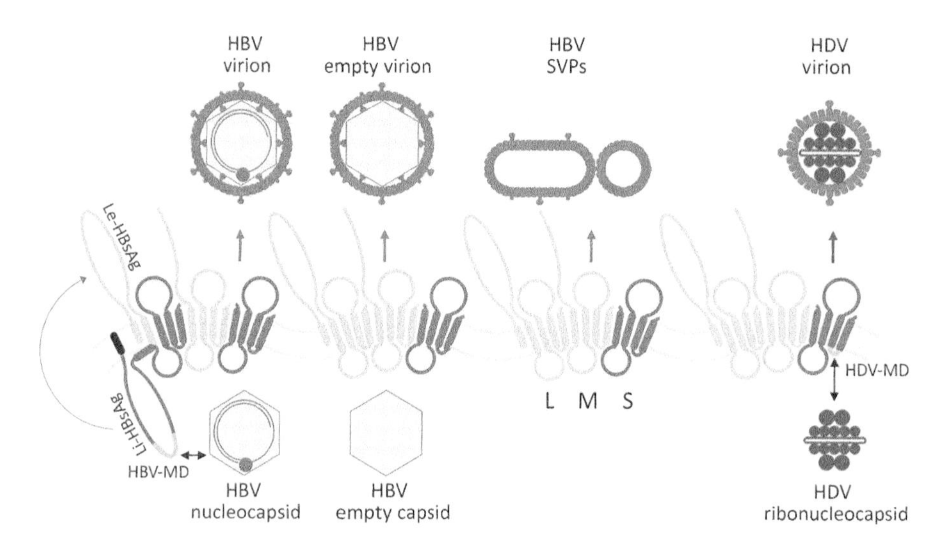

FIGURE 19.11 **Model for HDV and HBV virions assembly.** HBV and HDV particles assemble and bud into the lumen of the cellular intermediate compartment (IC) between ER and Golgi. Aggregates of HBV envelope protein bud spontaneously at the IC membrane. When aggregates include S-HBsAg proteins only, or S-HBsAg + M-HBsAg, it leads to secretion of spherical SVPs. When aggregates include L-HBsAg in the presence of HBV nucleocapsid, budding of HBV virions occurs in multi vesicular bodies. In case of HDV coinfection, the HDV RNP is addressed to the ER membrane and interacts with the HBV proteins, irrespective of the presence of L-HBsAg, leading to the release of HDV virion. Incorporation of the L-HBsAg protein in the HDV envelope confers infectivity. Alternative topologies of L-HBsAg are represented: N-terminal pre-S domain is cytosolic at the ER membrane (Li-HBsAg) for recruiting DNA-containing nucleocapsid in virion assembly, or luminal (Le-HBsAg), that is, external on secreted HBV virions for receptor-binding function. HDV-MD, HDV matrix domain in S-HBsAg. HBV-MD, HBV matrix domain in L-HBsAg.

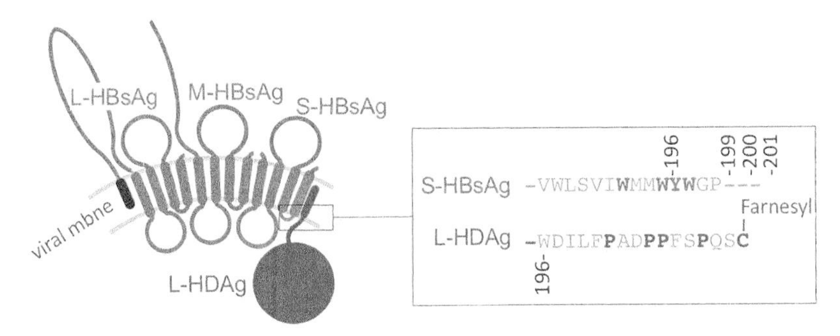

FIGURE 19.12 HBV–HDV interaction. The HDV matrix domain consists of tryptophan -196, -199, -201, and Tyr-200 in the S domain of the HBV envelope proteins. The matrix domain is assumed to interact (directly or indirectly) with the C-terminus of the RNP-associated L-HDAg protein. Within the C-terminus of L-HDAg, the CXXQ sequence is a signal for farnesylation at cysteine-211, which is essential for HDV virion assembly. Proline residues are important for interaction with HBV envelope proteins.

hepatitis virus (WHV). Furthermore, the envelope proteins of other *Orthohepadnaviruses*, such as the woolly monkey HBV (WMHBV), the tent-making bat HBV (TBHBV), or capuchin monkey hepatitis B virus (CMHBV) are competent for HDV virion production when tested in an *in vitro* culture model.[7,23,39,140,155] By contrast, the envelope proteins of the duck hepatitis B virus (DHBV) lack a HDV matrix domain, and, consequently, DHBV cannot serve as helper.[134]

The HDV matrix domain is conserved among all HBV genotypes, and even all *Orthohepadnaviruses* but paradoxically, it is dispensable for the HBV life cycle.[13] A likely explanation is that its conservation is a consequence of the overlap between ORFs for polymerase (*pol*) and envelope proteins (*env*) in the HBV genome (Fig. 19.13). As a matter of fact, the HBV DNA sequence that codes for the HDV matrix domain in *env* also encodes, in the minus-one frame, the reverse transcriptase catalytic domain (YMDD) in *pol*, and it is likely that the strict requirement of YMDD for reverse transcriptase activity imposes in *env* a tryptophan-rich domain that is used by HDV as a matrix domain.

HDV virions released in the extracellular space have an average diameter of 36 nm and a buoyant density of 1.25 g/cm^3 in CsCl.[148] The HDV envelope is identical to that of HBV SVPs, consisting of cell-derived lipids associated to HBV envelope proteins surrounding the inner RNP of approximately 20 nm in diameter and assumed to contain a single copy of genomic RNA.[17,62,70,148]

Since HDV RNA can replicate within cells of different species and tissues in the absence of HBV, there is a theoretical possibility that HDV could propagate using the envelope proteins of non-HBV. When this hypothesis was tested experimentally, it was found that envelope proteins of *Vesiculovirus*, *Flavivirus*, and *Hepacivirus* could, to some extent, package the HDV RNP and lead to the production and release of pseudotyped HDV particles. Moreover, HDV was shown to propagate in the liver of immune-deficient liver-humanized mice coinfected with HCV, suggesting that the latter could serve as a helper.[138] However, this hypothesis is supported by neither clinical observations nor serological testing.

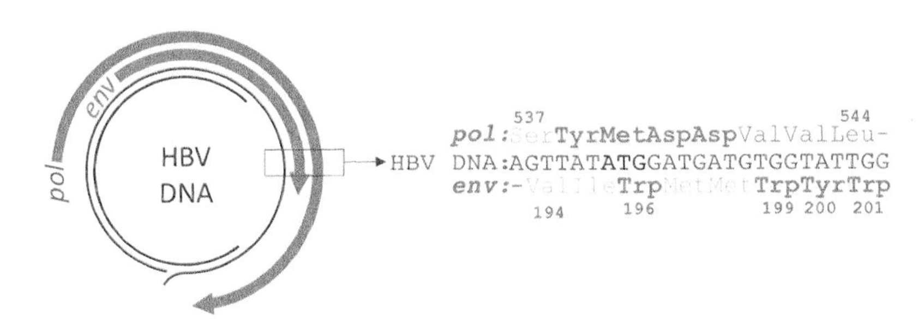

FIGURE 19.13 Conservation of the HDV matrix domain. The HDV matrix domain in HBV envelope proteins (env) consists of Trp-196, -199, -201, and Tyr-200. It is assumed to be conserved as a consequence of the HBV *env* and *pol* genes overlap in the HBV genome. The HBV DNA sequence that codes for the HDV matrix domain, also codes, in the minus-one reading, for the YMDD catalytic motif of HBV reverse transcriptase. It is hypothesized that the strict requirement for YMDD motif in *pol-RT* is at the origin of the HDV matrix domain conservation in HBV *env* proteins.

PATHOGENESIS AND PATHOLOGY

Natural Host and Animal Models

In nature, HDV infection occurs only in humans infected with HBV, but it was achieved experimentally in the chimpanzee model under both coinfection and superinfection settings (Fig. 19.14).[147] In this animal model, coinfection resulted in hepatitis characterized by a transient elevation of serum alanine aminotransferase (ALT); the infection was self-limited but progressed to chronicity in 50% of superinfected animals.[125] Superinfection in this model was characterized by a transient suppression of HBV replication at the acute phase of HDV infection.[172] As in humans, the liver was the only infected organ, but it was affected with a more severe disease in comparison to other viral hepatitis. In theory, HDV should be able to propagate in species susceptible to other *Orthohepadnaviruses*, as long as their envelope proteins contain the HDV matrix domain.[7,23,39,155] In reality, HDV infection has been achieved experimentally in woodchucks infected with WHV, causing acute hepatitis, with a high proportion of animals becoming chronically infected.[140]

In recent years, numerous mouse models have been developed, including immune competent mice inoculated with HDV, HDV cDNA, or HDV RNA, in which low levels of genome replication in the liver could be documented.[126] But, in the absence of helper HBV replication, HDV propagation was not possible. In transgenic mice created to express S- or L-HDAg, or to sustain HDV RNA replication, no cytopathic effect in the liver could be observed.[66] More recently, several immune-deficient liver-humanized mouse models have been established that are susceptible and permissive to HBV/HDV infection, but again without evidence of cytopathy for the human hepatocytes.[18,112,138] Finally, transgenic mice expressing hNTCP have been generated that are also readily susceptible to infection, leading to replication of HDV RNA in the liver. Yet the animals remained resistant to HBV for lacking cellular factor(s) required for productive HBV infection.[71] Further improvement is thus required to generate an immunocompetent mouse model that could sustain chronic HDV infection.

Entry Into the Host and Site of Primary Replication

HDV enters into the host following the same parenteral route of transmission as that used by the helper HBV, via blood or body fluids. As a highly vascularized organ, the liver is directly exposed to HBV/HDV circulating in the bloodstream. Infectious particles are assumed to reach the liver sinusoids through the portal vein or hepatic artery and the space of Disse through fenestrations of the sinusoid endothelium. It is then taken up by hepatocytes after an initial binding to HSPG at the basolateral membrane followed by a secondary interaction of L-HBsAg to the hNTCP.[195] Primary replication of HDV occurs in human hepatocytes that are either already infected with HBV—a superinfection setting characterized by short incubation period—or to become coinfected by HBV (Fig. 19.14). In all cases, the direct pathologic effects of infection are limited to the liver.

Release From Host and Transmission

Within the liver, HBV and HDV virions egress coinfected hepatocytes through the basolateral membrane to reach the space of Disse and the blood circulation through the central vein. At the peak of an acute infection, serum titers of HDV virions can reach 10^{11} per mL. Therefore, HDV infection occurs, as for HBV, through percutaneous exposure to infected blood or blood products. The most efficient transmission

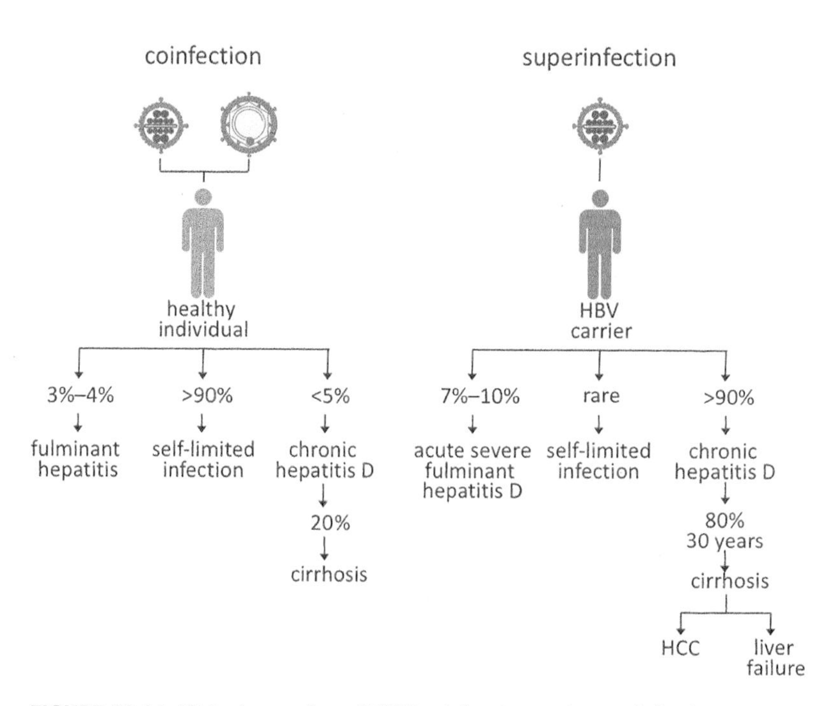

FIGURE 19.14 Clinical sequelae of HDV coinfection and superinfection. Comparison between coinfection of an individual by both HBV and HDV, and superinfection of a HBV-chronic carrier by HDV.

occurs in the context of HDV superinfection of HBsAg-positive individuals.[149]

Sexual transmission of HDV is suggested by the observation that infections are more prevalent in individuals under 40 years old in regions of high endemicity.[19] Furthermore, a recent meta-analysis study has shown a HDV seroprevalence in HBsAg carriers with high-risk sexual behavior at 17% in comparison with 10% in a population without risk factors.[33] By contrast, there is a low rate of mother-to-child transmission (MTCT) of HDV, which might correspond to the HDV suppressive effect on HBV viremia in coinfected mothers who, consequently, would not transmit HBV to their newborn.[162]

HDV transmission varies according to the prevalence in the general population. In industrialized countries, transmission occurs mainly through contact with infected blood, in particular among intravenous drug users (IVDUs).[33] Intrafamilial transmission has been documented in low-income communities through unapparent exchange of body fluids.[11,130] In Mongolia, the high HDV prevalence is attributed to horizontal transmission including inadequate dental/medical procedures in addition to sexual activity.[32]

Mechanisms of Liver Damage and Immune Response

HDV is strictly hepatotropic, inducing direct pathologic effects only in the liver. However, experiments conducted using *in vitro* and *in vivo* models could not demonstrate that HDAg proteins expression, or the production of HDV virions, were cytopathic.[35,66,114] In tissue culture, HDV RNA replication does not induce cytotoxicity *per se*, but may, at most, partially impair cell division. This effect could be detrimental to liver regeneration in the setting of CHD.[182] Because HBV is generally suppressed by HDV replication, liver damage is more likely induced by HDV rather than HBV. In CHD patients, the HDV and HBV markers fluctuate in alternation over time with repeated flares of hepatitis. Liver injury in CHD patients is, for the most part, immune-mediated, consisting essentially of hepatocyte necrosis and the presence of inflammatory infiltrates.[124] In a particular study of CHD patients selected for different stages of fibrosis, the levels of HDV replication in the liver could not be correlated to a specific histology pattern.[198] Instead, there was a correlation between an increase of HDAg-specific T-cell response and a decrease of liver disease.[133] In a cytokine profiling study, interleukin (IL)-2, IFN-gamma, IFN-inducible protein-10, and IL-10 responses were detectable in 53%, 35%, 65%, and 6% of CHD patients, respectively, with an HDV-specific IFN-gamma response occurring preferentially in patients with low-level HDV viremia.[56] Noteworthy, among all chronic viral hepatitis, the highest frequency of CD4+ cytotoxic T lymphocytes is found in CHD patients.[6]

Virus-specific CD8 T-cell response seems to play a role in the outcome of HDV infection. Yet, the HDV-specific T-cell epitope repertoire and mechanisms of CD8 T-cell failure have been poorly characterized. Only in a recent study, mutations within L-HDAg-specific CD8 T-cell epitopes of CHD patients could be associated with escape from the HLA-B27-restricted CD8 T-cell response and correlated with the clinical outcome.[87] In comparison to chronic hepatitis B (CHB) patients, CHD patients have lower levels of mucosa-associated invariant T (MAIT) cells in both peripheral blood and liver. MAIT cells appear as activated, functionally impaired, and severely depleted.[38] Overall, the HDV-specific adaptive immune responses in CHD patients fails to contain the infection.

In cell culture, the IFN signaling pathway is activated by HDV.[3,71,118,187] L-HDAg alone can activate the MxA ISG and inhibit HBV transcription.[188] But even if the IFN response of cells replicating HDV appears to be intact, IFN-alpha modestly inhibits HDV replication.[118]

In the liver-humanized mouse model, HDV infection can provoke a clear enhancement of the antiviral state in human hepatocytes, which might contribute to HBV suppression,[51] but the STAT1 ISG is barely detected in hepatocytes highly positive for HDAg, as if inhibited by the latter. This is in agreement with an *in vitro* study showing that HDV replication is associated with the inhibition of STAT1 and STAT2 response to IFN-alpha.[141] In the peripheral blood of CHD patients responding to IFN-alpha treatment, the number of NK cells is increased in comparison to healthy controls, suggesting a role of NK cells in HDV pathogenesis, but long-term treatments may cause changes in NK cell differentiation and functional impairment.[110]

Clinical Features and Natural History

Both coinfection and superinfection can induce the most aggressive form of hepatitis, although the severity of liver damage may vary from totally asymptomatic to acute liver failure and death.

Acute HDV Infection

The clinical course of acute hepatitis D is similar to that of an acute hepatitis B[164]; symptoms include fatigue, nausea, and hyporexia, accompanied by an elevation of serum ALT/AST levels.

Coinfection may lead to acute hepatitis D characterized by two sequential flares of liver enzymes and, occasionally, a cholestatic course. An icteric phase, characterized by an elevation of serum bilirubin, is not always observed. By contrast, in case of superinfection, the acute phase of HDV replication may lead to liver failure, especially when superinfection occurs in CHB patients already affected by massive necrosis of hepatocytes.[164] A study conducted in Taiwan reported a lesser frequency of acute liver failure related to hepatitis D in patients infected with HDV-2 genotype as compared to HDV-1.[191] By contrast, HDV-3, which prevails in South America, is associated with the highest risk of acute liver failure.[25] The aggressive course of HDV-3 has been tentatively assigned to a specific mutation in HDAg protein, but it is likely to also depend upon other factors, such as the genotype of the helper HBV.[173] Individuals simultaneously coinfected with HDV and HBV progress to chronicity for both viruses at a similar rate as in acute HBV monoinfection, that is, less than 5% in adults.

Chronic HDV Infection

HDV superinfection of HBV carriers leads to chronic HDV infection in the vast majority of patients and, eventually, to CHD (Fig. 19.14).[44] Once HDV chronicity is established, the preexisting liver disease worsen, even though HBV replication is typically, but not invariably, suppressed.[42,90] CHD is characterized by inflammatory infiltrates and progressive deposition of fibrosis often followed by cirrhosis through a wound-healing process. Accordingly, serum ALT/AST levels are persistently elevated in most cases. Longitudinal studies have shown that CHD patients are at a 3-fold higher risk of progression to cirrhosis in comparison to HBV monoinfection.[45] For CHD patients, the risk of cirrhosis was estimated to reach 77% after 30 years of infection.[196] Risk factors of disease progression include HDV genotypes 1 and 3 that are associated with more severe disease than that induced by HDV-2 and -4.[25,166] Severe liver damage in CHD patients is also observed when a high level of HBV replication is maintained during the chronic phase in the absence of, or despite, the HDV suppressive effect on the helper. To what extent HBV genotypes also play a role in the course of CHD remains to be explored.[196]

The fact that CHD-related cirrhosis may remain stable for long periods of time before progressing to liver decompensation or HCC was suggested to result from a decline in HDV replication over time.[154] In HDV-related cirrhosis, liver decompensation occurs at a rate twice that of HBV-related cirrhosis, with a probability of survival at 5 and 10 years estimated at 49% and 40%, respectively.[46,154]

Whether HDV infection increases the risk of developing HCC as compared to HBV monoinfection is still debated. Experiments conducted in mice transgenic for HDAg proteins failed to show any direct carcinogenic role.[66] Nonetheless, a retrospective study from the Eurohep cohort reported that patients with HDV-related cirrhosis had a 5-year risk of developing HCC of 13%, that is, 3.2-fold above that of HBV-related cirrhosis.[46] Subsequent studies pointed to liver decompensation and death, rather than HCC, as the major complication of CHD. In a large study conducted in Italy, the 5- and 10-year event-free survivals were at 83.9% and 59.4%, respectively, with a worse outcome among males. The cumulative probability of liver decompensation was at 75% at 17 years, with an incidence rate of complication of 2.47 per year. Cirrhosis evolved to HCC at a cumulative rate of 0.55 at 17 years, and an annual incidence rate of 1.0.[132] In another Italian study, the main cause of death among CHD patients with cirrhosis was liver failure in 59% of cases, whereas HCC occurred at a rate of 2.8% per year. Interestingly, HDV viremia was an independent predictor of HCC development and mortality.[153] A study from Sweden showed a standardized incidence ratio of 6.11 (95% CI = 2.77 to 11.65) for HCC in CHD as compared to HBV infection.[84] Although the above-mentioned studies indicate that HDV may indeed be a risk factor for HCC, there are discrepancies that may be explained by the very high genetic diversity of HDV and, to a lesser degree, that of coinfecting HBV strains. As shown by a Taiwanese study, the HDV-1/HBV-C coinfection correlated with more adverse outcomes of CHD than HDV-2/HBV-B.[166] In Asia, HDV-2 is associated with milder CHD compared to HDV-1, whereas in the Amazon region of South America, HDV-3 is associated with a particularly severe clinical presentation. In Africa where HDV-5 to -8 prevail, CHD patients are generally affected with a mild form of disease.

HDV Host Cell Interaction

HDV must interact with several components of the cell machinery to compensate for the lack of viral enzyme necessary to replication.[57] Furthermore, the accumulation at high levels of intracellular HDV RNA and proteins during the course of infection is likely to result in multiple host cell interactions and to impact cell metabolism. Numerous host proteins interacting with HDV RNA or proteins have been identified upon different screening approaches in HEK-293 or Huh-7 cell lines (for a review, see Goodrum and Pelchat[54]). Many of them are relevant to HDV replication, and some are likely to disrupt host processes related to nucleic acids and protein metabolism, transport, signal transduction, apoptosis, and cell growth. For instance, HDV replication was shown to increase histone H3 acetylation within the clusterin promoter, leading to an enhanced clusterin expression.[103] It is therefore conceivable that this epigenetic regulation contributes to carcinogenesis because clusterin overexpression has been reported in 89% of human HCC cases.[86] In that particular study, there was no mention of HDV markers, but 73% of clusterin-positive HCC were HBsAg-positive.

The observations concerning the relationship between HDV and cell proliferation are far from conclusive, because HDV replication has been shown to either impair cell proliferation in tissue culture,[182] or induce cell cycle arrest[28] and cell death.[35] By contrast, the expression of L-HDAg in cell culture led to activation of the serum response factor (SRF) and serum response element (SRE) signaling pathways, possibly in synergy with the HBV x (HBx) protein to activate cell proliferation.[55]

The analysis of the HEK-293 cell proteome changes upon expression of S-HDAg, or HDV RNP, identified differentially expressed proteins that, for the most part, were related to cell-cycle regulation and pyruvate metabolism. Interestingly, p53 was down-regulated, and the G2/M DNA damage checkpoint was among the most affected pathways, suggesting a possible mechanism of HCC induction by HDV.[119] In HEK-293 or Huh-7 cells, L-HDAg was shown to modulate the NF-kappaB signaling pathway.[136] NF-kappaB activation in L-HDAg-expressing cells may result from an increased ER stress or the production of reactive oxygen species.[187] In addition, L-HDAg may induce liver fibrogenesis by activating TGF-beta–induced signal transduction. In cell culture, L-HDAg has been shown to regulate TGF-beta–mediated signaling in a farnesylation-dependent manner, and the effect was synergistically activated by HBx.[34]

Finally, in a recent study, a screening of HDV-infected cells with siRNA and small molecules identified the carbamoyl-phosphatesynthetase 2, aspartate transcarbamylase and dihydroorotase (CAD), and estrogen receptor alpha (ESR1) as key host factors for HDV RNA replication. Since CAD and ESR1 inhibitors could suppress HDV replication, they may have potential as anti-HDV drugs.[179]

Persistence

In vivo, HDV RNA can survive in the absence of HBV, as demonstrated in the liver-humanized mouse model in which HDV RNA and proteins could be maintained for at least 6 weeks in absence of HBV.[52] In the same mouse model, HDV RNA could even persist during liver regeneration and be amplified through cell division.[4] HDV may thus cause latent, HBV-free infection as observed in the setting of liver transplantation.[135] Moreover, considering that HDV RNA and HDAg proteins accumulate at up to 300,000 and 6,000,000 copies per cell, respectively,[62] their persistence in the liver could even be maintained through several cell divisions without HDV RNA replication. Nevertheless, *de novo* infection of naive hepatocytes requires that the HBV envelope proteins be provided to assemble infectious particles.

Interference

HDV exerts a suppressive effect on HBV replication, which has been documented in both humans and animal models.[90,139,157] HDV is hence considered as dominant over HBV.[113] In a superinfection setting, HDV leads to a transient suppression of HBV markers in both serum and liver during the acute phase of HDV replication.[140,147,172] In CHD patients, longitudinal studies show a considerable variation of one or both viruses activities over time, including alternating predominance, fluctuation of both viruses in parallel, or stability of one virus with fluctuation of the other.[160] The underlying mechanism of interference is only partially understood, but it is likely to involve both a direct repression of HBV transcription exerted by HDAg proteins in coinfected cells[188,190] and an indirect, cytokine-mediated inhibition.[3,51] In Huh-7 cells, the sole expression of HDAg proteins could repress HBV enhancers 1 and 2, while activating transcription of the MxA ISG.[188] In differentiated HepaRG cells, HDV superinfection could activate the IFN pathway via MDA5, without change in the NF-kappaB pathway, and partially suppress HBV replication.[3,199] These findings are in agreement with the notion that HepaRG cells and primary cultures of human hepatocytes (PHH) do express innate immunity sensors and respond to IFN.[109] However, IFN-alpha–induced signaling might be repressed by HDV through a mechanism that inhibit the JAK/STAT signaling pathway.[141]

EPIDEMIOLOGY

Prevalence

HDV is always found in association with HBV infection. Until recently, it was estimated that 5% of the HBV carriers were coinfected with HDV, for a total of 15 to 20 million HDV carriers worldwide. Regions of highest prevalence include Central and West Africa, Central and Northern Asia, the Pacific Islands of Kiribati and Nauru, countries of the Middle East, Eastern Europe and the Mediterranean countries, the Amazonian basin, and Greenland.[40] Surprisingly, the HDV worldwide distribution does not exactly match that of HBV. Moreover, it is unclear why HDV prevalence may differ substantially between neighboring countries or even between neighboring regions, or villages, such as in Africa or the Amazon basin.[11,19] But one has to keep in mind that HDV prevalence has not been investigated, or reported, in many countries and hence, its global prevalence and geographic distribution remain incomplete.

To generate a better estimate of HDV prevalence, Chen and colleagues[33] performed a meta-analysis of studies published prior to 2017. They concluded that the pooled prevalence of HDV infection worldwide could be as high as 10% in the population of HBsAg carriers, that is, a rate double that reported in 2003.[40] Furthermore, seroprevalence—anti-HDAg antibodies—was estimated at 37% in the populations of HBsAg-positive IVDUs, and at 17% in the high-risk sexual behavior population. Based on this reassessment, HDV prevalence appears lower in asymptomatic HBsAg carriers compared to patients with active hepatitis, and the current HDV epidemics seem to mainly result from IVD use (37% of HBsAg carriers are anti-HDAg positive) and high-risk sexual behavior (17% of HBsAg carriers are anti-HDAg positive). Yet, this might not be true in countries such as Mongolia where iatrogenic infections are considered to play a major role. In a similar meta-analysis,[120] the pooled prevalence was reported at 13% among HBV carriers, corresponding to 48 to 60 million infections globally. HDV was most prevalent in HBV carriers suffering from fulminant hepatitis (26.7% HDV prevalence), cirrhosis (25.7%), and HCC (19.8%). In this study, the main risk factors for HDV transmission were IVDU and HIV or HCV coinfections. Even though, there were methodological weaknesses in both of the above-mentioned studies, they confirm that the global prevalence of HDV had been largely underestimated, and they agree on a real prevalence of 10% to 13% in the population of HBsAg carriers worldwide.

In Europe, because of universal HBV vaccination and improved socioeconomic conditions, there has been a significant decline in the incidence of HDV infection over the past two decades[145] and a consequential change of epidemiological data, with a preponderance of HDV-infected individuals with advanced cirrhosis.[154] However, recent HDV infections are still observed among high-risk groups such as IVDUs and immigrants from hepatitis D endemic countries.[145] Overall, the new data on HDV prevalence should advocate for all HBsAg-positive individuals to be tested for HDV as a public health measure aimed at reducing transmission and at providing better treatment to CHD patients.

Genetic Diversity

Eight different HDV clades, or genotypes (HDV-1 to -8), have been described (Fig. 19.15), and each has distinct geographic distribution. The classification has been extended from 1 to 4 subgenotypes per genotype.[96] HDV genotypes display an extensive divergence of their nucleotide sequences, with up to 40% divergence between genotypes 1 and 3, while maintaining the same genome structure and organization.[37] But despite a high divergence at the nucleotide sequence level, the functional domains of HDAg proteins are highly conserved.

HDV-1 is the most prevalent worldwide and predominant in Europe and North America. HDV-1 strains might have evolved for a long time from an ancient ancestor that spread to the rest of the world through human migrations. HDV-1 and -5-to-8 appear to originate from central and eastern Africa, emphasizing the wide diversity of HDV in the African continent.[96] HDV-1 is generally associated with mild-to-severe disease, often followed over time by liver cirrhosis and hepatocellular carcinoma.[166] HDV-2 is prevalent in East Asia and the Yakutia Republic of the Russian Federation. It generally causes a mild disease,[189] although in a particular population of Yakutia, it appears as aggressive as HDV-1.[81] HDV-3 is found almost exclusively in the north part of South America. It displays the highest genetic divergence compared to the other genotypes (30% to 40%), with an intragenotype divergence of approximately 10%. HDV-3 is the most aggressive genotype, often associated with fulminant hepatitis and death.[25] HDV-4 is present in Taiwan and Japan. A prospective study of HBsAg carriers in Taiwan revealed that HDV-4 was prevalent (72.2%) among IVDUs, whereas HDV-2 was predominant in the

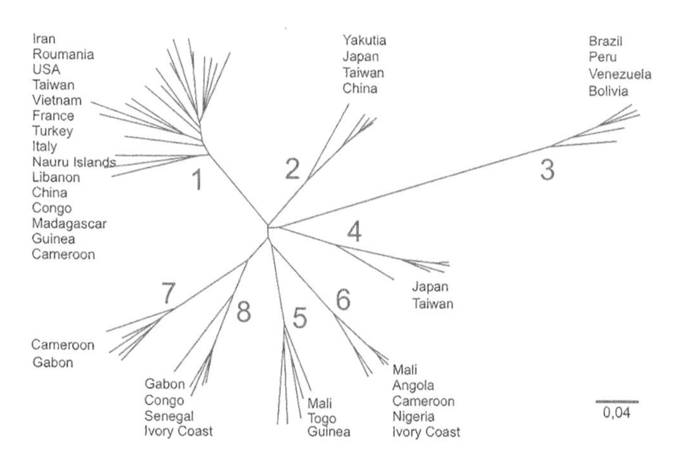

FIGURE 19.15 Unrooted phylogenetic network of HDV genomic sequences, computed with the SplitTree4 application using Clustal Omega, MAFFT, MUSCLE, T-COFFEE, and M-COFFEE alignments, with individual tree reconstruction. Results were obtained through Bayesian analyses using a general time reversible model with proportion of invariable sites and gamma distribution of four classes. At the end of analyses, 25% of the initial tree search was discarded. Note that all the eight genotypes are well defined.

non-IVDU population (73.3%).[106] In the Japanese Miyako Islands, HDV-4 appeared to cause a particularly severe disease.[183] With regard to the African strains, HDV-1 and HDV-5 to -8, the characterization of the associated disease is not yet well documented.

Finally, genetic diversity of HDV might also result from RNA recombination upon mixed infections, allowing the sudden emergence of new strains with functional genomic structure.[105] This phenomenon may add to the difficulty of detecting and quantifying HDV RNA, particularly in patients infected with African strains.[97]

CLINICAL FEATURES

As an obligate HBV satellite, HDV can establish an infection only in the presence of its helper and under circumstances of simultaneous coinfection with HBV, or superinfection of individuals already infected with HBV (Fig. 19.16).[40] In most immunocompetent adults, coinfection progresses to resolution of both HBV and HDV infections, evolving to chronicity in less than 5% of cases.[43] The clinical course of acute coinfection ranges from mild to fulminant hepatitis during which elevation of serum ALT/AST levels may follow a biphasic course,

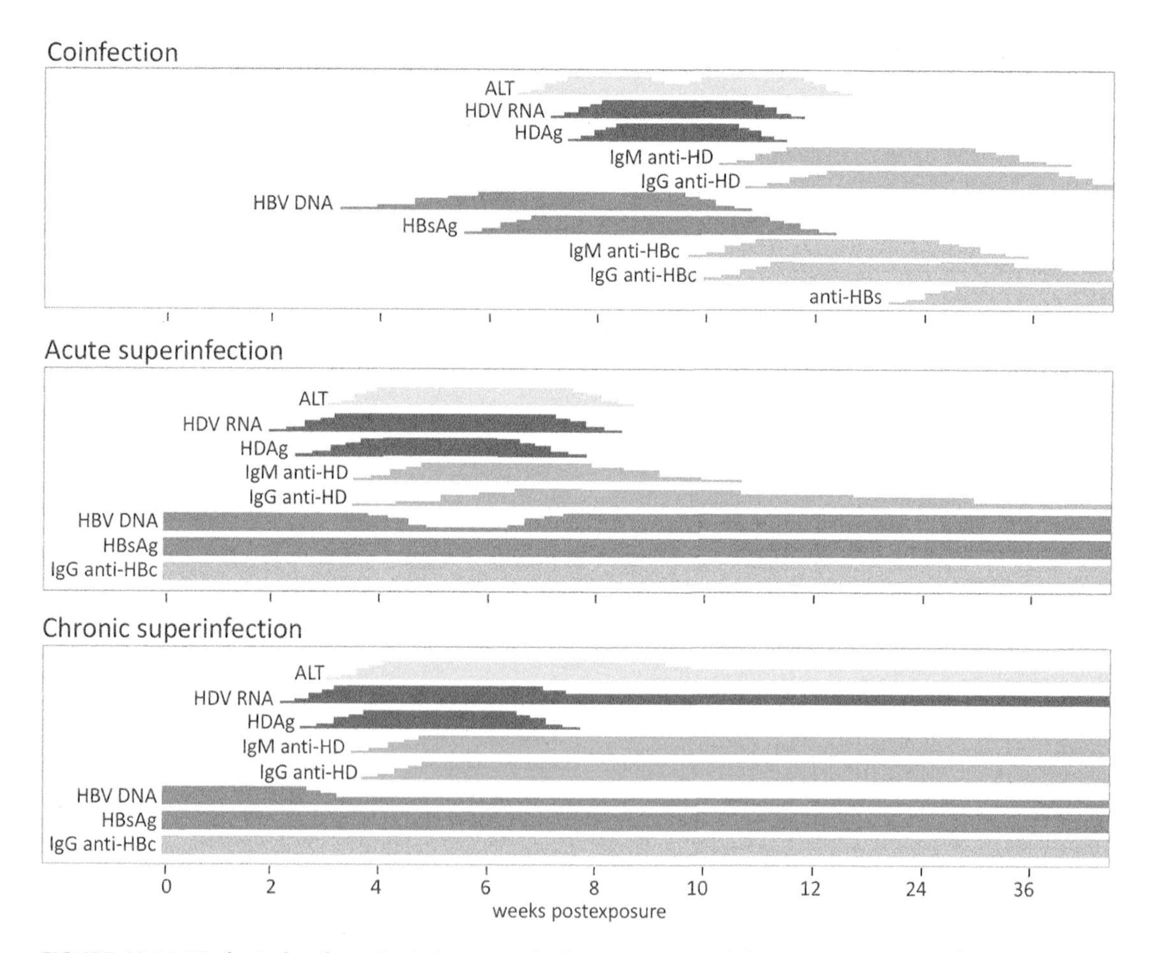

FIGURE 19.16 Virological and serological markers in the settings of coinfection, acute superinfection, and chronic superinfection. HBV markers are indicated in *red*; HDV markers in *blue*.

assumed to result from an initial HBV spread followed by HDV propagation.[164] Symptoms include episodes of fatigue, nausea, and hyporexia. The risk of acute liver failure—fulminant hepatitis—is nonetheless much higher than that observed during acute HBV monoinfection.[41,196]

Superinfection of a patient chronically infected with HBV is associated with an episode of acute hepatitis that occurs after a short incubation period and is associated with a high risk of fulminant hepatitis.[41] Strikingly, more than 90% of superinfected HBV carriers progress to chronic HDV infection.[41,196] The resulting CHD is considered the most severe form of chronic viral hepatitis, and it evolves more rapidly toward cirrhosis and liver failure in comparison to CHB.[46] Liver failure is the most frequent evolution of CHD,[132] with 10% to 15% of patients developing cirrhosis within 5 years, and 80% within 30 years.[45] The risk of HCC is also higher in CHD as compared to CHB.[46,84] Risk factors of disease progression are male sex, cirrhosis at presentation, and lack of antiviral therapy.[132] CHD patients with detectable HDV-RNA in the serum are also the most exposed to liver decompensation and HCC.[153] The clinical outcome of HDV infection depends also on the HBV- and HDV-respective genotypes as observed in populations of the Amazon Basin where the most severe form of acute hepatitis D is caused by HDV-3 associated to HBV-F.[25]

DIAGNOSIS

Screening for HDV infection is too often neglected. Ideally, it should be performed in all HBsAg carriers and in priority in IVDUs, in individuals with high-risk sexual behaviors and immigrants from endemic regions. For a very short period of time (2 to 3 weeks) at the acute phase of replication, and before clinical hepatitis, serum HDAg can be measured by enzyme-linked immunosorbent assay (ELISA) (Fig. 19.16). But, due to its lack of sensitivity, it is no longer in use for diagnosis. Intrahepatic detection of HDAg by immunohistochemistry can only be used when a liver biopsy sample is available. In immune-competent patients, immunoglobulins M and G (IgM and IgG) are the serological markers to test. IgM anti-HDAg appear 2 to 3 weeks after the onset of symptoms; they generally disappear 2 to 3 months after the acute phase of infection but may persist for months in chronically infected individuals. IgG anti-HDAg appear at later times in patients who resolve HDV infection or those who remain chronically infected. Testing for total anti-HDAg antibodies using commercial ELISAs is currently the first step for the detection of HDV infection. Recently, a highly sensitive assay revealed that 60% of HBsAg carriers in a Mongolian population were seropositive.[32] In case of positive serology, serum should be tested for HDV RNA, a procedure now accessible to diagnostic laboratories using commercially available quantitative real-time PCR assays to detect as few as 10 copies of HDV RNA per mL.[97] Still, the robustness of the HDV RNA assay with regard to highly divergent HDV genotypes remains to be confirmed. A WHO international HDV RNA standard has become available for reporting viremia in international units (IU).

PREVENTION AND CONTROL

Vaccine

No HDV-specific vaccine is currently available to protect the large population—estimated at 257 million worldwide—of HBV chronic carriers from becoming superinfected with HDV. An efficient HDV vaccine would be of great benefit to this population because 90% of HBV carriers become chronically infected with HDV and, consequently, at higher risk of liver disease progression to cirrhosis and HCC. Experiments on vaccine development for prevention of HDV superinfection have been conducted in the woodchuck model, but with only limited success. A DNA-prime/viral-vector-boost immunization approach was used that could induce an HDV-specific CD8 T-cell response and prevent coinfection. However, the T-cell response was considered insufficient to inhibit the spread of HDV in chronic HBV carriers.[152] Obviously, new strategies are needed to develop an HDV-specific vaccine.

Since HDV is an obligate satellite of HBV, HBV vaccination protects naive individuals against coinfection. At the population level, the HBV vaccination programs implemented in regions of high endemicity for HBV has helped contain the overall incidence of HDV infection, notably in Italy where circulation of HDV has decreased at a rate of 1.5% per year between 1987 and 1997 as a consequence of universal HBV vaccination in newborns and adolescents.[50]

Treatment

Current Treatment

Current guidelines do not mention specific treatment for acute hepatitis D, except for a liver transplantation in case of fulminant, end-stage liver disease.[131] For CHD patients, the elimination of both HDV and HBV is the ideal endpoint, yet not achievable in the absence of an efficient treatment to cure HBV infection. The major difficulty with HDV infection lies with its intrinsic characteristics; most of the genome replication mechanism is carried out by cellular enzymes that are essential for cell metabolism. Eventually, the HDV ribozymes could be targeted, but the presence of HDV-like ribozymes within host cells may limit the adequacy of such an antiviral approach.[185]

The only effective current treatment is a prolonged administration of IFN-alpha. Long-term IFN treatment decreases the risk of disease progression, irrespective of the on-treatment response pattern, but the rate of sustained virological response—that is, loss of serum HDV RNA—is low. The use of the more active pegylated IFN-alpha (pegIFN-alpha) has led to a more sustained viral response, but in only 25% to 30% of patients, 50% of whom eventually relapsed at 6-month follow-up. The currently recommended course of treatment is a weekly administration of pegIFN-alpha for a 48-week duration. The mechanism through which pegIFN suppresses HDV remains uncertain. When tested in PHH, or in the liver-humanized mouse model, IFN-alpha demonstrated an antiviral effect that appeared to occur at an early phase of infection, that is, viral entry, and/or initiation of replication.[53,67]

Future Treatments

Peg IFN-lambda, a type III interferon, is currently being evaluated in phase III clinical trials based on its better tolerability as compared to IFN-alpha for an equivalent efficacy.[20] In the United States, pegIFN-lambda benefits from an "Orphan Drug" designation that allows to fast-track its evaluation in clinical trials.

Myrcludex-B (also referred to as Bulevirtide) (Fig. 19.17) is a myristoylated pre-S1 peptide that inhibits HBV and HDV entry into human hepatocytes.[112] The receptor-blocking lipopeptide prevents HBV and HDV virions from binding to hNTCP at the basolateral hepatocyte membrane. Data from preclinical trials indicate that the antiviral effect is observed at doses 2 log10 lower than those required for inhibition of the bile acid transport activity of hNTCP. In Ib/IIa clinical trials, CHD patients who received Myrcludex B as monotherapy showed a significant reduction on serum HDV RNA and ALT levels. A combination of Myrcludex and pegIFN-alpha had a synergistic antiviral effect on HDV RNA and HBV DNA but no impact on serum HBsAg.[108]

Nucleic acid polymers (NAPs) are amphipathic phosphorothioate oligonucleotides that are able to establish interactions with a wide variety of integral membrane proteins in a sequence-independent manner. NAPs are assumed to interact with the hydrophobic alpha-helices such as transmembrane domains of viral glycoproteins. In tissue culture, NAPs were shown to interfere with the release of HBV SVPs (HBsAg),[12] and with HDV entry in susceptible cells.[10] In a phase II trial, a small cohort of CHD patients who received NAPs (REP 2139) for 15 weeks achieved a drastic reduction of circulating HBsAg and HDV RNA during the initial phase of NAPs-alone treatment. Combined with pegIFN, a high rate of HBsAg loss and anti-HBsAg seroconversion was observed, with clinical benefits to the patients.[8]

Lonafarnib is a farnesyl-transferase inhibitor that was developed as anticancer drug. When used *in vitro* on cells permissive for the production of HDV virions, it inhibits the farnesylation of L-HDAg, thereby preventing HDV RNP interaction with the HBV envelope proteins and the subsequent production of infectious HDV particles.[18] In a phase II clinical study, CHD patients treated with Lonafarnib for 4 weeks had a 1.5 log10 decline of serum HDV RNA at the end of treatment, but this was accompanied by significant adverse effects.[88] The combination of Lonafarnib with pegIFN-alpha achieved a better reduction of HDV-RNA as compared to pegIFN-alpha alone.[197]

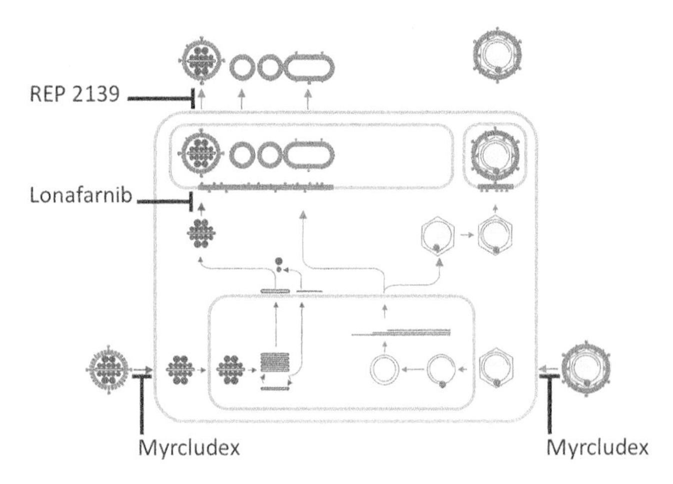

FIGURE 19.17 Novel treatments for HDV infection. Novel antiviral targets in the HDV replication cycle are at the steps of viral entry (Myrcludex), HDV virion assembly by HBV envelope proteins (Lonafarnib), and release of HDV virions and HBV SVPs (REP 2139).

PERSPECTIVES

HDV is unique among animal viruses in many aspects of its biology. It is a subviral agent with a small ssRNA genome and a single viral protein devoid of any enzymatic activity. Yet, with the help of HBV, it manages to cause the most severe form of viral hepatitis in humans.

We are still at the early stages of deciphering the mechanism of HDV RNA replication, and even though there is a growing consensus for genome and mRNA synthesis taking place in pol II–associated transcription factories in the nucleoplasm, and for antigenome synthesis restricted to the nucleolus, the identity of the enzyme(s) involved in antigenome production is still a matter of debate, and neither one of pol II, pol I, pol III, or even a cellular RdRp can be definitely excluded. However, the mechanism by which HDV usurps the cell transcription machinery for replication has begun to unravel when S-HDAg was shown to mimic the activity of acetylated histones in nucleosome as a means to recruit chromatin remodelers for HDV RNA synthesis by pol II. Progress in this area will undoubtedly help understand HDV persistence.

We know that in chimeric mice, HDV RNA can survive through cell division and even replicate in daughter cells in the absence of its helper. If true in humans, HDV RNA would then behave opposite to HBV circular covalently closed (ccc) DNA, by amplifying itself through cell division, while the latter would be lost in the process. Obviously, such distinctive features add a further degree of complexity to the interplay between HDV and its helper, especially in the context of CHD when hepatocyte turnover is increased, and upon antiviral treatment.

There are other gaps to fill in our knowledge of the complex relationship between HDV, the helper HBV, and the host immune system. To this end, the recent development of liver-humanized mouse models permissive for HBV/HDV coinfection has already provided insights into the interplay between the two viruses,[53,138] and it is expected that the forthcoming models of mice humanized for both liver and the immune system will broaden our understanding of the HDV/host interaction.[165]

Although progress has been made in the understanding of the interaction between HDV RNP and HBV envelope proteins, the binding—direct or indirect—between L-HDAg and S-HBsAg, which is at the center of the HBV/HDV interaction, should be further characterized as it may represent a new target for antiviral development.

The role of HDV in HCC development also requires further investigation as it is still questionable whether HDV plays a direct role in carcinogenesis. The long-lasting viral RNA replication and HDAg production in hepatocytes can either instigate cell transformation or induce cell death and compensatory proliferation.

With regard to virus taxonomy, the recent, and surprising, news is that HDV may not stand alone anymore in the classification of viruses. HDV and the recently identified

HDV-like RNAs may have arisen from a common ancestor.[30] But at this point, it is still questionable whether these circular RNAs are infectious agent, and eventually satellites of viruses in their respective hosts. Undoubtedly, more of such HDV-like RNAs will be discovered when metatranscriptomic analyses are extended to more species, and eventually to humans or other species susceptible to *Orthohepadnaviruses* infection. Since the latter have adapted to bats, a species known as a reservoir to many viral species, including *Hepadnaviruses*, it wouldn't be surprising to find HDV-like RNAs in the bat's transcriptome.

Finally, based upon the recent reevaluation of global prevalence of HDV infection at 10% to 13% of HBV-infected individuals,[33,120] HDV infection appears to be more frequent than previously thought, giving further incentive to screen all HBsAg-positive individuals for anti-HDAg and test for HDV RNA in case of positive serology. A larger population of HDV carriers may also indicate a greater diversity that could eventually preclude detection with the actual commercial assays. Taking into account the large number of HDV carriers worldwide, the severity of HDV-related disease, the absence of a specific HDV vaccine, and the scarcity of treatment options, HDV infection now rises as a major public health challenge that requires intensifying efforts to develop innovative antiviral strategies.

REFERENCES

1. Abeywickrama-Samarakoon N, Cortay J-C, Sureau C, et al. Hepatitis delta virus histone mimicry drives the recruitment of chromatin remodelers for viral RNA replication. *Nat Commun* 2020;11:419.
2. Abou-Jaoude G, Sureau C. Entry of hepatitis delta virus requires the conserved cysteine residues of the hepatitis B virus envelope protein antigenic loop and is blocked by inhibitors of thiol-disulfide exchange. *J Virol* 2007;81:13057–13066.
3. Alfaiate D, Lucifora J, Abeywickrama-Samarakoon N, et al. HDV RNA replication is associated with HBV repression and interferon-stimulated genes induction in super-infected hepatocytes. *Antiviral Res* 2016;136:19–31.
4. Allweiss L, Volz T, Giersch K, et al. Proliferation of primary human hepatocytes and prevention of hepatitis B virus reinfection efficiently deplete nuclear cccDNA in vivo. *Gut* 2018;67:542–552.
5. Alves C, Freitas N, Cunha C. Characterization of the nuclear localization signal of the hepatitis delta virus antigen. *Virology* 2008;370:12–21.
6. Aslan N, Yurdaydin C, Wiegand J, et al. Cytotoxic CD4 T cells in viral hepatitis. *J Viral Hepat* 2006;13:505–514.
7. Barrera A, Guerra B, Lee H, et al. Analysis of host range phenotypes of primate hepadnaviruses by in vitro infections of hepatitis D virus pseudotypes. *J Virol* 2004;78:5233–5243.
8. Bazinet M, Pantea V, Cebotarescu V, et al. Safety and efficacy of REP 2139 and pegylated interferon alfa-2a for treatment-naive patients with chronic hepatitis B virus and hepatitis D virus co-infection (REP 301 and REP 301-LTF): a non-randomised, open-label, phase 2 trial. *Lancet Gastroenterol Hepatol* 2017;2:877–889.
9. Beeharry Y, Goodrum G, Imperiale CJ, et al. The hepatitis delta virus accumulation requires paraspeckle components and affects NEAT1 level and PSP1 localization. *Sci Rep* 2018;8:6031.
10. Beilstein F, Blanchet M, Vaillant A, et al. Nucleic acid polymers are active against hepatitis delta virus infection in vitro. *J Virol* 2018;92(4):e01416–e01417.
11. Besombes C, Njouom R, Paireau J, et al. The epidemiology of hepatitis delta virus infection in Cameroon. *Gut* 2020 69(7):1294–1300. doi: 10.1136/gutjnl-2019-320027.
12. Blanchet M, Sinnathamby V, Vaillant A, et al. Inhibition of HBsAg secretion by nucleic acid polymers in HepG2.2.15cells. *Antiviral Res* 2019;164:97–105.
13. Blanchet M, Sureau C. Analysis of the cytosolic domains of the hepatitis B virus envelope proteins for their function in viral particle assembly and infectivity. *J Virol* 2006;80:11935–11945.
14. Blanchet M, Sureau C. Infectivity determinants of the hepatitis B virus pre-S domain are confined to the N-terminal 75 amino acid residues. *J Virol* 2007;81:5841–5849.
15. Blumberg BS, Alter HJ, Visnich S. A "new" antigen in leukemia sera. *JAMA* 1965;191:541–546.
16. Bonino F, Heermann KH, Rizzetto M, et al. Hepatitis delta virus: protein composition of delta antigen and its hepatitis B virus-derived envelope. *J Virol* 1986;58:945–950.
17. Bonino F, Hoyer B, Shih JW, et al. Delta hepatitis agent: structural and antigenic properties of the delta-associated particle. *Infect Immun* 1984;43:1000–1005.
18. Bordier BB, Ohkanda J, Liu P, et al. In vivo antiviral efficacy of prenylation inhibitors against hepatitis delta virus. *J Clin Invest* 2003;112:407–414.
19. Braga WS, Castilho Mda C, Borges FG, et al. Hepatitis D virus infection in the Western Brazilian Amazon—far from a vanishing disease. *Rev Soc Bras Med Trop* 2012;45:691–695.
20. Brancaccio G, Gaeta GB. Treatment of chronic hepatitis due to hepatitis B and hepatitis delta virus coinfection. *Int J Antimicrob Agents* 2019;54:697–701.
21. Brazas R, Ganem D. A cellular homolog of hepatitis delta antigen: implications for viral replication and evolution. *Science* 1996;274:90–94.
22. Bruss V. Envelopment of the hepatitis B virus nucleocapsid. *Virus Res* 2004;106:199–209.
23. de Carvalho Dominguez Souza BF, Konig A, Rasche A, et al. A novel hepatitis B virus species discovered in capuchin monkeys sheds new light on the evolution of primate hepadnaviruses. *J Hepatol* 2018;68:1114–1122.
24. Casey JL. Control of ADAR1 editing of hepatitis delta virus RNAs. *Curr Top Microbiol Immunol* 2012;353:123–143.
25. Casey JL, Brown TL, Colan EJ, et al. A genotype of hepatitis D virus that occurs in northern South America. *Proc Natl Acad Sci U S A* 1993;90:9016–9020.
26. Casey JL, Niro GA, Engle RE, et al. Hepatitis B virus (HBV)/hepatitis D virus (HDV) coinfection in outbreaks of acute hepatitis in the Peruvian Amazon basin: the roles of HDV genotype III and HBV genotype F. *J Infect Dis* 1996;174:920–926.
27. Chang MF, Chang SC, Chang CI, et al. Nuclear localization signals, but not putative leucine zipper motifs, are essential for nuclear transport of hepatitis delta antigen. *J Virol* 1992;66:6019–6027.
28. Chang J, Gudima SO, Tarn C, et al. Development of a novel system to study hepatitis delta virus genome replication. *J Virol* 2005;79:8182–8188.
29. Chang J, Nie X, Chang HE, et al. Transcription of hepatitis delta virus RNA by RNA polymerase II. *J Virol* 2008;82:1118–1127.
30. Chang WS, Pettersson JH, Le Lay C, et al. Novel hepatitis D-like agents in vertebrates and invertebrates. *Virus Evol* 2019;5:vez021.
31. Chao M, Hsieh SY, Taylor J. Role of two forms of hepatitis delta virus antigen: evidence for a mechanism of self-limiting genome replication. *J Virol* 1990;64:5066–5069.
32. Chen X, Oidovsambuu O, Liu P, et al. A novel quantitative microarray antibody capture assay identifies an extremely high hepatitis delta virus prevalence among hepatitis B virus-infected mongolians. *Hepatology* 2017;66:1739–1749.
33. Chen HY, Shen DT, Ji DZ, et al. Prevalence and burden of hepatitis D virus infection in the global population: a systematic review and meta-analysis. *Gut* 2019;68:512–521.
34. Choi SH, Jeong SH, Hwang SB. Large hepatitis delta antigen modulates transforming growth factor-beta signaling cascades: implication of hepatitis delta virus-induced liver fibrosis. *Gastroenterology* 2007;132:343–357.
35. Cole SM, Gowans EJ, Macnaughton TB, et al. Direct evidence for cytotoxicity associated with expression of hepatitis delta virus antigen. *Hepatology* 1991;13:845–851.
36. Daigh LH, Griffin BL, Soroush A, et al. Arginine-rich motifs are not required for hepatitis delta virus RNA binding activity of the hepatitis delta antigen. *J Virol* 2013;87:8665–8674.
37. Deny P. Hepatitis delta virus genetic variability: from genotypes I, II, III to eight major clades? *Curr Top Microbiol Immunol* 2006;307:151–171.
38. Dias J, Hengst J, Parrot T, et al. Chronic hepatitis delta virus infection leads to functional impairment and severe loss of MAIT cells. *J Hepatol* 2019;71:301–312.
39. Drexler JF, Geipel A, Konig A, et al. Bats carry pathogenic hepadnaviruses antigenically related to hepatitis B virus and capable of infecting human hepatocytes. *Proc Natl Acad Sci U S A* 2013;110:16151–16156.
40. Farci P. Delta hepatitis: an update. *J Hepatol* 2003;39(Suppl 1):S212–S219.
41. Farci P, Anna Niro G. Current and future management of chronic hepatitis D. *Gastroenterol Hepatol (N Y)* 2018;14:342–351.
42. Farci P, Karayiannis P, Lai ME, et al. Acute and chronic hepatitis delta virus infection: direct or indirect effect on hepatitis B virus replication? *J Med Virol* 1988;26:279–288.
43. Farci P, Niro GA. Clinical features of hepatitis D. *Semin Liver Dis* 2012;32:228–236.
44. Farci P, Smedile A, Lavarini C, et al. Delta hepatitis in inapparent carriers of hepatitis B surface antigen. A disease simulating acute hepatitis B progressive to chronicity. *Gastroenterology* 1983;85:669–673.
45. Fattovich G, Boscaro S, Noventa F, et al. Influence of hepatitis delta virus infection on progression to cirrhosis in chronic hepatitis type B. *J Infect Dis* 1987;155:931–935.
46. Fattovich G, Giustina G, Christensen E, et al. Influence of hepatitis delta virus infection on morbidity and mortality in compensated cirrhosis type B. The European Concerted Action on Viral Hepatitis (Eurohep). *Gut* 2000;46:420–426.
47. Ferre-D'Amare AR, Zhou K, Doudna JA. Crystal structure of a hepatitis delta virus ribozyme. *Nature* 1998;395:567–574.
48. Freitas N, Cunha C, Menne S, et al. Envelope proteins derived from naturally integrated hepatitis B virus DNA support assembly and release of infectious hepatitis delta virus particles. *J Virol* 2014;88:5742–5754.
49. Freitas N, Salisse J, Cunha C, et al. Hepatitis delta virus infects the cells of hepadnavirus-induced hepatocellular carcinoma in woodchucks. *Hepatology* 2012;56:76–85.
50. Gaeta GB, Stroffolini T, Chiaramonte M, et al. Chronic hepatitis D: a vanishing disease? An Italian multicenter study. *Hepatology* 2000;32:824–827.
51. Giersch K, Allweiss L, Volz T, et al. Hepatitis Delta co-infection in humanized mice leads to pronounced induction of innate immune responses in comparison to HBV mono-infection. *J Hepatol* 2015;63:346–353.
52. Giersch K, Helbig M, Volz T, et al. Persistent hepatitis D virus mono-infection in humanized mice is efficiently converted by hepatitis B virus to a productive co-infection. *J Hepatol* 2014;60:538–544.
53. Giersch K, Homs M, Volz T, et al. Both interferon alpha and lambda can reduce all intrahepatic HDV infection markers in HBV/HDV infected humanized mice. *Sci Rep* 2017;7:3757.
54. Goodrum G, Pelchat M. Insight into the contribution and disruption of host processes during HDV replication. *Viruses* 2019;11:21.
55. Goto T, Kato N, Yoshida H, et al. Synergistic activation of the serum response element-dependent pathway by hepatitis B virus x protein and large-isoform hepatitis delta antigen. *J Infect Dis* 2003;187:820–828.

56. Grabowski J, Yurdaydin C, Zachou K, et al. Hepatitis D virus-specific cytokine responses in patients with chronic hepatitis delta before and during interferon alfa-treatment. *Liver Int* 2011;31:1395–1405.
57. Greco-Stewart V, Pelchat M. Interaction of host cellular proteins with components of the hepatitis delta virus. *Viruses* 2010;2:189–212.
58. Griffin BL, Chasovskikh S, Dritschilo A, et al. Hepatitis delta antigen requires a flexible quasi-double-stranded RNA structure to bind and condense hepatitis delta virus RNA in a ribonucleoprotein complex. *J Virol* 2014;88:7402–7411.
59. Gripon P, Cannie I, Urban S. Efficient inhibition of hepatitis B virus infection by acylated peptides derived from the large viral surface protein. *J Virol* 2005;79:1613–1622.
60. Gripon P, Diot C, Guguen-Guillouzo C. Reproducible high level infection of cultured adult human hepatocytes by hepatitis B virus: effect of polyethylene glycol on adsorption and penetration. *Virology* 1993;192:534–540.
61. Gripon P, Rumin S, Urban S, et al. Infection of a human hepatoma cell line by hepatitis B virus. *Proc Natl Acad Sci U S A* 2002;99:15655–15660.
62. Gudima S, Chang J, Moraleda G, et al. Parameters of human hepatitis delta virus genome replication: the quantity, quality, and intracellular distribution of viral proteins and RNA. *J Virol* 2002;76:3709–3719.
63. Gudima S, Dingle K, Wu TT, et al. Characterization of the 5′ ends for polyadenylated RNAs synthesized during the replication of hepatitis delta virus. *J Virol* 1999;73:6533–6539.
64. Gudima S, He Y, Meier A, et al. Assembly of hepatitis delta virus: particle characterization, including the ability to infect primary human hepatocytes. *J Virol* 2007;81:3608–3617.
65. Gudima S, Wu SY, Chiang CM, et al. Origin of hepatitis delta virus mRNA. *J Virol* 2000;74:7204–7210.
66. Guilhot S, Huang SN, Xia YP, et al. Expression of the hepatitis delta virus large and small antigens in transgenic mice. *J Virol* 1994;68:1052–1058.
67. Han Z, Nogusa S, Nicolas E, et al. Interferon impedes an early step of hepatitis delta virus infection. *PLoS One* 2011;6:e22415.
68. Harichandran K, Shen Y, Stephenson Tsoris S, et al. Hepatitis delta antigen regulates mRNA and antigenome RNA levels during hepatitis delta virus replication. *J Virol* 2019;93: e01989-18.
69. Hartwig D. The large form of ADAR 1 is responsible for enhanced hepatitis delta virus RNA editing in interferon-α-stimulated host cells. *J Viral Hepat* 2006;13:150–157.
70. He LF, Ford E, Purcell RH, et al. The size of the hepatitis delta agent. *J Med Virol* 1989;27: 31–33.
71. He W, Ren B, Mao F, et al. Hepatitis D virus infection of mice expressing human sodium taurocholate co-transporting polypeptide. *PLoS Pathog* 2015;11:e1004840.
72. Heermann KH, Gerlich WH. Surface proteins of hepatitis B viruses. In: Maclachlan A, ed. *Molecular Biology of the Hepatitis B Virus.* Boca Raton, FL: CRC Press; 1991:109–144.
73. Hetzel U, Szirovicza L, Smura T, et al. Identification of a novel deltavirus in Boa constrictors. *MBio* 2019;10(2):e00014–e00019.
74. Hong SY, Chen PJ. Phosphorylation of serine 177 of the small hepatitis delta antigen regulates viral antigenomic RNA replication by interacting with the processive RNA polymerase II. *J Virol* 2010;84:1430–1438.
75. Hsieh SY, Chao M, Coates L, et al. Hepatitis delta virus genome replication: a polyadenylated mRNA for delta antigen. *J Virol* 1990;64:3192–3198.
76. Huang C, Chang SC, Yang HC, et al. Clathrin-mediated post-Golgi membrane trafficking in the morphogenesis of hepatitis delta virus. *J Virol* 2009;83:12314–12324.
77. Huang HC, Chen CC, Chang WC, et al. Entry of hepatitis B virus into immortalized human primary hepatocytes by clathrin-dependent endocytosis. *J Virol* 2012;86:9443–9453.
78. Huang WH, Chen CW, Wu HL, et al. Post-translational modification of delta antigen of hepatitis D virus. *Curr Top Microbiol Immunol* 2006;307:91–112.
79. Huang CR, Lo SJ. Evolution and diversity of the human hepatitis d virus genome. *Adv Bioinformatics* 2010;2010:323654.
80. Huang WH, Mai RT, Lee YH. Transcription factor YY1 and its associated acetyltransferases CBP and p300 interact with hepatitis delta antigens and modulate hepatitis delta virus RNA replication. *J Virol* 2008;82:7313–7324.
81. Ivaniushina V, Radjef N, Alexeeva M, et al. Hepatitis delta virus genotypes I and II cocirculate in an endemic area of Yakutia, Russia. *J Gen Virol* 2001;82:2709–2718.
82. Iwamoto M, Saso W, Sugiyama R, et al. Epidermal growth factor receptor is a host-entry cofactor triggering hepatitis B virus internalization. *Proc Natl Acad Sci U S A* 2019;116:8487–8492.
83. Jaoude GA, Sureau C. Role of the antigenic loop of the hepatitis B virus envelope proteins in infectivity of hepatitis delta virus. *J Virol* 2005;79:10460–10466.
84. Ji J, Sundquist K, Sundquist J. A population-based study of hepatitis D virus as potential risk factor for hepatocellular carcinoma. *J Natl Cancer Inst* 2012;104:790–792.
85. Julithe R, Abou-Jaoude G, Sureau C. Modification of the hepatitis B virus envelope protein glycosylation pattern interferes with secretion of viral particles, infectivity, and susceptibility to neutralizing antibodies. *J Virol* 2014;88:9049–9059.
86. Kang YK, Hong SW, Lee H, et al. Overexpression of clusterin in human hepatocellular carcinoma. *Hum Pathol* 2004;35:1340–1346.
87. Karimzadeh H, Kiraithe MM, Kosinska AD, et al. Amino acid substitutions within HLA-B*27-restricted T cell epitopes prevent recognition by hepatitis delta virus-specific CD8(+) T cells. *J Virol* 2018;92:e01891-17.
88. Koh C, Canini L, Dahari H, et al. Oral prenylation inhibition with lonafarnib in chronic hepatitis D infection: a proof-of-concept randomised, double-blind, placebo-controlled phase 2A trial. *Lancet Infect Dis* 2015;15:1167–1174.
89. Komla-Soukha I, Sureau C. A tryptophan-rich motif in the carboxyl terminus of the small envelope protein of hepatitis B virus is central to the assembly of hepatitis delta virus particles. *J Virol* 2006;80:4648–4655.
90. Krogsgaard K, Kryger P, Aldershvile J, et al. Delta-infection and suppression of hepatitis B virus replication in chronic HBsAg carriers. *Hepatology* 1987;7:42–45.
91. Lai MM. Hepatitis delta virus. In: Granoff A, Webster R, eds. *Encyclopedia of Virology.* London, UK: Academic Press; 1994:574–580.
92. Lai MM. The molecular biology of hepatitis delta virus. *Annu Rev Biochem* 1995;64:259–286.
93. Lamas Longarela O, Schmidt TT, Schoneweis K, et al. Proteoglycans act as cellular hepatitis delta virus attachment receptors. *PLoS One* 2013;8:e58340.
94. Lazinski DW, Taylor JM. Expression of hepatitis delta virus RNA deletions: cis and trans requirements for self-cleavage, ligation, and RNA packaging. *J Virol* 1994;68: 2879–2888.
95. Le Duff Y, Blanchet M, Sureau C. The pre-S1 and antigenic loop infectivity determinants of the hepatitis B virus envelope proteins are functionally independent. *J Virol* 2009;83:12443–12451.
96. Le Gal F, Brichler S, Drugan T, et al. Genetic diversity and worldwide distribution of the deltavirus genus: a study of 2,152 clinical strains. *Hepatology* 2017;66:1826–1841.
97. Le Gal F, Brichler S, Sahli R, et al. First international external quality assessment for hepatitis delta virus RNA quantification in plasma. *Hepatology* 2016;64:1483–1494.
98. Lee CH, Chang SC, Wu CH, et al. A novel chromosome region maintenance 1-independent nuclear export signal of the large form of hepatitis delta antigen that is required for the viral assembly. *J Biol Chem* 2001;276:8142–8148.
99. Lee CZ, Lin JH, Chao M, et al. RNA-binding activity of hepatitis delta antigen involves two arginine-rich motifs and is required for hepatitis delta virus RNA replication. *J Virol* 1993;67:2221–2227.
100. Lempp FA, Schlund F, Rieble L, et al. Recapitulation of HDV infection in a fully permissive hepatoma cell line allows efficient drug evaluation. *Nat Commun* 2019;10:2265.
101. Li Z, Kearse MG, Huang C. The nuclear export of circular RNAs is primarily defined by their length. *RNA Biol* 2019;16:1–4.
102. Li YJ, Stallcup MR, Lai MM. Hepatitis delta virus antigen is methylated at arginine residues, and methylation regulates subcellular localization and RNA replication. *J Virol* 2004;78:13325–13334.
103. Liao FT, Lee YJ, Ko JL, et al. Hepatitis delta virus epigenetically enhances clusterin expression via histone acetylation in human hepatocellular carcinoma cells. *J Gen Virol* 2009;90:1124–1134.
104. Lin BC, Defenbaugh DA, Casey JL. Multimerization of hepatitis delta antigen is a critical determinant of RNA binding specificity. *J Virol* 2010;84:1406–1413.
105. Lin CC, Lee CC, Lin SH, et al. RNA recombination in Hepatitis delta virus: identification of a novel naturally occurring recombinant. *J Microbiol Immunol Infect* 2017;50:771–780.
106. Lin HH, Lee SS, Yu ML, et al. Changing hepatitis D virus epidemiology in a hepatitis B virus endemic area with a national vaccination program. *Hepatology* 2015;61:1870–1879.
107. Lo K, Hwang SB, Duncan R, et al. Characterization of mRNA for hepatitis delta antigen: exclusion of the full-length antigenomic RNA as an mRNA. *Virology* 1998;250:94–105.
108. Loglio A, Ferenci P, Uceda Renteria SC, et al. Excellent safety and effectiveness of high-dose myrcludex-B monotherapy administered for 48 weeks in HDV-related compensated cirrhosis: a case report of 3 patients. *J Hepatol* 2019;71:834–839.
109. Luangsay S, Ait-Goughoulte M, Michelet M, et al. Expression and functionality of Toll- and RIG-like receptors in HepaRG cells. *J Hepatol* 2015;63:1077–1085.
110. Lunemann S, Malone DF, Grabowski J, et al. Effects of HDV infection and pegylated interferon alpha treatment on the natural killer cell compartment in chronically infected individuals. *Gut* 2015;64:469–482.
111. Luo GX, Chao M, Hsieh SY, et al. A specific base transition occurs on replicating hepatitis delta virus RNA. *J Virol* 1990;64:1021–1027.
112. Lutgehetmann M, Mancke LV, Volz T, et al. Humanized chimeric uPA mouse model for the study of hepatitis B and D virus interactions and preclinical drug evaluation. *Hepatology* 2012;55:685–694.
113. Lutterkort GL, Wranke A, Hengst J, et al. Viral dominance patterns in chronic hepatitis delta determine early response to interferon alpha therapy. *J Viral Hepat* 2018;25: 1384–1394.
114. Macnaughton TB, Gowans EJ, Reinboth B, et al. Stable expression of hepatitis delta virus antigen in a eukaryotic cell line. *J Gen Virol* 1990;71 (Pt 6):1339–1345.
115. Macnaughton TB, Lai MM. Genomic but not antigenomic hepatitis delta virus RNA is preferentially exported from the nucleus immediately after synthesis and processing. *J Virol* 2002;76:3928–3935.
116. Magnius L, Taylor J, Mason WS, et al. ICTV Virus Taxonomy Profile: Deltavirus. *J Gen Virol* 2018;99:1565–1566.
117. Manock SR, Kelley PM, Hyams KC, et al. An outbreak of fulminant hepatitis delta in the Waorani, an indigenous people of the Amazon basin of Ecuador. *Am J Trop Med Hyg* 2000;63:209–213.
118. McNair AN, Cheng D, Monjardino J, et al. Hepatitis delta virus replication in vitro is not affected by interferon-alpha or -gamma despite intact cellular responses to interferon and dsRNA. *J Gen Virol* 1994;75(Pt 6):1371–1378.
119. Mendes M, Perez-Hernandez D, Vazquez J, et al. Proteomic changes in HEK-293 cells induced by hepatitis delta virus replication. *J Proteomics* 2013;89:24–38.
120. Miao Z, Zhang S, Ou X, et al. Estimating the global prevalence, disease progression and clinical outcome of hepatitis delta virus infection. *J Infect Dis* 2020;221(10):1677–1687. doi: 10.1093/infdis/jiz633.
121. Modahl LE, Lai MM. The large delta antigen of hepatitis delta virus potently inhibits genomic but not antigenomic RNA synthesis: a mechanism enabling initiation of viral replication. *J Virol* 2000;74:7375–7380.
122. Moraleda G, Taylor J. Host RNA polymerase requirements for transcription of the human hepatitis delta virus genome. *J Virol* 2001;75:10161–10169.
123. Mu JJ, Tsay YG, Juan LJ, et al. The small delta antigen of hepatitis delta virus is an acetylated protein and acetylation of lysine 72 may influence its cellular localization and viral RNA synthesis. *Virology* 2004;319:60–70.
124. Negro F, Baldi M, Bonino F, et al. Chronic HDV (hepatitis delta virus) hepatitis. Intrahepatic expression of delta antigen, histologic activity and outcome of liver disease. *J Hepatol* 1988;6:8–14.
125. Negro F, Bergmann KF, Baroudy BM, et al. Chronic hepatitis D virus (HDV) infection in hepatitis B virus carrier chimpanzees experimentally superinfected with HDV. *J Infect Dis* 1988;158:151–159.

126. Netter HJ, Kajino K, Taylor JM. Experimental transmission of human hepatitis delta virus to the laboratory mouse. *J Virol* 1993;67:3357–3362.
127. Ni Y, Lempp FA, Mehrle S, et al. Hepatitis B and D viruses exploit sodium taurocholate co-transporting polypeptide for species-specific entry into hepatocytes. *Gastroenterology* 2014;146:1070–1083.
128. Ni Y, Zhang Z, Engelskircher L, et al. Generation and characterization of a stable cell line persistently replicating and secreting the human hepatitis delta virus. *Sci Rep* 2019;9:10021.
129. Nie X, Chang J, Taylor JM. Alternative processing of hepatitis delta virus antigenomic RNA transcripts. *J Virol* 2004;78:4517–4524.
130. Niro GA. Intrafamilial transmission of hepatitis delta virus: molecular evidence. *J Hepatol* 1999;30:564–569.
131. Niro GA, Rosina F, Rizzetto M. Treatment of hepatitis D. *J Viral Hepat* 2005;12:2–9.
132. Niro GA, Smedile A, Ippolito AM, et al. Outcome of chronic delta hepatitis in Italy: a long-term cohort study. *J Hepatol* 2010;53:834–840.
133. Nisini R, Paroli M, Accapezzato D, et al. Human CD4+ T-cell response to hepatitis delta virus: identification of multiple epitopes and characterization of T-helper cytokine profiles. *J Virol* 1997;71:2241–2251.
134. O'Malley B, Lazinski DW. Roles of carboxyl-terminal and farnesylated residues in the functions of the large hepatitis delta antigen. *J Virol* 2005;79:1142–1153.
135. Ottobrelli A, Marzano A, Smedile A, et al. Patterns of hepatitis delta virus reinfection and disease in liver transplantation. *Gastroenterology* 1991;101:1649–1655.
136. Park CY, Oh SH, Kang SM, et al. Hepatitis delta virus large antigen sensitizes to TNF-alpha-induced NF-kappaB signaling. *Mol Cells* 2009;28:49–55.
137. Patient R, Hourioux C, Sizaret PY, et al. Hepatitis B virus subviral envelope particle morphogenesis and intracellular trafficking. *J Virol* 2007;81:3842–3851.
138. Perez-Vargas J, Amirache F, Boson B, et al. Enveloped viruses distinct from HBV induce dissemination of hepatitis D virus in vivo. *Nat Commun* 2019;10:2098.
139. Pollicino T, Raffa G, Santantonio T, et al. Replicative and transcriptional activities of hepatitis B virus in patients coinfected with hepatitis B and hepatitis delta viruses. *J Virol* 2011;85:432–439.
140. Ponzetto A, Cote PJ, Popper H, et al. Transmission of the hepatitis B virus-associated delta agent to the eastern woodchuck. *Proc Natl Acad Sci U S A* 1984;81:2208–2212.
141. Pugnale P, Pazienza V, Guilloux K, et al. Hepatitis delta virus inhibits alpha interferon signaling. *Hepatology* 2009;49:398–406.
142. Radjef N, Gordien E, Ivaniushina V, et al. Molecular phylogenetic analyses indicate a wide and ancient radiation of African hepatitis delta virus, suggesting a deltavirus genus of at least seven major clades. *J Virol* 2004;78:2537–2544.
143. Riccitelli N, Luptak A. HDV family of self-cleaving ribozymes. *Prog Mol Biol Transl Sci* 2013;120:123–171.
144. Rizzetto M. The delta agent. *Hepatology* 1983;3:729–737.
145. Rizzetto M. Hepatitis D virus: introduction and epidemiology. *Cold Spring Harb Perspect Med* 2015;5:a021576.
146. Rizzetto M, Canese MG, Arico S, et al. Immunofluorescence detection of new antigen-antibody system (delta/anti-delta) associated to hepatitis B virus in liver and in serum of HBsAg carriers. *Gut* 1977;18:997–1003.
147. Rizzetto M, Canese MG, Gerin JL, et al. Transmission of the hepatitis B virus-associated delta antigen to chimpanzees. *J Infect Dis* 1980;141:590–602.
148. Rizzetto M, Hoyer B, Canese MG, et al. Delta agent: association of delta antigen with hepatitis B surface antigen and RNA in serum of delta-infected chimpanzees. *Proc Natl Acad Sci U S A* 1980;77:6124–6128.
149. Rizzetto M, Ponzetto A, Forzani I. Epidemiology of hepatitis delta virus: overview. *Prog Clin Biol Res* 1991;364:1–20.
150. Rizzetto M, Purcell RH, Gerin JL. Epidemiology of HBV-associated delta agent: geographical distribution of anti-delta and prevalence in polytransfused HBsAg carriers. *Lancet* 1980;1:1215–1218.
151. Rizzetto M, Shih JW, Gerin JL. The hepatitis B virus-associated delta antigen: isolation from liver, development of solid-phase radioimmunoassays for delta antigen and anti-delta and partial characterization of delta antigen. *J Immunol* 1980;125:318–324.
152. Roggendorf M. Perspectives for a vaccine against hepatitis delta virus. *Semin Liver Dis* 2012;32:256–261.
153. Romeo R, Foglieni B, Casazza G, et al. High serum levels of HDV RNA are predictors of cirrhosis and liver cancer in patients with chronic hepatitis delta. *PLoS One* 2014;9:e92062.
154. Rosina F, Conoscitore P, Cuppone R, et al. Changing pattern of chronic hepatitis D in Southern Europe. *Gastroenterology* 1999;117:161–166.
155. Ryu WS, Bayer M, Taylor J. Assembly of hepatitis delta virus particles. *J Virol* 1992;66:2310–2315.
156. Ryu WS, Netter HJ, Bayer M, et al. Ribonucleoprotein complexes of hepatitis delta virus. *J Virol* 1993;67:3281–3287.
157. Sagnelli E, Felaco FM, Rapicetta M, et al. Interaction between HDV and HBV infection in HBsAg-chronic carriers. *Infection* 1991;19:155–158.
158. Salehi-Ashtiani K, Luptak A, Litovchick A, et al. A genomewide search for ribozymes reveals an HDV-like sequence in the human CPEB3 gene. *Science* 2006;313:1788–1792.
159. Salisse J, Sureau C. A function essential to viral entry underlies the hepatitis B virus "a" determinant. *J Virol* 2009;83:9321–9328.
160. Schaper M, Rodriguez-Frias F, Jardi R, et al. Quantitative longitudinal evaluations of hepatitis delta virus RNA and hepatitis B virus DNA shows a dynamic, complex replicative profile in chronic hepatitis B and D. *J Hepatol* 2010;52:658–664.
161. Schulze A, Gripon P, Urban S. Hepatitis B virus infection initiates with a large surface protein-dependent binding to heparan sulfate proteoglycans. *Hepatology* 2007;46:1759–1768.
162. Sellier PO, Maylin S, Brichler S, et al. Hepatitis B virus-hepatitis D virus mother-to-child co-transmission: a retrospective study in a developed country. *Liver Int* 2018;38:611–618.
163. Shimura S, Watashi K, Fukano K, et al. Cyclosporin derivatives inhibit hepatitis B virus entry without interfering with NTCP transporter activity. *J Hepatol* 2017;66:685–692.
164. Smedile A, Farci P, Verme G, et al. Influence of delta infection on severity of hepatitis B. *Lancet* 1982;2:945–947.
165. Strick-Marchand H, Dusseaux M, Darche S, et al. A novel mouse model for stable engraftment of a human immune system and human hepatocytes. *PLoS One* 2015;10:e0119820.
166. Su CW, Huang YH, Huo TI, et al. Genotypes and viremia of hepatitis B and D viruses are associated with outcomes of chronic hepatitis D patients. *Gastroenterology* 2006;130:1625–1635.
167. Sureau C, Guerra B, Lanford RE. Role of the large hepatitis B virus envelope protein in infectivity of the hepatitis delta virion. *J Virol* 1993;67:366–372.
168. Sureau C, Jacob JR, Eichberg JW, et al. Tissue culture system for infection with human hepatitis delta virus. *J Virol* 1991;65:3443–3450.
169. Sureau C, Moriarty AM, Thornton GB, et al. Production of infectious hepatitis delta virus in vitro and neutralization with antibodies directed against hepatitis B virus pre-S antigens. *J Virol* 1992;66:1241–1245.
170. Sureau C, Negro F. The hepatitis delta virus: replication and pathogenesis. *J Hepatol* 2016;64:S102–S116.
171. Sureau C, Salisse J. A conformational heparan sulfate binding site essential to infectivity overlaps with the conserved hepatitis B virus A-determinant. *Hepatology* 2013;57:985–994.
172. Sureau C, Taylor J, Chao M, et al. Cloned hepatitis delta virus cDNA is infectious in the chimpanzee. *J Virol* 1989;63:4292–4297.
173. Tang JR, Hantz O, Vitvitski L, et al. Discovery of a novel point mutation changing the HDAg expression of a hepatitis delta virus isolate from Central African Republic. *J Gen Virol* 1993;74(Pt 9):1827–1835.
174. Taylor JM. Chapter 3. Replication of the hepatitis delta virus RNA genome. *Adv Virus Res* 2009;74:103–121.
175. Taylor J, Pelchat M. Origin of hepatitis delta virus. *Future Microbiol* 2010;5:393–402.
176. Tseng CH, Cheng TS, Shu CY, et al. Modification of small hepatitis delta virus antigen by SUMO protein. *J Virol* 2010;84:918–927.
177. Tseng CH, Lai MM. Hepatitis delta virus RNA replication. *Viruses* 2009;1:818–831.
178. Verrier ER, Colpitts CC, Bach C, et al. A targeted functional RNA interference screen uncovers glypican 5 as an entry factor for hepatitis B and D viruses. *Hepatology* 2016;63:35–48.
179. Verrier ER, Weiss A, Bach C, et al. Combined small molecule and loss-of-function screen uncovers estrogen receptor alpha and CAD as host factors for HDV infection and antiviral targets. *Gut* 2020;69:158–167.
180. Wang CJ, Chen PJ, Wu JC, et al. Small-form hepatitis B surface antigen is sufficient to help in the assembly of hepatitis delta virus-like particles. *J Virol* 1991;65:6630–6636.
181. Wang KS, Choo QL, Weiner AJ, et al. Structure, sequence and expression of the hepatitis delta (delta) viral genome. *Nature* 1986;323:508–514.
182. Wang D, Pearlberg J, Liu YT, et al. Deleterious effects of hepatitis delta virus replication on host cell proliferation. *J Virol* 2001;75:3600–3604.
183. Watanabe H, Nagayama K, Enomoto N, et al. Chronic hepatitis delta virus infection with genotype IIb variant is correlated with progressive liver disease. *J Gen Virol* 2003;84:3275–3289.
184. Watanabe T, Sorensen EM, Naito A, et al. Involvement of host cellular multivesicular body functions in hepatitis B virus budding. *Proc Natl Acad Sci U S A* 2007;104:10205–10210.
185. Webb CH, Riccitelli NJ, Ruminski DJ, et al. Widespread occurrence of self-cleaving ribozymes. *Science* 2009;326:953.
186. Wille M, Netter HJ, Littlejohn M, et al. A divergent hepatitis D-like agent in birds. *Viruses* 2018;10(12):720. doi: 10.3390/v10120720.
187. Williams V, Brichler S, Khan E, et al. Large hepatitis delta antigen activates STAT-3 and NF-kappaB via oxidative stress. *J Viral Hepat* 2012;19:744–753.
188. Williams V, Brichler S, Radjef N, et al. Hepatitis delta virus proteins repress hepatitis B virus enhancers and activate the alpha/beta interferon-inducible MxA gene. *J Gen Virol* 2009;90:2759–2767.
189. Wu JC. Functional and clinical significance of hepatitis D virus genotype II infection. *Curr Top Microbiol Immunol* 2006;307:173–186.
190. Wu JC, Chen PJ, Kuo MY, et al. Production of hepatitis delta virus and suppression of helper hepatitis B virus in a human hepatoma cell line. *J Virol* 1991;65:1099–1104.
191. Wu JC, Choo KB, Chen CM, et al. Genotyping of hepatitis D virus by restriction-fragment length polymorphism and relation to outcome of hepatitis D. *Lancet* 1995;346:939–941.
192. Xia YP, Yeh CT, Ou JH, et al. Characterization of nuclear targeting signal of hepatitis delta antigen: nuclear transport as a protein complex. *J Virol* 1992;66:914–921.
193. Yamaguchi Y, Filipovska J, Yano K, et al. Stimulation of RNA polymerase II elongation by hepatitis delta antigen. *Science* 2001;293:124–127.
194. Yamaguchi Y, Mura T, Chanarat S, et al. Hepatitis delta antigen binds to the clamp of RNA polymerase II and affects transcriptional fidelity. *Genes Cells* 2007;12:863–875.
195. Yan H, Zong G, Xu G, et al. Sodium taurocholate cotransporting polypeptide is a functional receptor for human hepatitis B and D virus. *Elife* 2012;1:e00049.
196. Yurdaydin C, Idilman R, Bozkaya H, et al. Natural history and treatment of chronic delta hepatitis. *J Viral Hepat* 2010;17:749–756.
197. Yurdaydin C, Keskin O, Kalkan C, et al. Optimizing lonafarnib treatment for the management of chronic delta hepatitis: The LOWR HDV-1 study. *Hepatology* 2018;67:1224–1236.
198. Zachou K, Yurdaydin C, Drebber U, et al. Quantitative HBsAg and HDV-RNA levels in chronic delta hepatitis. *Liver Int* 2010;30:430–437.
199. Zhang Z, Filzmayer C, Ni Y, et al. Hepatitis D virus replication is sensed by MDA5 and induces IFN-beta/lambda responses in hepatocytes. *J Hepatol* 2018;69:25–35.
200. Zuccola HJ, Rozzelle JE, Lemon SM, et al. Structural basis of the oligomerization of hepatitis delta antigen. *Structure* 1998;6:821–830.

CHAPTER

20 Mimiviridae

Matthias G. Fischer

INTRODUCTION AND HISTORY

Mimiviruses are double-stranded DNA viruses with genomes in the megabase range that infect a variety of eukaryotic hosts and are especially prominent among protists. Due to the size and complexity of their genomes and particles, giant viruses have challenged our definition of viruses and their roles in evolution. Whereas unusually large virus particles had been observed early in various protists by electron microscopy,[45,69,147] and algae-infecting DNA viruses with genome lengths exceeding those of herpes- and poxviruses were known since the 1980s,[106,164,165] the first giant virus with a genome longer than one million base pairs was described in 2004.[129] The serendipitous discovery of Acanthamoeba polyphaga mimivirus (APMV, mimivirus stands for mimicking microbe) followed the search for the causative agent of a 1992 pneumonia outbreak in Bradford, England. The team of Dr. T.J. Rowbotham isolated an obligate intracellular parasite of amoebae from the water of a cooling tower but failed to identify the pathogenic microorganism, which stained Gram positive and was named Bradford coccus.[128] The viral nature of this microbe was revealed only years later at the Unité des Rickettsies in Marseille, France, when electron micrographs showed isometric capsids with a diameter of approximately 500 nm.[95] DNA sequencing and bioinformatic analysis of the 1.2 megabase genome of mimivirus[129] heralded a new era in virology, and hundreds of giant viruses were isolated in subsequent years using the freshwater protist *Acanthamoeba polyphaga* as a host.[1,5,7,8,22,23,27,97,102,103,123] However, mimiviruses are not restricted to amoebae and infect many different protists[41,55,110,116,137,167] as well as animal hosts such as worms, sponges, and even vertebrates.[37,146]

CLASSIFICATION OF VIRUSES WITHIN THE FAMILY *MIMIVIRIDAE*

The family *Mimiviridae* was established in 2005 within the Nucleo-Cytoplasmic Large DNA Viruses (NCLDV), an unofficial grouping of several families of large dsDNA viruses that, at the time, included the *Poxviridae*, *Asfarviridae*, *Iridoviridae*, and *Phycodnaviridae*.[74,75,129] *Acanthamoeba polyphaga mimivirus* remained the only member of the sole genus *Mimivirus* until *Cafeteria roenbergensis virus* (CroV) was added to the family in 2011 within its own genus *Cafeteriavirus*.[55] With the 2020 reclassification of the global taxonomic framework of viruses, *Mimiviridae* are now found in the realm *Varidnaviria*, the kingdom *Bamfordvirae*, the phylum *Nucleocytoviricota*, the class *Megaviricetes*, and the order *Imitervirales*.[87] With this new classification scheme, previously proposed taxa such as the order Megavirales and the family *Megaviridae* have become obsolete.[8,40] Prompted by the serendipitous discovery of APMV, dozens of closely and more distantly related giant viruses were isolated in the following decade. Currently, hundreds of isolates and thousands of metagenomic sequences call for a refined classification within the family *Mimiviridae*.[22,34,59,64,97,143] Whereas the family was initially composed only of viruses that infected heterotrophic protists and had genome sizes upward of 600 kbp (APMV, CroV), it became soon apparent that algae-infecting viruses with shorter genomes (300 to 600 kbp) shared essential properties with the larger mimiviruses.[65,78,108,110,137,144,173]

These viruses would thus no longer be classified automatically within the family *Phycodnaviridae*, which until then exclusively harbored large algal DNA viruses. In addition to isolates, various metagenomic studies revealed a high diversity of mimiviruses in different environments such as open ocean, forest soil, and waste water.[72,117,141–143] These genomes helped to refine the taxonomic structure within the *Mimiviridae*, and the following subfamilies have been proposed (Fig. 20.1): the *Megamimivirinae* would comprise the *Acanthamoeba*-infecting mimiviruses[64]; the *Megamimivirinae* would group together algae-infecting mimiviruses with medium-sized genomes[34,64]; the *Klosneuvirinae* would contain various metagenome-assembled giant viruses as well as the cultured *Bodo saltans* virus (BsV-1) and Yasminevirus[10,41,141,142]; and finally, CroV and several related viruses[55,117,142] could constitute a separate subfamily. Furthermore, a genus-level classification is justifiable for the proposed *Megamimivirinae*, because this clade has been sampled in sufficient depth by dozens of isolates, which fall into four well-defined groups. The first group, also known as lineage A, comprises APMV and its close relatives, with genome lengths of 1.18 megabase pairs (Mbp) and a virion diameter of 750 nm (including fibers) and would correspond to the genus *Mimivirus*.[62,129] The second group (lineage B) comprises *Megavirus chilensis* and its relatives, with genome lengths of 1.26 Mbp and a virion diameter of 680 nm.[8] This group would be classified as the proposed genus Megavirus. The third group (lineage C) is made of *Acanthamoeba polyphaga* moumouvirus and its relatives, with genome lengths of 1.02 Mbp and a virion diameter of 620 nm, resulting in the proposed genus Moumouvirus.[174] The fourth proposed genus is called Tupanvirus and includes the tailed mimiviruses Tupanvirus soda lake and Tupanvirus deep ocean, with genome lengths of 1.4 to 1.5 Mbp and a virion length of approximately 1.2 μm (including fibers and tail structure).[5] Further subdivisions and rearrangements within the family *Mimiviridae* will be necessary as new isolates and metagenomes become available. In particular, the proposed subfamily *Mesomimivirinae* with giant viruses infecting mostly photosynthetic protists appears to harbor an enormous diversity that is yet to be explored.[143]

VIRION STRUCTURE

The infectious particles of mimiviruses are composed of multiple layers and substructures that involve hundreds of viral proteins. While all viruses in the family *Mimiviridae* have capsids with icosahedral symmetry that enclose the viral DNA genome in an internal lipid membrane, they differ remarkably in their diameter, triangulation number, exit portal structure, and other morphological features such as external fibers and tail structures (Fig. 20.2). The best-studied representative is APMV, whose virions have been examined by various techniques including thin-section electron microscopy, cryo-electron microscopy and tomography, scanning electron microscopy, STEM tomography, atomic force microscopy, and x-ray free electron lasers.[6,113–115,138,145,159,170,171,179] The APMV virion is a multilayered structure, composed of an external fiber layer, an outer capsid shell, an inner capsid shell, an internal membrane, and a core wall enclosing the genome and accessory proteins (Fig. 20.3). The outer protein shell of the capsid is 500 nm in diameter. The capsid has icosahedral symmetry and its 20 faces are composed of pseudo-hexagonal capsomers that contain trimers of the major capsid protein (MCP) encoded by gene *L425*. The MCPs of mimiviruses adopt a double jelly-roll fold, similar to other NCLDVs with icosahedral capsids.[81] Each jelly-roll consists of eight β-strands named A to H, which are connected by loops. The surface-exposed parts of the MCP between the DE and FG loops contain insertions of variable lengths that protrude from capsomers as tower-like structures.[171] APMV and CroV encode three additional capsid protein homologs with predicted double jelly-roll architecture.[57,171] The capsid vertices with their fivefold symmetry are made of pentameric capsomers formed by the penton protein. With recent advances in high-resolution imaging of macromolecular structures by cryo-electron microscopy, we have begun to understand the molecular machinery that determines the exact dimensions of large icosahedral capsids. Cryo-EM studies of the phycodnavirus PBCV-1 revealed a protein network beneath the outer capsid layer, which includes the minor capsid protein P2 that acts as a molecular ruler and is therefore called the tape-measure protein.[48] The P2 protein connects neighboring fivefold vertices and thus likely determines the PBCV-1 capsid size. Homologs of this tape-measure protein are present in other phycodnaviruses, in APMV (*L454* gene product) and CroV (*crov185* gene product), as well as in asfarviruses,[105,168] and the length of the tape-measure protein roughly correlates with the dimensions of the respective capsid: 566 aa and 190 nm for PBCV-1; 869 aa and 300 nm for CroV; and 1257 aa and 500 nm for APMV. These findings suggest that the capsid sizing mechanism is conserved in different families of viruses with icosahedral capsids in the phylum *Nucleocytoviricota*.

Members of the *Mimiviridae* have the largest icosahedral capsids that have been described so far and accordingly, these capsids possess the highest triangulation (*T*) numbers. The largest capsid for which a *T* number is currently known is that of CroV with $T = 499$ ($h = 7$, $k = 18$).[172] Based on the limited resolution of structural studies with larger mimiviruses, the *T* number of the APMV capsid has not been determined accurately, but it is estimated to be between 972 and 1,200 ($h = 19 \pm 1$, $k = 19 \pm 1$).[81]

Members of the *Mimiviridae* often exhibit a single modified vertex structure and various surface modifications on their capsids. A common feature of mimiviruses is an exit portal structure at one of the twelve vertices, where the nucleocapsid underneath the portal shows a characteristic concave depression (Fig. 20.4). In APMV, this unique vertex has been called the stargate, as it opens in a star-like formation to expose the lipid layer below.[179] The stargate portal is sealed by a large proteinaceous complex known as the starfish, because it consists of five 40-nm-thick and 50-nm-wide arms that extend about 200 nm toward the nearest fivefold vertices.[138,171] During phagocytosis of APMV and Tupanvirus particles, these structures enable a controlled opening of the capsid to release the genome into the host cytoplasm.

Whereas isometric viruses of eukaryotes generally lack recognizable tail structures, some mimiviruses such as Tupanvirus soda lake and Tupanvirus deep ocean present capsids with cylindrical tails that are typically approximately 550 nm long and approximately 450 nm thick.[5] The total length of a Tupanvirus particle amounts to approximately 1.2 μm, but variations in tail length can lead to particles that are up to 2.3 μm long.[132] In electron micrographs, Tupanvirus tails are attached to the capsid at the vertex opposite of the unique stargate vertex, but the tail is

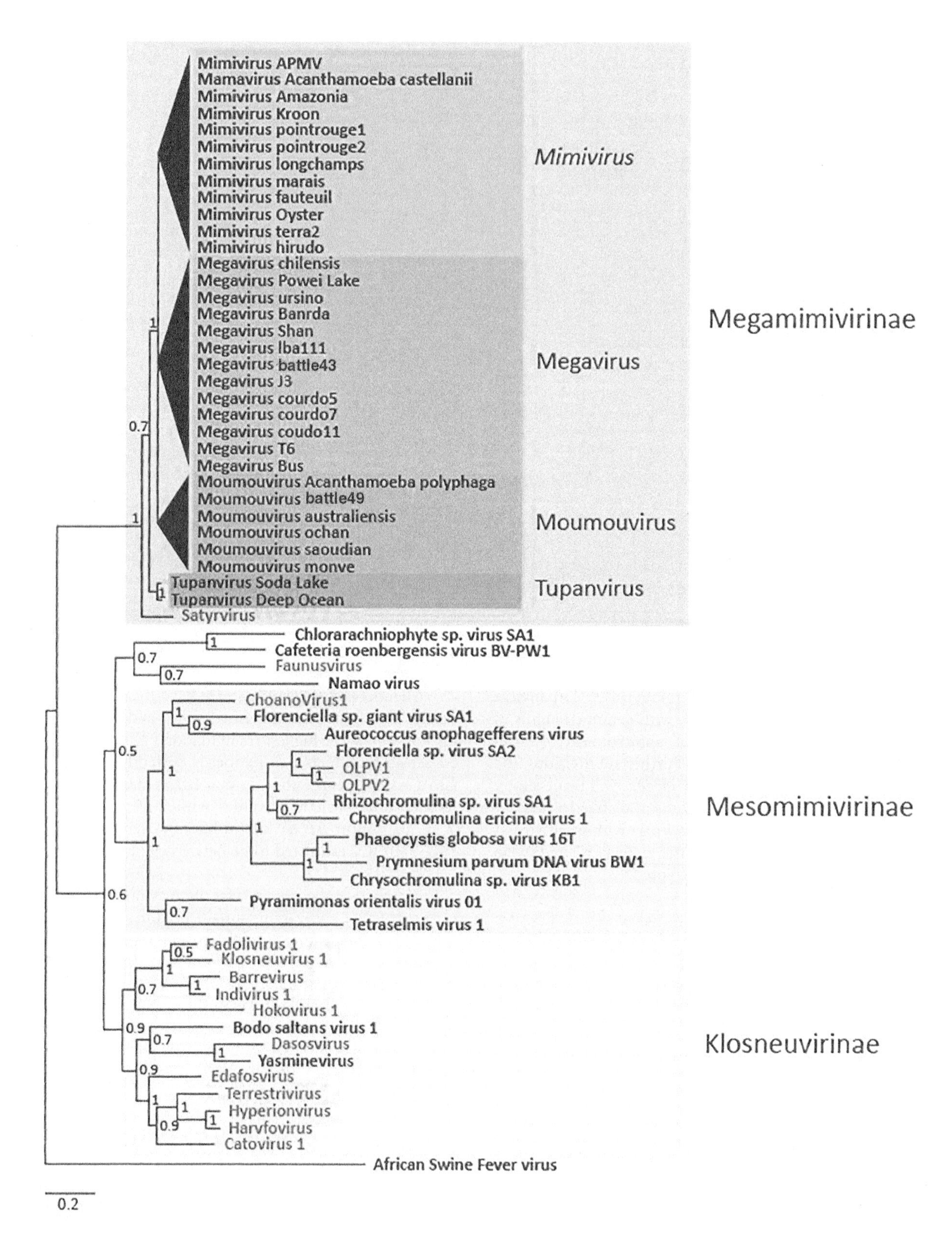

FIGURE 20.1 Phylogenetic relationship within the family *Mimiviridae* based on DNA polymerase B. This Bayesian tree shows the proposed substructure of viral clades within the family. Note that the only ICTV-approved taxon within the family *Mimiviridae* shown in this tree is the genus *Mimivirus* with its sole member *Acanthamoeba polyphaga mimivirus*; other taxa have not been approved and may be subject to changes. Genomes assembled from metagenomic data are printed in blue. Nodes are labeled with posterior probabilities. The unpublished genomes of Chlorarachniophyte sp. virus SA1, Florenciella sp. giant viruses SA1 and SA2, Rhizochromulina sp. virus SA1, and Chrysochromulina sp. virus KB1 were kindly provided by Dr. Christopher Schvarcz and Dr. Grieg Steward, Univ. of Hawai'i at Manoa, USA.

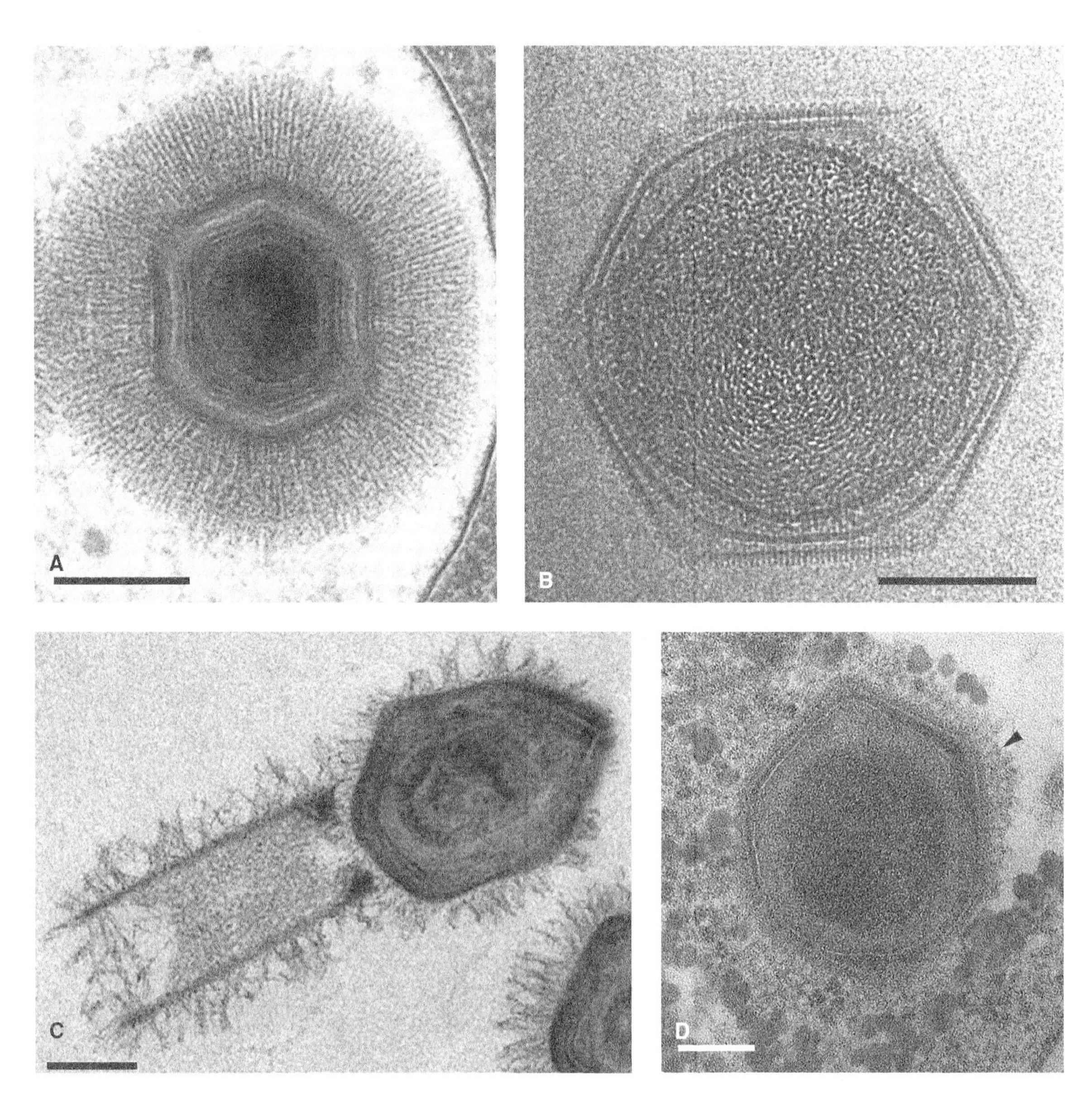

FIGURE 20.2 Morphological diversity among mimivirus particles. A: Transmission electron micrograph of *Acanthamoeba polyphaga* mimivirus (APMV). Scale bar 250 nm. (Adapted with permission from Mutsafi Y, Fridmann-Sirkis Y, Milrot E, et al. Infection cycles of large DNA viruses: emerging themes and underlying questions. *Virology* 2014;466–467: 3–14. Courtesy of Dr. Nathan Zauberman.) **B:** Cryo-EM image of Cafeteria roenbergensis virus (CroV). Scale bar 100 nm. (Image courtesy of Dr. Chuan Xiao, Univ. of Texas El Paso, USA.) **C:** Transmission electron micrograph of Tupanvirus soda lake. Scale bar 200 nm. (Adapted from Abrahão J, et al. Tailed giant Tupanvirus possesses the most complete translational apparatus of the known virosphere. *Nat Commun* 2018;9:749.) **D:** Transmission electron micrograph of Yasminevirus, a member of the proposed subfamily *Klosneuvirinae* that infects *Vermamoeba vermiformis*. The arrowhead points to a layer of short fibers. Scale bar 100 nm. (Adapted from Bajrai LH, et al. Isolation of yasminevirus, the first member of *klosneuvirinae* isolated in coculture with vermamoeba vermiformis. *J Virol* 2020;94:1–13.)

not continuous with the outer layer of the icosahedral capsid and appears to be partially filled with electron-dense material that may be released upon cell entry.[5] The biological role of this tail and its content remain to be studied.

The capsid surface of APMV and related mimiviruses of the proposed subfamily *Megamimivirinae* is decorated with a dense layer of fibers that spare only the starfish structure. In APMV, these outer capsid fibers are 120 to 140 nm long and approximately 1.4 nm thick, whereas *Megavirus chilensis* capsids feature shorter (approximately 75 nm) fibers with occasional patches of longer fibers named "cowlicks".[8,82,169,171] Tupanvirus fibers are slightly thicker and shorter than those of APMV and also cover the outside of the tail structures.[132] The fibers consist of heavily glycosylated proteins that form a peptidoglycan-like structure. As a result, the fiber layer stains Gram positive, which contributed to the initial misclassification of APMV as a bacterium.[95,128] Components of the fibers include APMV gene products R135, L725, and L829.[24] *R135* encodes a highly antigenic protein whose structure is similar to glucose–methanol–choline oxidoreductases.[83] However, despite the proteinaceous

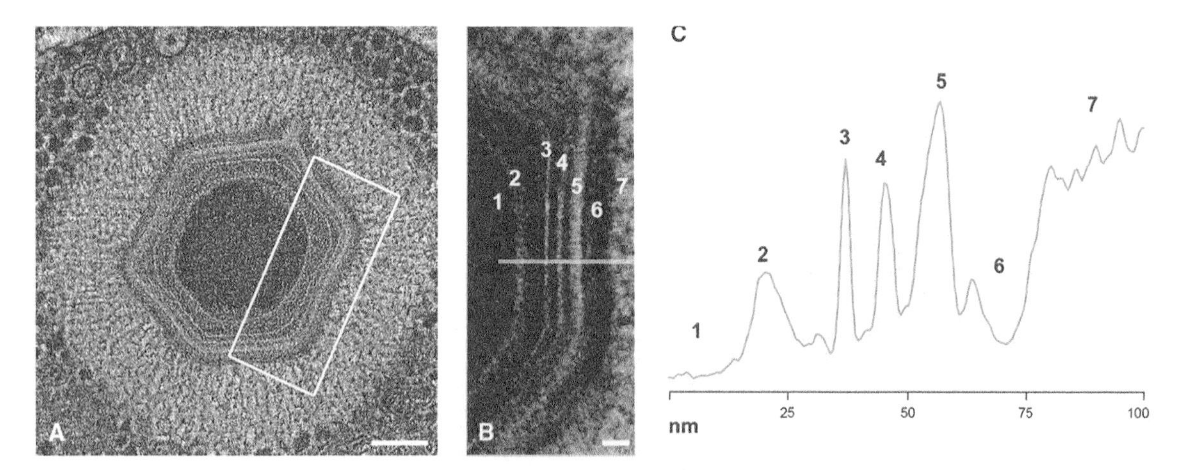

FIGURE 20.3 The APMV capsid is composed of multiple layers. A: Scanning transmission electron microscopy (STEM) tomography slice of an APMV particle. Scale bar 100 nm. **B:** Magnified representation of the region delineated in **(A)**. The layers constituting the APMV virion are (*1*) DNA genome; (*2*) core wall; (*3*) inner membrane; (*4*) a layer previously proposed to represent an additional membrane (From Xiao C, et al. Cryo-electron microscopy of the giant mimivirus. *J Mol Biol* 2005;353: 493–496.); (*5*) inner capsid shell; (*6*) outer capsid shell; (*7*) outer fiber shell. Scale bar 20 nm. **C:** Density plot of the various layers along the line drawn in **(B)**. Digits correspond to those depicted in **(B)**. (Adapted from Mutsafi Y, Shimoni E, Shimon A, et al. Membrane assembly during the Infection cycle of the giant mimivirus. *PLoS Pathog* 2013;9:e1003367.)

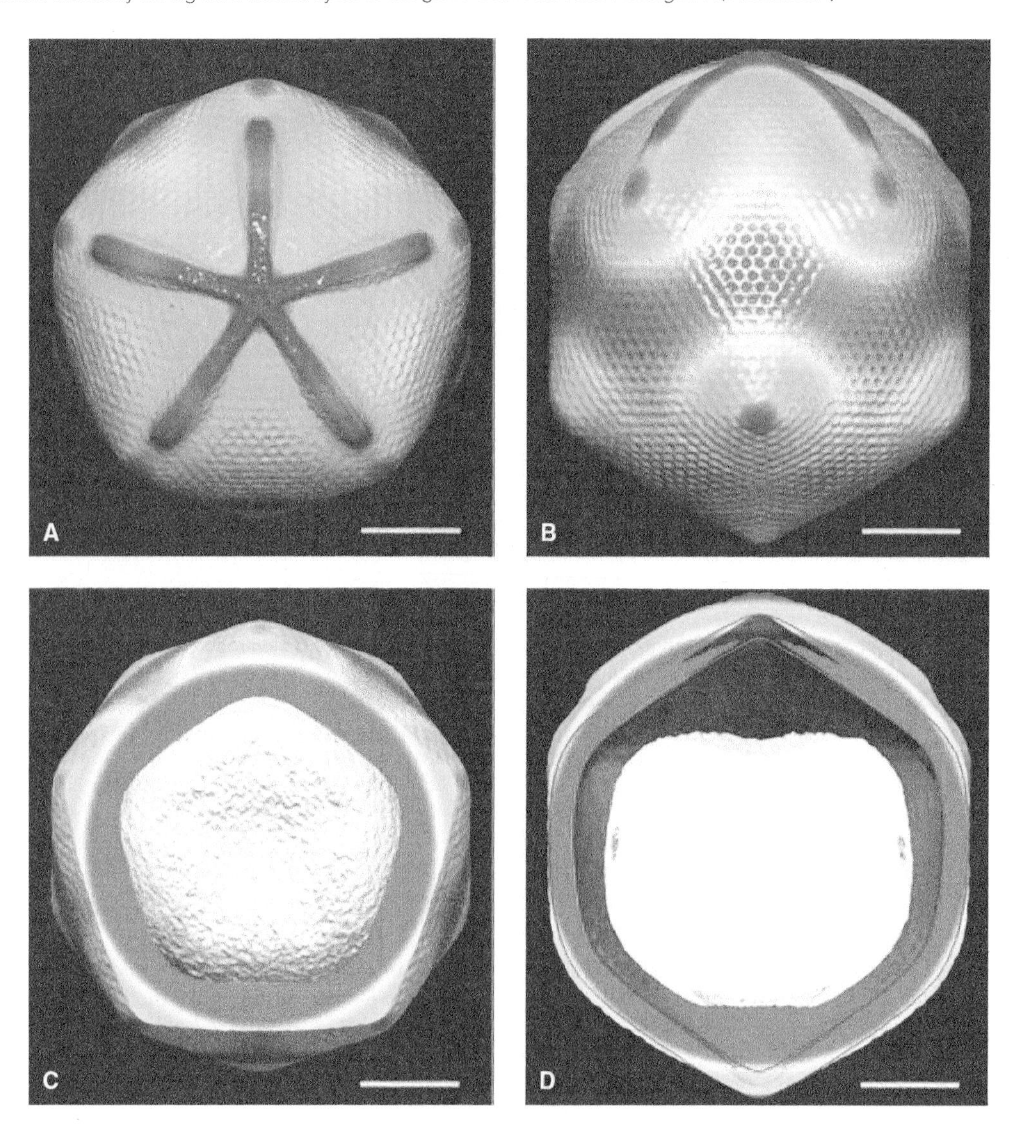

FIGURE 20.4 Cryo-electron microscopy reconstruction of the APMV capsid. Colors are based on the distance from the center of the capsid. **A:** Top-down view onto the unique pentameric vertex with the starfish structure (blue). **B:** Side view of the capsid with the unique vertex on top. **C and D:** Cross sections of the images shown in **(A)** and **(B)**, respectively, visualizing the concave depression of the nucleocapsid beneath the exit portal. **(C)** is sliced just below the stargate portal; **(D)** is a central cross section. All scale bars are 100 nm. (Adapted from Xiao C, et al. Structural studies of the giant mimivirus. *PLoS Biol* 2009;7:e92.)

nature of the fibers, proteolysis only occurs after treatment with lysozyme.[171] Several glycosyltransferases are involved in fiber formation and maturation, including the APMV *L136* gene that encodes a pyridoxal phosphate-dependent sugar aminotransferase that catalyzes the biosynthesis of UDP-viosamine, one of the major components of viral fibers.[124] Together with other sugar modifications, the fibers mediate adhesion of APMV virions to host sugars such as mannose and *N*-acetylglucosamine, which are present on the amoebal cell surface.[134] Overall, by mimicking the peptidoglycan layers of Gram-positive bacteria, the outer fiber layer of mimivirus capsids may facilitate recognition and uptake of virions by phagocytosis into the amoebal host. The fiber layer also contributes to the stability of the virion, making it resistant to most proteases.[92] The composition of the fiber layer may vary even within a genus, since fibers of the APMV-related Samba virus are resistant to lysozyme/proteinase K/bromelain treatment, whereas APMV fibers can be removed with this method.[139] Another role of the fiber layer has been proposed in connection with entry of the Sputnik virophage (see p.15), which may attach to the APMV fibers and enter the host cell as a composite with the giant virus.[24]

Virions of mimiviruses are composed of more than one hundred virus-encoded proteins, with 236 different proteins identified in APMV particles, 141 in CroV, and 127 in Tupanvirus.[5,35,57,61,107] Structural proteins[1] form the icosahedral shell, outer fibers, and tail structures (if present); they position the internal lipid membrane and compose the inner core layer. In addition, mimiviruses package a considerable number of nonstructural proteins with various enzymatic functions. Notably, this includes the presence of a presumably complete transcription machinery with six to eight DNA-dependent RNA polymerase subunits, homologs of vaccinia virus transcription factors A7, D6, and D11, a trifunctional mRNA capping enzyme, polyadenylate polymerase, and associated helicases.[5,57,131] Other functional categories are DNA repair, redox pathways, and protein modification.

Similar to poxviruses, whose infection cycles also take place exclusively in the cytoplasm,[140] enzymatic functions present in mimivirus capsids are probably essential for the initial infection stages, in particular viral genome maintenance and early gene expression. These enzymes are thus located in the inner nucleocapsid, also known as the viral core, which is embedded in the internal lipid layer of the virion. The structure of the viral core is mainly formed by the major core protein that is encoded by the APMV *L410* gene and its orthologs in other mimiviruses.[131]

GENOME STRUCTURE AND ORGANIZATION

Genome length varies considerably among different mimiviruses, currently ranging from 371 kbp in Aureococcus anophagefferens virus (AaV) to 1,516 kbp in Tupanvirus deep ocean (Table 20.1).[5,110] The DNA packaging density of APMV and other mimiviruses is low compared to other eukaryotic viruses and bacteriophages, prompting speculations about the upper genome size limits for giant viruses.[36] With the exception of Yasminevirus that has a GC content of 40.2% and Tetraselmis viridis virus 1, whose genome has a GC content of 41.2% and was assembled into a circular sequence, members of the *Mimiviridae* have linear genomes and low GC contents between 23% and 32%.[10,64,144] Their coding density is typically around 90% and the number of predicted proteins encoded by mimiviruses ranges from a few hundred (377 for AaV) to more than one thousand (1,359 for Tupanvirus deep ocean). Open reading frames (ORFs) are usually nonoverlapping, distributed approximately equally on both DNA strands, and separated by short intergenic regions (157 nt on average for APMV) that feature an elevated AT-content and harbor gene promoter and terminator elements.[26,121] The low GC content of the viral genome leads to a strong bias toward AT-rich codons and a shift in the amino acid composition toward asparagine, isoleucine, lysine, and other amino acids encoded by AT-rich codons.[39] In contrast to the AT-rich genomes of mimiviruses and their distinct codon usage profile, the genomes of their protist hosts often display high GC contents and opposing amino acid frequencies (Fig. 20.5).[71,129,148]

The best-studied genome of a *Mimiviridae* member is that of APMV.[129] Its 1,181,549 bp linear dsDNA genome is predicted to encode 1,018 genes, including 979 protein-coding genes, 6 tRNA genes, and 33 noncoding RNAs.[100,101] The genes lack spliceosomal introns, with the notable exception of the MCP *L425* gene that consists of three exons and two introns.[9,20] The APMV genome has no terminal inverted repeats as observed in other large DNA viruses but contains a 617-bp long inverted repeat at positions 22,515 and 1,180,529 that are suggested to be involved in genome replication through base pairing of these regions and loop formation into a Q-like configuration.[35]

Genes appear to be clustered by function, rather than by their temporal expression pattern.[125] Similar to poxviruses, the genome termini contain fewer conserved genes and are enriched in nonessential genes, horizontally acquired genes, and DNA repeats.[8,41,52,98] Proteins that are expressed during infection and present in the cytoplasmic viral factory are mostly encoded by the central part of the APMV genome.[61] Experimental evidence that the terminally located APMV genes are dispensable comes from passaging the virus 150 times under allopatric conditions, which led to the isolation of a deletion mutant called M4.[24] The M4 genome was only 993 kb long and contained two large deletions at either genome terminus, a 90.7-kb deletion starting at position 81,626 and a 95.6-kb deletion starting at position 1,074,695. These deletions removed 155 APMV genes, including several duplicated genes, as well as genes that are presumably involved in carbohydrate metabolism. Although the M4 mutant was still infective in cell culture, the M4 virions lacked the outer fiber layer that is present in wild-type virions. The deletions therefore affected fiber proteins and their glycosylation, leading to a bald mimivirus mutant.[24]

VIRAL TRANSLATION COMPONENTS AND THE EVOLUTIONARY ORIGIN OF GIANT VIRUSES

Arguably, the most striking feature about the coding potential of mimiviruses is their suite of protein biosynthesis genes

[1]Note that "structural proteins" is not synonymous with "virion proteins", that is, not every viral protein that is part of the virion is automatically classified as a structural protein. The difference is made between viral proteins that contribute to the architecture and integrity of the virus particle, and packaged viral proteins whose function is required during the intracellular stage of the viral replication cycle, often during early phase. This distinction is especially important for giant viruses, which package many nonstructural proteins with various enzymatic activities.

TABLE 20.1 Genome features of cultured *Mimiviridae* members

Virus	Genome Length (bp)	Genome Topology	GC Content	Predicted Genes	Coding Density	Reference
Aureococcus anophagefferens virus (AaV)	370,920	Linear	28.7%	377	88%	110
Acanthamoeba polyphaga mimivirus (APMV)	1,181,549	Linear	28.0%	979	90%	129
Acanthamoeba polyphaga moumouvirus	1,021,348	Linear	24.6%	930	91%	174
Bodo saltans virus (BsV-1)	1,385,869	Linear	25.3%	1,227	85%	41
Cafeteria roenbergensis virus (CroV BV-PW1)	691,790	Linear	23.3%	631	91%	55
Chrysochromulina ericina virus (CeV-1)	473,538	Linear	26.3%	512	91%	64
Megavirus chilensis	1,259,197	Linear	25.3%	1,120	90%	8
Phaeocystis globosa virus 16T (PgV-16T)	459,984	Linear	32.0%	434	91%	137
Tetraselmis viridis virus (TetV-1)	668,031	Circular	41.2%	663	94%	144
Tupanvirus deep ocean	1,439,508	Linear	29.4%	1,276	88%	5
Tupanvirus soda lake	1,516,267	Linear	27.8%	1,359	88%	5
Yasminevirus	2,126,343	Linear	40.2%	1,541	89%	10

(Table 20.2).[3,133] Translation is a hallmark of cells and as obligate intracellular parasites, viruses use the host ribosome and the associated translation machinery to produce viral proteins. Most viruses thus do not encode their own versions of translation proteins. It therefore came as a surprise to find four aminoacyl-tRNA synthetases (aaRS; namely *ArgRS*, *CysRS*, *MetRS*, and *TyrRS*) and five translation factors in the APMV genome.[129] Analysis of the Megavirus chilensis genome revealed the four aaRS genes previously seen in APMV, an *IleRS* gene also present in CroV, and two additional aaRS genes (*AsnRS*, *TrpRS*).[8] This striking pattern of scattered aaRS genes, some of them shared by different giant viruses, led to the hypothesis that the translation components encoded by mimiviruses could represent the remnants of a once complete machinery derived from a cellular ancestor that had undergone massive reductive evolution.[99] This so-called forth domain scenario was based on the hypothesis that deeper taxon sampling of the mimivirus clade will yield additional puzzle pieces that would allow reconstruction of the ancestral set of translation proteins. In 2017, the metagenome of Klosneuvirus was published and it contained 19 aaRS genes.[141] Finally, Tupanvirus and Yasminevirus were found to encode 20 aaRS genes, covering all 20 amino acid specificities.[5,10] A central underlying assumption

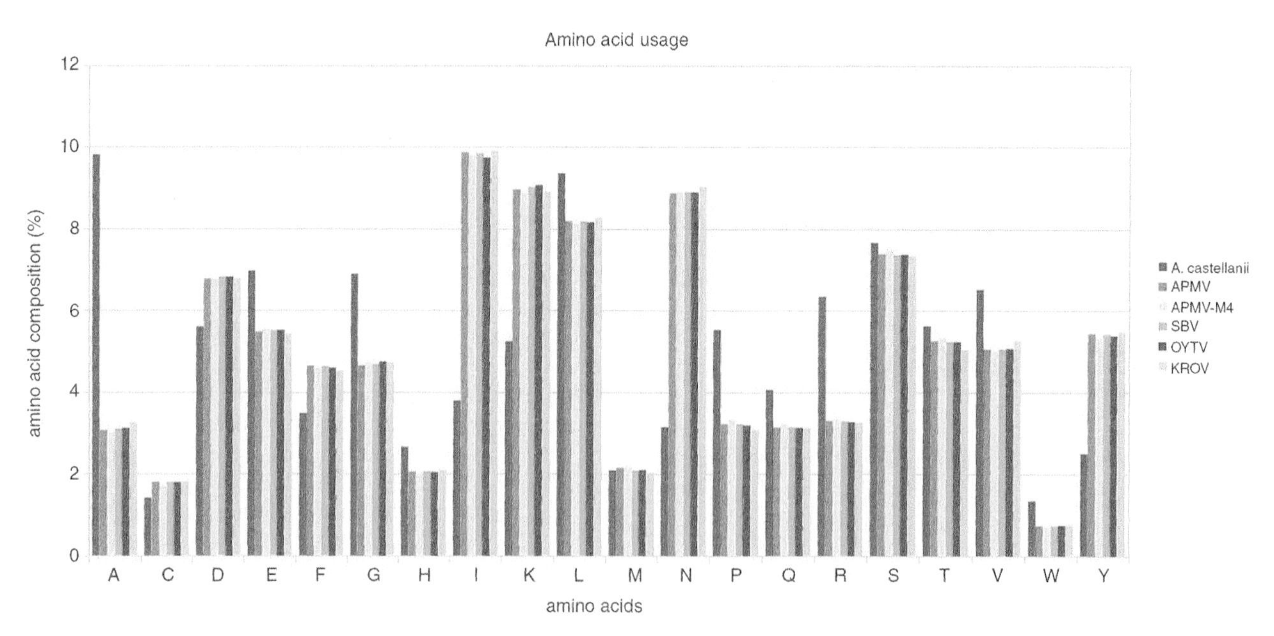

FIGURE 20.5 Amino acid frequencies of several mimivirus strains compared to their host *A. castellanii*. The amino acid usage profiles of APMV, the APMV deletion variant M4, Samba virus (SBV), oyster virus (OYTV), and Kroon virus (KROV) differ substantially from that of *A. castellanii*. (Adapted from Silva LCF, et al. Modulation of the expression of mimivirus-encoded translation-related genes in response to nutrient availability during Acanthamoeba castellanii infection. *Front Microbiol* 2015;6:539.)

TABLE 20.2 Translation components encoded by giant viruses of the family *Mimiviridae*

Virus	aaRS Genes	tRNA Genes	Translation Factors
APMV	4	6	5
Megavirus chilensis	7	3	4
Moumouvirus	5	3	3
CroV	1	57	8
Tupanvirus	20	70	11
Yasminevirus	20	70	7
BsV-1	5 (including 3 pseudogenes)	0	10
Klosneuvirus	19	25	2
Hokovirus	13	0	10
Indivirus	3	1	8
Catovirus	15	3	9

of the reductive evolutionary origin of giant viruses was that if mimiviruses were descendants of a lost cellular domain, then their translation genes should be deeply rooted and yield similar phyletic patterns. However, phylogenetic analysis of the viral aaRS proteins revealed a mixed pattern with some genes (e.g., IleRS) being monophyletic for mimiviruses, but the majority of viral aaRS genes were affiliated with various eukaryotic groups.[133,141] These results indicate that some aaRS genes have indeed resided for a long time in mimivirus genomes, whereas translation genes in general were transferred horizontally on multiple occasions from various hosts. Such scenarios are not in line with the forth domain hypothesis and current data rather suggest an evolutionary origin of mimiviruses from a smaller ancestor by net gene gain and gene duplications.[86] Evidence for loss of translation genes comes from genome analysis of BsV, a member of the proposed subfamily *Klosneuvirinae*.[41] In contrast to its relatives Yasminevirus with 20 aaRS genes and Klosneuvirus with 19 aaRS genes, BsV carries only five aaRS genes, three of which are pseudogenes with degenerated ORFs. These observations suggest that in BsV, aaRS genes are in the process of being lost, perhaps following a recent host switch that made these translation components obsolete.[41] The genomic flexibility of large dsDNA viruses was demonstrated in Vaccinia virus, where experimentally imposed selection pressure led to duplication of the K3L gene that encodes an antihost protein.[47] Subsequent genome reduction and retention of the best-adapted K3L copies resulted in a "gene accordion" scenario, where gene duplication, diversification, and selection, may help the virus to adapt rapidly to new environmental niches. This evolutionary mechanism may be a general feature of large and giant dsDNA viruses, as suggested by lineage-specific gene duplications in mimiviruses.[50,51] In APMV, genes encoding the 33 amino acid–long ankyrin repeat constitute the most prominent class of duplications, with up to 98 members identified.[61,155] Another example is the massive expansion in the CroV genome of genes that code for a 22-amino acid-long domain called FNIP or IP22 repeat.[55,60,118] Interestingly, both ankyrin and FNIP/IP22 repeats mediate protein–protein interactions, implying a possible function in targeting host proteins or contributing to intracellular protein networks during viral replication.

STAGES OF REPLICATION

Host Range

Members of the *Mimiviridae* infect eukaryotic hosts of different supergroups, including Amoebozoa (e.g., APMV), Archaeplastida (e.g., Tetraselmis viridis virus), Stramenopiles (e.g., CroV), Excavates (e.g., BsV), and presumably also Rhizaria (e.g., chlorarachniophytes) and Opisthokonts (e.g., choanoflagellates).[18,41,55,116,129,144] Few virus–host systems have been studied in sufficient detail to delineate specific steps of the viral infection cycle, and most data on viruses of the *Mimiviridae* family have been published on APMV and tupanviruses in their freshwater hosts *Acanthamoeba polyphaga*, *A. castellanii*, and *Vermamoeba vermiformis*. Despite the efficient infection of this host in the laboratory and the practical advantages of working with the amoebal system, it is not clear whether *Acanthamoeba* sp. represents the main natural host for viruses of the proposed subfamily *Megamimivirinae*. Although tupanviruses were not reported to replicate in protists other than *Acanthamoeba*, they are able to enter the ciliate *Tetrahymena* sp. and cause cytotoxicity at high multiplicities of infection.[5] The ecological role of mimiviruses in controlling natural protist populations is therefore an important area of research that is still in its beginnings. Mimiviruses are also part of the human microbiome as demonstrated by PCR detection, serological studies, and isolation of viruses such as Lentille virus from a keratitis patient.[43,97] APMV replicates in macrophages[66] and amoeba-associated mimiviruses have been suggested as opportunistic pneumonia agents,[80,94,127,136]; however, the clinical relevance of giant viruses remains controversial.[4,38]

Attachment and Entry

Attachment of APMV to the host cell is mediated by the outer 120- to 140-nm-thick fiber layer of the capsid, probably via the 25 kDa proteinaceous head group at the tip of the fibers.[92] Based on the peptidoglycan-mimicking surface and the large (750 nm) diameter of the virion, the APMV particle resembles bacteria that may fall within the prey scheme of the amoeba, resulting in uptake by phagocytosis. Virus particles attach either directly to the cell surface or to elongated cell protrusions, which then engulf the virion.[66] Within 30 minutes postinfection (p.i.), phagocytic vacuoles containing APMV particles are observed by transmission electron microscopy (TEM).[159] Infection studies in RAW 264.7 macrophages ruled out clathrin- and caveolin-mediated endocytosis and micropinocytosis, while inhibition of phagocytosis regulators reduced APMV entry.[66] Treatment with the phagocytosis inhibitor cytochalasin significantly reduced both APMV uptake by *Acanthamoeba* cells as well as viral titers, providing further evidence that phagocytosis is the preferred mode of entry for APMV.[6] Phagocytosis is not restricted to the uptake of single virions, and multiple APMV particles per phagosome can be observed.[179]

Similar to APMV, phagocytic entry has been proposed for Yasminevirus in the host *Vermamoeba vermiformis*. With a capsid of 330 nm in diameter and an outer 20- to 40-nm-thick fiber layer, the Yasminevirus particle is much smaller than that of APMV, yet virion-containing phagosomes are visible by TEM.[10] By contrast, no internalized capsids have been observed for CroV in the phagotrophic flagellate *Cafeteria burkhardae*. Instead, open empty capsid shell structures can be seen in close proximity to host cells, suggesting that CroV capsids open upon contact with the host cell and that the internal virion membrane fuses with the cytoplasmic membrane, releasing the genome-containing viral core into the cytoplasm (Fig. 20.6) (U. Mersdorf and M. Fischer, unpublished data). Phagocytosis thus appears to be the main entry mode for amoeba-infecting mimiviruses, whereas other entry mechanisms may be employed by different members of the family.

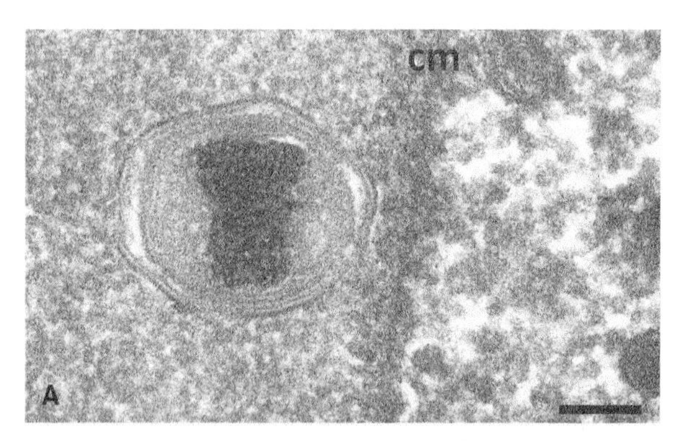

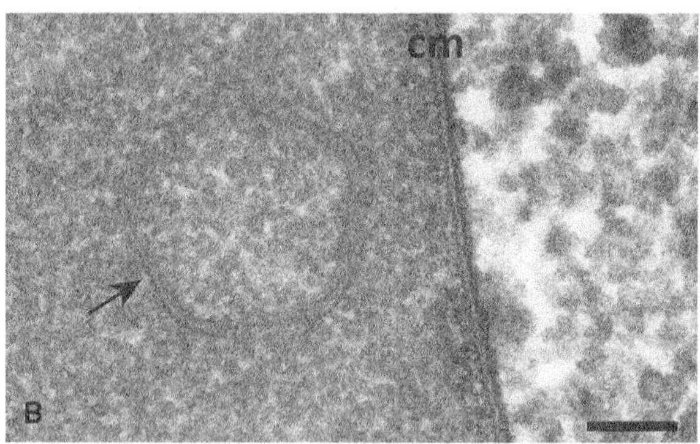

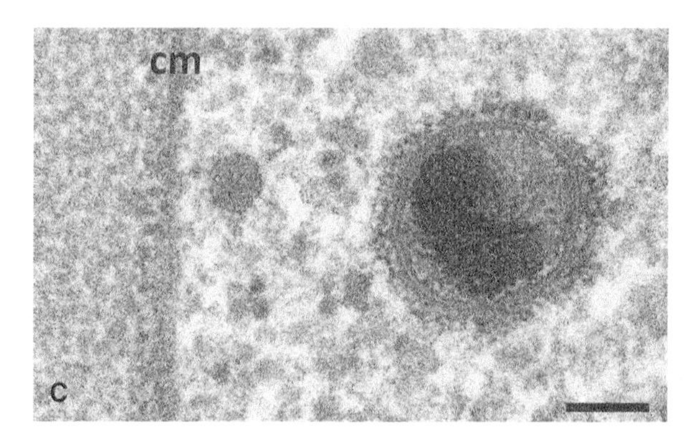

FIGURE 20.6 Pre- and postentry events of CroV. The thin-section transmission electron micrographs show early (approximately 15 minutes p.i.) events near the cytoplasmic membrane (cm) in the flagellate *Cafeteria burkhardae*. **A:** An extracellular CroV virion enclosed in its capsid shell attaches to the host cell membrane. **B:** Empty capsid shell (*arrow*) outside the host cell membrane. **C:** Early intracellular CroV nucleocapsid close to the cytoplasmic membrane. The outer capsid shell is missing, but the inner core layer is clearly visible. Fibers protrude from the nucleocapsid into the surrounding cytoplasm. Scale bars are 100 nm. (Images by Ulrike Mersdorf and Dr. Matthias Fischer, MPI for Medical Research, Germany.)

Uncoating and Virion Factory Formation

After internalization of the virus particle, APMV uncoating depends on acidification of the vacuole via fusion with lysosomes. When amoebae are treated with the vacuolar-type H^+-ATPase inhibitor Bafilomycin, APMV titers are greatly reduced.[6] Low pH conditions also trigger the opening of the viral capsid *in vitro*, as shown for Samba virus, APMV, and Tupanvirus.[138] The APMV capsid always opens at the unique stargate vertex. For this, the outer starfish seal must be removed, which probably occurs through an "unzipping" mechanism whereby the seal maintains contact with the capsid layer during opening.[138] The stargate portal then opens at the unique vertex with the five flanking trisymmetrons folding back like flower petals, exposing the internal virion lipid layer for fusion with the phagolysosome membrane (Fig. 20.7).[138,159,179] Little is known about the membrane fusion step and release of the viral core (also referred to as the nucleocapsid or the viral seed) into the host cytoplasm. However, stargate opening and fusion of viral and host membranes create a conduit for delivery of the genome-containing core. At this stage, the core is still surrounded by a layer that is presumably composed of the major core protein. Immediately after release from the capsid, early transcription commences in the viral core[115] and over the course of the first 4 hours, the core develops into a micrometer-sized pseudo-organelle termed the viral factory.[159] The early viral factory is visible after an eclipse phase of about 3 to 4 hours (Fig. 20.8).[32,95,149,160] Multiple cores can be present in a single cell, and each core will seed a separate factory, which may eventually fuse into a single large factory.[61,115] The viral factory is a hallmark structure of all mimiviruses studied so far and represents the subcellular location in which viral transcription, DNA replication, particle assembly, and various other viral enzymatic activities take place.

Transcription

The mode of gene expression in mimiviruses resembles that of poxviruses,[25] because viruses of both families package a multisubunit transcriptase complex into the viral particle and execute transcription in the cytoplasm of infected cells in a temporally regulated fashion.[25,115] Mimiviruses are therefore independent from the nuclear host transcription system, although it cannot be excluded that certain host factors are recruited for viral transcription. The genomes of APMV, CroV, and Bodo saltans virus encode a large number of proteins with predicted functions in transcription, including DNA-dependent RNA polymerase subunits Rpb1, Rpb2, Rpb3/11, Rpb5, Rpb6, Rpb7, Rpb9, and Rpb10.[41,55,100,129] In addition, mimiviruses encode at least six transcription factors involved in initiation, elongation, and termination, as well as RNA helicases and a catalytic subunit of polyadenylate polymerase.[125] Similar to poxviruses, mimiviruses encode a trifunctional mRNA capping enzyme that consists of RNA triphosphatase, guanylyltransferase, and guanine-N7 methyltransferase domains.[16] Mass spectrometric analysis of purified APMV and CroV virions revealed that most of these transcription components are packaged in the viral particle.[57,131] Following the release of the inner core into the cytoplasm, transcription of early viral genes commences.[115]

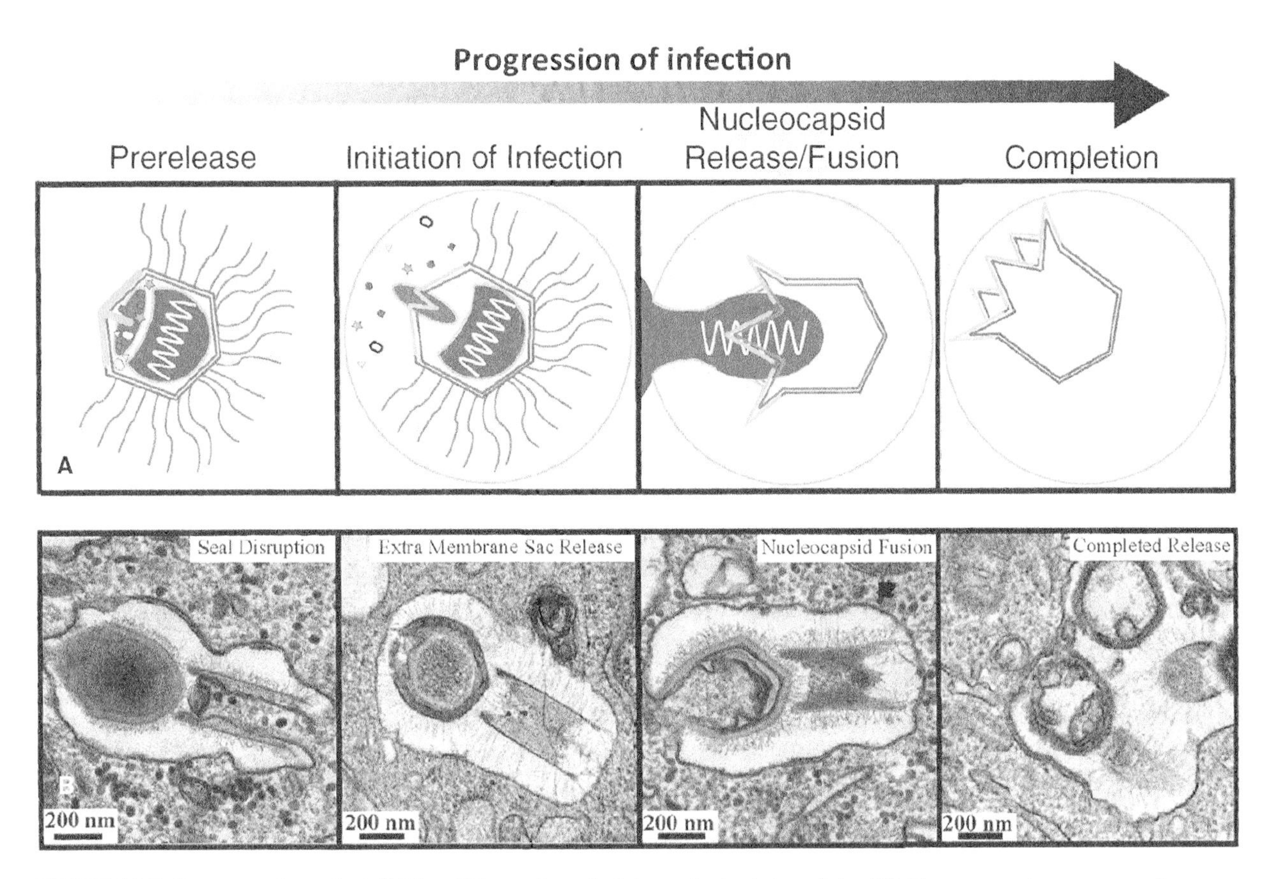

FIGURE 20.7 Genome release in APMV and Tupanvirus. A: Schematic depiction of the APMV genome release process from phagocytosed virions. The phagosome membrane and internal virion membrane are shown in *yellow*, the capsid layers in *red*, and the starfish structure in *light blue*. **B:** Thin-section transmission electron micrographs of capsid opening and genome release during Tupanvirus infection. (Adapted from Schrad JR, Abrahão JS, Cortines JR, et al. Structural and proteomic characterization of the initiation of giant virus infection. *Cell* 2020;181:1046–1061.e6 and Abrahão J, et al. Tailed giant Tupanvirus possesses the most complete translational apparatus of the known virosphere. *Nat Commun* 2018;9:749.)

Gene expression in mimiviruses follows a temporally regulated cascade similar to that described for poxviruses, with successive transcription of genes expressed during early, intermediate, and late phases. Early phase in APMV starts with the release of the viral core into the cytoplasm and ends around 3 hours p.i., followed by an intermediate phase proposed to last from 3 to 6 hours p.i., and a late phase that lasts from 6 to 12 hours p.i.[101] In CroV, early phase lasts approximately until 3 hours p.i. and late phase starts between 3 and 6 hours p.i.[55] Each temporal class is associated with its own set of transcription factors and gene regulatory sequences. Early gene products include transcription factors for intermediate phase, intermediate gene products include late transcription factors, and the early transcription factors are expressed during late phase and must be packaged in the capsid to initiate the expression of early genes in the next round of infection.[166] Indeed, proteins with homology to the Vaccinia virus early transcription factors A7 and D6 were found in the virion proteomes of APMV and CroV.[57,131] The early transcription factors may recognize the conserved "AAAATTGA" promoter motif that was found to be associated with early genes in the APMV genome.[101,156] This early promoter is conserved within the *Mimiviridae* family, including mega- and moumouviruses, AaV, BsV, CroV, and tupanviruses[8,41,55,109,132,174] and is similar to the early promoter motifs in pox- and iridoviruses.[121] Most of the early genes in APMV and CroV encode hypothetical proteins of unknown function, but RNA polymerase subunits are also found in this class. Some transcription genes have both early and late promoters, presumably for boosting viral gene expression during the onset of infection and for providing transcription proteins to be packaged into capsids during late phase. The intermediate phase is poorly defined in mimiviruses and has not been linked to specific regulatory signals. Intermediate gene products include the DNA polymerase and other associated replication proteins. Late gene products are involved in virion morphogenesis and include capsid proteins as well as assembly and packaging factors. In contrast to the widely conserved early gene promoter, the late gene promoters vary among different members of the *Mimiviridae*, with some viruses exhibiting a strong consensus sequence (e.g., "TCTA" in CroV), while others appear to have more degenerate late promoter motifs.[101,121] Nearly all APMV transcripts are polyadenylated at palindromic sequences that give rise to hairpin structures with a length of 26 to 46 nucleotides.[26] Polyadenylation is catalyzed by the highly processive virus-encoded poly(A) polymerase.[125] These hairpin structures have been proposed to act as transcription termination signals.[101] Two convergent genes may use the same hairpin and polycistronic mRNAs have also been observed.[26]

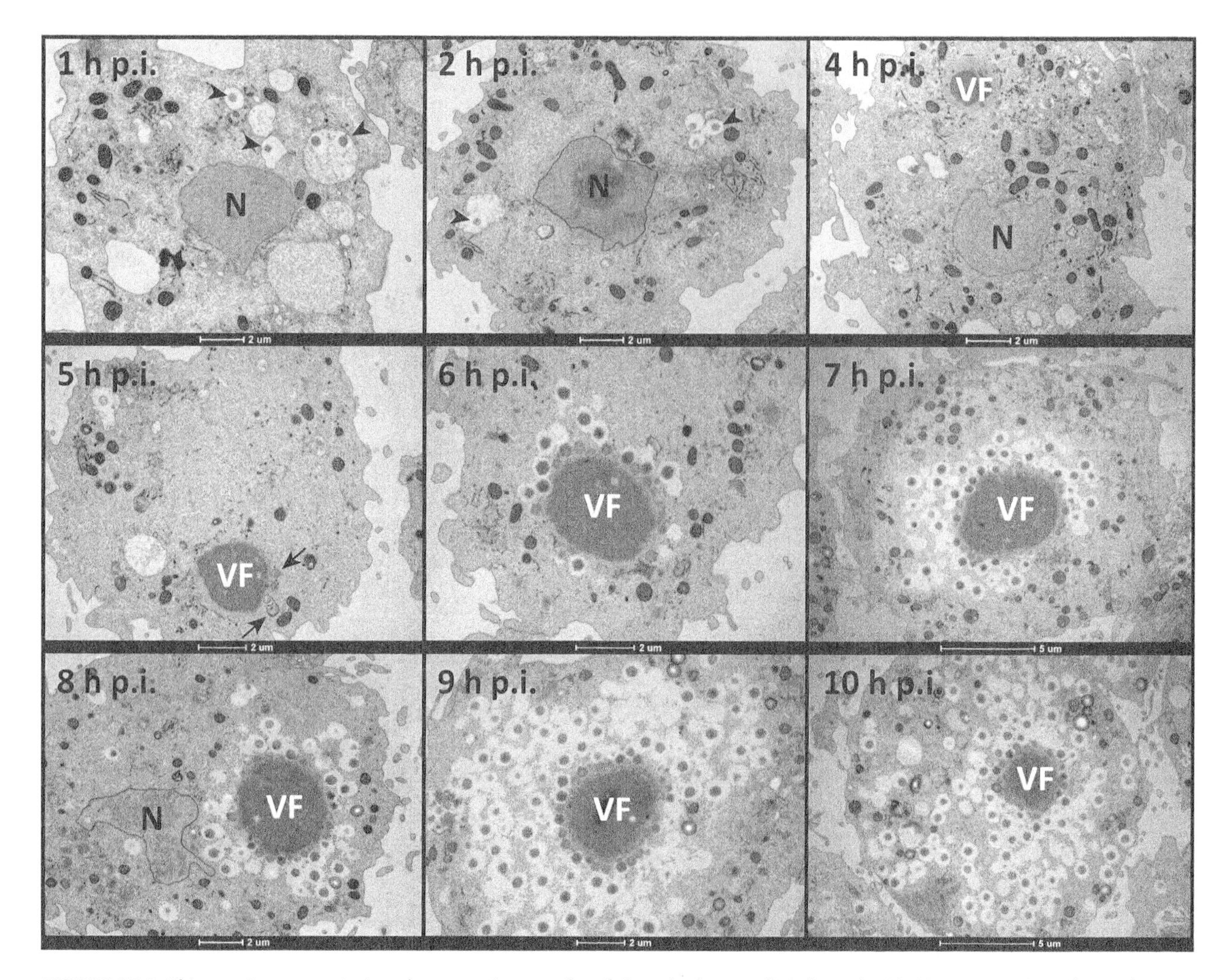

FIGURE 20.8 Thin-section transmission electron micrographs of *A. polyphaga* cells infected with Megavirus vitis. The nucleus (N) is visible during the early stages of infection and at 8 hours p.i. At 4 hours p.i., the first viral factories (VF) appear. Intermediate capsid structures are visible from 5 hours p.i. onward (*arrows*). From 6 hours p.i. on, the cytoplasm is increasingly filled with mature viral particles, displacing the cytoplasmic content. (Images courtesy of Dr. Sandra Jeudy and Dr. Lionel Bertaux, IGS UMR7256 CNRS-AMU.)

Translation

Translation-related genes are frequently encoded by mimiviruses and are particularly frequent in tupanviruses as well as in members of the proposed subfamily *Klosneuvirinae*.[5,10,141]

Despite the impressive number of virus-encoded translation genes, members of the *Mimiviridae* are still obligate intracellular parasites and thus depend on host ribosomes for protein biosynthesis. However, their extensive coding content and genomic flexibility may allow them to modulate many metabolic processes of the host to their advantage, including translation.[3,12] Given that APMV and its host *Acanthamoeba* sp. differ substantially in their GC contents and codon usages, viral substitution of translation components such as aaRS enzymes could lead to more efficient translation of viral proteins.[39] A comparative gene expression analysis of eight viral translation factors (4 tRNAs and 4 aaRS genes) during infection of *A. castellanii* with different members of the genus *Mimivirus* conducted under different nutrient conditions showed that expression levels were lowest in nutrient-replete conditions and highest when cells were starving.[148] Viral translation proteins could therefore provide a temporary selective benefit to host cells when competition for nutrients with other microorganisms is high. For instance, APMV translation initiation factor eIF4E was shown to be present in infected amoebae, where it was localized in the cytoplasm but not in the viral replication factory.[61] Functional assays conducted on selected viral translation proteins confirmed their predicted activity, such as for various mimivirus-encoded translational GTPases of the elongation factor 1 family[184] and two of the four APMV-encoded aaRS enzymes.[2] Experimental silencing of the APMV *R458*-encoded translation initiation factor eIF4a during viral infection resulted in changes of the APMV proteome and decreased viral fitness by delaying formation of the viral factory.[12] These experiments strongly suggest that mimivirus-encoded translation proteins perform important functions during infection.

Genome Replication and Repair

Viral genome replication takes place in the cytoplasmic viral factory. Bromodeoxyuridine (BrdU) labeling and DAPI staining of APMV-infected *A. polyphaga* cells showed that viral genome replication starts concomitantly with the release of the core from the phagosome and DNA decondensation.[115]

Members of the *Mimiviridae* encode multiple proteins involved in DNA replication. The B-family DNA polymerase is one of the few genes that are uniformly conserved among nucleocytoviruses, emphasizing its importance as the main processive enzyme in viral genome replication.[75] In addition to DNA polymerase B, the DNA replication core machinery of mimiviruses consists of a DNA helicase, primase, and a proliferating cell nuclear antigen (PCNA)-like DNA clamp. Further gene products involved in DNA replication are replication factor C subunits, RNase H, and topoisomerase II.[176] It is possible that additional proteins will be recognized as key players in viral replication. For instance, based on its primary sequence, APMV ORF *L537* was predicted to be a member of the archaeo-eukaryotic primase family.[76] Biochemical characterization revealed that this protein is a jack-of-all-trades, possessing terminal transferase, translesion synthesis, as well as DNA and RNA polymerase activities on DNA and RNA templates.[70] L437 is therefore a combined primase, polymerase, reverse transcriptase, and terminal transferase. Nothing is known about the molecular steps of DNA replication in mimivirus. Claverie, Abergel, and Ogata noted that the aforementioned 617-bp long inverted repeat of the APMV genome and the ORFs located at the 5′ terminus of the genome could be involved in DNA replication.[35] Mimiviruses encode up to three different DNA topoisomerases (types IA, IB, and II), which may reflect the need for topology control of such large DNA genomes. APMV topoisomerase IB was characterized biochemically and shown to relax supercoiled DNA.[15] This enzyme is structurally and functionally related to the vaccinia virus homolog, whereas its primary sequence suggests a closer relationship with bacteria.[15]

Owing to the bacterial-sized genomes of mimiviruses and their cytoplasmic replication, which separates them from host DNA maintenance mechanisms in the nucleus, mimiviruses encode DNA repair enzymes of several different pathways, namely base excision repair (BER), nucleotide excision repair (NER), mismatch repair, double-strand break repair, and direct damage reversal processes such as photocatalyzed repair.[19] BER is present in all three domains of life and involves recognition, excision, gap filling, and ligation of a damaged DNA base.[44] Recognition and base excision are catalyzed by glycosylases such as uracil-DNA glycosylase (UDG), resulting in an apurinic/apyrimidinic (AP) site. An AP endonuclease then cuts the DNA backbone and a family X DNA polymerase fills the cleaved gap with a nucleotide. Finally, a DNA ligase seals the repaired lesion site. Mimiviruses encode homologs of UDG,[93] AP endonuclease, DNA polymerase X, DNA ligase, and additional BER-related enzymes such as flap endonuclease.[130] Gene products found in *Mimiviridae* members that are predicted to function in other ATP-dependent DNA repair mechanisms include the NER-associated XPG protein,[19] DNA mismatch repair proteins MutS7 and MutS8,[119] and the double-strand break repair catalytic domains of Mre11 and Rad50 proteins.[175] Interestingly, viral DNA repair enzymes were found in the particles of APMV (DNA pol X, Alkylated DNA repair protein AlkB R406, repair endonuclease L687), Tupanvirus (AlkB homolog ORF72, DNA pol X, and 5′-3′ exonuclease ORF327), and CroV (DNA pol X, AP endonuclease, DNA ligase, 3′-5′ exonuclease CROV200, and a predicted DNA glycosylase).[5,35,57,131] CroV also packages a predicted (6–4) photolyase and encodes a CPD photolyase, indicating that DNA damage caused by ultraviolet light could be repaired in the particle, similar to observations in fowlpox virus.[151] In summary, mimiviruses appear to follow Drake's rule,[46] which states that the mutation rate is inversely proportional to the genome size of microorganisms, including DNA viruses. Accordingly, larger genomes require more DNA repair enzymes, which is confirmed by the large array of repair genes encoded by mimiviruses.[130]

Virion Assembly and Release

Capsid assembly of mimiviruses occurs at the periphery of the viral factory, visible in TEMs as a zone of lower electron density.[179] Within the periphery, distinct areas have been identified for membrane/capsid assembly, genome packaging, and fiber acquisition (Fig. 20.9). As each step of the assembly process

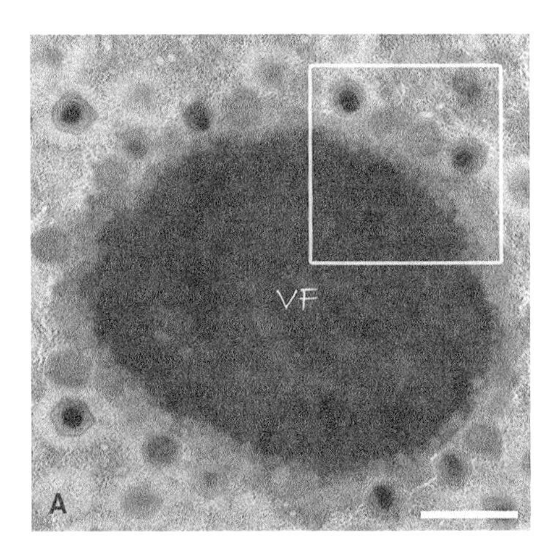

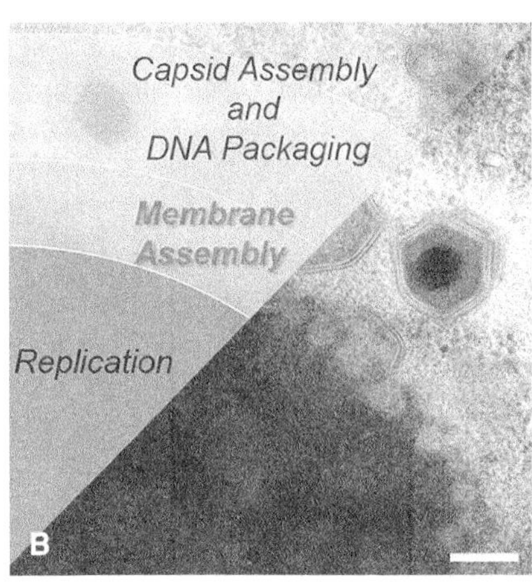

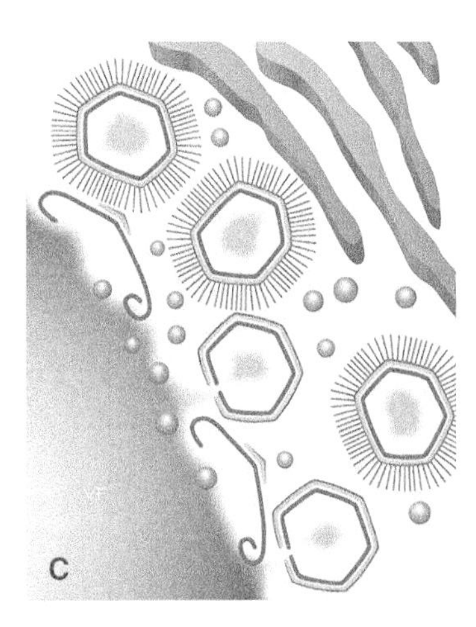

FIGURE 20.9 Spatial organization of the APMV factory in *Acanthamoeba*. A: Late-stage cytoplasmic viral factory (VF) with an electron-dense center and a translucent periphery. **B:** Magnification of the area shown in **(A)**, depicting distinct zones for replication, membrane assembly, and capsid assembly and maturation. **C:** Proposed sequence of events for APMV membrane assembly. Small membrane vesicles (*blue spheres*) that bud out from host ER cisternae (*elongated blue structures*) diffuse toward the VF and form multivesicular bodies that eventually rupture into open membrane sheets (*blue lines*). Icosahedral capsids (*yellow*) are assembled on top of these sheets. Scale bars are 2 μm for **(A)** and 500 nm for **(B)**. (**A and B** are adapted from Mutsafi Y, Fridmann-Sirkis Y, Milrot E, et al. Infection cycles of large DNA viruses: emerging themes and underlying questions. *Virology* 2014;466–467:3–14, **(C)** is adapted from Mutsafi Y, Shimoni E, Shimon A, et al. Membrane assembly during the Infection cycle of the giant mimivirus. *PLoS Pathog* 2013;9:e1003367.)

is completed, APMV particles move sequentially away from the center of the factory. The cytoplasmic factory is therefore ordered spatially and functionally, and a variety of biochemical pathways must be accommodated by its infrastructure. The viral factory has received considerable attention due to its organelle-like appearance, its dimensions, and the various viral enzymatic activities that take place within.[61,159] Conceptually, the viral factory has been considered the true living stage of the virus, in contrast to the seed-like capsid state that lacks metabolic activity.[32] The realization that the factories of large dsDNA viruses such as poxviruses concentrate viral enzymes whose cellular homologs are normally located in the nucleus has even inspired far-reaching evolutionary scenarios that postulate a viral origin for the eukaryotic nucleus ("viral eukaryogenesis").[13,14,161]

Yet, our understanding of viral factories remains superficial. Although the overall appearance is similar for viruses throughout the family *Mimiviridae*, they must differ according to the structural variety of mimivirus capsids that includes icosahedrons of various diameters with short fibers, long fibers, or no fibers, different exit portal architectures, tail structures, and more. Fridmann-Sirkis and colleagues purified APMV factories from different stages of infection in *A. polyphaga* and analyzed their morphologies and protein compositions.[61] Approximately one-third of the predicted APMV proteins were identified in purified factories by mass spectrometry, including 30 membrane proteins. Proteins involved in DNA replication and repair, transcription, and protein degradation were present in factories at all three time points sampled (4, 5.5., and 7 hours p.i.). Factories at 7 hours p.i. already contained most of the proteins that are packaged in the virions. They also noted that the viral factory is surrounded by ribosomes, although no ribosomes are present in the factory itself.

Particles assemble with the unique stargate portal facing away from the center of the factory[179] and newly synthesized particles with stargate structures first appear between 4 and 5.5 hours p.i. (Fig. 20.10).[61] Stargate formation may thus be involved in the symmetry-breaking early events of capsid assembly.[113] Capsid assembly initiates at a fivefold vertex and presumably involves the MCP as a scaffolding component.[114] After seeding a new capsid structure, capsomers could then be added in a spiral fashion around the first pentameric vertex, as suggested by cryo-EM studies of the CroV particle (Fig. 20.11).[172] The incorporation of other scaffolding proteins into the nascent capsid structure, such as the proposed tape-measure protein, remains to be studied.[48] The origin of the internal virion membrane in APMV was initially puzzling, because the viral factory was neither membrane bound nor connected to the endomembrane system of the host cell. A combination of diverse electron microscopy techniques revealed that the APMV membrane is derived from the endoplasmic reticulum (ER). Vesicles from the ER are transported to the viral factory, where they fuse into multivesicular bodies that then rupture to give rise to open membrane sheets. These open membrane intermediates have a diameter of approximately 90 nm for APMV.[114,153] Capsid and membrane assembly happen concomitantly as the growing capsid draws from the multivesicular bodies that feed membranes into the assembly zone, suggesting an early interaction between scaffolding proteins and the lipid layer. Upon completion of the icosahedral container, nonassembled open membrane overhang structures protrude from the residual capsid opening. These extra membranes are then trimmed in preparation for genome packaging.[114] Similar processes have been reported for poxviruses and asfarviruses, suggesting that membrane assembly via open membrane intermediates may be a common feature of nucleocytoviruses.[29,153,154]

As the nascent capsids move further from the center of the viral factory, they pass a zone that is characterized by lower electron density in thin-section TEMs and has been named the fibril acquisition area.[6] In this area, APMV capsids acquire the 120- to 140-nm-thick outer layer of glycosylated fibers (Fig. 20.9). Fiber-coated particles are first visible around 7 hours p.i.[61] Around the same time, the genome is delivered into the preassembled capsid via a transient 18- to 20-nm-wide portal that is located at an icosahedral face opposite of the stargate vertex (Fig. 20.12).[179] Viruses of the family *Mimiviridae* encode a DNA-pumping ATPase of the HerA-FtsK superfamily, which could catalyze the packaging of the viral genome into the preformed capsid. These viral motor proteins are similar to the bacterial apparatus for chromosome segregation.[28] At approximately 8 hours p.i., the viral factory of APMV is surrounded by fully assembled icosahedral capsids.[114] Mature virus particles are released from the infected amoeba by lysis at approximately 24 hours p.i. (Fig. 20.13).[160] The burst size of APMV is approximately 300 to 1,000 virions per cell, for Megavirus chilensis, and for CroV, the burst size is about 500 per cell.[8,35,163]

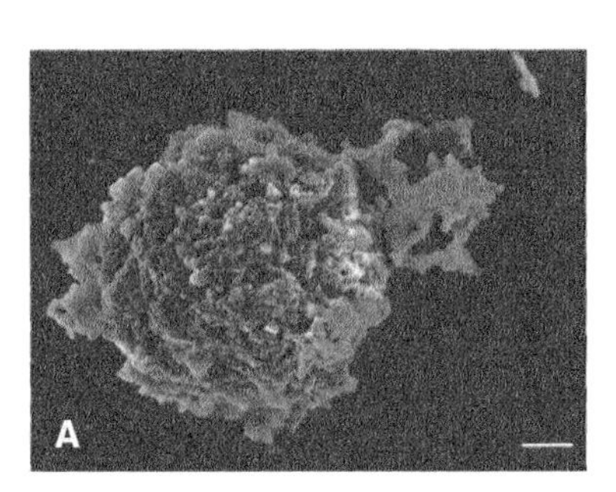

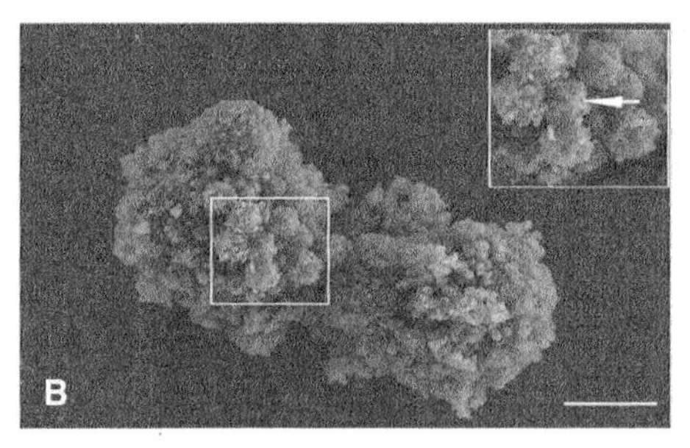

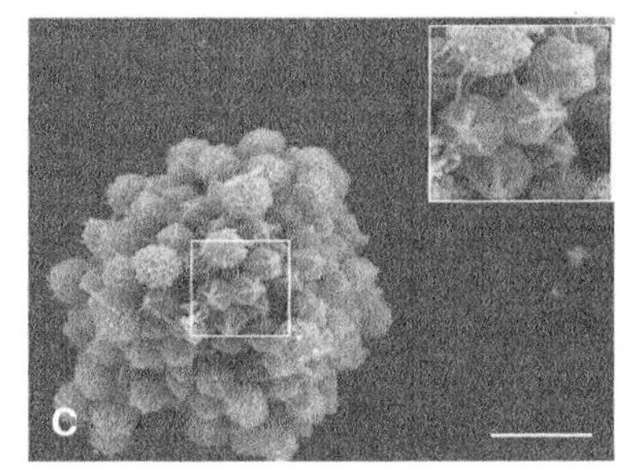

FIGURE 20.10 Scanning electron micrographs of isolated APMV factories from different stages of infection. A: At 4 hours p.i., replication centers have formed, but no capsid structures are visible yet. **B:** At 5.5 hours p.i., first capsids with stargate structures (*inset, arrow*) are discernible at the periphery of the viral factory. This image shows two fusing viral factories that are likely derived from two individual virus entry events. **C:** At 7 hours p.i., the factory is covered with newly synthesized APMV capsids; some are still naked with visible stargate portals (*inset*), and others have already acquired their fiber coat. Scale bars are 200 nm for **(A)** and 1 µm for **(B)** and **(C)**. (Adapted from Fridmann-Sirkis Y, et al. Efficiency in complexity: composition and dynamic nature of mimivirus replication factories. *J Virol* 2016;90:10039–10047.)

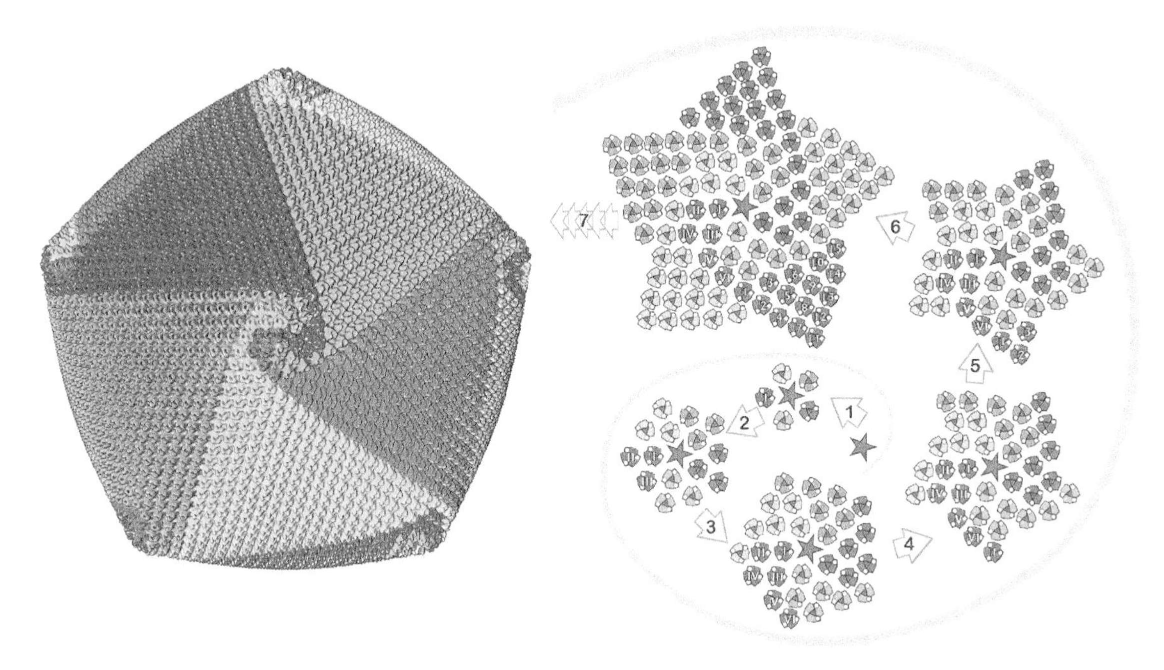

FIGURE 20.11 Cryo-electron microscopy reconstruction of the CroV capsid and proposed spiral assembly pathway. Capsomers are colored based on their orientation in *red*, *blue*, *green*, *cyan*, and *orange*. The pentameric capsomers are depicted as *purple stars*. The schematic on the right shows the proposed spiral assembly pathway. First, capsomers assemble in two layers around the pentameric capsomer (1+2). For the third layer, newly added capsomers spiral counterclockwise, according to their orientation (3+4), and will then seed the trisymmetron (forming one icosahedral face) by recruiting more capsomers of the same orientation (5–7). One set of capsomers (*red*) is labeled by Roman numerals if they are part of the pentasymmetron and by Arabic numerals if they are part of a trisymmetron. (Adapted from Xiao C, et al. Cryo-EM reconstruction of the Cafeteria roenbergensis virus capsid suggests novel assembly pathway for giant viruses. *Sci Rep* 2017;7:5484.)

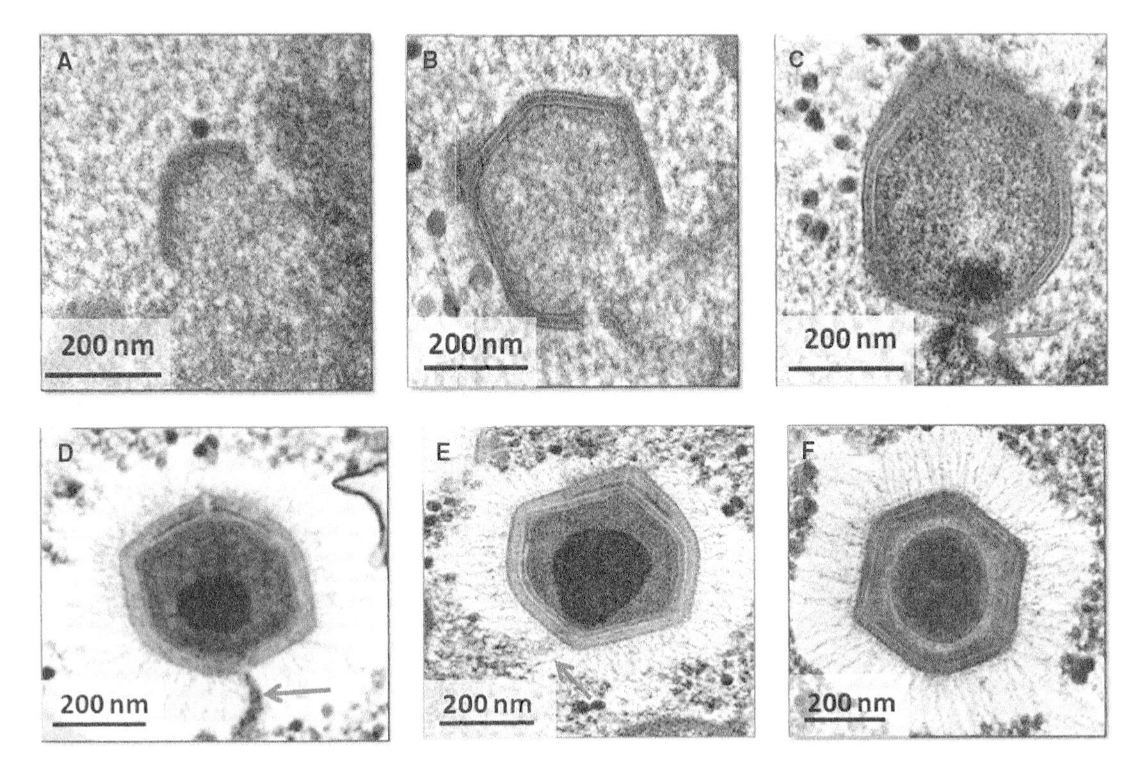

FIGURE 20.12 Transmission electron microscopy images showing stages of APMV particle formation. **A:** Initiation of capsid assembly at a pentameric vertex. **B:** Near-complete capsid shell prior to genome packaging. **C–E:** Capsids undergoing genome packaging (*red arrows*) through a portal opposite of the stargate vertex. Surface fibers are visible in **(D and E)**. **F:** Mature APMV particle. (Modified from Andrade ACDSP, et al. Filling knowledge gaps for mimivirus entry, uncoating, and morphogenesis. *J Virol* 2017;91:1–12.)

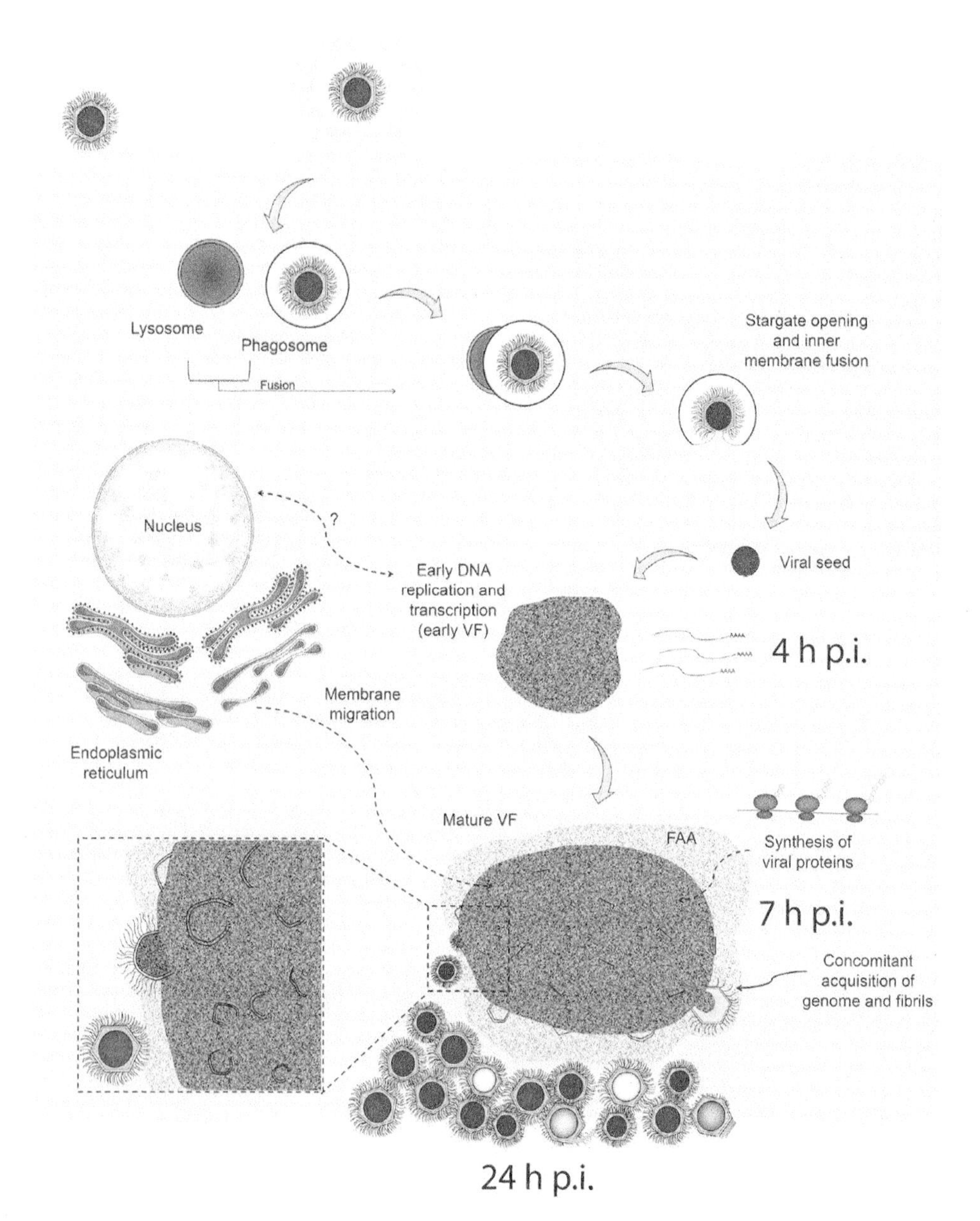

FIGURE 20.13 Schematic overview of the APMV replication cycle. Infectious APMV particles enter the amoebal host cell by phagocytosis. Fusion of the phagosome with a lysosome occurs and opening of the stargate is followed by release of the viral seed (nucleocapsid). An early viral factory (VF) is established at 3 to 4 hours p.i., and viral proteins are synthesized outside the factory. It is uncertain whether the cell nucleus is involved in mimivirus genome replication. Viral particle assembly commences at the periphery of the VF, and preformed capsids might acquire genomic material and fibers simultaneously. As the particles move further from the center of the VF, they enter the fibril acquisition area (FAA) where surface fibers are attached. Some of the newly synthesized viral particles may present with atypical morphologies and may not be infectious. The viral progeny are released by cell lysis at approximately 24 hours p.i. (Adapted from Andrade ACDSP, et al. Filling knowledge gaps for mimivirus entry, uncoating, and morphogenesis. *J Virol* 2017;91:1–12.)

VIROPHAGES AND OTHER MOBILE GENETIC ELEMENTS OF MIMIVIRUSES

Following the initial discovery of APMV in *Acanthamoeba* sp.,[95,129] a targeted search for additional giant viruses infecting amoebae was initiated. In 2008, La Scola et al. reported the isolation of an APMV strain named mamavirus.[96] Unexpectedly, they coisolated a smaller virus named Sputnik from the same sample. Sputnik was not able to replicate in host cells alone but required the presence of mamavirus, akin to several satellite-helper virus systems described previously.[30,91,96,150,183] A few other virophages have been isolated subsequently in culture, mostly in combination with *Acanthamoeba*-specific mimiviruses,[27,43,62,63,112,152] but also for the flagellate-infecting

CroV.[58] Based on these cultured representatives, thousands of virophage-like sequences were found in metagenomic datasets, indicating that virophages are widespread and diverse in the environment.[68,120,122,135,173,181,182]

Classification of Virophages in the Family *Lavidaviridae*

Based on their biological property of replicating exclusively in the presence of a coinfecting giant virus, Sputnik was initially grouped with satellite viruses in the obscure category of "subviral agents".[49] Following a debate on virophages versus traditional satellite viruses,[53,89,90] virophages and satellite viruses were eventually classified into their own families.[91] The family *Lavidaviridae* (large virus-depending or associated viruses) currently comprises two genera, *Sputnik* and *Mavirus*, although additional genera are likely to be added in the future.[135] The *Lavidaviridae* are part of the realm *Varidnaviria*, the kingdom *Bamfordvirae*, the phylum *Preplasmiviricota*, the class *Maveriviricetes*, and the order *Priklausovirales*.[87]

Structure of Virophage Particles

The virophages that have been cultured and studied so far have icosahedral particles with a diameter of 50 to 75 nm. In contrast to the much larger mimiviruses (Fig. 20.14), virophage particles lack a lipid component.[180] The capsid is composed of an MCP that folds into a double jelly-roll conformation and forms trimeric capsomers. The minor capsid protein, or penton protein, presents in a single jelly-roll conformation and occupies the fivefold vertices of the icosahedral particle.[158,180] Despite low primary sequence conservation, the overall structures of Sputnik and mavirus capsids are remarkably similar[21] and lavidaviruses have capsids with a quasisymmetry of $T = 27$.[180] Capsid modifications such as asymmetric portals or APMV-like fibers have not been reported.

Genomics of Virophages

Viruses of the family *Lavidaviridae* have linear or circular dsDNA genomes with lengths ranging from 17 kb to more than 30 kb for some metagenome-assembled representatives.[11,54] With some exceptions,[182] virophage genomes tend to have low GC contents of 27% to 37%. Terminal inverted repeats of several hundred bases flank the mavirus genome and are also found in metagenomic virophages.[56,177] Whereas the overall coding content of virophages varies considerably, most genomes share four core genes for capsid morphogenesis.[91,122] The *MCP* gene is typically adjacent to the *penton* gene, and these two gene products are sufficient for self-assembly of icosahedral mavirus-like capsids.[21] The capsid genes are complemented by an MCP-processing cysteine protease and a DNA-pumping ATPase of the FtsK-HerA family. Additional conserved functions found in lavidaviruses are genome integration and DNA replication/remodeling, which are represented by nonhomologous versions of integrases, DNA polymerases, and primase/helicases. The pan genome of virophages also includes a variety of accessory genes that may be derived from their hosts, associated giant viruses, or other mobile genetic elements.[85,122,135,173]

The Virophage Infection Cycle

Virophage particles enter their host cells either independently of their giant virus by endocytosis (e.g., mavirus) or as a composite with the giant virus by phagocytosis (e.g., Sputnik).[42,58,162] Upon cell entry, the viral genome is released into the cytoplasm and targeted to the virion factory of the giant virus, if present. Transcription and genome replication of the virophage then occur within the virion factory (Fig. 20.15), often clustered in a specific region thereof.[42,112] The molecular mechanism of virophage DNA replication has not been studied yet, but it is assumed that virophages are self-sufficient for this process since they encode their own DNA polymerases: Mavirus carries a predicted protein-primed B-family DNA polymerase and Sputnik encodes a superfamily A polymerase (TV-Pol) fused to a D5-like helicase.[73] Newly synthesized virophage particles then accumulate within or close to the virion factory (Fig. 20.14) and are released from the cell during lysis.

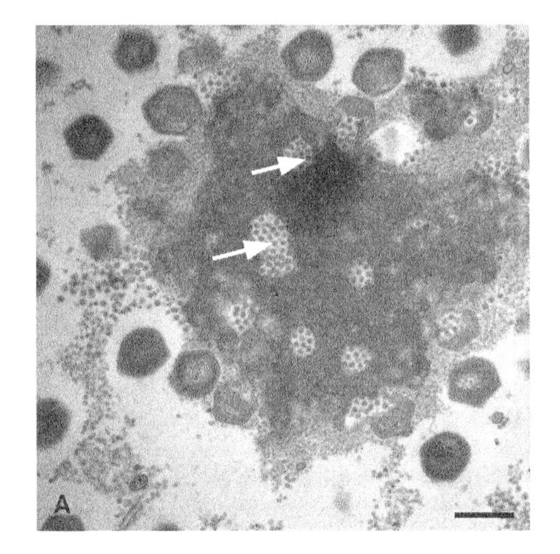

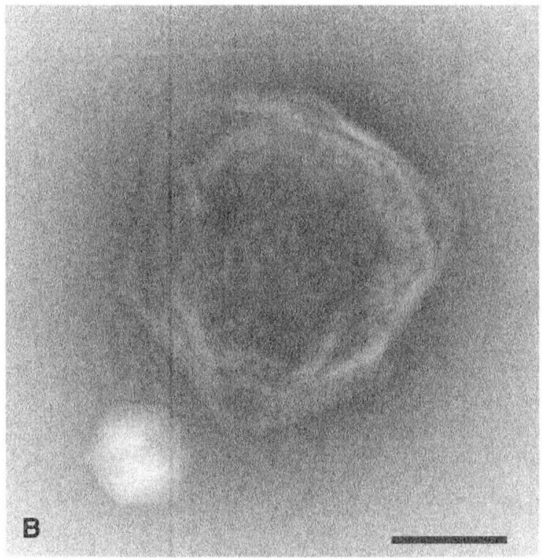

FIGURE 20.14 Mimiviruses and their virophages. A: Thin-section electron micrograph of a Megavirus vigne factory where giant virus particles co-assemble with their Zamilon particles (*arrows*). (Image courtesy of Dr. Sandra Jeudy and Dr. Lionel Bertaux, IGS UMR7256 CNRS-AMU.) **B:** Transmission electron micrograph of a CroV particle next to a mavirus capsid. Image by Ulrike Mersdorf and Dr. Matthias Fischer, MPI for Medical Research, Germany. Scale bars are 500 nm for **(A)** and 100 nm for **(B)**.

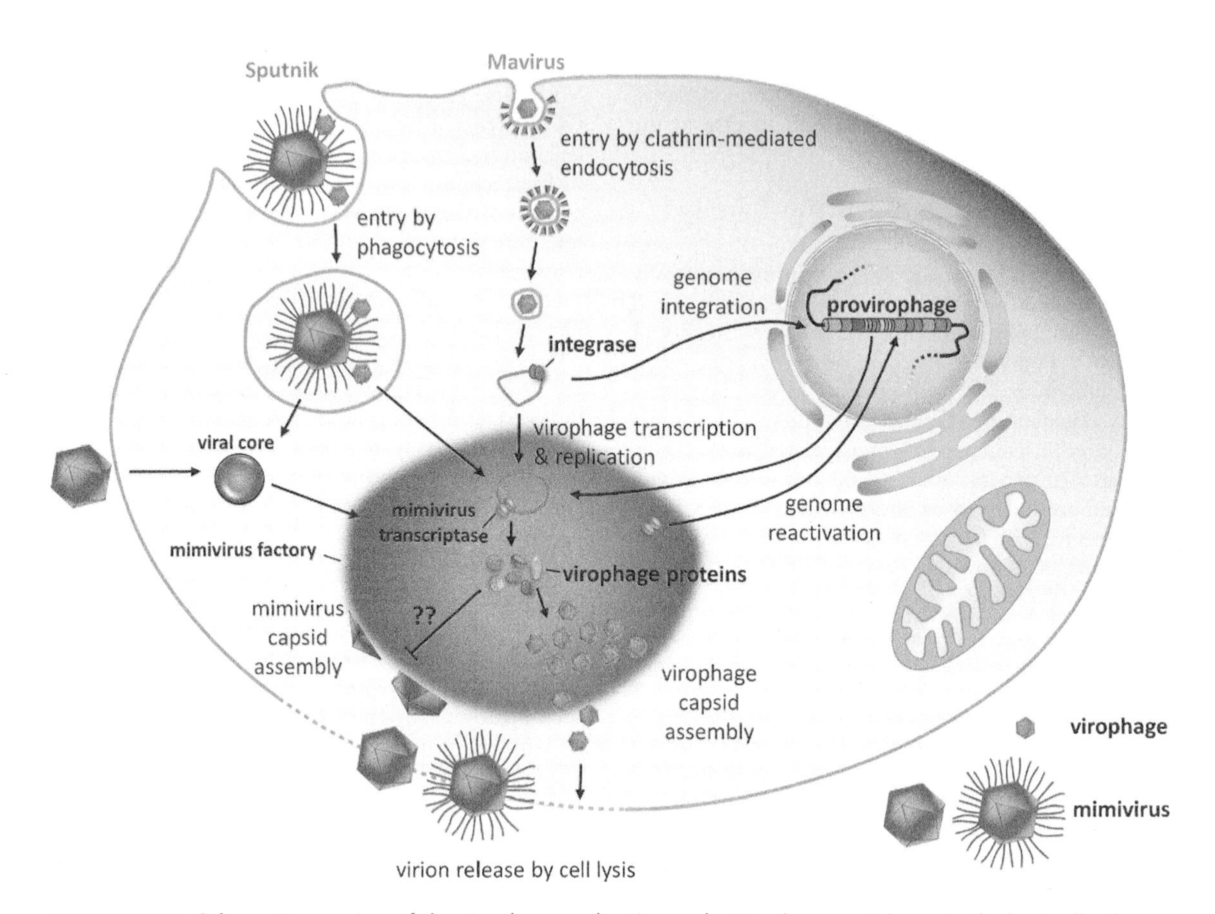

FIGURE 20.15 Schematic overview of the virophage replication cycle. Virophage particles enter the host cell either by endocytosis (mavirus) or by phagocytosis as a composite with an associated mimivirus (Sputnik). After release from the endosome, the virophage genome is translocated to the mimivirus factory where transcription, DNA replication, and capsid assembly occur. During these processes, the replication cycle of the mimivirus may be inhibited. Alternatively, mavirus can integrate into the host genome in the absence of a coinfecting giant virus, allowing persistence as an inactive provirophage. Reactivation of the provirophage occurs after infection of the host cell with a compatible mimivirus. (Adapted from Duponchel S, Fischer MG. Viva lavidaviruses! Five features of virophages that parasitize giant DNA viruses. *PLoS Pathog* 2019;15:e1007592.)

Although virophages do not actively replicate in the absence of a coinfecting mimivirus, their integrase enzymes allow them to enter a persistent state by coupling to another genome. Sputnik encodes a tyrosine recombinase and integration as a provirophage in the APMV genome has been reported.[43] Mavirus virions contain an rve-family integrase enzyme and this virophage is able to integrate into its eukaryotic host genome in the absence of a coinfecting giant virus.[21,56] The provirophage can resume active replication and horizontal transmission when the provirophage-bearing host cell is infected by a compatible mimivirus.

Virophages Depend on a Coinfecting Mimivirus

No virophage isolated to date is able to replicate on its own in a host cell. Sputnik and Guarani replicate in the presence of a virus of the genus *Mimivirus*, or of the proposed genera Moumouvirus and Megavirus.[112] Zamilon also replicates with the latter two, but not with members of the genus *Mimivirus*.[63] Mavirus requires a coinfection with CroV for active replication.[58] Given that virophages encode capsid and DNA polymerase genes, their dependence on a giant virus is not rooted in deficiencies regarding DNA replication or encapsidation. Instead, since gene expression occurs outside the nucleus and virophages lack their own RNA polymerase, they depend on the cytoplasmic transcription machinery provided by the mimivirus. Accordingly, the transcriptional initiation and termination signals were found to be highly similar between a virophage and its associated giant virus.[31,58,101] In particular, virophage gene promoters resemble those of giant virus late genes, and virophage gene expression thus would commence at the onset of late phase of the giant virus infection cycle. A Sputnik-related virophage strain named Guarani was shown to start replicating at 4 hours p.i. and to produce particles late (12 to 16 hours p.i.) during a coinfection with APMV, with virophage particles still absent at 12 hours p.i.[112] Virophages thus likely hijack the mimiviral factory at the onset of late phase, with the mimivirus-encoded transcriptase complex recognizing and expressing the virophage genes.

In theory, other large dsDNA viruses such as poxviruses that possess cytoplasmic transcription capacity could also be prone to parasitism by virophage-like entities.

Host–Virus Symbioses and Defense Systems Involving Giant Viruses

Compared to other viruses, mimiviruses have reached a remarkable degree of enzymatic autonomy and biological complexity. The viral transcription complex enables mimiviruses to express their genes independently of the host machinery, which may facilitate host switching and evasion of host defenses. At the same time, cytoplasmic transcription bears the potential cost of attracting a virophage that interferes with replication of the giant virus.

During a virophage–mimivirus coinfection, Sputnik reduces the yield of infectious mamavirus particles by about two-thirds, Guarani reduces APMV yields by up to 90%, and mavirus reduces CroV yields by more than 99%, depending on the multiplicity of infection.[56,96,112] Initially, the presence of Sputnik was linked to abnormal capsid structures of mimivirus, such as multiple capsid layers and open-ended capsid extensions.[96] However, Andrade et al. observed such structures also in *Acanthamoeba* cells infected with APMV only, in the absence of virophages.[6] Similarly, abnormal APMV particles were reported at a rate of approximately 1% for both, Guarani coinfected, and Guarani-free infections.[112] It appears thus rather unlikely that the presence of virophages induces structural anomalies in APMV. Instead, the virophage might suppress late gene expression of the mimivirus by recruiting its transcription machinery. Interestingly, the Zamilon virophage replicates with APMV in a commensal manner, because coinfection has no measurable negative impact on APMV production.[63] The symbiotic relationship between virophages and giant viruses thus ranges from commensalism to strong parasitism and has important implications for the infected host cell population. While a Zamilon–mimivirus coinfection does not reduce host mortality compared to a mimivirus infection,[63] Sputnik, Guarani, and mavirus significantly increase host population survival in the presence of their respective lytic giant viruses.[56,96,112] The latter virophages therefore act as mutualists of their host organisms.

The genome integration capacity of mavirus adds another level of ecological significance to the tripartite host–virus–virophage relationship. Mavirus not only integrates rather efficiently into the nuclear genome of *Cafeteria* sp. but is also reactivated in response to CroV infection.[56] By retaining a functional yet transcriptionally silent provirophage in the host genome, a population of protists may increase its survival chances when infiltrated by a lytic mimivirus, compared to a provirophage-naive population.[17] Mavirus protection of host populations may thus be regarded as a case of adaptive immunity in unicellular eukaryotes.[84]

Mimiviruses, on the other hand, are not defenseless against virophage parasitism. The "mimivirus virophage resistance element" (MIMIVIRE) in APMV consists of a gene cassette that involves a Cas4-like nuclease R354, a helicase–nuclease R350, and the *R349* gene that contains a 28 nt long sequence and four repeats of a 15 nt long sequence matching ORF4 of the Zamilon genome.[104] Presence of the MIMIVIRE system in members of the *Mimivirus* genus was linked to resistance of these viruses to Zamilon replication. Silencing the APMV *R349*, *R354*, and *R350* genes by RNA interference led to increased Zamilon replication with the otherwise nonpermissive mimivirus.[104] Furthermore, an *R349* knockout in APMV restored Zamilon replication, and Zamilon also replicated with a *Mimivirus* member that had only one of the four 15 nt repeats.[111] The proposed analogy of MIMIVIRE to CRISPR-Cas systems has been criticized[33] and the molecular basis for this defense system remains to be studied. However, defense systems of this or other types may exist in a variety of giant viruses to fend off genetic parasites.

Other Mobile Genetic Elements Associated With Mimiviruses

In addition to virophages, mimiviruses contain a diverse mobilome that includes transposases, self-splicing introns, inteins, and a class of linear plasmid-like elements called transpovirons.[43,137,178] Transpovirons are approximately 7 kb long and encode 6 to 8 genes, some of which are shared with other mobile genetic elements including Sputnik and linear yeast plasmids.[178] They replicate in extremely high copy numbers in the presence of a mimivirus, can integrate themselves into the mimivirus genome, and are packaged as episomes in both mimivirus and virophage particles.[43,77] Moreover, different versions of transpovirons are associated with specific mimivirus and virophage strains, suggestive of adaptive coevolution between these entities.[77] Phylogenetic analysis indicates that transpovirons may be evolutionarily derived from maverick/polinton elements (MPEs) or related polinton-like viruses.[85] The MPEs were originally described as eukaryotic self-replicating transposons,[79,126] but after two conserved MPE genes were identified as distant capsid protein homologs, it is likely that many of them represent endogenous viruses.[88] MPEs are genetically related to virophages, in particular those of the genus *Mavirus*. Indeed, MPEs and virophages not only share the same set of morphogenesis genes, the rve-family integrase, DNA polymerase B, and helicase genes of MPEs are homologous to those found in mavirus.[58] Moreover, MPEs are flanked by terminal inverted repeats and target site duplications very similar to those of integrated mavirus genomes.[56] The emerging picture of the mimivirus mobilome, and that of large and giant DNA viruses in general,[67,157] is an expansive gene-sharing network, where different types of genetic parasites interact and recombine with one another.[85]

PERSPECTIVE

Mimiviruses have profoundly changed our perception of viruses. Their genome lengths and particle sizes, coding content, structural and enzymatic complexity, and their entourage of various mobile genetic elements have pushed these viruses into the range of single-celled organisms and have blurred some of the boundaries that once firmly separated viruses from cells. Despite these fascinating features, however, they remain bona fide viruses based on their obligate dependence on a cellular host for propagation, and their mode of replication via de novo synthesis and structural discontinuity. The past two decades have revealed an astounding diversity of giant viruses, many of which have been isolated from *Acanthamoeba polyphaga*, and many more were identified by metagenomics. These combined findings prove that the serendipitous discovery of APMV was not just that of a freak virus, but representative of a widespread and ancient group of viruses that we had previously missed because of our own technical and conceptual limitations.

Despite the great advances made on the genetic diversity, structure, infection biology, and biochemistry of mimiviruses, much remains to be discovered. Their host range presumably covers all major eukaryotic supergroups, yet little is known about individual virus–host interactions. The ecological impact of their role in regulating natural protist populations has been hardly addressed so far, yet the implications must be far-reaching, from affecting species composition and controlling algal blooms to influencing global biogeochemical cycles. Owing to their tremendous genetic storage capacity, mimiviruses offer a window into the past through phylogenomic analysis, allowing us to reconstruct gene flows and ancient evolutionary events, but they also provide many opportunities to observe evolution in action. Detailed investigations into the diverse spectrum of mimivirus-associated mobile genetic elements such as virophages and transpovirons may uncover previously unknown types of symbiotic interactions, including novel types of defense systems.

ACKNOWLEDGMENTS

The author thanks the Max Planck Society for support, Dr. Sandra Jeudy and Dr. Lionel Bertaux for contributing electron micrographs, and Dr. Christopher Schvarcz and Dr. Grieg Steward for sharing unpublished DNA sequences.

REFERENCES

1. Abergel C, Legendre M, Claverie J-M. The rapidly expanding universe of giant viruses: Mimivirus, Pandoravirus, Pithovirus and Mollivirus. *FEMS Microbiol Rev* 2015;39:779–796.
2. Abergel C, Rudinger-Thirion J, Giegé R, et al. Virus-encoded aminoacyl-tRNA synthetases: structural and functional characterization of mimivirus TyrRS and MetRS. *J Virol* 2007;81:12406–12417.
3. Abrahão JS, Araújo R, Colson P, et al. The analysis of translation-related gene set boosts debates around origin and evolution of mimiviruses. *PLoS Genet* 2017;13:1–12.
4. Abrahão J, Silva L, Oliveira D, et al. Lack of evidence of mimivirus replication in human PBMCs. *Microbes Infect* 2018;20:281–283.
5. Abrahão J, et al. Tailed giant Tupanvirus possesses the most complete translational apparatus of the known virosphere. *Nat Commun* 2018;9:749.
6. Andrade ACDSP, et al. Filling knowledge gaps for mimivirus entry, uncoating, and morphogenesis. *J Virol* 2017;91:1–12.
7. Andreani J, et al. Orpheovirus IHUMI-LCC2: a new virus among the giant viruses. *Front Microbiol* 2018;8:1–11.
8. Arslan D, Legendre M, Seltzer V, et al. Distant Mimivirus relative with a larger genome highlights the fundamental features of Megaviridae. *Proc Natl Acad Sci U S A* 2011;108:17486–17491.
9. Azza S, Cambillau C, Raoult D, et al. Revised Mimivirus major capsid protein sequence reveals intron-containing gene structure and extra domain. *BMC Mol Biol* 2009;10:39.
10. Bajrai LH, et al. Isolation of yasminevirus, the first member of klosneuvirinae isolated in coculture with vermamoeba vermiformis. *J Virol* 2020;94:1–13.
11. Bekliz M, Colson P, La Scola B. The expanding family of virophages. *Viruses* 2016;8:E317.
12. Bekliz M, et al. Experimental analysis of mimivirus translation initiation factor 4a reveals its importance in viral protein translation during infection of acanthamoeba polyphaga. *J Virol* 2018;92:1–13.
13. Bell PJL. The viral eukaryogenesis hypothesis: a key role for viruses in the emergence of eukaryotes from a prokaryotic world environment. *Ann N Y Acad Sci* 2009;1178:91–105.
14. Bell PJL. Evidence supporting a viral origin of the eukaryotic nucleus. *Virus Res* 2020;289:198168.
15. Benarroch D, Claverie J-M, Raoult D, et al. Characterization of mimivirus DNA topoisomerase IB suggests horizontal gene transfer between eukaryal viruses and bacteria. *J Virol* 2006;80:314–321.
16. Benarroch D, Smith P, Shuman S. Characterization of a trifunctional mimivirus mRNA capping enzyme and crystal structure of the RNA triphosphatase domain. *Structure* 2008;16:501–512.
17. Berjón-Otero M, Koslová A, Fischer MG. The dual lifestyle of genome-integrating virophages in protists. *Ann N Y Acad Sci* 2019;1447:97–109.
18. Blanc G, Gallot-Lavallée L, Maumus F. Provirophages in the Bigelowiella genome bear testimony to past encounters with giant viruses. *Proc Natl Acad Sci U S A* 2015;112:E5318–E5326.
19. Blanc-Mathieu R, Ogata H. DNA repair genes in the Megavirales pangenome. *Curr Opin Microbiol* 2016;31:94–100.
20. Boratto PVM, et al. Analyses of the Kroon virus major capsid gene and its transcript highlight a distinct pattern of gene evolution and splicing among mimiviruses. *J Virol* 2017;92:e01782.
21. Born D, et al. Capsid protein structure, self-assembly, and processing reveal morphogenesis of the marine virophage mavirus. *Proc Natl Acad Sci U S A* 2018;115:7332–7337.
22. Boughalmi M, et al. High-throughput isolation of giant viruses of the *Mimiviridae* and *Marseilleviridae* families in the Tunisian environment. *Environ Microbiol* 2013;15:2000–2007.
23. Boyer M, et al. Giant Marseillevirus highlights the role of amoebae as a melting pot in emergence of chimeric microorganisms. *Proc Natl Acad Sci U S A* 2009;106:21848–21853.
24. Boyer M, et al. Mimivirus shows dramatic genome reduction after intraamoebal culture. *Proc Natl Acad Sci U S A* 2011;108:10296–10301.
25. Broyles SS, Knutson BA. Poxvirus transcription. *Future Virol* 2010;5:639–650.
26. Byrne D, et al. The polyadenylation site of Mimivirus transcripts obeys a stringent 'hairpin rule'. *Genome Res* 2009;19:1233–1242.
27. Campos RK, et al. Samba virus: a novel mimivirus from a giant rain forest, the Brazilian Amazon. *Virol J* 2014;11:95.
28. Chelikani V, Ranjan T, Zade A, et al. Genome segregation and packaging machinery in Acanthamoeba polyphaga mimivirus is reminiscent of bacterial apparatus. *J Virol* 2014;88:6069–6075.
29. Chlanda P, Carbajal MA, Cyrklaff M, et al. Membrane rupture generates single open membrane sheets during vaccinia virus assembly. *Cell Host Microbe* 2009;6:81–90.
30. Christie GE, Dokland T. Pirates of the caudovirales. *Virology* 2012;434:210–221.
31. Claverie J-M, Abergel C. Mimivirus and its virophage. *Annu Rev Genet* 2009;43:49–66.
32. Claverie J-M, Abergel C. Mimivirus: the emerging paradox of quasi-autonomous viruses. *Trends Genet* 2010;26:431–437.
33. Claverie J-M, Abergel C. CRISPR-Cas-like system in giant viruses: why MIMIVIRE is not likely to be an adaptive immune system. *Virol Sin* 2016;31:193–196.
34. Claverie JM, Abergel C. *Mimiviridae*: an expanding family of highly diverse large dsDNA viruses infecting a wide phylogenetic range of aquatic eukaryotes. *Viruses* 2018;10:8–15.
35. Claverie J-M, Abergel C, Ogata H. Mimivirus. *Curr Top Microbiol Immunol* 2009;328:89–121.
36. Claverie J-M, et al. Mimivirus and the emerging concept of 'giant' virus. *Virus Res* 2006;117:133–144.
37. Claverie J-M, et al. Mimivirus and *Mimiviridae*: giant viruses with an increasing number of potential hosts, including corals and sponges. *J Invertebr Pathol* 2009;101:172–180.
38. Colson P, Aherfi S, La Scola B, et al. The role of giant viruses of amoebas in humans. *Curr Opin Microbiol* 2016;31:199–208.
39. Colson P, Fournous G, Diene SM, et al. Codon usage, amino acid usage, transfer RNA and Amino-Acyl-tRNA synthetases in mimiviruses. *Intervirology* 2013;56:364–375.
40. Colson P, et al. 'Megavirales', a proposed new order for eukaryotic nucleocytoplasmic large DNA viruses. *Arch Virol* 2013;158:2517–2521.
41. Deeg CM, Chow CET, Suttle CA. The kinetoplastid-infecting Bodo saltans virus (BsV), a window into the most abundant giant viruses in the sea. *Elife* 2018;7:1–22.
42. Desnues C, Raoult D. Inside the lifestyle of the virophage. *Intervirology* 2010;53:293–303.
43. Desnues C, et al. Provirophages and transpovirons as the diverse mobilome of giant viruses. *Proc Natl Acad Sci U S A* 2012;109:18078–18083.
44. Dianov GL, Hübscher U. Mammalian base excision repair: the forgotten archangel. *Nucleic Acids Res* 2013;41:3483–3490.
45. Dodds JA, Cole A. Microscopy and biology of Uronema gigas, a filamentous eucaryotic green alga, and its associated tailed virus-like particle. *Virology* 1980;100:156–165.
46. Drake JW. A constant rate of spontaneous mutation in DNA-based microbes. *Proc Natl Acad Sci U S A* 1991;88:7160–7164.
47. Elde NC, et al. Poxviruses deploy genomic accordions to adapt rapidly against host antiviral defenses. *Cell* 2012;150:831–841.
48. Fang Q, et al. Near-atomic structure of a giant virus. *Nat Commun* 2019;10:388.
49. Fauquet CM, Mayo MA, Maniloff J, et al., eds. *Virus Taxonomy: Eighth Report of the International Committee on Taxonomy of Viruses*. London, UK: Elsevier; 2005:1163.
50. Filée J. Lateral gene transfer, lineage-specific gene expansion and the evolution of Nucleo Cytoplasmic Large DNA viruses. *J Invertebr Pathol* 2009;101:169–171.
51. Filée J. Route of NCLDV evolution: the genomic accordion. *Curr Opin Virol* 2013;3:595–599.
52. Filée J, Pouget N, Chandler M. Phylogenetic evidence for extensive lateral acquisition of cellular genes by Nucleocytoplasmic large DNA viruses. *BMC Evol Biol* 2008;8:320–333.
53. Fischer MG. Sputnik and Mavirus: more than just satellite viruses. *Nat Rev Microbiol* 2012;10:78; author reply 78.
54. Fischer MG. The virophage family lavidaviridae. *Curr Issues Mol Biol* 2020;40:1–24.
55. Fischer MG, Allen MJ, Wilson WH, et al. Giant virus with a remarkable complement of genes infects marine zooplankton. *Proc Natl Acad Sci U S A* 2010;107:19508–19513.
56. Fischer MG, Hackl T. Host genome integration and giant virus-induced reactivation of the virophage mavirus. *Nature* 2016;540:288–291.
57. Fischer MG, Kelly I, Foster LJ, et al. The virion of Cafeteria roenbergensis virus (CroV) contains a complex suite of proteins for transcription and DNA repair. *Virology* 2014;466–467:82–94.
58. Fischer MG, Suttle CA. A virophage at the origin of large DNA transposons. *Science* 2011;332:231–234.
59. Francis R, Ominami Y, Bou Khalil JY, et al. High-throughput isolation of giant viruses using high-content screening. *Commun Biol* 2019;2:216.
60. Frey S, Richter RP, Görlich D. FG-rich repeats of nuclear pore proteins form a three-dimensional meshwork with hydrogel-like properties. *Science* 2006;314:815–817.
61. Fridmann-Sirkis Y, et al. Efficiency in complexity: composition and dynamic nature of mimivirus replication factories. *J Virol* 2016;90:10039–10047.
62. Gaia M, et al. Broad spectrum of *Mimiviridae* virophage allows its isolation using a mimivirus reporter. *PLoS One* 2013;8:e61912.
63. Gaia M, et al. Zamilon, a novel virophage with *Mimiviridae* host specificity. *PLoS One* 2014;9:e94923.
64. Gallot-Lavallée L, Blanc G, Claverie J-M. Comparative genomics of chrysochromulina ericina virus and other microalga-infecting large DNA viruses highlights their intricate evolutionary relationship with the established *Mimiviridae* family. *J Virol* 2017;91:e00230.
65. Gallot-Lavallée L, et al. The 474-kilobase-pair complete genome sequence of CeV-01B, a Virus Infecting Haptolina (Chrysochromulina) ericina (Prymnesiophyceae). *Genome Announc* 2015;3:1–2.
66. Ghigo E, et al. Ameobal pathogen mimivirus infects macrophages through phagocytosis. *PLoS Pathog* 2008;4:e1000087.
67. Gilbert C, et al. Population genomics supports baculoviruses as vectors of horizontal transfer of insect transposons. *Nat Commun* 2014;5:3348.

68. Gong C, et al. Novel virophages discovered in a freshwater lake in China. *Front Microbiol* 2016;7:5.
69. Gowing MM. Large virus-like particles from vacuoles of Phaeodarian radiolarians and from other marine samples. *Mar Ecol Prog Ser* 1993;101:33–44.
70. Gupta A, Lad SB, Ghodke PP, et al. Mimivirus encodes a multifunctional primase with DNA/RNA polymerase, terminal transferase and translesion synthesis activities. *Nucleic Acids Res* 2019;47:6932–6945.
71. Hackl T, et al. Four high-quality draft genome assemblies of the marine heterotrophic nanoflagellate Cafeteria roenbergensis. *Sci Data* 2020;7:29.
72. Hingamp P, et al. Exploring nucleo-cytoplasmic large DNA viruses in Tara Oceans microbial metagenomes. *ISME J* 2013;7:1678–1695.
73. Iyer LM, Abhiman S, Aravind L. A new family of polymerases related to superfamily A DNA polymerases and T7-like DNA-dependent RNA polymerases. *Biol Direct* 2008;3:39.
74. Iyer LM, Aravind L, Koonin EV. Common origin of four diverse families of large eukaryotic DNA viruses. *J Virol* 2001;75:11720–11734.
75. Iyer LM, Balaji S, Koonin EV, et al. Evolutionary genomics of nucleo-cytoplasmic large DNA viruses. *Virus Res* 2006;117:156–184.
76. Iyer LM, Koonin EV, Leipe DD, et al. Origin and evolution of the archaeo-eukaryotic primase superfamily and related palm-domain proteins: structural insights and new members. *Nucleic Acids Res* 2005;33:3875–3896.
77. Jeudy S, et al. Exploration of the propagation of transpovirons within *Mimiviridae* reveals a unique example of commensalism in the viral world. *ISME J* 2020;14:727–739.
78. Johannessen TV, et al. Characterisation of three novel giant viruses reveals huge diversity among viruses infecting Prymnesiales (Haptophyta). *Virology* 2014;476C:180–188.
79. Kapitonov VV, Jurka J. Self-synthesizing DNA transposons in eukaryotes. *Proc Natl Acad Sci U S A* 2006;103:4540–4545.
80. Khan M, La Scola B, Lepidi H, et al. Pneumonia in mice inoculated experimentally with Acanthamoeba polyphaga mimivirus. *Microb Pathog* 2007;42:56–61.
81. Klose T, Rossmann MG. Structure of large dsDNA viruses. *Biol Chem* 2014;395:711–719.
82. Klose T, et al. The three-dimensional structure of mimivirus. *Intervirology* 2010;53:268–273.
83. Klose T, et al. A mimivirus enzyme that participates in viral entry. *Structure* 2015;23:1058–1065.
84. Koonin EV, Krupovic M. Virology: a parasite's parasite saves host's neighbours. *Nature* 2016;540:204–205.
85. Koonin EV, Krupovic M. Polintons, virophages and transpovirons: a tangled web linking viruses, transposons and immunity. *Curr Opin Virol* 2017;25:7–15.
86. Koonin EV, Yutin N. Evolution of the large nucleocytoplasmic DNA viruses of eukaryotes and convergent origins of viral gigantism. *Adv Virus Res* 2019;103:167–202.
87. Koonin EV, et al. Global organization and proposed megataxonomy of the virus world. *Microbiol Mol Biol Rev* 2020;84:1–33.
88. Krupovic M, Bamford DH, Koonin EV. Conservation of major and minor jelly-roll capsid proteins in Polinton (Maverick) transposons suggests that they are bona fide viruses. *Biol Direct* 2014;9:6.
89. Krupovic M, Cvirkaite-Krupovic V. Virophages or satellite viruses? *Nat Rev Microbiol* 2011;9:762–763.
90. Krupovic M, Cvirkaite-Krupovic V. Sputnik and Mavirus: not more than satellite viruses. *Nat Rev Microbiol* 2012;10:88.
91. Krupovic M, Kuhn JH, Fischer MG. A classification system for virophages and satellite viruses. *Arch Virol* 2016;161:233–247.
92. Kuznetsov YG, et al. Atomic force microscopy investigation of the giant mimivirus. *Virology* 2010;404:127–137.
93. Kwon E, Pathak D, Chang HW, et al. Crystal structure of mimivirus uracil-DNA glycosylase. *PLoS One* 2017;12:e0182382.
94. La Scola B, Marrie TJ, Auffray J-P, et al. Mimivirus in pneumonia patients. *Emerg Infect Dis* 2005;11:449–452.
95. La Scola B, et al. A giant virus in amoebae. *Science* 2003;299:2033.
96. La Scola B, et al. The virophage as a unique parasite of the giant mimivirus. *Nature* 2008;455:100–104.
97. La Scola B, et al. Tentative characterization of new environmental giant viruses by MALDI-TOF mass spectrometry. *Intervirology* 2010;53:344–353.
98. Lefkowitz EJ, Wang C, Upton C. Poxviruses: past, present and future. *Virus Res* 2006;117:105–118.
99. Legendre M, Arslan D, Abergel C, et al. Genomics of Megavirus and the elusive fourth domain of Life. *Commun Integr Biol* 2012;5:102–106.
100. Legendre M, Santini S, Rico A, et al. Breaking the 1000-gene barrier for Mimivirus using ultra-deep genome and transcriptome sequencing. *Virol J* 2011;8:99.
101. Legendre M, et al. mRNA deep sequencing reveals 75 new genes and a complex transcriptional landscape in Mimivirus. *Genome Res* 2010;20:664–674.
102. Legendre M, et al. Thirty-thousand-year-old distant relative of giant icosahedral DNA viruses with a pandoravirus morphology. *Proc Natl Acad Sci U S A* 2014;111:4274–4279.
103. Legendre M, et al. In-depth study of Mollivirus sibericum, a new 30,000-yold giant virus infecting Acanthamoeba. *Proc Natl Acad Sci U S A* 2015;112:E5327–E5335.
104. Levasseur A, et al. MIMIVIRE is a defence system in mimivirus that confers resistance to virophage. *Nature* 2016;531:249–252.
105. Liu S, et al. Cryo-EM structure of the African swine fever virus. *Cell Host Microbe* 2019;26:836–843.e3.
106. Meints RH, Lee K, Burbank DE, et al. Infection of a Chlorella-like alga with the virus, PBCV-1: ultrastructural studies. *Virology* 1984;138:341–346.
107. de Miranda Boratto PV, dos Santos Pereira Andrade AC, Araújo Lima Rodrigues R, et al. The multiple origins of proteins present in tupanvirus particles. *Curr Opin Virol* 2019;36:25–31.
108. Monier A, et al. Marine mimivirus relatives are probably large algal viruses. *Virol J* 2008;5:12.
109. Moniruzzaman M, Gann ER, Wilhelm SW. Infection by a giant virus (AaV) induces widespread physiological reprogramming in Aureococcus anophagefferens CCMP1984-A harmful bloom algae. *Front Microbiol* 2018;9:1–16.
110. Moniruzzaman M, et al. Genome of brown tide virus (AaV), the little giant of the Megaviridae, elucidates NCLDV genome expansion and host-virus coevolution. *Virology* 2014;466–467:60–70.
111. Mougari S, Abrahao J, Oliveira GP, et al. Role of the R349 gene and its repeats in the MIMIVIRE defense system. *Front Microbiol* 2019;10:1147.
112. Mougari S, et al. Guarani virophage, a new Sputnik-Like isolate from a Brazilian lake. *Front Microbiol* 2019;10:1003.
113. Mutsafi Y, Fridmann-Sirkis Y, Milrot E, et al. Infection cycles of large DNA viruses: emerging themes and underlying questions. *Virology* 2014;466–467:3–14.
114. Mutsafi Y, Shimoni E, Shimon A, et al. Membrane assembly during the Infection cycle of the giant mimivirus. *PLoS Pathog* 2013;9:e1003367.
115. Mutsafi Y, Zauberman N, Sabanay I, et al. Vaccinia-like cytoplasmic replication of the giant Mimivirus. *Proc Natl Acad Sci U S A* 2010;107:5978–5982.
116. Needham DM, et al. A distinct lineage of giant viruses brings a rhodopsin photosystem to unicellular marine predators. *Proc Natl Acad Sci U S A* 2019;116:20574–20583.
117. Needham DM, et al. Targeted metagenomic recovery of four divergent viruses reveals shared and distinctive characteristics of giant viruses of marine eukaryotes. *Philos Trans R Soc B Biol Sci* 2019;374:20190086.
118. O'Day DH, Suhre K, Myre MA, et al. E. Isolation, characterization, and bioinformatic analysis of calmodulin-binding protein cmbB reveals a novel tandem IP22 repeat common to many Dictyostelium and Mimivirus proteins. *Biochem Biophys Res Commun* 2006;346:879–888.
119. Ogata H, et al. Two new subfamilies of DNA mismatch repair proteins (MutS) specifically abundant in the marine environment. *ISME J* 2011;5:1143–1151.
120. Oh S, Yoo D, Liu WT. Metagenomics reveals a novel virophage population in a Tibetan mountain lake. *Microbes Environ* 2016;31:173–177.
121. Oliveira G, et al. Promoter motifs in NCLDVs: an evolutionary perspective. *Viruses* 2017;9:16.
122. Paez-Espino D, et al. Diversity, evolution, and classification of virophages uncovered through global metagenomics. *Microbiome* 2019;7:1–14.
123. Philippe N, et al. Pandoraviruses: amoeba viruses with genomes up to 2.5 Mb reaching that of parasitic eukaryotes. *Science* 2013;341:281–286.
124. Piacente F, et al. Giant DNA virus mimivirus encodes pathway for biosynthesis of unusual sugar 4-amino-4,6-dideoxy-D-glucose (Viosamine). *J Biol Chem* 2012;287:3009–3018.
125. Priet S, Lartigue A, Debart F, et al. MRNA maturation in giant viruses: variation on a theme. *Nucleic Acids Res* 2015;43:3776–3788.
126. Pritham EJ, Putliwala T, Feschotte C. Mavericks, a novel class of giant transposable elements widespread in eukaryotes and related to DNA viruses. *Gene* 2007;390:3–17.
127. Raoult D, Renesto P, Brouqui P. Laboratory infection of a technician by mimivirus. *Ann Intern Med* 2006;144:702–703.
128. Raoult D, La Scola B, Birtles R. The discovery and characterization of Mimivirus, the largest known virus and putative pneumonia agent. *Clin Infect Dis* 2007;45:95–102.
129. Raoult D, et al. The 1.2-megabase genome sequence of Mimivirus. *Science* 2004;306:1344–1350.
130. Redrejo-Rodríguez M, Salas ML. Repair of base damage and genome maintenance in the nucleo-cytoplasmic large DNA viruses. *Virus Res* 2014;179:12–25.
131. Renesto P, et al. Mimivirus giant particles incorporate a large fraction of anonymous and unique gene products. *J Virol* 2006;80:11678–11685.
132. Rodrigues RAL, Arantes TS, Oliveira GP, et al. The complex nature of tupanviruses. *Adv Virus Res* 2019;103:135–166.
133. Rodrigues RAL, da Silva LCF, Abrahão JS. Translating the language of giants: translation-related genes as a major contribution of giant viruses to the virosphere. *Arch Virol* 2020;165:1267–1278.
134. Rodrigues RAL, et al. Mimivirus fibrils are important for viral attachment to the microbial world by a diverse glycoside interaction repertoire. *J Virol* 2015;89:11812–11819.
135. Roux S, et al. Ecogenomics of virophages and their giant virus hosts assessed through time series metagenomics. *Nat Commun* 2017;8:858.
136. Saadi H, et al. First isolation of Mimivirus in a patient with pneumonia. *Clin Infect Dis* 2013;57:e127–e134.
137. Santini S, et al. Genome of Phaeocystis globosa virus PgV-16T highlights the common ancestry of the largest known DNA viruses infecting eukaryotes. *Proc Natl Acad Sci* 2013;110:10800–10805.
138. Schrad JR, Abrahão JS, Cortines JR, et al. Structural and proteomic characterization of the initiation of giant virus infection. *Cell* 2020;181:1046–1061.e6. doi:10.1016/j.cell.2020.04.032.
139. Schrad JR, Young EJ, Abrahão JS, et al. Microscopic characterization of the Brazilian giant samba virus. *Viruses* 2017;9:1–16.
140. Schramm B, Krijnse-Locker J. Cytoplasmic organization of Poxvirus DNA replication. *Traffic* 2005;6:839–846.
141. Schulz F, et al. Giant viruses with an expanded complement of translation system components. *Science* 2017;356:82–85.
142. Schulz F, et al. Hidden diversity of soil giant viruses. *Nat Commun* 2018;9:4881.
143. Schulz F, et al. Giant virus diversity and host interactions through global metagenomics. *Nature* 2020;578:432–436.
144. Schvarcz CR, Steward GF. A giant virus infecting green algae encodes key fermentation genes. *Virology* 2018;518:423–433.
145. Seibert MM, et al. Single mimivirus particles intercepted and imaged with an X-ray laser. *Nature* 2011;470:78–81.
146. Shinn GL, Bullard BL. Ultrastructure of meelsvirus: a nuclear virus of arrow worms (phylum Chaetognatha) producing giant "tailed" virions. *PLoS One* 2018;13:8–12.
147. Sicko-Goad L, Walker G. Viroplasm and large virus-like particles in the dinoflagellate Gymnodinium uberrimum. *Protoplasma* 1979;99:203–210.
148. Silva LCF, et al. Modulation of the expression of mimivirus-encoded translation-related genes in response to nutrient availability during Acanthamoeba castellanii infection. *Front Microbiol* 2015;6:539.
149. Silva LCF, et al. Microscopic analysis of the tupanvirus cycle in vermamoeba vermiformis. *Front Microbiol* 2019;10:1–9.

150. Simon AE, Roossinck MJ, Havelda Z. Plant virus satellite and defective interfering RNAs: new paradigms for a new century. *Annu Rev Phytopathol* 2004;42:415–437.
151. Srinivasan V, Tripathy DN. The DNA repair enzyme, CPD-photolyase restores the infectivity of UV-damaged fowlpox virus isolated from infected scabs of chickens. *Vet Microbiol* 2005;108:215–223.
152. Stough JMA, et al. Genome and environmental activity of a chrysochromulina parva virus and its virophages. *Front Microbiol* 2019;10:703.
153. Suarez C, et al. Open membranes are the precursors for assembly of large DNA viruses. *Cell Microbiol* 2013;15:1883–1895.
154. Suarez C, et al. African swine fever virus assembles a single membrane derived from rupture of the endoplasmic reticulum. *Cell Microbiol* 2015;17:1683–1698.
155. Suhre K. Gene and genome duplication in Acanthamoeba polyphaga Mimivirus. *J Virol* 2005;79:14095–14101.
156. Suhre K, Audic S, Claverie J-M. Mimivirus gene promoters exhibit an unprecedented conservation among all eukaryotes. *Proc Natl Acad Sci U S A* 2005;102:14689–14693.
157. Sun C, Feschotte C, Wu Z, et al. DNA transposons have colonized the genome of the giant virus Pandoravirus salinus. *BMC Biol* 2015;13:38.
158. Sun S, et al. Structural studies of the Sputnik virophage. *J Virol* 2010;84:894–897.
159. Suzan-Monti M, La Scola B, Barrassi L, et al. Ultrastructural characterization of the giant volcano-like virus factory of Acanthamoeba polyphaga Mimivirus. *PLoS One* 2007;2:e328.
160. Suzan-Monti M, La Scola B, Raoult D. Genomic and evolutionary aspects of Mimivirus. *Virus Res* 2006;117:145–155.
161. Takemura M. Poxviruses and the origin of the eukaryotic nucleus. *J Mol Evol* 2001;52:419–425.
162. Taylor BP, Cortez MH, Weitz JS. The virus of my virus is my friend: ecological effects of virophage with alternative modes of coinfection. *J Theor Biol* 2014;354:124–136.
163. Taylor BP, Weitz JS, Brussaard CPD, et al. Quantitative infection dynamics of cafeteria roenbergensis virus. *Viruses* 2018;10:468.
164. Van Etten JL, Burbank DE, Xia Y, et al. Growth cycle of a virus, PBCV-1, that infects chlorella-like algae'. *Virol J* 1983;125:117–125.
165. Van Etten JL, Lane LC, Meints RH. Viruses and viruslike particles of eukaryotic algae. *Microbiol Rev* 1991;55:586–620.
166. Walsh D. Poxviruses: slipping and sliding through transcription and translation. *PLoS Pathog* 2017;13:1–5.
167. Wilhelm SW, et al. A student's guide to giant viruses infecting small eukaryotes: from acanthamoeba to zooxanthellae. *Viruses* 2017;9:46.
168. Xian Y, Avila R, Pant A, et al. The role of tape measure protein in nucleocytoplasmic large DNA virus capsid assembly. *Viral Immunol* 2021;34:41–48.
169. Xiao C, et al. Cryo-electron microscopy of the giant mimivirus. *J Mol Biol* 2005;353:493–496.
170. Xiao C, et al. AFM and cryoEM studies of the giant Mimivirus. *Microsc Microanal* 2008;14:2007–2008.
171. Xiao C, et al. Structural studies of the giant mimivirus. *PLoS Biol* 2009;7:e92.
172. Xiao C, et al. Cryo-EM reconstruction of the Cafeteria roenbergensis virus capsid suggests novel assembly pathway for giant viruses. *Sci Rep* 2017;7:5484.
173. Yau S, et al. Virophage control of antarctic algal host-virus dynamics. *Proc Natl Acad Sci U S A* 2011;108:6163–6168.
174. Yoosuf N, et al. Related giant viruses in distant locations and different habitats: acanthamoeba polyphaga moumouvirus represents a third lineage of the *Mimiviridae* that is close to the megavirus lineage. *Genome Biol Evol* 2012;4:1324–1330.
175. Yoshida T, Claverie J-M, Ogata H. Mimivirus reveals Mre11/Rad50 fusion proteins with a sporadic distribution in eukaryotes, bacteria, viruses and plasmids. *Virol J* 2011;8:427.
176. Yutin N, Colson P, Raoult D, et al. *Mimiviridae*: clusters of orthologous genes, reconstruction of gene repertoire evolution and proposed expansion of the giant virus family. *Virol J* 2013;10:106.
177. Yutin N, Kapitonov VV, Koonin EV. A new family of hybrid virophages from an animal gut metagenome. *Biol Direct* 2015;10:19.
178. Yutin N, Raoult D, Koonin EV. Virophages, polintons, and transpovirons: a complex evolutionary network of diverse selfish genetic elements with different reproduction strategies. *Virol J* 2013;10:158.
179. Zauberman N, et al. Distinct DNA exit and packaging portals in the virus Acanthamoeba polyphaga mimivirus. *PLoS Biol* 2008;6:e114.
180. Zhang X, et al. Structure of Sputnik, a virophage, at 3.5-Å resolution. *Proc Natl Acad Sci U S A.* 2012;109:18431–18436.
181. Zhou J, et al. Diversity of virophages in metagenomic data sets. *J Virol* 2013;87:4225–4236.
182. Zhou J, et al. Three novel virophage genomes discovered from Yellowstone Lake metagenomes. *J Virol* 2015;89:1278–1285.
183. Ziegelin G, Lanka E. Bacteriophage P4 DNA replication. *FEMS Microbiol Rev* 1995;17:99–107.
184. Zinoviev A, Kuroha K, Pestova TV, et al. Two classes of EF1-family translational GTPases encoded by giant viruses. *Nucleic Acids Res* 2019;47:5761–5776.

Index

Note: Page number followed by "*f*" and "*t*" indicates figure and table respectively.

D

Q

R

S

T

W

X

Y

Z